Principles and Practice of

Geriatric Medicine

Fourth Edition

Volume 2

In memory of my wife, Norma Mary, for her enduring support and encouragement and to my children, Aidan, Anne, Sarah, Helen and Damian for graciously accepting the limitations of my time.

- M.S. John Pathy

In loving memory of my parents, to whom I owe so much, and to my wife, Caroline, for her unflinching support throughout these last two years during the preparation of this textbook.

- Alan J. Sinclair

To all my older friends and patients who have taught me geriatrics, to my wife Pat and my children Robert, Sue and Jacqueline who have supported me throughout my career and to my grandchildren Amanda, Conor, Katelyn, Nicole and Paige who are my eternal joy and my hope for the future of elder care.

- John E. Morley

Principles and Practice of

Geriatric Medicine

Fourth Edition

Volume 2

Editors

M.S. John Pathy

University of Wales, Cardiff, UK

Alan J. Sinclair

University of Warwick, Coventry, UK

John E. Morley

*Saint Louis University School of Medicine and
Saint Louis Veterans' Affairs Medical Center,
St Louis, MO, USA*

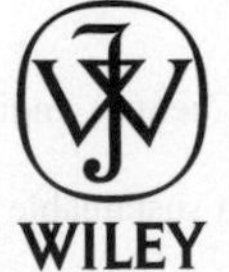

WILEY

The Atrium,
Southern Gate,
Chichester,
West Sussex,
PO19 8SQ, England

Telephone: (+44) 1243 779777

Email (for orders and customer service enquiries): cs-books@wiley.co.uk
Visit our Home Page on www.wiley.com

Other Wiley Editorial Offices

John Wiley & Sons Inc., 111 River Street,
Hoboken, NJ 07030, USA

Jossey-Bass, 989 Market Street,
San Francisco, CA 94103-1741, USA

Wiley-VCH Verlag GmbH, Boschstr. 12,
D-69469 Weinheim, Germany

John Wiley & Sons Australia Ltd, 42 McDougall Street,
Milton, Queensland 4064, Australia

John Wiley & Sons (Asia) Pte Ltd, 2 Clementi Loop #02-01,
Jin Xing Distripark, Singapore 129809

John Wiley & Sons Canada Ltd, 5353 Dundas Street West, Suite 400,
Etobicoke, Ontario, Canada M9B 6HB

Wiley also publishes its books in a variety of electronic formats. Some content that appears in print may not be available in electronic books.

British Library Cataloguing in Publication Data

A catalogue record for this book is available from the British Library

ISBN-13 978-0-470-09055-8
ISBN-10 0-470-09055-3

Typeset in 10/11.5 pt Times Roman by Laserwords Private Limited, Chennai, India.
Printed and bound by Grafos SA, Barcelona, Spain.
This book is printed on acid-free paper responsibly manufactured from sustainable forestry in which at least two trees are planted for each one used for paper production.

Contents of Volume 1

List of Contributors . . . xiii

Preface . . . xxiii

Preface to Third Edition . . . xxv

Preface to Second Edition . . . xxvi

Preface to First Edition . . . xxvii

1 Historical Perspectives . . . 1
Michael J. Denham

Part I Human Aging: A Biological Perspective

2 A Biological Perspective on Aging . . . 13
Thomas B.L. Kirkwood

3 Immunity and Aging . . . 19
Katsuiku Hirokawa, Masanori Utsuyama and Takashi Makinodan

4 Physiology of Aging . . . 37
Rafi Kevorkian

5 Aging of the Brain . . . 47
Charles Mobbs

6 Psychological Aspects of Aging . . . 53
Peggy A. Szwabo

7 Neurochemistry of Aging . . . 59
Alan M. Palmer and Paul T. Francis

8 Neuropathology of Aging . . . 69
Seth Love

Part II Human Aging: Social and Community Perspectives

9 The Demography of Aging . . . 87
Kenneth G. Manton

10 Social and Community Aspects of Aging . . . 101
Rodney M. Coe, John E. Morley and Nina Tumosa

11 Sexuality and Aging . . . 115
John E. Morley

12 Physical Fitness and Exercise . . . 123
Maria A. Fiatarone Singh

13 Transportation, Driving, and Older Adults . . . 141
Desmond O'Neill and David Carr

14 Smoking in the Elderly . . . 151
Norman J. Vetter

15 Alcohol Use and Abuse . . . 157
Mary C. Dufour

16 On the Evolution of All-cause and Cause-specific Mortality in the Age Class 75–84 years: a Worldwide Overview . . . 169
Hugo E. Kesteloot

17 Elder Abuse . . . 181
Jed Rowe

18 Smart Homes . . . 189
Roger D. Orpwood

Part III Medicine in Old Age

19 Preventive Geriatrics . . . 201
Joseph H. Flaherty and Antony J. Bayer

20 Polypharmacy, is this Another Disease? . . . 215
Oscar A. Cepeda and John E. Morley

21 **The Problem-Orientated Approach to Geriatric Medicine** . . . 223
Cameron G. Swift

Section 1 Eating Disorders and Nutritional Health

22 **Oral Health** . . . 239
Janet F. Griffiths

23 **Oral Disease** . . . 261
Donald Murray Walker

24 **Epidemiology of Nutrition and Aging** 279
Wija A. van Staveren and Lisette C.P.G.M de Groot

25 **Absorption of Nutrients** . . . 291
Akeeb Adedokun

26 **The Anorexia of Aging** . . . 297
Ian M. Chapman

27 **Weight Loss in Older Adults** . . . 309
David R. Thomas and Bruno Vellas

28 **Dehydration** . . . 321
Margaret-Mary G. Wilson

29 **Vitamins and Minerals in the Elderly** 329
Seema Joshi and John E. Morley

30 **Obesity in the Elderly** . . . 347
Richard Y.T. Chen and Gary A. Wittert

Section 2 Gastro Disorders

31 **Changes in Gastrointestinal Motor and Sensory Function Associated with Aging** . . . 357
Christopher K. Rayner and Michael Horowitz

32 **Gastrointestinal Bleeding** . . . 371
Syed H. Tariq

33 **Liver and Gall Bladder** . . . 381
Margaret-Mary G. Wilson

34 **Sphincter Function** . . . 395
Syed H. Tariq

35 **Constipation** . . . 407
Charlene M. Prather

36 **Diseases of the Pancreas** . . . 417
John S. Morris

Section 3 Hematological Disorders

37 **Anemia in Older Persons** . . . 427
David R. Thomas

38 **Disorders of Hemostasis** . . . 437
Kingsley K. Hampton

39 **Disseminated Intravascular Coagulation** . . . 445
Kingsley K. Hampton

40 **Anticoagulants in the Elderly** . . . 449
Hamsaraj G.M. Shetty and Philip A. Routledge

41 **Myelodysplasia** . . . 455
Martha Wadleigh, David S. Rosenthal and Richard M. Stone

42 **Management of Leukemia in the Elderly** . . . 465
Hussain Saba and Lodovico Balducci

Section 4 Cardiovascular Disease and Health

43 **Epidemiology of Heart Disease** . . . 475
Chris MacKnight and Colin Powell

44 **Cardiac Aging and Systemic Disorders** . . . 487
David J. Stott and Arun K. Singh

45 **Arrhythmias in the Elderly** . . . 493
A. John Camm and Laurence Nunn

46 **Ischemic Heart Disease in Elderly Persons** . . . 515
Wilbert S. Aronow

47 **Valvular Disease in the Elderly** . . . 529
Jeffrey S. Borer

48 **Hypertension** . . . 541
Ramzi R. Hajjar

49 **Mechanisms of Heart Failure** . . . 555
Michael P. Frenneaux and Lynne K. Williams

50 **Heart Failure in the Elderly** . . . 567
Michael W. Rich

51 **Management of Acute Cardiac Emergencies and Cardiac Surgery** . 585
Wilbert S. Aronow

52 **Cardiac Surgery in the Elderly** 593
Ulrich O. von Oppell and Adam Szafranek

53 **Pathogenesis of Atherosclerosis** 611
Andrew C. Newby

54 **Peripheral Vascular Disease in Elderly Persons** 623
Wilbert S. Aronow

55 **Venous Thromboembolism** 633
Gordon D.O. Lowe

56 **Cardiac Cachexia** 639
Gerhard-Paul Diller and Stefan D. Anker

57 **Cardiac Rehabilitation in Older People** 647
Niccolò Marchionni, Francesco Fattirolli, Lucio A. Rinaldi and Giulio Masotti

Section 5 Respiratory Diseases

58 **Epidemiology of Respiratory Infection** 665
Joseph M. Mylotte

59 **The Effect of Aging on the Respiratory Skeletal Muscles** 671
Meme Wijesinghe and Lindsey Dow

60 **Aspiration Pneumonia** 685
Takashi Ohrui and Hidetada Sasaki

61 **Respiratory Disease in the Elderly** . . 693
Martin J. Connolly

62 **Pulmonary Rehabilitation** 727
Peter Spiegler and Jonathan S. Ilowite

63 **Sleep Disorders in Elderly People** . . . 733
Paul Montgomery

Section 6 CNS Disorders

64 **Neurological Signs of Aging** 743
Andrew J. Larner

65 **Headache in the Elderly** 751
Stephen D. Silberstein and William B. Young

66 **Parkinson's Disease and Parkinsonism in the Elderly** 765
Jeremy R. Playfer

67 **Non Parkinsonian Movement Disorders in the Elderly** 777
Katie Kompoliti and Cynthia L. Comella

68 **Normal Pressure Hydrocephalus** 787
Dennis S. Oh and Peter McL. Black

69 **Epidemiology of Stroke** 795
Mitchell T. Wallin and John F. Kurtzke

70 **Management of Carotid Artery Stenosis** 805
Lucy J. Coward and Martin M. Brown

71 **Acute Stroke** 815
Peter Crome and Elliot F. Epstein

72 **Secondary Stroke** 827
Helen Rodgers

73 **Communication Disorders and Dysphagia** 841
Pamela M. Enderby

74 **Stroke Rehabilitation** 849
Lalit Kalra

75 **Clinical Psychology in Physical Rehabilitation** 859
Julie R. Wilcox and Janice Rees

76 **Epilepsy** 869
Pamela M. Crawford

77 **Syncope and Nonepileptic Attacks** . . 879
Richard C. Roberts

78 **Peripheral Neuropathy** 889
Bakri H. Elsheikh Mohamed and Miriam L. Freimer

79 **Disorders of the Neuromuscular Junction** 899
Ian K. Hart

80 **Sarcopenia and Sarcopenic-Obesity** . 909
Richard N. Baumgartner and Debra L. Waters

81 **Muscle Disorders** 935
David Hilton-Jones

82 **Motor Neurone Disease** 949
Hardev S. Pall

83 Abnormalities of the Autonomic Nervous System 969
Kenneth J. Collins

84 Control of Chronic Pain 981
Robert D. Helme and Benny Katz

85 Cervical and Lumbar Spinal Canal Stenosis 991
M.S. John Pathy

86 Spinovascular Insufficiency 1001
M.S. John Pathy

87 Subarachnoid Hemorrhage 1015
Jan van Gijn and Gabriel J.E. Rinkel

88 Acute and Chronic Subdural Hematoma 1027
Jonathan A. Vafidis

Appendix: Conversion of SI Units to Standard Units i

Index iii

Contents of Volume 2

List of Contributors xiii

Preface xxiii

Preface to Third Edition xxv

Preface to Second Edition xxvi

Preface to First Edition xxvii

Section 7 Dementia and Cognitive Disorders

89 Communication Disorders in Dementia 1037
Jennie A. Powell

90 Delirium 1047
Joseph H. Flaherty

91 Memory Clinics 1061
Antony J. Bayer

92 Cellular Changes in Alzheimer's Disease 1073
Jean-Pierre Brion

93 Clinical Aspects of Alzheimer's Disease 1083
Fatemeh Nourhashémi, Alan J. Sinclair and Bruno Vellas

94 Mild Cognitive Impairment 1095
Pieter Jelle Visser

95 Vascular Dementia 1103
Ingmar Skoog

96 Other Dementias 1111
Wee Shiong Lim and William A. Banks

97 Treatment of Behavioral Disorders . 1135
Ladislav Volicer

98 Geriatric Psychiatry 1149
Abhilash K. Desai and George T. Grossberg

99 Organization of Services in Geriatric Psychiatry 1163
Susan M. Benbow and David Jolley

100 Depression in Late Life: Etiology, Diagnosis and Treatment 1173
Natalie Sachs-Ericsson and Dan G. Blazer

101 The Older Patient with Down's Syndrome 1185
John E. Morley

102 Drug Misuse and the Older Person: A Contradiction in Terms? 1191
Ilana B. Crome

Section 8 Special Senses

103 Disorders of the Eye 1205
Nina Tumosa

104 The Epidemiology of Hearing in Aging Population 1211
Adrian C. Davis and Padma Moorjani

105 Auditory System 1219
R. Gareth Williams

106 Disorders of the Vestibular System . 1235
Linda M. Luxon and Charlotte Ågrup

107 Smell and Taste 1249
Richard L. Doty

Section 9 Bone and Joint Health

108 Age-related Changes in Calcium Homeostasis and Bone Loss 1261
Harvey James Armbrecht

109 Paget's Disease of Bone 1269
Sanjay Sharma and Kenneth W. Lyles

110 Epidemiology of Osteoporosis 1281
Horace M. Perry

111 Osteoporosis and its Consequences: a Major Threat to the Quality of Life in the Elderly 1285
René Rizzoli

112 Gait, Balance, and Falls 1299
Peter W. Overstall and Thorsten Nikolaus

113 Foot Problems in the Elderly 1311
Arthur E. Helfand and Donald F. Jessett

114 Hip Fracture and Orthogeriatrics 1329
Antony Johansen and Martyn Parker

115 Diseases of the Joints 1347
Terry L. Moore

116 Back Pain 1355
John V. Butler

Section 10 Endocrine and Metabolic Disorders

117 Water and Electrolyte Balance in Health and Disease 1369
Allen I. Arieff

118 Endocrinology of Aging 1389
John E. Morley and Moon J. Kim

119 The Pituitary Gland 1397
James F. Lamb and John E. Morley

120 Thyroid Disorders 1405
Rachel F. Oiknine and Arshag D. Mooradian

121 Ovarian and Testicular Function 1415
Syed H. Tariq

122 Type 2 Diabetes Mellitus in Senior Citizens 1431
Alan J. Sinclair and Graydon S. Meneilly

Section 11 Urogenital Disorders

123 Gynecology and the Older Patient 1449
Radha Indusekhar, F. O'Mahony and P.M.S. O'Brien

124 The Aging Bladder 1459
James M. Cummings and Kimberly C. Berni

125 Prostate Diseases 1469
Timothy D. Moon and Jennifer L. Maskel

126 Urinary Incontinence 1485
Margaret-Mary G. Wilson

127 Renal Diseases 1495
Carlos G. Musso and Juan F. Macías-Núnez

Section 12 Cancer

128 Cancer and Aging 1509
Claudia Beghe and Lodovico Balducci

129 Oncological Emergencies and Urgencies 1519
Samuel Spence McCachren

130 Breast Cancer in the Elderly 1531
R.E. Mansel and A. Srivastava

Section 13 Functional Disorders and Rehabilitation

131 Multidimensional Geriatric Assessment 1543
Laurence Z. Rubenstein and Andreas E. Stuck

132 Function Assessment Scales 1553
Fredric D. Wolinsky

133 Frailty 1565
John E. Morley

134 Rehabilitation 1571
Paul M. Finucane and Philip J. Henschke

Section 14 Special Issues

135 Skin Disorders in the Elderly 1589
Daniel S. Loo, Mina Yaar and Barbara A. Gilchrest

136 Pressure Ulceration 1605
Joseph E. Grey and Keith G. Harding

137 Perioperative and Postoperative Medical Assessment 1631
D. Gwyn Seymour

138 Anesthesia in Older People 1647
Suzanne Crowe

139 Health Issues in the Aging Female 1659
Carolyn Philpot

140 Antiaging 1665
Alfred L. Fisher

141 Ethical Issues 1681
Maureen Junker-Kenny and Davis Coakley

142 Restraints and Immobility 1689
Elizabeth A. Capezuti and Laura M. Wagner

143 Centenarians 1701
Thomas T. Perls and Dellara F. Terry

Section 15 Diagnostic Interventions

144 Diagnostic Imaging and Interventional Radiology 1711
J. Richard Harding

Section 16 Infectious Disorders

145 Infectious Diseases 1725
Ann R. Falsey

146 Tuberculosis 1739
Shobita Rajagopalan and Thomas T. Yoshikawa

147 Infective Endocarditis in the Elderly 1749
Philippe Moreillon, Alain Bizzini and Yok Ai Que

148 Infections of the Central Nervous System 1763
Michael Blank and Allan R. Tunkel

Part IV Health Care Systems

149 Geriatric Medicine Education in Europe 1783
Antonio Cherubini, Philippe Huber and Jean-Pierre Michel

150 Education in Geriatric Medicine in the United Kingdom 1789
Robert W. Stout

151 The Contribution of Family Doctors to the Primary Care of Older People: Lessons from the British Experience 1799
Steve Iliffe

152 Carers and the Role of the Family . 1809
Jo Moriarty

153 Nursing Home Care 1817
David R. Thomas and John E. Morley

154 Clinical Audit of Health Care 1827
Jonathan M. Potter and Michael G. Pearson

155 Improving Quality of Care 1837
Julie K. Gammack and Carolyn D. Philpot

156 Resident Assessment Instrument/ Minimum Data Set 1855
Brant E. Fries, Catherine Hawes, John N. Morris and Roberto Bernabei

157 Nursing (UK) 1867
Nicky Hayes

158 Geriatric Occupational Therapy: Focus on Participation in Meaningful Daily Living 1879
Karen F. Barney

159 Systems of Health Care: the United Kingdom, the United States, and Australia 1889
Julie K. Gammack, Gideon A. Caplan and Krishnendu Ghosh

160 Geriatric Day Hospitals 1907
Neil D. Gillespie and Irene D. Turpie

161 Health and Care for Older People in the United Kingdom 1915
Clive Bowman and Catherine Dixon

162 Geriatrics in the United States 1923
John E. Morley and Julie K. Gammack

163 Geriatrics and Gerontology in Japan 1935
Yuko Suda and Ryutaro Takahashi

164 Care of the Elderly in Israel: Old Age in a Young Land 1947
A. Mark Clarfield, Jenny Brodsky and Arthur Leibovitz

165 Geriatric Medicine in China 1953
Leung-Wing Chu

166 Aging in Developing Countries 1965
Luis M. Gutiérrez-Robledo

167 Geriatrics from the European Union Perspective 1977
Alfonso J. Cruz-Jentoft and Paul V. Knight

168 Delivery of Health Care in India . . . 1983
Om Prakash Sharma

169 Geriatrics in Latin America 1993
Fernando Morales-Martínez and Martha Pelaez

170 Management of the Dying Patient . . 2001
Ilora G. Finlay and Saskie Dorman

Appendix: Conversion of SI Units to Standard Units i

Index iii

Contributors

Akeeb Adedokun
Saint Louis University, St Louis, MO, USA

Charlotte Ågrup
University College of London Hospitals NHS Trust, London, UK

Stefan D. Anker
Applied Cachexia Research Unit, Charite, Campus Virchow – Klinikum, Berlin, Germany

Allen I. Arieff
University of California, San Francisco, CA, USA

Harvey James Armbrecht
Saint Louis University Health Sciences Center and Saint Louis Veterans' Affairs Medical Center, St Louis, MO, USA

Wilbert S. Aronow
Westchester Medical Center/New York Medical College, Valhalla, NY, USA, and Mount Sinai School of Medicine, New York, NY, USA

Lodovico Balducci
University of South Florida College of Medicine, Tampa, FL, USA and H. Lee Moffitt Cancer Center and Research Institute, Tampa, FL, USA

William A. Banks
Saint Louis University School of Medicine and Saint Louis Veterans' Affairs Medical Center, St Louis, MO, USA

Karen F. Barney
Saint Louis University, St Louis, MO, USA

Richard N. Baumgartner
University of Louisville, Louisville, KY, USA

Antony J. Bayer
Cardiff University, Cardiff, UK

Claudia Beghe
University of South Florida College of Medicine, Tampa, FL, USA and James A. Haley Veterans' Hospital, Tampa, FL, USA

Susan M. Benbow
University of Staffordshire, Staffordshire, UK

Roberto Bernabei
Hebrew Rehabilitation Center for Aged, Boston, MA, USA and Università Cattolica del Sacro Cuore, Rome, Italy

Kimberly C. Berni
Saint Louis University, St Louis, MO, USA

Alain Bizzini
University of Lausanne, Lausanne, Switzerland

Peter McL. Black
Brigham and Women's Hospital, Harvard Medical School, Boston, MA, USA

Michael Blank
Drexel University College of Medicine, Philadelphia, PA, USA

Dan G. Blazer
Duke University Medical Center, Durham, NC, USA

Jeffrey S. Borer
Weill Medical College of Cornell University, New York, NY, USA

Clive Bowman
BUPA Care Services, Leeds, UK

Jean-Pierre Brion
Université Libre de Bruxelles, Brussels, Belgium

Jenny Brodsky
JDC-Brookdale Institute, Jerusalem, Israel

Martin M. Brown
The National Hospital for Neurology and Neurosurgery, London, UK, and University College London, London, UK

John V. Butler
Caerphilly District Miners Hospital, Caerphilly, UK

A. John Camm
St George's Hospital Medical School, London, UK

Elizabeth A. Capezuti
New York University, New York, NY, USA

Gideon A. Caplan
Prince of Wales Hospital, Randwick, New South Wales, Australia

David Carr
Division of Geriatrics and Nutritional Science, Park Provence, St Louis, MO, USA

Oscar A. Cepeda
Saint Louis University School of Medicine, St Louis, MO, USA

Ian M. Chapman
University of Adelaide, Royal Adelaide Hospital, Adelaide, South Australia, Australia

Richard Y.T. Chen
University of Adelaide, Royal Adelaide Hospital, Adelaide, South Australia, Australia

Antonio Cherubini
Perugia University Medical School, Perugia, Italy

Leung-Wing Chu
University of Hong Kong and Hong Kong West Cluster Geriatrics Service, Queen Mary Hospital, Fung Yiu King Hospital, Tung Wah Hospital and Grantham Hospital, Hong Kong

A. Mark Clarfield
Ben Gurion University of the Negev, Beer Sheva, Israel, and McGill University, Montreal, QC, Canada

Davis Coakley
Trinity College, Dublin, Ireland

Rodney M. Coe
Saint Louis University Health Sciences Center, St Louis, MO, USA

Kenneth J. Collins
St Pancras and University College Hospitals, London, UK

Cynthia L. Comella
Rush University Medical Center, Chicago, IL, USA

Martin J. Connolly
University of Manchester & Manchester Royal Infirmary, Manchester, UK

Lucy J. Coward
The National Hospital for Neurology and Neurosurgery, London, UK, and University College London, London, UK

Pamela M. Crawford
York Hospital, York, UK

Ilana B. Crome
Keele University Medical School, Keele, UK

Peter Crome
Keele University Medical School, Keele, UK

Suzanne Crowe
Adelaide & Meath Hospital incorporating the National Children's Hospital, Dublin, Ireland

Alfonso J. Cruz-Jentoft
Hospital Ramón y Cajal, Madrid, Spain

James M. Cummings
Saint Louis University, St Louis, MO, USA

Adrian C. Davis
University of Manchester, Manchester, UK

Lisette C.P.G.M. de Groot
Wageningen University, Wageningen, The Netherlands

Michael J. Denham
Wellcome Trust Centre for the History of Medicine at UCL, London, UK

Abhilash K. Desai
Saint Louis University Health Sciences Center, St Louis, MO, USA

Gerhard-Paul Diller
National Heart and Lung Institute, London, UK

Catherine Dixon
BUPA Care Services, Leeds, UK

Saskie Dorman
Velindre Cancer Centre, Cardiff, UK

Richard L. Doty
University of Pennsylvania, Philadelphia, PA, USA

Lindsey Dow
Royal United Hospital NHS Trust, Bath, UK

Mary C. Dufour
CSR Incorporated, Arlington, VA, USA

Bakri H. Elsheikh Mohamed
Ohio State University College of Medicine, Columbus, OH, USA

Pamela M. Enderby
University of Sheffield, Sheffield, UK

Elliot F. Epstein
Walsall Manor Hospital, Walsall, UK

Ann R. Falsey
University of Rochester School of Medicine and Dentistry, Rochester, NY, USA

Francesco Fattirolli
University of Florence and Azienda Ospedaliero Universitaria Careggi, Florence, Italy

Maria A. Fiatarone Singh
University of Sydney, New South Wales, Australia, Hebrew Rehabilitation Center for Aged, Roslindale, MA, USA, and Tufts University, Boston, MA, USA

Ilora G. Finlay
Cardiff University, Cardiff, UK

Paul M. Finucane
University of Limerick, Limerick, Ireland

Alfred L. Fisher
University of California, San Francisco, CA, USA

Joseph H. Flaherty
Saint Louis University School of Medicine and Saint Louis Veterans' Affairs Medical Center, St Louis, MO, USA

Paul T. Francis
King's College London, London, UK

Miriam L. Freimer
Ohio State University College of Medicine, Columbus, OH, USA

Michael P. Frenneaux
University of Birmingham, Birmingham, UK

Brant E. Fries
University of Michigan and Ann Arbor Veterans' Affairs Medical Center, Ann Arbor, MI, USA

Julie K. Gammack
Saint Louis University School of Medicine, St Louis, MO, USA, and Geriatric Research Education and Clinical Center, St Louis, MO, USA

Krishnendu Ghosh
University Hospital, Coventry, UK

Barbara A. Gilchrest
Boston University School of Medicine, Boston, MA, USA

Neil D. Gillespie
University of Dundee, Dundee, UK

D. Grammatopoulos
University of Warwick, Warwick, UK

Joseph E. Grey
University of Wales College of Medicine, Cardiff, UK

Janet E. Griffiths
University Dental Hospital, Cardiff, UK

George T. Grossberg
Saint Louis University Health Sciences Center, St Louis, MO, USA

Luis M. Gutiérrez-Robledo
Instituto Nacional de Ciencias Médicas y Nutrición "Salvador Zubirán", México D.F., Mexico

Ramzi R. Hajjar
Saint Louis University Health Sciences Center, St Louis, MO, USA, and Saint Louis Veterans' Affairs Medical Center, St Louis, MO, USA

Kingsley K. Hampton
Royal Hallamshire Hospital, Sheffield, UK

J. Richard Harding
St Woolos and Royal Gwent Hospitals, Newport, UK

Keith G. Harding
University of Wales College of Medicine, Cardiff, UK

Ian K. Hart
Walton Centre for Neurology and Neurosurgery, Liverpool, UK

Catherine Hawes
Texas A&M University System Health Science Center, College Station, TX, USA

Nicky Hayes
King's College Hospital NHS Trust, London, UK

Arthur E. Helfand
Temple University, Philadelphia, PA, USA, and Thomas Jefferson University, Philadelphia, PA, USA

Robert D. Helme
Barbara Walker Centre for Pain Management, Fitzroy, Victoria, Australia

Philip J. Henschke
Repatriation General Hospital, Daw Park, South Australia, Australia

David Hilton-Jones
Radcliffe Infirmary NHS Trust, Oxford, UK, Milton Keynes Hospital NHS Trust, Buckinghamshire, UK, and Myasthenia Gravis Association Myasthenia Centre, Oxford, UK

Katsuiku Hirokawa
Tokyo Medical & Dental University, Tokyo, Japan

Michael Horowitz
University of Adelaide, Adelaide, South Australia, Australia

Philippe Huber
University Hospital of Geneva, Geneva, Switzerland

Steve Iliffe
Royal Free & UCL Medical School, London, UK

Jonathan S. Ilowite
Winthrop University Hospital, New York, NY, USA

Radha Indusekhar
University Hospital of North Staffordshire, Stoke-on-Trent, UK

Donald F. Jessett
Formerly of University of Wales, Cardiff, UK

Antony Johansen
University Hospital of Wales, Cardiff, UK

David Jolley
University of Staffordshire, Staffordshire, UK

Seema Joshi
Saint Louis University Health Sciences Center, St Louis, MO, USA

Maureen Junker-Kenny
Trinity College, Dublin, Ireland

Lalit Kalra
King's College London, London, UK

Benny Katz
Pain Management Clinic for the Elderly, Victoria, Australia

Hugo E. Kesteloot
Katholieke Universiteit Leuven, Leuven, Belgium

Rafi Kevorkian
Saint Louis University, St Louis, MO, USA

Moon J. Kim
Saint Louis University School of Medicine and Saint Louis Veterans' Affairs Medical Center, St Louis, MO, USA

Thomas B.L. Kirkwood
University of Newcastle, Newcastle-upon-Tyne, UK

Paul V. Knight
Royal Infirmary, Glasgow, UK

Katie Kompoliti
Rush University Medical Center, Chicago, IL, USA

John F. Kurtzke
Veterans' Affairs Medical Center and Georgetown University, Washington, DC, USA

James F. Lamb
Ohio State University College of Medicine and Public Health, Columbus, OH, USA

Andrew J. Larner
Walton Centre for Neurology and Neurosurgery, Liverpool, UK

Arthur Leibovitz
Shmuel Harofeh Medical Centre, Beer Yaacov, Israel

Wee Shiong Lim
Tan Tock Seng Hospital, Singapore

Daniel S. Loo
Boston University School of Medicine, Boston, MA, USA

Seth Love
University of Bristol, Bristol, UK

Gordon D.O. Lowe
University of Glasgow, Glasgow, UK, and Glasgow Royal Infirmary, Glasgow, UK

Linda M. Luxon
University College of London Hospitals NHS Trust, London, UK, and University College London, London, UK

Kenneth W. Lyles
Veterans' Affairs Medical Center, Duke University Medical Center, Durham, NC, USA

Juan F. Macías-Núnez
University Hospital of Salamanca, Salamanca, Spain

Chris MacKnight
Dalhousie University, Halifax, NS, Canada

Takashi Makinodan
University of California at Los Angeles School of Medicine, Los Angeles, CA, USA

Robert E. Mansel
Wales College of Medicine, Cardiff University, Cardiff, UK

Kenneth G. Manton
Duke University, Durham, NC, USA

Niccolò Marchionni
University of Florence and Azienda Ospedaliero Universitaria Careggi, Florence, Italy

Jennifer L. Maskel
University of Wisconsin and Veterans' Affairs Medical Center, Madison, WI, USA

Giulio Masotti
University of Florence and Azienda Ospedaliero Universitaria Careggi, Florence, Italy

Samuel Spence McCachren
Thompson Cancer Survival Center, Knoxville, TN, USA

Graydon S. Meneilly
University of British Columbia, Vancouver, BC, Canada

Jean-Pierre Michel
University Hospital of Geneva, Geneva, Switzerland

Charles Mobbs
Mount Sinai School of Medicine, New York, NY, USA

Paul Montgomery
University of Oxford, Oxford, UK

Timothy D. Moon
University of Wisconsin and Veterans' Affairs Medical Center, Madison, WI, USA

Arshag D. Mooradian
Saint Louis University, St Louis, MO, USA

Terry L. Moore
Saint Louis University Health Sciences Center, St Louis, MO, USA

Padma Moorjani
University of Manchester, Manchester, UK

Fernando Morales-Martínez
University of Costa Rica, San José, Costa Rica

Philippe Moreillon
University of Lausanne, Lausanne, Switzerland

Jo Moriarty
King's College London, London, UK

John E. Morley
Saint Louis University School of Medicine and Saint Louis Veterans' Affairs Medical Center, St Louis, MO, USA

John N. Morris
Hebrew Rehabilitation Center for Aged, Boston, MA, USA

John S. Morris
Princess of Wales Hospital, Bridgend, UK

Carlos G. Musso
Hospital Italiano de Buenos Aires, Buenos Aires, Argentina

Joseph M. Mylotte
University at Buffalo, Buffalo, NY, USA

Andrew C. Newby
University of Bristol, Bristol, UK

Thorsten Nikolaus
University of Ulm, Ulm, Germany

Fatemeh Nourhashémi
Toulouse University Hospital, Toulouse, France

Laurence Nunn
St George's Hospital Medical School, London, UK

P.M.S. O'Brien
University Hospital of North Staffordshire, Stoke-on-Trent, UK

Dennis S. Oh
Tufts University School of Medicine, Springfield, MA, USA

Takashi Ohrui
Tohoku University School of Medicine, Sendai, Japan

Rachel F. Oiknine
Saint Louis University, St Louis, MO, USA

F. O'Mahony
University Hospital of North Staffordshire, Stoke-on-Trent, UK

Desmond O'Neill
Adelaide & Meath Hospital incorporating the National Children's Hospital, Dublin, Ireland

Roger D. Orpwood
University of Bath, Bath, UK

Peter W. Overstall
County Hospital, Hereford, UK

Hardev S. Pall
University of Birmingham, Birmingham, UK, and University Hospital Birmingham Foundation Trust, Birmingham, UK

Alan M. Palmer
Pharmidex, London, UK

Martyn Parker
University Hospital of Wales, Cardiff, UK

M.S. John Pathy
University of Wales, Cardiff, UK

Michael G. Pearson
Royal College of Physicians, London, UK

Martha Pelaez
Pan American Health Organization, World Health Organization, Washington, DC, USA

Thomas T. Perls
Boston University School of Medicine, Boston, MA, USA

Horace M. Perry
Saint Louis University, St Louis, MO, USA

Carolyn D. Philpot
Saint Louis University School of Medicine, St Louis, MO, USA

Jeremy R. Playfer
Royal Liverpool University Hospital, Liverpool, UK

Jonathan M. Potter
Royal College of Physicians, London, UK

Colin Powell
Dalhousie University, Halifax, NS, Canada

Jennie A. Powell
Llandough Hospital, Cardiff, UK

Charlene M. Prather
Saint Louis University, St Louis, MO, USA

Yok Ai Que
Centre Hospitalier Universitaire Vaudois, Lausanne, Switzerland

Shobita Rajagopalan
Charles R. Drew University of Medicine and Science, Los Angeles, CA, USA

Christopher K. Rayner
University of Adelaide, Adelaide, South Australia, Australia

Janice Rees
St Woolos Hospital, Newport, UK

Michael W. Rich
Washington University School of Medicine, St Louis, MO, USA

Lucio A. Rinaldi
University of Florence and Azienda Ospedaliero Universitaria Careggi, Florence, Italy

Gabriel J.E. Rinkel
University Medical Centre, Utrecht, The Netherlands

René Rizzoli
University Hospitals, Geneva, Switzerland

Richard C. Roberts
University of Dundee, Dundee, UK

Helen Rodgers
University of Newcastle, Newcastle-upon-Tyne, UK

David S. Rosenthal
Dana-Farber Cancer Institute, Boston, MA, USA

Philip A. Routledge
Cardiff University, Cardiff, UK

Jed Rowe
Moseley Hall Hospital, Birmingham, UK

Laurence Z. Rubenstein
Geriatric Research Education and Clinical Center, UCLA – Greater Los Angeles Veterans' Affairs Medical Center, CA, USA

Hussain Saba
University of South Florida College of Medicine, Tampa, FL, USA, and James A. Haley Veterans' Hospital, Tampa, FL, USA

Natalie Sachs-Ericsson
Florida State University, Tallahassee, FL, USA

Hidetada Sasaki
Tohoku University School of Medicine, Sendai, Japan

D. Gwyn Seymour
University of Aberdeen, Aberdeen, UK

Om Prakash Sharma
Geriatric Society of India, New Delhi, India

Sanjay Sharma
Veterans' Affairs Medical Center, Duke University Medical Center, Durham, NC, USA

Hamsaraj G.M. Shetty
University Hospital of Wales, Cardiff, UK

Stephen D. Silberstein
Thomas Jefferson University, Philadelphia, PA, USA

Alan J. Sinclair
University of Warwick, Coventry, UK

Arun K. Singh
Glasgow Royal Infirmary, Glasgow, UK

Ingmar Skoog
University of Gothenburg, Gothenburg, Sweden

Peter Spiegler
Winthrop University Hospital, New York, NY, USA

Anurag Srivastava
Wales College of Medicine, Cardiff University, Cardiff, UK

Richard M. Stone
Dana-Farber Cancer Institute, Boston, MA, USA

David J. Stott
Glasgow Royal Infirmary, Glasgow, UK

Robert W. Stout
Queen's University Belfast, Belfast, UK

Andreas E. Stuck
Department of Geriatric Medicine, Spital Bern Ziegler, Bern, Switzerland

Yuko Suda
Toyo University, Tokyo, Japan

Cameron G. Swift
King's College London, London, UK

Adam Szafranek
University Hospital of Wales, Cardiff, UK

Peggy A. Szwabo
Saint Louis University School of Medicine, St Louis, MO, USA

Ryutaro Takahashi
Tokyo Metropolitan Institute of Gerontology, Tokyo, Japan

Syed H. Tariq
Saint Louis University School of Medicine, St Louis, MO, USA

Dellara F. Terry
Boston University School of Medicine, Boston, MA, USA

David R. Thomas
Saint Louis University Health Sciences Center and Saint Louis Veterans' Affairs Medical Center, St Louis, MO, USA

Nina Tumosa
Saint Louis University School of Medicine and Saint Louis Veterans' Affairs Medical Center, St Louis, MO, USA

Allan R. Tunkel
Drexel University College of Medicine, Philadelphia, PA, USA

Irene D. Turpie
McMaster University, Hamilton, ON, Canada

Masanori Utsuyama
Tokyo Medical & Dental University, Tokyo, Japan

Jonathan A. Vafidis
University Hospital of Wales, Cardiff, UK

Jan Van Gijn
University Medical Centre, Utrecht, The Netherlands

Wija A. van Staveren
Wageningen University, Wageningen, The Netherlands

Bruno Vellas
Toulouse University Hospital, Toulouse, France

Norman J. Vetter
University of Wales College of Medicine, Cardiff, UK

Pieter Jelle Visser
University of Maastricht, Maastricht, The Netherlands, and VU Medical Center, Amsterdam, The Netherlands

Ladislav Volicer
University of South Florida, Tampa, FL, USA

Ulrich O. von Oppell
University Hospital of Wales, Cardiff, UK

Martha Wadleigh
Dana-Farber Cancer Institute, Boston, MA, USA

Laura M. Wagner
Baycrest Centre for Geriatric Care, Toronto, ON, Canada

Donald Murray Walker
University of Sydney, Westmead, New South Wales, Australia

Mitchell T. Wallin
Veterans' Affairs Medical Center and Georgetown University, Washington, DC, USA

Debra L. Waters
University of Otago, Dunedin, New Zealand

Meme Wijesinghe
Royal United Hospital NHS Trust, Bath, UK

Julie R. Wilcox
Cardiff Royal Infirmary, Cardiff, UK

Lynne K. Williams
University of Birmingham, Birmingham, UK

R. Gareth Williams
University Hospital of Wales, Cardiff, UK

Margaret-Mary G. Wilson
Saint Louis University Health Sciences Center and Veterans' Affairs Medical Center, St Louis, MO, USA

Gary A. Wittert
University of Adelaide, Royal Adelaide Hospital, Adelaide, South Australia, Australia

Fredric D. Wolinsky
University of Iowa, Iowa City, IA, USA, and Center for Research in the Implementation of Innovative Strategies and Practices, Iowa City Veterans' Affairs Medical Center, Iowa City, IA, USA

Mina Yaar
Boston University School of Medicine, Boston, MA, USA

Thomas T. Yoshikawa
Charles R. Drew University of Medicine and Science, Los Angeles, CA, USA

William B. Young
Thomas Jefferson University, Philadelphia, PA, USA

Preface

"I offer no apology for the publication of this volume. The subject is one of the highest importance, and yet it has been strangely overlooked during the last half-century by the physicians of all countries."

-George Edward Day
(1815–1872)

George Day's introduction to his textbook *Disease of Advanced Life*, published in 1848, regrettably remains appropriate for textbooks published over 150 years later. Modern physicians can still fail to recognize the differences in disease presentation and management between middle-aged and older adults. It is our hope that this Fourth Edition of "Principles and Practice of Geriatric Medicine" will help increase the awareness of geriatric principles and improve the treatment of older individuals. John Pathy's original vision for the first edition was to provide, in a single volume, a comprehensive reference source for all those involved in the medicine of old age. We have endeavored to adhere to this vision, but inevitably the size of the textbook has grown. While in any text of this size some overlap with general texts of medicine will occur, the emphasis is on those assessments and disorders that are particularly of relevance to older persons.

Over the seven years since the last edition of this text was published, there have been dramatic advances in our understanding of the pathophysiology of disease as it interacts with the physiological processes of aging. There has been a continuing validation of assessment tools for older persons and the development of some new ones. Large-scale studies of the efficacy of various geriatric systems such as Acute Care for the Elderly Units, Geriatric Evaluation and Management Units, and Home Care Systems have been carried out. All of these have demonstrated the value and cost-effectiveness of the geriatric specialist approach to managing older people. In comparison, most studies assessing Coronary Care Units and Intensive Care Units have failed to come close to demonstrating the effectiveness that has been shown for geriatric units. Despite this, all major hospitals have highly expensive critical care units, while fewer have developed geriatric units. The last decade has also seen an increased awareness of the need to enhance the quality of long-term care. This increase in geriatric knowledge has been recognized by the addition of nearly 40 new chapters in this edition. In addition, many of the previous chapters have been totally rewritten to allow the recognition of the changes that have occurred in our understanding of the care of older persons.

Previous editions of this textbook were edited by a single person, John Pathy. With the rapid increase in geriatric knowledge and John's desire for the Fourth Edition to reflect the input of other academic minds, he has added two new editors to share the burden with him, namely, Alan Sinclair and John Morley. This has allowed a more even distribution of the editing tasks, though John Pathy has continued to carry the lion's share. In recognition of the globalization of the world, in general, and geriatrics, in particular, one of the new editors, John Morley, is from the United States, while Alan Sinclair draws on his European experiences. In addition, a major effort has been made at the end of the text to recognize the differences (as well as the similarities) of geriatrics as it is practiced around the world. The enormous good fortune the editors had in recruiting a stellar class of contributors from around the world has, we hope, allowed this text to be truly representative of a global view of geriatric medicine. From the beginning, John Pathy has made this a goal of his text, and the editors feel that this edition has truly achieved an international view of old-age medicine as originally developed by Marjorie Warren and her colleagues in the United Kingdom.

The general outline of the text still follows that of the first edition. The first sections provide a general perspective of old age, the processes of aging, and social and community perspectives. The chapter on preventive medicine now focuses on issues of particular importance to older persons. In Part III "Medicine in Old Age", the section "Eating Disorders and Nutritional Health" has been increased to recognize the increased importance and understanding of nutrition in old age. Chapters on frailty, sarcopenia, palliative care, and women's health have been added to recognize the increasing importance of these issues in older persons. The final part on "Health Care Systems" focuses first on the emergence of continuous quality improvement, geriatric systems and evidence-based medicine as the foundation of high-quality geriatric medicine. The development of novel education systems is discussed. Finally, unique aspects of geriatric care around the world are examined.

In an attempt to improve the readability of the text, we have asked the authors to make liberal use of tables and figures, and key points have been added at the end of each chapter. References have been limited, and at the beginning of the reference list, authors identify a few key references to allow for further reading. The new editors have tried to keep the easy reading style of the previous editions, but, as can be imagined, this has been a difficult task as we have increased the number of contributors from around the world.

Overall, we hope our readers enjoy and learn from this textbook; for the three of us, it has been a true labor of love. We particularly would like to thank our contributors for the excellent job they have done. We would also like to thank Layla Paggetti from John Wiley & Sons for her tireless efforts in making sure this book came to fruition. Finally, we would like to thank our families for their forbearance. This book is dedicated to all those who care for older persons.

M.S. John Pathy, Alan J. Sinclair, John E. Morley
December 2005

Preface to the Third Edition

With an increasingly aging population in both the industrialized and developing world, the health care needs of older people can no longer be dismissed by society.

A national provision for geriatric medical services was initially a British phenomenon that was later adopted by other European nations. On the other hand, the USA has long been at the forefront of much gerontological research. During the past decade, however, clinical practice and teaching in geriatric medicine has also moved forward at a phenomenal pace. The balance in this new edition reflects and emphasizes these changes.

Those familiar with the previous editions will note that this edition has been published as a two volume set. This has been necessitated by the addition of 27 new chapters and the reorganization of and increase in the number of clinical chapters. The original objective of providing an authoritative text on the medicine of old age has been maintained thanks to the distinguished panel of nearly 200 international contributors.

It is with deepest regret that I record the deaths of Professor Verna Wright and Professor Frank Benson.

Dr John Morris, Dr Arup Banergee and Dr Brian Williams have generously provided editorial advice on the gastroenterology, haematology and cardiology sections respectively.

The sustained support of Michael Osuch and Lewis Derrick of John Wiley & Sons is gratefully acknowledged.

It is hoped that these two volumes will encourage and inform all those whose clinical practice brings them into contact with elderly patients.

Preface to the Second Edition

In this new edition my priority was not only to revise and update, but to reorganize and restructure to make the information as accessible and useful to the reader as possible. The result is that not only have we included some 45 distinguished new contributors, and indeed several entirely new topics, but about 50% of the book has been rewritten almost from scratch, with the remainder heavily revised and updated, and the entire content radically reorganized into what I believe is a more practical and logical format. New subjects now considered to be at the forefront of practice, and some published here for the first time, are covered, and I am delighted to welcome the following group of new authors:

Professor D. Armstrong, Dr C.A. Bar, Dr W.H. Barker, Dr A.J. Bayer, Professor M. Bergman, Dr E.T. Bloom, Dr D.G. Clements, Dr K.J. Collins, Dr I.G. Finlay, Dr P. Finucane, Dr C. Freer, Dr S.R. Gambert, Professor A.M. Gelb, Ms J.E. Griffiths, Dr J.T. Hartford, Ms A.E. Helfand, Dr S.J. James, Mr D.F. Jessett, Dr R.A. Kane, Professor H. Katsunuma, Professor H. Kesteloot, Dr J. Lubinski, Dr L.M. Luxon, Professor W.J. Maclennan, Dr S.S. McCachren, Professor J.F. Macias-Nunez, Dr S.E. Mathers, Dr K. Morgan, Dr J.G. O'Brien, Dr M.E. Piper, Dr J. Powell, Ms H.G. Prince, Dr T. Pullar, Dr D.S. Rosenthal, Dr H.R. Silberman, Dr I.C. Stewart, Dr R. Strong, Professor M. Swash, Professor C.G. Swift, Professor W.A. Wallace, Dr M.F. Wilkins, Dr W.G. Wood, Dr A.M. Woods, Professor V. Wright.

It is with deepest regret, however, that I must record the death of three contributors:

Professor A.N. Exton-Smith, Dr R.A. Griffiths and Sir Alan Parks.

I express my sincere appreciation to Dr A.J. Bayer for his invaluable assistance with some of the chapters, to my secretary, Mrs Shirley Green, for her meticulous typing, checking of references and collating material, and to the Department of Medical Illustration, University of Wales College of Medicine, for undertaking the additional illustrations for the revised chapter on rehabilitation in the elderly. It is a pleasure to acknowledge the high standard of general editorial services provided by Dr Lewis Derrick, Desk Editor, and the continuing support of Mrs Verity Waite, Publishing Editor in Medicine, John Wiley & Sons.

Preface to the First Edition

In some parts of the world, notably Europe, North America and Japan, the impact of an expanding elderly population resulting from an era of unprecedented reduction in the diseases of early life has already had a dramatic effect on the epidemiology of disease. Within the foreseeable future no nation will escape a similar increase in the number of its elderly citizens with similar changes in the disease profile of its society. In the developed industrial nations Governments and medical schools, recognizing this phenomenon, are increasingly encouraging teaching and research in the medicine of later life. The objective of this textbook, written by authors of international repute, is to provide in a single volume a comprehensive reference source for all who are involved in the medicine of old age. Some overlap with textbooks of general medicine is inevitable but appropriate emphasis and attention is given to those disorders which are of particular relevance to the elderly.

Whilst this is primarily a clinical textbook, an account is given of the fundamental changes associated with aging which are so inextricably interlinked with diseases that their study is essential to our understanding and management of elderly sick and disabled people.

Equally important for those treating and caring for the old is an understanding of the influence, for good or ill, of the social environment within which the elderly have to function and its effect on their health.

Knowledge of programmes aimed at the promotion and maintenance of health, early detection of its impending breakdown and the organization and provision of services for health care are additional essential components of a complete account of the medicine of old age.

The early chapters of the book provide a general perspective of old age and the process of aging. Preventive aspects together with accounts of nutrition and sleep in the elderly and the interpretation of biochemical data in older patients, precede the main clinical section which occupies the greater part of the text. The later chapters cover rehabilitation, the management of the dying patient and aspects of the delivery of health care.

I acknowledge with gratitude the willing help of my colleagues, Dr Deirdre Hine and Dr D. Gwyn Seymour who read through much of the text and provided valuable criticisms and suggestions; and to my secretaries Mrs Lorraine Spriggs who did much of the typing and the arduous task of checking references, and Mrs Sylvia Bevan. I am indebted to Dr Ralph Marshall and his team in the Department of Medical Illustration at the University Hospital of Wales for preparing a number of figures and photographs.

PART III

Medicine in Old Age

Section 7

Dementia and Cognitive Disorders

89

Communication Disorders in Dementia

Jennie A. Powell

Llandough Hospital, Cardiff, UK

THE NORMAL COMMUNICATION PROCESS – A MODEL

Communication is the process through which an "idea" or "thought" is passed from one person to another. Ideas commonly are expressed through the use of words, and nonverbally, for example, through body language, gesture, or facial expression. The generation of an idea in the mind and its expression, or the appreciation of ideas received from an external source requires a complex interaction of many cognitive systems and processes. In order to account for the pattern of breakdown of communication in dementia, it is important first to consider some of the components that underlie verbal communication.

Three long-term memory stores are fundamental to the communication process. *Semantic memory (conceptual or "meaning" memory)* is knowledge of the environment that is common to everyone within that environment. For example, the concept "champagne" would be represented in long-term memory in a similar way from one person to another. It could be represented with "visual memories" of context (in a bottle, glass, party, bar, wedding), color (white, pink), and movement (within a glass, poured from a bottle), "gustatory memories" of how it tastes, "olfactory memories" of how it smells, "nonverbal acoustic memories" (cork popping), "emotional memories" (joy, celebration), "kinaesthetic memories" (lifting glass, pouring action), "tactile memories" (feeling of gaseous liquid in the mouth), and so on. These memories in combination form the concept of "champagne" represented in semantic memory.

Episodic memory is an individual's memory of the world that is personal to that individual. For example, whereas basic knowledge of what champagnes is common knowledge (stored in semantic memory), the fact that *you* drank champagne *yesterday* is personal knowledge which is stored in episodic memory. Episodic memory is therefore probably built up of elements of semantic memory with a personal context attached.

Lexical memory (word memory) is a mental dictionary or lexicon. The label "champagne", which represents the concept of champagne would be stored here. The label in itself is meaningless without reference to conceptual knowledge in semantic memory.

Working memory is a buffer that holds information in consciousness – it is in effect what you are thinking right now. Information stored in long-term memory is brought back into consciousness in working memory as and when it is needed – this creates an internally generated "thought". Information received into working memory from an external source is matched to information previously stored in semantic, episodic, and lexical memory in order to be "understood". If the information is new to the individual, for example, a new concept, word or event, it is transferred into semantic and/or episodic and/or lexical memory for long-term storage and future reference. Working memory incorporates executive functions, attention, concentration, extraction, reasoning, and so on.

The relationship between thought and language (lexical memory) is complex. An information-processing model of the normal communication process can provide a helpful framework for understanding how they may relate (Figure 1).

Thinking refers to the formation, generation, and manipulation of memories, concepts, and ideas in the mind. Semantic, episodic, and working memories are fundamental components. Thinking is heavily dependent on efficient working memory. We are all aware of times when we have trouble with thought – when our ideas are not well organized, when we have only vague, hazy, or wooly knowledge about something or when we lose track of what we are thinking.

The relationship of language to thought has been the subject of debate for centuries. Understanding some of the complexities of this relationship is important in order to understand communication breakdown in dementia. In considering the link between thought and words, it is helpful here to consider three subcomponents within lexical

Principles and Practice of Geriatric Medicine, 4th Edition. Edited by M.S. John Pathy, Alan J. Sinclair and John E. Morley.

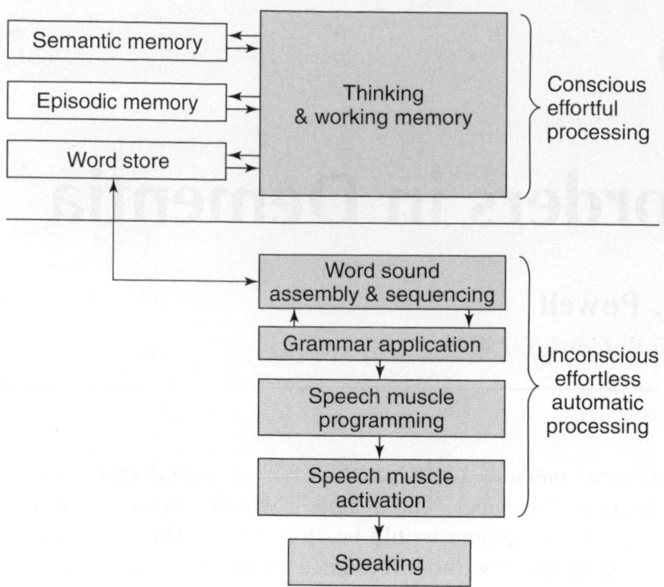

Figure 1 A model of the communication process – from internally generated thought to speech

memory – *word store, word sound assembly and sequencing, and grammar (syntax) application.*

The *word store* is the actual store that contains word memories. Semantic memory, thinking, and word store are closely intertwined. Concepts weakly established in semantic memory can give rise to "word-finding" difficulties in the normal person. For example, when first encountering a new exotic fruit, its name may not be recalled on a second occasion if the concept is too weakly represented in semantic memory. Further encounters with the fruit (its taste, texture, appearance, uses, etc.) help establish and strengthen the concept in semantic memory. Hearing and using the word strengthens the label of its name in the word store. Selection and retrieval of the name of the item is easier if its concept representation in semantic memory, its word memory representation in the word store and the connections between the two types of representations are strong.

A second subcomponent of lexical memory is *word sound assembly and sequencing. This* refers to the selection and sequencing of word sounds (phonemes) to form words. A third subcomponent of lexical memory is *grammar (syntax) application.* This is the ordering of words into meaningful phrases and sentences according to an internalized set of rules. It includes the application of morphemes (minimal grammatical units), for example, the addition of "ed" after "walk" to denote the past tense.

Speech muscle programming is the process of planning the pattern and sequence of movements to be made by the speech muscles. Finally, *speech muscle activation* refers to the physical enactment of the motor program.

Communication is, in reality of course, not a linear process – there is considerable overlap and interaction between its various components. Words loop back into thinking, thereby facilitating thought and becoming a part of thought in themselves. In addition, impairment within one component can give the impression of impairment within another component that is, in fact, intact. For example, when there are problems within thinking with holding onto and organizing ideas, grammar is consequentially affected with the use of half sentences as the person loses their train of thought. In reality, the grammar system may in itself be fully intact. Clinically, it can be a challenge to identify the primary locus of a presenting impairment. However, doing so can help in differential diagnosis of the dementias.

BREAKDOWN OF THE NORMAL COMMUNICATION PROCESS IN DEMENTIA

The concept of "*conscious effortful processing*" versus "*automatic processing*" is fundamental to understanding communication breakdown in dementia. Degree of effort required for each of the components in the communication process varies. *Thinking,* including accessing episodic, semantic, and lexical memory requires conscious effortful processing, whereas *word sound assembly and sequencing, grammar application, speech muscle programming*, and *speech muscle activation* are all normally automatic, unconscious, and effortless. Whereas we can be consciously aware of thinking of what to say and the words to say it, we are not normally aware of choosing word sounds or grammar or of programming and activating the speech muscles – these skills are, in effect, akin to "procedural memory" tasks like walking or riding a bicycle.

As a general rule, in dementia the more conscious and effortful a process is, the more likely that it will be affected. Unconscious, automatic processing is least affected.

Thinking in Dementia

In most dementias, the biggest problem is with thinking. Thinking requires highly effortful, conscious processing. It also involves a large number of cognitive components and processes spread over a wide area of the brain. Thinking is therefore particularly vulnerable to the brain damage that in itself gives rise to dementia. The quality, quantity, clarity, and relevance of "ideas" and the ability to manipulate these are impaired.

Alzheimer's Disease (AD) (see Chapter 93, Clinical Aspects of Alzheimer's Disease)

A problem with new learning often is the first reported symptom in Alzheimer's Disease (AD). This affects the ability to add new information to episodic, semantic, and word memory stores. The greatest impact of this is felt on episodic memory, since remembering what has happened in day-to-day life is so fundamental to effective thinking and functioning. The person may forget an event of the previous week or forget something he was told a few days earlier. Often this reflects more a registration deficit rather than a recall deficit – the person has not so much forgotten the new event as not recorded it in the first place. On the other hand, in the early stages of dementia, episodic memories from previous years are often retained, since they were laid down in long-term memory when the brain was still functioning effectively. This explains why memory for events of many years previously may be remembered when events of the previous week are not.

With reduced ability to form new memories, old memories tend to come to the forefront. The person may become repetitive and may talk frequently about the past. As the disease progresses, distant memories also are lost as the episodic memory store itself becomes degraded.

A deficit in working memory occurs in AD, with memory span and central executive function affected. There is impaired ability to "hold on" to information within working memory and the person may lose track of what they were saying. They may report getting stuck for words in conversation when it is actually the idea that has been forgotten. Problems with working memory also give rise to reduced ability to retrieve and manipulate information stored in other memory systems and a generalized "cognitive slowing" (Nebes and Madden, 1988; Nebes and Brady, 1992). This has a marked effect on thinking and thus on communication.

Semantic memory also is impaired. Ability to distinguish subtle differences between concepts diminishes. As the disease progresses, concepts themselves become degraded and merge. On a confrontation-naming test, the patient may call a "zebra" a "donkey" because knowledge of the fact that zebras have stripes and donkeys do not is inaccessible or has been lost. In its severest form, the patient has literally "forgotten" what the item is. As a result, there may appear to be problems with lexical memory, when in reality the problem here is semantic memory – it is not possible to produce an accurate name for an item when the underlying concept is unclear.

Degraded semantic memory results in "empty" speech, which is lacking in specificity and contains few content words – the patient tends to use many words that convey very little information.

Vascular Dementia (VD) (see Chapter 95, Vascular Dementia)

In Vascular Dementia (VD), thinking may be impaired in a way that is very similar to thinking in Alzheimer's disease. However, the picture can be more patchy with relative preservation or impairment of one function relative to another. This reflects the brain areas implicated in the individual vascular pathology. There may be significant insight into difficulties with consequential frustration.

Frontotemporal Dementias (FTD)

The frontal lobes are pivotal to thinking; they are the seat of adaptive behavior, abstract conceptual ability, set shifting, mental flexibility, problem solving, planning, personality, social awareness, social behavior, initiation, inhibition, drive, and motivation.

Thinking in the frontotemporal dementias (FTD) is dependent on the anatomic regions of the brain that are primarily affected. In the frontal dominant variant of FTD, "frontal" features emerge such as poor planning and reasoning, disinhibition, poor social awareness, tactlessness, and egocentricity. Pragmatic difficulties are common, whereby the person has difficulty judging the appropriateness of what they say in the situation.

In the early stage of primary progressive aphasia (PPA), thinking is unaffected. The person is able to carry out occupational tasks and activities of daily living (Tranel, 1992). However, whilst language impairment remains the prominent feature, other cognitive abilities eventually are compromised (Delecluse *et al.*, 1990; Graff-Radford *et al.*, 1990; Kempler *et al.*, 1990; Tyrell *et al.*, 1990).

In semantic dementia, there is breakdown in the conceptual database underlying thinking (Bayer and Reban, 2004). There is profound semantic loss, manifest in failure of word comprehension and naming and/or face and object recognition. Speech is fluent and empty (Neary *et al.*, 1998).

Word Store, Word Sound Assembly and Sequencing and Grammar Application in Dementia

Alzheimer's Disease

Difficulties with word finding are commonly reported in the early stages of AD. The names of people and places can be a particular problem. The locus of this problem may be within thinking and/or the semantic system rather than within the word store itself. Selecting names of people and places requires fine, discriminatory conceptual judgments and strong semantic representations. This requires effortful processing skill; lower-frequency words can also be a particular problem. This may be because lower-frequency words are used less often. They are therefore less available than higher frequency words and, as such, are harder to retrieve. Lower-frequency words may also require more complex semantic judgments. Thus word-finding difficulties in AD may be, in large part, a reflection of task difficulty level rather than a problem with the word store itself.

Typically in AD, as the disease progresses from early to middle stages, difficulty with word finding is reported less often and becomes less problematic for the person. This may be because, as thinking becomes more impaired, the ideas the person wishes to express are less complex and require fewer low frequency words. Also, as the disease progresses and insight is lost, the person may become less aware of any difficulty with word finding and thus less frustrated.

The characteristic pattern in AD is for word sound assembly and sequencing and grammar application to remain relatively preserved until the more advanced stages of the illness. This is because these functions require more automatic and effortless processing and can run on "autopilot".

The most obvious linguistic deficit in typical AD is a failure to use language to convey information (Hier *et al.*, 1985). In summary, the AD patient may be said to "speak well" but "convey little".

Some AD patients have greater atrophy in brain regions responsible for language and therefore present with language difficulties disproportionate to their overall cognitive impairment. These patients may exhibit aphasic features, with struggle to find words and phonemic (sound substitution) errors. They are more likely to be helped by phonemic cueing, which helps them access the words for concepts they are trying to express. However, even where there is a language bias to the AD, the presentation may be qualitatively different from classic aphasia. The impairment sometimes seems to occur at the interface of thought and language. It is as if the person has difficulty thinking and speaking at the same time. If thought load is reduced (for example, when the person is talking about something they are clear about in their mind or when describing a picture in front of them), the language difficulties often lessen.

Vascular Dementia

The pattern of deficit in VD with cortical involvement is similar to that observed in AD. Infarction in brain areas responsible for language, can give rise to specific problems with word store or word store access.

Frontotemporal Dementias

The onset of PPA is, heralded by progressive deterioration of language function in the absence of generalized cognitive decline (Mesulam, 1982). Aphasia is nonfluent (Neary *et al.*, 1998). There may be problems with any one or more lexical components – with word store, word sound assembly and sequencing or grammar application.

Speech Muscle Programming in Dementia

Problems with speech muscle programming give rise to speech apraxia. This does not generally occur in AD in the mild and moderate stages. In VD, problems here are rare but could arise if a vascular event occurred in area of the brain responsible for speech muscle programming. It can be a feature of PPA. Here it may also present as a problem with co-ordinating respiration with speech (a 'respiration-to-speech apraxia'). This may present superficially as hyperventilation or panic.

Speech Muscle Activation in Dementia

Dysarthria typically occurs in the dementias associated with motor signs. These include Parkinson's disease (PD; *see* **Chapter 66, Parkinson's Disease and Parkinsonism in the Elderly**), dementia with lewy bodies (DLB; *see* **Chapter 96, Other Dementias**), progressive supranuclear palsy (PSP), cortico-basal degeneration (CBD) and Huntington's disease (HD). It may also be associated with VD.

Clinical Presentation of Communication in Alzheimer's Disease

Table 1 contains a transcription of the responses of four AD patients who were asked to retell a short story straight after it was presented by the examiner (Bayles and Tomoeda, 1992). The patients varied in severity of dementia, as measured on the global deterioration scale (GDS) (Reisberg *et al.*, 1982). The performances reflect the typical pattern of communication breakdown in AD.

None of the four patients show evidence of specific difficulty with word sound assembly and sequencing, grammar application, speech muscle programming, or speech muscle activation. Grammatical structure is disturbed in the GDS 4, 5, and 6 patients but this appears to be a consequence of hesitancy in thinking rather than impairment within grammar application *per se*. The GDS 6 patient shows that when output is driven by an appropriate thought, grammar can be intact (e.g. "I don't believe I can do that").

On thinking and word store, the GDS 3 patient performs well. There are relevant units of information within sentences that flow freely. The performance of the GDS 4 patient shows inaccuracies and hesitancy. The hesitancy is probably due to uncertainty with the facts rather than specific problems with the word store. Inaccuracy is even

Table 1 Typical performances of AD patients of varying severity on story retelling in the immediate condition. Patient is told the story below and is asked to retell it immediately

While a lady was shopping, her wallet fell out of her purse but she did not see it fall. When she got to the checkout counter, she had no way to pay for her groceries. So she put the groceries away and went home. Just as she opened the door to her house, the phone rang and a little girl told her that she had found her wallet. The lady was very relieved.

GDS 3 patient (mild cognitive decline)

A lady went shopping at the grocery store. Oh. When she got to the counter with her groceries, she reached for her wallet and it was gone. She'd lost it. So she put the groceries back and when she got home the phone rang. Little girl told her she'd found the wallet.

GDS 4 patient (moderate cognitive decline)

A lady went to a um sho.. food store and uh when she went to pay for her food the uh money fell on the floor and someone, a little girl came and picked it up and gave it to her.

GDS 5 patient (moderately severe cognitive decline)

The little girl picked up her wallet that had fal.. fallen out of her carriage and uh she took more than she had planned on taking, her moving it from the ground.

GDS 6 patient (severe cognitive decline)

I don't I don't believe I can do that, let's see (unintelligible). The only the only thing I know of it of it is to to get get back and then up and then up to to up to to turn to another thing that's the only way that's the only thing that I can I can can do it right right now now I'm I'm completely out in in that.

Table 2 Typical performances of AD patients of varying severity on story retelling in the delayed condition. Patient is asked to retell the story a short time later

GDS 3 patient (mild cognitive decline)
Can't do it. Completely gone. I've been concentrating on what we've been doing. It's out the window.
GDS 4 patient (moderate cognitive decline)
Today you told me a short story? Oh my memory is really going.
GDS 5 patient (moderately severe cognitive decline)
Heavens I don't know what story you mea.. asked me (prompt) No.
GDS 6 patient (severe cognitive decline)
That was it and and there and I saw one right out here that that they they came they came came out here and into into the street and ...

greater in the description of the GDS 5 patient, who confabulates in an attempt to fill in the facts. There may, in addition, be problems with word store but this is difficult to disentangle from the problems with thinking that dominate. The GDS 6 patient is totally unable to recall the story reflecting marked impairment of thinking, including problems with attention and concentration. The patient is involved in his own thought. He demonstrates severe problems with thinking, and probably has problems with word store itself. However, again it is difficult to differentiate thinking problems from any specific problems with word store.

Table 2 contains a transcription of the same four patients' responses when asked to recall the same story a short time later. The GDS 3 patient, who repeated the story so well in the immediate condition, is now totally unable to recall the story. The GDS 4 and 5 patients appear to have forgotten the episode of having been told a story at all. The GDS 6 patient responds with totally inappropriate content, reflecting his egocentricity of thought and inability to attend to the task.

ASSESSMENT OF COMMUNICATION AND COMMUNICATION INTERVENTIONS IN DEMENTIA

Assessment of communication provides information that contributes to differential diagnosis of the dementias. Identification of relative strengths and weaknesses also helps in planning appropriate interventions and in guiding carers on management options and strategies that will optimize communication and quality of life. Formal assessment may, at times, seem threatening for the person with dementia. A basic principle therefore is to formally assess only to the extent required to guide diagnosis and management and within the patient's tolerance.

Assessing Communication Components and Processes

A primary focus of assessment is to determine to what extent the presenting problems are due to impairment within thought versus impairment within lexical components and processes. Assessment therefore aims to identify the locus of deficits, that is, where in the communication process the problems originate. The interdependency of thought and language can render this a challenge.

It is helpful again here to bear in mind the distinction between the conscious effortful processing required for thinking and word store access, and the normally unconscious automatic effortless processing needed for word sound assembly and sequencing, grammar application, speech muscle programming, and speech muscle activation.

General conversation allows preliminary evaluation of the more automatic components and processes. Speech muscle activation can be screened by noting any evidence of muscle weakness or dysarthria – slurred speech, indistinct speech, problems with volume control and problems with voice quality or pitch. Also note any problems with prosody resulting from poor motor control, that is, inability to employ or control intonation patterns. Problems with speech muscle programming (apraxia) may present with articulatory groping or awkwardness, struggle movements, or distorted speech.

Grammar application also may be evaluated in conversation. Sentence structure is best assessed when the person is talking about something with which they are familiar. This reduces load on thinking, thus filtering out as far as possible the knock-on effect of problems with thinking on sentence structure. Specific problems with grammar may present as "telegrammatic" speech output with paucity of function (noncontent) words plus/minus grammatical word part (morphological) errors (e.g. walk for "walked").

Any major problems with word sound assembly will show in conversation as phonemic paraphasias (sound substitution errors).

Reading aloud is a skill that can be carried out with automatic processing, bypassing the semantic system. This is demonstrated by our ability to read aloud while taking in nothing of what we have read. Asking the patient to read aloud can provide useful information on the more automatic components of speech and language.

It should, of course, be remembered that while word sound assembly and sequencing, grammar application, speech muscle programming, and speech muscle activation are normally unconscious automatic and effortless, pathology within specific brain areas can interrupt these normally effortless processes.

Word store and word sound assembly and sequencing should be assessed during conversation and on a confrontation picture-naming task comprising pictures with names of varying frequency levels. An analysis of naming errors on a naming task will help determine the locus of impairment. Table 3 lists features that might suggest specific problems with word store, word store access, or word sound assembly and sequencing. Typical naming errors suggestive of a semantic origin for word-finding difficulties would be naming a goat as a dog, for example. If only semantic or "visual" errors (e.g. naming a ruler as a "ladder") are present with none of the features listed in Table 3, the origin of the naming problem is more likely to be within thinking and/or the

Table 3 Features suggestive of specific problems with lexical components or processes

- Clear search or struggle (perhaps with frustration) to think of a word to express an apparently clear thought or idea.
- Clear acknowledgement, if a word is supplied, that this was the word they were trying to say.
- Giving a description that shows accurate concept knowledge, for example, "They come from Australia and they jump".
- Circumlocution around a word that demonstrates they know the concept behind the word they are trying to say, for example, "the soup was made of that thing that rabbits like".
- Self-cueing, for example, "I use it to open the door so it's ...... a key".
- Good response to phonemic cueing (being given the first sound of the word by someone else), for example, It's a k..."
- Use of gesture.
- Giving accurate information about the target word, for example, It begins with "b".
- Phonemic (sound substitution) errors, for example, "wartrode" for "wardrobe"; "flish" for "fish".

semantic system rather than within lexical processes and systems.

Routine psychometric assessments commonly use language to evaluate a range of cognitive skills – failure to identify those patients who have specific language or speech involvement out of proportion to overall generalized cognitive status can lead to false conclusions regarding the overall level of functioning and thus inappropriate decisions for management/placement.

A patient whose general conversation seems impaired by language difficulties but who does surprisingly well on confrontation tasks such as picture naming, may belong to that subset of dementia patients who have particular difficulty thinking and speaking at the same time (see earlier). If thought is assisted, for example, as in a picture-naming task where the concept they are expressing is visible, expressive language comes more easily.

An important element of the evaluation of the thinking component of the communication process is the evaluation of how the person manages with "nonlanguage" activities of daily living. Routine psychometric assessments can be used to obtain an overview of cognitive function in general, but allowances should be made for patients who have demonstrated specific difficulties with language.

Functional Assessment of Communication and Communication Interventions in Dementia

A commonly voiced objection to intervention in dementia is that the person will inevitably deteriorate and thus intervention constitutes an inefficient use of resources. However, the person with dementia has the right to receive interventions that will optimize strengths, compensate for weakness, reduce stress in both patient and carer and promote best possible quality of life. Failure to address the issues can have detrimental consequences for the mental health both of patients and carers. Communication in dementia is the responsibility of the whole multidisciplinary team, which should include a speech and language therapist whose role in empowering and educating others as well as providing direct specialist input is increasingly recognized (Position Paper, 2005).

Loss of meaningful interaction which results from communication breakdown in dementia is distressing for carers (Gilleard, 1984). In an evaluation of communication in 10 mild and moderate dementia patients (Ulatowska *et al.*, 1988), difficulty with staying on topic was reported in 25% of subjects. Sixty-three percent were reported to show memory deficits in conversation by repeating what they had just said, repeatedly asking for the same information or requiring instructions from others over and over again. Problems with communication have been reported by 68% of primary caregivers of dementia patients and were seen as problematic by 74% of these carers (Rabins *et al.*,1982). Bayles and Tomoeda (1991) found the most prevalent of 16 linguistic communication symptoms reported by carers of AD patients was difficulty finding the right word; the least prevalent was an increase in talkativeness.

In a study of the effects of dementia on functional communication (Powell *et al.*, 1995), the perceptions of the carers of 79 community-living dementia patients (59 probable AD; 20 vascular) were compared with the perceptions of family/close friends of a comparable group of 76 control subjects. Informants were asked to rate the prevalence of 32 symptoms of communication breakdown. Comparison of the magnitude of difference between the two groups for each question showed that each of the 32 symptoms was significantly more prevalent in the dementia group than in the control group. Table 4 shows the 32 symptoms, in order of frequency from most to least prevalent, that differentiated the two groups. These data demonstrate that the range of communication problems faced by carers of those with dementia is great.

The aims of communication interventions with people with dementia are many and varied (Powell, 2000a) (Table 5). The overriding aim should be quality of life for patient and carer.

The range of communication-based interventions promoted for people with dementia is wide (Powell, 2000a) Three commonly advocated approaches – reality orientation, validation, and reminiscence – have been the subject of recent systematic reviews (Spector *et al.*, 2005; Neal and Briggs, 2005; Woods *et al.*, 2005). Reality orientation involves the presentation of orientation information – time, place, and person related. It is thought to provide the person with greater understanding of their surroundings, possibly resulting in improved sense of control and self-esteem. Validation is an approach that involves verbalizing the feelings underlying confused behavior rather than reemphasizing facts. Reminiscence is the vocal or silent recall of the events of a person's life alone, with another person, or in a group. The reviews concluded that there is some evidence for the benefits of reality orientation on both cognition and behavior. No firm conclusions could be made about validation or reminiscence at present.

It is almost certain that there is merit in many of the approaches advocated – the challenge is to determine, on

Table 4 Symptoms of communication breakdown in dementia

1. Asks the same question a number of times
2. Struggles to think of the names of places
3. Trouble following television programs
4. Difficulty following a conversation when a group of people are talking
5. Struggles to think of people's names
6. Has trouble keeping a conversation going
7. Calls people by the wrong name
8. Starts to say something and then forgets what he or she was talking about
9. Tells you the same story or piece of information a number of times
10. Difficulty following a conversation with just you
11. Struggles to think of the names of objects
12. If asked to pass something that is nearer to him or her than to you, passes something else instead
13. Has trouble starting up a conversation
14. Drifts from the point during a conversation
15. When asked a question, gives an answer that has nothing to do with the question
16. Calls places by the wrong name
17. Trouble understanding the meaning of words when you talk to him or her
18. Calls objects by the wrong name
19. During conversation, changes the subject inappropriately
20. Deliberately avoids speaking to friends
21. Fails to say "Hello" to friends when meeting them
22. Talks to imaginary people or things
23. Stares at you too much during a conversation
24. Uses words like "thingey", "what's-a-name" or "thingumy-jig" instead of using a person's correct name
25. Uses words like "thingey", "what's-a-name" or "thingumy-jig" instead of using the correct name for an object
26. Uses words like "thingey", "what's-a-name" or "thingumy-jig" instead of using the correct name for a place
27. Talks too much at an inappropriate time
28. Uses a word in a conversation which sounds like the word you know he or she is trying to say but means something else
29. Uses "words" in conversation which are not real words
30. Talks out loud in an inappropriate place
31. Comes up too close to you when talking
32. Avoids looking at you during a conversation

Table 5 Some aims of communication interventions in dementia

- Improvement in functional memory skills, for example, the ability to remember to take medications
- Improvement in specific language skills, for example, comprehension and word finding
- Increased relevance of content of conversations
- Increased social interaction
- Delay in the progression of cognitive deficits
- Behavioral changes, for example, decreased agitation or anxiety
- Increased interest and responsiveness
- Improved well-being/comfort

an individual basis, who would benefit from which approach and when.

Planning effective programs of intervention requires that the clinician obtains a holistic profile of the patient, their carers, and environment. Alongside assessment of the communication components and processes (above), the following should be evaluated: hearing and vision; carer's perceptions of communication, carer–patient interaction, carer's management strategies and stress levels, daily lifestyle/activities/engagement opportunities, physical environment.

Hearing and Vision

Patients with dementia who, in addition, have problems with hearing and/or vision are highly vulnerable to the adverse effects of these sensory deprivations on communication. It is difficult for the person to capitalize on remaining cognitive abilities and they may become disproportionally handicapped relative to their underlying cognitive status. They are likely to have difficulty remembering that vision and hearing are a problem and may be unable to compensate, for example, by asking for a repeat when they have not heard. Remembering how to adjust and clean hearing aids and glasses and remembering when to use them becomes problematic. Carers often fail to recognize the person's deteriorating ability to cope with aids and are likely to require advice on aid maintenance. A nonfunctioning hearing aid or an aid blocked with wax simply acts as an ear plug, while glasses caked in debris may lead to misinterpretations and could increase risk of falls.

Carer's Perceptions of Communication, Carer–Patient Interaction, Carer's Management Strategies and Stress Levels

One of the most prevalent communication symptoms in dementia is a tendency to ask the same question a number of times. This behavior has been described as particularly stressful to caregivers (Quayhagen and Quayhagen, 1988). When carers are asked how they respond when faced with repetitiousness, replies vary: "I keep answering"; "I ignore it"; "I tell her she's already said that"; 'For the first five times I answer'; "I tend to walk away"; "I will get a piece of paper and write it down"; "I say that I'm not sure".

An interview with the carer will help identify communication difficulties that are most bothersome. Discussion of current management strategies may indicate alternative approaches that could be tried to enhance communication and limit distress (Tables 6–8). Some carers learn by trial and error what does and does not help in their situation, but timely discussion can help this process along. The relief carers feel from reassurance that their approaches to management are appropriate cannot be underestimated.

Daily Lifestyle, Activities, and Engagement Opportunities

Daily lifestyle can have positive or negative effects on communication. Impaired thinking often affects ability to take the initiative – this may make the person appear apathetic or deliberately negative. Thus, even in the early to middle stages of dementia, the person is likely to require direction and guidance in order to occupy time constructively and enjoyably and to maintain remaining abilities for as long as possible. Carers may need to be helped to understand this. It may be needed to be explained that, with appropriate

Table 6 General principles for managing communication problems in dementia

- React in a way that causes the least upset to patient and carer
- The most appropriate approach may differ among individuals
- An approach that works in one situation may not work for the same person in a different situation
- Use trial and error to find out what works best and when
- Avoid asking open-ended questions about recent events that set the person up for failure
- Supply missing words and names rather than let the person struggle
- Do not draw attention to mistakes
- Avoid confrontation – do not argue the point
- Try to think of practical ways around problem situations – for example, remove dirty clothing at night if this is a possible source of confrontation
- Try using a "validation"-type approach by responding to the patient's underlying emotion, for example, "You seem upset"
- Distract from repetition or perseveration
- Use a soothing, calm voice

Table 7 Practical strategies to help communication in dementia

- Memory aides, for example, diaries, notebooks, sticky notes
- Written instructions and written labeling of environment (e.g. contents of cupboard)
- Memory albums (Powell, 2000b; Bourgeois, 1992; Powell and Bayer, 1996)
- Timetables (see "daily lifestyle")
- Day-date-month clock for orientation
- Adapted radio with volume fixed and tuning set to favorite channel – only one large on/off switch visible and accessible
- Memory prompter with infrared motion detection that activates a prerecorded message. For example, placed near the door, motion activates "don't forget to take your keys"

Table 8 Helping communication where attention and comprehension are a problem

- Limit extraneous noise (TV/radio/trolleys in residential setting, etc.)
- When speaking, sit or stand close to the person with your face in clear view
- One to one is usually easier than a group
- Get eye contact (call name/touch arm)
- Use short simple sentences
- Speak slowly and clearly
- Give time for each short sentence to be understood
- Repeat and rephrase if necessary
- Point to objects or people as you mention them
- Be literal – do not use metaphors
- Break commands down into a series of individual steps (task segmentation)

prompts, the person may be able continue with many routine tasks or activities. For example, the person may no longer automatically select a CD to listen to, switch on and start the CD player. With the right prompts (e.g. "Shall we select a CD?") the occupation may be retained and enjoyed.

A routine and familiar structure to the day is helpful. In the early and middle stages, using a timetable or "weekly planner" may help provide structure and purpose to the day and promote confidence. A carer will need to help the patient fill in the timetable and use it. The timetable may record appointments (e.g. 11 o'clock hairdresser), essential tasks (e.g. sweep the path) and leisure activities (e.g. feed the birds). Checking the timetable regularly can help with orientation. Completed tasks could be marked off, giving a sense of achievement. Tasks and activities should capitalize on well-learned routines, especially those that are repetitive. This is because abilities based on more routine, automatic "procedural memory" are better preserved in dementia than abilities requiring more complex reasoning and planning skills.

Activities can help reestablish a sense of usefulness and pleasure and to reduce feelings of helplessness and futility (Mace, 1987). Carers should be guided by what the person may have enjoyed premorbidly, but should also consider new activities the person may now enjoy. It is a challenge to find activities that the person can enjoy with limited supervision.

The degree to which a relative carer should be asked to be involved in activities should be carefully assessed (Table 9). Carers are likely to be struggling to adjust emotionally to the illness and practically to the additional responsibilities of caring and may find organizing activities burdensome. Patient–carer support groups can allow the patient to explore new activities and friendships, while supporting the carer emotionally and practically. As the disease progresses, it often becomes appropriate to transfer some of the responsibility for activities/daily occupation to other agents, for example, volunteers, day centers, care workers committed to quality lifestyles.

In the middle and advanced stages of dementia, when the person may be in continuing care, it is just as important to find relevant activities and engagement opportunities. Failure to address the level of activity or engagement and to provide stimulation appropriate to the individual can have serious consequences. A lack of touch and attention, sensory impairments, and being deprived of conversation and mental stimulation may result in boredom, withdrawal, somatic complaints, visual distortions, hallucination and delusions, increased dependency, and a lower survival rate (Beisgen, 1989). On the other hand, too much stimulation can cause fear, anxiety, irritability, or panic. Many elderly people without dementia are happy to spend a large part of the day doing nothing or being passively rather than actively involved. Stimulation should therefore be appropriate to the individual and be designed to add pleasure and a sense of purpose in the moment, perhaps evoking pleasant memories, associations, and sensations. Care should be taken not to impose one's own needs or opinions on the person with dementia. It is important for professional caregivers to have available information concerning the individual's life history. It is helpful for extended care facility staff to remember that even though events, activities, and interactions may not be remembered explicitly, implicit memories of an interaction

Table 9 Points to consider when involving relatives in activity plan

- Carer's stress level
- Carer's cognitive status
- Realism of carer's expectations and ability to offer appropriate degree of encouragement
- Time, energy, and will of carer to be involved

Table 10 Ideas for adapting the environment to promote good communication

- Adequate lighting to limit misperceptions/"hallucinations"
- Good-sized window through which change of seasons and weather is visible
- Seasonal decorations for "absorbed" (not forced) orientation
- Photo and name on bedroom door
- Bright colors on door of bathroom and toilet for orientation
- Brightly colored tape on edges of steps
- Visually stimulating posters, pictures, mobiles, tropical fish
- Vibrant colors, for example, brightly colored plain furniture
- Multisensory environment that allows opportunity for appropriate tactile, auditory, olfactory, and visual stimulation
- Cover or remove mirrors if they cause distress
- Limit extraneous noises
- Rummage area or rummage box with miscellaneous items to search through may help with restlessness

or event can increase sense of well-being and raise level of alertness.

In an ideal setting, a range of communication approaches should be available and professionals should be trained formally to evaluate benefits and adverse reactions to interventions on an individual basis (Powell, 2000a). A tool such as the Cardiff lifestyle improvement profile for people in extended residential care (CLIPPER) can assist with this (Powell, 2000b). The profile aims to improve the lifestyle of people in continuing care who have difficulty communicating their needs and wishes. It encourages staff to develop greater awareness of verbal and nonverbal responses in order to identify pleasant and unpleasant activities and to plan effective interventions. Dementia care mapping is an observation tool designed to examine quality of care from the perspective of the person with dementia. It can be useful as part of a process of bringing about improvements within formal care settings (Kitwood and Bredin, 1992).

Physical Environment

People with dementia can have difficulty adapting to major changes within their physical environment. Carers should be advised to change the environment as little as possible. However, periodic removal of clutter can help patients discriminate the objects they need to carry out activities of daily life. The physical environment can be subtly adapted to promote optimum communication for moderately and severely impaired patients (Table 10).

KEY POINTS

- An information-processing model of communication provides a framework for understanding the relationship between thought and language.
- Understanding how impairments in thought and in language may present clinically can contribute to differential diagnosis of the dementias.
- Identification of relative strengths and weaknesses allows planning of appropriate interventions and guidance of carers on management options and strategies.
- The person with dementia has the right to receive interventions that will optimize strengths, compensate for weakness, reduce stress in both patient and carer and promote best possible quality of life.
- Failure to address communication issues can have detrimental consequences for the quality of life and mental health both of patients and carers.

KEY REFERENCES

- Kitwood T & Bredin K. A new approach to the evaluation of dementia care. *Journal of Advances in Health and Nursing Care* 1992; **1**(5):41–60.
- Neary D, Snowden JS, Gustafson L *et al.* Frontotemporal lobar degeneration: a consensus on clinical diagnostic criteria. *Neurology* 1998; **51**:1546–54.
- *Position Paper – Speech and Language Therapy Provision for People with Dementia* 2005; Royal College of Speech & Language Therapists, London.
- Powell JA. Communication interventions in dementia. *Reviews in Clinical Gerontology* 2000a; **10**:161–8.
- Powell J. *Care to Communicate – Helping the Older Person with Dementia* 2000b; Hawker Publications, London.

REFERENCES

Bayer A & Reban J (eds). *Alzheimer's Disease and Related Conditions. A Dementologist's Handbook* 2004; Medea Press, Czech Republic.

Bayles KA & Tomoeda CK. Caregiver report of prevalence and appearance order of linguistic symptoms in Alzheimer's patients. *The Gerontologist* 1991; **2**:210–6.

Bayles KA & Tomoeda CK. *The Effects of Alzheimer's Disease on Linguistic Communication* 1992; Telerounds Pilot 1, National Center for Neurogenic Communication Disorders, Tucson.

Beisgen BA. *Life-Enhancing Activites for Mentally Impaired Elders* 1989; Springer, New York.

Bourgeois MS. Evaluating memory wallets in conversations with persons with dementia. *Journal of Speech and Hearing Research* 1992; **35**:1344–57.

Delecluse F, Andersen AR, Waldemar G *et al.* Cerebral blood flow in progressive aphasia without dementia. *Brain* 1990; **113**:1395–404.

Gilleard C. *Living with Dementia* 1984; Croom Helm, London.

Graff-Radford NR, Damasio AR, Hyman BT *et al.* Progressive aphasia in a patient with Pick's disease: a neuropsychological, radiologic and anatomic study. *Neurology* 1990; **40**:620–6.

Hier DB, Hagenlocker K & Shindler AG. Language disintegration in dementia: effects of etiology and severity. *Brain and Language* 1985; **25**:117–33.

Kempler D, Matter EJ, Riege WH *et al.* Slowly progressive aphasia: three cases with language, memory, CT and PET data. *Journal of Neurology, Neurosurgery, and Psychiatry* 1990; **53**:987–93.

Kitwood T & Bredin K. A new approach to the evaluation of dementia care. *Journal of Advances in Health and Nursing Care* 1992; **1**(5):41–60.

Mace NL. Principles of activities for persons with dementia. *Physical & Occupational Therapy in Geriatrics* 1987; **5**(3):13–27.

Mesulam MM. Slowly progressive aphasia without generalised dementia. *Annals of Neurology* 1982; **11**:592–8.

Neal M & Briggs M. Cochrane Dementia and Cognitive Improvement Group. Validation therapy for dementia. [Systematic Review] *Cochrane Database of Systematic Reviews* 2005; 2.

Neary D, Snowden JS, Gustafson L *et al.* Frontotemporal lobar degeneration: a consensus on clinical diagnostic criteria. *Neurology* 1998; **51**:1546–54.

Nebes RD & Brady CB. Generalised cognitive slowing and severity of dementia in Alzheimer's disease: implications for the interpretation of response-time data. *Journal of Clinical and Experimental Neuropsychology* 1992; **14**:317–26.

Nebes RD & Madden DJ. Different patterns of cognitive slowing produced by Alzheimer's disease and normal aging. *Psychology and Aging* 1988; **3**:102–4.

Position Paper – Speech and Language Therapy Provision for People with Dementia 2005; Royal College of Speech & Language Therapists, London.

Powell JA. Communication interventions in dementia. *Reviews in Clinical Gerontology* 2000a; **10**:161–8.

Powell J. *Care to Communicate – Helping the Older Person with Dementia* 2000b; Hawker Publications, London.

Powell JA & Bayer EM. Using the past to make sense of the present: memory albums for people with dementia. *Signpost* 1996; **32**:10–2.

Powell JA, Hale MA & Bayer AJ. Symptoms of communication breakdown in dementia: carers' perceptions. *European Journal of Disorders of Communication* 1995; **30**:65–75.

Quayhagen MP & Quayhagen M. Alzheimer's stress: coping with the caregiving role. *The Gerontologist* 1988; **28**:391–6.

Rabins PV, Mace NL & Lucas MJ. The impact of dementia on the family. *The Journal of the American Medical Association* 1982; **248**:333–5.

Reisberg B, Ferris SH, de Leon MJ *et al.* The global deterioration scale for assessment of primary degenerative dementia. *The American Journal of Psychiatry* 1982; **139**:1136–9.

Spector A, Orrell M, Davies S & Woods B, Cochrane Dementia and Cognitive Improvement Group. Reality orientation for dementia. [Systematic Review] *Cochrane Database of Systematic Reviews* 2005; 2.

Tranel D. Neurology of language. *Current Opinion in Neurology and Neurosurgery* 1992; **5**:77–82.

Tyrell PJ, Warrington EK, Frackowiak RSJ *et al.* Heteogeneity in progressive aphasia due to focal cortical atrophy. *Brain* 1990; **113**:1321–36.

Ulatowska H, Allard L, Donnell A *et al.* Discourse performance in subjects of the Alzheimer type. In HA Whitaker (ed) *Neuropsychological Studies of Nonfocal Brain Damage* 1988; Springer, New York.

Woods B, Spector A, Jones C *et al.* Cochrane Dementia and Cognitive Improvement Group. Reminiscence therapy for dementia. [Systematic Review] *Cochrane Database of Systematic Reviews* 2005; 2.

90

Delirium

Joseph H. Flaherty

Saint Louis University School of Medicine and Saint Louis Veterans' Affairs Medical Center, St Louis, MO, USA

OVERVIEW

Delirium is a dangerous diagnosis. It is common; it is commonly missed; and it is associated with several adverse outcomes. Although most clinicians label patients with delirium as having an "acute change in mental status", the formal diagnostic criteria according to the *Diagnostic and Statistical Manual of Mental Disorders* (DSM-IV-Text Revision) paints a more complete and descriptive picture of these patients if put into sentence form: "A sudden onset of impaired attention, disorganized thinking, or incoherent speech. The patient usually has a clouded consciousness, perceptual disturbances, sleep-wake cycle problems, psychomotor agitation or lethargy, and is disoriented (American Psychiatric Association, 2000)."

PREVALENCE AND INCIDENCE FOR VARIOUS SITES AND SITUATIONS

In the hospital setting, using the available DSM criteria at the time, studies have found delirium in up to 22% of older patients on admission (prevalence), and up to 31% of older patients while hospitalized (incidence) (Francis *et al.*, 1990; Inouye *et al.*, 1993; Johnson *et al.*, 1990). Prevalence rates for confusion of any kind during admission have been found to be even higher (Levkoff *et al.*, 1992).

In general, surgical patients have been found to have higher rates of delirium than medical patients. In a review of primary data-collection studies, Dyer and colleagues found that rates are highest postoperatively among coronary artery bypass graft patients, ranging from 17 to 74% (>50% in five of the 14 studies reviewed). They also found that rates among orthopedic surgical patients ranged from 28–53% (>40% in five of the six studies). Of the two urologic studies reviewed, rates ranged from 4.5 to 6.8% (Dyer *et al.*, 1995). Past biases have blamed anesthesia agents for most cases, which wrongly have kept alive the belief, like that in the case of the intensive care unit (ICU), that delirium is unpreventable. Several studies have evaluated the association between routes of anesthesia (general, epidural, spinal, regional) and the risk of postoperative delirium. They found that the route of anesthesia was not associated with the development of delirium (Marcantonio *et al.*, 1998a; Williams-Russo *et al.*, 1996; Somprakit *et al.*, 2002).

One of the sites with the highest rates of delirium, but perhaps the most controversial because of so many complicating factors, is the ICU. Rates as low as 19% and as high as 80% have been found (Ely *et al.*, 2001a; Ely *et al.*, 2004a; Dubois *et al.*, 2001; McNicoll *et al.*, 2003). For years, however, people have ignored these facts, have called it inevitable and unpreventable, and have even labeled it "ICU-psychosis" so as to blame it on the ICU, which is something that cannot be changed. This may partly explain the high unrecognized rates of 66–84% (Ely *et al.*, 2004b).

Discharge or "transition" of patients out of the acute hospital setting has seen many changes over the past three decades (Makowski *et al.*, 2000). Data from postacute-care facilities (under such names as subacute-care facilities, skilled nursing facilities, rehabilitation centers, and long-term care facilities) reveal two major issues: patients are discharged from acute hospitals with persistent delirium and delirium at these sites persists for an extended period of time. Kelly and colleagues found that 72% of 214 nursing home patients who were hospitalized still had delirium at the time of discharge back to the nursing home. The delirium persisted for 55% of the patients at 1 month and 25% at 3 months after discharge (Kelly *et al.*, 2001). Marcantonio *et al.* (2000) found that 39% of 52 patients with hip fractures were discharged with delirium, which persisted for 32% of the patients at 1 month and 6% at 6 months after discharge.

In a large study of over 80 postacute-care facilities using the Minimum Data Set (MDS) to identify patients with any symptoms of delirium, Marcantonio *et al.* (2003) found a prevalence rate of 23% on admission. Using the Confusion

Principles and Practice of Geriatric Medicine, 4th Edition. Edited by M.S. John Pathy, Alan J. Sinclair and John E. Morley.

Assessment Method (CAM) as a screening tool (Inouye *et al.*, 1990), Kiely *et al.* (2003) found that 16% of 2158 patients at seven postacute-care facilities met the full criteria for delirium, 13% met two or more of the criteria, and 40% had one of the criteria. In the Marcantonio study, of the 23% who had symptoms of delirium, 52% still had the symptoms at 1 week follow-up (Marcantonio *et al.*, 2003).

While one could argue that delirium in postacute-care facilities should be expected to some extent because of pressures on acute facilities to shorten length of stays, two studies that looked at point of prevalence within nursing facilities discovered a similarly high rate of delirium. Mentes *et al.* (1999) evaluated 324 long-term nursing home patients using the MDS and found that 14% of patients had delirium. Cacchione *et al.* (2003) prospectively evaluated 74 long-term nursing home patients and identified 24 (33%) patients with delirium. While neither study could determine whether the delirium was a persistent one after a hospital stay, or was an incident (new episode of) delirium, it is evident that incidence of delirium was common.

Home Care is an understudied site concerning delirium. However, two studies (detailed under the Section "Prevention and Management Interventions") showed lower rates of delirium among ill, older persons cared for at home compared to similarly ill, older persons cared for in the hospital. It is unclear whether something positive is being done in the home that prevents delirium or whether something negative is occurring in the hospital that contributes to the development of delirium (Caplan *et al.*, 1999; Leff *et al.*, 2004).

ASSOCIATED ADVERSE OUTCOMES

Delirium is one of the most serious illnesses patients can have or develop and one that clinicians should not miss at the reported rate of 32–66% (Inouye, 1998). Data about the adverse outcomes associated with delirium mainly come from studies of older patients in the hospital setting. Here, delirium has been found to be associated with hospital complications, loss of physical function, increased length of stay in the hospital, increased instances of discharge to a long-term care facility, and even higher rate of mortality (Francis *et al.*, 1990; Pompei *et al.*, 1994; Cole *et al.*, 2003; McCusker *et al.*, 2002a,b; McCusker *et al.*, 2003; Rockwood, 1999; Inouye *et al.*, 1998; O'Keeffe and Lavan, 1997; Thomas *et al.*, 1988). Mortality rates for hospitalized delirious patients have been reported to be 25–33%, as high as the mortality rates for acute myocardial infarction and sepsis (Inouye, 2003).

There has been some question in the past whether delirium was independently associated with these adverse outcomes, or whether it was merely a marker of severe illness and physical frailty since most studies identified older age, underlying cognitive impairment, severe, acute and chronic illness, and functional impairment as the predisposing factors. However, when adjusting for these factors, delirium has been found to be independently associated with poor outcomes in most studies (O'Keeffe and Lavan, 1997; McCusker *et al.*, 2002a; Rockwood, 1999; Inouye *et al.*, 1998).

Associated adverse outcomes among delirious ICU patients have shown prolonged ICU stay, prolonged hospital stay, and increased mortality compared to patients without delirium (Ely *et al.*, 2001a; Ely *et al.*, 2004a). Emerging data from postacute facilities have also shown associated adverse outcomes, related to loss of physical function and mortality (Marcantonio *et al.*, 2003; Cacchione *et al.*, 2003; Kelly *et al.*, 2001).

THE COMPREHENSIVE APPROACH TO DELIRIUM

In order to improve the adverse outcomes associated with delirium, it is not enough just to improve our skills in diagnosing delirium and treating the underlying medical causes. The following are the necessary components of a comprehensive approach for those involved in the care of older persons, and health-care systems that interface with older persons.

1. *Awareness*: Be aware of how commonly delirium occurs, where it occurs, and get others involved in the care of older persons to do the same.
2. *Diagnosis*: Know why it is important to differentiate and how to differentiate between delirium and dementia.
3. *Evaluation*: Identify and treat the underlying causes of delirium.
4. *Prevention*: Implement strategies or care systems that can prevent delirium.
5. *Management*: Manage patients who develop delirium.

Although there are no available studies to date that implement all five interventions, a multifaceted approach is warranted because of the nature of this multifactorial problem (Inouye, 2001).

Awareness

Delirium should become part of the medical jargon for all who care for older persons (Flaherty *et al.*, 2003). Furthermore, given the frequency with which delirium is seen and the seriousness of this diagnosis, the rates of incidence and outcomes associated with delirium should be monitored (that is, they should become quality-of-care measures) at all sites where delirium occurs (Inouye *et al.*, 1999b).

Diagnosis

Delirium is not dementia. The latest version of the DSM is the DSM-IV-TR (American Psychiatric Association, 2000). There is no difference in the core features of delirium in the DSM-IV-TR version compared to the previous version, DSM-IV, except that the DSM-IV-TR version recognizes that delirium can arise during the course of dementia. Although this appears to be a minor detail, the message this gives to health-care professionals is a critically important one: "delirium is not dementia". Most types of dementia have a progressive downhill course. Delirium is reversible. A mislabeling, or lack of differentiation between these two diagnoses is thought to be the reason why delirium is missed by physicians at rates as high as 32–66% (Inouye, 1998) and by nurses up to 69% of the time (Inouye *et al.*, 2001). Misdiagnosis or late diagnosis may also partly explain why delirium is associated with adverse outcomes (Francis and Kapoor, 1992; Lyness, 1990). Table 1 details some of the differentiating characteristics between delirium and dementia, based on DSM criteria, keeping in mind that one of the criteria not in Table 1 is that delirium must occur in the context of a medical illness, metabolic derangement, drug toxicity, or withdrawal.

Altered level of consciousness (LOC) is an excellent clue in differentiating delirium and dementia because it is not always possible to know the patient's baseline mental status. Without ever having seen the patient before, one can determine whether the patient's LOC lies toward the agitated or vigilant side of the spectrum of LOC, or toward the lethargic, drowsy or stuporous side of the spectrum.

One can ask orientation questions, but since disorientation and problems with memory are present in both delirium and dementia, the key in determining delirium from dementia is *how* the patient answers. The delirious patient will often give disorganized answers, which can be described as rambling or even incoherent.

The classic identifiers of delirium are acute onset and fluctuating course, both of which are usually obtained by close caregivers (family or nurses). Although acute implies 24 hours, the term subacute is used to emphasize that subtle mental status changes can be overlooked by caregivers. Over a period of many days, the patient may appear to be slowly declining mentally due to the underlying dementia. If left unchecked, the initial delirium may impair other necessary functions, leading to further medical problems, such as dehydration and malnutrition, further complicating the delirium. This snow-ball effect explains in part why the etiology of delirium is typically multifactorial. Thus, if it is unclear how long the change has been occurring, patients should be put in the category of delirium and an evaluation should be done.

Table 1 Differentiating delirium from dementia

	Delirium	Dementia
Consciousness	Decreased or hyper alert "Clouded"	Alert
Orientation	Disorganized	Disoriented
Course	Fluctuating	Steady slow decline
Onset	Acute or sub acute	Chronic
Attention	Impaired	Usually normal
Psychomotor	Agitated or lethargic	Usually normal
Hallucinations	Perceptual disturbances May have hallucinations	Usually not present
Sleep-wake cycle	Abnormal	Usually normal
Speech	Slow, incoherent	Aphasic, anomic difficulty finding words

Attention is also one of the classic identifiers of delirium, which may often be helpful if the patient's baseline mental status is not known. It can be tested by having a conversation. Patients may have difficulty maintaining or following the conversation, perseverate on the previous question, or become easily distracted. Attention can also be tested with cognitive tasks such as days of the week backward, spelling backward, or digit span.

Psychomotor agitation or lethargy, hallucinations, sleep-wake cycle abnormalities and slow or incoherent speech can all be seen in patients with delirium, but these features are not necessary for the diagnosis.

Evaluation

General guidelines for the medical evaluation of patients are to consider all possible causes, proceed cautiously with appropriate testing, and keep in mind that delirium is usually caused by a combination of underlying causes.

After a physical check and ascertaining the history, which includes obtaining details from anyone considered a caregiver (e.g. family, nurse's aide) and a thorough medication list, the mnemonic D-E-L-I-R-I-U-M-S can be used as a checklist to cover most causes of delirium (Table 2).

Drugs are notorious for causing delirium. According to most authors in this area, "virtually any" (Carter *et al.*, 1996) and "practically every" (Lipowski, 1989) drug can be considered deliriogenic.

Several drugs have been found *in vitro* to have varying amounts of anticholinergic properties. However, since the pathophysiologic and neurotransmitter mechanisms of delirium go beyond anticholinergic mechanisms, a more practical approach is to remember certain categories of medications that have been reported to cause delirium, some more common than others. The mnemonic A-C-U-T-E C-H-A-N-G-E I-N M-S is long, as would be expected, but highlights why drugs are such a common cause of delirium (Table 3). In order to be as inclusive as possible, and because many older reports did not discuss strict delirium criteria, or such criteria were not commonly used, the following paragraphs describe not just delirium as a side effect, but psychiatric side effects that might indicate presence of delirium, such as hallucinosis, paranoia, delusions, psychosis, general confusion, aggressiveness, restlessness, and drowsiness.

Table 2 Causes of delirium

D	Drugs
E	Eyes, ears
L	Low O_2 state (MI, stroke, PE)
I	Infection
R	Retention (of urine or stool)
I	Ictal
U	Underhydration/undernutrition
M	Metabolic
(S)	Subdural

Table 3 Medications that can cause (have been reported to cause) an A-C-U-T-E C-H-A-N-G-E I-N mental status

A	Antiparkinson's
C	Corticosteroids
U	Urinary incontinence drugs
T	Theophylline
E	Emptying drugs (e.g. metoclopramide, compazine)
C	Cardiovascular drugs
H	H2 blockers
A	Antibiotics
N	NSAIDs
G	Geropsychiatry drugs
E	ENT drugs
I	Insomnia drugs
N	Narcotics
M	Muscle relaxants
S	Seizure drugs

Antiparkinsonian drugs probably cause delirium due to a tip in the tenuous balance of the neurotransmitters dopamine and acetylcholine, both implicated in the pathophysiology of delirium. Levodopa has been reported to cause mental status changes at a rate of 10–60% and include hallucinosis on a background of a clear sensorium, delusional disorders, and paranoia. Abnormal dreams and sleep disruption may precede the more frank delirium symptoms and may be an early clue to their onset. Selegiline has been reported to cause mental status changes described as psychosis, aggressiveness, even mania (Flaherty, 1998).

Corticosteroids have been reported to cause "psychiatric complications" in up to 18% of patients with doses above $80\,\mathrm{mg\,day^{-1}}$. The mental status changes seen have been described as depressive/manic, an organic affective disorder with associated paranoid-hallucinating features, and general "confusion". Withdrawal of corticosteroids may also cause delirium (Flaherty, 1998).

Drugs for urinary incontinence (specifically antispasmodics) have the potential to cause delirium by two mechanisms: through the anticholinergic properties of the drug, or through causing urinary retention, known as the *cytocerebral syndrome* (discussed in the following text) (Blackburn and Dunn, 1990). Although older short-acting antispasmodics have more of a potential to cause delirium, newer sustained-release agents have been reported as well (Edwards and O'Connor, 2002).

Theophylline "madness" probably meets delirium criteria, as one of the first case reports described it: "the blood level, toxic on admission but decreasing over 48 hours, correlated well with the number of episodes of hyperactive periods marked by flailing of limbs, intense emotional lability, incessant crying and ripping out of intravenous lines and nasogastric tubes. Not always is there a direct correlation between the presence or severity of side effects and the toxic serum level of theophylline" (Flaherty, 1998).

Emptying drugs, or motility agents, are a class of drugs that are intended to stimulate the upper gastrointestinal tract through cholinergic mechanisms. However, these agents also have peripheral and central antidopaminergic properties. Reported mental status side effects include restlessness, drowsiness, depression, and confusion (Flaherty, 1998).

Cardiovascular drugs rarely cause mental status problems, but because they are so commonly prescribed for older persons, it is worthwhile to remember that some are more likely to cause problems, as well as a few that have been reported in case-reports. One of the first reports of confusion due to digoxin toxicity was over 100 years ago. Since then, reports of confusion even at therapeutic levels have been published (Flaherty, 1998).

Methyldopa and reserpine are centrally acting antihypertensives that have been reported to cause depression, nightmares, psychosis, and delirium. The centrally acting alpha agonist clonidine may cause depression, delirium, and hallucinations (Flaherty, 1998).

Several antiarrhythmics have been reported to cause mental status changes, thought to be either idiosyncratic or dose-related. Reported culprits include disopyramide, procainamide, quinidine, lidocaine, amiodarone, flecainide, mexiletine, propafenone, and tocainamide (Flaherty, 1998).

Antihypertensive agents that may cause mental status changes have primarily been reported in the literature through case reports. However, since they are so commonly used, it is worthwhile being suspicious about a few of them. These include beta-blockers (including in the form of eye drops), angiotensin-converting enzyme inhibitors, and calcium channel antagonists (Flaherty, 1998).

H2 blockers, because they are primarily renal excreted and may have some H1 activity (antihistamine receptor subtype-1), may cause delirium, especially if patients have underlying risk factors such as renal insufficiency and dementia (Flaherty, 1998).

Antimicrobials, like cardiovascular drugs, rarely cause mental status changes, but are so commonly used; some examples are worth being aware of: penicillin, erythromycin, clarithromycin, gentamycin, tobramycin, streptomycin, trimethoprim-sulfamethoxazole, ciprofloxacin, some cephalosporins, and the antiviral acyclovir, particularly at high doses. Most of these reports propose that the mechanisms by which antimicrobials cause mental status changes are related to impaired renal function, drug–drug interaction, and occasionally idiosyncratic behavior (Flaherty, 1998).

Several types of nonsteroidal anti-inflammatory drugs have been reported to cause delirium, even the newer selective cyclooxygenase-2 inhibitors (Macknight and Rojas-Fernandez, 2001), and aspirin and salicylate compounds (Flaherty, 1998).

"Geropsychiatric" medications is too large a category to go in-depth about, but a few comments are warranted to create some balance between reflexively blaming these drugs for the delirium just because "any drug that works in the brain, can cause a problem in the brain" and understanding that while no centrally acting psychiatric medication is completely safe, certain ones may be safer than others and psychiatric illnesses, especially depression, need to be treated (Flaherty, 1998).

Tricyclic antidepressants (TCAs) can cause delirium with an overall incidence ranging from 1.5 to 20%. The highest rates, of course, seem to be among older, previously cognitively impaired, and medically ill patients. Delirium can be caused by low or therapeutic doses and may not be associated with signs of peripheral muscarinic blockade such as dilated pupils or urinary retention. Some TCAs are not as anticholinergic as others (e.g. desipramine) so that the risk of delirium is not an absolute contraindication to their use (Flaherty, 1998).

Serotonin selective reuptake inhibitor (SSRIs) antidepressants have a much safer side effect profile compared to the TCAs as far as delirium is concerned. However, one of the main side effects of SSRIs, hyponatremia, can present as delirium in older persons. This has been reported with fluoxetine, fluvoxamine, paroxetine, and sertraline. Although frank delirium due to SSRIs is rare, most reported cases seem to point toward drug interactions as a plausible cause (Flaherty, 1998). However, to emphasize that no centrally acting drug is completely safe, in a study of 10 healthy volunteers, paroxetine increased ratings of confusion and fatigue (Brauer *et al.*, 1995). There are also case reports of confusion due to antidepressants such as mirtazapine (Bailer *et al.*, 2000) and venlafaxine (Howe and Ravasia, 2003).

The serotonin syndrome, although rare, since the use of L-tryptophan and monoamine oxidase inhibitors are less nowadays, is a constellation of symptoms that may include confusion, agitation and restlessness, myoclonus and hyper-reflexia, involuntary movements, shivering, diaphoresis, tremor, and fever. However, SSRIs alone and combinations such as sertraline and tramadol (a mu-receptor pain medication), trazodone and buspirone, and trazodone and methylphenidate have been reported to cause symptoms similar to those described in the serotonin syndrome (Flaherty, 1998).

Benzodiazepines (BDZs) were introduced in the 1960s and are one of the most widely used psychoactive drugs in most communities. Unfortunately, their use is highest among the elderly. In one study of over 400 hospitalized patients, aged 58–88 years, who had normal mini-mental status examination scores on admission, the use of BDZs was associated with a relative risk of developing cognitive impairment of 3.5 (95% CI; 1.4–8.8) (Foy *et al.*, 1995). Postoperative use of BDZs has also been found to increase the risk of delirium. Short-acting BDZs, even in small doses, have been recorded to cause problems, and the clinician should be aware that withdrawal from BDZs in the elderly may also present as delirium, perhaps more so when discontinuing short-acting BDZs compared to long-acting ones. However, there are models of successfully withdrawing patients from BDZs and this should be attempted whenever possible (Petrovic *et al.*, 1999).

Antipsychotics can cause delirium. In one study of patients who were transferred from the psychiatric ward to a medical ward because of delirium, 31% of the cases were due to low potency antipsychotic agents (Popli *et al.*, 1997). Whether the antipsychotic prescribed is considered a typical antipsychotic or an atypical antipsychotic, the clinician needs to keep in mind that none of these drugs have pure mono-neurotransmitter activity. Rather, they have varying degrees of activity, either agonist or antagonist to many of the neurotransmitters implicated in the pathophysiology of delirium, such as dopamine, acetylcholine, serotonin, and histamine (Tandon *et al.*, 1999). Thus, like other geriatric psychiatric medications, antipsychotic drugs can and should be considered as a potential cause of delirium.

Two additional points need to be made concerning antipsychotics. The neuroleptic malignant syndrome is classically described as a triad consisting of fever, elevated creatinine kinase enzymes, and confusion. However, some authors believe that a variant, or rather a clinical spectrum of the neuroleptic malignant syndrome can be seen, wherein patients may only have one or two of the triad features and may only have a small degree of these features. For example, patients may have subtle confusion and muscle rigidity, which is intermittent but only mild, or no elevation of creatinine kinase enzymes (Reilly *et al.*, 1991).

Patients with Lewy-body dementia have an increased sensitivity to neuroleptics. The clinical challenge here is that sometimes it is difficult to differentiate between Alzheimer's dementia and Lewy-body-type dementia (McKeith *et al.*, 1992).

The ENT drugs in the mnemonic are a reminder of the multiple drugs, in particular, over the counter (OTC) medications that are taken for respiratory or sinus illnesses. This category should encompass decongestants, antihistamines, expectorants, and antitussins. Older persons use a disproportionate share of OTC drugs, and the average number of OTC drugs used by ambulatory older persons has increased. The most worrisome of these ENT medications are the combination formulas, which contain two, sometimes three, or even four active ingredients. Antihistamines, particularly the drug diphenhydramine, can cause problems at high doses, at moderately high doses, after a first time oral dose in compromised elderly patients, and even with topical use. Common OTC decongestants include sympathomimetics such as pseudoephedrine and phenylpropanolamine, which are found in most cough and cold remedies, and phenylephrine, which is found in OTC nasal sprays. Mental status changes have been reported to occur at high doses, low doses, and even from overuse of nasal inhalation. Expectorants are probably safe to use alone in older patients although their actual clinical benefit has been questioned. Antitussins are also probably safe as long as they are only used by themselves (Flaherty, 1998).

One of the most commonly used, if not overused ENT medications is meclizine. Although used for dizziness because of its mechanism of action to decrease excitability of the middle ear labyrinth and block conduction in the middle ear vestibular-cerebellar pathways, it has the potential to cause mental status changes because of its central anticholinergic action at the chemoreceptor trigger zone. The anticholinergic properties were thought to be the cause of confusion and steady cognitive as well as functional decline in an older patient who had been on meclizine for 3 years. Within 1 month off the drug, the patient's function and mentation improved. When rechallenged, the patient had cognitive and functional decline within 1 week (Molloy, 1987).

"I" is a reminder that medications used for insomnia because of their effect on sedation have potential to cause varying degrees of delirium. Nonpharmacological approaches should be used before medications for insomnia as well as a thorough evaluation of the causes of insomnia. Clinicians should be aware that most OTC sleeping aides come under a multitude of brand names without specifying the potentially dangerous deliriogenic medications, dyphenhydramine or scopolamine. Various herbal medicines, although thought to be safe, need to be evaluated to see whether they contain atropine or scopolamine (Flaherty, 1998).

Narcotics can be used safely in older persons with little risk of developing delirium, but a few important details need to be remembered. Meperidine is particularly risky in older persons, likely due to the anticholinergic activity of its active metabolite nor-meperidine. According to Lipowski's thorough review of drugs causing delirium, morphine and propoxyphene rarely appear to cause delirium, however, the latter drug can lead to dependence, abuse, and withdrawal symptoms. At the time of Lipowski's review, there were no reported cases of delirium due to codeine. The main problems associated with the use of narcotics are probably related to toxicity, overuse, or overdosage in patients with impaired hepatic or renal function (Lipowski, 1989).

Muscle relaxant is a misnomer because these medications act centrally in the brain, not locally at the muscles. Some of the commonly used muscle relaxants include cyclobenzaprine, methocarbamol, and carisoprodol, and have been reported to cause delirium (Flaherty, 1998).

Seizure medications have been reported to cause varying types of cognitive impairment including drowsiness, agitation, depression, psychosis, and delirium. The cognitive impairment is thought to be related to serum levels, but clinicians should keep in mind that most anticonvulsants are protein bound and if the patient's nutritional status is poor then there is potential that the amount of free drug will actually be higher than what is measured by the serum level (Flaherty, 1998).

In conclusion, although the list of medications that can cause delirium is long, the mnemonic, A-C-U-T-E C-H-A-N-G-E I-N M-S can help clinicians recognize some of the more common and some of the rare offenders. For patients who present with delirium or for patients who are at risk for delirium, the following general guidelines concerning medication management can be used.

1. Use nonpharmacological interventions whenever possible instead of a medication.
2. Do not treat vague symptoms with a medication (for example, do not routinely give H2 antagonists for vague gastrointestinal complaints).
3. Include an assessment of OTC medications as potential offenders.
4. Evaluate all drugs for drug–drug and drug–disease interactions.
5. If a drug is started, decide on how long that drug will be used. The old rule of "start low and go slow" needs to be expanded to "start low, go slow, and know when to stop".
6. The justification for prescribing medications should be based on therapeutic reasons and not on preventive reasons, and until the patient is no longer at risk for delirium or the delirium has resolved.
7. Do not treat adverse effects of drugs with another drug unless completely necessary (as may be the case with long-acting narcotics and laxatives).

The "E" in the D-E-L-I-R-I-U-M mnemonic stands for emotions and reminds the clinician that depression can have psychotic features and as such may present similar to patients with delirium. Although depression has classically been considered the masquerader of dementia, given some of the DSM-IV criteria for delirium such as disorganized thinking or psychomotor lethargy, depression should be considered a reversible cause of delirium.

Low O_2 (Oxygen) states in the mnemonic should highlight to the clinician that older patients with acute cardiovascular or pulmonary illnesses can present with delirium. It could be said that "delirium is as serious as a heart attack" because not only can the mortality rate of delirium be as high as that of myocardial infarction but also that the older delirious patients can have myocardial infarctions that are commonly missed or present atypically (Malone *et al.*, 1998). It is unclear whether patients, because of the delirium, cannot either describe or tell clinicians about chest pain, or whether there exists a cardiocerebral syndrome in which the stress of the myocardial infarction affects on the adrenergic system causing a stress on the balance in the central nervous system, that is, in cognition.

Not only are patients with stroke at risk of developing delirium as a complication of the stroke or the underlying comorbidities associated with the stroke but also delirium which may be the presenting feature of some stroke patients (Ferro *et al.*, 2002).

Infections are one of the most common underlying causes of delirium among older people. The most common types of infections that cause delirium are urinary tract infections and respiratory infections. However, subtle infections such as cholecystitis and diverticulitis should not be overlooked (Freeman and Kirdar, 1990). Although meningitis should be considered, it is not clear whether or not cerebrospinal fluid analysis is warranted in the initial work-up of delirious patients without other symptoms that point toward a central nervous system infection (Warshaw and Tanzer, 1993).

It is worth noting that because one of the risk factors identified for patients to develop delirium is hospitalization, procedures that seem to be standard and are carried out in hospitals should be questioned. One of these common procedures that occurs is the placement of an indwelling urinary catheter. It seems logical that the most common nosocomial infection for older patients is urinary tract infection because of the use of these indwelling urinary catheters. It has been reported that more than one-third of the attending physicians and more than one-quarter of the resident physicians at four academic medical centers did not know which of their patients at any one time had one of these indwelling urinary catheters. These catheters can also be considered as a one point restraint that limit mobility, thus adding to the complications of hospitalization (Saint *et al.*, 2002). Given these risks without any clear benefit, indwelling urinary catheters are not indicated for urinary incontinence, urinary retention that can be managed with straight intermittent catheterization, and should not be used to monitor input and output unless this monitoring is critical in decision making and outcomes related to this parameter.

Retention of urine and feces can both cause delirium although typically the presentations differ. Urinary retention causing delirium has been well reported in the literature under the term cystocerebral syndrome (Blackburn and Dunn, 1990; Ble *et al.*, 2001; Liem and Carter, 1991). The original report was of three cases, all were older men who became acutely agitated and nearly mute. All three patients had large volumes of urine in their bladder and in all three patients, the agitated delirium resolved within a short time after emptying the bladder. Liem and Carter have suggested that the adrenergic tension related to the urinary retension might increase in the central nervous system and the consequent increase in catecholamines might produce delirium. Although this pathophysiological explanation has not been proven, clinicians should be very aware of this syndrome. One of the best ways to quickly evaluate for urinary retention is with a hand held bladder ultrasound. Although these have a fairly high initial cost, cost savings from the reduction in use of straight catheterizations may help balance this issue (Frederickson *et al.*, 2000).

Fecal retention as a cause of delirium has not been reported in the literature. However, since older patients for multiple reasons are at risk for fecal impactions, clinicians should be suspicious of this problem when the delirium is of the lethargic type.

Ictal states are a rare cause of delirium and are not difficult to diagnose clinically for patients with tonic clonic seizures. However, patients who experience absence seizures may go unnoticed by caregivers and may only seem to have fluctuating mental status changes. Although an electroencephalogram (EEG) is not indicated in the initial medical evaluation of delirium, it should be considered when pertinent history is obtained.

Underhydration is used in the mnemonic, not only to emphasize the fact that dehydration can be one of the underlying causes of delirium but also to highlight the fact that those at risk for dehydration are at risk for delirium. Although there is much debate and consternation about which, if any, physical signs are pathomnemonic for dehydration among older persons, one quick method is to calculate the blood urea nitrogen (BUN) and creatinine ratio. Although there are several circumstances when the BUN/Creatinine ratio may not be accurate, there are data to suggest that a ratio of greater than 17 : 1 puts patients at risk for delirium (Inouye *et al.*, 1993). Given this easy and commonly accessible parameter and given the data supporting the use of dehydration or difficulty with hydration as a target for interventions as will be seen below, dehydration should be considered on the top of the list as a contributing cause and not as only a risk factor for delirium, and should be treated as aggressively as possible keeping in mind the limitations of each patient related to their cardiovascular status.

Undernutrition, or malnutrition is rather complex and difficult to understand as a cause of delirium, most likely because unlike other causes of delirium it is less likely to be reversed quickly. It is evident, though, that malnutrition among the hospitalized patient is not only common but is also associated with longer hospital stays, postoperative complications, and even higher mortality. Clinicians as well as all health-care providers in the hospital should be aware that restricted diets are likely to exacerbate malnutrition. According to one study of over 1000 consecutive hospitalized patients, over 400 were malnourished according to the body mass index, and almost 50% of these malnourished patients had an order by a physician for a restricted diet (Thomas and Kamel, 2004). Malnutrition is most directly related to delirium probably through the issue of medications that are protein bound. Patients who are malnourished may have lower protein stores and thus protein bound drugs will have a higher free concentration that puts the patient at risk for delirium. Other proposed relationships between malnutrition and delirium, which have yet to be fully elucidated, include those mechanisms looking at cytokines (Banks *et al.*, 2003).

Metabolic abnormalities that cause delirium are not difficult to identify because of the availability of commonly used laboratory tests. A complete metabolic panel usually will identify hyponatremia or hypernatremia, hypocalcemia or hypercalcemia, and abnormalities of liver function or renal function. Thyroid function tests and B12 are typically put in this category.

Although delirium is not spelled with an "s" in the end, using the mnemonic DELIRIUMS emphasizes to the clinician that delirium usually has more than one cause. The "s" also reminds the clinician that a subdural hematoma can cause a mental status change. Although the mortality rate of subdural hematomas among younger people is quite high, the prognosis for older people is quite good as long as the diagnosis is not missed (Tagle *et al.*, 2003). The other difference between older and younger patients with subdural hematomas is that older patients may develop the subdural hematoma over a period of a few hours or days. Although there could be some debate as to whether or not all older patients presenting to a hospital with delirium should have some sort of brain imaging, most would agree that because this is a very reversible problem and which would cease to be reversible if the diagnosis is delayed, imaging should be considered if there has been a history of head trauma or falls or any suspicion that there was an unwitnessed fall.

One of the other causes of delirium not represented in the mnemonic is pain. Recognition of pain is improving, now identified as the *5th vital sign*, and should be considered as a readily treatable cause of delirium, especially associated with elective surgery (Lynch *et al.*, 1998).

Prevention and Management Interventions

Before identifying which interventions are effective and which are not, it is important to understand the goals of interventions concerning delirium. They are: (1) to prevent the development of delirium; (2) to reduce the adverse outcomes associated with delirium in those patients for whom delirium is not prevented; and (3) to provide health-care professionals with alternatives to physical restraints and pharmacological methods in the management of delirium.

It is also important to emphasize that delirium is a complex issue related to the challenge of identifying who is at risk of developing it, diagnosing it if it does develop, and getting other health-care professionals to do the same. Interventions that are successful will involve several components, many of which are not easily measured. These include education about the risk factors and diagnosis of delirium, a "culture" change about how *not* to use what seems logical and protective (for example, physical restraints or pharmacological sedation), and a realization that multicomponent interventions are not simple but can be done.

The most consistent message about successful interventions is to use an interdisciplinary team approach and follow geriatric principles.

One of the most rigorous studies to date because of the assessment methods used and the close follow-up of patients was a prospective study of a multicomponent intervention to prevent the development of delirium in hospitalized older patients (Inouye *et al.*, 1999a). The study identified patients at risk for delirium on the basis of a previously developed predictive model (Inouye *et al.*, 1993). The study used the following six out of seven risk factors for the development of delirium: baseline cognitive impairment, eye or visual problems, altered sleep/wake cycle, dehydration, restricted or decreased mobility, or hearing impairment (Table 4). The seventh risk factor, addition of >3 medications, was not used in the study, but is included in Table 4 for completeness (B-E-W-A-R-E). The standardized intervention protocols that were used in the study included the first six targeted interventions as described in Table 4 (P-R-E-V-E-N-T).

Delirium developed in 15% of 426 usual care patients compared to only 9.9% of 426 intervention group patients (OR, 0.60, 95% CI, 0.39–0.92). The total number of days of delirium and the total number of episodes of delirium were also significantly lower in the intervention group, but the severity of delirium and recurrence rates were not significantly different. The interdisciplinary team included a specialist geriatric nurse, two specially trained persons familiar with the standardized intervention protocols, a certified therapeutic recreation specialist, a physical therapy consultant, a geriatrician, and trained volunteers.

The importance of this study is twofold. This study probably underestimates the success of a multicomponent intervention such as this because of the likely contamination that occurred throughout the hospital through implementing some of the standardized protocols. Since the study was done within one hospital, it was unable to randomize patients to separate floors and thus, some intervention patients were on floors that also included patients from the usual care group. This was evident based on the 15% rate of delirium in the usual care group, which is lower than previous studies. Although a multicomponent intervention such as this seems labor-intensive and costly, cost-effective analysis have been favorable (Rizzo *et al.*, 2001).

Table 4 Risk factors for delirium (B-E A-W-A-R-E) and targeted interventions (P-R-E-V-E-N-T) based on intervention trial to prevent delirium

B	Baseline dementia?
E	Eye problems?
A	Altered sleep/wake cycle?
W	Water or dehydration problems?
A	Adding >3 medications, especially sedating and psychoactive ones?
R	Restricted mobility?
E	Ear problems?
P	Protocol for sleep (back massage, relaxation music, decreased noise, warm milk, or caffeine-free herbal tea)
R	Replenish fluids and recognize volume depletion
E	Ear aids (amplifier or patient's own hearing aid)
V	Visual aids (patient's own glasses, magnifying lens)
E	Exercise or ambulation as soon as possible
N	Name person, place and time frequently for reorientation
T	Taper or discontinue unnecessary medications. Use alternative and less harmful medications.

A study that targets a very high risk group for delirium, older patients with surgical repair of hip fractures, was performed using a geriatric consultation as the primary mode of intervention (Marcantonio *et al.*, 2001). In this study, 126 patients who were 65 years or older and admitted for surgical repair of hip fracture were randomized to geriatric consultation or usual care. The geriatric consultation was "proactive", which meant that the consultation began preoperatively (for 61% of the patients) or within 24 hours of surgery, and a geriatrician made daily visits for the duration of the hospitalization. Targeted recommendations were made on the basis of a structured protocol emphasizing geriatric principles as well as postoperative medical care. Recommendations covered areas such as treatment of severe pain, elimination of unnecessary medications, regulation of bowel/bladder function (including discontinuing bladder catheters by postoperative day 2), adequate nutritional intake, and early mobilization. The overall adherence rate by the orthopedics team to the recommendations was 77%.

Delirium developed in 32% of the 62 consultation group patients compared with 50% of the 64 usual care group patients (OR, 0.64, 95% CI, 0.37–0.98). There was a greater reduction of severe delirium, occurring in 12% of the consultation group and 29% of the usual care group (OR, 0.40, 95% CI, 0.18–0.89). Median length of stay did not differ in the two groups (5 days).

Two studies of "home–hospital care" have shown lower rates of delirium among medical patients cared for in the home compared to similar patients cared for in the hospital (Caplan *et al.*, 1999; Leff *et al.*, 2004). In the study by Caplan and colleagues, 100 patients with a mean age of 76 years (71% from home, 25% from nursing homes and 4% from hostels) with medical illnesses such as acute infections requiring intravenous antibiotics, deep venous thrombosis, minor cerebrovascular accidents, or cardiac failure, were randomized within 24 hours of diagnosis to either home or hospital. Although the researchers used the term "confusion" instead of the formal diagnosis of delirium, they found a lower incidence of confusion (0 vs 20.4%; $P = 0.0005$), in the home group compared to the hospital group. Other geriatric complications were also found to be at a lower rate in the home group compared to the hospital group: urinary complications (incontinence or retention) (2.0% vs 16.3%; $P = 0.01$), and bowel complications (incontinence or constipation) (0 vs 22.5%; $P = 0.0003$) (Caplan *et al.*, 1999).

The study by Leff and colleagues identified older patients who required hospital level care for pneumonia, congestive heart failure, chronic obstructive pulmonary disease and cellulitis. Of those who went home for treatments associated with hospital care, compared to patients who completed their treatments in the hospital (average length of stay 2.9 days versus 4.9 days), the adjusted odds ratio for incident delirium was 0.25 (0.11, 0.58, adjusted 95% CI) (Leff *et al.*, 2004).

What about patients for whom delirium is not preventable or who already have delirium on admission to the hospital? The Delirium Room (DR) is a specialized four-bed room to provide 24-hour nursing care and observation by at least one nurse in the room and is completely free of physical restraints (Flaherty *et al.*, 2003). The hallmarks of the DR are the following. The four-bed DR is an integral part of an acute care for the elderly (ACE) unit. As such, the patients in the DR not only receive 24 hour close observation but also the benefits of the geriatric principles for which the ACE unit has been shown to be effective in preventing loss of functional decline (Landefeld *et al.*, 1995). Nursing inservices and protocols developed by nurses on how to identify and manage delirious patients are necessary. The DR is not isolated from the rest of the floor, rather it is the closest room to the main nurses' station. Having a location on the floor called the *Delirium Room* (see Figure 1) raises the awareness among health-care professionals that delirium is a serious diagnosis, with serious consequences. Putting delirious or potentially delirious patients together in a room does not increase agitation as previous literature might suggest.

Although the report of the Delirium Room was descriptive, it showed that over a 12-month consecutive time frame, out of the 69 patients with a diagnosis (according to the International Classification of Disease 9th edition) of delirium in the DR, negative associations found in other studies of delirious patients were minimized. No physical restraints were used and only 29% of the patients received new orders for medications considered to be pharmacological restraints (haloperidol, risperidone, or lorazepam), all at total

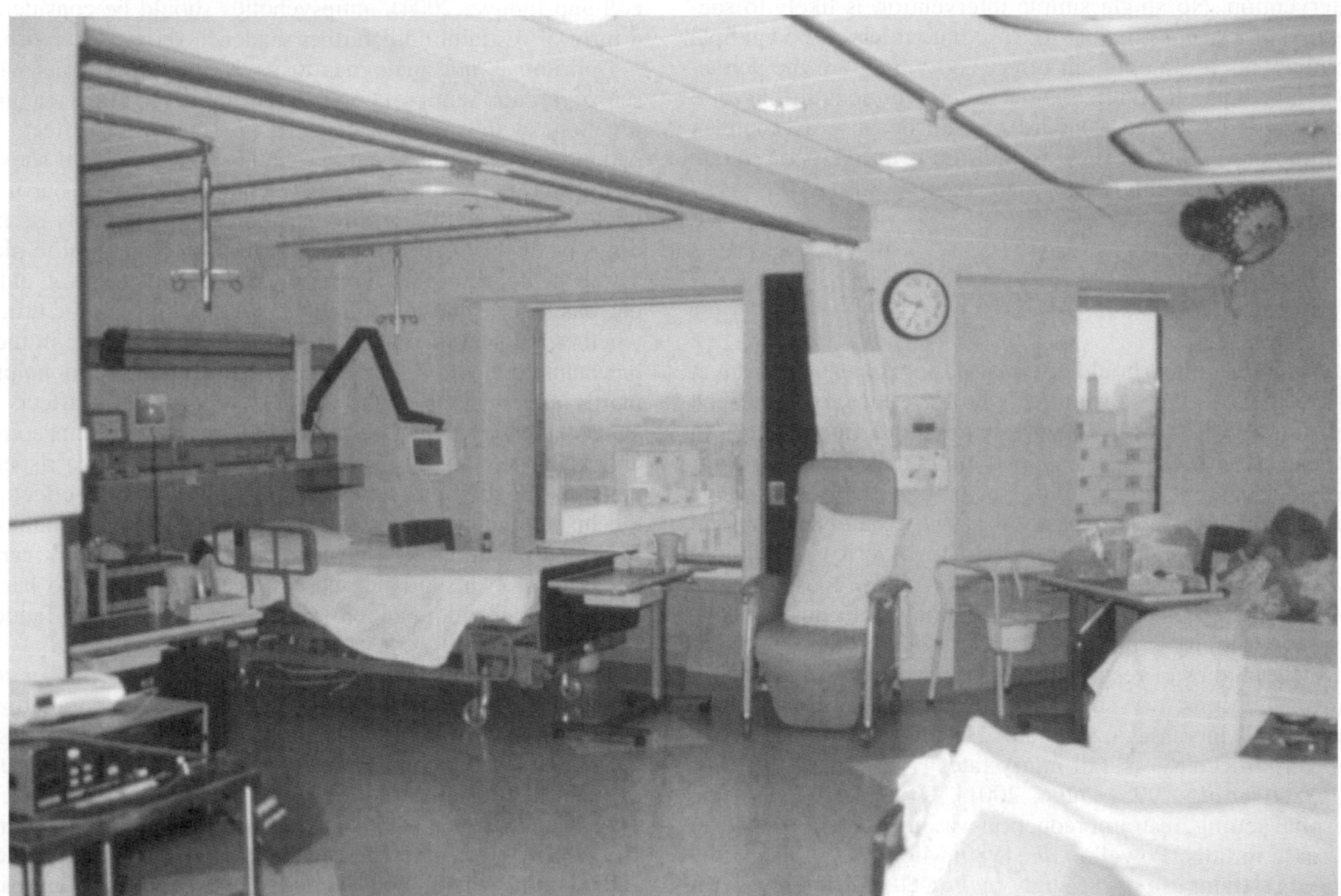

Figure 1 The Delirium Room, Saint Louis University Hospital, 1998

daily doses of less than 2.0 mg. Only 13% of the patients lost physical function and none of the 69 patients died during their stay in the hospital. Mean length of stay for these patients was not significantly different compared to the length of stay for all other patients over the age of 70 during the same time frame (Flaherty *et al.*, 2003).

The above studies have been highlighted because of their positive results. However, not all interventions have been successful. A thorough review of evidence concerning delirium management in the hospital setting by Boustani and colleagues looked at controlled clinical trials that used any intervention aimed at delirium among populations over the age of 55. They found 23 studies that met the inclusion criteria. Seven of the trials were among older hospitalized patients for medical conditions, eight trials among older hospitalized patients for surgical repair of hip fracture, six trials among older cardiac surgery patients, one trial for patients after bilateral knee replacement and one trial following gastrointestinal procedures. Most trials showed a lack of efficacy in reducing the severity or duration of delirium after its onset. However, overall, 86% of interdisciplinary team-based trials and 29% of nurse-based trials showed positive impact on delirium management (Boustani *et al.*, 2004).

The take-home message for delirium is that although this is a difficult problem to prevent, or manage when unpreventable, it can be done usually through a multicomponent intervention. No single simple intervention is likely to succeed, and it is not possible to tease out which of the multiple components are having an effect and which are the detractors. Nonetheless, multicomponent interventions still need to be considered as the standard of care because a "complex mutifactorial problem such as delirium is unlikely to respond consistently to a single approach (Inouye, 2001)".

PHYSICAL RESTRAINTS

Physical restraints should not be used for patients who are at risk of developing delirium or who have already developed delirium (*see* **Chapter 142, Restraints and Immobility**). In one study, physical restraints had the highest relative risk of five independent precipitating factors for delirium (Inouye and Charpentier, 1996), and another study found that physical restraints were significantly related to severity of delirium (McCusker *et al.*, 2001). Furthermore, the proposed reason for the use of physical restraints among delirious patients, to prevent injury primarily related to falls, is misconceived. Of three studies of restraint reduction programs in long-term care institutions, two showed no change in fall rate and one showed an increase in fall rate. However, all three studies showed a decrease in fall injury rates (Neufeld *et al.*, 1999; Capezuti *et al.*, 1998; Dunn, 2001). Of two studies in the hospital setting, restraint reduction was not associated with an increase in falls (Powell *et al.*, 1989; Mion *et al.*, 2001). The rate of restraint use in the study by Powell *et al.* (1989) went from 52 per 1000 patient-days to just 0.3 per 1000 patient-days. Although neither study reported injury rates before and after restraint reduction, the study by Mion and colleagues reported that injury rates after the restraint reduction program were low. Importantly, they were modestly successful ($\geq$20% reduction) in two of six intensive care units in restraint reduction and reported that no deaths occurred as a result of a fall or disruption in therapy, including in the case of intensive care unit patients on mechanical ventilators (Powell *et al.*, 1989; Mion *et al.*, 2001).

Furthermore, the fact that restraint-free environments can be achieved, as in some geriatric departments in European hospitals (De Vries *et al.*, 2004), ACE Units in United States hospitals (Flaherty *et al.*, 2003) and some nursing facilities (Gatz, 2000; Makowski *et al.*, 2000), adds to the evidence that restraint free care should be the standard of care.

PHARMACOLOGICAL RESTRAINTS

Currently, no antipsychotic or other pharmacological agent is approved by the US Food and Drug Administration (FDA) for the treatment of delirium. On the basis of the available data concerning medications used in the management of delirium and the commonly accepted reason to use them (for patients whose behavior interrupts the necessary medical care or puts themselves or others at risk of physical harm) (McNicoll and Inouye, 2004), antipsychotics should be considered a form of restraint until further evidence shows otherwise.

Delirium is not analogous to psychosis. In patients with schizophrenia, antipsychotics can improve behavior and function, with sedation being a common side effect. In patients with delirium, antipsychotics have not been shown to do this. It is argued that they control behavior, but it is unclear whether this is through the sedation effects of the drugs or their effect on the neurotransmitters thought to play a role in delirium. To further complicate matters for older persons, one of the main problems with antipsychotic drugs, whether atypical or typical, is that they are not pure in their mechanism of action. For example, although risperidone primarily affects serotonergic (5-HT_2A) receptors, it affects to some extent dopaminergic and alpha-1 receptors. Olanzapine, although it affects the 5-HT_2A receptors, similar to risperidone, its sedation properties are probably due to its effect on the histaminic receptors. Clozapine also affects histaminic as well as muscarinic receptors, and quetiapine has varying effects on histaminic and α-1 receptors and also has a small affect on dopaminergic and 5-HT receptors (Tandon *et al.*, 1999).

The available data for the use of antipsychotics in the management of delirium are poor because of the populations studied, types of studies done, or the presence of the common mistake of not including a placebo group in order to measure the natural course (duration) of delirium without pharmacological intervention. One randomized trial (Breitbart *et al.*, 1996) that is often referenced in review articles (Meagher, 2001; Burns *et al.*, 2004) condoning the use of antipsychotic medications compared haloperidol, chlorpromazine, and lorazepam in 30 delirious hospitalized patients with

AIDS, whose mean age was 39.2 years (range 23–56 years). Although the study by Nakamura *et al.* (1997) comparing haloperidol and mianserin included 60 patients with a mean age of 65 years, they did not have a control group either. Thus, when they reported improvement on a delirium rating scale at 1 week, one questions whether or not patients would have improved by this time anyway. Newer studies with atypical antipsychotics are also wrought with this error of not taking into account the duration of delirium without medication. One case report study using risperidone claims that the delirium cleared by day 14 (Sipahimalani and Masand, 1997). A prospective study of 64 patients with delirium who received risperidone reported improvement at day seven (Parellada *et al.*, 2004). Olanzapine was evaluated in a retrospective study of 11 delirious patients compared to 11 others who received haloperidol. It took 6.8 days and 7.2 days respectively for the peak clinical response (Sipahimalani and Masand, 1998). A case report of delirium due to olanzapine has been reported (Samuels and Fang, 2004).

The proper dosages of antipsychotics have also never been established. One recent text recommends that if severe agitation is present, haloperidol doses of 0.25–1.0 mg can be used as often as every 20–30 minutes with a maximum 24-hour dose of 3–5 mg. This dose is recommended because D2-dopaminergic receptors are saturated at low doses, and thus theoretically, doses above 5 mg over a 24-hour period are likely to only increase adverse events without providing additional clinical benefit. The goal should be an awake patient who is manageable, not a sedated patient, and the drug should be tapered and discontinued as soon as possible (McNicoll and Inouye, 2004). A recent study of mostly surgical delirious ICU patients, with an average age of 65 years, compared haloperidol and olanzapine. For patients over 60 years, haloperidol was initiated at 0.5–1.0 mg and olanzapine at 2.5 mg every eight hours. Younger patients were initiated at doses of 2.5–5.0 mg and 5 mg, respectively. The Delirium Index (measure of severity) decreased over time and clinical improvement was the same in both groups. The study did not detail what percentage of patients were mechanically ventilated (Skrobik *et al.*, 2004).

It is evident from the lack of evidence that randomized placebo controlled trials are needed. It should be noted that in a randomized controlled trial of a nonpharmacological intervention to prevent delirium, Inouye and colleagues found that even in the control group patients who developed delirium, the average total number of days of delirium was approximately 2.5 (Inouye *et al.*, 1999a). Although this study does not go into detail about the percent of delirious patients who received antipsychotics, or the dose, another study mentioned above (Flaherty *et al.*, 2003), found that only 29% of 69 delirious patients received any form of pharmacological restraint (antipsychotics, benzodiazepines, sedative/hypnotic), and this group had an average length of stay in hospital less than five days.

On the basis of the available current data the following conclusions can be made:

1. There is not enough evidence for the routine use of antipsychotic or other pharmacological approaches in the management of delirium.
2. On the basis of general geriatric principles, nonpharmacologic interventions that have no or less risk should be tried before any pharmacological approach is tried.
3. If pharmacological agents are used, the lowest possible dose should be tried first, keeping in mind the goal that is intended (manageable and awake, not over sedated).
4. On the basis of the very limited data, the category of drug of choice seems to be antipsychotics, not benzodiazepines or sedative-hypnotics.

KEY POINTS

- Delirium is common among older persons in the hospital, especially in surgical patients and patients in the intensive care unit (ICU), and in postacute-care settings, but not so common among patients with acute illnesses cared for at home.
- Delirium is a dangerous diagnosis and has been found to be associated with hospital complications, loss of physical function, increased length of stay in the hospital and ICU, increased incidence of discharge from the hospital to a long-term care facility, and even higher mortality.
- The comprehensive approach to delirium involves awareness, diagnosis, evaluation, prevention, and management. The causes of delirium can be remembered using the two mnemonics D-E-L-I-R-I-U-M-S and A-C-U-T-E C-H-A-N-G-E I-N M-S.
- Successful prevention and management interventions include a multicomponent intervention with protocols targeting risk factors to prevent the development of delirium, a geriatric consultation service for patients with hip fracture, and a specialized four-bed room to provide 24-hour nursing care, called *the Delirium Room*.
- Physical restraints should not be used in patients with delirium, and rarely should pharmacological restraints be used.

KEY REFERENCES

- Flaherty JH. Psychotherapeutic agents in older adults. Commonly prescribed and over-the-counter remedies: causes of confusion. *Clinics in Geriatric Medicine* 1998; **14**:101–27.
- Flaherty JH, Tariq SH, Raghavan S *et al.* A model for managing delirious older inpatients. *Journal of the American Geriatrics Society* 2003; **51**:1031–5.
- Inouye SK, Bogardus ST Jr, Charpentier PA *et al.* A multicomponent intervention to prevent delirium in hospitalized older patients. *New England Journal of Medicine* 1999a; **340**:669–76.

- Marcantonio ER, Flacker JM, Wright RJ & Resnick NM. Reducing delirium after hip fracture: a randomized trial. *Journal of the American Geriatrics Society* 2001; **49**:516–22.

REFERENCES

American Psychiatric Association. *Diagnostic and Statistical Manual of Mental Disorders: DSM-IV-TR*. 2000, 4th, rev. edn; The Association: Washington (DC).

Bailer U, Fischer P, Kufferle B *et al.* Occurrence of mirtazapine-induced delirium in organic brain disorder. *International Clinical Psychopharmacology* 2000; **15**:239–43.

Banks WA, Farr SA & Morley JE. Entry of blood-borne cytokines into the central nervous system: effects on cognitive processes. *Neuroimmunomodulation* 2003; **10**:319–27.

Blackburn T & Dunn M. Cystocerebral syndrome. Acute urinary retention presenting as confusion in elderly patients. *Archives of Internal Medicine* 1990; **150**:2577–8.

Ble A, Zuliani G, Quarenghi C *et al.* Cystocerebral syndrome: a case report and literature review. *Aging-Clinical and Experimental Research* 2001; **13**:339–42.

Boustani M, Heck D, Farlow M *et al.* Managing delirium in hospitalized elderly. *Journal of the American Geriatrics Society* 2004; **52**:S199.

Brauer LH, Rukstalis MR & deWit H. Acute subjective responses to paroxetine in normal volunteers. *Drug and Alcohol Dependence* 1995; **39**:223–30.

Breitbart W, Marotta R, Platt MM *et al.* A double-blind trial of haloperidol, chlorpromazine, and lorazepam in the treatment of delirium in hospitalized AIDS patients. *American Journal of Psychiatry* 1996; **153**:231–7.

Burns A, Gallagley A & Byrne J. Delirium. *Journal of Neurology, Neurosurgery and Psychiatry* 2004; **75**:362–7.

Cacchione PZ, Culp K, Laing J & Tripp-Reimer T. Clinical profile of acute confusion in the long-term care setting. *Clinical Nursing Research* 2003; **12**:145–58.

Capezuti E, Strumpf NE, Evans LK *et al.* The relationship between physical restraint removal and falls and injuries among nursing home residents. *Journals of Gerontology. Series A, Biological Sciences and Medical Sciences* 1998; **53**:M47–52.

Caplan GA, Ward JA, Brennan NJ *et al.* Hospital in the home: a randomised controlled trial. *Medical Journal of Australia* 1999; **170**:156–60.

Carter GL, Dawson AH & Lopert R. Drug-induced delirium. Incidence, management and prevention. *Drug Safety* 1996; **15**:291–301.

Cole M, McCusker J, Dendukuri N & Han L. The prognostic significance of subsyndromal delirium in elderly medical inpatients. *Journal of the American Geriatrics Society* 2003; **51**:754–60.

De Vries OJ, Ligthart GJ & Nikolaus Th. European Academy of Medicine of Ageing-Course III. Differences in period prevalence of the use of physical restraints in elderly inpatients of European hospitals and nursing homes. *Journals of Gerontology Series A-Biological Sciences and Medical Sciences* 2004; **59**(9):M922–3.

Dubois MJ, Bergeron N, Dumont M *et al.* Delirium in an intensive care unit: a study of risk factors. *Intensive Care Medicine* 2001; **27**:1297–304.

Dunn KS. The effect of physical restraints on fall rates in older adults who are institutionalized. *Journal of Gerontological Nursing* 2001; **27**:40–8.

Dyer CB, Ashton CM & Teasdale TA. Postoperative delirium. A review of 80 primary data-collection studies. *Archives of Internal Medicine* 1995; **155**:461–5.

Edwards KR & O'Connor JT. Risk of delirium with concomitant use of tolterodine and acetylcholinesterase inhibitors. *Journal of the American Geriatrics Society* 2002; **50**:1165–6.

Ely EW, Gautam S, Margolin R *et al.* The impact of delirium in the intensive care unit on hospital length of stay. *Intensive Care Medicine* 2001a; **27**:1892–900.

Ely EW, Shintani A, Truman B *et al.* Delirium as a predictor of mortality in mechanically ventilated patients in the intensive care unit. *Journal of the American Medical Association* 2004a; **291**:1753–62.

Ely EW, Stephens RK, Jackson JC *et al.* Current opinions regarding the importance, diagnosis, and management of delirium in the intensive care unit: a survey of 912 healthcare professionals. *Critical Care Medicine* 2004b; **32**:106–12.

Ferro JM, Caeiro L & Verdelho A. Delirium in acute stroke. *Current Opinion in Neurology* 2002; **15**:51–5.

Flaherty JH. Psychotherapeutic agents in older adults. Commonly prescribed and over-the-counter remedies: causes of confusion. *Clinics in Geriatric Medicine* 1998; **14**:101–27.

Flaherty JH, Tariq SH, Raghavan S *et al.* A model for managing delirious older inpatients. *Journal of the American Geriatrics Society* 2003; **51**:1031–5.

Foy A, O'Connell D, Henry D *et al.* Benzodiazepine use as a cause of cognitive impairment in elderly hospital inpatients. *Journals of Gerontology. Series A, Biological Sciences and Medical Sciences* 1995; **50**:M99–106.

Francis J & Kapoor WN. Prognosis after hospital discharge of older medical patients with delirium. *Journal of the American Geriatrics Society* 1992; **40**:601–6.

Francis J, Martin D & Kapoor WN. A prospective study of delirium in hospitalized elderly. *Journal of the American Medical Association* 1990; **263**:1097–101.

Frederickson M, Neitzel JJ, Miller EH *et al.* The implementation of bedside bladder ultrasound technology: effects on patient and cost postoperative outcomes in tertiary care. *Orthopaedic Nursing* 2000; **19**:79–87.

Freeman NJ & Kirdar JA. An unusual manifestation of a common illness in the elderly. *Hospital Practice (Office Edition)* 1990; **25**:91–4.

Gatz D. Moving to a restraint-free environment. *Balance* 2000; **4**:12–5.

Howe C & Ravasia S. Venlafaxine-induced delirium. *Canadian Journal of Psychiatry–Revue Canadienne de Psychiatrie* 2003; **48**:129.

Inouye SK. Delirium in hospitalized older patients: recognition and risk factors. *Journal of Geriatric Psychiatry and Neurology* 1998; **11**:118–25.

Inouye SK. Delirium after hip fracture: to be or not to be? *Journal of the American Geriatrics Society* 2001; **49**:678–9.

Inouye SK. Delirium. In CK Cassel, RM Leipzig, HJ Cohen *et al.* (eds) *Geriatric Medicine: An Evidence-Based Approach* 2003, pp 1113–22 Springer, New York.

Inouye SK, Bogardus ST Jr, Charpentier PA *et al.* A multicomponent intervention to prevent delirium in hospitalized older patients. *New England Journal of Medicine* 1999a; **340**:669–76.

Inouye SK & Charpentier PA. Precipitating factors for delirium in hospitalized elderly persons. Predictive model and interrelationship with baseline vulnerability. *Journal of the American Medical Association* 1996; **275**(11):852–7.

Inouye SK, Schlesinger MJ & Lydon TJ. Delirium: a symptom of how hospital care is failing older persons and a window to improve quality of hospital care. *American Journal of Medicine* 1999b; **106**:565–73.

Inouye SK, Foreman MD, Mion LC *et al.* Nurses' recognition of delirium and its symptoms: comparison of nurse and researcher ratings. *Archives of Internal Medicine* 2001; **161**:2467–73.

Inouye SK, Rushing JT, Foreman MD *et al.* Does delirium contribute to poor hospital outcomes? A three-site epidemiologic study. *Journal of General Internal Medicine* 1998; **13**:234–42.

Inouye SK, van Dyck CH, Alessi CA *et al.* Clarifying confusion: the confusion assessment method. A new method for detection of delirium. *Annals of Internal Medicine* 1990; **113**:941–8.

Inouye SK, Viscoli CM, Horwitz RI *et al.* A predictive model for delirium in hospitalized elderly medical patients based on admission characteristics. *Annals of Internal Medicine* 1993; **119**:474–81.

Johnson JC, Gottlieb GL, Sullivan E *et al.* Using DSM-III criteria to diagnose delirium in elderly general medical patients. *Journal of Gerontology* 1990; **45**:M113–9.

Kelly KG, Zisselman M, Cutillo-Schmitter T *et al.* Severity and course of delirium in medically hospitalized nursing facility residents. *American Journal of Geriatric Psychiatry* 2001; **9**:72–7.

Kiely DK, Bergmann MA, Murphy KM *et al.* Delirium among newly admitted postacute facility patients: prevalence, symptoms, and severity. *Journals of Gerontology. Series A, Biological Sciences and Medical Sciences* 2003; **58**:M441–5.

Landefeld CS, Palmer RM, Kresevic DM *et al.* A randomized trial of care in a hospital medical unit especially designed to improve the functional outcomes of acutely ill older patients. *New England Journal of Medicine* 1995; **332**:1338–44.

Leff B, Burton L, Guido S *et al.* Home hospital: a feasible and efficacious approach to care for acutely ill older persons. *Journal of the American Geriatrics Society* 2004; **52**:S194.

Levkoff SE, Evans DA, Liptzin B *et al.* Delirium. The occurrence and persistence of symptoms among elderly hospitalized patients. *Archives of Internal Medicine* 1992; **152**:334–40.

Liem PH & Carter WJ. Cystocerebral syndrome: a possible explanation. *Archives of Internal Medicine* 1991; **151**:1884–6.

Lipowski ZJ. Delirium in the elderly patient. *New England Journal of Medicine* 1989; **320**:578–82.

Lynch EP, Lazor MA, Gellis JE *et al.* The impact of postoperative pain on the development of postoperative delirium. *Anesthesia and Analgesia* 1998; **86**:781–5.

Lyness JM. Delirium: masquerades and misdiagnosis in elderly inpatients. *Journal of the American Geriatrics Society* 1990; **38**:1235–8.

Macknight C & Rojas-Fernandez CH. Celecoxib-and rofecoxib-induced delirium. *Journal of Neuropsychiatry and Clinical Neurosciences* 2001; **13**:305–6.

Makowski TR, Maggard W & Morley JE. The Life Care Center of St. Louis experience with subacute care. *Clinics in Geriatric Medicine* 2000; **16**:701–24.

Malone ML, Rosen LB & Goodwin JS. Complications of acute myocardial infarction in patients > or = 90 years of age. *American Journal of Cardiology* 1998; **81**(5):638–41.

Marcantonio ER, Flacker JM, Michaels M & Resnick NM. Delirium is independently associated with poor functional recovery after hip fracture. *Journal of the American Geriatrics Society* 2000; **48**:618–24.

Marcantonio ER, Flacker JM, Wright RJ & Resnick NM. Reducing delirium after hip fracture: a randomized trial. *Journal of the American Geriatrics Society* 2001; **49**:516–22.

Marcantonio ER, Goldman L, Orav EJ *et al.* The association of intraoperative factors with the development of postoperative delirium. *American Journal of Medicine* 1998a; **105**:380–4.

Marcantonio ER, Simon SE, Bergmann MA *et al.* Delirium symptoms in post-acute care: prevalent, persistent, and associated with poor functional recovery. *Journal of the American Geriatrics Society* 2003; **51**:4–9.

McCusker J, Cole M, Abrahamowicz M *et al.* Environmental risk factors for delirium in hospitalized older people. *Journal of the American Geriatrics Society* 2001; **49**:1327–34.

McCusker J, Cole M, Abrahamowicz M *et al.* Delirium predicts 12-month mortality. *Archives of Internal Medicine* 2002a; **162**:457–63.

McCusker J, Kakuma R & Abrahamowicz M. Predictors of functional decline in hospitalized elderly patients: a systematic review. *Journals of Gerontology. Series A, Biological Sciences and Medical Sciences* 2002b; **57**:M569–77.

McCusker J, Cole M, Dendukuri N *et al.* The course of delirium in older medical inpatients: a prospective study. *Journal of General Internal Medicine* 2003; **18**:696–704.

McKeith I, Fairbairn A, Perry R *et al.* Neuroleptic sensitivity in patients with senile dementia of Lewy body type. *British Medical Journal* 1992; **305**:673–8.

McNicoll L & Inouye SK. Delirium. In CS Landefeld, RM Palmer, MA Johnson *et al.* (eds) *Current Geriatric Diagnosis and Treatment* 2004, pp 53–9; Laonge Medical Books/McGraw Hill, New York.

McNicoll L, Pisani MA, Zhang Y *et al.* Delirium in the intensive care unit: occurrence and clinical course in older patients. *Journal of the American Geriatrics Society* 2003; **51**:591–8.

Meagher DJ. Delirium: optimising management. *British Medical Journal* 2001; **322**:144–9.

Mentes J, Culp K, Maas M & Rantz M. Acute confusion indicators: risk factors and prevalence using MDS data. *Research in Nursing & Health* 1999; **22**:95–105.

Mion LC, Fogel J, Sandhu S *et al.* Outcomes following physical restraint reduction programs in two acute care hospitals. *Joint Commission Journal on Quality Improvement* 2001; **27**:605–18.

Molloy DW. Memory loss, confusion, and disorientation in an elderly women taking meclizine. *Journal of the American Geriatrics Society* 1987; **35**:454–6.

Nakamura J, Uchimura N, Yamada S & Nakazawa Y. Does plasma free-3-methoxy-4-hydroxyphenyl(ethylene)glycol increase in the delirious state? A comparison of the effects of mianserin and haloperidol on delirium. *International Clinical Psychopharmacology* 1997; **12**:147–52.

Neufeld RR, Libow LS, Foley WJ *et al.* Restraint reduction reduces serious injuries among nursing home residents. *Journal of the American Geriatrics Society* 1999; **47**:1202–7.

O'Keeffe S & Lavan J. The prognostic significance of delirium in older hospital patients. *Journal of the American Geriatrics Society* 1997; **45**:174–8.

Parellada E, Baeza I, de Pablo J & Martinez G. Risperidone in the treatment of patients with delirium. *Journal of Clinical Psychiatry* 2004; **65**:348–53.

Petrovic M, Pevernagie D, Van Den Noortgate N *et al.* A programme for short-term withdrawal from benzodiazepines in geriatric hospital inpatients: success rate and effect on subjective sleep quality. *International Journal of Geriatric Psychiatry* 1999; **14**:754–60.

Pompei P, Foreman M, Rudberg MA *et al.* Delirium in hospitalized older persons: outcomes and predictors. *Journal of the American Geriatrics Society* 1994; **42**:809–15.

Popli AP, Hegarty JD, Siegel AJ *et al.* Transfer of psychiatric inpatients to a general hospital due to adverse drug reactions. *Psychosomatics* 1997; **38**:37.

Powell C, Mitchell-Pedersen L, Fingerote E & Edmund L. Freedom from restraint: consequences of reducing physical restraints in the management of the elderly. *Canadian Medical Association Journal* 1989; **141**:561–4.

Reilly JJ, Crowe SF & Lloyd JH. Neuroleptic toxicity syndromes: a clinical spectrum. *Australian and New Zealand Journal of Psychiatry* 1991; **25**:499–505.

Rizzo JA, Bogardus ST Jr, Leo-Summers L *et al.* Multicomponent targeted intervention to prevent delirium in hospitalized older patients: what is the economic value? *Medical Care* 2001; **39**:740–52.

Rockwood K. Educational interventions in delirium. *Dementia and Geriatric Cognitive Disorders* 1999; **10**:426–9.

Saint S, Lipsky BA & Goold SD. Indwelling urinary catheters: a one-point restraint? *Annals of Internal Medicine* 2002; **137**:125–7.

Samuels S & Fang M. Olanzapine may cause delirium in geriatric patients. *Journal of Clinical Psychiatry* 2004; **65**:582–3.

Sipahimalani A & Masand PS. Use of risperidone in delirium: case reports. *Annals of Clinical Psychiatry* 1997; **9**(2):105–7.

Sipahimalani A & Masand PS. Olanzapine in the treatment of delirium. *Psychosomatics* 1998; **39**(5):422–30.

Skrobik YK, Bergeron N, Dumont M & Gottfried SB. Olanzapine vs haloperidol: treating delirium in a critical care setting. *Intensive Care Medicine* 2004; **30**:444–9.

Sompraktit P, Lertakyamanee J, Satraratanamai C *et al.* Mental state change after general and regional anesthesia in adults and elderly patients, a randomized clinical trial. *Journal of the Medical Association of Thailand* 2002; **85**:S875–83.

Tagle P, Mery F, Torrealba G *et al.* Chronic subdural hematoma: a disease of elderly people. *Revista Medica de Chile* 2003; **131**(2):177–82.

Tandon R, Milner K & Jibson MD. Antipsychotics from theory to practice: integrating clinical and basic data. *Journal of Clinical Psychiatry* 1999; **60**:21–8.

Thomas RI, Cameron DJ & Fahs MC. A prospective study of delirium and prolonged hospital stay. Exploratory study. *Archives of General Psychiatry* 1988; **45**:937–40.

Thomas DR & Kamel H. Therapeutic diets among hospitalized patients. *Journal of Nutrition, Health & Aging* 2004; accepted for publication.

Warshaw G & Tanzer F. The effectiveness of lumbar puncture in the evaluation of delirium and fever in the hospitalized elderly. *Archives of Family Medicine* 1993; **2**:293–7.

Williams-Russo P, Sharrock NE, Haas SB *et al.* Randomized trial of epidural versus general anesthesia: outcomes after primary total knee replacement. *Clinical Orthopaedics and Related Research* 1996; **331**:199–208.

FURTHER READING

Agostini JV, Leo-Summers LS & Inouye SK. Cognitive and other adverse effects of diphenhydramine use in hospitalized older patients. *Archives of Internal Medicine* 2001; **161**:2091–7.

Cacchione PZ. Four acute confusion assessment instruments: reliability and validity for use in long-term care facilities. *Journal of Gerontological Nursing* 2002; **28**:12–9.

Caeiro L, Ferro JM, Albuquerque R & Figueira ML. Delirium in the first days of acute stroke. *Journal of Neurology* 2004; **251**:171–8.

Cole MG, McCusker J, Bellavance F *et al.* Systematic detection and multidisciplinary care of delirium in older medical inpatients: a randomized trial. *Canadian Medical Association Journal* 2002; **167**:753–9.

Dolan MM, Hawkes WG, Zimmerman SI *et al.* Delirium on hospital admission in aged hip fracture patients: prediction of mortality and 2-year functional outcomes. *Journals of Gerontology. Series A, Biological Sciences and Medical Sciences* 2000; **55**:M527–34.

Ely EW, Inouye SK, Bernard GR *et al.* Delirium in mechanically ventilated patients: validity and reliability of the confusion assessment method for the intensive care unit (CAM-ICU). *Journal of the American Medical Association* 2001b; **286**:2703–10.

Ely EW, Margolin R, Francis J *et al.* Evaluation of delirium in critically ill patients: validation of the Confusion Assessment Method for the Intensive Care Unit (CAM-ICU). *Critical Care Medicine* 2001c; **29**:1370–9.

Inouye SK, Bogardus ST Jr, Williams CS *et al.* The role of adherence on the effectiveness of nonpharmacologic interventions: evidence from the delirium prevention trial. *Archives of Internal Medicine* 2003; **163**:958–64.

Lundstrom M, Edlund A, Bucht G *et al.* Dementia after delirium in patients with femoral neck fractures. *Journal of the American Geriatrics Society* 2003; **51**:1002–6.

Marcantonio ER, Juarez G, Goldman L *et al.* The relationship of postoperative delirium with psychoactive medications. *Journal of the American Medical Association* 1994; **272**:1518–22.

Marcantonio ER, Michaels M & Resnick NM. Diagnosing delirium by telephone. *Journal of General Internal Medicine* 1998b; **13**:621–3.

O'Keeffe ST & Lavan JN. Clinical significance of delirium subtypes in older people. *Age and Ageing* 1999; **28**:115–9.

Rockwood K, Cosway S, Carver D *et al.* The risk of dementia and death after delirium. *Age and Ageing* 1999; **28**:551–6.

Sands LP, Yaffe K, Covinsky K *et al.* Cognitive screening predicts magnitude of functional recovery from admission to 3 months after discharge in hospitalized elders. *Journals of Gerontology. Series A, Biological Sciences and Medical Sciences* 2003; **58**:37–45.

Sipahimalani A & Masand PS. Olanzapine in the treatment of delirium. *Psychosomatics* 1998; **39**:422–30.

Sipahimalani A & Masand PS. Olanzapine in the treatment of delirium. Use of risperidone in delirium: case reports. *Annals of Clinical Psychiatry* 1998; **9**:105–7.

Skrobik Y. Haloperidol should be used sparingly. *Critical Care Medicine* 2002; **30**:2613–4.

Trzepacz PT & Francis J. Low serum albumin levels and risk of delirium. *American Journal of Psychiatry* 1990; **147**:675.

91

Memory Clinics

Antony J. Bayer
Cardiff University, Cardiff, UK

INTRODUCTION

Clinics specifically for the diagnosis and management of early dementia were first developed in the United States in the late 1970s. These were primarily research-based, linked to developing Alzheimer's disease (AD) and aging research centers and acted as a focus for expert assessment, investigation, treatment, and advice (Knopman *et al.*, 1985; Larrabee *et al.*, 1990). Initially described as "dementia clinics", the terminology soon changed to the more acceptable name of "memory clinic", or "memory disorders clinic". While the new title is less stigmatizing, it runs the risk of serving as a euphemism, avoiding an open and honest approach to the reality of dementia.

Predominantly service-oriented memory clinics were set up in the United Kingdom in the early 1980s (Bayer *et al.*, 1987; Van der Cammen *et al.*, 1987; Philpot and Levy, 1987), offering multidisciplinary, outpatient-based assessment and diagnosis for mainly older people with memory and other cognitive problems, in an acceptable and accessible environment. At first, many of these clinics were funded from outside the National Health Service and were based mainly in university departments of geriatric medicine or old age psychiatry. Existing services tended to consider memory clinics to be a luxury, allowing academics to indulge their narrow clinical interests away from the reality of budgetary considerations and the priorities of practical dementia care. However, this reflected the concentration of service provision on dealing with the behavioral and psychological symptoms of advanced dementia and on crisis intervention and institutional-based management. The first memory clinics played an important role in raising awareness of the value of elective intervention and interdisciplinary care for people with early dementia and acted as a focus for development of specialist knowledge and expertise in early diagnosis and management of people presenting with cognitive impairment.

Most of the early UK clinics were also very actively involved in research, especially recruiting into clinical trials of the emerging antidementia drugs. Largely thanks to the work of these centers, specific drug treatment for AD became available in the late 1990s and the focus of activity shifted toward provision of an effective clinical service for patients presenting with memory disturbances and best use of medication, together with psychosocial interventions and patient and carer support and education (Wilcock *et al.*, 1999). The evolution of hospital-based memory clinics into more community-based memory teams was the natural consequence, working alongside or as an independent part of traditional mental health teams for older people.

In 1993, a survey identified 20 active memory clinics in the British Isles (Wright and Lindesay, 1995), but considered them to be too academic and isolated from mainstream practice and also ill-equipped to provide for care after diagnosis. However, a follow-up survey just a few years later (Lindesay *et al.*, 2002) identified at least 58 active clinics and noted that the newer clinics were tending to be smaller, less academic and less involved in research than the more established clinics. In 2001, the UK government published two important documents. The National Institute of Clinical Excellence (NICE) guidance on use of drugs for treatment of AD (NICE, 2001) advocated the need for further development of memory clinics to support best use of the drugs and the National Service Framework (NSF) for Older People (Department of Health, 2001) recommended memory clinics as an essential component of hospital-based services.

While most clinics focus on diagnosis of mild cognitive impairment (MCI) and early dementia, others encompass all acquired cognitive disorders, including head injury and epilepsy (Kopelman and Crawford, 1996). A few specifically target people with purely subjective memory loss, or younger people with early-onset dementia, or people with learning disabilities (Hassiotis *et al.*, 2003). Many concentrate on diagnosis and assessment with a view to best use of available medication and those in academic centers continue to conduct a lot of research, including clinical trials of newer drug treatments. The emphasis on assessment for drug treatment and the powerful influence of the pharmaceutical industry

Principles and Practice of Geriatric Medicine, 4th Edition. Edited by M.S. John Pathy, Alan J. Sinclair and John E. Morley.

has tended to detract from the importance of additional or alternative perspectives and the provision of a holistic, multiprofessional and multiagency approach to dementia care should be central to the activity of all clinics.

Referral may be open access (those willing to see all-comers), or restricted to secondary or tertiary referrals, or to selected individuals who meet predetermined criteria. In general, patients referred by their general practitioners (GPs) seem more likely to have dementia than self-referrals, though the reassurance given to those without organic disease (the "worried well") should not be underestimated. Some so-called memory clinics are merely rebranded old age psychiatry outpatient clinics, or community-based services solely monitoring antidementia drugs. Others are innovative service developments, for example, clinics providing memory-screening tests in shopping malls or mobile clinics and telemedicine to aid evaluation and treatment in patients' homes.

DEVELOPMENTS AROUND THE WORLD

Memory clinics are now a feature of health services for older people in centers around the world, but they exist in various forms and are variously based in neurology, psychiatry, or geriatric secondary care services; most involve multiprofessional assessment, often with everyone coming together to share results in a diagnostic consensus meeting. Despite the differing needs and varied settings, the fundamental similarity between memory clinics across the world is striking.

In Switzerland, there is a collaborative group of 11 memory clinics enabling an active program of education and training for health professionals and clinical research. The GP plays an important role in initial assessment before comprehensive diagnosis and treatment recommendations are made in the memory clinic, including memory training and caregiver support activities. There is also close involvement with the National Alzheimer's Association (Monsch *et al.*, 1998).

In France, memory clinics are well established as expert centers for early diagnosis and management of dementia and have an important educational and research role (Mahieux, 2000). The multidisciplinary day hospital has been proposed as the ideal setting for a memory clinic, though some experts have questioned whether a single specialist in charge of adjusting examinations and management to particular situations would be preferable to a routine multispecialty approach (Derouesne, 1997).

In Italy, the "Progetto Memoria" provided what was effectively a mobile memory clinic, bringing memory testing to communities in a bus (Zappala *et al.*, 1995). A national project has also seen the development of regional centers for the diagnosis and care of people with AD. In other Northern European countries, memory clinics have become the centers of a broader model of care, with preliminary home visits by a nurse and/or psychologist before clinic attendance, and further home visits afterwards to discuss assessment results and plan future management.

In the southern hemisphere, memory clinics providing multidisciplinary assessment and management for community-living people with dementia are developing in every continent, from Brazil and Mexico, to Hong Kong and Singapore, to South Africa and Australia. The memory clinics in Australia are amongst the longest established (Ames *et al.*, 1992) and have developed into a coordinated network of clinics across the state of Victoria (Cognitive, Dementia and Memory Services (CDAMS) Clinics). These have highlighted the importance of clinics being sensitive to the needs of people from a range of cultural and linguistic backgrounds (LoGiudice *et al.*, 2001), a challenge also being addressed in many North American clinics.

WHY THE NEED?

The worldwide growth in memory clinics has largely developed because of increasing demand and expectations of patients and families, frustrated by the difficulties of obtaining informed diagnosis and advice from existing services. They are not a replacement or alternative to these, but rather a more focused service providing a consistent approach to assessment, more specific diagnosis and a single resource for expert information and support (Table 1). Demographic changes are rapidly leading to greater numbers of patients with age-related cognitive disorders and there is appropriate reluctance to attribute forgetfulness merely to age. The growing awareness that memory failure is not inevitable and that effective intervention is available has lead to a desire for

Table 1 Potential benefits of memory clinics

Benefits for patients and families

- Nonstigmatizing, specialist resource
- Expert multidisciplinary assessment and diagnosis of cognitive disorders
- Ensures treatable conditions are not overlooked
- Early identification of dementia and intervention
- Antidementia drugs are effectively targeted, monitored, and stopped as appropriate
- Education and practical support for patients and carers
- Empowers people with dementia while they are still able to maintain control over their lives
- Provides advice on memory aids and memory training
- Opportunities for counseling and psychosocial management
- Continuing care in the community may reduce need for institutionalization
- Access to research studies

Benefits for service provision

- Addresses growing demand for specialist diagnosis and treatment
- Encourages earlier referral and multidisciplinary management
- Develops awareness of dementia in primary care
- Provides standardized assessment and diagnosis
- Gateway to services
- Efficient targeting and monitoring of scarce resources (including medication and psychosocial interventions)
- Expertise in legal and ethical issues
- Facilitates audit, planning, and evaluation of services
- Elective decisions may help to avoid crises in care
- Postponement of institutionalization may reduce costs
- Focus for professional education and research activity

comprehensive assessment, diagnosis, advice, and treatment to be provided by professionals with specific expertise.

In many areas, existing services for diagnosis and management of memory disorders have been inadequate, with no clear professional responsibility and a widespread lack of specialist expertise and experience. There is a growing appreciation of the complexity of the needs of these patients and that optimal assessment and management requires a multidisciplinary rather than a monodisciplinary approach (Verhey *et al.*, 1993; Bayer *et al.*, 1990).

Even in expert hands, assessment and management of mild cognitive disturbance is not always straightforward, with a difficult differential diagnosis ranging from the trivial to the very serious and from the easily reversible to the irreversible. Not all forgetful old people have dementia and not all demented old people have AD. Comprehensive assessment reduces the chances of inappropriate labeling. There is a multiplicity of available assessment tools and investigations and some informed selection need to be made, without access to the definitive diagnostic test of histopathology. Once a working diagnosis has been reached, there is also a wide spectrum of available medical, psychological, and social interventions that need to be tailored according to the requirements of the individual.

The availability of specific drug treatment for AD and some other dementias and the need to identify suitable patients and to monitor drug efficacy is the most obvious justification for early diagnosis. However, the emphasis on a medical model of care and the perceived influence of the pharmaceutical industry in driving forward the expansion of memory clinics has attracted criticism. Wider benefits of early recognition and intervention are now better appreciated (Moniz-Cook and Woods, 1997).

While reversible dementia is uncommon, nearly all patients will have problems that can be helped and appropriate intervention can be instigated at a stage when it is likely to be most effective. A positive diagnosis reduces the risk of inappropriate management and avoids wrong assumptions being made. It empowers people with dementia to become involved in decision-making while they are still able to do so. The opportunities for forward planning may improve the psychosocial health of carers and also help to lessen the risk of crises in care at a later stage. Certainly, a proactive approach is likely to be more efficient as well as more humane than one that is crisis-driven.

ARE THEY EFFECTIVE?

The rapid growth in memory clinics has occurred despite lack of specific evidence from randomized controlled trials about their effectiveness. However, there is much indirect evidence from numerous clinical trials of anticholinesterase drugs for AD supporting early diagnosis and treatment for dementia (Bullock, 2002) and evidence that psychosocial support and caregiver education can also improve outcomes (Moniz-Cook and Woods, 1997).

One randomized controlled trial by LoGiudice *et al.* (1999) has looked at the quality of life for carers of 50 community-dwelling patients with mild to moderate dementia, randomized to attend a memory clinic or act as a control group. Those carers attending the memory clinic were found to have significant improvement in psychosocial health-related quality of life, particularly in the domains of alertness behavior and social interaction, which was maintained at 12 months. However, there was no significant improvement in carer burden or knowledge of dementia.

Luce *et al.* (2001) compared consecutive referrals to the memory clinic in Newcastle upon Tyne with referrals to the traditional and well established old age psychiatry service in the same city. Memory clinic patients were younger, had lower levels of cognitive impairment and a wider range of diagnoses, with those diagnosed as having dementia being at least 2 years earlier in the course of the disease than those seen in the standard service. The authors concluded that memory clinics target a distinct patient group compared to traditional old age psychiatry services, identifying cases of dementia much earlier and having the potential to make valuable contributions to patient care in terms of access to treatments, services, and support networks, and in terms of obtaining information and preparing for the future.

Another British study in the more rural area of Dorset (Simpson *et al.*, 2004) compared consecutive new referrals to a memory clinic with consecutive new domiciliary requests within the same old age psychiatry service over the same period of time. The clinic patients had fewer behavioral and psychological symptoms of dementia, but were otherwise similar in demographic and clinical characteristics. Subsequently, they were less likely to have a psychotropic drug prescribed, but were more likely to have documented risk management, care planning and follow-up, with a trend toward fewer moves into residential care and psychiatric ward admissions.

Surveys of memory clinic users' opinions of their experiences are generally very positive. van Hout *et al.* (2001) used questionnaires with patients, relatives, and general practitioners to measure their perception of the quality of care of an outpatient memory clinic. Positive opinions were recorded on the way the results were communicated, the usefulness of the assessment and attitude of the clinicians. In contrast to GPs and relatives, patients were less positive about the clarity of the diagnostic information received, and both relatives and GPs were negative on information and advice given to relatives. A subsequent study by the same researchers highlighted the importance of providing information not only on issues considered relevant by clinicians, but also tailored to the individual needs of patients and carers (Verooij-Dassen *et al.*, 2003). An Australian study of GPs' satisfaction with services provided by memory clinics also found them to be positive about the completeness and utility of the assessment and diagnostic information provided, but relatively less satisfied with advice regarding the family's coping and community support services for the patient (Gardner *et al.*, 2004). It was considered that the service enhanced the capacity of

GPs to provide ongoing care to people with dementia, but that the establishment of firmer communication and collaborative protocols between the clinics and GPs would improve their usefulness.

THE MEMORY CLINIC TEAM

In order to provide a comprehensive service, memory clinics are characteristically multidisciplinary in nature, with a number of different professionals, each offering a particular expertise. Involvement is often based less on possession of any specific subspecialist qualification than on interest and knowledge. In some centers, the medical input may be from a geriatrician, in others from a neurologist, and in others from a psychiatrist. Ideally, there should be all three specialties involved. The other constant member of the memory clinic team tends to be a psychologist, not just to carry out neuropsychological assessment to aid diagnosis and management, but also to advise on and to undertake psychosocial interventions with both patient and family. Another invaluable team member is a specialist nurse, who can help with both the medical and psychological assessment and management. This can be carried out beyond the physical confines of the clinic, facilitating and reinforcing the process in the patient's own environment. Finally, dedicated administrative help is essential, not only to ensure the efficient running of the clinic, but also to cope with the forgetful patients who phone repeatedly to check the time of their appointments.

Beyond these core team members, there needs to be easy access to other professionals, such as speech and language therapists, occupational therapists and social workers. Increasingly, there is also a need for someone competent to provide genetic counseling and advice to worried relatives. Developments in drug therapy suggest an important potential role for the pharmacist and newer diagnostic techniques may require greater involvement of radiologists and neurophysiologists. Volunteers and support workers from the local Alzheimer's Society are becoming closely associated with some clinics, providing additional practical support and counseling to newly diagnosed patients and their families.

The optimum size of the team is likely to be between four and seven, united by a common feeling of direction and purpose. While each member should be able to identify the specific and general contribution they can make, a flexible working style which crosses conventional professional boundaries will provide greatest job satisfaction and most effective care for patients.

As in other aspects of geriatric practice, getting the multidisciplinary team to work effectively is essential for the smooth running of the clinic. Good teamwork takes time to develop and whoever is the team leader (usually the senior physician or psychiatrist) needs to strike a balance between overstructuring clinic activities and allowing individuals to function totally independently. The team will not work effectively when one particular professional (or profession) considers the guarding of their perceived area of expertise as a priority, setting up artificial borders which others fear to cross. A belief in the importance of professional hierarchies, concerns over territory and differences in terminology will act as barriers to effective care delivery and can lead to wasteful duplication of effort and apparently contradictory management advice. Individual members should be encouraged to view the value of their contribution as depending on the functioning of the whole team.

WHAT HAPPENS IN A MEMORY CLINIC?

There would seem to be general agreement that a memory clinic can provide in one setting all the essential components of comprehensive assessment leading to diagnosis for older people presenting with memory problems. The assessment will include full history and medical examination, detailed neuropsychological and neurobehavioral assessment, and appropriate laboratory tests and neuroimaging (Knopman *et al.*, 2001). Some clinics have a totally standardized approach, where everyone gets everything, while others will tailor the assessments to what is specifically indicated and what has not been done before. While some clinics will restrict themselves to a one-off evaluation, confirming a diagnosis and perhaps recommending an appropriate intervention, others will aim to provide ongoing support and more comprehensive management. Certainly, diagnosis divorced from effective intervention is likely to be unsatisfactory for all.

Clinics should be held close to the community they serve. Holding them away from the stigmatizing settings of geriatric or psychiatric hospitals will help to encourage referral and attendance. Remembering to keep appointments is an obvious problem for this client group and sending reminders a few days before and asking people to confirm that they will be coming will help to reduce nonattendance. Forewarning people about how long the assessment will take is advisable. While in some clinics assessments take all day, moving from one professional to another, many patients find this tiring and cannot cooperate fully. Some psychometric tests need to be repeated at a set interval, so initial assessment will require more than one visit. Certainly, given the gravity of the potential diagnoses, a case can be made for all patients to be tested on at least two occasions a few weeks apart. We have found that a maximum of 60–90 minutes a visit (of which 30 minutes may be taken up with cognitive testing) is optimum.

Patients should be asked to come with someone who knows them well and can provide corroborative background. The presence of a close relative or carer will also help to ensure that advice and information provided in the clinic is acted upon. Ideally, there need to be two clinic rooms, allowing opportunity for patient and informant to talk separately to different team members.

History and Medical Examination

The essential first step in clinic assessment must be to obtain a detailed and accurate history. Cognitive impairment in elderly patients is often unrecognized. A patient who superficially appears alert, pleasant and cooperative, and denies any significant symptoms is too often assumed to have no problems and mild dementia is easily overlooked. Establishing the reason for referral is a good place to start.

The onset and duration of symptoms is crucial and claims that difficulties date from some seemingly relevant event such as an accident, bereavement, or hospital admission must not be accepted unquestioningly. Often, a sudden change in circumstances merely draws attention for the first time to preexisting problems. Changes in role are often of significance and questions should be asked about loss of competence in everyday skills and activities (e.g. driving, traveling away from home, handling correspondence and finances, taking medication regularly). The nature and progress of any changes should be established.

It is essential to take a history from both the patient and from a carer or friend (a neighbor may be of more value than an uninvolved relative) and specific examples of practical difficulties should be elicited. Associated mood disturbances, personality change, and behavioral difficulties must be sought. Specific questions should be asked about delusions and hallucinations. Present and past consumption of alcohol, use of prescribed and nonprescribed drugs, and the patient's general medical condition need to be established. A family history may give pointers to the diagnosis and sometimes explains a patient's excessive concern or apprehension. Much useful information is often available in previous medical records.

The Cambridge Mental Disorder of the Elderly Examination (CAMDEX) (Roth *et al.*, 1986) attempts to standardize the clinical information gathered in the course of a diagnostic interview with history being obtained from both the patient and a relative. Some details are therefore duplicated, but it serves as a useful starting place for those less confident in eliciting all the relevant issues. Questionnaires, such as an informant questionnaire on cognitive decline in the elderly (IQCODE) (Jorm and Jacomb, 1989), can be completed by relatives before clinic attendance as an aid to establishing their report of changes in everyday cognitive function compared with 10 years before. Numerous other assessment scales, for example, of neuropsychiatric symptoms, depression, activities of daily living, quality of life, and carer burden, are available (Burns *et al.*, 1999) and can be incorporated into clinic practice. They are valuable as an objective basis for documenting change and as a source of data for audit and research.

A medical examination, with particular attention to the cardiovascular system, central nervous system and special senses (eyes and ears) is also required. This may help to elucidate the cause of the memory problems, may identify physical consequences of the condition (poor nutrition, neglected personal hygiene, signs of physical abuse), or may identify coexisting morbidities. Focal neurological signs will suggest vascular disease or a space-occupying lesion, and extrapyramidal signs will raise the possibility of Parkinson's disease or dementia with Lewy bodies (DLB). Primitive reflexes (e.g. palmo-mental, grasp, pout, rooting) are common in most forms of dementia, though not always easy to elicit. Myoclonus may be seen in prion disease, Huntington's disease, and early-onset AD, and muscle fasciculation may suggest motor neurone disease associated with frontotemporal dementia (FTD).

Cognitive Assessment

Following the history, an objective assessment of cognitive functioning is required. This will aim at establishing strengths and weaknesses of a variety of functions relative to a standardized, norm-referenced scoring system. In this way the nature and extent of cognitive deficits can be determined, informing diagnosis and management, and acting as a comparator for past and future assessments. Ideally an experienced psychologist should undertake testing, though much useful information can still be obtained by any suitably trained professional, using screening tests such as the mini-mental state examination (MMSE) and clock face drawing. This combination was shown to be an easily administered, nonthreatening, and highly sensitive screening test for dementia in a memory clinic population (Schramm *et al.*, 2002). As most of these tests are designed for detecting cortical rather than subcortical deficits, they should be supplemented by a simple measure of executive function, such as verbal fluency or proverb interpretation. When possible, assessment should be made of premorbid intellectual status, to assist in the satisfactory interpretation of other test scores. Tests must also be appropriately selected to take account of limitations imposed by deficits such as language impairment and dyspraxia. For example, recognition memory tests may reduce the demand on expressive language, normally required in recall-memory tests. A standardized measure of mood is also desirable.

There is a very wide choice of psychometric tests suitable for use with memory clinic patients and choice will be governed by the main purpose of the examination and the time available, as well as personal preference and experience. Computer-based assessment of cognitive function is becoming more available and has the advantage of being sensitive to small changes in performance and allowing detailed assessment of attention and motor responses. At present, its use is still mainly confined to research settings. An outline of the assessments used routinely in the Cardiff memory clinics is shown in Table 2.

Whatever tests are chosen, they must be acceptable to the person being tested, and with no content that belittles their adult status. Consent to the assessment procedure needs to be obtained and the tester should spend some time in explanation of the purpose of specific tests, and be competent to answer queries regarding their usefulness and acceptability. Sensory and physical limitations should be accommodated as

Table 2 Cognitive tests used routinely in the memory clinics in Cardiff

- National Adult Reading Test (NART)
- Mini-mental State Examination (MMSE)
- Middlesex Elderly Assessment of Mental State (MEAMS)
- Story Recall (immediate and delayed)
- Irving Names Learning Test (NLT)
- Kendrick Object Learning Test (KOLT)
- Kendrick Digit Copying Test (DCT)
- Frontal Assessment Battery (FAB)
- Verbal Fluency (Animals and FAS)
- Trailmaking Task
- Graded Naming Test
- Clock drawing

much as possible, by the provision of adequate lighting, additional specialist earphone amplifiers, suitable seating, and minimum distractions. During testing, realistic reassurance should be provided, with feedback phrased positively to highlight strengths as much as weaknesses. At the end of testing, patients should be given an opportunity to make their own observations on their performance.

Observations of the person's concentration, cooperation, anxiety, and motivation during assessment should be carefully weighed against performance. The approach of the patient to each test and his or her satisfaction with the outcome is often as revealing as the particular score obtained. Results should be considered in the context of the patient's previous education and experience, their age and presence of sensory impairments and comorbidity, and diagnostic cutoffs for each score treated as guides rather than absolutes. In particular, a "normal" score does not exclude the possibility of significant problems, including dementia. In such cases, more detailed testing will often reveal minor detriments in a range of tests, which are inconsistent with the patient's expected level of functioning. It is nearly always desirable, and sometimes essential, for assessment to be repeated at a future date in order to detect any progressive deterioration. Longitudinal follow-up increases the accuracy of diagnosis, particularly in mild dementia.

Laboratory Tests

A routine screening battery of laboratory tests will be indicated in most patients when first seen (van Crevel *et al.*, 1999). These should include a full blood count, urea and electrolytes, liver function tests, calcium and phosphate, random blood glucose, thyroid function, and vitamin B12 and folate. A more extensive range of tests may be indicated in younger people with dementia and in those with atypical presentations or signs and evidence of systemic illness. These might include plasma viscosity or C-reactive protein and autoantibodies for inflammatory disease and tumor markers for malignancy and paraneoplastic syndromes. Syphilis serology is now less commonly carried out as a routine, but still needs to be considered. Genetic testing, for example, for apolipoprotein genotype, is not yet diagnostically useful, but may be rarely indicated when familial dementia is suspected. It should only be undertaken after appropriate counseling, preferably in collaboration with a specialist genetics service.

An electrocardiogram is desirable in any patient with possible vascular disease and in patients with a bradycardia or history of dysrhythmia who are being considered for AChE drug treatment. An electroencephalogram may be useful in suspected encephalitis, metabolic encephalopathy, seizures, or prion disease and in confirming the presence or absence of delirium, in which it is almost always abnormal. Lumbar puncture for examination of cerebrospinal fluid is not widely used, though it is useful in patients with suspected infectious, inflammatory, autoimmune or demyelinating disease. In normal pressure hydrocephalus (NPH), it may help in predicting the suitability for surgery. Rarely, nerve conduction studies may help to diagnose FTD associated with motor neurone disease, muscle biopsy may be useful in mitochondrial disorders and even cerebral biopsy may be justified in suspected primary cerebral vasculitis.

Neuroimaging

The role of neuroimaging in the routine management of memory clinic patients is still debated. Certainly neuroimaging no longer merely fulfils the negative role of excluding "treatable" conditions that mimic or cause dementia, but can positively contribute to differential diagnosis and provide useful prognostic information. Depending on availability, computed tomography (CT), magnetic resonance imaging (MRI) and single photon emission computed tomography (SPECT) may all contribute to clinical care. Various other techniques are available in research centers.

Recent diagnostic guidelines suggest that at least one structural CT or MRI examination should be made over the course of a dementing illness to rule out space-occupying or vascular lesions, and that SPECT (or PET) should be used in cases of significant diagnostic uncertainty. In practice, it may not be possible to perform neuroimaging in every memory clinic patient with suspected dementia. Indications for scanning have therefore been proposed, including presence of focal neurological signs, recent onset of epileptic fits or recent head injury, any suspicion of intracranial tumor, including raised intracranial pressure, or evidence of a source for metastases outside the brain, any suspicion of NPH and any suspicion of stroke disease. However, the clinical utility of such clinical predictors to select memory clinic patients most likely to benefit from neuroimaging has not been demonstrated (Condefer *et al.*, 2003).

Imaging with CT is probably the radiological investigation most used in memory clinic patients, owing to its wide availability. It can show good detail of the brain structure and is especially useful in identifying dementia due to space-occupying lesions, hydrocephalus or large cerebral infarcts. Smaller lacunar infarcts are less easily seen and absence of infarcts does not exclude the possibility of vascular disease. Generalized and localized cortical atrophy is a common finding in older patients, not necessarily associated with clinically abnormal brain function. Some patients with AD will have a normal scan. Nevertheless, the presence of atrophy is useful supportive evidence of degenerative brain disease. Overall, CT may be expected to impact on diagnosis and treatment in about 1 in 8 of dementia cases.

The use of magnetic resonance imaging is less widely available, less tolerated by patients, and more expensive than CT. However, contrast sensitivity and spatial resolution is better, even without use of contrast agents and it does not suffer from bone artefacts. Evidence of generalized atrophy is no more diagnostically useful than with CT, but measurement of the size of the hippocampus and entorhinal cortex plays an important role not only in diagnosis of AD, but also in identifying patients with mild cognitive impairment who are at risk of progressing to dementia. Smaller infarcts can be seen more clearly than with CT, and MRI has the potential to detect focal signal abnormalities that may assist the clinical differentiation between AD and vascular dementia (VaD). Severe temporal lobe atrophy and hyperintensities involving the hippocampal or insular cortex are more frequently noted in AD. Basal ganglionic/thalamic hyperintense foci, thromboembolic infarctions, confluent white matter, and irregular periventricular hyperintensities (leukoencephalopathy) are more common in VaD. Leukoencephalopathy involving at least 25% of the total white matter must be present to diagnose small vessel cerebrovascular disease.

Functional imaging using SPECT allows regional cerebral blood flow to be visualized and quantified. In established AD there is a reduction of flow in mainly temporoparietal regions, though this finding is inconsistent in the early stage of the disease when diagnosis is most problematic. In FTD, SPECT shows diminished perfusion anteriorly. In VaD, multiple focal deficits may be seen.

WHAT INTERVENTIONS CAN BE OFFERED?

At the very least, patients assessed in memory clinics should receive an informed discussion of their diagnosis and prognosis, with arrangements made for ongoing review, support, and management. In a few patients, there will be a reversible cause for their symptoms (e.g. medication side effects, hypothyroidism, vitamin B12 deficiency, cerebral vasculitis, Wernicke–Korsakoff's syndrome) which will respond to specific treatment. The proportion of patients with reversible dementia is probably less than 4%, but concurrent medical conditions causing mild cognitive disturbances are much more common and are potentially treatable (Hejl *et al.*, 2002). Depression, whether primary or secondary, is especially deserving of energetic treatment, generally using a selective serotonin reuptake inhibitor (SSRI) that is free of cognitive side effects. Even in patients with established dementia, appropriate medical intervention may help cognition and slow progression of the disease. Control of vascular risk factors may favorably influence the clinical course of degenerative as well as vascular cognitive impairment. Timely use of specific drug treatments for AD and probably VaD and DLB will give significant benefit to a majority of patients taking them.

Certainly, all patients with cognitive difficulties and their carers will benefit from informed discussion about their problems. Advice can be given on the appropriate use of memory aids, memory training, and specific psychological interventions for patients and families. Financial and legal advice will usually be appropriate and practical suggestions to help with problems of daily living and safety concerns, particularly the advisability of continued driving. Issues surrounding advanced directives are attracting growing attention. Meeting the needs of carers is also important, by providing information, individual counseling, access to support groups, and respite care through contact with local Alzheimer's organizations and relevant community services.

Diagnostic Disclosure and Meeting Information Needs

Most advocates for people with dementia and their carers now believe that, in most cases, patients should be told what is wrong with them, what the implications are, what can be done for them and what treatment is likely to involve. Breaking the news in a timely and tactful manner is an important role for memory clinic staff. Reactions of AD patients to being told their diagnosis include relief (as the diagnosis provides an explanation for their difficulties), disbelief (as they may lack insight and do not feel ill), loss (grieving for failing intellectual abilities and limitations in the future) and fear of becoming a burden. All these can be satisfactorily addressed.

Practice of diagnosis disclosure amongst specialists is changing (Gilliard and Gwilliam, 1996). In the 1990s, less than one-third of old age psychiatrists and geriatricians "usually told" people with mild dementia their diagnosis, whereas recent studies report that a majority of specialists now regularly disclose diagnosis. However, a recent survey of carers of people with AD or other dementia in 11 European countries found that in 46% of cases, diagnosis had been disclosed to the family only and not to the patient, 46% of carers found information provided to them was insufficient and 29% subsequently had no regular contact with any health professional (OPDAL, 2003).

Memory clinic patients should be given the opportunity to learn as much or as little as they want to know about their condition, with information provided in a sensitive and measured way (Table 3). Patients and carers both have individual needs and each should be addressed separately. As well as clearly describing diagnosis, specific attention should be given to comprehensible and practical information about coping strategies, care services, likely course of the disease and treatment, specific drug treatment and follow-up. Wald *et al.* (2003) has proposed the "rule of threes" for information provision to carers of people with dementia. At diagnosis, they want information about what dementia is, medications available, and behavioral and psychiatric

Table 3 Recommendations for telling a diagnosis of dementia to patients and family (OPDAL, 2003)

- Communication of the diagnosis should ordinarily occur in a joint meeting with patient and family
- Use simple language. Avoid technical jargon that may conceal the truth
- Use a graded approach which is patient led and allows the information given to be matched to what the patient wants to know
- Allow sufficient time to explain and to answer questions from the patient and family
- Assess the patient's and the family's understanding and arrange follow-up (to reinforce information provided, clarify misunderstandings, and answer questions that are outstanding)
- Use the term "Alzheimer's disease" (or other appropriate medical diagnosis) rather than just dementia and ensure that they understand the sense of both terms
- Mellow the bad news with the possibility of therapeutic approaches (not just drugs). Avoid conveying the feeling that "nothing more can be done"
- Make it clear that a reorganized family network can alleviate burden and maintain quality of life
- Inform the patient about the possibility to take decisions about his/her future

symptoms of dementia. In an early follow-up appointment they want information about services, the course of the illness and what to do in a crisis. In a later follow-up appointment they want information about support groups, benefits and financial and legal issues. At a later stage, they want information about psychological therapies, the effects of the illness on carers and complementary therapies.

Information giving is not only a medical responsibility. All members of the multidisciplinary team should consider every therapeutic encounter to be an opportunity for education and information provision. Dedicated time should be put aside during every memory clinic consultation for information provision – it should never be merely an after-thought at the end of the assessment. Verbal information should be backed up by written information, with recommendations for further reading. Increasingly, people are turning to the Internet for more detailed information and trustworthy websites should be recommended to those interested. Mention should be made of local support group and meetings and contact details of local Alzheimer support organizations. A telephone contact number for information and advice is always appreciated and unlikely to be abused.

Memory Aids

The most simple and effective methods of helping patients with cognitive difficulties are the establishment of regular routines, the careful organization of daily activities, and the use of environmental cues and external memory aids. None of these require the patient to learn new strategies of thinking or remembering and may thus be potentially useful in those with even moderately severe dementia. Written aids such as diaries, checklists and carefully positioned notes as reminders are often of benefit and reusable sticky note pads are ideal for sticking in conspicuous places. Labeling or color coding of switches and doors may sometimes be helpful. A timer, or digital alarm watch, may act as a reminder to take medication, to attend to cooking or other household tasks, or to refer to an appointments diary for guidance as to planned activities. In the kitchen, use of a microwave cooker may avoid food being incinerated in a conventional oven, red warning lights on electrical appliances may help to remind when they are on, and use of kettles that whistle may ensure that a planned cup of tea is made and prevent open pans boiling dry. More sophisticated electronic devices and programmable organizers are generally too unfamiliar to the present generation of older people to prove useful, but assistive technology that does not require the person to operate it is attracting much interest.

Memory Training

The idea of cognitive training as a method of improving, retaining, or regaining skills is attractive to those worried about memory loss and to relatives who hope that developing problems might be minimized. Recent evidence suggesting that education and continued intellectual activity may reduce the risk of developing AD has further increased interest in this area.

Experience of formal training programs designed to improve the cognitive skills of healthy elderly subjects and those with cognitive deficits is limited (Clare *et al.*, 2003; De Vreese *et al.*, 2001). Those most likely to gain appear to be well-motivated, healthy individuals wishing to conserve their mental faculties as a prophylactic measure. There is little evidence of sustained benefit or generalizability in those with established dementia and regular tests and "exercises" for the memory can easily become counterproductive. Positive benefits to patients may even be at the cost of increased distress to carers.

Specific approaches have included relaxation techniques, organization of material (e.g. with the use of categorization, associative cues, and mnemonics), regular and repeated practice sessions, using spaced retrieval to rehearse information, techniques for improving visual imagery (e.g. pegword methods, face-name association etc.), and verbal strategies (rhymes, first letter cueing, alphabet searching etc.). Computer-aided cognitive training is also being developed. Reactivating therapy, including manual and creative activities, self-management skills and orientation tasks, has been claimed to improve cognitive performance and psychosocial functioning of people with mild dementia. Training in groups with other people with memory impairment or with family members and carers may provide opportunities to harness a wider range of training resources and facilitate expression of mutual support. Another approach is to involve family members in providing the cognitive training at home.

Drug Treatments

Nearly all clinics would now see themselves as central to the effective prescribing of specific antidementia drug treatments. Careful initial assessment and diagnosis is essential before any pharmacological intervention is considered and the impact of treatment and the indication for its continuing use must be kept under regular review. The size of any drug effect that can be considered worthwhile is open to debate. Statistically significant improvement on psychometric tests does not necessarily equate with meaningful change in quality of life and a noticeable improvement or stabilization is more important than change in test score. Patients and carers tend to be more positive than professionals when assessing apparently small benefits of treatment, with three quarters believing that halting progression of symptoms of early dementia for about six months justifies intervention. Such modest effect would seem comparable to that achieved by the drugs now available (Bullock, 2002).

The acetylcholinesterase inhibitor (AChEI) drugs have become the mainstay of treatment for AD, and may also have benefits in VaD and DLB. They act by inhibiting the breakdown of acetylcholine within the synapse, increasing its availability to muscarinic and nicotinic receptors. In mild to moderate AD, the available AChEI (donepezil, rivastigmine, and galantamine) have all been shown to be statistically better than treatment with placebo, with improvements in cognition, ADL and overall clinical global impression and with positive effect on aspects of behavior such as apathy, anxiety, hallucinations, and agitation. There is also evidence of efficacy in more severe AD and suggestion of potential savings in health-care costs, carer time and burden, and delay in need for permanent institutional care. All AChEIs have qualitatively similar cholinergic adverse effects, including nausea, vomiting, diarrhea, fatigue, and dizziness. These are generally mild and short-lived, resolving despite continued therapy. Caution with use of AChEIs should be observed in the presence of bradycardia and atrial or ventricular conduction disorders. Muscle cramps, insomnia, and nightmares are more common with donepezil and can sometimes be reduced by administering the drug in the morning rather than at night. About 40–60% of AD patients respond to AChEIs. So far similarities appear to be greater than the differences between the available AChEIs, but it may be reasonable to consider switching drugs if patients do not tolerate or respond to the first drug used.

Memantine is a noncompetitive NMDA (glutamate) receptor antagonist that blocks pathologically elevated glutamate. Glutaminergic overstimulation and consequent calcium overload has been implicated in neurodegeneration and memantine offers neuroprotection, while still allowing physiological receptor activation. The drug has recently become available for treatment of moderately severe to severe AD and there is also preliminary evidence of efficacy in milder AD and VaD. In clinical trials in patients with severe AD, patients taking memantine showed significantly less deterioration in functional, cognitive, and global measures and need for institutionalization, and demands on caregiver time were significantly reduced. The addition of memantine to donepezil treatment appears to show benefit over donepezil alone.

Antioxidants are thought to reduce free radical production and the excessive lipid peroxidation that can lead to neuronal damage. This is thought to be the likely mechanism supporting the use of vitamin E, selegiline, and Ginkgo biloba in people with mild cognitive impairment and dementia, though proof of efficacy is very limited.

THE MEMORY CLINIC AS PART OF LOCAL DEMENTIA SERVICES

The WHO consensus statement on the organization of care for elderly people with mental health problems (World Health Organisation, 1998) highlighted specific principles that should underpin service development. Good-quality dementia care should be comprehensive, taking into account not just the medical aspects of the problem but also the psychological and social consequences. It should be accessible and user-friendly, minimizing obstacles to effective assessment and intervention. It should be responsive, listening to and understanding the problems brought to its attention, and able to act promptly and appropriately. Finally, assessment and care should be individualized, tailored to the needs of the patient and their family.

The consensus document emphasizes that a team approach is essential, not just multidisciplinary but transdisciplinary, going beyond traditional professional boundaries, and providing responsive, coordinated and community-orientated intervention. An effective memory clinic team can be the foundation of a comprehensive dementia service, encouraging early recognition and specialist referral, providing thorough initial assessment and careful diagnosis and ensuring appropriate high quality support and care which can be flexibly integrated with other local service providers.

KEY POINTS

- Recent years have seen a rapid growth in memory clinics offering specialist assessment, diagnosis, treatment and advice for people with memory disorders and their families. They also act as a center for professional education and research.
- Most clinics focus on diagnosis and management of dementia, emphasizing benefits of early presentation, psychometric assessment, differential diagnosis, appropriate use of drug treatments, and psychosocial interventions.
- They have a multidisciplinary approach, with medical, psychology and nursing input and close working relationships with other professionals and dementia services.
- Potential benefits include improved quality of life of patients, reduced carer burden and delayed institutionalization.

KEY REFERENCES

- Hejl A, Hogh P & Waldemar G. Potentially reversible conditions in 1000 consecutive memory clinic patients. *Journal of Neurology, Neurosurgery and Psychiatry* 2002; **72**:390–4.
- Knopman DS, DeKosky ST, Cummings JL *et al.* Practice parameter: diagnosis of dementia (an Evidence-based Review). *Neurology* 2001; **56**:1143–53.
- Moniz-Cook E & Woods RT. The role of memory clinics and psychosocial intervention in the early stages of dementia. *International Journal of Geriatric Psychiatry* 1997; **12**:1143–5.
- Verhey FRJ, Jolles J, Ponds RW *et al.* Diagnosing dementia: a comparison between a monodisciplinary and a multidisciplinary approach. *Journal of Neuropsychiatry and Clinical Neuroscience* 1993; **5**:78–85.
- Wilcock GK, Bucks RS & Rockwood K. *Diagnosis and Management of Dementia: A Manual for Memory Disorders Teams* 1999; Oxford Medical Publications, Oxford.

REFERENCES

Ames D, Flicker L & Helme RD. A memory clinic at a geriatric hospital: rationale, routine and diagnosis from the first 100 patients. *Medical Journal of Australia* 1992; **156**:618–22.

Bayer AJ, Pathy MS & Twining C. The memory clinic: a new approach to the detection of early dementia. *Drugs* 1987; **22**(suppl 2):84–9.

Bayer A, Richards V & Phillips G. The Community Memory Project: a multidisciplinary approach to patients with forgetfulness and early dementia. *Care of the Elderly* 1990; **2**:236–8.

Bullock R. New drugs for Alzheimer's disease and other dementias. *British Journal of Psychiatry* 2002; **180**:135–9.

Burns A, Lawlor B & Craig S. *Assessment Scales in Old Age Psychiatry* 1999; Martin Dunitz, London.

Clare L, Woods RT, Moniz-Cook ED *et al.* Cognitive rehabilitation and cognitive training for early-stage Alzheimer's disease and vascular dementia. *Cochrane Database of Systematic Reviews* 2003; **4**:CD003260.

Condefer KA, Haworth J & Wilcock GK. Prediction rules for computed tomography in the dementia assessment: do they predict clinical utility of CT? *International Journal of Geriatric Psychiatry* 2003; **18**:285–7.

Department of Health. *National Service Framework for Older People* 2001; Department of Health, London.

Derouesne C. Which memory clinic and for whom? *Therapie* 1997; **52**:477–80.

De Vreese LP, Neri M, Fioravanti M *et al.* Memory rehabilitation in Alzheimer's disease: a review of progress. *International Journal of Geriatric Psychiatry* 2001; **16**:794–809.

Gardner IL, Foreman P & Davis S. Cognitive dementia and memory service clinics: opinions of general practitioners. *American Journal of Alzheimer's Disease and Other Dementias* 2004; **19**:105–10.

Gilliard J & Gwilliam C. Sharing the diagnosis: a survey of memory disorder clinics, their policies on informing people with dementia on their families, and the support they offer. *International Journal of Geriatric Psychiatry* 1996; **11**:1001–3.

Hassiotis A, Strydom A, Allen K & Walker Z. A memory clinic for older people with intellectual disabilities. *Aging and Mental Health* 2003; **7**:418–23.

Hejl A, Hogh P & Waldemar G. Potentially reversible conditions in 1000 consecutive memory clinic patients. *Journal of Neurology, Neurosurgery and Psychiatry* 2002; **72**:390–4.

Jorm AF & Jacomb PA. An informant questionnaire on cognitive decline in the elderly (IQCODE): sociodemographic correlates, reliability, validity and some norms. *Psychological Medicine* 1989; **19**:1015–22.

Knopman DS, Deinard S, Kitto J *et al.* A clinic for dementia. Two years experience. *Minnesota Medicine* 1985; **68**:687–92.

Knopman DS, DeKosky ST, Cummings JL *et al.* Practice parameter: diagnosis of dementia (an Evidence-based Review). *Neurology* 2001; **56**:1143–53.

Kopelman M & Crawford S. Not all memory clinics are dementia clinics. *Neuropsychological Rehabilitation* 1996; **6**:187–202.

Larrabee GJ, Pathy MSJ, Bayer AJ & Crook TH. Memory clinics: state of development and future prospects. In M Bergener & SI Finkel (eds) *Clinical and Scientific Psychogeriatrics* 1990; Springer Verlag, New York.

Lindesay J, Marudkar M, van Diepen E & Wilcock G. The second Leicester survey of memory clinics in the British Isles. *International Journal of Geriatric Psychiatry* 2002; **17**:41–7.

LoGiudice D, Hassett A, Cook R *et al.* Equity of access to a memory clinic in Melbourne? *International Journal of Geriatric Psychiatry* 2001; **16**:327–34.

LoGiudice D, Waltrowicz W, Brown K *et al.* Do memory clinics improve the quality of life of carers? A randomized pilot trial. *International Journal of Geriatric Psychiatry* 1999; **14**:626–32.

Luce A, McKeith I, Swann A *et al.* How do memory clinics compare with traditional old age psychiatry services? *International Journal of Geriatric Psychiatry* 2001; **16**:837–45.

Mahieux F. Memory clinics: value and limitations. *Press Medicale* 2000; **29**:863–9.

Moniz-Cook E & Woods RT. The role of memory clinics and psychosocial intervention in the early stages of dementia. *International Journal of Geriatric Psychiatry* 1997; **12**:1143–5.

Monsch A, Ermini-Funfschilling D, Mulligan R *et al.* Memory clinics in Switzerland: collaborative group of Swiss Memory Clinics. *Annales De Medecine Interne* 1998; **198**:221–7.

National Institute for Clinical Excellence. *NICE Guidance on the Use of Donepezil, Rivastigmine and Galantamine for the Treatment of Alzheimer's Disease* 2001; *Technology Appraisal Guidance Number 19*, NICE, London.

OPDAL Study Group. *Optimisation of the Diagnosis of Alzheimer's disease* 2003; Alzheimer Europe, Luxembourg.

Philpot MP & Levy R. A memory clinic for the early diagnosis of dementia. *International Journal of Geriatric Psychiatry* 1987; **2**:195–200.

Roth M, Tym E, Mountjoy CQ *et al.* CAMDEX: a standardised instrument for the diagnosis of mental disorder in the elderly with special reference to the early detection of dementia. *British Journal of Psychiatry* 1986; **149**:698–709.

Schramm U, Berger G, Muller R *et al.* Psychometric properties of Clock Drawing Test and MMSE or Short performance Test (SKT) in dementia screening in a memory clinic population. *International Journal of Geriatric Psychiatry* 2002; **17**:254–60.

Simpson S, Beavis D, Dyer J & Ball S. Should old age psychiatry develop memory clinics? A comparison with domiciliary work. *Psychiatric Bulletin* 2004; **28**:78–82.

van Crevel H, van Gool WA & Walstra GJM. Early diagnosis of dementia: which tests are indicated? What are their costs? *Journal of Neurology* 1999; **246**:73–8.

Van der Cammen TJ, Simpson JM, Fraser RM *et al.* The Memory Clinic. A new approach to the detection of dementia. *British Journal of Psychiatry* 1987; **150**:359–64.

van Hout H, Vernooij-Dassen M, Hoefnagels W & Grol R. Measuring the opinions of memory clinic users: patients, relatives and general practitioners. *International Journal of Geriatric Psychiatry* 2001; **16**:846–51.

Verhey FRJ, Jolles J, Ponds RW *et al.* Diagnosing dementia: a comparison between a monodisciplinary and a multidisciplinary approach. *Journal of Neuropsychiatry and Clinical Neuroscience* 1993; **5**:78–85.

Verooij-Dassen MJ, van Hout HP, Hund KL *et al.* Information for dementia patients and their caregivers: what information does a memory clinic pass on, and to whom? *Aging and Mental Health* 2003; **7**:34–8.

Wald C, Fahy M, Walker Z & Livingston G. What to tell dementia caregivers – the rule of threes. *International Journal of Geriatric Psychiatry* 2003; **18**:313–7.

Wilcock GK, Bucks RS & Rockwood K. *Diagnosis and Management of Dementia: A Manual for Memory Disorders Teams* 1999; Oxford Medical Publications, Oxford.

World Health Organisation & World Psychiatric Association. Organisation of care in psychiatry of the elderly – a technical consensus statement. *Aging and Mental Health* 1998; **2**:246–52.

Wright N & Lindesay J. A survey of memory clinics in the British Isles. *International Journal of Geriatric Psychiatry* 1995; **10**:379–85.

Zappala G, Measso G, Cavarzeran F *et al.* Aging and memory: corrections for age, sex and education for three widely used memory tests. *Italian Jounal of Neurological Science* 1995; **16**:177–84.

92

Cellular Changes in Alzheimer's Disease

Jean-Pierre Brion

Université Libre de Bruxelles, Brussels, Belgium

INTRODUCTION

A considerable interest in Alzheimer's disease has developed in the last two decades among clinicians and basic researchers. This interest parallels the growing awareness in the medical community that this devastating disease is quite common in the aged population and that most cases of severe mental deterioration in aged people can be attributed to Alzheimer's disease and do not simply result from "normal" aging of the brain.

Although the neuropathological lesions of Alzheimer's disease were described around the beginning of the twentieth century, a controversy about the nosology of the disease was generated by psychiatrists and neurologists at the same time. Initially, Alzheimer's disease was often used to designate a relatively rare cause of presenile dementia, restricted to patients less than 65 years of age, as opposed to "senile dementia" affecting older patients. The realization that Alzheimer's disease and senile dementia constitute the same pathological entity can in some ways be traced back to detailed anatomic clinical studies (see, for example, reference (Tomlinson *et al.*, 1970)). Careful neuropathological examinations of large series of the brains of patients affected with dementing conditions showed that the cerebral lesions of Alzheimer's disease were present in about 50% of these patients. These studies also stressed two important findings: first, the neuropathological lesions of Alzheimer's disease are commonly found in patients affected with senile dementia (i.e. over 65 years) and, from the neuropathological point of view, there is no reason to distinguish between the two conditions; second, dementia resulting from vascular lesions, although not infrequent, is not the preponderant cause of dementia in the aged. Vascular dementia accounted for about 15% of all dementia cases, and in another 10%, vascular lesions were admixed with the cerebral lesions of Alzheimer's disease.

This chapter deals essentially with major facts related to our present knowledge of the neurobiology of Alzheimer's disease.

NEUROPATHOLOGY AND THE DIAGNOSIS OF ALZHEIMER'S DISEASE

The clinical diagnosis of Alzheimer's disease relies on the demonstration of a dementing syndrome and the exclusion of other possible causes of dementia (*see* **Chapter 93, Clinical Aspects of Alzheimer's Disease**). Diagnostic criteria based on clinical data have been introduced, such as the NINCDS–ADRDA criteria (National Institute of Neurological and Communicative Disorders and Stroke and the Alzheimer's Disease and Related Disorders Association), and the DSM-III-R criteria (*Diagnostic and Statistical Manual of Mental Disorders*, revised third edition). These diagnostic criteria include assessments of the cognitive functions of the patient and results of laboratory examinations and neuroimaging techniques. It is noteworthy that a definitive diagnosis of the disease cannot be made without neuropathological confirmation. Numerous clinicopathological correlation studies have been performed in Alzheimer's disease; using the NINCDS–ADRDA criteria, the clinical diagnosis of Alzheimer's disease has often been confirmed by postmortem neuropathological examination in more than 80% of cases (Tierney *et al.*, 1988).

NEUROPATHOLOGICAL LESIONS IN ALZHEIMER'S DISEASE

Brain atrophy, characterized by a decrease in brain weight, ventricular dilatation, and sulci widening, is often observed at the macroscopic level. This atrophy can, however, be moderate and can overlap significantly with brain atrophy observed in normal aged people.

The neuropathological diagnosis of Alzheimer's disease is based on the demonstration of two characteristic lesions, neurofibrillary tangles (NFT) and senile plaques, in sufficient numbers and in several selected areas. Neuropathological criteria have been proposed in several studies (Khachaturian, 1985; Braak and Braak, 1991; Mirra *et al.*, 1991) and

Principles and Practice of Geriatric Medicine, 4th Edition. Edited by M.S. John Pathy, Alan J. Sinclair and John E. Morley.

interrater reliability of neuropathological diagnosis assessed in collaborative studies (Duyckaerts *et al.*, 1990). NFT and senile plaques per se are not pathognomonic of Alzheimer's disease: both lesions increase in number during "normal" aging and NFT are found in a variety of other neurological diseases; however, NFT are never abundant in the brain of cognitively normal people.

NFT are fibrillary inclusions accumulating in neurones. In pyramidal neurones, NFT often adopt a "flame-shaped" form, filling the perikarya and the base of the apical dendrites (Figure 1a,b). Some NFT remain in the neuropil after neuronal death and are called *extracellular NFT*. NFT are composed of bundles of abnormal filaments, called *paired helical filaments* (PHF, due to their ultrastructural aspects, although their fine structure might be more complex); these 25-nm-wide filaments show regular constrictions, to 10 nm wide every 80 nm (Figure 2a and 2b). PHF are found in neuronal cell bodies, in dendrites, and even in axons and synapses.

NFT have been reported to appear first in the transentorhinal cortex, a transitional cortex located around the rhinal sulcus at the ventral part of the temporal lobe; in the next stage, they are found in the entorhinal cortex, the hippocampus, and other limbic areas; in the final stage of the disease, they spread to the associative cortex of temporal, frontal, parietal, and occipital lobes (Braak and Braak, 1991). NFT are also commonly found in some subcortical nuclei (nucleus of Meynert, thalamus) and in some brainstem nuclei, for example, in the locus ceruleus and in the raphe nuclei. In the entorhinal cortex, NFT predominate in layers II and IV; neurones in these layers provide major afferents (layer II) to the hippocampus and relay major hippocampal efferents (layer IV). It has been proposed that the dysfunction of these neurones destroys the main connections of the hippocampal formation, leading to the memory disorders frequently observed in the disease. In the cerebral cortex, NFT predominate in neurones in layers III and V (these neurones are involved in corticocortical connections). Some areas are relatively spared from the formation of NFT, for example, the primary motor and sensory cortex, the cerebellum, and the spinal cord. This relatively stereotyped and hierarchical

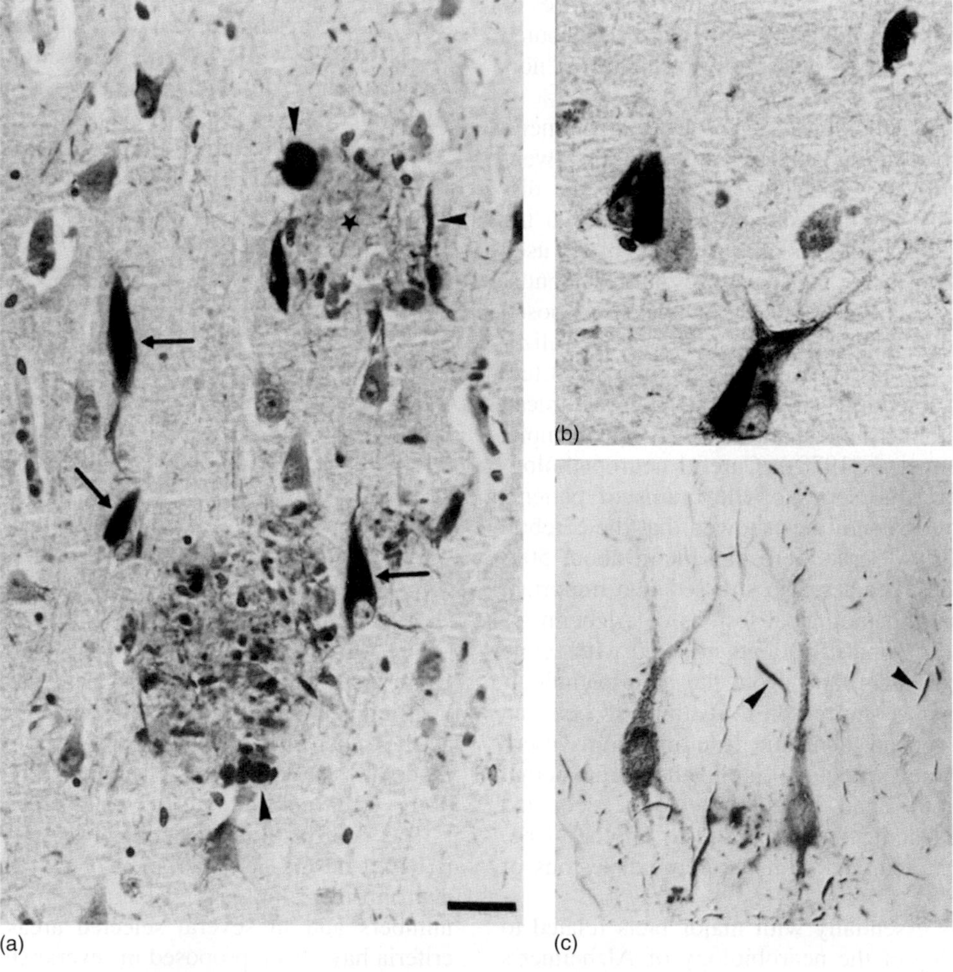

Figure 1 Tissue sections of the hippocampus in a case of Alzheimer's disease, immunolabeled with an anti-tau antibody. (a) Neurofibrillary tangles (arrows) and dystrophic neurites (arrowheads) in two senile plaques are labeled by the anti-tau antibody. The amyloid deposits (stars) in the core of the senile plaques are unlabeled. (b) Higher magnification showing two pyramidal neurones containing neurofibrillary tangles. (c) Two neurones show a diffuse and granular tau immunoreactivity, probably corresponding to an early stage of neurofibrillary tangle formation. Arrowheads point to neuropil threads, also immunolabeled by the anti-tau antibody. Sections in (a) and (b) were counterstained with haematoxylin-eosin. Scale bar: (a) 25 μm; (b), (c) 30 μm

spreading of NFT pathology has been confirmed by biochemical analysis (Delacourte *et al.*, 1999). Neuropil "threads" are small linear or curved neurites, which also contain abnormal filaments and are, as are NFT, immunolabeled by anti-tau antibodies (Figure 1c) (see the following). These neuropil threads are generally abundant in areas rich in NFT.

Neurones containing NFT seem to have a reduced level of protein synthesis and a lower metabolism, as they have been observed, among other things, to have a reduction in the size of their rough endoplasmic reticulum and a decrease in their content of RNA.

Apart from the human species, NFT are not or are rarely present in other species. The molecular basis of the selective susceptibility of neurones to develop NFT in different brain regions, and even in different architectonic areas inside these regions, is still poorly understood.

The other characteristic neuropathological lesion, the senile plaque, exists in several morphological types, which might constitute different developmental stages of this lesion. The "classical" senile plaque consists of a meshwork of dystrophic neurites (Figure 1a) surrounding an extracellular deposit of amyloid substance (Figures 3a and 4a); this amyloid substance can be stained by classical dyes for amyloid, such as thioflavine and Congo red, and is composed of 10-nm-wide amyloid fibers (Figure 4b). These dystrophic neurites in senile plaques contain accumulations of degraded membranous organelles and often-abnormal paired helical filaments. "Primitive" plaques are composed only of dystrophic neurites, and "burned-out" plaques only of a dense amyloid core. With the advent of sensitive immunocytochemical markers, "preamyloid" or "diffuse" plaques have been described: these plaques are made only of an extracellular deposit of Aβ peptide (the main component of plaque amyloid, see the following) not yet organized in the form of amyloid fibers (Figure 3a). These diffuse plaques are abundant at early stages of the disease and can also be found in normal people. It is believed that at least some diffuse plaques evolve to the stage of "classical" senile plaques during the progression of the disease. Fibrillary astrocytes and microglial cells are also found in classical senile plaques; microglial cells might be involved in the processing of the Aβ peptide (Dickson, 1997).

The distribution of senile plaques during the progression of the disease seems to vary from individual to individual. These lesions are initially found in the ventral part of the frontal and temporal lobes (including the hippocampus) and then they spread quickly to associative cortical areas; in advanced stages they can be found in high numbers in most regions of the cortex (predominantly in layers II and III), including primary areas. Senile plaques are also abundant in subcortical nuclei (thalamus, striatum) and in the brainstem, and amyloid deposits can be found in the cerebellum. In the cortex, Aß deposits precede NFT (Metsaars *et al.*, 2003). Unlike NFT, senile plaques have been evidenced in a variety of aged mammals.

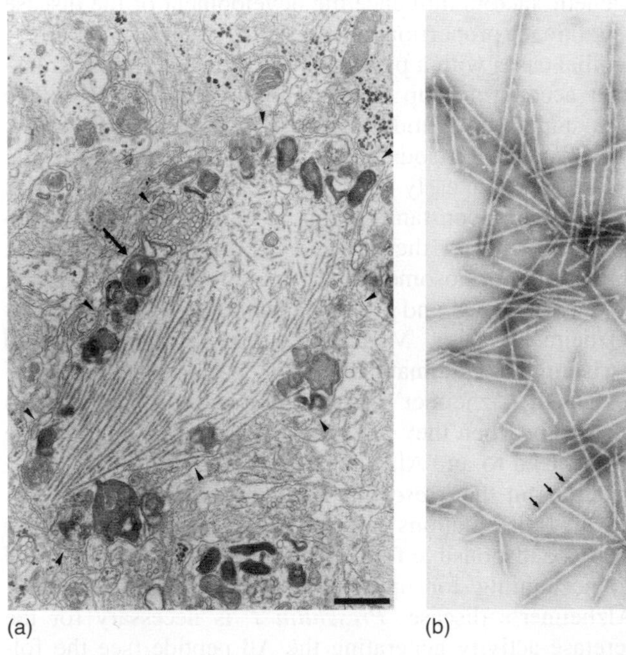

Figure 2 (a) Ultrathin section of cortical tissue (biopsy material) in a case of Alzheimer's disease, examined by transmission electron microscopy. An abnormal neurite (its limits are marked by arrowheads) contains numerous paired helical filaments (small arrow) and degraded membranous organelles (large arrow). The accumulation of these membranous organelles can result from disturbances of their axoplasmic transport. (b) Isolated paired helical filaments are shown by negative staining. These abnormal filaments exhibit regular constrictions (arrows). Scale bar: (a) 500 nm; (b) 200 nm

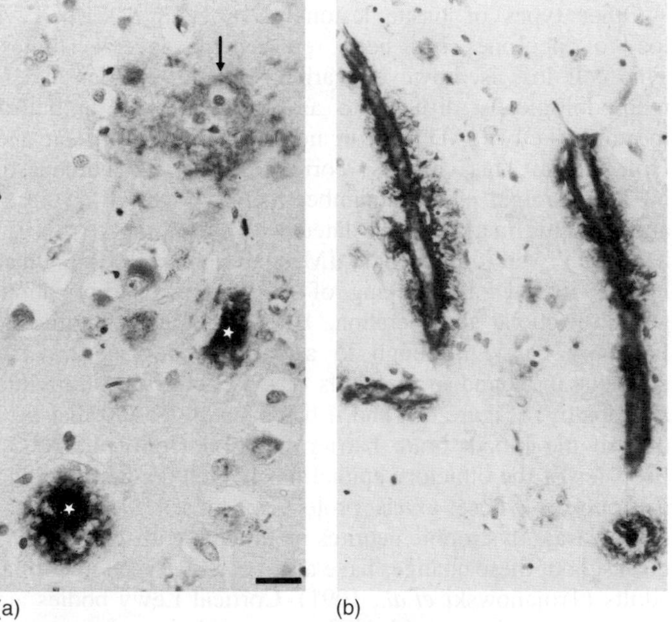

Figure 3 Tissue section of the cortex in a case of Alzheimer's disease, immunolabeled with an anti-A4/β-amyloid antibody and counterstained with haematoxylin-eosin. (a) A4/β-amyloid deposits in classical senile plaques (stars) are strongly labeled, whereas the A4/β-amyloid immunoreactivity in a diffuse plaque (arrow) is less intense. (b) These blood vessels show a strong A4/β-amyloid immunoreactivity in their walls. Some immunoreactivity is also visible in the adjacent neuropil. Scale bar: (a), (b) 30 µm

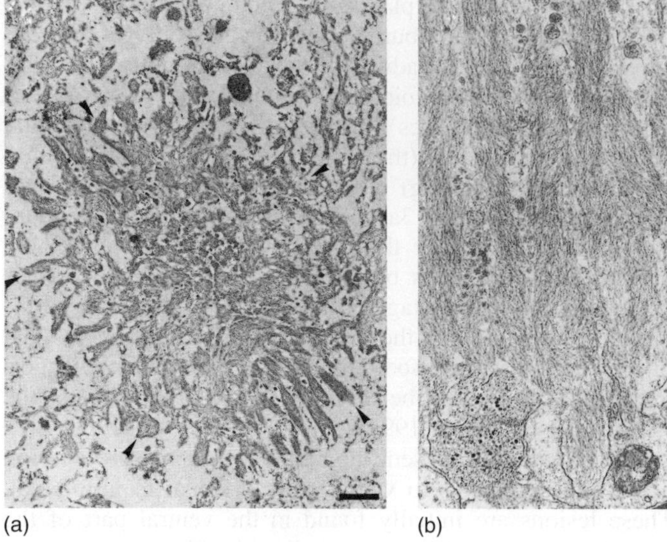

Figure 4 Ultrathin sections of cortical tissue in a case of Alzheimer's disease. (a) Low magnification of the amyloid core of a senile plaque (the general limits of the amyloid core are marked by arrowheads). (b) Higher magnification showing the bundles of amyloid fibers in the amyloid core of senile plaque. Scale bar: (a) 1 μm; (b) 80 mn

Many clinicopathological studies have established that the number of NFT in cortical areas is strongly correlated with the severity of dementia; this correlation is less strong with the number of senile plaques (Duyckaerts *et al.*, 1990; Arriagada *et al.*, 1992).

Other types of tissue lesions have been described. A loss of neurones has been reported in several studies. This cell loss is, however, variable among regions and is methodologically difficult to assess (Mann, 1991) but is more marked in AD than in normal aging (Morrison and Hof, 1997). This cell loss correlates with the number of NFT and might even outnumber them. A loss of synapses and synaptic markers (correlated with the number of NFT) has been well documented (Masliah *et al.*, 2001). Other lesions include a shrinking of the dendritic arborization, granulovacuolar degeneration, Hirano bodies, and gliosis. In many cases, although to a variable degree, amyloid deposits are found in the walls of small arterioles (amyloid angiopathy) (Figure 3b) and it has been suggested that they disturb the blood–brain barrier function (Jellinger, 2002). Biopsies of the olfactory epithelium (which contain dividing neuroblasts whose axons project to the olfactory bulbs) demonstrate dystrophic neurites in patients with Alzheimer's disease, but these changes have also been observed in normal adults (Trojanowski *et al.*, 1991). Cortical Lewy bodies are found in association with NFT in a population of demented patients, but this is probably more characteristic of a separate nosological entity (the so-called *diffuse Lewy body disease*). Many neurones also show various indices of metabolic dysfunction, even in the absence of NFT: reduction in nucleoli volume, disruption and loss of the Golgi apparatus (Stieber *et al.*, 1996), reduction in translational activity and global levels of messenger RNA, decrease in the activity of mitochondrial cytochrome oxidase (Hatanpää *et al.*, 1996) and so on.

A severe decrease in the level of acetylcholine and acetylcholinesterase in the cortex, but not of postsynaptic muscarinic receptors, has been repeatedly observed in the disease, reflecting the loss of cholinergic neurones in the nucleus of Meynert, whose axons project to cortical areas (Whitehouse *et al.*, 1982). This cholinergic deficit has generated many therapeutic attempts to correct it by the use of cholinergic agents and anticholinesterase drugs. Cortical neurones producing the neuropeptides somatostatin and corticotrophin-releasing factor are also frequently affected. Projection neurones producing noradrenalin and serotonin, and cortical neurones producing glutamate, gamma-aminobutyric acid (GABA) and various neuromodulators, have also been observed to be affected, although variable results have been published (Bowen, 1990). Dystrophic neurites in senile plaques and neurones containing NFT can be labeled by antibodies to different neuropeptides and different enzymes involved in the synthesis of neurotransmitters, suggesting that these lesions are not specific for a single type of neurotransmitter.

GENETIC ASPECTS

Although most cases of Alzheimer's disease appear to be "sporadic", it has become increasingly evident in recent years that genetic factors influence the development of the disease in a significant proportion of cases (Rocchi *et al.*, 2003).

Familial cases with a pattern of autosomal dominant transmission account for up to 10–15% of all cases. Genetic linkage studies have indicated that Alzheimer's disease is genetically heterogeneous; familial cases of Alzheimer's disease can have an early or a late onset, the age of onset being relatively constant within a family. Several mutations in the gene for the amyloid peptide precursor (APP), localized on chromosome 21 (16 mutations found to date), have been described and are responsible for 2–3% of familial Alzheimer's cases. Most interestingly, patients affected with trisomy 21 systematically develop the neuropathological lesions of Alzheimer's disease (NFT and senile plaques) and dementia when they age, suggesting that a gene dosage effect can lead to an "Alzheimer-like" phenotype.

Mutations in the *presenilin 1* gene localized on chromosome 14 (140 mutations found to date) have been demonstrated to be responsible for most cases of early onset familial cases, accounting for up to 80% of the cases of familial Alzheimer's disease. *Presenilin 1* is necessary for the γ-secretase activity generating the Aß peptide (see the following text). Mutations in the closely related *presenilin 2* gene present on chromosome 1 (10 mutations found to date) have been identified as being responsible for many of the remaining familial Alzheimer's cases. The presenilins are serpentine transmembrane proteins (Thinakaran, 1999) that have been localized in the endoplasmic reticulum and in the Golgi apparatus.

Apart from these genetic mutations, it has been discovered that the apolipoprotein E genotype affects the risk of developing Alzheimer's disease and its mean age of onset, acting as a susceptibility gene (Roses, 1996). Three main alleles of the apolipoprotein E gene exist (APOE2, E3, E4) and the gene is present on chromosome 19. Each inherited APOE4 allele increases the risk and lowers the mean age of onset, whereas the inheritance of an APOE2 decreases the risk and increases the mean age of onset of the disease. Homozygotes for APOE4 have a risk of developing the disease, which is eight times greater, and a mean age of onset of the disease (<70 years), which is 20 years shorter, than APOE2/3 individuals (>90 years). The mechanisms by which different apolipoprotein E isoforms can modulate the susceptibility to the disease are not yet clearly understood (Lahiri *et al.*, 2004), although it has been suggested that a differential binding of apolipoprotein E isoforms to Aβ and/or tau proteins might be one such mechanism (Roses, 1996).

Aß PEPTIDE AND THE AMYLOID PEPTIDE PRECURSOR

Many investigators have chosen to study senile plaques and NFT as a route to elucidating the pathogenesis of the disease, and important progress has been made in the molecular analysis of these lesions.

The amyloid deposits in senile plaques and in the cerebrovascular angiopathy have been found to be composed of a peptide of 39–43 amino acids (now called *Aβ peptide*) (Glenner and Wong, 1984; Masters *et al.*, 1985). This peptide is derived from a precursor, APP, expressed in neurones and in a variety of nonneuronal cells (including outside the central nervous system) (Octave, 1995; Ling *et al.*, 2003). APP is a transmembrane protein, which might play a role in contacts with the extracellular matrix and has been found to be concentrated at the level of synaptic contacts and in lipid rafts of the plasma membrane. Several isoforms of APP have been identified, which show differential tissue expression.

In one metabolic pathway, APP is cleaved by an enzyme ("α-secretase") and its N-terminal portion is secreted outside the cell. This cleavage occurs inside the sequence of the Aβ peptide and thus cannot generate the latter (hence this pathway is also called *non-amyloidogenic*). In another metabolic pathway the Aβ peptide is generated from APP by cleavage with two other enzymes: the ß-secretase generating its N-terminus and γ-secretase generating its C-terminus (Haass, 2004; Wilquet and De Strooper, 2004). The γ-secretase activity results from the assembly of a multiprotein complex containing *presenilin 1* (Takasugi *et al.*, 2003). This pathway is called *amyloidogenic*, and thus, all factors favoring it could potentially precipitate the disease. For instance, cells expressing APP with mutations at sites described in familial Alzheimer's disease produce more Aβ peptide or more of the longer Aβ peptide (which form amyloid fibers more readily). Transgenic mice overexpressing a mutated APP protein develop amyloid deposits (but not NFT) and coexpression of mutated APP and PS1 proteins greatly accelerates the formation of these Aß deposits (for a review, see (Gotz *et al.*, 2004)). Before forming extracellular deposits, the Aß peptide seems to accumulate intracellularly in neurones, an event that might be critical in the pathophysiology of the disease, for example, some transgenic mice overexpressing mutated APP develop neuronal deficits before developing extracellular amyloid deposits (Casas *et al.*, 2004). In Alzheimer's disease, however, there is no major overexpression of APP (contrary to what is observed in Down's syndrome).

In addition to the Aβ peptide, other components have been identified in the amyloid deposits: these include α_1-antichymotrypsin, apolipoprotein E, components of the complement pathway, various molecules of the extracellular matrix (proteoglycans, heparin sulfate), and so on. Molecules such as aluminum and zinc have also been identified in some studies. The physiopathological role of these additional components is still difficult to delineate, although some of them (e.g. α_1-antichymotrypsin, apolipoprotein E) have been observed to promote amyloid-like fibril formation *in vitro* and could thus act *in vivo* as "pathological chaperones", favoring amyloid fibrillogenesis. Transgenic mice overexpressing a mutated APP protein do not develop amyloid deposits if their APOE gene is invalidated. Quite interestingly, Aß vaccination has been successful in removing Aß deposits in transgenic mice (Morgan *et al.*, 2000). Initial attempts on AD patients have, however, resulted in mitigated results, due to serious side effects in a proportion of patients (Broytman and Malter, 2004).

NEUROFIBRILLARY TANGLES AND TAU PROTEINS

Neurofibrillary tangles have been found by immunochemical and biochemical methods to be composed of a microtubule-associated protein called *tau* (Brion *et al.*, 1985; Buée *et al.*, 2000; Lee *et al.*, 2001). This protein is expressed in neurones, where it probably plays a role in the maintenance of the stability of microtubules, particularly in the axons, by its ability to bind to tubulin. Microtubules are one of the three main fiber systems that form the cellular cytoskeleton. Microtubules are essential for the maintenance of the shape of the neurone and its extensions, and play a fundamental role in targeted intracellular transport of various molecules and organelles. One particular aspect of transport in neurones is the axoplasmic transport along axons, which provides energy-generating machinery and neurotransmitters at the synaptic level. Inactivation of the tau gene leads to developmental malformations in the central nervous system characterized by defects in the formation of long axonal tracts (Takei *et al.*, 2000). In the human central nervous system, six isoforms of tau proteins are generated by alternative splicing from a single gene localized on chromosome 17. Pathogenic mutations in the tau gene have been identified in familial forms of frontotemporal dementia (Rademakers *et al.*, 2004) and are often associated with the formation of tau-positive neurofibrillary lesions. Such mutations have, however, not been identified in Alzheimer's disease. Nevertheless, transgenic animals expressing mutant forms of tau develop NFT and constitute a powerful *in vivo* experimental model (for a review, see (Gotz *et al.*, 2004)). The existence of a tau pathology in several neurodegenerative diseases, including Alzheimer's disease, frontotemporal dementia, progressive supranuclear palsy, corticobasal degeneration, and so on, has led to their grouping under the term of *tauopathies* (Buée *et al.*, 2000; Lee *et al.*, 2001).

Tau proteins in PHF present several types of posttranslational modifications, resulting in several populations of modified tau proteins. Well-documented modifications are a high state of phosphorylation (Brion *et al.*, 1991; Delacourte, 1994), partial proteolysis (Wischik *et al.*, 1988), ubiquitination (Morishima-Kawashima *et al.*, 1993), and glycation (Yan *et al.*, 1995). These modified tau proteins have been called *PHF-tau* proteins (for a review, see (Buée *et al.*, 2000)). The accumulation of NFT in brain tissue is correlated with a decrease in the levels of normal, soluble tau and an increase in the PHF-tau proteins (Mukaetova-Ladinska *et al.*, 1993). A diffuse or granular accumulation of tau in neurones can represent an early stage, preceding the formation of bundles of PHF (Figure 1c) (Bancher *et al.*, 1989; Braak *et al.*, 1994).

The ability of tau proteins to interact with microtubules is decreased when the protein is phosphorylated at selected sites. Although tau is already significantly phosphorylated in the fetal (Brion *et al.*, 1993) and the adult (Matsuo *et al.*, 1994) normal brain, much of the tau protein present in neurofibrillary tangles is highly phosphorylated, and the presence of highly phosphorylated tau species in the brain of patients has led to the suggestion that these phosphorylated proteins would be unable to maintain a stable network of microtubules in affected neurones, leading to disturbances of cellular functions such as axoplasmic transport (Dustin and Flament-Durand, 1982; Brion, 1992; Roy *et al.*, 2005). Actually, decrease in the number of microtubules (Flament-Durand and Couck, 1979) in tubulin expression (Hempen and Brion, 1996) and in the ability of tubulin to polymerize in microtubules (Iqbal and Grundke-Iqbal, 1995) have been observed in the disease. Several protein kinases, for example, the glycogen synthase kinase-3ß (Leroy *et al.*, 2002), the cyclin dependant kinase 5 (Cruz and Tsai, 2004) and protein phosphatases have been identified as *potential candidate enzymes* involved in the regulation of tau phosphorylation (Anderton *et al.*, 2001; Planel *et al.*, 2002; Geschwind, 2003) and it has been suggested that a relative imbalance in their activities might play a role in the generation of the highly phosphorylated tau proteins found in the disease. Such an imbalance might also result from aberrant activation or inhibition of signal transduction pathways in Alzheimer's disease. Aberrant cell cycle activation in neurones is one of the evoked mechanisms (Arendt, 2003). An increased concentration of hyperphosphorylated tau proteins detached from microtubules would favor their aggregation in PHF and additional neuronal dysfunction. Experimental modulation of tau phosphorylation in culture systems and in transgenic animals is currently an active area of research, with the hope of interfering with the mechanisms of formation of abnormally phosphorylated PHF-tau species.

NFT have been reported to be immunoreactive *in situ* with antibodies to other molecules (ubiquitin, microtubule-associated protein 5 (MAP5), neurofilaments, APP, etc.), suggesting an *in situ* interaction between these molecules and the PHF components. Most consistent is the identification of the stress polypeptide ubiquitin (also identified by protein sequencing). Ubiquitin (also present in neuronal inclusions found in other neurodegenerative diseases, such as the Lewy bodies) is covalently conjugated to molecules destined to be proteolyzed by the proteasomal system.

RELATIONSHIP BETWEEN NEUROFIBRILLARY TANGLES AND SENILE PLAQUES AND PHYSIOPATHOLOGICAL CONCEPTS OF THE DISEASE

One leading physiopathological hypothesis (the "amyloid hypothesis") of Alzheimer's disease is that an abnormal processing of APP leads to an excessive generation of the Aβ peptide that is directly responsible for the development of the disease (Hardy, 2003; Selkoe and Schenk, 2003). According to this hypothesis, Aβ deposits would become toxic for surrounding neurones and their processes when they form amyloid fibers, and would induce the formation of abnormal tau proteins and NFT. The main support for this hypothesis comes from the observation that people affected by APP mutations develop full-blown Alzheimer's disease, including the classical neuropathological lesions (senile plaques and NFT tangles). Down's syndrome patients also offer strong support for this hypothesis, as the earliest lesions found in these patients are diffuse Aβ deposits, with NFT and senile plaques appearing later (*see* **Chapter 101, The Older Patient with Down's Syndrome**). In addition, the Aβ peptide has been observed to be neurotoxic in culture when it is aggregated in the form of amyloid fibers (Busciglio *et al.*, 1995). It has been postulated that the toxicity of the Aβ peptide is mediated by a variety of mechanisms: the Aβ peptide has been reported to induce oxidative damage, mediated by the generation of free radicals, to trigger apoptosis in neurones, to sensitize neurones to excitotoxic amino acids, to increase intracellular calcium, and so on (Atwood *et al.*, 2003).

On the other hand, in most studies it has been difficult to correlate dementia with the loading of Aβ peptide in the brain of patients, whereas many reports have pointed to the correlation between the number of NFT and synaptic loss and the degree of dementia. Some investigators have thus favored the hypothesis that early changes in the neuronal cytoskeleton and/or synaptic degeneration are key events in the development of neuronal dysfunction in the disease (Terry, 2000).

The relationship between the formation of senile plaques, and NFT remains a central issue for the understanding of the physiopathology of the disease. A link between abnormal processing of APP and the formation of NFT is quite probable (e.g. people affected by APP mutations also develop NFT). APP, Aβ and tau might directly interact (Giaccone *et al.*, 1996). APP is transported along axons by fast axoplasmic transport and any interference with this transport, as suggested in neurones developing NFT, might be expected to affect its metabolism (Hirokawa and Takemura, 2004). An abnormal metabolism of APP might also be secondary to alterations in its intracellular trafficking. It also seems possible that the formation of NFT and of amyloid deposits occur independently, as there is no complete chronological and topographical overlap in their evolution. For instance, NFT develop in transgenic animals expressing mutants' tau proteins, in the absence of amyloid deposits, but they do not develop in transgenic animals expressing mutants' APP proteins and developing Aß deposits, in the presence of a wild-type human tau (Boutajangout *et al.*, 2004). However, coexpression of mutants' tau and APP proteins enhances the formation of NFT (Lewis *et al.*, 2001). A current hypothesis is thus that Aß peptide could accelerate the formation of NFT that appear at low levels during normal aging.

Other physiopathological concepts of the disease are also currently being investigated. A lack of trophic factors would lead to the degeneration of selected neuronal populations, for example, a lack of nerve growth factor has been suggested to play a role in the degeneration of cholinergic neurones in the nucleus basalis (severely affected in Alzheimer's disease) (Lang *et al.*, 2004). Evidence of oxidative damage has been found in brain tissue of AD patients and could also play a pathogenic role (Perry *et al.*, 2002). An inflammatory reaction (suggested by the presence of microglial cells and inflammatory molecules in senile plaques) might also lead to neuronal insult (Eikelenboom and Van Gool, 2004). The roles played by apoptosis and excitotoxicity are two research avenues (among others) being actively investigated. Although aging is a major "risk factor" for the disease, it seems improbable that Alzheimer's disease is simply an exacerbation of normal aging mechanisms (Morrison and Hof, 1997).

Although these various hypotheses are not necessarily exclusive, it is, however, still difficult to discriminate between mechanisms that play an important role in the development of neuronal dysfunction and secondary processes that are rather a consequence of primary mechanisms but might nevertheless contribute to the evolution of tissue lesions.

Acknowledgment

This work was supported by grants from the Belgian F.R.S.M, Alzheimer Belgique, and the International Alzheimer Research Foundation.

KEY POINTS

- The definitive diagnosis of the disease relies on the neuropathological examination, showing the presence of neurofibrillary tangles and senile plaques.
- Neurofibrillary tangles are composed of hyperphosphorylated forms of the microtubule-associated protein tau and the Aß amyloid peptide is the main molecular component of senile plaques.
- According to the amyloid cascade hypothesis, the Aß peptide is neurotoxic and could accelerate the formation of neurofibrillary tangles. The latter lesions are, however, more strongly correlated to the severity of dementia.
- Neuronal and synaptic loss in selected brain areas occurs in the disease. This loss is more important in AD than during normal aging.
- A few cases of Alzheimer's disease have a familial transmission and are mostly due to pathogenic mutations in the presenilins and the amyloid peptide precursor genes.

KEY REFERENCES

- Braak H & Braak E. Neuropathological stageing of Alzheimer-related changes. *Acta Neuropathologica* 1991; **82**:239–59.
- Buée L, Bussière T, Buée-Scherrer V *et al.* Tau protein isoforms, phosphorylation and role in neurodegenerative disorders. *Brain Research Reviews* 2000; **33**:95–130.
- Hardy J. Alzheimer's disease: genetic evidence points to a single pathogenesis. *Annals of Neurology* 2003; **54**:143–4.
- Lee VMY, Goedert M & Trojanowski JQ. Neurodegenerative tauopathies. *Annual Review of Neuroscience* 2001; **24**:1121–59.
- Wilquet V & De Strooper B. Amyloid-beta precursor protein processing in neurodegeneration. *Current Opinion in Neurobiology* 2004; **14**:582–8.

REFERENCES

Anderton BH, Betts J, Blackstock W *et al.* Sites of phosphorylation in tau and factors affecting their regulation. *Neuronal Signal Transduction and Alzheimer's Disease* 2001, pp 73–80; Portland Press.

Arendt T. Synaptic plasticity and cell cycle activation in neurons are alternative effector pathways: the "Dr. Jekyll and Mr. Hyde concept" of Alzheimer's disease or the yin and yang of neuroplasticity. *Progress in Neurobiology* 2003; **71**:83–248.

Arriagada PV, Growdon JH, Hedley-Whyte ET & Hyman BT. Neurofibrillary tangles but not senile plaques parallel duration and severity of Alzheimer's disease. *Neurology* 1992; **42**:631–9.

Atwood CS, Obrenovich ME, Liu TB *et al.* Amyloid-beta: a chameleon walking in two worlds: a review of the trophic and toxic properties of amyloid-beta. *Brain Research Reviews* 2003; **43**:1–16.

Bancher C, Brunner C, Lassmann H *et al.* Accumulation of abnormally phosphorylated tau precedes the formation of neurofibrillary tangles in Alzheimer's disease. *Brain Research* 1989; **477**:90–9.

Boutajangout A, Authelet M, Blanchard V *et al.* Cytoskeletal abnormalities in mice transgenic for human tau and familial Alzheimer's disease mutants of APP and presenilin-1. *Neurobiology of Disease* 2004; **15**:47–60.

Bowen DM. Treatment of Alzheimer's disease. Molecular pathology versus neurotransmitter-based therapy. *British Journal of Psychiatry* 1990; **157**:327–30.

Braak H & Braak E. Neuropathological stageing of Alzheimer-related changes. *Acta Neuropathologica* 1991; **82**:239–59.

Braak E, Braak H & Mandelkow E-M. A sequence of cytoskeleton changes related to the formation of neurofibrillary tangles and neuropil threads. *Acta Neuropathologica* 1994; **87**:554–67.

Brion JP. The pathology of the neuronal cytoskeleton in Alzheimer's disease. *Biochimica Et Biophysica Acta* 1992; **1160**:134–42.

Brion JP, Hanger DP, Couck AM & Anderton BH. A68 proteins in Alzheimer's disease are composed of several tau isoforms in a phosphorylated state which affects their electrophoretic mobilities. *Biochemical Journal* 1991; **279**:831–6.

Brion JP, Passareiro H, Nunez J & Flament-Durand J. Mise en évidence immunologique de la protéine tau au niveau des lésions de dégénérescence neurofibrillaire de la maladie d'Alzheimer. *Archives of Biology* 1985; **95**:229–35.

Brion JP, Smith C, Couck AM *et al.* Developmental changes in tau phosphorylation: fetal-type tau is transiently phosphorylated in a manner similar to paired helical filament-tau characteristic of Alzheimer's disease. *Journal of Neurochemistry* 1993; **61**:2071–80.

Broytman O & Malter JS. Anti-abeta: the good, the bad, and the unforeseen. *Journal of Neuroscience Research* 2004; **75**:301–6.

Buée L, Bussière T, Buée-Scherrer V *et al.* Tau protein isoforms, phosphorylation and role in neurodegenerative disorders. *Brain Research Reviews* 2000; **33**:95–130.

Busciglio J, Lorenzo A, Yeh J & Yankner BA. β-amyloid fibrils induce tau phosphorylation and loss of microtubule binding. *Neuron* 1995; **14**:879–88.

Casas C, Sergeant N, Itier JM *et al.* Massive CA1/2 neuronal loss with intraneuronal and N-interminal truncated a beta(42) accumulation in a novel Alzheimer transgenic model. *American Journal of Pathology* 2004; **165**:1289–300.

Cruz JC & Tsai LH. Cdk5 deregulation in the pathogenesis of Alzheimer's disease. *Trends in Molecular Medicine* 2004; **10**:452–8.

Delacourte A. Pathological Tau proteins of Alzheimer's disease as a biochemical marker of neurofibrillary degeneration. *Biomedicine & Pharmacotherapy* 1994; **48**:287–95.

Delacourte A, David JP, Sergeant N *et al.* The biochemical pathway of neurofibrillary degeneration in aging and Alzheimer's disease. *Neurology* 1999; **52**:1158–65.

Dickson DW. The pathogenesis of senile plaques. *Journal of Neuropathology and Experimental Neurology* 1997; **56**:321–39.

Dustin P & Flament-Durand J. Disturbances of axoplasmic transport in Alzheimer's disease. In DG Weiss & A Gorio (eds) *Axoplasmic Transport in Physiology and Pathology* 1982, pp 131–6; Springer, Berlin.

Duyckaerts C, Delaère P, Hauw JJ *et al.* Rating of lesions in senile dementia of the Alzheimer type: concordance between laboratories. An European multicenter study under the auspices of Eurage. *Journal of Neurological Sciences* 1990; **97**:295–323.

Eikelenboom P & Van Gool WA. Neuroinflammatory perspectives on the two faces of Alzheimer's disease. *Journal of Neural Transmission* 2004; **111**:281–94.

Flament-Durand J & Couck AM. Spongiform alterations in brain biopsies of presenile dementia. *Acta Neuropathologica* 1979; **46**:159–62.

Geschwind DH. Tau phosphorylation, tangles, and neurodegeneration: the chicken or the egg? *Neuron* 2003; **40**:457–60.

Giaccone G, Pedrotti B, Migheli A *et al.* βPP and tau interaction – A possible link between amyloid and neurofibrillary tangles in Alzheimer's disease. *American Journal of Pathology* 1996; **148**:79–87.

Glenner GG & Wong CW. Alzheimer's disease: initial report of the purification and characterization of a novel cerebrovascular amyloid protein. *Biochemical and Biophysical Research Communications* 1984; **120**:885–90.

Gotz J, Streffer JR, David D *et al.* Transgenic animal models of Alzheimer's disease and related disorders: histopathology, behavior and therapy. *Molecular Psychiatry* 2004; **9**:664–83.

Haass C. Take five – BACE and the gamma-secretase quartet conduct Alzheimer's amyloid beta-peptide generation. *The EMBO Journal* 2004; **23**:483–8.

Hardy J. Alzheimer's disease: genetic evidence points to a single pathogenesis. *Annals of Neurology* 2003; **54**:143–4.

Hatanpää K, Brady DR, Stoll J *et al.* Neuronal activity and early neurofibrillary tangles in Alzheimer's disease. *Annals of Neurology* 1996; **40**:411–20.

Hempen BJ & Brion JP. Reduction of acetylated α-tubulin immunoreactivity in neurofibrillary tangle-bearing neurones in Alzheimer's disease. *Journal of Neuropathology and Experimental Neurology* 1996; **55**:964–72.

Hirokawa N & Takemura R. Molecular motors in neuronal development, intracellular transport and diseases. *Current Opinion in Neurobiology* 2004; **14**:564–73.

Iqbal K & Grundke-Iqbal I. Alzheimer abnormally phosphorylated tau is more hyperphosphorylated than the fetal tau and causes the disruption of microtubules. *Neurobiology of Aging* 1995; **16**:375–9.

Jellinger KA. Alzheimer disease and cerebrovascular pathology: an update. *Journal of Neural Transmission* 2002; **109**:813–36.

Khachaturian ZS. Diagnosis of Alzheimer's disease. *Archives of Neurology* 1985; **42**:1097–105.

Lahiri DK, Sambamurti K & Bennett DA. Apolipoprotein gene and its interaction with the environmentally driven risk factors: molecular, genetic and epidemiological studies of Alzheimer's disease. *Neurobiology of Aging* 2004; **25**:651–60.

Lang UE, Jockers-Scherübl MC & Hellweg R. State of the art of the neurotrophin hypothesis in psychiatric disorders: implications and limitations. *Journal of Neural Transmission* 2004; **111**:387–411.

Lee VMY, Goedert M & Trojanowski JQ. Neurodegenerative tauopathies. *Annual Review of Neuroscience* 2001; **24**:1121–59.

Leroy K, Boutajangout A, Authelet M *et al.* The active form of glycogen synthase kinase-3ß is associated with granulovacuolar degeneration in neurons in Alzheimer's disease. *Acta Neuropathologica* 2002; **103**:91–9.

Lewis J, Dickson DW, Lin WL *et al.* Enhanced neurofibrillary degeneration in transgenic mice expressing mutant tau and APP. *Science* 2001; **293**:1487–91.

Ling Y, Morgan K & Kalsheker N. Amyloid precursor protein (APP) and the biology of proteolytic processing: relevance to Alzheimer's disease. *The International Journal of Biochemistry & Cell Biology* 2003; **35**:1505–35.

Mann DMA. Is the pattern of nerve cell loss in ageing and Alzheimer's disease a real, or only an apparent, selectivity? *Neurobiology of Aging* 1991; **12**:340–3.

Masliah E, Mallory M, Alford M *et al.* Altered expression of synaptic proteins occurs early during progression of Alzheimer's disease. *Neurology* 2001; **56**:127–9.

Masters CL, Simms G, Weinman NA *et al.* Amyloid plaque core protein in Alzheimer's disease and down syndrome. *Proceedings of the National Academy of Sciences of the United States of America* 1985; **82**:4245–9.

Matsuo ES, Shin R-W, Billingsley ML *et al.* Biopsy-derived adult human brain tau is phosphorylated at many of the same sites as Alzheimer's disease paired helical filament tau. *Neuron* 1994; **13**:989–1002.

Metsaars WP, Hauw JJ, Van Welsem ME & Duyckaerts C. A grading system of Alzheimer disease lesions in neocortical areas. *Neurobiology of Aging* 2003; **24**:563–72.

Mirra SS, Heyman A, McKeel D *et al.* The consortium to establish a registry for Alzheimer's disease (CERAD). Part II. Standardization of the neuropathologic assessment of Alzheimer's disease. *Neurology* 1991; **41**:479–86.

Morgan D, Diamond DM, Gottschall PE *et al.* Aβ peptide vaccination prevents memory loss in an animal model of Alzheimer's disease. *Nature* 2000; **408**:982–5.

Morishima-Kawashima M, Hasegawa M, Takio K *et al.* Ubiquitin is conjugated with amino-terminally processed tau in paired helical filaments. *Neuron* 1993; **10**:1151–60.

Morrison JH & Hof PR. Life and death of neurons in the aging brain. *Science* 1997; **278**:412–9.

Mukaetova-Ladinska EB, Harrington CR, Roth M & Wischik CM. Biochemical and anatomical redistribution of tau protein in Alzheimer's disease. *American Journal of Pathology* 1993; **143**:565–78.

Octave JN. The amyloid peptide and its precursor in Alzheimer's disease. *Reviews in the Neurosciences* 1995; **6**:287–316.

Perry G, Nunomura A, Hirai K *et al.* Is oxidative damage the fundamental pathogenic mechanism of Alzheimer's and other neurodegenerative diseases? *Free Radical Biology & Medicine* 2002; **33**:1475–9.

Planel E, Sun XY & Takashima A. Role of GSK−3β in Alzheimer's disease pathology. *Drug Development Research* 2002; **56**:491–510.

Rademakers R, Cruts M & van Broeckhoven C. The role of tau (MAPT) in frontotemporal dementia and related tauopathies. *Human Mutation* 2004; **24**:277–95.

Rocchi A, Pellegrini S, Siciliano G & Murri L. Causative and susceptibility genes for Alzheimer's disease: a review. *Brain Research Bulletin* 2003; **61**:1–24.

Roses AD. Apolipoprotein E alleles as risk factors in Alzheimer's disease. *Annual Review of Medicine* 1996; **47**:387–400.

Roy S, Zhang B, Lee VMY & Trojanowski JQ. Axonal transport defects: a common theme in neurodegenerative diseases. *Acta Neuropathologica* 2005; **109**:5–13.

Selkoe DJ & Schenk D. Alzheimer's disease: molecular understanding predicts amyloid-based therapeutics. *Annual Review of Pharmacology and Toxicology* 2003; **43**:545–84.

Stieber A, Mourelatos Z & Gonatas NK. In Alzheimer's disease the golgi apparatus of a population of neurons without neurofibrillary tangles is fragmented and atrophic. *American Journal of Pathology* 1996; **148**:415–26.

Takasugi N, Tomita T, Hayashi I *et al.* The role of presenilin cofactors in the gamma-secretase complex. *Nature* 2003; **422**:438–41.

Takei Y, Teng JL, Harada A & Hirokawa N. Defects in axonal elongation and neuronal migration in mice with disrupted *tau* and *map1b* genes. *Journal of Cell Biology* 2000; **150**:989–1000.

Terry RD. Cell death or synaptic loss in Alzheimer disease. *Journal of Neuropathology and Experimental Neurology* 2000; **59**:1118–9.

Thinakaran G. The role of presenilins in Alzheimer's disease. *Journal of Clinical Investigation* 1999; **104**:1321–7.

Tierney MC, Fisher RH, Lewis AJ *et al.* The NINCDS-ADRDA work group criteria for the clinical diagnosis of probable Alzheimer's disease. *Neurology* 1988; **38**:359–64.

Tomlinson BE, Blessed G & Roth M. Observations on the brains of demented old people. *Journal of Neurological Sciences* 1970; **11**:205–42.

Trojanowski JQ, Newman PD, Hill WD & Lee VM-Y. Human olfactory epithelium in normal aging, Alzheimer's disease, and other neurodegenerative disorders. *Journal of Comparative Neurology* 1991; **310**:365–76.

Whitehouse PJ, Price DL, Struble RG *et al.* Alzheimer's disease and senile dementia. Loss of neurones in the basal forebrain. *Science* 1982; **215**:1237–9.

Wilquet V & De Strooper B. Amyloid-beta precursor protein processing in neurodegeneration. *Current Opinion in Neurobiology* 2004; **14**:582–8.

Wischik CM, Novak M, Thogersen HC *et al.* Isolation of a fragment of tau derived from the core of the paired helical filament of Alzheimer disease. *Proceedings of the National Academy of Sciences of the United States of America* 1988; **85**:4506–10.

Yan SD, Yan SF, Chen X *et al.* Non-enzymatically glycated tau in Alzheimer's disease induces neuronal oxidant stress resulting in cytokine gene expression and release of amyloid β-peptide. *Nature Medicine* 1995; **1**:693–9.

93

Clinical Aspects of Alzheimer's Disease

Fatemeh Nourhashémi[1], Alan J. Sinclair[2] *and* Bruno Vellas[1]

[1] Toulouse University Hospital, Toulouse, France, and [2] University of Warwick, Coventry, UK

INTRODUCTION

With the aging of the population, Alzheimer's disease has become a major public health problem. General awareness of the problems posed by this disease is increasing, but its overall cost for society, already very high, will no doubt continue to rise as its prevalence also increases exponentially with age. The advances in pathophysiology and clinical knowledge made in recent years, along with improvements in treatment, are considerable. One of the clinician's prime concerns at the present time is to diagnose the disease as early as possible, which implies that it is distinguished from other important causes of dementia, and institute rapid and appropriate management (including appropriate investigations). This will inevitably comprise a detailed account of the domestic and social situation, caregiver information, accompaniment, and support of the patient and his or her family throughout the duration of the illness.

THE DIAGNOSIS OF ALZHEIMER'S DISEASE

Alzheimer's disease is responsible for 75% of all dementias. It affects 5% of the population aged over 65 years and 30% of persons aged over 85. Dementia disorders are responsible for about 50% of cases of dependency in the elderly (Aguero-Torres *et al.*, 1998). Among the known risk factors are the following:

- age: increasing age is associated with exponential increase of the incidence of Alzheimer's disease;
- family history of the disease;
- presence of the e4 allele of the *apolipoprotein E* gene on chromosome 19: this increases the risk of development of dementia of Alzheimer type. This risk is greater and the onset of the disease is earlier in subjects who are homozygous for the e4 allele;
- gender: prevalence and incidence seem to be higher in women in the majority of studies;
- head injury;
- trisomy 21, but the family link between dementia of Alzheimer type and Down's syndrome is debated.

Hormone replacement therapy for the menopause, nonsteroidal anti-inflammatory drugs and certain nutritional factors such as the consumption of antioxidant agents may be protective factors against Alzheimer's disease.

Alzheimer's disease is characterized clinically by cognitive impairment, dominated by memory complaints, which may or may not be associated with a syndrome of aphasia, apraxia, and agnosia. All these lead to disorders of instrumental function, executive function, and judgment. The clinical presentation and the course of the disease may be extremely varied. The clinical disorders observed often differ widely from one subject to another, depending on factors such as age at onset, rapidity of progression and the diversity of cognitive and behavioral disturbances. For these reasons, clinical diagnosis may be a problem for the practitioner, who should refer to predetermined clinical criteria such as those of the DSM-IV and NINCDS-ADRDA (appendix 1) (American Psychiatric Association, 1995; McKhann *et al.*, 1984).

In Alzheimer's disease, memory impairment is constant and is a requisite for diagnosis; it is also very often the first sign. The onset of the disorder is generally insidious and difficult to detect, and the course slow and progressive. The early stage is usually marked by memory disturbance which may go unnoticed for some time by the family and friends, be attributed to normal aging or concealed by the patient. The majority of clinical evidence indicates that a considerable time may elapse – an average of −3 years – between the appearance of the first symptoms and establishing the diagnosis (Freels *et al.*, 1992; Knopman *et al.*, 2000).

Principles and Practice of Geriatric Medicine, 4th Edition. Edited by M.S. John Pathy, Alan J. Sinclair and John E. Morley.

Memory disorders primarily relate to recall of recent events or short-term memory, while older memories are better preserved. Later, the disease progresses and gradually affects other cognitive domains (language, attention, calculation, orientation in time and place) as well as more complex functions such as executive function that allows planning and performance of successive, organized tasks. The course of the disease is also marked by major disturbances of judgement and reasoning, which may result in behavioral problems. These problems have a progressive impact on the activities of daily living (ADL) function and on independence which may become apparent initially in domestic activities, and then in essential ADL, with the patient becoming progressively dependent. Problems of sphincter control, alteration of nutritional status, and disturbances of balance and gait accelerate the process of dependence.

Mood is often disturbed, with symptoms of depression or anxiety or excessive lability resulting in frequent swings from apathy to agitation. Although progress has been made in the diagnosis of the disease, many patients are still seen at a late stage when the neuropsychiatric symptoms have become unmistakable. Forms with slower progression have been described, characterized essentially by memory problems that evolve very slowly over 15 to 20 years, without physical complications; inversely, very rapid and serious forms exist, which lead to the death of the patient within a few years.

The principal factors of aggravation of cognitive disturbances are iatrogenic (psychotropic drugs) and intercurrent physical conditions. Nutritional and vitamin deficiencies, sensory deficits, hypothyroidism, vascular risk factors or stress linked with family relationships (a possible source of conflict) or the domestic environment (risk of falls) also intervene.

Psychological and behavioral signs and symptoms are frequent, but generally develop in the advanced stages of Alzheimer's disease (unlike frontotemporal dementia where they occur earlier). Their onset often requires emergency management. They affect cognitive performance and decrease the tolerance of family and friends toward the patient's problems. They may prompt the family to seek medical advice for the first time and allow a diagnosis to be made.

The advantages of early diagnosis include the avoidance of certain behavioral problems arising directly from the disease and which could have unfortunate consequences such as errors, which could financially embarrass the patient or his or her family, or patients continuing to drive when they have lost the ability to act safely.

Briefly, the diagnosis of Alzheimer's disease may be made in four main clinical situations:

1. An elderly patient who is seen because of memory difficulties: this may be a case of anxiety or depression, or it may be true early Alzheimer's disease, or mild cognitive impairment (MCI) (Petersen *et al.*, 1999). MCI corresponds to a memory complaint evidenced by psychometric tests (in particular, a short-term memory deficit that is not improved by cueing, together with globally normal cognitive function). Every year, a proportion of these patients progress to Alzheimer's disease.
2. A patient who is brought to the clinic by the family because they have noticed memory or behavior disturbances: in such cases cognitive function is often severely impaired.
3. An emergency call from an agitated or confused patient: here, among other causes we must exclude distended bladder, fecal impaction, or electrolyte or metabolic imbalances. Careful history-taking and interviews with the family are also important.
4. A patient whose performance has slowed, with fatigue or lack of energy: the differential diagnosis must include other neurological disorders: hypothyroidism, normal-pressure hydrocephalus, Parkinson's disease, vascular disorders, depression.

In each of these diagnostic situations, after a comprehensive examination, the following investigations should be made:

- neuropsychological investigation, whose nature depends on the complexity of the clinical picture;
- laboratory tests (hemoglobin, erythrocyte sedimentation rate (ESR), thyroid function, lipid profile, blood glucose, serum creatinine, electrolytes, etc.);
- brain CT scan (usually without contrast agent).

In the more difficult forms of the disease and in specialized facilities, more specific investigations can be carried out such as MRI, brain scintigraphy, or ApoE4 typing (these are not recommended as routine tests).

At the present time, the diagnosis of Alzheimer's disease is a positive diagnosis and not one of exclusion. The case history, the results of clinical, neuropsychological and psychiatric examination, supported by imaging findings make it possible to establish the diagnosis with a high degree of probability in most cases. It is still very important to make a precise diagnosis of Alzheimer's disease so that it is not confused with another type of degenerative dementia (e.g. frontotemporal dementia, Lewy body dementia, focal atrophy), or vascular dementia, which is sometimes associated with Alzheimer's dementia, but should not be missed.

BOX 1

The diagnosis of dementia is defined by the ICD-10 of the WHO and makes it possible to exclude:

- depressive syndromes,
- confusional syndrome,

- drug-related cognitive decline (mainly secondary to long-term abuse of neuroleptics),
- mental deficiency and social deprivation.

The following are the most frequent dementias other than dementia of Alzheimer type:

Nondegenerative dementias:

- vascular dementia: this is the second commonest cause of dementia syndromes after Alzheimer's disease; vascular lesions are the exclusive etiology in 15 to 20% of dementias and are associated with other etiologies (mixed dementias) in 15 to 20% of cases, so that nearly one-third of syndromes can be considered as having a vascular origin;
- hydrocephalus with normal pressure;
- metabolic disorders: thyroid disorders, vitamin B12 deficiency, hypercalcemia, hepatic encephalopathy;
- secondary to a brain tumor.

Non-Alzheimer degenerative dementias:

- Lewy body dementia: characterized by associated recurrent hallucinations (visual in particular), an unstable cognitive state and motor symptoms of Parkinson's disease;
- Frontotemporal dementia: where cognitive disturbances have a secondary role. Behavioral problems signal the onset of the disease and not memory complaints, unlike Alzheimer's disease;
- Focal atrophy: which causes cognitive dysfunction but which may remain isolated for a long period;
- Alcoholic dementia: characterized by slowed psychomotor performance, disturbances of language, and visual spatial coordination;
- Creutzfeldt-Jacob's disease: which is associated with psychiatric, cognitive, and neurological signs/symptoms.

Mixed dementias:

Cerebral vascular lesions are associated with degenerative dementia of Alzheimer type.

Alzheimer's disease is diagnosed increasingly early. The growing number of *memory clinics* plays an increasing role here; general practitioners who have become increasingly aware of the problems and issues in dementia and patient's families (who previously tended to consider a failing memory as the normal consequence of aging) are more prone to refer patients to these specialized centers. The complaints of the patients and of the family must be assessed, placing them in their social, cultural, and psychological context, and attention should be given to changes in relation to previous capacities.

In order to acquire a diagnosis of established Alzheimer's disease, in addition to the case history and clinical examination, global evaluation scales such as Folstein's Mini-Mental State Examination (MMSE) can be administered in a few minutes at the patient's bedside by the physician. Thus, for all cases of Alzheimer's disease that meet the DSM-IV criteria, the global scales are sufficient for diagnosis. The initial evaluation and then the follow-up of disease progression can be based on various parameters: decline of cognitive function, assessment of dependence, or decline related to changes in living arrangements. However, all these factors remain subordinate to others such as marital status, or quality of management at home, itself dependent on the level of resources and services available, which vary according to the country.

For evaluation of cognitive function, the MMSE remains the instrument generally used. It is a simple scale with 30 questions and can be administered in about 10 to 15 minutes. It objectively evaluates temporospatial orientation, a mental arithmetic task requiring working memory, recall of three words, reproduction of a complex design which detects constructive apraxia, and a simple language assessment (Folstein *et al.*, 1975). Among the global evaluation scales, the Clinical Dementia Rating (CDR) assesses six different domains: memory, orientation, judgement, community affairs, home and hobbies, and personal care. Each domain is scored from 0 to 3 (0: no impairment; 0.5: very mild, 1: mild; 2: moderate, and 3: severe (Hughes *et al.*, 1982; Morris, 1993). The dependence scales evaluate the ability to perform the various activities of daily living. Among them, the ADL scale explores, in six items (personal hygiene, dressing, toileting, mobility, continence, and eating) the basic activities of daily living. It is used to evaluate dependence of elderly persons in hospital, living in retirement homes, or being cared for in their own home (Katz *et al.*, 1970). The instrumental activities of daily living (IADL) scale evaluates more complex activities of daily life (such as using the telephone, doing housework, or managing money) (Lawton and Brody, 1969).

The MMSE and the IADL should systematically be used when an elderly person complains of memory problems. These scales allow the general practitioner either to reassure the patient or to refer him or her to a specialized center, bearing in mind that it is often only through repeated visits that cognitive disturbance or decreased independence can be detected at the start of the disease.

EVOLUTION OF ALZHEIMER'S DISEASE AND PATIENT FOLLOW-UP

Alzheimer's is a chronic disease. Various complications can cause the subject to lose his or her independence and eventually become permanently bedridden. Such a state is always accompanied by its own complications: pressure sores, infections, undernutrition, and therefore by high morbidity, loss of quality of life, and suffering, all of which result in high medical costs.

One of the essential aims of medical follow-up of Alzheimer's patients is to preserve satisfactory physical independence and a better quality of life. It is possible to maintain a patients' independence for activities of daily living even at very advanced stages of the disease. There appears to be no correlation between the histopathological lesions and the quality of life or independence of the patients.

We will now look in turn at

- our present knowledge of the natural history of Alzheimer's disease;
- the principal complications of the disease;
- the type of medical follow-up that we are able to propose at the present time.

The Evolution of Alzheimer's Disease

The natural history of Alzheimer's disease is now much better understood because of recently published long-term and retrospective studies. The study of Grossberg and colleagues retraces the history of 100 subjects with Alzheimer's disease confirmed by autopsy. The authors observed that the mean time elapsing between the onset of symptoms and the clinical diagnosis of the disease was 32.1 months (±37.9) and time elapsing between clinical diagnosis and institutionalization was 23.9 months (±33.6). Institutionalization therefore occurred at a mean of 56.5 months after the onset of the first symptoms. The mean duration of the disease after the onset of the first symptoms to the death of the patient was 101.3 months, or nearly 8.5 years. The longest duration of the disease was 252.1 months, or nearly 21 years, for one of these patients. The authors of this study reported that in typical Alzheimer's disease, the diagnosis was made at the age of 75 or 32 months after the onset of the first signs. Admission to a retirement home took place on average 24 months after diagnosis, or 57 months (4.5 years) after the onset of the first signs of the disease. The subject then spent about 44 months in the retirement home before dying (Jost and Grossberg, 1995).

Alzheimer's disease is one of the most frequent causes of death, even if this has long been unrecognized. Study of the causes of death in 1995 in the United States reveals that 7.1% of all deaths can be attributed to this disease, which is the third leading cause of death (Ewbank, 1999). A prospective study recently carried out in the state of Washington found concordant results, and revealed that certain factors decreased the duration of the patients' life and in particular, rapid decline of cognitive function, loss of independence, and falls were poor prognostic factors. Identification and follow-up of these factors may help the patient and his or her family to better plan their future (Larson *et al.*, 2004). Median survival also appears to depend on age at the time of diagnosis (Brookmeyer *et al.*, 2002).

Principal Complications

Three signs should attract the attention of the physician caring for a patient with Alzheimer's disease:

- weight loss;
- alteration in balance and gait/posture with an increased risk of falls;
- behavioral disturbances.

These are the basic essentials of noncognitive follow-up of these patients. Nevertheless, regular evaluation of the patient's neurocognitive function should not be neglected.

Weight Loss and Alzheimer's Disease

When he first described the disease in 1906, Alois Alzheimer emphasized the occurrence of weight loss in his patient. However, this weight loss has long been mistakenly considered as occurring at the late stages of the disease. We now know than it can occur as soon as the first symptoms of the disease appear.

The sooner a management strategy is set up, the more effective it will be. Otherwise, we may rapidly find ourselves confronted with undernourished, anorexic subjects, where there is very little room for maneuver between doing nothing (often seen as abandonment of treatment) or setting up enteral nutrition (which is then seen as artificial prolongation of life), whereas early on, especially in subjects who live alone at home, a visit from a home help will often be sufficient to assist these patients in doing their shopping and preparing their meals. It therefore appears to be essential to assess the nutritional status of each Alzheimer's patient, particularly if he or she lives alone or has little family support.

The pathophysiological mechanisms of weight loss are complex and have only partially been elucidated. Alteration of nutritional status may be secondary to the development of inability to perform the activities of everyday living or to disturbances of eating behavior. However, numerous studies have shown that weight loss is observed in the course of the disease even when the subjects still have a satisfactory energy intake. Certain authors suggest that atrophy of the internal temporal cortex or the effect of the e4 allele may play a role in weight regulation (Grundman *et al.*, 1996; Vanhanen *et al.*, 2001). Clinical practice shows that weight loss is accompanied by a variety of complications (decreased immunity, muscle atrophy, falls, and fractures) that affect the state of health and increase the risk of institutionalization and mortality.

Mobility Problems, Falls, and Risk of Accidents

In patients with Alzheimer's disease, posture rapidly becomes incorrect as a consequence of aging (arthritis, impaired vision, muscle wasting, etc.) but this may also be directly related to Alzheimer's disease (Kluger *et al.*, 1997; Franssen *et al.*, 1999) or to medication. Disturbances of equilibrium can lead to numerous falls and fractures, or to abusive use of restraint. Accidents generally occur in patients in whom Alzheimer's disease has not been diagnosed: drug-related accidents or accidents in the street or in the home. Balance and mobility problems have major psychological consequences leading to anxiety and a feeling of insecurity. They can result in decreased physical activity and loss of social contacts.

Psychological and Behavioral Signs and Symptoms

These problems are observed in the majority of patients with dementia, and in particular, in Alzheimer's disease. The Neuropsychiatric Inventory (NPI) (Cummings *et al.*, 1994) has helped clarify the definition of these disturbances. The NPI makes it possible to define the type of disturbance (it covers the field of the 10 most common neuropsychiatric symptoms) and also its frequency, severity, and emotional impact on the family and relatives. Of these symptoms, apathy is probably the most frequent. In the medical literature, apathy, considered as a deficiency syndrome, is reflected in lack of initiative and interest, social withdrawal, and flattening of affect.

The majority of studies show that "depressive symptoms" are an integral part of the classic picture of Alzheimer's disease. These symptoms are found in more than 80% of patients (Lyketsos *et al.*, 2001). Depression is also a frequent disorder in this population (Weiner *et al.*, 2002). The prevalence of anxiety symptoms varies depending on the authors. Anxiety may, in fact, be difficult to diagnose because of other symptoms masking the anxious patient. It can be the cause of agitated or inhibited behavior. Psychotic manifestations (delirium and hallucinations) can result in aggressive behavior and consequently affect the emotional state of the family and relatives, who often find it difficult to tolerate the persistence of such behavior and strongly press for symptomatic treatment to be given. It is therefore not surprising that numerous authors report a greater risk of institutionalization in these subjects.

Sleep disorders are a major problem in the medical follow-up of patients with Alzheimer's disease. Specific changes in sleep architecture have been described in the great majority of patients. Sleep becomes less and less restorative, which explains the high frequency of daytime sleep. These symptoms can rapidly make life intolerable for the family or the residents of a retirement home.

There are various types of sleep disorder. Typically, agitation and anxiety appear in the late afternoon. If the patient is not rapidly calmed, this state worsens; he or she refuses to go to bed and remains anxious and agitated for the best part of the night. It may be necessary to relieve this anxiety at the end of the afternoon by giving an anxiolytic, followed by appropriate use of a hypnotic with a short half-life to allow the patient to sleep. Hypnotics are even more effective if given to a patient who is already calm and not anxious. A second typical case is that of patients who have been given neuroleptics because they presented with behavioral disorders. They are then often somnolent during the day and may even be restrained in bed or in an armchair, so it is only to be expected that they should be agitated at night. Neuroleptics must be stopped during the day, and these patients must be mobilized and a normal sleep–wake rhythm restored. Walking or any kind of physical exercise, in particular in the late afternoon, is a good means to help prevent anxiety at this time of day as well as nocturnal agitation. Aberrant motor behavior and wandering, the irrepressible need to walk about, is a dysfunction that is peculiar to dementia states.

Agitation in the patient with Alzheimer's disease may also be related to associated pathologies that have not been diagnosed (e.g. infections). Poor interpretation of sensory stimuli may also be the cause of a number of episodes of agitation in these patients. Sometimes, no cause is found. Problems such weight loss, difficulty in walking, falls, and nocturnal agitation will develop in almost all Alzheimer's subjects at one time or another in the course of the disease. They sometimes occur simultaneously. Undernutrition increases the likelihood of muscle wasting and falls. Falls often lead staff to use restraint during the day, resulting in agitation at night. All these factors rapidly end in the patient becoming permanently bedridden.

Other Symptoms

Alzheimer's disease is one of the causes of epilepsy in the elderly subject. Numerous patients develop extrapyramidal symptoms. Resting tremor is rarer than in idiopathic Parkinson's disease or in drug-induced striatal syndromes. On the other hand, rigidity and bradykinesia or a "parkinsonian" gait are more frequent (Mitchell, 1999). An underlying brain disorder, in this instance Alzheimer's disease, is a risk factor for confusion in the elderly. Sphincter problems generally develop in advanced forms.

At a late stage of Alzheimer's disease, muscle and joint contractures may develop, leading to a permanently bedridden state and to death because of the complications of decubitus ulcers. The value of walking and passive mobilization of the joints to prevent such contractures must be stressed.

Medical Follow-up

Once the diagnosis has been established, patients can be followed by standardized gerontological evaluation (Rubenstein *et al.*, 1984). One of the principal aims of management is to postpone the period of loss of independence that precedes death. It is very important to provide therapeutic management for these patients and their families. This need is felt by the family, and if it is not met, they will often turn to alternative medicine. Standardized evaluation allows rapid and objective exploration of several facets of the elderly patient: dependence (ADL, IADL), memory deficit and the syndrome of aphasia/apraxia/agnosia (MMS), the risk of pressure sores (Norton's scale), nutritional status with the MNA (Mini Nutritional Assessment), study of walking and balance (Tinetti's test). Two other tools may also be useful: the NPI, which explores the psychiatric complications of the disease (as described earlier), and the Zarit scale (Zarit *et al.*, 1980) which assesses caregiver burden. These two questionnaires are administered to the family. The NPI quantifies the psychiatric aspects of the disease (which cause considerable distress to the family, distress they have difficulty in expressing). The Zarit scale, by exploring caregiver burden, makes it possible to adapt the services proposed or helps to pose the indication of admission to a retirement home when this seems necessary.

It is wise to have discussions about the possibility of the subject moving to a retirement home at an early stage and when the subject is relatively well, rather than wait until the last minute and then have to resort to emergency admission under poor conditions for all those concerned: the patient, the family, and those close to them.

Here we must stress that therapeutic management must be well organized. Apart from purely pharmacological treatment (specific treatments for Alzheimer's disease and treatment of the various symptoms), we propose the following management strategy:

Comprehensive clinical examination of the patient must be carried out initially and then every 3 months. This examination must be repeated if a new incident occurs (e.g. agitation, fever). In particular, bladder distension should be sought (in women and in men), as well as polyuria and altered general health. It should include examination of vision and hearing, and of the teeth and mouth to seek for poor dental condition or fungal infections. Signs of depression or anxiety and mobility problems should be sought. It is also important to look for fecal impaction, constipation, and gastric or abdominal pain especially in those patients who cannot adequately express their complaints. The same is true of rheumatological pain, which may be the cause of unexplained refusal to walk.

The interview should yield information on the living arrangements of the patient, the quality of support from his or her family and relatives and the impact of the disease on the couple, and there should be no hesitation in asking questions about any difficulties the subject may have in managing personal affairs.

Among the radiological examinations and biological tests a chest X ray is advisable (this is particularly useful for patients who attend a day center or who live in an institution, if a resident with whom the patient may have been in contact develops tuberculosis or a lung infection). It will serve as a reference.

Study of the cardiac silhouette can show associated heart failure. Plain abdominal X ray can exclude high faecal loading that could not be found by digital rectal examination. Lastly, a basic ECG is useful, as well as a battery of laboratory tests which should include a complete blood count/ESR, urea and electrolyte, glucose, thyroid-stimulating hormone (TSH), liver function tests, and urine culture.

The standardized gerontological evaluation should be carried out in all patients at the time of diagnosis and then every 6 months or when a change in circumstances occurs, whether social (death of a family member or relative, change of living arrangements, institutionalization, hospitalization), or the onset of an intercurrent disease. Social evaluation should look at the living arrangements of the patient (alone, with family, in institution), and the characteristics of family and relatives (availability, state of health, age). The family must also be fully informed about the services available and the possibilities of legal protection when this is necessary, bearing in mind that it is better to anticipate and prevent problems than have to suffer them.

Specific Pharmacological Treatments for Alzheimer's Disease

Treatment has a double aim: to stabilize or at least to delay the progression of the disease and to reduce the psychological and behavioral problems that often accompany it. These replacement therapies act on the consequences of the lesions, but not on their cause. They are prescribed to reduce neurotransmitter deficiency and so to improve the clinical signs or to delay the progression of the deficiencies observed. The improvement gained ceases after treatment is discontinued.

Anticholinesterase inhibitors are the first drugs to show proven efficacy in Alzheimer's disease. They increase the level of acetylcholine (ACh) in the synapse, by blocking acetylcholine esterase (AChE) which breaks down ACh in the synaptic cleft.

The undesirable side effects are cholinomimetic, that is, nausea, vomiting, diarrhea, agitation, and confusion. Because of these cholinergic properties, prudence is necessary, particularly in poorly controlled asthma, disorders of cardiac rhythm and repolarization, poorly controlled epilepsy, and duodenal ulcer.

Three drugs are now commercially available: donepezil, rivastigmine, and galantamine. Tacrine (Cognex*) is no longer used because of its liver toxicity. Donepezil chlorhydrate (Aricept*) is the second anticholinesterase inhibitor to have been marketed (in 1996 in the United States). It should be started initially at the effective dose of 5 mg (once daily); the optimal dose of 10 mg (once daily) is reached after 6 weeks of treatment. This progressive dose increase makes it possible to limit the side effects. Rivastigmine (Exelon*) is given twice daily. The treatment is begun with a gradually increasing dose: 1.5 mg morning and evening for 2 weeks, then 3 mg morning and evening (6 mg a day is the lowest effective dose), then 4.5 mg morning and evening and finally 6 mg morning and evening (12 mg daily is the maximum dose). The dose of galantamine (Reminyl*) must also be increased gradually. Treatment is started at a dose of 4 mg twice daily for about 1 month, then increased to 8 mg twice daily (and sometimes up to 24 mg a day).

In practice, treatment must be initiated by a physician experienced in the diagnosis of Alzheimer's disease. If there is no absolute contraindication (known hypersensitivity to the molecule, severe liver failure) or relative contraindication (cardiac rhythm disorders, atrioventricular block, sinoatrial block, active gastric or duodenal ulcer, severe asthma, severe decompensated obstructive airways disease), anticholinesterase treatment is indicated in the mild to moderate stages of the disease. Briefly, these stages correspond to MMS scores of 10 or more, associated with relatively good independence. However, these molecules also seem to have beneficial effects at the advanced stages of the disease, above all on behavior. It is necessary for a relative or friend to monitor compliance. Treatment is started gradually, with a clinical check-up 3 to 6 months later. Such intense biological surveillance appears not to be required for the new anticholinesterase inhibitors (rivastigmine, donepezil, galantamine).

Specific treatment for Alzheimer's disease can only be contemplated as part of a care plan which includes treatment of behavioral problems, nutritional problems and mood, appropriate social management (services delivered to relieve the informal caregiver), and psychological support. Treatment may be discontinued if there is major gastrointestinal intolerance, respiratory decompensation, worsening of cardiac rhythm disorders. If there is any doubt, treatment may be temporarily suspended. Adverse events often occur when doses are changed and regress in a few days. If they do not, it is advisable first of all to add a symptomatic treatment (for gastrointestinal problems, for example), then if this fails, to go back to a lower dose and attempt a more gradual increase.

Poor compliance is also a possible cause of discontinuation of treatment, as is the death or departure of the family member or person who was responsible for the patient's medication.

Lastly, treatment may be stopped if there is no improvement and/or stabilization after 6 months. But in this case, most authors emphasize that a similar drug of the same class should be tried for a sufficiently long period. It should be noted that entry to an institution is all too often the cause for unjustified discontinuation of treatment.

In practice, every patient with mild to moderate Alzheimer's disease should be able to benefit from specific treatment if there is no contraindication. In 2003, a new therapeutic class became available, the antiglutaminergic agents (*N*-methyl-D-aspartate (NMDA) antagonists). Among them, Ebixa* (memantine) is reserved for the time being for the moderately severe and severe forms of the disease.

MANAGEMENT STRUCTURES

The concern of the clinician at the present time must be to identify patients as early as possible in order to rapidly set up a medical and nonmedical intervention strategy, with the aim of maintaining as long as possible satisfactory independence for the patient and his or her family and friends.

Management at Home with Increased Support

Pharmacological and nonpharmacological management of the patient and support and assistance to family and relatives remain the decisive factors in postponing admission to an institution. The majority of patients with dementia live at home, and they are often cared for by the family alone, without any help from professionals.

However, intermediate solutions between care at home by the family and institutionalization have been developed in recent years: care at home with increased support, respite families, day care centers, or temporary care centers are possibilities that offer specific and appropriate management to persons with Alzheimer's disease. But families are still too often insufficiently informed, the facilities available differ widely depending on location, and the financial cost of the services proposed or of the accommodation are still an obstacle to appropriate management of the elderly person with dementia.

Management at home with increased support calls upon external professional help, working as a team with a common objective, and usually coordinated by the general practitioner. Various professionals and services intervene, which are adapted and modulated according to the needs of the patient and his or her family. The following assistance can be provided:

- *nursing care* for toileting, prevention of decubitus ulcers and distribution of medication. This is provided by a nurse in private practice or by a care association;
- *physiotherapy*;
- *the help of an occupational therapist* with, if necessary, *conversion of the accommodation* to reduce the risk of accidents in the home (increased security, prevention of the risk of falls, locking of doors and potentially dangerous places);
- *the services of a home nurse or a helper*, the latter trained in the physical and psychological management of dependent persons;
- *a home help* for the daily activities the person can no longer carry out (shopping, housework, meal preparation). Visits may be daily except for weekends and public holidays. These services are organized by the local health/social councils and the hourly cost depends on the beneficiary's financial resources; similar assistance may be provided by an independent home help;
- a *meal delivery service*, which some local councils provide and which is subject to the same conditions as domestic help;
- *provision of a tele-alarm*, a device that is indicated in mild to moderate dementia without marked temporospatial disorientation and above all without major behavioral disturbance.

Relatives and family also require support if maintenance at home is to be prolonged. Numerous studies have shown that the decisive factor in institutionalization of patients was less dependent on the severity of the disease than on the stamina of the caregiver, usually the spouse. The family need information and assistance if they are to react and adjust well to the disease. This information and support can be provided by the family doctor and the staff of specialized centers (day care center, day hospital, memory clinic) aided by the various associations.

Hospitalization at Home and Hospitalization in Medium- or Long-stay Units

The physician plays an essential role in detecting intercurrent disorders or complications of the disease. He may make it possible to avoid hospitalization by preventing or treating factors of aggravation such as urinary, bronchial or skin infections, foot care problems, constipation, dehydration, sensory deficits, and so on.

Hospital at home, usually planned for a limited period, is often a more beneficial alternative than hospitalization in a medium-stay unit or admission to a convalescent home. It comprises the intervention in the home of a genuine health-professional team with a doctor, nurse, and nursing auxiliary.

But admission to hospital may become necessary to manage an acute psychiatric or medical problem or to give the family some respite. The following structures all have as their primary aim the rehabilitation of the subject and discharge to his or her own home:

Departments of medicine (geriatrics, neurology, internal medicine, or psychiatry) offer specialized management of the problem that motivated the admission to hospital. But sometimes these facilities are not adapted to aged, demented patients (for example, in internal medicine departments the premises are not suited to management of a behavioral problem, while in psychiatry departments it may be difficult to give a physical complication the specialized medical management required).

The acute-care unit can take in Alzheimer patients whatever the stage of the disease and whatever the intercurrent or associated diseases for a stay lasting a few days. There are very few of these facilities.

Community Residences, Respite Families, and Short-stay Centers

Between the home and long-stay facilities (private retirement home or long-stay unit in a hospital), *community residences* offer patients some independence, with the possibility of access to catering services (restaurant, room service).

Retirement Homes and Long-stay Units

Admission to a long-stay unit may become indispensable when management at home becomes too heavy a burden for the family. Many innovative experiments are being carried out in the hospital setting. They all try to improve the quality of life and management of these patients. Specialized units are being developed; these may be day care units, sheltered units, or true units for diagnosis and rehabilitation. Unfortunately, such initiatives are still very rare and there are many difficulties in the way of their creation, due to lack of funding.

The general practitioner accompanies Alzheimer patients for perhaps 10 years, and copes, with the help of a specialized center, with all the complications that develop throughout the course of the disease. Some can be managed at home; others will require hospitalization. Hospitalization is known to be in itself a factor aggravating the problems of the elderly person in general (frequent episodes of confusion), and these are all the more likely when the care facility is not adapted to behavioral disturbances. This raises the problem of how these hospital facilities can be converted to meet the specific needs of this very particular population.

CONCLUSIONS

Alzheimer's disease has long been considered as an exaggerated manifestation of normal aging, an irremediable end-of-life phenomenon, about which nothing could be done. Over the last 10 years, through advances in our understanding, this view has been replaced by its recognition as a specific neurodegenerative disease state, partly amenable to treatment.

KEY POINTS

- Alzheimer's disease is the commonest cause of dementia.
- The prevalence of Alzheimer's disease is greater than 20% in subjects over the age of 90.
- In the early stages, the disease is characterized by memory and learning difficulties and then language, constructional deficits, apraxia, and dysphasia may intervene.
- Diagnosis is dependent on a thorough clinical evaluation supported by various objective tests for meeting the DSM-IV criteria or the ICD-10 definition.
- There are a range of anticholinesterase treatments available, but these must be viewed as part of an overall management strategy.

KEY REFERENCES

- Aguero-Torres A, Fratiglioni L, Guo Z *et al.* Dementia is the major cause of functional dependence in the elderly: 3-year follow-up data from a population-based study. *American Journal of Public Health* 1998; **88**:1452–6.
- Larson EB, Shadlen MF, Wang L *et al.* Survival after initial diagnosis of Alzheimer disease. *Annals of Internal Medicine* 2004; **140**:501–9.
- Petersen RC, Smith GE, Waring SC *et al.* Mild cognitive impairment. Clinical characterization and outcome. *Archives of Neurology* 1999; **56**:303–8.

- Weiner MF, Doody RS, Sairam R *et al.* Prevalence and incidence of major depressive disorder in Alzheimer's disease: findings from two databases. *Dementia and Geriatric Cognitive Disorders* 2002; **13**:8–12.

REFERENCES

Aguero-Torres A, Fratiglioni L, Guo Z *et al.* Dementia is the major cause of functional dependence in the elderly: 3-year follow-up data from a population-based study. *American Journal of Public Health* 1998; **88**:1452–6.

American Psychiatric Association. *Diagnostic and Statistical Manual of Mental Disorders* 1995, 4th edn; (DSM-IV), APA, Washington.

Brookmeyer R, Corrada MM, Curriero FC *et al.* Survival following a diagnosis of Alzheimer disease. *Archives of Neurology* 2002; **59**:1764–7.

Cummings JL, Mega M, Gray K *et al.* The neuropsychiatric inventory: comprehensive assessment of psychopathology in dementia. *Neurology* 1994; **44**:2308–14.

Ewbank DC. Deaths attributable to Alzheimer's disease in the United States. *American Journal of Public Health* 1999; **89**:90–2.

Folstein M, Folstein S & McHugh PR. "Mini-mental State". A practical method for grading the cognitive state patients for the clinician. *Journal of Psychiatric Research* 1975; **12**:189–98.

Franssen EH, Souren LE, Torossian CL *et al.* Equilibrium and limb coordination in mild cognitive impairment and mild Alzheimer's disease. *Journal of the American Geriatrics Society* 1999; **47**:463–9.

Freels S, Cohen D, Eisdorfer C *et al.* Functional status and clinical findings in patients with Alzheimer's disease. *The Journals of Gerontology. Series A, Biological Sciences and Medical Sciences* 1992; **47A**:M177–82.

Jost BC & Grossberg GT. The natural history of Alzheimer's disease: a brain bank study. *Journal of the American Geriatrics Society* 1995; **43**:1248–55.

Grundman M, Corey-Bloom J, Jernigan T *et al.* Low body weight in Alzheimer's disease is associated with mesial temporal cortex atrophy. *Neurology* 1996; **46**:1585–91.

Hughes CP, Berg L, Danziger WL *et al.* A new clinical scale for the staging of dementia. *The British Journal of Psychiatry* 1982; **140**:566–72.

Katz S, Downs TD, Cash HR *et al.* Progress in development of the index of ADL. *The Gerontologist* 1970; **10**:20–30.

Kluger A, Gianutsos JG, Golomb J *et al.* Patterns of motor impairment in normal aging, mild cognitive decline, and early Alzheimer's disease. *Journal of Gerontology* 1997; **52B**:P28–39.

Knopman D, Donohue JA & Gutterman EM. Patterns of care in the early stages of AD: impediments to timely diagnosis. *Journal of the American Geriatrics Society* 2000; **48**:300–4.

Larson EB, Shadlen MF, Wang L *et al.* Survival after initial diagnosis of Alzheimer disease. *Annals of Internal Medicine* 2004; **140**:501–9.

Lawton MP & Brody EM. Assessment of older people: self-maintaining and instrumental activities of daily living. *The Gerontologist* 1969; **9**:179–86.

Lyketsos CG, Sheppard JM, Steinberg M *et al.* Neuropsychiatric disturbances in Alzheimer's disease clusters into three groups: the cache county study. *International Journal of Geriatric Psychiatry* 2001; **16**:1043–53.

McKhann G, Drachman D, Folstein M *et al.* Clinical diagnosis of Alzheimer's disease: report of the NINCDS-ADRDA work group under the auspices of department of health and human services task force on Alzheimer's disease. *Neurology* 1984; **34**:939–44.

Mitchell SL. Extrapyramidal features in Alzheimer's disease. *Age and Ageing* 1999; **28**:401–9.

Morris JC. The Clinical Dementia Rating (CDR): current version and scoring rules. *Neurology* 1993; **43**:2412–4.

Petersen RC, Smith GE, Waring SC *et al.* Mild cognitive impairment. Clinical characterization and outcome. *Archives of Neurology* 1999; **56**:303–8.

Rubenstein LZ, Josephson KR, Wieland GD *et al.* Effectiveness of a geriatric evaluation unit. A randomised clinical trial. *The New England Journal of Medicine* 1984; **311**:1664–70.

Vanhanen M, Kivipelto M, Koivisto K *et al.* ApoE-epsilon4 is associated with weight loss in women with AD: a population-based study. *Neurology* 2001; **56**:655–9.

Weiner MF, Doody RS, Sairam R *et al.* Prevalence and incidence of major depressive disorder in Alzheimer's disease: findings from two databases. *Dementia and Geriatric Cognitive Disorders* 2002; **13**:8–12.

Zarit SH, Reever KE & Bach-Peterson J. Relatives of the impaired elderly: correlates of feelings of burden. *The Gerontologist* 1980; **20**:649–55.

FURTHER READING

Brickman AM, Riba A, Bell K *et al.* Longitudinal assessment of patient dependence in Alzheimer disease. *Archives of Neurology* 2002; **59**:1304–8.

Vellas B, Guigoz Y, Garry PJ *et al.* The Mini Nutritional Assessment (MNA) and its use in grading the nutritional state in elderly patients. *Nutrition* 1999; **15**:116–22.

APPENDIX 1

DSM IV : Dementia of the Alzheimer's Type

1. The development of multiple cognitive deficits manifested by both (1) memory impairment (impaired ability to learn new information or to recall previously learned information) (2) one (or more) of the following cognitive disturbances:
   (a) aphasia (language disturbance)
   (b) apraxia (impaired ability to carry out motor activities despite intact motor function)
   (c) agnosia (failure to recognize or identify objects despite intact sensory function)
   (d) disturbance in executive functioning (i.e. planning, organizing, sequencing, abstracting).
2. The cognitive deficits in Criteria A1 and A2 each cause significant impairment in social or occupational functioning and represent a significant decline from a previous level of functioning.
3. The course is characterized by gradual onset and continuing cognitive decline.
4. The cognitive deficits in Criteria A1 and A2 are not due to any of the following:
   (1) other central nervous system conditions that cause progressive deficits in memory and cognition (e.g. cerebrovascular disease, Parkinson's disease, Huntington's disease, subdural hematoma, normal-pressure hydrocephalus, brain tumor)
   (2) systemic conditions that are known to cause dementia (e.g. hypothyroidism, vitamin B or folic acid deficiency, niacin deficiency, hypercalcemia, neurosyphilis, HIV infection)
   (3) substance-induced conditions.
5. The deficits do not occur exclusively during the course of a delirium.
6. The disturbance is not better accounted for by another Axis I disorder (e.g. Major Depressive Episode, Schizophrenia).

With Early Onset: if onset is at age 65 years or below

With Delirium: if delirium is superimposed on the dementia
With Delusions: if delusions are the predominant feature
With Depressed Mood: if depressed mood (including presentations that meet full symptom criteria for a Major Depressive Episode) is the predominant feature. A separate diagnosis of Mood Disorder Due to a General Medical Condition is not given.
Uncomplicated: if none of the above predominates in the current clinical presentation

With Late Onset: if onset is after 65 years

With Delirium: if delirium is superimposed on the dementia
With Delusions: if delusions are the predominant feature
290. meet full symptom criteria for a Major Depressive Episode) is the predominant feature. A separate diagnosis of Mood Disorder Due to a General Medical Condition is not given.
290.0 Uncomplicated: if none of the above predominates in the current clinical presentation.

Clinical diagnosis of Alzheimer's disease: report of the NINCDS-ADRDA work group under the auspices of Department of Health and Human Services Task Force on Alzheimer's disease: Neurology, 1984; 34 : 939.

1. The criteria for the clinical diagnosis of probable Alzheimer's disease include
   Dementia established by clinical examination and documented by the Mini-Mental Test, Blessed Dementia Scale, or some similar examination, and confirmed by neuropsychological tests
   Deficits in two or more areas of cognition
   Progressive worsening of memory and other cognitive functions
   No disturbance of consciousness
   Onset between ages 40 and 90, most often after age 65
   Absence of systemic disorders or other brain diseases that in and of themselves could account for the progressive deficits in memory and cognition.

2. The diagnosis of probable Alzheimer's disease is supported by
   Progressive deterioration of specific cognitive functions such as language (aphasia), motor skills (apraxia), and perception (agnosia)
   Impaired activities of daily living and altered patterns of behavior

Family history of similar disorders, particularly if confirmed neuropathologically
Laboratory results of
Normal lumbar puncture as evaluated by standard techniques
Normal pattern or nonspecific changes in EEG, such as increased slow-wave activity
Evidence of cerebral atrophy on CT with progression documented by serial observation.

3. Other clinical features consistent with the diagnosis of probable Alzheimer's disease, after exclusion of causes of dementia other than Alzheimer's disease, include
Plateaus in the course of progression of the illness
Associated symptoms of depression, insomnia, incontinence, delusions, illusions, hallucinations, catastrophic verbal, emotional, or physical outbursts, sexual disorders, and weight loss
Other neurologic abnormalities in some patients, especially with more advanced disease and including motor signs such as increase muscle tone, myoclonus, or gait disorder
Seizures in advanced disease
CT normal for age.

4. Features that make the diagnosis of probable Alzheimer's disease uncertain or unlikely include
Sudden, apoplectic onset
Focal neurologic findings such as hemiparesis, sensory loss, visual field deficits, and incoordination early in the course of the illness; and seizures or gait disturbances at onset or very early in course of the illness.

5. Clinical diagnosis of possible Alzheimer's disease
May be made on the basis of the dementia syndrome, in the absence of other neurologic, psychiatric, or systemic disorders sufficient to cause dementia, and in the presence of variations in the onset, in the presentation, or in the clinical course
May be made in the presence of a second systemic or brain disorder sufficient to produce dementia, which is not considered to be the cause of the dementia
Should be used in research studies when a single, gradually progressive severe cognitive deficit is identified in the absence of other identifiable cause.

6. Criteria for diagnosis of definite Alzheimer's disease are
The clinical criteria for probable Alzheimer's disease
Histopathologic evidence obtained from a biopsy or autopsy.

7. Classification of Alzheimer's disease for research purposes should specify features that may differentiate subtypes of the disorder, such as
Familial occurrence
Onset before age of 65
Presence of trisomy 21
Coexistence of other relevant conditions such as Parkinson's disease.

94

Mild Cognitive Impairment

Pieter Jelle Visser

University of Maastricht, Maastricht, The Netherlands, and VU Medical Center, Amsterdam, The Netherlands

INTRODUCTION

The concept Mild Cognitive Impairment (MCI) has been introduced to describe cognitive impairment in nondemented subjects. The prevalence of MCI varies between 2 and 30% in the general population and between 6 and 85% in a clinical setting (average 40%) (Visser, 2000). Subjects with MCI are of major clinical importance because they have an increased risk of developing Alzheimer-type dementia. However, there is much confusion about the concept of MCI: there is no uniform definition, there is no single underlying cause, and the long-term outcome appears to be heterogeneous. In this chapter, definitions of MCI and terminology used, causes of MCI, outcome of MCI, and predictors of dementia will be discussed.

DEFINITIONS AND TERMINOLOGY OF MCI

MCI refers to the presence of cognitive impairment that is not severe enough to meet the criteria of dementia. It has been operationalized in many ways. In a review of the literature performed in 2004, we identified more than 40 definitions of MCI. On the basis of these different MCI definitions, six major concepts can be identified: MCI definitions based on cognitive complaints only, on the presence of mild functional impairment only, on the presence of impairment on cognitive tests only, on a combination of cognitive complaints and test impairment, on a combination of mild functional impairment and test impairment, and on mild functional impairment or test impairment (Table 1). Definitions that fall within the same concept can be further classified according to the cognitive domain that is impaired: impairment in at least the memory domain, in only the memory domain, in any domain, or in a combination of domains. Also, the definition of impairment on cognitive tests is variable and ranges from a score 1 standard deviation below the mean in healthy young subjects to a score 2 standard deviations below the mean in age-matched control subjects. As can be seen in Table 1, the terminology is variable because different terms refer to similar MCI concepts and the same terms are used for different MCI concepts. The MCI definition that is most widely used is that of amnestic MCI (Petersen *et al.*, 1999). It requires a memory complaint, impairment on a memory test after correction for age and education, preserved general cognitive functioning, intact activities of daily living, and absence of dementia. However, due to a lack of detailed criteria, this definition has been operationalized in many different ways. Another common MCI definition is that of Age-Associated Memory Impairment (AAMI) (Crook *et al.*, 1986). It requires a complaint of memory impairment, a score on a memory test one standard deviation below the mean performance of healthy young adults, adequate intellectual functioning, absence of dementia, and absence of diseases that may cause memory impairment. This definition was common in the period 1986–1995, but it is presently less often used.

The lack of standardization is confusing and limits the interpretation of MCI studies. In the remaining part of the chapter, the term MCI will be used for cognitive impairment that do not meet criteria for dementia. It does not refer to any specific definition.

CAUSES OF MCI

One of the most important causes of MCI is Alzheimer's disease. However, all somatic, other neurological, or psychiatric disorders that influence brain functioning can also cause MCI. From a diagnostic perspective, these conditions can be classified in three groups (Visser, 2003). The first group of conditions are obvious causes for MCI. This means that they are a sufficient cause for the impairments and can be identified by clinical examination and/or ancillary tests like laboratory tests or neuroimaging (see Table 2 part A for examples). The second group of conditions are sufficient causes for the MCI that can presently not be diagnosed by

Principles and Practice of Geriatric Medicine, 4th Edition. Edited by M.S. John Pathy, Alan J. Sinclair and John E. Morley.

Table 1 Main MCI concepts

1.	Cognitive complaints Examples: MCI (Tei *et al.*, 1997), minor cognitive impairment (Visser *et al.*, 2002a), questionable dementia (Thompson *et al.*, 2002), memory impairment (Tierney *et al.*, 1996).
2.	Mild functional impairment Examples: MCI or questionable dementia (a score of 0.5 on the Clinical Dementia Rating scale) (Morris *et al.*, 2001), MCI (a score of 3 on the Global Deterioration Scale) (Reisberg *et al.*, 1982), Minimal dementia (Roth *et al.*, 1986).
3.	Impairment on cognitive tests Examples: MCI (Bennett *et al.*, 2002), CIND (Conquer *et al.*, 2000).
4.	Cognitive complaints and test impairment Examples: Aging-associated cognitive decline (Levy, 1994), age-associated memory impairment (Crook *et al.*, 1986), age-related cognitive decline (Celsis *et al.*, 1997), amnestic MCI (Petersen *et al.*, 2001).
5.	Mild functional impairment and test impairment Examples: MCI (Larrieu *et al.*, 2002), CIND (Wu *et al.*, 2002).
6.	Mild functional impairment or test impairment Examples: CIND (Ebly *et al.*, 1995), MCI (Albert *et al.*, 1999), Questionable dementia (Devanand *et al.*, 1997).

MCI, mild cognitive impairment; CIND, cognitive impairment no dementia.

Table 2 Causes of mild cognitive impairment

A. Disorders that have a strong relationship with mild cognitive impairment and that can often be easily recognized by clinical examination and/or ancillary tests

Parkinson's disease, Huntington's disease, severe brain trauma, brain infections, large intracerebral tumors, cerebral bleeding, large cerebral infarcts, extensive white matter pathology, severe depression, psychotic disorders, longstanding and severe alcohol intoxication, drug intoxication (i.e. prolonged use of high doses of benzodiazepines), severe thiamine or vitamin B12 deficiency, unregulated diabetes mellitus or thyroid disorders.

B. Disorders that have a strong relationship with mild cognitive impairment, but that are difficult to recognize by clinical assessment and/or ancillary tests

Predementia or prodromal stage of Alzheimer's disease, Lewy body disease, frontotemporal dementia, vascular dementia, Parkinson's disease, multiple system atrophy, or Huntington's disease.

C. Disorders that have a weak relationship with mild cognitive impairment

Mild brain trauma, transient ischemic attack, epilepsy, disorders that chronically or temporarily impair brain perfusion (hyper/hypotension, stenosis of the carotid artery, generalized atherosclerosis, cardiac surgery), mild depression, bipolar disorders, anxiety disorders, regulated diabetes mellitus or thyroid disorders, mild thiamine or vitamin deficiency, heart failure, obstructive sleep apnea syndrome, chronic obstructional pulmonary diseases, anemia, severe liver or kidney disorders, hearing loss, "normal aging", fear of dementia, psychosocial problems in relation to work, relationships, life phase change, or somatic disorders.

clinical examination or ancillary tests (see Table 2 part B for examples). The third group of conditions have a weak relation with MCI, that is, subjects with such conditions may have MCI on a group level, but it is not clear whether the disorder is the cause for MCI in individual patients (see Table 2 part C for examples). In most studies on MCI, which will be discussed below, subjects with MCI due to obvious causes have been excluded.

OUTCOME OF MCI

MCI is not a stable condition. Depending on the cause, subjects may progress to dementia, may continue to have MCI, or may improve. A meta-analysis of studies with a short to intermediate follow-up period (average 3.1 years, range 1.1–5 years) indicated that on average 10% (range 2–31%) of the subjects with MCI developed dementia at each year of follow-up (Bruscoli and Lovestone, 2004). The conversion rate to dementia appeared to be higher in a clinical setting than in a population-based setting. Similar data were obtained from another meta-analysis (Visser, 2000). This meta-analysis also showed that about 90% of the subjects who converted to dementia had Alzheimer-type dementia. Studies with a follow-up longer than 5 years indicated that subjects continued to convert to dementia at longer follow-up intervals. After 8–10 years, 50 to 80% of the subjects had become demented (Morris *et al.*, 2001; Petersen *et al.*, 2001). Figure 1 shows the long-term outcome of subjects older than 60 years with cognitive complaints and amnesic MCI from the Maastricht Memory Clinic. This figure shows that the conversion rate is dependent on the way MCI is defined. It is noteworthy that the annual conversion rates decline with longer follow-up intervals and that even after 10 years of follow-up a substantial number of subjects have not become demented.

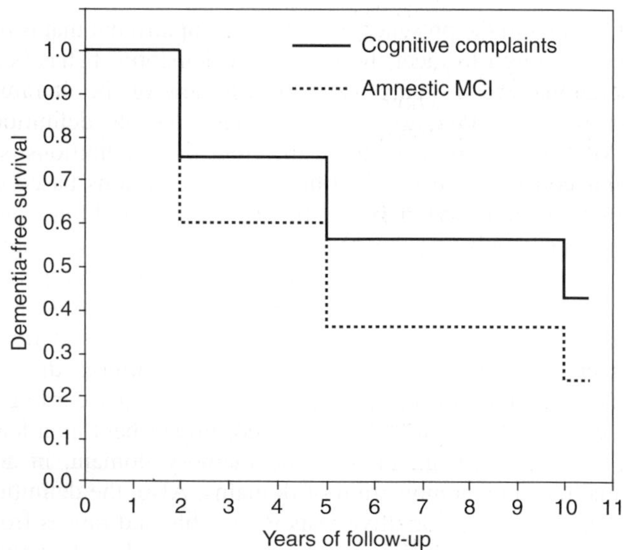

Figure 1 Long-term outcome of subjects older than 60 years with cognitive complaints ($N = 56$, straight line) and amnestic MCI ($N = 33$, dotted line) from the Maastricht Memory Clinic. Follow-up evaluations were performed after 2, 5, and 10 years. The average age at baseline was 69 years (range 60–84 years). 96% of the subjects with dementia had probable AD

PREDICTORS OF DEMENTIA IN SUBJECTS WITH MCI

It is of major importance to identify subjects with MCI who become demented, in order to give them a prognosis and to allow for starting treatment in an earlier phase than is possible now. Many variables have been tested as predictors of dementia in subjects with MCI (DeCarli, 2003). Since the majority of the subjects with dementia have Alzheimer's Disease-type (AD-type) dementia, these predictor variables can be regarded as predictors of AD-type dementia, rather than of dementia in general. Most of the studies discussed below had a follow-up period of 5 years or less (3 years on average). We will first discuss studies that tested predictive accuracy of single variables and then studies that tested predictive accuracy of a combination of variables.

Predictive Accuracy of Single Variables

Predictors Tested in More than Four Studies with a Similar Design

Age, mini-mental state examination (MMSE) score, functional impairment, memory impairment, medial temporal lobe atrophy, and the apolipoprotein E (APOE) genotype have been tested as predictor in more than four studies with a similar design. We have pooled data from these studies (Table 3). Age, the MMSE score, medial temporal lobe atrophy, and the APOE genotype were weak predictors with the odds ratios between 2 and 5 (the odds ratio is a global measure of diagnostic accuracy – an odds ratio of 25 of more indicates a good diagnostic accuracy). Functional impairment and memory impairment were moderately strong predictors with odds ratios between 5 and 8. None of the variables combined a high sensitivity (i.e. the percentage of subjects with dementia at follow-up in whom the predictor was present) with a high positive predictive value (PPV) (i.e. the percentage of subjects in whom the predictor was present and who had dementia at follow-up).

Other predictor Variables

Cognitive predictors. Impairments on neuropsychological tests in domains other than memory such as language function (as measured for example by the Boston Naming Test or verbal fluency), executive functions (as measured for example by the Stroop Color Word test card 3 or the Trail Making Test B), or attention (as measured for example by the Symbol Digit Substitution Test) were also predictors for dementia, but the predictive accuracy was generally less compared to that of tests of memory (Visser, 2003).

Neuroimaging predictors. One study found that the presence of white matter lesions was predictive of dementia (Wolf *et al.*, 2000), but this finding was not replicated in other studies (Korf *et al.*, 2004; Maruyama *et al.*, 2004). Several studies have shown that Single-Photon Emission Computed Tomography (SPECT) hypoperfusion in the parietal–temporal region or posterior cingulate gyrus may be predictive for dementia, but findings have been conflicting (Celsis *et al.*, 1997; McKelvey *et al.*, 1999; Huang *et al.*, 2002; Okamura *et al.*, 2002; Encinas *et al.*, 2003). Also, hypometabolism in the posterior cingulate gyrus or parietal–temporal area as measured with Positron Emission Tomography (PET) scanning was associated with an increased risk for dementia although not in all studies (Berent *et al.*, 1999; Arnaiz *et al.*, 2001; Chetelat *et al.*, 2003; Drzezga *et al.*, 2003; Nestor *et al.*, 2004).

Electrophysiological predictors. A combination of different background frequencies accurately identified subjects with dementia at follow-up with an overall accuracy of 82% in one small study (Jelic *et al.*, 2000). Another small study showed that event-related potentials may be useful for the prediction of dementia with an overall diagnostic accuracy of 85% (Olichney *et al.*, 2002).

Biochemical predictors. The most promising biochemical predictors of dementia are the levels of tau protein (either total tau or phosphorylated tau) and β-amyloid ending at amino acid 42 (Abeta42) in the cerebrospinal fluid. These proteins are thought to reflect the neurodegeneration caused by AD (Blennow and Hampel, 2003). An elevated concentration of total tau protein had a high sensitivity for detecting subjects with Alzheimer-type dementia at follow-up (Arai *et al.*, 1997; Maruyama *et al.*, 2004). The sensitivity of the combination of an elevated concentration of total tau protein and a decreased concentration of Abeta42 for AD-type dementia at follow-up was about 90% (Andreasen *et al.*, 1999; Riemenschneider *et al.*, 2002). The odds ratio

Table 3 Pooled estimates of predictive accuracy for dementia

	OR	Sensitivity (%)	Specificity (%)	PPV (%)	NPV (%)
Age (>75 versus 60–75)	2.0	47	70	54	67
Functional impairment (mild versus very mild)	6.8	77	66	51	86
MMSE (<27 versus >26)	3.8	57	73	49	81
Memory (impairment *yes* versus *no*)	7.6	74	73	59	85
MTL atrophy (*yes* versus *no*)	4.6	59	79	61	81
APOE (e4 allele carrier versus *no* e4 allele carrier)	3.4	61	67	45	81

OR, odds ratio; PPV, positive predictive value; NPV, negative predictive value; MMSE, mini-mental state examination; MTL, medial temporal lobe; APOE, apolipoprotein E genotype.
Data are based on a meta-analysis of prospective MCI studies from a clinical setting with a follow-up of on average 3 years (Visser *et al.*, unpublished data).

of this combination for AD-type dementia at follow-up was between 18 and 64 and the positive predictive value between 60 and 94% (Riemenschneider *et al.*, 2002; Zetterberg *et al.*, 2003). In one study, the level of tau phosphorylated at threonine 231 was predictive of dementia (Buerger *et al.*, 2002). Preliminary data indicate that an elevated level of F2-isoprostane 8,12-iso-iPF$_{2\alpha}$-VI in cerebrospinal fluid, plasma, or urine and the level of sulfatide in cerebrospinal fluid may be predictors of dementia as well (Pratico *et al.*, 2002; Han *et al.*, 2003).

It can be concluded that there is no single variable that can accurately identify subjects with dementia at follow-up from among subjects with mild cognitive impairment that will not become demented. The meta-analysis of variables that have been investigated in at least five studies indicated that no variable has an Odds Ratio (OR) higher than 8. Several new promising predictors of dementia have been investigated in small studies, but larger studies are needed to further assess the diagnostic value of these predictors.

Predictive Accuracy of a Combination of Variables

In the previous section, we showed that there is no single variable that can accurately predict progression to dementia. Several studies have suggested that a combination of variables may have a higher accuracy for Alzheimer's disease in subjects with MCI than a single variable (Okamura *et al.*, 2002; Visser *et al.*, 2002b). In the present section, we will discuss one of these multivariable approaches in more detail: the Predementia Alzheimer's disease Scale (PAS) (Table 4) (Visser *et al.*, 2002b). The PAS combines six markers for Alzheimer's disease: age, MMSE score, degree of functional impairment, cognitive test performance, medial temporal lobe atrophy, and the apolipoprotein E genotype. Each variable is scored on a three- to four-point scale and the total sum score indicates the risk for predementia Alzheimer's disease. A retrospective validation study of the PAS in two samples of subjects with MCI who were older than 55 years indicated that the best cutoff score was 6 for the full PAS and 5 for the PAS without the neuroimaging variable. The odds ratio at the best cutoff score was 25, the sensitivity 82% and the positive predictive accuracy 75%. Subjects with a score of 7 or higher had a very high risk (93%) for Alzheimer's disease in both samples, subjects with a score lower than 4 had a very low risk (7%) for Alzheimer's disease, while subjects with a score between 3 and 7 had an intermediate risk for Alzheimer's disease (46%). These intermediate scores were seen in 38% of the subjects. This means that the diagnosis remains uncertain in a substantial number of subjects.

CONCLUSIONS

MCI is a heterogeneous condition. The risk for dementia, typically Alzheimer-type dementia, is high but at longer follow-up intervals, a subset of patients do not develop dementia.

Table 4 Predementia Alzheimer's disease scale (PAS)

	−1	0	1	2	Score
A. *Age*	≤59	60–64	65–74	≥75	
B. *MMSE*[a]	–	≥28	26,27	≤25	
C. *Functional impairment*[b]					
C.1 GDS					
C.2 CDR	–	GDS 1	GDS 2	GDS 3	
C.2.1. Total box score	–	<0.5	0.5–1	≥1.5	
C.2.2. Final score	–	CDR = 0	–	CDR = 0.5	
C.3 CAMDEX		–	–	Min Dem	
D. *Neuropsychological tests*[c]	Memory ≥50 perc	Other	1 test impaired	2 tests impaired	
E. *MTL atrophy*[d]					
E.1 Qualitative rating					
Age <75 years	–	0	1	2	
Age ≥75 years	0	1	2	3	
E.2 Volumetry	≥66 perc	33–66 perc	10–33 perc	≤10 perc	
F. *ApoE genotype*	–	Other	e2e4/e3e4	e4e4	
				TOTAL SCORE	

The table indicates which score corresponds with the test result. The total score is an indication for the risk of predementia AD. More information can be found in (Visser *et al.*, 2002b), and at www-np.unimaas.nl/scales/pas.

MMSE, mini-mental state examination; GDS, Global Deterioration Scale (Reisberg *et al.*, 1982); CDR, Clinical Dementia Rating scale (Morris, 1993); MTL, medial temporal lobe; ApoE, apolipoprotein E; Min Dem, minimal dementia; perc, percentile; CAMDEX, Cambridge Mental Disorders of the Elderly Examination (Roth *et al.*, 1986).

[a]The MMSE should be corrected for age and education: if age is 75 or higher or if the period of education has been 8 years or less, one point should each time be added to the observed score; if the period of education has been 14 years or more, one point should be subtracted from the observed score. [b]One option should be used. The CDR can be scored using the Sum of Boxes score (preferred) or the final rating. [c]At least two and maximal four tests including one memory test for delayed recall or learning. An impairment is a score below the 10th percentile or above the 90th percentile (for speed related tasks) after correction for age, sex, and education. [d]One option should be used. A qualitative score can be performed on a CT scan or a MRI scan (Scheltens *et al.*, 1992; de Leon *et al.*, 1993). Volumetry should measure the hippocampus (preferred), parahippocampal gyrus, or entorhinal cortex. The percentile score is relative to age, sex, and intracranial volume.

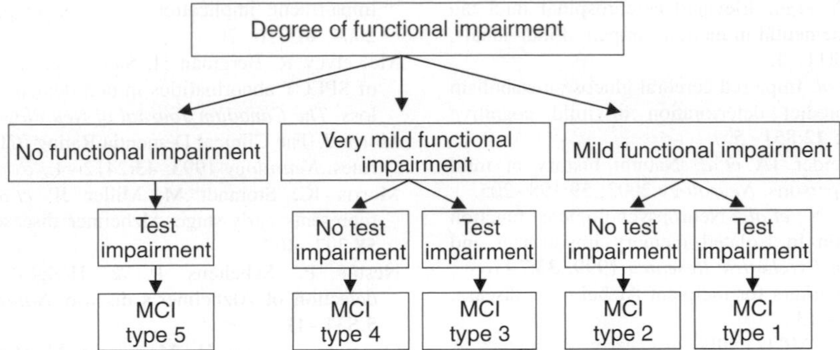

Figure 2 Classification scheme for subjects with mild cognitive impairment. The classification should be performed for each cognitive domain separately (examples of cognitive domains are memory, language, executive function, abstract reasoning/problem solving, and attention). See also www-np.unimaas.nl/scales/cirs. The functional rating is based on a clinical assessment of the performance in daily living. Very mild functional impairments mean that complaints are present and that more effort may be needed to perform tasks. The overall presentation, however, is not impaired and there is no notable deficit in employment or social situation as observed by colleagues or family members. Mild functional impairments mean that complaints are present, impairments are noticeable to colleagues, family members, or the physician, impairments may slightly affect social or occupational functioning, but does affect self-care and does not cause need for assistance from others. The impairment indicates a decrease in functioning that cannot be attributed to normal aging. Test impairment means that performance on cognitive tests is not normal as evidenced by a mild but consistent impairment on a number of tests or a severe impairment on one or more tests

Therefore, MCI should be considered as a description of the severity of cognitive impairment rather as a specific disease.

The lack of standardization of MCI definitions and terminology is confusing and makes it difficult to compare studies. In clinical practice, it may be more informative to classify subjects within the MCI spectrum instead of using a specific MCI definition. An approach for such a classification is shown in Figure 2. More information regarding this classification system can be found at www-np.unimaas.nl/scales/cirs.

There is no single predictor of Alzheimer's disease, but a multivariable approach such as the PAS may provide good diagnostic accuracy. Low-risk and high-risk subjects can be accurately identified by a multivariable approach, but there remains a substantial group of subjects with an intermediate risk for Alzheimer's disease in whom the diagnosis remains uncertain. It is expected that the diagnostic accuracy for these subjects will increase if new predictors for Alzheimer's disease such as the concentration of tau and Abeta42 in cerebrospinal fluid are included in the multivariable approach.

In clinical practice, it seems advisable to keep subjects at intermediate or high risk for dementia under clinical supervision. There is no evidence that subjects at high risk for dementia will benefit from pharmacological treatment. Preliminary data from trials that aimed to prevent progression from MCI to Alzheimer-type dementia with acetylcholine esterase inhibitors, vitamin E, piracetam, or rofecoxib showed lack of efficacy (data presented at the 9th International Conference on Alzheimer's Disease and related disorders in Philadelphia, 19–22 July 2004).

Since subjects continue to develop dementia at longer follow-up studies, studies that investigate predictors of long-term outcome are needed to improve the identification of subjects with MCI who will become demented.

KEY POINTS

- There are no standard criteria for MCI.
- MCI is not related to one specific disorder.
- Subjects with MCI have a high risk for Alzheimer-type dementia, but even in the long term, a substantial number of subjects do not develop dementia.
- A combination of variables may be useful to identify subjects with MCI who are at high risk for Alzheimer-type dementia.
- MCI should be considered as a syndrome rather than as a disease.

KEY REFERENCES

- DeCarli C. Mild cognitive impairment: prevalence, prognosis, aetiology, and treatment. *Lancet. Neurology* 2003; **2**:15–21.
- Nestor P, Scheltens P & Hodges J. Advances in the early detection of Alzheimer's disease. *Nature Reviews. Neuroscience* 2004; **5**:S34–41.
- Petersen RC, Doody R, Kurz A *et al.* Current concepts in mild cognitive impairment. *Archives of Neurology* 2001; **58**:1985–92.
- Visser PJ. *Predictors of Alzheimer Type Dementia in Subjects with Mild Cognitive Impairments* 2000; Neuropsych Publishers, Maastricht.

REFERENCES

Albert SM, Michaels K, Padilla M *et al.* Functional significance of mild cognitive impairment in elderly patients without a dementia diagnosis. *The American Journal of Geriatric Psychiatry* 1999; **7**:213–20.

Andreasen N, Minthon L, Vanmechelen E *et al.* Cerebrospinal fluid tau and A-beta-42 as predictors of development of Alzheimer's disease in patients with mild cognitive impairment. *Neuroscience Letters* 1999; **273**:5–8.

Arai H, Nakagawa T, Kosaka Y *et al.* Elevated cerebrospinal fluid tau protein level as a predictor of dementia in memory-impaired individuals. *Alzheimer's Research* 1997; **3**:211–3.

Arnaiz E, Jelic V, Almkvist O *et al.* Impaired cerebral glucose metabolism and cognitive functioning predict deterioration in mild cognitive impairment. *Neuroreport* 2001; **12**:851–5.

Bennett DA, Wilson RS, Schneider JA *et al.* Natural history of mild cognitive impairment in older persons. *Neurology* 2002; **59**:198–205.

Berent S, Giordani B, Foster N *et al.* Neuropsychological function and cerebral glucose utilization in isolated memory impairment and Alzheimer's disease. *Journal of Psychiatric Research* 1999; **33**:7–16.

Blennow K & Hampel H. CSF markers for incipient Alzheimer's disease. *Lancet. Neurology* 2003; **2**:605–13.

Bruscoli M & Lovestone S. Is MCI really just early dementia? A systematic review of conversion studies. *International Psychogeriatrics* 2004; **16**:129–40.

Buerger K, Teipel SJ, Zinkowski R *et al.* CSF tau protein phosphorylated at threonine 231 correlates with cognitive decline in MCI subjects. *Neurology* 2002; **59**:627–9.

Celsis P, Agniel A, Cardebat D *et al.* Age related cognitive decline: a clinical entity? A longitudinal study of cerebral blood flow and memory performance. *Journal of Neurology, Neurosurgery, and Psychiatry* 1997; **62**:601–8.

Chetelat G, Desgranges B, De La Sayette V *et al.* Mild cognitive impairment: can FDG-PET predict who is to rapidly convert to Alzheimer's disease? *Neurology* 2003; **60**:1374–7.

Conquer JA, Tierney MC, Zecevic J *et al.* Fatty acid analysis of blood plasma of patients with Alzheimer's disease, other types of dementia, and cognitive impairment. *Lipids* 2000; **35**:1305–12.

Crook T, Bartus RT, Ferris SH *et al.*, Report of the National Institute of Mental Health Work Group. Age-associated memory impairment: proposed criteria and measures of clinical change. *Developmental Neuropsychology* 1986; **2**:261–76.

DeCarli C. Mild cognitive impairment: prevalence, prognosis, aetiology, and treatment. *Lancet. Neurology* 2003; **2**:15–21.

de Leon MJ, George AE, Convit A *et al.* The radiologic prediction of Alzheimer disease: the atrophic hippocampal formation. *American Journal of Neuroradiology* 1993; **14**:897–906.

Devanand DP, Folz M, Gorlyn M *et al.* Questionable dementia: clinical course and predictors of outcome. *Journal of the American Geriatrics Society* 1997; **45**:321–8.

Drzezga A, Lautenschlager N, Siebner H *et al.* Cerebral metabolic changes accompanying conversion of mild cognitive impairment into Alzheimer's disease: a PET follow-up study. *European Journal of Nuclear Medicine and Molecular Imaging* 2003; **30**:1104–13.

Ebly E, Hogan D & Parhad I. Cognitive impairment in the nondemented elderly. Results from the Canadian study of health and aging. *Archives of Neurology* 1995; **52**:612–9.

Encinas M, De Juan R, Marcos A *et al.* Regional cerebral blood flow assessed with 99mTc-ECD SPET as a marker of progression of mild cognitive impairment to Alzheimer's disease. *European Journal of Nuclear Medicine and Molecular Imaging* 2003; **30**:1473–80.

Han X, Fagan AM, Cheng H *et al.* Cerebrospinal fluid sulfatide is decreased in subjects with incipient dementia. *Annals of Neurology* 2003; **54**:115–9.

Huang C, Wahlund LO, Svensson L *et al.* Cingulate cortex hypoperfusion predicts Alzheimer's disease in mild cognitive impairment. *BMC Neurology* 2002; **2**:9.

Jelic V, Johansson SE, Almkvist O *et al.* Quantitative electroencephalography in mild cognitive impairment: longitudinal changes and possible prediction of Alzheimer's disease. *Neurobiology of Aging* 2000; **21**:533–40.

Korf E, Wahlund L-O, Visser P & Scheltens P. Medial temporal lobe atrophy on MRI predicts dementia in patients with mild cognitive impairment. *Neurology* 2004; **63**:94–100.

Larrieu S, Letenneur L, Orgogozo JM *et al.* Incidence and outcome of mild cognitive impairment in a population-based prospective cohort. *Neurology* 2002; **59**:1594–9.

Levy R Chairperson. Aging-associated cognitive decline. *International Psychogeriatrics* 1994; **6**:63–8.

Maruyama M, Matsui T, Tanji H *et al.* Cerebrospinal fluid tau protein and periventricular white matter lesions in patients with mild cognitive impairment: implications for 2 major pathways. *Archives of Neurology* 2004; **61**:716–20.

McKelvey R, Bergman H, Stern J *et al.* Lack of prognostic significance of SPECT abnormalities in non-demented elderly subjects with memory loss. *The Canadian Journal of Neurological Sciences* 1999; **26**:23–8.

Morris J. The Clinical Dementia Rating (CDR): current version and scoring rules. *Neurology* 1993; **43**:2412–4.

Morris JC, Storandt M, Miller JP *et al.* Mild cognitive impairment represents early-stage Alzheimer disease. *Archives of Neurology* 2001; **58**:397–405.

Nestor P, Scheltens P & Hodges J. Advances in the early detection of Alzheimer's disease. *Nature Reviews. Neuroscience* 2004; **5**:S34–41.

Okamura N, Arai H, Maruyama M *et al.* Combined analysis of CSF tau levels and [(123)I] Iodoamphetamine SPECT in Mild cognitive impairment: implications for a novel predictor of Alzheimer's disease. *American Journal of Psychiatry* 2002; **159**:474–6.

Olichney JM, Morris SK, Ochoa C *et al.* Abnormal verbal event related potentials in mild cognitive impairment and incipient Alzheimer's disease. *Journal of Neurology, Neurosurgery, and Psychiatry* 2002; **73**:377–84.

Petersen R, Smith G, Waring S *et al.* Mild cognitive impairment. Clinical characterization and outcome. *Archives of Neurology* 1999; **56**:303–8.

Petersen RC, Doody R, Kurz A *et al.* Current concepts in mild cognitive impairment. *Archives of Neurology* 2001; **58**:1985–92.

Pratico D, Clark CM, Liun F *et al.* Increase of brain oxidative stress in mild cognitive impairment: a possible predictor of Alzheimer disease. *Archives of Neurology* 2002; **59**:972–6.

Reisberg B, Ferris SH, De Leon MJ & Crook T. The global deterioration scale for assessment of primary degenerative dementia. *American Journal of Psychiatry* 1982; **139**:1136–9.

Riemenschneider M, Lautenschlager N, Wagenpfeil S *et al.* Cerebrospinal fluid tau and beta-amyloid 42 proteins identify Alzheimer disease in subjects with mild cognitive impairment. *Archives of Neurology* 2002; **59**:1729–34.

Roth M, Tym E, Mountjoy CQ *et al.* A standardized instrument for the diagnoses of mental disorder in the elderly with special reference to the early detection of dementia. *British Journal of Psychiatry* 1986; **149**:698–709.

Scheltens P, Leys D, Barkhof F *et al.* Atrophy of medial temporal lobes on MRI in "probable" Alzheimer's disease and normal ageing: diagnostic value and neuropsychological correlates. *Journal of Neurology, Neurosurgery, and Psychiatry* 1992; **55**:967–72.

Tei H, Miyazaki A, Iwata M *et al.* Early-stage Alzheimer's disease and multiple subcortical infarction with mild cognitive impairment: neuropsychological comparison using an easily applicable test battery. *Dementia and Geriatric Cognitive Disorders* 1997; **8**:355–8.

Thompson SA, Graham KS, Patterson K *et al.* Is knowledge of famous people disproportionately impaired in patients with early and questionable Alzheimer's disease? *Neuropsychology* 2002; **16**:344–58.

Tierney MC, Szalai JP, Snow WG *et al.* A prospective study of the clinical utility of ApoE genotype in the prediction of outcome in patients with memory impairment. *Neurology* 1996; **46**:149–54.

Visser PJ. *Predictors of Alzheimer Type Dementia in Subjects with Mild Cognitive Impairments* 2000; Neuropsych Publishers, Maastricht.

Visser PJ. Diagnosis of predementia AD in a clinical setting. In RW Richter & B Zoeller-Richter (eds) *Alzheimer's Disease. A Physician's Guide to Practical Management* 2003, pp 157–64; Humana Press, New Jersey.

Visser PJ, Verhey FRJ, Hofman PAM *et al.* Medial temporal lobe atrophy predicts Alzheimer's disease in subjects with minor cognitive impairment. *Journal of Neurology, Neurosurgery, and Psychiatry* 2002a; **72**:491–7.

Visser PJ, Verhey FRJ, Kester A, Jolles J *et al. Predictors of Dementia in Subjects with Mild Cognitive Impairment- a Quantitative Meta-Analysis* unpublished data.

Visser PJ, Verhey FRJ, Scheltens P *et al.* Diagnostic accuracy of the Preclinical AD Scale (PAS) in cognitively mildly impaired subjects. *Journal of Neurology* 2002b; **249**:312–9.

Wolf H, Ecke GM, Bettin S *et al.* Do white matter changes contribute to the subsequent development of dementia in patients with mild cognitive impairment? A longitudinal study. *International Journal of Geriatric Psychiatry* 2000; **15**:803–12.

Wu CC, Mungas D, Petkov CI *et al.* Brain structure and cognition in a community sample of elderly Latinos. *Neurology* 2002; **59**:383–91.

Zetterberg H, Wahlund LO & Blennow K. Cerebrospinal fluid markers for prediction of Alzheimer's disease. *Neuroscience Letters* 2003; **352**:67–9.

95

Vascular Dementia

Ingmar Skoog
University of Gothenburg, Gothenburg, Sweden

BACKGROUND

Cognitive function declines with increasing age. This decline differs between individuals probably due to genetic predisposition, and educational, and professional background. The decline may be accelerated by different insults to the brain, such as Alzheimer's disease (AD), cerebrovascular disease (CVD), other brain disorders, and different peripheral disorders such as cardiovascular diseases. When the cognitive function reaches a certain threshold, giving rise to difficulties in everyday life, the term dementia is used. The two most common causes of dementia are AD and cerebrovascular disorders. The latter cause of dementia is often subsumed under the term vascular dementia (VaD). AD and CVD often coexist in the same patient, and is then labeled mixed dementia (Langa *et al.*, 2004).

Current criteria for dementia and its subtypes are old, more than 10 years, and often show inconsistencies in their descriptions (Skoog and Copeland, 2002). Criteria such as those of the ICD-10 (World Health Organization, 1993) and diagnostic and statistical manual of mental disorders (DSM-IV) (American Psychiatric Association, 1994), describe dementia as a global decline in intellectual function affecting memory, orientation, visuospatial abilities, executive function, language, and thinking. It is often accompanied by changes in personality and emotions. These criteria also state that the decline in cognitive function must include significant memory dysfunction. This concept is based on the symptoms seen in AD. However, CVD may cause significant cognitive dysfunction with relatively preserved memory function. The term vascular cognitive impairment has therefore been introduced during recent years (Bowler and Hachinski, 1995). This term includes both VaD and other forms of cognitive decline caused by cerebrovascular and cardiovascular diseases.

VaD can thus be regarded as one manifestation of CVD, together with, for example, focal motor and sensory symptoms. There are many different etiologies of VaD, including stroke, silent infarcts, ischemic white-matter lesions (WMLs), hereditary cerebral hemorrhage with amyloidosis, granular cortical atrophy, hypertensive encephalopathy, cerebral amyloid angiopathy, and cerebral vasculitis. Most cases of VaD exhibit a combination of vascular changes (Munoz, 1991). The two most common causes of VaD are, however, stroke and WMLs. Cerebrovascular disorders are also associated with the overall cognitive decline observed in elderly populations (Breteler *et al.*, 1994a,b,c; Skoog *et al.*, 1996). Several causes of VaD or vascular cognitive impairment are potentially preventable, and can even be treated.

Diagnostic Criteria

The Hachinski Ischemic Score (Hachinski *et al.*, 1975) was the most widely used instrument for the diagnosis of VaD, or multi-infarct dementia (MID) as it was called, from the 1970s to the early 1990s. It comprises a symptom check list which incorporates some symptoms that are believed to be essential in the stroke-related form of VaD, such as abrupt onset, stepwise deterioration, fluctuating course, a history of stroke, and focal neurological symptoms and signs. It also incorporates risk factors such as hypertension and cardiovascular diseases. The assumption was that MID was caused by embolic phenomena, so that the onset would be sudden and acute. Subsequent further emboli would produce other sudden deteriorations, perhaps followed by some improvement.

Memory impairment is mandatory for the diagnosis of VaD in the ICD-10 (World Health Organization, 1993), DSM-III-R (American Psychiatric Association, 1987) and DSM-IV (American Psychiatric Association 1994) criteria. This is not ideal as cognitive dysfunction in CVD may be substantial while memory dysfunction is mild (Bowler and Hachinski, 1995). The ICD-10 requires that "deficits in higher cognitive functions are unevenly distributed" and DSM-III-R that there is "a patchy distribution of deficits (i.e. affecting some functions, but not others) early in the course." The latter was, however, no longer included in the DSM-IV.

Principles and Practice of Geriatric Medicine, 4th Edition. Edited by M.S. John Pathy, Alan J. Sinclair and John E. Morley.

Although stroke increases the risk of developing dementia several-fold (Tatemichi *et al.*, 1992; Pohjasvaara *et al.*, 1997; Linden *et al.*, 2004), the contributions of a stroke or an infarct for the clinical symptoms of dementia are not always easy to elucidate. Most criteria leave it to the clinician to make the decision whether the CVD "may be judged to be etiologically related to the dementia" (Skoog and Copeland, 2002).

In most criteria for VaD, the definition of CVD is based on the history or findings of focal neurological motor symptom/signs, or brain imaging findings of CVD. DSM-IV gives examples of signs, while the ICD-10 specifically requires that at least one should be (1) unilateral spastic weakness of the limbs, (2) unilateral increased tendon reflexes, (3) extensor plantar response, or (4) pseudobulbar palsy.

The DSM-IV specifies that there should be signs AND symptoms OR laboratory evidence indicative of CVD (e.g brain imaging findings of multiple infarctions involving the cortex and subcortical white matter) that are judged to be etiologically related to the disturbance, while ICD-10 requires that there should be evidence from history, examination OR tests of a significant CVD, which may be reasonably judged to be etiologically related to the dementia (e.g history of stroke or evidence of cerebral infarction). In the National Institute of Neurological Disorders and Stroke and the Association Internationale pour la Recherche et l'Enseignement en Neurosciences (NINDS-AIREN) criteria (Román *et al.*, 1993), a diagnosis of probably VaD requires that focal signs consistent with stroke AND relevant CVD by brain imaging should be present. Tatemichi, one of the authors of the NINDS-AIREN criteria published a modified version (Tatemichi *et al.*, 1994b) in which this criterion was changed to focal signs consistent with stroke OR relevant CVD by brain imaging. The first criterion is probably too strict and underestimates the occurrence of VaD (Skoog and Copeland, 2002), especially since individuals with silent infarcts or WMLs without stroke symptoms will not be considered. In a study on 85-year-olds (Skoog *et al.*, 1993), 13% of the demented had VaD based on the criteria "focal signs consistent with stroke AND relevant CVD by brain imaging" while 47% had VaD with the criterium "focal signs consistent with stroke OR relevant CVD by brain imaging". The NINDS-AIREN criteria allows a diagnosis of "possible" VaD in the presence of dementia with focal neurological signs in patients in whom brain imaging studies are missing; or in the absence of a clear temporal relationship between dementia and stroke; or in patients with subtle onset and variable course. This means that if CVD is present in a patient with dementia, a diagnosis of VaD will be made. Furthermore, the interpretation of a single stroke leading to dementia likely differs between centers, and may be one reason for the disparate results regarding the prevalence of VaD.

The temporal relationship between stroke and the onset of dementia is often thought to strengthen the possibility that the two disorders are etiologically related. The NINDS-AIREN criteria suggest an arbitrary limit of 3 months for the onset of dementia after stroke. However, a stroke which occurred years before may still indicate the presence of CVD.

Epidemiology

Almost all epidemiological studies reporting on the frequency of VaD are concerned with the subtype related to clinically manifest stroke or transitory ischemic attacks (TIA). As may be seen in Table 1, the proportion of VaD vary widely between studies. The differences might be due to differences in diagnostic criteria, differences in the rate of cerebrovascular disorders, or constitutional or environmental factors. It may also reflect the efforts done to diagnose CVD and whether brain imaging has been used. Although the prevalence of dementia is similar in most parts of the world, there are differences regarding the type of dementia. MID is reported to be more common in Finland, the former Soviet Union, and Asian countries, including Japan and China, than in western Europe and the United States, where AD is generally reported to be the most common type of dementia. However, more recent studies from China and Japan report similar proportions of VaD as in western countries (Zhang *et al.*, 2005). Also, the proportion diagnosed with VaD in autopsy studies vary (Table 2), probably due to different samples and the importance given to CVD as a cause of the dementia. It is noteworthy that few patients in autopsy studies were regarded as having pure VaD.

Table 1 Proportion of vascular dementia in population studies

	Country	Sex	Proportion (%) with vascular dementia among the demented
Fratiglioni *et al.* (1991)	Sweden	Male	26
		Female	24
Ott *et al.* (1995)	Holland	Male	18
		Female	15
Rocca *et al.* (1990)[a]	Italy	Male	40
		Female	35
O'Connor *et al.* (1989)	Britain	All	21
Aevarsson and Skoog (1997)[a]	Sweden	Male	44
		Female	45
Livingston *et al.* (1990)			
Manubens *et al.* (1995)	Spain	Male	16
		Female	11
Brayne and Calloway (1989)	Britain	Female	31

[a]CT, scan aided in diagnosis of vascular dementia.

Table 2 Proportion of vascular dementia in autopsy studies

Study	Sample size	VaD%	Pure VaD, %	Setting
Galasko *et al.* (1994)	170	9	2	AD research centers
Ince *et al.* (1995)	69	6	NA	Nursing home
Drach *et al.* (1997)	59	27	12	Nursing home
Holmes *et al.* (1999)	80	29	9	Dementia register
Lim *et al.* (1999)	134	34	3	AD patient registry
Barker *et al.* (2002)	384	18	3	Memory clinics, GP

Stroke-related Dementia

All criteria for VaD include history of stroke due to cerebral infarcts. Most cerebral infarcts are due to thromboembolism from extracranial arteries and the heart, and are often related to large vessel disease. The typical patient has a history of stroke or TIA with acute focal neurological symptoms and signs. The main risk factors for stroke are hypertension, diabetes mellitus, atherosclerosis, atrial fibrillation, smoking, and hypercholesterolemia (Qiu *et al.*, 2002). All these risk factors are potentially treatable.

Stroke is a component of most criteria for VaD or vascular cognitive impairment, but is stroke related to an increased frequency of dementia? According to Tatemichi *et al.* (1992, 1993, 1994a), subjects with ischemic stroke had at least nine times greater risk for dementia than stroke-free controls. Pohjasvaara *et al.* (1997) also reported an increased prevalence of dementia in stroke victims, as well as a decrease in independent living for those with dementia. Linden *et al.* (2004) recently reported that stroke victims had 2–3 times increased risk for dementia. The relative risk for dementia compared to population controls was larger in younger age-groups, but the frequency of dementia was higher after the age of 80, approximately 35%. Furthermore, 60% of nondemented stroke victims had some cognitive dysfunction. In the population studies from Gothenburg, Sweden, Liebetrau *et al.* (2003) reported that stroke increased the risk for dementia 2–3 times in 85-year-olds.

However, cerebral infarcts may occur without focal symptoms, so-called silent infarcts. Silent infarcts become more common with increasing age (Vermeer *et al.*, 2002). Silent infarcts have long believed to be benign incidental findings on brain imaging. Recently, researchers from the Rotterdam Study reported that individuals with silent infarcts have an increased risk for clinical stroke (Vermeer *et al.*, 2002) or dementia (Vermeer *et al.*, 2003) during follow-up. Liebetrau *et al.* (2004) reported that 10% of 85-year-olds had silent infarcts on computerized tomography (CT) and that these lesions were related to a twofold increased prevalence of dementia.

If focal symptoms occur in connection with the onset of dementia, it is considered to strengthen the diagnosis of VaD (Román *et al.*, 1993). However, the recent reports that silent infarcts are common in the elderly and that they are related to an increased risk for dementia may question this statement. The typical clinical course of VaD includes sudden onset, stepwise deterioration, and a fluctuating course. In the early stages, the cognitive impairment may have a large variability depending on the site of the lesions. However, a large group of patients with CVD have a gradual onset of dementia with a slowly progressive course (Fischer *et al.*, 1990) and without focal signs or infarcts on brain imaging, which makes it difficult to differentiate from AD. It has been suggested that individuals with cortical strokes show less decline in cognitive function than those with subcortical CVD (Gunstad *et al.*, 2005). Other cardiovascular manifestations, including myocardial infarction and hypertension, are common in the patients.

The pathogenesis behind stroke-related dementia is not clear. It has been suggested that the dementia may be related to the location or the volume of the infarcts, but there are also other possibilities. The risk factors suggested for VaD are similar to those in stroke, including male sex, hypertension, diabetes mellitus, smoking, and cardiac diseases (Skoog, 1998). Non-stroke-related risk factors are similar to those found in AD (Skoog, 1998), including higher age, lower level of formal education, family history of dementia, and the presence of cerebral atrophy, supporting the view that "poststroke dementia" is a combination of the direct consequences of stroke, and preexisting AD pathology. Pure VaD, without any AD brain changes, is probably rare.

Subcortical White-matter Lesions

The other dominating CVD associated with dementia and cognitive decline are subcortical WMLs (Fernando and Ince, 2004), which has been suggested to be the most common form of VaD. The neuropathological findings include marked or diffuse ischemic demyelination and moderate loss of axons with astrogliosis and incomplete infarction in subcortical structures of both hemispheres and arteriosclerotic changes with hyalinization or fibrosis and thickening of the vessel walls and narrowing of the lumina of the small penetrating arteries and arterioles in the WM (Román, 1987; Brun and Englund, 1986). The cortex is generally well preserved, as are the subcortical U fibers and corpus callosum, probably due to a different blood supply.

The main hypothesis regarding the cause of WMLs is that long-standing hypertension causes lipohyalinosis and thickening of the vessel walls with the narrowing of the lumen of the small perforating arteries and arterioles that nourish the deep WM (Román, 1987). Episodes of hypotension, related to, for instance, aging, drugs, or cardiac failure, may lead to hypoperfusion and hypoxia-ischemia, leading to loss of myelin in the WM. The deep WM has few collaterals, which makes it more vulnerable to ischemia than the cortex when a penetrating vessel occludes. Furthermore, myelin is probably more vulnerable to ischemia than axons are (Englund and Brun, 1990). It has been suggested that the arterial changes are due to exposure of vessel walls to increased pressure over time. The greater the pressure and/or lifespan, the more likely are these changes to be present. This may be one reason for the observed increase with age reported in most studies.

WMLs appear as low density areas on CT scans and as hyperdense areas on magnetic resonance imaging (MRI). In 15 studies or case reports on the clinicopathologic correlations of subjects with WMLs on CT, the histopathologic picture described above had been reported in 53 out of 55 autopsied cases (Skoog *et al.*, 1994). WMLs on MRI are often reported as being the same entity as WMLs on CT. However, WMLs on MRI correspond to several different histological findings, most often état crible, and often show no correlation with cognitive decline and dementia. MRI is more sensitive than CT to detect changes in the white matter, but has a lower specificity, and WMLs on MRI may bear little relationship to the hypodensities seen on CT.

MRI studies have generally reported substantially higher rates of WMLs than CT studies. The population study from Rotterdam (Breteler *et al.*, 1994b) reported that 11% in the age strata 65–69 years, 21% in those aged 70–74 years, 27% in 70–79-year-olds and 54% in those aged 80–84 years had WMLs, and the Helsinki Aging Brain Study (Ylikoski *et al.*, 1995) reported periventricular hyperintensities in 21% of those aged 55–75 years and 65% in those above that age. In the latter two studies severity also increased with age. A recent population-based neuropathological study reported that 94% of demented subjects had WMLs (Fernando and Ince, 2004).

The cognitive decline in subjects with WMLs has been suggested to be caused by a disconnection of subcortical–cortical pathways, producing a decline in abilities related to subcortical or frontal lobe structures. Individuals with WMLs generally exhibit psychomotor slowness (Skoog *et al.*, 1996; Junqué *et al.* 1990; Ylikoski *et al.*, 1993; Breteler *et al.*, 1994c) and deficiencies in frontal lobe skills (Boone *et al.*, 1992), such as executive dysfunction.

Dementia associated with WMLs often has an insidious onset and a slowly progressive course (Román, 1987; Gunstad *et al.*, 2005), which makes it difficult to distinguish from AD. In the initial stage, there may be transient and fleeting attacks of focal neurological deficits, with a subacute accumulation of focal deficits. The typical picture includes subcortical symptoms with extrapyramidal signs, especially psychomotor retardation, and a frontal lobe syndrome with executive dysfunction, apathy, loss of drive, and emotional blunting. Other features may include bilateral or unilateral pyramidal tract signs, and hemi- or motoranesthesia, pseudobulbar palsy, urinary incontinence, and gait dysfunction. However, WMLs seldom occurs as the sole cause of dementia, and the clinical picture may vary depending on what other causes contribute to the dementia. Recently, it was reported that punctate WMLs on MRI do not progress, while confluent white-matter abnormalities are progressive, and thus more malignant in the long-time (Schmidt *et al.*, 2003).

The main risk factor for WMLs is hypertension, and hypertension-clustering factors.

Mixed Dementias

The common coincidence of AD and VaD is becoming increasingly recognized (Langa *et al.*, 2004; Fernando and Ince, 2004), and this may even be the most common form of dementia. Although CVD increases the risk of developing dementia (Tatemichi *et al.*, 1992; Pohjasvaara *et al.*, 1997; Linden *et al.*, 2004; Liebetrau *et al.*, 2003; Skoog *et al.*, 1994), the contribution of CVD for the clinical symptoms of dementia are not always easy to elucidate. CVD may be the main cause of dementia in an individual, it may be the event that finally overcomes the brain's compensatory capacity in a subject whose brain is already compromised by Alzheimer pathology, albeit not yet clinically manifest, and in many instances minor manifestations of both disorders which individually would not be enough to produce dementia may produce it together (Erkinjuntti and Hachinski, 1993a,b). On a clinical basis, it is, however, difficult to differentiate mixed dementia from VaD. CVD as a contributing cause of dementia may be under-diagnosed as sometimes the onset is insidious, the course gradual, the infarctions clinically silent, and the infarcts not detectable by CT or MRI of the brain (Skoog, 1994; Fischer *et al.*, 1990). Pure VaD may also be overdiagnosed as the presence of stroke, WMLs, or other CVD does not necessarily mean that they are the only cause of the dementia (Skoog, 1994). Often AD becomes a diagnosis by exclusion, and the diagnosis of VaD will be assigned if the patient has a history of CVD. This leads to a situation where the dementias will not infrequently be divided into one group with stroke and one without. Even the histopathological diagnoses of AD and VaD are uncertain. Extensive histopathological signs of AD (Tomlinson *et al.*, 1970; Arriagada *et al.*, 1992) and CVD (Del Ser *et al.*, 1990; Tomlinson *et al.*, 1970) have been found in persons who show no clinical signs of dementia during life. In fact, the MRC-FAS study (Neuropathology Group. Medical Research Council Cognitive Function and Aging Study, 2001), and the Nun Study (Snowdon *et al.*, 1997) reported that only about 50% of those fulfilling neuropathological criteria for AD were demented during life. This shows that AD alone does not always lead to dementia. A considerable proportion of subjects fulfilling the diagnosis of probable NINCDS-ADRDA criteria for AD or probable NINDS-AIREN for VaD have mixed pathologies (Holmes *et al.*, 1999; Lim *et al.*, 1999). WMLs have been described on both brain imaging and at autopsy in cases of Alzheimer's disease (Brun and Englund, 1986; De la Monte, 1989; Skoog *et al.*, 1994). The Nun Study showed that CVD increased the possibility that individuals with AD lesions in their brains will express a dementia syndrome (Snowdon *et al.*, 1997). Furthermore, patients with VaD may exhibit cholinergic deficits, similar to that seen in AD, due to ischemia of basal forebrain nuclei and of cholinergic pathways (Erkinjuntti *et al.*, 2004; Roman, 2005). Also other markers of AD, such as cerebrospinal tau (Skoog *et al.*, 1995) and β-amyloid (Skoog *et al.*, 2003) may show similar patterns in VaD as in AD. In addition, vascular risk factors may also be important for the development of AD (Skoog and Gustafson, 2003).

DIAGNOSIS

The first step in the diagnostic work-up is to determine whether the patient has cognitive dysfunction, and to evaluate the nature of this dysfunction. Such examination should be performed on all elderly patients with a recent stroke. For this purpose, a simple screening instrument may be used, for example, the widely used Mini Mental State Examination. Examples of other tests include examinations of executive function, the clock test, word fluency, naming ability, and five-items memory test. Individuals with dementia related to CVD may often be difficult to test because of language dysfunction.

In the second phase, a possible cerebrovascular cause of the dementia is identified. Auxiliary investigations, including brain imaging are necessary in this step, not only to identify CVD but also to diagnose other conditions that might contribute to the cognitive decline, for example, cardiovascular diseases, low-pressure hydrocephalus, subdural hematoma, brain tumors, deficiency states, infections, and depression. It is important to note that in the elderly there are often multiple causes of dementia, and that every contributing treatable cause that can be diagnosed may be important in the treatment of the patient. The examinations include careful history-taking, neurological, psychiatric, and physical examinations, interview of a close informant, brain imaging such as CT scan or MRI of the head, a chest X ray, ECG and biochemical screening including vitamin B12 level, a thyroid function test and, in selected cases, cerebrospinal fluid examinations. Brain imaging is important to detect WMLs and cerebral infarcts. An ECG should be performed to detect arrhythmias. Traditionally, AD has been a diagnosis of exclusion and the diagnosis of VaD has often been assigned if the patient has a history of stroke thought to be related to dementia onset. However, from a clinical standpoint, it is neither important nor possible to differentiate between AD and VaD in most cases. Most cases of VaD are probably of a mixed etiology (see Table 2), and older patients with AD may often have concomitant CVD, which needs treatment. Therefore, treatment should be directed both to the CVD and the AD.

TREATMENT POSSIBILITIES

The general strategy in the treatment of VaD is to prevent new strokes or infarcts. Although no formal studies have been performed, the use of anticoagulant agents, for example, low-dose treatment with salicylates, is often used. Treatment of cardiac arrhythmias, high blood pressure, and hypercholesterolemia is also essential. Regarding white-matter dementia, antihypertensive treatment may potentially prevent the changes in the small vessels. VaD often have concomitant AD. In these cases, one should initiate treatment with an acetylcholinesteras inhibitor (Erkinjuntti *et al.*, 2002, 2004).

KEY POINTS

- Vascular cognitive impairment is a relatively new term that embraces both vascular dementia and other forms of cognitive decline caused by cerebrovascular and cardiovascular diseases.
- Stroke-related dementia is likely to be more common than previously reported and may occur in patients with silent cerebral infarcts and the absence of focal symptoms.
- Subcortical white-matter lesions (WML) linked to long-standing hypertension appear to be an important pathogenetic mechanism in vascular dementia.

REFERENCES

Aevarsson O & Skoog I. Dementia disorders in a birth cohort followed from age 85 to 88. The influence of mortality, non-response and diagnostic change on prevalence. *International Psychogeriatrics/IPA* 1997; **9**:11–23.

American Psychiatric Association. *Diagnostic and Statistical Manual of Mental Disorders* 1987, 3rd edn, revised; American Psychiatric Association, Washington.

American Psychiatric Association. *Diagnostic and Statistical Manual of Mental Disorders* 1994, 4th edn; American Psychiatric Association, Washington.

Arriagada P, Marzloff K & Hyman B. Distribution of Alzheimer-type pathologic changes in nondemented elderly individuals matches the pattern in Alzheimer's disease. *Neurology* 1992; **42**:1681–8.

Barker WW, Luis CA & Kashuba A. Relative frequencies of Alzheimer disease, Lewy body, vascular and frontotemporal dementia, and hippocampal sclerosis in the State of Florida Brain Bank. *Alzheimer Disease and Associated Disorders* 2002; **16**:203–12.

Boone KB, Miller BL, Lesser BL *et al.* Neuropsychological correlates of white-matter lesions in healthy elderly subjects. A threshold effect. *Archives of Neurology* 1992; **49**:549–54.

Bowler JV & Hachinski V. Vascular cognitive impairment: a new approach to vascular dementia. *Bailliére's Clinical Neurology* 1995, pp 357–76; Bailliére Tindall.

Brayne C & Calloway P. An epidemiological study of dementia in a rural population of elderly women. *The British Journal of Psychiatry* 1989; **155**:214–21.

Breteler MMB, Claus JJ, Grobbee DE & Hofman A. Cardiovascular disease and distribution of cognitive function in elderly people: the Rotterdam study. *British Medical Journal* 1994a; **308**:1604–8.

Breteler MMB, van Swieten JC, Bots ML *et al.* Cerebral white matter lesions, vascular risk factors, and cognitive function in a population-based study: the Rotterdam study. *Neurology* 1994b; **44**:1246–52.

Breteler MMB, van Amerongen NM, van Swieten JC *et al.*, The Rotterdam Study. Cognitive correlates of ventricular enlargement and cerebral white matter lesions on Magnetic Resonance Imaging. *Stroke* 1994c; **25**:1109–15.

Brun A & Englund E. A white matter disorder in dementia of the Alzheimer type: a pathoanatomical study. *Annals of Neurology* 1986; **19**:253–62.

De la Monte SM. Quantitation of cerebral atrophy in preclinical and end-stage Alzheimer's disease. *Annals of Neurology* 1989; **25**:450–9.

Del Ser T, Bermejo F, Portera A *et al.* Vascular dementia. A clinicopathological study. *Journal of the Neurological Sciences* 1990; **96**:1–17.

Drach LM, Steinmetz HE, Wach S & Bohl J. High proportion of dementia with Lewy bodies in the postmortems of a mental hospital in Germany. *International Journal of Geriatric Psychiatry* 1997; **12**:301–6.

Englund E & Brun A. White matter changes in dementia of Alzheimer's type. The difference in vulnerability between cell compartments. *Histopathology* 1990; **16**:433–9.

Erkinjuntti T & Hachinski V. Dementia post stroke. *Physical Medicine and Rehabilitation: State of the Art Reviews* 1993a, vol 7, pp 195–212; Hanley & Belfus, Philadelphia.

Erkinjuntti T & Hachinski V. Rethinking vascular dementia. *Cerebrovascular Diseases* 1993b; **3**:3–23.

Erkinjuntti T, Kurz A, Gauthier S *et al.* Efficacy of galantamine in probable vascular dementia and Alzheimer's disease combined with cerebrovascular disease: a randomised trial. *Lancet* 2002; **359**:1283–90.

Erkinjuntti T, Roman G & Gauthier S. Treatment of vascular dementia–evidence from clinical trials with cholinesterase inhibitors. *Journal of the Neurological Sciences* 2004; **226**:63–6.

Fernando MS & Ince PG, MRC Cognitive Function and Ageing Neuropathology Study Group. Vascular pathologies and cognition in a population-based cohort of elderly people. *Journal of the Neurological Sciences* 2004; **226**:13–7.

Fischer P, Gatterer G, Marterer A *et al.* Course characteristics in the differentiation of dementia of the Alzheimer type and multi-infarct dementia. *Acta Psychiatrica Scandinavica* 1990; **81**:551–3.

Fratiglioni L, Grut M, Forsell Y *et al.* Prevalence of Alzheimer's disease and other dementias in an elderly urban population: relationship with age, sex and education. *Neurology* 1991; **41**:1886–92.

Galasko D, Hansen LA, Katzman R *et al.* Clinical-neuropathological correlations in Alzheimer's disease and related dementias. *Archives of Neurology* 1994; **51**:888–95.

Gunstad J, Brickman AM, Paul RH *et al.* Progressive morphometric and cognitive changes in vascular dementia. *Archives of Clinical Neuropsychology* 2005; **20**:229–41.

Hachinski VC, Iliff LD, Phil M *et al.* Cerebral blood flow in dementia. *Archives of Neurology* 1975; **32**:632–7.

Holmes C, Cairns N, Lantos P & Mann A. Validity of current clinical criteria for Alzheimer's disease, vascular dementia and dementia with Lewy bodies. *The British Journal of Psychiatry* 1999; **174**:45–50.

Ince PG, McArthur FK, Bjertness E *et al.* Neuropathological diagnoses in elderly patients in Oslo: Alzheimer's disease, Lewy body disease, vascular lesions. *Dementia* 1995; **6**:162–8.

Junqué C, Pujol J, Vendrell P *et al.* Leuko-araiosis on magnetic resonance imaging and speed of mental processing. *Archives of Neurology* 1990; **47**(2):151–6.

Langa KM, Foster NL & Larson EB. Mixed dementia. Emerging concepts and therapeutic implications. *The Journal of the American Medical Association* 2004; **292**:2901–8.

Liebetrau M, Steen B & Skoog I. Stroke in 85-year-olds. Prevalence, incidence, risk factors and relation to mortality and dementia. *Stroke* 2003; **34**:2617–22.

Liebetrau M, Steen B, Hamann GF & Skoog I. Silent and symptomatic infarcts on cranial computerized tomography in relation to dementia and mortality. A population-based study in 85-year-olds. *Stroke* 2004; **35**:1816–2.

Lim A, Tsuang D, Kukull W *et al.* Clinico-neuropathological correlation of Alzheimer's disease in a community-based case series. *Journal of the American Geriatrics Society* 1999; **47**:564–9.

Linden T, Skoog I, Fagerberg B *et al.* Cognitive impairment and dementia 20 months after stroke. *Neuroepidemiology* 2004; **23**:45–52.

Livingston G, Sax K, Willison J *et al.* The Gospel Oak study stage II: the diagnosis of dementia in the community. *Psychological Medicine* 1990; **20**:881–9.

Manubens JM, Martinez-Lage JM, Lacruz F *et al.* Prevalence of Alzheimer's disease and other dementing disorders in Pamplona, Spain. *Neuroepidemiology* 1995; **14**:155–6.

Munoz DG. The pathological basis of multi-infarct dementia. *Alzheimer Disease and Associated Disorders* 1991; **5**:77–90.

Neuropathology Group. Medical Research Council Cognitive Function and Aging Study. Pathological correlates of late-onset dementia in a multicentre, community-based population in England and Wales. *Lancet* 2001; **357**:169–75.

O'Connor DW, Pollitt PA, Hyde JB *et al.* The prevalence of dementia as measured by the Cambridge Mental Disorders of the Elderly Examination. *Acta Psychiatrica Scandinavica* 1989; **79**:190–8.

Ott A, Breteler MMB, van Harskamp F *et al.*, The Rotterdam Study. Prevalence of Alzheimer's disease and vascular dementia: association with education. *British Medical Journal* 1995; **310**:970–3.

Pohjasvaara T, Erkinjuntti T, Vataja R & Kaste M. Dementia three months after stroke. Baseline frequency and effect of different definitions of dementia in the Helsinki Stroke Aging Memory (SAM) cohort. *Stroke* 1997; **28**:785–92.

Qiu C, Skoog I & Fratiglioni L. Occurrence and determinants of vascular cognitive impairment. In T Erkinjuntti & S Gauthier (eds) *Vascular Cognitive Impairment* 2002, pp 61–83; Martin Dunitz.

Rocca WA, Bonaiuto S, Lippi A *et al.* Prevalence of clinically diagnosed Alzheimer's disease and other dementing disorders: a door-to-door survey in Appignano, Macerata Province, Italy. *Neurology* 1990; **40**:626–31.

Román GC. Senile dementia of the Binswanger type. A vascular form of dementia in the elderly. *The Journal of the American Medical Association* 1987; **258**:1782–8.

Roman GC. Cholinergic dysfunction in vascular dementia. *Current Psychiatry Reports* 2005; **7**:18–26.

Román GC, Tatemichi TK, Erkinjuntti T *et al.* Vascular dementia: diagnostic criteria for research studies. Report of the NINDS-AIREN international workshop. *Neurology* 1993; **43**:250–60.

Schmidt R, Enzinger C, Ropele S *et al.*, Austrian Stroke Prevention Study. Progression of cerebral white matter lesions: 6-year results of the Austrian Stroke Prevention Study. *Lancet* 2003; **361**:2046–8.

Skoog I. Risk factors for vascular dementia. A review. *Dementia* 1994; **5**:137–44.

Skoog I. Guest editorial. Status of risk factors for vascular dementia. *Neuroepidemiology* 1998; **17**:2–9.

Skoog I, Berg S, Johansson B *et al.* The influence of white matter lesions on neuropsychological functioning in demented and non-demented 85-year-olds. *Acta Neurologica Scandinavica* 1996; **93**:142–8.

Skoog I & Copeland JRM. Nosology of dementia. In JRM Copeland, MT Abou-Saleh & DG Blazer (eds) *Principles and Practice of Geriatric Psychiatry* 2002, 2nd edn, pp 185–9; John Wiley & Sons, Chichester.

Skoog I & Gustafson D. Hypertension, hypertension-clustering factors and Alzheimer's disease. *Neurological Research* 2003; **25**:675–8.

Skoog I, Davidsson P, Aevarsson O *et al.* Cerebrospinal fluid beta-amyloid 42 is reduced before the onset of sporadic dementia: a population-based study in 85-year-olds. *Dementia and Geriatric Cognitive Disorders* 2003; **15**:169–7.

Skoog I, Nilsson L, Palmertz B *et al.* A population-based study of dementia in 85-year-olds. *The New England Journal of Medicine* 1993; **328**:153–8.

Skoog I, Palmertz B & Andreasson L-A. The prevalence of white matter lesions on computed tomography of the brain in demented and non-demented 85-year-olds. *Journal of Geriatric Psychiatry and Neurology* 1994; **7**:169–75.

Skoog I, Vanmechelen E, Andreasson L-A *et al.* A population-based study of tau protein and ubiquitin in cerebrospinal fluid in 85-year-olds: relation to severity of dementia and cerebral atrophy, but not to the apolipoprotein E4 allele. *Neurodegeneration* 1995; **4**:433–42.

Snowdon DA, Greiner LH, Mortimer JA *et al.*, The Nun Study. Brain infarction and the clinical expression of Alzheimer disease. *Journal of the American Medical Association* 1997; **277**:813–7.

Tatemichi TK, Desmond DW, Mayeux R *et al.* Dementia after stroke: baseline frequency, risks, and clinical features in a hospitalized cohort. *Neurology* 1992; **42**:1185–93.

Tatemichi TK, Desmond DW, Paik M *et al.* Clinical determinants of dementia related to stroke. *Annals of Neurology* 1993; **33**:568–75.

Tatemichi TK, Paik M, Bagiella E *et al.* Dementia after stroke is a predictor of long-time survival. *Stroke* 1994a; **25**:1915–191.

Tatemichi TK, Sacktor N & Mayeux R. Dementia associated with cerebrovascular disease, other degenerative diseases, and metabolic disorders. In RD Terry, R Katzman & KL Bick (eds) *Alzheimer Disease* 1994b; Raven Pressd, New York.

Tomlinson BE, Blessed G & Roth M. Observations on the brains of demented old people. *Journal of the Neurological Sciences* 1970; **11**:205–42.

Vermeer SE, Koudstaal PJ, Oudkerk M *et al.* Prevalence and risk factors of silent brain infarcts in the population-based Rotterdam Scan Study. *Stroke* 2002; **33**:21–5.

Vermeer SE, Prins ND, Den Heijer T *et al.* Silent brain infarcts and the risk of dementia and cognitive decline. *The New England Journal of Medicine* 2003; **348**:1215–22.

World Health Organization. *The ICD-10 Classification of Mental and Behavioural Disorders. Diagnostic Criteria for Research* 1993; WHO, Geneva.

Ylikoski A, Erkinjuntti T, Raininko R *et al.* White matter hyperintensities on MRI in the neurologically non-diseased elderly. Analysis of cohorts of consecutive subjects aged 55 to 85 years living at home. *Stroke* 1995; **26**:1171–7.

Ylikoski R, Ylikoski A, Erkinjuntti T *et al.* White matter changes in healthy elderly correlate with attention and speed of mental processing. *Archives of Neurology* 1993; **50**:818–24.

Zhang ZX, Zahner GE, Roman GC *et al.* Dementia subtypes in China: prevalence in Beijing, Xian, Shanghai, and Chengdu. *Archives of Neurology* 2005; **62**:447–53.

FURTHER READING

Hachinski VC, Potter P & Merskey H. Leuko-araiosis. *Archives of Neurology* 1987; **44**:21–3.

Tatemichi TK, Foulkes MA, Mohr JP *et al.* Dementia in stroke survivors in the Stroke Data Bank cohort. Prevalence, incidence, risk factors, and computed tomographic findings. *Stroke* 1990; **21**:858–66.

96

Other Dementias

Wee Shiong Lim[1] *and* William A. Banks[2]

[1] Tan Tock Seng Hospital, Singapore, and [2] Saint Louis University School of Medicine and Saint Louis Veterans' Affairs Medical Center, St Louis, MO, USA

INTRODUCTION

Dementia is an acquired syndrome in which there is impairment of cognitive abilities, severe enough to interfere with the individual's occupational, social, and functional abilities. As conventionally used, the term dementia implies "degenerative" and "progressive", but it is also often used in the context of static conditions (such as poststroke cognitive impairment) or reversible conditions (such as depression or medication-related cognitive impairment). Table 1 provides a list of the many causes of dementing illnesses that can occur in older individuals.

Results of different epidemiological studies indicate that Alzheimer's disease (AD) is by far the commonest cause of dementia worldwide (Green, 2001). It may be tempting for clinicians to routinely make this diagnosis without systematically considering alternative or additional diagnoses. Such a practice is time-saving and probably fortuitously correct most of the time. However, it risks a great disservice to a significant proportion of patients as it fails to detect reversible diseases affecting cognition (which often occur concomitantly with degenerative diseases like AD) and by extension, fails to provide appropriate treatment and accurate prognoses.

In population-based studies, the commonest reported dementia etiology after AD is vascular dementia (VaD) (Lobo *et al.*, 2000; von Strauss *et al.*, 1999; Andersen *et al.*, 2000), especially in Asian populations like the Japanese (Ikeda *et al.*, 2001) and Chinese (Wang *et al.*, 2000). Recent reports also indicate that when actively sought for with standard criteria, the prevalence of dementia with Lewy bodies (DLB) and frontotemporal dementia (FTD) may be higher than previously thought. For example, the Islington study of dementia subtypes in community-dwelling elderly revealed the following distribution of dementia subtypes: AD–31.3%; VaD–21.9%; DLB–10.9%; and FTD–7.8% (Stevens *et al.*, 2002).

Specialized memory clinic–based estimates differ somewhat from population-based studies in having a relatively higher prevalence of non-AD etiologies, and concomitant potentially reversible conditions, especially depression and metabolic abnormalities. Larson *et al.* (1986) evaluated 200 older persons with dementia and found that 33.7% had metabolic abnormalities. Generally, however, only a small percentage of these have been found to be completely reversible (Clarfield, 1988; Walstra *et al.*, 1997; Siu, 1991), most notably in conditions such as hypothyroidism and vitamin B12 deficiency. The prevalence of etiologies in demented patients presenting to private practitioners has not been estimated, but would likely reflect values intermediate between population and specialized outpatient-based estimates (Green, 2001).

The rest of this chapter seeks to discuss some conditions that are commonly encountered in clinical practice, and concludes with a general approach to the evaluation of dementia in older persons.

VASCULAR DEMENTIA

One of the most controversial and difficult areas in the pathology of dementing disorders is the role of cerebrovascular disease (CVD) in dementia. In the early 1900s, it was erroneously held that the most frequent cause of late-onset dementia was arteriosclerosis (arteriosclerotic insanity). Pioneering work in the 1960s and early 1970s challenged this assumption, establishing that only stroke-related loss of brain tissue exceeding 50 to 100 ml resulted in dementia, and that Alzheimer pathological changes were important in the majority of cases (Tomlinson *et al.*, 1970). In 1974, the term *multi-infarct dementia* (MID) was coined to reflect dementia due to multiple large and small strokes (Hachinski *et al.*, 1974). It has since been realized that the contribution of CVD to VaD is more than MID, since VaD can arise from a single

Principles and Practice of Geriatric Medicine, 4th Edition. Edited by M.S. John Pathy, Alan J. Sinclair and John E. Morley.

Table 1 Causes of dementia other than Alzheimer's disease

1. Other degenerative dementias
   a. Dementia with parkinsonism
      i. Diffuse Lewy body disease
      ii. Parkinson's disease dementia
      iii. Progressive supranuclear palsy
      iv. Others for example, corticobasal degeneration, multiple system atrophy
   b. Frontotemporal dementia
   c. Huntington's disease
   d. Hallervorden–Spatz disease
   e. Kufs' disease
2. Vascular dementia
3. Other CNS causes
   a. Normal pressure hydrocephalus
   b. Epilepsy
   c. Traumatic dementia
      i. Acute and chronic subdural hematoma
      ii. Dementia pugilistica
      iii. Craniocerebral injury
   d. Tumors
      i. Primary CNS tumors: gliomas, meningiomas
      ii. Metastatic tumors, lymphoma, leukemia
      iii. Paraneoplastic limbic encephalitis
4. Psychiatric disorders
   a. Depression
   b. Others: schizophrenia, mania, other psychoses
5. Inflammatory
      i. Cerebral vasculitis
         - Primary angiitis of the CNS
         - Part of systemic involvement: disseminated lupus erythematosus, temporal arteritis, Behcet's, Wegener's granulomatosis, Churg–Strauss disease
      ii. Multiple sclerosis
6. Metabolic
   a. Endocrinopathies
      i. Hyper- and hypothyroidism
      ii. Glucose disorders: HHNK
      iii. Cushing's disease
      iv. Addison's disease
   b. Electrolyte abnormalities
      i. Hypo- and hypernatremia
      ii. Hypercalcemia
   c. Inherited
      i. Wilson's disease
      ii. Mitochondrial disorders
      iii. Adult lysosomal diseases (particularly metachromatic leukodystrophy)
      iv. Peroxisomal disorders
7. Nutritional deficiency
      i. Thiamine deficiency
      ii. Vitamin B12 deficiency
      iii. Folate deficiency
      iv. Vitamin B6 deficiency (pellagra)
8. Infective
   a. Neurosyphilis
   b. Human prion disease
   c. HIV-associated dementia
   d. Progressive multifocal leukoencephalopathy
   e. Postmeningitic/postencephalitic dementia
9. Drugs (remembered by the mnemonic: ACUTE CHANGE IN MS[a])
   a. **A**ntiparkinsonian drugs
   b. **C**orticosteroids
   c. **U**rinary incontinence drugs
   d. **T**heophylline
   e. **E**mptying (motility) drugs
   f. **C**ardiovascular drugs

Table 1 *(continued)*

   g. **H**2 blockers
   h. **A**ntimicrobials
   i. **N**SAIDs
   j. **G**eropsychiatric drugs
   k. **E**NT drugs
   l. **I**nsomnia drugs
   m. **N**arcotics
   n. **M**uscle relaxants
   o. **S**eizure drugs
10. Toxins
   a. Alcohol
   b. Heavy metals: lead, aluminum, mercury
   c. Carbon monoxide poisoning
11. Others
   a. Obstructive sleep apnea
   b. Whipple's disease
   c. Neurosarcoidosis

HHNK, hypoglycemia, hyperglycemic hyperosmolar nonketotic syndrome.
[a]Flaherty JH. Clin Geriatr Med 1998;14(1): 101–27.

strategic stroke, lacunar infarcts, or incomplete white matter ischemia.

Epidemiological studies in the West indicate that VaD is second in prevalence to AD, accounting for 12–20% of dementia cases (Roman, 2003a). The incidence of VaD increased with age, but much less steeply than AD. Unlike AD, men are disproportionately more affected, especially at the younger ages. Interestingly, international comparative studies reveal a comparatively higher frequency of VaD in some Asian countries, especially Japan and China. Among ethnic Japanese, the ratio of AD to VaD ranged from 0.5 in Japan to 1.5 in Hawaii, indicating possible interactions between genes and environment (Chui, 2000). The ratio of AD to VaD varied from 1.4 in Beijing, China, to 2.8 in Korea, compared with the ratio of 3.4 in Europe (Morris *et al.*, 2004).

Dementia may occur in 25–33% of ischemic stroke cases at ages 65 and older. Predictors of the occurrence of dementia following stroke include: older age, lower education level, non-White race, preexisting cognitive decline, diabetes, lower blood pressure or orthostatic hypotension, "silent" infarcts on neuroimaging, ischemic rather than hemorrhagic strokes, hemispheric rather than brainstem or cerebellar lesions, left rather than right hemispheric lesions, larger and recurrent strokes, a more severe neurological deficit on admission, and complications of acute stroke, including hypoxic and ischemic events (seizures, cardiac arrhythmias, aspiration pneumonia, hypotension) (Roman, 2003b). In addition, periventricular white matter lesions of significant size and hippocampal atrophy have been associated with increased risk of VaD (Liu *et al.*, 1992; Mungas *et al.*, 2001). Interestingly, apolipoprotein $\varepsilon 4$ has been associated with increased risk for AD, but not VaD (Frank *et al.*, 2002).

VaD encompasses several clinicopathologic subtypes, ranging from hemorrhagic (including hypertension, cerebral amyloidal angiopathy, subarachnoid hemorrhage, posthemorrhagic obstructive hydrocephalus, subdural hematoma, and hematological causes) to ischemic, and combinations of ischemia and hemorrhage (such as cortical vein and sinus

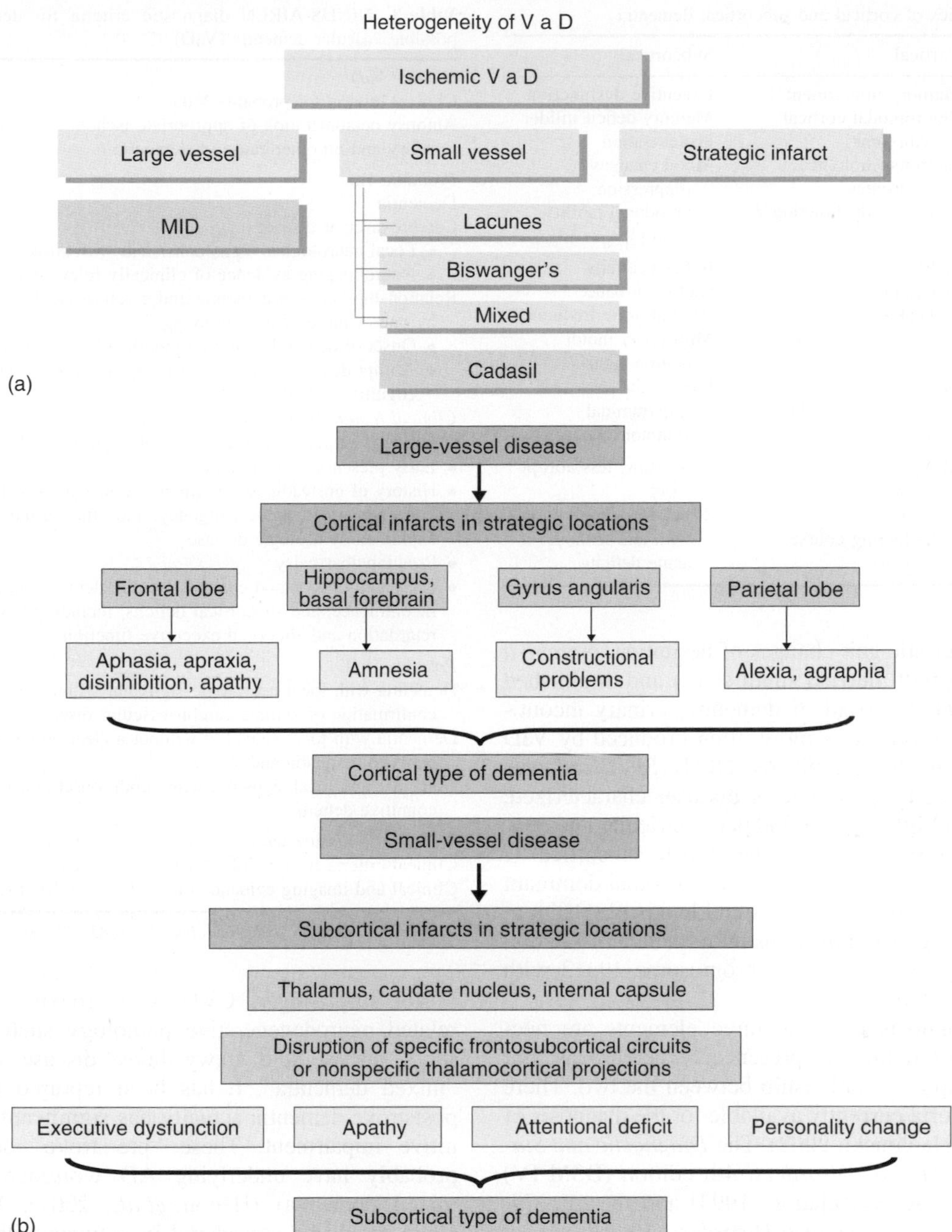

Figure 1 Heterogeneity of clinical presentation of vascular dementia. (a) Heterogeneity of ischemic vascular dementia and (b) differentiation of clinical features by vessel size

thromboses). The ischemic forms of VaD can be further divided into large-vessel, small-vessel, and strategic infarct subtypes (Figure 1a). Strategic stroke VaD results from a single stroke in a strategic location critical to cognitive function, and can occur in large-vessel (usually right posterior cerebral artery, anterior cerebral artery or left gyrus angularis) or small-vessel arterial territory (in the capsular genu, intraluminary nuclei of the thalamus, or head of caudate nucleus). The term *multi-infarct dementia* is now reserved for the combination of multiple cortical and subcortical vascular lesions.

Although there is some degree of overlap, large-vessel strokes tend to yield a clinical picture of cortical dementia, as opposed to the subcortical dementia of small-vessel forms (Figure 1b). These can be reasonably differentiated by a combination of cognitive features, neurological features, and clinical course (Table 2) (Roman, 2002). Subcortical ischemic vascular dementia (SIVD) typically causes a clinically slow, subacute-onset dementia, that is characterized by executive dysfunction, impaired attention, and impaired processing speed, with a comparatively milder memory deficit (Looi and Sachdev, 1999). There may be "lower-half parkinsonism"

Table 2 Characteristics of cortical and subcortical dementia

	Cortical	Subcortical
Cognitive deficits	Memory impairment Heteromodal cortical symptoms Neuropsychological syndromes Executive dysfunction	Executive dysfunction Memory deficit milder Perseveration Mood changes (depression, emotional lability, apathy)
Neurological symptoms	Field cut Lower facial weakness Upper motor neuron signs Dominant/ nondominant lobe signs	Imbalance/falls Gait disturbance Altered urine frequency Mild upper motor neuron signs Dysphagia Extrapyramidal symptoms
Clinical course	Abrupt onset, stepwise deterioration, fluctuating course, plateaus	60%: slow, less abrupt onset 80%: slow progression with and without acute deficits

producing characteristic gait changes of hesitation, *marche a petit pas* (walking with hurried small steps) and diminished step height. In fact, the triad of dementia, urinary incontinence, and gait disturbance is more often produced by VaD than normal pressure hydrocephalus (NPH). SIVD includes the lacunar state and Binswanger's disease, characterized, respectively, by multiple lacunes and periventricular leukoencephalopathy that typically spares the arcuate subcortical U fibers. Included in this group is cerebral autosomal dominant arteriopathy with subcortical infarcts and leukoencephalopathy (CADASIL), a genetically transmitted small-vessel disorder which has been mapped to chromosome 19q12 with mutations in the Notch 3 gene.

To make a diagnosis of VaD, three elements are necessary: presence of dementia, presence of cerebrovascular lesions, and a temporal relationship between the two. There are two sets of criteria currently available for the diagnosis of VaD (Bowler and Hachinski, 2002). The *Diagnostic and Statistical Manual of Mental Disorders*, 4th edition (DSM-IV) (American Psychiatric Association, 1994) and the *Classification of Mental and Behavioural Disorders*, 10th Revision, under the International Classification of Diseases (ICD-10) (World Health Organization, 1993) are general diagnostic tools that outline criteria without operationalizing them. The second set, such as the National Institute of Neurological Disorders and Stroke and the Association Internationale pour la Recherche at L'Enseignement en Neurosciences (NINDS-AIREN) (Roman *et al.*, 1993) criteria (Table 3), is a development of the first two and offers operational criteria. Autopsy studies (Gold *et al.*, 1997; Gold *et al.*, 2002) have shown that while these criteria are generally able to exclude about 90% of AD, they have only modest sensitivity (50–70%) in diagnosing VaD. There is also a tendency to misclassify mixed dementia (AD with CVD) as VaD (54% for ADDTC and 29% for NINDS-AIREN), especially in the "possible VaD" category (Gold *et al.*, 1997).

Table 3 NINDS-AIREN diagnostic criteria for definite, probable, and possible vascular dementia (VaD)

Definite VaD
Clinical criteria for probable VaD
Autopsy demonstration of appropriate ischemic or hemorrhagic brain injury and no other cause of dementia

Probable VaD
Dementia
Cerebrovascular disease
- Focal neurological signs consistent with stroke
- Neuroimaging evidence of clinically relevant vascular lesions

Relationship between dementia and cerebrovascular disease, as evidenced by one or more of the following:
- Onset of dementia within 3 months of a recognized stroke
- Abrupt deterioration or fluctuating or stepwise progression of the cognitive deficit

Clinical features consistent with diagnosis:
- Subtle onset and variable course of cognitive deficits
- Early presence of gait disturbance
- History of unsteadiness, frequent and unprovoked falls
- Early urinary frequency, urgency, and other urinary symptoms not explained by urologic disease
- Pseudobulbar palsy
- Personality and mood changes, abulia, depression, emotional incontinence, and subcortical deficits, including psychomotor retardation and abnormal executive function

Possible VaD
Dementia with focal neurologic signs but without neuroimaging confirmation of definite cerebrovascular disease
Dementia with focal signs but without a clear temporal relationship between dementia and stroke
Dementia and focal signs but with subtle onset and variable course of cognitive deficits

Alzheimer's disease with cerebrovascular disease
Clinical criteria for possible Alzheimer's disease
Clinical and imaging evidence of cerebrovascular disease

Reference: Roman GC *et al. Neurology* 1993; **43**:250–60.

Not surprisingly, CVD often coexists with other age-related neurodegenerative pathology such as AD, Parkinson's disease and Lewy body disease (LBD), to yield "mixed dementia". It has been reported that 10–15% of poststroke dementia actually has significant preexisting cognitive impairment. These "pre-stroke" dementia patients probably have underlying AD worsened by stroke (i.e. mixed dementia) (Hénon *et al.*, 2001). Mixed AD with CVD should be considered in patients with a prior diagnosis of AD or amnestic mild cognitive impairment (MCI), or if there is preexisting insidiously progressive cognitive impairment. The Nun Study showed that patients with lacunar strokes had 20 times increased risk of clinical dementia and required fewer senile plaques and neurofibrillary tangles to exhibit signs of dementia (Snowdon *et al.*, 1997). Thus, in patients with AD plus CVD, both conditions require treatment, even if the vascular component appears trivial (for example, one or two lacunes).

Nonetheless, VaD and AD can often be distinguished on the basis of differences in onset, progression, domains of cognitive impairment, and gait disturbances (Table 4) (Roman, 2003b). The features that best distinguish VaD from AD are stepwise deterioration, fluctuating course, history of stroke,

Table 4 Characteristics of vascular dementia and Alzheimer's disease

Characteristic	Vascular dementia	Alzheimer's disease
Onset	Sudden or gradual	Gradual
Progression	Slow, stepwise fluctuation	Constant insidious decline
Neurological findings	Evidence of focal deficits	Subtle or absent
Memory	Mildly affected	Early and prominent deficit
Executive dysfunction	Early and severe	Later and less severe
Neuroimaging	Infarcts and/or white matter lesions	Normal; hippocampal atrophy
Gait	Often disturbed early	Usually normal
Cardiovascular history	Transient ischemic attacks, strokes, vascular risk factors	Less common

Source: Modified from Roman GV. *J Am Geriatr Soc* 2003; **51**:S296–304 with permission of Blackwell Publishing Ltd.

and focal neurological symptoms (Moroney *et al.*, 1997). Neuropsychiatric disturbances such as depression, anxiety, agitation, disinhibition, and apathy are more common in VaD than in AD, and delusions tend to be less common in VaD. Depression in the acute phases following stroke is associated with left frontal lesions, while depression in more chronic poststroke patients is more likely to occur with right posterior lesions (Shimoda and Robinson, 1999). Brain imaging, typically magnetic resonance imaging (MRI) or computed tomography (CT), usually demonstrates with varying degrees of sensitivity, vascular lesions such as a single strategic stroke, multiple cortico-subcortical strokes, and periventricular white matter ischemia. Neuroimaging has come to play such an important role in diagnosing and evaluating VaD that the absence of vascular lesions identified on neuroimaging virtually excludes the diagnosis.

Nomenclature-wise, there has been a recent movement to more accurately define the contribution of CVD in cognitive disorders (Roman *et al.*, 2004). The term *vascular cognitive impairment* (VCI) is now proposed to refer to the subset with ischemic brain injury producing less severe cognitive impairment that do not meet the criteria for VaD (i.e. vascular cognitive impairment no dementia, VCI-ND), analogous to the concept of amnestic MCI, currently considered the earliest clinically diagnosable stage of AD. This is to emphasize the preventable nature of VaD, and the importance of early diagnosis. In addition, the current requirement of memory loss as the *sine qua non* for the diagnosis of VaD may result in oversampling of patients with AD worsened by stroke (i.e. mixed dementia). Thus, the definition of dementia in VaD has been proposed to be modified to the presence of *executive dysfunction* of sufficient degree to interfere with social or occupational functioning. Lastly, the term, *vascular cognitive disorder* (VCD) (Sachdev, 1999), has been proposed as the global diagnostic category for cognitive impairment of vascular origin, ranging from VCI to VaD. It includes specific disease entities such as poststroke VCI, poststroke VaD, CADASIL, Binswanger's disease, and AD plus CVD.

Pharmacologic management of VaD involves a multiprong approach addressing specific treatment for cognition, management of neuropsychiatric disturbances, management of stroke-related disabilities such as spasticity, parkinsonism and incontinence, and prevention strategies centered around the prevention of stroke. The latter involves anticoagulation in patients at risk of cardioembolism, antiplatelet agents, and targeting modifiable risk factors such as hypertension, diabetes, hyperlipidemia, negative lifestyle factors (habitual cigarette smoking, inactivity, obesity), and hyperhomocysteinemia. There is some evidence that treatment of hypertension may reduce the risk of dementia (Pantoni *et al.*, 2000; PROGRESS Collaborative Group, 2001). Despite the benefit of statins in reducing stroke by 30%, this did not translate into benefits in cognition in a recent trial with cognition as the primary endpoint (Shepherd *et al.*, 2002).

It has been postulated that there is a cholinergic deficit in VaD, akin to AD, resulting from interruption of cholinergic pathways by vascular lesions. This hypothesis has been borne out in the results of recent randomized controlled trials of cholinesterase inhibitors, which show modest benefits in global response, cognition, activities of daily living and behavior after 24 weeks, compared with placebo (Erkinjuntti *et al.*, 2004). These benefits were seen in both mixed dementia and VaD patients. Interestingly, the cognitive scores in untreated patients with VaD did not deteriorate over the study period, in contrast to the worsening typically observed in the control group in AD trials, suggesting that VaD patients may be distinct from AD (Figure 2) (Wilkinson *et al.*, 2003). More importantly, it suggests that the treatment aims in the two groups may possibly differ. In VaD, the cognitive effect is dependent on absolute improvement over baseline, representing an *improvement* in cognition, unlike the *stabilization* of cognition observed in AD, where the cognitive effect is mostly dependent on continuing deterioration in the placebo group. There is also evidence that memantine, an *N*-methyl-D-Aspartate (NMDA) receptor antagonist that protects against glutamate-mediated excitotoxicity, shows modest benefits in mild to moderate VaD (Orgogozo *et al.*, 2002).

DEMENTIA WITH PARKINSONISM

General Approach

The concomitant presentation of cognitive impairment with Parkinsonism is not uncommonly encountered in clinical practice, and presents a diagnostic conundrum to most clinicians. The principal causes in the elderly are listed in Table 5. A detailed clinical history and physical examination, coupled with relevant investigations, is indispensable in navigating through the labyrinth of differential diagnoses.

It is important to ascertain the onset, duration, and progression of the illness. A younger age of onset would alert

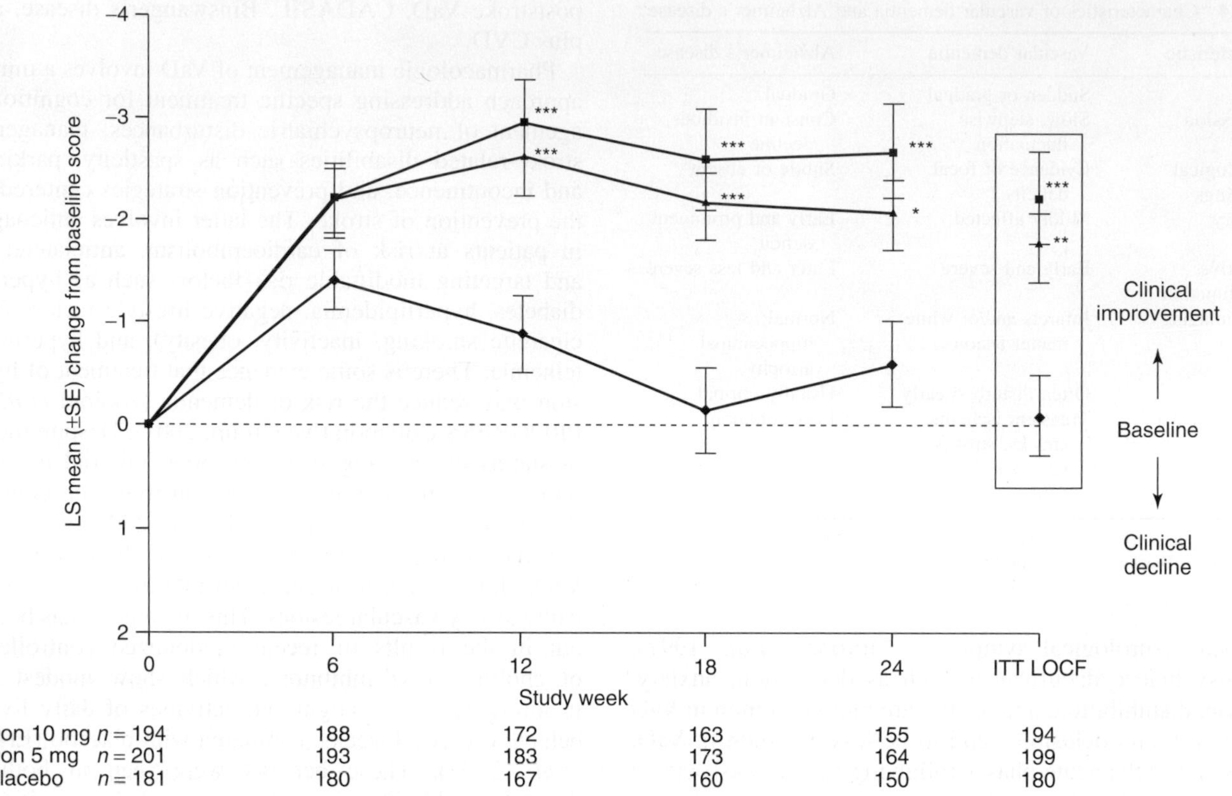

Figure 2 Alzheimer disease assessment scale–cognitive subscale least squares mean change from baseline score in donepezil- and placebo-treated patients. $*p < 0.05$, $**p < 0.01$, $***p < 0.001$ versus placebo. —■— = Donepezil 10 mg/day; —▲— = donepezil 5 mg/day; —◆— = placebo (Reproduced from Wilkinson D, *et al.*, Donepezil in vascular dementia, *Neurology*, **61**, 479–86, Copyright 2003, with permission from Lippincott Wiliams and Wilkins)

Table 5 Principal causes of parkinsonism with cognitive impairment in the elderly

Parkinson's disease
- Idiopathic
- Familial

Parkinsonism in other neurodegenerative diseases
- Dementia with Lewy bodies
- Progressive supranuclear plasy
- Frontotemporal dementia with parkinsonism
- Multiple system atrophy
  - Olivopontocerebellar degeneration
  - Shy–Drager syndrome
  - Striatonigral degeneration
- Corticobasal degeneration
- Hallervorden–Spatz disease

Vascular dementia with parkinsonism

Postencephalitic parkinsonism
- Encephalitis lethargica
- Other encephalitides eg, syphilis

Secondary parkinsonism
- Pharmacologic: antipsychotic agents, especially the high potency conventional agents, and other dopamine blocking drugs
- Toxins: carbon monoxide intoxication, cyanide poisoning, methanol, ethanol
- Postanoxic parkinsonism
- Dementia pugilistica
- Normal pressure hydrocephalus
- Space-occupying lesions: tumors, blood clot, abscess, and so on
- Metabolic, for example, Wilson's disease

the clinician to familial syndromes, hereditary illnesses (e.g. Wilson's disease), and certain neurodegenerative causes (e.g. FTD and multiple system atrophy). Cognitive decline without significant progression for several years, is not, in general, likely to be secondary to a neurodegenerative disease since once symptomatic, these tend to be progressive. Chronology of presenting symptoms, in particular, the temporal relationship between the onset of Parkinsonism and dementia, can yield useful information. For instance, dementia onset more than 12 months after the initial motor symptoms of Parkinsonism, favors the diagnosis of Parkinson's Disease dementia (PDD) rather than DLB (McKeith *et al.*, 1996). Marked fluctuations in cognition, attention, and alertness are pathognomonic of DLB and PDD, although it is prudent to exclude delirium and its myriad causes if the duration is short. A history of frequent falls early in the course of disease suggest progressive supranuclear palsy (PSP), although this can also be seen in idiopathic Parkinson's disease (PD), DLB, multiple system atrophy (MSA) and NPH. Early dysphagia or dysarthria is characteristic of PSP. Compared to AD, the degree of memory impairment in the group of dementias with Parkinsonism is comparatively milder by disease stage, and there are usually more neuropsychiatric features at the time of presentation. Frontotemporal dementia patients are more likely to manifest euphoria and disinhibition, while visual hallucinations, delusions, and misidentifications are more common in DLB and PDD. A detailed family history and medication review cannot be overemphasized. Other relevant history includes occupational history (e.g. dementia pugilistica results from recurrent significant head trauma and this typically occurs in boxers), ethanol ingestion, and significant illnesses (e.g. strokes, encephalitis).

Pertinent pointers during physical examination include examination of the eyes (impairment of vertical gaze with intact oculocephalic reflex in PSP, and nystagmus suggestive of olivopontocerebellar degeneration), cerebellar signs (olivopontocerebellar degeneration), pattern of extrapyramidal involvement (PSP is characterized by predominantly axial as opposed to distal rigidity), postural blood pressure (orthostatic hypotension from autonomic dysfunction is a feature of MSA, but can also occur in DLB and PD; it can also be secondary to drug treatment with levodopa and dopamine agonists), higher cortical function (asymmetrical limb apraxia and cortical sensory loss in corticobasal degeneration), and gait (apraxic gait typically in NPH, but also seen in Binswanger's disease and SIVD).

Structural neuroimaging with CT or MRI can yield useful information about the differential diagnosis: hydrocephalus; space-occupying lesions; evidence of vascular parkinsonism such as lacunar infarcts, periventricular, and white matter hyperintensities; midbrain atrophy which is typical of PSP; pontine and cerebellar changes evident in olivopontocerebellar degeneration; and mixed low and high signal intensity in the putamen evident in striatonigral degeneration. Hypointensity of the striatum on MRI is generally against the diagnosis of idiopathic Parkinson's disease (Cummings, 2003).

In summary, the cardinal task of the clinician when confronted with a patient with Parkinsonism and cognitive impairment is first, to exclude easily identified secondary causes, and then determine if the clinical picture supports a diagnosis of Parkinson's plus syndrome as opposed to idiopathic Parkinson's disease. Useful discriminating features in favor of Parkinson's plus syndrome are symmetrical onset of Parkinsonism, absence of resting tremors, and the presence of concomitant atypical features (history of poor response to levodopa, predominantly axial involvement, early severe dementia, early marked autonomic disturbance, gaze palsies, and upper motor neuron findings). When patients with two out of the three classic signs of parkinsonism (tremors, rigidity, and bradykinesia) were compared with postmortem pathologic diagnosis of Parkinson's disease (Hughes *et al.*, 1992), the strongest additional bedside argument for PD (positive likelihood ratio = 4.1; negative likelihood ratio = 0.4) is the combination of (1) asymmetrical onset, (2) no atypical features, and (3) no alternative diagnosis. This can then direct the clinician to further investigations and management.

DEMENTIA WITH LEWY BODIES

There is growing appreciation that LBD may be a single disease spectrum comprising DLB at one end and PDD at the other (Figure 3). Accumulating evidence favors this unified school of thought, as opposed to the thinking that they are independent diseases ending in a similar common pathway (McKeith and Mosimann, 2004). The hallmark of both diseases is the presence of Lewy bodies, which contain α-synuclein and suggest neurobiological links with other synucleinopathies such as MSA (Baba *et al.*, 1998). In Parkinson's disease, Lewy bodies are prominent in the brain stem and rare in the cortex, whereas in DLB, they are common in the brainstem, limbic system, and neocortex. Although concomitant AD pathology (β-amyloid plaques, and to a lesser degree, neurofibrillary tangles) may be present, clinicopathologic correlations reveal that the severity of cognitive impairment is significantly associated with α-synuclein rather than AD pathology (Gomez-Tortosa *et al.*, 1999). In DLB, cortical LB density has been associated with cognitive impairment and visual hallucinations, while better correlates with visual hallucinations are found with Lewy neurites (LN), neurone loss, dopaminergic, and cholinergic deficits (Perry *et al.*, 2003). The cholinergic deficit in DLB is better defined and more pronounced then AD.

Onset of DLB is between 50 and 90 years of age, and the duration of illness varies between 6 and 10 years. Risk factors include older age, male sex, and the presence of apolipoprotein-ε4 allele. DLB accounts for approximately 15–20% in autopsy series. Clinically, DLB is marked by a progressive dementia syndrome with fluctuating cognition and alertness, recurrent, well formed visual hallucinations and parkinsonism (Table 6). Autopsy validation studies have shown the criteria for DLB to have high specificity (80–100%), but more limited sensitivity (35–80%)

Table 6 Concensus guidelines for the clinical diagnosis of probable and possible dementia with Lewy bodies (DLB)

Central feature
Progressive cognitive decline of sufficient magnitude to interfere with normal social and occupational function
Core features (two core features essential for a diagnosis of probable, one for possible DLB)
Fluctuating cognition with pronounced variations in attention and alertness
Recurrent visual hallucinations that are typically well formed and detailed
Spontaneous motor features of parkinsonism
Supportive features
Repeated falls
Syncope
Transient loss of consciousness
Neuroleptic sensitivity
Systematized delusions
Hallucinations of other modalities
REM sleep behavior disorder
Depression
Features less likely to be present
History of stroke
Any other physical illness or brain disorder sufficient enough to interfere with cognitive performance

Source: Modified from McKeith IG *et al.* Consensus guidelines for the clinical and pathologic diagnosis of dementia with Lewy bodies (DLB), *Neurology* 1996; **47**:1113–24, with permission of Lippincott Williams & Wilkins.

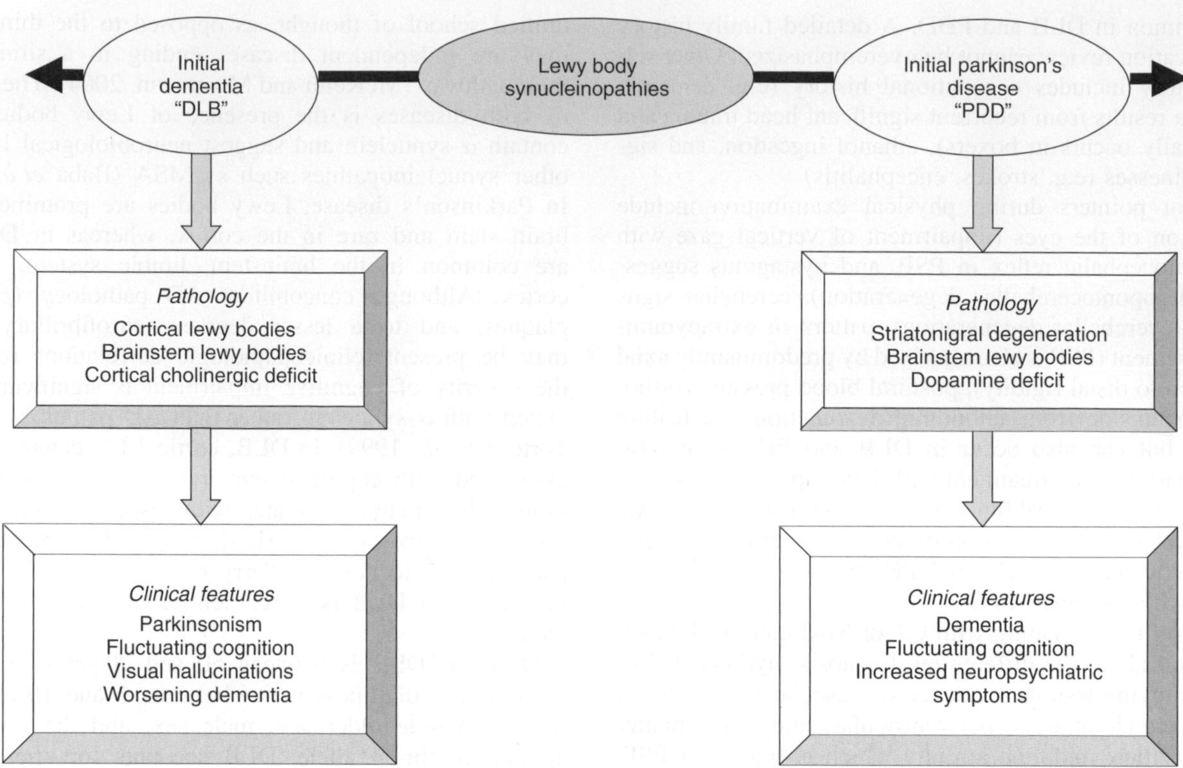

Figure 3 Schematic representation of the spectrum of clinical presentation of dementia Lewy bodies, based on the premise that Parkinson's disease dementia (PDD) and dementia with Lewy bodies (DLB) are actually different representations of the same neurobiological process with different initial manifestations

(McKeith, 2002). It is the identification of cognitive fluctuation that poses clinicians the greatest difficulty, and the most frequent clinical misdiagnosis of DLB is AD.

Prominent or persistent memory impairment may not necessarily occur in the early stages, but is usually evident with progression. The characteristic neuropsychological profile in early LBD is that of prominent executive, attentional, and visuospatial dysfunctions with relatively preserved memory functions. Fluctuation in cognitive performance, attention, and level of consciousness is the most characteristic feature of DLB. The marked amplitude between best and worst performances distinguishes it from the minor day-to-day variations that commonly occur in dementia of any cause. Transient disturbances of consciousness in which patients are found mute and unresponsive for periods of several minutes, may represent the extreme of fluctuation in arousal, but are often mistaken for transient ischemic attacks, despite a lack of focal neurological signs. One study (Ferman *et al.*, 2004) reported that informant endorsement of at least three items out of four composite features of fluctuations (daytime drowsiness and lethargy, daytime sleep of 2 or more hours, staring into space for long periods, episodes of disorganized speech) yielded a positive predictive value of 83% for DLB against the alternate diagnosis of AD.

Prominent neuropsychiatric symptoms at time of presentation are among the defining features of DLB. Although not unique to DLB, the behavioral alterations occurring in DLB are present at a much higher frequency than in other dementias (Cummings, 2003). The visual hallucinations typical of DLB are typically recurrent, well formed and detailed, and usually involve people and animals that appear to be real but make no noise. Depressive symptoms are common and 40% have a major depressive episode, which is significantly greater than in AD (McKeith, 2002). Other common behavioral manifestations include hallucinations in other modalities, misidentifications (such as Capgras syndrome), systematized delusions, and rapid eye movement (REM) sleep disorders.

Extrapyramidal motor symptoms (EPS) of DLB, present in about 80% of DLB patients, consist primarily of bradykinesia and rigidity, with resting tremors seen in less than 50%. When present, these symptoms can be as severe as in PD, although progression of EPS is uncommon. It is reported that 70% of DLB patients have at least a transient beneficial response to levodopa treatment (Louis *et al.*, 1997). Recurrent falls and syncope occur in a third, presumably reflecting autonomic dysfunction.

Differential diagnosis include other dementia syndromes such as AD and VaD; other causes of delirium; other neurological syndromes such as Parkinson's disease, PSP, or Creutzfeld–Jakob disease; and other psychiatric disorders such as late-onset delusional disorders, depressive psychosis, and mania. There are as yet no clinically applicable genotypic or cerebrospinal fluid (CSF) markers to support a DLB diagnosis, though neuroimaging investigations may be helpful.

These include relative preservation of hippocampal and medial temporal lobe volume on MRI, and occipital hypoperfusion on single photon emission computerized tomography (SPECT), compared with posterior parietal-temporal hypoperfusion in AD (Lobotesis *et al.*, 2001).

Forty percent to 50% of DLB patients show neuroleptic sensitivity reactions with a 2–3-fold increase in mortality (McKeith *et al.*, 1992). These range from sedation, increased confusion, and worsening of parkinsonism, to more deleterious effects like irreversible parkinsonism, impaired consciousness, and marked autonomic disturbances *à la* neuroleptic malignant syndrome. Conventional neuroleptic medications are best avoided, while atypical newer agents (such as clozapine, olanzepine, risperidone, and quetiapine) should be used judiciously. In addition, medications with anticholinergic or dopaminergic antagonism (e.g. tricyclic antidepressants, low potency neuroleptics, antiparkinsonian anticholinergic drugs and antispasmodics) should be avoided, as they have the potential to impair cognition, exacerbate psychotic symptoms and may be associated with orthostatic hypotension. There is evidence that cholinesterase inhibitors are effective and relatively safe for the treatment of neuropsychiatric and cognitive symptoms in DLB, with major side effects similar to those reported in AD; mainly gastrointestinal symptoms with nausea, vomiting, and diarrhea (McKeith *et al.*, 2000).

PARKINSON'S DISEASE DEMENTIA

It is now recognized that crude prevalence figure of 20–40% from earlier cross-sectional surveys of movement-disorder clinic populations, underestimated the frequency of PDD. Subsequent long-term follow-up studies showed that 60–80% of PD patients will develop dementia, typically after 10–15 years of motor disability (Aarsland *et al.*, 2003). Older age, at PD onset, duration of motor symptoms, akinetic-rigid profile (as opposed to the tremor-predominant subtype), reduced verbal fluency (naming number of items belonging to a specific category, for example, animals, in 1 minute), early hallucinations, and depression are predictive factors of dementia development (Emre, 2003).

There are four pertinent issues related to the management of PDD. Firstly, from a diagnostic standpoint, there is a need to review the current concept of the dementia syndrome, such as those found in the DSM-IV and ICD-10, which often are heavily AD-based (McKeith, 2004). Unlike AD, the initial impairment in PDD typically involves attention, executive function, and visuospatial performance with only mild memory impairment in the initial stages. Moreover, it can be difficult to judge the extent to which functional impairment is attributable to cognitive dysfunction rather than motor disability.

Secondly, it is imperative for the managing clinician to be cognizant of attendant sleep and neuropsychiatric issues, and to actively screen for their presence. The former consists of longer sleep latency, poor quality sleep with frequent awakenings, restless leg syndrome, excessive daytime sleepiness and REM sleep disorders. The latter is more common in PD patients with dementia than those without, and corresponds with the severity of cognitive impairment. In a study of community-dwelling PD patients, the most common behavioral issues were dysphoric mood (38%), hallucinations (27%) and anxiety (20%) (Cummings *et al.*, 1994). Risk factors for depression include early onset of PD, presence of hallucinations or delusions, the akinetic-rigid clinical syndrome, greater degree of cognitive impairment, and right-sided parkinsonism (due to greater left brain involvement) (Tandberg *et al.*, 1997). Anxiety disorders are common in PD, especially in the "off" period of treatment, and usually coexist with depression. Mood fluctuations are also common in PD patients with the "on–off" phenomenon, with increased depression and anxiety during the "off" state and increased elation during the "on" state (Richard *et al.*, 2001).

Thirdly, managing clinicians should be mindful of treatment-associated neuropsychiatric symptoms, occurring with levodopa, dopamine agonists, anticholinergic agents, and amantadine. These include sleep disturbances, hallucinations, delusions, mania/euphoria, and hypersexuality/sexual paraphilias. The most important determinant of which individuals will develop psychiatric phenomena following therapy initiation, is individual susceptibility (the presence of cognitive impairment is the most influential among these factors), rather than drug dosage. The syndrome of *hedonistic homeostatic dysregulation* (HHD) has been described, typically in men with early onset PD who exhibit drug induced dyskinesias. HHD is an addiction syndrome to levodopa characterized by excessive use beyond that required to alleviate motor impairment, increasing dose requirements as drug tolerance develops, withdrawal reactions, and classic substance abuse behaviors of drug hoarding and denial. Frequently associated symptoms include punding (this refers to repetitive, purposeless motor acts), hypersexuality, psychomotor restlessness, pathological gambling and shopping, and anorexia.

Lastly, with regard to therapeutic options, there is evidence from three randomized controlled trials of PDD patients (Emre *et al.*, 2004; Aarsland, 2002; Leroi *et al.*, 2004) that cholinesterase inhibitors can offer modest improvements in memory mirroring the degree seen in AD, as well as attention and neuropsychiatric features (especially hallucinations). Tremors occurred more frequently with treatment, but the overall motor function did not decline. Further trials are needed to ascertain which subgroup responds best to cholinergic enhancement, and at which stage cholinesterase inhibitors should be offered. Although improved cognition has been reported in patients with mild Parkinson's disease following the administration of levodopa, mixed results have been found in moderately to severely affected PD patients (Morrison *et al.*, 2004). In an evaluation of 800 patients studied in the Deprenyl and Tocopherol Antioxidant Therapy of Parkinsonism (DATATOP) trial, no clear benefit was noted with either deprenyl or tocopherol, alone or in combination

(Kieburtz *et al.*, 1994). Finally, the role of memantine, a novel NMDA receptor antagonist, needs to be established; it has been shown to improve cognition in moderate to severe AD (Reisberg *et al.*, 2003), and may also ameliorate motor symptoms (the parkinsonian drug, amantadine, is a related compound) and apathy.

PROGRESSIVE SUPRANUCLEAR PALSY

Progressive supranuclear palsy is a tauopathy characterized neuropathologically by marked midbrain atrophy, neurofibrillary tangles, or neuropil threads in the basal ganglia and brainstem, as well as tau-positive astrocytes. Clinically, it is the degenerative disorder most commonly confused with PD. According to the National Institute of Neurological Diseases and Stroke-Society for Progressive Supranuclear Palsy (NINDS-SPSP) criteria, key clinical features for probable PSP are onset at age 40 or later, a gradually progressive course, paralysis of vertical gaze, and prominent postural instability with falls in the first year of disease onset (Litvan *et al.*, 1996). Typically, there are limitations of volitional vertical downgaze followed by decreased vertical upgaze, with vertical pursuit and lateral movements affected next. Oculocephalic reflexes remain intact through most of the disease course. There is symmetrical rigidity that is predominantly axial with extensor posturing resulting in retrocollis. Other pertinent features include early dysphagia and dysarthria leading to unintelligibility of speech, and poor response of parkinsonism to levodopa therapy. Cognitive impairment is primarily one of the executive dysfunctions involving the frontal-subcortical circuits, with slower processing speed, diminished free recall but relatively preserved recognition memory, impairment in abstract thought and verbal fluency (Bak and Hodges, 1998). Compared with PD patients, those with PSP have significantly more apathy and disinhibition while those with PD exhibit more delusions, hallucinations, and depression (Aarsland *et al.*, 2001). Sleep abnormalities are common in PSP, and include shortened sleep time, lower percentage of time spent in REM sleep, and awakenings. Unfortunately, PSP is a treatment resistant condition and prognosis is generally poor (Kompoliti *et al.*, 1998). Parkinsonism may respond to dopaminergic agents, especially dopamine receptor agonists in some cases (Jackson *et al.*, 1983). Patients are intolerant of anticholinergic compounds, which should be avoided. Local treatment with botulinum toxin injections may relieve blepharospasm or painful spasms in affected limbs (Polo and Jabbari, 1994).

CORTICOBASAL DEGENERATION

Corticobasal degeneration (CBD) is a tauopathy which has substantial overlap with FTD (Kertesz *et al.*, 2000). The cardinal neuropathological features are asymmetrical cortical degeneration involving primarily the frontal and parietal regions, severe neuronal loss in the substantia nigra, ballooned achromatic cells as well as tau-positive neurofibrillary tangles and neuropil threads in the cortex, subcortex, and brainstem (Schneider *et al.*, 1997). Patients have a parkinsonian syndrome manifested by asymmetrical rigidity, dystonia, and reflex myoclonus. Cognitive features include apraxia, cortical sensory loss and alien limb phenomenon, which refers to actions performed by the affected limb that are not consciously intended by the patient. The apraxia of CBD is of the ideomotor type, referring to inability to perform movements on command that is not explained by motor or sensory abnormalities. The apraxia is typically most severe in the limb affected by dystonia or myoclonus, and rarely, can involve buccofacial structures. The low sensitivity but relatively high specificity of the diagnosis of CBD means that most patients with a clinical diagnosis of CBD have the diagnosis confirmed at autopsy, but autopsy also detected many cases not suspected clinically (Riley and Lang, 2000). CBD has a unique cognitive profile of combined cortical and frontal-subcortical cognitive deficits that is marked by executive dysfunction, visuospatial disturbances, retrieval memory deficit, and aphasia. Behaviorally, depression and apathy are frequent and often prominent, while most other symptoms are less common. MRI may reveal asymmetrical frontoparietal atrophy, while functional neuroimaging such as positron-emission tomography (PET), show asymmetrical changes that are most severe on the side contralateral to the affected limb (Hirono *et al.*, 2000).

MULTIPLE SYSTEM ATROPHY

Multiple system atrophy is a synucleinopathy characterized by α-synuclein containing cytoplasmic inclusions in glial cells and affected neurons. It is a sporadic, progressive, adult-onset disorder that includes striatonigral degeneration (when parkinsonian features predominate), olivopontocerebellar atrophy (when cerebellar features predominate) and Shy–Drager syndrome (when autonomic failure is predominant) (Concensus Committee of the American Autonomic Society and the American Academy of Neurology, 1996). Cognitive changes are typically mild and represent executive dysfunction. Diagnostic features for MSA have high specificity but low sensitivity and many patients go unrecognized; it is most commonly misdiagnosed as PD or PSP (Litvan *et al.*, 1997). The features that discriminate MSA from PD are an earlier age of onset (50–55 years of age), rapid progression, and the presence of autonomic dysfunction preceeding or within 2 years of the onset of the motor symptoms. Progression is more rapid than idiopathic PD, with 40% of patients markedly disabled or wheelchair-bound within 5 years of onset (Wenning *et al.*, 1994). Treatment is mainly supportive. Fludrocortisone or midodrine may be used for treating symptomatic postural hypotension.

FRONTOTEMPORAL LOBAR DEGENERATION

Frontotemporal lobar degeneration (FTLD) denotes a progressive dementia syndrome characterized by behavioral change, prominent aphasia, or both. It is the commonest form of primary degenerative dementia in middle age after AD, accounting for up to 20% of presenile dementia cases (Snowden *et al.*, 2002). Only a minority of patients exhibit Pick-type histological changes, hence the more generic term FTLD is preferred to "Pick's disease". FTLD is superior to "dementia" as a generic term for this group of disorders, since patients may have progressive neurological dysfunction for substantial periods of time before meeting criteria for a dementia syndrome.

Onset occurs most commonly between the ages 45 and 65, although the disorder can present before the age of 30 as well as in the elderly. There is an equal gender distribution. The mean duration is 8 years, ranging from 2 to 20 years. A family history of dementia is present in about 40% of first-degree relatives. Ten percent of the familial cases and 0–3% of sporadic cases have been linked to specific mutations. Most of these mutations occur in the tau gene on chromosome 17, although rare cases of both familial motor neurone disease with FTLD and familial FTLD, have been linked to chromosome 9 and 3 respectively (Brown *et al.*, 1995; Hosler *et al.*, 2000).

Three main neuropathological findings have been identified in FTLD (Lund and Manchester Groups, 1994; McKhann *et al.*, 2001). The most common (microvacuolar) type, accounting for 60% of cases, displays microvacuolation, neuronal loss, mild gliosis, and the lack of distinctive changes (swellings or inclusions). In this disorder, there is a loss of tau protein function ("tauless tauopathy") (Zhukavera *et al.*, 2001), which may be functionally related to abnormal tau aggregation. The second histological pattern (Pick-type) is seen in 25% of cases, including Pick's disease and FTLD with parkinsonism linked to chromosome 17; it is characterized by neuronal loss with widespread gliosis, minimal or no microvacuolation, inclusions that are positive for both tau and ubiquitin, and greater involvement of the limbic system, and striatum. Tau-positive inclusions are also evident in CBD and PSP. In about 15% of cases, neuronal loss and gliosis with ubiquitin positive and tau-negative inclusions are present. These changes have been described in FTLD with motor neurone disease and FTLD with marked striatal degeneration.

There are three distinct clinical syndromes in FTLD (Neary *et al.*, 1998): the commonest (at least 70%) is FTD, followed by semantic dementia (SD) (about 15%), and progressive nonfluent aphasia (PNA) (about 10%). There can be substantial overlap between the three syndromes, as well as with other clinical disorders, notably CBD and PSP. Motor neurone disease has been seen in combination with all three subtypes, but is most common with FTD and PNA (Neary *et al.*, 1998). All eventually worsen and produce a dementia syndrome. The clinical syndrome does not predict histological type, so that clinical distinctiveness itself does not imply etiological difference.

In general, three behavioral subtypes of FTD have been described (Snowden *et al.*, 2002). The *disinhibited* type is characterized by jocularity, unconcern, breakdown of social and interpersonal behaviors, easy distractability, and purposeless overactivity. At the other extreme is the *apathetic* subtype, featuring inertia, aspontaneity, loss of volition, unconcern, mental rigidity and perseveration; the *stereotypic* type has pronounced behavioral stereotypes, compulsions, and ritualistic behavior. These broad behavioral subtypes reflect regional involvement. The disinhibited subtype corresponds to orbital frontal and anterior temporal dominance; the apathetic form occurs when there is extensive frontal involvement extending into the dorsolateral frontal cortex, and the stereotypic type is most strongly related to marked striatal changes with variable cortical involvement, often with emphasis on temporal rather than frontal lobe pathology. Clinical presentation often reflects asymmetrical hemispheric involvement, with the right-sided disorders manifesting primarily marked neuropsychiatric disturbances, whereas the left-sided disorders tend to exhibit more language dysfunction.

Frontotemporal Dementia

The salient clinical characteristic is an early and profound alteration in personality and social conduct, occurring in the context of relative preservation of memory, spatial skills, and praxis. Clinical features are summarized in Table 7 (Neary *et al.*, 1998).

There is difficulty modulating behavior to the social demands of a situation, and is often associated with disinhibition, impulsivity, undue jocularity, inappropriate sexual behavior, distractability, and impersistence. Rigidity and inflexibility are common, and often accompanied by repetitive and compulsive behaviors, ranging from simple verbal or motor mannerisms to more elaborate routines, such as tapping each wall twice upon entering a room, rereading the same book, walking to the same location repeatedly, as well as clock-watching and adherence to a fixed routine. However, FTD patients do not typically experience the feelings of anxiety and release from anxiety characteristic of obsessive-compulsive disorder. Dietary changes typically take the form of overeating, food fads, and a preference for sweet foods. There is a loss of concern for one's personal appearance, and the patient may be increasingly unkempt early in the disease. Utilization and imitation behaviors are common in the later stages; the former refers to stimulus-bound behavior in which patients grasp and use an object in their visual field, despite its contextual inappropriateness (e.g. drinking from an empty cup). All of this occurs in the setting of loss of insight, indifference, and unconcern for one's actions. Although there may be memory complaints, cognitive changes reflect frontal lobe dysfunction (inattention, poor abstraction, difficulty shifting mental set, and perseverative tendencies) rather than a true amnestic syndrome. Speech output is attenuated, with progressive reduction of speech to

Table 7 Clinical diagnostic features of frontotemporal dementia

Character change and disordered social conduct are the dominant features initially and throughout the disease course. Instrumental functions of perception, spatial skills, praxis, and memory are intact or relatively well preserved

Core features
Insidious onset and gradual progression
Early decline in social interpersonal conduct
Early impairment in regulation of personal conduct
Early emotional blunting
Early loss of insight

Supportive features
Behavioral disorder

- Decline in personal hygiene and grooming
- Mental rigidity and inflexibility
- Distractibility and impersistence
- Hyperorality and dietary changes
- Perseverative and stereotyped behavior
- Utilization behavior

Speech and language

- Altered speech output:
  - Aspontaneity and economy of speech
  - Pressure of speech
- Stereotype of speech
- Echolalia
- Perseveration
- Mutism

Physical signs

- Primitive reflexes
- Incontinence
- Akinesia, rigidity, and tremor
- Low and labile blood pressure

Investigations

- Neuropsychology: significant impairment on frontal lobe tests in the absence of severe amnesia, aphasia, or perceptuospatial disorder
- Electroencephalography: normal on conventional electroencephalography despite clinically evident dementia
- Brain imaging (structural and/or functional): predominant frontal and/or temporal abnormality

Source: Modified from Neary D *et al.* Frontotemporal lobar degeneration: a concensus on clinical diagnostic criteria. *Neurology* 1998; **51**:1546–54, with permission from Lippincott Williams & Wilkins.

a mute state. Also common are verbal stereotypies, involving repeated use of a word, phrase, or complete theme. Patients may tell the same joke over and over again, or retell the same story many times a day.

Table 8 summarizes the distinguishing features of FTD from AD. In one study, the behavioral features of loss of social awareness, hyperorality, stereotyped and perseverative behavior, reduced speech output, and preserved spatial orientation had good specificity (97–100%), but lower sensitivity (63–73%) for the diagnosis of FTD compared with AD (Miller *et al.*, 1997). Other useful discriminating features include dietary changes and loss of affective response (generalized blunting of emotions), which is typically more severe than in AD.

Physical examination-wise, primitive reflexes, such as grasping, pouting, and sucking reflexes, occur earlier in the course of FTD then AD. Parkinsonian signs of akinesia, rigidity, and tremor develop with disease progression. A minority of FTD patients develop fasiculations, wasting, and weakness typical of motor neurone disease. Structural imaging with MRI is more sensitive then computed tomography in showing atrophy of the frontal and anterior temporal lobes. In some cases, these alterations show a striking asymmetry, which is most sensitively picked up by functional imaging techniques such as SPECT.

Table 8 Distinguishing features between frontotemporal dementia (FTD) and Alzheimer's disease (AD)

Clinical feature	Frontotemporal dementia	Alzheimer's disease
Cognitive		
Amnesia	Delayed until later in the course	Occurs early, *sine qua non* of AD
Executive dysfunction	Early, progressive	Less early in most cases
Language	Reduction of speech output	Anomia with fluent aphasia; speech output preserved
Visuospatial skills	Relatively preserved	Involved early
Calculation	Relatively preserved	Involved early
Behavioral		
Disinhibition	Common	Occurs, but is less severe
Euphoria	Common	Rare
Stereotyped behavior	Common and marked	Less common
Apathy	Common and severe with marked emotional blunting	Common, less severe
Dietary changes	Hyperorality and food fads (high carbohydrates) common	Anorexia more common then overeating
Self-neglect	Common	Rare until late
Psychosis	Occurs, but is less common	Delusions and hallucinations more common

Rational treatments for FTD are currently limited. The cholinergic system is not implicated in FTD in neurochemical studies, unlike in AD (Wenning *et al.*, 1994). Nonetheless, there is some evidence that behavioral symptoms such as disinhibition, overeating, and compulsions may benefit from treatment with selective serotonin reuptake inhibitors (SSRIs), suggesting that a modicum of symptomatic improvement can be achieved at least in some cases (Swartz *et al.*, 1997).

Progressive Nonfluent Aphasia

Progressive nonfluent aphasia is the FTLD syndrome corresponding to degeneration of the left frontal cortex. The dominant feature initially and throughout the course is disorder of expressive language, presenting as progressively worsening nonfluent spontaneous speech with agrammatism (omission or incorrect use of grammatical terms including articles, prepositions, etc.), phonemic paraphasia with sound-based errors, and anomia (Neary *et al.*, 1998). There is often accompanying stuttering, impaired repetition with paraphasic intrusions, alexia, and agraphia. In the early stages, comprehension is preserved for word meaning, but impaired for syntactic relationships. Behaviorally, there is early preservation of social skills, although evolution to dementia with behavioral features of FTD is common after several years of progressive linguistic changes (Weintraub *et al.*, 1990). PNA can usually be distinguished from the fluent aphasia of AD. Unlike AD, amnesia and perceptuospatial disorders are also noticeably absent in the early stages.

Semantic Dementia

The term semantic dementia typically refers to patients with progressive fluent aphasia associated with visual agnosia (Neary *et al.*, 1998). These patients have impaired inability to understand the meaning of words (semantics), manifested by impaired word naming and comprehension, such that speech, although fluent, is progressively devoid of content. Semantic paraphasic errors are common, and there may be associated surface dyslexia and dysgraphia, although syntax and phonology, visual perceptual and visuo-skills, single-word repetition, calculation, and nonverbal problem-solving abilities are often preserved. In fact, an unusual number of SD patients have an emergence of artistic talent in their dementia syndrome, reflecting the integrity and possibly, disinhibition of right hemispheric activity (Miller *et al.*, 1998). Other cognitive functions such as episodic memory are relatively well preserved in the early stages; typically, there is preservation of episodic events and semantic facts from very recent life compared with other time periods. Perceptual disorders are characterized by prosopagnosia (impaired recognition of identity of familiar faces) and/or associative agnosia (impaired recognition of object identity).

The main differential diagnosis is AD, which can also manifest as a progressive fluent aphasic disorder. However, AD patients exhibit a greater degree of amnesia, and concomitant visuospatial and calculation dysfunction. In addition, although both groups exhibit medial temporal lobe atrophy, there is asymmetrical hippocampal atrophy (left greater than right) and greater atrophy of the temporal poles in SD patients compared with AD (Galton *et al.*, 2001).

DEPRESSION

Depression is common among the elderly. The term *pseudodementia* was coined to reflect the impairment in thinking and memory that frequently accompany depression. The cognitive domains affected in depression include slowed mental processing and deficits in attention and executive function (Porter *et al.*, 2003). Individuals with late-onset depression have more significant cognitive impairment (van Reekum *et al.*, 1999).

Confirming the diagnosis of depression in a patient presenting with cognitive impairment can be difficult, since the patient may not complain of classical mood changes or have comorbid medical conditions that confound interpretation of "physical" symptoms of sleep, appetite/weight, psychomotor change, and energy disturbance. Although certain clinical features can be helpful in the differential diagnosis of dementia and depression (Table 9), none are diagnostic and frequent exceptions and overlaps exist. This is confounded by three possible relationships that can exist between depression and dementia.

Firstly, the two conditions often coexist. Epidemiological data indicates prevalence rates of 30–50% for depressive symptoms among AD patients, especially in the earlier stages of dementia where insight is often retained (Olin *et al.*, 2002). Studies have generally found an absence of effect of depression on cognitive performance in early stage AD (Powlishta *et al.*, 2004). Thus, it is often the experience that while antidepressant treatment of concomitant depression in dementia can result in impressive improvement in mood and

Table 9 Comparison of clinical presentations of depression (presenting as memory difficulties) and mild Alzheimer's Disease

Feature	Depression without underlying dementia	Alzheimer's disease without depression
Age of onset	Common below and above age 60	Uncommon below age 60
Onset	Subacute or insidious	Insidious
Course	Fluctuations may be present	Progressive decline
Insight	Almost always present	Sometimes present, usually in earlier stages
Cognitive domains		
Memory	Less prominent	Prominent and early
Executive function/ psychomotor speed	Prominent and early, proportional to dementia severity	Less prominent in earliest stages
Language/praxis	Uncommon unless depression is severe	Uncommon in mild stages but common in moderate and severe stages
Mood	Sad, stoic, or agitated	Sad, stoic, agitated or euthymic
Sleep-wake cycle	Often disturbed; early morning awakening	Sometimes disturbed
Response to cholinesterase inhibitor	Improvement in cognitive status not expected	Modest improvement in cognitive status can occur
Response to antidepressant	Significant improvement likely	Mild improvement in mood or behavior may occur

Source: Modified from Green RC. *Diagnosis and management of Alzheimer's Disease and other dementias.* Caddo, OK: Professional Communications, Inc; 2001, with permission.

quality of life, the cognitive impairment remains relatively unchanged.

Secondly, there is a growing body of evidence that depression at baseline is a risk factor for incident dementia and cognitive decline (Jorm, 2000). Thus, dementia needs to be entertained as a differential diagnosis in cases of long-standing depression where there is lack of cognitive improvement, despite adequate treatment of the underlying affective disorder.

Thirdly, owing to the considerable overlap in symptoms, some individuals with dementia may be erroneously diagnosed as having depression instead. Features of depression such as loss of interest, decreased energy, psychomotor changes, and decreased concentration lose diagnostic specificity in the presence of dementia (Burke and Wengel, 2003). Affective symptoms such as guilt, expressions of worthlessness and suicidal thoughts, if present, are more useful in distinguishing depression from dementia. It is also important to give appropriate consideration to the proxy informant's subjective reports of symptoms of depression in a demented patient, as the latter tends to minimize or underreport depressive symptoms, particularly when there is lack of insight into the underlying cognitive deficits (Burke *et al.*, 1998).

Since depression in the elderly is not always easily recognizable, many clinicians maintain an appropriate readiness to try antidepressants empirically or even as a therapeutic challenge to evaluate the response. A 6–8-week treatment trial of an appropriate antidepressant without significant anticholinergic properties, such as the SSRIs, is relatively safe and can sometimes provide considerable improvement (Green, 2001).

HUMAN PRION DISEASES

Prion diseases (also known as *transmissible spongioform encephalopathies*) are progressive and invariably fatal neurodegenerative diseases occurring in a wide range of mammals, including humans. They are defined by four cardinal neuropathological features: spongioform change, neuronal loss, reactive gliosis, and accumulation of the prion protein (PrP). According to the prion hypothesis, the infectious agent (termed PrP^{sc}) is an altered form of prion protein (termed PrP^{c}). PrP^{sc} results from the conversion of PrP^{c}, a host-encoded soluble protein of as-yet indeterminate function (Prusiner, 1982).

Prion diseases are unique amongst human neurodegenerative disorders in that they occur in sporadic, familial, and acquired forms (Table 10). Several point mutations and insertional mutations of the human prion protein gene (PRNP) on the short arm of chromosome 20 have been described in the familial forms. In the sporadic forms, either spontaneous somatic mutations or conformational change to PrP^{sc} occurs. The polymorphisms at codon 129 (methionine/valine) and 219 (glutamic acid/lysine) are thought to influence disease susceptibility in sporadic and variant Creutzfeld–Jakob disease (CJD) (Windl *et al.*, 1996). With regard to the iatrogenic forms, transmission can occur via inoculation of PrP^{sc} from contaminated surgical instruments, tissue grafts (corneal and dural) and human pituitary gland extracts from affected donors.

Table 10 Classification of human prion diseases

Idiopathic
Sporadic Creutzfeld–Jakob disease
Sporadic fatal insomnia
Inherited
Familial Creutzfeld–Jakob disease
Gerstmann–Straussler--Scheinker (classical and variant forms)
Fatal familial insomnia
Acquired
Human source: kuru
Iatrogenic Creutzfeld–Jakob disease
Bovine source: variant Creutzfeld–Jakob disease

Sporadic Creutzfeld–Jakob disease (sCJD) is the commonest form of human prion disease, occurring in a worldwide distribution with an annual incidence of 0.5–1.0 per million population. Most cases occur in the elderly, with peak onset in the 70s. Homozygotes for the codon 129 genotype, tend to have a significantly younger age of onset (Alperovitch *et al.*, 1999). Males and females are equally affected. The median duration of sCJD is 4 months and around 65% of cases have an illness duration of less than 6 months. In 14% of cases, there is a relatively long duration of 12 months or more; durations of more than 2 years are rare (5% of cases). Clinically, the classical triad of rapidly progressing dementia, myoclonic jerks, and characteristic electroencephalographic (EEG) findings should alert the clinician to consider the possibility of CJD. Other commonly associated symptoms include pyramidal and extrapyramidal signs, visual manifestations (restriction of visual field, homonymous hemianopsia, metamorphosia, palinopsia, and optic atrophy), and cerebellar gait disturbances. However, there can be a wide spectrum of clinical presentation, including (1) nonspecific symptoms such as asthenia, disturbances of sleep and eating patterns, (2) mental deterioration only, (3) predominantly neurological symptoms, usually of visual (the Heidenhain variant) or cerebellar (the Brownell–Oppenheimer variant) origin. Conditions that can mimic the initial presentation of CJD include Hashimoto's encephalitis, intracranial vasculitis, paraneoplastic limbic encephalitis, AIDS dementia complex, chronic meningitis, subacute sclerosing panencephalitis and myoclonic epilepsy with Lafora bodies.

Characteristic EEG findings in CJD, consisting of periodic lateralized or generalized bursts of spike-wave complexes, may be absent in the initial stages of the disease. However, as the disease evolves, periodic activity often becomes apparent. Periodic EEG activity is not specific to CJD, but can also be seen in postanoxic encephalopathy, Hashimoto's encephalitis, AIDS dementia complex, MELAS (mitochondrial myopathy, encephalopathy, lactic acidosis, and stroke) syndrome, severe metabolic derangement, multiple cerebral abscesses, and AD.

Among the brain associated proteins in CSF, 14-3-3 has high sensitivity and specificity of 90–97% and 84–96%

respectively (Zerr *et al.*, 2000). False-positive results can be found in patients with extensive central nervous system (CNS) damage, including recent stroke, subarachnoid hemorrhage, viral encephalitis, paraneoplastic CNS syndromes, AD and dementia with Lewy bodies. The CSF picture is otherwise bland, aside from occasional elevated total protein. MR brain imaging shows increased signals in the basal ganglia, (particularly caudate nucleus and the putamen), in the diffusion weighted image (DWI), fluid-attenuated inversion recovery (FLAIR), and T2-weighted sequences. In particular, diffusion weighted changes may be seen as early as 1 month after symptom onset (Bahn *et al.*, 1999).

Neuropathological examination is required for a definite diagnosis of CJD. Brain biopsy is carried out less frequently nowadays, largely due to the better-defined clinical diagnostic criteria for human prion diseases (Table 11). However, accurate and definitive diagnosis from brain biopsy can exclude an underlying treatable condition, aid caregivers in planning of care, as well as facilitate community surveillance of future transmission (See *et al.*, 2004). Biopsy of the nasal epithelium has recently been reported as a reliable and less invasive way of obtaining tissue (Zanusso *et al.*, 2003).

In 1996, a new variant form of CJD (vCJD) was reported in the United Kingdom, which, on the basis of epidemiologic, biochemical, and experimental transmission evidence, is strongly linked to human exposure to bovine spongioform encephalopathy (BSE), indicating that vCJD is the first example of a zoonotic form of prion disease in humans (Ironside and Head, 2004). There are distinct clinical features from sporadic CJD. It occurs in a younger age-group (mean age 28 years) with a prolonged duration of illness (mean 13 months), and is characterized by marked neuropsychiatric features (depression, anxiety, apathy, withdrawal, delusions) at onset and the prominence of sensory abnormalities (dysesthesias involving the face, arms, back, or legs), in addition to ataxia, movement disorders (myoclonus, dystonia or chorea), and dementia (Will *et al.*, 1999). Investigation-wise, the characteristic EEG changes of sCJD are absent, while the CSF 14-3-3 protein is elevated in only 50%, although it retains its specificity (Green *et al.*, 2001). The MRI scans show hyperintensities mainly in the posterior thalamus. Microscopic examination of the brain shows widespread spongioform change characterized by numerous florid plaques throughout the cerebrum and cerebellum.

Table 11 Clinical diagnostic criteria for sporadic and iatrogenic Creutzfeld–Jakob disease (CJD) and familial prion disease (from www.cjd.ed.ac.uk)

1. Sporadic
   - a. Rapidly progressive dementia
   - b. i) Myoclonus
     - ii) Visual or cerebellar problems
     - iii) Pyramidal or extrapyramidal features
     - iv) Akinetic mutism
   - c. Typical EEG
2. Iatrogenic
   - 2.1 Definite:
     Definite CJD with a recognized risk
   - 2.2 Probable
     - 2.2.1 Progressive cerebellar syndrome in human pituitary hormone recipients
     - 2.2.2 Probable CJD with recognized risk
3. Familial prion diseases[a]
   - 3.1 Definite
     Definite TSE plus definite or probable TSE in a first-degree relative
   - 3.2 Probable
     - 3.2.1 Probable TSE plus definite or probable TSE in a first-degree relative
     - 3.2.2 Progressive neuropsychiatric disorder plus disease-specific mutation

TSE, transmissible spongioform encephalopathy.
[a]Includes Gerstmann–Straussler–Scheinker and familial fatal insomnia.

HUNTINGTON'S DISEASE

The prevalence of Huntington's disease in Europe is approximately 0.5–8/100 000 (Harper, 1992). It is caused by the expansion of a CAG trinucleotide repeat sequence on the huntington gene located on the short arm of chromosome 4. The number of repeats correlates inversely with age of onset, with 40 repeats being the pathological threshold, beyond which disease will most likely develop (Harper, 1996). Inheritance is autosomal dominant with complete penetrance. New mutations are rare and most apparently sporadic cases in fact reflect either an incomplete family history or nonpaternity. Histopathologically, it is characterized by neuronal loss and gliosis mainly affecting the frontal lobes and caudate nucleus, and the presence of polyglutamine nuclear inclusions.

Onset is generally in middle life (mean age 40 years). The course is one of inexorable progression of cognitive, behavioral and motor decline, with death occurring 12–15 years from the time of symptomatic onset. Neuropsychiatric symptoms of depression, apathy, aggression, disinhibition, and social disintegration are common, and may predate the hallmark chorea, other extrapyramidal signs, and gaze apraxia (Paulsen *et al.*, 2001). A subcortical dementia marked by executive dysfunction, cognitive slowing, apathy, and typically, inattention develops. Bilateral atrophy of the head of caudate nucleus may be seen on brain imaging. Genetic testing is a powerful diagnostic tool that should be offered only if recommended provisions can be followed (International Huntington Association and the World Federation of Neurology Research Group on Huntington's Chorea, 1994).

CEREBRAL VASCULITIS

Vasculitis can affect the CNS, usually as part of a systemic involvement. The differential diagnosis is wide and includes primary vasculitides such as Wegener's granulomatosis, temporal arteritis, Churg–Strauss syndrome and polyarteritis nodosa; systemic diseases that can produce vasculitis such as systemic lupus, sarcoidosis, Henoch–Schonlein papura and Behcet's disease; infectious agents such as Lyme's disease; and other rare conditions such as intravascular lymphoma. These conditions can be easily distinguished by the clinical picture, elevated inflammatory markers, autoantibodies, and histopathological findings. However, it is important to be aware of the condition of primary angiitis of the CNS, where there is isolated CNS involvement. Pathologically, it is characterized by patchy inflammation (granulomatous, necrotizing, or lymphocytic), preferentially affecting small leptomeningeal and parenchymal vessels. Clinical presentations range from acute confusion to relapsing-remitting fluctuations to an indolent subcortical dementia. Headache is common but not universal, and seizures may occur. Inflammatory markers and autoantibodies are usually negative, however. Besides mild pleocytosis, the CSF is otherwise bland. MRI may show nonspecific white matter lesions. Cerebral angiogram can be useful, although beading of vessels is found in only approximately a third of patients with histologically confirmed CNS vasculitis, as well as in CNS infection, atherosclerosis, cerebral embolism, and vasospasm; multiple microaneurysms, often seen on visceral angiography in systemic vasculitis, are distinctly rare in CNS vessels (Younger, 2004). In many cases, the definitive diagnosis is clinched by histopathology, and unconfirmed suspicion of cerebral vasculitis remains one of the few indications for brain biopsy before committing the patient to immunosuppressive therapy.

ALCOHOL-RELATED DEMENTIA

The Liverpool Longitudinal Study of mental health of community-dwelling elderly, found that dementia was 4.6 times more likely to occur in men aged 65 and above who had a lifetime history of heavy drinking (Saunders *et al.*, 1991). However, the concept of a distinct entity of alcohol-related dementia remains a source of nosological confusion because of the considerable overlap with concomitant conditions, such as Wernicke–Korsakoff syndrome (thiamine deficiency), other nutritional deficiencies (e.g. B12 deficiency, pellagra), and hepatic encephalopathy. Nonetheless, the observation in epidemiological studies of the considerable number of demented alcoholics, even when these causes have been excluded, supports a case for the direct vindicative role of alcohol on the development of dementia (Harper and Scolyer, 2004). Diagnostic criteria for alcohol-related dementia have been proposed (Oslin *et al.*, 1998).

Histopathological findings reveal region-specific neuronal loss (the frontal lobe, hypothalamus, and cerebellum) and white matter–associated brain atrophy. Some of the white matter loss appears to be reversible in that, after prolonged abstinence, the brain shrinkage reverts towards normality (Liu *et al.*, 2000). There is a wide spectrum of effects of alcohol on the brain, depending on individual susceptibility, drinking pattern, and comorbid factors like recurrent head injury, seizures, and polydrug abuse. Typically, chronic alcohol abuse can lead to progressive intellectual deterioration resulting in long-term cognitive and neuropsychiatric sequelae. Executive function and autobiographical memory appear especially vulnerable, and confabulation may occur. Brain imaging shows nonspecific generalized cerebral atrophy with frontal predominance.

HUMAN IMMUNODEFICIENCY VIRUS–ASSOCIATED DEMENTIA

The spectrum of human immunodeficiency virus (HIV) cognitive involvement range from the nonspecific "aseptic meningitis" during the viremia of primary infection, to "minor cognitive motor disorder" which confers a worse prognosis for a similar HIV disease stage, to the most severe form, HIV-associated dementia (HAD) (Working Group of the American Academy of Neurology AIDS Task Force, 1991). HAD is believed to be the direct result of central nervous HIV infection, and it is a diagnosis of exclusion in patients with known AIDS who develop cerebral symptoms. It generally presents as a subcortical dementia with cognitive and motor slowing, and accompanying behavioral changes, seizures, and gait ataxia. Brain MRI reveals diffuse cerebral atrophy and white matter hyperintensities. It is associated with a relatively low CD4 count and the control of HIV viral load through intensive combination antiretroviral therapy is associated with significantly lower risk of progression to HAD (Childs *et al.*, 1999). Recent comparisons of neuropsychiatric performance with the addition of protease inhibitor (PI) drugs demonstrate better performance in subjects treated with a PI compared to those receiving less intensive HIV therapy (Ferrando *et al.*, 1998). Epidemiologic studies support the declining incidence of HAD with the advent of more effective and intensive retroviral therapy (Clifford, 2000). More recent studies have focused on the role of neuroprotective strategies (nimodipine, antioxidant agents, *N*-methyl-D-aspartate antagonist, tumor necrosis factor antagonist) in the treatment of HAD.

PARANEOPLASTIC LIMBIC ENCEPHALITIS

This condition arises from the autoimmune response to tumor antigens, and usually precedes the diagnosis of the underlying malignancy. The most commonly associated primaries are in the lung, testis, and breast. The characteristic histopathological finding is that of inflammatory infiltrates and neuronal loss typically in the mesial temporal area, and also the extralimbic areas such as the hypothalamus and brainstem. Clinically, it is characterized by changes in mood and personality, hallucinations, seizures, and cognitive impairment.

There may be symptoms and signs referable to other areas of the CNS, such as ataxia and sensory neuropathy. Supportive features include focal temporal lobe abnormalities on MRI and electroencephalography, and an inflammatory CSF yield; the presence of oligoclonal bands in the CSF but not the serum indicates local immunoglobulin synthesis, in a high proportion. It is associated with positive antineuronal antibodies (predominantly anti-Hu) in about 60% of cases (Gultekin *et al.*, 2000). An underlying primary may be uncovered by an exhaustive workup, usually including thoracoabdominal computed tomography or whole-body positron-emission tomography, if available. Therapeutic options are limited but some patients improve after treatment of the underlying malignancy.

NORMAL PRESSURE HYDROCEPHALUS

The underlying pathophysiology in NPH is believed to be due to impaired CSF absorption and increased intraventricular pulse pressure. The resultant increase in ventricular size exerts a pressure on surrounding white matter tracts to produce the classical triad of gait instability, urinary incontinence, and cognitive impairment. The diagnosis is clinched by the radiological finding of enlarged ventricles out of proportion to the degree of cerebral atrophy. Estimated to cause no more than 5% of cases of dementia, NPH is often treatable, and careful evaluation of symptoms coupled with radiographic evidence yields vital information of likely responders to shunting. A good prognosis is indicated by short duration of symptoms, onset of gait abnormality before or at same time as dementia, duration of cognitive impairment of less than 2 years, the presence of secondary causes (e.g. subarachnoid hemorrhage, meningitis, head injury, previous brain surgery), the absence of aphasia and alcohol abuse, and an improvement in gait following drainage of 30–50 cc of CSF (Graff-Radford, 1999). Radiologically, less favorable prognostic factors include concomitant sulcal enlargement and hippocampal atrophy (which may indicate underlying AD), and extensive white matter lesions. MRI flow void studies and cisternography have not been proven to reliably predict shunting outcome (Verrees and Selman, 2004). CSF diversion by ventriculoperitoneal shunting remains the treatment of choice, although, the highly variable success rate of 33–90% emphasizes the importance of careful patient selection. In one review (Hebb and Cusimano, 2001), 59% of NPH patients reported improvement after shunting with a persistent improvement in only 29%.

MEDICATIONS

Strictly speaking, medications cause a state of cognitive impairment secondary to chronic confusion or delirium rather than an actual dementia. As with depression, cognitive impairment due to medications is often superimposed upon other dementing disorders. Virtually any medication, including many over-the-counter drugs, has been implicated. The commonest culprits are drugs affecting the cholinergic, dopaminergic, serotonergic, and noradrenergic systems, and can be remembered by the mnemonic ACUTE CHANGE IN MS (mental status) (Flaherty, 1998). (refer Table 1) Medications are potentially reversible causes of cognitive impairment, hence a high index of suspicion is required, especially if there is a clear temporal relationship between the onset of symptoms and change in type or dosage of medications. Removing or reducing unnecessary medications may improve cognition, even in patients with underlying neurodegenerative diseases such as AD.

APPROACH TO THE DIAGNOSIS OF DEMENTIA IN OLDER PERSONS

The evaluation of dementia should be targeted at patients in whom there is some suspicion of cognitive impairment. These include: subjects with memory and other cognitive complaints (such as forgetfulness and confusion), either self-reported or by a reliable collateral source; subjects who arouse suspicion of cognitive impairment during the clinical encounter despite absence of memory complaints; those who are at increased risk of dementia (such as those with a strong family history of dementia); and medico-legal situations where the subject's mental competency is called into question (such as financial matters or making a will).

A four-step evidence-based approach is recommended in the evaluation (Chong and Sahadevan, 2003). *Firstly*, it is imperative to determine whether the cognitive symptoms are acute or chronic in onset. If acute, delirium needs to be ruled out using a well-validated instrument like the confusion assessment method (CAM) (Inouye *et al.*, 1993).

Secondly, if the forgetfulness or confusion is of a chronic nature, the clinician needs to determine if this is due to underlying dementia, or other conditions such as depression, late-onset psychiatric disorders, or partial epilepsy. Dementia is a clinical diagnosis, and the DSM-IV (American Psychiatric Association, 1994) criteria are useful for this purpose. The criteria require the presence of memory impairment, as well as deficits in one other cognitive domain (aphasia, apraxia, agnosia, and executive dysfunction), which should be of sufficient severity to cause perceptible impairment in social or occupational functioning. Table (12a) gives examples of questions that can be asked to elicit these criteria. It cannot be overemphasized that the clinical diagnosis of dementia is established purely by history-taking, and therefore, a corroborating history from a reliable collateral source should always be obtained. Objective tests like mental status tests (brief cognitive screening instruments) or more detailed neuropsychological tests administered by psychologists, can yield useful adjunct information in the diagnosis of dementia. These tests, however, are prone to floor and ceiling effects, require subject cooperation, can be difficult to administer with concomitant hearing impairment and aphasia, and

Table 12 Approach to assessment of dementia
(a) DSM-IV clinical criteria for diagnosis of dementia

Symptom	Questions
Amnesia	Is there forgetfulness? Was onset sudden or gradual? Is there a progressive course? If so, is the decline gradual, stepwise or fluctuating? Does amnesia affect short (e.g. appointments, misplacing, medications) or long-term domains? Is there undue repetition?
Plus impairment in at least one of the following domains:	
Aphasia	Any difficulty in word-finding, comprehension (e.g. conversations, television programs), or reading?
Apraxia	Any difficulties with buttoning, dressing, brushing teeth? Any problems using utensils during mealtimes?
Agnosia	Any difficulty recognizing familiar faces or familiar items?
Executive dysfunctioning	Any problems handling money (e.g. loose change, tip, paying bills, balancing accounts)? Any change in general problem-solving abilities? Is one's "work" (occupation, social activities, housework) getting more disorganized?
The above cognitive deficits, if present, must represent:	
A decline from a previously higher level of functioning	Does the cognitive deficit (e.g. forgetfulness) represent a change from one's baseline level, and is this change a decline?
Sufficient severity to cause significant impairment in social or occupational functioning	As a result of the above, is one therefore less independent in his community affairs, home and hobbies, and personal care?

Source: Reprinted with permission from the Diagnostic and Statistical Manual of Mental Disorders, Fourth Edition, Text Revision, Copyright 2000. American Psychiatric Association.

(b) Behavioral, functional, and social assessment in dementia

Variable	Questions
Behavioral	
Depression	Has patient been noted to be sad, tearful, having thoughts of worthlessness or inappropriate guilt, exhibiting diminished interest in work, hobbies, or recreational activities? Is there poor sleep, early morning awakening, change in appetite/weight, or impaired concentration?
Anxiety	Does patient get worried easily?
Agitation	Is patient easily agitated or irritable? Is there undue restlessness, overactivity, or aggressive behavior? Is the agitation related to certain times of the day (sundowning pattern)?
Paranoia	Is patient suspicious of others, accusing others of causing him harm or stealing his possessions (when in fact they have been misplaced)?
Hallucinations	Does patient see, hear, or smell things that are not present?
Sleep problems	Does patient have problems falling asleep or have sleep-wake reversals?
Functional	
Community functioning	Can patient find his way around in unfamiliar surroundings, manage his finances, shop, or participate in social activities independently?
Home-care functioning	Can he prepare his own food, help in housework and cooking? Is he able to choose proper attire to dress himself? Is he safe to be left at home alone?
Self-care functioning	Is he able to bathe and dress himself? Is he able to go to toilet, transfer, or feed himself? Is he continent of bladder and bowels?
Social	
Coping difficulties	How are caregivers coping? What is their level of stress? Are they also depressed? Are there features of elder abuse?
Financial issues	Are the financial costs of care manageable?
Legal issues	Are there any legal issues that require the assessment of decision-making capacity for example, will-making, placement decisions
Driving safety	Can the patient be persuaded not to drive? (Otherwise, he may require regular assessments of fitness to drive)

Table 12 *(continued)*

(c) Canadian consensus conference criteria[a] for performing cranial CT in patients with dementia

Criteria:
<60-years old
Rapid (e.g. over 1 to 2 months), unexplained decline in cognition or function
Dementia of relatively short duration (<2 years)
Recent, significant head trauma
Unexplained neurologic symptoms (e.g. new onset of severe headache or seizures)
History of cancer, especially of a type or at a site associated with metastasis to the brain
Use of anticoagulants or history of bleeding disorder
History of urinary incontinence and gait disturbance early in the disease (suggestive of normal pressure hydrocephalus)
Presence of any new localizing signs on physical examination (hemiparesis, Babinski's sign)
Unusual or atypical cognitive symptom or presentation (e.g. progressive aphasia)
Gait disturbance
CT is recommended if one or more of these criteria are present

Source: Modified from Chong MS, S Sahadevan. *Ann Acad Med Singapore* 2003; **32**:740–8.
CT, computed tomography.
[a]Patterson CJ *et al.* CMAJ 1999;160:S1–5.

require adjustments for age and education. It should be appreciated that these tests can only identify cognitive impairment and not dementia *per se* – the definitive diagnosis of dementia is still clinical.

Thirdly, if dementia is present, what are the complications? Behavioral, functional, and social problems are often amenable to treatment or palliation and should be assessed in all patients with dementia. These areas can be evaluated by a semistructured clinical approach (refer Table 12b) or by the use of validated scales such as the Geriatric Depression Scale (GDS) (Yesavage *et al.*, 1983), the Cornell Depression Scale in Dementia (Alexopoulos *et al.*, 1988), the neuropsychiatric inventory (NPI) (Cummings *et al.*, 1994), and the Bristol Activities of Daily Living Scale (Bucks *et al.*, 1996). The reader is referred to the excellent review article by Burns *et al.*, (2002), for more information on commonly used rating scales in geriatric psychiatry.

Lastly, if dementia is present, what is the etiology? The main aim of determining the etiology is to rule out potentially reversible causes of dementia and it begins with a focused history and physical examination, followed by selected laboratory tests and neuroimaging.

The most commonly recommended hematological tests are easy to perform and of a relatively low cost: complete blood count, urea and electrolytes, liver function test, serum calcium, serum glucose, thyroid function tests, vitamin B12 level, and sedimentation rate. Given the problems in interpreting the serum and CSF serology for neurosyphilis, routine testing is not advocated. Serum Venereal Disease Research Laboratory (VDRL) testing detects only 75% of cases of tertiary syphilis and CSF VDRL may be negative in 30–70% of neurosyphilis. Thus, the diagnostic utility of serum VDRL and treponemal antibody is optimized in situations where patients are already manifesting some of the clinical features of neurosyphilis (i.e. the "pretest probability" is sufficiently high to warrant a confirmatory test) (Jacobs, 2000).

The principal value of neuroimaging in the evaluation of dementia is the identification of cerebral infarcts and clinically important surgical brain lesions (SBLs), such as subdural hematomas, cerebral tumors, and NPH (Engel and Gelber, 1992). There is currently no consensus with regard to routine neuroimaging for all patients, versus selective usage based on judicious application of certain clinical indicators. One reasonable approach is to use a well-validated criteria like the Canadian Consensus Conference on the Assessment of Dementia (CCCAD) criteria (Table 12c) (Patterson *et al.*, 1999), with the additional consideration of the functional stage of dementia (Chong and Sahadevan, 2003). In cases of advanced dementia, caregivers are often not looking to the doctor for a precise etiological diagnosis; rather, they seek the doctor's help in managing the attendant's behavioral, functional, and social problems. Thus, in a patient with advanced dementia of a long duration (>2 years based on the CCCAD recommendation) not fulfilling any of the CCCAD criteria, a brain scan is of limited benefit. Conversely, if the dementia is of mild to moderate severity (even after 2 years), there is still a role for neuroimaging evaluation of dementia.

KEY POINTS

- Non-Alzheimer dementias constitute a significant proportion of dementia etiologies in epidemiologic studies. The major degenerative subtypes are vascular dementia (VaD), dementia with Lewy bodies (DLB), Parkinson's disease dementia (PDD), and frontotemporal dementia (FTD). These conditions have distinct clinical features and can often be reliably distinguished clinically from Alzheimer's disease (AD) through the use of standard criteria.
- It is important to accurately diagnose non-Alzheimer's dementia, as they often carry different prognoses, and entail different treatment considerations from AD. For instance, FTD generally carries a worse prognosis and is not amenable to cholinesterase

inhibitor treatment, unlike AD. Accurate diagnosis of DLB would alert the physician to the dangers of neuroleptic sensitivity when deciding on the course of treatment for the management of attendant neuropsychiatric problems. Aggressive treatment of vascular risk factors and secondary stroke prevention may impede progression of cognitive decline in VaD, even if the stroke lesions appear insignificant.

- In patients presenting with confusion of forgetfulness, it is important to exclude delirium, either in isolation (acute/subacute presentation) or in combination with an underlying neurodegenerative process (acute on chronic presentation).
- In the evaluation of dementia, it is vital to evaluate the behavioral, functional, and social complications, as these are often amenable to treatment or palliation.
- Through a four-step systematic approach involving comprehensive history-taking, targeted physical examination, and selected investigations, the clinician can confidently evaluate the diagnosis, complications, and etiology of older persons presenting with memory problems or confusion.

KEY REFERENCES

- Chong MS & Sahadevan S. An evidence-based clinical approach to the diagnosis of dementia. *Annals of the Academy of Medicine, Singapore* 2003; **32**:740–8.
- McKhann GM, Albert MS, Grossman M *et al.* Clinical and pathological diagnosis of frontotemporal dementia. Report of the Work Group on Frontotemporal Dementia and Pick's disease. *Archives of Neurology* 2001; **58**:1803–9.
- McKeith IG & Mosimann UP. Dementia with Lewy bodies and Parkinson's disease. *Parkinsonism & Related Disorders* 2004; **10**:S15–8.
- Roman GV. Vascular dementia: distinguishing characteristics, treatment, and prevention. *Journal of the American Geriatrics Society* 2003b; **51**:S296–304.
- Siu AL. Screening for dementia and investigating its causes. *Annals of Internal Medicine* 1991; **115**:122–32.

REFERENCES

Aarsland D. Donepezil for cognitive impairment in Parkinson's disease: a randomised controlled study. *Journal of Neurology, Neurosurgery, and Psychiatry* 2002; **72**:708–12.

Aarsland D, Andersen K, Larsen JP *et al.* Prevalence and characteristics of dementia in Parkinson's disease – an 8 year prospective study. *Archives of Neurology* 2003; **60**:387–92.

Aarsland D, Litvan I & Larsen JP. Neuropsychiatric symptoms of patients with progressive supranuclear palsy and Parkinson's disease. *The Journal of Neuropsychiatry and Clinical Neurosciences* 2001; **13**:42–9.

Alexopoulos GS, Abrams RC, Young RC *et al.* Cornell scale for depression in dementia. *Biological Psychiatry* 1988; **23**:271–84.

Alperovitch A, Zerr I, Pocchiari M *et al.* Codon 129 genotype and sporadic Creutzfeld-Jakob disease. *Lancet* 1999; **353**:1673–4.

American Psychiatric Association. *Diagnostic and Statistical Manual of Mental Disorders* 1994, 4th edn; American Psychiatric Association, Washington.

Andersen K, Lolk A, Nielsen H *et al.* Prevalence and incidence of dementia in Denmark. The Odense study. *Ugeskrift for Laeger* 2000; **162**:4386–90.

Baba M, Nakajo S, Tu P-H *et al.* Aggregation of alpha-synuclein in Lewy bodies of sporadic Parkinson's disease and dementia with Lewy bodies. *American Journal of Clinical Pathology* 1998; **152**:879.

Bahn MN, Kido DK, Lin W *et al.* Brain magnetic resonance diffusion abnormalities in Creutzfeld-Jakob disease. *Archives of Neurology* 1999; **56**:577–83.

Bak TH & Hodges JR. The neuropsychology of progressive supranuclear palsy. *Neurocase* 1998; **4**:89–94.

Bowler JV & Hachinski V. In JRM Copeland, MT Abou-Saleh & DG Blazer (eds) *Principles and Practice of Geriatric Psychiatry* 2002, p 249; John Wiley and Sons.

Brown J, Ashworth A, Gydesen S *et al.* Familial non-specific dementia maps to chromosome 3. *Human Molecular Genetics* 1995; **4**:1625–8.

Bucks RS, Ashworth DI, Wilcock GK *et al.* Assessment of activities of daily living in dementia: development of the Bristol Activities of Daily Living scales. *Age and Ageing* 1996; **25**:113–20.

Burke WJ, Roccaforte WH, Wengel SP *et al.* Disagreement in the reporting of depressive symptoms between patients with dementia of Alzheimer type and their collateral sources. *The American Journal of Geriatric Psychiatry* 1998; **6**(4):308–19.

Burke WJ & Wengel SP. Late life mood disorders. *Clinics in Geriatric Medicine* 2003; **19**:777–97.

Burns A, Lawlor B & Craig S. Rating scales in old age psychiatry. *The British Journal of Psychiatry* 2002; **180**:161–7.

Childs EA, Lyles RH, Selnes OA *et al.* Plasma viral load and CD4 lymphocytes predict HIV-associated dementia and sensory neuropathy. *Neurology* 1999; **52**:607–13.

Chong MS & Sahadevan S. An evidence-based clinical approach to the diagnosis of dementia. *Annals of the Academy of Medicine, Singapore* 2003; **32**:740–8.

Chui HC. Vascular dementia, a new beginning: shifting focus from clinical phenotype to ischemic brain injury. *Neurologic Clinics* 2000; **18**:951–77.

Clarfield AM. The reversible dementia: do they reverse? *Archives of Internal Medicine* 1988; **109**:476–86.

Clifford DB. Human immunodeficiency virus-associated dementia. *Archives of Neurology* 2000; **57**:321–4.

Concensus Committee of the American Autonomic Society and the American Academy of Neurology. Concensus statement on the definition of orthostatic hypotension, pure autonomic failure, and multiple system atrophy. *Neurology* 1996; **46**:1470.

Cummings JL. *The Neuropsychiatry of Alzheimer's Disease and Related Dementias* 2003; Martin Dunitz, London.

Cummings JL, Mega M, Gray K *et al.* The Neuropsychiatry Inventory: comprehensive assessment of psychopathology in dementia. *Neurology* 1994; **44**:2308–14.

Emre M. Dementia associated with Parkinson's disease. *Lancet. Neurology* 2003; **60**:387–92.

Emre M, Aarsland D, Albanese A *et al.* Rivastigmine for the dementia associated with Parkinson's disease. *The New England Journal of Medicine* 2004; **351**:2509–18.

Engel PA & Gelber J. Does computed tomographic brain imaging have a place in the diagnosis of dementia? *Archives of Internal Medicine* 1992; **152**:1437–40.

Erkinjuntti T, Roman G & Gauthier S. Treatment of vascular dementia–evidence from clinical trials with cholinesterase inhibitors. *Journal of the Neurological Sciences* 2004; **226**:63–6.

Ferman TJ, Smith GE, Boeve BF *et al.* DLB fluctuations: specific features that reliably differentiate DLB from AD and normal aging. *Neurology* 2004; **62**:181–7.

Ferrando S, van Gorp W, McElhiney M *et al.* Highly active antiretroviral treatment in HIV infections: benefits for neuropsychological function. *AIDS* 1998; **12**(8):F65–70.

Flaherty JH. Psychotherapeutic agents in older adults. Commonly prescribed and over-the-counter medications: causes of confusion. *Clinics in Geriatric Medicine* 1998; **14**(1):101–27.

Frank A, Diez-Tejedor E, Bullido MJ *et al.* APOE genotype in cerebrovascular disease and vascular dementia. *Journal of the Neurological Sciences* 2002; **203-4**:173–6.

Galton CJ, Patterson K, Graham KS *et al.* Differing patterns of temporal lobe atrophy in Alzheimer's disease and semantic dementia: diagnostic and theoretical implications. *Neurology* 2001; **57**:216–25.

Gold G, Bouras C, Canuto A *et al.* Clinicopathological validation study of four sets of clinical criteria for vascular dementia. *The American Journal of Psychiatry* 2002; **159**(8):1439–40.

Gold G, Giannakopoulos P, Montes-Paixao C *et al.* Sensitivity and specificity of newly proposed clinical criteria for possible vascular dementia. *Neurology* 1997; **49**:690–4.

Gomez-Tortosa E, Newell K, Irizarry MC *et al.* Clinical and quantitative pathological correlates of dementia with Lewy bodies. *Neurology* 1999; **53**:1248–91.

Graff-Radford NR. Normal pressure hydrocephalus. *The Neurologist* 1999; **5**:194–204.

Green RC. *Diagnosis and Management of Alzheimer's Disease and Other Dementias* 2001; Professional Communications.

Green AJE, Thompson EJ, Stewart GE *et al.* Use of 14-3-3 and other brain-specific proteins in the diagnosis of variant Creutzfeld-Jakob disease. *Journal of Neurology, Neurosurgery, and Psychiatry* 2001; **70**:744–8.

Gultekin SH, Rosenfeld MR, Voltz R *et al.* Paraneoplastic limbic encephalitis: neurological symptoms, immunological findings and tumour association in 50 patients. *Brain* 2000; **123**:1481–94.

Hachinski V, Lassen N & Marshall J. Multi-infarct dementia. A cause of mental deterioration in the elderly. *Lancet* 1974; **14**:207–10.

Harper PS. The epidemiology of Huntington's disease. *Human Genetics* 1992; **89**:365–76.

Harper PS. *Huntington's Disease. Major Problems in Neurology* 1996, vol. 31, 2nd edn; WB Saunders Company, London.

Harper C & Scolyer RA. In M Esiri, VMY Lee & JQ Trojanowski (eds) *The Neuropathology of Dementia* 2004, 2nd edn, pp 427–41; Cambridge University Press, Cambridge.

Hebb AO & Cusimano MD. Idiopathic normal pressure hydrocephalus: a systematic review of diagnosis and outcome. *Neurosurgery* 2001; **49**:1166–84.

Hénon H, Durieu I, Gueronaou D *et al.* Poststroke dementia. Incidence and relationship to prestroke cognitive decline. *Neurology* 2001; **57**:1216–22.

Hirono N, Ishii K, Sasaki M *et al.* Features of regional cerebral glucose metabolism abnormality in corticobasal degeneration. *Dementia and Geriatric Cognitive Disorders* 2000; **11**:39–46.

Hosler BA, Siddique T, Sapp PC *et al.* Linkage of familial amyotrophic lateral sclerosis with frontotemporal dementia to chromosome 9q21-q22. *The Journal of the American Medical Association* 2000; **284**:1664–9.

Hughes AJ, Ben-Shlomo Y, Daniel SE *et al.* What features improve the accuracy of clinical diagnosis in Parkinson's disease: a clinico-pathologic study. *Neurology* 1992; **42**:1142–6.

Ikeda M, Hokoishi K, Maki N *et al.* Increased prevalence of vascular dementia in Japan: a community-based epidemiological study. *Neurology* 2001; **57**:839–44.

Inouye SK, Viscoli CM, Horwitz RI *et al.* A predictive model for delirium in hospitalized elderly medical patients based on admission characteristics. *Annals of Internal Medicine* 1993; **119**:474–81.

International Huntington Association and the World Federation of Neurology Research Group on Huntington's Chorea. Guidelines for the molecular genetics predictive test in Huntington's disease. *Neurology* 1994; **44**:1533–6.

Ironside JW & Head MW. Human prion diseases. In M Esiri, VMY Lee & JQ Trojanowski (eds) *The Neuropathology of Dementia* 2004, 2nd edn, pp 402–26; Cambridge University Press, Cambridge.

Jackson JA, Jankovic J & Ford J. Progressive supranuclear palsy: clinical features and response to treatment in 16 patients. *Annals of Neurology* 1983; **13**:273–8.

Jacobs RA. Infectious diseases: spriochetal. In L Tierney, SJ McPhee & MA Papadakis (eds) *Current Medical Diagnosis and Treatment* 2000, 39th edn, pp 1376–86; McGraw-Hill.

Jorm AF. Is depression a risk factor for dementia or cognitive decline? *Gerontology* 2000; **46**:219–27.

Kertesz A, Martinez-Lage P, Davidson W *et al.* The corticobasal degeneration syndrome overlaps progressive aphasia and frontotemporal dementia. *Neurology* 2000; **55**:1368–75.

Kieburtz K, McDermott M, Como P *et al.*, The Parkinson Study Group. The effect of deprenyl and tocopherol on cognitive performance in early untreated Parkinson's disease. *Neurology* 1994; **44**:1756–9.

Kompoliti K, Goetz CG, Litvan I *et al.* Pharmacological therapy in progressive supranuclear palsy. *Archives of Neurology* 1998; **55**:1099–102.

Larson EB, Reifler BV, Sumi SM *et al.* Diagnostic tests in the valuation of dementia. A prospective study of 200 elderly outpatients. *Archives of Internal Medicine* 1986; **146**:1917–20.

Leroi I, Brandt J, Reich SG *et al.* Randomized placebo-controlled trial of donepezil in cognitive impairment in Parkinson's disease. *International Journal of Geriatric Psychiatry* 2004; **19**:1–8.

Litvan I, Agid Y, Calne D *et al.* Clinical research criteria for the diagnosis of progressive supranuclear palsy (Steele-Richardson-Olszewski syndrome): report of the NINDS-SPSP International Workshop. *Neurology* 1996; **47**:1–9.

Litvan I, Goetz CG, Jankovic J *et al.* What is the accuracy of the clinical diagnosis of multiple system atrophy? A clinicopathologic study. *Archives of Neurology* 1997; **54**:937–44.

Liu RS, Lemieux L, Shorvon SD *et al.* Association between brain size and abstinence from alcohol. *Lancet* 2000; **355**:1969–70.

Liu CK, Miller BL, Cummings JL *et al.* A quantitative MRI study of vascular dementia. *Neurology* 1992; **42**:138–43.

Lobo A, Launer AJ, Fratiglioni L *et al.* Prevalence of dementia and major subtypes in Europe: a collaborative study of population based cohorts. *Neurology* 2000; **54**(5):S4–9.

Lobotesis K, Fenwick JD, Phipps A *et al.* Occipital hypoperfusion on SPECT in dementia with Lewy bodies but not AD. *Neurology* 2001; **56**:643–9.

Looi JCL & Sachdev PS. Differentiation of vascular dementia from AD on neuropsychological tests. *Neurology* 1999; **53**:670–8.

Louis ED, Klatka LA, Liu Y *et al.* Comparison of extrapyramidal features in 31 pathologically confirmed cases of diffuse Lewy body disease and 34 pathologically confirmed cases of Parkinson's disease. *Neurology* 1997; **48**:376–80.

Lund and Manchester Groups. Concensus Statement. Clinical and neuropathological criteria for frontotemporal dementia. *Journal of Neurology, Neurosurgery, and Psychiatry* 1994; **57**:416–8.

McKeith IG. Dementia with Lewy bodies. *British Journal of Health Psychology* 2002; **180**:144–7.

McKeith IG. Dementia in Parkinson's disease: common and treatable. *Lancet. Neurology* 2004; **3**:456.

McKeith IG, Del Ser T, Spano P *et al.* Efficacy of rivastigmine in dementia with Lewy bodies a randomized, double-blind, placebo-controlled international study. *Lancet* 2000; **356**:2031–6.

McKeith IG, Fairbairn AF, Perry R *et al.* Neuroleptic sensitivity in patients with senile dementia of Lewy body type. *British Medical Journal* 1992; **305**:673–8.

McKeith IG, Galasko D, Kosaka K *et al.* Consensus guidelines for the clinical and pathologic diagnosis of dementia with Lewy bodies (DLB): report of the consortium on DLB international workshop. *Neurology* 1996; **47**:1113–24.

McKeith IG & Mosimann UP. Dementia with Lewy bodies and Parkinson's disease. *Parkinsonism & Related Disorders* 2004; **10**:S15–8.

McKhann GM, Albert MS, Grossman M *et al.* Clinical and pathological diagnosis of frontotemporal dementia. Report of the Work Group on Frontotemporal Dementia and Pick's disease. *Archives of Neurology* 2001; **58**:1803–9.

Miller BL, Cummings J, Mishkin F *et al.* Emergence of artistic talent in frontotemporal dementia. *Neurology* 1998; **51**:978–82.

Miller BL, Ikonte C, Ponton M *et al.* A study of the Lund-Manchester research criteria for frontotemporal dementia: clinical and single-photon emission CT correlations. *Neurology* 1997; **48**:937–42.

Moroney JT, Bagiella E, Desmond DW *et al.* Meta-analysis of the Hachinski Ischemic Score in pathologically verified dementias. *Neurology* 1997; **49**:1096–105.

Morris JH, Kalimo H & Viitanen M. In M Esiri, VMY Lee & JQ Trojanowski (eds) *The Neuropathology of Dementia* 2004, 2nd edn, pp 289–327; Cambridge university Press, Cambridge.

Morrison CE, Borod JC, Brin MF *et al.* Effects of levodopa on cognitive functioning in moderate-to-severe Parkinson's disease. *Journal of Neural Transmission* 2004; **111**:1333–41.

Mungas D, Jagust WJ, Reed BR *et al.* MRI predictors of cognition in subcortical ischemic vascular disease and Alzheimer's disease. *Neurology* 2001; **57**:2229–35.

Neary D, Snowden JS, Gustafson L *et al.* Frontotemporal lobar degeneration: a concensus on clinical diagnostic criteria. *Neurology* 1998; **51**:1546–54.

Olin JT, Katz IR, Meyers BS *et al.* Provisional diagnostic criteria for depression of Alzheimer disease. *The American Journal of Geriatric Psychiatry* 2002; **10**:120–41.

Orgogozo J-M, Rigaud A-S, Stöffler A *et al.* Efficacy and safety of memantine in patients with mild to moderate vascular dementia: a randomized, placebo-controlled trial (MMM 300). *Stroke* 2002; **33**:1834–9.

Oslin D, Atkinson RM, Smith DM *et al.* Alcohol related dementia: proposed clinical criteria. *International Journal of Geriatric Psychiatry* 1998; **13**:203–12.

Pantoni L, Rossi R, Inzitari D *et al.* Efficacy and safety of nimodipine in subcortical vascular dementia. A subgroup analysis of the Scandinavian Multi-Infarct Dementia Trial. *Journal of the Neurological Sciences* 2000; **175**:124–34.

Patterson CJ, Gauthier S, Bergman H *et al.* The recognition, assessment and management of dementing disorders: conclusions from the Canadian Consensus Conference on Dementia. *Canadian Medical Association Journal* 1999; **160**:S1–15.

Paulsen JS, Ready RE, Hamilton JM *et al.* Neuropsychiatric aspects of Huntington's disease. *Journal of Neurology, Neurosurgery, and Psychiatry* 2001; **71**:310–4.

Perry EK, Piggott MA, Johnson M *et al.* Neurotransmitter correlates of neuropsychiatric symptoms in dementia with Lewy bodies. In M-A Bedard, Y Agid, S Chouinard *et al.* (eds) *Mental and Behavioural Dysfunction in Movement Disorders* 2003, pp 285–91; Humana Press, Totowa.

Polo KB & Jabbari B. Botulinum Toxin-A improves the rigidity of progressive supranuclear palsy. *Annals of Neurology* 1994; **35**:237–9.

Porter RJ, Gallagher P, Thompson JM *et al.* Neurocognitive impairment in drug-free patients with major depressive disorder. *The British Journal of Psychiatry* 2003; **182**:214–20.

Powlishta KK, Storandt M, Mandernach TA *et al.* Absence of effect of depression on cognitive performance in early-stage Alzheimer disease. *Archives of Neurology* 2004; **61**:1265–8.

PROGRESS Collaborative Group. Randomized trial of perindopril-based blood-pressure lowering regimen among 6105 individuals with prior stroke or transient ischemic attack. *Lancet* 2001; **358**:1033–41.

Prusiner SB. Novel proteinaceous particles cause scrapie. *Science* 1982; **216**:136–44.

Reisberg B, Doody R, Stöffler A *et al.*, Memantine Study Group. Memantine in moderate-to-severe Alzheimer's disease. *The New England Journal of Medicine* 2003; **348**(14):1333–41.

Richard JH, Justus AW & Kurlan R. Relationship between mood and motor fluctuations in Parkinson's disease. *The Journal of Neuropsychiatry and Clinical Neurosciences* 2001; **13**:35–41.

Riley DE & Lang AE. Clinical diagnostic criteria. In I Litvan, CG Goetz & AE Lang (eds) *Corticobasal Degeneration and Related Disorders* 2000, pp 29–34; Lippincott & Williams, Philadelphia.

Roman GC. Vascular dementia revisited. Diagnosis, pathogenesis, treatment and prevention. *The Medical Clinics of North America* 2002; **86**:477–99.

Roman GC. Stroke, cognitive decline and vascular dementia: the silent epidemic of the 21st century. *Neuroepidemiology* 2003a; **22**(3):161–4.

Roman GV. Vascular dementia: distinguishing characteristics, treatment, and prevention. *Journal of the American Geriatrics Society* 2003b; **51**:S296–304.

Roman GC, Sachdev P, Royall DR *et al.* Vascular cognitive disorder: a new diagnostic category updating vascular cognitive impairment and vascular dementia. *Journal of the Neurological Sciences* 2004; **226**:81–7.

Roman GC, Tatemichi TK, Erkinjuntti T *et al.* Vascular dementia: diagnostic criteria for research studies. Report of the NINDS-AIREN international workshop. *Neurology* 1993; **43**:250–60.

Sachdev P. Vascular cognitive disorder. *International Journal of Geriatric Psychiatry* 1999; **14**:402–3.

Saunders PA, Copeland JR, Dewey ME *et al.* Heavy drinking as a risk factor for depression and dementia in elderly men. *The British Journal of Psychiatry* 1991; **159**:213–6.

Schneider JA, Watts RL, Gearing M *et al.* Corticobasal degeneration: neuropathological and clinical heterogeneity. *Neurology* 1997; **48**:959–69.

See SJ, Pan A, Seah A *et al.* Case reports of two biopsy proven patients with Creutzfeld-Jakob disease in Singapore. *Annals of the Academy of Medicine, Singapore* 2004; **33**:651–5.

Shepherd J, Blauw GJ, Murphy MB *et al.* Pravastatin in elderly individuals at risk of vascular disease (PROSPER): a randomized controlled trial. *Lancet* 2002; **360**:1623–30.

Shimoda K & Robinson RG. The relationship between poststroke depression and lesion location in long-term follow up. *Biological Psychiatry* 1999; **45**:187–92.

Siu AL. Screening for dementia and investigating its causes. *Annals of Internal Medicine* 1991; **115**:122–32.

Snowdon DA, Greiner LH, Mortimer JA *et al.* Brain infarction and the clinical expression of Alzheimer disease. The Nun study. *The Journal of the American Medical Association* 1997; **277**:813–7.

Snowden JS, Neary D, Mann DMA *et al.* Frontotemporal dementia. *The British Journal of Psychiatry* 2002; **180**:140–3.

Stevens T, Livingston G, Kitchen G *et al.* Islington study of dementia subtypes in the community. *The British Journal of Psychiatry* 2002; **180**:270–6.

Swartz JR, Miller BL, Lesser IM *et al.* Frontotemporal dementia: treatment response to serotonin selective reuptake inhibitors. *The Journal of Clinical Psychiatry* 1997; **58**:212–6.

Tandberg E, Larsen JP, Aarsland D *et al.* Risk factors for depression in Parkinson's disease. *Archives of Neurology* 1997; **54**:625–30.

Tomlinson BE, Blessed G & Roth M. Observations on the brains of demented people. *Journal of the Neurological Sciences* 1970; **11**:205–42.

van Reekum R, Simard M, Clarke D *et al.* Late life depression as a possible predictor of dementia: cross-sectional and short-term follow-up results. *The American Journal of Geriatric Psychiatry* 1999; **7**:151–9.

Verrees M & Selman WR. Management of normal pressure hydrocephalus. *American Family Physician* 2004; **70**:1071–8.

von Strauss E, Viitanen M, De Ronchi D *et al.* Aging and the occurrence of dementia: findings from a population based cohort with a large sample of nonagenarians. *Archives of Neurology* 1999; **56**:587–92.

Walstra GJ, Tenuisse S, van Gool WA *et al.* Reversible dementia in elderly patients referred to a memory clinic. *Journal of Neurology* 1997; **224**:17–22.

Wang W, Wu S, Cheng X *et al.* Prevalence of Alzheimer's disease and other dementing disorders in an urban community of Beijing, China. *Neuroepidemiology* 2000; **19**:194–200.

Weintraub S, Rubin N, Mesulam MM *et al.* Primary progressive aphasia, longitudinal course, neuropsychological profile and language features. *Annals of Neurology* 1990; **31**:174–83.

Wenning GK, Ben Shlomo Y, Magalhaes M *et al.* Clinical features and natural history of multiple system atrophy. An analysis of 100 cases. *Brain* 1994; **117**:835–45.

Wilkinson D, Doody R, Helme R *et al.* Donepezil 308 Study Group. Donepezil in vascular dementia: a randomized, placebo-controlled study. *Neurology* 2003; **61**:479–86.

Will RG, Alpers MP, Dormont D *et al.* Infectious and sporadic prion diseases. In SB Prusiner (ed) *Prion Biology and Diseases* 1999, pp 465–508; Cold Spring Harbour Laboratory Press, Cold Spring Harbour.

Windl O, Dempster M, Estibeiro P *et al.* Genetic basis of Creutzfeld-Jakob disease in the United Kingdom: a systematic analysis of predisposing mutations and allelic variation in the PRNP gene. *Human Genetics* 1996; **98**:259–64.

Working Group of the American Academy of Neurology AIDS Task Force. Nomenclature and research case definitions for neurologic manifestations of human immunodeficiency virus type 1 (HIV-1) infection. *Neurology* 1991; **41**:778–85.

World Health Organization. *The ICD-10 Classification of Mental and Behavioural Disorders. Diagnostic Criteria for Research* 1993; World Health Organization, Geneva.

Yesavage J, Brink T, Rose T *et al.* Development and validation of a geriatric depression scale. *Journal of Psychiatric Research* 1983; **17**:37–49.

Younger DS. Vasculitis of the nervous system. *Current Opinion in Neurology* 2004; **17**:317–36.

Zanusso G, Ferrari S, Cardone F *et al.* Detection of pathologic prion protein in the olfactory epithelium on sporadic Creutzfeld-Jakob disease. *The New England Journal of Medicine* 2003; **348**:711–9.

Zerr I, Pocchiari M, Collins S *et al.* Analysis of EEG and 14-3-3 proteins as aids to the diagnosis of Creutzfeld-Jakob disease. *Neurology* 2000; **55**:811–5.

Zhukavera V, Vogelsberg-Ragaglia V, Van Deerlin VMD *et al.* Loss of brain tau defines novel sporadic and familial tauopathies with frontotemporal dementia. *Annals of Neurology* 2001; **49**:165–75.

Treatment of Behavioral Disorders

Ladislav Volicer
University of South Florida, Tampa, FL, USA

INTRODUCTION

Behavioral disorders in elderly individuals are most commonly caused by a dementing process. Individuals who suffered from lifelong psychiatric diseases, such as schizophrenia, might continue to exhibit symptoms of these diseases even in old age, but management of these symptoms follows general psychiatric practice. Therefore, this chapter will concentrate on behavioral disorders caused by a progressive degenerative dementia.

Problem behavior is a serious problem in progressive dementias and is the most common reason for institutionalization (Phillips and Diwan, 2003). The most common progressive dementias are Alzheimer's disease, vascular dementia, dementia with Lewy bodies, and frontotemporal dementia. A behavioral disorder may also be caused by a delirium that is induced by an acute medical or surgical condition (e.g. infections, dehydration, metabolic disorder) or by adverse effects of medications (e.g. drugs that have anticholinergic effect such as diphenhydramine, thioridazine, and benztropine, by cardiac medications such as digoxin and antihypertensive agents, and by drugs used to treat peptic ulcers such as cimetidine). Individuals with dementia are more sensitive to development of delirium and occurrence of delirium in cognitively intact individuals is an indication that the individual is at high risk of developing dementia.

Delirium is characterized by an acute onset of mental status change, fluctuating course, decreased ability to focus, sustain and shift attention, and either disorganized thinking or an altered level of consciousness that resolves if the precipitating causes are removed (*see* **Chapter 90, Delirium**). However, diagnosis of delirium is not easy because some of these diagnostic criteria are not unique for delirium. Acute onset of mental status change may be caused also by a vascular dementia, and fluctuating course of cognitive impairment is an important clinical diagnostic feature of dementia with Lewy bodies (McKeith *et al.*, 1996). Delirium is also not always a transient cognitive impairment because cognitive impairment resolves within 3 months in only 20% of patients with diagnosis of delirium. The specific symptoms of reversible dysfunction include plucking at bedclothes, poor attention, incoherent speech, abnormal associations, and slow vague thoughts. Delirium superimposed on dementia ranges from 22%–89% of hospitalized and community populations aged 65 and older with dementia and has several adverse effects including accelerated decline, need for institutionalization, and increased mortality. Therefore, the possibility that delirium is responsible for the onset of new behavioral symptoms should be always considered.

The diagnostic criteria for Alzheimer's disease include multiple cognitive deficits manifested by both memory impairment and at least one other cognitive disturbance (aphasia, apraxia, agnosia, or disturbance of executive functioning). These cognitive deficits have to be severe enough to cause significant impairment in social or occupational functioning and has to represent a significant decline from a previous level of functioning. The course of the Alzheimer's disease is characterized by a gradual onset and continuing cognitive decline. The cognitive impairment cannot be due to other brain disease, to systemic disturbances that can cause dementia, or to drug-induced effects. Clinical diagnosis of the Alzheimer's disease is tentative and needs to be supported by neuropathological examination of the brain after the patient dies. Thus, the most definite clinical diagnosis of Alzheimer's disease is "Probable Alzheimer's disease", which is made when there are no other possible etiological factors and "Possible Alzheimer's disease" when other possible etiological factors are also present.

There are several diagnostic sets of criteria for vascular dementia and they differ from each other (Verhey *et al.*, 1996) (*see* **Chapter 95, Vascular Dementia**). Most criteria require an abrupt onset of dementia, focal neurological findings (abnormal reflexes or nerve functions), low-density areas (indicating vascular changes in the white matter) and/or the presence of multiple strokes on CT (computerized tomography) or MRI (magnetic resonance imaging) scans. Other criteria also include fluctuation of impairment, unchanged personality, emotional lability, and a temporal relation between

Principles and Practice of Geriatric Medicine, 4th Edition. Edited by M.S. John Pathy, Alan J. Sinclair and John E. Morley.

a stroke and development of dementia. However, it has to be recognized that vascular changes are often present together with Alzheimer changes during brain autopsy. Thus, it is difficult to exclude the possibility that a patient has Alzheimer's disease even when several criteria for vascular dementia are met.

Dementia with Lewy bodies (also sometimes called *diffuse Lewy body disease*) is characterized by a fluctuating course of cognitive impairment that includes episodic confusion with lucid intervals similar to delirium (McKeith *et al.*, 1996) (*see* **Chapter 96, Other Dementias**). In addition, there must be at least one of the following: (1) visual and/or auditory hallucinations resulting in paranoid delusions, (2) mild extrapyramidal symptoms (muscle rigidity, slow movements) or adverse extrapyramidal response to standard doses of antipsychotics, or (3) repeated unexplained falls. The clinical features of dementia with Lewy bodies persist over a long period of time in contrast to delirium that is usually shorter and usually does not progress to severe dementia. As with Alzheimer's disease, other causes of the progressive cognitive decline have to be excluded.

The diagnosis of frontotemporal dementia is based on personality changes and the presence of atrophy of the frontal brain areas in neuroimaging studies (CT scan, or MRI). The personality changes in frontotemporal dementia are similar to changes induced by the damage of frontal lobes by other causes (injury, stroke) and include behavioral disinhibition, loss of social or personal awareness, or disengagement with apathy. Patients with frontotemporal dementia differ from Alzheimer patients because they maintain some abilities (e.g. elementary drawing and calculations) into the later stages of dementia. Pick's disease is a pathological subtype of frontotemporal dementia, which is characterized by specific neuropathological findings: Pick bodies inside nerve cells and ballooned nerve cells.

PHYSICAL CAUSES OF BEHAVIORAL SYMPTOMS

Before any behavioral symptoms are ascribed to underlying dementia, possible physical causes have to be eliminated. Behavioral symptoms may be induced by an acute illness or an exacerbation of a chronic condition. These conditions include cardiovascular disease, brain tumors, sensory deprivation (*see* **Chapter 103, Disorders of the Eye**; **Chapter 105, Auditory System**), metabolic disorders, chronic obstructive pulmonary disease, and anemia. Acute illness can be an infection, acute abdominal conditions, or an injury. Unrecognized pain is a common cause of behavioral symptoms and treatment of behavioral symptoms with acetaminophen may decrease the inappropriate use of psychoactive medications (*see* **Chapter 84, Control of Chronic Pain**). The pain could result from fecal impaction, urinary retention, or unrecognized fracture, but the most common cause of chronic pain in nursing home residents is arthritis, followed by old fractures, neuropathy, and malignancy. Detection of pain is difficult in individuals with dementia who cannot describe the pain and its location. A comprehensive evaluation of pain in noncommunicative individual relies on the observation of facial expression, vocalization, and body movements and tension and may use a recently developed scale (Warden *et al.*, 2003).

CONCEPTUAL FRAMEWORK OF BEHAVIORAL SYMPTOMS OF DEMENTIA

Although progressive degenerative dementias differ in their early presentation, the behavioral disorders that they cause in later stages of dementia are very similar. Several conceptual frameworks were developed to classify and describe behavioral symptoms of dementia on the basis of nursing, psychological, or psychiatric concepts (Volicer and Hurley, 2003). A model integrating all these approaches postulates a hierarchy of causes of behavioral symptoms (Figure 1). At the core of these symptoms is the dementing process itself that may be modified by the underlying personality of the individual. Primary consequences of dementia are functional impairment, mood disorders, and delusions/hallucinations. These primary consequences, alone or in combination, lead to secondary consequences that are inability to initiate meaningful activities, dependence in activities of daily living (ADLs), spatial disorientation, and anxiety. Primary and secondary consequences of dementia cause peripheral symptoms: agitation, apathy, insomnia, interference with other residents, resistiveness to care, food refusal, and elopement. Peripheral symptoms may be caused by more than one of the primary and secondary consequences, and each primary and secondary consequence can generate several peripheral symptoms. For instance, functional impairment may lead to an inability to initiate meaningful activities, dependence in

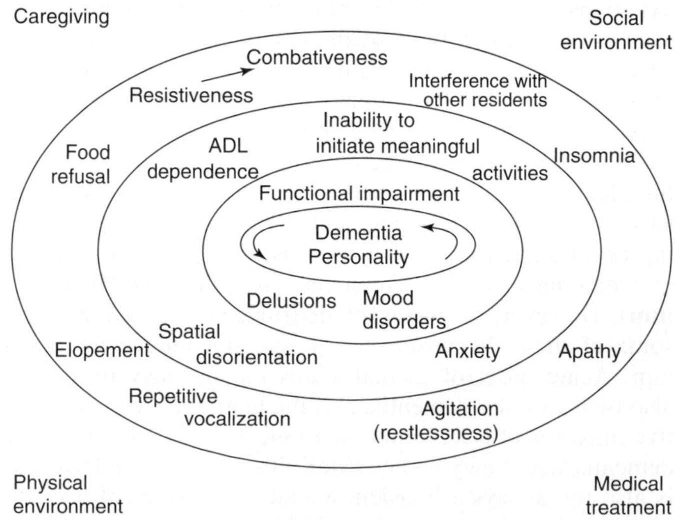

Figure 1 Comprehensive model of psychiatric symptoms of progressive degenerative dementias. (From Mahoney, Volicer and Hurley (2000). *Management of challenging behaviors in dementia* (p. 2). Baltimore: Health Professions Press; reprinted by permission)

ADLs, and anxiety and agitation if stressful demands are made, or agitation/apathy and repetitive vocalization if meaningful activities are not provided. Similarly, depression may lead to anxiety, worsening of the ability to initiate meaningful activities and to engage in ADLs, to food refusal, agitation, insomnia, and worsening of resistiveness to care. Therefore, it is important to analyze the cause(s) of peripheral behavioral symptoms of dementia and treat effectively the primary or secondary consequences that are causing these symptoms instead of treating each peripheral symptom in isolation.

Behavioral symptoms of dementia are influenced by four environmental factors. Caregiving approaches are most important for the resistiveness/combativeness continuum (see below). Social environment is important because it eliminates problems related to interaction with cognitively intact nursing home residents. Physical environment should prevent elopement and provide for safe ambulation and wandering. And finally, medical interventions may aggravate behavioral symptoms because demented individuals do not understand the need for these interventions and do not cooperate with diagnostic and therapeutic procedures. The rest of this chapter will describe in more detail elements of this model and therapeutic approaches that can be used.

DEMENTIA AND PERSONALITY

Dementia is at the core of behavioral disorders. There is some evidence that premorbid personality traits are related to subsequent psychiatric symptoms. Patients who were more neurotic and less assertive before developing dementia are more likely to become depressed, while patients who were more hostile before developing dementia are more likely to have paranoid delusions. Patients who were neurotic and extroverted before developing dementia are more likely to engage in aggressive behavior while previous agreeableness decreases the probability of aggression.

Unfortunately, there is no treatment currently available that would stop or reverse the course of progressive degenerative dementias. However, there are currently two classes of medications approved for the treatment of Alzheimer's disease (Table 1). There is some evidence that cholinesterase inhibitors may be also useful for treatment of vascular dementia (Kumar *et al.*, 2003) and dementia with Lewy bodies (Wesnes *et al.*, 2002). Although the primary effect of cholinesterase inhibitors is the improvement of cognitive function, their administration also leads to some improvement in behavioral symptoms of dementia. Metanalysis of published reports regarding the efficacy of cholinesterase inhibitors showed that the behavior of patients treated with cholinesterase inhibitors improved significantly according to the Neuropsychiatric Inventory (Trinh *et al.*, 2003). There was no difference in efficacy among cholinesterase inhibitors. Memantine was found to decrease agitation (Areosa and Sherriff, 2003).

Table 1 Drugs for treatment of dementia

Drug	Mechanism of action	Daily doses (mg)	Maintenance dose
Donepezil (Aricept)	Inhibition of AChE	5, 10[a]	10 mg QD
Galantamine (Reminyl)	Inhibition of AChE Nicotinic receptor modulation	8, 16, 24[b]	8–12 mg BID
Rivastigmine (Exelon)	Inhibition of AchE Inhibition of BChE	3, 6, 9, 12[b]	4.5–6 mg BID
Memantine (Namenda)	Modulation of NMDA receptors	5, 10, 15, 20[c]	10 mg BID

AChE, acetylcholine esterase; BChE, butyrylcholine esterase; NMDA, *N*-methyl-d-aspartate.
[a]The dose should be increased after 4–6 weeks. [b]The dose should be increased if lower dose is tolerated for 4 weeks. [c]The dose should be increased every week.

Cholinesterase inhibitors may not be effective enough to control all behavioral symptoms of dementia, but they may be useful as a first line treatment. Donepezil was found to potentiate the antipsychotic effect of perphenazine (Bergman *et al.*, 2003) and caregivers of individuals with dementia treated with donepezil report lower level of behavioral disturbances than caregivers of individuals not receiving this treatment. Donepezil patients were described as significantly less likely to be threatening, destroy property, and talk loudly. Cholinesterase inhibitors are usually well tolerated, with diarrhea and nausea being the most common adverse effects.

FUNCTIONAL IMPAIRMENT

Presence of functional impairment that interferes with daily activities is necessary for the diagnosis of dementia. Functional impairment is a result of several deficits affecting both cognitive and physical functions. Memory impairment causes inability to remember appointments and prevents the individual from participating in social games, for example, bridge. Speech impairment interferes with social contact and may result in an inability to understand spoken or written language. Apraxia leads to the inability to use tools and continue engagement in previous hobbies. Spatial disorientation leads to the inability to take independent walks. Executive dysfunction leads to deficits in problem solving and judgment and prevents the individual from planning and executing an activity.

Functional impairment may cause three secondary consequences of dementia: dependence in ADLs, inability to initiate meaningful activities, and anxiety if a person with dementia recognizes his/her limitations, or if a caregiver has unrealistic expectations about abilities of the care recipient. These secondary consequences may cause several peripheral symptoms: resistiveness to care, agitation, repetitive vocalization, apathy, and insomnia. Functional impairment may involve both cognitive and physical components.

Treatment of cognitive component of functional impairment involves both behavioral and pharmacological approaches. Because of the progressive nature of dementia, the deficits cannot be reversed. However, they can be minimized and the function maintained for as long as possible by creating an environment in which the individual with dementia can experience positive emotions and by preventing excess disability that may be induced either by expecting too much or by expecting too little from the individual (*see* **Chapter 158, Geriatric Occupational Therapy: Focus on Participation in Meaningful Daily Living**). In the mild to moderate stage of dementia, memory aids may be helpful. Cueing and creating connections to familiar things, and simplifying and breaking tasks into small parts may be useful to maintain dressing behavior (Beck *et al.*, 1997). Practice may also help maintain cognitive skills. Patients who performed exercises that included word fluency, immediate and long-term verbal and nonverbal recall and recognition, and problem solving, improved their cognitive function and had less behavioral problems while control group continued to decline. These results indicate that procedural learning can occur in individuals with dementia and that the rate of decline can be slowed by the prevention of excess disability. Individuals may also maintain ability to perform an activity (e.g. playing dominoes) even after they lose the ability to explain the rules.

Pharmacological management of cognitive component of functional impairment involves drugs used for treatment of dementia described above. There is good evidence that both cholinesterase inhibitors and memantine improve temporarily functional abilities or slow down the rate of their loss. Multifactorial approaches to maintenance of cognitive function were also developed. In a study involving administration of ginkgo biloba, vitamin C, vitamin E, and low fat diet, and including meditation, mind-body exercises, physical exercises, stress reduction techniques and cognitive rehabilitation exercises, experimental group improved in verbal fluency, controlled oral word association test, and paired association (Bender *et al.*, 2002).

Physical component of functional impairment includes decreased ability to ambulate and eat. Individuals with dementia become unable to ambulate independently because they cannot recognize objects in their path and because neurological impairment leads to unsteady or narrow-based gait (*see* **Chapter 112, Gait, Balance, and Falls**). Both of these consequences lead to an increased risk for falls. If the risk for falls is managed by restraints, the individuals deteriorate further because of deconditioning and forgetting how to walk. It is important to maintain ambulatory ability for as long as possible because walking represents meaningful activity and because inability to walk increases the risk of intercurrent infections and pressure ulcers. Ability to walk can be promoted by a regular walking program and by assistive devices, such as Merry Walker (Trudeau *et al.*, 2003).

MOOD DISORDERS

Mood disorders that can occur in individuals with dementia include depressive disorders and bipolar disorder. Depressive disorders are major depression with or without psychosis, dysthymic disorder, and minor depressive disorder (*see* **Chapter 100, Depression in Late Life: Etiology, Diagnosis and Treatment**). Depression is very common in community dwelling individuals with dementia and should be considered even in individuals with advanced dementia. Depression can cause or aggravate the inability to initiate meaningful activity and dependence in ADLs, and often has an anxiety component. These secondary consequences may lead to several peripheral symptoms, such as apathy, agitation, food refusal, and repetitive vocalization. Depression may also aggravate resistiveness to care because depressed individuals ignore ADLs. Depression also increases the propensity for escalation of resistiveness into combativeness because even cognitively intact depressed individuals are angry and do not tolerate others. Depression was significantly more common among residents with dementia who manifested physical or verbal aggression than in those without such behaviors (Menon *et al.*, 2001). Depressive symptomatology may be improved by providing sufficient meaningful activities, but often requires treatment with antidepressants.

The first line drugs to use for treatment of depression in individuals with dementia are selective serotonin reuptake inhibitors (SSRIs) (Table 2). These medications are usually well tolerated with the most common adverse effect being diarrhea. Since many individuals with dementia suffer from

Table 2 Selected antidepressants for treatment of depression in individuals with dementia

Drug class[a]	Name (trade name)	Dose range (mg)	Frequency[b]	Elimination half-life (hours)
Tricyclics	Amitryptyline (Elavil, Endep)	25–100	TID	24
	Nortryptyline (Aventyl, Pamelor)	25–50	BID–QID	26
SSRIs	Citalopram (Celexa)	20–60	QAM/HS	35
	Escitalopram (Lexapro)	10–20	QAM/HS	27–32
	Fluoxetine (Prozac)	10–40	QAM	168
	Fluvoxamine (Luvox)	50–300	QHS	15
	Paroxetine (Paxil)	20–50	QHS	24
	Sertraline (Zoloft)	50–200	QAM	24
Other	Bupropion (Wellbutrin)	150–300	BID–TID	14
	Mirtazepine (Remeron)	15–45	QHS	30
	Trazodone (Desyrel)	50–300	TID, QHS	8
	Venlafaxine (Effexor)	25–75	BID–TID	11

[a]SSRIs, selective serotonin reuptake inhibitors; [b]QD, once a day; BID, twice a day; TID, three times a day; QID, four times a day; QAM, every morning; QHS, every evening.

constipation, this usually is not a problem. SSRIs have some differences in their effects. Fluoxetine is the most stimulating of them and may result in increased agitation while paroxetine is sedating. Both fluoxetine and paroxetine, and to a lesser extent sertraline affect cytochrome P450 isoenzymes and interfere with metabolism of several drugs. Escitalopram may be an improvement over the first generation SSRIs because it is faster acting than citalopram (Valuck, 2004).

In individuals who do not tolerate SSRIs, venlafaxine, or bupropion may be used. Another option is mirtazepine, which may promote food intake in individuals with decreased appetite. Tricyclic antidepressants are used infrequently because they cause significant adverse effects that are partly mediated by an anticholinergic activity. Because of this activity, they are contraindicated in individuals treated with cholinesterase inhibitors. Trazodone is a relatively weak antidepressant but is useful for treatment of insomnia as will be discussed below. Electroshock therapy is effective in the treatment of depression in elderly individuals but may increase memory loss caused by dementia. Treatment of psychotic depression requires addition of antipsychotics to the antidepressant therapy. However, addition of an antipsychotic may be also effective in the treatment of resistant depression without psychotic features (Shelton *et al.*, 2001).

The prevalence of manic episodes in individuals with Alzheimer's disease and other dementias is relatively low and most of the individuals who exhibit them have a history of mania before the onset of Alzheimer's disease. Manic episodes are more common in people with cerebrovascular disease, especially when it involves the right hemisphere and orbitofrontal cortex. Manic symptomatology can be a significant cause of agitation and may also lead to interference with other residents, for example, unwelcome sexual advances.

Manic symptomatology is best treated with mood stabilizers (Table 3). Lithium is a drug of choice for the treatment of bipolar disorder in young individuals but its use in older individuals is questionable because the elderly may have age-related decreased kidney function or diseases and drug treatments that affect lithium excretion. Lithium is less effective in older adults with "organic manic disorder"; dementia, or mania complicated by serious medical conditions or by other psychiatric diagnoses. Carbamazepine is effective in the treatment of agitation in nursing home residents with dementia, but it has significant adverse effects that include rash, sedation, ataxia, agranulocytosis, hepatic dysfunction, and electrolyte disturbance.

The most commonly used mood stabilizers in dementia are valproic acid and gabapentin. Valproic acid, or its better tolerated enteric-coated derivative, divalproex sodium, was shown to be effective in dementia in several trials and this effect may be partly mediated by a neuroprotective effect (Tariot *et al.*, 2002). However, a recent metanalysis of these trials concluded that low doses of valproate may not be effective and high doses are associated with unacceptable rate of adverse effects, mainly sedation (Lonergan *et al.*, 2004). Other potential adverse effects of valproic acid include weight gain, hair loss, thrombocytopenia, and hepatic dysfunction.

Gabapentin is used increasingly in the management of behavior problems in individuals with dementia despite lack of randomized control studies. An open label study found that gabapentin was well tolerated and decreased caregiver stress. The advantages of gabapentin over other mood stabilizers are the relative lack of adverse effects and no need to monitor plasma levels. Several newer anticonvulsants are also sometimes used for treatment of behavioral symptoms of dementia but there are no data about their effectiveness and side effect profiles.

DELUSIONS AND HALLUCINATIONS

Delusion is a false belief, based on incorrect inference about an external reality that is firmly sustained despite evidence to the contrary. Delusions are often combined with hallucinations, which are sensory perceptions occurring without the appropriate stimulation of the corresponding sensory organ. Delusions occur in about half of individuals with Alzheimer's disease. Most of them have only delusions, some have both delusions and hallucinations, while isolated hallucinations are rare. Isolated hallucinations are more common in dementia with Lewy bodies. Delusions and hallucinations could be caused by other conditions. The most common one is delirium, which was described above.

Delusions may be divided into two types: simple persecutory delusions and complex, bizarre, or multiple delusions (*see* **Chapter 98, Geriatric Psychiatry**). Simple persecutory delusions include delusions of theft or suspicion. Suspicions involve beliefs such as being watched or having an unfaithful spouse. Complex delusions may include a conviction about a family member or a pet being injured, about plots against individuals of certain religious faith, and about wild parties happening on a nonexisting floor of the

Table 3 Selected mood stabilizers used in dementia

Name (trade name)	Dose range (mg)	Frequency[a]	Elimination half-life (hours)	Therapeutic level
Lithium (Eskalith, Lithobid, etc.)	100–300	BID–QID	22	$0.6-1.2\ mEq\ l^{-1}$
Valproic acid (Depakene); divalproex sodium (Depakote)	100–300	BID–QID	9–16	$50-125\ \mu g\ ml^{-1}$
Carbamazepine (Tegretol)	100–200	BID	25–65 (12–17)[b]	$4-12\ \mu g\ ml^{-1}$
Gabapentin (Neurontin)	300–900	TID[c]	5–7	Not measured

[a]BID, twice a day; TID, three times a day; QID, four times a day; [b]After chronic administration. [c]After titration phase (during titration, 300 mg once a day of BID).

nursing home. An example of complex delusion is Capgras syndrome that consists of a false belief that significant people have been replaced by identical-appearing impostors. Complex delusions may also present as grandiose delusions often connected with euphoria and hypomanic mood.

The most common delusions in Alzheimer patients are paranoid delusions, and the most common of those are delusions of theft that occurred in 28% of patients. The cause of these delusions may be memory problem of the patient, who forgets where he or she has put personal belongings. Delusions of suspicion were seen in 9% of the patients and more complex delusions in 3.6%. A common delusion of suspicion is that other patients in a long-term care facility are criticizing the patient behind his or her back. A stimulus for this delusion may be an innocent conversation in the hallway that is not heard very well by the patient and is misinterpreted. A very common delusion is the belief that the patient is much younger than his or her actual age. This delusion may be connected with misidentification, for example, of the patient's wife as his mother.

Onset of hallucinations in Alzheimer's disease is usually later in the disease progression, more than 5 years after the onset of dementia or more than a year after diagnosis. In approximately half of the patients the hallucinations are temporary, while in other patients hallucinations persist until death. Therefore, it is important to frequently reevaluate the need for pharmacological treatment in demented individuals. Hallucinations and delusions are associated with greater functional impairment and are more common in individuals who have extrapyramidal signs, such as muscle rigidity, and in individuals who have myoclonus.

Delusions and hallucinations may cause several secondary and peripheral behavioral symptoms of dementia. They may induce anxiety and spatial disorientation, and they may also interfere with ADLs because the individual does not believe that the activity is needed. Delusions and hallucinations are related to resistiveness to care and "aggression" (Kunik *et al.*, 1999), and agitation (Haupt *et al.*, 1998). They may also lead to food refusal if the individual believes that the food is poisoned and to attempts to leave a home or facility if the individual believes that he/she has to go to work or go "home". Misidentification of other residents and staff may lead to interference with other residents or inappropriate behavior toward the staff.

Treatment of delusions and hallucinations should consider their relationship to other behavioral symptoms of dementia. Some individuals with dementia have many delusions or hallucinations but are not bothered by them and they do not affect them behaviorally. In that case, no treatment is necessary. Otherwise, it is important to attempt nonpharmacological management of delusions and hallucinations before initiating treatment with antipsychotic medications. Nonpharmacological management should include attention to sensory perceptions, environmental modifications, and behavior strategies. Improvement of vision or hearing may decrease auditory delusions or visual hallucinations. Increased lighting, decreased noise, safe space for ambulation, and social environment of a dementia special care unit will decrease the need to treat delusions and hallucinations, which cause behaviors that may be distressing to other cognitively intact residents. Behavior strategies should recognize that reasoning cannot change behavior because the individual with dementia does not understand reasoning and does not remember what he/she was told; therefore, caregivers have to change their behavior. Caregivers should avoid the word "no" and instead of arguing, distract the individual from undesirable activity. It is better to accept the individual's reality than to try to orient them to reality. And the person with dementia should always be made comfortable by smiling, by a positive tone of voice, and by answering in a positive way even if the individual's speech does not make sense.

Pharmacological treatment of delusions and hallucinations utilizes administration of antipsychotics (Table 4). Older antipsychotics, represented by haloperidol, were potent antagonists of dopamine receptors. This led to a high incidence of extrapyramidal side effects and akathisia. These drugs are mostly replaced by newer (atypical) antipsychotics that have more beneficial adverse effect profile. This improvement is due to their effect on other than dopamine receptors. The most significant is blockade of the serotonin 2A receptors that prevents extrapyramidal side effects and may also lead to improvement in apathy. This activity is present in risperidone and olanzapine. However, activity at other receptors may lead to other adverse effects. Olanzapine and quetiapine block histamine 1 receptors, resulting in sedation and weight gain. The weight gain is especially troublesome in olanzapine, because it could lead to development of diabetes. Blockade of noradrenergic alpha 1 receptors, that is present in quetiapine and risperidone, may lead to orthostatic hypotension. Aripiprazole has a novel mechanism of action because it is a partial agonist on dopamine receptors. This effect prevents excessive dopamine activity while preserving normal dopamine function.

Table 4 Selected antipsychotics used for treatment in dementia

Name (trade name)	Dose range (mg)	Frequency[a]	Elimination half-life (hours)	Most common adverse effects
Aripiprazole (Abilify)	10–15	QD	75 (94)[b]	Insomnia, somnolence
Haloperidol (Haldol)	0.5–1	QD–TID	18	EPS[a], tardive dyskinesia
Olanzapine (Zyprexa)	2.5–10	QD	30	Weight gain, anticholinergic, sedation
Quetiapine (Seroquel)	25–100	BID–TID	6	Sedation, hypotension
Risperidone (Risperdal)	0.25–1	QD–BID	3–20 (21–30)[a]	EPS, hypotension

[a]QD, once a day; BID, twice a day; TID, three times a day; EPS, extrapyramidal side effects; [b]active metabolite.

Most clinical studies in dementia involved risperidone but usually used agitation or aggression as an outcome because delusions and hallucinations are difficult to measure in individuals with dementia who have limited communication ability (Brodaty *et al.*, 2003). Risperidone administration resulted in lower risk for falls and weight gain than olanzapine. Quetiapine has a broad dose range and its efficacy is somewhat unpredictable although it was found to be effective in an open label study (Tariot *et al.*, 2004). Risperidone was associated with slightly increased incidence of cerebrovascular incidents and other antipsychotics may also increase the risk of strokes. Therefore, it is important to avoid the use of antipsychotics if possible and use the lowest effective dose when they are being used.

DEPENDENCE IN ACTIVITIES OF DAILY LIVING

ADLs are the activities that are needed for self-care and independent living. They include instrumental activities of daily living (IADLs) and physical activities of daily living (PADLs) sometimes called *basic ADLs*. Dependence in ADLs is the result of functional impairment induced by dementia, but depression or delusions may aggravate the dependence, resulting in excess disability. Therefore, it is important to determine carefully the reasons for dependence. If the individual is dependent in PADLs, physical care has to be provided. The individual with dementia might not recognize the reason for this care and might resist the care. This resistiveness may escalate into combative behavior as will be described below. Thus, ADL dependence may lead to significant behavioral changes.

IADLs include shopping, preparing meals, traveling, doing housework and laundry, using telephone, taking medications, and managing money. Continued participation in ADLs is important for the self-esteem of the individual with dementia but safety and stress induced by these activities have to be considered. IADLs should be simplified because the individual with dementia may still be able to participate in some steps but not in the entire activity (Table 5). Supportive services, such as a homemaker or Meals on Wheels, may allow an individual with dementia to continue living in his/her own home. Assistance may come in many forms: encouragement, verbal cues, visual cues (gestures), and physical guidance.

Table 5 Examples of IADL adaptations for individuals with dementia

IADL	Suggested adaptations
Shopping	Plan and go shopping with others Continue to help choosing purchases
Meal preparation	Prepare one dish, with steps presented one at a time
Using telephone	Help person list things to talk about before making a call Help person call relatives and friends Put pictures of people on preprogramed telephone buttons
Money management	Simplify bill-paying routine Carry small amount of money Make small purchases with assistance on shopping trips

Source: (Adapted from Stehman *et al.*, *Handbook of dementia care* (1996)).

PADLs include bathing, dressing, grooming, toileting, walking, and eating. PADL functional abilities decline in a predictable temporal order according to the complexity of the ADL – bathing, dressing, grooming, toileting, walking, and eating. Bathing is an activity that most often results in resistive behavior. Strategies for bathing dependence will be described below. Dressing is the ADL that has been studied most extensively. A significant improvement in dressing performance can be achieved by implementing strategies that promote independence in dressing by nursing assistants (Beck *et al.*, 1997). Strategies for toileting difficulties include behavioral interventions (prompted voiding), establishing a routine, clothing modifications, making going to the bathroom easier, becoming familiar with and watching for cues indicating that the individual needs to use the bathroom, preserving dignity, and physical assistance to reach a bathroom. Independent eating is promoted by encouraging independence while providing supervision and assistance, by creating a social mealtime environment and by simplifying the eating process. Walking ability can be maintained for as long as possible by the use of assistive devices, such as Merry Walker (Trudeau *et al.*, 2003).

INABILITY TO INITIATE MEANINGFUL ACTIVITIES

This inability is caused by functional impairment but may also be aggravated by depression. Lack of meaningful activities may result in apathy or agitation, repetitive vocalization and insomnia, if the individual with dementia sleeps during the day. Involvement in meaningful activities is important for maintenance of functional abilities, social involvement, feeling of success and accomplishment, improvement in mood, and reduction of disruptive behavior (Volicer and Bloom-Charette, 1999).

Individuals with dementia live in the moment, and there is a widespread agreement among experts that the moment should be pleasurable. Management goals for people with the inability to initiate meaningful activity, therefore, are to prevent disability and to improve their interaction with the environment and their quality of life. Individuals with dementia who are unable to initiate meaningful activities may be unoccupied and appear bored or not engaged with the environment, sitting motionless, or wandering around aimlessly. They spend more time in a state of inner retreat, and this withdrawn behavior may manifest itself as lack of behavior, somnolence, perseveration, or nondirected verbal agitation.

The goal of management of the inability to initiate meaningful activities is to create environment with optimal stimulation and a steady flow of meaningful activities that are adapted to the functional capacity of the individual with

Table 6 Guidelines for planning activities for people with dementia

Principle	Rationale
Focus on enjoyment, not achievement	The goals of therapeutic program are to prevent excess disability and help the person "feel good"
Create "failure-free" environment	Helps person maintain self-esteem
Design therapeutic activities to stimulate multiple senses(Trudeau, 1999)	The ability to experience a range of human responses (emotions, behavior) continues across mild, moderate, and severe stages of dementia
Make activities part of daily routine	Maintain homelike routines Make all activities (including ADLs) meaningful Not an extra burden for the caregiver
Plan structured activities that employ previously learned motor patterns	These tasks require no new learning, yet can make the person feel useful and productive

Source: (Simard, 1999; Stehman *et al.*, 1996).

dementia. Engaging the individual in meaningful activities throughout the course of Alzheimer's disease or any other type of progressive dementia is challenging. Individuals with dementia do not ask for something to do as the more alert residents will, and as their dementia progresses they are increasingly difficult to keep engaged during activities because of their short attention span. An activity program that provides continuous programing throughout the majority of the residents' waking hours is not only an effective way to reduce psychotropic medication, reduce falls and social isolation, but it also helps individuals with dementia to live with some purpose and meaning in spite of the disease. General guidelines for planning activities for individuals with dementia are listed in Table 6.

In an institution, the programming should take into consideration the routine the individual had before admission for long-term care. The continuous programming for moderate dementia should begin with a morning routine that may include the Pledge of Allegiance, patriotic song, newspaper, or weather report discussion. Exercise programs, food and beverages served in a social atmosphere, word games, and spelling bees should follow. All these programs should be "no fail" opportunities to have fun. An individualized program that was found to decrease agitation and improve mood is Simulated Presence Therapy (Camberg *et al.*, 1999). At the end of the day, active participants are tired and ready for a video or a movie, a snack, and a peaceful sleep.

As dementia progresses into the severe stage, it becomes more challenging to engage individuals in meaningful activities. They tend to sleep during programs and may have difficulty communicating. Another level of programming, one that has more individual attention and has less physical activities helps meet their needs at this stage. Activity staff provides more touch, respects when the resident needs to take short "naps" and uses more visual cues. Physical exercise may require the activity staff standing in front of the resident and modeling the movement, or assisting the resident to move their arms or legs. Fewer programs are scheduled but the activity professional is in the room with the residents so that when they are awake, they can be engaged. Music, old musicals, sensory stimulation, and showing items from the past are some ways to engage residents in the severe stage of dementia.

Meaningful activities should be provided even for individuals in the terminal stage of dementia because Alzheimer's disease rarely, if ever, progresses to the persistent vegetative state (Volicer *et al.*, 1997a). Activities useful in that stage include pet therapy, massage, and Snoezelen (Brown, 1999).

ANXIETY

Anxiety is defined as a vague, uneasy feeling, the source of which is often nonspecific or unknown to the individual who is experiencing it. Anxiety is a feeling of distress, subjectively experienced as fear or worry, and objectively expressed through autonomic and central nervous system responses. Anxiety can be a symptom of depression or caused by disturbing delusions and hallucinations. It also can be caused by a primary anxiety disorder such as generalized anxiety disorder, phobia, posttraumatic stress disorder, and obsessive-compulsive disorder. However, new onset primary anxiety disorders are unusual in older adults. In most instances, older people with primary anxiety disorders have a history of them, and it is therefore important to obtain complete personal and family psychiatric history.

Anxiety may be also a symptom of physical illness or caused by medications. It may be induced by decreased delivery of oxygen to the brain caused by cardiac or pulmonary disease and by endocrine disorders such as hyperthyroidism and hypoglycemia. Medications that may cause anxiety as an adverse effect include anticholinergic drugs, caffeine, steroids, decongestants, bronchodilators, alcohol, narcotics, sedative-hypnotics and other psychotropic medications. Anxiety also may be a withdrawal symptom in individuals dependent on alcohol, benzodiazepines, or sedatives/hypnotics.

Anxiety is very common in Alzheimer's disease occurring in 52% of patients in mid and late stages of the disease (Hart *et al.*, 2003). The prevalence of anxiety increases with the progression of the disease (Porter *et al.*, 2003) but it is present together with suspiciousness even in individuals with mild cognitive impairment. Anxiety is even more common in individuals with vascular dementia and frontotemporal dementia than in individuals with Alzheimer's disease (Porter *et al.*, 2003).

Presence of anxiety is associated with reduced functional status in performing ADLs (Schultz *et al.*, 2004) and with sleep disturbances. Over a half of individuals with Alzheimer's disease who were experiencing anxiety woke up their caregivers at least once at night during the past week. The awakenings were associated with higher levels of patient anxiety and impairment in ADLs (McCurry *et al.*, 2004). Anxiety may also lead to agitation and repetitive vocalization.

Table 7 Selected medication for treatment of anxiety

Drug class	Name (trade name)	Dose range and frequency[a]	Elimination half-life (hours)	Side effects
Benzodiazepines	Alprazolam (Xanax) Lorazepam (Ativan) Oxazepam (Serax)	0.25–0.5 mg TID 0.5–1 mg BID or TID 10–20 mg TID or QID	12 15 8	Sedation, impaired motor coordination, risk of falls, memory loss, respiratory depression, dependence, paradoxical reaction
Azapirone	Buspirone (busPIRone)	5–20 mg TID	Onset of action 3–6 weeks	Headache, nausea, drowsiness, lightheadedness
Antidepressants	See Table 2			
Antipsychotics	See Table 4			

Source: Data from Raskind (1998).

Nonpharmacological management of anxiety is based on decreasing the stress level to which the individual with dementia is exposed. This may be accomplished by rest periods that prevent fatigue, positive communication strategies, prevention of overstimulation by providing low stimulation environment, and avoiding unfamiliar situations. Pharmacological management should first consider treatment of the primary consequences of dementia that may cause anxiety: mood disorders and delusions/hallucinations. Only if this approach is not effective or there is a strong evidence that the anxiety is caused by a primary anxiety disorder, anxiolytic medications should be used. These medications include administration of benzodiazepines and buspirone (Table 7). Only short-acting benzodiazepines should be used, and they may be useful also for a short-term treatment of an anxiety-induced catastrophic reaction that usually causes extreme agitation. Trazodone is another medication that may be useful on an as-needed basis because of its antidepressant and sedative effects.

SPATIAL DISORIENTATION

Spatial disorientation is the misperception of immediate surroundings, not being aware of one's setting, or not knowing where one is in relation to the environment. Spatial disorientation may cause misunderstanding of the environment and lead to development of fear, anxiety, suspicions, delusions, and safety problems such as getting lost. Getting lost may also lead to interference with other residents occurring if an individual with dementia invades their space, and the inability to find a bathroom contributes to ADL deficit. In the early stages of dementia, the individual may become confused when in unfamiliar place. In the later stages, the individual becomes confused even in previously familiar places.

Spatial disorientation may be related to a damage of specific brain area-posterior cingulate gyrus, because hypofunction of this area measured by positron-emission tomography was associated with disorientation for place. Another brain area that is necessary for place navigation, and is damaged severely in Alzheimer's disease, is the hippocampus. A healthy hippocampus uses two mechanisms for spatial orientation: cognitive mapping and cue navigation. Cognitive mapping requires cognitive processing to identify and store mental images of the most frequently encountered elements in a particular environment and the ability to make the connections among those elements. Cue navigation works by selection of a single landmark that directs an individual toward a specific location in the environment. Individuals retain these cues longer when they are familiar and are strongly associated with an environmental landmark. Another factor that participates in spatial disorientation in Alzheimer's disease is impaired depth perception. Because of this impairment, a change in color of a carpet or tile may be perceived as a step or obstacle.

Management of spatial disorientation utilizes information from these studies by using pop-up cues and environmental landmarks. Pop-up cues strategy attempts to simplify detection of the cue by providing one salient feature and color contrasts. If the cue is complex, it requires more cognitive processing than a simple cue. Individuals with dementia, who have impaired attention span and cognitive processing, may not recognize complex cues. Color contrast improves detection of the cue. Thus, a white toilet in a red bathroom is easier to find than a white toilet in a white bathroom. Environmental landmark strategy utilizes long-term memory by either keeping the environment unchanged or by using familiar objects as landmarks in a new environment. Personal or emotionally charged objects should be used as orientation devices. It is also important to simplify the environment by removing clutter and scatter rugs. Spatial orientation is promoted by signs on doors of common rooms, personal pictures or effects by the door of individual rooms, adequate lighting that does not cast shadows that may be misinterpreted, and by establishing a walking area with color contrasting borders.

RESISTIVENESS TO CARE

Resistiveness to care is defined as the repertoire of behaviors with which individuals with dementia withstand or oppose the efforts of a caregiver (Mahoney *et al.*, 1999). These behaviors occur primarily during hands-on care that includes bathing, dressing, toileting, eating, and administering medication. They can also occur when the caregiver attempts to redirect the individual with dementia. Resistiveness to care is caused by either misperception of the need for care activity or by misperception of the caregiver's intent (*see* **Chapter 89, Communication Disorders in Dementia**). Thus, an individual who does not recognize that he/she has soiled clothing will resist caregiver's attempt to change his/her clothes. Communication difficulties may prevent the individual with dementia from recognizing what the caregiver's intent is. In both cases, the individual with dementia does not cooperate with the caregiver but actively resists the caregiver's approach. If the caregiver insists on providing care, the individual with dementia may defend him/herself from this unwanted attention, becomes combative and even strikes out. Such an individual may be labeled "aggressive". However, the patient perceives the caregiver as the aggressor and just defends him/herself. Most individuals with dementia are not aggressive unless provoked and most "aggressive" behaviors reported in the literature occur in the context of personal care.

Several factors increase probability of resistive behavior. Delusions and hallucinations may prevent recognition of the need for care or lead to misidentification of a staff person. Depression increases resistiveness to care because depressed individuals are angry and do not tolerate others. Spatial disorientation may result in increased need for toileting because the individual cannot find a bathroom. Management of these factors may decrease resistiveness to care but the most important factor for its management is the caregiver approach. Therefore, caregiver behavior should always be evaluated when resistiveness of care occurs before initiation of any pharmacological therapy.

The goal of care is to prevent escalation of resistive behavior into combative behavior. The approach used by the caregiver is crucial. Relaxed and smiling caregiver behavior is related to calm and functional behavior of the individual with dementia. It is important to avoid making demands that create stress or are beyond the ability of the individual with dementia, avoid rushing through ADL, avoid touching without warning, avoid painful procedures, avoid overstimulating the individual, and to express respect for the individual with dementia by allowing him/her to maintain some control. Distraction may be also used to direct the individual's attention away from the stressful stimulus. Engaging an individual in conversation on a favorite topic or reminiscing about happy memories that are retained takes the focus away from the task and places it on the person. This person-centered approach is effective even with individuals who have significant cognitive and language impairment. In an institutional setting, distraction may be accomplished by using two caregivers. While one caregiver engages the individual's attention by talking or singing, a second caregiver performs the ADL care.

Another important factor is the environment in which the care is provided. This is especially important for bathing. The bathroom should feel private and personal, it should be warm, have relaxing music, soft light, low noise level, homelike furnishings, aromas to evoke memories, set mood and make the bathing experience pleasant, and the bathing equipment should be comfortable and functional. Very effective strategy for decreasing resistiveness to care is the modification of care procedures. Some individuals prefer to bathe in the morning and some in the afternoon or evening. It is also possible to replace shower or tub bath with a bed bath that is much less stressful for an individual with dementia (Sloane *et al.*, 1995).

Pharmacological management should take into account the possible causes of resistiveness to care. A possibility that resistiveness is induced by pain that the individual experiences during care procedures should be considered and if pain is present premedication with analgesics before a care episode should be instituted. If symptoms of depression are present, antidepressant treatment often decreases the resistive behavior. Delusions are a common cause of resistive behavior and if the behavior cannot be managed by behavioral strategies, antipsychotic therapy may be useful.

FOOD REFUSAL

One important goal of dementia care is to provide adequate nutrition by promoting eating and preventing food refusal. Food refusal may have several causes (*see* **Chapter 26, The Anorexia of Aging**; **Chapter 27, Weight Loss in Older Adults**; **Chapter 73, Communication Disorders and Dysphagia**). An individual with dementia may dislike institutional food especially if he/she is of different ethnic background and was used to eating different food. Food refusal may also be caused by physical reasons, such as fatigue, overstimulation, constipation, medication-induced nausea, dehydration, toothache, or ill-fitting dentures. Food refusal is an important symptom of depression and may be also caused by delusions about food being poisoned. In advanced dementia, when individuals develop swallowing difficulties, food refusal may be a consequence of choking on food and liquids. Finally, in the terminal stage of dementia, some individuals are unable to open mouth and swallow.

Food refusal may lead to weight loss and malnutrition although very often it is only occasional and the individual with dementia makes up for decreased food intake one day by eating more the next day. Management of food refusal should first consider personal and behavioral factors that may contribute to food refusal. It is important to obtain information about foods that the individual with dementia likes or dislikes although sometimes food preferences are significantly changed as dementia progresses. Environmental factors are chaotic or noisy dining area, inadequate staff time or knowledge of how to promote eating, unappealing food presentation, and improper utensils. As dementia progresses, individuals become unable to use utensils and their failure to eat may not indicate food refusal. Serving finger food may allow them to eat independently much longer.

If the behavioral and environmental interventions are ineffective, pharmacological management may be initiated. The most important is to eliminate depression and delusion as causes of food refusal by appropriate treatment with antidepressants or antipsychotics. If that approach is not appropriate or effective, food intake may be enhanced by administration of megestrol acetate or dronabinol. Megestrol acetate is a progesterone derivative with androgenic properties. It is used for treatment of anorexia and cachexia in cancer and AIDS. Megestrol acetate improved appetite and well-being in nursing home patients but a weight gain occurred only after discontinuation of the treatment (Yeh *et al.*, 2000). Dronabinol is a cannabinoid derivative that is used for treatment of anorexia in AIDS and prevention of vomiting after chemotherapy for cancer. Dronabinol increased body weight of institutionalized individuals with Alzheimer's disease and also improved their problem behaviors (Volicer *et al.*, 1997b).

Tube feeding is not an appropriate strategy for management of food refusal in individuals with advanced dementia. Tube feeding does not have any benefits on these individuals (Finucane *et al.*, 1999). Tube feeding does not prevent malnutrition or infections and it does not increase survival in individuals with progressive degenerative dementia (*see* **Chapter 60, Aspiration Pneumonia**). Nasogastric tube may cause infections of sinuses and middle ear, and gastrostomy tubes may cause cellulitis, abscesses, and even necrotizing fasciitis and myositis. Contaminated feeding solution may cause gastrointestinal symptoms and bacturiuria. Insertion of a tube may actually cause death from arrhythmia during insertion of a nasogastric tube and from perioperative mortality in percutaneous endoscopic gastrostomy tube placement. Occurrence of pressure ulcer is not decreased by tube feeding and it may actually be increased because of the use of restraints and increased production of urine and stool (*see* **Chapter 142, Restraints and Immobility**). There is also no evidence that tube feeding promotes healing of pressure ulcers or improves functional status of individuals with advanced dementia (Finucane *et al.*, 1999).

INSOMNIA

Sleep disturbances are common in elderly and probably even more common in individuals with dementia (*see* **Chapter 63, Sleep Disorders in Elderly People**). A survey of individuals 65 years old or older who were living at home showed that 28% had difficulty falling asleep and 42% had difficulty both in falling asleep and staying asleep. Aging affects sleep structure, resulting in less time spent in deep sleep and slightly more time spent in lighter stages of sleep. The elderly experience frequent nighttime awakenings and fragmentation of sleep. They also sleep less efficiently with their actual time asleep being only 70–80% of the total time spent in bed (Folks and Fuller, 1997).

Insomnia could be a primary condition but it also may be caused by other factors. These factors include medical and psychiatric illness, medication use, specific sleep disorders, psychosocial factors, and circadian rhythm changes. Insomnia is associated with respiratory symptoms, physical disabilities, use of nonprescription medications, depressive symptoms, and poor self-perception of health (Folks and Fuller, 1997). Many medications that are used for treatment of chronic conditions may affect sleep. These medications include decongestants, antiasthmatics, corticosteroids, antihypertensives, alcohol, caffeine, nicotine, and thyroid preparations. Sleep disorders include sleep apnea and periodic limb movement in sleep. Both of these conditions are very common in the elderly (Ancoli-Israel, 2000). Psychosocial factors include loneliness, bereavement, and the lack of physical activity. Circadian rhythm changes differently in normal aging and in Alzheimer's disease. In normal aging, there is an advance of the sleep phase with early evening sleepiness and early morning awakenings. Even if elderly go to bed later, they may wake up early in the morning and be unable to go back to sleep (Ancoli-Israel, 2000).

In Alzheimer's disease, there is a delay in circadian rhythm resulting in inability to go to sleep in the evening. This rhythm shift may be so pronounced that it results in complete reversal of day and night activities with the individual with dementia sleeping during the day and staying up during the night. The delay in circadian rhythm may also participate in increased behavioral disturbances in the afternoon and evening that are often called *sundowning* (Volicer *et al.*, 2001). In contrast, individuals with frontotemporal dementia have no change in circadian rhythm of body temperature but an advanced rhythm of motor activity (Harper *et al.*, 2001). Institutionalized individuals with dementia have extremely fragmented sleep, barely sleeping full hour and barely staying awake for a full hour throughout the day and night.

Management of insomnia should first utilize behavioral modifications. This includes avoiding caffeine, heavy meals, and excessive amount of alcohol before going to sleep, avoiding nocturia by decreased fluid intake in the evening, reviewing medications, and limiting day naps to 30 minutes. If behavioral modifications are not effective in reducing insomnia, use of hypnotic medications may be considered (Table 8). Antihistamines should not be used because they have strong anticholinergic effects that can aggravate memory problems and can also cause other adverse effects. Most common agents used in the management of insomnia are benzodiazepines. Only short-acting benzodiazepines should be used to avoid daytime sedation and increased risk for falls. The shortest acting agent, zaleplon, is especially useful in individuals who have difficulty falling asleep. Trazodone is a nontricyclic sedative antidepressant. Although there are few data to support the use of trazodone in nondepressed individuals (James and Mendelson, 2004), trazodone is useful in the treatment of insomnia

Table 8 Drugs for treatment of insomnia

Name (trade name)	Dose range (mg)	Elimination half-life (hours)
Trazodone	50–300	4–9
Triazolam (Halcion)	0.125–0.25	2–3
Zaleplon (Sonata)	5–10	1
Zolpidem	5–10	1.5–3.5

associated with administration of stimulating antidepressants (Kaynak *et al.*, 2004). Melatonin was not found to be an effective sleep agent in individuals with Alzheimer's disease.

APATHY AND AGITATION

Agitation is sometimes used as a term to label all behavioral symptoms of dementia. However, such a use of this term does not take into consideration the context in which a behavior happens and does not differentiate between behavioral symptoms induced by caregiving activity (resistiveness to care) and symptoms that occur without provocation or environmental triggers. Therefore, it is more useful to limit the term "agitation" to behaviors that communicate to others that the individual with dementia is experiencing an unpleasant state of excitement and that are observable without subjective interpretation, are not strictly behaviors that are invoked by caregiving activities, are unrelated to known physical needs of the patient that can be remedied, and are without known motivational intent (Hurley *et al.*, 1999).

Apathetic individuals appear passive, demonstrate inattention to the external environment (e.g. fixed staring or immobility), and are uninterested in what is happening around them. Apathy and depression are not synonymous and there is no significant correlation between them. Apathy and depression also result in a different pattern of brain blood flow changes.

Both agitation and apathy denote a lack of psychological well-being. The most common cause of agitation and apathy is functional impairment, resulting in inability to initiate meaningful activities. If these activities are not provided, the individuals with dementia experience boredom and become apathetic. Alternatively, the individuals attempt to stimulate themselves and that may result in repetitive behaviors or repetitive vocalization. Therefore, the most important intervention for both apathy and agitation is the availability of meaningful activities. Because lack of meaningful activities may induce both apathy and agitation, both of these symptoms are often present in the same individuals. Treatment of agitation with sedating medications results in an even more apathetic individual.

However, agitation may persist even in the presence of these activities and may actually interfere with participation in activities. In that case, the agitation may be a symptom of depression or a consequence of anxiety that may be induced by delusions or hallucinations. Therefore, careful analysis of the likely causes of agitation and a treatment of the underlying cause is necessary. Agitation may also be induced by changes of circadian rhythms. Delay in circadian rhythm is related to agitation in the afternoon and evening, which is called *sundowning* (Volicer *et al.*, 2001). Resetting of the circadian rhythm by bright light exposure may improve sundowning, although the effect is not very strong (Ancoli-Israel *et al.*, 2003).

ELOPEMENT AND INTERFERENCE WITH OTHERS

Unsupervised wandering away from a home or institution may have severe consequences for the individual with dementia. Elopement exposes the individual to a risk of injury if they walk into traffic, to hypothermia in cold climates, and hyperthermia with dehydration in warm climates. Wandering into rooms of other residents leads to conflict between residents, especially if the other resident is cognitively intact and resents the intrusion.

Wandering commonly describes the ambulating behavior of a person with dementia when that person walks away from one area or walks into an area "without permission". Wandering may be caused by spatial disorientation, or by delusions and hallucinations. An individual may be searching for something, attempting to fulfill unmet needs, escaping a threatening situation, reacting to reminders of departure near an exit, or carrying out a predementia lifestyle function. Wandering occurs in one-third of individuals with dementia living in a community and two-thirds of individuals with dementia living in an institution. It was reported that 26% of nursing home residents elope during the course of their institutionalization and 69% of individuals with dementia living at home experience at least one elopement episode. However, 81% of them do elope repeatedly (G. Flaherty, personal communication).

Some individuals with dementia walk back and forth as if following a rhythm or pattern. In that case, their activity is called *pacing*. Pacing often occurs with speed and a sense of urgency and may seem to represent hyperactivity or restlessness. Pacing may pose a problem for the individual with dementia if it occupies so much walking time that the individual becomes overtired. Pacing may also interfere with sitting down to eat and may result in weight loss. Pacing actually consumes considerable amount of energy and it was estimated that up to additional 1600 calories are required to maintain adequate nutrition in individuals who pace. Another adverse effect of pacing may be foot problems, such as blisters.

Both wandering and pacing should not be a problem if they occur in a safe environment and may actually provide beneficial physical exercise. Interference with other residents may be avoided by providing care for individuals with dementia in a dementia special care unit, where residents may not mind the intrusion because they themselves have spatial orientation difficulties. Thus, the most important intervention for these behaviors is environmental modification. These modifications should provide a safe walking path away from exits, and secure exits by disguising them or by a touch padlocking device. Wandering and pacing may also be a consequence of lack of meaningful activities. Engaging an individual in activity might distract them from seeking an exit from a home or institution. Because an individual with dementia living in a community may wander away from a caregiver in public places and because the individual may elope from a home despite safety measures, it is important to register the individual with both the Alzheimer's Association Safe Return Program and the Medic Alert Program.

KEY POINTS

- Interaction of dementia with personality results in three main consequences: functional impairment, mood disorders, and delusions/hallucinations.
- Continuous programing providing meaningful activities prevents many behavioral symptoms of dementia.
- Environmental influences affecting behavioral symptoms of dementia include caregiving strategies, social environment, physical environment, and medical interventions.
- Caregiving strategies are most important in preventing escalation of resistive behavior into a combative behavior that is sometimes labeled "aggression".
- Medical interventions should be congruent with goals of care and avoid unnecessary aggressive procedures that increase behavioral symptoms of dementia.

KEY REFERENCES

- Finucane TE, Christmas C & Travis K. Tube feeding in patients with advanced dementia: a review of the evidence. *Journal of the American Medical Association* 1999; **282**(14):1365–70.
- James SP & Mendelson WB. The use of trazodone as a hypnotic: a critical review. *The Journal of Clinical Psychiatry* 2004; **65**(6):752–5.
- Lonergan ET, Cameron M & Luxenberg J. Valproic acid for agitation in dementia. *Cochrane Database of Systematic Reviews* 2004; (2):CD003945.
- Trinh NH, Hoblyn J, Mohanty SU & Yaffe K. Efficacy of cholinesterase inhibitors in the treatment of neuropsychiatric symptoms and functional impairment in Alzheimer disease – a meta-analysis. *Journal of the American Medical Association* 2003; **289**(2):210–6.
- Volicer L & Hurley AC. Management of behavioral symptoms in progressive degenerative dementias. *The Journals of Gerontology. Series A, Biological Sciences and Medical Sciences* 2003; **58**(9):837–45.

REFERENCES

Ancoli-Israel S. Insomnia in the elderly: a review for the primary care practitioner. *Sleep* 2000; **23**(suppl 1):S23–30.

Ancoli-Israel S, Martin JL, Gehrman P *et al.* Effect of light on agitation in institutionalized patients with severe Alzheimer's disease. *The American Journal of Geriatric Psychiatry* 2003; **11**(2):194–203.

Areosa SA & Sherriff F. Memantine for dementia. *Cochrane Database of Systematic Reviews* 2003; CD003154.

Beck C, Heacock P, Mercer SO *et al.* Improving dressing behavior in cognitively impaired nursing home residents. *Nursing Research* 1997; **46**:126–32.

Bender RL, Moore R, Russell D *et al.* Multifaceted approach to cognitive decline. *Brain Aging* 2002; **2**:44–7.

Bergman J, Brettholz I, Shneidman M & Lerner V. Donepezil as add-on treatment of psychotic symptoms in patients with dementia of the Alzheimer's type. *Clinical Neuropharmacology* 2003; **26**(2):88–92.

Brodaty H, Ames D, Snowdon J *et al.* A randomized placebo-controlled trial of risperidone for the treatment of aggression, agitation, and psychosis in dementia. *The Journal of Clinical Psychiatry* 2003; **64**(2):134–43.

Brown EJ. Snoezelen. In L Volicer & L Bloom-Charette (eds) *Enhancing Quality of Life in Advanced Dementia* 1999, pp 168–85; Taylor & Francis, Philadelphia.

Camberg L, Woods P, Ooi WL *et al.* Evaluation of simulated presence: a personalized approach to enhance well-being in persons with Alzheimer's disease. *Journal of the American Geriatrics Society* 1999; **47**(4):446–52.

Finucane TE, Christmas C & Travis K. Tube feeding in patients with advanced dementia: a review of the evidence. *Journal of the American Medical Association* 1999; **282**(14):1365–70.

Folks DG & Fuller WC. Anxiety disorders and insomnia in geriatric patients. *The Psychiatric Clinics of North America* 1997; **20**:137–64.

Harper DG, Stopa EG, McKee AC *et al.* Differential circadian rhythm disturbances in men with Alzheimer disease and frontotemporal degeneration. *Archives of General Psychiatry* 2001; **58**(4):353–60.

Hart DJ, Craig D, Compton SA *et al.* A retrospective study of the behavioural and psychological symptoms of mid and late phase Alzheimer's disease. *International Journal of Geriatric Psychiatry* 2003; **18**(11):1037–42.

Haupt M, Jänner M, Ebeling S *et al.* Presentation and stability of noncognitive symptom patterns in patients with Alzheimer disease. *Alzheimer Disease and Associated Disorders* 1998; **12**(4):323–9.

Hurley AC, Volicer L, Camberg L *et al.* Measurement of observed agitation in patients with Alzheimer's disease. *Journal of Mental Health and Aging* 1999; **5**(2):117–33.

James SP & Mendelson WB. The use of trazodone as a hypnotic: a critical review. *The Journal of Clinical Psychiatry* 2004; **65**(6):752–5.

Kaynak H, Kaynak D, Gozukirmizi E & Guilleminault C. The effects of trazodone on sleep in patients treated with stimulant antidepressants. *Sleep Medicine* 2004; **5**(1):15–20.

Kumar V, Anand R, Messina J *et al.* An efficacy and safety analysis of Exelon in Alzheimer's disease patient with concurrent vascular risk factors. *European Journal of Neurology* 2003; **7**:159–69.

Kunik ME, Snow-Turek AL, Iqbal N *et al.* Contribution of psychosis and depression to behavioral disturbances in geropsychiatric inpatients with dementia. *Journals of Gerontology Series A: Biological Sciences and Medical Sciences* 1999; **54A**(3):m157–61.

Lonergan ET, Cameron M, & Luxenberg J. Valproic acid for agitation in dementia. *Cochrane Database of Systematic Reviews* 2004; (2):CD003945.

Mahoney EK, Hurley AC, Volicer L *et al.* Development and testing of the resistiveness to care scale. *Research in Nursing & Health* 1999; **22**:27–38.

Mahoney EK, Volicer L, & Hurley AC. *Management of Challenging Behaviors in Dementia* 2000, p 2; Health Professions Press Baltimore.

McCurry SM, Gibbons LE, Logsdon RG & Teri L. Anxiety and nighttime behavioral disturbances. Awakenings in patients with Alzheimer's disease. *Journal of Gerontological Nursing* 2004; **30**(1):12–20.

McKeith IG, Galasko D, Kosaka K *et al.* Consensus guidelines for the clinical and pathologic diagnosis of dementia with Lewy bodies (DLB): report of the consortium on DLB international workshop. *Neurology* 1996; **47**(5):1113–24.

Menon AS, Gruber-Baldini AL, Hebel JR *et al.* Relationship between aggressive behaviors and depression among nursing home residents with dementia. *International Journal of Geriatric Psychiatry* 2001; **16**(2):139–46.

Phillips VL & Diwan S. The incremental effect of dementia-related problem behaviors on the time to nursing home placement in poor, frail, demented older people. *Journal of the American Geriatrics Society* 2003; **51**(2):188–93.

Porter VR, Buxton WG, Fairbanks LA *et al.* Frequency and characteristics of anxiety among patients with Alzheimer's disease and related dementias. *The Journal of Neuropsychiatry and Clinical Neurosciences* 2003; **15**(2):180–6.

Raskind MA. Psychopharmacology of noncognitive abnormal behaviors in Alzheimer's disease. *The Journal of Clinical Psychiatry* 1998; **59**(suppl 9):28–32.

Schultz SK, Hoth A & Buckwalter K. Anxiety and impaired social function in the elderly. *Annals of Clinical Psychiatry* 2004; **16**(1):47–51.

Shelton RC, Tollefson GD, Tohen M *et al.* A novel augmentation strategy for treating resistant major depression. *The American Journal of Psychiatry* 2001; **158**(1):131–4.

Simard J. Making a positive difference in the lives of nursing home residents with Alzheimer disease: the lifestyle approach. *Alzheimer Disease and Associated Disorders* 1999; **13**(suppl 1):S67–72.

Sloane PD, Rader J, Barrick A-L *et al.* Bathing person with dementia. *The Gerontologist* 1995; **35**:672–8.

Stehman JM, Strachan GI, Glenner JA & Glenner GGNJK. *Handbook of Dementia Care* 1996; The Johns Hopkins University Press, Baltimore.

Tariot PN, Loy R, Ryan JM *et al.* Mood stabilizers in Alzheimer's disease: symptomatic and neuroprotective rationales. *Advanced Drug Delivery Reviews* 2002; **54**(12):1567–77.

Tariot PN, Profenno LA & Ismail MS. Efficacy of atypical antipsychotics in elderly patients with dementia. *The Journal of Clinical Psychiatry* 2004; **65**(suppl 11):11–5.

Trinh NH, Hoblyn J, Mohanty SU & Yaffe K. Efficacy of cholinesterase inhibitors in the treatment of neuropsychiatric symptoms and functional impairment in Alzheimer disease – a meta-analysis. *Journal of the American Medical Association* 2003; **289**(2):210–6.

Trudeau SA. Bright eyes: a structured sensory-stimulation intervention. In L Volicer & L Bloom-Charette (eds) *Enhancing the Quality of Life in Advanced Dementia* 1999, pp 93–106; Taylor & Francis, Philadelphia.

Trudeau SA, Biddle S & Volicer L. Enhanced ambulation and quality of life in advanced Alzheimer's disease. *Journal of the American Geriatrics Society* 2003; **51**(3):429–31.

Valuck R. Selective serotonin reuptake inhibitors: a class review. *P & T* 2004; **29**(4):234–43.

Verhey FRJ, Lodder J, Rozendaal N & Jolles J. Comparison of seven sets of criteria used for the diagnosis of vascular dementia. *Neuroepidemiology* 1996; **15**:166–72.

Volicer L, Berman SA, Cipolloni PB & Mandell A. Persistent vegetative state in Alzheimer disease – Does it exist? *Archives of Neurology* 1997a; **54**(11):1382–4.

Volicer L & Bloom-Charette L. *Enhancing the Quality of Life in Advanced Dementia* 1999; Taylor & Francis, Philadelphia.

Volicer L, Harper DG, Manning BC *et al.* Sundowning and circadian rhythms in Alzheimer's disease. *The American Journal of Psychiatry* 2001; **158**:704–11.

Volicer L & Hurley AC. Management of behavioral symptoms in progressive degenerative dementias. *The Journals of Gerontology. Series A, Biological Sciences and Medical Sciences* 2003; **58**(9):837–45.

Volicer L, Stelly M, Morris J *et al.* Effects of dronabinol on anorexia and disturbed behavior in patients with Alzheimer's disease. *International Journal of Geriatric Psychiatry* 1997b; **12**:913–9.

Warden V, Hurley AC & Volicer L. Development and psychometric evaluation of the PAINAD (Pain Assessment in Advanced Dementia) Scale. *Journal of the American Medical Directors Association* 2003; **4**:9–15.

Wesnes KA, McKeith IG, Ferrara R *et al.* Effects of rivastigmine on cognitive function in dementia with Lewy bodies: a randomised placebo-controlled international study using the Cognitive Drug Research computerised assessment system. *Dementia and Geriatric Cognitive Disorders* 2002; **13**(3):183–92.

Yeh S-S, Wu S-Y, Lee T-P *et al.* Improvement in quality-of-life measures and stimulation of weight gain after treatment with megestrol acetate oral suspension in geriatric cachexia: results of a double-blind, placebo-controlled study. *Journal of the American Geriatrics Society* 2000; **48**(5):485–92.

98

Geriatric Psychiatry

Abhilash K. Desai *and* George T. Grossberg
Saint Louis University Health Sciences Center, St Louis, MO, USA

Based in part on the chapter 'Psychiatry' by Susan Jolley and David Jolley, which appeared in *Principles and Practice of Geriatric Medicine*, 3rd Edition.

INTRODUCTION

Over the last two decades, geriatric psychiatry has emerged as an organized subspecialty within psychiatry. Multiple textbooks and subspecialty journals have emerged, such as International Psychogeriatrics, the American Journal of Geriatric Psychiatry and the International Journal of Geriatric Psychiatry. Also, an impressive body of evidence-based clinical knowledge specific to the behavioral health care of older adults is now increasingly available. Psychiatric disorders are profound in their impact upon the economic well-being and quality of life among older adults and their families. Interventions may avoid or delay onset, reduce the initial burden of symptoms and reduce functional impairment over time. Older adults with psychiatric disorders are often precluded from adequate mental health care due to inadequate funding of research, training, and service provision. Clinical and biological complexity is the rule rather than the exception in geriatric psychiatric syndromes. Moreover, behavioral abnormalities, cognitive deficits, and physical symptoms and signs are often manifested by more than one psychiatric, neurological, or medical condition. The quality of psychiatric services for older persons lags behind services for younger adults, despite a growing evidence-base supporting the effectiveness of a variety of interventions and services for late-life psychiatric disorders (Bartels, 2003a). The evidence-base is most developed for interventions addressing late-life depression and dementia, although effective treatments and service models have been identified for a variety of disorders (Bartels *et al.*, 2002).

EPIDEMIOLOGY

One in four older adults has a significant psychiatric disorder (Bartels, 2003a). Most of these individuals have anxiety disorders, followed by mood disorders, cognitive disorders, and alcohol abuse. Future growth of the population of older adults with mental illness in conjunction with the projected shortfall in providers with expertise in geriatrics and the inadequate financing for geriatric mental health services is predicted to create a future health-care crisis (Jeste *et al.*, 1999). Generalized anxiety disorder (GAD) is highly prevalent in older adults with rates of 7.3% reported in the older population. Prevalence rates of phobia range from 3.1 to 12%. Dementia affects around 7% of the general population older than 65 years and 30% of people older than 80 (O'Brien *et al.*, 2003). Twice as many people have cognitive impairment that falls short of diagnostic criteria for dementia (O'Brien *et al.*, 2003). Depression affects about one in 10 people over the age of 65 (Mellow *et al.*, 2003). Approximately 2% of the population older than 54 years have a chronic psychiatric disorder (such as schizophrenia, bipolar disorder, chronic depression) other than dementia (Jeste *et al.*, 1999). Older adults account for 13% of the population but almost a fifth of all suicides. Thirty-three out of every 100 000 older white men commit suicide compared to national rate of 11 for every 100 000. Four older adults attempt suicide for each who succeeds. This compares with 200 attempts per completed suicide among young adults. The prevalence of psychotic disorders in older adults ranges from 0.2 to 5.7% in community-based samples to 10% in a nursing home population. A more recent study found an even higher prevalence (10%) of psychotic symptoms in nondemented individuals aged 85 and older (Ostling and Skoog, 2002). 12 to 25% of healthy older adults report chronic insomnia, with higher rates among those with coexisting medical or psychiatric illness (Montgomery, 2002). 65 to 90% of residents in long-term care (LTC) have a significant psychiatric disorder (American Geriatrics Society and American Association for Geriatric Psychiatry, 2003). Moreover, the majority (89%) of older adults with severe and

Principles and Practice of Geriatric Medicine, 4th Edition. Edited by M.S. John Pathy, Alan J. Sinclair and John E. Morley.

Table 1 CAGE questionnaire

C	"Have you ever felt you ought to CUT DOWN on your drinking?"
A	"Have people ANNOYED you by criticizing your drinking?"
G	"Have you ever felt bad or GUILTY about your drinking?"
E	"Have you ever had a drink first thing in the morning (EYE OPENER) to steady your nerves or get rid of a hangover?"

persistent psychiatric disorder who receive institution-based care are in nursing homes. The prevalence of psychiatric disorders in older adults is expected to double over the next 30 years, making them a priority for health-care and social-care services (Jeste *et al.*, 1999).

THE PSYCHIATRIC INTERVIEW OF AN OLDER ADULT

The foundation of the diagnostic workup of the older adult experiencing a psychiatric disorder is the diagnostic interview. Input from a reliable informant who is familiar with the patient is often crucial for accurate diagnosis. To supplement the clinical interview, use of structured interview schedules and rating scales such as the Confusion Assessment Method (CAM) for delirium (Inouye, 1990), the Mini-Mental State Examinaton (MMSE) (Folstein *et al.*, 1975) for dementia, the CAGE questions (Table 1) for alcohol abuse, the Beck Anxiety Inventory (BAI) (Beck *et al.*, 1988) for anxiety and the Geriatric Depression Scale (GDS) (Yesavage *et al.*, 1983) for depression may be helpful. Because age-related cognitive changes, mood changes, or behavioral changes may signal treatable medical conditions, it is important to take any complaint seriously. Risk factors which should trigger a cognitive and/or depression screen include age older than 65 years, illnesses that increase the possibility of diagnosis of cognitive or mood disorders, for example, diabetes, Parkinson's disease, cerebrovascular disease and so on, a past history of depression or a family history of dementia. A simple screening question asking about the patient's memory and mood state is often informative. Every person aged 65 and older is recommended to be screened for alcohol and prescription drug use/abuse as part of regular medical and psychiatric care and patients should be screened again yearly if certain physical or emotional symptoms emerge or if the person is undergoing major life changes or transitions.

DEPRESSION

Depression can be reliably and easily distinguished from normal aging but is often overlooked. It is extremely treatable if appropriate pharmacotherapy and/or psychotherapeutic interventions are prescribed and accepted by patients and their caregivers. The outcome of depressive disorder in older adults is as good as in other age groups. It is important to follow-up depressed older patients with cognitive impairment for later signs of dementia. Depression is recognized in only a fraction of older primary care patients, and an even smaller fraction of those identified receive appropriate antidepressant treatment (Alexopoulos, 2001). The major impediment to recognition and treatment of depression in older adults is the limited time of general practitioners. Many older adults with clinically significant depressive symptoms do not meet diagnostic criteria for major depressive disorder. However, the cumulative functional morbidity of these subsyndromal disorders actually exceeds that of major depression among the older adults (Lyness, 2004a). Also, evidence to date suggests that major depression may not be pathogenetically distinct from less-severe forms of depression (Lyness, 2004a). Within the emerging concept of vascular depression there is some evidence of a lower response rate to antidepressant monotherapy but the response rate to electroconvulsive therapy (ECT) may be as favorable as for other patients but with an increased risk of ECT-induced delirium (Baldwin *et al.*, 2002).

BEREAVEMENT

Bereavement is associated with declines in health, inappropriate health service use, and increased risk of death (Prigerson and Jacobs, 2001). Identifying and intervening on behalf of bereaved patients may help address these increased risks. Complicated bereavement may be distinct from major depression and formal criteria have been proposed (Prigerson and Jacobs, 2001). Complicated bereavement includes symptoms such as extreme levels of "traumatic distress", numbness, feeling that part of oneself has died, assuming symptoms of the deceased, disbelief, or bitterness, and symptoms endure for 6 months. Immediate attention from a mental health professional should be sought if suicidality is suspected at any time post-loss. For bereaved patients diagnosed with major depression and complicated bereavement, treatment should follow general guidelines including prescription of antidepressants. Brief dynamic psychotherapy, traumatic grief therapy, crisis intervention, and support groups can significantly reduce grief symptoms (Prigerson and Jacobs, 2001).

BIPOLAR AFFECTIVE DISORDER

Most older adults with bipolar disorder have the disorder from their young adulthood although onset as late as in the ninth and tenth decades has been reported (Umapathy *et al.*, 2000). Late-onset bipolar disorder (onset after age 50) is commonly associated with comorbidities such as hypertension, diabetes or coronary artery disease, and neurological disorders. It is less likely to be associated with a family history of mood disorders. Bipolar elderly patients in outpatient treatment were found to use four times the total amount of mental health services and are four times more likely to have had a psychiatric hospitalization over the previous 6 months compared to older outpatients with unipolar depression (Bartels *et al.*, 2000). Older manic patients seldom display the euphoric or elated mood characteristic of younger adults, and are more likely to appear irritable, angry, paranoid, and disorganized. Older adults often have more frequent episodes of mania and depression, with a shorter (e.g. rapid cycling) duration of symptoms than younger patients. A significant proportion of older bipolar patients exhibit neuropsychological deficits when they are clinically euthymic. Lithium and divalproex have been most studied in older adults, and both may be efficacious in acute treatment of mania, but there are no controlled efficacy or effectiveness trials (Young *et al.*, 2004). Despite lack of systematic data, atypical antipsychotics may be useful in the treatment of older adults with bipolar disorder. There are no systematic studies of the treatment of bipolar depression in older adults and there are no systematic studies using psychosocial interventions to treat bipolar disorder in older adults. Nonetheless, psychopharmacologic treatment of older adults with bipolar depression and use of psychosocial interventions based on extrapolation of research from younger adults can improve functional outcomes in older adults with bipolar disorder. Adjunctive psychotherapy is recommended to help increase adherence to medication, enhance social and occupational functioning, and improve detection of an impending mood episode. Psychosocial interventions that focus on reducing stressful life events and maintaining a stable living environment are helpful for older adults with bipolar disorder. Electroconvulsive therapy (ECT) should be considered in all older adults with severe bipolar depression or mania, especially in those with a history of previous good response to ECT.

LATE-LIFE PSYCHOSES

There is an increased incidence of psychotic symptoms (delusions and hallucinations) in older adults in contrast to younger adults (Desai and Grossberg, 2003). Psychotic disorders in old age have more toxic (e.g. drugs), metabolic (e.g. laboratory abnormalities), and structural (e.g. brain lesions, tumors) associations and a greater association with dementia. New onset of psychotic symptoms in the background of cognitive impairment are most likely to be due to delirium or dementia. Schizophrenia makes up the majority of the diagnoses of older adults with severe and persistent psychotic disorder.

SCHIZOPHRENIA

Although schizophrenia is less prevalent than dementing disorders and depression, the total health expenditures for individuals aged 65 and above with schizophrenia exceed those for individuals aged 65 and above with depression, dementia, or all medical disorders (Bartels *et al.*, 2003b). Onset of illness typically begins in early adulthood, with a small but distinct subgroup of older adults developing the disease after the age of 55. Late-onset schizophrenia has a higher prevalence of the paranoid type, less-severe negative symptoms, overrepresentation of women and requires lower doses of antipsychotic medications as compared to early-onset schizophrenia. The course of schizophrenia in late life appears stable, but most elderly patients remain symptomatic and impaired. In spite of considerable ongoing disability, most older adults with schizophrenia continue to function in the community. Long-term studies have begun to erode the belief that most patients with schizophrenia have a downward course. At least 50 to 60% of early-onset schizophrenia patients over two to three decades significantly reclaimed their lives (Harding, 2003). Many older adults with schizophrenia have spent lengthy periods in hospitals and do not have community living skills. Sustained remission can occur even in older adults with chronic schizophrenia, but its prevalence is lower than that previously thought. Significant cognitive and functional deficits are also commonly seen in older adults with schizophrenia, particularly those whose lifetime course of illness has been chronic. Older adults with schizophrenia are more impaired in most domains of functioning and less impaired in memory than are patients with dementia. Cognitive decline is not uniform across older adults with schizophrenia, with some showing cognitive and functional decline even in brief follow-up periods. Risk factors for decline include less education, advanced age, and more severe positive symptoms of schizophrenia at the time of initial assessment. Poor outcome over the course of the entire life span may be a risk factor for further decline in later life.

Although older adults with schizophrenia may not have more physical problems than age-matched peers, the severity of their medical conditions may be greater (Schoos and Cohen, 2003). It should be remembered that older adults with schizophrenia are even more a group of survivors than are their same-age peers in the general population. Many of these patients have difficulty complying with care regimens for chronic medical conditions such as diabetes and hypertension and have poor dietary habits. Most of the older adults with schizophrenia have been active smokers for many years. Mortality rates among older adults with schizophrenia are higher than those of their same-age peers.

For most adults with schizophrenia, there is evidence of adaptation and compensation with aging. However, countervailing factors such as cognitive deficits, poor physical health, and movement disorders can worsen adaptive functioning. Cognitive impairment, negative symptoms, and social isolation, rather than psychosis, appear to predict the level of care needed. Atypical antipsychotics are the primary form of intervention and have tremendous advantages over older drugs in terms of side effects (Cohen *et al.*, 2000). Psychosocial treatments for older adults with schizophrenia such as cognitive-behavioral therapy, health management intervention, social skills training, and residential alternatives are also recommended. Assertive community treatment and case management greatly increase the success of pharmacological and psychosocial interventions.

COGNITIVE DISORDERS

These primarily include dementing disorders, delirium, cognitive impairment no dementia (CIND), mild cognitive impairment (MCI) and vascular cognitive impairment (VCI).

Dementing Disorders

The dementias are a growing problem in an aging world. Cognitive impairment and functional decline associated with dementia can be reliably differentiated clinically from normal effects of aging in most older adults. Primary care physicians are the first medical contact for most patients with early-stage dementia. Physicians often underdiagnose dementia, and, when dementia is detected, some physicians choose not to disclose the diagnosis to the patient. It is important to formally diagnose the type of dementia. A trial of a cholinesterase inhibitor or/and memantine is recommended for the treatment of Alzheimer's disease and vascular dementia (Cummings, 2003; Doody *et al.*, 2004). Cholinesterase inhibitors may also be useful for dementia with Lewy bodies and Parkinson's dementia. Empirical evidence supports the value of psychosocial interventions in addressing behavioral symptoms of dementia, but there is less agreement on the effectiveness of antipsychotics, anticonvulsant, and antidepressant agents (Bartels *et al.*, 2002). Better matching of the available nonpharmacologic interventions for behavioral symptoms of dementia to patient's needs and capabilities is necessary for consistently successful outcomes (Cohen-Mansfield, 2001). The Clinical Antipsychotic Trials of Intervention Effectiveness (CATIE) protocol for Alzheimer's disease (AD), a trial developed in collaboration with the National Institute of Mental Health (NIMH), assessing the effectiveness of atypical antipsychotics for psychosis and agitation occurring in AD outpatients has just been completed and its results are expected to clarify the role of atypical antipsychotics in the treatment of psychosis and agitation in older adults with AD.

Delirium

The incidence and prevalence of delirium among hospitalized elderly, those in intensive care units and in emergency departments is high. Postoperative delirium is particularly common among older adults. Preexisting cognitive impairment is a major risk factor for postoperative delirium. Delirium is frequently superimposed on dementia. Although there are many potential causes for delirium, a "final common pathway" involving a concomitant decrease in cholinergic tone and increase in dopaminergic tone in relevant brain regions has been hypothesized (Trzepacz, 2000). Finding and treating the cause of delirium and reducing anticholinergic burden of drug regimens are key to successful functional outcome of older adults with delirium. Management of behavioral disturbances associated with delirium is primarily nonpharmacological using multicomponent interventions such as improved sleep hygiene, range-of-motion exercises, ambulation, reorientation, and cognitive stimulation (Inouye *et al.*, 2003). Low-dose antipsychotics such as parenteral haloperidol may be needed to control severe agitation.

Mild Cognitive Impairment (MCI) and Cognitive Impairment, No Dementia (CIND)

Many conditions cause cognitive impairment, which does not meet current criteria for dementia. Within this heterogenous group, termed *Cognitive Impairment, No Dementia* (CIND), there are disorders associated with an increased risk of progression to dementia (Davis and Rockwood, 2004). MCI describes older adults with subjective complaints of memory loss and objective psychometric measures of memory impairment compared with individuals of the same age. However, these individuals do not have pronounced impairments in daily function and generally do not have impairment of other cognitive functions such as language or abstract thinking. Amongst patients with MCI, especially its amnestic form, many will progress to AD. The occurrence of neuropsychiatric symptoms in MCI and the similarity of these symptoms to those of early AD suggest that these symptoms may assist in identifying patients in the earlier stages of AD and distinguishing them from patients with other disorders. In contrast to clinic-based studies, where progression is more uniform, population-based studies suggest that the MCI classification is unstable in that context. In addition to Amnestic MCI, other syndromes exist and can progress to dementia. For example, an identifiable group with vascular cognitive impairment without dementia shows a higher risk of progression to vascular dementia, AD, and mixed dementia. Also, in some cases, mild vascular cognitive impairment can be reversible if appropriately treated (Borroni *et al.*, 2004).

Vascular Cognitive Impairment (VCI)

Cerebrovascular disease is the second most common cause of acquired cognitive impairment and dementia and contributes to cognitive decline in the neurodegenerative dementias (O'Brien *et al.*, 2003). The current narrow definitions of vascular dementia needs to be broadened to recognize the important part cerebrovascular disease plays in several cognitive disorders, including the hereditary vascular dementias, multi-infarct dementia, poststroke dementia, subcortical ischemic vascular disease and dementia, MCI, and degenerative dementias (including Alzheimer's disease, frontotemporal dementia, and dementia with Lewy bodies). The term Vascular Cognitive Impairment (VCI), which is characterized by a specific cognitive profile involving preserved memory with impairments in attentional and executive functioning has been proposed. Important noncognitive features of VCI include depression, apathy, and psychosis. Diagnostic criteria have been proposed for some subtypes of VCI, and there is a pressing need to validate and further refine these. Evidence from the available studies support the benefit of cholinesterase inhibitors for the treatment of VCI.

SUBSTANCE ABUSE

Substance use and abuse in older adults is a growing public health issue. Primary care physicians and emergency care providers can play a crucial role in early identification and initial management of addiction problems in older persons. Alcohol use/abuse is the most common form of substance abuse in older adults. Heavy drinking is a well-established factor in causing disability and excessive mortality. However, among elders with chronic medical and emotional health disorders, even modest alcohol consumption can lead to excessive disability and poorer perceived health. Alcohol abuse in older adults is a hidden epidemic because its symptoms often mimic or are masked by common physical and mental infirmities of aging and because health-care providers rarely ask about when and how much their older patients drink or what effect alcohol may have on their lives. In addition, older adults and their relatives are often in denial about the extent and effects of their drinking habits and because the amount of alcohol now causing trouble had no untoward social or physical effects in middle age. Use of screening tools such as the CAGE questionnaire and Short Michigan Alcoholism Screening Test-Geriatric Version (SMAST-G) (Blow *et al.*, 1998) are recommended to minimize this oversight. Older adults with alcohol abuse also face greater risk for suicide (Blow and Oslin, 2003). Alcohol abuse is seen in older men as well as women. Older adults with alcohol abuse are more likely to present with physical symptoms and to be admitted to medical or surgical wards than younger patients with alcohol abuse. A nonjudgmental and tactful approach is recommended in asking about and attempting to treat alcohol abuse, especially in aging women.

There is insufficient evidence to endorse pharmacological interventions for geriatric alcohol abuse (Bartels *et al.*, 2002). In contrast, psychosocial interventions are likely to be effective for older persons with alcohol use disorders. Brief interventions (5 minutes for five brief sessions) targeting a specific health behavior (at-risk drinking) by primary care providers are quite effective. As the post–World War II baby-boom generation ages, providers may begin to see a greater number of elderly patients who use illicit drugs than has been seen in previous cohorts. The abuse of narcotics is rare among older adults, except if they have a history of abuse at a younger age, or in the presence of alcoholism. Older heroin abusers are usually life-long addicts who have survived. With the current epidemic of acquired immunodeficiency syndrome (AIDS) and hepatitis C among illicit drug users, all older adults with illicit drug use (current or past) should be screened for these conditions. The need for treatment may diminish as in some individuals, addiction wanes with age.

Misuse and inappropriate use of prescription medications (especially benzodiazepines but also opiates) is a substantial issue in this population. Presence of a psychiatric disorder is a risk factor for prescription drug dependence in older adults. Benzodiazepine use increases with age, and older adults tend to be on higher doses. Depression in older individuals often presents with features of anxiety and may be inappropriately treated with benzodiazepines rather than an antidepressant or *referred* for psychotherapy. Signs of prescription drug abuse in older people include loss of motivation, memory loss, family or marital discord, new difficulty with activities of daily living, trouble with sleeping, drug seeking behavior, and doctor shopping. The long-term treatment of older adults who have misused or abused prescription drugs should be individualized. Most misuse can be treated outside of specialized substance abuse treatment programs through education of patients, families, and providers. Self-help groups (e.g. narcotic anonymous) is unlikely to benefit an older adult with prescription opioid abuse. Groups specific for older adults should be sought. Primary care provider involvement is essential, both for counseling and for coordination of a treatment plan. In older adults, safe withdrawal may take weeks to months as compared with days to weeks in younger adults. Implementation of nonpharmacologic methods for treating chronic pain or insomnia can play an essential role in long-term treatment. Specific advice about the dangers of combining alcohol with prescription and over-the-counter (OTC) medications, especially psychoactive agents, should be given and regularly reinforced (Blow and Oslin, 2003). Effective screening and intervention can prevent and reverse morbidity.

ANXIETY DISORDERS

Although anxiety disorders are the most prevalent disorders among older adults, we know far less about the clinical characteristics, course, treatment, and prognosis of these disorders (Mellow *et al.*, 2003). Substantial comorbidity of medical and anxiety disorders with the possibility that physiologic symptoms of anxiety can be a manifestation of a medical condition or adverse effects of a drug further confound and complicate proper detection of anxiety disorders in older adults. Despite these challenges, parsing anxiety symptoms from medical conditions can be accomplished by a thorough clinical assessment, the use of self-report inventories, and laboratory findings.

GAD is one of the most common psychiatric syndrome in older adults. Half of older adults with GAD have had symptoms for most of their lives, whereas the remaining half report developing GAD within the last 5 years. Anxiety symptoms are also common features of late-life depression and dementia. Preliminary evidence indicates that many older patients with onset of panic attacks in early life continue experiencing symptoms in later life, with few receiving adequate treatment over the years. Less common are new onset cases of panic disorder in old age. Phobic disorders are highly prevalent, chronic, and persist into old age.

posttraumatic stress disorder (PTSD) symptoms may recur later in life and recent losses or dementia may trigger a recurrence of symptoms.

Anxiety commonly is associated with medical illness (such as chronic obstructive pulmonary disease, coronary artery disease, Parkinson's disease) in older adults. Anxiety disorders occasionally may be due to an underlying medical condition (such as hyperthyroidism or pheochromocytoma), drug-induced (such as due to theophylline, OTC sympathetomimetics, steroids, thyroid preparations) or drug-withdrawal states (such as caffeine withdrawal, alcohol withdrawal, sedative hypnotic withdrawal).

Treatment of anxiety in elderly persons has typically involved the use of benzodiazepines, which are often effective but problematic because they are associated with increased risk of cognitive impairment, falls, and fractures (Desai, 2003). Pharmacological alternatives such as antidepressants (especially selective serotonin reuptake inhibitors and serotonin norepinephrine reuptake inhibitors) and buspirone are recommended for the treatment of anxiety disorders in older persons. Because it may take 2 to 4 weeks for the onset of therapeutic action with these compounds, use of an adjunctive short acting benzodiazepine for the first few weeks may be considered in severe cases. Cognitive-behavioral therapy may also be useful for treatment of anxiety disorders in older adults. Collaborative care models that address physician, patient, and health-care service delivery barriers also hold promise for adequately treating anxiety disorders experienced by older adults.

GERIATRIC PSYCHIATRY EMERGENCIES

1. **Suicide:**

Suicide rates are highest in older adults; the majority of older adults who die by suicide have seen a primary care physician in preceding months (Maris, 2002). Older white men are the most at risk. In contrast, older black women have the lowest rate of suicide. Although reasons for this difference are not clear, strong ties to social and religious support networks may be the key protection for older black women. Depression is the strongest risk factor for late-life suicide and for suicide's precursor, suicidal ideation. Chronic medical illness, psychiatric disorders, physical disability, unrelenting pain/discomfort, alcohol abuse, psychosocial stressors, and poor social support are some of the other major risk factors for late-life suicide. Older adults are more likely to be socially isolated and have more physical illnesses than younger adults. They are also more likely to use highly lethal methods of suicide, such as firearms. Health-care providers are less apt to determine that suicidal thinking in an older adult is a serious condition that might respond to treatment. With novel interventions in community-based primary care, suicidal ideation can be reduced regardless of depression severity (Bruce *et al.*, 2004). Such interventions include utilizing depression case managers, education of primary care providers on assessment and management of suicide and incorporation of such education into clinical practice. Psychiatrists must take prominent, central roles in this training and work more integrally with primary care physicians.

2. **Elder abuse:**

Elderly men and women of all socioeconomic and ethnic backgrounds are vulnerable to abuse and neglect, and most often it goes undetected. Physical abuse is most recognizable, yet neglect is most common. Psychological and financial abuse may be more easily missed. Awareness of the risk factors (cognitive impairment, depression, frailty, caregiver stress, institutionalization) and clinical manifestations (bruises, fractures, malnutrition) allows primary care physicians to provide early detection and intervention for elder neglect and abuse (Levine, 2003). Interdisciplinary collaboration between physicians, social workers, and mental health professional is crucial. Health-care providers should have a high index of suspicion for abuse and neglect in older adults at risk. Physical and verbal abuse by older adults with dementia toward their family members and other caregivers (many of whom are elderly themselves) is a growing problem and needs to be inquired into and addressed during the visit to primary health-care provider.

DRUG-INDUCED PSYCHIATRIC DISORDERS

Psychotropic side effects of commonly prescribed medications in the elderly are prevalent and, in most instances, predictable and preventable (Desai, 2004). They are also associated with considerable morbidity and mortality. Delirium, mood changes, and psychotic symptoms are the most serious categories of psychotropic side effects. Anticholinergics, antihistaminics, psychotropics, and many OTC drugs are the usual suspects. Long-acting benzodiazepines are the most common cause of drug-induced cognitive impairment in older adults. Herbal medicine use is prevalent in the older adult population and is associated with high risk of serious herb–drug interactions (Desai and Grossberg, 2003). Psychotropics are one of the most common class of drugs prescribed inappropriately in older adults (Curtis *et al.*, 2004). Avoiding potentially inappropriate medications and performing a routine evaluation of the drug regimen in question (including OTC drugs, herbal, and nonherbal supplements) are some of the key interventions for preventing psychotropic side effects of commonly prescribed medications (Fick *et al.*, 2003).

INSOMNIA

Insomnia is highly prevalent in older adults (Ancoli-Israel, 2000). However, few mention their sleep problems to their primary care providers and most self-medicate with OTC medications. Many OTC sleep-aides (such as diphenhydramine) have considerable risk of cognitive and behavioral toxicity (Desai, 2004). Those who receive treatment typically receive benzodiazepines, which have known side effects including tolerance, addiction, daytime sedation, cognitive impairment, associated falls, hip fractures, and motor vehicle accidents – especially from preparations with a long half-life – and impaired sleep due to long-term use. Initial assessment of insomnia involves evaluating the cause. Causes of insomnia in older adults include: medical, psychiatric, and drug issues; circadian rhythm changes; sleep disorders; and psychosocial factors. Sleep apnea occurs in 4% of middle-aged men and 2% of middle-aged women. In males over 65, the figure rises to 28%; for women, the number climbs to 24%. Nonpharmacological interventions such as cognitive-behavioral interventions for psychophysiological insomnia, bright light treatments for problems related to timing of sleep, and physiological interventions such as exercise for insomnia may be considered. Pharmacotherapy should be limited to short-term use of agents least likely to cause daytime sedation such as zolpidem, zaleplon, trazodone, and perhaps valerian. A systematic review of the efficacy of acupuncture and acupressure is currently underway.

PERSONALITY DISORDERS

Late-life personality disorders (PDs) have not been well studied. The most commonly identified PDs in late life include obsessive-compulsive, dependent, and mixed. Research indicates gradual improvement of several PDs in middle age, most notably borderline and antisocial PDs. Studies of behavioral traits in late life have consistently found decreased levels of activity, extroversion, impulsivity, aggression, and increased levels of introversion and suspiciousness. All PDs in late life are particularly vulnerable to the reemergence or exacerbation of maladaptive traits, or to the development of secondary psychopathology as a result of acute stress or the accumulation of age-related losses and other stressful experiences. Longitudinal research relative to PD's has not looked beyond middle age. Owing to limited information and lack of awareness, many health-care providers often end up deferring the diagnosis of a PD. But there is a cost to this: patients may consequently be labeled as treatment-resistant when short-term psychotherapy or pharmacotherapy fails to alleviate distressing or disruptive behaviors, which actually reflect long-standing personality characteristics. Treatments of PDs in late life utilize the same basic approaches as with younger patients, but clinicians must incorporate a much broader understanding of the impact of age-related stressors and comorbid conditions. The overall goal of treatment is not to cure the disorder, but to decrease the frequency and intensity of disruptive behaviors. It may be necessary to convey a basic formulation of the patient's behaviors to caregivers and affiliated health-care professionals, such as primary care providers, social workers, and visiting nurses (Agronin and Maletta, 2000).

SEXUAL DISORDERS

Sexual function is a very important life issue for older adults but is often overlooked. Psychosocial factors such as societal attitude and lack of available partners (especially for older women) can negatively impact sexual functioning. Medical conditions such as diabetes, hypothyroidism, neuropathy, cardiovascular disease, adverse drug effects and psychiatric conditions such as depression, dementia, and chronic alcoholism often negatively impact sexual functioning. Many of these conditions are treatable. The critical first step to address sexual disorders for health-care providers is to start talking about sex with their older patients.

SPECIAL POPULATIONS IN GERIATRIC PSYCHIATRY

1. **LTC residents:**

Psychiatric disorders account for at least one-half of the morbidity in LTC and are the prime reason for admission to LTC facilities. The LTC setting is unique relative to patient characteristics and systems issues. Depression and behavioral and other psychiatric symptoms associated with dementia are the most common psychiatric problems in nursing homes. Nursing directors report substantial limitations in the competence of staff at all levels in managing behaviorally disturbed patients and a broad-based need for improvement in skills. Nursing assistants report low confidence in their ability to prevent agitation or aggression in LTC residents and report an even lower confidence in their ability to decrease resident's agitation and aggression once they become agitated or aggressive (Gates *et al.*, 2004). Education and training of mental health professionals working in nursing homes and of nursing home staff in the recognition, assessment, treatment, and monitoring of behavioral symptoms in nursing home residents is thus essential.

Depression screening instruments should be used for the identification and assessment of depressed residents and evaluation of treatment effectiveness. Verbal, nonverbal, and physical behavioral symptoms should be described and quantified as current tools are not adequate in identifying all residents with behavioral symptoms. Violence by residents against other residents and health-care providers is highly prevalent and one of the most serious issues in LTC. There is an immediate need for violence prevention education and for developing violence prevention programs in nursing homes. Major depression in LTC residents can be effectively treated with nonpharmacological or pharmacological interventions and minor depression can be effectively treated with nonpharmacological intervention although data regarding pharmacological intervention for minor depression in LTC residents is limited. Atypical antipsychotics are the first line pharmacological intervention for severe behavioral disturbances with psychotic features in LTC residents and may even be effective for severe agitation without psychotic symptoms. Neither pharmacological nor nonpharmacological interventions totally eliminate behavioral symptoms, but both types of interventions decrease the severity of symptoms (Snowden *et al.*, 2003).

2. **Older inmates:**

As the prison population grows, so does the number of older inmates. 8.6% of all inmates are aged 50 years or older. The age 50 cutoff is important in understanding prison health care. A 50-year-old inmate may have a physiological age that is 10 to 15 years older, because inmates generally age faster because of such factors as abuse of illicit drugs and alcohol and limited lifetime access to preventive care and health services. Up to 20% of inmates older than 55 have a significant mental illness (Mitka, 2004). Ethnic minorities are overrepresented in prison population. About one-third of the prison population tests positive for hepatitis C. Almost all inmates are released back to their family and community. Treatment inside the institution needs to address this transition. Involving clinical faculty and staff from academic medical centers to provide health care (including mental health care) to the aging prison population can produce significant improvements in access to care and health outcomes (Raimer and Stobo, 2004).

3. **Caregivers:**

Families are now the major caregivers and lifetime support systems to the majority of older adults with dementia or chronic mental disorders. The majority of the caregivers are wives or daughters. Caregiving can take a toll on the mental health of caregivers and has been associated with an increased risk of depression, poor health, and substance abuse in the caregivers. Living with older adults suffering from dementia or chronic mental illness is about learning to "bend without breaking" (Gwyther, 1998). These disorders affect multiple generations within the family and each family responds in its own unique ways. Transition to institutional care is particularly difficult for spouses, almost half of whom visit the patient daily and continue to provide help with physical care during their visits. Symptoms of depression and anxiety do not diminish after institutional placement, use of anxiolytic medications increase, and nearly half the caregivers are at risk for clinical depression following placement of their loved one in long-term facilities (Schulz *et al.*, 2004). Clinical interventions that prepare the caregiver for a placement transition and treat their depression and anxiety following placement are recommended.

Living with older adults with chronic psychiatric disorders implies a permanent imbalance in the normal give-and-take of family relationships. Health-care providers must help families work toward effectively coping with the disease, decreasing the harmful effects on the family, and keeping family conflicts to a minimum (Gwyther, 1998). Interventions such as counseling, support groups, psychoeducational groups, training in contingency planning, respite services, skills training, and family-directed treatments can alleviate caregiver stress, prevent caregiver depression, and improve coping skills.

4. **Ethnic/minority elderly:**

Psychiatric disorders in ethnic/minority elders are underrecognized and undertreated (Charney *et al.*, 2003). Older African-American patients with bipolar disorder are more likely to receive diagnoses of schizophrenia (Kilbourne *et al.*, 2004). Differential response to psychotropic medications by ethnicity (besides age and gender) is an important factor when choosing a potential pharmacotherapy regimen for an older minority adult. Inclusion criteria for clinical dementia trials have been shown to preferentially select subjects who are not ethnic minorities (Schneider *et al.*, 1997). Also, values of many older adults with psychiatric illness are often not reflected in research objectives and methods. There has been a proclivity for western research to reflect assumptions of individualism and personal advancement rather than mutuality and social equity. Health-care providers extrapolating current evidence-based practice recommendations for late-life mental disorders need to be aware of this bias when they treat patients from a different cultural background and must make appropriate intuitive adjustments in treatment recommendations. Clinical practice and research need to tailor their approach to reflect sensitivity to cultural, race, and ethnic issues in older adults with psychiatric disorders.

5. **Oldest old:**

One of the most critical areas of neglect in geriatric psychiatry to date is the neglect of the oldest old. This term refers to the 85 plus age group, which is the fastest growing age group in our society. This group remains difficult to study and is poorly understood by psychiatrists. Though function varies widely among the oldest old, once people reach this age they frequently experience serious medical and/or psychiatric illness along with physical and social impairments, which coalesce and cascade, often resulting in the condition described by geriatricians as frailty. After the age of 85, nearly half of all elders living in the community are frail despite their apparent functional well-being. Geriatric psychiatry might take a lesson from geriatric medicine and recognize that syndromes such as frailty may be critical to formulating appropriate care for all older adults and especially for the oldest old, the most vulnerable of the older adult population.

END-OF-LIFE CARE

80% of deaths in developed countries now occur among persons age 65 and older (Lyness, 2004b). Majority of death in older adults occur in the context of chronic illnesses and are too often accompanied by potentially remediable emotional or physical suffering. Conversations with patients and family about end-of-life care; the evaluation and treatment of suffering, including pain, depression, suicidality,

(Cole and Bellavance, 1997) of the prognosis of elderly medical inpatients with depression, researchers found that at three months, 18% of patients were well, 43% were depressed, and 22% were dead. At 12 months or more, 19% were well, 29% were depressed, and 53% were dead. Factors associated with worse outcomes included more severe depression and more serious physical illness. Among those older depressed adults without significant comorbid medical illness or dementia and who were treated optimally, the outcome was much better, with over 80% recovering and remaining well throughout follow-up (Reynolds *et al.*, 1992).

Medical comorbidity, functional impairment, and comorbid dementing disorders all adversely influence outcome of depression (Blazer, 2003). Depression also adversely affects the outcome of the comorbid problems such as cardiovascular disease (Frasure-Smith *et al.*, 1993) in which, depressive disorder is associated with an increase in mortality (Romanelli *et al.*, 2002), particularly for women but less so for men (McGuire *et al.*, 2002; Williams *et al.*, 2002a).

NONSUICIDE MORTALITY

Psychiatric disorders in general and severe depressive disorders increase the risk of nonsuicide related mortality (Bruce *et al.*, 1994; Blazer, 2003). For example, in a review of 61 reports of this relationship from 1997 to 2001, 72% demonstrated a positive association between depression and mortality in elderly people (Schulz *et al.*, 2002). Both the severity and duration of depressive symptoms predict mortality in the elderly population in these studies (Geerlings *et al.*, 2002). Other studies, however, have suggested that the association between depression and mortality is related to the high correlation between depression and other medical problems. That is, depression impacts nonsuicide mortality through intermediate risk factors.

SUICIDE

The association of depression and suicide across the life cycle has been well established (Goldstein *et al.*, 1991; Conwell *et al.*, 2002; Turvey *et al.*, 2002). Older adults are at a higher risk for suicide than any other age-groups. While older Americans comprise about 13% of the US population, they account for 18% of all suicide deaths (Arias *et al.*, 2001). Increased risk for suicide attempts in late life is associated with being a widow or a widower, living alone, perception of poor health status, poor sleep quality, lack of a confidant, and experience of stressful life events, such as financial and interpersonal discord (Conwell *et al.*, 2002; Turvey *et al.*, 2002) (see Table 2).

The most common means of committing suicide in the elderly are use of a firearm (Goldstein *et al.*, 1991) and drug ingestion (Blazer, 2003). Women attempt suicide more than men do; however, men completed suicide more often than women (Sachs-Ericsson, 2000). Though completed suicides increase with age, suicidal behaviors do not increase (De Leo *et al.*, 2001). This is consistent with the contention that older adults are more intent in their efforts to commit suicide (Conwell *et al.*, 1998).

Table 2 Demographic characteristics, symptoms, and behaviors associated with increased risk factors for suicide

Demographic characteristics	Symptoms and behaviors	Suicidal thoughts or behaviors
Widow(er)	Depressive symptoms	History of suicide attempts
Living alone	Pervasive hopelessness	Resolved plans regarding suicide
Male	Feelings of being a burden	Courage and/or competence regarding suicide
Caucasian	Self-harming behaviors	Access to means of suicide (e.g. gun or pills)
Over age 65	Social isolation	
	Poor social support	
	Marked impulsivity	Acute desire for death
	Substance abuse	
	Personality disorder	

There are many risk factors for suicide. Depression is the strongest risk factor (Bruce *et al.*, 2004). Perhaps the most well studied factor is pervasive feelings of hopelessness (Rifai *et al.*, 1994). Other psychological constructs include emotional pain (Shneidman, 1992), feelings of being a burden, and social isolation (Alexopoulos *et al.*, 1999). The lack of social networks and their disruption are significantly associated with risk for suicide in later life (Conwell *et al.*, 2002).

Older persons with mental disorders rarely seek help from mental health professionals, preferring to visit their primary care physician instead (Goldstrom *et al.*, 1987). The majority of older adults who die by suicide have seen a primary care physician in preceding months, underscoring the physicians potential role in intervention. Suicide prevention strategies rely on the identification of specific, observable risk factors. Depression, hopelessness, and self-harming behaviors (such as food refusal) are possible indicators of suicide risk (Pearson and Brown, 2000; Conwell *et al.*, 2002).

Individuals with a previous history of suicide are more likely to attempt suicide again (Goldstein *et al.*, 1991). Increased risk is also associated with resolved plans, a sense of courage and/or competence regarding suicide, and access to means of suicide (e.g. pills or gun) (Joiner *et al.*, 1999). Other variables that increase suicide risk include substance abuse (Conwell and Brent, 1995), marked impulsivity, and personality disorder (Duberstein, 1995).

ETIOLOGY

Biological

As noted above, increased rates of depression are associated with many medical conditions including dementing disorders

(Sachs-Ericsson and Blazer, In Press), cardiovascular disease (Schulz *et al.*, 2000), hip fractures (Whooley *et al.*, 1999), and Parkinson's disease (Starkstein *et al.*, 1990). Depression has been associated with pain in institutionalized elderly people (Parmelee *et al.*, 1991) and is also common among homebound elders with urinary incontinence (Endberg *et al.*, 2001). Therefore, any exploration of the etiology of late-life depression must begin with the possibility that the depression is caused in part, or perhaps in whole, by physical illness.

The role of heredity, that is, genetic susceptibility, has been of great interest in exploring the origins of depression across the life cycle (Barondes, 1998). Among elderly twins, genetic influences accounted for 16% of the variance in total depression scores on the CES-D and 19% of psychosomatic and somatic complaints. In contrast, genetics contributed a minimal amount to the variance of depressed mood and psychological well-being (Gatz *et al.*, 1992). Attention has been directed to specific genetic markers for late-life depression. For example, a number of studies have focused on the susceptibility gene apolipoprotein E (APOE; the e4 allele) for Alzheimer's disease. No association was found in a community sample between e4 and depression (Blazer *et al.*, 2002). In another study, hyperintensities in deep white matter but not in the periventricular white matter were associated with depressive symptoms, especially in elders carrying the e4 allele (Nebes *et al.*, 2001).

Much attention has been directed to vascular risk for late-life depression, dating back at least 40 years, although the advent of MRI increased interest considerably (Kumar *et al.*, 2002a,b). Vascular lesions in some regions of the brain may contribute to a unique variety of late-life depression. MRI of depressed patients has revealed structural abnormalities in areas related to the cortical–striatal–pallidal–thalamus–cortical pathway (George *et al.*, 1994), including the frontal lobes (Krishnan *et al.*, 1993), caudate (Krishnan *et al.*, 1992), and putamen (Husain *et al.*, 1991). These circuits are known to be associated with the development of spontaneous performance strategies demanded by executive tasks. Recent serotonin activity, specifically 5 HT2A receptor binding, decreases dramatically in a variety of brain regions from adolescence through midlife, but the decline slows from midlife to late life. Receptor loss occurred across widely scattered regions of the brain (anterior cingulated, occipital cortex, and hippocampus). Serotonin depletion can also be studied indirectly by the study of radioisotope-labeled or tritiated imipramine binding (TIB) sites. There is a significant decrease in the number of platelet-TIB sites in elderly depressed patients, compared with elderly controls and individuals.

Late-life depression is also associated with endocrine changes. Although the dexamethasone suppression test was long ago ruled out as a diagnostic test for depression, nonsuppression of cortisol is associated with late-life depression compared with age-matched controls (Davis *et al.*, 1984). Depression is also associated with increase of corticotrophin releasing factor (CRF), which mediates sleep and appetite disturbances, reduced libido, and psychomotor changes (Arborelius *et al.*, 1999). Aging is associated with an increased responsiveness of adrenocorticotropic hormone (ACTH), cortisol, and dehydroepiandrosterone sulfate (DHEA-S) to CRF (Luisi *et al.*, 1998). Low levels of DHEA have been associated with higher rates of depression and a greater number of depressive symptoms in community-dwelling older women (Yaffe *et al.*, 1998). Total testosterone levels have been found to be lower in elderly men with dysthymic disorder than in men without depressive symptoms (Seidman *et al.*, 2002). However, the efficacy of testosterone in treating depression has not been established (Seidman *et al.*, 2001).

Psychological and Social

A variety of different psychological origins have been theorized for depression in later life including behavioral, cognitive, developmental, and psychodynamic theories. Among the behavioral explanations, learned helplessness (Seligman and Maier, 1967) was originally used to describe the increasingly passive behavior of dogs who were exposed to inescapable shock. The theory has been expanded, suggesting that one cause of depression is learning that initiating action in an environment that cannot be changed is futile (Seligman, 1972; Blazer, 2002). As individuals face new challenges associated with aging, coping strategies that were once useful may become less effective. Within this context, behavioral interventions (described below) encourage the individual to find new ways to successfully cope with environmental stress.

The most dominant current psychological model of depression is that of cognitive distortions (Beck, 1987). Several researchers have found consistent differences in the cognitive styles of depressed individuals compared to nondepressed individuals. Beck and others have described the cognitive schema of depressed persons as having logical errors that promote depression (Beck, 1963; Kovacs and Beck, 1978; Beck, 1987). Cognitions may be distorted such that the elder has expectations that are not realistic, overgeneralizes or overreacts to adverse events, and personalizes events. Thus, in reaction to a negative life event (loss of a loved one, move into a nursing home), an individual's cognitive style may increase the likelihood of an episode of depression.

A developmental theory of aging, the *disengagement theory* of aging (Adams, 2001) contends that there is a mutual social and affective withdrawal between older adults and their social environment. Similarly, *Gerotranscendence* (Tornstam, 1989) is a concept in which the older individuals are thought to narrow their personal social world and to have a decreased investment in activities that were once important. Others have conceptualized this withdrawal as a subtype of geriatric depression that has been termed *depletion* (Johnson and Barer, 1992). A more recent, yet controversial theory complements the depletion theory, suggesting that successful aging is associated with *selective optimization with compensation* (Baltes and Baltes, 1990). This model is based on the recognition by the elder of the realities of aging, especially the losses. Such recognition leads to selection of realistic activities, optimization of those activities, and compensation for lost activities, which in turn leads to a reduced and transformed life. More recently, *socioemotional selectivity theory* (Frederickson and Carstensen, 1990; Carstensen, 1992) posits that decreasing rates of social contact reflect a greater selectivity in social partners. Other factors being equal, it is probable that elders who are less socially engaged are more depressed. For example, elders who stopped driving had a greater risk of worsening depressive symptoms (Fonda *et al.*, 2001).

The association between late-life depression and impaired social support has been established for many years. Poor social support is strongly associated with depression in the elderly (Goldberg *et al.*, 1985; DuPertuis *et al.*, 2001). The quality of social support networks has been identified as an important factor in predicting relapse in depressive episodes and future levels of depressive symptoms (Holahan *et al.*, 1999; Joiner and Coyne, 1999). Further, among the elderly, social support may serve as a buffer against disability (Mendes de Leon *et al.*, 2003) while social disengagement may be a risk factor for cognitive impairment (Bassuk *et al.*, 1999).

Perceived negative interpersonal events are also associated with depression among individuals in general, as well as among elders, particularly in those who demonstrate a high need for approval and reassurance in the context of interpersonal relationships. Ironically, the interpersonal behaviors (e.g. excessive reassurance seeking) of individuals who become depressed are often associated with the withdrawal of social support from friends and family (Joiner and Metalsky, 1995).

DIAGNOSIS

The diagnostic workup of late-life depression derives predominantly from what we know about symptom presentation and etiology. The diagnosis is made on the basis of a history augmented with a physical examination and supplemented with laboratory studies. Importantly, there is no biological marker or test that makes the diagnosis of depression. However, for some subtypes of depression, such as vascular depression, the presence of subcortical white matter hyperintensities on MRI scanning are critical to confirming the diagnosis (Kraaij and de Wilde, 2001; Blazer, 2002).

There are several standardized screening measures for depression often used by primary care physicians (Williams *et al.*, 2002b). Examples of such instruments includes the Geriatric Depression Scale (GDS) or the CES-D (Yesavage *et al.*, 1983; Koenig *et al.*, 1995). Screening in primary care is critical. Not only is the frequency of depression high, but suicidal ideation can be detected by screening as well.

Despite the centrality of the clinical interview, other diagnostic tools must be employed to assess the depressed elder. Cognitive status should be assessed with the Mini-Mental State Examination (MMSE) or a similar instrument, given the high likelihood of comorbid depression and cognitive dysfunction (Sachs-Ericsson and Blazer, In Press). Height, weight, history of recent weight loss, lab tests for hypoalbuminemia, and cholesterol are markers of nutritional status and are critical to assess, given the risk for frailty and failure to thrive in depressed elders, especially the very old (Fried, 1994; Blazer, 2000). General health perceptions as well as functional status (activities of daily living) should be assessed for all depressed elderly patients (Fillenbaum, 1988). Assessment of social functioning (Blazer, 1982), medications (many prescribed drugs can precipitate symptoms of depression), mobility and balance, sitting and standing blood pressure, blood screen, urinalysis, chemical screen (e.g. electrolytes, which may signal dehydration), and an electrocardiogram if cardiac disease is present (especially if antidepressant medications are indicated) round out the diagnostic workup.

Dementia and depression have considerable overlap in symptoms (Aarsland *et al.*, 1999). Thus, distinguishing between late-life depression and neurological disorders is one of the more challenging problems facing health-care professionals treating the elderly (Karlawish and Clark, 2003) (see Table 3). There are a cluster of cognitive deficits that are common to both dementia and depression. Memory impairment is the most frequent symptom that is common to both (Knott and Fleminger, 1975; Blazer, 2002). Apathy is also a common symptom among individuals with dementia including those with and without comorbid depression, as well as among nondemented elderly individuals with depression (Starkstein *et al.*, 2001).

Clinicians often have difficulty in their attempt to distinguish a primary mood disorder from other problems associated with depressed mood, in particular, what some have referred to as *pseudodementia* (Blazer, 2002, p 349–372). Pseudodementia is a syndrome in which dementia is mimicked; however, the underlying cause is a psychiatric disorder, which is typically but not always depression (Wells, 1979).

Table 3 Characteristics distinguishing depression from dementia (adapted from Wells, 1979)

Clinical characteristics	Dementia	Depression
Onset	Indeterminate	Rapid
Duration of symptoms	Long	Short
Mood	Consistently depressed	Fluctuating course
Mental status exam	Tries to answer, but typically incorrect	"Don't know" answers
Presentation	Tries to conceal disabilities	Highlights disabilities
Cognitive impairment	Stable	Fluctuates

TREATMENT

Biological

There is clear and mounting evidence for the efficacy of antidepressant medications (both alone and in combination with psychotherapy) in the treatment of older adults with major depression as well as for the treatment of dysthymia (Unützer *et al.*, 2003) Antidepressant medications have become the foundation for the treatment of moderate to severe depression in older adults (Blazer, 2003). While antidepressant medications are equally effective for treating serious major depression across the life cycle (Forlenza *et al.*, 2000; Salzman *et al.*, 2002), differences in side effects make some antidepressants more desirable. That is, while studies that compare tricyclic antidepressants (TCAs) and selective serotonin reuptake inhibitors (SSRIs) usually find equal efficacy, there are fewer side effects with SSRIs (Mulsant *et al.*, 2001) which make them the first choice for treatment of older adults. Therefore, SSRIs are the treatment of choice (Callahan *et al.*, 1996). The antidepressants even appear to be efficacious in subjects with AD and vascular depression (Reifler *et al.*, 1989; Lyketsos *et al.*, 2000) (see Table 4).

Interestingly, antidepressants appear less efficacious in treating less severe depression in older adults (Ackerman *et al.*, 2000). The overall evidence suggests that antidepressants and counseling have relatively small benefits in these less severe conditions (Oxman and Sungupta, 2002). However, in a study conducted in a primary care setting, paroxetine (compared with problem-solving therapy) was found to have moderate benefits for depressive symptoms in elderly patients with dysthymia and more severely impaired elderly patients with minor depression (Williams *et al.*, 2000). Most of the currently available SSRIs have been demonstrated to be efficacious in elderly people, including fluoxetine (Feighner and Cohn, 1985), sertraline (Cohn *et al.*, 1990), paroxetine (Mulsant *et al.*, 2001), citalopram (Nyth *et al.*, 1992), and fluvoxamine (Rahman *et al.*, 1991). Escitalopram, recently entering the antidepressant market, has not been shown to be specifically efficacious in the elderly population. Other new-generation antidepressants that have been shown to be efficacious include venlafaxine (Mahapatra and Hackett, 1997), mirtazapine (Schatzberg *et al.*, 2002), and buproprion (Weihs *et al.*, 2001). To date there has been no study of the drug in the elderly population of nefazodone (Baldwin *et al.*, 2001).

In a recent consensus of practicing geriatric psychiatrists, the SSRIs along with psychotherapy were identified as the treatments of choice for late-life depression, along with venlafaxine. Buproprion and mirtazapine are alternatives, as was electroconvulsive therapy (ECT) in severe depression. Medication (SSRI plus an antipsychotic, with risperidone and olanzapine being the antipsychotics most commonly recommended) and/or ECT are the preferred treatments for major depression with psychotic features. Psychotherapy in combination with medications is recommended for dysthymic disorder. Education plus watchful waiting are recommended for minor depression that lasts for less than two weeks (antidepressant medication plus psychotherapy are recommended for minor depression if symptoms persist).

The preferred antidepressant for treating both major and minor depression, according to the consensus report, is citalopram (20–30 mg) followed by sertraline (50–100 mg) and paroxetine (20–30 mg), with fluoxetine (20 mg) as an alternative (escitalopram was not in the market when this survey was conducted). Nortriptyline (40–100 mg) is the preferred tricyclic agent, with desipramine (50–100 mg) as the alternative. The consensus group recommended continuing the antidepressant for three to six weeks before a change in medications is made because of the first choice medication not being effective. If little or no response is observed, the consensus is to switch to venlafaxine (75–200 mg) (Blazer, 2003). For a first episode of depression with recovery following antidepressant therapy, one year of continual therapy is recommended. For two episodes, two years of continual therapy and for three or more episodes, three years of continual therapy are recommended (Alexopoulos *et al.*, 2001).

The new-generation antidepressants inhibit a number of the cytochrome P450 enzymes that metabolize most medications, such as CYP3A, CYP2D6, DYP2C, CYP1A2, and CYP2E1. The CYP3A enzymes metabolize 60% of the medications used today. Fluoxetine is a moderate inhibitor of CYP3A4. Approximately 8–10% of adults lack the CYP2dD6 enzyme, and paroxetine is a potent inhibitor of this enzyme (which

Table 4 Treatment choices and alternatives associated with depressive disorders

Diagnoses	First choice	Alternative
Late-life depression	SSRIs plus psychotherapy Citalopram (20–30 mg) Sertraline (50–100 mg) Paroxetine (20–30 mg) Fluoxetine (20 mg)	Tricyclic agents: Nortriptyline (40–100 mg) Desipramine (50–100 mg)
More severe depression	Venlafaxine. Buproprion Mirtazapine	Electroconvulsive therapy
Depression with psychotic features	SSRI plus an antipsychotic (risperidone or olanzapine)	Electroconvulsive therapy
Dysthymic disorder	Psychotherapy in combination with medications	
Minor depression (less than 2 weeks)	Education plus watchful waiting	
Minor depression (that persists)	Antidepressant medication plus psychotherapy	

may explain, among some patients treated with paroxetine, the lack of efficacy of analgesics such as codeine that are metabolized by this enzyme). Citalopram and venlafaxine are the "cleanest" of the medications in terms of inhibition of the cytochrome P450 enzymes (Greenblatt *et al.*, 1998; Pollock, 2000).

Hyponatremia (39% in one study) is a clear risk for the elderly on SSRIs or venlafaxine. Frail older adults and those with medical illness should have sodium levels checked before and after commencement of antidepressant medications (Kirby *et al.*, 2002). The safest practice is to monitor all elders for sodium levels who are on these medications. This hyponatremia is due to the syndrome of inappropriate secretion of antidiuretic hormone (SIADH). Other serious side effects reported with the SSRIs include the risk of falls (no less risk than with the tricyclics in one study) (Thapa *et al.*, 1998), the serotonin syndrome (lethargy, restlessness, hypertonicity, rhabdomyolysis, renal failure, and possible death) (Gillman, 1999), and gastrointestinal bleeding (de Abajo *et al.*, 1999). Less serious side effects include weight loss, sexual dysfunction, anticholinergic effects (most pronounced with paroxetine), agitation, and difficulty in sleeping.

Psychotic depression in late life responds poorly to antidepressants but well to ECT (Godber *et al.*, 1987; Flint and Rifat, 1998). In one study using bilateral ECT versus pharmacotherapy, the older age-group had a better response to ECT than younger age-groups (O'Conner *et al.*, 2001). Memory problems remain the major adverse effect of ECT that affects quality of life. Memory problems are usually transient and clear within weeks following treatment.

A repetitive transcranial magnetic stimulation (rTMS) could replace ECT in some situations (McNamara *et al.*, 2001). rTMS does not require anesthesia and seizure induction is avoided. Though not studied specifically in elderly people, in one outcome study, patients treated with rTMS, compared with those treated with ECT, responded equally well and their clinical gains lasted just as long (Dannon *et al.*, 2002). In another study, executive function improved in both middle-aged and elderly depressed subjects with rTMS compared with sham treatments (Moser *et al.*, 2002).

A variety of adjunct physical therapies may alleviate depression. In a community-based study, among subjects who were not depressed at baseline, those who reported a low activity level were at significantly greater risk for depression at follow-up (Camacho *et al.*, 1991). Aerobic exercise training programs may be considered an alternative to antidepressants for treatment of depression in older persons with mild to moderate symptoms. (Blumenthal *et al.*, 1999). However, the advantages of exercise are not limited to aerobic activities. Unsupervised weight lifting has been found to decrease depressive symptoms up to 20 weeks after induction (Singh *et al.*, 2001). Light therapy may also be beneficial, especially if the depression follows a seasonal pattern. Thirty minutes of bright light a day improved depression among institutionalized elders in one controlled study (Sumaya *et al.*, 2001).

Psychological

Cognitive behavioral therapy (CBT) and interpersonal therapy (IPT) have been shown to be efficacious in the treatment of depression for the elderly, especially in combination with medications. Given that these therapies are short-term (12–20 sessions), they are attractive to third-party payers. In addition, the educational (as opposed to a reflective) posture of the therapist employing such therapies is attractive to elders (Blazer, 2003).

Cognitive behavioral therapies focus on the patient's cognitions surrounding a given negative life event and assist the person to cognitively restructure their thought processes in a more realistic manner. The evidence is clear that treatments aimed at changing cognitive distortions can be quite effective in decreasing depressive symptoms and even in preventing future relapse. Treatments that focus on problem solving and behavioral activation have also been found to be effective in the treatment of depression. For example, in a study to determine the effectiveness of a home-based program for treating minor depression or dysthymia among older adults, patients were randomly assigned to a in-home based treatment (Program to Encourage Active, Rewarding Lives for Seniors, PEARLS) or usual care (Frasure-Smith *et al.*, 1993). The PEARLS intervention consisted of problem-solving treatment, social and physical activation, and recommendations to patients' physicians regarding antidepressant medications. The intervention was found to significantly reduce depressive symptoms and improved health status in chronically ill older adults with minor depression and dysthymia.

Another frequently used treatment for depression is IPT (Klerman *et al.*, 1984; Frank *et al.*, 1993) and it has been adapted for older adults (Frank and Spanier, 1995). IPT focuses on four components hypothesized to lead to or maintain depression: grief (e.g. death of a loved one); interpersonal disputes (e.g. conflict with adult children); role transitions (e.g. retirement); and interpersonal deficits (e.g. lack of assertiveness skills). In a study of IPT and elderly depressed patients, clinicians determined that the most common problem areas in therapy were role transition (41%), interpersonal disputes (34.5%), and grief (23%) (Miller *et al.*, 1998). Miller and colleagues (Miller *et al.*, 2001) found that IPT was an effective treatment not only with elderly patients with depression but also including those with moderate cognitive impairment.

It is important to note that most studies of depression have found a combination of psychotherapy and pharmacotherapy to have a better outcome than with either treatment taken alone (Reynolds *et al.*, 1999; Thompson *et al.*, 2001).

SUMMARY

Depression has a profound negative impact on older adults, significantly decreasing quality of life, functioning, and increasing both medical morbidity and mortality. While rates of depressive disorders are no greater among the elderly than in the general population, significant rates of depressive symptoms have been identified in elderly populations. Older persons with mental disorders rarely seek help from mental health professionals, preferring to visit their primary care physician instead. Nonetheless, depression among the elderly often goes unrecognized and untreated. However, when identified and addressed, depression, regardless of age, is a highly treatable illness. There are several psychotherapies that have been specifically developed for the treatment of depression, the most effective being CBT and IPT. There are antidepressant medications that are efficacious in treating the depressed elderly patient; moreover, a combination of medication and psychotherapy has been shown to produce the most positive outcomes.

KEY POINTS

- Depression, the most frequent cause of emotional suffering in later life is associated with significant losses in health-related quality of life.
- Depression is often comorbid with other disorders including dementia and medical problems.
- Etiological determinants of depression include psychological, biological, and developmental life-span theories.
- There is an association of suicide with depression.
- Depression often goes undetected and untreated; however, when identified, it is a highly treatable illness.

KEY REFERENCES

- Alexopoulos GS, Katz IR, Reyonalds CF *et al.* The expert consensus guideline series: pharmacotherapy of depressive disorders in older patients. *Postgraduate Medicine* 2001; **110**(Oct Special Issue):1–86.
- Blazer D. Psychiatry and the oldest old. *American Journal of Psychiatry* 2000; **157**:1915–24.
- Blazer D. Depression in late life: review and commentary. *Journals of Gerontology Series A-Biological Sciences and Medical Sciences* 2003; **58**(3):M249–65.
- Hays J, Saunders W, Flint E & Blazer D. Social support and depression as risk factors for loss of physical function in late life. *Aging and Mental Health* 1997; **1**:209–20.
- Sachs-Ericsson N & Blazer DG. Depression and anxiety associated with dementia. In G Maletta (ed) *Geriatric Psychiatry: Evaluation and Management*; Lippincott Williams & Wilkins (in press).

REFERENCES

Aarsland D, Larsen JP, Lim NG *et al.* Range of neuropsychiatric disturbances in patients with Parkinson's disease. *Journal of Neurology Neurosurgery and Psychiatry* 1999; **67**:492–6.

Aarsland D, Tandberg E, Larsen JP *et al.* Frequency of dementia in Parkinson disease. *Archives of Neurology* 1996; **53**:538–42.

Ackerman D, Greenland S, Bystritsky A & Small GW. Side effects and time course of response in a placebo-controlled trial of fluoxetine for the treatment of geriatric depression. *Journal of Clinical Psychopharmacology* 2000; **20**:658–65.

Adams KB. Depressive symptoms, depletion, or developmental change? Withdrawal, apathy, and lack of vigor in the geriatric depression scale. *Gerontologist* 2001; **41**(6):768–77.

Alexopoulos GS. Clinical and biological interactions in affective and cognitive geriatric syndromes. *American Journal of Psychiatry* 2003; **160**(5):811–4.

Alexopoulos GS, Bruce ML, Hull J *et al.* Clinical determinants of suicidal ideation and behavior in geriatric depression. *Archives of General Psychiatry* 1999; **56**(11):1048–53.

Alexopoulos GS, Katz IR, Reyonalds CF *et al.* The expert consensus guideline series: pharmacotherapy of depressive disorders in older patients. *Postgraduate Medicine* 2001; **110**(Oct Special Issue):1–86.

Alexopoulos G, Meyers B, Young RC *et al.* Recovery in geriatric depression. *Archives of General Psychiatry* 1996; **53**:305–12.

APA. *DSM-IV: Diagnostic and Statistical Manual of Mental Disorders* 1994; American Psychiatric Association, Washington.

Arborelius L, Owens M, Plotsky PM & Nemeroff CB. The role of corticotropin-releasing factor in depression and anxiety disorders. *Journal of Endocrinology* 1999; **160**:1–12.

Arias E, Anderson RN, Murphy S *et al. Deaths: Final Data for 2001* 2001, p 1120; DHHS publication (DHS), National Center for Health Statistics, Hyattsville; *National Vital Statistics Reports* **52**(3):2003.

Baldwin D, Hawley C & Mellors K. A randomized, double-blind controlled comparison of nefazodone and paroxetine in the treatment of depression: safety, tolerability and efficacy in continuation phase treatment. *Journal of Psychopharmacology* 2001; **15**:161–5.

Ballard C, Bannister C, Solis M *et al.* The prevalence, associations and symptoms of depression amongst dementia sufferers. *Journal of Affective Disorders* 1996; **36**(3–4):135–44.

Baltes P & Baltes M (eds) *Successful Aging: Perspectives from the Behavioral Sciences* 1990; Cambridge University Press, Cambridge.

Barondes S. *Mood Genes: Hunting for Origins of Mania and Depression* 1998; W.H. Freeman and Company, New York.

Bassuk SS, Glass TA & Berkman LF. Social disengagement and incident cognitive decline in community-dwelling elderly persons. *Annals of Internal Medicine* 1999; **3**:165–73.

Beck AT. Thinking and depression. *Idiosyncratic Content and Cognitive Distortions* 1963; **14**:324–33.

Beck A. Cognitive model of depression. *Journal of Cognitive Psychotherapy* 1987; **1**:2–27.

Beekman A, Deeg D, Van Tilberg T *et al.* Major and minor depression in later life: a study of prevalence and risk factors. *Journal of Affective Disorders* 1995; **36**:65–75.

Berkman L, Berkman C, Kasl S *et al.* Depressive symptoms in relation to physical health and functioning in the elderly. *American Journal of Epidemiology* 1986; **124**:372–88.

Blazer D. Social support and mortality in an elderly community population. *American Journal of Epidemiology* 1982; **115**:684–94.

Blazer D. Dysthymia in community and clinical samples of older adults. *American Journal of Psychiatry* 1994; **151**:1567–9.

Blazer D. Psychiatry and the oldest old. *American Journal of Psychiatry* 2000; **157**:1915–24.

Blazer D. *Depression in Late Life* 2002; Springer, New York.

Blazer D. Depression in late life: review and commentary. *Journals of Gerontology Series A-Biological Sciences and Medical Sciences* 2003; **58**(3):M249–65.

Blazer D, Bachar J & Hughes DC. Major depression with melancholia: a comparison of middle-aged and elderly adults. *Journal of the American Geriatrics Society* 1987; **35**:927–32.

Blazer D, Burchett B, Fillenbaum G *et al.* APOE E4 and low cholesterol as risks for depression in a biracial elderly community sample. *American Journal of Geriatric Psychiatry* 2002; **10**:515–20.

Blazer D, Burchett B, Service C & George LK. The association of age and depression among the elderly: an epidemiologic exploration. *Journal of Gerontology: Medical Sciences* 1991; **46**:M210–5.

Blazer D, Hybels C, Simonsick EM & Hanlon JT. Marked differences in antidepressant use by race in an elderly community sample: 1986 – 1996. *American Journal of Psychiatry* 2000; **157**:1089–94.

Blazer D, Landerman L, Hays JC *et al.* Symptoms of depression among community-dwelling elderly African-American and white older adults. *Psychological Medicine* 1998; **28**:1311–20.

Blazer D, Swartz M, Woodbury M *et al.* Depressive symptoms and depressive diagnoses in a community population. *Archives of General Psychiatry* 1988; **45**:1078–84.

Blumenthal J, Babyak M, Moore KA *et al.* Effects of exercise training on older patients with major depression. *Archives of Internal Medicine* 1999; **159**:2349–56.

Bruce ML, Leaf P, Rozal G *et al.* Psychiatry status and 9-year mortality data in the New Haven Epidemiologic Catchment Area Study. *American Journal of Psychiatry* 1994; **51**:716–21.

Bruce ML, Ten Have TR, Reynolds CF *et al.* Reducing suicidal ideation and depressive symptoms in depressed older primary care patients: a randomized controlled trial. *Journal of the American Medical Association* 2004; **291**(9):1081–91.

Callahan C, Hendrie H, Nienaber NA *et al.* Suicidal ideation among older primary care patients. *Journal of the American Geriatrics Society* 1996; **44**:1205–9.

Camacho T, Roberts R, Lazarus NB *et al.* Physical activity and depression: evidence from the Alameda County Study. *American Journal of Epidemiology* 1991; **134**:220–31.

Carstensen L. Motivation for social contact across the life span: a theory of socioemotional selectivity. *Nebraska Symposium on Motivation* 1992; **40**:209–54.

Charles S, Reynolds C, Gatz MJ *et al.* Age-related differences and changes in positive and negative affect over 23 years. *Journal of Personality and Social Psychology* 2001; **80**:136–51.

Cochran D, Brown DR & McGregor KC. Racial differences in the multiple social roles of older women: Implications for depressive symptoms. *Gerontologist* 1999; **39**(4):465–72.

Cohn C, Shrivastava R, Mendels J *et al.* Double-blind multicenter comparison of sertraline and amitriptyline in elderly depressed patients. *Journal of Clinical Psychiatry* 1990; **51**:28–33.

Cole MG & Bellavance F. Depression in elderly medical inpatients: a meta-analysis of outcomes. *Canadian Medical Association Journal* 1997; **157**(8):1055–60.

Cole MG & Dendukuri N. Risk factors for depression among elderly community subjects: a systematic review and meta-analysis. *American Journal of Psychiatry* 2003; **160**:1147–56.

Cole MG & Yaffe K. Pathway to psychiatric care of the elderly with depression. *International Journal of Geriatric Psychiatry* 1996; **11**:157–61.

Conwell Y & Brent D. Suicide and aging. I: patterns of psychiatric diagnosis. *International Psychogeriatrics* 1995; **7**(2):149–64.

Conwell Y, Duberstein PR & Caine ED. Risk factors for suicide in later life. *Biological Psychiatry* 2002; **52**(3):193–204.

Conwell Y, Duberstein PR, Cox C *et al.* Age differences in behaviors leading to completed suicide. *American Journal of Geriatric Psychiatry* 1998; **6**:122–6.

Cummings SM, Neff JA & Husaini BA. Functional impairment as a predictor of depressive symptomatology: the role of race, religiosity, and social support. *Health and Social Work* 2003; **28**:23–32.

Dannon P, Dolberg O, Schreiber S & Grunhaus L. Three and six-month outcome following courses of either ECT or rTMS in a population of severely depressed individuals – preliminary report. *Biological Psychiatry* 2002; **51**:687–90.

Davis K, David B, Mathe A *et al.* Age and the dexamethasone suppression test in depression. *American Journal of Psychiatry* 1984; **141**:872–4.

de Abajo F, Rodriguez L & Montero D. Association between selective serotonin reuptake inhibitors and upper gastrointestinal bleeding: population based case-control study. *British Medical Journal* 1999; **319**:1106–9.

De Leo D, Padoani W, Scocco P *et al.* Attempted and completed suicide in older subjects: results from the WHO/EURO Multicentre study of suicidal behaviour. *International Journal of Geriatric Psychiatry* 2001; **16**:300–10.

Duberstein PR. Openness to experience and completed suicide across the second half of life. *International Psychogeriatrics* 1995; **7**:183–98.

DuPertuis LL, Aldwin CM, Bosse R *et al.* Does the source of support matter for different health outcomes? Findings from the Normative Aging Study. *Journal of Aging and Health* 2001; **13**:495–510.

Endberg S, Sereika S, Weber E *et al.* Prevalence and recognition of depressive symptoms among homebound older adults with urinary incontinence. *Journal of Geriatric Psychiatry and Neurology* 2001; **14**:130–9.

Fabrega H, Mulsant BM, Rifai AH *et al.* Ethnicity and psychopathology in an aging hospital-based population: a comparison of African-American and Anglo-European patients. *Journal of Nervous and Mental Disease* 1994; **182**(3):136–44.

Feighner J & Cohn J. Double-blind comparative trials of fluoxetine and doxepin in geriatric patients with major depression. *Journal of Clinical Psychiatry* 1985; **46**:20–5.

Fillenbaum G. *Multidimensional Functional Assessment of Older Adults: The Duke Older Americans Resources and Services Procedures* 1988; Erlbaum, Hillsdale.

Flint A & Rifat S. The treatment of psychotic depression in later life: a comparison of pharmacotherapy and ECT. *Journal of Geriatric Psychiatry* 1998; **13**:23–8.

Fonda S, Wallace R & Herzog AR. Changes in driving patterns and worsening depressive symptoms among older adults. *Journal of Gerontology:Series B Psychological and Social Sciences* 2001; **56**:S343–51.

Forlenza O, Junior A, Hirata ES & Ferreira RC. Antidepressant efficacy of sertraline and imipramine for the treatment of major depression in elderly outpatients. *Sao Paolo Medical Journal* 2000; **118**:99–104.

Frank E, Frank N, Cornes C *et al.* Interpersonal psychotherapy in the treatment of late life depression. In G Klerman & M Weissman (eds) *New Applications of Interpersonal Psychotherapy* 1993; American Psychiatric Press, Washington.

Frank E & Spanier C. Interpersonal psychotherapy for depression: overview, clinical efficacy, and future directions. *Clinical Psychology-Science and Practice* 1995; **d2**:349–65.

Frasure-Smith N, Lesperance F & Talajic M. Depression following myocardial infarction. Impact on 6-month survival. *Journal of the American Medical Association* 1993; **270**:1819–25.

Frederickson BL & Carstensen LL. Choosing social partners: how old age and anticipated endings make people more selective. *Psychology and Aging* 1990; **5**:335–47.

Fried L. Frailty. In W Hazzard, E Bierman, J Blass *et al.* (eds) *Principles of Geriatric Medicine and Gerontology* 1994, pp 1149–56; McGraw Hill, New York.

Gallo J, Cooper-Patrick L, Lesikar S *et al.* Depressive symptoms of whites and African Americans aged 60 years and older. *Journals of Gerontology Series B-Psychological Sciences and Social Sciences* 1998; **53**(5):P277–86.

Gallo J, Rabins P & Anthony JC. Sadness in older persons: 13-year follow-up of a community sample in Baltimore, Maryland. *Psychological Medicine* 1999; **29**:341–50.

Gatz M, Pedersen N, Plomin R *et al.* Importance of shared genes and shared environments for symptoms of depression in older adults. *Journal of Abnormal Psychology* 1992; **101**:701–8.

Geerlings S, Beekman A, Deeg D *et al.* Duration and severity of depression predict mortality in older adults in the community. *Psychological Medicine* 2002; **32**:609–18.

Geerlings M, Schoevers R, Beekman A *et al.* Depression and the risk of cognitive decline and Alzheimer's disease: results of two prospective community-based studies in the Netherlands. *British Journal of Psychiatry* 2000; **176**:568–75.

George M, Ketter T, Post R *et al.* Prefrontal cortex dysfunction in clinical depression. *Depression* 1994; **2**:59–72.

Gillman P. The serotonin syndrome and its treatment. *Journal of Psychopharmacology* 1999; **13**:100–9.

Godber C, Rosenvinge H, Wilkinson DG & Smithies J. Depression in old age: prognosis after ECT. *International Journal of Geriatric Psychiatry* 1987; **2**:19–24.

Goldberg EL, Van Natta P & Comstock GW. Depressive symptoms, social networks and social support of elderly women. *American Journal of Epidemiology* 1985; **121**:448–56.

Goldstein RB, Black DW, Nasrallah A *et al.* The prediction of suicide. Sensitivity, specificity, and predictive value of a multivariate model applied to suicide among 1906 patients with affective disorders. *Archives of General Psychiatry* 1991; **48**:418–22.

Goldstrom ID, Burns BJ, Kessler LG *et al.* Mental health services use by elderly adults in a primary care setting. *Journal of Gerontology* 1987; **42**:147–53.

Greenblatt D, van Moltke L, Harmatz JS & Shader RI. Drug interactions with newer antidepressants: role of human cytochromes P450. *Journal of Clinical Psychiatry* 1998; **59**(suppl 15):19–27.

Hays J, Saunders W, Flint E & Blazer D. Social support and depression as risk factors for loss of physical function in late life. *Aging and Mental Health* 1997; **1**:209–20.

Holahan CJ, Moos RH, Holahan CK & Cronkite RC. Resource loss, resource gain, and depressive symptoms: a 10-year model. *Journal of Personality and Social Psychology* 1999; **77**:620–9.

Husain M, McDonald W, Doraiswamy PM *et al.* A magnetic resonance imaging study of putamen nuclei in major depression. *Psychiatry Research* 1991; **40**:95–9.

Hybels C, Blazer D & Pieper C. Toward a threshold for subthreshold depression: an analysis of correlates of depression by severity of symptoms using data from an elderly community survey. *Gerontologist* 2001; **41**:357–65.

Johnson CL & Barer BM. Patterns of engagement and disengagement among the oldest old. *Journal of Aging Studies* 1992; **6**:351–64.

Joiner T & Coyne JC. *The Interaction Nature of Depression: Advances in Interpersonal Approaches* 1999; American Psychological Association, Washington.

Joiner T & Metalsky G. A prospective test of an integrative interpersonal theory of depression: a naturalistic study of college roommates. *Journal of Personality and Social Psychology* 1995; **69**(4):778–88.

Joiner T, Walker R, Rudd MD & Jobes D. Scientizing and routinizing the outpatient assessment of suicidality. *Professional Psychology- Research and Practice* 1999; **30**:447–53.

Karlawish J & Clark C. Diagnostic evaluation of elderly patients with mild memory problems. *Annals of Internal Medicine* 2003; **138**(5):411–9.

Kim J, Lyons D, Shin IS & Yoon JS. Differences in the behavioral and psychological symptoms between Alzheimer's disease and vascular dementia: are the different pharmacologic treatment strategies justifiable? *Human Psychopharmacology* 2003; **18**(3):215–20.

Kirby D, Harigan S & Ames D. Hyponatremia in elderly psychiatric patients treated with selective serotonin reuptake inhibitors and venlafaxine: a retrospective controlled study in an inpatient unit. *International Journal of Geriatric Psychiatry* 2002; **17**:231–7.

Klerman GL, Weissman MM, Rounsaville BJ *et al. Interpersonal Psychotherapy of Depression* 1984; Basic Books, New York.

Knott P & Fleminger J. Presenile dementia: the difficulties of early diagnosis. *Acta Psychiatrica Scandinavica* 1975; **51**:210–7.

Koenig H, Cohen H, Blazer DG *et al.* Cognitive symptoms of depression and religious coping in elderly medical patients. *Psychosomatics* 1995; **36**:369–75.

Kovacs M & Beck A. Maladaptive cognitive structures in depression. *American Journal of Psychiatry* 1978; **135**(5):525–33.

Kraaij V & de Wilde E. Negative life events and depressive symptoms in the elderly: a life span perspective. *Aging and Mental Health* 2001; **5**:84–91.

Krishnan K, McDonald W, Doraiswamy PM *et al.* Neuroanatomical substrates of depression in the elderly. *European Archives of Psychiatry and Clinical Neuroscience* 1993; **243**:41–6.

Krishnan K, McDonald W, Escalona R *et al.* Magnetic imaging of the caudate nuclei in depression: preliminary observation. *Archives of General Psychiatry* 1992; **49**:553–7.

Kumar A, Mintz J, Warren B & Gary G. Autonomous neurobiological pathways to late-life depressive disorders: clinical and pathophysiological implications. *Neuropsychopharmacology* 2002a; **26**:229–36.

Kumar A, Thomas A, Lavretsky H *et al.* Frontal white matter biochemical abnormalities in late-life major depression detected with proton magnetic resonance spectroscopy. *American Journal of Psychiatry* 2002b; **159**:630–6.

Lopez OL, Jagust WJ, Dulberg C *et al.* Risk factors for mild cognitive impairment in the cardiovascular health study cognition study: part 2. *Archives of Neurology* 2003; **60**(10):1394–9.

Luisi S, Tonetti A, Brnardi F *et al.* Effect of acute corticotropin releasing factor on pituitary-adrenocortical responsiveness in elderly women and men. *Journal of Endocrinological Investigation* 1998; **21**:449–53.

Lyketsos C, Sheppard J, Steel CD *et al.* A randomized placebo-controlled, double-blind, clinical trial of sertraline in the treatment of depression complicating Alzheimer disease: initial results from the Depression in Alzheimer Disease Study (DIADS). *American Journal of Psychiatry* 2000; **157**:1686–9.

Mahapatra S & Hackett D. A randomized, double-blind, paralleled-group comparison of venlafaxine and dothiepin in geriatric patients with major depression. *International Journal of Clinical Practice* 1997; **51**:209–13.

McGuire L, Kiecolt-Glaser J & Glaser R. Depressive symptoms and lymphocyte proliferation in older adults. *Journal of Abnormal Psychology* 2002; **111**:192–7.

McNamara B, Ray J, Arthurs J *et al.* Transcranial magnetic stimulation for depression and other psychiatric disorders. *Psychological Medicine* 2001; **31**:1141–6.

Meller I, Fichter MM, Schroppel H, *et al.* Incidence of depression in octo- and nonagenerians: results of an epidemiological follow-up community study. *European Archives of Psychiatry and Clinical Neuroscience* 1996; **246**(2):93–9.

Mendes de Leon CF, Glass TA & Berkman LF. Social engagement and disability in a community population of older adults: the New Haven EPESE. *American Journal of Epidemiology* 2003; **157**:633–42.

Miller MD, Cornes C, Frank E *et al.* Interpersonal psychotherapy for late-life depression: past, present, and future. *Journal of Psychotherapy Practice and Research* 2001; **10**(4):231–8.

Miller MD, Wolfson L, Frank E *et al.* Using Interpersonal Psychotherapy (IPT) in a combined psychotherapy/ medication research protocol with depressed elders: a descriptive report with case vignettes. *Journal of Psychotherapy Practice and Research* 1998; **7**(1):47–55.

Moser D, Jorge R, Manes F *et al.* Improved executive functioning following repetitive transcranial magnetic stimulation. *Neurology* 2002; **58**:1288–90.

Mulsant B, Pollock B, Nebes R *et al.* A twelve-week, double -blind, randomized comparison of nortriptyline and paroxetine in older depressed inpatients and outpatients. *American Journal of Geriatric Psychiatry* 2001; **9**:406–14.

Nebes R, Vora I, Meltzer CC *et al.* Relationship of deep white matter hyperintensities and apolipoprotein E genotype to depressive symptoms in older adults without clinical depression. *American Journal of Psychiatry* 2001; **158**:878–84.

Nyth A, Gottfried C, Lyby K *et al.* A controlled multicenter clinical study of citalopram and placebo in elderly depressed patients with and without concomitant dementia. *Acta Psychiatrica Scandinavica* 1992; **86**:138–45.

O'Conner M, Knapp R, Husain M *et al.* The influence of age on the response of major depression to electroconvulsive therapy: a C.O.R.E. Report. *American Journal of Geriatric Psychiatry* 2001; **9**:382–90.

Olin J, Schneider L, Katz IR *et al.* Provisional diagnostic criteria for depression of Alzheimer disease. *American Journal of Geriatric Psychiatry* 2002; **10**:125–8.

Oxman T & Sungupta A. Treatment of minor depression. *American Journal of Geriatric Psychiatry* 2002; **10**:256–64.

Parker G, Roy K, Hadzi-Pavlovic D *et al.* The differential impact of age on the phenomenology of melancholia. *Psychological Medicine* 2001; **31**:1231–6.

Parmelee P, Katz I & Lawton MP. The relation of pain to depression among institutionalized aged. *Journal of Gerontology* 1991; **46**:15–21.

Pearson JL & Brown GK. Suicide prevention in late life: directions for science and practice. *Clinical Psychology Review* 2000; **20**(6):685–705.

Pollock B. Geriatric psychiatry: psychopharmacology: general principles. In B Sadock & V Sadock (eds) *Kaplan & Sadock's Comprehensive Textbook of Psychiatry/VII* 2000, pp 3086–90; Williams and Wilkins, Baltimore.

Radloff L. The CES-D scale: a self-report depression scale for research in the general population. *Applied Psychological Measurement* 1977; **1**:385–401.

Rahman M, Akhton M, Savla NC *et al.* A double-blind, randomized comparison of fluvoxamine and dothiepin in the treatment of depression in the elderly. *British Journal of Clinical Practice* 1991; **45**:255–8.

Reifler B, Teri L, Raskind M *et al.* Double-blind trial of imipramine in Alzheimer's disease patients with and without depression. *American Journal of Psychiatry* 1989; **146**:45–9.

Reynolds C, Frank E, Perel JM *et al.* Combined pharmacotherapy and psychotherapy in the acute and continuation treatment of elderly patients with recurrent major depression: a preliminary report. *American Journal of Psychiatry* 1992; **149**:1687–92.

Reynolds C, Frank E, Perel JM *et al.* Nortriptyline and interpersonal psychotherapy as maintenance therapies for recurrent major depression: a randomized controlled trial in patients older than 59 years. *Journal of the American Medical Association* 1999; **281**:39–45.

Rifai AH, George CJ, Stack JA *et al.* Hopelessness in suicide attempters after acute treatment of major depression in late-life. *American Journal of Psychiatry* 1994; **151**:1687–90.

Ritchie K, Gilham C, Ledesert B *et al.* Depressive illness, depressive symptomology and regional cerebral blood flow in elderly people with sub-clinical cognitive impairment. *Age and Ageing* 1999; **28**:385–91.

Romanelli J, Fauerbach J, Bush DE *et al.* The significance of depression in older patients after myocardial infarction. *Journal of the American Geriatrics Society* 2002; **50**:817–22.

Sachs-Ericsson N. *Gender, Social Roles and Suicidal Ideation and Attempts in a General Population Sample* 2000; Kluwer Academic Publishers, Norwell.

Sachs-Ericsson N & Blazer DG. Depression and anxiety associated with dementia. In G Maletta (ed) *Geriatric Psychiatry: Evaluation and Management*; Lippincott Williams & Wilkins (in press).

Salzman C, Wong E & Wright B. Drug and ECT treatment of depression in the elderly, 1996–2001: a literature review. *Biological Psychiatry* 2002; **52**:265–84.

Schatzberg A, Kremer C, Rodrigues HE *et al.* Double-blind, randomized comparison of mirtazapine and paroxetine in elderly depressed patients. *American Journal of Geriatric Psychiatry* 2002; **10**:541–50.

Schulz R, Beach S, Ives DG *et al.* Association between depression and mortality in older adults: The Cardiovascular Health Study. *Archives of Internal Medicine* 2000; **160**:1761–8.

Schulz R, Drayer R & Rollman BL. Depression as a risk factor for non-suicide mortality in the elderly. *Biological Psychiatry* 2002; **52**:205–25.

Seidman S, Araujo A, Roose SP *et al.* Low testosterone levels in elderly men with dysthymic disorder. *American Journal of Psychiatry* 2002; **159**:456–9.

Seidman S, Spatz E, Rizzo C & Roose SP. Testosterone replacement therapy for hypogonadal men with major depressive disorder: a randomized, placebo-controlled clinical trial. *Journal of Clinical Psychiatry* 2001; **62**:406–12.

Seligman MEP. Learned helplessness. *Annual Review of Medicine* 1972; **23**:407.

Seligman M & Maier S. Failure to escape traumatic shock. *Journal of Experimental Psychology* 1967; **74**:1–15.

Shneidman E. *What do Suicides have in Common? A Summary of the Psychological Approach. Suicide: Guidelines for Assessment, Management and Treatment* 1992; Oxford University Press, New York.

Singh N, Clements K & Singh MA. The efficacy of exercise as a long-term antidepressant in elderly subjects: a randomized controlled trial. *Journal of Gerontology: Medical Sciences* 2001; **56**:M497–504.

Snaith R. The concepts of mild depression. *British Journal of Psychiatry* 1987; **150**:387–93.

Starkstein SE, Petracca G, Chemerinski E & Merello M. Prevalence and correlates of parkinsonism in patients with primary depression. *Neurology* 2001; **57**(3):553–5.

Starkstein S, Preziosi T, Bolduc PL & Robinson RG. Depression in Parkinson's disease. *Journal of Nervous and Mental Disorders* 1990; **178**:27–31.

Steffens DC, Skook I, Norton MC *et al.* Prevalence of depression and its treatment in an elderly population: the Cache County Study. *Archives of General Psychiatry* 2000; **57**:601–7.

Sumaya I, Rienzi B, Deegan JF II & Moss DE. Bright light treatment decreases depression in institutionalized older adults: a placebo-controlled crossover study. *Journal of Gerontology Medical Sciences* 2001; **56**:M356–60.

Teresi J, Abrams R, Holmes D *et al.* Influence of cognitive impairment, illness, gender, and African-American status on psychiatric ratings and staff recognition of depression. *American Journal of Geriatric Psychiatry* 2002; **10**:506–14.

Thapa P, Gideon P, Cost T *et al.* Antidepressants and the risk of falls among nursing home residents. *New England Journal of Medicine* 1998; **339**:918–20.

Thompson L, Coon D, Gallagher-Thompson D *et al.* Comparison of desipramine and cognitive/behavioral therapy in the treatment of elderly outpatients with mild-to-moderate depression. *American Journal of Geriatric Psychiatry* 2001; **9**:225–40.

Tornstam L. Gero-transcendence: a reformulation of disengagement theory. *Aging* 1989; **1**:55–63.

Turvey C, Conwell Y, Jones M *et al.* Risk factors for late-life suicide: a prospective, community-based study. *American Journal of Geriatric Psychiatry* 2002; **10**:398–406.

Unützer J, Katon W, Callahan CM *et al.* Depression treatment in a sample of 1,801 depressed older adults in primary care. *Journal of the American Geriatrics Society* 2003; **51**(4):505–14.

Unützer J, Patrick DL, Diehr P *et al.* Quality adjusted life years in older adults with depressive symptoms and chronic medical disorders. *International Psychogeriatrics* 2000; **12**:15–33.

Watkins L, Schneiderman N, Blumenthal JA *et al.* Cognitive and somatic symptoms of depression are associated with medical comorbidity in patients after acute myocardial infarction. *American Heart Journal* 2003; **146**(1):48–54.

Weihs K, Settle E, Batey S *et al.* Buproprion sustained release versus paroxetine for the treatment of depression in the elderly. *Journal of Clinical Psychiatry* 2001; **61**:196–202.

Weissman M, Bruce M, Leaf PJ *et al.* Affective disorders. In DA Regier & LN Robins (eds) *Psychiatric Disorders in America* 1991, pp 53–80; The Free Press, New York.

Wells C. Pseudodementia. *American Journal of Psychiatry* 1979; **136**:895–900.

White L & Blazer D. Related health problems. In J Cornoni-Huntley, D Blazer, M Lafferty *et al.* (eds) *Established Populations for Epidemiologic Studies of the Elderly* 1990, pp 70–85; National Institute on Aging, Bethesda.

Whooley MA, Kip KE, Cauley JA *et al.* Depression, falls, and risk of fracture in older women. *Archives of Internal Medicine* 1999; **159**(5):484–90.

Williams J, Barrett J, Oxman T *et al.* Treatment of dysthymia and minor depression in primary care: a randomized controlled trial in older adults. *Journal of the American Medical Association* 2000; **284**:1519–26.

Williams S, Kasl S, Krumholz HM *et al.* Depression and risk of heart failure among the elderly: a prospective community-based study. *Psychosomatic Medicine* 2002a; **64**:6–12.

Williams JW Jr, Noel PH, Cordes JA *et al.* Is this patient clinically depressed? *Journal of the American Medical Association* 2002b; **287**(9):1160–70.

Yaffe K, Ettinger B, Presseman A *et al.* Neuropsychiatric function and dehydroepiandrosterone sulfate in elderly women: a prospective study. *Biological Psychiatry* 1998; **43**:694–700.

Yesavage J, Brink T, Rose TL *et al.* Development and validation of a geriatric depression screening scale: a preliminary report. *Journal of Psychiatric Research* 1983; **17**:37–49.

Zubenko GS, Zubenko WN, McPherson S *et al.* A collaborative study of the emergence and clinical features of the major depressive syndrome of Alzheimer's disease. *American Journal of Psychiatry* 2003; **160**(5):857–66.

101

The Older Patient with Down's Syndrome

John E. Morley

Saint Louis University School of Medicine and Saint Louis Veterans' Affairs Medical Center, St Louis, MO, USA

INTRODUCTION

The association between trisomy 21 and Down's syndrome was first recognized in 1959 by Lejeune, Gautier, and Tarpin. In recent times, the number of fetuses conceived with Down's syndrome has increased, but prenatal screening has resulted in a decline in the number of children conceived with this condition. Thus, the occurrence of Down's syndrome has decreased from 1 in 700 to 1 in 1000 live births (Roizen and Patterson, 2003).

In modern times, it is not unusual to see persons with Down's syndrome in their 60s. From 1983 to 1997, the median age of death of persons with Down's syndrome increased from 25 years of age to 49 years (Yang *et al.*, 2002). Another study suggested that the average life expectancy for Down's syndrome was in the mid-50s. The oldest reported person with Down's syndrome lived until 83 years of age. Three factors make the persons with Down's syndrome of interest to the geriatrician viz (1) the increasing life span; (2) the fact that these persons tend to develop early frailty and functional decline in their 40s; and (3) the early onset of Alzheimer's disease.

GENES AND DOWN'S SYNDROME

Three hundred and twenty-nine genes are predicted to be on chromosome 21. Sixteen of these genes play a role in mitochondrial energy metabolism or the generation of free radicals. Abnormalities in these genes are thought to lead to increased free radical production leading to premature aging.

At least ten genes on chromosome 21 play a role in brain development and neuronal loss. Two of these are associated with Alzheimer's disease, namely, the amyloid precursor protein and the S100 calcium binding protein. Overproduction of amyloid precursor protein and, thus, beta amyloid, is thought to play a key role in the early onset of Alzheimer's disease in persons with Down's syndrome. In addition, excess production of beta amyloid has been shown to lead to problems with learning and memory, which may contribute to the cognitive problems seen in persons with Down's syndrome.

There are six genes that are involved in folate and methyl group metabolism on chromosome 21. Elevated levels of homocysteine, which are seen in folate deficiency, are associated with Alzheimer's disease. In our clinical experience, elevated homocysteine levels are not rare in younger adults with Down's syndrome.

THE PHYSICIAN, AND THE PATIENT WITH DOWN'S SYNDROME

Older persons with Down's syndrome are usually easily recognized when they present to the physician, because of the classical facial features (brachycephaly, epicanthal folds, and flat nasal bridge) and short stature. These persons also often have broad hands, lax ligaments, and wide gap between the first and second toes, brachydactyly, and mental retardation. The majority of persons with Down's syndrome live in the community. They may live in group housing and work in sheltered workshops. Physicians need to identify the person who accompanies the individual with Down's to the office. This person often provides supervisory care for the individual with Down's and can provide useful historical information on behavioral and other changes that may be occurring. We recommend office visits every 6 months for healthy persons with Down's and every 3 to 4 months when functional or mental decline is present. This allows the patient to become comfortable with the health-care provider. Many patients enjoy hugging and this can further increase trust in the physician. However, the physician must remember to ask the patient first if they wish to hug. The physician should always discuss the patient's work and how it is progressing. Also, note should be made of their recreational activities, and how they are interacting with other persons within a group home.

Principles and Practice of Geriatric Medicine, 4th Edition. Edited by M.S. John Pathy, Alan J. Sinclair and John E. Morley.

Always address the person with Down's directly, before hearing the caregiver's story. This gains their confidence and allows observation of their language ability. Finally, never assume that changes in persons with Down's syndrome are due to Down's itself before excluding other common medical causes.

For some medical examinations, for example, pap smears, and special tests, for example, MRI or CT scan, or procedures such as dental care, persons with Down's may require sedation. We have found that 0.5–1 mg of lorazepam orally is usually sufficient for this purpose and produces no adverse effects. Low dose intravenous lorazepam can also be used in more difficult situations. Others have recommended oral ketamine and midazolam, given under the supervision of an anesthetist (Smith, 2001). Before undergoing a procedure requiring sedation, a risk benefit evaluation should always be undertaken. Informed consent needs to be obtained from the patient or, where applicable, the court appointed guardian.

Preventive measures should be similar for Down's syndrome patients as for the general adult population. This includes screening for hypertension and heart disease. Because obesity is a common problem in this population, regular counseling on the need for exercise is mandatory. While, in our experience, most of the Down's patients do not smoke or drink alcohol, this should be confirmed both from the patient and the caregiver.

Down's adults tend to complain of pain, even when present, less often than other persons. Therefore, it is important to utilize facial expressions during the examination to obtain input concerning presence of pain. Also, such patients may stop using a limb when it is painful. Rocking and "head banging" behaviors occur as visceral pain proxies. As is the case with older adults, middle-aged adults with Down's often manifest medical problems as a delirium or other behavioral problem.

Persons with Down's are a vulnerable population, and thus, like children and older people, are at increased risk for abuse. When adults with Down's become withdrawn, this may suggest abuse or an unrecognized pain syndrome or depression. Presence of unexplained bruises, skin tears or fractures must increase the physician's suspicion of abuse. New onset falls can suggest delirium, functional deterioration or abuse.

Health counseling includes decisions on advanced directives and guardianship. Financial support questions need to be addressed, and relatives need to be aware of local resources. Estate planning, for example trusts, need to be created where appropriate, as Down's syndrome persons are now regularly outliving their parents and other close relatives. Parent (caregiver) support groups can be invaluable as caregiver stress is common, particularly as the parent ages. Local and national societies for Down's syndrome or for persons with developmental disabilities are an important resource. The physician needs to look for excess stress and/or depression in caregivers, and advise treatment where appropriate.

Functional ability using at least basic activities of daily living (ADLs) and instrumental activities of daily living (IADLs) should be assessed yearly. Where possible, mental status screening using the Mini-Mental Status Examination (MMSE) or the Saint Louis University Mental Status Examination and the Geriatric Depression Scale or the Cornell Depression Inventory should be done yearly.

Table 1 Conditions that occur commonly in adults with Down's syndrome

Obesity
Periodontal disease
Hearing loss
Visual problems including early cataracts
Aortic valvular disease
– Mitral valve prolapse
– Aortic regurgitation
Arthritis
Hypogonadism (male)
Hypothyroidism
Hyperthyroidism
Diabetes mellitus
Early menopause
Osteoporosis
Celiac disease
Sleep apnea
Atlantoaxial subluxation
Testicular cancer
Seizures
Dermatological abnormalities
Depression
Alzheimer's disease
Delirium
Agitated behavior
Foot problems
Seizures

There are a number of disease conditions that occur more commonly in adults with Down's syndrome than in the general population (Table 1). "Health-Care Guidelines for Individuals with Down Syndrome" were developed by a consensus panel of the Down Syndrome Medical Interest Group (Smith, 2001). There is a lack of evidence in this area and so physician-substituted judgment is important in deciding which health-care screening approaches are most efficacious in this population.

DISORDERS ASSOCIATED WITH DOWN'S SYNDROME

Endocrinological

Congenital hypothyroidism occurs in 1 in 141 neonates with Down's and the prevalence increases with age. In adults with Down's between 15 and 40% of persons have hypothyroidism (Karlsson *et al.*, 1998). Its presentation is often insidious, and many of the early signs and symptoms are difficult to detect in patients with Down's. All patients with a recent decline in mental function need to be screened for hypothyroidism. Because of the frequency of hypothyroidism in this population, it is recommended that adult patients are screened by having a TSH measured every year. All patients with a TSH greater than $10\,\mathrm{mU\,l^{-1}}$ should be treated, regardless of whether or not the thyroxine level is normal. Goiter and thyroiditis also occur commonly in this population. No studies have determined the utility of examining thyroid antibodies to determine which patients will progress to hypothyroidism. Thyroid cancer is extremely rare in this population.

Type 1 diabetes mellitus occurs in over 1% of young persons with Down's syndrome. No studies have examined the prevalence of type 2 diabetes mellitus in adults with Down's syndrome. However, in view of the high prevalence of obesity, it is generally believed that there is a higher prevalence. Similarly, the metabolic syndrome (insulin resistance, hypertension, hypertriglyceridemia, and hyperuricemia) is not rare in this group of patients. Uric acid levels are increased in the serum of most patients with Down's.

Male hypogonadism occurs fairly commonly in males in their 40s with Down's syndrome. It is predominantly of the secondary hypogonadism type, with low lueinizing hormone as well as low testosterone and bioavailable testosterone. Treatment with testosterone can stabilize mood and prevent loss of muscle and bone. Males with trisomy 21 have reduced fertility. Females have a premature menopause of 47.1 years compared to 51 years for the woman without developmental disabilities. At present, based on the findings of the Women's Health Initiative, we are not utilizing estrogen replacement in postmenopausal women with Down's.

Persons with Down's syndrome have lower peak bone mass and, therefore, are more likely to develop osteopenia and osteoporosis (Angelopoulou *et al.*, 1999). This is aggravated by the high use of anticonvulsant medicines in this age-group. Bone mineral density should be measured in all patients with Down's at the age of 50. Calcium and vitamin D administration should be initiated at age 40 for women. The use of hip pads should be considered in Down's patients who have frequent falls.

Otolaryngolic Conditions

Hearing loss occurs in up to two-thirds of persons with Down's syndrome (Venail *et al.*, 2004; Van Buggenhout *et al.*, 1999). This can worsen with aging. In addition, many middle-aged patients have further hearing deterioration because of common impaction. Hearing loss can aggravate speech problems and make the person appear more cognitively impaired than they are or to appear unresponsive to simple requests.

As many as half of the adults with Down's syndrome can have sleep apnea (Dahlqvist *et al.*, 2003). It is related, in part, to mid-facial hypoplasia and also to their short neck and obesity. While in patients it is of the obstructive type, central sleep apnea can also occur. Sleep apnea presents with daytime fatigue and somnolence and nighttime snoring with apneic periods. Behavioral changes such as irritability or withdrawal can result from sleep apnea. Diagnosis is made with a sleep study. Some patients will tolerate continuous positive airways pressure, but this is often rejected. Surgical approaches can help, but the failure rate is relatively high.

Table 2 Presentation of spinal cord compression in persons with Down's syndrome who have atlantoaxial subluxation

Neck pain
Gait disturbance
Clumsiness of hands
Torticollis
Incontinence
Hyperreflexia
Clonus
Quadriplegia/paresis
Positive Hoffman's and Babinski reflexes

Joint Problems

Children with Down's syndrome can develop a condition similar to juvenile rheumatoid arthritis. It is associated with subluxation of joints. The diagnosis is often delayed. Similarly, arthritis is often only diagnosed late in adults with Down's syndrome.

Atlantoaxial instability occurs in Down's syndrome, where there is excessive movement of the first cervical vertebra (atlas) on the second one (axis) (Ferguson *et al.*, 1997). The diagnosis is made when there is increased space between the posterior segment of the anterior arch of C1 and the anterior segment of the odontoid process. This occurs in 15% of patients with Down's syndrome. About 1–2% will have subluxation with neurological signs and symptoms consistent with spinal cord compression (Table 2). When this occurs, it is a neurosurgical emergency. However, outcomes of surgery are often poor.

Severe cervical and lumbar-sacral osteoarthritis are fairly common. This is associated with pain, gait disturbance, sometimes hand clumsiness, difficulty in moving and associated behavioral disturbances.

Celiac Disease

Celiac disease is a malabsorption syndrome that occurs in response to the ingestion of gluten products. It occurs in as many as 7% of Down's syndrome patients (Carnicer *et al.*, 2001). It is screened for at 24 months of age. Symptoms include diarrhea and weight loss. Diagnosis is made by serum antibodies and intestinal biopsy. Celiac disease can present for the first time later in life, and should be considered as the diagnosis in any Down's patients with unexplained weight loss or diarrhea.

Dermatological Conditions

Vitiligo and alopecia are seen in adults with Down's syndrome. Dry skin is extremely common and often associated with pruritus. Fungal infections are common and often difficult to eradicate. Seborrheic and atopic dermatitis also occur frequently. A fissured or geographic tongue is present in almost a third of patients with Down's syndrome.

Cardiovascular Disorders

Congenital heart disease occurs in about half the children born with Down's syndrome (Howells, 1989). Some of these, such as isolated secundum atrial septal defects, may have been missed in childhood and present for the first time in adults. Mitral valve prolapse occurs in about half of patients and aortic regurgitation in 17%. In the presence of signs or symptoms, an echocardiogram should be carried out. Alterations in cardiac conduction are not rare and should be considered in those with new onset falls with or without syncope. In those with valvular defects, antibiotic prophylaxis needs to be given before dental care or other instrumentation.

In view of the high prevalence of insulin resistance in this population, atherosclerotic heart disease is not rare and occurs at a younger age. Angina often goes unreported in this population.

Dental Problems

Gingivitis and periodontal disease are common and lead to tooth loss. Orthodontic problems are common and may not have been able to be corrected during childhood. Bruxism is not rare.

Cancer

In children, both acute lympoblastic and myeloid leukemia occur with increased frequency (Roizen and Patterson, 2003). While most cancers occur with a decreased frequency in persons with Down's syndrome (Roberge *et al.*, 2001; Goldacre *et al.*, 2004), testicular cancers appear to be more common.

Foot Problems

These include hallux valgus, hammer toe deformities, plantar fasciitis, and early onset of foot arthritis. All of these can result in unstable gait and increased falls. Feet should be examined regularly and the services of a podiatrist utilized when necessary.

Gynecological Problems

Where possible, as in any other adult, papanicolau smear and pelvic examination should be carried out. This is often extremely difficult and may need to be deferred. Similarly, mammography should be carried out when feasible. Breast examinations should be done yearly.

Table 3 Approximate prevalence of Alzheimer's disease in persons with Down's syndrome

Age (years)	% Alzheimer's
31–40	10
41–50	20
51–60	40
61–70	75

Eye Disorders

Refractive errors are present in 40% of adults. Cataracts occur in 3% of patients and keratoconus is present in 15% of patients.

Alzheimer's Disease

Alzheimer's disease occurs commonly in Down's syndrome patients, starting at the age of 30 (Table 3) (Lott and Head, 2001; Schweber, 1989). Over three-quarters of patients, by the time they reach 70 years of age, will have some symptoms of Alzheimer's disease. The diagnosis of Alzheimer's disease is very difficult to make in persons with Down's syndrome. Common early changes are memory loss, loss of conversational skills, withdrawal and functional decline. The diagnosis requires the careful exclusion of other causes of dementia such as drugs, depression, hypothyroidism, vitamin B_{12} deficiency, visual and auditory problems, space occupying lesions, for example, bilatent subdural hematomas following a fall, or infections. Late presentations associated with Alzheimer's disease include seizures, apathy, focal neurological signs and personality changes.

Epilepsy

Seizures occur in about 8% with half occurring with the first year of life and half in the third decade or later (Stafstrom, 1993). We are particularly impressed with the ease of use of kepra, compared to dilantin, in these patients.

Behavior Disorders

Depression occurs commonly. Loss of a parent or caregiver can precipitate depression, as can change in a familiar environment. Problems within the social environment of a group house can also precipitate depression. Most of those who are depressed are treated with selective serotonin reuptake inhibitors. These agents can cause hyponatremia, leading to delirium.

Aggressive behavior occurs in about 6% of adults with Down's syndrome. Management is difficult. Valproic acid, trazadone, lorazepam, and antipsychotics have all been tried with limited success. Oversedation is often a complication of these treatments.

CONCLUSION

Middle-aged persons with Down's syndrome often present with all the special needs of frail-older adults. For this reason, geriatricians are the ideal physicians for this group. In addition, some of the special needs of this population make it preferable for them to utilize a physician who cares for a number of patients with Down's syndrome. The physician needs to work closely with the interdisciplinary team that provides day-to-day care for these individuals.

KEY POINTS

- Down's syndrome (trisomy 21) is associated with early onset of frailty and Alzheimer's disease.
- Sleep apnea occurs commonly in Down's syndrome.
- Hypothyroidism, diabetes mellitus, osteoporosis and celiac disease occur more commonly in Down's syndrome.
- Subluxation of the cervical spine can lead to spinal cord damage in Down's syndrome and is a neurosurgical emergency.

KEY REFERENCES

- Dahlqvist A, Rask E, Rosenqvist CJ *et al.* Sleep apnea and Down's syndrome. *Acta Oto-Laryngologica* 2003; **123**:1094–7.
- Howells G. Down's syndrome and the general practitioner. *The Journal of the Royal College of General Practitioners* 1989; **39**:470–5.
- Roizen NJ & Patterson D. Down's syndrome. *Lancet* 2003; **361**:1281–9.
- Smith DS. Health care management of adults with Down syndrome. *American Family Physician* 2001; **64**:1031–8.
- Yang Q, Rasmussen SA & Friedman JM. Mortality associated with Down's syndrome in the USA from 1983 to 1997: a population-based study. *Lancet* 2002; **359**:1019–25.

REFERENCES

Angelopoulou N, Souftas V, Sakadamis A & Mandroukas K. Bone mineral density in adults with Down's syndrome. *European Radiology* 1999; **9**:647–51.

Carnicer J, Farre C, Varea V *et al.* Prevalence of celiac disease in Down's syndrome. *European Journal of Gastroenterology & Hepatology* 2001; **13**:263–7.

Dahlqvist A, Rask E, Rosenqvist CJ *et al.* Sleep apnea and Down's syndrome. *Acta Oto-Laryngologica* 2003; **123**:1094–7.

Ferguson RL, Putney ME & Allen BL Jr. Comparison of neurologic deficits with atlanto-dens intervals in patients with Down syndrome. *Journal of Spinal Disorders* 1997; **10**:246–52.

Goldacre MJ, Wotton CJ, Seagroatt V & Yeates D. Cancers and immune related diseases associated with Down's syndrome: a record linkage study. *Archives of Disease in Childhood* 2004; **89**:1014–7.

Howells G. Down's syndrome and the general practitioner. *The Journal of the Royal College of General Practitioners* 1989; **39**:470–5.

Karlsson B, Gustafsson J, Hedov G *et al.* Thyroid dysfunction in Downs syndrome – relation to age and thyroid autoimmunity. *Archives of Disease in Childhood* 1998; **49**:242–5.

Lott IT & Head E. Down syndrome and Alzheimer's disease: a link between development and aging. *Mental Retardation & Developmental Disabilities Research Reviews* 2001; **7**:172–8.

Roberge D, Souhami L & Laplante M. Testicular seminoma and Down's syndrome. *The Canadian Journal of Urology* 2001; **8**:1203–6.

Roizen NJ & Patterson D. Down's syndrome. *Lancet* 2003; **361**:1281–9.

Schweber MS. Alzheimer's disease and Down syndrome. *Progress in Clinical and Biological Research* 1989; **317**:247–67.

Smith DS. Health care management of adults with Down syndrome. *American Family Physician* 2001; **64**:1031–8.

Stafstrom CE. Epilepsy in Down syndrome: clinical aspects and possible mechanisms. *American Journal of Mental Retardation* 1993; **98**(suppl 1):12–26.

Van Buggenhout GJCM, Trommelen JCM, Schoenmaker A *et al.* Down syndrome in a population of elderly mentally retarded patients: genetic-diagnostic survey and implications for medical care. *American Journal of Medical Genetics* 1999; **85**:376–84.

Venail F, Gardiner Q & Mondain M. ENT and speech disorders in children with Down's syndrome: an overview of pathophysiology, clinical features, treatments, and current management. *Clinical Pediatrics* 2004; **43**:783–91.

Yang Q, Rasmussen SA & Friedman JM. Mortality associated with Down's syndrome in the USA from 1983 to 1997: a population-based study. *Lancet* 2002; **359**:1019–25.

102

Drug Misuse and the Older Person: A Contradiction in Terms?

Ilana B. Crome

Keele University Medical School, Keele, UK

INTRODUCTION

This chapter will provide a description of the terminology and classificatory systems for drug problems. The epidemiology of drug misuse will then be outlined. There will be a summary of associated psychological and physical complications. Most importantly, attention will be drawn to the effectiveness of treatment interventions in both the pharmacological and psychosocial domains. Some suggested options for ways forward in service delivery and policy are presented.

WHY IS THIS IMPORTANT TO THE CLINICIAN?

No major specialty or subspecialty in medical practice can *avoid* drug misusers. Accident and emergency units, and departments of cardiology, dermatology, gastroenterology, neurology, infectious diseases, and general surgery, as well as those of trauma and orthopedic surgery, will generate their share of older patients with drug-related problems, as will psychiatric specialities such as liaison psychiatry (Fingerhood, 2000). It is well worth noting that even if the patient presents with a drug problem, this may not be his or her major problem. This is because older people may present with abstinence syndromes, convulsions, acute disturbance (psychosis, panic, confusion, perceptual dysfunction), trauma, cancer, or cardiovascular conditions.

Brennan *et al.* (2000) have conducted a study of the characteristics and predictors of hospital readmissions over a 4-year period in elderly medicare inpatients with substance-use disorders. This group found that elderly substance misusers make costly, relatively heavy use of inpatient health services. Elderly women and blacks more often have prior substance-related hospitalizations, psychiatric comorbidities, and accidents (falls, adverse drug reactions, poisoning). Diagnosis at baseline discharge can identify high-risk patients, and plans can be made accordingly.

WHAT IS A DRUG?

In the context of this chapter, the term "drug" will be used to cover illicit substances, central nervous system depressants such as opiates and opioids (for example, heroin and methadone) stimulants such as cocaine, crack, amphetamine and ecstasy, and LSD, khat and magic mushrooms. It will also be used to describe street-use and noncompliant use of prescription drugs such as benzodiazepines, and noncompliance in the use of over-the-counter preparations such as codeine-based products, for example, cough medicines, decongestants.

Although tobacco and alcohol are beyond the scope of this chapter, it should be noted that clinical experience and a growing literature base indicate that people may use a combination of licit and illicit substances, as well as prescribed and over-the-counter medications (used compliantly and noncompliantly). This so-called *polypharmacy* or *polydrug misuse* is a particular issue in older people who have physical or psychological comorbidity. This is what makes this work challenging and stimulating! Patients may borrow, share, not report all medications, use out-of-date drugs, take foods and drugs that interact, and store drugs inappropriately.

Of course, "misuse" may be the result of lack of judgment, misconceptions about the drug(s), inability to purchase medications, inability to manage the combination of medications (due to memory problems, for instance), or they may be intentionally using medications for purposes other than they should.

Principles and Practice of Geriatric Medicine, 4th Edition. Edited by M.S. John Pathy, Alan J. Sinclair and John E. Morley.

EPIDEMIOLOGY – DRUG MISUSERS DO SURVIVE INTO OLD AGE

It has been reported that one in ten older people are receiving a drug that is potentially inappropriate (Gottlieb, 2004). Older people not only receive most of the prescriptions in the United Kingdom but are also being dispensed multiple medications. Multiple analgesic drug use is a particular problem (Chrischilles *et al.*, 1990). The prevalence of psychotropic drug misuse is four times greater in women than in men, and the risk of dependence is enhanced if the woman happens to be widowed, less educated, of lower income, in poor health and with reduced social support (Kelly *et al.*, 2003).

Opiate-dependent people do survive into old age (Lynskey *et al.*, 2003). In the United States the lifetime prevalence rates for illicit drug dependence are 17% for 18–29 years old, 4% for 30–59 years old and less than 1% for the over-60 age-group (Hinkin *et al.*, 2002). Older women drink less, smoke less, and use less illicit drugs than other age–gender groups (Graham *et al.*, 1995).

The Office for National Statistics study of psychiatric morbidity (Coulthard *et al.*, 2002) utilized a number of questions to measure drug use (frequency, started dependence, inability to cut down, need for larger amounts, withdrawal symptoms). Dependence on cannabis only, on another drug, and nondependence were gauged. Age of first use, overdose, injecting, and treatment sought were additional. Data on ages 16–74 were reported. This report indicated that lifetime experience of any illicit drug was 84/1000 in the 55–59 age-group, 65/1000 in the 60–64 age-group, 24/1000 in the 65–69 age-group, and 34/1000 in the 70–74 age-group. Comparable figures for illicit drug use over the last year are 19, 10, 6, and 11 per thousand, and for the last month 7, 7, 2, and 2 per thousand respectively. Over the previous month and year, older people tended to use cannabis and tranquilizers, with some lifetime use of stimulants, magic mushrooms and heroin (Figure 1). In addition, 9% of those in the 55–59 age-group who had ever taken drugs had experienced an overdose, as had 5% of those over 60 who had ever taken drugs. Thus, drug misuse is a problem in older people, which is captured by national datasets.

It has also been established that around half of all elderly people have seen their GP in the last three months, with one-quarter seeing a hospital doctor. Many older people have contact with primary care as well as many other health service providers, who are in a position to assess their substance use. Furthermore, in an epidemiological study of psychiatric illness and substance misuse in primary care, a 27% increase in comorbidity occurred in those aged 75–84. This was due to dependence on licit substances, that is, benzodiazepines, and resulted in confusional states (Frischer *et al.*, 2003). These recent studies demonstrate that there may be some differences in rates of different types of comorbid conditions in older people compared to younger people (Speer and Bater, 1992), and further underline the cumulative effects of benzodiazepines reported earlier (Morgan *et al.*, 1988).

DRUG USE AND MENTAL HEALTH

Psychiatric Comorbidity

In this section the term comorbidity is used to describe the co-occurrence of psychiatric disorder and substance misuse

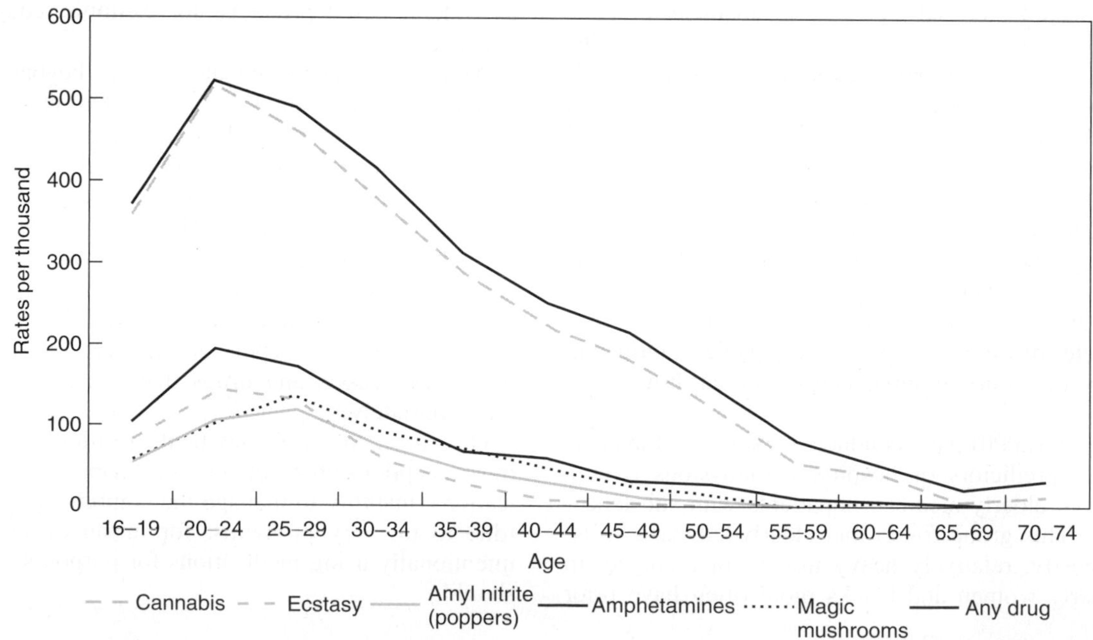

Figure 1 Proportion in each age-group reporting ever using each of the five most commonly used drugs by age (From Coulthard *et al.*, (2002) *Tobacco, Alcohol, and Drug Use, and Mental Health.* London: The Stationery Office.)

(Day and Crome, 2002; Crome and Day, 2002; Banerjee *et al.*, 2002; Waller and Rumball, 2004). Psychoactive substances have differing psychological effects, including those caused by intoxication and withdrawal. Chronic use, intoxication with depressant drugs, and withdrawal from stimulants produce symptoms similar to depressant drugs, while acute intoxication from stimulants and cannabis may mimic a schizophrenic illness. Withdrawal from depressant drugs may result in symptoms of anxiety, panic, and even confusional states. These complex interactions have implications in that not only does drug use interfere with emotional, cognitive, and social behavior but the combination of disorders also results in poorer treatment compliance and both short- and longer-term outcomes.

An association between drug use and psychiatric conditions has been consistently documented in substance-misusing clinical populations, psychiatric populations, the general population, prisons, and the homeless. Indeed, in the well-known Epidemiological Catchment Area (ECA) study, drug addiction was associated with a 53.1% lifetime rate of an additional mental disorder (Regier *et al.*, 1990).

Furthermore, the interrelationships between physical health, mental health, and drug misuse are well documented. Apart from the direct effects of drugs on general health (see later), there are indirect effects such as dietary neglect, impoverishment, trauma, bereavement, and loss. Malnutrition, for instance, may emanate from drug-induced anorexia, malabsorption, and economic deprivation. Liver dysfunction, for example, HIV, Hepatitis B and C, produces psychological as well as physical problems.

Psychiatric conditions such as anxiety, depression, posttraumatic stress disorder, drug-induced psychosis, schizophrenia, delirium, and dementia may lead to, be a consequence of, or coincide with drug misuse. Withdrawal from barbiturates and benzodiazepines leads to delirium, whereas head injuries and serious infections are associated with dementia. The differing mechanisms and types of relationship demand careful history-taking and judicious interpretation. Depression, dementia, delirium, and a heightened risk of suicide are probably the problems most commonly faced by clinicians. Of course, some of these conditions are associated with chronic pain and sleep disorders, which may make patients vulnerable and lead to them seeking relief from prescription and nonprescription medications in a noncompliant fashion.

Because there are effective medications and psychosocial interventions available for many psychiatric conditions, correct diagnosis, and treatment or referral have tangible benefits.

Physical Comorbidity

The health risks which drug use poses include the pharmacological action, for example, toxicity of the drug itself, the route of use, blood-borne pathogens, contaminants, unknown purity, and quantity. The adverse effects are summarized in the following section (Banerjee *et al.*, 2002).

Benzodiazepines

In the short term, users may experience tiredness, depressed respiration, dizziness, and unsteadiness. With other depressants, for example, alcohol and opiates, overdose can be fatal. Dependence can develop on low doses, and convulsions occur with withdrawal. Rebound symptoms such as insomnia, anxiety, and tension can occur.

Opiates and Opioids

Diverted pharmaceutical opiates and opioids may be formulated for injection or oral use, or as suppositories. Tablets may be crushed and injected.

Heroin may be inhaled, snorted, smoked, or injected intravenously, intramuscularly, or subcutaneously. Dependence can develop rapidly, that is, within weeks. Since tolerance also develops rapidly, but diminishes quickly after abstinence, relapse can lead to overdose and death. This is also the case for methadone.

Opiates and opioids depress coughing, breathing, and heart rate, dilate blood vessels, reduce bowel activity, and produce constipation. Overdose usually occurs in combination with other drugs. Injecting carries the risk of HIV and Hepatitis B and C, as well as septicemia and infective endocarditis, which can lead to heart failure.

Cannabis

Cannabis use can lead to depression, anxiety, and paranoia. Panic attacks are a feature, and there is controversy as to whether cannabis "causes" an enduring schizophrenia-like psychosis or simply exacerbates it. Memory and learning are affected. Cannabis is smoked, and evidence is accumulating of the risk of lung cancer, and cancers of the head and neck.

Amphetamines and Cocaine

Use of stimulants may lead to anxiety, exhaustion, depression, and weight loss. A paranoid and/or confusional state may also occur. Hypertension, cardiac arrhythmias, stroke, hepatic and renal damage, and abscesses are the result of heavy use, especially if injecting. Violent and aggressive behavior may ensue. Snorting of cocaine leads to nasal septal perforation and damage to the nasal passages.

Despite all these complications, an early study by McInnes and Powell (1994) demonstrated that most patients assessed by medical staff were not being accurately diagnosed with problematic substance misuse. The main implication was that treatment would, therefore, be denied.

THE IMPORTANCE OF A THOROUGH ASSESSMENT

A Very High Index of Suspicion is Necessary

In order to get to grips with the way in which older people may be affected by substances, the two most important elements are a very high index of suspicion that older people are using and/or misusing several different substances *and* a thorough history (King *et al.*, 1994).

A Comprehensive History is Fundamental

Although several instruments specifically developed for the assessment of older people have evolved in the clinical situation, there is no substitute for a comprehensive history. A detailed protocol is included in this chapter, but a highly personal style may develop on this foundation. As long as key components are incorporated, potentially related to the patient's clinical condition, any permutation is up to the individual clinician. There are some complaints or symptoms that might alert the physician, especially if the patient is undergoing some life transitions, for example, retirement, bereavement, or new carer responsibilities.

Diagnosis is Based on a Set of Established Criteria

In order to reach a "diagnosis", the two systems that have emerged are the International Classification of Diseases (ICD-10) (World Health Organisation, 1992) and the American Psychiatric Association's Diagnostic and Statistical Manual (DSM IV) (American Psychiatric Association, 1994). The criteria required to reach a diagnosis of either harmful use or dependent use are to be found in Tables 1 and 2. These systems have similarities, but they are not identical.

Table 1 Criteria for substance abuse (DSM IV) and harmful use (ICD10)

DSM IV (APA, 1994)	ICD10 (WHO, 1992)
(A) A maladaptive pattern of substance use leading to clinically significant impairment or distress, as manifested by one (or more) of the following occurring within a 12-month period 1. Recurrent substance use resulting in a failure to fulfill major role obligations at work, school, or home 2. Recurrent substance abuse in situations that are physically hazardous 3. Recurrent substance-abuse-related legal problems 4. Continued substance abuse despite having persistent or recurrent social or interpersonal problems caused or exacerbated by the effects of the substance (B) Has never met the criteria for substance dependence for this class of substance	(A) A pattern of psychoactive substance use that is causing damage to health; the damage may be to physical or mental health

Distinction Between Dependence and Harmful Use

However, from the perspective of the clinician, *the* most important issue is to be able to determine with regard to the range of substances, whether patients are dependent on them, or are engaging in harmful use. This differentiation is critical

Table 2 Criteria for dependence syndrome in DSM IV and ICD10

DSM IV (APA, 1994)	ICD10 (WHO, 1992)
(A) Diagnosis of dependence should be made if three (or more) of the following have been experienced or exhibited at any time in the same 12-month period	(A) Diagnosis of dependence should be made if three or more of the following have been experienced or exhibited at some time during the last year
1. Tolerance defined by either need for markedly increased amount of substance to achieve intoxication or desired effect or markedly diminished effect with continued use of the same amount of the substance	1. A strong desire or sense of compulsion to take the substance
2. Withdrawal as evidenced by either of the following: the characteristic withdrawal syndrome for the substance or the same (or closely related) substance is taken to relieve or avoid withdrawal symptoms	2. Difficulties in controlling substance-taking behavior in terms of its onset, termination, or levels of use
3. The substance is often taken in larger amounts over a longer period of time than was intended	3. Physiological withdrawal state when substance use has ceased or been reduced, as evidenced by either of the following: the characteristic withdrawal syndrome for the substance or use of the same (or closely related) substance with the intention of relieving or avoiding withdrawal symptoms
4. Persistent desire or repeated unsuccessful efforts to cut down or control substance use	4. Evidence of tolerance, such that increased doses of the psychoactive substance are required in order to achieve effects originally produced by lower doses
5. A great deal of time is spent in activities necessary to obtain the substance, use the substance, or recover from its effects	5. Progressive neglect of alternative pleasures or interests because of psychoactive substance use and increased amount of time necessary to obtain or take the substance or to recover from its effects
6. Important social, occupational, or recreational activities given up or reduced because of substance use	6. Persisting with substance use despite clear evidence of overly harmful consequences (physical or mental)
7. Continued substance use despite knowledge of having had a persistent or recurrent physical or psychological problem that was likely to have been caused or exacerbated by the substance	

in terms of decisions around the selection of appropriate treatment interventions (in terms of type and intensity) and suitability of settings.

Ongoing Process That Aids Communication and Coordination

Thus, assessment is an ongoing process, the summation of each phase of which can be communicated to the patient, carers, and other professionals. A phasic assessment can be utilized to monitor change, establish to what extent goals have been achieved, and coordinate care with other disciplines or agencies.

The Use of Investigations

In order to corroborate the verbal history provided by the patient, carers and professionals, and clinical findings, biochemical tests on blood, saliva, sweat, urine, and hair can be undertaken (Wolff *et al.*, 1999). In clinical practice, urinalysis, and more recently saliva, are most commonly used to test for drugs. Cannabis, methadone, and long-acting benzodiazepines may remain in the urine for a week or longer, but other drugs may not be found after 48–72 hours. Thus, if drugs are *not* detected, this does not necessarily indicate that the patient has *not* been using. If a patient is assessed as being dependent, the clinical picture may be that of a withdrawal syndrome: every drug has a specific set of criteria by which withdrawal can be diagnosed (Tables 3–6).

Since these criteria were established on the basis of an adult population, some may not apply to older people. For instance, older people may have substance-related problems without the development of tolerance; they may not develop dependence; cognitive impairment may interfere with noticing whether they need to take larger amounts over a longer period; negative effects may take a shorter time to develop; they may have fewer activities to give up; they may not appreciate that their problems are related to substance use.

Table 3 Symptoms of intoxication and withdrawal

Benzodiazepine intoxication	*Benzodiazepine withdrawal*
Euphoria, disinhibition, lability of mood	Confusion and convulsions
Apathy, sedation	Tremor, postural hypotension
Abusiveness and aggression	Nausea and vomiting
Impaired attention, amnesia	Agitation
Impaired psychomotor performance	Paranoid ideation
Unsteady gait, slurred speech, nystagmus	Tachycardia
Decreased level of consciousness, hypothermia	Rebound insomnia, tension
Opiate intoxication	*Opiate withdrawal*
Apathy, sedation, disinhibition, psychomotor retardation, impaired attention, impaired judgment	Craving
Interference with personal functioning	Sneezing, yawning, runny eyes
Drowsiness, slurred speech, pupillary constriction	Muscle aches, abdominal pains
Decreased level of consciousness	Nausea, vomiting, diarrhea
	Pupillary dilatation
	Goose flesh, recurrent chills
	Restless sleep
Cannabis intoxication	*Cannabis withdrawal*
Euphoria and disinhibition	Anxiety
Anxiety and agitation	Irritability
Suspiciousness and paranoid ideation	Tremor
Impaired reaction time	Sweating
Impaired judgment and attention	Muscle aches
Hallucinations with preserved orientation	
Depersonalization and derealization	
Increased appetite	
Dry mouth	
Conjunctival injection	
Tachycardia	
Stimulant intoxication	*Stimulant withdrawal*
Euphoria and increased energy	Lethargy
Hypervigilance; repetitive stereotyped behaviors	Psychomotor retardation or agitation
Grandiose beliefs and actions	Craving
Paranoid ideation	Increased appetite
Abusiveness, aggression, and argumentativeness	Insomnia or hypersomnia
Auditory, tactile, and visual hallucinations	Bizarre and unpleasant dreams
Sweats, chills, muscular weakness	
Nausea or vomiting, weight loss	
Pupillary dilatation, convulsions	
Tachycardia, arrhythmias, chest pain, hypertension	
Agitation	

TREATMENT INTERVENTIONS

Pharmacological Interventions

Pharmacotherapies are available to treat a variety of situations, such as:

- emergencies, for example, overdose, fits, dehydration, hypothermia;
- detoxification and withdrawal syndromes, for example, lofexidine, methadone, buprenorphine;
- substitution, for example, methadone, buprenorphine;
- relapse prevention, for example, naltrexone;
- comorbid substance problems;
- comorbid psychiatric disorders;
- comorbid physical disorders, for example, HIV, Hepatitis C, diabetes.

Readers are advised to access recent guidelines from the British Association of Psychopharmacology (BAP), which summarize the evidence base for the pharmacological treatment of substance misuse and comorbid conditions. The findings which follow are drawn from this document (Lingford-Hughes *et al.*, 2004).

Summary Recommendations from the BAP Guidelines

There is considerable evidence for the use of methadone, buprenorphine, and α-2 agonists (clonidine and lofexidine)

Table 4 Suggested outline for schedule of issues to be covered in assessment

Demographic characteristics	Age Gender Employment, retired, unemployment Nationality, religious affiliation, ethnicity, and culture Living arrangements, for example, with parent(s), spouse, relatives, friends, homeless, institutional care General environment, for example, deprivation, affluence, violence
Presenting complaint(s) or problems	May or may not be a substance problem or mental health issue
Each substance should be discussed separately: Alcohol Amphetamines Benzodiazepines Cannabis Cocaine Ecstasy Heroin and other opiates Methadone Nicotine Over-the-counter medication Prescribed medication	Age of initiation "first tried" Age of onset of weekend use Age of onset of weekly use Age of onset of daily use Pattern of use during each day Route of use, for example, oral, smoking, snorting, intramuscular, intravenous Age of onset of specific withdrawal symptoms and dependence syndrome features Current use over previous day, week, month Current cost of use Maximum use ever How is the substance use being funded? Periods of abstinence Triggers to relapse Preferred substance(s) and reasons
Treatment episodes for substance problems	Dates, service, practitioner details, treatment interventions, success or otherwise, triggers to relapse
Family history	Parents, siblings, children. History of substance misuse and related problems History of psychiatric problems, for example, suicide, deliberate self harm, depression, anxiety, psychotic illness History of physical illness Separation, divorce, death Family relationships, conflict, support Occupational history
Medical history	Episodes of acute or chronic illnesses: respiratory, infective, HIV, hepatitis, injury including accidents, surgery Admission to hospital, dates, problems, treatment, and outcome
Psychiatric history	Assessment by general practitioner for any "minor" complaints, for example, anxiety, depression Treatment by general practitioner with any psychoactive drugs Referral to specialist psychiatric services: dates, diagnosis, treatment, and outcome Mental Health Act assessments
Personal history	Occupational, sexual, marital relationships
Educational background	Age started and left school Achievements and aspirations
Vocational history	Ongoing activities and plans
Criminal activities	Involvement in criminal activities preceding or directly related to substance problems Cautions, charges, convictions Shoplifting, violence, prostitution
Social services	Child abuse and neglect Social service involvement
Social environment	Level of community support and network
Social activities	Sports, hobbies, community work, religious affiliation and activities
Financial situation	Debt to finance substance problems
Useful information	Current address Phone number including mobile phone General practitioner's name, address, and phone number Details of other professionals involved
Investigations	Biochemical, hematological, urinary, salivary, sweat, hair Special investigations
Collateral information	Family and friends Occupational colleagues, if appropriate Social services Criminal justice agencies Health services Voluntary agencies
Consent and confidentiality	

Table 4 *(continued)*

Current stressors	Bereavement, marriage, divorce, ongoing legal problems
How the client perceives the problems and what they want	Belief systems
Profile of strengths and risks	
Readiness to engage in treatment	
Mental state examination	
Physical examination	

Table 5 Testing for current drug use (maximum range)

Drug	Maximum range
Cocaine	12–72 hours
Amphetamines	2–4 days
Heroin	2–4 days
Codeine	2–4 days
Cannabis	30 days
Diazepam	30 days

Source: Adapted from Banerjee *et al.*, (2002) *Coexisting Problems of Mental Disorder and Substance Misuse*. London: Royal College of Psychiatrists Research Unit.

Table 6 Some features of withdrawal that necessitate immediate medical attention

- Ingestion of unknown quantities of substances
- Trauma
- Confusion or delirium
- Fever
- Tachycardia
- Tremulousness
- Hallucinations
- Paranoid behavior

Source: Adapted from Banerjee *et al.*, (2002) *Coexisting Problems of Mental Disorder and Substance Misuse*. London: Royal College of Psychiatrists Research Unit.

in the management of withdrawal states. However, *all* this available evidence relates to younger adults. There are differences in choice of medication, depending on the priorities around duration of treatment, adverse effects (brachycardia and hypotension due to α-2 adrenergic agonists), and withdrawal severity. Obviously, the patient's clinical condition, degree of dependence, preference, and practitioner experience will determine which drug to use.

Similarly, there is an established evidence base for methadone maintenance treatment and, more recently, for buprenorphine. Once again, this relates to younger people.

There is inadequate evidence for treatment with naltrexone and injectable opioids, and for using coercive methods.

For stimulant drugs such as cocaine and amphetamine, the guidelines do *not* recommend the use of dopamine agonists, antidepressants, or carbamazepine. Furthermore, there is no clear evidence to support substitute prescribing of dexamphetamines. In fact, "psychosocial" interventions are considered the "mainstay" of treatment, although the evidence is limited.

The guidelines also make recommendations for benzodiazepine dependence, whether licitly used on a prescription, or its illicit use. In early or mild dependence, "minimal" interventions, for example, relaxation or general practitioner advice are suggested. For more severe dependence, graded discontinuation is advised.

For "illicit" misusers, there is no evidence that continued prescribing is beneficial, other than to reduce illicit use.

It must be reiterated that the above advice is related to an adult population.

Psychological Interventions

The majority of interventions are based on learning theory models, but there is also the recognition that there are non-treatment routes to improvement (Crome and Bloor; 2005; Crome and Ghodse; in press). Furthermore, information-based approaches, for example, health education and information, are useful in less complex situations. These might include education about harm minimization, immunization, and vaccination.

In the addiction literature, the term counseling is used to incorporate brief or intensive interventions, be they supportive, directive, or motivational counseling, individual, family, or group behavioral treatments, as well as social network behavioral therapy. Counseling may aim to reduce the use of alcohol and drugs, as well as the negative consequences or related problems.

The term may encompass assessment, engagement and support, together with the development of therapeutic relationships. The nonjudgmental and empathic method of challenging decisions and assumptions in motivational interviewing is included in the gamut of techniques.

Important common objectives may include:

- problem solving: developing competence in dealing with a specific problem;
- acquisition of social skills: mastery of social and interpersonal skills by assertiveness or anger control;
- cognitive change: modification of irrational beliefs and maladaptive patterns of thought;
- behavior change: modification of maladaptive behavior;
- systemic change: introducing change into family systems.

Counseling is a widely used term and is a form of therapy or intervention, which includes a wide range of theoretical models. There are many different definitions, each emphasizing specific aspects of the counseling role and processes practiced in a multiplicity of settings. It embodies psychodynamics, cognitive, behavioral, and person-centered approaches.

There are various options, the choice of which depends on the nature and extent of the problems and which approach may appear more appropriate and suitable for a particular drug user. The options include:

counseling
cognitive behavioral therapy
family dynamics
group therapy
motivational enhancement.

Nondirective counseling comprises the following components. The patient determines the content and direction of the counseling and explores conflict and emotions at the time. While allowing empathic reflection, the counselor does not offer advice and feedback.

A cognitive behavioral approach assumes that the patient would like to change, and analyzes situations that cause drug use, so that these can be altered. Problem-solving techniques, self-monitoring, anger management, relapse prevention, assertiveness training and the acquisition of social skills, and modification of irrational beliefs or patterns of thought or behavior are used. Individual, group, and family therapies used in the treatment of addiction problems are often based along cognitive behavioral lines.

Social network behavior therapy considers the social environment as being important in the development, maintenance, and resolution of substance problems. It maximizes positive social support, which is central to the process. The therapist offers advice and feedback and thereby facilitates change in the patient's social world; behavior is not interpreted, and engagement with significant others is the key in bringing about change and achieving goals.

Family therapy involves attempts to understand and interpret the family dynamics in order to change the psychopathology. Substance use is perceived as a symptom of family dysfunction and, therefore, altering the dynamics brings about change in substance misuse. Family members are viewed as contributory to the problems. Behavioral techniques may be used in family therapy as well as psychodynamic techniques.

Group therapies and 12-step programs. Participation in self-help groups is an important feature of many treatment programs where participants receive support from recovering members who often take members back to the negative consequences of substance misuse. A variant of group therapy is the 12-step approach. Central to the 12-step philosophy is the idea that recovery from addiction is possible only if the individual recognizes his or her problem, and admits that he or she is unable to use substances in moderation. Alcoholics Anonymous and Narcotics Anonymous are examples of the "12-step" philosophy where drug users have to abstain completely.

Recently, the most influential and popular form of treatment has been a "brief" or "minimal" intervention, designated *motivational interviewing*.

Motivational interviewing aims to build motivation for change. The focus is on a nonjudgmental approach and the patient's concerns about, and choices regarding future drug use, and it elicits strategies from the patient. Motivational enhancement directs the patient to motivation for change by offering empathic feedback and advice and information and selectively reinforces certain discrepancies that emerge between current behavior and goals in order to enhance motivation for change. Significant others play some role in the treatment but not a central role. It is, by and large, a personal therapeutic situation where the individual's motivation is seen as central. It aims to alter the decisional balance so that patients themselves direct the process of change.

The key characteristics are best described by the acronym FRAMES (Miller and Sanchez, 1994):

- personalized **f**eedback or assessment results detailing the target behavior and associated effects and consequences on the individual;
- emphasizing the individual's personal **r**esponsibility for change;
- giving **a**dvice on how to change;
- providing a **m**enu of options for change;
- expressing **e**mpathy through behaviors conveying caring, understanding, and warmth;
- emphasizing **s**elf-efficacy for change and instilling hope that change is not only possible, but also within reach.

This technique has not been evaluated in older substance misusers but evidence is accumulating with regard to the benefits and cost-effectiveness of this type of intervention (Dunn *et al.*, 2001; Project MATCH Research Group, 1997, 1998).

Treatment Effectiveness

Adult Population

The first relatively long-term, prospective, observational study on outcome in drug misusers in the United Kingdom, the National Treatment Outcome Research Study (NTORS), has been under way since 1995 (Gossop *et al.*, 2003). This study follows up 1075 drug misusers in two types of residential services (inpatient and residential units), and two kinds of community services (methadone reduction and methadone maintenance). The age range was 16–58, half of whom were responsible for caring for children. The older age-group has not been analyzed or reported on, separately.

Most important to note is that the specific nature of the treatment modalities provided has not been identified or described in any depth or in detail. Opiates, amphetamines, cocaine, nonprescription benzodiazepines and alcohol were assessed. The impact of treatment on psychological health, suicide, mortality, and crime was evaluated. In summary, the study reported that drug use as well as injecting and sharing needles was reduced. Crime also decreased with concurrent improvement in physical and psychological health. However, 20% of the study population continued to use daily, and 40% continued to use once a week. Over the 5-year period, 62 people died, alcohol use remained at a constantly high level, and 80 were using two or more illicit drugs and were long-term users. There was a history of treatment for psychiatric disorder in the 2 years prior to treatment, and in the 3 months prior to treatment 30% had suicidal ideation.

At 5 years, between 33.3% and 50% of users achieved abstinence in community and residential services respectively. However, 20% were still using daily. While 40% used illicit drugs regularly, this had reduced from 66% at intake in the residential services and 80% in community services.

In summary, daily and regular use was found in 20–40% respectively. Likewise, injecting reduced from 60–40%, criminal activity halved, and 25% were drinking above safe limits. This evidence is encouraging despite the limitations in design described above. The study points to some value in the treatment programs, which are currently being implemented in the United Kingdom. Of course, this study was on an adult population.

Older People

Recently, Satre *et al.*, (2004) reported a 5-year alcohol and drug treatment outcome study as a comparative study of older adults (aged 55–77) versus younger and middle-aged people. They found that older adults were less likely to be drug dependent at baseline than younger (aged 18–39) and middle-aged (aged 40–54) adults, and had longer retention in treatment than younger adults. At 5 years, older adults were less likely than younger adults to have close family or friends who encouraged alcohol or drug use. Fifty-two percent of older adults had been totally abstinent from alcohol and drugs in the past 30 days, versus 40% of younger adults. Older women had higher 30-day abstinence rates than older men or younger women. Thus, although older adults had a favorable long-term outcome, these differences may be accounted for by variables associated with age, for example, type of substance dependence, treatment retention, social network, or gender. This data provides valuable information on which to base service provision, for example, persistence in treatment has long lasting benefits, the need for adequate social support, less likelihood of encouragement to use substances from family and friends.

Satre *et al.* (2003) also demonstrated that older patients are more likely to have an abstinence goal and a lower rate of psychiatric symptoms than younger people. This view has been substantiated by Oslin *et al.* (2002).

A further study by Brennan *et al.* (2003) indicated that older substance misusers are obtaining specialized outpatient mental health services, as are younger patients. In this study, older patients were less likely to be experiencing drug problems and psychiatric problems, but more likely to report alcohol and medical problems. This equality of gaining access was despite the fact that older people perceived the relative importance of treatment for psychological problems as less than younger people. Thus, the authors raise the interesting question of why older people appear to be more robust than younger people. Indeed, in this study, older patients had better outcomes than a matched sample of younger patients.

It is also worth mentioning in this context a study on the effects on mortality of brief interventions for problem drinking. In this meta-analysis Cuijpers *et al.* (2004), demonstrated that brief interventions appear to reduce mortality. This has far-reaching implications for public health measures, the role of primary care and, potentially, application to the drug-misusing population.

POLICY

There has been a plethora of policy initiatives around drugs in the United Kingdom. These include the following:

- Clinical guidelines on the management of drug misuse and dependence (1999).
- Tackling drugs to build a better Britain (1998).
- The national drugs strategy (Cabinet Office, 2000a,b).
- Models of care (NTA, 2002).

Attention should also be drawn to the Misuse of Drugs Act (1971) and the Misuse of Drugs Regulations (2001) (see Tables 7 and 8).

It is fair to say that these have been targeted at young people, with little or even *no* mention of older people. Furthermore, the National Service Framework for Older People (Department of Health, 2001) did not even raise the real possibility of dependence and addiction in older people, although some attention was given to the problem of prescription drugs. Hence, *no* suggestions about service delivery, training, and research in this invisible group were made.

To my knowledge, there is no designated service provider for older people with drug problems in the United Kingdom, and few elsewhere. The United States Department of Health and Human Services has published a useful guide on the assessment and treatment of substance use in older people (US Dept of Health & Human Services, 1998). This outlines guidance for treatment interventions and service delivery for older people. The key characteristics include availability, accessibility, and multidisciplinary team working across agencies. In this framework, geriatricians and primary care physicians and their teams have a vital role in the assessment and provision of brief interventions and onward referral (Crome and Day, 1999).

There is evidence that, as drug misuse increases in young people, and the elderly population increases, the drug problem in older people is likely to rise. There are unresolved questions about the types of service models that might be developed and evaluated (Gfroerer *et al.*, 2003). At present, this is a vision and a speculation. There is every reason why provision for this invisible, neglected, and stigmatized group should be established as mainstream.

Table 7 Summary of the classes of the misuse of drugs act, 1971

Class	Main drugs in each class	Maximum penalties for possession	Maximum penalties for possession with intent to supply
A	Heroin, cocaine (and crack cocaine); ecstasy, LSD, methadone, morphine, opium, dipipanone, pethidine, cannabinol, and cannabinol derivatives. Class B drugs when designed for injection become Class A.	6 months or a fine of £5000 or both (in a magistrate's court) Or, in a trial by jury 7 years or an unlimited fine or both	6 months or a fine of £5000 or both (in a magistrate's court) Or, in a trial by jury Life or an unlimited fine or both.
B	Amphetamines, barbiturates, cannabis[a] (herbal and resin), codeine, dihydrocodeine, and methylamphetamine.	3 months or a fine of £2500 or both (in a magistrate's court) Or, in a trial by jury 5 years or an unlimited fine or both.	6 months or a fine or of £5000 or both (in a magistrate's court) Or, in a trial by jury 14 years or an unlimited fine or both.
C	Benzodiazepines, buprenorphine, diethylpropion, anabolic steroids	3 months or a fine of £1000 or both (in a magistrate's court) Or, in a trial by jury 2 years or an unlimited fine or both.	3 months or a fine of £2500 or both (in a magistrate's court) Or, in a trial by jury 5 years or an unlimited fine or both.

Source: Reprinted from Young People and Substance Misuse, Crome I *et al.*, Copyright 2004, with permission from Royal College of Psychiatrists.
The tables have not been amended in light of the changes to (or relaxation of) the cannabis legislation, which took place on 29 January 2004, as the evidence on which this legislation was changed is currently undergoing review.
[a]Cultivation of the cannabis plant carries a maximum penalty of six months or a fine of £5000 or both in a magistrate's court, or in a trial by jury, 14 years or an unlimited fine or both.

Table 8 Summary of schedules of the misuse of drugs regulations, 2001

Schedule	Main drugs included	Restrictions
1	LSD, ecstasy, raw opium, psilocin, cannabis (herbal and resin)	Import, export, production, possession, and supply only permitted under Home Office licence for medical or scientific research. Cannot be prescribed by doctors or dispensed by pharmacists
2	Heroin, cocaine, methadone, morphine, amphetamine, dexamphetamine, pethidine, and quinalbarbitone	May be prescribed and lawfully possessed when on prescription. Otherwise, supply, possession, import, export, and production are offences except under Home Office licence. Particular controls on their prescription, storage, and record keeping apply
3	Barbiturates, temazepam, flunitrazepam, buprenorphine, pentazocine, and diethylpropion	May be prescribed and lawfully possessed when on prescription. Otherwise, supply, possession, import, export, and production are offences except under Home Office licence. Particular controls on their prescription and storage apply. Temazepam prescription requirements are less stringent than those for the other drugs in this schedule
4 Part 1	Benzodiazepines (except flunitrazepam and temazepam) and pemoline	May be prescribed and lawfully possessed when on prescription. Otherwise, supply, possession, import, export, and production are offences except under Home Office licence
4 Part 2	Anabolic steroids	May be lawfully possessed by anyone even without a prescription, provided they are in the form of a medical product
5	Compound preparations such as cough mixtures which contain small amounts of controlled drugs such as morphine. Some may be sold over the counter	Authority needed for their production or supply but can be freely imported, exported, or possessed (without a prescription)

Source: Reprinted from Young People and Substance Misuse, Crome I *et al.*, Copyright 2004, with permission from Royal College of Psychiatrists.
The tables have not been amended in light of the changes to (or relaxation of) the cannabis legislation, which took place on 29 January 2004, as the evidence on which this legislation was changed is currently undergoing review.

KEY POINTS

- Drug misuse in older people poses a considerable problem, which is likely to rise.
- There are substantial associated physical and mental health problems, which geriatricians are in a position to assess.
- Treatment interventions for substance misuse are effective and cost-effective.
- Models of service delivery comprise multidisciplinary teams working across agencies.
- The policy agenda must now take account of the current prevalence, projected increase, associated comorbidity, and cost-effectiveness, so as to implement the staff training and provision.

KEY REFERENCES

- Crome IB & Day E. Substance misuse and dependence: older people deserve better services. *Reviews in Clinical Gerontology* 1999; **9**:327–42.
- Lingford-Hughes AR, Welch S & Nutt DJ. Evidence-based guidelines for the pharmacological management of substance misuse, addiction and comorbidity: recommendations from the British association for psychopharmacology. *Journal of Psychopharmacology* 2004; **18**:293–335.
- Satre DD, Mertens JR, Arean PA *et al.* Five year alcohol and drug treatment outcomes of older adults versus middle aged and younger adults in a managed care program. *Addiction* 2004; **99**:1286–97.
- US Dept of Health & Human Services. *Substance Abuse Among Older Adults Treatment Improvement Protocol (TIP) Series No. 26* 1998; US Dept of Health & Human Services, Rockville.
- Waller T & Rumball D. *Treating Drinkers and Drug Users in the Community* 2004; Blackwell Publishing, Oxford.

REFERENCES

American Psychiatric Association. *Diagnostic and Statistical Manual of Mental Disorders IV* 1994; American Psychiatric Association, Washington.

Banerjee S, Clancy C & Crome IB. *Coexisting Problems of Mental Disorder and Substance Misuse* 2002; Royal College of Psychiatrists Research Unit, London.

Brennan PL, Kagay CR, Geppert JJ *et al.* Elderly medicare in patients with substance use disorders: characteristics and predictors of hospital readmissions over a four-year interval. *Journal of Studies on Alcohol* 2000; **61**:891–5.

Brennan PL, Nichol AC & Moos RH. Older and younger patients with substance use disorders: outpatient mental health service use and functioning over a 12-month interval. *Psychology of Addictive Behaviors* 2003; **17**.42–8.

Cabinet Office. *The United Kingdom's Anti-drug Coordinator's Annual Report 1999/2000* 2000a; Cabinet Office, London.

Cabinet Office. *The United Kingdom's Anti-Drug Coordinator's Second National Plan* 2000b; Cabinet Office, London.

Chrischilles EA, Lemke JH, Wallace RB *et al.* Prevalence and characteristics of multiple analgesic drug use in an elderly study group. *Journal of the American Geriatrics Society* 1990; **38**:979–84.

Coulthard M, Farrell M, Singleton N *et al. Tobacco, Alcohol, and Drug Use and Mental Health* 2002; The Stationery Office, London.

Crome IB & Bloor R. Substance misuse and psychiatric comorbidity in adolescents. *Current Opinion in Psychiatry* 2005; **18**:435–9.

Crome IB & Day E. Substance misuse and dependence: older people deserve better services. *Reviews in Clinical Gerontology* 1999; **9**:327–42.

Crome IB & Day E. Substance misuse. In A Elder & J Holmes (eds) *Mental Health in Primary Care* 2002, pp 221–40; Oxford University Press, Oxford.

Crome I, Ghodse H, Gilvarry E *et al.* (eds). *Young People and Substance Misuse* 2004; Gaskell, London.

Crome IB & Ghodse A-H. Drug misuse in medical patients. In G Lloyd & E Guthrie (eds) *Handbook of Liaison Psychiatry* in press; Cambridge University Press, Cambridge.

Cuijpers P, Riper H & Lemmers L. The effects on mortality of brief interventions for problem drinking: a meta-analysis. *Addiction* 2004; **99**:839–45.

Day E & Crome IB. Physical health problems. In T Petersen & A McBride (eds) *Working with Substance Misusers* 2002, pp 174–89; Routledge, London.

Department of Health. *National Service Framework for Older People* 2001; Department of Health, London.

Dunn C, Deroo L & Rivara F. The use of brief interventions adapted from motivational interviewing across behavioural domains: a systematic review. *Addiction* 2001; **96**:1725–42.

Fingerhood M. Substance abuse in older people. *Journal of the American Geriatrics Society* 2000; **48**:985–95.

Frischer M, Crome I, Croft P *et al. A National Epidemiological Study of Comorbid Substance Abuse and Psychiatric Illness in Primary Care Using the General Practice Research Database (Report to the Department of Health)* 2003, Executive summary available at http://www.mdx.ac.uk/www/drugsmisuse/execsummary.html.

Gfroerer J, Penne M, Pemberton M *et al.* Substance abuse treatment need among older adults in 2020: the impact of the aging baby boom cohort. *Drug and Alcohol Dependence* 2003; **69**:127–35.

Gossop M, Marsden J, Stewart D *et al.* The National Treatment Outcome Research Study (NTORS): 4–5 year follow-up results. *Addiction* 2003; **98**:291–303.

Gottlieb S. Inappropriate drug prescribing in elderly people is common. *British Medical Journal* 2004; **329**:367.

Graham K, Carver V & Brett PJ. Alcohol and drug use by older women: results of a national survey. *Canadian Journal on Ageing* 1995; **14**:769–91.

Hinkin C, Castellin S, Dickinson-Fuhrman E *et al.* Screening for drug and alcohol abuse among older adults using a modified version of CAGE. *American Journal on Addictions* 2002; **10**:319–26.

Kelly KD, Pickett W, Yiannakoulias N *et al.* Medication use and falls in community dwelling older persons. *Age and Ageing* 2003; **32**:503–9.

King C, Van Hesselt VB, Segal D *et al.* Diagnosis and assessment of substance abuse in older adults: current strategies and issues. *Addictive Behaviours* 1994; **19**:41–55.

Lingford-Hughes AR, Welch S & Nutt DJ. Evidence-based guidelines for the pharmacological management of substance misuse, addiction and comorbidity: recommendations from the British association for psychopharmacology. *Journal of Psychopharmacology* 2004; **18**:293–335.

Lynskey MT, Day C & Hall W. Alcohol and other drug use disorders among older people. *Drug and Alcohol Review* 2003; **22**:125–33.

McInnes E & Powell J. Drug and alcohol referrals: are elderly substance abuse diagnoses and referrals being missed? *British Medical Journal* 1994; **308**:444–6.

Miller WR & Sanchez VC. Motivating young adults for treatment and lifestyle change. In G Howard (ed) *Issues in Alcohol Use and Misuse by Young Adults* 1994, pp 55–81; University of Notre Dame Press, Notre Dame.

Morgan K, Dallusso H, Ebrahim S *et al.* Prevalence, frequency, and duration of hypnotic drug use among the elderly living at home. *British Medical Journal* 1988; **296**:601–2.

National Treatment Agency for Substance Misuse (NTA). *Models of Care for the Treatment of Drug Misusers: Promoting Quality, Efficiency and Effectiveness in Drug Misuse Treatment Services in England* 2002; National Treatment Agency for Substance Misuse, London.

Oslin DW, Pettinati H & Volpicelli JR. Alcoholism treatment adherence: older age predicts better adherence and drinking outcomes. *American Journal of Geriatric Psychiatry* 2002; **10**:740–7.

Project MATCH Research Group. Matching alcoholism treatments to client heterogeneity: project MATCH posttreatment drinking outcomes. *Journal of Studies on Alcohol* 1997; **58**:7–29.

Project MATCH Research Group. Therapist effects in three treatments for alcohol problems. *Psychotherapy Research* 1998; **8**:455–74.

Regier DA, Farmer ME, Rae DS *et al.* Comorbidity of mental disorders with alcohol and other drug abuse: results from the Epidemiological Catchment Area (ECA) study. *Journal of the American Medical Association* 1990; **264**:2511–8.

Satre DD, Mertens J, Arean PA *et al.* Contrasting outcomes of older versus middle-aged and younger adult chemical dependency patients in a managed care program. *Journal of Studies on Alcohol* 2003; **64**:520–30.

Satre DD, Mertens JR, Arean PA *et al.* Five-year alcohol and drug treatment outcomes of older adults versus middle-aged and younger adults in a managed care program. *Addiction* 2004; **99**:1286–97.

Speer DC & Bater K. Comorbid mental and substance disorders among older psychiatric patients. *Journal of the American Geriatrics Society* 1992; **40**:886–90.

US Dept of Health & Human Services. *Substance Abuse Among Older Adults Treatment Improvement Protocol (TIP) Series No. 26* 1998; US Dept of Health & Human Services, Rockville.

Waller T & Rumball D. *Treating Drinkers and Drug Users in the Community* 2004; Blackwell Publishing, Oxford.

Wolff K, Farrell M, Marsden J *et al.* A review of biological indicators of illicit drug use, practical considerations and clinical usefulness. *Addiction* 1999; **94**:1279–98.

World Health Organisation. *ICD 10 Classification of Mental and Behavioural Disorders* 1992; World Health Organisation, Geneva.

FURTHER READING

Cabinet Office. *Tackling Drugs to Build a Better Britain: The Government's 10-Year Strategy for Tackling Drug Misuse* 1998; The Stationery Office, London.

Department of Health. *Guidelines on Clinical Management: Drug Misuse and Dependence* 1999; The Stationery Office, Norwich.

PART III

Medicine in Old Age

Section 8

Special Senses

Disorders of the Eye

Nina Tumosa

Saint Louis University School of Medicine and Saint Louis Veterans' Affairs Medical Center, St Louis, MO, USA

INTRODUCTION

Age is the leading risk factor for visual impairment and blinding disorders of the eye. Five major disorders cause the greatest visual disability: cataracts, refractive error, macular degeneration, glaucoma, and diabetic retinopathy. The overall prevalence of refractive error caused by these five causes of visual impairment is remarkably consistent around the world. Figure 1 shows average values for the prevalence of these disorders in people aged 75 and over in the American population gleaned from multiple studies (AAO PPP, 2001; 2003a; 2003b; 2003c) (http://www.aao.org/aao/education/library/ppp/index.cfm).

Visual impairment is often described as a person's most feared disability, and with good reason. In the elderly, visual impairment is particularly devastating because it has been associated with dramatic reduction in quality of life (Lee and Coleman, 2004). As vision declines, people are forced to curtail driving. People who can no longer see clearly report having a reduction in mobility, and having difficulty walking and leaving their homes to participate in social and religious activities. They report a loss of ability to perform activities of daily living (ADL) such as dressing, shopping, and getting in and out of bed safely. Poor vision interferes with the ability to take medications properly. It is also a leading risk factor for falls and fractures which, in turn, are risk factors for placement in a nursing home and for loss of independence. In addition, other conditions appear to be strongly comorbid with low vision. These include dementia, depression, and delirium and other sensory losses, such as hearing and balance deficits. Thus, vision impairment has profound effects on the elderly and it is incumbent upon health-care providers to identify people at risk for leading causes of visual impairment, and to initiate treatments in a timely manner.

DEFINITIONS, TREATMENTS, AND RISK FACTORS

Refractive Error

Refractive error can be described as visual acuity with best lens prescription worse than 20/40. It is the most frequent eye problem and is usually corrected with prescription eyewear. The percentage of people whose visual acuity cannot be improved beyond 20/40 increases dramatically with age: 0.8% for those between 43 and 54 years old, 0.9% for those between 55 and 64, 5% for those between 65 and 74, and 21.1% for those 75 and older. This increasing degree of uncorrected refractive error is due to a number of variables. For example, there is normally an increase in the against-the-rule astigmatism with age and it is often exacerbated during surgery that breaches the conjunctiva such as cataract and glaucoma (Egrilmez *et al.*, 2004) surgeries. The long-term effects of refractive surgeries such as laser-assisted *in situ* keratomileusis (LASIK) that many people are now undergoing for the correction of myopia, hyperopia, and presbyopia are still unknown.

There is also a normal hyperopic shift in older adults that may be altered by cataract surgery (Guzowski *et al.*, 2003). Contrast sensitivity decreases with age, in part due to the increased prevalence of dry eye with age, and in part due to the smaller pupil size found in the elderly. Dark adaptation also decreases with age and with diseases such as diabetic retinopathy and cancer. Finally, cataracts, yellow lenses, and aberrations of the cornea, all of which increase with age, produce glare, or excess light scattered within the eye. This glare can be debilitating. It can cause difficulty with driving and other tasks conducted in bright light. It can also cause headaches. As people who have been faithful contact lens wearers for decades enter their 70s and 80s, it will be interesting to determine whether the rate of corneal aberrations rises.

There are many risk factors for refractive errors in the elderly. Many of the medical and social risk factors are listed in Tables 1 and 2.

Principles and Practice of Geriatric Medicine, 4th Edition. Edited by M.S. John Pathy, Alan J. Sinclair and John E. Morley.

Incidence rate of eye disorders in persons age 75 and older

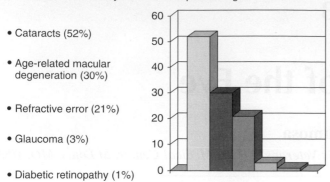

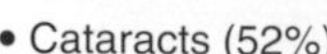

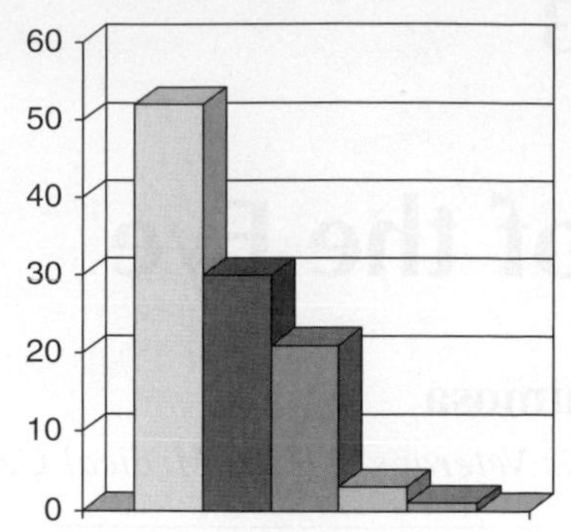

Figure 1 Over 50% of Americans aged 75 and older will suffer from visual impairment due to cataracts, 30% will lose central vision from age-related macular degeneration, 21% will have uncorrected refractive errors, 3% will report visual field loss due to optic nerve damage from glaucoma, and 1% will suffer vision loss due to diabetic retinopathy

Table 1 Medical risk factors for refractive errors

- Dry eye
- Increased glare
- Cataracts
- Yellowing of lenses
- Reduction in dark adaptation
- Decreased pupil size (miosis)
- Decreased contrast sensitivity
- Normal hyperopic shift with age
- Increasing against-the-rule astigmatism with age

Table 2 Social risk factors for refractive errors

- Cost of care
- Lack of access to care
- Living in a nursing home
- Lower expectations of patients and providers with age

Age-related Macular Degeneration

Age-related macular degeneration (AMD) is a disorder of the macula characterized by the presence of drusen, hypo- or hyper-pigmentation of the retinal pigment epithelium (RPE), local atrophy of the RPE and choriocapillaris, neovascularization of the macula, and a reduction or loss of central vision. AMD is the leading cause of severe, irreversible vision impairment in developed countries. Ninety percent of the AMD cases are of the nonexudative (dry or atrophic) type. Ten percent are of the exudative (or wet) type. Nonexudative AMD is characterized by the presence of drusen and loss of RPE and photoreceptors. Sight in the central visual field is lost gradually. Exudative AMD is characterized by a much more rapid loss of central vision due to neovascularization of the choroid and its accompanying hemorrhages that lead to retinal and RPE detachments and scarring. Although nonexudative AMD is more prevalent, most of the people with severe vision loss have exudative AMD.

Currently, there are no pharmaceutical treatments for AMD. However, there are several recommendations that can be made to people with AMD. Patients with early AMD should receive regular dilated fundus eye exams and should increase the consumption of antioxidants. They should be educated about how to use an Amsler grid to screen for the progression and encouraged to seek medical attention at the first sign of new symptoms. Dietary consumption of fresh fruits and vegetables is encouraged because they contain antioxidants such as Vitamin C, Vitamin E, carotenoids, selenium, and zinc, which neutralize damage caused by free radicals. Those who have unilateral AMD should be encouraged to take supplements in order to reduce their chances of developing AMD in the other eye. Results from the National Eye Institute Age-related Eye Disease Study (AREDS) showed that supplements containing high levels of antioxidants and zinc significantly reduce the risk of advanced AMD and its associated vision loss (Higginbotham *et al.*, 2004). The same nutrients had no significant effect on the development or progression of cataract.

There are surgical treatments for AMD. Two well-proven strategies for preserving residual vision are laser photocoagulation and photodynamic therapy. Other promising methods that are currently under study are submacular surgery, transpupillary thermotherapy, and pharmacological modalities like angiostatic steroids (Mohan *et al.*, 2003). These techniques target the more progressive disease that is no longer responsive to diet and supplements. Research into new treatments of AMD is ongoing. For example, apheresis, which is used to treat microcircuitry disorders such as myasthenia-gravis, is currently being tested for safety and effectiveness for treating nonexudative AMD. The hypothesis being tested is that decreasing blood plasma viscosity and red blood cell (RBC) aggregation might improve blood flow through the choriocapillaris and improve perfusion of the macula and preserve RPE and photoreceptors.

Understanding of both old and new risk factors is constantly being investigated and refined. Sunlight, long suspected to be a risk factor, is slowly yielding its complicated relationship with the onset of AMD (Tomany *et al.*, 2004) as is dietary fat consumption (Seddon *et al.*, 2003). Estrogens, despite extensive scrutiny, have not been implicated in the risk for AMD (Abramov *et al.*, 2004). Finally, researchers are in the process of uncovering molecular interventions for the treatment and eventual cure of AMD. Transgenic and knockout mice studies are providing new insights into choroidal neovascularization, the principal cause of vision loss in AMD, and gene searches are close to identifying genes such as the *fibulin 5* gene (Stone *et al.*, 2004) that may be responsible for the pathogenesis of AMD.

People with advanced AMD may be classified as legally blind and often require assistance with ADL even if the AMD is monocular because contrast sensitivity is affected, thereby reducing visual acuity in the unaffected eye. They are also at significant risk for depression. Vision can often be enhanced by the use of low vision aids such as magnifiers and bright lights. Motivated patients can be taught to read with the peripheral retina. Because functional status and quality of life are related, every effort should be made to encourage patients to seek rehabilitation.

Table 3 Confirmed risk factors for age-related macular degeneration

- Smoking
- Female sex
- Advanced age
- Caucasian race
- Low levels of antioxidants
- Exposure to sunlight in early adulthood

Table 4 Factors associated with AMD

- High fat diet
- Alcohol use
- Hormonal status
- Family history of AMD
- High levels of C-reactive protein
- High intake of saturated fats and cholesterol

Risk factors for and other factors associated with AMD are listed in Tables 3 and 4.

Diabetic Retinopathy

Diabetic retinopathy (DR) is the most frequent cause of blindness among adults aged 20 to 74 years. DR is a disorder of the retinal vasculature in which retinal changes such as waxy exudates, punctuate hemorrhages, and microaneurysms may occur as a result of uncontrolled systemic diabetes. DR can occur with both type I (insulin deficient) and type 2 (non-insulin dependent) diabetes mellitus. Despite the fact that type 1 diabetics develop the disease at an earlier age, a greater number of type 2 diabetics will develop DR because more than 90% of diabetics have type 2 diabetes. DR progresses from its mild, nonproliferative stage with increased vascular permeability, to severe, nonproliferative DR which is characterized by vascular closure, to proliferative DR with neovascularization in the retina and on the vitreous humour which tends to produce vitreal hemorrhages and resultant vision loss, retinal detachment, and possibly, glaucoma. Vision loss can result in several ways: (1) central vision can be lost due to macular edema or capillary loss; (2) neovascularization can lead to retinal detachment; (3) pre-retinal or vitreal hemorrhages can obstruct vision; (4) glaucoma can result in response to the damage caused by DR.

The retinal damage caused by DR cannot be cured. However, DR does respond favorably to early detection and treatment of diabetes and to case management of the disease (Norris *et al.*, 2002). Annual dilated fundus examinations are recommended for early detection and management of DR. Laser photocoagulation significantly reduces vision loss (ETDRS, 1991). Finally, for those who have experienced vision loss, low vision care and rehabilitation is recommended. These recommendations on how to minimize vision loss associated with DR are particularly significant in light of the research that shows that vision loss contributes significantly to poorer health, more disability, and increased frequency of falls in diabetics (Miller *et al.*, 1999) as well as restrictions in reading, mobility, work, and leisure activities (Lamoureux *et al.*, 2004).

Table 5 Risk factors for diabetic retinopathy

- Duration of diabetes
- Late diagnosis of diabetes
- No perception of vision problems
- Lack of frequent evaluation of vision
- Uncontrolled or poorly controlled blood sugar level (Hemoglobin A_{1c})
- Presence of other systemic diseases such as hypertension and hyperglycemia

Table 6 Factors associated with diabetic retinopathy

- Age
- Clotting factors
- Renal disease
- Use of angiotensin-converting enzyme inhibitors

Diabetics are at greater risk for comorbid conditions. The presence of diabetes mellitus increases the risk for the development of cataracts. In turn, the presence of cataracts complicates both the patient's and the provider's abilities to monitor vision changes due to DR. In addition, diabetics are at greater risks for complications during cataract surgery. Finally, comorbid conditions such as hypertension and hyperglycemia can worsen DR and should be treated (Fong *et al.*, 2003). Risk factors of and other factors associated with diabetic retinopathy are listed in Tables 5 and 6.

Glaucoma

Glaucoma is a general term that refers to a number of disorders of the optic nerve that are often accompanied by increased intraocular pressure (IOP) (ocular hypertension) and that results in a gradual and progressive visual field loss when the optic nerve is damaged. Glaucoma is the second leading cause of legal blindness in the United States and the leading cause of legal blindness in African-Americans. The destruction of the optic nerve that occurs as glaucoma progresses causes gradual loss of peripheral vision. As the disease progresses, the field of vision gradually narrows and blindness can result. Glaucoma has no early symptoms so about half of the people who are affected are unaware they have the disease. By the time people experience problems with their vision, they usually have a significant amount of optic nerve damage.

Early detection of glaucoma is critical. If glaucoma can be controlled, serious vision loss can be prevented. Comprehensive dilated eye examinations are recommended at least once every two years for African-Americans over age 40 and all people over age 60. Primary open-angle glaucoma (POAG) is the most common form of glaucoma and one of the nation's leading causes of vision loss. POAG has a characteristic loss of retinal ganglion cells and atrophy of the optic nerve that occurs in the presence of an open and normal looking angle. The visual field loss may be monocular but if it is binocular, it may well be asymmetric (AAO PPP, 2003c), (http://www.aao.org/aao/education/library/ppp/index.cfm). Although there is a dearth of convincing evidence about causal relationships, there is evidence that macular degeneration, pseudo exfoliation, diabetes, and hypertension (Hennis *et al.*, 2003; Le *et al.*, 2003; Racette *et al.*, 2003) often occur in people with glaucoma, perhaps because all of these diseases represent increased risks of increased IOP. It may be that glaucoma is one more consequence of circulatory diseases.

Treatment to control IOP is helpful in reducing the visual field losses associated with glaucoma, regardless of whether the patient has elevated or normal (low-tension) glaucoma (Lee and Coleman, 2004). Drug therapy, in the form of eye drops, is normally initiated first, in large part due to the development of new drug therapies such as prostaglandins to lower IOP. The older drug therapy for glaucoma treatment, β-blockers, had so many side effects that surgery was often considered to be a reasonable alternative, despite the increased risk of infections and the large failure rate with its concomitant need to repeat the surgery several times. With the advent of prostaglandins, which have very few side effects (other than a tendency to darken iris and lash color), and of α-adrenergic drugs (which have some of the significant side effects of β-blockers) for the treatment of the more intractable cases, pharmaceutical control of IOP has become the standard of treatment. Even though African-Americans respond differently to eye drops than do Caucasians, the NEI (National Eye Institute) Ocular Hypertension Treatment Study (OHTS) showed that daily pressure-lowering eye drops reduced the development of primary open-angle glaucoma in African-Americans by almost 50% (www.nei.nih.gov/glaucomaeyedrops/).

Surgery is recommended if a patient becomes intolerant of the drugs or is not compliant with the drug schedule. Surgical procedures for glaucoma have become much more standardized in the past 10 years. Although glaucoma surgery can be done with manual or laser incisions, the most common types of surgery are done with lasers. The most common laser techniques are argon laser trabeculoplasty, argon or neodymium:YAG (Nd:YAG) laser iridotomy, and trans-scleral laser cyclophotocoagulation. The argon laser trabeculoplasty involves removing part of the trabecular meshwork in order to improve the outflow of aqueous humor from the anterior chamber. This technique works well in the treatment of POAG.

For patients with narrow anterior chamber angles or who have a closed angle, then surgery to open a hole in the iris is often recommended. This iridotomy surgery can be made manually or with either argon or Nd:YAG lasers. Care must be taken to not damage the corneal endothelium, which lies close to the iris.

When other surgical methods have failed to reduce IOP and the advancement of optic nerve damage, trans-scleral laser cyclophotocoagulation can be tried. This surgery selectively destroys the ciliary body, where aqueous humor is produced, thereby lowering IOP by reducing the amount of aqueous humor produced.

Table 7 Risk factors for glaucoma

- Age greater than 60
- Central corneal thickness
- Elevated intraocular pressure
- African descent over age of 40
- Family history (parent or sibling)

Table 8 Other factors associated with glaucoma

- Late onset menarche
- Migraine headaches
- Peripheral vasospasm
- Low diastolic perfusion pressure
- Presence of AMD, hypertension or diabetes
- High ratio of n-3 to n-6 polyunsaturated fat
- Suspicious optic nerve appearance (cup-to-disc ratio greater than 0.5)

The efficacy of surgical interventions, the number of times each of the surgeries needs to be repeated, and the order in which the surgery types are offered in combination, differ for black and white patients (Ederer *et al.*, 2004). Further study will undoubtedly fine-tune future surgical interventions.

Before determining whether the disease will be treated with eyedrops or surgery, an effort must be made to determine patient's health status and life expectancy, how difficult daily treatment of eyedrops will be, how expensive the drugs costs are, and what the possible side effects will be.

The use of marijuana as a complementary therapy for POAG glaucoma is not recommended. NEI studies have demonstrated that some derivatives of marijuana do result in lowering IOP for 3 to 4 hours when administered orally, intravenously, or by smoking. However, potentially serious side effects included increased heart rate, a decrease in blood pressure, impaired memory of recent events, and impaired motor coordination.

Efforts to better understand the pathogenesis of glaucoma have led to attempts to locate gene anomalies associated with glaucoma. Defects in the *myocilin* gene (MYOC) have been associated with POAG and defects in PITX2, FOXC1, and CYP1B1 are associated with anterior segment development (WuDunn, 2002).

The risk factors for and other factors associated with glaucoma are summarized in Tables 7 and 8.

Cataracts

Cataracts are a leading cause of blindness worldwide. They are opacities of the lens or the lens capsule. Cataracts are *named* by the location of the opacity; the opacity may occur in the nucleus (nuclear cataract), in the lens cortex (cortical cataract), or in the lens periphery (coronary cataract), or posterior (posterior subcapsular, posterior cortical, and posterior polar cataracts).

Cataracts are caused by the hardening of the lens that occurs as a part of normal aging. They also may occur as a result of blunt trauma, but the history of this type of cataract is a rapid onset and a rapid rate of progression. Normal cataracts progress slowly and may be present for years before they are noticed.

Cataracts are not normally life threatening. No effective medical treatment for cataract exists, but a diet rich in lutein and zeaxanthin, carotene, and Vitamin A and long-term Vitamin C supplementation are thought to slow the progression of cataracts.

Once the patient reports a decreased quality of life or impaired function, elective surgery can correct the visual impairment. For patients with glaucoma, AMD, or diabetes, where visualization of the fundus is necessary for continuing management and treatment, surgery may be indicated before the patient reports a decline in functional status (AAO PPP, 2003a; 2003b; 2003c), (http://www.aao.org/aao/education/library/ppp/index.cfm).

When vision becomes cloudy enough to bother the patient, surgery can remove the clouded lens and replace it with an intraocular lens implant (IOL). Surgery is normally an outpatient procedure using local anesthetic. Phacoemulsification (ultrasonic cataract removal) is used to emulsify the lens for easy removal (although promising research on the use of lasers to break up the lens is ongoing (Bowman and Allen, 2003)). An IOL is then implanted within the empty lens capsule to serve as the new lens. Normally the incision is self-sealing. The surgical procedure is so safe that it has changed little in the past 10 years although lens implants of differing powers can reduce dependence upon glasses for either reading or distance work.

Many risk factors have been associated with cataracts although the studies have been largely observational. General risk factors for cataracts are listed in Table 9 and specific risk factors for cortical, nuclear, and posterior subcapsular cataracts are listed in Tables 10 to 12.

Table 9 General risk factors for all cataracts

- Age
- Diabetes
- Cost of treatment
- Low socioeconomic status
- Diet low in lutein and zeaxanthin
- Lack of education about cataracts

Table 10 Risk factors specific for cortical cataracts

- Iris color
- Hypertension
- Hyperglycemia
- Family history
- Abdominal obesity
- Low body mass index
- Exposure to UV-B radiation

Table 11 Risk factors specific for nuclear cataracts

- Smoking
- Iris color
- Family history
- Low education level
- Nonprofessional occupation
- Occupational sun exposure in third decade of life

Table 12 Risk factors specific for posterior subcapsular cataracts

- Smoking
- Hyperglycemia
- Inhaled corticosteroid use
- Systemic corticosteroid use
- Alcohol consumption
- Exposure to UV-B radiation

SUMMARY

Each type of eye disorder discussed above has unique risk factors, ranging from diet to environment. Increased age is associated with all of the eye disorders, that is, the frequency of the disorder in the population increases with age. In addition, some of the risk factors are shared by two of the eye disorders. Excessive exposure to sunlight is a risk factor for both cataracts and macular degeneration. Additionally, a particular symptom may have more than one cause. For example, glare may be caused by corneal aberrations or by the development of cataracts. A decrease in contrast sensitivity may be the result of decreased illumination to the retina because of a decreased pupil size, but it may also be caused by AMD, glaucoma or diabetic retinopathy. A decrease in dark adaptation may be caused by a miotic pupil or it may also be caused by cataracts. Thus, treatment of a specific visual deficit may require more than one approach because due consideration must be given to how different disorders contribute to the resulting morbidity.

In addition to having shared risk factors, there is some degree of comorbidity between the eye disorders. Either cataracts or glaucoma may often co-occur with DR and AMD often co-occurs with glaucoma. Interactions between diseases may complicate the treatments needed to prevent visual impairment and blindness. Finally, although there is little research about how comorbid eye disorders affect an already decreased level of function and quality of life, the quality of life of patients is dependent upon better understanding of the interactions between diseases and between their treatments.

For people who become blind from an eye disorder, there is some hope. Research on artificial vision techniques is ongoing. Artificial vision through the use of cortical implants is a promise of the future (Dobelle, 2000), although it is designed to promote mobility, not reading. These cortical implants are contraindicated for people with severe chronic infections and for those blinded by stroke or cortical trauma. However, cortical models for patients without viable optic nerves (e.g. glaucoma patients) and retinal prostheses for those without viable photoreceptors (e.g. AMD patients) are under development. Research such as this should considerably brighten the future of visually impaired people.

KEY POINTS

- Increasing age is a risk factor for loss of vision due to the following eye disorders: cataract, age-related macular degeneration, refractive error, glaucoma, and diabetic retinopathy.
- Poor vision due to refractive error and cataracts is often reversible.
- Loss of vision due to diabetic retinopathy, glaucoma, and age-related macular degeneration is not recoverable.
- Vision impairment caused by these eye disorders has a negative impact on functional status, mobility, independence, and cognitive status of elders.
- Education and visual rehabilitation play important roles in improving the quality of life of persons with visual impairments.

KEY REFERENCES

- AAO PPP (American Academy of Ophthalmology Preferred Practice Patterns). *Cataracts*, 2001; http://www.aao.org/aao/education/library/ppp/index.cfm.
- AAO PPP (American Academy of Ophthalmology Preferred Practice Patterns). *Age-related Macular Degeneration*, 2003a; http://www.aao.org/aao/education/library/ppp/index.cfm.
- AAO PPP (American Academy of Ophthalmology Preferred Practice Patterns). *Diabetes*, 2003b; http://www.aao.org/aao/education/library/ppp/index.cfm.
- AAO PPP (American Academy of Ophthalmology Preferred Practice Patterns). *Primary Open Angle Glaucoma*, 2003c; http://www.aao.org/aao/education/library/ppp/index.cfm.
- Lee AG & Coleman AL. Geriatric ophthalmology. In DH Solomon, J LoCicero 3rd & RA Rosenthal (eds) *New Frontiers in Geriatric Research: An Agenda for Surgical and Related Medical Specialties* 2004, pp 177–202; American Geriatrics Society, New York.

REFERENCES

AAO PPP (American Academy of Ophthalmology Preferred Practice Patterns). *Cataracts*, 2001; http://www.aao.org/aao/education/library/ppp/index.cfm.

AAO PPP (American Academy of Ophthalmology Preferred Practice Patterns). *Age-related Macular Degeneration*, 2003a; http://www.aao.org/aao/education/library/ppp/index.cfm.

AAO PPP (American Academy of Ophthalmology Preferred Practice Patterns). *Diabetes*, 2003b; http://www.aao.org/aao/education/library/ppp/index.cfm.

AAO PPP (American Academy of Ophthalmology Preferred Practice Patterns). *Primary Open Angle Glaucoma*, 2003c; http://www.aao.org/aao/education/library/ppp/index.cfm.

Abramov Y, Borik S, Yahalom C *et al.* The effect of hormone therapy on the risk for age-related maculopathy in postmenopausal women, *Menopause* 2004; **11**:62–8.

Bowman DM & Allen RC. Erbium:YAG laser in cataract extraction. *Journal of Long Term Effects of Medical Implants* 2003; **13**:503–8.

Dobelle WH. Artificial vision for the blind by connecting a television camera to the visual cortex. *American Society for Artificial Internal Organs* 2000; **46**:1–7.

Ederer F, Gaasterland DA, Dally LG *et al.* AGIS Investigators. The Advanced Glaucoma Intervention Study (AGIS): 13. Comparison of treatment outcomes within race: 10-year results. *Ophthalmology* 2004; **11**:651–64.

Egrilmez S, Ates H, Nalcaci S *et al.* Surgically induced corneal refractive change following glaucoma surgery: nonpenetrating trabecular surgeries versus trabeculectomy. *Journal of Cataract Refractive Surgery* 2004; **30**:1232–39.

ETDRS (Early Treatment Diabetic Retinopathy Study Research Group). Early photocoagulation for diabetic retinopathy. ETDRS Report Number 9. *Ophthalmology* 1991; **98**:766–85.

Fong DS, Aiello L, Gardner TW *et al.* Diabetic retinopathy. *Diabetes Care* 2003; **26**:S99–S102.

Guzowski M, Wang JJ, Rochtchina E *et al.* Five-year refractive changes in an older population: the blue mountains eye study. *Ophthalmology* 2003; **110**:1364–70.

Hennis A, Wu SY, Nemesure B & Leske MD. the Barbados Eye Studies Group. Hypertension, diabetes, and longitudinal changes in intraocular pressure. *Ophthalmology* 2003; **110**:908–14.

Higginbotham EJ, Gordon MO, Beiser JA *et al.* for the Ocular Hypertension Treatment Study Group. The ocular hypertension treatment study. Topical medication delays or prevents primary open-angle glaucoma in african american individuals, *Archives of Ophthalmology* 2004; **122**:813–20.

Lamoureux EL, Hassell JB & Keeffe JE. The impact of diabetic retinopathy on participation in daily living. *Archives of Ophthalmology* 2004; **122**:84–8.

Le A, Mukesh BN, McCarty CA & Taylor HR. Risk factors associated with the incidence of open-angle glaucoma: the visual impairment project. *Investigative Ophthalmology and Visual Science* 2003; **44**:3783–89.

Lee AG & Coleman AL. Geriatric ophthalmology. In DH Solomon, J LoCicero 3rd & RA Rosenthal (eds) *New Frontiers in Geriatric Research: An Agenda for Surgical and Related Medical Specialties* 2004, pp 177–202; American Geriatrics Society, New York.

Miller DK, Lui LY, Perry MD 3rd *et al.* Reported and measured physical functioning in older inner-city diabetic african americans. *The Journals of Gerontology Series A, Biological Sciences and Medical Sciences* 1999; **54**:M230–39.

Mohan KC, Shukla D, Namperumalsamy P & Kim R. Management of age-related macular degeneration. *Journal of the Indian Medical Association* 2003; **101**:471–76.

Norris SL, Nichols PJ, Caspersen CJ *et al.* Task Force on Community Preventive Services. The effectiveness of disease and case management for people with diabetes. *American Journal of Preventive Medicine* 2002; **22**(Supp 1):15–38.

Racette L, Wilson MR, Zangwill LM *et al.* Primary open-angle glaucoma in blacks: A review. *Survey of Ophthalmology* 2003; **48**:295–313.

Seddon JM, Cote J & Rosner B. Progression of age-related macular degeneration: association with dietary fat, transunsaturated fat, nuts, and fish intake. *Archives of Ophthalmology* 2003; **121**:1728–37.

Stone EM, Braun TA, Russell SR *et al.* Missense variations in the fibulin 5 gene and age-related macular degeneration. *The New England Journal of Medicine* 2004; **351**:346–53.

Tomany SC, Cruickshanks KJ, Klein R *et al.* Sunlight and the 10-year incidence of age-related maculopathy: the beaver dam eye study. *Archives of Ophthalmology* 2004; **122**:750–57.

WuDunn D. Genetic basis of glaucoma. *Current Opinions in Ophthalmology* 2002; **13**:55–60.

104

The Epidemiology of Hearing in Aging Population

Adrian C. Davis *and* **Padma Moorjani**

University of Manchester, Manchester, UK

SCOPE

Epidemiology is defined as "the study of how often diseases occur in different groups of people and why". The public health context needs a through consideration of the epidemiology of hearing impairment and disabilities as well as good, independent information on the current service provision for those with a genuine health need. To assess public-health priorities for the prevention, early identification of need and rehabilitation, a national and a local epidemiology of hearing impairment and disability are required. It is estimated that hearing impairment is the most prevalent disability in the developed countries (Davis, 1997). In some studies, it has been estimated to affect approximately 15% of adults, and its prevalence is expected to increase up to 25% by the year 2020 (Rosenhall *et al.*, 1999; Sorri *et al.*, 2001). According to some estimates, the current proportion of those suffering from hearing impairment is even higher than that comprising up to 18–20% of the adult population. (Uimonen *et al.*, 1999; Davis, 1989; Gates *et al.*, 1990; Quaranta *et al.*, 1996). Within the United Kingdom, it is estimated that 3.5% of the population have hearing aids (Taylor and Paisley, 2000).

The ongoing change in the society, for example, the fact that much of the workforce is changing from manual to communication work, where good hearing ability is a necessity, influences future needs for hearing services. Independent of the profession, present-day working requires good communication abilities. In the urban population, it is estimated that as high as 87.5% of the entire workforce is dependent on communications skills. The challenge presented to the health-care service is, with appropriate management, to maintain the hearing-disabled at work.

The aim of this chapter is to show that hearing disorders are a major and under-reported disability and handicap, underestimated in terms of their burden on society and traditionally undersupplied with appropriate health services to ameliorate that burden through improving quality of life.

Most of the data presented here was collected during the 1980s and 1990s in Great Britain and, therefore, has limitations in terms of its generality. However, the major conclusions are probably similar for most developed countries and there are some aspects that can be applied to developing countries as well. The main limitation to the work described was the very great difficulty in conducting rigorous work with populations that were very elderly, because of the difficulties in obtaining proper random samples in this population and in the restriction of mobility that makes laboratory-based studies difficult. In this context, "very elderly" means 80 years and over.

INTRODUCTION

There are three major disorders that arise from auditory-based pathology, (i) hearing impairment, (ii) tinnitus, and to a lesser extent (iii) vestibular dysfunction (*see* **Chapter 105, Auditory System** and **Chapter 106, Disorders of the Vestibular System**). While the first of these has been documented by some systematic population studies (Davis, 1995, 1989; Salomon, 1986; Brooks, 1989) and also by investigation of the elderly in nursing homes or residential settings (Alpiner, 1963; Martin and Peckford, 1978; Schow and Norbonne, 1989; Tolson *et al.*, 1992), tinnitus has been relatively underdocumented (Reich and Vernon, 1995) in the elderly, and vestibular dysfunction rarely documented (Davis, 1997). The consequences of our lack of knowledge concerning the extent of those who could benefit from rehabilitation for their disorder is a lack of prioritization of services for those people at a primary and secondary level of health care. Hearing impairment and tinnitus are not visible to society and their effects are therefore under-recognized.

Principles and Practice of Geriatric Medicine, 4th Edition. Edited by M.S. John Pathy, Alan J. Sinclair and John E. Morley.

However, the effects exist and are suffered by the relatives and carers who try to communicate with the hearing impaired or tinnitus sufferer, on a regular basis. In addition to this chronic and long-term breakdown in communication facility, when there is an exacerbation of the disorders by an accompanied vestibular dysfunction or lack of orientation, the effects may indirectly be manifest in a greater number of accidents requiring emergency treatment or surgery and hospitalization (Davis, 1996). Hence, apart from social and mental health implications for the nuclear family, there may be indirect effects on physical functioning and vitality at a population level. A major challenge for current research is to separate the effect of hearing on quality of life from the effects due to other comorbidity factors.

Hearing disability should have a major public health priority because of the extent and nature of its impact on individuals and their families. The knowledge base concerning the need in the community has expanded over the last 20 years (Davis, 1995), and there has been a systematic attempt to develop outcome measures that reflect the impact of hearing impairment to guide and evaluate rehabilitation (Gatehouse, 1994; Dillon *et al.*, 1997). However, a major omission in that work concerns the very elderly population. Indeed, the perceived lack of rehabilitative success (Tolson *et al.* 1992; Hart, 1980) with this very elderly population has shifted the emphasis, in terms of personal rehabilitation in this group, to secondary prevention in the younger generations by fitting hearing aids 10–20 years earlier than is presently the case. Consequently, the subsequent generation should have benefited from earlier use *per se*, and, in addition, by adapting to the changes, should be better equipped, both cognitively and ergonomically, to cope with the demands of using hearing aid technology (Davis *et al.*, 1992; Stephens *et al.*, 1990). In addition, the complexities and cost of providing a thorough service to the very elderly have led to the idea that it would be more cost-effective to educate the carers to provide better acoustic environments and promote the use of good hearing tactics (Haggard, 1993) than to concentrate solely on increasing the provision of personal hearing aids, which, without proper rehabilitation and support, or an individual care plan, are likely to accumulate unused in drawers. There appears to be little systematic research into the most appropriate and cost-effective form of rehabilitation for this very elderly population. For instance, what are the communications needs of the very elderly and their carers? What would these people accept and how could their needs be met in a sustainable and cost-effective fashion? These are questions that need to be addressed but which will be given only the lowest level of input in terms of our knowledge base in this chapter.

The main data used in this review comes from the National Study of Hearing (Davis, 1995, 1989). This is a major population study carried out using random samples of the population by means of postal questionnaires ($n = 48\,313$) and clinical interviews expanded by audiological assessment of a representative subsample ($n = 2708$) during 1980–1986. This is supplemented by a more recent study carried out by Medical Research Council (MRC) Institute of Hearing Research (Gray, 1995) in Glasgow and Nottingham in 1994–1996, asking similar questions but in addition more details concerning the service received ($n = 11\,471$ at the postal questionnaire phase, $n = 1301$ people interviewed in their own homes including 546 people who had audiological assessment). In the Nottingham and Glasgow study, sampling was based on households, while the National Study drew its sample from individual electors.

Where comparisons are made between the samples over time, only those people living in Glasgow or Nottingham in the first study are used ($n = 12\,549$ at the postal phase).

PREVALENCE OF HEARING DISORDERS

The prevalence of hearing impairment is the number of people who have a specific degree of hearing impairment at a given time. This can also be expressed as a percentage of the relevant population. When generalizing between populations, care has been taken to ensure that the assumptions underpinning such generalizations are valid in terms of congruence of age, gender, and occupational distribution, together with an assessment of whether there are particular risk factors present in one of the sample populations. In terms of hearing impairment, it is particularly important to define the degree of impairment or disability, enabling comparison of like with like. Terms such as deaf or deafness should be avoided, as these tend to give rise to misleading and emotive statements. As hearing impairment is a chronic and progressive problem, often accompanied by tinnitus, and, sometimes, by vestibular dysfunction, the *incidence* of hearing impairments, which is the number of new cases of a given degree of severity of hearing impairment that arise in a year, is difficult to establish (Davis *et al.*, 1991). The prevalence is the important consideration for service provision. Given that the prevalence far outweighs the provision, the question becomes "the prevalence of what form of hearing impairment deserves our consideration?"

Figure 1 shows the broad extent of hearing impairment and reported hearing disability in the adult population (aged 18 and over) in the United Kingdom. It can be seen from this figure that almost 1 in 3 of UK adults has, at least, a mild hearing impairment in one ear, with 1 in 5 showing a bilateral hearing impairment. Great difficulty in hearing what is said in a background of noise is reported by 1 in 4 people, with 1 in 10 reporting that they have prolonged spontaneous tinnitus (PST) (Coles *et al.*, 1990). At a moderate degree of hearing impairment in the better ear, 7% of the adult population is impaired (Davis, 1995). This means a substantial number of people in the United Kingdom who may have the need for some associated services, that is, who may benefit from the provision of hearing services. Supplying those services is a substantial public health problem, substantial enough to warrant considerable debate. This has been discussed by several authors (Haggard, 1993; Davis *et al.*, 1992; Stephens *et al.*, 1990), and revolves around criteria concerning the extent to which the population

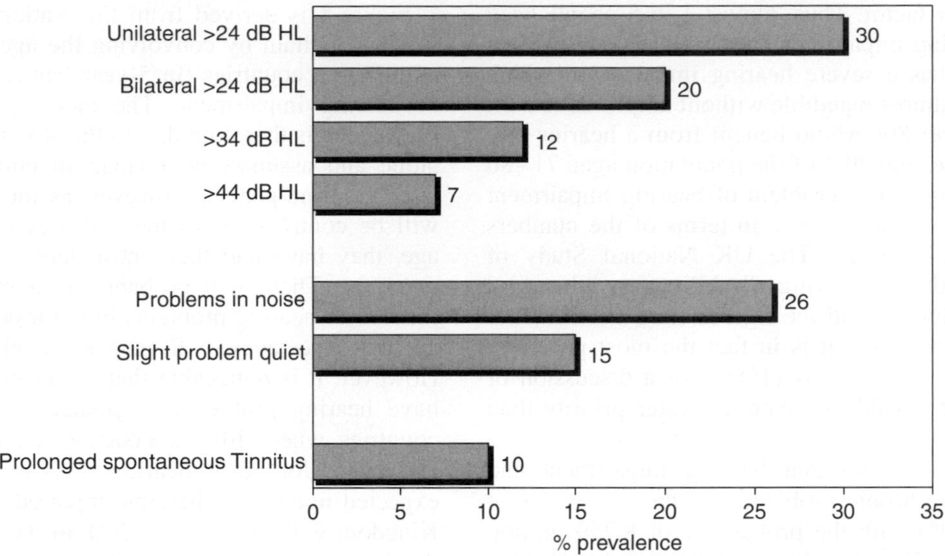

Figure 1 The prevalence of hearing impairment at different degrees of severity, hearing disability as shown by finding it "very difficult" to hear what someone says if there is a background of noise and also by having at least a slight difficulty hearing in quiet. The prevalence of tinnitus that is not only after loud sounds and which lasts for 5 minutes or more (PST, prolonged spontaneous tinnitus) is also shown

can benefit from intervention and a cost-effective analysis of such an intervention; obviously, hearing disability and handicap are the major targets of rehabilitation, both present and future. However, the extent of hearing impairment is the best predictor of need that can be assessed quantitatively. Both aspects will be presented in this chapter. Some authors (Davis *et al.* 1992; Stephen *et al.* 1990) think that the low threshold for provision of hearing aids should be set at about 25 dB HL in the better ear, measured as an average over the frequencies 0.5, 1, 2, and 4 kHz. Other authors (Haggard, 1993) consider more complex schemes and higher thresholds, but the differences are actually quite small operationally and relate mainly to the degree of impairment in the better ear.

Using the lower threshold definition, the prevalence in the adult population aged 18 and over of a hearing impairment in the better ear of 25 dB HL or greater is 20%. Taking more severe criteria, 12 and 7% are the prevalences for impairments of 35 dB HL or greater and 45 dB HL or greater, respectively. The pattern of hearing impairment does change with age (Davis, 1995), with the higher frequencies being more susceptible to aging and noise.

Figure 2 shows the prevalence of hearing impairment as a function of age-group (see Davis (1995) for the confidence intervals and a more detailed description). Within the figure, the data are derived from the National Study of Hearing 18–80 age-group and from a number of studies for the aged over 80 years (Davis *et al.*, 1992; Hart, 1980). These do not disagree widely with the estimates made by Soucek and Michaels (1987) and by Tolson *et al.* (1992). The estimates for the 71–80 age-groups are reasonably accurate in terms of their relatively bias-free derivation. Those for the over 80s have been derived from 862 people using a variety of testing procedures, and are thus more open to criticism. Gatehouse and Davis (1992) suggest that at least some of the prevalence in the elderly may be due to central response-based processes rather than peripheral perceptual processing (i.e. it takes a stronger signal for an elderly person to give a response). For public health purposes, this makes very little difference until differential rehabilitation is considered. In any case, it is unlikely that a response bias would make over 10 dB difference to the hearing thresholds in the over-80-year olds.

The major effects on the prevalence of hearing impairment have been shown by Davis (1989). By far the most important was the age-group, with occupational group and occupational noise exposure having major effects throughout the severity range. In terms of gender, at mild–moderate impairments, men have a higher prevalence at 25 dB HL (odds ratio 1.4 : 1). The effect of age-group, as seen in Figure 2, is large and

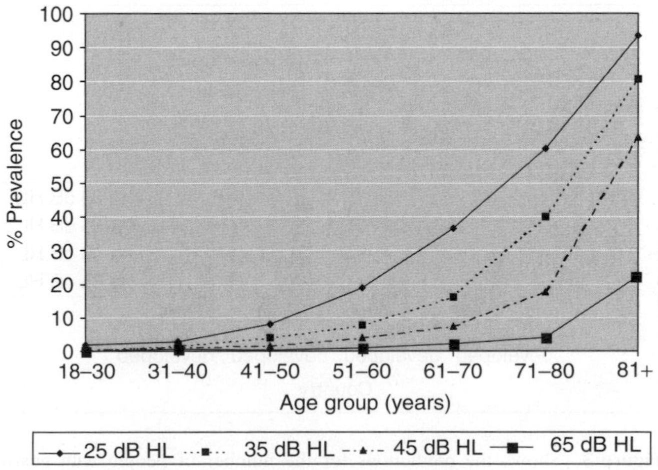

Figure 2 The prevalence (%) of different degrees of hearing impairment as a function of age in the Great Britain population

dominates any other factor. Thus, almost 1 in 5 people aged 51–60 have a hearing impairment in the better ear and 1 in 5 of the over 80s has a severe hearing impairment, which will render speech almost inaudible without amplification. At least 80% of the over 80s would benefit from a hearing aid, if they could use one, and 40% of the population aged 71–80 would benefit likewise. The problem of hearing impairment in the elderly is thus a major issue in terms of the numbers of people that are involved. The UK National Study of Disability estimated that hearing disability was the third most prevalent disability, and the figures from the National Study of Hearing show that it is in fact the most prevalent disability in the aged (see Davis (1989) for a discussion of this difference) and should be given a greater priority than at present.

While there is no doubt that hearing impairment and disability are major chronic problems for the population at present (Davis, 1995) with the probability of 8.759 million people in the United Kingdom having a hearing impairment as described previously, the situation may deteriorate because of demographic changes in the population (Davis, 1997, 1991). Figure 3 shows an extract of the predictions for the number of people with hearing impairment in the United Kingdom, United States, developed countries and developing countries for 1995 and 2015.

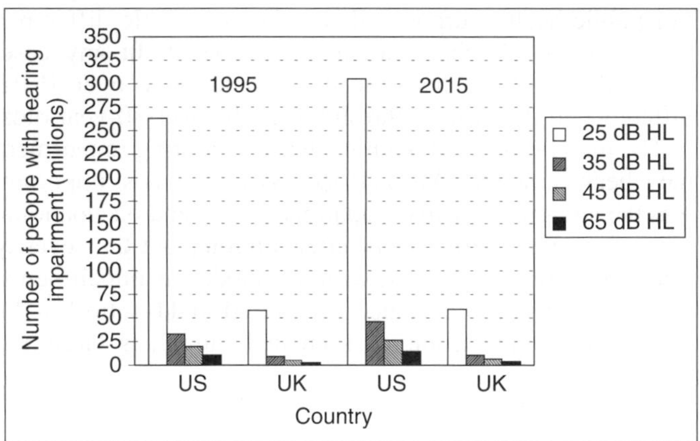

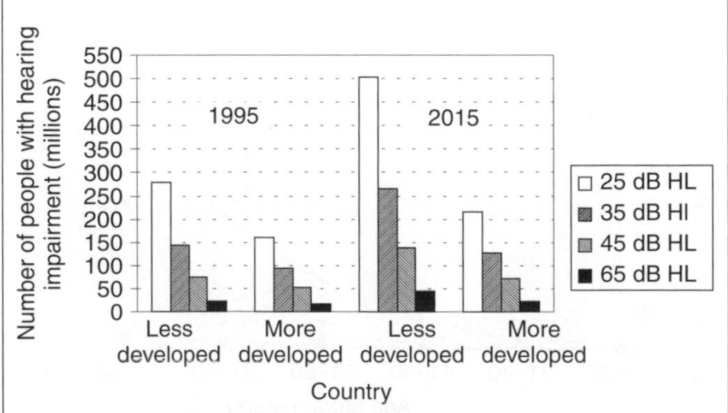

Figure 3 Shows the predictions for the number of people with hearing impairment as a function of country and severity of hearing impairment using the 1994 revision of the UN projected world populations in 1995 and 2015

Figure 3 is derived from the National Study of Hearing in Great Britain by convolving the age and sex distribution of different countries (in 5-year bands) with the prevalence of hearing impairment. The increase seen in the overall prevalence is therefore due to the structure of the population alone and assumes no change in etiology or risk factors over the time period. However, as most of the people who will be contributing to the statistics are already in middle age, they have had their most dangerous time for noxious exposure. There will probably be a more rapid growth in those with hearing problems in the less developed countries, as life expectancy will increase over the next 20 years. However, it is noticeable that the proportion of people who have hearing problems is greater in the more developed countries where life expectancy is already high. Another key factor for health/hearing services planning is that the expected number of hearing-impaired people in the United Kingdom will rise by over 20% in the next 20 years. Using the data for Great Britain, with 8.58 million hearing impaired in 1994, the numbers who were aged 18–60 were 2.131 m, aged 61–80 years were 4.486 m and aged over 80 years were 1.963 m. At ≥45 dB HL there were 0.471 m, 1.132 m and 1.337m, and at ≥65 dB HL there were 0.136 m, 0.294 m and 0.469 m respectively for 18–60, 61–80 and over 80 (Davis, 1995). Thus, as the severity criterion increases, there is a larger and larger proportion of the very elderly in the hearing-impaired group.

Figure 4 shows the prevalence of reported hearing disability in the population (Davis, 1995) in the 1980s. The question "How well can you hear someone talking to you when that person is sitting on your left-/right-hand side in a quiet room" was used with responses "No, slight, moderate and great difficulty" and an option for "Can't hear at all". A response of slight difficulty in hearing in an ear relates to a median hearing impairment of about 35 dB HL, the moderate and worse to 50 dB HL and the great and worse to 75 dB HL (averaged over 0.5, 1, 2, and 4 kHz). Figure 4 shows that at all degrees of reported hearing disability, there is an increase with age. Thus, at 61–70 years, about 15% report difficulty on the better ear, with about 25% at 71–80 and 40% for the over 80s. Comparing the reported hearing disability to the measured hearing impairment, it is noticeable that far fewer people have a reported better-ear hearing disability compared with a measured hearing impairment. Furthermore, the ratio of reported problem to measured impairment is not constant across age, giving fair correspondence up to 50 years and then giving progressive discrepancies. Thus, older people are far less likely to report a hearing disability for a given level of hearing impairment. However, it could be argued that they are less likely to benefit from rehabilitation unless they recognize that problem.

Figure 4 also reports the prevalence of tinnitus that lasts for five minutes or more and was not only after loud sounds, adjusted for the proportion of the sample who did not complete all three parts of the question (this was particularly so in the elderly). It is noticeable that the prevalence of tinnitus increases with age until 60 years of age, when it reaches a peak of 1 in 5 people. The factors that influence

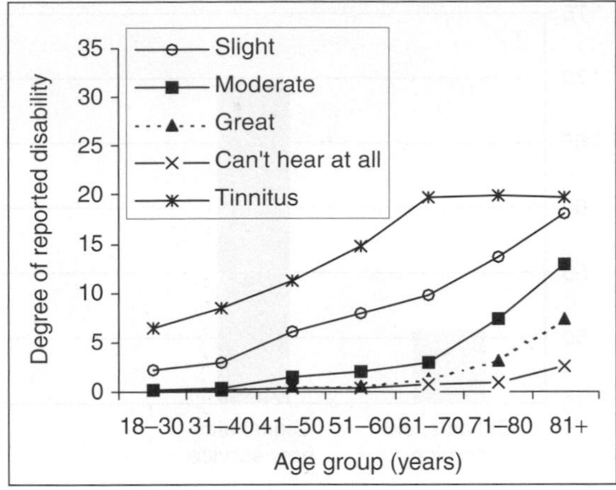

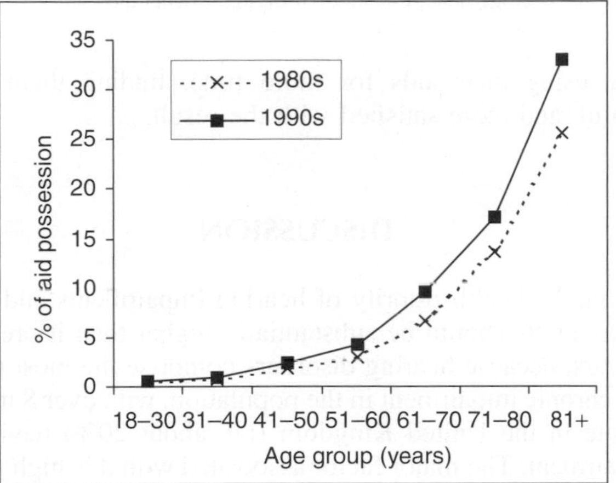

Figure 4 Prevalence (%) of different degrees of reported hearing disability, tinnitus, and hearing-aid possession as a function of age in the population of Great Britain

tinnitus report are systematically explored in Davis *et al.* (1992). Davis and Roberts (1996) explored the quality-of-life implications for those with prolonged spontaneous tinnitus and/or a reported hearing disability. They examined the scores on the SF-36 and showed that both reported hearing disability and tinnitus affect the scores on the SF-36 in a differential way, with tinnitus that is severe giving the largest deficits, particularly in terms of the vitality, social function, and mental health. Using the 1990s sample, the largest effect of reported hearing disability was concerned with the social function score and is shown in Figure 5.

The terms "hearing difficulty" and "disability/handicap" were obtained from the subject- and situation-specific hearing questionnaire devised by Gatehouse and Davis (1992), and the factor effect shown here is for a shift in 10% of the scores on this questionnaire that only uses items that are relevant to individual patients/hearing aid users. Figure 5 shows that the effect of a slight reported hearing disability is a deficit in 6 points of the social function score (range 0–100%), and that a moderate reported disability is a deficit of 14% with about 30 points for a great disability. However, those who use their hearing aids most or all of the time do get this deficit from the hearing disability offset by up to 12%. Those who use the hearing aid only some of the time do not get a significant benefit. This may be for a number of reasons including the fact that there needs to be a reasonable amount of time to adapt to the input from the aid (cognitive plasticity). Also, there were significant beneficial effects of "using a hearing aid most or all of the time" for body pain and mental health scores.

SERVICE PROVISION (*see* Chapter 105, Auditory System)

Services for hearing-impaired people have very different modes of organization and service delivery in different countries, and are very much a function of the ways in which health care is funded, structured, and delivered. In the United Kingdom, for example, hearing aid services are located in hospitals and are free at the point of delivery as

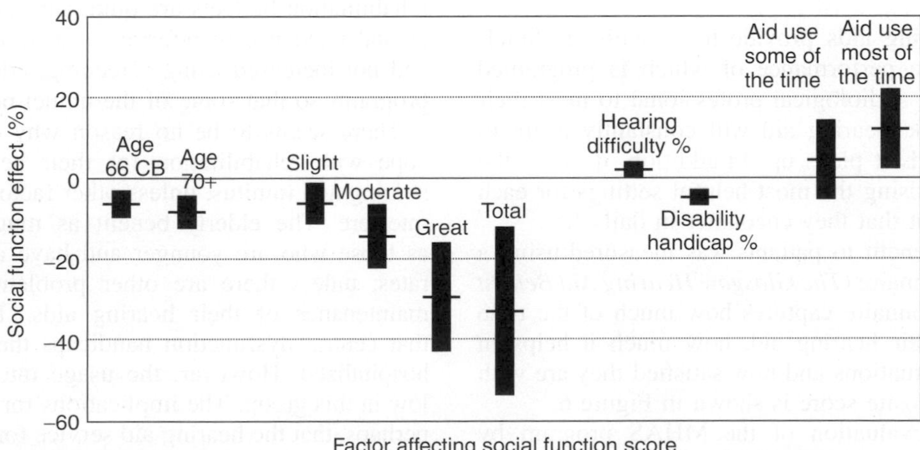

Figure 5 The effect (with confidence interval) of age, hearing disability, difficulty handicap, and hearing-aid use on the social function score of the SF-36 using a general linear model to estimate the effects

part of the UK National Health Service (NHS), funded by direct taxation. Prior to the Modernisation of NHS Hearing Aid Services (MHAS) program, four basic analog models accounted for more than half of the aids distributed, and only 2% were digital. Ten to fifteen percent of hearing aid users have a bilateral aid in the United Kingdom, compared to up to 60% in other European countries (Barton *et al.*, 2001). It has also been estimated that 150 000 people have a private aid in the United Kingdom (Taylor and Paisley, 2000), over 25% of the number estimated to be provided by the NHS. This figure is higher than that in the European countries (Barton *et al.*, 2001) and it has been argued as too high, as private aids enable people to receive the benefits of private technology and avoid having to wait as long as they might with the NHS while providing the option of a hearing aid in both ears (Audit Commission, 2000).

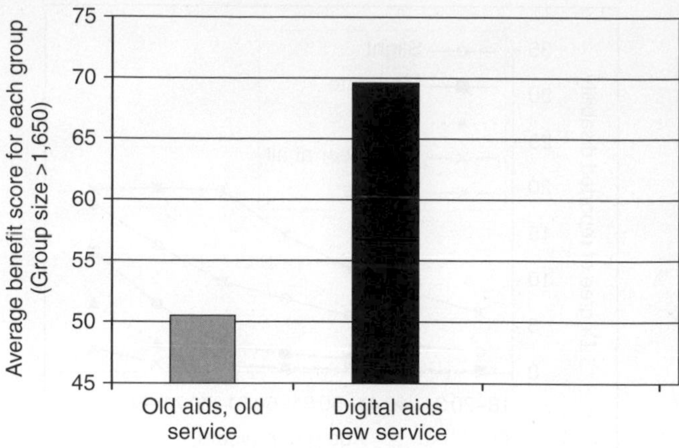

Figure 6 Average benefit of modern digital hearing aids

THE NEW SERVICE

As a result of the MHAS program, patients are fitted to nationally agreed protocols that ensure that the technology is used to specifically tailor the hearing aid to each individual's hearing loss. The audiologist spends longer with each patient, and there are now standardized national systems to monitor patient outcomes.

In addition to the equipment and hearing aids, NHS services were given additional funding to recruit extra staff to fit the new hearing aids; furthermore, in order to be able to fit the new hearing aids to their patients, a comprehensive national training package was delivered, including hands-on training within the individual hearing aid department. This has effectively meant that every audiologist in England has been fully trained to fit digital hearing aids to NHS patients.

EVIDENCE-BASED CHANGE

Modern digital hearing aids provide users with an "intelligent" amplifier, the performance of which is programed and fine-tuned by an audiological professional to meet their individual needs. The hearing aid will constantly adapt to changes in the sounds it picks up. In addition, it offers the user a means of choosing the most helpful settings for each listening environment that they encounter in daily life.

The differential benefit to patients was measured using a standardized questionnaire (*The Glasgow Hearing Aid Benefit Profile*). This questionnaire captures how much of the time each person uses their hearing aid, how much it helps in different everyday situations and how satisfied they are with the result. The composite score is shown in Figure 6.

An independent evaluation of the MHAS program by the MRC found that people fitted with high-quality digital hearing aids in the modernized service reported 41% greater overall benefit compared to those with analog aids. They were using their aids for more time, finding them more helpful, and more satisfied with the result.

DISCUSSION

The public health priority of hearing impairments and tinnitus in adults should be substantially higher than it presently appears, because hearing disorders comprise the most prevalent chronic impairment in the population, with over 8 million people in the United Kingdom (i.e. about 20%) having an impairment. The major factor associated with this high prevalence is age, with noise being the major preventable factor, especially in young people. Because age is the major factor, prevalence of hearing impairments in the whole population will increase over the next 20 years by up to 20% because of the change in demographics (Doyle and Gough, 1991). The data show that the need is great at most levels of severity of hearing impairment and particularly for the over-60s. Demand and supply seem to be increasing, which will be driven by the changing demographics of the aging population over the next 20 years. The implications for hearing-aid and rehabilitation budgets are quite substantial even if the same annual incidence of referral for a hearing aid is maintained and not increased using screening, education, or awareness programs so that some of the unmet need can be fulfilled.

There seems to be no reason why elderly people cannot cope with rehabilitation for their hearing disorders, both hearing and tinnitus, unless other factors affecting morbidity interfere. The elderly benefit as much from hearing aids as those who are younger and have about the same usage rates, unless there are other problems that interfere with maintenance of their hearing aids. There is no evidence that central dysfunction handicaps the elderly who are not hospitalized. However, the usage rates are disappointingly low in this group. The implications for service provision are, perhaps, that the hearing aid service for the elderly should be situated increasingly in the community and thought should be given as to how individual care plans can be enacted, which take a client-oriented approach to individual facets of the disability that are presented by clients. There is little evidence on the effectiveness of different styles of rehabilitation on their costs and benefits. The comments received from the 318 individuals who had a hearing aid in the 1990's study suggest that more thought should be given to meeting specific needs (including detailed training in tactics and handling skills) and less emphasis be placed on technology as the primary means to these ends.

In terms of research requirements, there is an urgent need to build up a better evidence base in order to suggest guidelines for better and more acceptable rehabilitation services for the elderly who have a hearing problem. There are very few studies of whole population samples or randomized control trials on which to base good practice. Such trials should be given an urgent priority to consider why take-up and access are so poor and also to determine what factors can increase systematic use of hearing aids for example, early detection and intervention.

KEY POINTS

- Prevalence of hearing impairment is expected to increase by up to 25% by 2020.
- The major factor associated with its high prevalence is age.
- A study of the prevalence is most important for service provision.
- The quality of digital hearing aids in the modernized service in the United Kingdom reported 41% greater overall benefit compared to analog aids.
- The elderly benefit as much from hearing aids as those who are younger and have same usage, unless there are other problems that interfere with maintenance of their hearing aids.

KEY REFERENCES

- Davis AC. The prevalence of hearing impairment and reported hearing disability among adults in Great Britain. *International Journal of Epidemiology* 1989; **18**:911–7.
- Davis AC. Epidemiology. In SDG Stephens (ed) *Scott-Brown's Otolaryngology* 1997, vol 2, chapter 3, Adult Audiology, 6th edn; Butterworth-Heineman, Oxford.
- Sorri M, Jounio-Ervasti K, Uimonen S & Huttunen K. Will hearing health care be affordable in the next millennium? *Scandinavian Audiology* 2001; **30**:203–4.
- Taylor R & Paisley S. *The Clinical and Cost Effectiveness of Advances in Hearing Aid Technology*. 2000; Report to the national Institute for Clinical Excellence United Kingdom. (www.nice.org.uk).

REFERENCES

Alpiner JG. Audiological problems of the aged. *Geriatrics* 1963; **18**:19–27.

Audit Commission. *Fully Equipped: the provision of equipment to older or disabled people by the NHS and Social Services in England and Wales* 2000, http://www.audit-commission.gov.uk/reports/NATIONAL-REPORT.asp.

Barton GR, Davis AC, Mair IWS & Pa M. Provision of hearing aid services: a comparison between the Nordic countries and the United Kingdom. *Scandinavian Audiology. Supplementum* 2001; **30**:16–20.

Brooks D. *Adult Auditory Rehabilitation* 1989; Chapman and Hall, London.

Coles RRA, Smith P & Davis AC. The relationship between noise induced hearing loss and tinnitus and its management. In B Berglund & T Lundvall (eds) *Noise as a Public Health Problem* 1990, pp 87–112; Swedish Council for Building Research, Stockholm.

Davis AC. The prevalence of hearing impairment and reported hearing disability among adults in Great Britain. *International Journal of Epidemiology* 1989; **18**:911–7.

Davis AC. Epidemiological profile of hearing impairments: the scale and nature of the problem with special reference to the elderly. *Acta Otolaryngologica (Stockholm)* 1991; (suppl 476):103–9.

Davis AC. *Hearing Impairment in Adults* 1995; Whurr, London.

Davis AC. The aetiology of tinnitus: risk factors for tinnitus in the UK population – a possible role for conductive pathologies? In GE Reich & JA Vernon (eds) *Proceedings of the Fifth International Tinnitus Seminar* 1996; American Tinnitus Association, Portland.

Davis AC. Epidemiology. In SDG Stephens (ed) *Scott-Brown's Otolaryngology* 1997, vol 2, chapter 3, Adult Audiology, 6th edn; Butterworth-Heineman, Oxford.

Davis AC, Ostri B & Parving A. Longitudinal study of hearing. *Acta Otolaryngologica* 1991; (suppl 482):103–9.

Davis AC & Roberts H. Tinnitus and health status: SF-36 profile and accident prevalance. In GE Reich & JA Vernon (eds) *Proceedings of the Fifth International Tinnitus Seminar* 1996; American Tinnitus Association, Portland.

Davis A, Stephens D, Rayment A & Thomas K. Hearing impairments in middle age: the acceptability, benefit and cost detection (ABCD). *British Journal of Audiology* 1992; **26**:1–14.

Dillon H, James A & Ginis J. Client orientated scale of improvement (COSIE) and its relation to several other methods of hearing aid benefit and satisfaction. *Journal of the American Academy of Audiology* 1997; **8**:27–43.

Doyle L & Gough I. *A Theory of Human Need* 1991; Macmillan Education, Basingstoke.

Gatehouse SG. Application of quality standards to hearing aid services. Outcome measures should be based on listeners' needs. *British Medical Journal* 1994; **308**:1454.

Gatehouse SG & Davis AC. Clinical pure-tone vs three-inferred forced choice thresholds: effects of hearing level and age. *Audiology* 1992; **31**:30–44.

Gates GA, Cooper JC, Kannel WB & Miller NJ. Hearing in the elderly: the Framingham cohort, 1983–1985. *Ear and Hearing* 1990; **11**:247–56.

Gray R. *Surveys of Hearing: Technical Report* 1995, Published by: NatCen, p 1401 http://www.natcen.ac.uk.

Haggard MP. *Research in the Development of Effective Services for Hearing-Impaired People* 1993; Nuffield Provincial Hospitals Trust, London.

Hart FS. *The Hearing of Residents in Homes for the Elderly – South Glamorgan (Report)* 1980; University of Wales.

Martin D & Peckford B. Hearing impairment in homes for the elderly. *Social Work Service* 1978; **17**:52–62.

Quaranta A, Asennato G & Sallustio V. Epidemiology of hearing problems among adults in Italy. *Scandinavian Audiology* 1996; **25**(suppl 42):7–11.

Reich GE & Vernon JA. In GE Reich & JA Vernon (eds) *Proceedings of the Fifth International Tinnitus Seminar, Portland, Oregon* 1995; American Tinnitus Association, Portland.

Rosenhall U, Jönsson R & Söderlind O. Self-assessed hearing problems in Sweden: a demographic study. *Audiology* 1999; **38**:328–34.

Salomon G. Hearing problems and the elderly. *Danish Medical Bulletin* 1986; **33**(suppl 3):1–22.

Schow RL & Norbonne MA. *Introduction to Aural Rehabilitation* 1989; 2nd edn; Pro-Ed, Texas.

Sorri M, Jounio-Ervasti K, Uimonen S & Huttunen K. Will hearing health care be affordable in the next millennium? *Scandinavian Audiology* 2001; **30**:203–4.

Soucek S & Michaels L. *Hearing Loss in the Elderly* 1987; Springer-Verlag, London.

Stephens SDG, Callaghan DE, Hogan S *et al.* Hearing disability in people 50–65: effectiveness and acceptability of early rehabilitation intervention. *British Medical Journal* 1990; **300**:508–11.

Taylor R & Paisley S. *The Clinical and Cost Effectiveness of Advances in Hearing Aid Technology*. 2000; Report to the national Institute for Clinical Excellence United Kingdom. (www.nice.org.uk).

Tolson D, McIntosh J & Swan IRC. Hearing impairment in elderly hospital residents. *British Journal of Nursing* 1992; **1**(14):705–10.

Uimonen S, Huttunen K, Jounio-Ervasti K & Sorri M. Do we know the real need for hearing rehabilitation at the population level? Hearing impairments in the 5- to 75- year-old cross-sectional Finnish population. *British Journal of Audiology* 1999; **33**:53–9.

FURTHER READING

Davis AC, Spencer H & Paulson J. Cost implications in setting a target for hearing aid provision in England and Wales. Poster presented at *The Scientific Basis of Health Services, International Conference*, London, 2–4th October 1995.

Davis AC & Thornton ARD. The impact of age on hearing impairment: some epidemiological evidence. In JH Jenson (ed) *Proceedings of 14th Danavox Symposium. Presbyacusis and Other Age-Related Aspects* 1990, pp 69–89; Danavox Jubilee Foundation, Copenhagen.

Gatehouse S. Rehabilitation: identification of needs, priorities and expectations, and the evaluation of benefit. *International Journal of Audiology* 2003; **42**:2S77–2S83.

Haggard MP & Gatehouse SG. Candidature for hearing aids: justification for the concept and a two-part audiometric criterion. *British Journal of Audiology* 1993; **27**:303–18.

Reeves D, Mason L, Prosser H & Kiernan C. *Direct Referral Systems for Hearing Aid Provision* 1994; HMSO, London.

105

Auditory System

R. Gareth Williams
University Hospital of Wales, Cardiff, UK

INTRODUCTION

The auditory system is one of the special senses, which, together with the visual system, is largely responsible for the way in which we perceive our environment. In addition to audition, the system encompasses the vestibular apparatus with special senses for the detection of gravity and movement (*see also* **Chapter 106, Disorders of the Vestibular System**). The auditory system is responsible for the detection of sound energy, its effective transfer from the surrounding air to the inner ear fluid and the subsequent conversion of this physical stimulus to a psychoacoustic sensation, which we perceive as sound.

Abnormalities of the auditory system can result in a variety of symptoms, the most frequent of which are hearing impairment and tinnitus. Assessment of the auditory system is directed toward

1. the identification of the pathological processes and their anatomical location;
2. quantifying the impairment and disability;
3. reducing the handicap by the most appropriate means.

ACOUSTICS AND HEARING

The transmission of sound through air involves the oscillation of air molecules, producing regions of alternating pressure changes traveling away from the sound source. If these sound waves reach a normal functioning ear, a noise is heard. The human ear is capable of detecting sound wave oscillations of varying frequency and amplitude. Variations in frequency of vibrations are perceived as variations in pitch of sound; similarly, variations in amplitude of vibrations are perceived as a variation in loudness.

Pitch

The frequency of sound wave vibration is measured in Hertz (Hz or cycles per second). Some human ears are able to detect a sound frequency as low as 20 Hz, but hearing is not normally tested for sounds below about 100 Hz. Similarly, sound is not easily detected at frequencies above 10 000 Hz although some individuals can hear up to 20 000 Hz. Pure-tone audiometry (PTA) assesses the ability to hear tones presented to each ear individually and is normally done using between 7 and 11 pure tones in the range between 125 and 8000 Hz.

Loudness

Sound pressure is a physical measure that relates to the perception of loudness. The sound pressure level at which the human ear is able to detect sound is approximately 10 million times smaller than the loudest level that can be tolerated. As a result, it is not practical to refer to actual sound pressure levels when measuring the variations in the threshold and tolerance of sound amongst the human population. The alternative and more practical method is the decibel (dB) scale. The basis of this scale is the comparison of a sound pressure to a reference sound pressure level, usually that at the threshold of normal human hearing (2×10^{-4} dynes cm^{-2}), and converting the ratio into a logarithmic scale (the Bel), then dividing by 10 (the decibel). Using this scale, a sound pressure at the threshold of normal hearing is represented by a decibel score of 0 dB. If the sound pressure being tested is less than the reference level, such that the test to reference ratio is less than 1, the resulting decibel score will be negative. A 10-fold increase in sound pressure level equates to an increase of 20 dB.

Sound frequencies in the midrange of normal human hearing are heard better than those at the extreme ends of the range. In order to simplify the graphical representation of normal hearing levels, a decibel scale is used that uses different reference sound pressure levels for each frequency tested, thus providing a means of representing normal hearing as a horizontal line on an audiogram chart. The decibel scale

Principles and Practice of Geriatric Medicine, 4th Edition. Edited by M.S. John Pathy, Alan J. Sinclair and John E. Morley.

used is known as the *Hearing Level scale* (dB HL) and was initially achieved by testing otologically normal, young adults.

MEASUREMENT OF HEARING LOSS

Clinical assessment of hearing usually begins with free-field voice tests and tuning fork tests. The approximate loudness of the whispered voice is 15 dB at 2 ft and 35 dB at 6 in. Similarly, a conversational voice is approximately 50 dB at 2 ft and 60 dB at 6 in. A loud voice is about 75 dB at 2 ft. Using these figures as a guide, it is possible to estimate the hearing loss by simple voice tests, presenting simple words or numbers to one ear at a time and occluding the opposite ear and rubbing the tragus to help mask the nontest ear.

Tuning Fork Tests

Common tuning fork test that can be helpful in differentiating conductive from sensorineural deafness are the Rinne and Weber tests.

Rinne Test

This test compares the effective transmission of sound through the normal route of the outer and middle ear (air conduction) against the transmission through bone. A tuning fork placed onto the mastoid bone transmits sound to the cochlea through the skull. In the presence of a functioning cochlea, a sound will be heard until the loudness of the tone reduces to the individual's hearing threshold. If the tuning fork is then placed next to the ear canal and heard, it indicates that the normal conductive mechanism is intact. Alternatively, the perceived loudness of sound is compared by alternating the position of the tuning fork between the mastoid and ear canal. In the presence of a conductive deafness, the sound may appear louder by bone conduction than by air conduction. The magnitude of conductive deafness at which the perceived loudness shifts from air to bone conduction is about 20 dB HL (Browning and Swan, 1988). By convention, the "normal" result (air conduction perceived as louder than bone conduction) is a Rinne positive result. If bone conduction sounds louder than air conduction, the result is Rinne negative.

Sound transmission through bone means that sound presented anywhere on the skull will travel to both ears. If a sound source is placed on the right mastoid bone, sound will be transmitted to the right and left cochlea. Therefore, even if the right cochlea is not functioning, the sound will be heard – by the left ear. When the sound is presented to the right ear by air conduction, no sound will be heard because the left ear will not detect the sound. In this situation, the sound will appear louder by bone conduction than air conduction, by virtue of the fact that the opposite ear has detected sound transmitted across the skull. This can be mistaken for a conductive loss and is known as a *false Rinne negative* result.

Weber Test

When a tuning fork is placed centrally on the skull, sound is transmitted to both ears equally. Whether the sound is perceived equally depends on the sensitivity of hearing in both ears. The transmission of sound to the cochlea by bone conduction is not only directly through the skull vault to the cochlea, but also via the skull to the middle ear and then through the ossicular chain to the cochlea. As a result, the transmission of sound by bone conduction is affected by abnormalities of the middle ear. When sound reaches the middle ear through the skull, it will travel through the ossicular chain in both directions, resulting in some loss of sound outwards through the ear canal. Any process that affects the transmission of sound through the middle ear (i.e. a conductive deafness) will reduce the loss of sound from the middle and outer ear. This is one explanation for the phenomenon of increased loudness in the ear with a conductive deafness when the sound of a tuning fork is presented to the vertex of the skull. The magnitude of conductive deafness at which the perceived loudness shifts from midline to the affected ear is about 12 dB(HL) (Stankiewicz and Mowry, 1979).

In the absence of a conductive deafness, the loudness of the tone will be determined by the relative sensitivities of both cochlea. Therefore, the lateralization of the Weber test may be because of a conductive loss in the affected ear or a sensorineural loss in the opposite ear.

Pure-tone Audiometry

Hearing thresholds can be assessed using audiometry. The commonest method used is pure-tone audiometry (PTA), which measures the subjective threshold of hearing of various pure-tone frequencies. The results are usually presented graphically and normally include both air conduction and bone conduction. Air conduction refers to the detection of sound as presented through the normal anatomical pathway, via the outer ear. The sound may be presented either through standard earphones, or alternatively through insert earphones or using free-field sound from speakers. Bone conduction measures the threshold of sound applied directly to the skull.

The pure-tone audiogram graphically represents the magnitude of hearing loss at different frequencies. It is convenient to summarize the average hearing loss as a single figure, and by convention, the thresholds over the midrange of 0.5, 1, 2, and 4 kHz are used. On this basis, hearing impairment can be described according to the severity of the average loss (see Table 1; Browning, 1998).

In healthy state, the air conduction is similar to bone conduction. In broad terms, hearing loss may be due to abnormalities of the sound conduction mechanisms affecting the outer or middle ear, resulting in a conductive deafness, or

Table 1 Classification of deafness based on pure-tone average hearing thresholds at 0.5, 1, 2, and 4 kHz)

Pure-tone average (dB)	Description
0–24	Normal
25–50	Mild
51–70	Moderate
71–90	Severe
91–110	Profound
>110	Total

alternatively, may be due to abnormalities of the cochlea or neural pathways resulting in a sensorineural deafness. Differentiation between conductive and sensorineural deafness identifies the anatomical part of the auditory pathway at fault and in turn allows a suitable management plan to be made. Most conductive losses are associated with identifiable changes affecting the outer and middle ear, including the tympanic membrane.

Acoustic Admittance and Tympanometry

The ability to measure the ease with which sound energy travels through the middle ear has been developed into a clinical application that is easily used to assess so-called acoustic admittance of the ear. Acoustic tympanometers are used to measure admittance, a parameter that is influenced by changes in the stiffness, mass, and resistance of the tympanic membrane and middle ear. The test is performed automatically using a sealed probe inserted into the ear canal, which measures the changes in intensity to an 85 dB SPL (sound pressure level) tone at 226 Hz as the pressure in the ear canal between probe tip and drum are adjusted from −400 daPa to +200 daPa, relative to atmospheric pressure. Acoustic admittance will vary as the pressure changes, because of the splinting effect of the increase or decrease in pressure on the eardrum. When the pressure in the outer ear is similar to the middle ear pressure, the acoustic admittance will be highest. A graphical representation of this series of measurements is the tympanogram, and is clinically useful because it provides information about middle ear pathologies and can identify normal and abnormal contraction of middle ear muscles. Examples of different tympanograms are shown in Figure 1.

The normal pattern, known as a *type A curve*, has a distinctive peak in the vicinity of atmospheric pressure. The height of the peak represents the acoustic admittance of the middle ear and is affected by changes in stiffness and mass. A low peak is seen in conditions that fix the ossicles such as otosclerosis. A flat curve is known as a *type B tympanogram*, and is seen in the presence of middle ear fluid, but can also occur if there is a perforated drum or impacted wax. If the peak of the tympanogram is shifted to the left, it indicates that acoustic admittance is best when the pressure in the outer ear canal has been reduced below atmospheric, and, by inference, corresponds to the middle ear pressure. A peak below −100 daPa is a type C tympanogram and may occur in the presence of Eustachian tube obstruction associated with

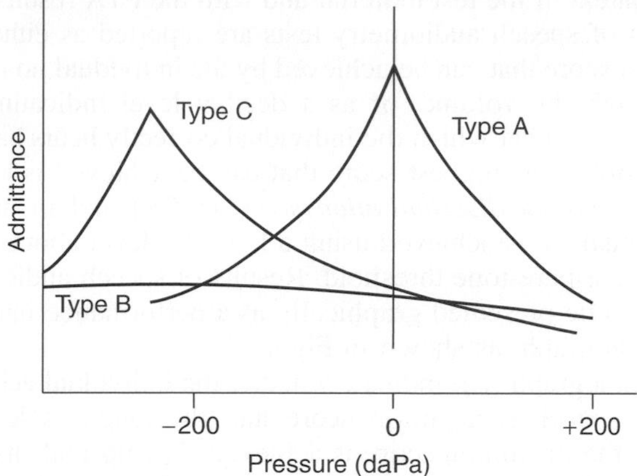

Figure 1 Classification of tympanogram shapes. (a) Normal tympanogram with peak centred at atmospheric pressure. (b) Flat curve due to middle ear fluid. (c) Negative peak due to eustachian tube dysfunction associated with a negative middle ear pressure

a negative middle ear pressure due to a failure to replace middle ear air lost by absorption through the middle ear mucosa.

Tympanometry can be used to assess the integrity of the stapedius muscle contraction by virtue of the fact that this muscle can be made to contract in response to a loud sound; contraction alters the middle ear mechanics, resulting in reduced acoustic admittance. The introduction of a loud sound and measurement of acoustic admittance constitutes an acoustic reflex test, the afferent arm of which is the stimulation of the acoustic nerve and the efferent arm is triggered by a bilateral brain stem (superior olivary complex) reflex to the facial nerve, which supplies the stapedius muscle. The test will assess the integrity of both the 7th and 8th cranial nerves and can be performed ipsilaterally (stimulus and tympanometry in same ear) or contralaterally (stimulus and tympanometry probe in opposite ears).

Speech Audiometry

The assessment of speech perception is perhaps a more appropriate test of hearing than PTA when assessing impairment. A speech audiometer can assess the ability to perceive and understand the complex and rapidly changing spectrum of sound that constitute speech. The test is usually performed using headphones and asking the patient to repeat words presented at varying loudness levels. Words may be presented as single words from standard word lists (e.g. Boothroyd word lists) or as sentences. When using sentences, key words in the sentence are used for scoring. The ability to understand words presented within the context of a meaningful sentence is easier than words presented in isolation. Speech audiometry can also be assessed using visual presentation as well, combining the speech signal with a recorded image of the speaker in a standard audiovisual test.

Because of the varied ways in which speech tests are performed and reported, the results must be interpreted within the context of the test material and with the PTA results. The results of speech audiometry tests are reported as either the highest score that can be achieved by the individual no matter how high the volume, or as a decibel level indicating the loudness level at which the individual correctly hears half the test words. The highest score that can be achieved is known as the *optimal discrimination score* (*ODS*) and in normal individuals, it is achieved using a loudness level about 30 dB above the pure-tone threshold. Results of speech audiometry can also be presented graphically as a performance-intensity function graph, as shown in Figure 2.

Such a graph will indicate whether the individual achieves 100% speech recognition score and the loudness level at which the maximum score is achieved. The normal shape to the speech audiogram performance-intensity graph is a rapid increase in speech recognition over a 20–30 dB increase in loudness, to the maximum speech recognition level of 100%. Two common abnormalities are seen using this type of graph, a shift to the right in the presence of a conductive loss or a reduced speech recognition score seen in sensorineural deafness.

Speech audiometry is particularly useful when assessing hearing disability and the value of interventions such as hearing aids or surgery. Because speech recognition is a phenomenon largely regulated by neural processing beyond the cochlea, abnormalities affecting the cochlear nerve or central auditory pathways will have a greater affect on speech recognition than on the detection of pure tones, which is a much more basic audiological function. Therefore, hearing loss caused by a retrocochlear pathology will result in a greater-than-expected loss of speech discrimination, than that predicted by the pure-tone audiogram. With retrocochlear pathology, the discrimination of speech may in fact deteriorate with increasing loudness, resulting in another type of speech audiogram curve where the speech recognition score decreases after reaching its peak, so-called rollover (Figure 2). Speech audiometry is therefore useful in that it reflects the site of the disorder as well as degree of disability.

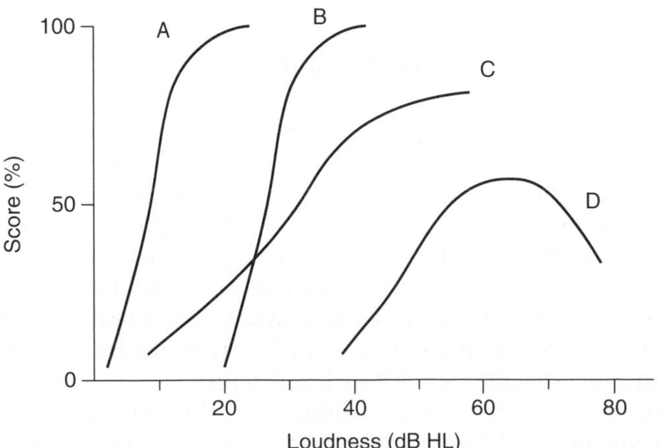

Figure 2 Speech audiometry, examples of various performance-intensity curves. (a) normal hearing individual reaching maximum score of 100%. (b) conductive deafness causing displacement of curve to the right by 25 dB. (c) sensory deafness in a patient whose score reaches 80% at 50 dB. (d) neural deafness in a patient with rollover, representing deterioration in discrimination with increasing loudness

THE SYMPTOMS OF EAR DISEASE

Hearing Loss

One of the commonest symptoms of ear disease is hearing loss. The broad classification of hearing loss is conveniently categorized according to the anatomical site within the auditory pathway affected. Deafness caused by any abnormality affecting the transmission of sound to the cochlear is a conductive deafness, whereas abnormalities of the cochlea or subsequent neural pathways result in sensorineural deafness. The distinction is useful as it conveniently allows the clinician to focus on the different potential pathological processes and management approaches that are required for the two types of deafness.

Conductive Hearing Loss

Most causes of conductive deafness can be identified on otoscopy. Common causes are listed in Table 2.

Wax (Cerumen)

Wax is an uncommon cause of deafness because it either has to completely occlude the ear canal or impinge against the eardrum. Wax is produced by the ceruminous glands, found in the outer third of the ear canal. Wax will become impacted if attempts are made to clean ears using blunt objects such as cotton tipped probes or tissues. Wax can become impacted by hearing aid molds if there is excessive wax production.

Wax should be removed either by syringing or manual removal using suitable wax hooks, ear forceps, or microsuction. Hard occlusive wax is best softened first, using oil or sodium bicarbonate. Syringing should not be performed in the presence of a known perforation or if the ear is effectively the only hearing ear, in which case, patients are best referred to an otologist for careful manual removal (Aung and Mulley, 2002).

Table 2 Causes of conductive deafness according to site

Site	Description
Pinna	Atresia, perichondritis
Ear canal	Wax occlusion, otitis externa, osteoma, foreign body, tumor ("ceruminoma")
Tympanic membrane	Myringitis, perforation, calcification (tympanosclerosis)
Middle ear	Otitis media, ossicular fixation (otosclerosis or ankylosis), ossicular disruption, tumor (e.g. glomus)

Otitis Externa

The accumulation of infected debris and soft tissue occlusion of the ear canal in otitis externa may result in conductive deafness. Infection may be bacterial, viral, or fungal. Acute bacterial otitis externa is a very painful condition. Discomfort and irritation of the ear canal precedes the most severe period of pain, and discharge often precedes the onset of deafness. The mainstay of treatment is removal of debris and wax, usually by gently syringing or microsuction, and instillation of topical antibiotic and steroid drops. Ear swabs for bacteriology should be taken beforehand so that recalcitrant infection can be treated appropriately. The commonest bacterial pathogens are Staphylococcal and Pseudomonas (Roland and Stroman, 2002), over 90% of which remain sensitive to aminoglycosides and quinolones. Therefore, topical gentamicin or ciprofloxacin (0.3% solution) is often effective. Topical treatments are only effective after the removal of infected debris and discharge.

Fungal otitis externa is most often seen following prolonged antibiotic treatment. Careful cleaning and removal of fungal hyphae and spores will maximize the chances of resolution. Topical antifungal treatments using clotrimazole or clioquinol are important adjuncts. Systemic treatment is only needed in invasive infection in immunocompromised patients.

Myringitis

Inflammation or infection of the tympanic membrane is not uncommon, and tends to be mistaken for otitis media by virtue of the fact that the appearances can be similar.

Acute myringitis is usually viral in origin and may be accompanied by bullae on the outer surface of the drum. A common form of myringitis is characterized by hemorrhagic bullae associated with severe, sudden onset otalgia and conductive hearing loss, so-called *myringitis haemmorhagica bullosa*. It may be associated with sensorineural deafness in up to 40% cases. Granular myringitis has the typical appearance of vascular granulations on the outer surface of a de-epithelialized drum. This may respond to the application of topical steroid, repeated cauterization using silver nitrate carefully applied using an otological microscope or it may require surgical skin grafting (Blevins and Karmody, 2001).

Otitis Media

Infection or inflammation of the middle ear cleft is a common cause of conductive deafness. The distinction between inflammatory and infective otitis media is useful in that treatment options and symptoms differ between the two pathologies, although both coexist much of the time. Infective otitis media is usually followed by an inflammatory process before full resolution, characterized by a middle ear effusion that may take a few weeks to fully resolve. Conversely, inflammatory otitis media is characterized by the production of a sterile middle ear effusion, which may become secondarily infected.

Acute Infective Otitis Media

Acute infection of the middle ear cleft is usually viral. This may take the form of infection of the middle ear cleft itself or nasopharyngeal infection affecting Eustachian tube function. Secondary bacterial infection can occur, resulting in a prolonged episode requiring systemic antibiotics. Viral to bacterial conversion in acute otitis media occurs in about 10–20% of cases. In the majority of cases, therefore, all that is required is analgesia until the acute viral episode resolves after 2–3 days. Bacterial otitis media is characterized by increasing pain and toxicity, often culminating in tympanic membrane perforation and mucopurulent discharge from the ear. Common bacterial pathogens are *Streptococcus pneumoniae, Hemophilus influenzae*, and *Moraxella catarrhalis*. First-line treatment should be with amoxicillin or erythromycin for 5 days (O'Neill, 1999).

Chronic Otitis Media

Chronic middle ear infections are conveniently divided into those associated with cholesteatoma and those associated with middle ear mucosal disease and tympanic membrane perforations, the latter type is referred to as *tubotympanic otitis media*. The distinction between these types of chronic infection is not absolute and both may coexist. Historically, a distinction was made because cholesteatoma was thought to have a greater likelihood of leading to intracranial infection, but this is not the case. The serious complications of facial nerve palsy and meningitis are just as common with mucosal disease (Sing and Maharaja, 1993). The actual risk of developing intracranial infection from active chronic otitis media is between 0.5 and 1% over a 60-year period (Nunez and Browning, 1989).

Conductive deafness in chronic otitis media has a number of potential mechanisms. A number of causes may coexist, requiring a combined medical and surgical approach (see Table 3).

Management of Chronic Otitis Media

Examination of the ear should begin by carefully looking for a postaural scar. Acute mastoid infections were much more common years ago, and many elderly patients will have undergone mastoid surgery as children. Many of these will have been cortical mastoidectomies, whereby infection in the

Table 3 Pathological causes of conductive deafness in chronic otitis media and the otological procedures for their correction

Pathology	Treatment
Perforated drum	Myringoplasty
Disrupted ossicular chain	Ossiculoplasty
Mucosal edema	Topical steroid
Active infection	Antibiotics
	Mastoid surgery with Tympanoplasty
Tympanosclerosis and fixed ossicular chain	Ossiculoplasty

mastoid was drained through a postaural incision removing bone from the outer table of the mastoid, but not opening the cavity into the ear canal. Surgery to deal with cholesteatoma usually leaves an open cavity communicating with the ear canal, allowing inspection and cleaning of the cavity.

Findings on otoscopy direct the investigations and management principles. It is usually possible on inspection to determine if there is active infection or not. With inactive chronic otitis media, the commonest findings are: dry perforations of the tympanic membrane, patchy calcification of the drum (tympanosclerosis), retraction of the tympanic membrane. Retraction of the pars tensa may occur in the central portion of the drum or near the margin, most often the posterior margin. Deep retractions can mimic perforations, the distinction being that retractions are lined with a thin layer of dry squamous epithelium, whereas moist middle ear mucosa can be seen through perforations. Retraction of the pars flaccida in the upper part of the drum (the attic) is more often associated with accumulation of squamous epithelium and recurrent infection and may be the precursor of cholesteatoma or the only external feature of an extensive mastoid cholesteatoma. It is advisable to inspect the ear with an otological microscope where there is a marginal or attic retraction.

Purulent discharge should be cultured and treated using systemic antibiotics such as amoxicillin initially. Persistent infection usually signifies loculations of infected debris, inappropriate antibiotic, or poor penetrance into the middle ear cleft. Careful cleaning and removal of debris from the ear is essential in these cases. The outer ear canal can be dry mopped using cotton wool wrapped/mounted on a probe such as a Jobson Horne probe. It is much more difficult to clean debris lying against the drum or in the middle ear cleft, and this usually requires microsuction using the otoscopic microscope. Topical antibiotics can then be administered. Many of these contain potentially ototoxic antibiotics and are not recommended by manufacturers or the Committee on Safety of Medicines (CSM) in the presence of a perforation. Nevertheless, specialists have used topical aminoglycosides for many years to good effect and consider the presence of pus and active infection in the middle ear to be a greater risk to the hearing than the short-term use of these drops (Lundy and Graham, 1993). A nonototoxic alternative is ciprofloxacin 0.3% or ofloxacin 0.3% (both available as ophthalmic solutions but unlicensed for otitis media), especially as *Pseudomonas* is a common pathogen in chronic otitis media (Ghosh *et al.*, 2000).

Referral to a specialist is recommended in the presence of persistent granulations on the tympanic membrane or middle ear mucosa, or if there is continued drainage despite topical antibiotics.

Complications of Otitis Media

Complications of otitis media are uncommon but can be serious. They fall into two broad groups – extracranial and intracranial.

Extracranial Complications

Acute Mastoiditis. Because the mastoid air cells are confluent with the middle ear space, infection within the mastoid is almost inevitable following otitis media. Improvements in imaging over the last few years have highlighted the frequency of mastoiditis and serve as a reminder that most cases of mastoiditis go undiagnosed and are successfully treated along with the otitis media. Treatment should be modified if there is involvement of the periosteum of the postauricular area with associated erythema and protrusion of the pinna. These features indicate spreading infection and demand a change in antibiotic therapy as well as consideration of intravenous administration. If the tympanic membrane is intact, a myringotomy with drainage of middle ear pus will aid resolution and provide material for microbiology. Progress beyond this stage with osteitis results in increasing fever, postauricular swelling, and downward protrusion of the pinna and requires surgical drainage (mastoidectomy).

Chronic Mastoiditis. Chronicity following simple acute otitis media is uncommon. A more common scenario is an acute infection on a background of chronic disease. Bacterial infection in chronic mastoiditis is more often mixed, anaerobic bacteria can be isolated in the majority of cases, and *Pseudomonas* is quite prevalent.

Acute Labyrinthitis. The pathological progress of inner ear infection allows a distinction to be made between so-called serous labyrinthitis and suppurative labyrinthitis. Serous labyrinthitis results from bacterial toxins and other chemical changes disrupting the normal chemical equilibrium within the perilymph of the inner ear. It is potentially reversible and therefore results in temporary vertigo and a fluctuating sensorineural hearing loss. Conversely, suppurative labyrinthitis refers to bacterial invasion and manifests itself with severe vertigo and profound hearing loss. Meningitis may develop if infection spreads along perilymph channels to the internal auditory canal or through the cochlear aqueduct to reach the CSF. Labyrinthitis secondary to otitis media is today a very rare occurrence, in contrast to a reported 4% incidence at the turn of the last century (Whitehead, 1904).

Facial Palsy in Otitis Media. Only about 5% of all facial palsies are caused by otitis media (Table 4 – causes of facial palsy). Facial weakness rarely occurs in acute otitis media,

Table 4 Causes and incidence of acute facial palsy, excluding true idiopathic ("Bell's palsy"), which still accounts for about 20% of facial palsies (Reproduced from Peitersen E, Bell's palsy, *Acta Otolaryngol Suppl*. (2002) **549**, 4–30, by permission of Taylor & Francis)

Causes	Incidence (%)
Herpes simplex virus type 1	75
Herpes zoster virus	15
Trauma	4
Otitis media or cholesteatoma	5
Rare and unusual conditions	1

but it may occur when the facial nerve canal is dehiscent in the middle ear. In chronic otitis media, the thin bone overlying the facial nerve may be eroded by osteoclastic activity resulting in neuropraxia. The overall incidence of facial nerve palsy increases with age, from approximately 1 per 10 000 at the age of 20 to about 6 per 10 000 at age 60. Facial nerve weakness resulting from middle ear infection will sometimes respond to the treatment targeted toward the middle ear infection.

One of the most important prognostic predictors is the degree of paralysis. Over 90% of partial palsies make a full recovery, whereas the likelihood of recovery reduces to about 60% if the palsy is complete. The rate of recovery of complete facial palsy secondary to middle ear infection improves with surgical intervention. In acute otitis media, a myringotomy should be performed to aspirate middle ear mucopus, sending pus for microbiology. In chronic otitis media, surgery should be performed after radiological investigations, with CT being the most appropriate as it demonstrates bone erosion and cholesteatoma; surgery can then be targeted appropriately.

Petrositis. Extension of infection into the petrous part of the temporal bone may be a cause of persistent otorrhea associated with deep otalgia. Irritation of the trigeminal nerve as it crosses the apex of the petrous temporal bone results in orbital pain and more extensive involvement of the ophthalmic division of the trigeminal nerve. The abducent nerve may also be involved, resulting in a lateral rectus palsy. The combination of trigeminal pain, 6th nerve palsy and deep otalgia constitutes Gradenigo's Syndrome. Diagnosis is confirmed by radiology and requires immediate antibiotic therapy, although the duration of medical treatment before considering surgery is controversial. Access to the petrous apex is difficult and therefore surgery should only be considered if there is a deterioration clinically and radiologically, despite appropriate medical treatment.

Intracranial Complications

Intracranial complications are rare in otitis media, occurring in about 0.3% of all cases (Kangsanarak *et al.*, 1995). When intracranial complications do occur, they are often multiple.

Meningitis (see Chapter 148, Infections of the Central Nervous System). This is the commonest intracranial complication of otitis media, accounting for about a half of all intracranial complications. Treatment must be directed primarily toward the meningitis (Heyderman *et al.*, 2003), using intravenous cefotaxime or cefriaxone. A CT scan will determine whether there are associated complications and whether surgery to drain the ear or mastoid is necessary.

Intracranial Abscess (see Chapter 148, Infections of the Central Nervous System). Subdural, extradural, and parenchymal brain abscesses are less common than meningitis and require the input of neurosurgeons. The mortality of patients with intracranial abscess formation following chronic otitis media is close to 10%.

Lateral Sinus Thrombosis. Thrombosis of the lateral (sigmoid) sinus is diagnosed by MRI or CT scan. Thrombosis may extend into the internal jugular vein and very rarely results in septic emboli. It requires aggressive antibiotic treatment and may require surgery to deal with the mastoid infection and infected clot if symptoms persist. Altered venous drainage may result in raised intracranial pressure and so-called "otitic hydrocephalus", with papilloedema, vomiting, headache, and 6th nerve palsy. It is a misnomer as the ventricles are reduced in volume because of the generalized raised intracranial pressure. It occurs more often in younger patients and is treated by CSF drainage and anticoagulation.

Sensorineural Deafness

Hearing loss in the elderly is predominantly a form of degenerative deafness to which the term "presbycusis" applies. The potential causes of sensorineural deafness increase with increasing age by virtue of the fact that many of the causes are more likely to have occurred in the older population. With increasing age, people are more likely to have been exposed to noise, ototoxic drugs, ear infections, vascular disorders, neural disorders, and trauma. The term presbycusis is reserved for those cases of hearing loss for which there is no identifiable cause and in whom the cause is thought to be related to a degenerative change associated with aging.

What is "Normal" in the Aging Population?

Various epidemiological studies have examined the pattern of hearing loss in the aging population (*see* **Chapter 104, The Epidemiology of Hearing in Aging Population**). Age-related hearing loss (ARHL) affects virtually all people to a varying degree. Studies have shown that the loss with age is greater in men than in women and greater in manual workers even after allowing for noise exposure (Davis, 1989). Figure 3 illustrates the mean hearing thresholds in the typical UK adult male and female population based on the MRC National Study of Hearing (Davies, 1995).

The greatest change in hearing with age disproportionately affects the higher frequency hearing thresholds. The audiograms in Figure 4 illustrate the expected range of hearing in the cohort of men aged 40–49 years compared to the 70–79 year age-group. The shaded areas represent the range of hearing in the 25–75th percentile of these population cohorts (data from MRC National Study of Hearing (NSH) database).

These audiograms demonstrate how the individuals with the least amount of ARHL in the 70–79 year age-group have similar hearing to those individuals with the worst ARHL in the 40–49 year age-group.

The pathological processes responsible for ARHL have been divided into four main groups – sensory, neural, strial, and cochlear conductive (Schuknecht, 1993).

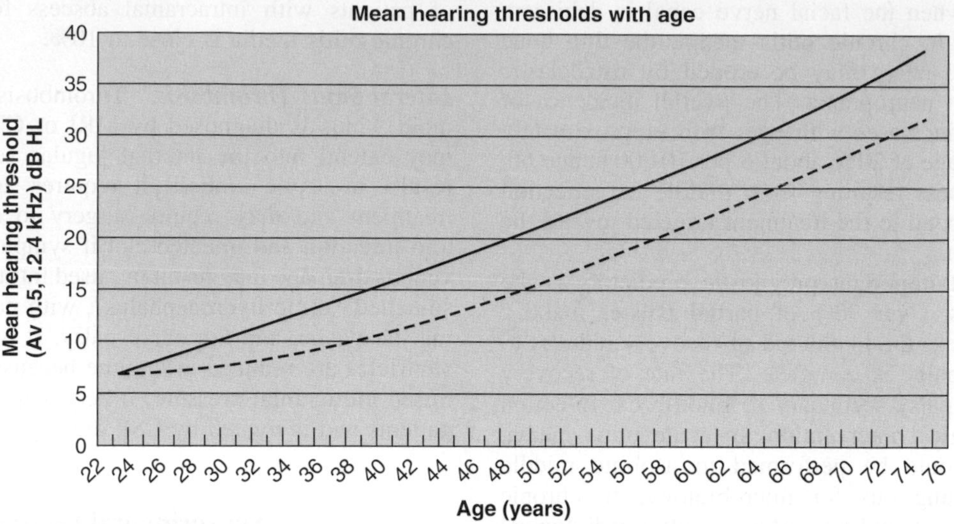

Figure 3 Graph showing mean hearing thresholds against age for men (solid line) and women (dashed line); data from UK MRC National Study of Hearing

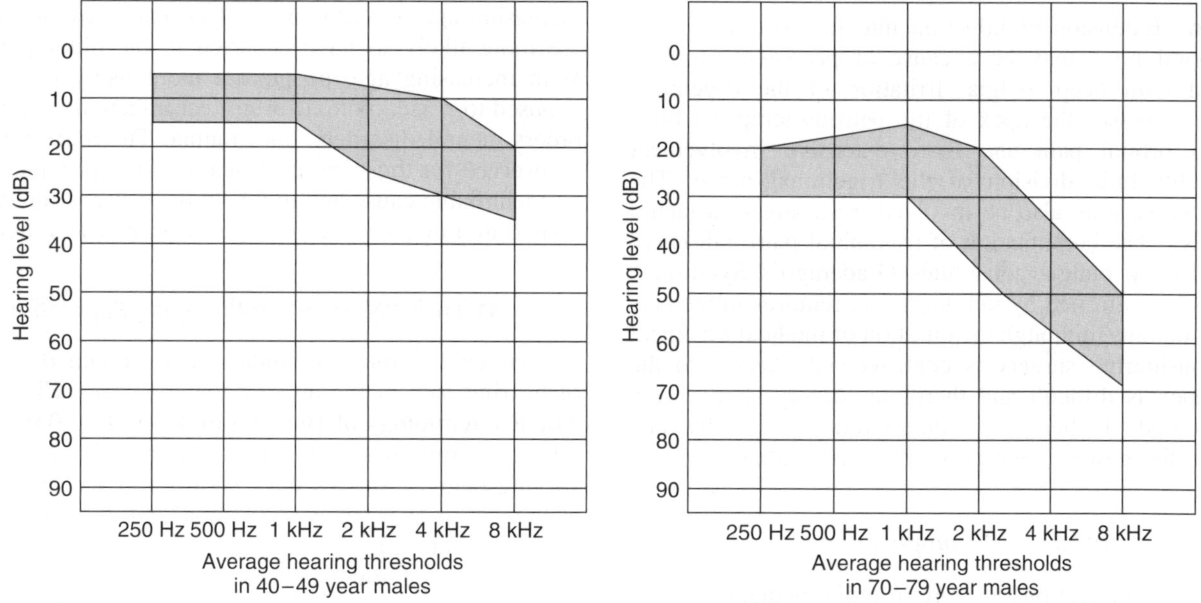

Figure 4 Audiograms illustrating the range of hearing (25th – 75th centiles) in two 10-year cohorts of men, aged 40–49 years and 70–79 years (based on MRC National Study of Hearing)

The different types are based on patterns of histological change associated with characteristic patterns of hearing loss. This is a useful classification in that it helps with the understanding of pathophysiology and may be useful in explaining why similar magnitudes of hearing loss can result in markedly different degrees of discriminatory loss.

Sensory Presbycusis

Sensory presbycusis is predominantly caused by loss of sensory epithelium within the organ of Corti. Most of the loss tends to occur near the basal end of the cochlea, accounting for high-frequency loss. There is relative sparing of the neuronal and supportive elements within the cochlear, which accounts for the reason why many of these types of hearing loss may have quite good speech discrimination.

Neural Presbycusis

Neural presbycusis, on the other hand, is associated with a loss of speech discrimination, which is more marked for a given loss in pure-tone threshold compared to sensory presbycusis. Loss of cochlear neurones is almost inevitable with increasing age, although pure-tone threshold appears not to be affected until about 90% have disappeared. The commonest pattern of pure-tone loss is similar to that seen in sensory presbycusis, a high-frequency loss.

Strial Presbycusis

Degeneration and atrophy of the stria vascularis is believed to affect the homeostatic control of inner ear endolymph and glucose metabolism and has been described as a pathological feature in some forms of familial hearing loss. The pattern of hearing loss affects all frequencies equally, producing a so-called flat loss on PTA. Preservation of the neuronal population results in good speech discrimination relative to the pure-tone hearing loss.

Cochlear Conductive Presbycusis

A fourth pathological variety of presbycusis is proposed on the basis that some individuals with a significant hearing loss have no obvious histopathological changes other than changes to the cochlear likely to result in changes to its mechanical properties, such as fat deposition and calcification in the basilar membrane. Altered electromechanical properties affecting the outer hair cells, which are responsible for the cochlear amplification process, may contribute to this type of hearing loss. These changes are proposed as an explanation for some cases of high-frequency loss without significant loss of sensory epithelium or neuronal population.

Patterns in Hearing Loss

Progressive Bilateral Loss

Overall, it is estimated that about half of all patients with progressive bilateral sensorineural deafness have a genetic cause, and of these, the majority are nonsyndromic (70 vs 30% syndromic), and the majority of these are autosomal recessive (75 vs 25% autosomal dominant). In the remaining patients, environmental factors and certain diseases may be implicated, for instance, noise-induced deafness, ototoxic drug exposure (e.g. aminoglycosides) and viral or bacterial infections. Progressive bilateral deafness is the commonest pattern of hearing loss seen in the adult population. In the majority of cases, the etiology is unknown, but because the prevalence of this type of impairment increases with age, the cause is often thought to be an age-related degeneration ("presbycusis"). Age-related deafness tends to affect the higher frequencies first, the commonest pattern of hearing loss on a pure-tone audiogram being a sloping line downward to the right, which, if severe, is sometimes referred to as a *ski-slope* loss.

The loss of predominantly low frequency hearing is unusual, although it is associated with Meniere's syndrome. The term Meniere's syndrome refers to the triad of sensorineural hearing loss, tinnitus, and episodic vertigo, and has been associated with the pathological changes of endolymphatic hydrops in which the endolymph compartments within the inner ear are expanded relative to the perilymph compartments. Although Meniere's syndrome often affects both ears, it does so in a varied way such that some patients will have an asymmetric loss (see the following text).

Very few general diseases have a proven association with bilateral sensorineural deafness, but they include diabetes (Tay *et al.*, 1995), Paget's disease, and neurosyphilis.

Asymmetrical Hearing Loss

In most individuals with a hearing impairment, there is no noticeable difference between the two ears. An average difference of about 15 dB between ears will be detectable by most people, and the majority of cases of asymmetric hearing loss in the population are due to a conductive deafness. The incidence in the UK population of asymmetric sensorineural deafness is about 3% (MRC NSH data). In the majority of cases, the cause of the hearing loss cannot be identified even after extensive investigations. In about 5% of cases, the deafness can be attributed either to a congenital cause, head injury, previous labyrinthitis, or noise exposure, or to ototoxic drugs. Rather surprisingly, ototoxicity from aminoglycoside drugs predominantly affects one ear in 60% of cases (Lerner *et al.*, 1983).

A small number of patients with asymmetrical sensorineural deafness will have an acoustic neuroma. This benign tumor arising from shwann cells of the vestibular nerve is more correctly termed *vestibular schwannoma* and accounts for 6% of all intracranial tumors. The peak incidence is in the 7th decade, with a slightly higher incidence in females compared to males in the 8th decade. The commonest presenting symptom is an asymmetric hearing loss (90%), or unilateral tinnitus (70%). As the tumor enlarges, it may compress the facial nerve or affect the trigeminal nerve resulting in some facial weakness or paresthesia. Some tumors will enlarge, so as to become life threatening, and, therefore, this is a condition that needs to be identified and treated if necessary. Age alone should not dictate whether or not a patient with appropriate symptoms is investigated. Knowledge of the diagnosis, even if no treatment is offered, may help in patient management. Once established, the most appropriate investigation of a patient with asymmetrical hearing loss is an MRI scan. Specialized audiometric investigations such as auditory brainstem responses (ABR) have a high sensitivity and specificity (over 90%) in the diagnosis of acoustic neuromas; however, the false negative rate of ABR, especially for small neuromas, is unacceptably high and approaches 17% (Wilson *et al.*, 1997). Nevertheless, it may be useful in patients who cannot undergo MRI. CT may not detect small tumors (<10 mm), but may be useful in elderly patients in whom the aim is limited to detecting larger space-occupying lesions. Once diagnosed, management options are interval scanning, surgery, or radiotherapy. Up to two-thirds of acoustic neuroma remains stable over a follow-up period of 35 months (Tschudi *et al.*, 2000) and about 1 in 10 will regress (Luetje, 2000). No study exists that systematically compares the different modalities of management (surgery, radiosurgery, interval scanning). Although surgery will achieve total removal in well over 90% of cases, radiosurgery appears to achieve control of tumor growth in most cases. With both modalities, damage to adjacent neural structures is possible, facial nerve palsy being one of the commonest complications. Operative mortality remains at about 1%.

Sudden Hearing Loss

Sudden hearing loss should be considered a medical emergency if the loss is sensorineural, although for the majority of cases the definitive diagnosis will remain unknown. A sudden loss is defined as 30 dB or more sensorineural hearing loss over at least three adjacent audiometric frequencies occurring within 3 days or less. About one in every 10 000 to 15 000 people will suffer from this condition, with the highest incidence occurring between 50 and 60 years.

Suggested causes of idiopathic sudden sensorineural hearing loss include viral infections, immunologic, vascular compromise, and intracochlear membrane breaks. Serial audiometric testing provides documentation of the progression or resolution of the hearing loss and response to treatment. Few laboratory studies have been shown to be helpful, although initial screening tests should be directed based on history and suspected conditions and aim to identify potentially treatable conditions. Test might include: full blood count, erythrocyte sedimentation ratio (ESR), glucose, cholesterol/triglycerides, T3, T4, TSH, VDRL, and Lyme titer. MRI is useful in evaluating for acoustic tumors, multiple sclerosis, and cerebrovascular accidents. About 10% of all acoustic neuroma present with a sudden hearing loss.

Autoimmune hearing loss may be associated with or part of systemic autoimmune diseases such as Cogan's syndrome, Wegener's granulomatosis, polyarteritis nodosa, temporal arteritis, Buerger's disease (thromboangitis obliterans), and systemic lupus erythomatosis.

Traumatic breaks in the membranous labyrinth are accepted causes of sudden hearing loss. Cochlear membrane breaks may be either intracochlear, as is thought to occur in Meniere's syndrome, or involve the labyrinthine oval and/or round windows with a resultant perilymph fistula. The patient's history will usually elicit an inciting event such as a blow to the head, sneezing, bending over, lifting a heavy object, exposure to sudden changes in barometric pressure (such as during flying or diving), or exposure to a loud noise. Initial treatment should include 5 days of strict bed rest with the head of bed elevated 30°. The patient should avoid straining or forceful nose blowing. Stool softeners may be given. If no improvement is seen after 5 days, surgical therapy, including middle ear exploration with patching of the perilymphatic fistula should be considered.

Because the majority of cases of sudden sensorineural deafness are idiopathic, treatment options are limited. Despite this, there is a long list of suggested options described, which include steroids, cyclophosphamide, methotrexate, diuretics, antiviral agents, vasodilators, and low-molecular-weight dextran, although there is little supportive evidence for their use (Wilkins *et al.*, 1987). Some studies have found that steroids had a significant effect on the recovery of hearing in patients with hearing loss between 40 and 90 dB (Moskowitz *et al.*, 1984; Wilson *et al.*, 1980), whereas patients with profound hearing loss do not appear to benefit significantly from steroid use.

Tinnitus

Although a common symptom, tinnitus rarely becomes a significant clinical problem, but when it does, it requires careful evaluation and a combination of counseling and consideration of various management strategies.

Tinnitus is a symptom whereby an individual has a conscious perception of sound originating from within the individual. The perceived sound varies considerably between patients. One useful characteristic that may indicate the source of the tinnitus is that of pulsation, which may represent transmitted vascular sounds indicative of cardiovascular pathology. Another unusual description that suggests a physical origin to the tinnitus is that of a repetitive clicking or "a chirping cricket" that may occur in myoclonus of middle ear muscles (usually tensor tympani) or palatal muscles.

Physiological tinnitus accounts for less than 5% of all cases presenting to a tinnitus clinic, and the majority of these result from the perception of vascular sounds. A pulsation or humming noise may originate from arterial or venous flow in or around the ear, or from stenosis of the carotid artery. Occasionally, transmitted cardiac sounds, especially murmurs associated with aortic stenosis, can cause troublesome pulsatile tinnitus. Rarely, vascular malformations or tumors such as glomus tumors of the middle ear (*glomus tympanicum*) or jugular fossa (*glomus jugulare*) will present with pulsatile tinnitus.

Pathophysiological tinnitus occurs in situations where auditory function is temporarily disturbed by external factors. The three commonest factors are noise exposure, pharmacological, and toxemic. Excessive noise exposure has long been associated with tinnitus. Short-term noise exposure can result in temporary tinnitus as a result of probable chemical and neurological effects within the cochlear. The duration of noise exposure that may produce tinnitus varies according to the noise level, typically from being a few hours exposure to noise at 90 dB to a few milliseconds of high-intensity explosive sounds. Prolonged and repetitive exposure to loud sound may result in longer periods of temporary tinnitus, eventually leading to permanent tinnitus and hearing loss, with the greatest loss being close to 4 kHz.

Drug-induced tinnitus may be temporary or permanent. Although there are a large number of drugs associated with tinnitus, most cases of drug-induced tinnitus are associated with those listed in Table 5. They broadly fall into two groups, those associated with permanent tinnitus and deafness as a result of ototoxic effects and those producing

Table 5 Drugs capable of causing either permanent or temporary tinnitus

Permanent tinnitus	Temporary tinnitus
Aminoglycosides	*Nonsteroidal anti-inflammatory drugs*
Gentamicin	Ibuprofen
Neomycin	Diclofenac
Streptomycin	Indomethacin
Tobramycin...	
Other antibiotics	*Antidepressants*
Rifampicin	Venlafaxine
Vancomycin	
Chloramphenicol	
Erythromycin	
Polymyxin	
Cytotoxic agents	*Hypnotics*
Cisplatin	Benzodiazepine
Vincristine	
Loop diuretics	*Antimalarials*
Frusemide	Quinine
Bumetanide	Primaquine

temporary tinnitus, often as a result of effects on the central nervous system.

As well as inducing tinnitus as a result of pharmacological changes to the auditory system itself, some drugs are associated with tinnitus as a consequence of a hyperexcitable state brought on during rapid drug withdrawal. This is not uncommon with benzodiazepines.

Tinnitus may occur in patients with systemic illness, who are toxic and in whom the illness causes a temporary tinnitus. Many of these individuals have an underlying abnormality predisposing them to tinnitus.

Pathological tinnitus occurs as a result of physical or psychological disorders, which can broadly be divided into disorders of the auditory pathway, or disorders affecting other associated systems. Auditory disorders can be further classified as those affecting the conductive mechanism, the cochlea, the peripheral neural pathway or the central auditory pathway. The associated systems that can give rise to tinnitus include transmitted sounds from muscular structures (e.g. palatal myoclonus in which there is episodic twitching of the soft palate), respiratory sounds transmitted through a patulous Eustachian tube and vascular sounds. Vascular tinnitus may be "physiological" or may be secondary to turbulent blood flow through normal or abnormal structures adjacent to the ear. A history of pulsatile tinnitus, which is synchronous with the pulse, requires further radiological investigations including carotid assessment and, if the carotids are normal, magnetic resonance angiography if a skull base vascular tumor or vascular malformation is suspected.

The auditory disorders giving rise to tinnitus are usually associated with hearing loss, the identification and investigation of which usually locates the site of the abnormality. Conductive tinnitus may result from the reduction of ambient background noise consequent to the conductive deafness. Tinnitus is an uncommon association with isolated conductive losses; it is more often seen in sensorineural deafness. Individuals with sensorineural deafness and tinnitus may experience a deterioration in the tinnitus if they develop an additional conductive loss, as a result of accumulation of wax or debris in the ear canal, for instance.

Tinnitus arising from disorders of the cochlea and/or cochlear nerve account for the majority of tinnitus cases. An association between the severity of hearing loss and the prevalence of tinnitus means that tinnitus is more likely to occur in the aging population, with up to 70% of patients with presbycusis attending audiology clinics admitting to having some degree of tinnitus (Spoendlin, 1987). There is also a broad association between the perceived loudness of the tinnitus and the severity of the hearing loss. Despite these associations, not everyone with a sensorineural deafness suffers from tinnitus. Various studies have estimated the prevalence of tinnitus within different groups and populations. The NSH in the United Kingdom found that 7% of the adult population consult their family doctor at some point of time because of tinnitus. The commonest group that seek advice are aged 55–65 years (MRC Institute of Hearing Research, 1987), about 40% of patients attending tinnitus clinics are aged over 60 years, and a quarter of these (10% of attendances) are aged over 70 years (Hazell *et al.*, 1985). Many of the reports and studies of tinnitus prevalence gather data from specialist clinics and therefore from a highly selected population, which tends to bias the data. Unselected epidemiological studies have indicated that less than 0.5% of the UK population suffer troublesome tinnitus, whereas 35% of the adult population have suffered nontroublesome tinnitus (MRC Institute of Hearing Research, 1987).

Investigation

The history may direct the examination and subsequent investigations, which should include general examination of the cardiovascular and neurological systems, concentrating on the head and neck. This should include auscultation of the neck and ears and, cranial nerve examination including baseline audiology. Assessment of the tinnitus is of some value in that pitch and loudness matching using an audiometer will give an indication of the characteristics complained of.

Although a variety if blood tests have been advocated in the investigation of tinnitus, they must be interpreted with caution; there are no specific blood investigations necessary for the investigation of tinnitus in isolation. Radiological investigations may be necessary where there is clinical evidence or suspicion of a vascular cause or pathology within the temporal bone affecting the VIIIth nerve.

Treatment

In the vast majority of cases, tinnitus cannot be eliminated, and treatment is directed toward ameliorating the effects, with only about 5% of cases having an identifiable cause that can be treated. The majority of patients with tinnitus also have a hearing loss and anything that can be done to reduce this may also benefit the tinnitus by virtue of increasing the awareness of ambient background noise. For the time being, there is no routine specific medical treatment for tinnitus. It has been known for sometime that intravenous lidocaine can reduce or eliminate tinnitus and there have been reports of its use in severe tinnitus (Marzo *et al.*, 2004), but its effects are temporary and the potential risks outweigh its benefits for routine use. These reports have increased interest in the local application of similar drugs to the round window membrane or middle ear cavity via a small catheter inserted into the middle ear (Adunka *et al.*, 2003; Schwab *et al.*, 2004), the results of which indicate little or no benefit on the tinnitus, although there does appear to be a short-term benefit in the control of vertigo in Meniere's disease.

The mainstay of tinnitus therapy is psychological support and counseling, once treatable causes have been eliminated. Professional counseling is usually available at local audiology departments, with much of the work now being done by audiological physicians supported by hearing therapists. Counseling can be supported by literature and there are many suitable booklets and information leaflets on this subject. The availability of material on the Internet has also enabled patients to understand more about tinnitus and access useful self-help advice. The quality and suitability of this information is varied, and should not be recommended unless appropriate. Some information may be difficult to understand and can lead to rather negative and pessimistic conclusions. In the United Kingdom, patients can be encouraged to join local self-help groups, which are often set up by local members of the British Tinnitus Association. The association also provides useful information on the Internet (http://www.tinnitus.org.uk) and can provide support material and audio recordings for relaxation in the form of tapes and CDs. Additional help is sometimes provided by way of tinnitus maskers. These devices provide a source of noise that the patient finds more acceptable than the tinnitus; they do not (as the name suggests) cancel the tinnitus sound. Complete masking is unusual, most patients report being able to perceive the sound of the tinnitus as well as the masking noise. The use of environmental sounds to relieve the tinnitus may seem an obvious alternative, yet many elderly patients will not have thought of this. Tinnitus is often more troublesome in a quiet environment and can be particularly troublesome at night. The presence of background noise from a clock, fan, or radio can be beneficial, and the use of a flat under-pillow speaker to deliver low volume sounds can help in relaxation and sleep. Many tinnitus support associations provide recordings of sounds that can be useful in relaxation.

Surgical treatment of tinnitus is very limited, although many patients with both profound deafness and tinnitus who have received a cochlear implant have reported improvements in the tinnitus. The prevalence of tinnitus amongst these patients is high (approximately 80% have significant tinnitus), but between 50 and 70% report improvements or resolution of tinnitus after implant surgery (Tyler, 1995; Ito and Sakakihara, 1994).

The Management of Hearing Loss in the Elderly

The nature of progressive hearing loss in the elderly, by virtue of its slow relentless progress, results in a degree of adaptation. This may be all that is needed in the early stages, when the odd misunderstanding creeps into conversation and may be followed by a simple explanation. Also, the listener may be able to modify the listening environment, for example by sitting closer to family and friends, especially in noisy environments.

As hearing loss worsens, adaptations occur that become more noticeable to others. The volume of the television and radio increase, people are asked to repeat themselves more and more; slowly but surely, frustration grows and situations with difficult listening environments are avoided. Group conversations become an ordeal. Frustration turns to embarrassment or, worse, bitterness, and loneliness.

The magnitude of the hearing loss does not in itself determine the disability caused by the loss because this is also determined by the patients' listening requirements. Various self-assessment questionnaires have been used to assess disability and are useful in assessing the benefit of any intervention.

Amplification

Apart from hearing aids (detailed below) there are many other sources of amplification to help hearing-impaired adults. These include personal listening devices that can be used in isolation or act as a link between a hearing aid and television, radio, or other sound sources. Many of these are available on the NHS in the United Kingdom and are provided through audiology departments on the advice of various professionals, including hearing therapists, audiologists, otologists, and audiological physicians.

Hearing Aids

Hearing aids are amplification devices that allow the users to perceive sounds that would otherwise have been at intensity levels below their auditory thresholds. The basic components of most simple hearing aids are a microphone, a transducer and amplifier, and a receiver or loudspeaker. Most hearing aids are powered using a small battery housed in a hidden battery compartment. Air conduction hearing aids have a custom-made earmold taken from an impression of the patient's ear. Rarely, earmolds cannot be tolerated or used, in which case a bone conducting hearing aid can be used. These transmit sound to the mastoid bone through a bone conduction vibrator held in place by either a spring headband or surgically implanted attachments.

Air Conduction Hearing Aids

These are hearing aids that deliver sound to the ear through a receiver or speaker in the ear canal, the sound traveling through the air of the ear canal. The commonest variety is the "behind the ear" (BTE) configuration, which consists of a small hearing aid behind the pinna onto which a custom-made earmold is fitted. Most hearing aids fitted in the United Kingdom on the NHS are of this type.

Some patients prefer small discrete aids that fit into the ear canal. The hearing aid components are fitted within the hearing aid mold. These aids vary in size with some small enough to fit well within the ear canal ("in the canal" (ITC)); others are slightly larger, sitting in the conchal bowl of the pinna ("in the ear" (ITE) or modular hearing aids) and still being visible. ITE and modular aids tend to need more frequent repairs than BTE hearing aids, with the added disadvantage that patients often have to have another ear mold made in order to manufacture a new aid. The BTE aids can be replaced off the shelf and immediately fitted onto the patient's existing ear mold.

Digital hearing aids are those that process the sound signal digitally before converting it back into an analog sound signal. They too come as BTE, ITE, or ITC types. They can process and adjust sounds in various ways, providing additional benefits for some patients. Analog hearing aids may still be preferable to digital aids in some situations; for instance, there appears to be little benefit in using digital over analog aids in many cases of conductive deafness.

The external features of a typical BTE hearing aid is shown in Figure 5. The introduction of digital aids has increased the variety of aids available and in use by patients. Most aids have a battery compartment, which, in small aids, may serve as the on/off switch. The aid may have a separate selection switch including the on/off control. Analog aids with conventional control switches will have three positions: M, T, and O. "M" is used to select the microphone (i.e. switching on the aid), "T" for using the induction loop in the aid, and "O" for Off. When set to the "T" setting, the aid can pick up a signal from an induction loop system and will

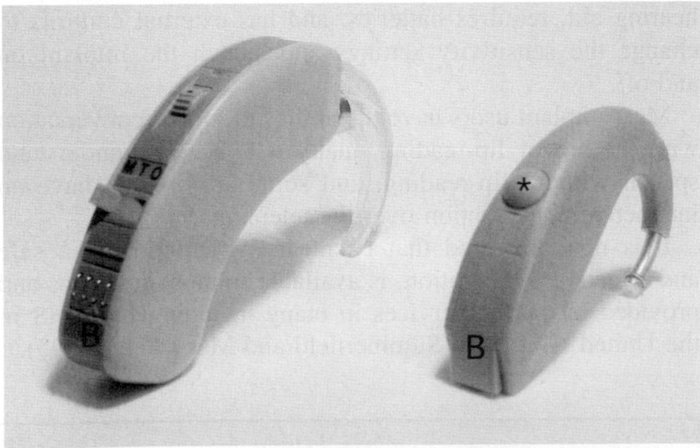

Figure 5 Modern, behind the Ear (BTE) hearing aids. On the left is one with conventional patient controls including a volume control wheel. On the right is a digital aid that can be programed to a number of different settings. The button marked with an asterix is used to cycle through the different programs. B indicates the battery compartments

inactivate the external hearing aid microphone. This has the advantage of cutting out any background noise. The presence of a "loop system" is normally indicated in public places such as banks and post offices; they are often used in churches, theaters, and cinemas. Hearing aid–compatible telephones also use a loop system and can improve the clarity of sound when using the "T" setting.

Digital aids have the capacity to be programed to manipulate sounds to the advantage of the listener according to the magnitude and frequency location of the hearing loss. Two or more programs can be loaded into the aid, so an additional feature on digital aids is the ability to select different programs, for instance, one for common everyday use and another for listening to music.

Most hearing aids have a volume control wheel, although many digital aids will automatically adjust volume and some will not have a manual volume control. With some digital aids, it is possible to disable the volume control wheel (useful in confused elderly patients who "fiddle" with their aids), a point to remember if patients report an apparent fault with this control.

Candidature

Any patient with hearing difficulty is a potential candidate for a hearing aid. A simple predictor of hearing aid use is the degree of disability for everyday speech (Davies *et al.*, 1991). Also, those patients unable to hear a forced whisper at 70 cm in their worst ear are likely to accept a hearing aid. The mean hearing threshold at which patients seek amplification is about 45 dB HL, and over 50% of patients with an average loss of 55 dB HL or more will accept and use bilateral hearing aids. That is not to say that hearing aids cannot provide significant benefit to those with lower hearing thresholds, but reluctance to use hearing aids for various reasons means fewer people than predicted ask for aids. It is estimated that only about 35% of patients with hearing thresholds of 45–55 dB HL have hearing aids (Davies, 1997).

The UK National Study of Hearing, carried out by the MRC Institute of Hearing Research (Davies, 1995) found that approximately 20% of individuals in the age bracket 71–80 years had hearing thresholds worse than 45 dB. The overall prevalence of individuals reporting hearing difficulties in the United Kingdom population is 16%, but in the 75-and-over age-group, 52% report difficulties with their hearing (General Household Survey, 2002; Office of National Statistics, UK). Less than half of these wear hearing aids (23%) (see Figure 6).

Approximately 1 in 10 people given a hearing aid are, for various reasons, nonusers. The percentage of hearing aid users who continue to have hearing difficulties despite using hearing aids is not age dependant, with about 60% of all age-groups reporting some ongoing difficulties. This is perhaps a reflection that patient expectations are often unreasonable, many expect hearing aids to restore hearing to near normal. This will never be achieved by amplification alone, especially where there is associated central neural degeneration affecting discrimination and central processing.

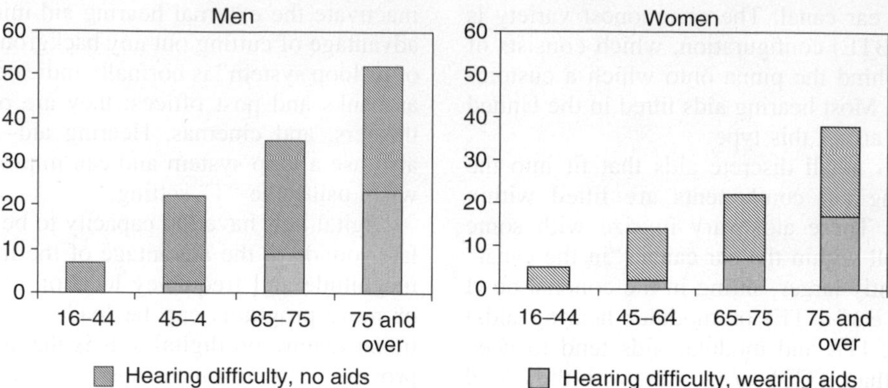

Figure 6 Percentage by age of men and women reporting some difficulty with hearing. Based on: Living in Britain, General Household Survey 2002, Office of National Statistics

Part of the process of hearing aid fitting should involve careful counseling and support in other ways so as to reduce the residual disability after appropriate hearing aid fitting. With this type of approach, about 95% of patients fitted with hearing aids will continue to use them on a regular basis.

Other Types of Hearing Aids

Bone conducting hearing aids provide a means of directing sound to the ear through the skull. They can be attached either to a headband or on the end of spectacle arms, directing sound to the mastoid bone behind the pinna. They are used only if air conduction aids cannot be used because of atresia of the ear canal or a chronic persistent discharge from the ear.

Bone anchored hearing aids work in similar situations, but are attached to a surgically implanted receiver (abutment). The abutment is a metal stud onto which the custom-made hearing aid attaches. This is useful if the need for a bone conducting aid is a long-term one.

Cochlear Implants

In situations where the hearing loss is so severe that there is little residual hearing, and the patient is unable to benefit from conventional hearing aids, cochlear implants may be used. Cochlear implants consist of an internal component, which has to be surgically implanted, and an external processor worn behind the ear or as a body worn device. The internal component consists of a receiver placed under the skin behind the ear and an electrode array inserted into the cochlear itself. The number of electrodes on the array varies according to the design of the device, most commonly used implants having between 12 and 22. The external component consists of an external coil that transmits the signal to the internal receiver, a speech processor and microphone. In the BTE variety of cochlear implants, the microphone is situated on the speech processor and is similar to a BTE hearing aid.

In order to benefit from a cochlear implant, the auditory nerve must be intact, and there must be a residual population of spiral ganglion cells within the cochlea. Insertion of the electrode into the cochlea is only possible if the cochlea is patent, although obliteration by disease (labyrinthitis following meningitis, or otosclerosis) is not a contraindication, a specially designed split electrode being used in such circumstances.

The outcomes from cochlear implantation are varied and can be difficult to predict beforehand. Suitable candidates are adults who have lost their hearing in both ears and gain little or no benefit from the most appropriate, properly fitted, and adjusted hearing aids. Adults with speech recognition scores on speech audiometry of less than 30% may be considered. One of the best predictors of successful outcome is the period of deafness, with those deafened for over 20 years unlikely to do well.

Not only must patients be well enough to undergo the surgery, which lasts about 2 hours, they should have realistic expectations and the ability to attend regular rehabilitation sessions. The implant itself functions like a complex hearing aid, requires batteries, and has external controls to change the sensitivity settings and switch the implant on and off.

Most implant users have the ability to follow conversation with the aid of lip-reading, many will learn to understand speech without lip-reading, and some are able to have an interactive conversation over the telephone.

It is now accepted that cochlear implantation is a safe and effective intervention, is available in most countries and provided by public services in many including the NHS in the United Kingdom (Summerfield and Marshfield, 1995).

KEY POINTS

- Hearing assessment should be performed using clinical evaluation, supplemented by audiometry; speech audiometry will provide a better indication of disability than PTA. PTA will indicate the likely site of pathology.

- Conductive hearing losses are usually associated with identifiable conditions on otoscopy and may be treated by a number of methods, including medical, surgical, and amplification.
- Sensorineural deafness is common in the elderly population and requires investigation if asymmetrical or sudden in onset.
- Mild forms of tinnitus are common, are most often associated with a hearing impairment. Most require limited investigations, counseling, and amplification.
- Hearing aid technology has improved the quality of rehabilitation of deafened adults; some complex and severe hearing losses may be treated using bone anchored hearing aids or cochlear implants.

KEY REFERENCES

- Browning GG. *Clinical Otology & Audiology. Second Edition.* 1998; Butterworth Heinemann, Oxford.
- Davies AG. Epidemiology. In *Adult Audiology* Scott-Brown's Otolaryngology, 1997, vol 2, Chapter 3, 6th edn; Butterworth-Heinemann, Oxford.
- Davis AC. The prevalence of hearing impairment and reported hearing disability amongst adults in Great Britain. *International Journal of Epidemiology* 1989; **18**:911–917.
- O'Neill P. Acute otitis media. *British Medical Journal* 1999; **319**:833–835.
- Schuknecht HF. *Pathology of the Ear* 1993, 2nd edn; Lea & Febiger, Philadelphia.

REFERENCES

Adunka O, Moustaklis E & Weber A *et al.* Labyrinth anesthesia – a forgotten but practical treatment option in Meniere's disease. *Journal of Oto-Rhino-Laryngology and Its Related Specialties* 2003; **65**:84–90.

Aung T & Mulley GP. Removal of ear wax. *British Medical Journal* 2002; **325**:27.

Blevins NH & Karmody CS. Chronic myringitis: prevalence, presentation, and natural history. *Otology & Neurotology* 2001; **22**:3–10.

Browning GG. *Clinical Otology & Audiology. Second Edition.* 1998; Butterworth Heinemann, Oxford.

Browning GG & Swan IRC. Sensitivity and specificity of the Rinne tuning fork test. *British Medical Journal* 1988; **297**:1381–2.

Davies A. *Hearing in Adults* 1995; Whurr Publishers, London.

Davies AG. Epidemiology. In *Adult Audiology* Scott-Brown's Otolaryngology, 1997, vol 2, Chapter 3, 6th edn; Butterworth-Heinemann, Oxford.

Davies JE, John DG & Stephens SDG. Intermediate hearing tests as predictors of hearing aid acceptance. *Clinical Otolaryngology* 1991; **16**:76–83.

Davis AC. The prevalence of hearing impairment and reported hearing disability amongst adults in Great Britain. *International Journal of Epidemiology* 1989; **18**:911–17.

Ghosh S, Panarese A, Parker AJ & Bull PD. Quinolone ear drops for chronic otitis media. *British Medical Journal* 2000; **321**:126–7.

Hazell JWP, Wood SM & Cooper HR *et al.* A clinical study of Tinnitus maskers. *British Journal of Audiology* 1985; **19**:65–146.

Heyderman RS, Lambert HP & O'Sullivan I *et al.* Early management of suspected bacterial meningitis and meningococcal septicaemia in adults. *Journal of Infection* 2003; **46**:75–7.

Ito J & Sakakihara J. Tinnitus suppression by electrical stimulation of the cochlear wall and by cochlear implantation. *Laryngoscope* 1994; **104**:752–4.

Kangsanarak J, Navacharoen N, Fooanant S & Ruckphaopunt K. Intracranial complications of suppurative otitis media: 13 years' experience. *American Journal of Otology* 1995; **16**:104–9.

Lerner AM, Cone AL & Jansen W *et al.* Randomised, controlled trial of the comparative efficacy, auditory toxicity, and nephrotoxicity of tobramycin and Netilmicin. *Lancet* 1983; **i**:1123–5.

Luetje C. Spontaneous involution of acoustic neuromas. *American Journal of Otology* 2000; **21**:393–8.

Lundy LB & Graham MD. Ototoxicity and ototopical medications: a survey of otolaryngologists. *Otology & Neurotology* 1993; **14**:141–7.

Marzo S, Stankiewicz JA & Consiglio AP. Lidocaine for the relief of incapacitating tinnitus. *Ear, Nose, & Throat Journal* 2004; **83**(4):236–8.

MRC Institute of Hearing Research. Epidemiology of tinnitus in adults. In JWP Hazell (ed) *Tinnitus* 1987, chapter 3; Churchill Livingstone.

Moskowitz D, Lee KJ & Smith HW. Steroid use in idiopathic sudden sensorineural hearing loss. *Laryngoscope* 1984; **94**:664–6.

Nunez D & Browning GG. The risks of developing an otogenic intracranial abscess. *Journal of Laryngology and Otology* 1989; **104**:468–72.

Office of National Statistics, UK; Living in Britain 2002 General Household Survey, National Statistics website: www.statistics.gov.uk Chapter 11, Hearing & Hearing aids: http://www.statistics.gov.uk/CCI/nugget.asp?ID=831&Pos=1&ColRank=2&Rank=880.

O'Neill P. Acute otitis media. *British Medical Journal* 1999; **319**:833–5.

Peitersen E. Bell's palsy: the spontaneous course of 2,500 peripheral facial nerve palsies of different etiologies. *Acta Oto-laryngologia Supplementum* 2002; **549**:4–30.

Roland PS & Stroman DW. Microbiology of acute otitis externa. *Laryngoscope* 2002; **112**:1166–77.

Schuknecht HF. *Pathology of the Ear* 1993, 2nd edn; Lea & Febiger, Philadelphia.

Schwab B, Lenarz T & Heermann R. Use of the round window micro cath for inner ear therapy – results of a placebo-controlled, prospective study on chronic tinnitus. *Laryngo- Rhino- Otologie* 2004; **83**:164–72.

Sing B & Maharaja TJ. Radical mastoidectomy: its place in otitic intracranial complications. *Journal of Laryngology and Otology* 1993; **107**:113–8.

Spoendlin H. Inner ear pathology and tinnitus. In H Feldmann. (ed) *Proceedings of the Third International Tinnitus Seminar, Munster* 1987, p 42–51; Karlsruhe, Harsch Verlag.

Stankiewicz JA & Mowry HS. Clinical accuracy of tuning fork tests. *Laryngoscope* 1979; **89**:1956–63.

Summerfield AQ & Marshfield DH. *Cochlear Implantation in the UK 1990–1994* 1995; HSMO Publications, London. Report by the MRC Institute of the Hearing Research in the evaluation of the national cochlear implant programme.

Tay HL, Ray N, Ohri R & Frootko NJ. Diabetes mellitus and hearing loss. *Clinical Otolaryngology* 1995; **20**:130–4.

Tschudi DC, Linder T & Fisch U. Conservative management of unilateral acoustic neuromas. *American Journal of Otology* 2000; **21**:722–8.

Tyler RS. Tinnitus in the profoundly hearing-impaired and the effects of cochlear implants. *Annals of Otology, Rhinology, & Laryngology – Supplement* 1995; **165**:25–30.

Wilkins SA, Mattox DE & Lyles A. Jr Evaluation of a "shotgun" regimen for sudden hearing loss. *Otolaryngology Head and Neck Surgery* 1987; **97**:474–80.

Wilson WR, Byl FM & Laird N. The efficacy of steroids in the treatment of idiopathic sudden hearing loss. *Archives of Otolaryngology* 1980; **106**:772–6.

Wilson DF, Talbot M & Mills L. A critical appraisal of the role of auditory brainstem response and magnetic resonance imaging in acoustic neuroma diagnosis. *American Journal of Otology* 1997; **18**(5):673–81.

Whitehead AL. Suppuration in the labyrinth. *Journal of Laryngology Rhinology and Otology* 1904; **19**:242–5.

106

Disorders of the Vestibular System

Linda M. Luxon[1,2] *and* **Charlotte Ågrup**[1]

[1] *University College of London Hospitals NHS Trust, London, UK, and* [2] *University College London, London, UK*

INTRODUCTION

Man has developed a sophisticated system for maintaining balance, which requires the integration and modulation of visual, vestibular, and proprioceptive information within the central nervous system (CNS) (Figure 1). Pathology of any one of the three sensory inputs or of the central vestibular pathways may give rise to disequilibrium, as may many pathological processes that affect directly or indirectly the systems essential for perfect balance (Table 1). Dizziness is a frequent complaint in elderly, and the prevalence of balance problems at age 70 has been reported in 36% of women and 29% of men, increasing with advanced age to 45–51% at ages 88–90 (Jonsson *et al.*, 2004). Dizziness and vestibular abnormalities are reported to be a major risk factor predisposing to falls among the elderly (O'Loughlin *et al.*, 1993) and the significance of this lies in the high morbidity and mortality associated with falls in this age-group (Downton, 1993). In addition, fear of falling may constitute an independent risk factor for disability, leading older people to unnecessarily restrict their daily living activity (Burker *et al.*, 1995; Staab and Ruckenstein, 2003). However, with the correct diagnosis many vestibular disorders are treatable, leading to improved quality of life. Thus for the geriatrician, an understanding of the pathophysiology of the vestibular system and its central connections is particularly important if the common complaint of disequilibrium is to be managed successfully.

VESTIBULAR ANATOMY

The inner ear is a minute, complex, fluid-filled structure surrounded by a bony labyrinth located deep in the temporal bone. The cochlea corresponds to the acoustic end-organ, whereas the vestibular end-organs consist of the three semicircular canals, the saccule, and the utricle. The semicircular canals are called the *horizontal* (or *lateral*), the *posterior*, and the *superior canal*. The two ends of all semicircular canals open into the vestibule, near the utricle. One end of each semicircular canal has a dilated portion, called the *ampulla*, containing the sensory epithelium, that is, the hair cells. The utricle and the saccule correspond to the otolith organs and both contain a small area of sensory epithelium, called *maculae*. All vestibular sensory epithelium is covered with a gelatinous mass, which, in the saccule and the utricle, contains calcium carbonate–rich crystals termed *otoconia*.

A force parallel to the surface of the sensory epithelium provides the maximal stimulus. The semicircular canals with their ampullary tissue sense angular acceleration, whereas the saccule and the utricle sense linear acceleration. The planes of the two otolith organs lie approximately at right angles to each other. The utricular macula is oriented roughly horizontally and the saccular macula is roughly vertical. Accordingly, the saccule is well equipped to sense vertical head acceleration and the constant pull of gravity, whereas the utricle senses linear head motion in the horizontal plane. The utricle also plays an important role in signaling the spatial upright when the head is tilted with regard to gravity. The ampullae in the semicircular canals are insensitive to the static gravitational vector or position of the head in space. However, when an appropriate angular force is introduced, the fluid in the semicircular canal is displaced along the lumen of the canal leading to changed activity in the sensory epithelium of the ampullae.

PHYSIOLOGY AND AGING OF THE VESTIBULAR APPARATUS

In a normal subject holding the head in the anatomical position, the sensory epithelium in each ear generates resting neural activity, which passes via the VIIIth cranial nerve and the vestibular nuclei within the brainstem to the cortex.

Principles and Practice of Geriatric Medicine, 4th Edition. Edited by M.S. John Pathy, Alan J. Sinclair and John E. Morley.

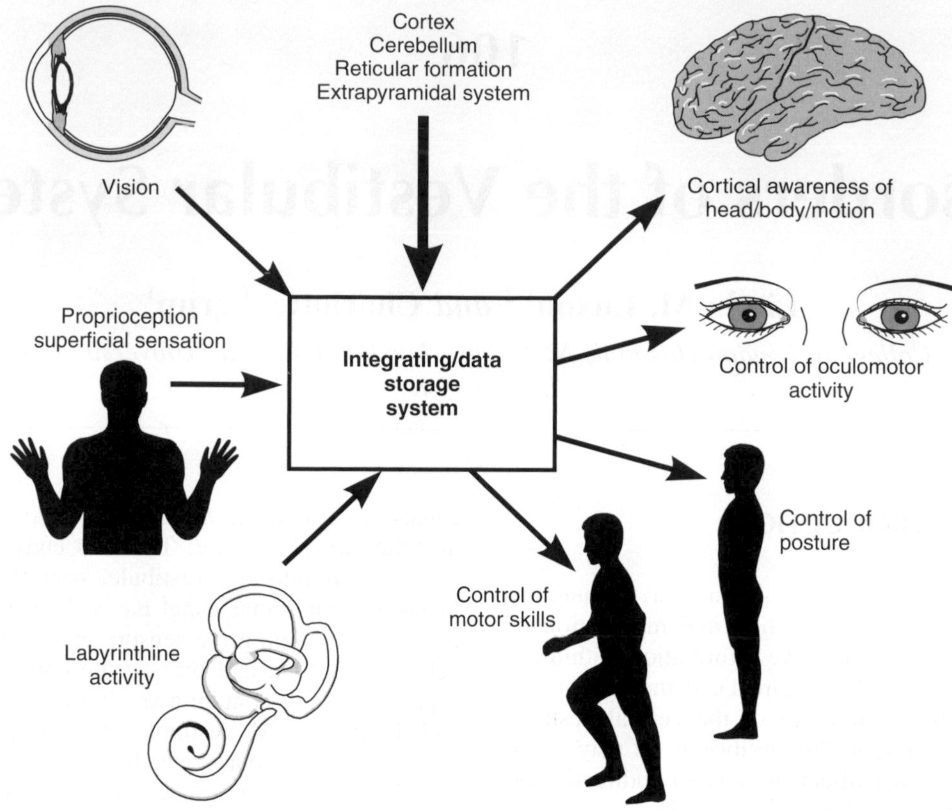

Figure 1 Mechanisms subserving balance in man (Reproduced from Savundra P and Luxon LM, 1997. Copyright Elsevier)

Head movements result in linear and/or angular accelerations, which stimulate the vestibular sensory epithelium and modulate the neural activity in an equal but opposite manner in each ear (Figure 2). Hence, an asymmetry of information is generated, which passes into the CNS. This asymmetric vestibular input allows cortical awareness of head position in space and provides the stimulus for compensatory eye and body movement (Savundra and Luxon, 1997). Pathology involving the peripheral labyrinth, VIIIth cranial nerve, or central vestibular connections may result in an asymmetry of vestibular information, which is "misinterpreted" by the brain and perceived as vertigo and instability.

The incidence of vertigo has been reported to rise with advancing age, in parallel with the incidence of hearing loss (Enrietto *et al.*, 1999). Histopathologic age-related changes reported in the human vestibular sensory organs include progressive hair-cell degeneration, otoconial degeneration in the otolith organs, and decreasing number of vestibular nerve fibers (Rauch *et al.*, 2001; Nadol and Schuknecht, 1990). In addition, age-dependent changes in both caloric and rotation-test responses have been demonstrated (Enrietto *et al.*, 1999; Kazmierczak *et al.*, 2001). However, vestibular symptoms result from an asymmetry of afferent information arising within the vestibular apparatus and degenerative changes tend to occur symmetrically. It is therefore unlikely that disequilibrium in the elderly is solely consequent upon vestibular degenerative changes and is more probably multifactorial in origin (Baloh, 1992). Accordingly, dizziness in the elderly is often the result of central pathology and/or sensory deficits: visual impairment (not correctable); neuropathy; vestibular deficits; cervical spondylosis; and orthopedic disorders, interfering with joint mechanoreceptors.

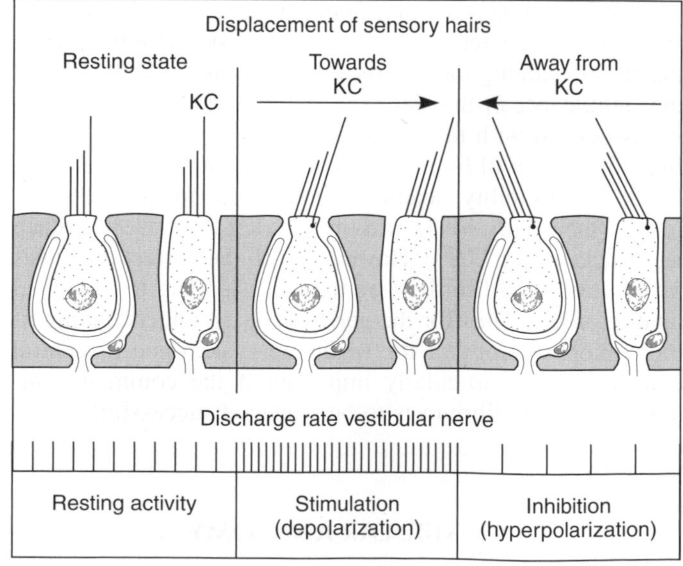

Figure 2 Schematic illustration of the relation between hair-cell orientation and the pattern of stimulation of the innervating fibers in the mammalian crista. KC = kinocilium (Reproduced from Wersall J *et al.*, 1967. Copyright Elsevier)

Table 1 Causes of dizziness in the elderly

General medical	
Hematological	Anemia
	Polycythemia
	Hyperviscosity syndromes
Cardiovascular	Postural hypotension
	Carotid sinus syndrome
	Dysrhythmias
	Mechanical dysfunction
	Shock
Metabolic/endocrine	Hypo- and hyperglycemia
	Thyroid disease
	Chronic renal failure
	Alcohol
Neurological	
Supratentorial	Trauma
	Neoplasia
	Epilepsy
	Cerebrovascular disease
	Syncope
	Psychogenic
Infratentorial	Vertebrobasilar insufficiency
	Subclavian steal syndrome
	Wallenberg's syndrome
	Anterior inferior cerebellar artery syndrome
	Degenerative disorders including neuropathy
	Tumor, including those of the vestibulocochlear nerves
Infective disorders	Ramsay–Hunt
	Neurosyphilis
	Tuberculosis
Foramen magnum abnormalities	
Cerebellar degeneration	
Basal ganglion disease	
Multiple sclerosis	
Otological	
Drug-induced/ototoxic	
Degenerative (e.g. positional vertigo)	
Posttraumatic syndrome	
Infection	
Vascular	
Tumors	
Menière's syndrome	
Otosclerosis and Paget's disease	
Autoimmune disorders	
Others	
Migraine	
Multisensory dizziness syndrome	

Following an acute unilateral vestibular upset, the patient experiences vertigo, but usually the symptoms are relatively short lived and resolve in 6–12 weeks, as a result of processes collectively known as *cerebral compensation*. Functional recovery depends on the degree of vestibular loss and cerebral compensation. The restoration of perfect balance involves reduction or abolition of the asymmetry in postural and ocular motor tone and recalibration of the gain of dynamic vestibular reflexes, in order to ensure symmetrical compensatory vestibulospinal and vestibulo-ocular reflex action during movement of the head and body. However, in some patients recovery does not occur. The persisting symptoms are usually less dramatic

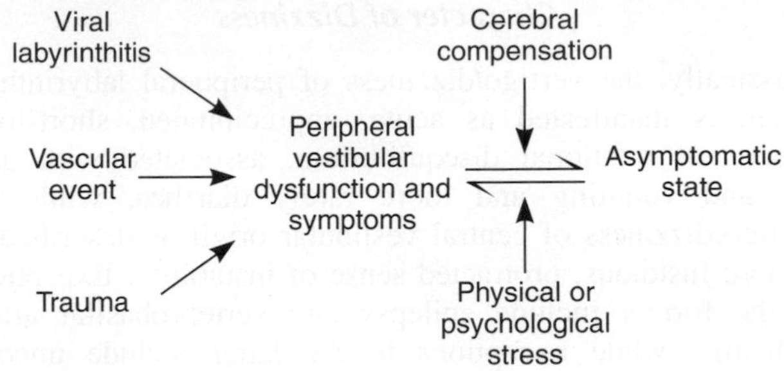

Figure 3 Diagram to illustrate normal sequence of events leading to recovery from a peripheral vestibular abnormality and factors relevant in decompensation

and the vertigo may not be rotational, but may consist of more vague symptoms of floating, rocking, or a sense of depersonalization. Such symptoms may be continuous, but may also present as episodic attacks of disequilibrium frequently triggered by an intercurrent illness or a psychological upset such as bereavement (Figure 3). It is well established that vestibular compensation is dependent on a variety of brainstem, cerebellar, and cortical structures, together with sensory inputs including vision, somatosensory afferents, and remaining labyrinthine input, which are involved in the normal perception of space, body posture, and locomotion. The causes of failure of compensation or intermittent decompensation are not clear, but cerebellar damage, impairment of proprioception, visual impairment, mild cerebral dysfunction, and psychological disorders have all been cited as possible contributing factors. Thus, the age-dependent changes in sensory inputs and CNS function noted above would suggest that central compensation for vestibular deficits in the elderly is likely to be less efficient.

CLINICAL ASPECTS AND DIAGNOSTIC STRATEGY

Vertigo defined as "an hallucination of movement" is a cardinal manifestation of a disordered vestibular system; while dizziness is a lay term, defined in the *Concise Oxford Dictionary* as "a feeling of being in a whirl, or in a daze, or as if about to fall", associated commonly with a multiplicity of general medical disorders. This semantic distinction is volunteered rarely by the elderly patient who more frequently complains of feeling faint, swimmy, or lightheaded. Hence, for practical purposes, all complaints of disorientation are considered most easily within a single diagnostic approach.

History

In the history, the character, time course, and associated symptoms of the dizziness/vertigo are valuable pointers in elucidating the underlying diagnosis.

Character of Dizziness

Classically, the vertigo/dizziness of peripheral labyrinthine origin is manifested as acute, unprecipitated, short-lived attacks of rotational disequilibrium, associated with nausea and vomiting and more rarely diarrhea, while the vertigo/dizziness of central vestibular origin is described as a more insidious, protracted sense of instability. Exceptions to the former include epilepsy and vertebrobasilar artery ischemia, while exceptions to the latter include uncompensated peripheral vestibular disorders, bilateral vestibular failure, and psychogenic disequilibrium. Additional common symptoms with peripheral vestibular dysfunction are a sensation of being pulled downward or sideways or of the room tilting and a sensation of swimming, floating, and lightheadedness. However, if a clear description of subjective or objective motion is given, the suspicion of vestibular pathology is raised, whereas symptoms of lightheadedness, swimminess, or faintness are more likely to be attributable to a general medical/neurological disorder.

Time Course

Acute rotational vertigo of less than 1-minute duration is most commonly associated with the diagnosis of benign positional vertigo or paroxysmal type (see the following text), while acute rotational vertigo of less than 1-hour duration may suggest the diagnosis of vertebrobasilar insufficiency. Vertigo of several hours' duration (less than 24 hours) is most commonly associated with migraine and Ménière's disease (see the following text). Acute rotational vertigo of several days' duration, with gradual resolution of symptoms, points to a viral or vascular vestibular neuritis, although persistence of such symptoms in the elderly patient may indicate poor compensation from a peripheral vestibular insult or a fixed neurological deficit as a result of a vascular event within the brainstem.

Apart from the duration of the vertigo the time course of the episodes is also of diagnostic value. A single acute episode with gradual resolution over days or weeks would point to a peripheral vestibular pathology, such as a viral neuritis or an ischemic event. In the elderly patient, cerebral plasticity is reduced, as noted previously, and hence compensation from such a single insult may be protracted and intercurrent illness may result in an exacerbation of symptoms. Repeated short episodes with complete and rapid recovery in-between would suggest migraine, Menière's disease, or, most commonly, benign positional vertigo. It should be emphasized that in these conditions, the episodes also tend to occur in clusters, with intervals of months, or even years, of freedom.

Associated Symptoms

Within the labyrinth and VIIIth cranial nerve, the vestibular and cochlear elements are in close anatomical proximity. Hence pathology in these sites gives rise commonly to both cochlear and vestibular symptoms. Frequently, the elderly patient will not volunteer a complaint of tinnitus or hearing loss, as they attribute the symptoms to their age, and it is therefore important to enquire specifically. Within the CNS, the vestibular and auditory pathways diverge, and vestibular symptoms of brainstem or cerebellar origin are rarely associated with cochlear symptoms, but commonly associated with neurological symptoms and signs. Loss of vestibular function leads to impaired gaze stabilization during fast head movements, that is, oscillopsia (Bronstein, 2004). Typically, the patients complain of blurred vision or bouncing images while walking or riding in a car. The vestibular system is sensitive to fast, high-frequency head movements (1–10 Hz) and cortical–optokinetic reflexes are too slow to compensate for this functional loss above 2–3 Hz. Many patients with vestibular dysfunction report a worsening or triggering of dizziness with certain visual stimuli, such as rapidly changing images, fast-moving traffic, crowds, and striped material. This symptom is called *visual vertigo* (Bronstein, 2004). In addition, anxiety disorders, depression, and panic attacks have been described in association with peripheral vestibular disease and it is likely that in some patients vestibular dysfunction may play an important role in the etiology of these disorders (Burker *et al.*, 1995; Staab and Ruckenstein, 2003).

Examination

A full general examination is essential with special reference to the fundi, visual fields and acuity, a general neurological examination, and examination of the cardiovascular and peripheral vascular systems. On the basis of a comprehensive history and a thorough examination, the diagnosis of many neurological and general medical disorders will be excluded. The diagnosis of vestibular disorders giving rise to vertigo/dizziness is based on a neuro–otological examination, which may be divided into:

- an examination of the external ear and tympanic membrane together with clinical tests of auditory acuity/whispered-voice tests and tuning-fork tests;
- an assessment of vestibulo-ocular function;
- an assessment of vestibulospinal function, as part of the overall balance.

Otological Examination

In all patients with vertigo, particularly in ethnic minorities, immigrants, and immunosuppressed patients, it is essential to exclude active, chronic middle-ear disease with labyrinthine erosion. A labyrinthine fistula should be suspected in all patients with vertigo and previous surgery for middle-ear disease. Clinical tests of auditory function, including tuning-fork tests, are important when attempting to localize pathology, since the presence of an auditory deficit may suggest an underlying labyrinthine or VIIIth nerve pathology.

Vestibulo-ocular Examination

A detailed account of vestibular physiology and pathophysiology is beyond the scope of this chapter, but a clear understanding of these subjects is essential if an informed assessment of vestibular function and vestibular investigations are to be made (Eggers and Zee, 2003).

As has been outlined earlier, an asymmetry of vestibular activity may result from unilateral peripheral vestibular, VIIIth nerve, or brain-stem pathology. This asymmetry is "monitored" by the brain and, via the pathways subserving the vestibulo-ocular reflex, results in a slow vestibular-induced drift of the eyes in the same direction as the peripheral labyrinthine lesion. For reasons that are not fully understood, this slow drift is interrupted by rapid saccadic eye movements, which are generated within the brainstem in the opposite direction. This combination of slow and fast eye movements is known as *spontaneous vestibular nystagmus* and is characteristic of acute peripheral vestibular lesions. Initially, the nystagmus present with fixation but is more prominent without fixation. As a general rule, nystagmus with fixation (nystagmus seen on routine neurological examination) disappears within 1–2 weeks after the acute lesion. By contrast, spontaneous nystagmus can be recorded in the dark for as long as 5–10 years after the acute episode. Spontaneous vestibular nystagmus will usually beat away from the affected side, unless the lesion is irritative.

By definition, the direction of the nystagmus is defined by the fast phase, for clinical purposes. Thus, a right peripheral vestibular lesion gives rise to horizontal left beating nystagmus, which obeys Alexander's law. This states that the nystagmus is always in one direction irrespective of direction of gaze and that the intensity of the nystagmus is greatest when the eyes are deviated in the direction of the fast phase.

For purposes of accurate record keeping, nystagmus should be described in the following terms: 1° nystagmus describes nystagmus which is beating in the same direction as gaze deviation; 2° nystagmus describes nystagmus in the midposition of gaze; and 3° nystagmus describes nystagmus which is beating in the opposite direction to the direction of gaze (e.g. to the right, when the eyes are deviated to the left).

Bidirectional nystagmus (e.g. first degree nystagmus to the right on looking to the right and first degree nystagmus to the left on looking to the left), vertical nystagmus (i.e. upbeat nystagmus and/or downbeat nystagmus), and dysconjugate nystagmus (a differing nystagmic response in each eye) indicate CNS disease, requiring further investigation.

Clinically, *spontaneous nystagmus* should be sought in every patient complaining of dizziness/vertigo. The eyes should be examined in the midposition of gaze, with eyes 30° to the right and 30° to the left. Care must be taken that this angle is not exceeded, otherwise physiological end-point nystagmus may be observed and this may be confused with pathological nystagmus. In addition, vertical nystagmus with the eyes 30° upwards and 30° downward should be sought.

The presence of *positional nystagmus* is a most valuable and most frequently overlooked sign, and should be sought by a briskly performed Hallpike maneuver (Figure 4). The patient is made to sit close to the top end of a flat examination couch. The head is held firmly between the examiner's hands and turned 30–45° to the right or left. The patient is then carried rapidly backward with the head over the edge of the couch and the eyes carefully observed. If nystagmus develops, it is observed until it disappears, or for 2 or 3 minutes, until it is clear that the nystagmus is persistent. The patient is then returned to the upright position and the procedure repeated in the opposite direction. In broad clinical terms, the positional nystagmus which may develop can be divided into two main types, as identified in Table 2, although there are cases which do not clearly fit into either category, and those should be investigated, as should the "central" category, for neurological disease. If the positional nystagmus is of peripheral labyrinthine origin, after a latent period of a few seconds in the head-back position, severe vertigo develops which lasts for less than a minute, but during which the patient may feel extremely distressed and nauseated. The nystagmus is rotatory in nature and directed toward the undermost ear. Symptoms and signs adapt and fatigue on repeated testing. Thus, care must be taken that the procedure is carried out correctly at the first attempt. Moreover, it is important to establish this condition, as it is a troublesome cause of vertigo for which highly effective treatment is available (see the following text).

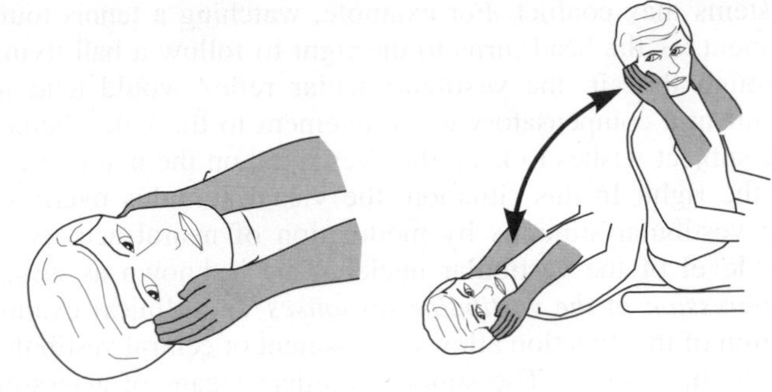

Figure 4 The Hallpike maneuver for inducing positional nystagmus

The vestibular system, via the vestibulo-ocular reflex (VOR), provides one system for the control of eye movements and gaze stability. Visual stimuli provide another mechanism for stabilizing gaze, that is, smooth pursuit and optokinetic reflexes, and under certain circumstances the two

Table 2 Characteristics of positional nystagmus

	Benign paroxysmal type	Central type
Latent period	2–20 seconds	None
Adaptation	Disappears in 50 seconds	Persists
Fatigue ability	Disappears on repetition	Persists
Vertigo	Always present	Typically absent
Direction of nystagmus	To undermost ear	Variable
Incidence	Relatively common	Relatively uncommon

systems may conflict. For example, watching a tennis tournament, as the head turns to the right to follow a ball flying through the air, the vestibulo-ocular reflex would tend to result in a compensatory eye movement to the left, whereas the subject wishes to keep the eyes fixed on the ball moving to the right. In this situation, the visual stimulus overrides the vestibular stimulus by modulation of neural activity at the level of the vestibular nuclei. This is known as *visual suppression of the vestibular responses* and clinical examination of this function allows assessment of central vestibular integrating ability. The simplest clinical means of assessing vestibulo-ocular reflex suppression is by observing the effect of optic fixation upon rotationally induced vestibular nystagmus. This may be simply accomplished in the clinic by observing the patient's eyes, while the patient is oscillated on an office chair while fixating his/her own thumbs (Bronstein, 2004). If the eyes remain fixated on the target, VOR suppression is intact. On the contrary, if clear nystagmus is elicited by the rotation, VOR suppression is abnormal indicating CNS pathology.

Vestibulospinal Assessment

Vestibulospinal function cannot be assessed in isolation and tests are nonspecific and insensitive, compared with tests of vestibulo-ocular function, but they may provide an indication of the extent of the patient's disability and interaction of vestibulospinal activities with other systems. The *Romberg test* is performed by asking the patient to stand in the upright position with feet together, arms by the side, and eyes closed. A tendency to sway to one side usually suggests peripheral vestibular pathology, while an inability to stand with the feet together is more characteristic of cerebellar ataxia. Baloh *et al.*, (1998) have demonstrated that there is a marked increase in postural sway in elderly patients with unilateral vestibular hypofunction, in comparison with younger patients with the same disorder. Anxious elderly patients frequently tend to fall backward like a wooden soldier and this is indicative of a nonorganic component to their symptoms, but it must be emphasized that this is almost always observed in the presence of an underlying abnormality, which will be elucidated on full examination.

Gait testing is assessed by asking the patient to walk toward a fixed point in a normal manner, but with eyes closed. Again, a tendency to veer in one direction is most commonly the result of an ipsilateral peripheral vestibular disturbance, but may on occasions be observed with cerebellar disease. This latter diagnosis is most commonly associated with a broad-based, ataxic gait.

Having briefly reviewed vestibular physiology and pathophysiology and outlined the aspects in the history and examination, which may enable the clinician to identify a vestibular abnormality, the remainder of this chapter will be devoted to a review of the more common causes of vestibular pathology in the elderly and the therapeutic options available.

PERIPHERAL VESTIBULAR DISORDERS

Viral Vestibular Neuritis

Single episodes of acute rotational vertigo associated with nausea and vomiting and with or without cochlear symptoms, are a common occurrence in all age-groups. The attacks are usually unprecipitated, but may be preceded by an upper-respiratory-tract infection, and are therefore presumed to be of viral origin, although there is little definitive evidence for this (Nadol, 1995). Additional possible causes of vestibular neuritis include other infectious agents, vascular, or immune-mediated disorders.

The vertigo may last for a few hours or several days, and the patient may then be extremely unsteady for a period of weeks, during which time cerebral compensation produces a degree of symptomatic recovery. However, in the elderly patient, the plasticity of the CNS is compromised, and recovery is often slower and is rarely complete.

Ramsay–Hunt Syndrome (*see* Chapter 148, Infections of the Central Nervous System)

The Ramsay–Hunt syndrome, or herpes zoster oticus is an example of a mononeuritis of the VIIth cranial nerve. The patient experiences a deep burning pain in the ear, which is followed within a few days by a vesicular eruption in the external auditory canal and on the concha. The patient often develops facial paralysis. In addition, some patients present with hearing loss, tinnitus, vomiting, vertigo, and nystagmus indicating VIIIth nerve involvement (Sweeney and Gilden, 2001).

Bacterial Infection

Chronic middle-ear disease is a prevalent condition in the elderly, and it cannot be overemphasized that in any patient with vestibular symptoms in whom there is the slightest suspicion of middle-ear disease or history of previous middle-ear surgery, the presumptive diagnosis must be of labyrinthine erosion. Labyrinthine fistulae are often the result of bony erosion by cholesteatoma with the lateral semicircular canal being the most commonly affected site (Minor, 2003). Rarely, labyrinthine fistulae may be caused by syphilitic osteitis, tuberculous otitis media, chronic perilabyrinthine osteomyelitis, or glomus jugulare tumor.

Otitis externa is a common benign disorder, but in debilitated elderly patients, particularly diabetics and other immunosuppressive conditions, it may present in a more malignant form (Rubin Grandis *et al.*, 2004). The causative organism is mainly *Pseudomonas aeruginosa*. The disease spreads rapidly, invading surrounding soft tissues, cartilage, and bone structures with occasional involvement of adjacent cranial nerves causing hearing loss and vertigo. Prolonged treatment with effective antibiotics, carbenicillin, or gentamicin, has improved the previously poor prognosis.

Neoplasia

Vestibular disorders as a direct result of neoplasia are uncommon, even in the elderly. The nonmetastatic complications of carcinomatous encephalomyelitis may involve the vestibular nerve (Gulya, 1993), while cochlear and vestibular symptoms have been reported in 10% of patients with carcinomatous meningitis (Alberts and Terrence, 1978).

Secondary tumor involvement of the inner ear by blood-borne metastases from hypernephroma, lung-, prostate-, breast-, and uterine carcinoma have been reported and direct extension of nasopharyngeal carcinoma may occur. Aural tumors are rare, with the exception of cholesteatoma, as outlined previously. Morrison (1975) reported that 20% of patients with acoustic neurinoma were over the age of 60 at the time of presentation. Cochlear symptoms (tinnitus and hearing loss) are the most common presenting symptoms of acoustic neurinoma, but 10% of patients complain of vertigo, dizziness, and/or unsteadiness. A unilateral asymmetric hearing loss must be investigated, and brain-stem auditory-evoked responses provide the best screening technique. If these are abnormal, a computed tomography (CT) scan or, preferably, a magnetic resonance (MR) scan, should be obtained.

The diagnosis and management of this condition in the elderly does not differ from that of any other patient, but early diagnosis is essential, as excellent surgical results are achieved with small tumors (below 20 mm in size) (Tos *et al.*, 2003). However, it has been shown that small tumors do not invariably enlarge with time (Piazza *et al.*, 2003) and the high sensitivity of MR scanning may mean that clinically insignificant tumors may be detected. In the elderly patient, it is reasonable to monitor growth of small acoustic neuromas, but this must be balanced against the significantly decreased mortality/morbidity associated with surgery for smaller tumors.

Vascular Disorders

Both the peripheral and central vestibular apparatus are supplied by the vertebrobasilar circulation and, as cerebrovascular disease is common in developed countries (the risk factors being diabetes mellitus, hypertension, and a raised hematocrit), disequilibrium in the elderly is commonly ascribed to vascular pathology. Ischemia of the internal auditory artery may give rise to three differing clinical syndromes: vestibular disorders alone, cochlear disorders alone, or combined vestibulocochlear symptomatology. An isolated acute episode of rotational vertigo, as outlined in the description of viral vestibular neuritis, may be of vascular origin. The diagnosis is usually presumptive and is based on evidence of vestibular dysfunction in a patient with other manifestations of vascular disease. Risk factors (diabetes mellitus, hyperlipidemia, hypertension, myxedema) should be sought and treated appropriately.

Trauma

The elderly are particularly prone to falls (O'Loughlin *et al.*, 1993), and vestibular abnormalities as a result of even trivial head injury are now well recognized (Luxon, 1996). Damage to the vestibular system may be the result of direct injury, for example, labyrinthine concussion and/or temporal bone fracture, or of secondary shearing forces in the brainstem and cerebellum. Falls may cause cervical trauma in the elderly, which may also give rise to vestibular disturbances (Luxon, 1996).

Two posttraumatic vestibular syndromes may be identified.

Unilateral Auditory and Vestibular Failure

This is associated with transverse fractures of the temporal bone, in which severe vertigo and hearing loss are accompanied by bleeding from the ear, nausea, and vomiting. The patient prefers to lie completely still with the affected ear uppermost. Over a period of 6–12 weeks there is marked improvement in the disequilibrium, although in the elderly patient, as noted earlier, this may be slower and less complete than in a younger person. There is no recovery of the auditory deficit.

Benign Positional Vertigo of Paroxysmal Type

This is the most common clinical syndrome after head injury, but may also be seen in the elderly as an idiopathic disorder or secondary to vestibular neuritis. Recent work has led to the theory of canalithiasis (Figure 5), which explains the majority of the characteristic features of benign positional nystagmus (Brandt and Steddin, 1993; Baloh, 1996). This theory proposes that debris from the otolith organ lies in the most dependent portion of the posterior canal and, upon assuming the critical head position, the clot moves in an ampullofugal direction and, thus, has a "plunger" effect within the narrow posterior semicircular canal. This causes

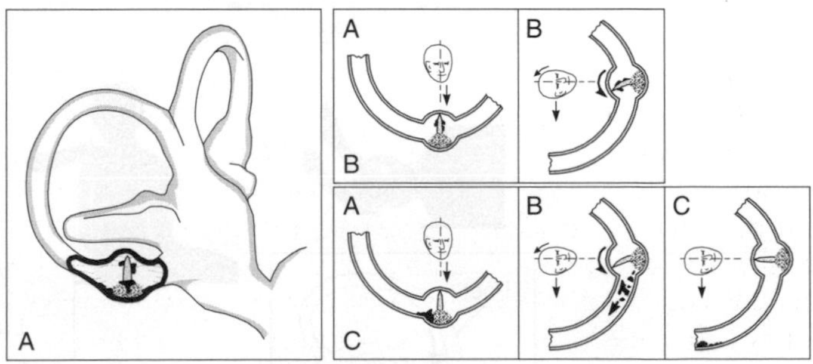

Figure 5 Diagram to illustrate the pathophysiological mechanisms of cupulolithiasis and canalithiasis. (A) Illustration of cupula in ampulla of posterior semicircular canal, with debris attached to and surrounding the cupula. (B) Illustration of the effect of gravity on the cupula and debris as proposed by the theory of cupulolithiasis. (C) Illustration of the effect of gravity on the cupula and debris as proposed by the theory of canalithiasis. (Reproduced from *Vestibular Research*, vol 3, Brandt T and Steddins S, pp 373–82, Copyright 1993, with permission from IOS Press)

movement of the cupula in an ampullofugal direction, with a brief paroxysm of vertigo and nystagmus as a result.

The clinical course of posttraumatic benign positional vertigo is that some days or weeks after even a trivial head injury, momentary, short-lived episodes of vertigo occur, on assuming specific head positions, particularly associated with neck extension. Frequently, the only abnormal clinical sign is benign positional nystagmus of paroxysmal type on performing the Hallpike maneuver (see earlier text). The vertigo associated with this condition is particularly severe and the elderly patient is frequently extremely afraid, as the attacks are very sudden and may cause drop to the ground and vomiting. This leads to anxiety, partly from fear of embarrassment if this should happen in a public place, and partly from fear of being incapacitated at home, unable to reach help. Not infrequently, this diagnosis is overlooked and the clinician merely observes an extremely anxious elderly patient, who finds difficulty explaining such brief yet severe symptoms. It is therefore extremely important that the Hallpike maneuver is performed and a clear explanation of the benign nature of the condition given.

In 1980, Brandt and Daroff (1980) reported complete relief of symptoms in 66 or 67 patients with benign positional vertigo as a result of precipitating head positions "on a repeated and serial basis". They suggested that the mechanism of improvement using this therapy lay in rapid and aggressive vertigo-provocative movements, which loosened and dispersed otholitic debris from the cupula of the posterior semicircular canal (cupulolithiasis) (Figure 5). However, on the basis of our current knowledge, it seems more likely that these maneuvers cleared debris from the most dependent part of the posterior semicircular canal into the utricle, where they no longer interfered with semicircular canal dynamics.

More recently, single positional maneuvers (Epley, 1992) have been described in which specific movements of the head allow the offending debris in the posterior canal to be moved by gravitation into the utricle (Figure 6). The patient is instructed to sit upright for 48 hours after this procedure, which has been reported to be effective in 80–85% of patients on the first attempt at treatment and in a further 10% upon a second attempt. Relapses may occur, but the maneuver should then be repeated. Pretreatment sedation is not required except for the most anxious of patients, and the maneuver is as effective in older people as in younger people.

In a small percentage of patients it would appear that the particle repositioning procedures are not effective and, in intractable cases, plugging of the posterior semicircular canal (Ludman, 1984) or section of the posterior and ampullary nerve (Ludman, 1984) should be considered.

Menière's Disease

Menière's disease was first described in 1861 by Prosper Menière and is characterized by episodic vertigo,

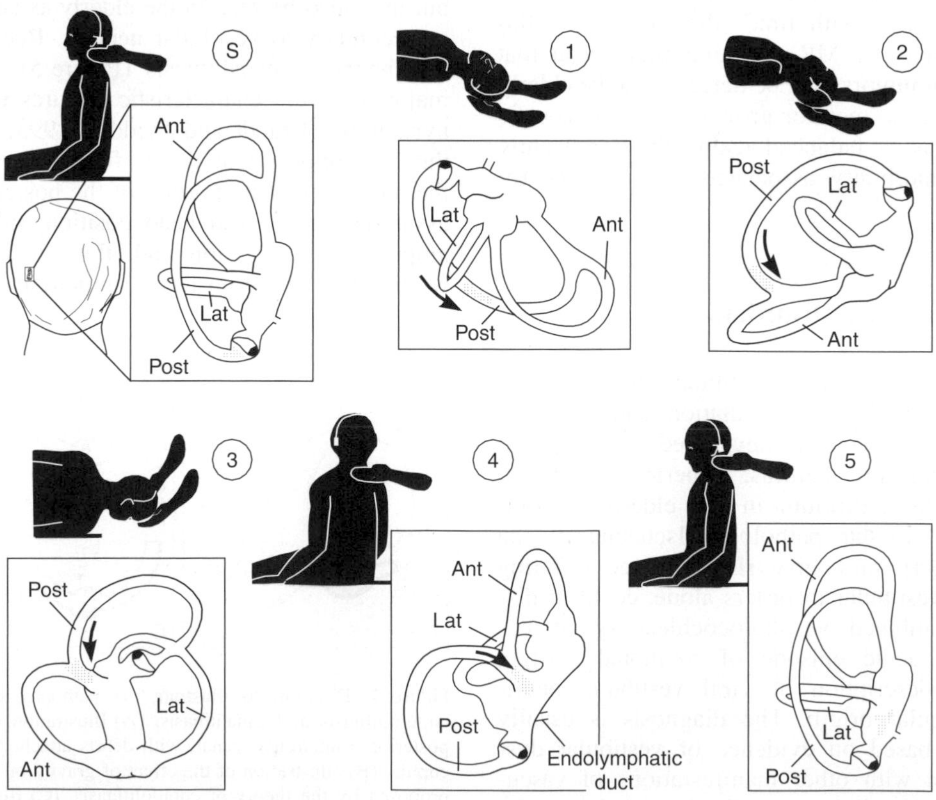

Figure 6 Diagram to illustrate particle repositioning procedure for canalithiasis of lest posterior semicircular canal, as described by Epley (1992). S = sitting. 1–5 = Stages of maneuver. Semicircular canals: Ant = anterior, Post = posterior, Lat = lateral (Reproduced from Epley JM., 1992. Copyright Elsevier)

low-frequency hearing loss with tinnitus, and fullness. Menière's disease does occur in the elderly (Ballester *et al.*, 2002) and the pathological underlying process is thought to be due to increase in endolymph volume, that is, endolymphatic hydrops (Paparella and Djalilial, 2002). If the Menière-like episodes of vertigo cannot be controlled by diuretics and a salt-free diet, the treatment of choice is labyrinthectomy, provided that there is no usable hearing.

Iatrogenic Vestibular Dysfunction

Iatrogenic dizziness may be surgical or medical in origin and it is well established that otological surgery carries a risk of inducing dizziness/vertigo postoperatively. Moreover, vestibular disturbances after nonotological surgery have been documented (O'Mahoney *et al.*, 1995).

Drug-induced dizziness is a very significant problem in the elderly and many, if not all, drugs may produce dizziness, although it is often impossible to identify the underlying mechanism causing disequilibrium. Anemia secondary to gastrointestinal bleeding, hypoglycemia, cardiovascular effects including reduction in cardiac output, dysrhythmias, and postural hypotension, and ototoxicity should all be considered. The most common drugs giving rise to dizziness in the elderly are shown in Table 3.

Ototoxic damage is of particular importance, as it is irreversible. The vestibulotoxic effect of the aminoglycoside antibiotics is common knowledge, and in the elderly, they should be used only as a lifesaving measure. It is well established that age is an important factor in the susceptibility to aminoglycoside ototoxicity, and for this reason blood levels of these drugs should be measured meticulously in the elderly, especially in the presence of concurrent diuretic therapy and/or any change in the overall medical state. Moreover, although standard vestibular tests are not feasible in a severely ill patient, recent methods of assessing vestibular function at the bedside have been developed and are of particular value in potential ototoxicity (Bronstein, 2004; Schubert and Minor, 2004).

Table 3 Drugs causing dizziness/vertigo

Psychotropic drugs	
Antidepressants	Tricyclics, MAOIs, SSRIs
Tranquilizers	Benzodiazepines, phenothiazines
Anticonvulsants	Phenytoin, carbamazepine, gabapentine, lamotrigine
Analgesics	Paracetamol, acetylsalicylate, NSAIDs, opioids
Cardiovascular drugs	
Antihypertensives	Diuretics (thiazides and loop), β-blockers, calcium-channel blockers, ACE inhibitors, methyldopa, hydralazine
Antiarrhythmic	β-Blockers, verapamil, mexiletine, flecainide, amiodarone, disopyramide
Antiangina	Nitrates, calcium-channel blockers, β-blockers, potassium-channel activators
Antimicrobials	Aminoglycosides, tetracyclines, macrolides, chloroquine, isoniazid
Antiallergic drugs	Nonsedating and sedating antihistamines
Hormone replacement/substitute	Hypoglycemics, corticosteroids, HRT
Chemotherapeutic agents	Cisplatin, busulfan, cyclophosphamide, vinblastine, methotrexate

MAOI, monoamine oxidase inhibitor; SSRI, selective serotonin re-uptake inhibitor; NSAID, non-steroidal anti-inflammatory drugs; ACE, angiotensin-converting enzyme inhibitors; HRT, hormone replacement therapy.

CENTRAL VESTIBULAR DISORDERS

Cerebrovascular Disease

Cerebrovascular disease is most commonly secondary to atheroma, although giant cell arteritis should be considered in the elderly. The vertebrobasilar circulation supplies the peripheral vestibular apparatus as described earlier, but also supplies the vestibular nuclei. These nuclei occupy a large area in the lateral zone of the brainstem and are particularly susceptible to a reduction in the blood flow of the main basilar artery and the cerebellum, which is extremely important in modulating information required for balance at the level of the vestibular nuclei. The vertebral and internal carotid arteries provide the brain with a rich blood supply and the terminal branches anastomose to form the circle of Willis. This forms an anatomical safeguard against ischemia arising from narrowing of one vessel and, in addition, there are autoregulatory mechanisms within the cerebral circulation protecting it from fluctuations in the systemic blood pressure. Nonetheless, cerebrovascular disease is one of the most common causes of chronic disability and death. In addition, white-matter changes due to vascular ischemic damage produce gait disorders as well as cognitive impairment, both of which predispose to falls.

Vertebrobasilar Artery Ischemia

Episodic vertigo in an elderly patient is ascribed commonly to vertebrobasilar insufficiency, in the knowledge that cerebrovascular disease is common in the elderly and also on the basis that vertigo and/or dizziness has been reported as the first and most frequent symptom of this condition (Luxon, 1990; Caplan, 2003).

The classical symptoms of vertebrobasilar insufficiency include dizziness/vertigo, dysarthria, numbness of the face, hemiparesis, headache, dysphagia, sensory disturbance cerebellar ataxia, and visual disturbances. The diversity of symptoms and signs reflects the close proximity of cranial nerve nuclei and motor and sensory tracts, within the small confines of the brainstem. The duration of transient ischemic attacks in the vertebrobasilar territory may be variable, but by definition must be without actual infarction and less than 24 hours. They may recur at variable intervals and may or may not be stereotyped.

Classical attacks of vertebrobasilar artery ischemia associated with vertigo do not present a diagnostic problem. However, a study of 50 patients, of whom two-thirds were over the age of 60 with well-defined episodes of vertebrobasilar insufficiency, failed to identify episodic vertigo in isolation as a frequent occurrence in this condition (Luxon, 1990). In this context, it is important to emphasize that dizziness or vertigo, accompanied by only VIIIth nerve manifestations, is unlikely to be of vascular origin. Moreover, tinnitus and deafness are unusual manifestations of vertebrobasilar ischemia and, if present, are accompanied almost always by other symptoms and signs of brain-stem involvement. Despite the presence of vestibular and oculomotor abnormalities in vertebrobasilar ischemia, no characteristic pattern of neuro–otological findings has emerged in this disorder (Luxon, 1990). Hence, isolated episodes of rotational vertigo in an elderly patient should not be ascribed to vertebrobasilar insufficiency, unless there is other neurological evidence to support this diagnosis.

Completed Strokes (see Chapter 71, Acute Stroke)

Completed strokes in the vertebrobasilar territory may involve the vestibular nuclei and there are a number of well-recognized syndromes. The Wallenberg or lateral medullary syndrome may result from occlusion of the posterior inferior cerebellar artery or the vertebral artery (Fisher, 1967). The syndrome is characterized by acute rotational vertigo with nausea and vomiting and ipsilateral dissociated sensory loss in the distribution of the facial nerve, together with contralateral truncal loss and ipsilateral cerebellar ataxia, bulbar palsy, and Horner's syndrome. Specific visuo–vestibular abnormalities have been identified with Wallenberg's syndrome, including spontaneous rotatory nystagmus, with the fast phase directed toward the normal side; tonic deviation of the eyes toward the side of the lesion, with loss of fixation; voluntary and involuntary saccades of larger amplitude in the direction of the lesion; and asymmetry of smooth pursuit, optokinetic, and vestibular responses as a result of the interaction between spontaneous nystagmus and/or slow eye movements.

Pontine/medullary and cerebellar hemorrhages may involve the vestibular apparatus. In the former, there are multiple brain-stem signs and vertigo is usually a fleeting event, although a common presenting symptom, before the patient becomes unconscious (Barinagarrementeria and Cantu, 1994). Cerebellar hemorrhage presents with acute vertigo, vomiting, and an inability to stand, in the presence of cerebellar signs. The importance of rapid diagnosis lies in the ability to correct this condition surgically. Without rapid intervention, the patient dies from brain-stem compression.

Cervical Vertigo

Cervical vertigo is defined as vertigo induced by changes of position of the neck in relation to the body (Brandt, 1996). There is much controversy as to the underlying pathophysiology of cervical vertigo, but sympathetic irritation resulting in vertebrobasilar ischemia, intermittent vertebral artery compression by osteophytes caused by cervical spondylosis and deranged sensory input from the cervical kinesthetic receptors have been postulated.

It is a widely held belief, particularly in the elderly, that vertigo and nystagmus may result from vertebrobasilar ischemia, secondary to compression of blood vessels, as a result of arthritic changes in the neck. This seems unlikely noting the observations that unilateral, or indeed bilateral, compression of the vertebral arteries in the presence of a normal circle of Willis and internal carotid arteries produces only minimal brain-stem ischemia. It should be emphasized that radiological findings may prove misleading, as 75% of people over the age of 50 years show osteoarthritic changes in the cervical vertebrae, which are not directly related to symptomatology (Pallis *et al.*, 1954). Neuro–otological tests in patients suspected of having cervical vertigo are frequently normal and no specific assessment objectively defines the condition. The diagnosis will be facilitated with the development of a specific test defining specific abnormalities.

Neoplasia

Dizziness and/or vertigo are early or initial symptoms in 25% of brain-stem tumors. In later life, metastases are the most common neoplasms involving the brainstem and/or cerebellum, which give rise to vestibular dysfunction. Brain-stem lesions typically present with progressive cranial nerve palsies together with long tract signs, while midline cerebellar lesions give rise to truncal ataxia and oculomotor abnormalities, including impaired smooth pursuit, saccadic dysmetria, and rebound nystagmus (Savundra and Luxon, 1997). Hemispheric cerebellar lesions cause ataxia of the ipsilateral limbs with truncal ataxia.

Temporal-lobe tumors give rise to "disequilibrium" more frequently than in any other cortical site. This is not surprising in view that the temporal lobes exert a modifying influence upon the vestibular nuclei.

Cerebellopontine angle lesions and, in particular, acoustic neurinomas have been mentioned above, but are a rare cause of vestibular symptoms. Acoustic neurinomas, despite the misnomer, arise mainly on the vestibular division of the VIIIth cranial nerve. As they expand in the cerebellopontine angle, there is involvement of the Vth and VIIth cranial nerves, together with ipsilateral cerebellar signs and ultimately lower cranial nerve involvement. If surgical intervention is not undertaken, brain-stem compression results in death.

Infection

Although tuberculosis is no longer a common disorder in developed countries, the possibility of a tuberculoma in the brainstem, cerebellopontine angle, or temporal lobe should be borne in mind, especially in elderly immigrants and in elderly, debilitated, or alcoholic patients.

Neurosyphilis may involve the vestibular apparatus at all stages of the disease and a review of neurosyphilis reported that 30% of patients were over the age of 60 at the time of presentation (Luxon *et al.*, 1979). A high index of suspicion is necessary if rare cases in the elderly are not to be missed.

Neurological Conditions

Many neurological disorders may affect the central vestibular connections, and a discussion of each is beyond the scope of this chapter. The reader is referred to a more extensive review of causes of balance disorders (O'Mahoney and Luxon, 1997). In the elderly, of special note are Parkinson's disease, cerebellar disease, and multisystem atrophies.

Migraine is an important cause of various forms of episodic vertigo and may occur at any time throughout life (Dieterich and Brandt, 1999). The vertigo may last a few minutes or several hours, and in 32% of patients vertigo and headache are not contemporaneous. The symptoms often resolve with effective antimigrainous treatment.

The importance of the cerebellar connections on the vestibular system in terms of maintaining balance and eye position has been emphasized. Neuro-otological abnormalities in cerebellar disease are well defined (Baloh *et al.*, 1986). Cerebellar degeneration may be seen in the elderly in association with malignancy (paraneoplastic syndrome), phenytoin intoxication, hereditary ataxias, alcoholism, and myxedema. Early diagnosis may lead to effective treatment in these groups.

Of importance in the elderly, Paget's disease may give rise to basilar impression which may be accompanied by vertigo (Davies, 1968). The neurological symptoms produced by spinal cord and cerebellar compression together with obstruction of the fourth ventricle usually overshadow the vestibular disorder.

This review of vestibular disorders in the elderly has concentrated on the more common vestibular pathologies affecting this age-group, but it must be emphasized that any vestibular disorder may occur and conditions such as endolymphatic hydrops, migraine, and multiple sclerosis should not be overlooked.

MANAGEMENT

The initial management of a patient must be directed at establishing the presence of an underlying diagnosis for which specific treatment may be instituted. A number of elderly patients will be found to have minor visual impairment, which should be corrected if possible. If there is proprioceptive impairment that is predominantly in the lower limbs, it may be helpful to provide a walking stick to provide additional proprioceptive information through the upper limbs. In addition, assistive devices and interventions for preventing falls should be considered. The management of peripheral vestibular dysfunction consists of counseling and vestibular rehabilitation exercises. Drug therapy may be of value in the management of acute vertigo, but has no place in the long-term management of chronic vestibular symptoms, as it delays compensation.

Symptoms of disequilibrium are especially disturbing for the elderly not only because they fear some sinister pathology but also because they are terrified of the consequences of repeated attacks of vertigo during which they may be unable to summon outside assistance. It is therefore extremely important to obtain a detailed history, carry out a full examination and appropriate investigations, and give a simple and clear explanation of the underlying cause of symptoms of disequilibrium and the therapeutic options that are available.

Chronic vestibular symptoms may be caused by central vestibular pathology or uncompensated peripheral vestibular disorders. The management of central vestibular dysfunction remains poorly understood, but a trial of cinnarizine, clonazepam, or carbamazepine may prove of value. The sedative side effects of these drugs should be recalled in the elderly and the dose titrated against sedation. In patients with a sense of instability and falls, which are frequently associated with basal ganglia disorders and cerebellar disease, physiotherapy to teach alternative gait strategies may prove invaluable in enabling the patient to regain a sense of confidence and improve their mobility.

Vertigo associated with peripheral vestibular disorders may either be attributable to specific conditions, for which there is a recognized treatment regime, or a specific etiology may not be identified despite the evidence of peripheral vestibular dysfunction on standard vestibular tests. The treatment of specific otological disorders is no different in the elderly to any other age-group and the reader is referred to standard otology texts.

Persistent vestibular symptoms due to peripheral labyrinthine dysfunction are frequently amenable to vestibular rehabilitation, and it cannot be overemphasized that destructive surgical procedures should not be considered, particularly in the elderly, until detailed neuro-otological investigation determining site of lesion and exhaustive medical management have been tried. There is no reason to assume that a patient will compensate more efficiently from a total labyrinthine destruction than from a partial impairment of vestibular function, particularly when it is likely that the failure of compensation in the elderly may be due to mild central processing disorders or unsuspected psychological factors.

Acute vertigo associated with nausea and vomiting requires immediate treatment with an antiemetic such as prochlorperazine, by buccal absorption, intramuscularly or by suppository, or metoclopramide intramuscularly, such that nausea and vomiting are alleviated. This enables the administration of a vestibular sedative, of which cinnarizine 15 mg 8-hourly is the treatment of choice. Again, in the elderly patient, sedative side effects must be carefully monitored and the dose adjusted accordingly.

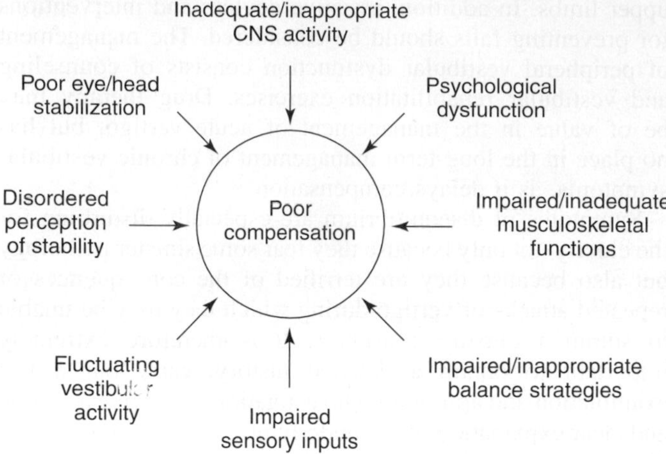

Figure 7 Factors predisposing to decompensation (After Shumway-Cook and Horak, 1990)

Chronic or recurrent vertigo, associated with poorly compensated peripheral pathology (Figure 7), is frequently accompanied by secondary symptoms of psychological distress (anxiety, depression, and phobic symptoms), malaise, fatigue, and cervical pain related to tension in neck muscles, as a result of conscious or subconscious limitation of neck movements, which are likely to precipitate an increase in vertiginous symptoms. The development of psychological symptoms in patients with disequilibrium is now well recognized (Burker *et al.*, 1995; Staab and Ruckenstein, 2003), and appropriate psychological support in the form of behavioral therapy or psychiatric care is essential for patients who manifest psychological symptoms if optimal vestibular compensation is to be achieved. This is particularly important in the elderly age-group, who are more likely to be susceptible than their younger counterparts and are therefore deeply concerned by disorders that impair their physical abilities and threaten their independence.

As early as the mid-1940s, physical exercise regimes (the Cawthorne Cooksey exercises) were introduced as a means of expediting recovery from peripheral vestibular disorders. These exercises are a graduated series of exercises aimed at encouraging head and eye movements, which provokes dizziness in a systematic manner and facilitates vestibular compensation. The exercises are not an endurance test, and for the elderly patient it is important to modify the regime within the limits of the patient's physical abilities. The passage of time has supported the efficacy of these exercises (Norre, 1987) and successful vestibular rehabilitation improves activities of daily living and reduces fall risk. Significant improvement has been shown in patients with peripheral vestibular dysfunction, but also in patients with central balance disorders. Moreover, there is no evidence that age is a negative prognostic factor (Whitney *et al.*, 2002).

Recent work has suggested that "customized" exercises, tailored to the individual patient, are equally effective (Herdman, 1994). Specific positional maneuvers for the management of benign positional vertigo have been described earlier and form an important element of vestibular management. A combination of canalith repositioning maneuver and vestibular rehabilitation has been shown to improve benign positional vertigo in the elderly. Although repositioning maneuver is the most effective treatment, vestibular rehabilitation can be added to improve the results in the treatment.

As noted previously, vestibular sedatives such as cinnarizine are of value in the management of acute vertigo, but have a very limited role in the management of chronic vestibular syndromes. In particular, antiemetics such as prochlorperazine should be avoided, because of the rare but irreversible syndrome of extrapyramidal dysfunction. Moreover, psychotropic drugs should be administered only for specific psychiatric indications, as such medication may interfere with compensatory mechanisms for peripheral vestibular disorders.

In the elderly, the indications for otological surgery for vestibular disorders must be carefully weighed against the general medical state of the patient and the likely extent of recovery postoperatively. Ludman's (1984) excellent review of the surgical treatment of vertigo outlines the various techniques available. As has already been noted, compensation may be prolonged or indeed incomplete as a result of dysfunction of the integrating ability of the CNS and/or other sensory modalities. The risk of a persisting imbalance after vestibular destruction must therefore be borne in mind.

KEY POINTS

- Do not attribute vertigo to "age".
- A thorough history and examination will often provide a clear direction as to diagnosis.
- Correct diagnosis allows treatment of many of the peripheral and central vestibular disorders.
- Introduce vestibular rehabilitation/gait strategy exercises in the elderly early and aggressively.
- Destructive surgical procedures should not be considered, until detailed neuro-otological investigation and medical management have been tried exhaustively.

KEY REFERENCES

- Baloh RW. Dizziness in older people. *Journal of the American Geriatrics Society* 1992; **40**:713–21.
- Eggers SD & Zee DS. Evaluating the dizzy patient: bedside examination and laboratory assessment of the vestibular system. *Seminars in Neurology* 2003; **23**:47–58.
- Nadol JB Jr. Vestibular neuritis. *Otolaryngology and Head and Neck Surgery* 1995; **112**:162–72.
- Nadol JB Jr & Schuknecht HF. Pathology of peripheral vestibular disorders in the elderly. *American Journal of Otolaryngology* 1990; **11**:213–27.
- Schubert MC & Minor LB. Vestibulo-ocular physiology underlying vestibular hypofunction. *Physical Therapy* 2004; **84**:373–85.

REFERENCES

Alberts MC & Terrence CF. Hearing loss in cases of Carcinomatous meningitis. *The Journal of Laryngology and Otology* 1978; **92**:233–41.

Ballester M, Liard P, Vibert D & Hausler R. Meniere's disease in the elderly. *Otology & Neurotology* 2002; **23**:73–8.

Baloh RW. Dizziness in older people. *Journal of the American Geriatrics Society* 1992; **40**:713–21.

Baloh RW. Benign positional vertigo. In RW Baloh & M Halmagyi (eds) *Handbook of Neuro-otology/Vestibular System* 1996, pp 328–39; Oxford University Press, New York.

Baloh RW, Jacobson KM, Enrietto JA *et al.* Balance disorders in older persons: quantification with posturography. *Otolaryngology and Head and Neck Surgery* 1998; **119**:89–92.

Baloh RW, Yee RD & Honrubia V. Late cortical cerebellar atrophy. Clinical and oculographic features in 240 cases. *Neurology* 1986; **37**:371–8.

Barinagarrementeria F & Cantu C. Primary medulla haemorrhage. Report of four cases and review of the literature. *Stroke* 1994; **25**:1684–7.

Brandt T. Cervical vertigo-reality or fiction? *Audiology & Neuro-Otology* 1996; **1**:187–96.

Brandt T & Daroff RB. Physical therapy for benign positional vertigo. *Archives of Otolaryngology* 1980; **106**:484–844.

Brandt T & Steddin S. Current view of the mechanism of benign paroxysmal positioning vertigo: cupulolithiasis or canalolithiasis. *Journal of Vestibular Research* 1993; **3**:373–82.

Bronstein AM. Vision and vertigo; some visual aspects of vestibular disorders. *Journal of Neurology* 2004; **251**:381–7.

Burker EJ, Wong H, Sloane PD *et al.* Predictors of fear of falling in dizzy and nondizzy elderly. *Psychology and Aging* 1995; **10**:104–10.

Caplan LR. Vertebrobasilar disease. *Advances in Neurology* 2003; **92**:131–40.

Davies DG. Paget's disease of the temporal bone. *Acta Oto-Laryngologica* 1968; **242**:7–47.

Dieterich M & Brandt T. Episodic vertigo related to migraine (90 cases): vestibular migraine? *Journal of Neurology* 1999; **246**:883–92.

Downton JH.*Falls in the Elderly* 1993; Edward Arnold,London.

Eggers SD & Zee DS. Evaluating the dizzy patient: bedside examination and laboratory assessment of the vestibular system. *Seminars in Neurology* 2003; **23**:47–58.

Enrietto JA, Jacobson KM & Baloh RW. Aging effects on auditory and vestibular responses: a longitudinal study. *American Journal of Otolaryngology* 1999; **20**:371–8.

Epley JM. The canalith repositioning procedure: for treatment of benign paroxysmal positional vertigo. *Otolaryngology and Head and Neck Surgery* 1992; **107**:399–404.

Fisher CM. Vertigo in cerebrovascular disease. *Archives of Otolaryngology* 1967; **85**:529–34.

Gulya AJ. Neurologic paraneoplastic syndromes with neurotologic manifestations. *The Laryngoscope* 1993; **103**:754–61.

Herdman SJ. *Vestibular Rehabilitation* 1994; F. A. Davis Company, Philadelphia.

Jonsson R, Sixt E, Landahl S & Rosenhall U. Prevalence of dizziness and vertigo in an urban elderly population. *Journal of Vestibular Research* 2004; **14**:47–52.

Kazmierczak H, Pawlak-Osinska K & Osinski P. Visuoocular reflexes in presbyvertigo. *The International Tinnitus Journal* 2001; **7**:112–4.

Ludman H. Surgical treatment of vertigo. In MR Dix & JD Hood (eds) *Vertigo* 1984, pp 113–32; John Wiley & Sons, Chichester.

Luxon LM. Signs and symptoms of Vertebrobasilar insufficiency. In B Hofferberth (ed) *Vascular Brainstem Diseases* 1990; Karger, Basel.

Luxon LM. Post-traumatic vertigo. In RW Baloh & M Halmagyi (eds) *Handbook of Neuro-otology/Vestibular System* 1996, pp 381–95; Oxford University Press, New York.

Luxon LM, Lees AJ & Greenwood RJ. Neurosyphilis today. *Lancet* 1979; **1**:90–3.

Minor LB. Labyrinthine fistulae: pathobiology and management. *Current Opinion in Otolaryngology & Head and Neck Surgery* 2003; **11**:340–6.

Morrison AW. Acoustic neuroma. *Management of Sensorineural Deafness* 1975; Butterworth, London.

Nadol JB Jr. Vestibular neuritis. *Otolaryngology and Head and Neck Surgery* 1995; **112**:162–72.

Nadol JB Jr & Schuknecht HF. Pathology of peripheral vestibular disorders in the elderly. *American Journal of Otolaryngology* 1990; **11**:213–27.

Norre ME. Rationale of rehabilitation treatment for vertigo. *American Journal of Otolaryngology* 1987; **8**:31–5.

O'Mahoney C & Luxon LM. Causes of balance disorders. In AG Kerr (ed) *Scott-Brown's Otolaryngology* 1997, vol 9, 6th edn; Butterworth, London.

O'Loughlin JL, Robitaille Y, Boivin JF & Suissa S. Incidence of and risk factors for falls and injurious falls among the community dwelling elderly. *American Journal of Epidemiology* 1993; **1**:342–54.

O'Mahoney C, Gatland D & Luxon LM. Audiovestibular complications of non-otological surgery. *Clinical Otolaryngology and Allied Sciences* 1995; **20**:510–7.

Pallis C, Jones AM & Spillane JD. Cervical spondylosis. *Brain* 1954; **77**:274–89.

Paparella MM & Djalilial HR. Etiology, pathophysiology of symptoms and pathogenesis of Meniere's disease. *Otolaryngologic Clinics of North America* 2002; **35**:529–45.

Piazza F, Frisina A, Gandolfi A *et al.* Management of acoustic neuromas in the elderly: retrospective study. *Ear, Nose, & Throat Journal* 2003; **82**:374–8.

Rauch SD, Velazquez-Villasenor L, Dimitri PS & Merchant SN. Decreasing hair cell counts in aging humans. *Annals of the New York Academy of Sciences* 2001; **942**:220–7.

Rubin Grandis J, Branstetter BF IV & Yu VL. The changing face of malignant (necrotising) external otitis: clinical radiological and anatomic correlations. *The Lancet Infectious Diseases* 2004; **4**:34–9.

Savundra P & Luxon LM. The physiology of equilibrium and its application in the dizzy patient. In AG Kerr (ed) *Scott-Brown's Otolaryngology* 1997, vol 1, 6th edn; Butterworth, London.

Schubert MC & Minor LB. Vestibulo-ocular physiology underlying vestibular hypofunction. *Physical Therapy* 2004; **84**:373–85.

Shumway-Cook A & Horak FB. Rehabilitation strategies for patients with vestibular deficits. *Neurology Clinics of North America* 1990; **8**:441–57.

Staab JP & Ruckenstein MJ. Which comes first? Psychogenic dizziness versus otogenic anxiety. *The Laryngoscope* 2003; **113**:1714–8.

Sweeney CJ & Gilden DH. Ramsay Hunt syndrome. *Journal of Neurology, Neurosurgery, and Psychiatry* 2001; **71**:149–54.

Tos T, Caye-Thomasen P, Strangerup SE *et al.* Long-term socio-economic impact of vestibular schwannoma for patients under observation and after surgery. *The Journal of Laryngology and Otology* 2003; **117**:955–64.

Wersall J, Gleisner L & Lundquist PG. *Symposium on Myostatic, Kinaesthetic and Vestibular Mechanisms* 1967; JA Churchill, London.

Whitney SL, Wrisley DM, Marchetti GF & Furman JM. The effect of age on vestibular rehabilitation outcomes. *The Laryngoscope* 2002; **112**:1785–90.

FURTHER READING

Dix MR, Harrison MJG & Lewis PB. Progressive supranuclear palsy (the Steel-Richardson-Olszewski syndrome). *Journal of the Neurological Sciences* 1971; **13**:237–56.

Reichert WH, Doolittle J & McDowell SH. Vestibular dysfunction in Parkinson's disease. *Neurology* 1982; **32**:1133–8.

107

Smell and Taste

Richard L. Doty
University of Pennsylvania, Philadelphia, PA, USA

INTRODUCTION

Since 1900, the percentage of Americans over the age of 65 has more than tripled (4.1% in 1900 to over 12% in 2000) and their number has increased over 11 times (from 3.1 to 34.9 million) (Facts for Features, 2004). Given the fact that the ability to perceive odors and tastes decreases markedly with age (Doty, 1995), it is not surprising that increasing numbers of elderly patients are seeking medical help for their chemosensory problem. Indeed, over half the population between the ages of 65 and 80 years, and over three-quarters beyond 80 years, have significant olfactory loss. The implications of such age-related chemosensory losses are far-reaching. Aside from being unable to appreciate fragrances, the taste of food, and the freshness of spring and the seashore, elderly persons suffering from chemosensory disorders are compromised in their ability to detect fire, leaking natural gas, toxic fumes, and spoiled food. Many become depressed, and a disproportionate number die in accidental gas poisonings (Chalke *et al.*, 1958). Others lose their lives or are severely burned in the hundreds of butane and propane gas explosions that occur each year. Clearly, it is incumbent upon both the physician and patient to be aware of this problem, and for the physician to employ the most modern means available to evaluate, counsel, and treat such patients whenever possible.

This chapter provides the gerontologist with an up-to-date overview of the nature and cause of age-related chemosensory disturbances, means for evaluating such disturbances, and approaches useful for counseling and treating the underlying dysfunction.

CHARACTERIZATION OF CHEMOSENSORY PROBLEMS

The general term for inability to smell is anosmia, and for lessened smell function, hyposmia. The corresponding terms for taste are ageusia and hypogeusia. In the older medical literature, anosmia is sometimes referred to as *olfactory anesthesia* or *anosphrasia*. In some nosological schemes, anosmia and hyposmia are classified under the general term dysosmia (distorted smell function), whereas ageusia and hypogeusia are classified under the term dysgeusia (distorted taste function). In this scheme, dysosmia includes forms of dysfunction in addition to anosmia, such as distorted smell sensations (parosmia, cacosmia) and smell hallucinations (phantosmia). Dysgeusia similarly includes both ageusia and distortions in taste function, such as sweet, salty, or sour sensations in the absence of appropriate stimulation. Today, however, it is more common that anosmia, ageusia, dysosmia, and dysgeusia are classified separately from one another, with the first two terms signifying losses, and the second two distortions of smell and taste sensations, respectively.

ANATOMY OF THE OLFACTORY SYSTEM

To be sensed, odorants must enter the nose and reach specialized receptors within the olfactory neuroepithelium, a patch of tissue a few square centimeters in size that lines the upper recesses of the nasal vault, including the cribriform plate and sectors of the nasal septum, middle turbinate, and superior turbinate (Menco and Morrison, 2003) (Figure 1). When activated, the odorant receptors open or close (e.g., via second-messenger systems) membrane channels on the cilia, resulting in a flux of ions and an alteration of the cell's resting potential that ultimately leads to an axonal action potential (Moon and Ronnett, 2003).

Odorant receptor genes, whose discovery by Buck and Axel in 1991 led to the Nobel Prize for Medicine or Physiology in 2004 (Buck and Axel, 1991), represent the largest of all mammalian gene families, comprising nearly 3% of the more than 30 000 genes in the mouse and human genomes. Interestingly, only one type of receptor is expressed

Principles and Practice of Geriatric Medicine, 4th Edition. Edited by M.S. John Pathy, Alan J. Sinclair and John E. Morley.

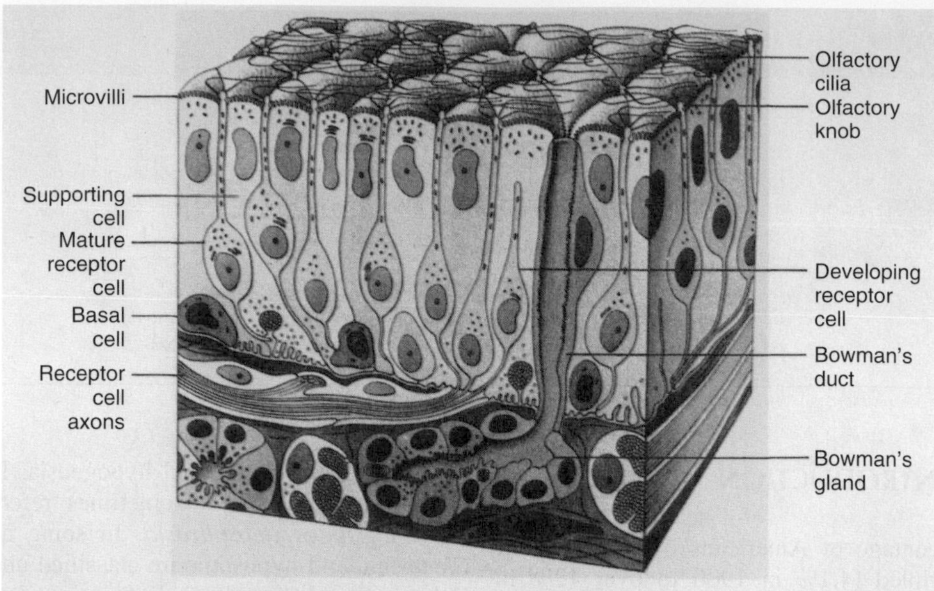

Figure 1 Schematic of the cellular organization of the human olfactory neuroepithelium. Not pictured are the microvillar cells, which are small goblet-shaped cells interspersed among the other cell types at the surface of the epithelium in a ratio to the mature receptor cells of 1 : 10 (Reprinted from Gray's Anatomy, Warwick R and Williams PL, Copyright 1973, with permission from Elsevier)

on the surface of the cilia of a given receptor cell, and odorants typically bind to more than one type of receptor. The olfactory receptor cells number from 6–10 million in the adult human and are insulated from one another at the epithelial surface by sustentacular cells (Menco and Morrison, 2003). A blanket of mucus, which contains a number of enzymes (e.g. cytochrome P-450), covers the olfactory neuroepithelium and deactivates or filters materials that are absorbed into the mucus, including some odorants (Ding and Dahl, 2003). This mucus also aids in protecting the epithelium from desiccation, heat, and xenobiotic insult, and serves as a solvent and carrier for odorant binding proteins – proteins that facilitate the transport of some lipophilic molecules to the receptors through aqueous phases of the mucus.

The unmyelinated axons of the bipolar olfactory receptor cells collect into 15–20 fascicles (fila olfactoria) that collectively make up the olfactory nerve (cranial nerve (CN) I). These axons course through the cribriform plate and synapse within spherical masses of neuropile within the olfactory bulb termed *glomeruli*. Second-order connections with the dendrites of mitral and tufted cells are made within these structures. The latter cells extend processes that project to higher centers, including the anterior olfactory nucleus, the entorhinal cortex, the prepiriform cortex, the olfactory tubercle, and the corticomedial nucleus of the amygdala. In turn, a number of these areas have extensive connections between hippocampus, mediodorsal thalamus, hypothalamus, and other brain regions (Doty and Bromley, 2000).

Ultimately, the perception of smell is the result of a complex series of electrochemical events extending from the surface of the olfactory epithelium to cortical brain structures. The pattern of neuronal activity set up by a given stimulus results in its intensity, duration, and quality. While only certain populations of receptor cells respond to a specific odorant, considerable overlap is present among odorants, and most odorants stimulate a broad range of receptor cells. The pattern of the projection of receptor cells suggests that the coding of odor quality relies on the activation of spatially overlapping projections of the olfactory receptor cells to various loci among and within the glomeruli.

In addition to the sensory innervation of the olfactory nerve, free nerve endings of the trigeminal nerve (CN V) are distributed throughout the nasal mucosa. The ophthalmic and maxillary divisions of CN V carry information regarding irritation, temperature, and pungency. Sensations mediated by non-CN I nerves are those of the "common chemical sense" and do not encode the qualitative perception of "odor" *per se* (Doty and Cometto-Muñz, 2003).

ANATOMY OF THE GUSTATORY SYSTEM

Taste receptor cells are located within taste buds on the tongue, soft palate, uvula, epiglottis, rostral esophagus, and mucous membranes of the laryngeal cartilages. Most lingual taste buds are found imbedded in the surface of protuberances termed *papillae*. Fungiform papillae are prevalent on the anterior tongue, circumvallate papillae within the chevron of the posterior tongue, and foliate papillae within the lateral margins of the medial tongue separating the anterior and posterior sectors (Shepherd, 1994) (Figure 2).

The sense of taste is supplied by three CNs: the facial nerve (CN VII), the glossopharyngeal nerve (CN IX), and vagus nerve (CN X). As shown in Figure 2, the taste buds

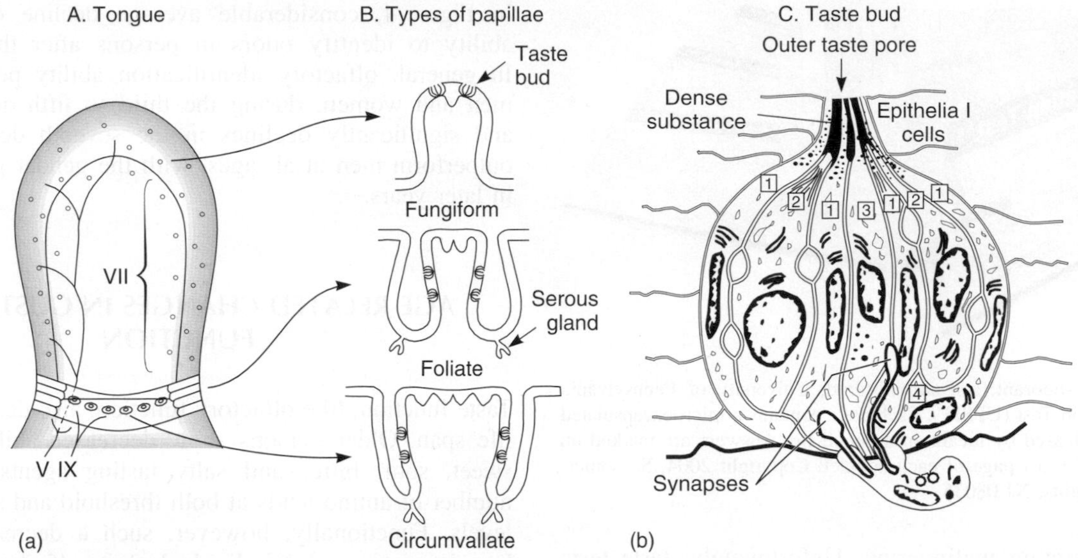

Figure 2 (a and b) Schematic of the distribution of taste buds on the human tongue. Taste buds of the fungiform and foliate papillae are innervated by CN VII. Those of the circumvallate papillae are innervated by CN IX. CN V carries nontaste somatosensory sensations. See text for details. (c) Schematic of fine structure of taste bud. (1) and (2) are presumably supporting cells that secrete materials into the lumen of the bud. (3) is a sensory receptor cell; and (4) a basal cell from which other cell types arise (Reproduced from Murray RG, 1973. Copyright Murray RG)

on the fungiform papillae are supplied by the chorda tympani branch of CN VII, whereas the taste buds on the other types of papillae are supplied by the lingual branch of CN IX. Taste buds located on the soft palate send their projections centrally via the greater superficial petrosal branch of CN VII and those on the epiglottis, esophagus, and larynx transmit taste information by way of the superior laryngeal branch of CN X. As in the case of olfaction, trigeminal (CN V) free nerve endings, distributed throughout the oral cavity, mediate somatosensory sensations (e.g. pungency, burning, sharpness). All branches of the gustatory nerves enter the brainstem and terminate in the rostral part of the nucleus of the solitary tract. The subsequent projections are not thoroughly understood in humans; however, connections are made with the ventral posteromedial thalamus and insular cortex. In rodents, fibers from the pons also travel to areas involved in feeding and autonomic regulation, including the lateral hypothalamus, central amygdala, and stria terminalis (Pritchard, 1991).

CLINICAL TESTS OF OLFACTORY AND GUSTATORY FUNCTION

The physician of the past assessed the ability to smell by asking a patient to sniff vials containing one or two odorants such as coffee or tobacco, and to report whether or not an odor is perceived. The analogous taste test was to sprinkle grains of sugar or salt onto the tongue, and ask about the corresponding sensations. Unfortunately, such procedures are akin to testing vision by shining a flashlight into the eye, or audition by sounding a bullhorn next to the ear. This problem is not corrected, in the case of olfaction, by having the patient attempt to identify the presented odorants, since without cuing, even normal subjects have difficulty identifying most odorants. In the case of taste, nonsolubilized tastants are often not recognized by patients whose mouths are dry, or who have little time to dissolve the tastants into saliva.

During the last 25 years, remarkable progress has been made in the development of reliable, valid, and clinically practical olfactory tests. Physicians and insurance carriers are now aware, more than ever, that objective chemosensory assessment is essential for (1) establishing the validity of a patient's complaint, (2) characterizing the specific nature of a chemosensory problem, (3) accurately monitoring medical or surgical interventions, (4) detecting malingering, (5) counseling patients to help cope with their problem, and (6) assigning disability compensation. Importantly, accurate assessment decreases the costs of continuing treatment seeking on the part of patients, who are usually assumed as having a problem even in the absence of objective data.

Several commercially available tests of olfactory function are now available, including tests of odor detection and identification (for review, see Doty, 2001). The most widely used of these tests (the University of Pennsylvania Smell Identification Test or UPSIT: commercially termed *the Smell Identification Test*™, Sensonics. Inc., Haddon Hts, NJ) was developed at our center and evaluates the ability of patients to identify, from sets of four descriptors, each of 40 "scratch and sniff" odorants (Doty, 1995; Figure 3). The number of items correctly identified out of 40 items serves as the test score. This measure is compared with norms based upon data from a large number of individuals sampled from the community at large and a percentile rank is determined, depending upon the age and gender of the patient. This test, which correlates strongly with traditional threshold tests, is amenable to self-administration and provides a

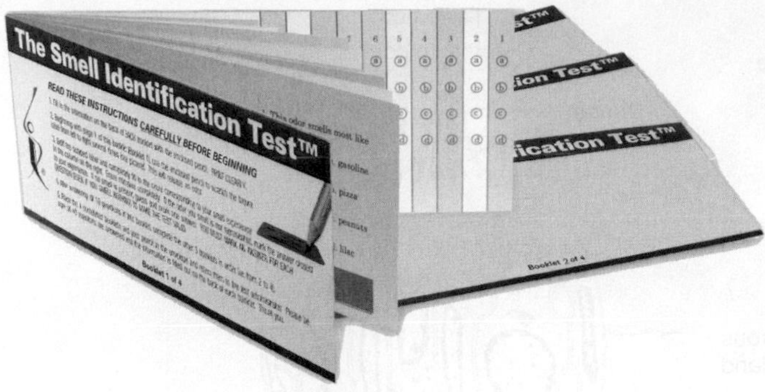

Figure 3 The 40-odorant, self-administered, University of Pennsylvania Smell Identification Test (UPSIT). Each page contains a microencapsulated odorant that is released by means of a pencil tip. Answers are marked on the columns on the last page of each booklet. Copyright 2004, Sensonics, Inc., Haddon Heights, NJ 08035

means for detecting malingering. Unfortunately, taste tests with similar reliability, validity, and practicality to that of the UPSIT do not exist, although electrogustometry can provide quantitative assessments of taste function that are correlated with the number of underlying taste elements (Miller *et al.*, 2002).

Traditionally, physicians have assumed that if a patient presenting with the complaint of anosmia fails to report the presence of an irritating vapor via CN V, he or she is malingering. However, this test is not foolproof, as even the most ardent malingerer rarely denies not perceiving a strong irritating substance, particularly one which leads to reflexive mucous secretion or eye watering. Furthermore, trigeminal thresholds to chemicals can be quite variable among individuals. Thus, a more valid means for detecting malingering is to determine the percentage of responses to stimuli that are correct in a forced-choice situation where chance responding can be calculated. When significantly fewer correct responses than expected on the basis of chance responding are demonstrated, malingering is suspected (Doty, 1995).

AGE-RELATED CHANGES IN OLFACTORY FUNCTION

It is not known to what extent age-related changes in olfactory function represent the process of aging *per se*, or alterations in the chemosensory systems brought about by factors correlated with age (i.e. cumulative viral insults, repeated exposures to environmental agents and air pollutants, alterations in trophic factors, the early progression of neurodegenerative disease pathology, etc.). Whatever the cause, however, the elderly evidence marked olfactory loss, as discussed in the beginning of this chapter. Such loss appears to occur in all cultures and is found using any one of a wide range of nominally distinct olfactory tests (e.g. odor threshold, detection, discrimination, and memory tests). However, large individual differences are present.

The age-related decline in olfactory function is exemplified by scores on the UPSIT (Doty, 1995). As can be seen in Figure 4, considerable average decline occurs in the ability to identify odors in persons after the age of 60. In general, olfactory identification ability peaks, for both men and women, during the third to fifth decades of life and significantly declines in the seventh decade. Women outperform men at all ages, with the gender gap increasing in later years.

AGE-RELATED CHANGES IN GUSTATORY FUNCTION

Taste function, like olfactory function, also declines over the life span. Older persons show decreased ability to discern sweet, sour, bitter and salty tasting agents, including a number of amino acids at both threshold and suprathreshold levels. Functionally, however, such a decrease has much less impact on the individual than olfactory loss, since whole-mouth tests often show only moderate declines in age-related function (Weiffenbach *et al.*, 1986). This is due, in part, to the fact that the taste buds in different regions of the mouth are innervated by several different sets of CNs. Such nerves are less susceptible to insult than the fine olfactory filaments. In the case of head trauma, for example, total ageusia, as measured by whole-mouth testing, is rare ($<0.5\%$), compared to total anosmia (Deems *et al.*, 1991). Nevertheless, studies that have tested well-defined localized regions of the tongue to brief presentations of stimuli report marked age-related dysfunction (Matsuda and Doty, 1995) (Figure 5). Such losses may be particularly significant for foodstuffs that minimally leach chemicals during mastication.

It is important for the clinician to be aware that complaints of loss of "taste" usually reflect the loss of flavor sensations derived from retronasal stimulation of the olfactory receptors (Deems *et al.*, 1991; Burdach and Doty, 1987). Thus, other than basic sweet, sour, salty, and bitter sensations (or possibly metallic or "Umami" sensations), or temperature or textural sensations (sharpness, pungency, burning, etc.), the rich experiences attributed to "taste" are actually due to molecules that enter the nose from the oral cavity via the nasal pharynx. Among the hundreds of "tastes" which are really due to stimulation of CN I are banana, chocolate, strawberry, pizza sauce, vanilla, root beer, cola, licorice, steak sauce, steak, fried chicken, apples, and lemon.

CAUSES OF SMELL DYSFUNCTION IN THE ELDERLY

The olfactory receptors are rather directly exposed to the outside environment, making them susceptible to insult from bacteria, viruses, toxic agents, and other nosogenic stimuli. For this reason, it is not surprising that environmentally induced damage to the olfactory epithelium appears to be the most common cause of age-related decrements in the ability to smell. Indeed, cumulative destruction of the olfactory

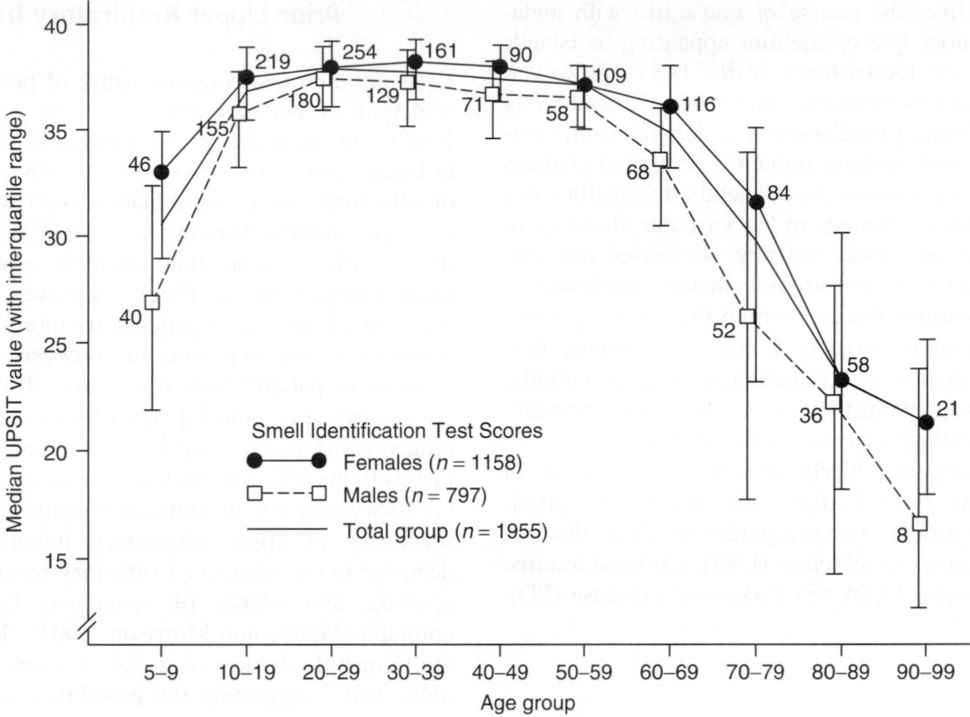

Figure 4 Scores on the University of Pennsylvania Smell Identification Test (UPSIT) as a function of age in a large heterogeneous group of subjects. Numbers by data points indicate sample sizes (Reprinted with permission from Doty RL *et al.*, Smell identification ability: changes with age. *Science*, **226**:1441–1443. Copyright 1984 AAAS.)

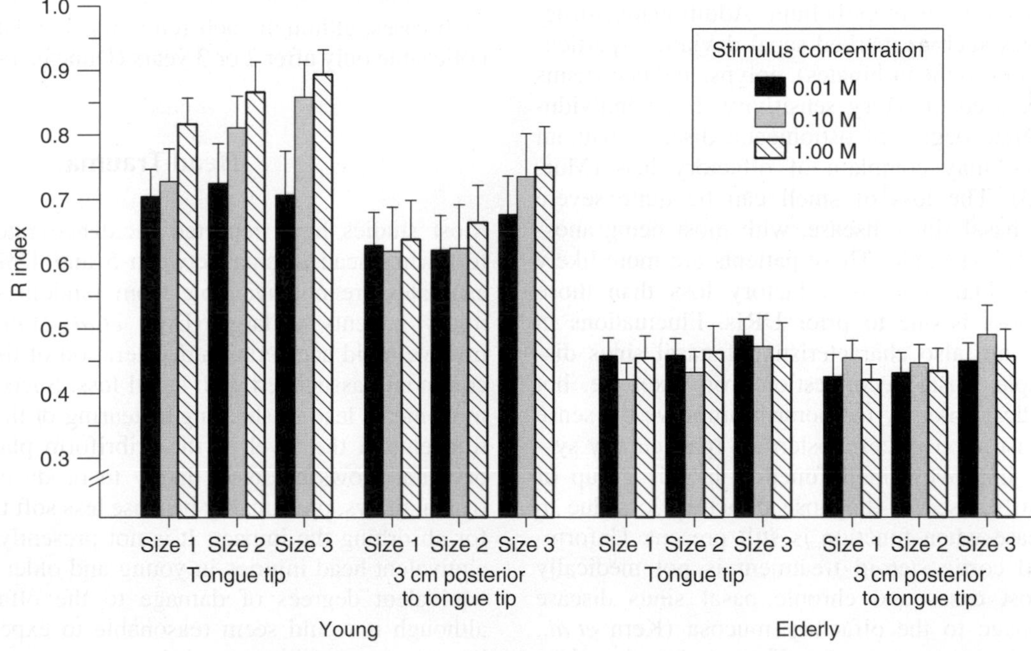

Figure 5 Mean (±SEM) sensitivity values (R index) obtained from 12 young and 12 elderly subjects for sodium chloride stimuli presented to the tongue tip and to a medial tongue region 3 cm posterior to the tongue tip for three stimulation areas (12.5. 25, 50 mm^2) and three stimulus concentrations. Note that the sensitivity of the elderly subjects was approximately chance and that the sensitivity did not increase as either a function of the stimulus area or concentration. Note also that, unlike the case with the young subjects, the tongue tip of the elderly subjects was no more sensitive than the tongue region 3 cm posterior to the tongue tip (Reproduced from Matsuda T, Doty RL. Regional taste sensitivity to NaCl:relationship to subject age, tongue locus and area of stimulation. Chem Senses 1995; **20**: 283–90, by permission of Oxford University Press)

epithelium occurs over the course of one's life with metaplasia from respiratory-like epithelium appearing as islands within the membrane (Nakashima *et al.*, 1984). However, age-related functional or structural changes may also directly damage the epithelium or predispose it to damage from environmental insults, such as from influenza. Potential changes include reduced protein synthesis or metabolic insufficiency (as in hypothyroidism), changes in the vascular elasticity of the epithelium, altered airway patency, decreased intramucosal blood flow, loss of neurotrophic factors, occlusion of cribriform plate foramina through which the olfactory nerve axons project, increased viscosity of the nasal mucus, atrophy of secretory glands and lymphatics, and, potentially, decreases in enzyme systems that deactivate xenobiotic materials within the olfactory mucosa (Doty, 1994).

The vast majority of elderly patients complaining of a smell deficit can be classified into one of six proximal etiologic categories: (1) nasal/paranasal sinus disease; (2) prior upper respiratory infection (URI); (3) head trauma; (4) Alzheimer's disease (AD); (5) Parkinson's disease (PD); or (6) idiopathic.

Nasal/Paranasal Sinus Disease

Inflammation of the nasal cavity and sinuses (e.g. chronic sinusitis, allergic rhinitis, bacterial rhinitis, viral rhinitis) reduces upper airway patency, thereby restricting odorant access to the olfactory neuroepithelium. Additionally, structural abnormalities such as marked sepal deviation (particularly with adhesions to the turbinates), polyps, and neoplasms can lead to decreased olfactory sensitivity. Even individuals with a moderate degree of ostiomeatal disease, without intranasal polyps, may complain of olfactory loss (Murphy *et al.*, 2003). The loss of smell can be quite severe in patients with nasal sinus disease, with most being anosmic or profoundly hyposmic. These patients are more likely to describe a gradual onset of olfactory loss than those patients whose loss is due to prior URIs. Fluctuations in smell sensitivity are also characteristic of nasal sinus disease. For example, nasal decongestion from exercise, hot showers, or medications may temporarily improve the sense of smell. Administration of corticosteroids (particularly systemic) typically improves smell function in this group of patients and can be used to diagnose olfactory loss due to nasal sinus disease when function is still present. Unfortunately, sustained corticosteroid treatment is not medically indicated in most cases and chronic nasal sinus disease can lead to damage to the olfactory mucosa (Kern *et al.*, 2004). Once such damage occurs, olfactory function does not improve by administration of an anti-inflammatory agent. It is encouraging, however, that olfactory dysfunction arising from nasal sinus disease is often amenable to treatment (Doty and Mishra, 2001). Management of allergies, sinusitis, and structural abnormalities through medication or endoscopic surgery can alleviate smell loss in a number of these patients.

Prior Upper Respiratory Infections

URIs are the most common cause of permanently decreased olfaction in persons older than 50 years (Deems *et al.*, 1991). The diagnosis of viral-induced olfactory dysfunction is based upon a history of a viral illness prior to the onset of olfactory loss in combination with the absence of other etiologic factors. Patients will often describe an olfactory deficit during a "cold" that was more severe than usual. After recuperation from the illness, however, the sense of smell does not return. These patients are more likely to experience a nonfluctuating hyposmia in comparison to the fluctuating anosmia of patients with nasal sinus disease.

Whether viral-induced smell loss is reflective of the age-related resistance to viral insult or a culmination of repeated insults to the olfactory neuroepithelium (or both) is unknown. Olfactory biopsies in individuals with olfactory dysfunction secondary to upper respiratory infections demonstrate a decrease in the number of olfactory receptor cells, extensive scarring, and islands of metaplasia from respiratory-like epithelia (Menco and Morrison, 2003). These characteristics are frequently evidenced in the olfactory epithelia of elderly individuals, suggesting the possibility that cumulative viral insults over time may be one reason for their overall loss, even if a precipitating event cannot be identified or differs from a viral infection.

Currently, no treatment is available for viral-induced chronic anosmia or hyposmia. Nevertheless, some authors have reported spontaneous remission in at least a few such cases, although such remission is relatively minor and noticeable only after 2 or 3 years (Duncan and Seiden, 1995).

Head Trauma

Most studies have reported incidence rates of smell loss following head trauma between 5 and 15%, although such estimates are not available from random samples of head injury patients at large (Doty *et al.*, 1997). Injuries that involve rapid acceleration/deceleration of the brain are most commonly associated with smell loss. Such coup/contrecoup movements lead to shearing or tearing of the olfactory nerve filaments at the level of the cribriform plate. Interestingly, occipital blows are more likely to produce smell loss than frontal blows, presumably because less soft tissue is available for absorbing the impact. It is not presently known whether equivalent head injuries in young and older persons produce equivalent degrees of damage to the olfactory pathways, although it would seem reasonable to expect the elderly to be more susceptible to such loss.

Smell loss in head trauma patients tends to be severe, as most are anosmic rather than hyposmic under objective testing. Unfortunately, such individuals rarely regain olfactory function and scar tissue at the level of the cribriform plate often precludes entry of axons from regenerating olfactory neurons through the cribriform plate into the central nervous system.

Alzheimer's Disease (*see* Chapter 93, Clinical Aspects of Alzheimer's Disease)

Most individuals with even mild AD demonstrate decreased olfactory function relative to age-matched controls. Physiological changes associated with normal aging may be responsible, in part, for some of the AD-related olfactory dysfunction. However, even relatively young and early-stage AD patients with mild dementia score markedly lower on olfactory tests than do age-matched controls. Thus, on the 40-item UPSIT, 50% of the items, on average, cannot be identified by early-stage AD patients. In a picture identification test analogous to the odor identification test (except that pictures, rather than odors, need to be identified), only 5% of the items are similarly misidentified by the same AD patients.

It now appears that olfactory dysfunction – particularly in conjunction with other risk factors – may be a predictor of the subsequent development of AD in older persons (Devanand *et al.*, 2000; Bacon *et al.*, 1998; Graves *et al.*, 1999). In one study, for example, a standardized 12-item odor identification test was administered to 1604 nondemented community-dwelling senior citizens aged 65 years and older (Graves *et al.*, 1999). The olfactory test scores were found to be a better predictor of cognitive decline over the following 2 years than scores on a global cognitive test. Persons who were anosmic and possessed at least one APOE-4 allele exhibited 4.9 times the risk of having cognitive decline than normosmic persons not possessing this allele. This was in contrast to a 1.23 times greater risk for cognitive decline in normosmic individuals possessing at least one such allele. A sex difference was noted. Thus, women who were anosmic and possessed at least one APOE-4 allele were 9.71 times more likely to experience cognitive decline than their normosmic nonallele possessing counterparts. The corresponding figure for men was 3.18. Women and men who were normosmic and possessed at least one allele were only 1.9 and 0.67 times more likely, respectively, than their normosmic nonallele possessing counterparts.

Although the olfactory system-related neuropathology of AD may involve the neuroepithelium, most likely central structures are the most heavily involved (Esiri and Wilcock, 1984; Hyman *et al.*, 1991; Kovacs *et al.*, 1999; Smutzer *et al.*, 2003; Davies *et al.*, 1993; Tsuboi *et al.*, 2003). There is evidence that AD pathology begins in olfactory regions within the medial temporal lobe, most notably, layer II of the entorhinal cortex (Brouillet *et al.*, 1994; Gomez-Isla *et al.*, 1996), and progresses from there to neocortical regions, although involvement of the olfactory bulbs early in the disease process has also been demonstrated (Kovacs *et al.*, 2001; Braak and Braak, 1998). A 40% decrease in the cross-sectional area of the olfactory tract and a 52% loss of myelinated axons has been reported in AD. Neurofibrillary tangle formation occurs earlier than amyloid deposition within the olfactory bulb of AD patients, and the presence of more than 10 neurofibrillary tangles per olfactory bulb section is associated with a 93.3% AD diagnostic accuracy rate (Kovacs *et al.*, 1999).

Parkinson's Disease

Idiopathic PD is another age-related neurodegenerative disorder characterized by olfactory dysfunction (Doty, 2003). As in AD, patients with PD evidence olfactory deficits on a wide variety of olfactory tests. Importantly, the proportion of early-stage PD patients with olfactory dysfunction appears to be equal to or greater than the proportion of early-stage PD patients exhibiting a number of the cardinal signs of PD (e.g. tremor) (Doty *et al.*, 1988).

The following important observations have been made: (1) PD-related smell loss is bilateral and present very early in the disease process; (2) the magnitude of olfactory dysfunction is unrelated to disease stage, severity of motor dysfunction or use of antiparkinsonian medications; (3) the olfactory loss is stable over time, even when other elements of the disease progress; (4) olfactory evoked potentials are abnormal in PD patients, demonstrating a prolonged latency, or in most cases, an absent response; and (5) among the major motor disorders, the olfactory loss of PD is relatively specific (Doty *et al.*, 1988; Doty, 2003). Thus, decreased ability to smell is absent, or present infrequently or only to a minor degree, in progressive supranuclear palsy (a condition that shares a number of signs with PD), essential tremor, multiple system atrophy, amyotrophic lateral sclerosis, multiple sclerosis, and parkinsonism induced by intravenous administration of the proneurotoxin 1-methyl-4-phenyl-1,2,3,6-tetrahydropyridine (MPTP) (Doty *et al.*, 1993; Wenning *et al.*, 1995; Sajjadian *et al.*, 1994; Doty *et al.*, 1992).

While the basis for the olfactory deficit in idiopathic PD is unknown, it appears to be indistinguishable from that observed in AD, suggesting the possibility that these two disorders may share a common neuropathological substrate (Doty *et al.*, 1991). As with AD, both olfactory vector and degenerative hypotheses could explain the dysfunction. Tangential support for the olfactory vector hypothesis comes from evidence that (1) certain viruses (e.g. encephalitis lethargica) have been epidemiologically associated with PD, (2) a number of viruses, including ones associated with encephalitis, enter the central nervous system via the primary olfactory neurons, and (3) patients whose parkinsonism is due to the intravenous administration of MPTP have a relatively normal olfactory function (Doty, 2003). Recent data suggest the possibility that the olfactory dysfunction of AD and PD may be secondary to the damage to the anterior olfactory nucleus, a relay station within the core of the olfactory bulb. Thus, intraneuronal pathology related to the protein τ is clearly marked in the anterior olfactory nucleus of neurodegenerative diseases such as AD and PD that are associated with olfactory loss, but nearly absent in such disorders as progressive supranuclear palsy, corticobasal degeneration, and frontal temporal dementia (disorders with little or no olfactory dysfunction) (Tsuboi *et al.*, 2003; Braak *et al.*, 2003; Doty, 1991).

Idiopathic Factors

A number of individuals presenting with an olfactory complaint lack a clear etiology for their dysfunction. It is possible that subclinical manifestations of disorders that alter the sense of smell are responsible for some of these cases. For example, we have observed patients presenting to our clinic with complaints of distorted olfactory function of unknown origin who came down with influenza a week or two later. The olfactory losses of a disproportionate number of idiopathic cases occur during the influenza season; thus, some of these cases may reflect influenza that culminates in no other noticeable clinical manifestations.

CAUSES OF TASTE DYSFUNCTION IN THE ELDERLY

As discussed in detail earlier in this chapter, the subjective complaint of "taste" loss, a common complaint of the elderly is often not verified by whole-mouth taste testing. A number of such patients are undoubtedly confusing "taste" with "flavor", and upon careful testing, exhibit major olfactory, rather than major gustatory, deficits (Deems *et al.*, 1991).

As with olfactory dysfunction, a broad array of age-related changes may predispose the taste system to damage from environmental insults or other factors, including reduced protein synthesis or metabolic insufficiency, changes in epithelial vascularity, decreased blood flow, loss of neurotrophic factors, and atrophy of secretory glands and lymphatics (Doty, 1994). Common conditions seen in the elderly that may interfere with the access of the tastant to the taste bud (transport loss) include inflammatory processes of the oral cavity, bacterial and fungal colonization of the taste pore, and xerostomia. Poor oral hygiene may also contribute to taste dysfunction.

Viral infections, medications, and radiation therapy to the oral cavity and pharynx represent the most common causes of sensory gustatory loss. The chorda tympani is particularly susceptible to viral or bacterial insult as it courses through the middle ear. In turn, the middle ear is connected to the eustachian tube and nasopharynx which provide a portal of entry for infectious agents. Thus, it is not surprising that taste loss or distortion has been associated with upper respiratory and middle ear infections. Numerous drugs have been suggested to alter the ability to taste, including antihypertensives and antilipidemics (Doty *et al.*, 2003), and drugs affecting cell turnover, such as antineoplastic, antithyroid, and antirheumatic agents (Doty and Bromley, 2004).

Neural gustatory loss results from head trauma, neoplasms, and a variety of dental and otologic operations that may damage the facial nerve or glossopharyngeal nerve. Injury in this patient population can be to the taste nerves or to more central structures.

In addition to the aforementioned causes of altered taste perception in the elderly, several other conditions are important. Diabetics often experience a loss in taste perception, especially for glucose. This loss can be progressive and eventually extend to other taste stimuli (Settle, 1991). Burning mouth syndrome is a poorly characterized disorder in which patients describe an intraoral burning sensation that commonly occurs in combination with dysgeusia (Ship *et al.*, 1995). This problem is prevalent in postmenopausal women. Although no clear etiologic factor has been identified, hormone replacement and tricyclic antidepressant are effective in alleviating the oral sensations in some cases. The limited data suggest that neurodegenerative disorders such as AD do not influence the ability to taste to any major degree.

EVALUATING AND MANAGING ELDERLY PATIENTS WITH CHEMOSENSORY DYSFUNCTION

In general, a thorough medical history will identify the proximal cause of most smell and taste problems. During this history, the clinician should question the patient as to whether there is loss (e.g. anosmia) or a decrease (e.g. hyposmia) in function and whether the symptoms are unchanging, progressive, or fluctuant. The degree to which the loss or distortion is localized to one nostril or the other, or to one section of the tongue or the other, is useful in establishing whether a given nerve is involved. Antecedent events (i.e. prior URI, head trauma, medications, surgery) leading up to the dysfunction as well as the duration of symptoms are important pieces of information to be gathered from the history. For example, fluctuating olfactory deficits suggest interference with the transport of the odorant to the olfactory neuroepithelium (e.g. nasal sinus disease) rather than a sensorineural disorder.

After obtaining a thorough medical history, it is critical to evaluate the patient objectively, so as to characterize the nature of the dysfunction. In most cases, olfactory dysfunction is the problem. Thus, even when the patient reports that smell is all right and only taste is problematic, quantitative olfactory testing should be performed. If unilateral dysfunction is suspected, the olfactory test can be administered to each half of the nose separately while occluding the contralateral naris using a piece of Microfoam™ tape (3M Corporation, Minneapolis, MN). Contemporaneously, a thorough upper airway examination, ideally using endoscopic procedures, should be performed along with appropriate imaging of the sinuses and higher brain structures. If nasal or intracranial disease is found, appropriate medical or surgical treatment should be initiated, and olfactory testing should be repeated some time after the completion of the treatment regimen to ascertain whether improvement has occurred. Obviously, the basic diseases associated with aging should be ruled out by the physician to preclude their possible association with the chemosensory dysfunction. Importantly, a review of the medications taken by the elderly should be undertaken, particularly if dysgeusia is the presenting symptom.

If the medical tests prove negative, it is likely that the dysfunction is due to neural damage for which no treatment is available (e.g. damage to the olfactory receptors proper). In this case, it is still prudent to assess the chemosensory function quantitatively and obtain a percentile score for the patient. While an older person may evidence, in an absolute sense, considerable olfactory loss, it is still important to characterize this person relative to his or her peer group. Thus, an 85-year-old man may have olfactory loss indicative of marked hyposmia; however, he may still be at the 75th percentile of his normative group, indicating that he is outperforming three-quarters of his peers. Simply telling him this fact would be highly therapeutic, as elderly persons expect some degree of decline in their function, but appreciate it when their decline is still not as great as that seen in most of their peers. This simple strategy is very therapeutic and ensures that at least half the patients complaining of chemosensory function loss can receive meaningful psychological benefit.

In cases where borderline dysfunction is present in menopausal women, the astute clinician can explore whether hormone or vitamin replacement therapy may be indicated in an attempt to return function. This is particularly the case in burning mouth syndrome, where such treatments have been found effective in some cases (Grushka and Sessle, 1991). Although zinc therapy has been suggested in the literature, double-blind studies indicate that zinc is no more effective than a placebo in helping patients with chemosensory disorders (unless, of course, frank zinc deficiency is present) (Henkin *et al.*, 1976). One study reporting effectiveness of the antioxidant α-lipoic acid had no controls and the number reporting resolution was of the same magnitude as would be expected from spontaneous resolution (Hummel *et al.*, 2002). Some cases of taste dysfunction may represent age-related xerostomia, and, therefore, this condition should be addressed and, if present, treated as well as possible.

Acknowledgment

Supported, in part, by research grants RO1 DC 04278 and RO1 DC 02974 from the National Institute on Deafness and Other Communication Disorders, and RO1 AG 17496 from the National Institute on Aging, National Institutes of Health, Bethesda, MD, USA. Disclosure: Dr. Doty is a major shareholder in Sensonics, Inc., the manufacturer and distributor of tests of taste and smell function.

KEY POINTS

- Taste and smell are critical for determining the flavor of foods and beverages and for protection from leaking natural gas, fire, toxic agents, and spoiled beverages and foodstuffs.
- Smell dysfunction is the norm, not the exception, for persons over the age of 65.
- It is important for the physician and patient to have an accurate understanding of a patient's abilities to taste and smell, and easy-to-administer quantitative tests of smell function are widely available.
- Smell loss is among the very earliest signs of Alzheimer's disease and idiopathic Parkinson's disease.
- The most common cause of *permanent* smell loss in the elderly is an upper respiratory infection.

KEY REFERENCES

- Braak H, Del Tredici K, Rub U *et al.* Staging of brain pathology related to sporadic Parkinson's disease. *Neurobiology of Aging* 2003; **24**:197–211.
- Buck L & Axel R. A novel multigene family may encode odorant receptors: a molecular basis for odor recognition. *Cell* 1991; **65**:175–87.
- Deems DA, Doty RL, Settle RG *et al.* Smell and taste disorders, a study of 750 patients from the University of Pennsylvania Smell and Taste Center. *Archives of Otolaryngology–Head & Neck Surgery* 1991; **117**:519–28.
- Doty RL, Deems DA & Stellar S. Olfactory dysfunction in parkinsonism: a general deficit unrelated to neurologic signs, disease stage, or disease duration. *Neurology* 1988; **38**(8):1237–44.
- Graves AB, Bowen JD, Rajaram L *et al.* Impaired olfaction as a marker for cognitive decline: interaction with apolipoprotein E epsilon4 status. *Neurology* 1999; **53**:1480–7.
- Menco BPM & Morrison EE. Morphology of the mammalian olfactory epithelium: form, fine structure, function, and pathology. In RL Doty (ed) *Handbook of Olfaction and Gustation* 2003; 2nd edn; Marcel Dekker, New York.
- Pritchard TC. The primate gustatory system. In TV Getchell, RL Doty, LM Bartoshuk & JB Snow Jr (eds) *Smell and Taste in Health and Disease* 1991; Raven Press, New York.

REFERENCES

Bacon AW, Bondi MW, Salmon DP & Murphy C. Very early changes in olfactory functioning due to Alzheimer's disease and the role of apolipoprotein E in olfaction. *Annals of the New York Academy of Sciences* 1998; **855**:723–31.

Braak H & Braak E. Evolution of neuronal changes in the course of Alzheimer's disease. *Journal of Neural Transmission* 1998; **53**(suppl 105):127–40.

Braak H, Del Tredici K, Rub U *et al.* Staging of brain pathology related to sporadic Parkinson's disease. *Neurobiology of Aging* 2003; **24**:197–211.

Brouillet E, Hyman BT, Jenkins BG *et al.* Systemic or local administration of azide produces striatal lesions by an energy impairment-induced excitotoxic mechanism. *Experimental Neurology* 1994; **129**:175–82.

Buck L & Axel R. A novel multigene family may encode odorant receptors: a molecular basis for odor recognition. *Cell* 1991; **65**:175–87.

Burdach KJ & Doty RL. The effects of mouth movements, swallowing, and spitting on retronasal odor perception. *Physiology & Behavior* 1987; **41**:353–6.

Chalke HD, Dewhurst JR & Ward CW. Loss of smell in old people. *Public Health* 1958; **72**:223–30.

Davies DC, Brooks JW & Lewis DA. Axonal loss from the olfactory tracts in Alzheimer's disease. *Neurobiology of Aging* 1993; **14**:353–7.

Deems DA, Doty RL, Settle RG *et al.* Smell and taste disorders, a study of 750 patients from the University of Pennsylvania Smell and Taste Center. *Archives of Otolaryngology–Head & Neck Surgery* 1991; **117**:519–28.

Devanand DP, Michaels-Marston KS, Liu X *et al.* Olfactory deficits in patients with mild cognitive impairment predict Alzheimer's disease at follow-up. *The American Journal of Psychiatry* 2000; **157**:1399–405.

Ding X & Dahl AR. Olfactory mucosa: composition, enzymatic localization, and metabolism. In RL Doty (ed) *Handbook of Olfaction and Gustation* 2003, 2nd edn; Marcel Dekker, New York.

Doty RL. Olfactory dysfunction in neurogenerative disorders. In TV Getchell, RL Doty, LM Bartoshuk & JB Snow Jr (eds) *Smell and Taste in Health and Disease* 1991; Raven Press.

Doty RL. Smell and taste in the elderly. In ML Albert & JE Knoefel (eds) *Clinical Neurology of Aging* 1994, 2nd edn; Oxford University Press.

Doty RL. *The Smell Identification Test*™ *Administration Manual* 1995, 3rd edn; Sensonics, Inc., Haddon Heights, New Jersey.

Doty RL. Olfaction. *Annual Review of Psychology* 2001; **52**:423–52.

Doty RL. Odor perception in neurodegenerative diseases. In RL Doty (ed) *Handbook of Olfaction and Gustation* 2003, 2nd edn; Marcel Dekker, New York.

Doty RL & Bromley SM. Olfaction and taste. In A Crockard, R Hayward & JT Hoff (eds) *Neurosurgery: The Scientific Basis of Clinical Practice* 2000; Blackwell Science, London.

Doty RL & Bromley SM. Effects of drugs on olfaction and taste. *Otolaryngologic Clinics of North America* 2004; **37**:1229–54.

Doty RL & Cometto-Muñz JE. Trigeminal chemosensation. In RL Doty (ed) *Handbook of Olfaction and Gustation* 2003, 2nd edn; Marcel Dekker, New York.

Doty RL, Deems DA & Stellar S. Olfactory dysfunction in parkinsonism: a general deficit unrelated to neurologic signs, disease stage, or disease duration. *Neurology* 1988; **38**(8):1237–44.

Doty RL, Golbe LI, McKeown DA *et al.* Olfactory testing differentiates between progressive supranuclear palsy and idiopathic Parkinson's disease. *Neurology* 1993; **43**:962–5.

Doty RL & Mishra A. Olfaction and its alteration by nasal obstruction, rhinitis, and rhinosinusitis. *The Laryngoscope* 2001; **111**:409–23.

Doty RL, Perl DP, Steele JC *et al.* Olfactory dysfunction in three neurodegenerative diseases. *Geriatrics* 1991; **46**(suppl 1):47–51.

Doty RL, Philip S, Reddy K & Kerr KL. Influences of antihypertensive and antihyperlipidemic drugs on the senses of taste and smell: a review. *Journal of Hypertension* 2003; **21**:1805–13.

Doty RL, Shaman P, Applebaum SL *et al.* Smell identification ability: changes with age. *Science* 1984; **226**:1441–3.

Doty RL, Singh A, Tetrude J & Langston JW. Lack of olfactory dysfunction in MPTP-induced parkinsonism. *Annals of Neurology* 1992; **32**:97–100.

Doty RL, Yousem DM, Pham LT *et al.* Olfactory dysfunction in patients with head trauma. *Archives of Neurology* 1997; **54**:1131–40.

Duncan HJ & Seiden AM. Long-term follow-up of olfactory loss secondary to head trauma and upper respiratory tract infection. *Archives of Otolaryngology–Head & Neck Surgery* 1995; **121**:1183–7.

Esiri MM & Wilcock GK. The olfactory bulbs of Alzheimer's disease. *Journal of Neurology, Neurosurgery, and Psychiatry* 1984; **47**:56–60.

Facts for Features 2004; US Census Bureau, Washington.

Gomez-Isla T, Price JL, McKeel DW Jr *et al.* Profound loss of layer II entorhinal cortex neurons occurs in very mild Alzheimer's disease. *The Journal of Neuroscience* 1996; **16**:4491–500.

Graves AB, Bowen JD, Rajaram L *et al.* Impaired olfaction as a marker for cognitive decline: interaction with apolipoprotein E epsilon4 status. *Neurology* 1999; **53**:1480–7.

Grushka M & Sessle BJ. Burning mouth syndrome. In TV Getchell (ed) *Smell & Taste in Health & Disease* 1991, chapter 42; Raven Press.

Henkin RI, Schecter PJ, Friedewald WT *et al.* A double blind study of the effects of zinc sulfate on taste and smell dysfunction. *The American Journal of the Medical Sciences* 1976; **272**:285–99.

Hummel TM, Heilmann SM & Huttenbriuk KBM. Lipoic acid in the treatment of smell dysfunction following viral infection of the upper respiratory tract. *The Laryngoscope* 2002; **112**:2076–80.

Hyman BT, Arriagada PV & van Hoesen GW. Pathologic changes in the olfactory system in aging and Alzheimer's disease. *Annals of the New York Academy of Sciences* 1991; **640**:14–9.

Kern RC, Conley DB, Haines GK III & Robinson AM. Pathology of the olfactory mucosa: implications for the treatment of olfactory dysfunction. *The Laryngoscope* 2004; **114**:279–85.

Kovacs T, Cairns NJ & Lantos PL. Beta-amyloid deposition and neurofibrillary tangle formation in the olfactory bulb in ageing and Alzheimer's disease. *Neuropathology and Applied Neurobiology* 1999; **25**:481–91.

Kovacs T, Cairns NJ & Lantos PL. Olfactory centres in Alzheimer's disease: olfactory bulb is involved in early Braak's stages. *Neuroreport* 2001; **12**:285–8.

Matsuda T & Doty RL. Regional taste sensitivity to NaCl: relationship to subject age, tongue locus and area of stimulation. *Chemical Senses* 1995; **20**:283–90.

Menco BPM & Morrison EE. Morphology of the mammalian olfactory epithelium: form, fine structure, function, and pathology. In RL Doty (ed) *Handbook of Olfaction and Gustation* 2003; 2nd edn; Marcel Dekker, New York.

Miller SL, Mirza N & Doty RL. Electrogustometric thresholds: relationship to anterior tongue locus, area of stimulation, and number of fungiform papillae. *Physiology & Behavior* 2002; **75**:753–7.

Moon C & Ronnett GV. Molecular neurobiology of olfactory transduction. In RL Doty (ed) *Handbook of Olfaction and Gustation* 2003; Marcel Dekker, New York.

Murphy C, Doty RL & Duncan HJ. Clinical disorders of olfaction. In RL Doty (ed) *Handbook of Olfaction and Gustation* 2003, 2nd edn; Marcel Dekker, New York.

Murray RG. The ultrastructure of taste buds. In I Friedman (ed) *The Ultrasructure of Sensory Organs* 1973, pp 1–81; Elsevier, New York.

Nakashima T, Kimmelman CP & Snow JB Jr. Structure of human fetal and adult olfactory neuroepithelium. *Archives of Otolaryngology* 1984; **110**:641–6.

Pritchard TC. The primate gustatory system. In TV Getchell, RL Doty, LM Bartoshuk & JB Snow Jr (eds) *Smell and Taste in Health and Disease* 1991; Raven Press, New York.

Sajjadian A, Doty RL, Gutnick DN *et al.* Olfactory dysfunction in amyotrophic lateral sclerosis. *Neurodegeneration* 1994; **3**:153–7.

Settle RG. The chemical senses in diabetes mellitus. In TV Getchell, RL Doty, LM Bartoshuk & JB Snow Jr (eds) *Smell and Taste in Health and Disease* 1991; Raven Press, New York.

Shepherd GM. *Neurobiology* 1994; Oxford University Press, New York.

Ship JA, Grushka M, Lipton JA *et al.* Burning mouth syndrome: an update. *Journal of the American Dental Association* 1995; **126**:842–53.

Smutzer GS, Doty RL, Arnolds SE & Trojanowski JQ. Olfactory system neuropathology in Alzheimer's disease, Parkinson's disease, and schizophrenia. In RL Doty (ed) *Handbook of Olfaction and Gustation* 2003, 2nd edn, pp 503–23; Marcel Dekker, New York.

Tsuboi Y, Wszolek ZK, Graff-Radford NR *et al.* Tau pathology in the olfactory bulb correlates with Braak stage, Lewy body pathology and apolipoprotein epsilon 4. *Neuropathology and Applied Neurobiology* 2003; **29**:503–10.

Warwick R & Williams PL. *Gray's Anatomy* 1973; W.B. Saunders, Philadelphia.

Weiffenbach JM, Cowart BJ & Baum BJ. Taste intensity perception in aging. *Journal of Gerontology* 1986; **41**:460–8.

Wenning GK, Shephard B, Hawkes C *et al.* Olfactory function in atypical parkinsonian syndromes. *Acta Neurologica Scandinavica* 1995; **91**:247–50.

PART III

Medicine in Old Age

Section 9

Bone and Joint Health

108

Age-related Changes in Calcium Homeostasis and Bone Loss

Harvey James Armbrecht

Saint Louis University Health Sciences Center and Saint Louis Veterans' Affairs Medical Center, St Louis, MO, USA

INTRODUCTION

Serum calcium (Ca) must be maintained within narrow limits for the proper functioning of nerve, muscle, and bone. In general, the diurnal variation of serum Ca is plus or minus 3%. The major organs involved in Ca homeostasis are the intestine, bone, and kidney. The intestine absorbs Ca from the diet, the bone serves as a large reserve for Ca, and the kidney reabsorbs filtered Ca. These organs work together so that Ca loss is balanced by Ca intake.

Serum Ca does not change with age, but the mechanism by which it is maintained changes markedly with age. This fact has important implications for bone mass in older adults. This review will first describe the changes that take place with age in regard to Ca metabolism. It will then describe age-related changes in the levels and actions of the major calcium-regulating hormones, vitamin D, and parathyroid hormone (PTH). The implication of these changes for the maintenance of bone mass with age and possible causes for bone loss will be discussed. Finally, the efficacy of Ca and vitamin D supplementation will be examined. In general, the results of clinical studies will form the basis of this review. However, animal studies will be cited where relevant, particularly in the discussion of mechanisms.

DESCRIPTION OF CALCIUM METABOLISM

A typical daily Ca balance for a young adult is shown in Table 1. If 1000 mg of Ca is taken in the diet during the day, then the intestine will absorb about 300 mg. This assumes a 30% absorption efficiency in a young person. About 700 mg will be unabsorbed and lost in the feces, along with about 200 mg secreted into the intestine. Thus, the net Ca loss via the intestine is 900 mg. The kidney filters large amounts of Ca, but it reabsorbs about 98–99%. A typical daily loss of Ca in the urine is about 100 mg. Thus, under normal circumstances, the loss of Ca in the feces and urine (900 + 100 mg) is just balanced by the intake of dietary Ca (1000 mg). Serum Ca levels are buffered by a constant exchange of the Ca in bone with the Ca in the extracellular fluid. This exchange has been estimated to be about 250 mg. Normally, the amount of Ca deposited in the bone equals the amount reabsorbed, so that there is no net gain or loss of bone mineral.

A number of changes take place in Ca metabolism with age, even though serum Ca levels themselves do not change with age (Table 2). First, the amount of Ca in the diet tends to decline with age. Second, there is a decline in the efficiency of Ca absorption with age. Third, with regard to bone, Ca resorption tends to exceed Ca deposition, so that the net loss of Ca from bone increases with age. On the other hand, there is no evidence that the amount of Ca secreted into the intestine or that the amount of Ca excreted in the urine changes with age. The net effect of the decreased absorption of dietary Ca and the increased loss of Ca from bone is for Ca balance to become more negative with age. These age-related changes in Ca balance are also summarized in Table 1 (right column). The mechanisms responsible for these changes in Ca balance will be described in greater detail in the rest of the chapter.

REGULATION OF CALCIUM METABOLISM

The regulation of Ca homeostasis by intestine, bone, and kidney is coordinated by vitamin D and PTH (Holick, 2003) (Figure 1). When serum Ca falls below 10 mg/100 ml, this decrease is sensed by the parathyroid glands, which secrete

Principles and Practice of Geriatric Medicine, 4th Edition. Edited by M.S. John Pathy, Alan J. Sinclair and John E. Morley.

Table 1 Daily calcium balance in young adults

Parameter	Calcium (mg day^{-1})		Age changes
Dietary Ca		+1000	Decreases
Intestine			
Ca unabsorbed	−700		Increases
Ca secreted	−200		Unchanged
NET		−900	
Kidney			
Ca excreted	−100		Unchanged
NET		−100	
Bone			
Ca deposited	+250		Ca deposited less than Ca reabsorbed
Ca reabsorbed	−250		
NET		0	
Balance		0	Becomes negative

Table 2 Age-related changes in calcium metabolism

- Decreased amount of Ca in diet.
- Decreased efficiency of intestinal Ca absorption.
- Resorption of Ca from bone greater than deposition.
- RESULT: Net Ca balance becomes negative.

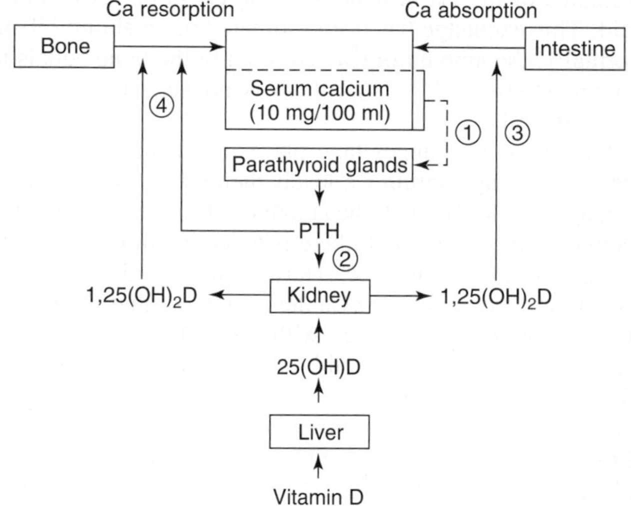

Figure 1 Regulation of serum calcium by vitamin D and PTH. A decrease in serum Ca is detected by the parathyroid glands, which respond by secreting PTH (step 1). PTH acts on the kidney to increase the conversion of 25(OH)D to $1,25(OH)_2D$, the active metabolite of vitamin D (step 2). $1,25(OH)_2D$ acts on the intestine to increase absorption of dietary Ca (step 3). $1,25(OH)_2D$ and PTH act together on bone to increase resorption of Ca from bone (step 4). These actions normalize serum Ca and reduce PTH secretion by the parathyroid glands

PTH in proportion to the fall in serum Ca (Figure 1, step 1). PTH acts on the kidney to increase the synthesis of the active form of vitamin D_3, 1,25-dihydroxyvitamin D_3 ($1,25(OH)_2D$) (Figure 1, step 2). Vitamin D_3 by itself has very little biological activity. The biologically active form is produced by first hydroxylating vitamin D_3 in the liver to form 25-hydroxyvitamin D_3 (25(OH)D), and 25(OH)D is then hydroxylated in the kidney to produce $1,25(OH)_2D$. The $1,25(OH)_2D$ then acts on the intestine to stimulate Ca absorption (Figure 1, step 3). In addition, PTH and $1,25(OH)_2D$ work in concert to stimulate Ca resorption from bone (Figure 1, step 4). The increased Ca absorption by the intestine and increased Ca resorption from bone tend to increase serum Ca levels. As serum Ca rises toward normal levels, PTH secretion by the parathyroid glands decreases.

AGE-RELATED CHANGES IN CALCIUM METABOLISM

In general, serum Ca does not change with age. Most clinical studies have reported that total serum Ca does not change with age (Fujisawa *et al.*, 1984; Insogna *et al.*, 1981; Tsai *et al.*, 1984), although some have reported a slight decline in serum ionized Ca (Wiske *et al.*, 1979). This maintenance of serum Ca is all the more remarkable since dietary intake of Ca tends to decline with age.

Changes in Intestinal Ca Absorption

There have been a number of clinical studies on the effect of age on intestinal Ca absorption (Gallagher *et al.*, 1979; Bullamore *et al.*, 1970; Ebeling *et al.*, 1992; Kinyamu *et al.*, 1997). Many of these studies have found a gradual decrease in Ca absorption with age (Gallagher *et al.*, 1979). The decrease in Ca absorption tended to parallel the decrease in serum $1,25(OH)_2D$ levels with age. One study (Bullamore *et al.*, 1970) found no decrease until after 60 years. One study, which found no age-related decrease in Ca absorption, reported an increase in serum $1,25(OH)_2D$ levels with age (Ebeling *et al.*, 1992). This suggested an age-related decrease in intestinal responsiveness to $1,25(OH)_2D$.

Changes in Bone Ca Deposition and Resorption

There is a progressive bone loss with age in both men and women. This bone loss results from the rate of resorption of Ca from bone exceeding the rate of Ca deposition during remodeling (Riggs and Melton, 1986). One possibility is that the activity of osteoblasts, the cells involved in bone formation, decreases with age relative to the activity of osteoclasts, the cells involved in bone resorption. In support of this, it has been reported that the osteoblasts of older individuals fail to completely refill the resorption cavities created by osteoclasts (Eriksen *et al.*, 1985). In addition, bone turnover (rate of formation and deposition) tends to increase with age (Eastell *et al.*, 1988). Thus, any discrepancy between bone formation relative to bone resorption tends to be magnified in older individuals who have rapid bone turnover.

Changes in Ca Balance

Ca balance is Ca ingested minus Ca excreted in the feces and urine. It must be zero or slightly positive to avoid chronic loss of bone mineral. Ca balance studies are difficult to perform because they generally require measuring the difference between two large numbers – Ca ingested in the diet and Ca excreted in the feces. However, when examined as a group, balance studies suggest that Ca balance decreases (becomes more negative) with age. Heaney (Heaney *et al.*, 1982) tabulated a number of balance studies, and they found that the mean Ca requirement was 668 mg day^{-1} for young and adult subjects and 1040 mg day^{-1} for elderly subjects.

AGE-RELATED CHANGES IN CALCIUM-REGULATING HORMONES

Changes in Serum $1,25(OH)_2D$

Most clinical studies have found a decline in serum $1,25(OH)_2D$ levels with age. Studies which have focused on older adults have reported a decrease in serum $1,25(OH)_2D$ between the ages of 50 and 65 (Fujisawa *et al.*, 1984; Gallagher *et al.*, 1979). This decrease in serum $1,25(OH)_2D$ levels could be due to several factors. These include decreased intake and absorption of dietary vitamin D, decreased synthesis of vitamin D in the skin (MacLaughlin and Holick, 1985), and decreased production of $1,25(OH)_2D$ by the kidney (Tsai *et al.*, 1984) (Table 3). In some of these studies, there was a decrease in serum $1,25(OH)_2D$ levels with age despite constant levels of 25(OH)D (Tsai *et al.*, 1984; Gallagher *et al.*, 1979). This suggests that there is a progressive decrease in the capacity of the kidney to hydroxylate 25(OH)D and form $1,25(OH)_2D$ with age. One study found no age-related change in serum $1,25(OH)_2D$ levels in men whose glomerular filtration rate was not reduced (Halloran *et al.*, 1990). This suggests that decreased renal function may contribute to decreased serum $1,25(OH)_2D$ levels.

Changes in Serum PTH

Numerous clinical studies have documented increases in serum immunoreactive PTH with age (Insogna *et al.*, 1981; Wiske *et al.*, 1979; Gallagher *et al.*, 1980; Forero *et al.*, 1987). The increased amount of PTH appears to be biologically active, since there is a concurrent increase in urinary cAMP and a decrease in tubular reabsorption of phosphorus with age (Insogna *et al.*, 1981; Forero *et al.*, 1987). These are both well-known actions of PTH in the kidney. It has been suggested that the age-related increase in serum immunoreactive PTH is due to decreased renal function. However, PTH levels increase with age even when decreased renal function is taken into account (Gallagher *et al.*, 1980). The increase in serum immunoreactive PTH appears to be due to increased PTH secretion by the parathyroid gland with age.

Table 3 Age-related changes in vitamin D metabolism

- Decreased intake and absorption of dietary vitamin D.
- Decreased vitamin D production by the skin.
- Decreased $1,25(OH)_2D$ production by the kidney.
- RESULT: Decreased serum $1,25(OH)_2D$ levels.

AGE-RELATED CHANGES IN THE REGULATION OF CALCIUM METABOLISM

There are a number of changes in the mechanism by which serum Ca is maintained throughout the lifespan (Table 4). Taken together, these changes tend to put older individuals at risk for age-related bone loss. In the following sections, these changes and their genesis will be discussed.

Decreased Renal $1,25(OH)_2D$ Production in Response to PTH

In the young, PTH stimulates renal $1,25(OH)_2D$ production (Figure 1, step 2). However, with age, serum $1,25(OH)_2D$ levels decline despite a progressive increase in serum PTH levels (see previous text). Refractoriness to PTH is also suggested by a study that found that maintenance of normal $1,25(OH)_2D$ production in elderly men required increased levels of serum PTH (Halloran *et al.*, 1990). The effect of age on renal responsiveness to PTH has been tested directly in several clinical studies. Two of these studies showed that the capacity of PTH to increase serum $1,25(OH)_2D$ declines with age (Tsai *et al.*, 1984; Kinyamu *et al.*, 1996). The third study found that the action of PTH was delayed with age, but that comparable levels were eventually achieved (Halloran *et al.*, 1996).

With regard to mechanisms, in the rat, the capacity of PTH to stimulate $1,25(OH)_2D$ production also declines with age (Armbrecht *et al.*, 1987). However, the capacity of PTH to stimulate second messenger signals does not change with age (Friedlander *et al.*, 1994). Likewise, the capacity of PTH to stimulate transcription of the gene for the enzyme that makes the $1,25(OH)_2D$, the renal 1alpha-hydroxylase, does not change with age (Armbrecht *et al.*, 2003). This suggests that there are age-related changes distal to the PTH receptor. However, an age-related decrease in PTH receptor number has also been reported (Hanai *et al.*, 1990).

Table 4 Age-related changes in Ca metabolism regulation

- Decreased renal $1,25(OH)_2D$ production in response to PTH.
- Decreased intestinal Ca absorption in response to $1,25(OH)_2D$.
- Decreased sensitivity of the parathyroid glands to serum Ca.
- Decreased bone deposition relative to resorption.

Decreased Intestinal Ca Absorption in Response to $1,25(OH)_2D$

In the young, $1,25(OH)_2D$ stimulates intestinal absorption of Ca (Figure 1, step 3). There are several clinical studies suggesting that intestinal responsiveness to $1,25(OH)_2D$ declines with age. In one study, increased levels of serum $1,25(OH)_2D$ were required to maintain Ca absorption in older individuals (Ebeling *et al.*, 1992). In a second study, serum $1,25(OH)_2D$ levels were manipulated over a wide range in young and elderly women (Pattanaungkul *et al.*, 2000). It was found that there was a relative resistance to $1,25(OH)_2D$ in elderly women with regard to Ca absorption.

The mechanisms responsible for this decreased intestinal responsiveness to $1,25(OH)_2D$ are still under investigation. In humans, some studies have found a correlation between decreased intestinal responsiveness and a decrease in intestinal vitamin D receptors (VDR) (Ebeling *et al.*, 1992). A decreased number of receptors could contribute to the decreased intestinal responsiveness to $1,25(OH)_2D$ with age. However, this has not been seen in all studies (Kinyamu *et al.*, 1997). In the rat, there is also an age-related decline in the capacity of $1,25(OH)_2D$ to stimulate intestinal Ca absorption (Wood *et al.*, 1998; Armbrecht *et al.*, 1999). This is correlated with the decreased capacity of $1,25(OH)_2D$ to stimulate key proteins involved in the intestinal transport of Ca (Armbrecht *et al.*, 1999; Armbrecht *et al.*, 1998). As in human studies, there is lack of agreement as to whether there is a decline in rat intestinal VDR with age. Some studies report a decline (Horst *et al.*, 1990) while others do not (Wood *et al.*, 1998).

Decreased Sensitivity of the Parathyroid Glands to Serum Ca

In the young, PTH secretion by the parathyroid glands is regulated by Ca levels in the blood (Figure 1, step 1). Numerous clinical studies have reported that serum PTH levels increase with age (see previous text), and one study correlated this with age-related bone loss (Ledger *et al.*, 1995). This rise in serum PTH is seen even when age-related changes in renal clearance are taken into account (Gallagher *et al.*, 1980), suggesting that there is an increase in PTH secretion by the parathyroid glands with age. Several studies have found that basal and stimulated PTH secretion was higher in older women compared to that in younger women (Ledger *et al.*, 1994; Portale *et al.*, 1997). However, the set point, which is the serum Ca concentration that inhibits half of the PTH secretion, did not change with age (Ledger *et al.*, 1994).

Since the rat also show studies in an age-related increase in serum PTH levels, it has been studied with regard to possible mechanisms. Perfusion studies have found that secretion of PTH increases with age in the rat (Uden *et al.*, 1992; Fox, 1991). One study attributed this to an increase in the set point with age (Uden *et al.*, 1992), but another did not (Fox, 1991). In molecular terms, the parathyroid gland senses external Ca levels via a Ca-sensing receptor. However, the expression of the Ca-sensing receptor in the parathyroid gland of the rat actually increases with age (Autry *et al.*, 1997).

PRIMARY VERSUS SECONDARY CHANGES IN Ca METABOLISM

Owing to the high degree of integration of the Ca regulating system, it is difficult to determine which age-related change (or changes) is primary and which changes are compensatory in response to the primary event(s). Two age-related changes that are often cited as explanations of age-related bone loss are (1) decreased stimulation of renal $1,25(OH)_2D$ production by PTH (Figure 1, step 2) and (2) decreased stimulation of intestinal Ca transport by $1,25(OH)_2D$ (Figure 1, step 3). Decreased production of $1,25(OH)_2D$ by the kidney would result in the observed decrease in serum $1,25(OH)_2D$ levels and in decreased intestinal Ca absorption with age. This would lead to a slight drop in serum Ca which would then result in increased secretion of PTH by the parathyroid glands.

On the other hand, decreased stimulation of the intestine by $1,25(OH)_2D$ could also explain the observed changes. Decreased Ca absorption would result in a slight drop in serum Ca, which would result in the observed increase in serum PTH with age. However, this model would predict a subsequent rise in serum $1,25(OH)_2D$ to overcome the intestinal resistance, unless there were also renal refractoriness to the action of PTH.

CHANGES IN Ca METABOLISM AND AGE-RELATED BONE LOSS (*see* Chapter 110, Epidemiology of Osteoporosis; Chapter 111, Osteoporosis and its Consequences: a Major Threat to the Quality of Life in the Elderly)

Postmenopausal Bone Loss

Bone mass declines with age in both men and women. There is a decline in skeletal mass that begins about the fourth or fifth decade and continues throughout life in both men and women. In women, there is an additional loss of bone during the first 5 years after menopause, which is superimposed on the age-related decline (Gallagher *et al.*, 1987). This has led to the concept that there are two types of bone loss – postmenopausal and age-related osteoporosis (Table 5) (Riggs and Melton, 1986). Postmenopausal (Type I) osteoporosis occurs earlier (51–75 years) and is seen in women. This type of osteoporosis is related to the loss of estrogen at menopause. The bone loss seen in postmenopausal osteoporosis is mainly trabecular, and it results in vertebral crush fractures and fractures of the distal radius. In postmenopausal osteoporosis, the primary event is excessive

Table 5 The two types of osteoporosis

	Postmenopausal (Type I)	Age-related (Type II)
Age (years)	51–75	70+
Sex	Female	Female/male
Fracture sites	Vertebrae (crush) Distal radius	Vertebrae (wedge) Hip
Ca absorption	Decreased	Decreased
Serum $1,25(OH)_2D$	Decreased	Decreased
Serum PTH	Decreased	Increased

Source: Adapted with permission from Riggs BL, Melton LJ, III, Involutional osteoporosis, *New England Journal of Medicine*, Copyright 1986, Massachusetts Medical Society.

resorption of bone due to the loss of the protective effect of estrogen at menopause. The excess Ca released from bone suppresses PTH secretion by the parathyroid glands, which reduces serum PTH levels (Figure 1). Decreased PTH levels then result in decreased renal production of $1,25(OH)_2D$ and decreased absorption of dietary Ca.

Age-related Bone Loss

Age-related (Type II) osteoporosis (sometimes referred to as *senile osteoporosis*) occurs later (after 70 years) and is found in men as well as in women (Table 5). The bone loss is cortical as well as trabecular, and it results in vertebral wedge fractures and hip fractures. Major contributors to age-related bone loss are the age-related changes in Ca metabolism described previously (Table 4). A decreased capacity of PTH to stimulate $1,25(OH)_2D$ production may lead to a decline in serum $1,25(OH)_2D$. A decreased action of $1,25(OH)_2D$ on the intestine tends to increase serum PTH levels. This rise in serum PTH is reinforced by the fact that the sensitivity of the parathyroid glands to Ca declines with age. The age-related rise in serum PTH levels results in a greater resorption of Ca from bone relative to deposition. It has also been proposed that a decline in estrogen plays a role in age-related bone loss – even in men (Riggs *et al.*, 1998). Possible mechanisms for this include the loss of estrogen action on the intestine and kidney, although these actions have not been well characterized.

Mechanisms of Age-related Bone Loss

Age-related bone loss is the culmination of multiple factors both extrinsic and intrinsic to bone (Seeman, 2003). The extrinsic factors include age-related changes in systemic hormones such as $1,25(OH)_2D$ and PTH (discussed above), estrogen, and growth hormone. Recent studies in rats have shown that at certain doses, $1,25(OH)_2D$ blocks the effect of PTH on bone resorption (Suda *et al.*, 2003). Thus, a decline in serum $1,25(OH)_2D$ levels may make the effect of PTH on bone even more pronounced in older animals. This may explain why chronic PTH administration increased the percent of bone-forming surface to a greater degree in aged rats than in young rats (Hock *et al.*, 1995). It has also been proposed that a decline in estrogen plays a role in age-related bone loss in both men and women (Riggs *et al.*, 1998). Finally, growth hormone and the insulin-like growth factors have been implicated in age-related bone loss (Geusens and Boonen, 2002).

In addition to hormonal changes, there are intrinsic changes within the bone itself that contribute to bone loss. There is increasing evidence that the responsiveness of bone cells to certain hormones and cytokines changes with age. Human osteoblast-like cells isolated from donors of different ages show a decreased responsiveness to insulin-like growth factor I (d'Avis *et al.*, 1997) and estrogen (Ankrom *et al.*, 1998). The response of osteoblastic cells to $1,25(OH)_2D$ has also been reported to decline with donor age (Martinez *et al.*, 2001). In osteoblast-like cells isolated from human trabecular bone, responsiveness to several growth factors declined as the age of the donor increased (Pfeilschifter *et al.*, 1993). In addition to changes in function, there also may be age-related changes that favor the production of osteoclasts over osteoblasts from bone marrow cells (Manolagas, 1998).

In general, the action of osteoblasts and osteoclasts is tightly coupled, but in age-related (and postmenopausal) osteoporosis, there is a loss of this coupling. Recently, the molecular basis of this coupling has been elucidated in the form of the RANK/RANKL/OPG regulatory system (see review by Boyle *et al.*, 2003). In mice, expression of RANKL (receptor activator of NF-kappaB ligand) and OPG (osteoprotegerin) correlates with age-related bone loss (Cao *et al.*, 2003). In humans, bone levels of RANKL increase with age (Fazzalari *et al.*, 2001), and this could mediate age-related bone loss. The RANK/RANKL/OPG system is regulated by many factors, including PTH and $1,25(OH)_2D$ (Suda *et al.*, 2003). It is also modulated by numerous hormones, growth factors, and cytokines. Changes in the local production and action of these factors, along with PTH and $1,25(OH)_2D$, may modulate the RANK/RANKL/OPG system and play an important role in age-related bone loss (see review by Troen, 2003).

DIETARY Ca AND VITAMIN D SUPPLEMENTATION (*see* Chapter 29, Vitamins and Minerals in the Elderly)

The roles of vitamin D supplementation (Lips, 2001) and Ca supplementation (Heaney, 2001) in reducing age-related bone loss have recently been reviewed. Since alterations in Ca and vitamin D metabolism contribute to age-related osteoporosis, Ca and vitamin D supplementation would be expected to be effective. This is in contrast to postmenopausal osteoporosis where there is an excess of Ca due to excessive resorption of mineral from bone. In a study by Dawson-Hughes *et al.*, (1990), Ca supplements had no effect on bone loss in the spine of women within 5 years of menopause. However, Ca supplementation retarded bone loss in women who were more than 5 years past menopause. Vitamin D and Ca supplementation together have been shown to reduce bone loss in both men and women over the age of 65 (Dawson-Hughes *et al.*, 1997). Significantly, in addition to reducing bone loss, vitamin D and Ca supplementation have been shown to reduce hip and other nonvertebral fractures (Chapuy *et al.*, 1992). Vitamin D and Ca supplementation have also been shown to reduce the seasonal variation in bone loss that is seen in more northern climates (Meier *et al.*, 2004). Finally, antiresorptive drug therapies are more effective in the presence of adequate dietary Ca (Nieves *et al.*, 1998).

Acknowledgment

This work was supported by the Geriatric Research, Education, and Clinical Center and the Medical Research Service of the Department of Veterans Affairs.

KEY POINTS

- Intestinal absorption of dietary Ca declines with age.
- Serum PTH increases with age while serum 1,25 $(OH)_2D$ stays the same or declines.
- Resorption of Ca from bone gradually exceeds deposition with age.
- These changes contribute to age-related bone loss after the age of 70.
- Age-related bone loss can be reduced by dietary Ca and/or vitamin D.

KEY REFERENCES

- Heaney RP. Calcium needs of the elderly to reduce fracture risk. *Journal of the American College of Nutrition* 2001; **20**:192S–7S.
- Holick MF. Vitamin D: a millenium perspective. *Journal of Cellular Biochemistry* 2003; **88**:296–307.
- Lips P. Vitamin D deficiency and secondary hyperparathyroidism in the elderly: consequences for bone loss and fractures and therapeutic implications. *Endocrine Reviews* 2001; **22**:477–501.
- Seeman E. Invited review: pathogenesis of osteoporosis. *Journal of Applied Physiology* 2003; **95**:2142–51.
- Suda T, Ueno Y, Fujii K & Shinki T. Vitamin D and bone. *Journal of Cellular Biochemistry* 2003; **88**:259–66.

REFERENCES

Ankrom MA, Patterson JA, d'Avis PY *et al.* Age-related changes in human oestrogen receptor alpha function and levels in osteoblasts. *The Biochemical Journal* 1998; **333**((Pt 3)):787–94.

Armbrecht HJ, Boltz MA, Christakos S & Bruns ME. Capacity of 1,25-dihydroxyvitamin D to stimulate expression of calbindin D changes with age in the rat. *Archives of Biochemistry and Biophysics* 1998; **352**:159–64.

Armbrecht HJ, Boltz MA & Hodam TL. PTH increases renal 25(OH)D_3-1alpha-hydroxylase (CYP1alpha) mRNA but not renal 1,25$(OH)_2D_3$ production in adult rats. *American Journal of Physiology Renal Physiology* 2003; **284**:F1032–6.

Armbrecht HJ, Boltz MA & Kumar VB. Intestinal plasma membrane calcium pump protein and its induction by 1,25$(OH)_2D_3$ decrease with age. *The American Journal of Physiology* 1999; **277**:G41–7.

Armbrecht HJ, Wongsurawat N & Paschal RE. Effect of age on renal responsiveness to parathyroid hormone and calcitonin in rats. *Journal of Endocrinology* 1987; **114**:173–8.

Autry CP, Kifor O, Brown EM *et al.* $Ca2^+$ receptor mRNA and protein increase in the rat parathyroid gland with advancing age. *The Journal of Endocrinology* 1997; **153**:437–44.

Boyle WJ, Simonet WS & Lacey DL. Osteoclast differentiation and activation. *Nature* 2003; **423**:337–42.

Bullamore JR, Gallagher JC, Wilkinson R & Nordin BEC. Effect of age on calcium absorption. *Lancet* 1970; **II**:535–7.

Cao J, Venton L, Sakata T & Halloran BP. Expression of RANKL and OPG correlates with age-related bone loss in male C57BL/6 mice. *Journal of Bone and Mineral Research* 2003; **18**:270–7.

Chapuy MC, Arlot ME, Duboeuf F *et al.* Vitamin D_3 and calcium to prevent hip fractures in the elderly women. *The New England Journal of Medicine* 1992; **327**:1637–42.

d'Avis PY, Frazier CR, Shapiro JR & Fedarko NS. Age-related changes in effects of insulin-like growth factor I on human osteoblast-like cells. *The Biochemical Journal* 1997; **324**(Pt 3):753–60.

Dawson-Hughes B, Dallal GE, Krall EA *et al.* A controlled trial of the effect of calcium supplementation on bone density in postmenopausal women. *The New England Journal of Medicine* 1990; **323**:878–83.

Dawson-Hughes B, Harris SS, Krall EA & Dallal GE. Effect of calcium and vitamin D supplementation on bone density in men and women 65 years of age or older. *The New England Journal of Medicine* 1997; **337**:670–6.

Eastell R, Delmas PD, Hodgson SF *et al.* Bone formation rate in older normal women: concurrent assessment with bone histomorphometry, calcium kinetics, and biochemical markers. *The Journal of Clinical Endocrinology and Metabolism* 1988; **67**:741–8.

Ebeling PR, Sansgren ME, DiMagno EP *et al.* Evidence of an age-related decrease in intestinal responsiveness to vitamin D: relationship between serum 1,25-dihydroxyvitamin D_3 and intestinal vitamin D receptor concentrations in normal women. *The Journal of Clinical Endocrinology and Metabolism* 1992; **75**:176–82.

Eriksen EF, Mosekilde L & Melsen F. Trabecular bone resorption depth decreases with age: differences between normal males and females. *Bone* 1985; **6**:141–6.

Fazzalari NL, Kuliwaba JS, Atkins GJ *et al.* The ratio of messenger RNA levels of receptor activator of nuclear factor kappaB ligand to osteoprotegerin correlates with bone remodeling indices in normal human cancellous bone but not in osteoarthritis. *Journal of Bone and Mineral Research* 2001; **16**:1015–27.

Forero MS, Klein RF, Nissenson RA *et al.* Effect of age on circulating immunoreactive and bioactive parathyroid hormone levels in women. *Journal of Bone and Mineral Research* 1987; **2**:363–6.

Fox J. Regulation of parathyroid hormone secretion by plasma calcium in aging rats. *The American Journal of Physiology* 1991; **260**:E220–5.

Friedlander J, Janulis M, Tembe V *et al.* Loss of parathyroid hormone-stimulated 1,25-dihydroxyvitamin D3 production in aging does not involve protein kinase A or C pathways. *Journal of Bone and Mineral Research* 1994; **9**:339–45.

Fujisawa Y, Kida K & Matsuda H. Role of change in vitamin D metabolism with age in calcium and phosphorus metabolism in normal human subjects. *The Journal of Clinical Endocrinology and Metabolism* 1984; **59**:719–26.

Gallagher JC, Goldgar D & Moy A. Total bone calcium in normal women: effect of age and menopause status. *Journal of Bone and Mineral Research* 1987; **2**:491–6.

Gallagher JC, Riggs BL, Eisman J *et al.* Intestinal calcium absorption and serum vitamin D metabolites in normal subjects and osteoporotic patients. *The Journal of Clinical Investigation* 1979; **64**:729–36.

Gallagher JC, Riggs BL, Jerpbak CM & Arnaud CD. The effect of age on serum immunoreactive parathyroid hormone in normal and osteoporotic women. *The Journal of Laboratory and Clinical Medicine* 1980; **95**:373–85.

Geusens PP & Boonen S. Osteoporosis and the growth hormone-insulin-like growth factor axis. *Hormone Research* 2002; **58**(suppl 3):49–55.

Halloran BP, Lonergan ET & Portale AA. Aging and renal responsiveness to parathyroid hormone in healthy men. *The Journal of Clinical Endocrinology and Metabolism* 1996; **81**:2192–7.

Halloran BP, Portale AA, Lonergan ET & Morris RC. Production and metabolic clearance of 1.25-dihydroxyvitamin D in men: effect of advancing age. *The Journal of Clinical Endocrinology and Metabolism* 1990; **70**:318–23.

Hanai H, Brennan DP, Cheng L *et al.* Downregulation of parathyroid hormone receptors in renal membranes from aged rats. *The American Journal of Physiology* 1990; **259**:F444–50.

Heaney RP. Calcium needs of the elderly to reduce fracture risk. *Journal of the American College of Nutrition* 2001; **20**:192S–7S.

Heaney RP, Gallagher JC & Johnston CC. Calcium nutrition and bone health in the elderly. *The American Journal of Clinical Nutrition* 1982; **36**:986–1013.

Hock JM, Onyia J & Bidwell J. Comparisons of *in vivo* and *in vitro* models of the response of osteoblasts to hormonal regulation with aging. *Calcified Tissue International* 1995; **56**(suppl 1):S44–7.

Holick MF. Vitamin D: a millenium perspective. *Journal of Cellular Biochemistry* 2003; **88**:296–307.

Horst RL, Goff JP & Reinhardt TA. Advancing age results in reduction of intestinal and bone 1,25-dihydroxyvitamin D receptor. *Endocrinology* 1990; **126**:1053–7.

Insogna KL, Lewis AM, Lipinski BA *et al.* Effect of age on serum immunoreactive parathyroid hormone and its biological effects. *The Journal of Clinical Endocrinology and Metabolism* 1981; **53**:1072–5.

Kinyamu HK, Gallagher JC, Petranick KM & Ryschon KL. Effect of parathyroid hormone (hPTH[1–34]) infusion on serum 1,25-dihydroxyvitamin D and parathyroid hormone in normal women. *Journal of Bone and Mineral Research* 1996; **11**:1400–5.

Kinyamu HK, Gallagher JC, Prahl JM *et al.* Association between intestinal vitamin D receptor, calcium absorption, and serum 1,25 dihydroxyvitamin D in normal young and elderly women. *Journal of Bone and Mineral Research* 1997; **12**:922–8.

Ledger GA, Burritt MF, Kao PC *et al.* Abnormalities of parathyroid hormone secretion in elderly women that are reversible by short term therapy with 1,25-dihydroxyvitamin D_3. *The Journal of Clinical Endocrinology and Metabolism* 1994; **79**:211–6.

Ledger GA, Burritt MF, Kao PC *et al.* Role of parathyroid hormone in mediating nocturnal and age-related increases in bone resorption. *The Journal of Clinical Endocrinology and Metabolism* 1995; **80**:3304–10.

Lips P. Vitamin D deficiency and secondary hyperparathyroidism in the elderly: consequences for bone loss and fractures and therapeutic implications. *Endocrine Reviews* 2001; **22**:477–501.

MacLaughlin J & Holick MF. Aging decreases the capacity of human skin to produce vitamin D3. *The Journal of Clinical Investigation* 1985; **76**:1536–8.

Manolagas SC. Cellular and molecular mechanisms of osteoporosis. *Aging (Milano)* 1998; **10**:182–90.

Martinez P, Moreno I, De Miguel F *et al.* Changes in osteocalcin response to 1,25-dihydroxyvitamin D_3 stimulation and basal vitamin D receptor expression in human osteoblastic cells according to donor age and skeletal origin. *Bone* 2001; **29**:35–41.

Meier C, Woitge HW, Witte K *et al.* Supplementation with oral vitamin D_3 and calcium during winter prevents seasonal bone loss: a randomized controlled open-label prospective trial. *Journal of Bone and Mineral Research* 2004; **19**:1221–30.

Nieves JW, Komar L, Cosman F & Lindsay R. Calcium potentiates the effect of estrogen and calcitonin on bone mass: review and analysis. *The American Journal of Clinical Nutrition* 1998; **67**:18–24.

Pattanaungkul S, Riggs BL, Yergey AL *et al.* Relationship of intestinal calcium absorption to 1,25-dihydroxyvitamin D [$1,25(OH)_2D$] levels in young versus elderly women: evidence for age-related intestinal resistance to $1,25(OH)_2D$ action. *The Journal of Clinical Endocrinology and Metabolism* 2000; **85**:4023–7.

Pfeilschifter J, Diel I, Pilz U *et al.* Mitogenic responsiveness of human bone cells *in vitro* to hormones and growth factors decreases with age. *Journal of Bone and Mineral Research* 1993; **8**:707–17.

Portale AA, Lonergan ET, Tanney DM & Halloran BP. Aging alters calcium regulation of serum concentration of parathyroid hormone in healthy men. *The American Journal of Physiology* 1997; **272**:E139–46.

Riggs BL, Khosla S & Melton LJ III. A unitary model for involutional osteoporosis: estrogen deficiency causes both type I and type II osteoporosis in postmenopausal women and contributes to bone loss in aging men. *Journal of Bone and Mineral Research* 1998; **13**:763–73.

Riggs BL & Melton LJ III. Involutional osteoporosis. *The New England Journal of Medicine* 1986; **314**:1676–86.

Seeman E. Invited review: pathogenesis of osteoporosis. *Journal of Applied Physiology* 2003; **95**:2142–51.

Suda T, Ueno Y, Fujii K & Shinki T. Vitamin D and bone. *Journal of Cellular Biochemistry* 2003; **88**:259–66.

Troen BR. Molecular mechanisms underlying osteoclast formation and activation. *Experimental Gerontology* 2003; **38**:605–14.

Tsai KS, Heath H, Kumar R & Riggs BL. Impaired vitamin D metabolism with aging in women. Possible role in pathogenesis of senile osteoporosis. *The Journal of Clinical Investigation* 1984; **73**:1668–72.

Uden P, Halloran B, Daly R *et al.* Set-point for parathyroid hormone release increases with postmaturational aging in the rat. *Endocrinology* 1992; **131**:2251–6.

Wiske PS, Epstein S, Bell NH *et al.* Increases in immunoreactive parathyroid hormone with age. *The New England Journal of Medicine* 1979; **300**:1419–21.

Wood RJ, Fleet JC, Cashman K *et al.* Intestinal calcium absorption in the aged rat: evidence of intestinal resistance to $1,25(OH)_2$vitamin D. *Endocrinology* 1998; **139**:3843–8.

109

Paget's Disease of Bone

Sanjay Sharma *and* Kenneth W. Lyles
Veterans' Affairs Medical Center, Duke University Medical Center, Durham, NC, USA

INTRODUCTION

Paget's disease of the bone, also known as *Osteitis deformans* is a common chronic focal disorder of the skeleton characterized by an abnormal rate of bone turnover and disorganized osteoid formation. The disorder was first described by Sir James Paget in 1877 (Paget, 1877). He described six cases of slowly progressive deforming bone disorder, which he termed *Osteitis deformans*. He considered the disease to be a chronic inflammation of the bone. The disease is characterized by accelerated skeletal remodeling due to abnormal osteoclasts, which can involve a single bone (monostotic) or multiple bones (polyostotic). This leads to bony hypertrophy, expansion of the bone cortex and resultant abnormal bone structure responsible for bone pain, deformity, and skeletal fragility. Complications of this disease can involve bones (deformity, fracture, and neoplastic degeneration), joints (osteoarthritis), the nervous system, and the vascular system (Delmas and Meunier, 1997). The abnormal bone has increased metabolic activity and blood flow, which in itself may contribute to pain, and can also increase neurological complications as a part of vascular steal syndrome. The disease usually affects people older than 50 years and has characteristic geographic distribution.

EPIDEMIOLOGY

The epidemiology of Paget's disease is unusual because of its distinctive geographic distribution throughout the world. It is commonly seen in the United Kingdom, Australia, United States, New Zealand, and central Europe. It is less common in Switzerland, Scandinavia, southern Europe, and Ireland, and is conspicuously rare in countries like India, Japan, China, the Middle East, and black Africa (Barker, 1984; Collins, 1956). Both environmental and genetic factors have been thought to play a role and have been studied for more than 20 years. There is still no definite answer to the disorder's etiology (Collins, 1956).

Since the disorder mostly affects older individuals, the disease is rarely seen before the age of 40; however, the prevalence doubles each decade from the age of 50 onwards (Kanis, 1998) to reach 10% in the ninth decade. The incidence of disease is difficult to estimate because most of the patients remain asymptomatic. A study from the Netherlands reports that 1 in 43 asymptomatic people over the age of 50 have Paget's disease, while 1 in 5 people over the age of 50 with an elevated alkaline phosphatase level have Paget's disease. In the United Kingdom, prevalence is 2.5% in men and 1.6% in women aged 55 years and older. However, there is also a marked variation in the prevalence of the disease in Great Britain itself, with rates ranging from 8.3% in parts of northwest England to 4.6% in southern areas. In the United States, it occurs in 1.5–3.0% of people over 60 years and the prevalence is slightly higher in northeast than in south (Ankrom and Shapiro, 1998). The disorder affects men and women equally (Polednak, 1987). Also, recent epidemiologic studies suggest a decline in the prevalence and the severity of the disorder in New Zealand and the United Kingdom (Ankrom and Shapiro, 1998; Polednak, 1987; Cundy *et al.*, 1997; Kanis, 1991; Cooper *et al.*, 1999; Baker *et al.*, 1997, 1980).

ETIOLOGY

The etiology of Paget's disease remains unknown (Delmas and Meunier, 1997). Several familial and pathologic studies suggest genetic susceptibility (Barry, 1969). Viral infections play a pathogenetic role. Several Paramyxoviruses (measles virus, respiratory syncytial virus, and canine distemper virus) have been thought to play a role in the etiology of Paget's disease but this hypothesis still remains controversial (Rebel *et al.*, 1974; Mills and Singer, 1976; Basle *et al.*, 1986; Gordon *et al.*, 1991, 1992; Ralston *et al.*, 1991; Birch *et al.*,

Principles and Practice of Geriatric Medicine, 4th Edition. Edited by M.S. John Pathy, Alan J. Sinclair and John E. Morley.

1994). These observations were based upon findings of intranuclear inclusion of nucleocapsid-like structures and antigens in the osteoclast nuclei and cytoplasm. In addition, Paramyxovirus transcripts also have been identified in the osteoclast precursor cells (Basle *et al.*, 1986; Gordon *et al.*, 1991, 1992; Ralston *et al.*, 1991; Birch *et al.*, 1994; Reddy *et al.*, 1995, 1996). However, attempts to isolate or culture the viruses from pagetic cells remain unsuccessful. Hence, the role of Paramyxovirus in the etiology of Paget's disease remains controversial. Some of the studies have also found elevated levels of Interleukin-6 (IL-6, a peptide produced by bone cells) in the marrow, plasma, and blood from patients with Paget's disease, which increases differentiation of monocyte/macrophage cells to osteoclasts. IL-6 has been shown to promote osteoclast formation when added to the marrow cells (Roodrnan *et al.*, 1992); however, elevated productions of cytokines have not been confirmed by all reports and hence still remains a subject of interest. It has also been postulated that viral infection upregulates the IL-6 gene and the IL-6 receptors in Paget's disease (Hoyland *et al.*, 1994). However, elevated levels of cytokines have not been consistently shown in all the studies. It still remains unknown what triggers the initial lesions.

Paget's disease also appears to have a significant genetic component, as approximately 15–30% of patients have a positive family history of the disorder (McKusick, 1972; Sins *et al.*, 1991; Morales-Piga *et al.*, 1995). An autosomal pattern of transmission has also been described. In families with apparent autosomal dominant inheritance of Paget's disease, four susceptibility loci have been identified, one on chromosome 18, one on chromosome 6 and two on chromosome 5 (Haslam *et al.*, 1998; Good *et al.*, 2001; Laurin *et al.*, 2001). Patients with a positive family history have an earlier onset of the disease and a greater prevalence of bone deformity than those with a negative family history. Various histocompatibility antigens (HLA) have also been associated with Paget's disease; however, these results have not been replicated (Tilyard *et al.*, 1982; Foldes *et al.*, 1991; Singer *et al.*, 1985, 1996).

PATHOPHYSIOLOGY

The disease is characterized by the formation of abnormal bone. In the early stages, there is increase resorption of the bone at localized areas caused by recruitment of large and numerous osteoclasts. These osteoclasts are large and may have up to 100 nuclei. These areas of localized resorption on radiographs are seen as advancing lytic wedge or "blade of grass" lesion in the long bones or as a resorptive wave or "osteoporosis circumscripta" in the skull. This phase of resorption is followed by a compensatory increase in bone formation with recruitment of osteoblasts in the areas of bone resorption. The osteoblasts form new osteoid tissue at a rapid rate and this is deposited in a disorganized, woven, or mosaic pattern that replaces the normal lamellar pattern seen in bone remodeling units. This result in the formation of a woven pattern of bone that is of poor quality and can bow and fracture easily (Meunier *et al.*, 1980). Different stages of the disease processes can be seen at the same time in different areas of bone. Furthermore, the bone marrow becomes infiltrated with an excess of fibrous connective tissue and blood vessels, leading to hypervascularity. Over time, the remodeling activity at a pagetic site decreases and leaves sclerotic or mosaic bone.

CLINICAL PRESENTATION

Most patients with Paget's disease are asymptomatic. It is commonly accepted that approximately 5% of the patients have symptoms but the estimates vary considerably. Most of the patients at the time of diagnosis are usually more than 45 years old. In the majority of cases, the diagnosis is made incidentally when the routine chemistry shows an elevated serum alkaline phosphatase level or an incidental lesion is noted on the X rays of the pelvis or spine, obtained for a different reason. Symptoms depend on the bone(s) and the part of the bone involved as well as the activity of the bone remodeling. Bone pain and deformity remain the two most common clinical manifestations of the disease. Most of the patients have one or several bones affected by Paget's disease. The areas commonly involved include the pelvis, vertebrae, skull, femur, and tibia. However, any bone may be affected. The bones of upper extremity, clavicle, and scapula are not commonly involved.

Bone deformity remains a hallmark of the disease. It is usually manifested as an increase in size and/or abnormal shape of bone. Progressive painless bowing of the weight-bearing, lower-extremity long bones is a feature. Deformity is most commonly seen in the femur, tibia, humerus, and ulna. The bowing seen in the femur and tibia are often associated with fissure (incomplete) fractures seen on the convex surface of the bowed bone. The most serious fractures involve the femoral shaft or subtrochanteric area. The femoral fractures may have a higher rate of nonunion, between 10 and 40%. Bone deformity can cause joint destruction and lead to osteoarthritis in joints proximate to bones with Pagetic lesions. There can be an increase in the skin temperature over the affected long bone, especially tibia. This is a sign of increased vascularity of the surrounding soft tissue and the bone, which is characteristic of active Paget's disease. Other bones in which deformity can occur are the skull, jaws, and the clavicles.

Bone pain is another well-recognized feature of Paget's disease that often appears late, rather than early, in the course of disease. Pain is usually described as dull but may be the sharp shooting type as well. It is often present at rest and worsen by weight bearing, especially if the disease involves the weight-bearing bones. Periarticular bone pain sometimes can be the presenting feature and is an important diagnostic problem because Paget's disease commonly affects bones around major weight-bearing joints as well as the spine. Acute pain may develop at times because of the consequence of pathologic fractures. It is thought that the pain arises because of periosteal stretching caused by bone enlargement, hyperemia, and often because of microfractures. The pain may be due to the pagetic lesion itself or from its complications caused by the abnormal bone, such as degenerative arthritis, nerve impingement, and rarely due to osteosarcoma. These complications have a striking impact on the overall quality of life for many patients (Gold *et al.*, 1996).

Neurological symptoms may arise due to the involvement of the axial skeleton, depending upon the site of involvement. The symptoms may be progressive and often overlooked in elders. The involvement of skull may cause nonspecific headaches, conductive hearing loss due to the involvement of the temporal bone, or the ossicles of the inner ear itself, which is a disabling complication (Sparrow and Duvall, 1967). Other cranial nerves including the optic, trigeminal, and facial nerves may also be involved, rarely resulting in visual loss, tic douloureux, and facial palsy. Enlargement of the skull may cause frontal bossing (enlargement of the vault) and the resultant change is the hat size. Deformity of the base of the skull can cause brainstem compression and sometimes obstructive hydrocephalus. Involvement of the spine can cause symptoms due to radiculopathy, spinal stenosis, and ischemia of the spinal cord due to "vascular steal" syndrome, resulting in ischemic myelitis. The symptoms associated with spinal stenosis are much less common despite the high prevalence of the pagetic involvement of the vertebrae. Patients may develop paraplegia or quadriplegia depending upon the extent of the disease.

A variety of cardiac disorders can be associated with Paget's disease and are usually seen if there is an involvement of more than one-third of the skeleton. Patients can develop calcific aortic stenosis (Hultgren, 1998), conduction abnormalities, and congestive heart failure. Cardiac output increases with increasing extent of the disease (Haworth, 1953) because of an increased vascularity of the bone and surrounding tissue; however, documented occurrences of the high output failure is uncommon.

A much higher incidence of bone tumors is seen in patients with Paget's disease compared to age-matched individuals. The most common tumor associated with Paget's disease is Osteosarcoma which is seen in less than 1% of patients (Haibach *et al.*, 1985; Hadjipavlou *et al.*, 1992). It is more commonly seen in the polyostotic form of Paget's. The prevalence of sarcoma gradually increases with age and the mean age at the time of diagnosis is usually 68 years. These are commonly found in the femur, pelvis, humerus, skull, and facial bones. The prognosis associated with sarcoma remains very poor and most of the patients die within 12 months of diagnosis. Other types of tumors associated with Paget's disease are chondrosarcomas, fibrosarcomas, and tumors of mixed histological characters. When malignant neoplasms occur, they tend to be very aggressive and may be fatal unless the neoplasm is completely removed (usually requiring limb amputation). Giant cell tumors of the bone are seen in a much smaller percentage of patients and are usually benign (Singer and Mills, 1993).

Other fibrosing or inflammatory disorders that are also sometimes seen with Paget's disease are Dupuytren's contracture, Peyronie's disease, and Hashimoto thyroiditis. It is not known whether these are caused by the release of cytokines from the areas of increased bone turnover or are just associated with Paget's disease.

Generally, levels of serum, calcium, and phosphorus do not change in Paget's disease; however, hypercalcemia can sometimes be seen due to prolonged immobilization or fractures. Nephrolithiasis can occur but is unusual. Occasionally, hyperuricemia and gout may be seen.

DIAGNOSTIC EVALUATION

As most of the patients with Paget's disease remain asymptomatic, the diagnosis is usually made on the basis of the radiological and biochemical abnormalities that are detected incidentally. A thorough history and physical examination remains the key to the diagnosis.

Radiology and Radionuclide Bone Scanning

The most sensitive means of detecting Paget's disease in the skeleton is by means of radionuclide bone scan. All patients with Paget's disease should have a total body bone scan using technetium-labeled bisphosphonate tracer (Fogelman *et al.*, 1981) to define the disease activity and its distribution. (Figure 1) The agent after administration is preferentially concentrated in areas of increased blood flow and high levels of bone formation, common characteristic of Paget's disease. These rapidly remodeling areas appear as hot spots. Even though there are characteristic patterns of tracer uptake, plain X rays are required to confirm the diagnosis of Paget's disease. In approximately 15–30% of the patients, the bone scan may pick up lesions not seen on the X rays. Rarely, a sclerotic lesion in an untreated patient exhibits no tracer uptake presumably because disease activity is negligible or "burned out". Generally, the bone scans are not used for follow-up of patients but primarily to establish the disease activity and extent of the skeletal involvement. However, in patients with localized disease, monostotic form, and normal biochemical indices, serial quantitative bone scans may be used to determine the objective response to the therapy.

The diagnosis of Paget's disease is primarily made by radiographic examination of the skeleton (Resnick, 1995). Plain radiographs are useful for diagnosis as well as detection of complications associated with the disease process (Figures 2, 3 and 4). In the early stages the disease is characterized by lytic areas that may be seen as V-shaped "cutting cone" lesions that are first seen at one end, gradually progressing toward the other end. The V-shaped lesion can grow at a speed of up to 1 cm $year^{-1}$. In the skull, the lytic areas are seen as osteoporosis circumscripta (well-defined lucent areas), which commonly involves the frontal, parietal, and occipital bones. In the later stages, the scleroticchanges also

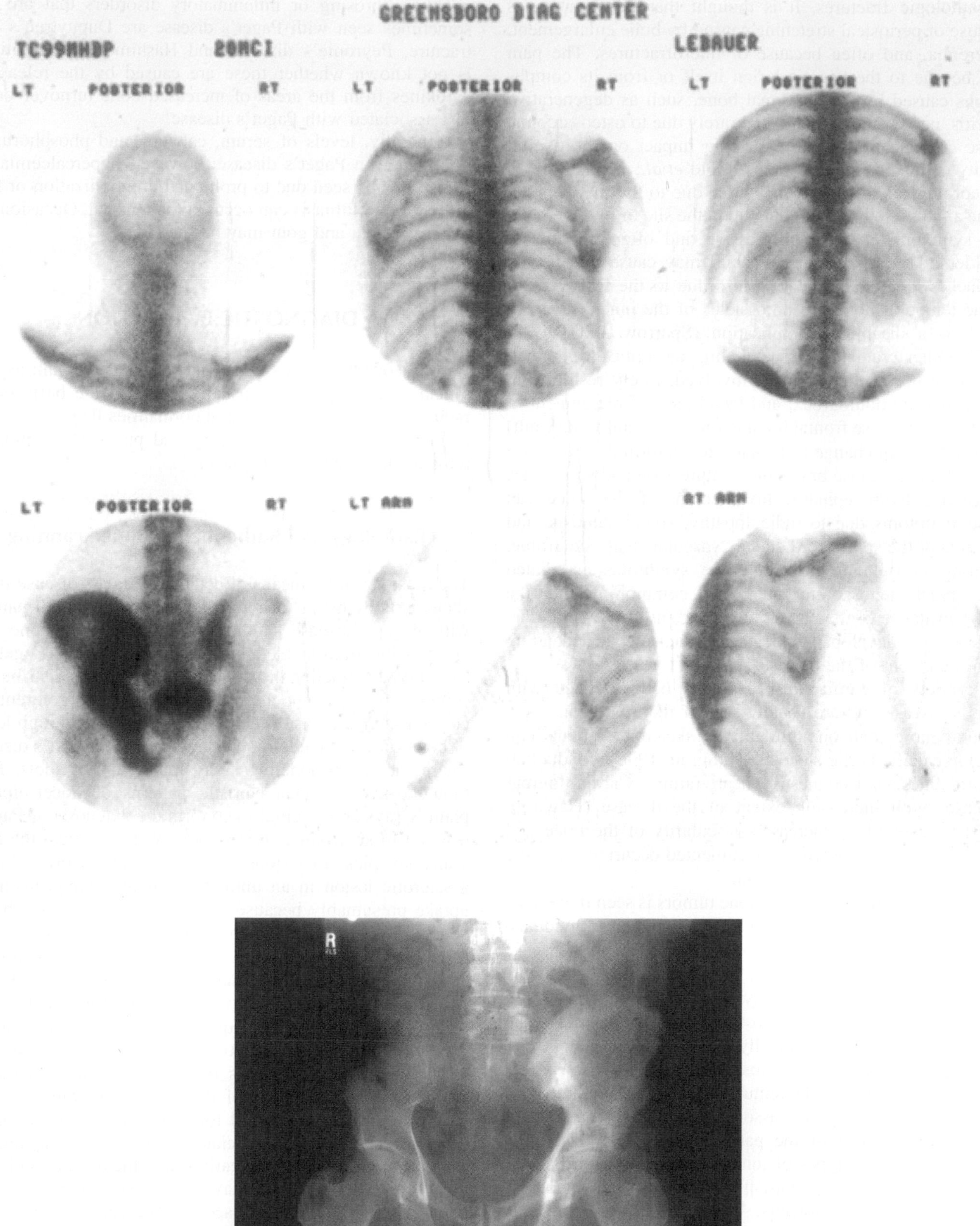

Figure 1 and 2 This 57-year-old man had an elevated alkaline phosphatase of 257 IU (normal 30–135) found on an annual physical examination. He had no symptoms and had a normal physical examination. Total body bone scan and pelvic radiographs confirmed Paget's disease of the bone on the left Ileum

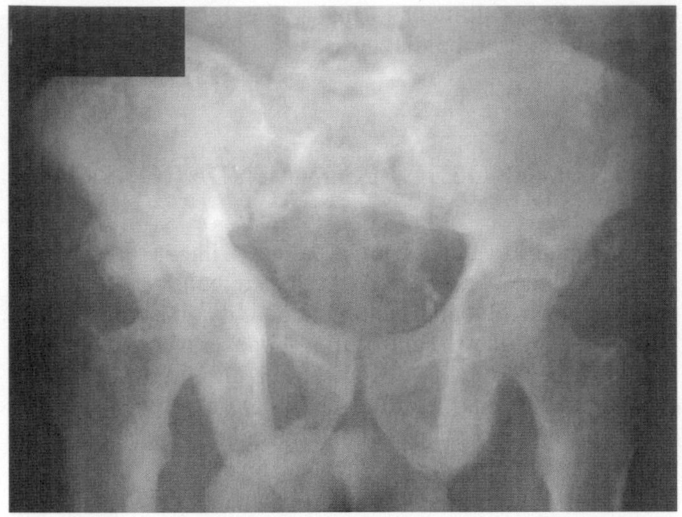

Figure 3 This 45-year-old man has polyostotic Paget's disease involving his pelvis, sacrum, and right femur. He has developed osteoarthritis in the right hip

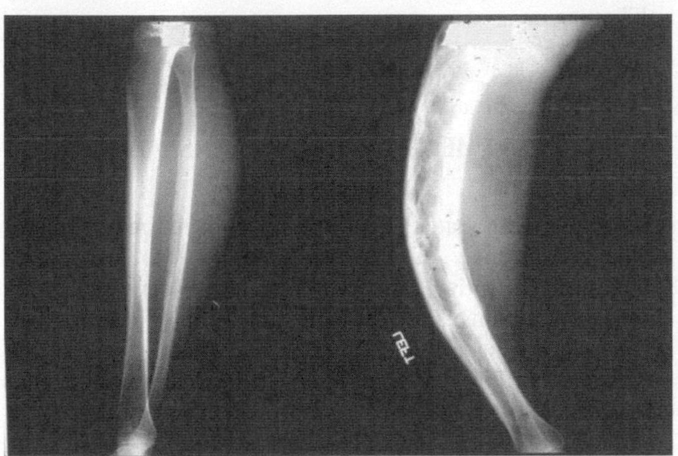

Figure 4 This 82-year-old lady had untreated Paget's disease of the bone in the left tibia. Notice the bowing compared to a normal tibia. Also the affected tibia is larger in size, has thickened cortices, evidence of thickened trabeculae and loss of trabeculae

appear along with the lytic changes resulting in thickening of the cortex and loss of distinction at the corticomedullary junction. Plain X rays can reveal both osteolytic and sclerotic changes in the same bone if taken at this stage. In the last and final stages of the disease, the sclerotic phase predominates, which is characterized by thickening and increase of bone size and marked sclerosis. The radiographs have a definite advantage over the bone scan as they can help decide if the process is predominantly osteolytic, osteoblastic, or mixed.

In selected patients, computerized tomography or magnetic resonance imaging may be helpful to define the atypical lesions, especially when sarcomatous changes are suspected. It may also be helpful in assessing back pain due to spinal stenosis, hydrocephalous, or brain stem compression from basilar skull invagination. Magnetic resonance imaging is also of value in detecting a soft tissue component of a tumor arising in a pagetic bone lesion.

If there is uncertainty about the diagnosis, a bone biopsy is a definite means of establishing the diagnosis. This is occasionally useful to differentiate from the metastatic osteoblastic lesions or osteosarcoma. However, biopsy specimen should be avoided in the weight-bearing bone because of the risk of fracture or of complications.

BIOCHEMICAL MARKERS IN PAGET'S DISEASE

A number of biochemical markers have been designed, which can predict the disease activity. These include the markers of bone formation and markers of bone resorption, which in turn reflect the activity of osteoblasts and osteoclasts.

Markers of Bone Formation

The most useful and standard biochemical index of Paget's disease activity is the measurement of the total serum alkaline phosphatase level, which has a sensitivity of 74% (Alvarez *et al.*, 1995). The enzyme is found on the plasma membrane of osteoblasts and its levels are elevated in more than 90% of affected patients. Its serum level provides a clinically useful index of osteoblastic activity in the absence of significant liver disease or pregnancy. The levels, however, may be normal in up to 15% of symptomatic patients as well as in some patients with monostotic form of Paget's disease. The enzyme can be used both in diagnosis and in monitoring of therapy. With the institution of treatment of Paget's disease, alkaline phosphatase levels fall more slowly than bone resorption parameters, but within 4–8 weeks, a clear response is usually noted. The levels correlate well with the extent of skeletal involvement as established by the radionuclide bone scan; however, the lesions in the skull may produce much higher levels of serum alkaline phosphatase. Serum alkaline phosphatase activity changes from day to day and hence to be clinically significant, the levels should increase or decrease by 25%. The specificity of the assay is limited because serum alkaline phosphatase includes isoenzymes derived from the liver, kidney, placenta, intestine, and spleen, as well as certain tumors.

Recently, assays for the bone-specific alkaline phosphatase have been developed. However, this test is more expensive, less readily available, and there are no convincing data to indicate that there is an advantage of this test over the cheaper, standard alkaline phosphatase assays in the average patient. This test may be of value in patients with monostotic Paget's disease, patients with liver disease, and in patients with Paget's disease without any elevation of total plasma alkaline phosphatase activity. Approximately 60% of patients with normal total alkaline phosphatase have increased bone-specific alkaline phosphatase.

Serum osteocalcin, another product of osteoblast may be increased in patients with Paget's disease, but its levels do not correlate well with disease activity (Calvo *et al.*, 1996). It has a sensitivity of approximately 35%. It is not recommended as a standard means of evaluating Paget's disease. The carboxy-terminal propeptide of type 1 procollagen in the serum of patients with Paget's disease may be evaluated, but it has not been proven to be a particularly useful clinical index of the disease. It is elevated in approximately 45% of patients with active Paget's disease.

Markers of Bone Resorption

A variety of biochemical tests reflecting bone matrix resorption provide good indices of disease activity including measurement of 24-hour or second morning void urinary hydroxyproline/creatinine as an index of bone collagen absorption. Other specific tests of bone collagen resorption include urinary and serum deoxypyridinoline, *N*-telopeptide, and *C*-telopeptide, and are not affected by dietary intake. Of all the markers, urinary excretion of pyridinium cross-link pyridinoline is a good measure of bone resorption than hydroxyproline, because pyridinoline molecules and the related *N*- and *C*-telopeptide of collagen are more specific components of bone matrix than is hydroxyproline. Markers of bone resorption change within a day or 1 week after the initiation of the therapy, whereas it may take 1–2 months before the alkaline phosphatase levels show a response to therapy.

Generally, the serum and urinary calcium and phosphorus levels remain normal during the course of disease unless the patient has a large amount of skeletal disease. Urinary calcium levels can be elevated in patients with active disease in multiple skeletal sites.

DIFFERENTIAL DIAGNOSIS

The differential diagnosis of Paget's disease consists of the conditions that can cause elevated alkaline phosphatase or the radiological lesions that are similar to Paget's disease (Table 1). With a careful analysis of the history, physical examination, biochemical studies and judicious use of radiological studies, in the vast majority of the patients, the diagnosis is not difficult to make. Rarely a bone biopsy is needed to confirm the diagnosis.

Table 1 Differential diagnosis of Paget's disease of bone

Osteoarthritis
Osteoporosis
Metastatic malignancy with osteoblastic lesions (Prostate, breast, lymphoma)
Metastatic malignancy with osteolytic lesions (Multiple myeloma, breast, lung)
Primary malignancy of bone
Ricketts/osteomalacia
Congenital syphilis
Other osteoblastic skeletal lesions
Other osteolytic lesions

Source: Lyles K., PIER, *Amer. College of Physicians*, 2002.

DIAGNOSTIC RECOMMENDATIONS

The minimum evaluation of a patient with Paget's disease should include X rays of the affected bones and at least one parameter of bone metabolic activity. In patients with lytic lesions in the weight-bearing bones, serial radiography should be performed to document healing. In most patients, changes in the total alkaline phosphatase activity are adequate to determine changes in the overall disease activity, but the total serum alkaline phosphatase level in any patient is a reflection of both the total bone surface affected by Paget's disease and the total activity of the disease at those sites. Consequently, serum alkaline phosphatase can be normal in patients with a small focus of symptomatic Paget's disease. A bone scan is valuable in defining the full extent of the diseases and identify still asymptomatic lesions located in "at risk" areas.

TREATMENT OF PAGET'S DISEASE

All patients with Paget's disease do not require treatment, as the disease may be localized and may not cause any symptoms. Thus, it is important to do a careful assessment of symptoms and physical and radiological findings before a decision is made to treat the patient. None of the treatments currently available cure the disease. The specific goals of the treatment are to alleviate pain, prevent complications and stop the resorptive process, and restore normal bone remodeling. Treatment reduces the extension of lytic fronts and progression of deformity and restores the normal pattern of bone deposition (Meunier and Vignot, 1995). In general, treatment is initiated in patients with metabolically active Paget's disease, causing persistent pain, fractures, and headaches. Involvements of weight-bearing long bones and presence of disease in proximity to major weight-bearing joints, as well as involvement of the axial skeleton are also some of the indications to initiate therapy. Treatment is also indicated in patients who are planning to undergo elective surgery on a pagetic site such as hip replacement, in an attempt to reduce the hypervascularity of the pagetic lesion and hence the intraoperative blood loss. Treatment is also offered in patients who have high output cardiac failure, hypercalcemia due to immobility and severe hypercalciuria, with or without renal stones. Treatment with alendronate and risedronate is associated with the reduction of elevated indices of bone turnover from active Paget's disease to the normal range in the majority of patients (Harinck *et al.*, 1987; Cantrill *et al.*, 1986; Reid *et al.*, 1996; Sins *et al.*, 1996).

Nonpharmacological Measures

Patients with bowing deformity of a limb, gait alterations, chronic back pain, or difficulties from spinal stenosis may be helped by walking aids such as canes, shoe lifts, or other orthotics devices. An external fixation device (Ilizarov) has been useful in patients with Paget's disease involving the tibia, which allows an osteotomy to be performed, and then a gradual change in external pressure is used to straighten the bowed tibia. It can also be used to heal a nonunion fracture seen in Paget's disease. Physical therapy may well be indicated to improve muscle strength and preserve function.

Pharmacological Measures

Treatment of Paget's disease has undergone significant improvement in the last three decades as more potent therapeutic agents continue to be available. Because the primary defect appears to be related to resorptive process, the treatment focuses on decreasing osteoclast-mediated bone resorption.

BISPHOSPHONATES

Bisphosphonates are analogs of inorganic pyrophosphates and are currently considered the drugs of choice for the treatment of Paget's disease. The main action of bisphosphonates is to induce marked and prolonged inhibition of bone resorption by decreasing osteoclastic activity (Felisch *et al.*, 1969; Zimolo *et al.*, 1995). Bisphosphonates are made of a phosphorus–carbon–phosphorus chain in which the hydrogen atoms can be replaced by various groups. They can be nitrogen containing such as pamidronate, alendronate, and risedronate or non-nitrogen containing such as etidronate, clodronate, and tiludronate. Currently, only four of them are registered in the United States for the treatment of Paget's disease; these include pamidronate, alendronate, tiludronate, and risedronate. Bisphosphonates bind to the hydroxyapatite crystal within the bone and decrease bone resorption by disrupting osteoclast recruitment and cellular activity. In addition, they also decrease the number of osteoclasts by perturbing cellular metabolism and inducing their apoptosis. These effects may last for several months in contrast to calcitonin which has short-lived effects (Felisch, 1993). The potency depends upon the structure of the attached side chain. In the order of increasing potency, these include etidronate, tiludronate, pamidronate, alendronate, and risedronate. Bisphosphonates, in general, are poorly absorbed from the gastrointestinal tract, and have to be taken in an empty stomach, and are not metabolized *in vivo*; approximately half of the orally administered dose is cleared by the kidney, and they are rapidly taken up by the bones. Patients should concurrently receive 1000 mg of oral calcium and 800 units of Vitamin D supplement in order to reduce the chances of hypocalcemia and secondary hyperparathyroidism, which can occur with bisphosphonate therapy. Approximately 20% of patients treated with bisphosphonates may experience exacerbation of pain in their pagetic lesions that can be well managed with acetaminophen, but sometimes short-term use of narcotic-based analgesics may be needed.

Etidronate was the first bisphosphonate to be used for the treatment of Paget's disease. It can be administered in doses of 5 mg kg^{-1} (average dose of 200–400 mg) daily, and is usually given for a period of 6 months. Treatment with etidronate shows moderate improvement in disease activity and lowers the alkaline phosphatase by 40–70% (Altman *et al.*, 1973). Higher doses are associated with gastrointestinal upset and focal osteomalacia. Approximately 25% of patients treated with etidronate develop resistance to etidronate with repeated courses (Siris *et al.*, 1981). Etidronate is contraindicated in presence of renal failure, preexistent osteomalacia, or known lytic lesions

Tiludronate is administered by the oral route as 200 mg twice daily for 3 months and is slightly more potent than etidronate. It has to be taken 2 hours before or after eating food with 6–8 oz of water. It is fairly well tolerated in the usual dose. It may also improve pagetic bone pain. Unlike etidronate, tiludronate does pose problems with mineralization deficits at the therapeutic doses. Approximately a third of the patients do achieve normal indices with the first course of etidronate or tiludronate, and the majority will have a 50% decrease in serum alkaline phosphatase (Canfield *et al.*, 1977; MdChmg *et al.*, 1995; Roux *et al.*, 1995). Patients who have gastrointestinal side effects with newer bisphosphonates, etidronate and possibly tiludronate may be an option to consider.

Pamidronate is administered by the intravenous route only and is more potent than etidronate. The dosing and the number of infusions depend upon the individual patient. Mild diseases can be successfully treated with one or two 60-mg infusions; however, more severe diseases may require several infusions of 60–90 mg given on a weekly or twice weekly basis. Once the required numbers of infusions are provided, the serum alkaline phosphatase should be measured in 2–3 months. Treatment results in the reduction of plasma alkaline phosphatase activity by 50–80%. If values after the treatment stabilize at a near normal level, retreatment is appropriate once the nadir level rises by 25%. The biochemical response may last 12–18 months posttreatment. One-third of the patients may experience mild flu-like episodes after the first dose, consisting of fever, myalgias, headache, and malaise. Uveitis, episcleritis, and ototoxicity have also been reported.

Alendronate administered orally as 40 mg is given daily for 6 months. Administration of alendronate can result in the reduction of the biochemical markers of turnover into the normal range in more than 50% of patients (Reid *et al.*, 1996; Sins *et al.*, 1996). The biochemical markers may remain stable for up to 6–18 months or longer before retreatment is considered. Gastrointestinal disturbances can occur in up to 17% of the patients and may result in discontinuation of the medication.

Risedronate has also been approved for the treatment of Paget's disease in the United States as a 30-mg tablet administered orally, once daily for 2 months. In an open label, multicenter study at the aforementioned dose, risedronate showed a 60–70% reduction in alkaline phosphatase levels (Sins *et al.*, 1998; Miller *et al.*, 1999). Another randomized double-blind controlled trial with etidronate showed that 73% of the patients had normalization of alkaline phosphatase, whereas only one out of seven in the etidronate group did normalize their alkaline phosphatase activity. The gastrointestinal side effects with risedronate appear to be less compared to alendronate and this may be better tolerated.

Both alendronate and risedronate are taken as a single daily dose with a 40-mg dose of alendronate or a 30-mg tablet of risedronate on rising after an overnight fast, with 6–8 oz of plain water and nothing by mouth (except more water) for the next 30 minutes. The patient may not lie down to avoid esophagitis, which is seen more in patients on alendronate than on risedronate.

Secondary resistance to bisphosphonates has been reported (Trdmbetti *et al.*, 1999). The exact biochemical mechanism of bisphosphonate resistance is unknown. It has been proposed that in patients treated with bisphosphonate therapy a certain group of osteoclasts gradually become resistant to apoptotic effect of the drug. Continued therapy with bisphosphonate may induce a series of enzymes that confer resistance to a subset of osteoclasts or their precursor cells. However, more studies are needed to provide further insights into osteoclasts biology and the action of bisphosphonates to better understand the true mechanism of resistance. It has also been shown that patients who become resistant to one type of bisphosphonate may respond well to another bisphosphonate (Trdmbetti *et al.*, 1999; Gutteridge *et al.*, 1999).

OTHER BISPHOSPHONATES

Several other newer bisphosphonates have been used in the treatment of Paget's disease and are currently under development and trials. These include neridronate, olpadronate, ibandronate, and zoledronate. The preliminary studies with zoledronic acid appear to have encouraging results and this could become a potential therapy for the treatment for Paget's disease; however, it is currently not approved by the US Food and drug administration (FDA) for the treatment of Paget's disease.

Calcitonin

Calcitonin is a 32-amino acid hormone secreted by the C-cells of the thyroid gland. It was the mainstay of treatment for Paget's disease in the 1970s and 1980s and now its use has been largely replaced by more potent bisphosphonates. Salmon calcitonin is available for use daily at doses of 100 units by subcutaneous route, which after 1 to 2 months can be changed to 3 times a week. Nasal formulation of calcitonin is available, but its use in Paget's disease is not approved in the United States, as only 40% of the drug is bioavailable after nasal administration. Calcitonin does inhibit osteoclast activity and rapidly decreases bone resorption. It reduces elevated indices of bone turnover by 50%, decreases symptoms of bone pain (by centrally mediated analgesic effects), reduces warmth over affected bone areas, and also promotes healing of lytic lesions. Today, its use probably is limited to those patients who are not able to tolerate bisphosphonates. The major drawbacks are its weaker activity, high cost and shorter duration of action, adverse side effect profile, and resistance that develops in approximately 20% of patients (Singer *et al.*, 1972). Patients also develop neutralizing antibodies, but it is not known if these play a role in its resistance. Downregulation of calcitonin receptors may lead to secondary hyperparathyroidism. Side effects include nausea, vomiting, polyuria, hypercalciuria, and facial or palmer flushing that is seen in approximately 20–30%. This may require the drug to be started at a dose of 25 units, with a gradual increase in dose every few days to the full 100 units. The suppression of disease activity does not persist long after the withdrawal of calcitonin treatment, which is the limiting factor to the use of such a treatment. Secondary resistance to salmon calcitonin can occur necessitating a change to bisphosphonate therapy.

Plicamycin

Formerly called *mithramycin*, plicamycin is a cytotoxic agent that inhibits the synthesis of ribonucleic acid. It was used in the management of hypercalcemia of malignancy (for which it is FDA approved) and as an early experimental agent in Paget's disease. At doses of 10 to 25 $mg\,kg^{-1}$ body weight daily for 10 days or 15–25 $mg\,kg^{-1}$ weekly, it may decrease bone pain and induce remission that may last several months. It is rarely indicated at this time because of its associated dose-dependent toxicity to the liver, bone marrow, skin, and kidney and the availability of potent newer bisphosphonates, which are relatively much safer to use.

Gallium Nitrate

Gallium nitrate has been approved for the treatment of hypercalcemia of malignancy. It inhibits bone resorption by inhibiting the adenosine triphosphate (ATP)-dependent proton pump of the osteoclasts. It has been proven to be effective in the treatment of Paget's disease; however, side effects such as renal failure preclude its use, and hence it is not currently approved by the FDA in the United States.

MONITORING OF THERAPY AND FOLLOW-UP

The ultimate goal of treatment of Paget's disease is to relieve the symptoms and prevent associated complications. The effect of treatment is usually evident in 3 to 6 months and if the patient has not responded by then, a second course of therapy should be offered. If the patient fails to respond to the second course of therapy, a different bisphosphonate should be tried. The frequency and extent of follow-up depends upon the severity of the disease. The disease activity can be efficiently monitored by the serial measurement of alkaline phosphatase levels every 3 to 6 months. In patients with monostotic form of Paget's disease, measurement of bone-specific alkaline phosphatase and sometimes urinary excretion of pyridinoline and related peptides may be necessary. Patients should also be monitored for bone pain, articular function, and any new neurological signs or symptoms every 3 to 6 months. Treatment regimen should be aimed at normalizing biochemical markers. The markers reach a nadir level several months after the completion of therapy and then the level needs to be followed every 6 months. Retreatment should be considered if the level of alkaline phosphatase rises by more than 20–30% above the nadir level. Routine radiographic follow-up of all the involved sites is not necessary; however, the involvement of the base of the skull and the weight-bearing bones requires imaging every 6 to 12 months.

ANALGESIC AGENTS

Patients with Paget's disease often experience bone pain related to the pagetic process. Pain can be successfully controlled with the use of acetaminophen, nonsteroidal anti-inflammatory drugs (NSAIDS), or the newer cox-2 inhibitors in addition to anti-osteoclastic agents. Care should be taken to monitor for renal, gastrointestinal, and hepatic toxicity, as many of the patients are elderly. Judicious use of narcotic analgesics may also be needed if the pain is not well controlled with the above regimen and is not contraindicated.

SURGERY

Orthopedic interventions may be required in several situations in patients with Paget's disease (Singer *et al.*, 1972). Pathological fractures and bony deformities are well-known complications of Paget's disease. Surgery may provide significant relief of pain and can improve mobility. Total hip or knee arthroplasty may be indicated for patients with severe arthritic pain, refractory to medical therapy. Complete pathological fracture of long bones may require internal fixation for early mobilization. Control of Paget's disease activity in these patients is recommended to minimize the chance of loosening of the prosthesis. Corrective proximal tibial osteotomies are sometime needed to realign the knee and decrease mechanical pain, especially if medical therapy is unsuccessful in managing severe pain symptoms. Spinal stenosis, focal nerve compression (in the spine or cranium), and resultant radiculopathies caused by pagetic and nonpagetic changes in vertebrae, skull, or facet joints, may require orthopedic or neurosurgical interventions. Prolonged treatment with bisphosphonates or calcitonin sometimes reverses the signs of nerve compression and hence should be tried to improve the symptoms before surgery is undertaken (Walpine and Singer, 1979; Ravichandran, 1979). In any case of surgical intervention, pretreatment with bisphosphonate or calcitonin is needed for several months prior to elective surgery to reduce hypervascularity and to significantly reduce the risk of excessive operative blood loss. In emergent situations, patient can receive intravenous pamidronate or calcitonin.

KEY POINTS

- The disease is unusual before the age of 40 with increasing prevalence after the age of 50.
- Pathophysiology is that of increased osteoclastic activity coupled with increased bone formation.
- Many patients with this disorder have no symptoms.
- In the last 30 years, there has been development of effective therapies.

KEY REFERENCES

- Cundy T, McAnulty K, Wattie D *et al.* Evidence for secular change in Paget's disease. *Bone* 1997; **20**:69–71.
- Gold DT, Boisture J, Shipp KM *et al.* Paget's disease of bone and quality of life. *Journal of Bone and Mineral Research* 1996; **11**:1897–904.
- Miller PD, Brown JP, Sins ES *et al.*, Paget's Risedronate/Etidronate Study Group. A randomized, double-blind comparison of risedronate and etidronate in the treatment of Paget's disease of bone. *The American Journal of Medicine* 1999; **106**:513–20.
- Reid I, Nicholson GC, Weinstein RS *et al.* Biochemical and radiologic improvement in Paget's disease of bone treated with alendronate: a randomized placebo-controlled trial. *The American Journal of Medicine* 1996; **101**:341–8.
- Sins ES, Ottman R, Raster E & Kelsey IL. Familial aggregation of Paget's disease of bone. *Journal of Bone and Mineral Research* 1991; **6**:495–500.

REFERENCES

Altman RD, Johnston CC, Khairi MR *et al.* Influence of disodium etidronate on clinical and laboratory manifestation of Paget's disease of bone (Osteitis deformans). *The New England Journal of Medicine* 1973; **289**:1379–84.

Alvarez L, Guanabens N, Peris P *et al.* Discriminative value of biochemical markers of bone turn over in assessing the activity of Paget's disease. *Journal of Bone and Mineral Research* 1995; **10**:458–65.

Ankrom MA & Shapiro JR. Paget's disease of bone (Osteitis deformans). *Journal of the American Geriatrics Society* 1998; **46**:1025–33.

Baker DJP, Chamberlain AT, Guyer PB & Gardner MJ. Paget's disease of bone: the Lancashire focus. *British Medical Journal* 1980; **280**:1105–7.

Baker DJP, Clough PWL, Guyer PB & Gardner MJ. Paget's disease of bone in 14 British towns. *British Medical Journal* 1997; **1**:1181–3.

Barker DJP. The epidemiology of Paget's disease of bone. *British Medical Journal* 1984; **40**:396–400.

Barry HC. *Paget's Disease of Bone* 1969; Churchill-Livingston, Edinborough.

Basle MF, Fournier JG, Rozenblatt S *et al.* Measles virus RNA detected in Paget's disease bone by in situ hybridization. *The Journal of General Virology* 1986; **67**:907–13.

Birch MA, Taylor W, Fraser WD *et al.* Absence of Paramyxo virus RNA in culture of pagetic bone cells and in pagetic bone. *Journal of Bone and Mineral Research* 1994; **9**:11–6.

Calvo MS, Eyre DR & Gundberg CM. Biological markers of bone turnover. *Endocrine Reviews* 1996; **17**:333–68.

Canfield RE, Rosner W, Skinner J *et al.* Diphosphonate therapy of Paget's disease of bone. *The Journal of Clinical Endocrinology and Metabolism* 1977; **44**:96–106.

Cantrill IA, Buckler HM & Anderson DC. Low dose iritrave nous 3-amino-l-hydroxypropylidene-1,I-bisphosphonate (ADP) for the treatment of Paget's disease of the bone. *Annals of the Rheumatic Diseases* 1986; **45**:1012–8.

Collins DH. Paget's disease of bone – incidence and subclinical forms. *Lancet* 1956; **2**:51–7.

Cooper C, Schafheutle K, Dennison E *et al.* The epidemiology of Paget's disease in Britain: is the prevalence decreasing? *Journal of Bone and Mineral Research* 1999; **14**:192–7.

Cundy T, McAnulty K, Wattie D *et al.* Evidence for secular change in Paget's disease. *Bone* 1997; **20**:69–71.

Delmas PD & Meunier PJ. The management of Paget's disease of bone. *The New England Journal of Medicine* 1997; **336**:558–66.

Felisch H. Bisphosphonates: mechanism of action and clinical use. In GR Mundy & TJ Martin (eds) *1993 Physiology and Pharmacology of Bone. Handbook of Experimental Pharmacology* 1993, vol 107, pp 377–418; Springer-Verlag, Berlin.

Felisch H, Russell RGG & Francis MD. Diphosphonates inhibit hydroxyapatite dissolution *in vitro* and bone resorption in tissue culture *in vivo*. *Science* 1969; **165**:1262–4.

Fogelman I, Carr D & Boyle IT. The role of bone scanning in Paget's disease. *Metabolic Bone Disease & Related Research* 1981; **3**:243–54.

Foldes I, Sharnir S, Brautbar C *et al.* HLA-D antigens and Paget's disease of bone. *Clinical Orthopaedics and Related Research* 1991; **266**:301–3.

Gold DT, Boisture J, Shipp KM *et al.* Paget's disease of bone and quality of life. *Journal of Bone and Mineral Research* 1996; **11**:1897–904.

Good D, Busfield F & Duffey D. Familial Paget's disease of bone: non linkage to the PDB1 and PDB2 loci on chromosome 6p and 18q in a large pedigree. *Journal of Bone and Mineral Research* 2001; **16**:33.

Gordon MT, Anderson DC & Sharpe PT. Canine distemper virus localized in bone cells of patient's with Paget's disease. *Bone* 1991; **12**:195–201.

Gordon MT, Mee AP, Anderson DC & Sharpe PT. Canine distemper virus transcripts sequenced from pagetic bone. *Bone and Mineral* 1992; **19**:159–74.

Gutteridge DH, Ward LC, Stewart GO *et al.* A randomized treatment trial of intravenous pamidronate and oral alendronate in Paget's disease: early results. *Bone* 1999; **24**(67S):(abstract).

Hadjipavlou A, Lander P, Srolovitz H & Enker IP. Malignant transformation in Paget's disease of bone. *Cancer* 1992; **70**:2802.

Haibach H, Farrell C & Dittrich FJ. Neoplasms arising in Paget's disease of bone: a study of 82 cases. *American Journal of Clinical Pathology* 1985; **83**:594–600.

Harinck HI, Papapoulos SE, Blanksma HI *et al.* Paget's disease of bone: early and late responses to three different modes of treatment with aminohydroxypropylidene-l,1-biphosphoriate (APD) for the treatment of Paget's disease of the bone. *Annals of the Rheumatic Diseases* 1987; **45**:1012–8.

Haslam SI, Van Hul W, Morales-Piga A *et al.* Paget's disease of. bone: evidence for a susceptibility locus on chromosome. lSq and for genetic heterogeneity. *Journal of Bone and Mineral Research* 1998; **13**:911–7.

Haworth S. Cardiac output in osteitis deformans. *Clinical Science* 1953; **12**:271–5.

Hoyland JA, Freemont AJ & Sharpe PT. Interleukin-6(IL-6), IL-6 receptor and IL-6 nuclear factor gene expression in Paget's disease. *Journal of Bone and Mineral Research* 1994; **9**:75–80.

Hultgren HN. Osteitis deformans(Paget's disease) and calcific disease of heart valves. *The American Journal of Cardiology* 1998; **81**:1461.

Kanis JA. Radiological features. In JA Kanis (ed) *Pathophysiology and Treatment of Paget's Disease of Bone* 1991, pp 41–8; Martin Dunitz, London.

Kanis JA. *Pathophysiology and Treatment of Paget's Disease of Bone* 1998, 2nd edn; Martin Dunitz, London.

Laurin N, Brown JP & Lemainque A. Paget's disease of bone: mapping of two loci at 5q35-qter and 5q31. *American Journal of Human Genetics* 2001; **69**:528.

McKusick VA. Pagets disease of bone. In VA McKusick (ed) *Heritable Disorders of Connective Tissue* 1972, pp 718–23; CV Mosby, St. Louis.

MdChmg MR, Tou CPK, Goldstein NH & Picot C. Tiludr onate therapy for Paget's disease of bone. *Bone* 1995; **17**:493S–6S.

Meunier PJ, Coindre I, Edouard CM & Arlot ME. Bone histomorphometry in Paget's disease: quantitative and dynamic analysis of pagetic and non-pagetic bone tissue. *Arthritis and Rheumatism* 1980; **23**:1095–103.

Meunier PJ & Vignot E. Therapeutic strategy in Paget's disease of bone. *Bone* 1995; **17**:489S–91S.

Miller PD, Brown JP, Sins ES *et al.*, Paget's Risedronate/Etidronate Study Group. A randomized, double-blind comparison of risedronate and etidronate in the treatment of Paget's disease of bone. *The American Journal of Medicine* 1999; **106**:513–20.

Mills BG & Singer FT. Nuclear inclusions in Paget's disease of Bone. *Science* 1976; **194**:201–2.

Morales-Piga AA, Rey-Rey IS, Corres-Gonzalez J *et al.* Frequency and characteristics of familial aggregation of Paget's disease of bone. *Journal of Bone and Mineral Research* 1995; **10**:663–70.

Paget J. On a form of chronic inflammation of bones. *Medico-Chirurgical Transactions* 1877; **60**:37–63.

Polednak AP. Rates of Paget's disease of bone among hospital discharges, by age and sex. *Journal of the American Geriatrics Society* 1987; **35**:550.

Ralston SH, Digiovine FS, Gallacher SJ *et al.* Failure to detect Paramyxo sequence in Paget's disease of bone using the polymerase chain reaction. *Journal of Bone and Mineral Research* 1991; **6**:1243–8.

Ravichandran G. Neurologic recovery of paraplegia following use of salmon calcitonin in a patient with Paget's disease of spine. *Spine* 1979; **4**:37–40.

Rebel A, Malkani K & Basle M. Anomalies nuclearies des osteoclasts de la maladie osseous de Paget. *La Nouvelle Presse Medicale* 1974; **3**:1299–301.

Reddy SV, Singer SV, Mallett L & Roodman GD. Detection of measles virus nucleocapsid transcripts in circulating blood cells from patients with Paget's disease. *Journal of Bone and Mineral Research* 1996; **11**:1602–7.

Reddy SV, Singer FR & Roodman GD. Bone marrow mononuclear cells from patient's with Paget's disease contain measles virus nucleocapsid messenger ribonucleic acid that has mutations in a specific region of the sequence. *The Journal of Clinical Endocrinology and Metabolism* 1995; **80**:2108–11.

Reid I, Nicholson GC, Weinstein RS *et al.* Biochemical and radiologic improvement in Paget's disease of bone treated with alendronate: a randomized placebo-controlled trial. *The American Journal of Medicine* 1996; **101**:341–8.

Resnick D. Paget's disease. In D Resnick (ed) *Diagnosis of Bone and Joint Disorders* 1995, 3rd edn, pp 1923–68; Saunders, Philadelphia.

Roodrnan GD, Kurihara N, Ohsalci Y *et al.* Interleukin 6: a potential autocrine/paracrine factor in Paget's disease of bone. *The Clinical Investigator* 1992; **89**:46–52.

Roux C, Gennari C, Farrerons J *et al.* Comparative prospective, double-blind,' multicenter study of the of tiludronate and etidronate in the treatment of Paget's disease of bone. *Arthritis and Rheumatism* 1995; **38**:851–8.

Singer FR, Alfred P, Neer RM *et al.* An evaluation of antibodies and clinical resistance to salmon calcitonin. *The Journal of Clinical Investigation* 1972; **51**:2331–8.

Singer FR & Mills BG. Giant cell tumor arising in page;'s disease of bone. Recurrences after 36 years. *Clinical Orthopaedics and Related Research* 1993; **293**:293–301.

Singer FR, Mills BG, Park MS *et al.* Increased HLA-DQW1 antigen pattern in Paget's disease. *Clinical Research* 1985; **33**:574A.

Singer FR, Sins ES, Knieriem A *et al.* The HLA DRB 1*1104 gene frequency is increased in Ashkenazi Jews with Paget's disease of bone. *Journal of Bone and Mineral Research* 1996; **11**:S369.

Sins ES, Chines AA, Altman ED *et al.* Risedronate in the treatment of Paget' s disease: an open-label, multicenter study. *Journal of Bone and Mineral Research* 1998; **13**:1032–8.

Sins ES, Ottman R, Raster E & Kelsey IL. Familial aggregation of Paget's disease of bone. *Journal of Bone and Mineral Research* 1991; **6**:495–500.

Sins B, Weinstein RS, Altman R *et al.* Comparative study of alendronate versus etidronate for the treatment of Paget's disease of bone. *The Journal of Clinical Endocrinology and Metabolism* 1996; **81**:961–7.

Siris E, Canfield RE, Jacobs TP *et al.* Clinical and biochemical effects of EHDP treatment of Paget's disease of bone: patterns of response to initial treatment and to long term therapy. *Metabolic Bone Disease & Related Research* 1981; **3**:301–8.

Sparrow NL & Duvall AJ. Hearing loss and Paget's disease. *The Journal of Laryngology and Otology* 1967; **81**:601–11.

Tilyard MW, Gardner RIM, Milligan L *et al.* A probable linkage between familial Paget's disease and the HLA loci. *Australian and New Zealand Journal of Medicine* 1982; **12**:498–500.

Trdmbetti A, Arlot M, Thevenon J *et al.* Effects of multiple intravenous pamidronate courses in Paget's disease of bone. *Revue du Rhumatisme* 1999; **66**:467–76.

Walpine LA & Singer FR. Paget's disease: reversal of severe paraparesis with calcitonin. *Spine* 1979; **4**:213–5.

Zimolo Z, Wesolowski G & Rodan GA. Acid extrusion is induced by osteoclast attachment to bone: inhibition by alendronate and calcitonin. *The Journal of Clinical Investigation* 1995; **96**:2277–83.

110

Epidemiology of Osteoporosis

Horace M. Perry
Saint Louis University, St Louis, MO, USA

INTRODUCTION

Osteoporosis is a condition of structural deterioration of skeletal tissue and low bone mass. Osteoporosis is associated with increased risk of fracture (Woolf and Pfleger, 2003; Klibanski *et al.*, 2001). Skeletal tissue may be readily divided into two types, cortical and trabecular. Cortical bone has a characteristic formation, layer wrapped around layer of bone. It occurs on the outermost portion of the skeleton and is only minimally reactive to metabolic stimuli. Trabecular bone, on the other hand, is the sponge-like inner portion of the bone. It is lined with osteoclasts (bone reabsorbing cells) and osteoblasts (bone forming cells) with pockets of marrow or fat distributed throughout. Trabecular bone is also much more metabolically active. Certain diseases, including Paget's and the osteomalacic phase of vitamin D Resistant Ricketts may result in the loss of the clear demarcation between these two types of bone, but it is otherwise generally maintained.

Skeletal mass peaks in the late second or early third decade of life and remains stable for 15–20 years after that. Peak bone mass has an obvious genetic component (Albagha and Ralston, 2003; Pocock *et al.*, 1987). Men have greater bone mass than women. Short individuals have less bone mass than tall individuals. Further, African or African-American individuals have greater mean bone mass than Caucasian individuals of the same gender and similar built (Melton, 2003). Finally certain genetic diseases, for example, cystic fibrosis (Conway *et al.*, 2000) or lactose intolerance (Kudlacek *et al.*, 2002) may prevent afflicted individuals from attaining their maximum (peak) bone mass.

Peak skeletal bone mass is also effected by behavior. Individuals who do not take or absorb adequate calcium or vitamin D intake, smoke or abuse alcohol as they are obtaining their peak bone mass will generally have lower peak skeletal mass, then might otherwise be expected.

In about the fifth decade of life, skeletal mass begins to decrease at a rate of about 4% per decade. Without intervention, this rate continues throughout the remaining life span. In women, this rate accelerates as menopause supervenes and then slowly returns to normal, so that women may lose as much as 5–15% of their previous bone mass in the 5 years surrounding menopause.

In the United States, 10 million Americans (8 million women and 2 million men) are estimated to have osteoporosis and an additional 34 million are estimated to have low bone mass (osteopenia) with an increased risk for developing osteoporosis. (US Department of Health and Human Services, 2004) One in two women over the age of 50 and one in four men of the age of 50 will have a fracture in their remaining life span because of differences in longevity in women, compared to men. Four out of five individuals with osteoporosis are women. Despite differences of bone mass related to gender and ethnicity, osteoporosis fractures occur in both genders and all ethnicities. Morbidity and mortality may be different in men versus women and Caucasians versus African-Americans. Thus, Caucasian women have the lowest mortality after hip fracture, with African-American women and Caucasian men having about twice and African-American men about three times the risk of death after hip fracture than men in the United States and who are over 50.

There is general widespread agreement about the cut points of bone density measurement for osteoporosis and osteopenia in Caucasian women. Osteopenia in Caucasian women is a bone mass between one and two and a half standard deviation below mean bone mass of young women. Osteoporosis in Caucasian women is a bone mass more than the two and a half standard deviations below mean bone mass of young women. This formal agreement of cut points does not exist at this time for women of other ethnicities or men of any ethnicity. Most reports have generally extended the same cut points in Caucasian women to other ethnicities and/or in men; comparing bone mass in older individuals to a mean young bone mass (Table 1). Using this methodology, 20% of Caucasian women, 20% of Asian women, 10% of Hispanic women and 5% of African-American women are estimated to have osteoporosis in the United States. Over the age of 50, 52% of Caucasian and Asian women, and 49% of Hispanic and 35% African-American women are estimated

Principles and Practice of Geriatric Medicine, 4th Edition. Edited by M.S. John Pathy, Alan J. Sinclair and John E. Morley.

Table 1 Risk for osteoporosis or osteopenia by gender and ethnicity over the age of 50

	Osteoporosis (%)	Osteopenia (%)
Women		
Caucasian/Asian	20	52
African-American	05	35
Hispanic	10	49
Men		
Caucasian/Asian	07	35
African-American	04	19
Hispanic	03	23

Table 2 Risk for future fragility fractures in individuals over the age of 50

	Men	Women
Overall risk of fracture	1 in 4	1 in 2
Risk of femur fracture	1 in 6	1 in 3
Risk of mortality	1 in 11	1 in 11
Placement	1 in 30	1 in 10

to have osteopenia with its concomitant increased risk for developing osteoporosis. It must be noted that the definition of osteoporosis includes a deterioration of skeletal integrity, which is generally poorly quantified. Attempts to quantify structural deterioration in trabecular bone are ongoing. These studies demonstrate loss of "struts" of trabecular bone but do not (cannot) quantify deterioration of skeletal integrity. Thus, the best (only) measure of osteoporosis at this time is bone mass (Klibanski *et al.*, 2001).

In the United States, in men over the age of 50, 7% of Caucasian men, 7% of Asian men, 3% of Hispanic men and 4% of African-American men are estimated to have osteoporosis. For osteopenia, the estimate for men over the age of 50 are 35% of Caucasian men, 35% of Asian men, 23% of Hispanic men, and 19% of African-American men.

The presence of certain risk factors can dramatically increase the risk for osteoporosis. These include medications like glucocorticoids and antiseizure medications (Lukert and Raisz, 1990), thin athletic build, early or surgical menopause in women without estrogen replacement, secondary amenorrhea (related to anorexia nervosa, excessive exercise, but not pregnancy), low testosterone in men, smoking, alcohol abuse or heavy use, low calcium intake and/or inadequate vitamin D intake.

The primary risk associated with osteoporosis is fracture. Essentially the incidence of all fractures increases with age (Table 2). Since trabecular bone is more metabolically active then cortical bone, the incidence of fractures of bone thought to be mostly trabecular (distal radius, vertebrae) increase earlier than those bones throughout cortical (femur). Fractures of either distal radius or vertebra are not easily studied, since some Colles fractures are seen in the office and a major portion of (perhaps two-thirds) of vertebral fracture are silent. On the other hand, hip fractures generally require hospitalization and are much easier to track. It is estimated that osteoporosis is responsible for about 1.5 million fractures each year. Of these approximately 300 000 are femoral fractures costing about 18 billion dollars in 2002 in direct expense for hospitals and nursing homes. The indirect cost to the families of the patients in the time lot to care for individuals transitioning back to independent living or to those unable to completely return to previous function is not known but estimated to be as much as twice the figure for direct cost.

Generally, after a hip fracture, most individuals perceive that they return to their previous ambulatory status in one year. Some, however, do not. These are reported to be those with marginal ambulatory status or dementia prior to fracture. Within the first year after fracture, however, many require ambulatory assistance. Thus, 6 months after fracture, 85% may require ambulatory assistance (walker, cane, or wheelchair). About one-quarter of those who were ambulatory prior to hip fracture require long-term placement no matter what their ambulatory status.

Other fractures have significant sequelae also. In particular, vertebral fractures often have significant sequelae. Kyphoscoliosis accounts for most of these. Permanent deformities related to collapsed vertebra (e) are associated with arthritic pain. Loss of vertebral height can compromise lung function, altering ventilation perfusion ratios throughout the lung fields, cause localized areas of emphysema and change pulmonary clearance of pathogens. Loss of vertebral height in the abdomen causes abdominal protrusion and discomfort. It has been associated with constipation. Generally compression fractures are associated with loss of body image, self-esteem, and more frequent pain (Ettinger *et al.*, 1988). Fractures of the distal forearm cause long-term osteoarthritis and deformities with some loss of function (Warwick *et al.*, 1993).

Present guidelines for assessing risk of osteoporosis using a direct measure of bone mass have been published by the National Osteoporosis Foundation and others. These recommendations include a bone mass measurement in all women of the age of 65. Secondly, a bone mass measurement is recommended for all postmenopausal women with a risk factor for osteoporosis in addition to being Caucasian or Asian (Table 3). These include their aesthenic habitus, primary relative with osteoporotic fracture, smoking, excessive alcohol use, early or surgical menopause and chronic use of medications (glucocoticoids or antiseizure) associated with osteoporosis. A series of other lifestyle differences also effects bone mass, but the epidemiologic effect is probably small. Vegetarians have a small increase in bone mass compared to similar individuals who eat meat. Soda (carbonated beverages) may decrease bone mass slightly (Wyshak *et al.*, 1989). Caffeine intake may have an adverse effect on bone mass (Lloyd *et al.*, 1997) and vitamin B12 levels are associated with low bone mass (Tucker *et al.*, 2005).

MEASUREMENT OF BONE MINERAL DENSITY

A series of machines provide localized measurement of bone mineral density measures, which may be used to estimate

Table 3 Risk factors for osteoporosis

Major		Moderate		Small	
Gender	Female	Habitus	Slender	Vegetarian	Lower
Ethnicity	Caucasian	Vitamin D/Calcium	Low	Caffeine intake	Higher
Age	Older	Smoke		Soda	Higher
		Heavy or abuse of alcohol			
		Medication			
		Glucocorticoid	Higher		
		Antiseizure	Higher		
		Thiazide	Lower		
		Premature or early menopause			

hip or spine bone density. The extrapolation is not exact, however, and these machines are most useful in determining who does not need further follow-up. Screening machines are much more widely available. These technologies include peripheral dual energy absorptiometry (pDXA) which measures distal forearms, calcaneus or metacarpals, single energy X-ray absorptionmetry (SXA) which measures distal forearm, calcaneus, quantitative ultrasound (QUS) which uses ultrasound to measure vibration at the calcaneus, tibia, and patella, peripheral quantitative tomography (pQCT) which measures the distal forearm, radiologic absorptiometry which compares metacarpal bone thickness to a standard; and single photon densitometry (SPA) which is not in general use and measures distal forearm. Individuals who screen positively and are to be treated or individuals with osteoporotic fractures who are to be treated should have basal quantitative computerized tomography (QCT) or DXA measurements of spine and/or hip prior to treatment. Individuals who screen positively should also be screened for primary hyperparathyroidism, hyperthyroidism, and tumors including multiple myeloma since therapies for any of these conditions may be significantly different from therapy for primary osteoporosis. Endogenous glucorticoid excess also causes osteoporosis and appropriate individuals should be screened for this. Secondary causes may be easy or difficult to deal with. Poor calcium intake is relatively easy to deal with, but glucorticoid therapy or antiseizure therapy, for example, are generally more difficult to treat. Definitive measurements of the hip or spine bone density may be performed by DXA (dual energy X-ray absorptiometry) which is generally performed at a center. It has relatively low radiation exposure and is widely accepted. Secondly, QCT is also generally performed at a center, is usually more expensive than DXA, and has more radiation exposure. It is widely accepted but much less frequently available than DXA. Thirdly, dual photon absorptiometry (DPA) has little radiation exposure. It is a precursor of DXA and is not generally available.

MANAGEMENT STRATEGIES

The cornerstone of treatment for osteoporosis is adequate calcium and vitamin D intake. Most studies of calcium intake indicate improvement in bone mass and/or decrease in fractures (Dawson-Hughes *et al.*, 1997). This is particularly true in older institutionalized women, but has not always been as easy to demonstrate in the younger, free-living senior. In the study of older institutionalized women 800 IU of vitamin D and 1200 mg of calcium significantly reduced fractures (Chapuy *et al.*, 1992). In the United States, the inclusion of vitamin A (10 000 IU/tablet) makes the use of the multiple vitamins problematic for vitamin D therapy. This dose of vitamin A has been associated with increased risk of fracture, presumably related to vitamin A toxicity (Michaelsson *et al.*, 2003).

A number of therapies in addition to vitamin D and calcium supplementation have been demonstrated to provide additional benefit. Bisphosphonates decrease bone reabsorption without apparently decreasing bone formation (except etidronate) and further decrease incidence of compression fractures, hip fractures, and all fractures (Black *et al.*, 1998; Harris *et al.*, 1999). These medications include alendronate and risidronate. Others are likely to be available shortly. Their major drawback is poor absorbability. They must be taken orally on an empty stomach. Because of gastrointestinal side effects, the patients must remain upright after taking the medication. Even in the best circumstances, about one-quarter of the patients still have gastrointestinal side effects which require withdrawal of the medication. Other bisphosphonates may be given intravenously to minimize this side effect. Biophosphonates improve bone density and reduce fracture incidence, but appear to require about 6 months of therapy, before onset of effect. At this time, alendronate is approved for primary osteoporosis in men and women. Alendronate and risidronate are approved for steroid-induced osteopenia in men and women.

Calcitonin has been used to improve bone density and decrease compression fracture incidence (Body, 2002). It is administered via a nasal inhaler and is approved for primary osteoporosis.

A parathyroid hormone derivative (amino acid residue 1–34) is also available in an injectable form for treatment of osteoporosis.

Selective estrogen receptor modulators (e.g. raloxifen) are demonstrated to decrease fracture risk (Delmas *et al.*, 1997). Estrogen has long been used to treat osteoporosis in postmenopausal women. The recent results from the Women's Health Initiative have cast the future of this therapy into grave doubt. The use of testosterone in older

Table 4 Control risk of trauma

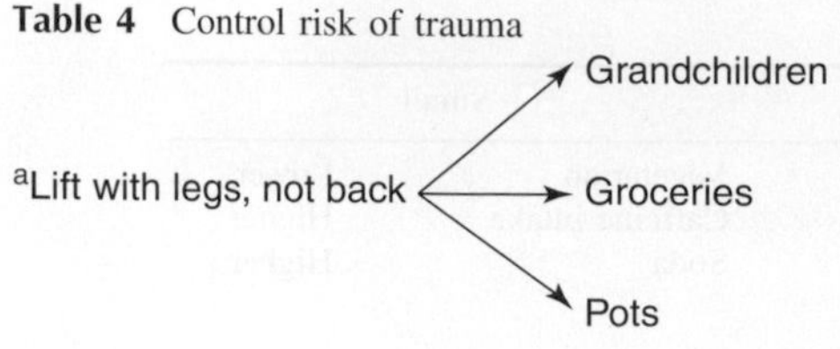

[a]Wear Safe Shoes.
Use lights and hand rails on stairs; remove low furniture and loose rugs.

(hypogonadal) men has been demonstrated to increase bone density, but not as yet to decrease fracture incidence. It has similar effects in women.

Lastly, there are a series of nonpharmacologic recommendations for all patients (Table 4). First, adequate weight-bearing exercise improves bone mass as long as the exercise is maintained. Secondly, falls or other fractures frequently are associated with fractures. Patients should be advised to review their surroundings to minimize the risk for falls. Thus, they should remove loose throw rugs, low furniture, and wires. They should ensure adequate lighting, particularly at night, and get up slowly from bed. Use of rails or grab bars on stairs and bathrooms will decrease the risk of falling. Restricting pet access from the bedroom decreases the risk of patients falling over them when they get up at night. Outdoor activity should be restricted as much as possible when ice or snow is present. Wearing high heels is a risk for falling. Lastly, patients should be taught to lift groceries, grandchildren, and so forth with their legs and not their backs. (i.e. bend knees and not back to pick up things.)

KEY POINTS

- Osteoporosis or low bone mass is one of the most common diseases of aging.
- Osteoporosis is defined as a bone mass more than two and a half standard deviations below that of young women.
- Males over the age of 50 have a 1 in 4 risk of fracture and females a 1 in 2 risk.

KEY REFERENCES

- Melton LJ III. Epidemiology worldwide. *Endocinology and Metabolism Clinics of North America* 2003; **32**:1–13.
- U.S. Department of Health and Human Services. *Bone Health and Osteoporosis: A Report of the Surgeon General* 2004; U.S. Department of Health and Human Services, Office of the Surgeon General, Rockville.

REFERENCES

Albagha OM & Ralston SH. Genetic determinants of susceptibility to osteoporosis. *Endocinology and Metabolism Clinics of North America* 2003; **32**:65–81.

Black DM, Cummings SR, Karpf DB *et al.*, The Fracture Intervention Trial Research Group. Randomized trial of effect of alendronate on risk of fracture in women with exiting vertebral fractures. *Journal of the American Medical Association* 1998; **280**:2077–82.

Body JJ. Calcitonin for the long-term prevention and treatment of postmenopausal osteoporosis. *Bone* 2002; **30**:75S–9S.

Chapuy MC, Arlot ME, Duboeuf F *et al.* Vitamin D3 and calcium to prevent hip fractures in the elderly women. *The New England Journal of Medicine* 1992; **327**:1637–42.

Conway SP, Morton AM & Oldroyd B. Osteoporosis and osteopenia in adults and adolescents with cystic fibrosis: prevalence and associated factors. *Thorax* 2000; **55**:798–804.

Dawson-Hughes B, Harris SS, Krall EA & Dallal GE. Effect of calcium and vitamin D supplementation on bone density in men and women 65 year of age or older. *The New England Journal of Medicine* 1997; **337**:670–6.

Delmas PD, Bjarnason NH, Mitlak BH *et al.* Effects of raloxifene on bone mineral density, serum cholesterol concentration and uterine endometrium in postmenopausal women. *The New England Journal of Medicine* 1997; **337**:1641–947.

Ettinger B, Block JE, Smith R *et al.* An examination of the association between vertebral deformities, physical disabilities and phychosocial problems. *Maturitas* 1988; **10**:283–96.

Harris ST, Watts NB, Genant HK *et al.*, The Vertebral Efficacy with Risedronate Therapy (VERT) Study Group. Effects of risedronate treatment on vertebral nonvertebral fractures in women with postmenopausal osteoporosis. *Journal of the American Medical Association* 1999; **282**:1344–52.

Klibanski A, Adams-Campbell L, Bassford T *et al.* Osteoporosis prevention, diagnosis, and therapy. *Journal of the American Medical Association* 2001; **285**:785–95.

Kudlacek S, Freudenthaler O, Weissboeck H *et al.* Lactose intolerance: a risk factor for reduced bone mineral density and vertebral fractures? *Journal of Gastroenterology* 2002; **37**:1014–9.

Lloyd T, Rollings N, Eggli DF *et al.* Dietary caffeine intake and bone status of postmenopausal women. *The American Journal of Clinical Nutrition* 1997; **65**:1826–30.

Lukert BP & Raisz LG. Glucocorticoid-induced osteoporosis. *Annals of Internal Medicine* 1990; **112**:352–64.

Melton LJ III. Epidemiology worldwide. *Endocinology and Metabolism Clinics of North America* 2003; **32**:1–13.

Michaelsson K, Lithell H, Vessby B & Melhus H. Serum retinol levels and the risk of fracture. *The New England Journal of Medicine* 2003; **348**:287–94.

Pocock NA, Eisman JA, Hopper JL *et al.* Genetic determinants of bone mass in adults. *The Journal of Clinical Investigation* 1987; **80**:706–10.

Tucker KL, Hannan MT & Qiao N. Low plasma vitamin B12 is associated with lower BMD: the framingham osteoporosis study. *Journal of Bone and Mineral Research* 2005; **20**:152–8.

U.S. Department of Health and Human Services. *Bone Health and Osteoporosis: A Report of the Surgeon General* 2004; U.S. Department of Health and Human Services, Office of the Surgeon General, Rockville.

Warwick D, Field J & Prothero D. Function ten years after colles' fracture. *Clinical Orthopaedics and Related Research* 1993; **295**:270–4.

Woolf AD & Pfleger B. Burden of major musculoskeletal conditions. *Bulletin of the World Health Organization* 2003; **81**:646–56.

Wyshak G, Frisch RE, Albright TE *et al.* Nonalcoholic carbonated beverage consumption and bone fractures among women former college athletes. *Journal of Orthopaedic Research* 1989; **7**:91–9.

111

Osteoporosis and its Consequences: a Major Threat to the Quality of Life in the Elderly

René Rizzoli

University Hospitals, Geneva, Switzerland

INTRODUCTION

Osteoporosis is defined as a systemic skeletal disease characterized by low bone mass and microarchitectural deterioration of bone tissue, with a consequent increase in bone fragility and susceptibility to fracture risk (World Health Organization, 2003). The diagnosis of the disease relies on the quantitative assessment of bone mineral mass/density, which represents so far one major determinant of bone strength and thereby of fracture risk. Thus, the diagnosis of osteoporosis is not based on the demonstration of fracture, which constitutes a complication, or the clinical expression of the disease, but on parameters capable of reliably predicting the risk of fracture. Indications to treatment are based on the evaluation of fracture risk, which also integrates other factors than osteoporosis diagnosis.

EPIDEMIOLOGY

Bone mass decreases and the risk of osteoporotic fracture increases as people age. Fractures of the vertebrae, proximal femur, distal forearm, and proximal humerus are considered to be typical of osteoporotic origin when they occur following a low-energy trauma (*see* **Chapter 110, Epidemiology of Osteoporosis**).

Hip fracture is the best studied osteoporotic fracture, because it cannot remain unrecognized, being nearly always treated in hospitals and thereby more precisely recorded. Most, if not all, hip fractures associated with osteoporosis result from a fall from standing height. The age-related increase in fracture risk depends on the progressive decrease in bone mass, and on the rising risk of falling. However, only a minority of falls in the elderly (less than 2%) result in hip fracture (Cummings and Melton, 2002; (*see* **Chapter 112, Gait, Balance, and Falls**)).

Vertebral fracture risk is less clearly studied than hip fracture. Only a fraction of all X-ray-determined vertebral fractures comes to clinical attention and diagnosis. Furthermore, even if the criteria used to define vertebral fracture may vary, deformities of vertebral body on conventional X-ray examination remain largely underrecognized, or not mentioned in the radiologist's report (Gehlbach *et al.*, 2000).

The incidence of osteoporotic fractures increases exponentially with age. After the age of 80, one-third and one-fourth of women and men respectively experience a fracture over a 5-year period (Center *et al.*, 1999) (Figure 1). At the age of 50, the lifetime risk of sustaining an osteoporotic fracture is close to 50% and more than 20% for women and men, respectively (Johnell and Kanis, 2005).

Osteoporosis and osteoporotic fractures have so far been a predominantly women's disease. Indeed, the women-to-men ratio for hip fracture risk is between 3 and 5. Several reasons can explain the lower age-adjusted incidence in men: a higher bone mass and larger bone size at the end of the growth period, the absence of accelerated bone loss occurring at the time of sex hormone deprivation, that is, after menopause, and a shorter life expectancy. In the framework of the progressive aging of the population, there is a particularly marked increase of life expectancy in men. Thus, fracture-related problems will become major public health issues for both genders in many countries.

The incidence of osteoporotic fractures varies from region to region, and may be related to population age distribution, genetic background, or lifestyle conditions. For instance, it appears that hip fracture incidence is higher in urban

Principles and Practice of Geriatric Medicine, 4th Edition. Edited by M.S. John Pathy, Alan J. Sinclair and John E. Morley.

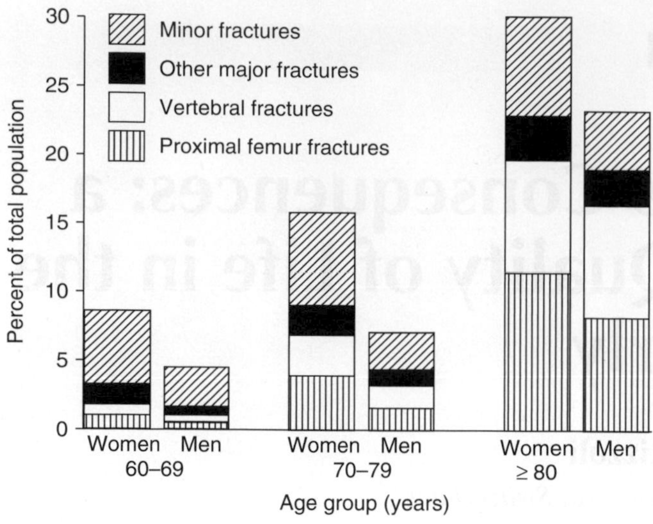

Figure 1 Fracture risk according to age and gender. In the Dubbo osteoporosis epidemiology study, fracture risk was recorded during a five-year cohort prospective follow-up. The results are presented per class of age and for each gender (Reprinted from Center *et al.*, 1999 with permission from Elsevier (The Lancet, 1999, Vol 353, pp 878–882))

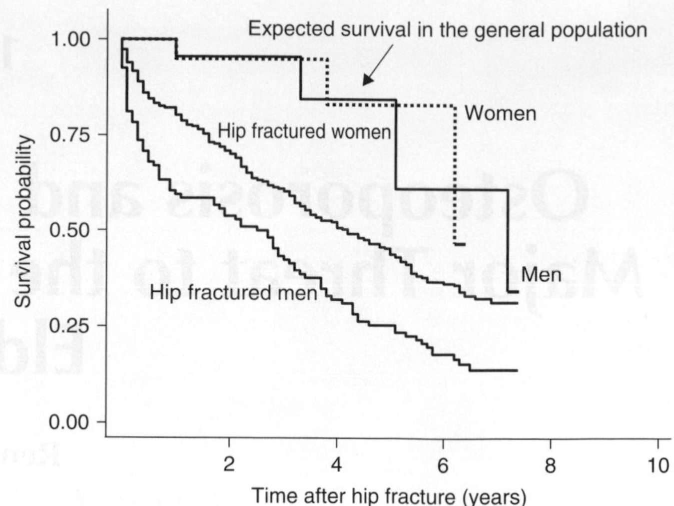

Figure 2 Survival estimate for age-matched men and women with hip fracture, and the expected survival in the general population (Reproduced from Trombetti A *et al.*, Survival and potential years of life lost after hip fracture in men and age-matched women, Osteoporosis International, 13, pp 731–737, Copyright 2002, with kind permission of Springer Science and Business Media)

Table 1 Age-standardized mortality ratio

Fracture	Women	Men
Proximal femur	2.2	3.2
Vertebral	1.7	2.4
Other major	1.9	2.2
Other minor	0.8	1.5

The mortality after major types of osteoporotic fracture was obtained in a 5-year prospective cohort study.
Source: Adapted from Center *et al.*, 1999.

than in rural areas in a given population (Chevalley *et al.*, 2002a). Up to 40% of hip fractures concern patients living in nursing homes (Schurch *et al.*, 1996). This is probably related to their advanced age and to a high prevalence of comorbidities requiring long-term care (*see* **Chapter 133, Frailty**). Moreover, this population is at high risk of repeated falls.

Among the complications of osteoporosis, increased mortality has been clearly demonstrated after hip or vertebral fracture (Table 1) (Center *et al.*, 1999). There is no increased mortality after forearm fracture. During the first year after hip fracture, mortality rate of the patients is around 25%, whereas, mortality rate in the nonfractured population of the same age remains around 5%. Hip fracture is thereby associated with a 20% increase in mortality (Schurch *et al.*, 1996). Mortality is nearly twice as high in men as in women, because of a higher prevalence of comorbidities (Trombetti *et al.*, 2002). Mortality is higher in the general male population, with a life expectancy approximately 7 years shorter. Given the reduction of life expectancy as a consequence of hip fracture, the proportion of the years of life lost is significantly higher in men than in women (70 vs. 59%) (Figure 2) (Trombetti *et al.*, 2002). Thus, among the complications of osteoporosis, hip fracture represents the most dramatic expression of the disease, in terms of morbidity, mortality, and medical costs. For vertebral fracture, reduced survival cannot be attributed directly to the fracture, but to underlying cardiovascular or pulmonary diseases that might become decompensated because of the fracture event. By the prolonged handicaps they cause, fractures are a major threat for the quality of life of the elderly and represent a significant reason of increased health costs. By one year after hip fracture, close to 20% of the patients still require rehabilitation in hospital. The burden is expected to worsen, since the number of hip fractures, for instance, is likely to quadruple worldwide during the first half of the twenty-first century. This will markedly increase the demand for health care, with treatment and consequences of osteoporotic fractures potentially compromising the economy and social equilibrium in many countries where the proportion of the elderly population is exploding.

DIAGNOSIS

Dual-energy Absorptiometry

There are many techniques available to assess bone mass, measure bone mineral content, or areal bone mineral density (BMD), which is the amount of bone mineral per projected bone scanned area. Dual X-ray absorptiometry (DXA) techniques are now validated for this measurement not only at the two skeletal sites particularly at risk of osteoporotic fracture, such as lumbar spine and proximal femur but also at the peripheral skeleton such as the forearm. For the diagnosis of osteoporosis, hip and/or spine are mainly to be considered (Cummings *et al.*, 2002; Kanis, 2002). Areal BMD accounts for more than two-thirds of the variance of bone strength as determined *in vitro* on isolated skeletal pieces (Ammann *et al.*, 1996). There is an inverse relationship between incidence of osteoporotic fracture and DXA-provided BMD values. Long-term longitudinal studies have demonstrated that a decrease of 1 SD in lumbar spine BMD (in anteroposterior view) is associated with a more than 2.5-fold increase in fracture risk, comparable with a 10–17-year increase in years after menopause (Marshall *et al.*, 1996). Areal BMD integrates the size of the bone and its thickness, as well as its true volumetric density.

With the progressive development of degenerative joint diseases, spine BMD values could be largely overestimated, particularly in the elderly. Lumbar spine BMD measurements in lateral view could theoretically offer an advantage over conventional anteroposterior projection by avoiding osteophytes and posterior elements osteoarthritis. However, measurement of lateral spine is not routinely advocated because of the superposition of ribs and/or pelvis, reducing the number of vertebrae analyzable, and because of the lower accuracy and precision of this measurement. Indeed, lateral BMD, at least with present technology, does not appear to be of clinical advantage, since the error of the measurement is more than double the annual bone loss after menopause. Thus, it does not seem to be superior in diagnostic sensitivity, except possibly for corticosteroid-induced bone loss. Above the age of 65, osteoarthritis makes the measurement of lumbar spine BMD highly unreliable for diagnostic purposes.

Femoral neck BMD appears to be a better predictor of fracture of the proximal femur. This is based on long-term prospective longitudinal studies with fracture as an outcome. Since this measurement seems to be influenced by osteoarthritis to a much lower extent than the measurement of the spine, it would be the most suitable one for the diagnosis of osteoporosis in the elderly. However, proximal femur measurements are influenced by a variety of factors likely to impair accuracy and decrease the precision of the measurement. The size of the region of interest as well as its location along the hip axis and the degree of leg rotation can affect proximal femur BMD measurement. The potential for error in terms of both accuracy and precision of dual X-ray absorptiometry measurements of lumbar spine and proximal femur emphasizes the need for strictly controlled conditions of measurements.

A World Health Organization (WHO) panel has proposed the limit of −2.5 standard deviations below the mean values recorded in young healthy individuals of the same gender as the diagnostic criterion for osteoporosis (T-Score; T-Score = [measured BMD − young adult BMD]/young adult SD). The fracture rate in this reference population is very low. This approach is very similar to the measurement of blood pressure for the diagnosis of hypertension. This constitutes a diagnosis threshold, which should not be automatically translated into a therapeutic threshold. Indeed, other factors such as age, concomitant risk factors, bone turnover, or treatment cost/benefits, should be included into the treatment

Table 2 Lifetime risk of fragility fracture in the Swedish population at the age of 50

	Women (%)	Men (%)
Proximal femur	23	11
Distal forearm	21	5
Vertebral (clinical)	15	8
Proximal humerus	13	5
Any site	46	22

Source: Adapted from Johnell and Kanis, 2005.

decision. The prevalence of subjects with bone mass values below this limit increases with age, reaching approximately 50% at the age of 80. Indeed, this prevalence corresponds to the lifetime risk of any skeletal fracture in a 50-year old woman (Johnell and Kanis, 2005) (Table 2). However, it should be remembered that there is no BMD threshold value for the risk of osteoporotic fracture, but the relationship is characterized by a continuous increasing gradient of risk with the decrease of BMD. Z-score compares a patient's value with the mean BMD of age- and gender-matched healthy subjects (Z-score = [measured BMD − age-matched mean BMD]/age-matched SD).

Other Skeletal Determinants of Osteoporotic Fractures

Macro- and Microarchitecture

In the proximal femur, the hip axis length has been shown to be a BMD-independent predictor of fracture risk. The bending strength of bones is influenced not only by the amount of bone within the bone, but also by its geometrical distribution. In cortical bone, mechanical strength is influenced by the histological structure, that is, primary versus osteonal bone, the orientation of the collagen fibers, the number and orientation of the cement lines, and the presence of microdamage or microcracks. In trabecular bone, mechanical strength is affected by the microstructural arrangement of trabeculae, which includes their orientation, their degree of connection, the mean trabecular thickness, and the trabecular interspace. Other important determinants of bone strength for both cortical and trabecular bone include the cross-linking between collagen fibers, the degree of mineralization of the matrix, as well as the crystal characteristics. Macro- and microarchitectural components of bone strength can explain, at least in part, clinical observations in which variations in bone mineral mass were not closely correlated to changes in fracture rate.

Bone Remodeling and Bone Fragility

The degree of bone remodeling, as assessed by the measurement of biochemical markers of bone resorption, has been shown to be a BMD-independent predictor of osteoporotic hip fractures (Delmas *et al.*, 2000). This observation suggests that increased bone resorption also increases skeletal fragility

Table 3 Biochemical markers of bone turnover

Bone formation markers (serum)	Bone resorption markers (serum and urine)
Osteocalcin	Hydroxyproline
Bone specific alkaline phosphatase	Deoxypyridinoline
Procollagen type 1 *N*-propeptide (P1NP)	Bone sialoprotein
Procollagen type 1 *C*-propeptide (P1CP)	Tartrate resistant acid phosphatase
	Peptide-bound pyridinoline cross-links (CTX, NTX)

To avoid the variations due to circadian rhythm and food intake, serum, and/or urine samples have to be collected in fasting state (Delmas *et al.*, 2000).

by an increase in bone loss, leading to a DXA detectable decrease in bone mineral mass and a deterioration of microarchitecture due to an increased trabecular plate perforation. The potential use of biochemical markers of bone turnover includes the prediction of bone loss (the higher the bone turnover, the greater the postmenopausal bone loss), the prediction of fracture risk, and the monitoring of therapy with anticatabolic agents (prediction of response and improvement of compliance) (Table 3).

Extraskeletal Determinants of Osteoporotic Fractures

A fracture represents a structural failure of the bone whereby the forces applied to the bone exceed its load-bearing capacity (Figure 3). Therefore, besides the size, geometry, and material property of the bone tissue, the direction and magnitude of the applied load will determine whether a bone will fracture. Almost all fractures, even those qualified as "low-trauma" fractures, occur as the result of some injury. Usually this is the result of a fall, or the application of a specific loading event in some cases of vertebral fractures, as bending forward to lift a heavy object with the arms extended.

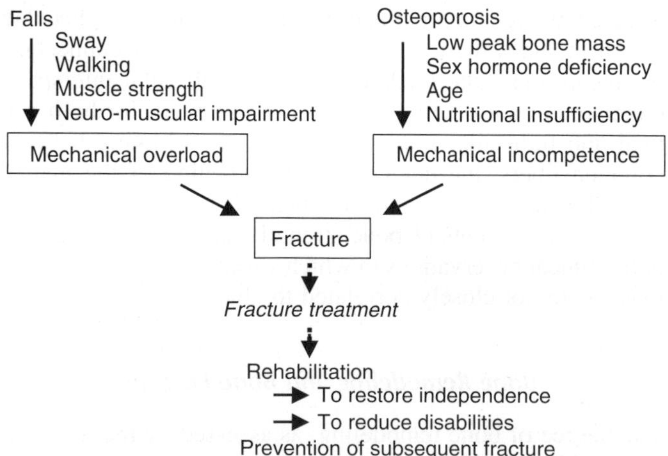

Figure 3 Pathogenesis and management of osteoporotic fracture. Fracture results from mechanical load and incompetence. Once fracture has occurred, the main goal is to prevent a subsequent one

Table 4 Risk factors associated with falls

1. Impaired mobility, disability
2. Impaired gait and balance
3. Neuromuscular or musculoskeletal disorders
4. Age
5. Impaired vision
6. Neurological, heart disorders
7. History of falls
8. Medication
9. Cognitive impairment

Source: Adapted from Myers *et al.*, 1996.

Risk Factors for Falls

The risk of falling increases with age (*see* **Chapter 112, Gait, Balance, and Falls**). Most falls in the elderly are due to intrinsic and extrinsic, or environmental factors (Table 4). Among the intrinsic factors, the risk of falling increases with the number of disabilities. Impairment of gait, mobility, and balance are the most consistently identified risk factors for falls and fall-related injuries. The ability to maintain postural control and avoid environmental obstacles depends on proprioceptive, vestibular, and visual input translated into appropriate motor responses. Thus, the risk of falling increases with reduced visual acuity or diminished sensory perception of the lower extremities. Chronic illnesses such as various neurological disorders, heart diseases, stroke, urinary incontinence, depression, and impaired cognitive functions increase the risk of falling. Medications such as hypnotics, antidepressants, or sedatives are associated with falls. Environmental factors include potential hazards that can be found in the home, such as slippery floors, unstable furniture, or insufficient lighting. The orientation of falls influences the consequences of falling. Indeed, the points of impact of a fall determine the type and extent of injury. When falling, the elderly tend to land on their hip. In contrast, middle-aged adults tend to fall forward with the main impact on their wrist. Several reflexes and postural responses are initiated during a fall, which can prevent or reduce the injury. The effectiveness of reflex actions depends on speed of execution and strength of the muscle initiating the protective movement. The impact of falls can be absorbed by surrounding soft tissue. The apparent protective effect of higher body weight may be due, at least in part, to the local shock-absorbing capacity of muscle and fat.

PATHOPHYSIOLOGY OF BONE LOSS

The onset of substantial bone loss occurs around the age of 50 and 65 years in women and men, respectively. In contrast with bone mineral accrual during adolescence, bone size varies little throughout life, other than the continuous and slight expansion of bone outer dimensions, which is mainly found in men, and which affects both the axial and the peripheral skeleton. This periosteal expansion is less than the increase in bone marrow space, which results from a continuous endosteal resorption. Under these conditions, bone cortex becomes thinner. This phenomenon, together with an increment in cortical porosity and a destruction of trabeculae through thinning and perforation, account for age-dependent bone loss. Thus, this modeling process could be interpreted as a response to bone loss, in an attempt to compensate for a reduction in mechanical resistance (Seeman, 2002).

Hormonal Causes of Bone Mass Loss

Sex Hormone Deficiency

Female sex hormones appear to be mandatory not only to the maximal acquisition of bone mass in both males and females, but also to the maintenance of bone mass by controlling bone remodeling during the reproductive life in females and in aging men (Riggs *et al.*, 2002; Seeman, 2002). Other pathological conditions associated with premature estrogen deficiency, such as anorexia nervosa, secondary amenorrhea due to strenuous exercise, or the use of inhibitors of gonadotropin secretion, support the concept of a causal link between estrogen deficiency and accelerated bone loss. By increasing bone turnover and uncoupling bone formation from resorption, estrogen deficiency appears to be the main cause of osteoporosis observed in women after the fifth decade, and possibly also in men, and thus is directly implicated in the age-related increase in the incidence of fragility fractures. It is now clearly established that bone loss does not attenuate with age, but continues throughout the whole life, at least in the peripheral skeletal sites.

Increased bone turnover, with an imbalance between bone formation and resorption as a consequence of estrogen deficiency, involves the production and action of a variety of cytokines released in the bone marrow environment. There is evidence that Tumor Necrosis Factor-alpha (TNF-alpha), Interleukin-1, Interleukin-6, and Receptor Activator Nuclear Kappa-b Ligand (RANKL), cytokines that stimulate bone resorption *in vitro* and *in vivo*, may affect the initial step leading to bone loss induced by estrogen deficiency. A critical role for TNF-alpha in bone loss induced by estrogen deficiency has been demonstrated in a model of transgenic mice in which the activity of TNF-alpha is permanently prevented by the constitutive presence of high levels of circulating soluble TNF-alpha-receptor 1 (Ammann *et al.*, 1997). In this model, the decrease in bone mass and the increase in bone turnover observed after ovariectomy in control mice were not observed in transgenic mice, which appeared to be fully protected.

Other Endocrine Causes of Bone Loss

Apart from gonadal deficiency, which is an important cause of osteoporosis in both genders, a number of other endocrine diseases can also lead to bone loss. The effect of primary hyperparathyroidism on bone is to increase the activation frequency of bone remodeling. This increase in bone turnover is associated with a reduction in cancellous bone volume as observed by histomorphometric technique. Osteodensitometry indicates a decrease in BMD at both axial and appendicular sites. An excess of thyroid hormones also increases the rate of bone remodeling. Thus, bone loss can occur in hyperthyroidism and in patients under long-term thyroid replacement therapy at doses suppressing thyroid stimulating hormone (TSH). The major net effect of glucocorticoid excess is the reduction of bone formation. In addition, there is some evidence that the administration of glucocorticoids in pharmacological excess decreases the intestinal absorption of calcium and perhaps the tubular reabsorption of calcium (Pennisi *et al.*, 2006). These latter two effects would lead to a negative calcium balance and consecutive increased bone resorption.

Nutritional Causes of Bone Mass Loss

Calcium Intake, Vitamin D, and Osteoporosis

Calcium contributes to the preservation of the bony tissue during adulthood, particularly in the elderly. Without an appropriate supply of vitamin D, from cutaneous and/or exogenous source, the bioavailability and metabolism of calcium is disturbed (Heaney, 2000). This results in accelerated bone loss.

In the elderly, several alterations contribute toward a negative calcium balance (*see* **Chapter 108, Age-related Changes in Calcium Homeostasis and Bone Loss**). Indeed, with aging there is a decrease in the calcium intake because of reduction in dairy products consumption, in the intestinal absorption of calcium, in the absorptive capacity of the intestinal epithelium to adapt to a low-calcium intake, in the exposure to sunlight and the capacity of the skin to produce vitamin D, and in the renal reabsorption of calcium, as well as in the tubular calcium reabsorptive capacity to respond to the stimulatory effect of parathyroid hormone (PTH). Furthermore, the mild renal insufficiency regularly observed in the elderly can contribute to a state of chronic hyperparathyroidism that favors negative bone mineral balance and thereby osteoporosis. Increasing calcium intake is certainly an important strategy that appears to be relatively easier to implement as compared to other possible preventive measures.

Protein Malnutrition

Nutritional deficiencies play a significant role in osteoporosis in the elderly. Indeed, undernutrition is often observed in the elderly, and it appears to be more severe in patients with hip fracture than in the general aging population. A low protein intake could be particularly detrimental for both the acquisition of bone mass during childhood and adolescence, and for the conservation of bone integrity with aging (Rizzoli and Bonjour, 1999; Rizzoli *et al.*, 2001a). Protein undernutrition can favor the occurrence of hip fracture by increasing the propensity to fall as a result of

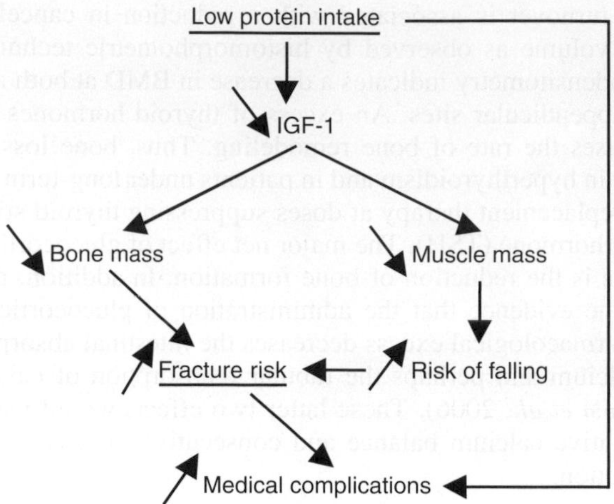

Figure 4 Protein undernutrition in the elderly. Possible role of IGF-I in bone mass, muscle mass, risk of fracture, and outcome after hip fracture

muscle weakness and impairment in movement coordination, by affecting protective mechanisms such as reaction time and muscle strength, thus reducing the energy required to fracture an osteoporotic proximal femur, and/or by decreasing bone mass (Rizzoli and Bonjour, 2004) (Figure 4). Furthermore, a reduction in the protective layer of soft tissue padding decreases the force required to fracture an osteoporotic hip.

Protein and Osteoporotic Fracture

Various studies have found a relationship between the level of protein intake and calcium phosphate or bone metabolism, and have come to the conclusion that either a deficient or an excessive protein supply could negatively affect the balance of calcium (Rizzoli and Bonjour, 2004). An indirect argument in favor of a potential deleterious effect of high protein intake on bone is that hip fracture appears to be more frequent in countries with high protein intake of animal origin. But, as expected, the countries with the highest incidence of hip fracture are those with the longest life expectancy. In a prospective study carried out on more than 40 000 women in Iowa, a higher protein intake was associated with a reduced risk of hip fracture. The association was particularly evident with protein of animal rather than vegetal origin (Munger *et al.*, 1999).

Protein and Bone Mass

Regarding the relation with bone mineral mass, there is a positive correlation with spontaneous protein intake in premenopausal women (Rizzoli *et al.*, 2001b). In a survey carried out in hospitalized elderly patients, low protein intake was associated with reduced femoral neck areal BMD and poor physical performances (Geinoz *et al.*, 1993). The group with high protein intakes and a greater BMD, particularly at the femoral neck level, had also a better improvement of bicipital and quadricipital muscle strength and performance, as indicated by the increased capacity to walk and climb stairs, after four weeks of hospitalization. In a longitudinal follow-up in the frame of the Framingham study, the rate of bone mineral loss was inversely correlated to dietary protein intake (Hannan *et al.*, 2000). Increasing protein intake has a favorable effect on BMD in the elderly receiving calcium and vitamin D supplements (Dawson-Hughes and Harris, 2002). Taken altogether, these results indicate that a sufficient protein intake is mandatory for bone health, particularly in the elderly. Thus, whereas a gradual decline in calorie intake with age can be considered as an adequate adjustment to the progressive reduction in energy expenditure, the parallel reduction in protein intake may be detrimental for maintaining the integrity and function of several organs or systems, including skeletal muscles and bone (Figure 4).

Relation with IGF-I

In association with the progressive age-dependent decrease in both protein intake and bone mass, several reports have documented a decrement in insulin-like growth factor-I (IGF-I) plasma levels. Experimental and clinical studies suggest that dietary proteins, by influencing both the production and action of growth factors, particularly the Growth Hormone (GH)–Insulin-like Growth Factor (IGF) system, could influence bone homeostasis. The hepatic production and plasma level of IGF-I are under the influence of dietary proteins. Protein restriction has been shown to reduce IGF-I plasma levels by inducing a resistance to the action of GH at the hepatic level. Decreased serum IGF-I has been found in states of undernutrition such as marasmus, anorexia nervosa, celiac disease, or HIV-infected patients. In addition, protein restriction could render the target organs less sensitive to IGF-I. When IGF-I is given to rats maintained under a low protein diet, at doses even higher than those normalizing its plasma levels, it failed to restore bone formation (Bourrin *et al.*, 2000). In addition, GH treatment was even associated with a decreased bone strength under conditions of a low protein diet (Ammann *et al.*, 2002).

Protein Replenishment and Osteoporosis

A state of undernutrition on admission, which is consistently documented in elderly patients with hip fracture, followed by an inadequate food intake during hospital stay can adversely influence their clinical outcome (Delmi *et al.*, 1990). Intervention studies using supplementary feeding by nasogastric tube or parenteral nutrition, or even a simple oral dietary preparation that normalizes protein intake, can improve the clinical outcome after a hip fracture. The latter way of correcting the deficient food intake has obvious practical and psychological advantages over nasogastric tube feeding or parenteral nutrition. An oral protein supplement, which brought the intake from low to a level still below Recommended Dietary Allowances (RDA) (i.e. $0.8\,\mathrm{g\,kg^{-1}}$ body weight), avoiding thus the risk of an excess of dietary protein, improved the clinical course in the rehabilitation hospitals by significantly lowering the rate of complications,

Table 5 Protein supplements in elderly persons with hip fracture

	Changes from baseline (%)		
	Placebo	*Protein*	*p*
Prealbumin	+56 ± 9	+86 ± 14	0.07
IGF-I	+34 ± 7	+86 ± 15	0.01
IgM	+40 ± 6	+66 ± 9	0.02
Proximal femur BMD	−4.7 ± 0.8	−2.3 ± 0.7	0.03
Median length of stay in rehabilitation hospital (in days)	54	33	0.02

The results are taken from Schürch *et al.*, 1998.

such as bedsore, severe anemia, intercurrent lung, or renal infections. The duration of hospital stay of elderly patients with hip fracture is not only determined by their present medical condition, but also by domestic and social factors. The total length of stay in the orthopedic ward and rehabilitation hospitals was significantly shorter by 25% in the case of supplemented patients than in controls (Delmi *et al.*, 1990; Schurch *et al.*, 1998; Tkatch *et al.*, 1992). Normalization of protein intake, independent of energy, calcium, and vitamin D intake, was in fact responsible for this more favorable outcome (Tkatch *et al.*, 1992). Finally, this normalization of protein intake was found to increase IGF-I, and even IgM concentrations (Table 5) (Schurch *et al.*, 1998). Thus, the lower incidence of medical complications with the correction of protein intake insufficiency is also compatible with the hypothesis of IGF-I improving the immune status, as this growth factor can stimulate the proliferation of immunocompetent cells and modulate immunoglobulins secretion (Auernhammer and Strasburger, 1995).

Besides the production and action of the growth hormone–IGF-I system, protein undernutrition can be associated with alterations of cytokines secretion, such as interferon gamma, TNF-alpha, or transforming growth factor beta. TNF-alpha and Interleukin-6 generally increase with age. In a situation of cachexia, such as in chronic heart failure, an inverse correlation between BMD and TNF-alpha levels has been found, further implicating a possible role of uncontrolled cytokines production in bone loss. Increased TNF-alpha can be a crucial factor in the sex hormone deficiency-induced bone loss, but it also plays a role in the target organ resistance to insulin, and possibly to IGF-I. The modulation by nutritional intakes of cytokines production and action, and the strong implication of various cytokines in the regulation of bone remodeling suggest a possible role of certain cytokines in the nutrition-bone link.

Vitamin K and Osteoporosis

A low level of vitamin K_1 and K_2 has been reported in patients sustaining hip fracture (Booth *et al.*, 2003). Vitamin K is essential for the production of gamma-carboxylated glutamyl residues present in several coagulation factors and bone proteins, particularly osteocalcin. The degree of vitamin K deficiency in humans can be assessed by measuring the undercarboxylated fraction of osteocalcin. This fraction increases with age and therefore is negatively related to BMD in elderly women. Hence, undercarboxylated osteocalcin was found to be a predictor of hip fracture. Energy-protein undernutrition is usually associated with various vitamin deficiencies. To what extent vitamin K deficiency *per se* contributes to bone loss in undernourished patients sustaining hip fracture is still not known.

Other Nutrients

By interfering with both the production and action of PTH, magnesium could indirectly affect bone metabolism. However, its specific role in the maintenance of bone mass during adulthood has not been yet identified. Several trace elements are required for normal bone metabolism. Various animal and/or ecological human studies suggest that aluminum, zinc, manganese, copper, boron, silicon, and fluoride at doses lower than that used in the treatment of osteoporosis, and vitamins B_6, B_{12}, and C, could play a positive role in the normal metabolism of bone tissue. Selective intervention studies are still required to delineate their respective role in the maintenance of bone mass, particularly in the elderly.

Mechanical Causes of Bone Mass Loss

Immobilization is an important cause of bone loss (*see* **Chapter 142, Restraints and Immobility**). The effect of "disuse" on bone mass is far greater than that of adding "walking" to an already ambulatory subject. Enforced immobilization in healthy volunteers results in a decrease in bone mineral mass. Motor deficit due to neurological disorders such as hemiplegia or paraplegia is a cause of bone loss. Bone mineral mass decreases during space flights despite forceful physical exercise. This observation underlines the importance of weight bearing in the maintenance of bone mass. At the tissue level, immobilization results in a negative balance, the amount of bone resorbed being greater than that formed. At the cellular level, immobilization results in an increased osteoclastic resorption associated with a decrease in osteoblastic formation. The nature of the molecular signal(s) perceiving the reduced mechanical strain has not yet been clearly identified.

Toxic Causes of Bone Mass Loss

Excessive alcohol consumption appears to be a significant risk factor for osteoporosis particularly in men (Kanis *et al.*, 2005a). Reduced rates of bone formation have been associated with alcohol abuse. High intake of alcohol is often associated with marked dietary disturbance such as low protein intake, other changes in lifestyle, liver disease, and decrease in testosterone production. These alterations can contribute to the osteoporosis observed in heavy drinkers. Use of tobacco appears to be associated with an increased risk of both axial and appendicular osteoporotic fractures in women and men (Kanis *et al.*, 2005b). This risk emerges with age. Smoking reduces the protective effects of obesity and of estrogen exposure. Reduced rate of bone formation and increased bone resorption might be responsible for bone loss, through a reduction in the production and acceleration in the degradation of estrogens.

PREVENTION AND TREATMENT

The ultimate goal of osteoporosis therapy is to prevent fractures, and thus pain, handicaps, and altered quality of life consecutive to fractures. The level of evidence and how convincing the results of clinical trials are, vary substantially among therapeutic strategies. To assess the quality of evidence provided by published clinical trials, evidence-based medicine offers a method to evaluate the strength of the evidence. Evidence-based medicine is the conscientious, explicit, and judicious use of current best evidence from clinical research in making decisions about the care of individuals (Guyatt, 1998). However, as in most domains of medicine, it appears that only a small percentage of the therapeutic decisions taken in the daily medical practice can be determined according to evidence-based medicine criteria. This is particularly true for the elderly, in whom trials are difficult to undertake, and the high prevalence of comorbidities impairs the interpretation of the results.

The strength of a study design is of major importance, because randomized controlled studies with homogeneous results are considered more valuable than randomized controlled studies with inconsistent results, and offer a higher level of evidence than observational studies. In the hierarchy in the level of evidence, the opinion of experts and/or the personal clinical experience are at the bottom. To attenuate the interaction with confounding variables, and the influence of subgroups selection susceptible to introducing significant bias, randomized trials should include an appropriate blinding of both the investigator and the subjects. This is the only way to avoid a preferential assignment of patients into a group, and an imbalance in the characteristics of the patients or of other factors influencing the outcome between the studied agent and the control groups.

Another important condition is that the outcome variable should be a predefined endpoint, since there is the risk in *post-hoc* analysis of trials with small sample size of detecting drug efficacy only by chance. Since the ultimate goal of osteoporosis treatment is the prevention of fracture, regulation authorities are considering fracture rate as the reliable endpoint. The type of fracture, as well as the diagnosis criteria should thus be clearly defined. Since a substantial number of vertebral fractures may not be accompanied by complaints, morphometric fractures (i.e. objectively documented on repeated X-ray examinations) may be considered as less clinically relevant than those with an overt clinical expression. Moreover, the definition of vertebral deformity can vary from one trial to the other. The conditions retained for fracture definition will thus influence the response to therapy and thus the outcome of clinical trials.

Regarding antifracture efficacy, an important criterion is that the occurrence of one event does not increase the probability of occurrence of another event. Thus, patients with fracture instead of fracture rates should be reported. In the former, a patient with fracture is censored once the event has occurred, whereas in the latter, the number of fractures *per sum* of observation times is given; thus, the same patient can be recorded several times if the individual experiences more than one event.

Attention should also be paid to the strength of the outcome. Indeed, this outcome could be of a direct and major importance for the patient (pain, disability and functional limitation in the case of fracture of long bones), or of some importance (for instance, vertebral fractures, since some could remain unrecognized), or of indirect importance, such as changes in BMD or in bone turnover. Finally, a clear trade-off between the benefits and adverse effects should be unequivocally specified. The role of costs/effectiveness analysis is also becoming an important factor to consider in relation with the limitations on health budget appearing in many countries.

Population Studied

Fracture rate exponentially increases from about the age of 60 onward. However, the incidence of fracture does not display the same kinetics at each skeletal site. For instance, the increase in the incidence of vertebral fracture mostly occurs during the sixth and seventh decades in women, whereas the mean age for hip fracture is around 82 years. Therefore, age, gender, the severity of osteoporosis, and the selective alteration of a specific skeletal site will influence the response to an antiosteoporotic therapy. A quite often misused concept is the so-called number needed to treat (NNT). This number represents the number of patients who should be treated to avoid the occurrence of one event. It corresponds to the inverse of the reduction of the absolute risk, that is, the event rate in the placebo group minus the event rate in the treated group. For the same reduction in the relative risk, this NNT is primarily determined by the event rate in the placebo group (Figure 5). Furthermore, with the same reduction in relative risk for a given agent, differences in the inclusion criteria, influencing thereby the fracture rate in the population studied, will be associated with different NNTs. This indicates that NNT cannot be used for comparing the efficacy of different drugs, unless fracture rates in the placebo groups are very similar. In the oldest old with a very high fracture rate, NNT may be much lower than in subjects in the 7th decade, as prevailing in many trials.

General Management

The general measures to apply are based on the following reasons (Table 6):

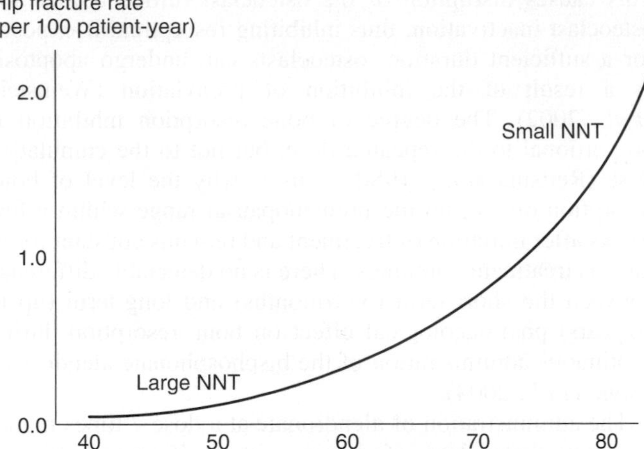

Figure 5 Number needed to treat to avoid one hip fracture in relation to age. NNT is calculated as the inverse of the absolute risk reduction observed for a given treatment. NNT is thus highly dependent on the fracture risk in the target population to be treated with a given treatment known to reduce the relative risk of fracture. The greater the fracture risk, the smaller the NNT

Table 6 General management

- Treatment of any disease causing bone loss
- Ensure dietary calcium intake of 1000 mg day^{-1} or greater
- Ensure adequate dietary protein intake (1 g kg^{-1} body weight)
- Correct and prevent vitamin D insufficiency (800 IU/day)
- Promote weight-bearing physical exercise
- Reduce the risk of falling
- Reduce the consequences of falls (hip protectors)

There is a high prevalence of calcium, protein, and vitamin D insufficiency in the elderly (Heaney, 2000; Rizzoli *et al.*, 2001a). Calcium and vitamin D supplements decrease secondary hyperparathyroidism and, particularly in the elderly living in nursing homes, reduce the risk of proximal femur fracture (Chapuy *et al.*, 1992). Sufficient protein intakes are necessary not only for the homeostasis of the musculoskeletal system but also to decrease the complications occurring after an osteoporotic fracture (Rizzoli and Bonjour, 1999, 2004; Schurch *et al.*, 1998). Under these conditions, intakes of at least 1000 mg day^{-1} of calcium, 800 IU of vitamin D, and of 1 g kg^{-1} body weight of protein can be recommended for the general management of patients with osteoporosis. Regular physical exercise helps to maintain bone health, not only by stimulating bone formation and by retarding bone resorption, but also through a favorable influence on the muscle function (Kelley *et al.*, 2000; Wolff *et al.*, 1999). These measures, together with the correction of decreased visual acuity, the reduction in consumption of drugs that alter wakefulness and balance, and the improvement of the home environment (slippery floor, obstacles, insufficient lighting) are important steps aimed at preventing falls (Myers *et al.*, 1996; Tinetti, 2003; (*see* **Chapter 12, Physical Fitness and Exercise**, **Chapter 112, Gait, Balance, and Falls**)). However, these have not been verified in randomized controlled trials fulfilling the requirements of evidence-based medicine. Wearing hip protectors is able to significantly and specifically reduce hip fracture risk (Kannus *et al.*, 2000). This has been shown in randomized controlled trials and seems to be particularly efficient in the elderly living in nursing homes. This population is at very high risk, since close to 40% of hip fractures are occurring in this kind of setting (Schurch *et al.*, 1996).

Pharmacological Intervention

The definition of osteoporosis, according to the number of standard deviations in areal BMD as compared with values observed in young healthy individuals, is an operational definition that should be clearly distinguished from a therapeutic threshold. An improved understanding of the pathophysiology of osteoporosis has led to the development of treatments with effects on BMD, bone turnover, and/or fracture risk (Delmas, 2002; Hauselmann and Rizzoli, 2003). The agents can be classified as anticatabolic or anabolic (Riggs and Parfitt, 2005). In the first category, there are calcium, hormone replacement therapy (HRT), bisphosphonates, estrogen analogs, tibolone or calcitonin, whereas PTH belongs to the second category. The mode of action of vitamin D analogs, anabolic steroids, and recently reported strontium ranclate, is not clearly established. Particular attention should be paid to the influence of the disease on the quality of life and as to whether the treatment applied improves it (Nevitt *et al.*, 2000). It is quite likely that over the next few years the impact of any kind of treatment against osteoporosis on the quality of life will become a highly relevant issue.

Applying rigorous criteria according to the principles of evidence-based medicine, a certain level of evidence can be attributed to each of these agents, depending on whether their effect on fracture risk has been studied in several randomized controlled trials with consistent results, in at least one controlled trial, or in observational studies (Table 7). If one considers only randomized controlled double-blind trials, with vertebral fracture or hip fracture as outcome, it appears

Table 7 Evidence of antifracture efficacy from randomized controlled trials

Agent	Evidence for reduction of vertebral fracture[a]	Evidence for reduction of hip fracture[a]
Alendronate	++	+
Anabolic steroids	o	o
Etidronate	+	o
Intranasal calcitonin	+	o
PTH	++	o
Raloxifene	++	o
Risedronate	++	+
Strontium ranelate	++	+
Tibolone	o	o
Vitamin D analogs	±	o

[a]In addition to calcium and vitamin D. ++, strong evidence (several trials with homogeneous results); +, some evidence (one or two trials); o, insufficient evidence; ±, variable effects

that the bisphosphonates alendronate and risedronate administered to osteoporotic women during the sixth and seventh decades, are able to decrease the incidence of both vertebral and hip fractures (Delmas, 2002; Hauselmann and Rizzoli, 2003). Raloxifene, clodronate, ibandronate, or PTH favorably influence vertebral fracture risk. Calcium and vitamin D supplements can decrease the incidence of hip fracture in institutionalized elderly women. The new generation bisphosphonates ibandronate have demonstrated unequivocal effectiveness for reducing the risk of fractures, including those of the hip. However, a number of potential concerns regarding bone health during long-term bisphosphonates administration have been raised. In particular, some have speculated that accumulation of bisphosphonates in bone might lead to excessive suppression of bone turnover, impairing the repair of defective bone tissue and thereby increasing fracture risk. Continuous administration of earlier bisphosphonates such as etidronate has been associated with defective bone mineralization and increased fracture risk in animal studies, but this has not been reported for nitrogen-containing bisphosphonates that are largely used nowadays. Recent studies on dogs have reported that high doses of alendronate or risedronate may affect a potential indicator of bone quality (microcracks), but the significance of this finding remains uncertain, since no additional risk was associated with this observation. Furthermore, bone strength did not appear to be dependent on microcracks density (Mashiba *et al.*, 2001).

Bisphosphonates Mechanism of Action Predicts Similar Short- and Long-term Effects

On the basis of the mechanism of action, there are essentially no significant differences between short- and long-term effects of nitrogen-containing bisphosphonates administered continuously, for example, daily or weekly (Rodan *et al.*, 2004; Rizzoli, 2006). This is because bisphosphonates must be present on the bone surface in order to produce their pharmacological action. At the minimal dose that produces maximal effects, they should be repeatedly administered to achieve fully effective pharmacological levels. The bisphosphonates moiety, two phosphate groups linked by a geminal carbon, is responsible for bisphosphonates localization on the bone surface through binding to the bone mineral calcium phosphate salt, hydroxyapatite. This moiety is also responsible for the low intestinal absorption of these compounds and the lack of penetration into most of the cells in the body.

Osteoclasts attach to exposed bone mineral surfaces, initiate bone resorption, and take-up the bisphosphonate along with the other resorption products, calcium and digested matrix. Inside the osteoclasts, nitrogen-containing bisphosphonates inhibit farnesyl diphosphate synthase, an enzyme in the mevalonate to cholesterol pathway. As a consequence, there is a reduction in the level of the lipids farnesyl diphosphate and geranylgeranyl diphosphate required for prenylation of GTPases, which are crucial enzymes for cytoskeletal organization and vesicular traffic. This causes disruption of the osteoclast ruffled border and osteoclast inactivation, thus inhibiting resorption. If exposed for a sufficient duration, osteoclasts can undergo apoptosis as a result of the inhibition of prenylation (Weinstein *et al.*, 2002). The degree of bone resorption inhibition is proportional to the repeated dose, but not to the cumulative dose (Reitsma *et al.*, 1980). This is why the level of bone resorption drops into the premenopausal range within a few weeks after initiation of treatment and remains constant for as long as treatment continues. There is no detectable difference between the short term (3–6 months) and long-term (up to 10 years) pharmacological effect on bone resorption during continuous administration of the bisphosphonate alendronate (Bone *et al.*, 2004).

The administration of alendronate at a dose 7 times higher than the daily dose of 10 mg with antifracture efficacy, but once a week, has the same effects on BMD and bone turnover, and seems to be associated with a greater convenience and possibly a better profile of adverse events (Rizzoli *et al.*, 2002). Risedronate at a weekly dose of 35 mg is equivalent to the daily dose of 5 mg. Though intravenous infusion of pamidronate or ibandronate increases BMD, there is no data indicating any favorable influence on fracture rate, so this treatment cannot be recommended for fracture prevention at the present time, according to the criteria of evidence-based medicine. Phase III therapeutic trials are under way to assess whether the annual administration of the bisphosphonate zoledronate reduces the incidence of osteoporotic fractures (Reid *et al.*, 2002).

More than 150 studies have addressed the issue of the effects of calcium on bone (Heaney, 2000). There are only 4 randomized controlled trials conducted in patients with osteoporosis with fracture as the outcome (Chapuy *et al.*, 1992; Chevalley *et al.*, 1994; Dawson-Hughes *et al.*, 1997; Recker *et al.*, 1996). The reduction in the risk of vertebral fracture seen with dietary calcium alone is based on a subgroup analysis of the patients with fracture at baseline and with a low dietary calcium ($<500\,\mathrm{mg\,day^{-1}}$) (Recker *et al.*, 1996). The risk of nonvertebral fracture is decreased by calcium and vitamin D supplements (Chapuy *et al.*, 1992; Dawson-Hughes *et al.*, 1997).

It is well established that sex hormone deficiency increases bone remodeling and leads to an accelerated bone loss. HRT corrects bone remodeling, prevents bone loss, and reduces fracture risk (Writing Group for the Women's Health Initiative Investigators, 2002). Two recently published meta-analyses have shown that HRT reduces vertebral and nonvertebral fractures by 33% and 27%, respectively (Torgerson and Bell-Syer, 2001a,b). However the risk/benefit ratio of such a treatment is the subject of strong debate (Petitti, 2002; Writing Group for the Women's Health Initiative Investigators, 2002).

The Selective Estrogen Receptor Modulators (SERMs) display agonistic properties in some tissues and antagonistic properties in others. For instance, raloxifene increases BMD and decreases vertebral fracture rate in patients with postmenopausal osteoporosis (Ettinger *et al.*, 1999). Nonvertebral fractures are not significantly influenced by this treatment. However, a *post-hoc* analysis suggests that raloxifene could also be efficacious on nonvertebral fractures in patients with severe vertebral deformities (Delmas *et al.*, 2003). One major benefit of raloxifene is undoubtedly the prevention of breast cancer.

Tibolone is transformed into various metabolites acting on either estrogen or on androgen receptors. Postmenopausal bone loss is prevented by tibolone. However, there are no available results on fracture rate at the present time.

Parathyroid hormone increases both bone formation and bone resorption. A chronic elevation of serum PTH levels is associated with a negative bone balance, with decreased BMD and increased fracture risk (Rubin *et al.*, 2002). Intermittent administration of PTH augments BMD, as well as bone strength in various animal models (Rubin *et al.*, 2002). In a large trial undertaken in patients with osteoporotic fracture, the daily injection of the aminoterminal fragment of PTH reduced the vertebral fracture incidence by 65% (Neer *et al.*, 2001).

Very recently, a "newcomer" appeared in the armentarium against osteoporosis. Strontium ranelate leads to a reduction in vertebral fracture rate (Meunier *et al.*, 2004). Hip fracture risk was decreased in patients older than 74 years and with osteoporosis. This agent appears to be well tolerated and efficacious on vertebral and nonvertebral fractures in patients older than 80 years.

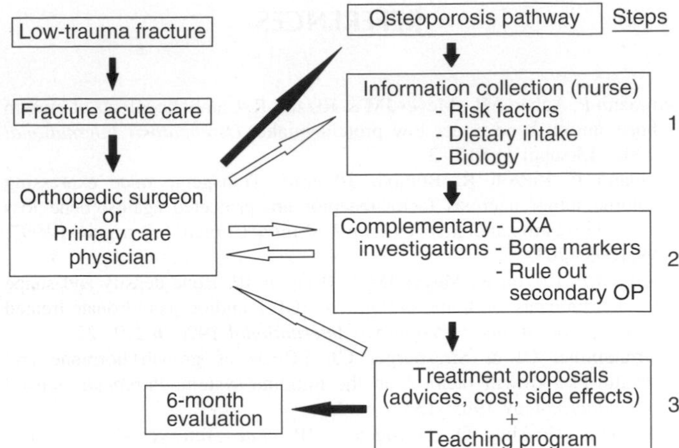

Figure 6 Course of an osteoporosis clinical pathway. The patients with a recent low-energy fracture enter this pathway in which clinical and biochemical data are completed. Then, a treatment is suggested to the medical team directly in charge of the patients. The latter is asked to attend a teaching program on osteoporosis. Filled arrows represent the patient's track after a low-trauma fracture. Open arrows represent a constant interaction between the physician in charge of the patient and the multidisciplinary team of the osteoporosis clinical pathway (Reproduced from Chevalley T *et al.*, An osteoporosis clinical pathway for the medical management of patients with low-trauma fracture, Osteoporosis International, 13, pp 450–455, Copyright 2002, with kind permission of Springer Science and Business Media)

PERSPECTIVES

The fundamental aim of the treatment of patients with osteoporosis is to rebuild bone to a normal quality and structure in order to restore a normal bone strength, reducing thereby the rate of low-trauma fracture to a level similar to that observed in young healthy people. Numerous agents are under development, such as anti-integrins, cathepsin K inhibitors, osteoprotegerin, statins, bone morphogenetic protein-like substances, or anabolic drugs. However, one of the main problems in the management of patients with osteoporosis is the identification of the patient who is at a high risk of fracture and likely to respond to the treatment. A patient with fracture has already a more than twofold risk of experiencing another one (Klotzbuecher *et al.*, 2000). This risk is as high as 20% within one year after a vertebral fracture (Lindsay *et al.*, 2001). A fracture thus constitutes the first priority to antiosteoporotic treatment. A medical pathway for the management of patients with osteoporosis provides an interaction between the medical team and the patients, as well as a teaching program on the disease (Chevalley *et al.*, 2002b) (Figure 6). It is never too late to take in charge and treat patients with osteoporosis.

Acknowledgment

The studies of our group quoted in this chapter were supported by the Swiss National Science Foundation (grants nos. 32–49757.96, 32–58880.99 and 3200B0-100714).

KEY POINTS

- Osteoporosis is a devastating disease for the elderly;
- Important signs like a history of low-trauma fracture are largely unrecognized;
- Patients at high risk can be detected, thanks to a pattern of various clinical risk factors;
- Nutritional aspects are highly important for the prevention of falls and osteoporosis;
- Treatment is rapidly efficacious in reducing fracture risk; thus it is never too late for treating a patient at high risk of fracture.

KEY REFERENCES

- Delmas PD, Eastell R, Garnero P *et al.*, Committee of Scientific Advisors of the International Osteoporosis Foundation. The use of biochemical markers of bone turnover in osteoporosis. *Osteoporosis International* 2000; **11**(suppl 6):S2–17.
- Hauselmann HJ & Rizzoli R. A comprehensive review of treatments for postmenopausal osteoporosis. *Osteoporosis International* 2003; **14**:2–12.
- Kanis JA, Borgstrom F, De Laet C *et al.* Assessment of fracture risk. *Osteoporosis International* 2005a; **16**:581–9.
- Rizzoli R & Bonjour JP. Dietary protein and bone health. *Journal of Bone and Mineral Research* 2004; **19**:527–31.
- Seeman E. Pathogenesis of bone fragility in women and men. *Lancet* 2002; **359**:1841–50.

REFERENCES

Ammann P, Aubert ML, Meyer JM & Rizzoli R. Catabolic effects of growth hormone on bone under low protein intake. *Osteoporosis International* 2002; **13**(suppl 1):S12–3.

Ammann P, Rizzoli R, Bonjour JP *et al.* Transgenic mice expressing soluble tumor necrosis factor-receptor are protected against bone loss caused by estrogen deficiency. *The Journal of Clinical Investigation* 1997; **99**:1699–703.

Ammann P, Rizzoli R, Meyer JM & Bonjour JP. Bone density and shape as determinants of bone strength in IGF-I and/or pamidronate-treated ovariectomized rats. *Osteoporosis International* 1996; **6**:219–27.

Auernhammer CJ & Strasburger CJ. Effects of growth hormone and insulin-like growth factor I on the immune system. *European Journal of Endocrinology* 1995; **133**:635–45.

Bone HG, Hosking D, Devogelaer JP *et al.* Ten years' experience with alendronate for osteoporosis in postmenopausal women. *The New England Journal of Medicine* 2004; **350**:1189–99.

Booth SL, Broe KE, Gagnon DR *et al.* Vitamin K intake and bone mineral density in women and men. *The American Journal of Clinical Nutrition* 2003; **77**:512–6.

Bourrin S, Ammann P, Bonjour JP & Rizzoli R. Dietary protein restriction lowers plasma insulin-like growth factor I (IGF-I), impairs cortical bone formation, and induces osteoblastic resistance to IGF-I in adult female rats. *Endocrinology* 2000; **141**:3149–55.

Center JR, Nguyen TV, Schneider D *et al.* Mortality after all major types of osteoporotic fracture in men and women: an observational study. *Lancet* 1999; **353**:878–82.

Chapuy MC, Arlot ME, Duboeuf F *et al.* Vitamin D3 and calcium to prevent hip fractures in the elderly women. *The New England Journal of Medicine* 1992; **327**:1637–42.

Chevalley T, Hermann FR, Delmi M *et al.* Evaluation of the age-adjusted incidence of hip fractures between urban and rural areas: the difference is not related to the prevalence of institutions for the elderly. *Osteoporosis International* 2002a; **13**:113–8.

Chevalley T, Hoffmeyer P, Bonjour JP & Rizzoli R. An osteoporosis clinical pathway for the medical management of patients with low-trauma fracture. *Osteoporosis International* 2002b; **13**:450–5.

Chevalley T, Rizzoli R, Nydegger V *et al.* Effects of calcium supplements on femoral bone mineral density and vertebral fracture rate in vitamin-D-replete elderly patients. *Osteoporosis International* 1994; **4**:245–52.

Cummings SR, Bates D & Black DM. Clinical use of bone densitometry. Scientific review. *The Journal of the American Medical Association* 2002; **288**:1889–97.

Cummings SR & Melton LJ. Epidemiology and outcomes of osteoporotic fractures. *Lancet* 2002; **359**:1761–7.

Dawson-Hughes B & Harris SS. Calcium intake influences the association of protein intake with rates of bone loss in elderly men and women. *The American Journal of Clinical Nutrition* 2002; **75**:773–9.

Dawson-Hughes B, Harris SS, Krall EA & Dallal GE. Effect of calcium and vitamin D supplementation on bone density in men and women 65 years of age or older. *The New England Journal of Medicine* 1997; **337**:670–6.

Delmas PD. Treatment of postmenopausal osteoporosis. *Lancet* 2002; **359**:2018–26.

Delmas PD, Eastell R, Garnero P *et al.*, Committee of Scientific Advisors of the International Osteoporosis Foundation. The use of biochemical markers of bone turnover in osteoporosis. *Osteoporosis International* 2000; **11**(suppl 6):S2–17.

Delmas PD, Genant HK, Crans GG *et al.* Severity of prevalent vertebral fractures and the risk of subsequent vertebral and nonvertebral fractures: results from the MORE trial. *Bone* 2003; **33**:522–32.

Delmi M, Rapin CH, Bengoa JM *et al.* Dietary supplementation in elderly patients with fractured neck of the femur. *Lancet* 1990; **335**:1013–6.

Ettinger B, Black DM, Mitlak BH *et al.* Reduction of vertebral fracture risk in postmenopausal women with osteoporosis treated with raloxifene: results from a 3-year randomized clinical trial. Multiple Outcomes of Raloxifene Evaluation (MORE) Investigators [see comments] [published erratum appears in JAMA 1999 Dec 8;282(22):2124]. *The Journal of the American Medical Association* 1999; **282**:637–45.

Gehlbach SH, Bigelow C, Heimisdottir M *et al.* Recognition of vertebral fracture in a clinical setting. *Osteoporosis International* 2000; **11**:577–82.

Geinoz G, Rapin CH, Rizzoli R *et al.* Relationship between bone mineral density and dietary intakes in the elderly. *Osteoporosis International* 1993; **3**:242–8.

Guyatt GA. Evidence-based management of patients with osteoporosis. *Journal of Clinical Densitometry* 1998; **1**:395–402.

Hannan MT, Tucker KL, Dawson-Hughes B *et al.* Effect of dietary protein on bone loss in elderly men and women: The Framingham Osteoporosis Study. *Journal of Bone and Mineral Research* 2000; **15**:2504–12.

Hauselmann HJ & Rizzoli R. A comprehensive review of treatments for postmenopausal osteoporosis. *Osteoporosis International* 2003; **14**:2–12.

Heaney RP. Calcium, dairy products and osteoporosis. *Journal of the American College of Nutrition* 2000; **19**:83S–99S.

Johnell O & Kanis J. Epidemiology of osteoporotic fractures. *Osteoporosis International* 2005; (suppl 2):S3–7.

Kanis JA. Diagnosis of osteoporosis and assessment of fracture risk. *Lancet* 2002; **359**:1929–36.

Kanis JA, Borgstrom F, De Laet C *et al.* Assessment of fracture risk. *Osteoporosis International* 2005a; **16**:581–9.

Kanis JA, Johnell O, Oden A *et al.* Smoking and fracture risk: a meta-analysis. *Osteoporosis International* 2005b; **16**:155–62.

Kannus P, Parkkari J, Niemi S *et al.* Prevention of hip fracture in elderly people with use of a hip protector. *The New England Journal of Medicine* 2000; **343**:1506–13.

Kelley GA, Kelley KS & Tran ZV. Exercise and bone mineral density in men: a meta-analysis. *Journal of Applied Physiology* 2000; **88**:1730–6.

Klotzbuecher CM, Ross PD, Landsman PB *et al.* Patients with prior fractures have an increased risk of future fractures: a summary of the literature and statistical synthesis. *Journal of Bone and Mineral Research* 2000; **15**:721–39.

Lindsay R, Silverman SL, Cooper C *et al.* Risk of new vertebral fracture in the year following a fracture. *The Journal of the American Medical Association* 2001; **285**:320–3.

Marshall D, Johnell O & Wedel H. Meta-analysis of how well measures of bone mineral density predict occurrence of osteoporotic fractures. *British Medical Journal* 1996; **312**:1254–9.

Mashiba T, Turner CH, Hirano T *et al.* Effects of suppressed bone turnover by bisphosphonates on microdamage accumulation and biomechanical properties in clinically relevant skeletal sites in beagles. *Bone* 2001; **28**:524–31.

Meunier PJ, Roux C, Seeman E *et al.* The effects of strontium ranelate on the risk of vertebral fracture in women with postmenopausal osteoporosis. *The New England Journal of Medicine* 2004; **350**:459–68.

Munger RG, Cerhan JR & Chiu BC. Prospective study of dietary protein intake and risk of hip fracture in postmenopausal women. *The American Journal of Clinical Nutrition* 1999; **69**:147–52.

Myers AH, Young Y & Langlois JA. Prevention of falls in the elderly. *Bone* 1996; **18**:87S–101S.

Neer RM, Arnaud CD, Zanchetta JR *et al.* Effect of parathyroid hormone (1–34) on fractures and bone mineral density in postmenopausal women with osteoporosis. *The New England Journal of Medicine* 2001; **344**:1434–41.

Nevitt MC, Thompson DE, Black DM *et al.*, Fracture Intervention Trial Research Group. Effect of alendronate on limited-activity days and bed-disability days caused by back pain in postmenopausal women with existing vertebral fractures. *Archives of Internal Medicine* 2000; **160**:77–85.

Pennisi P, Trombetti A & Rizzoli R. Glucocorticoid-induced osteoporosis and its treatment. *Clinical Orthopaedics and Related Research* 2006; (in press).

Petitti DB. Hormone replacement therapy for prevention: more evidence, more pessimism. *The Journal of the American Medical Association* 2002; **288**:99–101.

Recker RR, Hinders S, Davies KM *et al.* Correcting calcium nutritional deficiency prevents spine fractures in elderly women. *Journal of Bone and Mineral Research* 1996; **11**:1961–6.

Reid IR, Brown JP, Burckhardt P *et al.* Intravenous zoledronic acid in postmenopausal women with low bone mineral density. *The New England Journal of Medicine* 2002; **346**:653–61.

Reitsma PH, Bijvoet OL, Verlinden-Ooms H & van der Wee-Pals LJ. Kinetic studies of bone and mineral metabolism during treatment with (3-amino-1-hydroxypropylidene)-1,1-bisphosphonate (APD) in rats. *Calcified Tissue International* 1980; **32**:145–57.

Riggs BL, Khosla S & Melton LJ III. Sex steroids and the construction and conservation of the adult skeleton. *Endocrine Reviews* 2002; **23**:279–302.

Riggs BL & Parfitt AM. Drugs used to treat osteoporosis: the critical need for a uniform nomenclature based on their action on bone remodeling. *Journal of Bone and Mineral Research* 2005; **20**:177–84.

Rizzoli R. Long-term outcome of weekly bisphosphonates. *Clinical Orthopaedics and Related Research* 2006; (in press).

Rizzoli R, Ammann P, Chevalley T & Bonjour JP. Protein intake and bone disorders in the elderly. *Joint Bone Spine* 2001a; **68**:383–92.

Rizzoli R, Ammann P & Bourrin S. Protein intake and bone homeostasis. In P Burckhardt, B Dawson-Hughes & RP Heaney (eds) *Nutritional Aspects of Osteoporosis* 2001b, pp 219–35; Academic Press, San Diego.

Rizzoli R & Bonjour JP. Nutritional approaches to healing fractures in the elderly. In CJ Rosen, J Glowacki & JP Bilezikian (eds) *The Aging Skeleton* 1999, pp 399–409; Academic Press, San Diego.

Rizzoli R & Bonjour JP. Dietary protein and bone health. *Journal of Bone and Mineral Research* 2004; **19**:527–31.

Rizzoli R, Greenspan SL, Bone G III *et al.*, Two-year results of once-weekly administration of alendronate 70 mg for the treatment of postmenopausal osteoporosis. *Journal of Bone and Mineral Research*, 2002; **17**:1988–96.

Rodan G, Reszka A, Golub E & Rizzoli R. Bone safety of long-term bisphosphonate treatment. *Current Medical Research and Opinion* 2004; **20**:1291–300.

Rubin MR, Cosman F, Lindsay R & Bilezikian JP. The anabolic effects of parathyroid hormone. *Osteoporosis International* 2002; **13**:267–77.

Schurch MA, Rizzoli R, Mermillod B *et al.* A prospective study on socioeconomic aspects of fracture of the proximal femur. *Journal of Bone and Mineral Research* 1996; **11**:1935–42.

Schurch MA, Rizzoli R, Slosman D *et al.* Protein supplements increase serum insulin-like growth factor-I levels and attenuate proximal femur bone loss in patients with recent hip fracture. A randomized, double-blind, placebo-controlled trial. *Annals of Internal Medicine* 1998; **128**:801–9.

Seeman E. Pathogenesis of bone fragility in women and men. *Lancet* 2002; **359**:1841–50.

Tinetti ME. Clinical practice. Preventing falls in elderly persons. *The New England Journal of Medicine* 2003; **348**:42–9.

Tkatch L, Rapin CH, Rizzoli R *et al.* Benefits of oral protein supplementation in elderly patients with fracture of the proximal femur. *Journal of the American College of Nutrition* 1992; **11**:519–25.

Torgerson DJ & Bell-Syer SE. Hormone replacement therapy and prevention of nonvertebral fractures: a meta-analysis of randomized trials. *The Journal of the American Medical Association* 2001a; **285**:2891–7.

Torgerson DJ & Bell-Syer SE. Hormone replacement therapy and prevention of vertebral fractures: a meta-analysis of randomised trials. *BMC Musculoskeletal Disorders* 2001b; **2**:7.

Trombetti A, Herrmann F, Hoffmeyer P *et al.* Survival and potential years of life lost after hip fracture in men and age-matched women. *Osteoporosis International* 2002; **13**:731–7.

Weinstein RS, Chen JR, Powers CC *et al.* Promotion of osteoclast survival and antagonism of bisphosphonate-induced osteoclast apoptosis by glucocorticoids. *The Journal of Clinical Investigation* 2002; **109**:1041–8.

Wolff I, van Croonenborg JJ, Kemper HC *et al.* The effect of exercise training programs on bone mass: a meta-analysis of published controlled trials in pre- and postmenopausal women. *Osteoporosis International* 1999; **9**:1–12.

World Health Organization. *Prevention and Management of Osteoporosis. Report of a Scientific Group*, Technical Report Series, No 921, 2003, WHO.

Writing Group for the Women's Health Initiative Investigators. Risks and benefits of estrogen plus progestin in healthy postmenopausal women. *The Journal of the American Medical Association* 2002; **288**:321–33.

112

Gait, Balance, and Falls

Peter W. Overstall[1] ***and*** **Thorsten Nikolaus**[2]

[1] County Hospital, Hereford, UK, and [2] University of Ulm, Ulm, Germany

INTRODUCTION

Falls once thought to be an inevitable consequence of aging are now known to be the result of multiple pathological and social factors. A number of risk factors have been identified, notably muscle weakness, gait and balance abnormalities, and previous falls. The more risk factors a person has, the greater their likelihood of falling. Evidence-based guidelines for the prevention of falls have been jointly published by the American and British Geriatric Societies and the American Academy of Orthopedic Surgeons (AGS/BGS/AAOS Panel on Falls Prevention, 2002) and these emphasize the importance of assessment, identification of risk factors, and multifactorial interventions. However, less than half of the older fallers report any associated contact with the health services, and out of those who are seen by a health professional, only a tiny proportion are being prescribed treatment to prevent osteoporosis. This suggests that implementing an effective falls and bone health service will present a considerable challenge. In England a start has been made with the introduction of the National Service Framework for Older People, which requires the establishment of specialized falls services working in collaboration with local primary care and social services. The high cost of falls in terms of injury, loss of confidence and functional decline, and the effectiveness of interventions justify a widespread preventative strategy.

EPIDEMIOLOGY

About one-third of people over the age of 65 living in the community fall each year, and half of these fall repeatedly. Most studies report a higher rate in women and a rising incidence with increasing age. The incidence of falls among men living at home is 368/1000 person years (py) and in women is 611/1000 py. The incidence rate in institutions is much higher, with the falls experienced by men being 2021/1000 py and women 1423/1000 py. There is a decline in fall rate among the very elderly living in institutions, suggesting that these residents are very frail and probably chair- or bed-bound, thus reducing the opportunities for falling.

Falls at home most commonly occur in the day during periods of maximal activity, usually indoors or within the immediate environs of the house. Most falls occur when walking and result from slips and trips. Falls on stairs usually occur when descending and there are many more falls on straight single flights than on U-shaped two-flight stairs.

In institutions, falls are most common in the first week after admission and are usually associated with going to or from the toilet, although falls from a chair are also common. In hospital, risk factors for falls include gait instability, agitated confusion, urinary incontinence or frequency, falls history, and the prescription of sedative drugs (Oliver *et al*., 2004).

Serious injury following a fall is comparatively rare, with fractures occurring in about 5% of older people living at home. Accident and Emergency attendance rates following a fall per 10 000 population are 273 for those aged 60–64 years, rising to 945 in those aged 75 years and over. The percentage admitted to a hospital is 13% and 39% respectively. Recurrent fallers have a threefold increased risk of going in to institutional care compared with nonfallers.

BALANCE

Balance is a complex process that depends on the integration of vision, vestibular and peripheral sensation, central coordination, and the neuromuscular response – especially muscle strength and reaction times. When standing, any changes in orientation are perceived by proprioceptive and cutaneous sensors in the feet. Vision detects linear and angular motions of the visual field and the vestibular apparatus detects sway related linear and angular accelerations of the head. When the support surface is irregular or in motion vestibular inputs

Principles and Practice of Geriatric Medicine, 4th Edition. Edited by M.S. John Pathy, Alan J. Sinclair and John E. Morley.

become essential, but when the surface is fixed and level, sensory information from the feet is predominant. An age-related decline in function can be demonstrated in all parts of this system.

An individual maintains balance by keeping the vertical projection of the center of mass (COM) on the ground (often called *the center of gravity*) within specific boundaries known as *stability limits*. These are determined by the ability to control posture without altering the base of support. During normal quiet standing, the COM is kept within the support base provided by the feet. Maintenance of this upright position is associated with body sway mainly in the anterior/posterior (AP) direction and this sway can be measured in a variety of ways: typically, as displacements of the body at waist level or, using a force platform, as the excursions of the center of pressure. Both A/P sway velocity and the area are seen to increase in normal older subjects (i.e. those who report that their balance is normal and are functionally independent). This difference is more obvious if the difficulty of the test is increased by using a moving platform or when the eyes are closed. Indeed, many experiments have shown that loss of any sensory afferents (e.g. tilting the head to reduce vestibular inputs; standing on a compliant surface or in ice cold water to reduce somatosensory inputs) increases sway.

Increases in A/P sway has been correlated with spontaneous falls, but a better predictor of falls is mediolateral sway. Falls depend on the relationship between the COM and the base of support. In older people, postural reactions controlling the COM are slowed and there appears to be particular difficulty in controlling lateral instability. Moreover, unexpected perturbations require an adjustment of the base of support through compensatory stepping, and older fallers often have problems controlling these compensatory stepping movements. Lateral falls may increase the risk of hip fractures. Experiments with a movable platform that can produce multidirectional perturbations show that the young controls react with a rapid compensatory hinging at the hips and trunk, thus keeping their COM away from the direction of tilt. They also abduct their arms uphill when tilted sideways. In older subjects, compensatory trunk movements are reduced (probably due to stiffening) and their arms are stretched in the direction of the fall (Allum *et al.*, 2002).

Peripheral sensation (proprioception and touch) is the most important afferent in the control of standing balance in healthy older people. Other factors that are highly correlated with increased sway are reduced muscle strength in the legs, poor near visual acuity, and slowed reaction time. Vision can partially compensate for loss of other sensory inputs, and with increasing age as the postural task gets harder so the reliance on vision becomes greater. Thus, patients with proprioceptive or vestibular impairments are easily upset if the visual field is faulty or misleading in any way.

There is no doubt that some individuals maintain good postural control, even into extreme old age, indicating that age-related changes alone have only a minor effect and that imbalance is largely the result of pathology. Of major importance is the slowing of central coordination due to cerebrovascular or Alzheimer's disease. In its early stages, this is often unrecognized, and the diagnosis is not made until the patient is seen in a falls clinic. Minor and even major cognitive impairment is commonly uncovered for the first time among recurrent fallers. Balance depends on cognitive processes and attention, which may be affected by anxiety and depression as well as brain pathology. The ability to recover balance demands more attention even for healthy older people when compared with young adults. Older people appear less able to weigh and select appropriate responses quickly when the environment changes suddenly. Even a modest 10% increase in the mean response time can result in a five- to sixfold increase in the number of critically slow responses with an ensuing fall.

Doing two things at once ("dual tasking") becomes more difficult in old age and this was highlighted by a report from Scandinavia, which noted that institutionalized older people who were unable to keep up a conversation while walking had a high risk of falls ("stops walking when talking"). Subsequent investigations have shown that dual tasking impairs not only gait but also static and dynamic balance. A variety of cognitive and motor secondary tasks have been examined and all show similar adverse effects on gait and balance. The difficulties increase as the tasks become more complex, and both the young and the old tend to prioritize gait performance over the secondary cognitive task (Bloem *et al.*, 2001). Interestingly, patients with Parkinson's disease (PD) are less able to prioritize and try to perform all tasks simultaneously, regardless of complexity. As a result, their gait and balance performance is poor. Dual task impairment is not a good predictor of falls in a general older population or even in patients with PD. Among people over the age of 85 it predicts falls, but no better than a simple timed walking test. It is mainly a marker of falls in cognitively impaired individuals.

Fear of falling may adversely affect postural control by causing stiffening. This may be beneficial when standing still, but reduces flexibility and the ability to respond to perturbations.

GAIT

The same changes in physiological systems that impair balance also affect gait. Follow-up for 8–10 years of healthy people in their late eighth decade shows a decline in the Tinetti gait and balance scale test (maximum score, 28) of 0.5 units per year. Even relatively fit older people with a low fall risk adopt a more conservative gait pattern: they walk more slowly due to reduced step length, although cadence (steps per minute) remains unaltered, and stance time and double support time increase. These differences are more pronounced when walking on an irregular surface. This appears to be a compensatory strategy to ensure that the head and pelvis remain stable, so that the risk of falling is reduced (Menz *et al.*, 2003). The best single predictor of falling is stride-to-stride variability in velocity, but variability in step width also predicts falling.

An exaggeration of this compensatory strategy, the senile gait disorder, is characterized by caution, a wide base, shorter and more frequent steps, hesitation, and unstable turns. It occurs in nearly a quarter of older people, the incidence rising with increasing age, and is likely to be due to underlying neuro-degenerative syndromes and stroke. These patients have a twofold increased risk of cardiovascular death compared with age matched subjects with a normal gait. Although cerebrovascular disease is a major cause of gait abnormalities several other processes may contribute.

Cerebrovascular Disease

Cerebral MRI (magnetic resonance imaging) studies show an association between impaired gait and balance and an age-related decrease in white matter volume and increased white matter signal hyperintensities, which are not age related but correlate with vascular risk factors. These white matter lesions can be found, most commonly in the periventricular region, in 95% of a largely healthy older population with no history of stroke. The pathogenesis is unclear, but it has been suggested that the underlying mechanism is an impairment of cerebrospinal fluid dynamics caused by small vessel disease and it may be progressive. Subcortical/deep white matter lesions, periventricular lesions, and brain stem lesions are associated with poor balance. These lesions have a general deleterious effect on higher motor and cognitive functions since it has been found that mental ability is strongly related to gait speed and there appears to be a concordance between motor skills and intellect in old age (Starr *et al.*, 2003). The severity of the gait and balance disturbance is likely to depend on where the white matter lesions are situated and this is further discussed in the following text.

Apraxic Gait

This is defined as the loss of ability to use the lower limbs for walking in the absence of demonstrable sensory impairment or motor weakness. It is a feature of frontal lobe disease, but there have been criticisms of the use of the word apraxia to describe the gait abnormalities in these patients on the grounds that many of them have postural disturbances as the main feature and may walk normally with no other evidence of apraxia. Over the years many different names (senile gait disorder, marche à petits pas, vascular Parkinsonism, lower-half Parkinsonism etc.) have been given to the same pattern of gait abnormality resulting in much confusion. The most helpful classification is one that divides patients into whether they have a gait abnormality characterized by ignition failure, shuffling and freezing (ignition apraxia), or have poor balance and falls (equilibrium apraxia). A combination of the gait abnormality and poor balance is a mixed gait apraxia (Liston *et al.*, 2003).

The hypothesis behind this classification reflects current thinking on the role of the basal ganglia. Symptoms of PD such as start and turn hesitation and bradykinesia result from loss of internal cues from the basal ganglia to the supplementary motor area (SMA). However, the pathway linking the sensory cortex, the premotor area, and the motor cortex is intact and this allows PD patients to walk normally (at least for a short distance) in response to visual cues. In vascular Parkinsonism, the periventricular white matter lesions disrupt the pathway from the basal ganglia to the SMA and this produces the characteristic start and turn hesitation and wide-based gait. In fact, this hesitation (or freezing) is more common in vascular Parkinsonism than in idiopathic PD. However, some patients with vascular disease do not have problems with gait ignition or turn hesitation and instead suffer mainly from disequilibrium. It is suggested that these patients have white matter lesions affecting the sensory cortex, premotor area, and motor cortex pathway. Their ability to use visual, auditory, and proprioceptive information is impaired and their balance suffers. Their walking remains reasonably normal and they would not be expected to benefit from visual or environmental cues. Thus, with ignition apraxia the lesions are in the SMA, basal ganglia or its connections and patients are able to respond to visual cues. With equilibrium apraxia, the lesions are in the premotor area or its connections and there is no response to visual or auditory cues. With mixed gait apraxia, the lesions are in the premotor area or connections and the SMA, basal ganglia or connections.

Peripheral Mechanisms

The increased risk of falling in patients with peripheral neuropathy is well recognized. Annual fall rates are nearly 50% and the risk is highest in patients with a high body mass index and relatively severe neuropathy. Two-thirds of diabetics with prior foot ulcers report falls and although having insensate feet increases the risk, comorbid conditions also contribute. Most falls occur when walking, which suggests that these patients have difficulty maintaining dynamic balance. Relatively normal walking rhythms are maintained despite an increase in gait variability, and the increased risk of falling is due to an inability to respond appropriately when faced with an unexpected obstacle or perturbation. Patients compensate by reducing their walking speed.

Muscle strength is highly related to gait. The stronger the knee extension and flexion and ankle dorsiflexion are, the higher the walking speed and the longer the step. Muscle weakness is closely correlated with arthritis and results from reflex inhibition of anterior horn cells secondary to joint pathology. Disuse atrophy and lumbar nerve root lesions also contribute. Foot problems such as calluses, hallux valgus, and retracted toes may impair stability by reducing joint mobility and displacing the COM.

Cervical Myelopathy (*see* Chapter 85, Cervical and Lumbar Spinal Canal Stenosis)

This is a common cause of gait disorder in older people and is largely caused by degenerative changes in the cervical spine resulting from intervertebral disc decay. The first symptom is often weakness, with or without stiffness, in one leg alone. The weakness is distal and there is a tendency to drag the foot. Patients are aware that their balance is impaired and compensate by producing a protective gait pattern. Gait velocity, step length, and cadence are reduced, and step width is increased. Most patients complain of some neck stiffness and pain, although it is rarely severe. C5 and C6 nerve roots are most commonly involved and sensory symptoms and abnormal reflexes are often present in the upper limbs. In advanced cases, there is spasticity and hyper-reflexia in the legs with posterior column signs and a positive Romberg. Bladder problems consist of frequency and urgency. Urinary retention is rare.

Normal Pressure Hydrocephalus (*see* Chapter 68, Normal Pressure Hydrocephalus)

This produces the classical syndrome of dementia of insidious onset, unsteadiness of gait, and incontinence. Patients complain of a general slowing up and may describe feeling unsteady. Weakness and tiredness of the legs is commonly mentioned. Drop attacks may occur and there may be a number of vague complaints such as headaches, sleeplessness, and forgetfulness. Eventually a mixed gait apraxia develops (see preceding text) due, it is thought, to pressure on descending motor tracts as they pass close to the lateral ventricles before entering the internal capsule.

CLINICAL PRESENTATION

When people are asked why they fell, by far the commonest explanation is that they tripped or slipped. Other causes include a misplaced step, such as stepping into a hole, loss of balance, their legs giving way, or being knocked over. Many attribute their fall to hurrying too much or not looking where they were going. Although the patient's account of the circumstances of the fall is a vital part of the history, it is not a particularly helpful way of classifying falls and a more useful approach is to divide falls into intrinsic and extrinsic.

Intrinsic falls often leave the patient at a loss to explain why they fell. Remarks such as "it just happened", "down I went", or "I lost my balance" are often heard. Often they will say that they felt giddy at the time, but are usually describing a sense of unsteadiness and a fear of falling rather than true vertigo. Common causes of intrinsic falls are weakness of the leg muscles, gait and balance disorders, visual deficits, and cognitive and functional impairment. The relative risk posed by these various factors is shown in Table 1. There is likely to be synergism between multiple risk factors, since the more risk factors a person has the greater their likelihood of falling. Nearly 80% of community-living older people with four or more risk factors report falls. Urge incontinence (but not stress incontinence) carries an increased risk for women of both falls and fractures. Rushing to the toilet can be hazardous for frail-older people, and the fall may be the result of dual tasking (see preceding text) in someone with limited attentional resources who is so focused on avoiding wetting themselves that they fail to concentrate sufficiently on walking safely. An additional explanation is that falls and urinary incontinence both occur in functionally dependent patients who have multiple pathologies. They have the same predisposing risk factors and share a common multifactorial etiology.

Table 1 Results of univariate analysis of the most common risk factors for falls identified in 16 studies that examined risk factors

Risk factor	Mean Significant/Total[a]	RR-OR[b]	Range
Muscle weakness	10/11	4.4	1.5–10.3
History of falls	12/13	3.0	1.7–7.0
Gait deficit	10/12	2.9	1.3–5.6
Balance deficit	8/11	2.9	1.6–5.4
Use assistive device	8/8	2.6	1.2–4.6
Visual deficit	6/12	2.5	1.6–3.5
Arthritis	3/7	2.4	1.9–2.9
Impaired ADL	8/9	2.3	1.5–3.1
Depression	3/6	2.2	1.7–2.5
Cognitive impairment	4/11	1.8	1.0–2.3
Age > 80 years	5/8	1.7	1.1–2.5

[a]Number of studies with significant odds ratio or relative risk ratio in univariate analysis/total number of studies that included each factor. [b]Relative risk ratios (RR) calculated for prospective studies. Odds ratios (OR) calculated for retrospective studies (see AGS/BGS/AAOS Panel on Falls Prevention, 2002) (Reproduced by permission of Blackwell Publishing Ltd.)

Extrinsic falls are the result of drugs and environmental hazards. A number of hazards are recognized: trailing wires, loose mats, poor lighting, low toilet seat, lack of grab rails by the bath and toilet, shelves that are too high or too low, and stairs that are too steep, in need of repair or lack a handrail. Nearly all homes occupied by older people have at least two hazards, with the bathroom and stairs having the greatest potential for accidents. Sheltered housing designed for older people is less hazardous, but by no means as safe as one might assume. However, does any of this matter? Despite the home environment being blamed for up to a half of all falls, there is little evidence of a causal relationship between most potential hazards and falls, and no association with an increased risk of an injurious fall among most older people (Sattin *et al.*, 1998). Older, frailer people are more likely to have an intrinsic than an extrinsic fall and it is probable that people adapt to their hazardous homes. Indeed, what might appear to be a home alarmingly cluttered with furniture turns out to be a carefully placed series of handholds that aid mobility.

Drop Attacks

These were first described nearly 60 years ago as falls due to a sudden collapse or the legs giving way. There is no warning. One minute the patient is on her feet, the next she is on the ground without knowing why. Typically there is no loss of consciousness and patients often remark on their feeling of helplessness, almost paralysis, when lying on the floor, with immediate recovery once they are helped back onto their feet. However, after any type of fall about a half of older fallers, especially if they are also frail, are unable to get up without help. Women are affected more frequently than men and most studies note a rising incidence with increasing age: from, say, 2% in the 65–74 age-group to 15% in those aged over 75. Because there is no clear definition of a drop attack, the reported incidence varies widely and one study of nearly 600 falls did not recognize a single patient with classic drop attacks.

One of the early explanations of the attacks was that they were caused by brain stem ischemia, resulting in a temporary interruption of the cerebellar descending pathways, which control the efferents from cord to muscle, leading to loss of postural tone. From this developed the view that drop attacks were the result of vertebral artery compression by cervical osteophytes, particularly during rotation and extension of the neck. There are other explanations as to why falls may occur with head movements, and vertebro-basilar insufficiency should be regarded as a rare cause of drop attacks and then also only if accompanied by other symptoms such as vertigo, diplopia, bilateral simultaneous visual loss, weakness or sensory disturbance, and crossed sensory or motor loss. Many other causes have been described such as normal pressure hydrocephalus, frontal tumors, Meniere's disease, cervical cord compression due to a disc protrusion, and even overreliance on a faulty visual framework in someone with impaired postural feedback. In many patients, these are probably best regarded as a type of intrinsic fall where there may be a single explanation, but more often there are multiple postural defects.

However, in recent years, it has become clear that cardiac syncope must be considered in these patients, now that it has been shown that carotid sinus sensitivity is a common cause of unexplained falls, dizziness, and drop attacks.

Falls Associated with Loss of Consciousness

There are only two common causes: cardiac syncope and epilepsy. Hypoglycemia, usually due to long-acting hypoglycemic drugs, rarely leads to diagnostic difficulties. Transient ischemic attacks do not usually cause loss of consciousness and then only if there are accompanying focal neurological symptoms. The causes of cardiac syncope include orthostatic hypotension (OH), vasovagal syncope, carotid sinus sensitivity, arrhythmias, and aortic stenosis. Because patients are amnesic for the event, they may deny loss of consciousness.

Although OH affects 14% of the older population, it has not been found to be as good a predictor of falls as postural dizziness. This may be because the usual method of measuring lying and standing blood pressure in the clinic is too imprecise and underestimates the true prevalence of OH. However, using a tilt table with continuous blood pressure measurement, the finding of a large drop in systolic blood pressure and an unstable pressure in the three minutes after tilting predicts a twofold increased fall rate over the ensuing year (Heitterachi *et al.*, 2002).

Epilepsy is a frequent cause of "funny turns" although falls are uncommon. The type that causes diagnostic difficulty is complex partial seizures. Clues are the stereotyped symptoms and postictal drowsiness, although a reliable witness is invaluable (*see* **Chapter 76, Epilepsy**). Patients with apparent epilepsy who do not respond to treatment should undergo tilt table testing to exclude convulsive vasovagal syncope.

Vertigo and Dizziness

Dizziness is associated with impaired balance, functional decline, and falls. It is a complaint of 30% of the older people living in the community and it is often provoked by postural change and movements of the head and neck. Dizziness in most patients is multifactorial and 85% of chronically dizzy patients have more than one diagnosis: cerebrovascular and cardiovascular disease, cervical spondylosis, anxiety, and poor vision are some of the commonest. At 1-year follow-up there is an increased incidence of falls and syncope. Indeed, 46% of older people presenting in primary care with dizziness also have syncope and falls (Lawson *et al.*, 1999).

Dizziness or a sense of imbalance on head movement is most often due to cervical spondylosis. It results from an imbalance in the flow of stimuli from damaged mechanoreceptors in the cervical spine. However, it is important to consider the possibility of benign paroxysmal positional vertigo (BPPV) in patients complaining of vertigo provoked by head movements (typically, sitting up or rolling over in bed) since this is one of the few disorders of balance for which there is a simple, safe, and effective treatment (*see* **Chapter 106, Disorders of the Vestibular System**). BPPV is often unrecognized as yet, and has a prevalence of 9% in the older population. Eighty percent of older people presenting to an Accident and Emergency department with unexplained falls have symptoms of vestibular impairment (Pothula *et al.*, 2004).

Vision (*see* Chapter 103, Disorders of the Eye)

Vision is necessary for optimal balance. On its own, visual loss is not a particularly strong risk factor for falls, but when there are other postural defects, such as impaired lower limb proprioception, there is increased reliance on vision, especially depth perception and stereopsis (i.e. perception of spatial relationships). Regular users of multifocal glasses are at increased risk of tripping and have twice the fall rate of nonusers. The blurring of the lower visual field produced by multifocal glasses impairs contrast sensitivity and depth perception at critical distances, which is required for detecting obstacles when walking. Misleading information is even more disruptive than no vision at all. Visual loss (acuity 6/18 or worse) detected by standard tests of visual acuity is associated with falls and hip fracture, but simple acuity testing is not the best way of identifying an increased fall risk. The ability to accurately judge distances and detect hazards such as curbs and uneven pavements is critical, and the visual factors that are most strongly predictive of falls are impaired depth perception, contrast sensitivity, and low-contrast visual acuity (Lord and Dayhew, 2001). Fall rates are also increased in people with good vision in one eye but only poor or moderate vision in the other.

Drugs

Drugs are often implicated in causing falls, although the results from studies are inconsistent. The best evidence for an increased falls risk is for psychotropic drugs, particularly hypnotics and antidepressants, and withdrawing the medication reduces the risk of falling. None of the studies linking psychotropic drugs and falls has been a randomized controlled trial, and observational studies have fundamental weaknesses including the possibility that the underlying condition contributes to the risk of falling. Nonetheless, a critical meta-analysis showed that there is a small but consistent association between most classes of psychotropic drugs and falls. The odds ratio for one or more falls with any psychotropic drug use is 1.73 and fall risk is increased in those taking more than one psychotropic drug or having other fall risk factors (Leipzig *et al.*, 1999). There is also a weak association between falls and digoxin, type 1A antiarrhythmics (e.g. quinidine and disopyramide), and diuretics. There is an increased risk of recurrent falls in old people taking more than three or four drugs of any type.

Dementia

Patients with dementia have twice the annual incidence of falls compared with cognitively normal older people; their risk of fall-related injuries is high and they have a threefold increase in fractures. Patients are particularly vulnerable during dual tasking and even a simple additional task impairs postural control.

Parkinson's Disease (*see* Chapter 66, Parkinson's Disease and Parkinsonism in the Elderly)

Falls are not usually an early feature of PD, but eventually up to 90% of patients become fallers. The main determinant of falling is postural instability, particularly impairment in the response to perturbations. Although the increased stiffness of the PD patient improves standing balance, the loss of flexibility increases fall risk. The tendency to walk on the ball of the foot reduces stability, and the reduced height of the foot from the ground during the swing phase increases the risk of tripping. Freezing when turning causes the patient to often overbalance.

MAIN POINTS

- Falls occur in one-third of people over 65 years; rates rise with increasing age and are higher in women.
- Impaired peripheral sensation, reduced muscle strength in the legs, poor vision, and slowed reaction times are the key factors affecting balance.
- Unrecognized cerebrovascular disease is an important cause of gait and balance problems.
- Falls associated with loss of consciousness are most commonly due to cardiac syncope.
- The visual factors that best predict falls are impaired depth perception, contrast sensitivity, and low-contrast visual acuity.

CONSEQUENCES OF FALLS

Falls in older people are a leading cause of disability, distress, admission to supervised care, and death; it is these consequences that make falls important. Approximately one in ten falls results in a serious injury such as hip fracture, other fractures, subdural hematoma, other serious soft tissue injury, or head injury. Falls are responsible for approximately 10% of visits to the emergency department and 4–6% of urgent admissions among elderly persons. Other consequences are more subtle and less apparent although equally disabling. Fear of falling is a widespread problem for many elderly people and is as common as falls themselves. Although fallers are more likely to be frightened of further falls, up to a third of nonfallers limit their activity because of the fear of falling. The fear of going out can restrict people to their homes, decrease their social contacts, and lead to further functional decline. Falls or rather the consequences of falls are commonly cited as a reason for institutionalization. Restricted activities lead to a decline in the ability to carry out activities such as dressing, bathing, shopping, or housekeeping.

Death as a result of a fall seems to be relatively uncommon, but there is good evidence that deaths due to falls are probably underreported. Death certification is well known to be inaccurate and whether a person dies from pneumonia or hypothermia is often not recognized as a complication of a fall. In addition, old people dying from falls are less likely to have an autopsy than those dying from other accidents. In summary, death-rates from injuries due to falls in the elderly are likely to be substantially more than those suggested by death-certificate data.

Standardized comparisons of hip fracture incidence per total population in different European countries and in the United States show a typical picture of an exponential increase in fractures of the proximal femur, humerus and the pelvis with advancing age, which is much more marked in women than men. Fractures of the proximal femur are most frequent followed by proximal humerus and then pelvic-fractures. There is a different pattern for distal forearm-fracture (Colle's-fracture). The incidence in women begins to rise at an earlier age and levels-off in the sixties to seventies rather than continuing to increase as does the incidence of the other age-related fractures. A possible explanation is that distal forearm-fractures are a marker for the beginning of balance disturbance with aging, whereas the other fractures with increasing incidence rates in the very elderly are a result of ongoing deterioration of postural responses. These are associated with loss of the protective reaction of using the arms to break a fall and gait abnormalities with increased lateral instability.

Another consequence of falling is the "long lie", that is, remaining on the ground or floor for more than one hour. This consequence indicates frailty, illness, and social isolation, and is associated with increased mortality.

ASSESSMENT OF FALLERS

There are some falls that have a single cause, but the majority result from the interactions of two or more risk factors. The risk of falling consistently increases as the number of these risk factors increases. The risk of falling increases in a cohort of elderly persons living in the community, for example, from 8% among those with no risk factors to 78% among those with four or more risk factors. Many of these risk factors are interrelated as preliminary path analytical models have shown. A unidimensional classification of intrinsic versus extrinsic risk is an oversimplification. A better understanding of falls results from an appreciation of all the risk factors affecting a patient.

All risk factors are derived from the findings of population studies. In clinical practice, many medical conditions and disorders, in addition to those listed in Table 1, can play an important role in an individual's fall and may require investigation.

Although falls may result from various combinations of factors, a clinically sensible strategy can be extrapolated from the available clinical trial data augmented by observational data from well-designed studies.

The first and the most important step is to ask elderly patients on a regular basis about any falls or difficulties with balance and gait. If there is a positive answer, a more detailed assessment should be carried out. A multifactorial assessment must be the first step. It has been shown that assessments not linked to targeted interventions are ineffective in preventing falls. Thus, interventions must follow the identification of risk factors.

After history taking and asking about the circumstances of previous falls, a full general examination is required, with focus on the cardiovascular, neurological, and musculo-skeletal system. A neurological examination can reveal impaired proprioception, impaired cognition, and decreased muscle strength. A targeted musculo-skeletal examination should include an examination of the legs (joints and range of motion) and feet. Cardiovascular examination should include postural blood pressure and a more detailed investigation is required where syncope is suspected (see following text). A standard electrocardiogram may demonstrate arrhythmias as a possible explanation for falls and should be a routine part of the examination. The assessment of vision is also important and the examination should focus on visual acuity, depth perception and contrast sensitivity, as well as cataracts. The assessment is completed by a review of medication use with special emphasis on high-risk medications (e.g. benzodiazepines, hypnotics, neuroleptics, antidepressants, anticonvulsants and class 1a antiarrhythmics) and the overall number of medications. The assessment should be completed by a home-visit for home-hazard evaluation.

Inspection of gait and balance is essential. It is recommended that mobility and balance be assessed in a structured way. Persons reporting a single fall should be observed as they stand up from a chair without using their arms, walk a short distance and return (i.e. the "Timed up and go" test). Those demonstrating difficulty or unsteadiness need further assessment.

The often used 6-minute walk measures the walking distance (in meters) in 6 minutes at normal pace. In older people, the distance covered in the 6-minute walk depends on multiple physiological, psychological, and health factors and provides a measure of the overall mobility and physical functioning rather than a specific measure of cardiovascular fitness (Lord and Menz, 2002).

As shown in several studies, decreased lower limb muscle strength is associated with increased risk of falling. One recommended test is the sit to stand functional strength test, which is easy to administer and has been found to be a good predictor of falls. Another modification of this test is the five-chair-rise, where the patient is asked to sit in a chair and then stand up without using his arms for assistance five times.

Reaction time declines with increasing age and it has been shown that slow reaction time is associated with an increased risk of falls. Most tests of reaction time require specialized equipment and thus cannot be used in a broad range of settings.

One test to administer is the rod-catch-test. Patients while seated are asked to catch a wooden rod that is dropped vertically from just above the top of the hand. The point where the patient catches the rod is recorded as a method of simple reaction time.

TO ASSESS BALANCE

Numerous balance tests have been described in the literature. One recommended test is the sharpened Romberg Test, in which the subject stands with one foot in front of the other, referred to as *the tandem position*. However, a lot of older people are unable to perform the test. Thus, we use in our hospital the modified Romberg test with three standing positions and eyes open: both feet parallel for 10 seconds, feet in a tandem position with one foot half of the foot length in front of the other, and the tandem position with one foot in front of the other. The modified Romberg test is more sensitive and good at predicting falls. Another new measure of standing balance is a test developed by Lord. This test requires patients to stand in a near tandem position for 30 seconds with eyes closed and with the feet separated by 2.5 cm and the heel of the front foot 2.5 cm anterior to the toe of the back foot. An inability to hold the standing position without taking a protective step in the 30-second test-period indicates impaired balance.

Dynamic standing balance can be measured by the functional reach test, where the subject stands and stretches the arm forward against a fixed scale. This has been shown to correlate with other methods of balance and mobility and also has a relationship with the risk of falls and performance in activities of daily living (ADL). Various other methods of balance and gait have been developed for research, but most of them are complex and not appropriate for clinical situations.

TO EVALUATE GAIT

The modified "Get up and go Test" is recommended (refined as the "Timed up and go Test"). The test requires the subject to get up from a chair, walk a short distance, turn around and return to the chair, and sit down again. A more complex assessment test is the "performance-oriented mobility assessment (POMA)" developed by Tinneti for research purposes. The test provides more specific information about balance and gait abnormalities and has been shown to correlate with laboratory gait and balance measures and predict falls, death, and nursing home placement.

However, it is complex to administer and score, and difficult for frailer elderly subjects to perform.

DIZZINESS AND SYNCOPE

Fallers often complain of dizziness, but it is frequently unclear what is meant by dizziness. The term dizziness can include true vertigo, presyncope/syncope, unsteadiness, and some less-specific sensations. There are many problems because the loss of consciousness may not be recalled, and in the absence of a witness, important diagnostic features maybe overlooked. There is often an element of rationalization in the patient's explanation of their fall. Some elderly persons fall because of carotid sinus syncope; in these cases, an in-depth assessment is required. This will usually include tilt table testing with carotid sinus massage and possibly Holter monitoring if the episodes are very frequent, and electrophysiological studies if initial evaluation has shown a myocardial infarct or structural heart disease. Some falls that have a cardiovascular cause may be amenable to intervention strategies such as a medication change or cardiac pacing (*see* **Chapter 45, Arrhythmias in the Elderly**).

The role of these cardiac investigations and treatment is not yet clear. Preliminary studies suggested that patients with recurrent unexplained falls and a bradycardiac response to carotid sinus stimulation experience fewer falls after implantation of a permanent cardiac pacemaker. However, these results have not been confirmed, and pacemaker therapy cannot be recommended for unexplained falls at present.

FALLS CLINICS

Because of the growing evidence base relating to risk factors and intervention strategies, falls clinics are being established in several European countries and in the United States and Canada. Equipment and staff make an in-depth examination and assessment of fallers so that relevant physiological and pathological problems can be identified and appropriate interventions organized.

In such units, the diagnostic accuracy is considerably higher than in nonspecialized clinics. This is also true for the effects of the interventions.

REHABILITATION FOLLOWING FRACTURE

There is still a lack of evidence regarding how best to rehabilitate a faller. A part of the rehabilitation process is the prevention of future falls. The rehabilitation process per se has to address some very important points:

- fear of falling
- ability to get up after a fall
- behavioral changes (coping at home with declining functional abilities)

The rehabilitation program must be targeted on the problems of the individual faller. There may be a need for gait reeducation, particularly if the fall has resulted in a period of immobilization. Improving balance with graded balance exercises may be helpful. Another important issue is training and practice in getting up independently after a fall. If the faller can get up on his or her own after a fall in a relatively safe and supervised situation, this may help him or her to face a return home with more confidence. Exercise programs to increase muscle strength are an important part of the rehabilitation process. Teaching and education should accompany the process in order to initiate behavioral changes if decreasing functional capabilities have contributed to the fall. Education on the risk factors for falling and how to avoid them may increase confidence and reduce the fear of falling.

PREVENTION

The best evidence for the efficacy of interventions to prevent falling emerges from large well-conducted randomized controlled trials. It has been clearly demonstrated that the most consistently successful approach to prevention is multifactorial assessment followed by interventions targeting the identified risk factors (Tinetti, 2003). In a study of community-dwelling elderly people presenting to an accident and emergency department with a fall, an intervention with a detailed medical and occupational-therapy assessment and referral to relevant services when indicated resulted in a reduction in the rate of falls by 39% (Close *et al.*, 1999).

Pooled data of multidisciplinary, multifactorial intervention programs show a risk reduction of more than 25% for older people with a history of falling. Successful components of these interventions include review and possible reduction of medications, balance and gait training, muscle strengthening exercise, evaluation of postural blood pressure followed by strategies to reduce any falls in postural blood pressure, and targeted medical and cardiovascular assessments and treatments (Tinetti *et al.*, 1994; Fiatarone *et al.*, 1994; Hauer *et al.*, 2001). In these studies there are some shortcomings. Most studies evaluating the multifactorial interventions were conducted in community-settings, neglecting the high-risk population in the settings of long-term care, assisted living, and acute hospitals.

The individual elements of the interventions were described inconsistently and the relative efficacy of the different components is not always clear; taking these flaws into consideration some specific recommendations can be derived for multifactorial interventions. Among community-dwelling older persons, multifactorial interventions should include strength and balance training, home-hazard assessment and intervention, vision assessment and referral, review and modification of medication especially psychotropic medication, and treatment of cardiovascular disorders including cardiac arrhythmias.

In long-term care and assisted living settings, multifactorial interventions should include staff education programs, gait training and advice on the appropriate use of assistive devices, and review and modification of medications especially psychotropic medications. In a prospective, cluster-randomized study with 981 long-stay residents, a staff and resident education program on fall prevention, advice on environmental adaptations, progressive balance and resistance training, and hip protectors resulted in a 45% reduction rate of falls. The number of frequent fallers was reduced by 44% (Becker *et al.*, 2003).

Single intervention programs do not show such consistent results. Although exercise has many proven benefits, the evidence for the effectiveness of group exercise interventions remains limited (Lord *et al.*, 2003). Furthermore, the optimal type, duration, and intensity of exercise for falls prevention remain unclear. There is strong evidence that an individually tailored exercise program of progressive muscle strengthening, balance retraining, and a walking plan is effective in reducing falls. The program should be prescribed and monitored by a trained health-care professional. Tai-Chi has demonstrated effectiveness in reducing falls in one study (Wolf *et al.*, 1996), but before it can be recommended generally it requires further evaluation. In general, there is a dearth of studies involving men. In the long time care settings, there is no evidence of benefit for exercise alone.

Despite its face validity, modification of home hazards shows no clear effect in reducing falls. The results of studies published so far remain controversial. Modification of the home environment without the other components of multifactorial interventions showed no beneficial effect. However, two studies found that for a subgroup of older patients with recurrent falls, a facilitated home modification program after hospital discharge was effective in reducing falls. In one of these studies, (Nikolaus and Bach, 2003) a home intervention based on home visits to assess the home for environmental hazards, providing information about possible changes, facilitating any necessary modifications, and training in the use of technical and mobility aids showed a reduction in the rate of falls and the number of frequent fallers by more than 30% in the subgroup of subjects with a history of recurrent falls. It is hypothesized that the beneficial effect in the cited studies is caused not only by home modifications alone but also by behavioral changes.

The role of footwear in falls prevention remains unclear. There is some preliminary evidence derived from epidemiological studies for an association between footwear and falls. A clear causal relationship between wearing a particular style of shoe and falling cannot be established as there are clearly a multitude of other factors involved.

In a small randomized controlled intervention study with 26 subjects (median age 87 years), habitual shoes and two types of newly designed senior shoes differing in heel height were investigated with respect to static balance and gait. There was no difference found in static balance and gait with the habitual shoes when compared to either of the new footwear offered (Lindemann *et al.*, 2003).

Although behavioral and educational programs are often included in multifactorial interventions, cognitive and/or behavioral interventions alone do not show an effect in reducing the frequency of falls in elderly people.

MEDICATIONS

For all settings, there is a consistent association between the use of psychotropic medication and falls. Thus, it is astonishing that there has been only one placebo-controlled trial of medication withdrawal for fall prevention (Campbell *et al.*, 1999). The reduction of medication is a prominent component of many multifactorial studies in community-based and long-term care settings, and there should be a stronger evidence base to justify any recommendation to review medications or stop them as considered appropriate. The problem is that we do not know whether the risk of falls outweighs the benefits of psychotropic drugs. Shortly after the study by Campbell *et al.* was over, most patients had restarted the medications that had been withdrawn, indicating the dilemma faced by patients and their doctors. The association between taking four or more drugs and falls also needs closer examination in the light of modern recommendations for the prescriptions for ischemic heart disease, hypertension, and so on.

ASSISTIVE DEVICES

Several studies of multifactorial interventions have shown that assistive devices (e.g. bed alarms, canes, walkers, and hip protectors) are beneficial in reducing fall-related injuries although they do not appear to affect the risk of falling. On the basis of cluster-randomized trials, the use of hip protectors for prevention of hip fractures in high-risk individuals living in extended care settings can be supported. In a cluster-randomized controlled trial of 49 nursing homes with 942 participants, an intervention of a single education session by the nursing staff who educated residents and the provision of three hip protectors per resident resulted in a relative risk reduction of hip fractures by 43% (Meyer *et al.*, 2003). However, trials that have used individual patient randomization have produced no evidence to show that hip protectors are effective for older people living either in extended care settings or in their own home. Until further trials clarify the situation, the use of hip protectors should probably be restricted to carefully evaluated high-risk individuals.

Other potential interventions like bone-strengthening medications have proven effective in reducing fracture-rates. However, these agents do not reduce rates of falls *per se*. Whether vitamin D supplementation has a potential effect on muscle strength and can thus reduce the risk of falling remains to be clarified.

Visual acuity, reduced contrast sensitivity, decreased visual field, posterior subcapsular cataract, and nonmyotic glaucoma medication is clearly associated with an increased risk of falling. Multifocal glasses impair edge-contrast sensitivity and depth perception at critical distances for detecting obstacles in the environment and increase the risk of falling (Lord *et al.*, 2002). Despite this clear evidence of increased risk, there are no randomized control studies demonstrating that referral for correction of vision as a single intervention for community-dwelling older people is effective in reducing falls. However, it is a valuable component of multifactorial falls prevention programs.

Restraints have been traditionally used as a falls prevention approach. However, there is no evidence to support the use of restraints for the prevention of falls taking into account that they have major drawbacks and can contribute to serious injuries. Thus, restraint use should be strictly avoided.

AREAS OF FUTURE RESEARCH

It remains uncertain whether the interventions that are effective in reducing falls are equally effective in reducing fractures or other serious injuries. In Europe, a network of researchers plans to design and perform a study to answer this question. The first step of the Prevention of Falls Network Europe (ProFaNE) is to harmonize assessment tools and to standardize assessment, management, and intervention strategies considering the cultural differences and including the different clinical approaches across the European countries included in the study.

Additional information on the prevention of falls in hospital settings is necessary. So far, no randomized controlled trials exist.

The exercise programs found to be effective have been short term and usually lasting 1 year or less. Most of the improvements last only as long as physical exercises are carried out on a regular basis. Thus, it is important to design programs for enhancing long-term adherence. Furthermore, it is not clear as to what are the effective elements of the exercise programs, such as type, duration, intensity, and frequency.

There is some preliminary data suggesting that patients who have had recurrent unexplained falls and presenting with a carotid-sinus-syndrome may have fewer falls with cardiac pacing (Kenny *et al.*, 2001). These findings need to be confirmed in further clinical trials.

Another open field is how to best intervene in reducing medications. In the only placebo-controlled trial published so far, gradual withdrawal of psychotropic medication significantly reduced the risk of falling, but participants in this study were reluctant to comply permanently.

Other areas of uncertainty are how falls can be prevented in patients with cognitive impairments, whether treatment of visual problems alone will prevent falls, and for whom and when a home-hazard assessment should be carried out.

MAIN POINTS

1. As previous falls are one of the most important risk factors for future falls, all older persons should be asked at least once a year about falls.
2. Persons with previous falls and who are shown on physical examination to have gait and balance problems require a further assessment addressing all the major risk factors for falls.
3. Multifaceted interventions have shown benefits in reducing falls in older community-dwelling people.
4. Home assessment of older people at risk of falls without referral or direct intervention is not recommended. Home assessment has only shown benefit in a selected group of frail-older subjects with a history of recurrent falling.
5. Assessment of high-risk residents in nursing homes with relevant referral has demonstrated positive effects on fall rates.
6. Multifaceted interventions that include an exercise component are effective in preventing falls in institutionalized elderly people.
7. Hip protectors may be of benefit to high-risk individuals in preventing hip fractures, but their effectiveness remains controversial.
8. A pacemaker is not currently recommended for patients with unexplained falls and cardioinhibitory carotid sinus hypersensitivity.

KEY POINTS

- Falls occur in one-third of people over 65 years; rates rise with increasing age and are higher in women.
- Impaired peripheral sensation, reduced muscle strength in the legs, poor vision, and slowed reaction time are the key factors affecting balance.
- Since previous falls are one of the most important risk factors for future falls, all older persons should be asked at least once a year about falls.
- Persons with previous falls who are shown on physical examination to have gait and balance problems require a further assessment addressing all major risk factors for falls.
- Individualized multifaceted interventions that include strength and balance exercises have shown benefits in reducing falls in older community-dwelling people.

KEY REFERENCES

- AGS/BGS/AAOS Panel on Falls Prevention. Guideline for the prevention of falls in older persons. *Journal of the American Geriatrics Society* 2002; **49**:664–72.
- Becker C, Kron M, Lindemann U *et al.* Effectiveness of a multifaceted intervention on falls in nursing home residents. *Journal of the American Geriatrics Society* 2003; **51**:306–13.
- Campbell AJ, Robertson MC, Gardner MM *et al.* Psychotropic medication withdrawal and a home-based exercise program to prevent falls: a randomized, controlled trial. *Journal of the American Geriatrics Society* 1999; **47**:850–3.
- Close J, Ellis M, Hooper R *et al.* Prevention of Falls in the Elderly Trial (PROFET): a randomised controlled trial. *Lancet* 1999; **353**:93–7.
- Tinetti ME, Baker DI, McAvay G *et al.* A multifactorial intervention to reduce the risk of falling among elderly people living in the community. *The New England Journal of Medicine* 1994; **331**:821–7.

REFERENCES

AGS/BGS/AAOS Panel on Falls Prevention. Guideline for the prevention of falls in older persons. *Journal of the American Geriatrics Society* 2002; **49**:664–72.

Allum JH, Carpenter MG, Honegger F *et al.* Age-dependent variations in the directional sensitivity of balance corrections and compensatory arm movements in man. *The Journal of Physiology* 2002; **542**(Pt 2):643–63.

Becker C, Kron M, Lindemann U *et al.* Effectiveness of a multifaceted intervention on falls in nursing home residents. *Journal of the American Geriatrics Society* 2003; **51**:306–13.

Bloem BR, Valkenburg VV, Slabbekoorn M & Willemsen MD. The multiple tasks test: development and normal strategies. *Gait & Posture* 2001; **14**(3):191–202.

Campbell AJ, Robertson MC, Gardner MM *et al.* Psychotropic medication withdrawal and a home-based exercise program to prevent falls: a randomized, controlled trial. *Journal of the American Geriatrics Society* 1999; **47**:850–3.

Close J, Ellis M, Hooper R *et al.* Prevention of Falls in the Elderly Trial (PROFET): a randomised controlled trial. *Lancet* 1999; **353**:93–7.

Fiatarone MA, O'Neill EF, Ryan ND *et al.* Exercise training and nutritional supplementation for physical frailty in very elderly people. *The New England Journal of Medicine* 1994; **330**:1769–75.

Hauer K, Rost B, Rütschle K *et al.* Exercise training for rehabilitation and secondary prevention of falls in geriatric patients with a history of injurious falls. *Journal of the American Geriatrics Society* 2001; **49**:10–20.

Heitterachi E, Lord SR, Meyerkort P *et al.* Blood pressure changes on upright tilting predict falls in older people. *Age and Ageing* 2002; **31**(3):181–6.

Kenny RA, Richardson DA, Stehen N *et al.* Carotid sinus syndrome: a modifiable risk factor for nonaccidential falls in older adults (SAFE PACE). *Journal of the American College of Cardiology* 2001; **38**:1491–6.

Lawson J, Fitzgerald J, Birchall J *et al.* Diagnosis of geriatric patients with severe dizziness. *Journal of the American Geriatrics Society* 1999; **47**(1):12–7.

Leipzig RM, Cumming RG & Tinetti ME. Drugs and falls in older people: a systematic review and meta-analysis: I. Psychotropic drugs. *Journal of the American Geriatrics Society* 1999; **47**(1):30–9.

Lindemann U, Scheible S, Sturm E *et al.* Elevated heels and adaption to new shoes in frail elderly women. *Zeitschrift Fur Gerontologie Und Geriatrie* 2003; **36**:29–34.

Liston R, Mickelborough J, Bene J & Tallis R. A new classification of higher level gait disorders in patients with cerebral multi-infarct states. *Age and Ageing* 2003; **32**(3):252–8.

Lord SR, Castell S, Corcoran J *et al.* The effect of group exercise on physical functioning and falls in frail older people living in retirement villages: a randomized controlled trial. *Journal of the American Geriatrics Society* 2003; **51**:1685–92.

Lord SR & Dayhew J. Visual risk factors for falls in older people. *Journal of the American Geriatrics Society* 2001; **49**(5):508–15.

Lord SR, Dayhew J & Howland A. Multifocal glasses impair edge-contrast sensitivity and depth perception and increase the risk of falls in older people. *Journal of the American Geriatrics Society* 2002; **50**:1760–6.

Lord SR & Menz HB. Physiologic, psychologic, and health predictors of 6-minute walking performance in older people. *Archives of Physical Medicine and Rehabilitation* 2002; **83**:907–11.

Menz HB, Lord SR & Fitzpatrick RC. Age-related differences in walking stability. *Age and Ageing* 2003; **32**(2):137–42.

Meyer G, Warnke A, Bender R & Muhlhauser I. Effect on hip fractures of increased use of hip protectors in nursing homes: cluster randomised controlled trial. *British Medical Journal* 2003; **326**:76.

Nikolaus T & Bach M. Preventing falls in community-dwelling frail older people using a Home Intervention Team (HIT): results from the randomized Falls-HIT trial. *Journal of the American Geriatrics Society* 2003; **51**:300–5.

Oliver D, Daly F, Martin FC & McMurdo ME. Risk factors and risk assessment tools for falls in hospital in-patients: a systematic review. *Age and Ageing* 2004; **33**(2):122–30.

Pothula VB, Chew F, Lesser TH & Sharma AK. Falls and vestibular impairment. *Clinical Otolaryngology* 2004; **29**(2):179–82.

Sattin RW, Rodriguez JG, DeVito CA & Wingo PA, Study to Assess Falls Among the Elderly (SAFE) Group. Home environmental hazards and the risk of fall injury events among community-dwelling older persons. *Journal of the American Geriatrics Society* 1998; **46**(6):669–76.

Starr JM, Leaper SA, Murray AD *et al.* Brain white matter lesions detected by magnetic resonance [correction of resonance] imaging are associated with balance and gait speed. *Journal of Neurology, Neurosurgery, and Psychiatry* 2003; **74**(1):94–8.

Tinetti ME. Preventing falls in elderly persons. *The New England Journal of Medicine* 2003; **348**:42–9.

Tinetti ME, Baker DI, McAvay G *et al.* A multifactorial intervention to reduce the risk of falling among elderly people living in the community. *The New England Journal of Medicine* 1994; **331**:821–7.

Wolf SL, Barnhart HX, Kutner NG *et al.* Reducing frailty and falls in older person: an investigation of Tai Chi and computerized balance training. *Journal of the American Geriatrics Society* 1996; **44**:489–97.

113

Foot Problems in the Elderly

Arthur E. Helfand[1] ***and*** **Donald F. Jessett**[2]

[1] *Temple University, Philadelphia, PA, USA, and Thomas Jefferson University, Philadelphia, PA, USA, and*
[2] *Formerly of University of Wales Institute, Cardiff, UK*

INTRODUCTION

The human foot is unique. It has been evolved to serve as an interface between man and whatever territory he or she most commonly traverses. As a consequence, feet will demonstrate a wide range of adaptations to use. Those whose footwear is minimal because of climatic conditions or the nature of territory require little or no covering; have feet that are different than city dwellers. Within these groups, there will be considerable variation, which also relates to the needs of society and custom. In all cases though, the feet share certain common features that are of significance to the clinician (Helfand and Jessett, 1998; Jessett and Helfand, 1991).

Feet are required to withstand stress imposed by activities and occupations, which are extremely variable. The forces of pressure, the adaptations required for ambulation, prior care, and the effects of disease and aging, present different problems in the elderly, which makes comprehensive podogeriatric assessment an essential in patient evaluation (Helfand, 1981, 1987, 1993a).

At one extreme may be the long periods of limited movement experienced by those who work on a production line or operate machinery, which presents a particular occupational risk. At the other end of the scale may be those occupations, activities and/or interests involving great variability of movement, such as ballet dancing, delivery men, sports related activities, and weight/stress related involvements. All these leave their mark upon the foot in the form of a wide range of morbidities, which usually manifest in later life and produce residual disability in the elderly. Some may produce discomfort or temporary disability. Others will produce insidious but cumulative effects that cause pain, ambulatory dysfunction, and limit activities (Helfand, 1993b).

As age increases, problems that may have been tolerated in earlier years will limit the mobility of the individual and decrease the quality of life. One also needs to remember that the focus in the management of the older patient many times, turns from cure to comfort and providing a means to maintain ambulation in order to retain one's independence and dignity (Helfand, 2002).

To all of these functional adaptations to life must be added the consequences of age and disease, such as bone and joint diseases, arthropathies, neuropathies, and also atrophy of soft tissue and integument. These invariably occur to a greater or lesser degree in every individual as age advances. All of these conditions, collectively, serve to diminish activity and increase the need for the regular assessment and examination of the feet and related structures, followed by appropriate care, management, surveillance, health education, and preventive strategies.

The foot is that part of the human body at the greatest extremity of circulatory and neurologic systems. In addition, the ambient temperature of the feet is lower than that of most other parts of the body (Helfand and Motter, 2004).

The feet are covered with hosiery and then thrust into coverings that hide them from view for long periods of time. Footwear, either hosiery or shoes, does not always compliment the size and/or shape or function of the foot. Extremes in width, length, or depth of the foot will complicate shoe fitting, even with a relatively wide range of mass-produced footwear. This potential incompatibility between anatomy and coverings potentiates problems, which become more evident and pronounced in later life. Congenital and/or acquired disease processes may deform feet in a variety of ways which will result in difficulties throughout life and require proper care over long periods of time to manage these chronic diseases and impairments. The primary treatment goals include the relief of pain, restoring the individual to a level of maximum function, and maintaining that function once achieved.

Fashion in footwear cannot be disregarded. When style predominates over fit and function, foot problems are again initiated and/or exacerbated due to this functional incompatibility, that is many times, with a foot to shoe last (model, design, or shape) incompatibility.

It also should to be noted that foot problems and their management are not regarded as a part of many general health

Principles and Practice of Geriatric Medicine, 4th Edition. Edited by M.S. John Pathy, Alan J. Sinclair and John E. Morley.

programs or even being related to general health. It is significant but regrettable, that many believe that feet are part of the body that are designed to hurt. This is true for patients, other elements of the health-care systems, and in the field of occupational health. A majority of patients expect to be able to pursue their normal activities and occupations despite the presence of foot conditions that require rest, but not necessarily hospitalization. With advancing age and the changes in older adult lifestyle, these concerns magnify and may be the difference between living life with some quality and sedentary institutionalization. In addition, because of age-related changes and disease, patients are frequently unable to reach their feet because of arthritis, failing eyesight, obesity, postural hypotension, or some other related disorder. Continuing assessment, evaluation, and appropriate care is most essential for the "at-risk" older patients. Tables 1 and 2 identify some of the primary risks associated with the development of foot problems in the older population (Brodie, 2001).

DISORDERS WITH PEDAL MANIFESTATIONS

The primary risk diseases that present with significant pedal manifestations as identified by Medicare are summarized in, but not limited to, Table 3 as follows:

Table 1 Generalized risks (Collet, 2000; Crausman and Glod, 2004)

The process of aging
History of diabetes
Poor glucose control
History of prior amputation
Impaired vision
Inability to bend
Patients who live alone
Tobacco use (smoking)
Dementia and Alzheimer's disease
History of alcohol use
Risk taking behavior
Obesity
Sensory loss, loss of protective sensation, and neuropathy
Altered biomechanics and pathomechanics
Structural abnormalities including:
Limited joint mobility
Hallux Valgus
Digiti flexi (hammertoes)
Prominent metatarsal heads and prolapse (declination)
Altered Gait, Ambulatory Dysfunction, and Fall Risk
Abnormal or excessive foot pressure
Soft tissue and plantar fat pad atrophy
Subkeratotic and/or subungual hematoma
History of previous foot ulcers
Peripheral arterial and venous disease
Toenail pathology
Xerosis and fissures
Other related chronic diseases and complications
Cardiovascular disease
Renal disease
Retinal disease
Osteoarthritis
Rheumatoid arthritis
Gout

Table 2 Other related risks

The Degree of ambulation
The duration of prior hospitalization
Limitation of activity
Prior institutionalization
Episodes of social segregation
Prior care
Emotional adjustments to disease and life in general
Multiple medications and drug interactions
Complications and residuals associated with risk diseases

Table 3 Primary risk diseases

ALS
Arteriosclerosis obliterans (A.S.O., arteriosclerosis of the extremities, occlusive peripheral arteriosclerosis)
Arteritis of the feet
Buerger's disease (thromboangiitis obliterans)
Chronic indurated cellulitis
*Chronic thrombophlebitis
Chronic venous insufficiency
*Diabetes mellitus
Intractable edema – secondary to a specific disease (e.g. CHF, kidney disease, hypothyroidism)
Lymphedema – secondary to a specific disease (e.g. Milroy's disease, malignancy)
Peripheral neuropathies involving the feet
*Associated with malnutrition and vitamin deficiency
Malnutrition (general, pellagra)
Alcoholism
Malabsorption (celiac disease, tropical sprue)
Pernicious anemia
*Associated with carcinoma
*Associated with diabetes mellitus
*Associated with drugs and toxins
*Associated with multiple sclerosis
*Associated with uremia (chronic renal disease)
Associated with traumatic injury
Associated with leprosy or neurosyphilis
Associated with hereditary disorders
Hereditary sensory radically neuropathy
Angiokeratoma corporis diffusum (Fabry's)
Amyloid neuropathy
Peripheral vascular disease (Arterial and Venous)
Raynaud's disease

Note: ALS, Amyotrophic lateral sclerosis.
Those conditions marked with an asterisk (*), require medical evaluation and care within 6 months of their primary foot care service.

A secondary list of systemic "at-risk" conditions are summarized but not limited to, in Table 4, as follows:

There are also specialized risks identified in, but not limited to, Table 5.

The joint diseases such as, the arthroses, gout, rheumatoid arthritis, and osteoarthritis frequently manifest in the feet. Their primary clinical findings are noted but not limited to those listed in Table 6 (gout), Table 7 (rheumatoid arthritis) Figure 1, Table 8 (osteoarthritis or degenerative joint disease), and Figure 2.

In the older patient, the consequences of these diseases usually result in deformity, swollen joints, impaired foot function, and an altered and potentially podalgic gait. In many cases, the foot may be the primary site of deformity, disability, and limitation of activity. Each tends to

Table 4 Secondary risk conditions

Collagen vascular disease
Malignancy
Lymphedema
Postphlebitic syndrome
Venous (peripheral) insufficiency
Acromegaly
Cerebral palsy
Coagulopathies
Poststroke
Sarcoidosis
Sickle-cell Anemia
Reflex sympathetic dystrophy
Chronic obstructive pulmonary disease
Hypertension
Mental illness
Mental retardation
Hemophilia
Patients on anticoagulant therapy
Paralysis
Ambulatory dysfunction
Parkinson's disease
Immunosuppressed states (HIV, AIDS)

Table 5 Specialized risks

Vascular grafts
Joint implants
Heart valve replacement
Active chemotherapy
Renal failure – dialysis
Anticoagulant therapy
Hemorrhagic disease
Chronic steroid therapy

Table 6 Gout

Acute
Inflammation
Painful
Swelling
Redness
High uric acid levels
Podalgia
Limitation of motion
Ambulatory dysfunction
Chronic tophaceous gout
Deformity
Pain
Stiffness
Soft tissue tophi
Atrophy of soft tissue
Loss of bone substance
Gouty arthritis
Joint deformity
Excessive pain associated with the acute episodes and exacerbations

produce deformities that make weight bearing difficult and cause significant problems in obtaining adequate footwear to compensate for the residuals of these diseases (Robbins, 1994).

Variable and wide-ranging effects accompany endocrinopathies, such as diabetes mellitus, in the cardiovascular and

Table 7 Rheumatoid arthritis

Hallux limitus
Hallux rigidus
Hallux valgus
Hallux abducto valgus
Cystic erosion
Sesamoid erosion
Sesamoid displacement
Metatarsophalangeal subluxation
Metatarsophalangeal dislocation
Interphalangeal subluxation
Interphalangeal dislocation
Digiti flexi (hammertoes)
Ankylosis (fused joints)
Phalangeal reabsorption
Talonavicular arthritis
Extensor tenosynovitis
Rheumatoid nodules
Bowstring extensor tendons
Tendon displacement
Ganglions
Rigid pronation
Subcalcaneal bursitis
Retrocalcaneal bursitis
Retroachillal bursitis
Calcaneal ossifying enthesopathy (spur)
Prolapsed metatarsal heads
Atrophy of the plantar fat pad
Soft tissue displacement
Digiti quinti varus
Tailor's bunion
Early morning stiffness
Pain
Fibrosis
Spurs
Periostitis
Bursitis
Plantar fasciitis
Nodules
Contracture
Deformity
Impairment of function
Loss or reduction of normal ambulation

neurologic systems. Many of the symptoms and complications associated with the disease are manifested in the feet and produce potential and serious complications in the older patient. The changes involving the foot are the cause for a significant number of potentially life threatening hospitalizations. In addition, it has been estimated in the United Kingdom and United States, that 50–75% of all amputations relating to the complications associated with diabetes mellitus could be prevented and reduced with an appropriate program of preventive foot care and foot health education.

The most common clinical findings relating to the diabetic foot are listed but not limited to those in Figure 3 and Table 9.

To these problems one must add the effects of repeated microtrauma from footwear, environmental surfaces, lifestyle, neglect, and heat-reflecting surfaces, which produce hyperkeratosis and subcallosal hemorrhage, a predisposing factor for ulceration. Diabetic foot problems in the elderly are characterized by paresthesias, sensory impairment, motor weakness, reflex loss, neurotrophic arthropathy, absence of

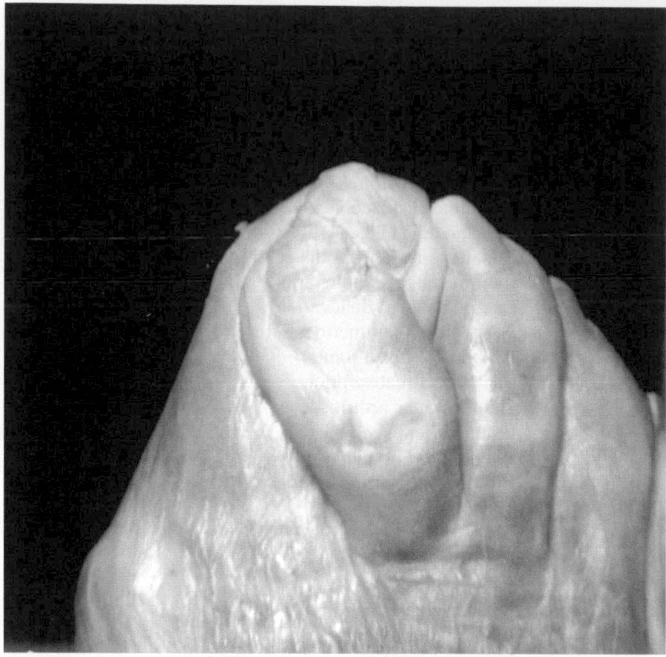

Figure 1 Overriding second toe, hallux valgus, pressure ulcer second toe, interphalangeal joint, onychodystrophy, and arterial insufficiency

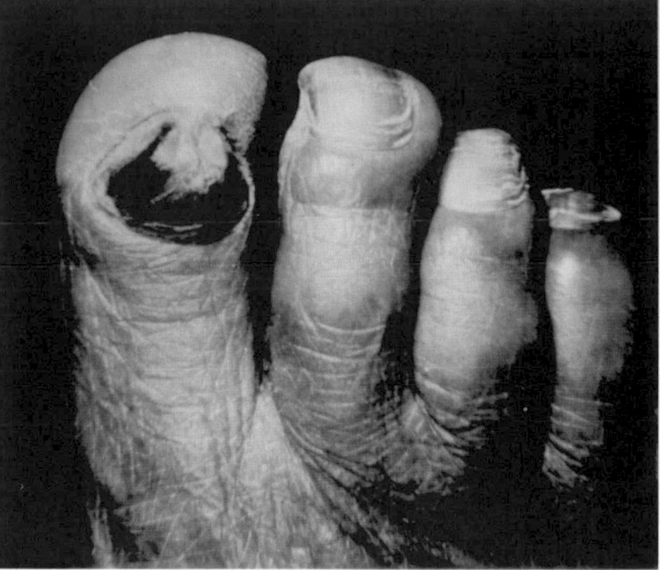

Figure 2 Multiple hammertoes, subungual hematoma, onychodysplasia (marked involution of hallux toe nail) xerosis, and onychauxis with onychomycosis

Table 8 Degenerative joint diseases – osteoarthritis

Pain related to minimal trauma
Inflammation
Strain
Plantar fasciitis
Spur formation
Periostitis
Myofascitis
Decalcification
Stress fractures
Tendonitis
Tenosynovitis
Residual deformities
Pes planus
Pes cavus
Hallux valgus
Digiti flexus (hammertoes)
Rotational digital deformities
Joint swelling
Increase pain
Limitation of motion
Reduced ambulatory status

pedal pulses, atrophy, infection, dermopathy, angiopathy, neuropathy, ulceration, and necrosis/gangrene.

Clinically, the most marked change perhaps for the elderly diabetic is sensory neuropathy. Where it is combined with poor eyesight, the elderly can be completely unaware of their feet. As Bloom has written, the elderly diabetic may be "divorced from his feet since he can neither see them or feel them properly". Paralysis of muscles due to motor neuropathy will result in deformities of the toes, claw toes. The bony prominences thus formed on the dorsum of the toes and the plantar aspect of the metatarsophalangeal joints may be the site of skin lesions, such as hyperkeratosis (tyloma and/or heloma, i.e. corns and calluses) and/or the sites of ulceration, due to pressure, residual subkeratotic hemorrhage, and local tissue ischemia.

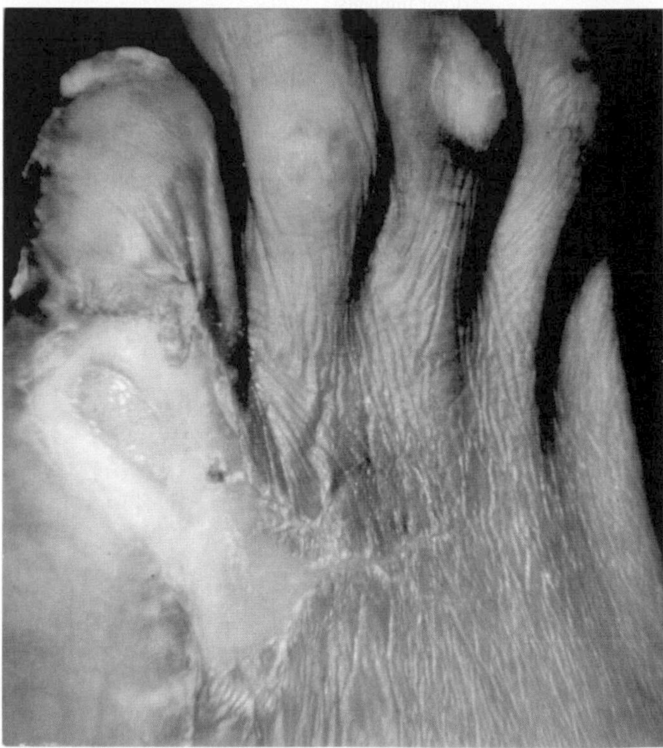

Figure 3 Diabetic ulcer, arteriosclerotic changes, multiple hammertoes, bow string tendons, heloma, and soft tissue atrophy

Table 9 Diabetic foot changes (ACFAS, 2000; ADA, 2003)

Vascular impairment
Degenerative changes related to aging
Neuropathy
Dermopathy
Atrophy
Deformity
Insensitivity
Pain
Fatigue
Paresthesia
Sensory impairment to pain and temperature
Motor weakness
Diminished or lost Achilles and patellar reflexes
Decreased or vibratory sense (pallesthesia)
Loss of proprioception
Neuropathy
Loss of protective sensation
Blebs
Excoriation
Hair loss
Xerosis
Anhidrosis
Neurotrophic arthropathy
Neurotrophic ulcers
Disparity in foot size and shape
Higher prevalence of infection
Necrosis
Gangrene
Pallor
Absence or decrease in posterior tibial and dorsalis pedis pulses
Dependent rubor
Decreased venous filling time
Coolness of the skin
Trophic changes
Numbness
Tingling
Claudication
Pigmentation
Cramps
Pain
Loss of the plantar metatarsal fat pad
Hyperkeratotic lesions
Tendon contractures
Claw toes (hammertoes)
Ulceration
Foot drop
Diabetic dermopathy (pretibial lesions – shin spots)
Necrobiosis
Arthropathy
Deformity
Radiographic
Thin trabecular patterns
Decalcification
Joint position change
Osteophytic formation
Osteolysis
Deformities
Osteopenia
Osteoporosis
Pruritus
Cutaneous infections
Dehydration
Trophic changes
Fissures
Onychial changes
Onychodystrophy
Diabetic onychopathy (nutritional and vascular changes)
Onychorrhexis (longitudinal striations)
Subungual hemorrhage (bleeding in the nail bed)
Onychophosis (keratosis)
Onychauxis (thickening with hypertrophy)
Onychogryphosis (thickening with gross deformity)
Onychia
Paronychia
Onychomycosis (fungal infection)
Subungual ulceration (ulceration in the nail bed)
Deformity
Hypertrophy
Incurvation or involution (onychodysplasia)
Splinter hemorrhage (nontraumatic)
Onycholysis (freeing from the distal segment)
Onychomadesis (freeing from the proximal segment)
Autoavulsion

The plantar surface of the foot has been the most common site for the development of diabetic ulceration, which is trophic in character. These ulcers develop underneath keratosis with pressure and thus the skilled and proper débridement of the keratosis is a prerequisite to the successful management of the diabetic ulcer and in the prevention of ulcer development. Appropriate weight diffusion and dispersion procedures are also essential elements to management, particularly in the elderly.

Skin texture and sweating patterns are also markedly altered in the elderly diabetic, due to autonomic neuropathy. It is probably also implicated as an additional and local factor in edema. The consequent enlargement of the foot is another cause of epidermal abrasions of the skin from footwear and other forms of trauma and pressure. In addition, with infection, management of infection becomes complicated unless appropriate metabolic management is instituted and maintained early in the disease process. The resulting sepsis can lead to necrosis, gangrene, and amputation of the limb, which additionally complicates the management of the disease in the elderly as well as necessitating changes in the patient's lifestyle (Alexander, 1997).

Varicose veins are a common manifestation in the legs and feet of the elderly. Varices may be observed on the dorsum of the foot sometimes extending as far as the toes, and also along the medial plantar arch area. Hemosiderin deposited in the skin over the lower one-third of the leg and the foot, giving them a freckled appearance and sometimes imparting a coppery hue where the change becomes marked. Edema of the foot and ankle also are a frequent accompaniment of varicose veins. Accidental damage to these vessels can produce hemorrhage. The diminished blood flow resulting from the presence of varicose veins impairs wound healing and causes trophic changes in the skin and nails. Adhesive dressings, even though they may be hypoallergenic, are not well tolerated by such skin for prolonged periods of time. Appropriate treatment may be required to improve both the appearance and function of the extremity.

Complicating factors of venous disease in the elderly include thrombophlebitis, deep venous thrombosis, and postphlebitic syndrome, which produce an "at-risk" status for the patient with foot problems.

The more common arterial diseases that can be observed in the elderly include the residuals of vasospastic disease, such as Raynaud's Disease or Phenomenon, acrocyanosis, livedo reticulosis, pernio, and erythromelalgia. Occlusive diseases such as arteriosclerosis obliterans, the residuals of thromboangiitis obliterans and related diseases, such as arteritis, periarteritis nodosa, polymyalgia rheumatica, systemic lupus erythematous, erythema nodosum, erythema induratum, nodular vasculitis, and hypertensive arteriolar disease. The primary risk factors for the development of peripheral arterial diseases in older patients include smoking, diabetes mellitus, hypertension, Buerger's, and Raynaud's diseases. With inadequate perfusion, nonhealing wounds, infection, tissue loss, and amputation are complications. The primary clinical findings associated with arterial insufficiency are summarized but not limited to those listed in Figures 4 and 5 and Table 10.

In the geriatric patient, arterial insufficiency is heralded by rest pain or nocturnal cramps and/or intermittent claudication. Although it is usually brought on by exercise or use, it may also occur at rest in severe cases of arterial occlusion, especially when bedclothes warm the foot, for example. One also needs to remember that any muscle may claudicate and thus foot pain in the elderly may be related to arterial insufficiency rather than biomechanics or pathomechanics. Painful ulcerations may occur over bony prominences and result from minor trauma and/or pressure. To desist from smoking is a significant contribution to management and the prevention of complications. Appropriate vascular studies, such as; imaging (arteriography, digital subtraction angiography, MRI, CT arteriography, and Doppler imaging), noninvasive studies (Doppler, oscillometric, ankle-brachial index, segmental pressure measurement, plethysmographic waveform analysis, pulse volume recording, skin perfusion pressure, laser Doppler pressure, color Doppler, ultrasonography, transcutaneous oxygen content (TcPO3), cutaneous oximetry, and treadmill exercise testing), and surgical consideration should be provided when pain is uncontrolled and/or when ulceration is significant.

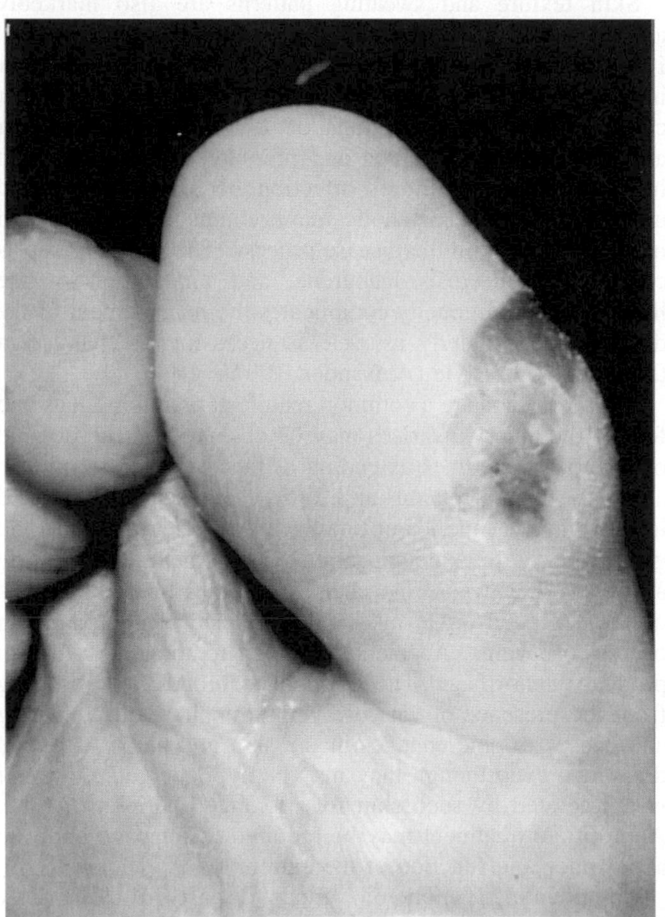

Figure 4 Subkeratotic hematoma, osseous deformity of the hallux with predisposition to ulceration

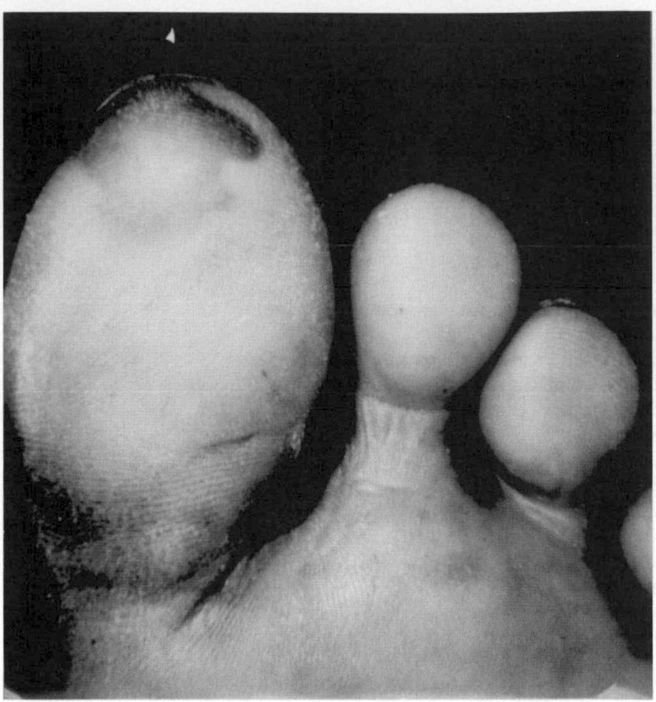

Figure 5 Distal thrombosis associated with arteriosclerotic changes and xerosis

CLINICAL ASSESSMENT (Merriman and Tollafield, 1995; Merriman and Turner, 2002)

Because of the risk involved in the geriatric patient and the relationship to multiple chronic diseases, assessment, examination, and evaluation of the feet of the elderly is essential. Essential as elements of this process include needs, relationships to ambulation and activities of daily living (ADL), and the fact that foot pain can result in functional disability, dysfunction, and increased dependency.

A Comprehensive Podogeriatric Assessment Protocol (Helfand Index), as developed by the Pennsylvania Department of Health is included as Table 11.

Table 10 Primary clinical vascular findings

Fatigue
Rest pain
Coldness
Decreased skin temperature
Burning
Color changes
Absent or diminished digital hair
Tingling
Numbness
Ulceration
History of phlebitis
Cramps
Edema
Claudication
History of repeated foot infections
Diminished or absent pedal pulses
Popliteal and/or femoral pulse change
Color changes – rubor – erythema and/or cyanosis
Temperature changes – cool – gradient
Xerosis, atrophic, and dry skin
Atrophy of soft tissue
Superficial infections
Onychial changes
Onychopathy
Onychodystrophy
Nutritional changes
Subungual hemorrhage
Discoloration
Onycholysis
Onychauxis (thickening)
Onychorrhexis (longitudinal striations)
Subungual keratosis
Deformity
Edema
Blebs
Varicosities
Delayed venous filling time
Prolonged capillary filling time
Femoral bruits
Ischemia
Necrosis and gangrene

In addition, Medicare in the United States has three additional sets of criteria for Class Findings required to qualify for primary foot care (Table 12); Criteria for Therapeutic Shoes for Diabetics (Table 13); Criteria of the Loss of Protective Sensation (LOPS) (Table 14); Criteria for Onychomycosis (Table 15).

A systems review of known chronic and risk diseases is a key element in the assessment process. Conditions such as diabetes mellitus, arteriosclerosis, anemia, chronic renal disease, CHF, arthritis, stroke, neurologic deficits are examples of these risk conditions. The patients' living conditions should also be noted as they are a relationship to care and needs. The chief complaint of the patient should be identified in the patient's own words and related to their daily lives in terms of activity and social needs. The duration, location, severity, prior treatment, and results should also be identified in relation to the presented condition. A social history is also a part of this assessment process.

The dermatologic symptoms and signs and the onychial findings are listed but not limited to Tables 16 and 17 and Figures 6 and 7.

The neurologic symptoms and signs are included but not limited to Table 18. The vascular findings are noted in Table 10.

A drug history and summary of findings, clinical impressions, and special notations for some of the primary basics for assessment, as anticoagulants, steroids, and medications to control diabetes mellitus present additional risk.

The primary musculoskeletal clinical findings are noted but not limited to Table 19 and Figures 8 and 9.

There are biomechanical and pathomechanical factors that combine with structural abnormalities and deformities to increase the risk for pedal ulceration. They are listed but not limited to Table 20 and Figure 10.

The forefoot (metatarsals and phalanges) is the most mobile part of the foot and the majority of problems that develop, occur in this area. Pressure from deformities and shoe to foot incompatibility, will give rise to keratotic lesions (corns and callosities) an initial response to pressure and friction, but footwear is by no means the only cause of painful lesions in the feet nor the prime etiologic factor. Congenital and acquired deformities will result in malfunction and dysfunction and give rise to secondary lesions as the body attempts to compensate for pain and deformity. Alteration in shape and function can arise from accidental trauma, paralysis, changes in function as a result of surgical revision and/or diseases, such as arthritis, which embarrass normal function. The mobility of the foot has a great influence on the type and extent of painful secondary foot lesions.

Rigid feet usually have circumscribed areas of hyperkeratosis. Mobile feet have more extensive areas of keratotic development. Where the foot is deficient in fibro-fatty padding or where the stress is chronic, constant, and severe, the so-called neurovascular heloma or tyloma may develop, creating a disruption in the normal dermal – epidermal relationship. Small blood vessels and nerve endings then extend into the epidermis and are enveloped in the keratotic lesion, creating excessive pain and complicating management. Such lesions may be completely disabling and in some patients, result in distressing hyperesthesia, which is difficult to relieve. Many practitioners will not believe that the patient is suffering so severely as they claim.

To the practiced eye, footwear can also reveal a great deal about disease and dynamic foot function. Neglected footwear generally demonstrates neglected foot care and may indicate social poverty. It may also demonstrate poor eyesight. Urine splashes that have dried on the uppers of shoes are sometimes the first indication of occult diabetes mellitus. Thus, the foot is a mirror of health and disease.

KERATOTIC LESIONS

The presence of hyperkeratotic lesions, such as tyloma and/or heloma (callous or corns) on the foot is symptomatic of some degree of malfunction of the foot, especially in the elderly. Elimination and/or management of the underlying cause are the principle objective of the podiatrist's treatment.

Table 11 Podogeriatric assessment protocol (Helfand, 1999, 2003a, 2003b, 2004a, 2004b)

Date of visit		MR#
Patient's name		Age
Date of birth		Social security #
Address		
City	State	Zip code
Phone number		
Sex M F	Race B W A L NA	
Weight LBS	Height IN	
Social status M S W D SEP		
Name of primary physician/health-care facility		
Date of last visit		
History of present illness		
Swelling of feet	Location	
Painful feet	Quality	
Hyperkeratosis	Severity	
Onychial Changes	Duration	
Bunions	Context	
Painful toe nails	Modifying factors	
Infections	Associated signs and symptoms	
Cold feet		
Other		
Past history		
Heart disease	Diabetes mellitus	
High blood pressure	* IDDM	
Arthritis	* NIDDM	
* Circulatory disease	Hypercholesterol	
Thyroid	Gout	
Allergy	History: Smoking: OH	
	Family – Social	
Systems review		
Constitutional		
ENT	Card/Vasc	GU
Eyes	Musculo-	Neurologic
Skin/Hair	Skeletal	Endocrine
Respiratory	GYN	GI
Psychiatric	Allergic	Immunologic
Hematologic	Lymphatic	
Medications		
Dermatologic		
* Hyperkeratosis	Xerosis	
Onychauxis B-2-b	Tinea pedis	
Infection	Verruca	
* Ulceration	Hematoma	
Onychomycosis	Rubor	
Onychodystrophy	* Preulcerative	
* Cyanosis B-2-e	Discolored	
Foot orthopedic		
* Hallux valgus	* Hallux rigidus-limitus	
* Anterior imbalance	* Morton's syndrome	
* Digiti flexus	Bursitis	
* Pes planus	* Prominent met head	
* Pes valgoplanus	* Charcot joints	
* Pes cavus	Other	
Vascular evaluation		
* Coldness C-2	* Claudication C-1	
* Trophic changes B-2-a	Varicosities	
* DP absent B-3	Other	
* PT absent B-1	* Amputation	
* Night cramps	* AKA BKA FF T A-1	
* Edema C-3	Atrophy B-2-d	
Neurologic evaluation		
* Achilles	Superficial plantar	
* Vibratory	* Joint position	
* Sharp/Dull	* Burning C-5	

Table 11 *(continued)*

* Paresthesia C-4 Other

Risk category – neurologic
0 = No Sensory loss
* 1 = Sensory loss
* 2 = Sensory loss and foot deformity
* 3 = Sensory loss, Hx ulceration, and deformity

Risk category – vascular
0 – 0 No change
* I – 1 Mild claudication
* I – 2 Moderate claudication
* I – 3 Severe claudication
* II – 4 Ischemic rest pain
* III – 5 Minor tissue loss
* III – 6 Major tissue loss

Class findings
A1 Nontraumatic amputation
B1 Absent posterior tibial
B2 Advanced trophic changes
B2a Hair growth (decrease or absent)
B2b Nail changes (thickening)
B2c Pigmentary changes (discoloration)
B2d Skin texture (thin, shiny)
B2e Skin color (rubor or redness)
B3 Absent dorsalis pedis
C1 Claudication
C2 Temperature changes (cold)
C3 Edema
C4 Paresthesia
C5 Burning

Onychomycosis: Documentation of mycosis/dystrophy causing secondary infection and/or pain, which results or would result in marked limitation of ambulation.
Discoloration
Hypertrophy
Subungual debris
Onycholysis
Secondary infection
Limitation of ambulation and pain

Classification of mechanical or pressure hyperkeratosis

Grade Description
0 No lesion
1 No specific tyloma plaque, but diffuse or pinch hyperkeratotic tissue present or in narrow bands
2 Circumscribed, punctate oval, or circular, well defined thickening of keratinized tissue
3 Heloma miliare or heloma durum with no associated tyloma
4 Well-defined tyloma plaque with a definite heloma within the lesion extravasation, maceration, and early breakdown of structures under the tyloma or callus layer
5 Complete breakdown of structure of hyperkeratotic tissue, epidermis, extending to superficial dermal involvement

Plantar keratomata pattern
LT 5 4 3 2 1 RT 1 2 3 4 5

Ulcer classification
Grade – 0 – Absent skin lesions
Grade – 1 – Dense callus but not preulcer or ulcer
Grade – 2 – Preulcerative changes
Grade – 3 – Partial thickness (superficial ulcer)
Grade – 4 – Full thickness (deep) ulcer but no involvement of tendon, bone, ligament or joint
Grade – 5 – Full thickness (deep) ulcer with involvement of tendon, bone, ligament or joint
Grade – 6 – Localized infection (abscess or osteomyelitis)
Grade – 7 – Proximal spread of infection (ascending cellulitis or lymphadenopathy)
Grade – 8 – Gangrene of forefoot only
Grade – 9 – Gangrene of majority of foot

Onychial grades at risk
Grade I Normal
Grade II Mild hypertrophy
Grade III Hypertrophic

(continued overleaf)

Table 11 (*continued*)

	Dystrophic
	Onychauxis
	Mycotic
	Infected
	Onychodysplasia
Grade IV	Hypertrophic
	Deformed
	Onychogryphosis
	Dystrophic
	Mycotic
	Infected
Footwear satisfactory	*Hygiene satisfactory*
Yes No	Yes No
Stockings: Nylon Cotton Wool Other None	
Assessment	
Plan	
Podiatric referral	
Patient education	
Medical referral	
Special footwear	
Vascular studies	
Clinical lab	
Imaging	
Rx	

Notes: B, Black; W, White, A, Asian; L, Latino/Hispanic; N/A, Native American; S, Single; M, Married; W, Widow/Widower; D, Divorced; S, Separated; DP, Dorsalis pedis pulse; PT, Posterior tibial pulse; AKA, Above the knee amputation; BKA, Below the knee amputation; FF, Forefoot amputation; T, Toe amputation; Hx, History of; Rx, Prescription for treatment as a part of the key to data analysis and risk stratification, the key notes of number and letter (i.e. 2-a) indicate Medicare Class Findings as risk factors and those noted with an asterisk (*) identify risk factors to qualify patients for Therapeutic Shoes under Medicare.

Table 12 Medicare class findings (CMS, 2002a)

Class findings
Class A findings
– Nontraumatic amputation of foot or integral skeletal portion thereof
Class B findings
– Absent posterior tibial pulse
– Absent dorsalis pedis pulse
– Advanced trophic changes as (three required):
Hair growth (decrease or absence)
Nail changes (thickening)
Pigmentary changes (discoloration)
Skin texture (thin, shiny)
Skin color (rubor or redness)
Class C findings
– Claudication
– Temperature changes (e.g. cold feet)
– Edema
– Paresthesias (abnormal spontaneous sensations in the feet)
– Burning

Table 13 Therapeutic shoe criteria (CMS, 2002b)

History of partial or complete amputation of the foot
History of previous foot ulceration
History of preulcerative callus
Peripheral neuropathy with evidence of callus formation
Foot deformity
Poor circulation

This is a goal that is more easily achieved in younger groups due to the wider range of treatment options available. In the elderly, continuing surveillance, monitoring, and primary management is the chief form of therapy, as is the approach for any other chronic condition, such as hypertension, arthritis, and/or diabetes mellitus.

Table 14 Onychomycosis Dauber *et al.*, 2001

Onychomycosis: Documentation of mycosis/dystrophy causing secondary infection and/or pain, which results or would result in marked limitation of ambulation
Discoloration
Hypertrophy
Subungual debris
Onycholysis
Secondary infection
Limitation of ambulation and pain
Dystrophic
Onychodysplasia
Onychauxis
Onychogryphosis

The normal response of the epidermis to intermittent, chronic pressure, and/or stress is to increase in thickness. The resulting excrescence is called *hyperkeratosis* (*tyloma* or *callous*) and may be both hyperplastic as well as hypertrophic. These commonly occur on the plantar aspect of the metatarsophalangeal joints, the hallux, and around the heel. Callous may also occur on the dorsum of the toes, especially with contracture and in the nail grooves. Atrophy of the adjacent dermis and soft tissue, is a common accompaniment in the case of chronic callosities, especially in the patient demonstrating a LOPS. With continuing pressure, vascular and neurologic elements become involved and the development of associated fibrous tissue may also occur. In

Table 15 Loss of protective sensation (Edmonds *et al.*, 2004; Frykberg, 1991)

Services furnished for the evaluation and management of a diabetic patient with diabetic sensory neuropathy, resulting in a LOPS must include the following:

1. a diagnosis of LOPS
2. a patient history
3. a physical examination consisting of findings regarding at least the following elements:
   (a) visual inspection of the forefoot, hindfoot, and toe web spaces
   (b) evaluation of protective sensation
   (c) evaluation of foot structure and biomechanics
   (d) evaluation of vascular status
   (e) evaluation of skin integrity
   (f) evaluation and recommendation of footwear
4. patient education

LOPS, loss of protective sensation.

Table 16 Dermatologic findings

Exquisitely painful or painless wounds
Slow healing or nonhealing wounds
Trophic ulceration
Necrosis
Skin color changes such as cyanosis or redness
Changes in texture and turgor
Pigmentation
- Hemosiderin deposition

Chronic itching – pruritus
Neurogenic, and/or emotional dermatoses
Contact dermatitis
Stasis dermatitis
Atopic dermatitis
Nummular eczema
Scaling
Xerosis or dryness
Excoriations
Recurrent infections
- Paronychia
- Tinea pedis
- Onychomycosis
- Pyoderma
- Cellulitis

Keratin dysfunction
Keratotic lesions without hemorrhage or hematoma
- Tyloma (callus)
- Heloma durum (hard corn)
- Heloma miliare (seed corn)
- Heloma molle (soft corn)
- Heloma neurofibrosuum (neuritic)
- Heloma vasculare (vascular)
- Onychophosis (callus in the nail groove)
- Intractable plantar keratosis

Keratotic lesions with hemorrhage or hematoma (preulcerative)
Verruca
Psoriasis
Fissures
Hyperhidrosis
Bromidrosis
Maceration
Diminished or absent hair growth
Diabetic dermopathy
Necrobiosis lipoidica diabeticorum
Bullous diabeticorum
Poroma
Absence of hair
Ulceration

Table 17 Onychial findings

Onychoatrophia (atrophy)
Onychia sicca (dryness)
Onycholysis (freeing from the free edge)
Subungual hyperkeratosis
Onychexallis (degeneration)
Diabetic onychopathy
Onychauxis (hypertrophy)
Onychogryphosis (hypertrophy and deformity)
Onychomycosis (fungal infection)
Onychia
Paronychia
Onychitis (inflammation)
Onychalgia (pain)
Subungual abscess
Subungual heloma (keratosis)
Subungual exostosis
Periungual verruca
Onychophyma (painful degeneration with hypertrophy)
Onychomadesis (freeing from the proximal portion)
Onychoschizia (splitting)
Onychyphemia (hemorrhagic)
Onychoclasis (cracking)
Onychomalacia (softening)
Onychoptosis (shedding)
Subungual spur
Onychophosis (hyperkeratosis in the nail groove)
Subungual hematoma
Splinter hemorrhage
Onychocryptosis (ingrown toenail)
Periungual ulcerative granulation tissue
Onychodysplasia (involuted or pincer nails)
Onychodystrophy (trophic changes)
Onychorrhexis (longitudinal ridging)
Beau's lines (transverse growth cessation)
Pterygium (hypertrophy of eponychium)
Onychoclasis (breaking of the nail)
Diabetic onychopathy (trophic diabetic changes)
Hypertrophic onychodystrophy

some instances, the fibrous tissues bind the skin to the underlying joint capsule and/or tissues.

Hemorrhagic spots indicate where blood has been forced from vessels and is indicative of extensive pressure and/or a complication of an associated systemic disease, such as diabetes mellitus. Occasionally, this makes a "lake" in the area and produces a moist, shallow ulceration, which dries and heals when the area is débrided of keratosis and appropriately managed. In some instances, a frank ulceration may develop, as in the case of a diabetic. Management including débridement of the keratosis is essential if healing is to be generated (Baran *et al.*, 1996).

The characteristic of a heloma durum (corn) is the presence of a nucleus. Heloma appear to represent a reaction to more localized stress than is the case with tyloma (callosity), although heloma are frequently found established in a much larger area of callous. The nucleus is 1 – 2 mm in diameter and may be circular or even crescentic in shape. It is harder due to increased density than the surrounding callous. The nucleus may represent parakeratotic changes histologically, similar to that which occurs in psoriasis.

Like tyloma, heloma are essentially epidermal in origin but may become more complex because of alteration in the

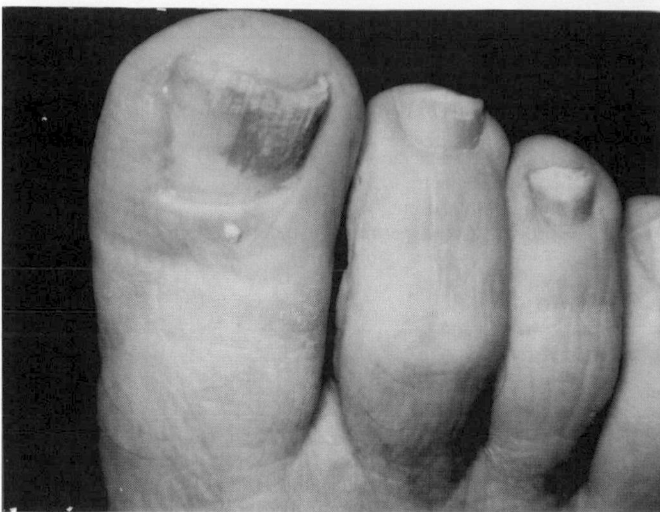

Figure 6 Onychocryptosis (ingrown toenail) with onychia, onychodysplasia (involuted hallux toenail, subungual hematoma, onychomycosis, hammertoes, and hypertrophy of the unguilabia (nail lip)

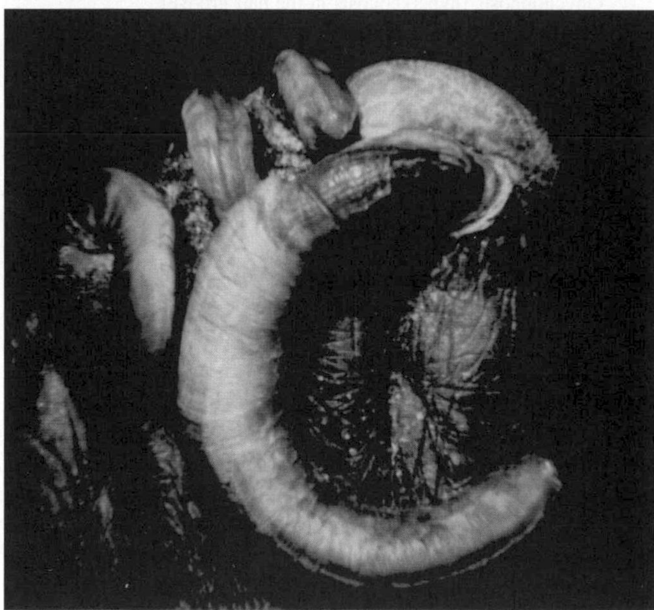

Figure 7 Onychogryphosis (Ram's Horn Toenails), marked hypertrophic and deformity, onychomycosis, and xerosis

dermis, frequently overlooked, and a source of considerable intractable chronic pain. This is due to the imbalance created in the normal chemo-epidermal function and the development of hyperkeratotic lesions with neural and vascular components, many times encapsulated, giving rise to much pain and discomfort. The resulting neurovascular lesion, heloma neurovarsculare, usually signifies a long-standing lesion. Not infrequently, these result from improper and inappropriate treatment or repeated self-treatment, resulting in hemorrhage and inadequate follow-up care. Sites where broken chilblains have occurred may also become calloused with

Table 18 Neurologic findings

Sensory changes
Burning
Tingling
Clawing sensations
Pain and hyperactivity
Two-point discrimination
Motor changes
Weakness
Foot drop
Autonomic
Diminished sweating
Hyperhidrosis
Sensory deficits
Vibratory
Proprioceptive
Loss of protective sensation
Changes in pain and temperature perception
Hyperesthesia
Diminished to absent deep tendon reflexes (Achilles and Patellar)
Hypohidrosis with perfusion
Diabetic dermopathy or pretibial lesions (shin spots)
Thickened skin with calluses under high-pressure areas, demonstrating an intrinsic minus foot (marked digital contractures, metatarsal prolapse, prominent metatarsal heads, and plantar fat pad atrophy and displacement)
Bowstring tendons
Charcot Foot

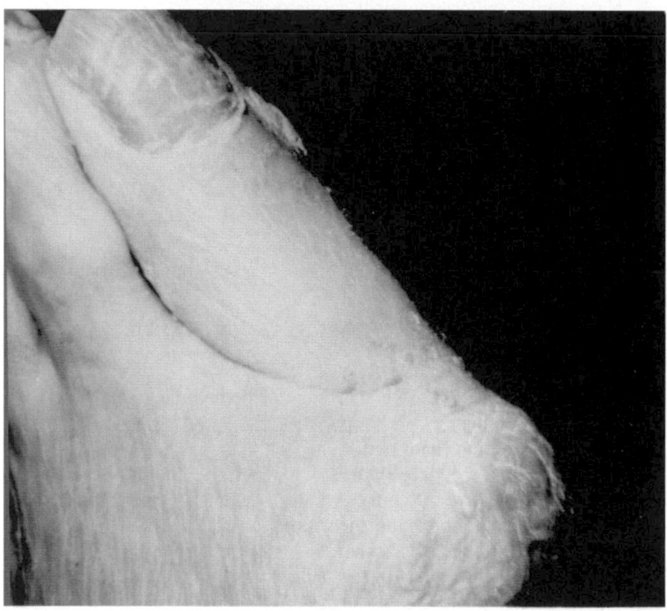

Figure 8 Hallux valgus, rotation of the hallux, onychomycosis, onychauxis, joint deformities, enlargement of the first metatarsal phalangeal joint, degenerative changes, and xerosis

accompanying neurovascular changes in the dermis, are further complicated by the presence of one or more of such nuclei. Heloma (corn) may arise anywhere on the skin where a bony prominence provides resistance to external pressure. The resulting intermittent stress – a combination of pressure, friction, and shearing – provokes changes in the skin which are not yet well understood, but which are readily recognized

Table 19 Musculoskeletal findings

Gradual change in shape or size of the foot
A sudden and painless change in foot shape with swelling and no history of trauma
Cavus feet with claw toe
Drop foot
"Rocker bottom foot" or Charcot foot
Neuropathic arthropathy
Elevated plantar pressure
Decreased muscle strength
Decreased ranges of motion
Multiple foot deformities
Limited joint mobility
Abnormal foot pressure and subsequent ulceration
Structural abnormalities or foot deformities
- Hammertoes
- Claw
- Prominent metatarsal heads
- Atrophy of plantar fat pad
- Plantar fat pad displacement
- Foot muscle atrophy
- Hallux valgus
- Hallux limitus
- Hallux rigidus
- Tailor's bunion
- Plantar Fasciitis
- Spur formation
- Calcaneal spurs
- Bursitis
- Periostitis
- Decalcification
- Stress fractures
- Tendonitis
- Tenosynovitis
- Metatarsalgia
- Morton's syndrome
- Joint swelling
- Bursitis
- Haglund's deformity
- Neuritis
- Entrapment syndrome
- Neuroma
- Sesamoid erosion
- Sesamoid displacement
- Tendo-Achilles contracture
- Digital amputation
- Partial foot amputation
- Charcot's joints
- Phalangeal reabsorption
- Functional abnormalities
- Pes cavus

Equinus
Pes planus
Residuals of arthritis (degenerative, rheumatoid, and gouty)
Biomechanical and pathomechanical variations
Gait evaluation
Shoe evaluation
- Type of shoe
- Fit and size
- Shoe wear and patters of wear
- Shoe lining wear
- Foreign bodies
- Insoles
- Orthoses

even by a laymen. In the elderly, atrophy of soft tissue and a reduction in the fluidity and elasticity of the soft tissues predispose the elderly to the development of these lesions.

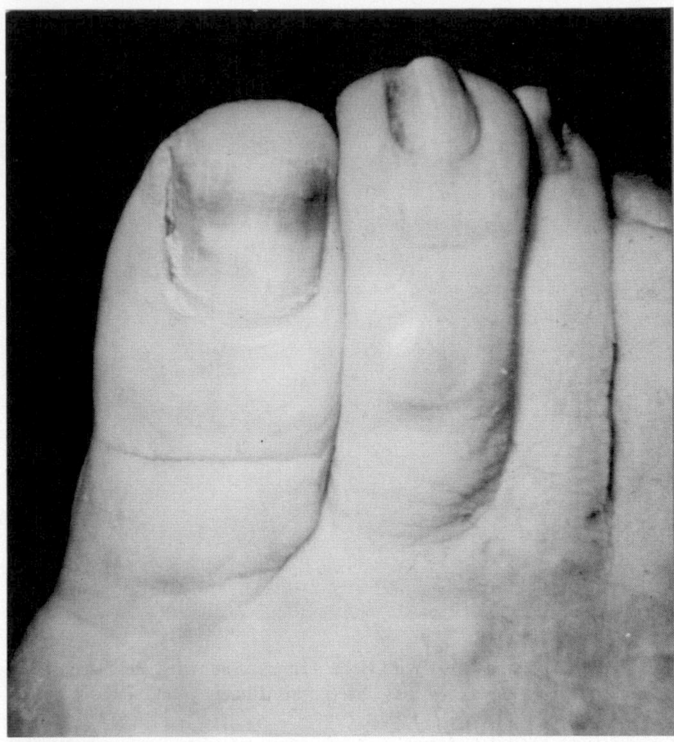

Figure 9 Subungual hematoma, xerosis, pterygium, early keratosis (heloma), and trophic changes

Table 20 Factors leading to ulceration

Body mass
Gait
Ambulatory speed
Tissue trauma
Weight diffusion
Weight dispersion
Pathomechanics, defined as structural change in relation to function
Biomechanics, defined as forces that change and affect the foot in relation to function
Imbalance, defined as the inability to adapt to alterations of stress
- Force – alteration in physical condition, either shape or position
- Compression stress – one force moves toward another
- Tensile stress – a pulling away of one part against another
- Shearing stress – a sliding of one part on the other
- Friction – the force needed to overcome resistance and usually associated with a sheering stress
- Elasticity – weight diffusion and weight dispersion
- Fluid pressure – soft tissue adaptation and conformity to stress

Bursae may occur in the tissues adjacent to a heloma. Localized pinpoint lesions, heloma miliare, or seed corns, occur with extreme localization of pressure, such as a protruding irregularity in a shoe. Heloma molle or soft corns are found between the toes and are macerated and soft due to excessive moisture. Their etiology is usually due to digital compression accompanied by bony abnormality and/or digital deformities, such as hammertoes and rotational deformities.

Management in the elderly is essential to prevent infection, particularly from improper débridement. Given the atrophy of soft tissue in the elderly, localized pressure from keratotic

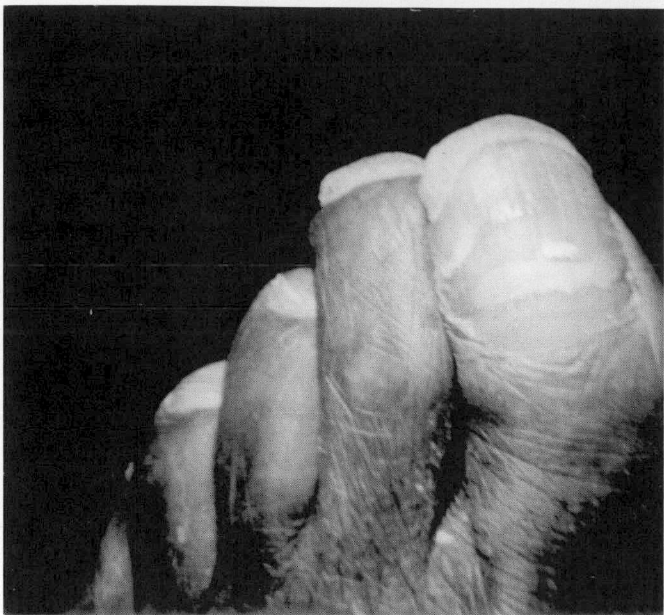

Figure 10 Onychomycosis with Beau's Lines, contracted and rotated toes, onychodystrophy, onychorrhexis, arterial insufficiency, and xerosis

lesions, may produce ulceration and can lead to osteomyelitis, with chronicity and intractable states.

Treatment includes initial débridement, the use of emollients such as 20% urea or 12% ammonium lactate, and materials to reduce pressure are essential elements in the management of the elderly. Silicone molds to compensate for deformity, padding materials to provide weight diffusion, orthotics to provide stability and weight dispersion, and shoe modifications as needed are also considerations in a long-range approach to the management of these lesions in the elderly.

ULCERS

Diabetes mellitus, peripheral arterial insufficiency, and vasculitis are probably the most common predisposing etiologies in the development of ulcerations in feet. Ulcerations resulting from vasculitis are usually superficial and treatment involves the relief of pressure. Healing is usually rapid and a resolution of the ulcer can be maintained with periodic management to prevent excessive localized pressure to stressful areas of the feet. The underlying cause should also be appropriately treated (Bild *et al.*, 1989; Cavanagh *et al.*, 2000).

Diabetic ulceration commonly occurs on weight bearing areas of the foot, although the tissue overlying any bony prominence exposed to pressure may breakdown and ulcerate. Even bed-ridden patients may develop ulcers due to the weight of bed-cloths or that of one limb upon another. Diabetic ulcers (perforating) may penetrate to involve deeper structures. Surgical intervention will then be required for more extensive débridement of tissue, drainage, and some times, skin grafting. The use of contact casts or removable cast walkers can be considered, but the patient's ability to adapt to these ambulatory changes must be part of the consideration for their use (Kozak *et al.*, 1995).

Ulcers that are due to arterial insufficiency are usually very painful and present with pending necrosis and gangrene. The changes are usually dry and at some point, the decision to manage and/or amputate will need to be considered. Decisions are based on the total clinical picture and the needs of the patient.

Ulcer etiology and assessment are initial considerations. Location, wound size, and shape, wound bed, color, drainage, wound edges, pain, periwound area, odor, edema, and the signs of infection are important issues. Management includes removing devitalized tissue by débridement, autolytic enzymes, mechanical, chemical, and cleansing are considerations. Managing the potential for an infection are critical issues. Preventing local injury and supporting the repair process are equally important. Vascular complications require indication, consultation, and possible surgical intervention. Topical recombinant platelet – derived growth factor can assist in wound care. Continuing evaluation, local wound care, management, and prevention are continuing issues, particularly in the older patient.

Management should include relief of pressure, control of infection, and appropriate débridement (Bottomley and Lewis, 2003). Note should be made of the duration of the ulcer, size of the ulcer, depth of the ulcer, and the amount of necrotic tissue present. Treatment parameters also include assessment of the patient's mental status, mobility, infection, tissue oxygenation, chronic pressure, arterial insufficiency (small vessel ischemia), venous stasis, edema, type of dressings, and chronic illnesses such as diabetes mellitus, uremia, COPD (chronic obstructive pulmonary disease), malnutrition, CHF (congestive heart failure), anemia, iron deficiency, and immune deficiency disorders. In addition, signs and symptoms, other medical conditions, the wound status, the patient's response to treatment, and early consultation are also important factors to preserve the patient's limb and life (Bolton *et al.*, 2000; Bowker and Pfeifer, 2001).

TOENAILS

As appendages of the skin, nails very readily reflect its state, becoming hard, dry, and brittle as age advances. Not infrequently, the nail plate is thinner than usual due to atrophy. In other instances, the toenails become so thickened and deformed that the patient cannot cut them and they are ashamed to show their nails to another person. The resulting discomfort may prevent them from wearing any other footwear than a house slipper, making the patient housebound. In addition, the deformity may present a podalgic gait and produce a degree of ambulatory dysfunction, making the patient partially functionally disabled.

Trauma is a precipitating factor in the development of thickening of the nail plate. The trauma may have been acute and marked or may be chronic and minimal, such as the constant friction or impaction of the toenail against the inferior portion of the toe box of the shoe. The nail plate may grow and twist across the foot. This is onychogryphosis or "Ram's horn nail". It also presents as a residual of inappropriate or no treatment. The danger of this condition is that the nail may penetrate the skin and provide a portal of entry for pathogens, resulting in infection (Evans *et al.*, 2000).

Toenails sometimes assume a claw-like appearance due to a dramatic increase in the transverse curvature (involution or convolution). They may also become thickened (onychauxis). Unskilled and inappropriate attempts to "dig out" the corners of this so-called ingrown toenail, because it is painful, very often lead to inflammation (onychia) and infection (paronychia). Temporary relief may be obtained but skin retraction usually results in increased pain and infection a short time after this attempt. Patients who have poor peripheral arterial supply may face serious consequences from the improper management of this condition. Very thin nail plates may also penetrate the skin of adjacent toes, with similar results.

Hyperkeratosis in the nail grooves (onychophosis) or under the free edge of the nail also creates pain. Periodic débridement of the thickness and length of the toe nail then permits débridement of the keratotic tissue. This is achieved with the use of a nail forceps, curette, and drill, and an appropriate burr. Suitable dressings of chamois, leather, ointments, or silicones, such as Viscogel can be utilized as nail packing under the nail plate to prevent it from digging into the surrounding tissue. The use of emollients such as 20% urea or 12% ammonium lactate also helps as a preventive measure. Depending on the patient's general health and the pain and deformity, avulsion of the whole nail or part of the nail plate, under local or regional anesthesia may be considered.

Another relatively common cause of thickening of the nail plate is mycotic infection. Streaks of yellow or brown discoloration may extend from the free edge, proximally to the lunula. One or more nails are usually involved, become thickened, brittle, and produce a characteristic musty odor. The patient's concern may be the unsightly nail that makes a hole in hosiery and sometimes the uppers of their foot wear. Pain is associated with deformity. However, this chronic infection may produce a mycotic onychia and may serve as a focus of infection (Baran *et al.*, 1999).

The most common organism producing these changes is *Trichophyton rubrum*. Although it is generally confined to the nails, the surrounding skin, and interdigital spaces may become scaly and itch intensely. Sometimes the infection spreads more extensively over the so-called moccasin area. Miconazole nitrate is an example of an antifungal agent that is effective in the treatment of mycotic infections of the skin. Oral terbinafine hydrochloride, itraconazole, and topical ciclopirox are available for the management of onychomycosis. Forty percent urea gel is also utilized as a topical application to assist in local onychial débridement. The appearance of the nail plate can be improved and the patient's comfort increased by reducing the thickness of the nail plate and providing a smooth surface to the plate.

BURSITIS

Bursae are found in a number of situations in the foot. The adventitious bursa over the medial aspect of the first metatarsophalangeal joint frequently becomes inflamed when the joint it overlies is deformed and enlarged, as in hallux valgus. Bursae are also found superficial and deep to the Achilles tendon, the plantar aspect of the heel and the lateral aspect of the fifth metatarsal-phalangeal joint (tailor's bunion). If for any reason, a superficial bursa is ruptured, secondary infection can ensue. A sinus may be formed and chronic subacute bursitis is then a persistent problems.

Enforced rest for long periods due to debilitating illness or accidental injury may lead to laxity and atrophy of the plantar calcaneal fibro-fatty padding, associated with dehydration. The plantar calcaneal bursa is then vulnerable due to overuse and bursitis results. Plantar calcaneal spurs and plantar myofascitis may also become troublesome in these circumstances (Birrer *et al.*, 1998).

The immediate treatment for bursitis is to reduce the inflammation and to manage any secondary infection that may be present. Pressure on the areas can be reduced with padding and shoe modifications. Physical modalities, such as heat and ultrasound can be of assistance if properly utilized. Local steroid injections as the use of nonsteroidal anti-inflammatory drugs are indicated, when appropriate, in the elderly.

In the long term, stress on the bursae has to be reduced to minimize an exacerbation of the condition, once the acute symptoms are resolved. This may involve modification to footwear an/or the wearing of an appropriate shield (orthotic), such as a silicone mold. Plantar bursitis can be improved with the use of heel cups, silicone heel pads, and/or orthosis that provide weight diffusion and modify the weight/pressure relationships in a superior, lateral, and posterior direction. Insoles from Plastazote, PPT, and other similar materials can aid in weight diffusion and dispersion. The normal warmth of the foot, even in the geriatric patient, will help mold the Plastazote. The resulting wear marks can be a good guide when constructing a more durable orthotic from materials such as Vitrathane. Plastazote as an insole or lining material in combination with Vitrathane will relieve the patient of the feeling that they are walking on pebbles, which is the result of soft tissue atrophy and atrophy of the plantar fat pad.

SCARRING

Scarring of the plantar surface of the foot may result from accidental injury, for example, penetration of a foreign body, when walking barefoot. It is not infrequently iatrogenic in origin, that is, following surgery. The plantar metatarsal is the commoner site for painful scars on the foot, which in the geriatric, is already deficient in fibro-fatty padding. This can be completely disabling. Patients will require primary podiatric care to débride the keratotic lesions (callous and corns) that usually develop within the scar tissue. Appropriate orthotics and insoles as noted above, should be employed to reduce friction and pressure by weight diffusion and dispersion.

FISSURES

Moist or dry skin may develop fissures. In either case, the fissuring may extend into the dermis and create hemorrhage in the soft tissues. In the geriatric, stress marks along the outer portion of the heel also serve as an etiologic factor and form the initial stages of pressure ulcerations. Fissures around the heel are usually dry and vertically oriented. Secondary infection is always an added risk. Interdigitally, fissures are usually moist and follow the flexures of the skin. Infection of the interdigital fissures may penetrate the fascial planes and require surgical drainage. The edges of the fissures usually become hyperkeratotic and indurated in the elderly patient, which prevents healing and can be extremely painful.

Moist fissures respond well to simple antiseptic dressings and when healed, the skin should be carefully washed daily. The hard edges of the dry fissures should be débrided. This may be aided by the use of 12.5% salicylic acid in collodion. Its action is to soften the hyperkeratosis and make débridement easier and less painful for the patient. Tissue stimulants can also be employed, once débridement is completed. Bland emollients that help soften keratosis and maintain skin integrity can also be suggested, such as 20% urea creams and 12% ammonium lactate lotion, in addition to daily hygiene (Lorimer *et al.*, 2002).

MANAGEMENT CONSIDERATIONS

Since healthy feet are essential for mobility and independence, as well as a catalyst to maintain patient dignity, none who are concerned with health and well-being of older persons should disregard foot care. The particular knowledge and skills of the podiatrist are vital for the multidisciplinary team caring for the geriatric patient. Regular assessment and inspection of the feet are an effective means of monitoring the preventive aspects of the complications of diabetes mellitus and arthritis for example. Other symptoms and overt abnormalities are many times detected during a foot evaluation, with appropriate referral for care to justify the secondary preventive aspects of chronic disease. The period evaluation also provides an appropriate time for health education. For the diabetic, this may be the difference between dignity and ulceration, gangrene and amputation. Projected changes in Medicare Regulations in the United States will mandate appropriate foot care as a Condition of Participation and quality assurance as a condition for approval (Helfand, 2000; Strauss and Spielfogel, 2003; Tollafield and Merriman, 1997).

FOOTCARE

Advice regarding foot care will benefit all elderly people whatever their state of general health. Daily washing of the feet should be encouraged. The skin should be dried carefully, dabbing rather than rubbing – especially between the toes. Extreme care should be taken to check that the temperature of wash water does not exceed 40 °C. An appropriate thermometer is best for this purpose. Immediately after bathing, emollients may be applied to the skin to increase hydration and lubrication. This helps in minimizing the drying out of the skin.

Toenails must not be picked or torn, but carefully trimmed, without cutting back the corners. Patients, who have any degree of abnormality, disease, or who cannot bend, see or maintain manual dexterity, should seek professional care. This is especially true for the "at-risk" patient. Ingrown toe nails (onychocryptosis) can readily result from badly trimmed or torn nail plates penetrating otherwise healthy skin.

The application of patent "corn cures", plasters, or paints must be avoided. These preparations contain salicylic acid and can create a second-degree chemical burn, initially; infection, ulceration, necrosis, and gangrene may result for their use in the "at-risk" patient, such as diabetics.

Any minor cut or abrasion should be covered with a sterile dressing. If healing of any breach in the skin is delayed, this should be brought to the attention of the attending practitioner or nurse. Sudden changes in skin color or pain should also be reported. Sitting too close to open fires or radiant heaters of any kind should be strongly discouraged. During winter months, adequate and appropriate warm clothing should be worn, such as long johns, thick tights, or socks.

Hot water bottles or electric blankets may be used to heat the bed but not the individual. Bottles should be removed from the bed and electric blankets switched off before retiring. Loose-fitting bed socks help maintain warmth. Garters should not be used where the circulation of the limb is compromised.

Patients should avoid footwear with pointed toe boxes. This is a frequent cause of impaired circulation in the toes. Hosiery should be free of darns and ridges. Shoes should be inspected before wearing for any roughness, nails, or even foreign bodies that have dropped into the shoe. Neuropathic feet will be insensitive to such problems and may cause significant and serious damage.

Foot health information and preventive strategies for the older patient, particularly with an "at-risk" concern can be found in the *FEET FIRST* and *IF THE SHOE FITS* booklets and videos, available from the Pennsylvania Department of Health, Diabetes Control Program, Harrisburg, PA (USA).

A professional education program entitled *Assessing the Older Diabetic Foot* is also available from the same source (Helfand, 2001).

FOOTWEAR

The treatment and long-term management of foot morbidities cannot be successful without the foot being adequately accommodated in footwear. The shoe or boot must have adequate width, depth, and length, especially in the region of the toes. A lace-up shoe ensures that the foot and shoe are held in the correct relationship as well as having the added virtue that the lace is infinitely adjustable – important where the foot may enlarge because of edema. The Thermold shoe is an example of such a shoe. The Darco Shoe, Hotter, or Walker style is ideal when specific dressing changes are required. High arched feet do sometimes have difficulty with a high lacing shoe. Here a slip-on shoe with an elasticized gusset may be more acceptable. An alternative may be an elastic lace. This is also useful when the patient is unable to tie his/her shoes. A broad heel with a maximum height of 1/5 in. (38 mm) will provide stability. The cobbler, floating it out or flaring the heel on one side or the other to further enhance stability, can modify such a heel (Burns, 2002; Cailliet, 1997).

The upper of boots or shoes should be plain – devoid of fancy stitching or designs, which involve the overlapping of several pieces of the upper material. These all limit the "give" of the material and the footwear fails to mold and accommodate minor foot deformities, such as hammer toes and bunion deformities.

Traditionally, leather has been the best material for the uppers of footwear, but very satisfactory man-made materials can provide lighter and economical made-to-measure footwear for patients with feet deformed by disease or altered in shape as a result of surgical intervention.

Synthetic materials used for the sole and heels of modern footwear have good wearing qualities. Their thickness provides a surface, which is shock absorbing and insulating. Modern manufacturing processes easily produce shoes that are relatively waterproof. Flexion of the first metatarsal-phalangeal joint can be limited by the addition of a steel splint or rocker sole. This can also be helpful in the management of osteoarthrosis of the first metatarsal-phalangeal joint or in incipient rigidity of this joint. Patients should be encouraged to keep all footwear in good repair. Serious injuries to the ligaments of the ankle and subtalar joints are frequently the result of badly worn heels (Helfand, 1995, 1996, 1998).

ORTHOTICS

The prolonged application to the foot of adhesive pads and dressings is undesirable, even with modern hypoallergic adhesives. It is also aesthetically unacceptable. The warmth and moisture resulting from occlusion of the skin may provoke contact dermatitis or infection, particularly in the elderly. Because of the fact that for many elderly patients, correction or cure is not possible, comfort becomes a primary goal. Deformities may need to remain but care should be directed to relieving pain, restoring a maximum level of function, and maintaining that restored degree of pain free activity. Many forms of orthotics are available. Some include the chairside fabrication of silicone molds. Others include devices that can be made to prescription and fabricated from man-made materials of varying thickness and density. Thermoplastic materials may be combined in one orthotic to give cushioning or support or redistribute the pressure load. These are all fabricated to meet the individual needs of individual patients and the presenting condition. The resulting appliance is more desirable and aesthetically more pleasing since it can be removed, cleaned, and utilized in many pairs of footwear (Helfand and Bruno, 1984).

Where patients are unable to fit and remove these devices themselves, relatives or neighbors can help. A molded shoe, made from light microcellular material and able to accommodate the most bizarre deformities is the only other alternative, if need be. Sandals may be a satisfactory alternative also, where the condition and climate are suitable.

KEY POINTS

- Podogeriatrics is that special area of podiatric medical practice that focuses on health promotion, prevention, and the treatment and management of foot and related problems, disability, deformity, and the pedal complications of chronic diseases in later life.
- Foot problems are common in the older population as a result of disease, deformity, complications, and neglect, resulting from a lack of preventive service, at the primary, secondary, and tertiary levels. They contribute to disability and can reduce an older persons independence and quality of life.
- It has been estimated in the United States, that 50%–75% of all amputations relating to the complications associated with diabetes mellitus could be prevented and reduced with an appropriate program of preventive foot care and foot health education.
- Because of the risk involved in the geriatric patient and the relationship to multiple chronic diseases, assessment, examination, and evaluation of the feet of the elderly is essential. Essential as elements of this process include needs, relationships to ambulation and activities of daily living, and the fact that foot pain can result in functional disability, dysfunction, and increase dependency.
- For the older patient, the ability to prevent complications, maintain mobility, and continue to ambulate will be reflected in the quality of life and permit older individuals to live life, to the end of life.

KEY REFERENCES

- Helfand AE. In BJ Goldstein & D Muller-Wieland (eds) *Diabetic Foot – Assessment, Management, and Prevention, Textbook of Type 2 Diabetes* 2003a; Martin Dunitz, London.
- Helfand AE. *Clinical Podogeriatrics: Assessment, Education, and Prevention* 2003b; W. B. Saunders Company, Philadelphia.
- Lorimer D, French G, O'Donnell M & Burrow JG. *Neale's Disorders of the Foot, Diagnosis and Management* 2002, 6th edn; Churchill Livingstone, New York.
- Merriman LM & Turner W. *Assessment of the Lower Limb* 2002, 2nd edn; Churchill Livingstone, London.
- Robbins JM. *Primary Podiatric Medicine* 1994; W. B. Saunders Company, Philadelphia.
- Tollafield DR & Merriman LM. *Clinical Skills in Treating the Foot* 1997; Churchill Livingstone, New York.

REFERENCES

Alexander IJ. *The Foot: Examination and Diagnosis* 1997, 2nd edn; Churchill Livingstone, New York.

American College of Foot & Ankle Surgeons. *Diabetic Foot Disorders – A Clinical Practice Guideline* 2000; Park Ridge.

American Diabetes Association. Preventive foot care in people with diabetes. *Diabetes Care* 2003; **26**(suppl 1):S78–9.

Baran R, Dawber RPR, Tosti A *et al. A Text Atlas of Nail Disorders, Diagnosis and Treatment* 1996; Mosby, St. Louis.

Baran R, Hay R, Haneke E *et al. Onychomycosis, the Current Approach to Diagnosis and Therapy* 1999; Martin Dunitz, London.

Bild DE, Selby JV, Sinnock P *et al.* Lower extremity amputation in people with diabetes, epidemiology and prevention. *Diabetes Care* 1989; **12**(1):23–31.

Birrer RB, Dellacorte MP & Grisafi PJ. *Common Foot Problems in Primary Care* 1998, 2nd edn; Henley & Belfus, Philadelphia.

Bolton AJM, Connor H & Cavanagh PR. *The Foot in Diabetes* 2000, 3rd edn; John Wiley & Sons, Chichester.

Bottomley JM & Lewis CB. *Geriatric Rehabilitation: A Clinical Approach* 2003; Prentice Hall, Upper Saddle River.

Bowker JH & Pfeifer MA. *Levin's & Oneal's the Diabetic Foot* 2001, 6th edn; Mosby, St. Louis.

Brodie BS. Health determinants and podiatry. *Journal of the Royal Society for the Promotion of Health* 2001; **121**(3):174–6.

Burns SL. Older people and ill-fitting shoes. *Postgraduate Medical Journal* 2002; **78**(920):344–6.

Cailliet R. *Foot and Ankle Pain* 1997, 3rd edn; F. A. Davis Company, Philadelphia.

Cavanagh PR, Boone EY & Plummer DL. *The Foot in Diabetes: A Bibliography* 2000; Pennsylvania State University, State College.

Centers for Medicare & Medicaid Services. *Program Manual, Foot Care and Supportive Devices for Feet* 2002; Baltimore, Chapter H, Section 2323, 03/27/2002; and Highmark Government Services. *Medicare Report, Coverage Requirements for Routine Foot Care (June 2, 2002)* 2002a; pp 33–6, Camp Hill.

Centers for Medicare & Medicaid Services. *Transmittal AB-02-096: Coverage and Billing of the Diagnosis and Treatment of Peripheral Neuropathy With Loss of Protective Sensation in People With Diabetes* 2002b; Baltimore, 07/17/2002.

Collet BS. Foot disorders. In BH Beers & R Berkow (eds) *The Merck Manual of Geriatrics* 2000, 17th edn; Merck & Company, Rathway.

Crausman RS & Glod DJ. Special topics in internal medicine and geriatrics. *Journal of the American Podiatric Medical Association* 2004; **94**(2):85–209.

Dauber R, Bristow I & Turner W. *Text Atlas of Podiatric Dermatology* 2001; Martin Dunitz, London.

Edmonds ME, Foster AVM & Saunders LJ. *A Practical Manual of Diabetic Footcare* 2004; Blackwell Publishing, Malden.

Evans JG, Williams TF, Michel J-P & Beattie B. *Oxford Textbook of Geriatric Medicine* 2000, 2nd edn; Oxford University Press, England.

Frykberg RG. *The High Risk Foot in Diabetes Mellitus* 1991; Churchill Livingstone, New York.

Helfand AE (ed). *Clinical Podogeriatrics* 1981; Williams and Wilkins, Baltimore.

Helfand AE (ed). *Public Health and Podiatric Medicine* 1987; Williams and Wilkins, Baltimore.

Helfand AE (ed). *The Geriatric Patient and Considerations of Aging, Clinics in Podiatric Medicine and Surgery* 1993a, vols I, II; W.B. Saunders Company, Philadelphia, PA, USA.

Helfand AE. Geriatric overview: Part I. *The Foot* 1993b; **3**:58–61;and Geriatric overview: Part II. *The Foot* 1995; **5**:19–23.

Helfand AE. *Feet First* 1995; Pennsylvania Diabetes Academy, Harrisburg.

Helfand E. What you need to know about therapeutic footwear. *Practical Diabetology* 1996; **15**(4):4–9.

Helfand AE. *IF the Shoe Fits* 1998; Pennsylvania Diabetes Academy, Harrisburg.

Helfand AE. Public health strategies to develop a comprehensive chronic disease and podogeriatric protocol. *National Academies of Practice Forum* 1999; **1**(1):49–57.

Helfand AE. A conceptual model for a geriatric syllabus for podiatric medicine. *Journal of the American Podiatric Medical Association* 2000; **90**(5):258–67.

Helfand AE. *Assessing the Older Diabetic Patient, CD* 2001; Pennsylvania Diabetes Academy, Pennsylvania Department of Health, Temple University, School of Medicine, Office for Continuing Medical Education, Temple University, School of Podiatric Medicine, Harrisburg.

Helfand AE. *Disorders and Diseases of the Foot, Geriatric Review Syllabus, A Core Curriculum in Geriatric Medicine* 2002, 5th edn, pp 287–94; Blackwell Publishing Company, Malden.

Helfand AE. In BJ Goldstein & D Muller-Wieland (eds) *Diabetic Foot – Assessment, Management, and Prevention, Textbook of Type 2 Diabetes* 2003a; Martin Dunitz, London.

Helfand AE. *Clinical Podogeriatrics: Assessment, Education, and Prevention* 2003b; W. B. Saunders Company, Philadelphia.

Helfand AE. Foot problems in older patients, a focused podogeriatric assessment study in ambulatory care. *Journal of the American Podiatric Medical Association* 2004a; **94**(3):293–304.

Helfand AE. Clinical assessment of podogeriatric patients. *Podiatry Management* 2004b; **23**(2):145–52.

Helfand AE & Bruno J (eds). *Rehabilitation of the Foot, Clinics in Podiatry* 1984, vol 1, number 2; W. B. Saunders Company.

Helfand AE & Jessett DF. Foot problems. In MSJ Pathy (ed). *Principles and Practice of Geriatric Medicine* 1998, 3rd edn; John Wiley & Sons, Edinburgh.

Helfand AE & Motter DF. *Podogeriatric Assessment, Geriatric Secrets* 2004, 3rd edn, pp 146–9; Hanley & Belfus, Philadelphia.

Jessett DF & Helfand AE. Foot problems in the elderly. In MSJ Pathy (ed) *Principles and Practice of Geriatric Medicine* 1991, 2nd edn; John Wiley & Sons, Edinburgh.

Kozak GP, Campbell DR, Frykberg RG *et al. Management of Diabetic Foot Problems* 1995, 2nd edn; W.B. Saunders Company, Philadelphia.

Lorimer D, French G, O'Donnell M & Burrow JG. *Neale's Disorders of the Foot, Diagnosis and Management* 2002, 6th edn; Churchill Livingstone, New York.

Merriman LM & Tollafield DR. *Assessment of the Lower Limb* 1995; Churchill Livingstone, New York.

Merriman LM & Turner W. *Assessment of the Lower Limb* 2002, 2nd edn; Churchill Livingstone, London.

Robbins JM. *Primary Podiatric Medicine* 1994; W. B. Saunders Company, Philadelphia.

Strauss H & Spielfogel WD. *Foot Disorders in the Elderly, Clinical Geriatrics* 2003, pp 595–602; The Parthenon Publishing Company, New York.

Tollafield DR & Merriman LM. *Clinical Skills in Treating the Foot* 1997; Churchill Livingstone, New York.

114

Hip Fracture and Orthogeriatrics

Antony Johansen *and* Martyn Parker
University Hospital of Wales, Cardiff, UK

BACKGROUND

Fractures affecting elderly people are a major and increasing health problem in the Western world. Over 40% of women and 13% of men will sustain an osteoporotic fracture during their lifetime (Melton *et al.*, 1992). The incidence and cost of osteoporotic fractures will rise by 1% per year – simply as a result of aging of the population (Burge *et al.*, 2001).

Fracture risk is multifactorial and reflects general frailty and falls-risk as much as it does bone fragility. Each year, 8% of women over 85 years of age will suffer a fracture. Hip fracture is the predominant injury in these older women with an annual fracture risk of 4% at the hip compared to 1.5% at the wrist and forearm, 0.6% at the upper arm, and 0.4% each at spine, hand, foot, and ankle (Johansen *et al.*, 1997). People living in residential and nursing homes are at nine times greater risk than the general population (Brennan *et al.*, 2003).

Patient frailty is reflected in the outcome of the injury, with around 10% of people dying in hospital within a month of their fracture. Over one-third of people will die during the year after fracture. The hip fracture can be shown to be responsible for less than half of these deaths (Parker and Anand, 1991), but the patient and their family will often identify the hip fracture as playing a central part in their final illness. A quarter of hip fractures affect residents in institutional care, and the distress of this illness can be compounded by recrimination in respect of failure to prevent the fall and fracture in the first place.

Only half of those who survive hip fracture will return to their previous level of independence. Most who survive the injury can expect to be left with at least some hip discomfort, and around half will suffer deterioration in their walking ability such that they will need an additional walking aid or physical help with mobility. 10–20% of people will need to move to a more supportive residence such as residential or nursing care. Such a move is greatly feared by patients, and in a study of quality of life 80% of elderly women indicated that they would prefer to die, rather than lose their independence as a result of a "bad hip fracture" that required their placement in a nursing home (Salkeld *et al.*, 2000).

Figures vary considerably between units, but length of stay in the orthopedic ward averages between 2 and 3 weeks, and overall hospital stay may average as much as 5 weeks. This leads to a cost of operation and hospital stay of around £7000 per case. The cost of complex home and institutional care for those individuals who make a poor recovery can be very high, leading to a mean cost of medical and social aftercare in the first 2 years of £13 000 and a cost of hip fracture of £20 000 overall (Torgerson and Dolan, 2000).

This profile of mortality, morbidity, loss of independence, and the resulting clinical and financial burden on health and social services underpins the need for effective management of this injury. The complexity of multiprofessional cooperation that is necessary for effective hip fracture care makes this condition an ideal tracer condition for the hospital care of frail and elderly people in general.

DIAGNOSIS

The typical presentation of a patient with a hip fracture is an elderly woman, who has tripped and fallen while walking within her own home (Parker *et al.*, 1997). Her symptoms are pain in the hip and inability to walk. Clinical examination reveals a shortened and externally rotated limb with any attempt at moving the hip-causing pain. The diagnosis is readily confirmed by x-ray.

Unfortunately in about 10–15% of patients the diagnosis is missed or delayed (Pathak *et al.*, 1997). The reasons for this may be:

- patient or carers do not seek medical help
- patients seen by doctor but no xray requested
- x-rays undertaken, but misinterpreted as not showing a fracture

Principles and Practice of Geriatric Medicine, 4th Edition. Edited by M.S. John Pathy, Alan J. Sinclair and John E. Morley.

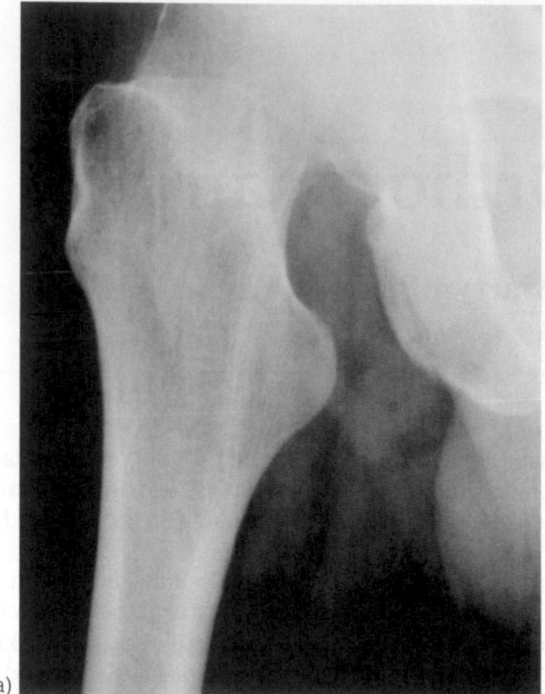

(a)

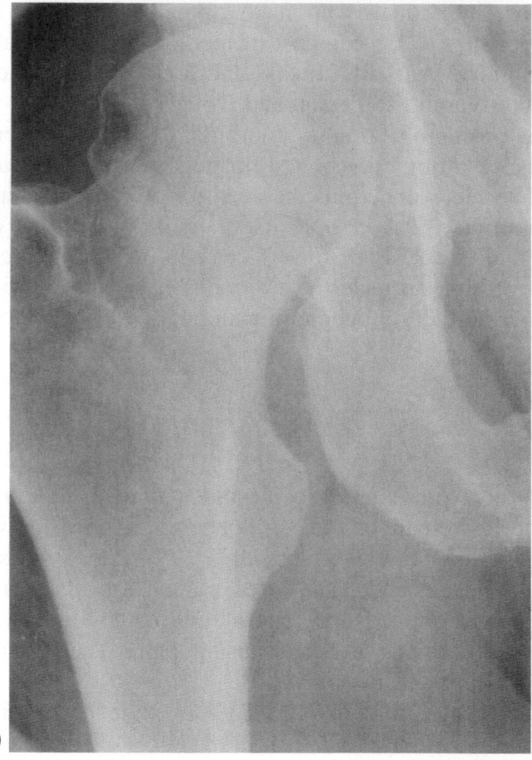

(b)

Figure 1 (a,b) An undisplaced intracapsular fracture, which only becomes apparent on an x-ray take in 10° internal rotation

- x-rays of such poor quality such that the fracture was missed
- fracture not visible on x-rays even with hindsight.

Factors contributing to missing the diagnosis include absence of a history of a fall in 5% of patients (Pathak *et al.*, 1997). The fracture may very rarely occur spontaneously or be related to a pathological weakness of the bone. Confusion and dementia may make the history and interpretation of physical finding more difficult. Approximately 15% of fractures are undisplaced which will mean there is no shortening or external rotation of the limb, hip movements, although painful, may be possible, and the patient may even be able to walk, albeit with difficulty. The x-ray changes of an undisplaced fracture may be minimal or even completely absent in about 1% of hip fractures.

Some experience is necessary in interpreting hip x-rays for suspected fractures. Firstly, two views must always be taken; an anterioposterior (AP) and a lateral view. The basic AP view is of the pelvis with hips at the bottom corners of the film. The x-ray beam is not centered on the hip. In addition, for a person with a painful hip, the leg is generally in external rotation. This external rotation means the greater trochanter lies posterior to the femoral neck obscuring details for this area (Figure 1). For an ideal hip AP view, the limb should be in 10 degrees of internal rotation so that the femoral neck is at right angles to the x-ray beam. Such a film will enable a "hidden" fracture to become visible (Figure 1).

No patient can have a hip fracture excluded without a lateral x-ray. The correct exposure of such films may be difficult in order to get good clarity of detail in the femoral neck. For those patients in whom the pelvis and lateral x-rays appear normal but a hip fracture is suspected, a third view is indicated. This is an AP with the film centered on the hip in question with 10 degrees internal rotation.

If doubt about the diagnosis of a fracture persists, additional investigations are indicated. An MRI scan is currently the investigation of choice. Alternative investigations are an isotope bone scan or CT scan of the hip. Another management option is to repeat the x rays after a delay of 1 to 2 weeks. Any invisible fracture or those with minimal radiographic changes will become apparent. The physician must be aware that the presence of apparent normal initial x-rays does not exclude a hip fracture.

In addition to the unnecessary pain caused by missing a fracture, an undisplaced fracture generally displaces if left untreated. The outcome for an undisplaced fracture is better than that for a displaced fracture, particularly if the fracture is intracapsular. Prolonged delays in diagnosis may have devastating consequences for the patient. Treatment for a late diagnosed fracture is more complex, and recovery of function is less likely.

CLASSIFICATION

Once the diagnosis has been established, the fracture may be classified depending on the site of the femur in which the fracture line is predominately located (Figure 2). The blood supply to the femoral head enters along the line of the hip capsule's attachment and this explains the importance of drawing a distinction between intracapsular and extracapsular fractures in terms of diagnosis and management.

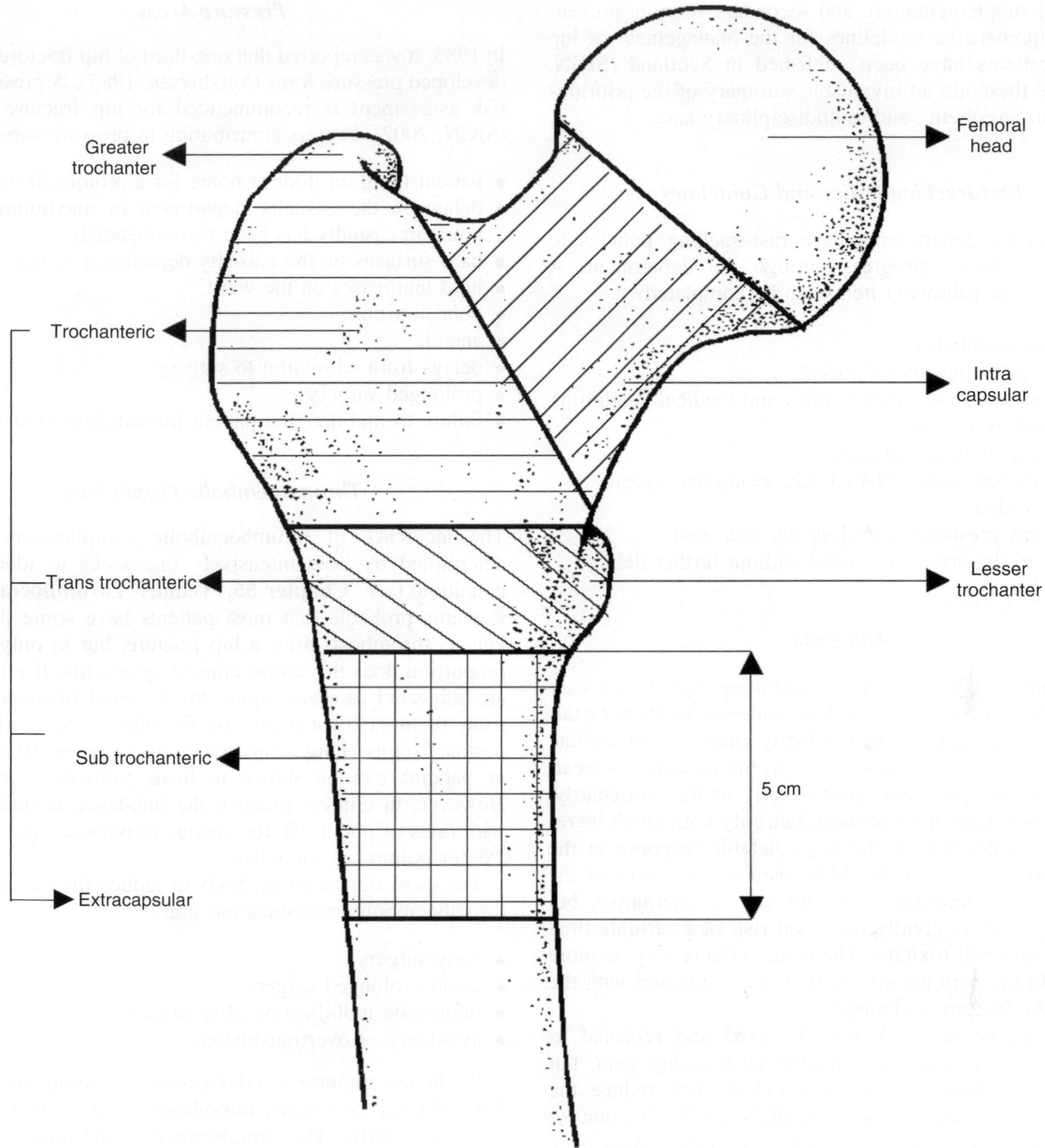

Figure 2 Radiographic classification of hip fractures

Intracapsular fracture may be subdivided into those which are essentially undisplaced (Figure 1) and those which are displaced. Extracapsular fractures are divided into trochanteric and subtrochanteric. Basal fractures are two-part fractures in which the fracture line runs along the intertrochanteric line. These fractures are uncommon and best thought of as two part trochanteric fractures. Trochanteric fractures may be subdivided into two part fractures, which are also termed *stable fractures*, and comminuted or multifragmentary, which may be termed *unstable fractures*. Subtrochanteric fractures are those in which the fracture is predominately in the 5 cm of bone immediately distal to the lesser trochanter.

INITIAL MANAGEMENT

The Cochrane collaboration has considered the published evidence in respect of hip fracture care, and has identified a number of key interventions that can be shown to improve outcome. These include perioperative prophylaxis against infection and thromboembolism, attention to nutritional supplementation, and secondary fracture prevention. Comprehensive guidelines for the management of hip fracture patients have been published in Scotland (SIGN, 2002), and these are an invaluable summary of the priorities of surgical, anesthetic, and multidisciplinary care.

Fast-tracking Policy and Guidelines

Many casualty departments have fast-tracking policies to speed the patient's progress through the department. A checklist of the following items can be completed:

- diagnosis established
- pressure relieving mattress used
- patient assessed for other injuries and medical conditions
- pain relief as appropriate
- intravenous fluids commenced
- routine bloods taken (FBC, U&E, group and save)
- ECG recorded
- chest x-ray presurgery, if clinically indicated
- transfer to the orthopedic ward without further delay.

Analgesia

The amount of pain experienced after a hip fracture can vary from moderate to severe. Therefore analgesia needs to be tailored to the individual patient. Initially and in the immediate postoperative period opiates still form the mainstay of treatment. These are preferably given orally or intramuscularly. Intravenous opiates may be used, but only with small incremental doses because of the unpredictable response in the elderly. Other analgesia should be paracetamol and codeine phosphate. Nonsteroidal analgesics are an alternative, but older people are at greatly increased risk of gastrointestinal bleeding and renal toxicity. These side effects may be more common in the perioperative period in conjunction with the stress of the fracture and surgery.

A femoral nerve block may be used and repeated as required. Such blocks are effective in reducing pain, but it remains unproven as to what extent they reduce the complications related to analgesia (SIGN, 2002). Traction for a hip fracture prior to surgery is no longer used, having been shown to have no benefit in reducing pain (SIGN, 2002).

Fluid Balance and Resuscitation

At the time of admission to hospital the patient may be dehydrated from lack of fluid intake, particularly if they have been unable to seek help for some time. In addition, there will be a variable amount of blood loss from the fracture site. This loss will vary from a few milliliters for an undisplaced intracapsular fracture to over a liter for a multifragmentary or subtrochanteric fracture. Intravenous saline should be started from the time of admission in casualty; the rate of infusion adjusted according to the estimated blood loss and degree of dehydration.

Pressure Areas

In 1985, it was reported that one-third of hip fracture patients developed pressure sores (Versluysen, 1985). A pressure sore risk assessment is recommended for hip fracture patients (SIGN, 2002). Factors contributing to pressure sores are:

- patient lying on floor at home for a prolonged time;
- delays in the casualty department (a maximum of two hours in casualty has been recommended)
- hard surfaces on the casualty department trolleys
- hard mattresses on the ward
- poor nutrition
- anemia
- delays from admission to surgery
- prolonged surgery
- failure to mobilize the patient immediately after surgery.

Thromboembolic Prophylaxis

The incidence of thromboembolic complication will be determined by how intensively one seeks to identify the condition (*see* **Chapter 55, Venous Thromboembolism**). It seems probable that most patients have some degree of venous thrombosis after a hip fracture, but in only a small proportion does this cause clinical symptoms. If all patients are subjected to venography, the reported incidence varies from 19 to 91% for deep vein thrombosis. Similarly, when routine isotope lung scans are used, between 10 and 14% of patients can be shown to have pulmonary embolism. However, in clinical practice the incidence is much lower with rates of about 3% for venous thrombosis and of about 1% for pulmonary embolism.

The most important methods to reduce the occurrence of thromboembolic complications are:

- early surgery
- avoid prolonged surgery
- immediate mobilization after surgery
- avoidance of overtransfusion.

Cyclic leg compression devices or foot pumps may reduce the incidence of venous thrombosis from 19 to 6% (Handoll *et al.*, 2004). They are, however, quite time-consuming to use and can be expensive. Controversy continues over whether any pharmacological prophylaxis should be given, what is the best pharmacological agent, and the duration of prophylaxis. The incidence of clinically significant thrombosis has declined as a result of earlier surgery and mobilisation. These changes may now mean that the adverse effects of therapy outweigh any benefits from the reduced thromboembolic complications.

Heparins reduced the incidence of venographic thrombosis from 39 to 24%, but in a systematic review of randomized trials (Handoll *et al.*, 2004), overall mortality showed a trend to be increased with heparin (8 vs. 11%). Warfarin, while popular in the United States has not been adequately assessed within randomized trials. Low dose aspirin has been studied in one large randomized trial (PEP Trial, 2000). 28 days of 150 mg aspirin reduced clinical endpoints of deep vein thrombosis from 1.5 to 1.0%, nonfatal pulmonary embolism from 0.6 to 0.4% and fatal pulmonary embolism from 0.6 to 0.3%. The incidence of wound healing complications was increased in the aspirin group (2.4 to 3.0%), as was gastrointestinal hemorrhage (2.1 to 3.1%). There was no difference in mortality between groups.

Nutrition

Poor nutritional state is a powerful risk factor for hip fracture, and practical problems with feeding and nutrition commonly pose a major threat to recovery following the injury. Many people do not eat and drink adequate amounts while in hospital, putting their health and recovery from illness at risk (*see* **Chapter 24, Epidemiology of Nutrition and Aging**). Dietary insufficiency is a significant problem, with many frail elderly inpatients achieving only half their recommended daily energy, protein, and other nutritional requirements (Duncan *et al.*, 2001). Nutrition is an interdisciplinary concern that requires effective liaison and communication between all members of the clinical and operational services teams. A number of approaches to nutritional support have been studied (Avenell and Handoll, 2004).

The strongest evidence for the effectiveness of nutritional supplementation exists for oral protein and energy feeds, but the evidence is still very weak as the quality of trials to date is poor. Oral multinutrient feeds (providing energy, protein, vitamins, and minerals), evaluated by seven trials, may reduce the risk of death or complications (Avenell and Handoll, 2004). Four randomized trials examining nasogastric feeding showed no evidence for an effect on mortality. The effect of protein in an oral feed, tested in three trials, showed no evidence for any effect on mortality, but may have reduced the number of long-term complications and days spent in rehabilitation wards.

In practical terms it is unrealistic to impose nasogastric feeding as a routine approach to nutritional supplementation, and patients' acceptance of supplement drinks is often poor. It is therefore crucial that all staff dealing with patients recovering from hip fracture understand the importance of adequate dietary intake and that specific attention is given to helping people to eat at meal times. Simple practical measures can be very effective in this respect (Duncan *et al.*, 2002).

FRACTURE REPAIR

Conservative or Operative Treatment

Historically, hip fractures were managed conservatively by traction, bed rest, or "skillful neglect". Clinical studies including some randomized trials have indicated improved outcomes for those treated operatively. This is particularly true for displaced intracapsular fractures, where conservative treatment leads to nonunion of the fracture and a painful hip of limited function. With the appropriate medical facilities and surgical and anesthetic expertise, the vast majority of hip fractures will be managed surgically.

Undisplaced intracapsular fracture may be treated conservatively with a regime of bed rest followed by gentle mobilization. The risk of nonunion of the fracture treated conservatively is about 30 to 50%. This falls to about 5–10% after internal fixation. Nonunion generally requires treatment with a replacement arthroplasty; therefore most surgeons elect to treat this type of fracture surgically by internal fixation.

For displaced intracapsular fractures, nonunion is inevitable after conservative treatment. This means that the hip cannot be used for weight bearing and is generally painful on all movements. Conservative treatment may be employed for those with very limited life expectancy or the immobile, but even for those of limited mobility, surgery is useful to relieve pain and provide a limb that can be used for limited walking or transfers (Hay and Parker, 2003).

Extracapsular fractures may be managed conservatively using traction. Traction will reduce the fracture, enabling it to heal in a reasonable position. Conservative treatment will inevitably result in a markedly increased hospital stay and an increase in the number of patients who are unable to return back to their original residence, in comparison with operative treatment (Hornby *et al.*, 1989). Conservative treatment for extracapsular fractures is therefore recommended for only those patients of a very limited life expectancy, those who refuse surgery, and in the absence of appropriate surgical facilities.

The presence of specialized medical staff in the acute orthopedic ward is of benefit in improving preoperative medical assessment so that surgery is not unnecessarily delayed. Many frail older people presenting with hip fractures will need to undergo surgery while their medical state remains suboptimal. The decision as to whether hip fracture surgery can go ahead is not the same as that appropriate for elective orthopedic surgery, where postponement carries little risk to the patient's long-term functional outcome and survival. In the setting of hip fracture the question is whether there is anything that can be done that will immediately improve the patient's operative risk so that surgery can go ahead. Judgment of whether surgery is appropriate despite the presence of acute and chronic medical problems can be difficult, and is eased by the involvement of clinical staff familiar with the assessment and treatment of older people.

Operative Care

Undisplaced Intracapsular Fractures

Undisplaced intracapsular fractures, as illustrated in Figure 1, may be managed conservatively as discussed earlier, but to reduce the risk of the fracture displacing, internal fixation is recommended. This is a relatively minor surgical procedure, which can even be undertaken using local nerve blocks

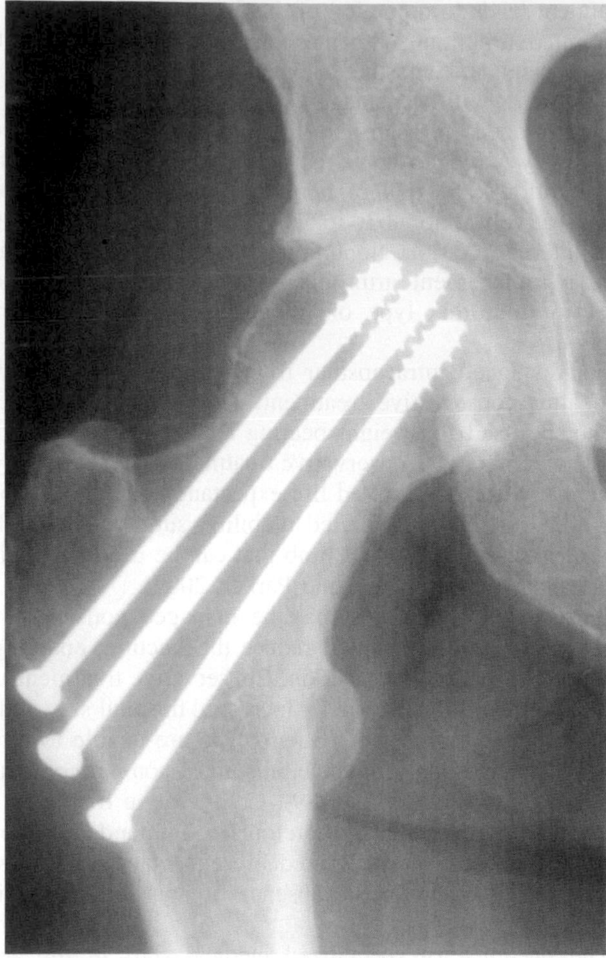

Figure 3 An intracapsular fracture fixed with three screws

and a percutaneous procedure. There are many different implants used, the most frequently used being two or three parallel screws (Figure 3) or a sliding hip screw (SHS). Postoperatively, most patients recover quickly with hospital stays of 7–10 days. Arthroplasty is not an appropriate method of treatment for this fracture type because of the increased surgical trauma and risk of postoperative complications.

Displaced Intracapsular Fractures

Surgical management of this fracture is either by internal fixation as illustrated in Figure 3 or using an arthroplasty (Figure 4). The main advantages and disadvantages of internal fixation and their approximated incidences of complications are:

- patients are able to retain their own femoral head
- less surgical trauma giving marginally lower mortality and morbidity
- low risk of wound sepsis (up to 1%)
- low risk of wound hematoma (1–2%)
- risk of nonunion incurred (20–33%)

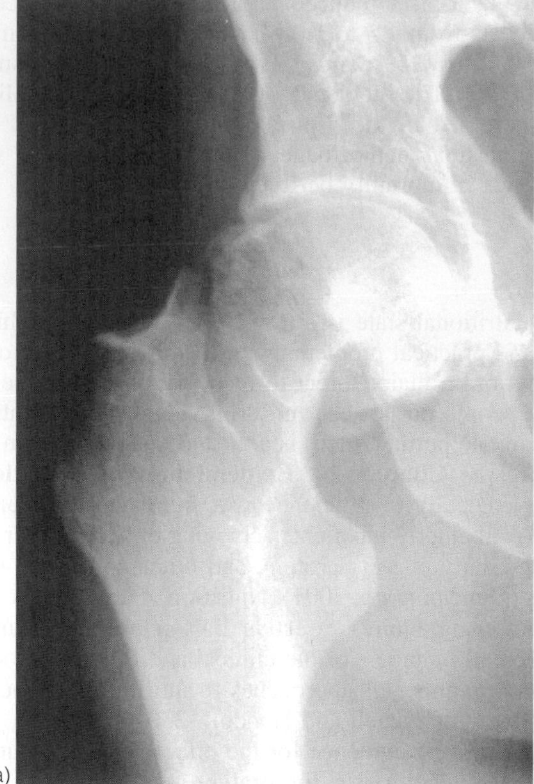

(a)

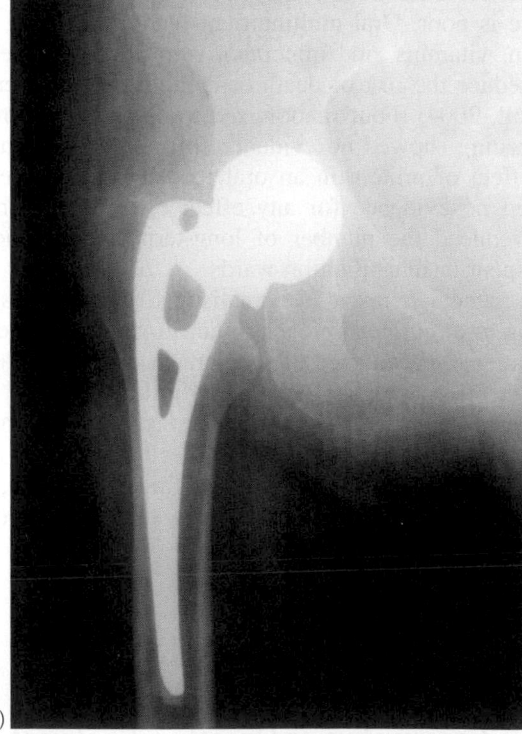

(b)

Figure 4 (a,b) A displaced intracapsular fracture treated with an uncemented Austin Moore hemiarthroplasty

- risk of avascular necrosis incurred (10–20%)
- risk of fracture around the implant (1–2%)
- markedly increased reoperation rate (20–36%).

For arthroplasty the advantages and disadvantages are:

- lower reoperation rate (6–18%)
- larger surgical procedure than internal fixation
- increased risk of deep infection around the implant (3%)
- increased risk of superficial wound infection (5–15%)
- increased risk of wound hematoma (2–5%)
- risk of dislocation incurred (2–5%)
- risk of fracture around implant (1–3%)
- later risk of prosthesis loosening (2–10%)
- later risk of acetabular wear (4–20%).

The main factor influencing choice of treatment is the risk of nonunion. Factors that will increase this risk are delays from fracture occurrence to fixation, pathological lesions of the bone such as tumor or Paget's disease, metabolic bone disease, and rheumatoid arthritis. Table 1 details the recommended treatment methods for the different situations.

Considerable controversy still exists about the optimum choice of treatment for an elderly patient with a displaced intracapsular fracture. By "elderly" one is referring to someone of around the age of 70 years, although others may choose a more functional assessment such as, an elderly patient is one who has some restriction in mobility or activities of daily living. The Cochrane review on this topic (Masson *et al.*, 2003) concludes that both treatment methods produce similar final function results of pain and regain of function. Internal fixation has a tendency to a lower mortality but an increased reoperation rate.

If arthroplasty is chosen as the method of treatment, a "partial" hip replacement may be used with only the femoral head being replaced (hemiarthroplasty) (Figure 4). Alternatively, a total hip replacement can be used, in which the acetabular articular surface is also replaced. The hemiarthroplasties entail a less complicated surgical procedure than a total hip arthroplasty and have a lower risk of dislocation. Therefore, they tend to be preferred to a total hip arthroplasty for the frail elderly patient, but controversy still exists about the final functional results and later requirement for revision surgery. The limited randomized trials to date on this topic have been summarized in a Cochrane review on this topic (Parker and Gurusamy, 2004).

An arthroplasty may be either cemented in place or uncemented as a press fit. No clear consensus exists which is better. Cementing does add the possibility of additional operative problems and should a later revision arthroplasty be necessary, it is more difficult for a cemented implant. However using cement may make the hip less painful with better function (Parker and Gurusamy, 2004).

Table 1 Possible treatment methods for displaced intracapsular fractures

	Internal fixation	Arthroplasty
Rheumatoid arthritis	Occasionally	Generally
Delay in treatment	Rarely	Generally
Pathological fractures	Rarely	Generally
Chronic renal failure	Rarely	Generally
Metabolic bone disease	Rarely	Generally
Arthritis of joint	Rarely	Generally
Paget's disease	Never	Always
Age less than about 70 years	Generally	Rarely
Age more than about 70 years	Occasionally	Generally

Trochanteric Fractures

A variety of implant are available for the treatment of this fracture. The SHS remains the foremost implant and should be regarded as the gold standard (Figure 5). It is also termed the *dynamic hip screw, compression hip screw* or *Abmi hip screw*. Numerous case series reports and randomized trials have all demonstrated the superiority of this implant over other designs. The more recently developed implants are the short intramedullary nails, which have shown considerable developments over the last 10 years. These include the Gamma nail, intramedullary hip screw (IMHS), proximal femoral nail (PFN), Holland nail, and Targon nail. Comparisons of these implants against the SHS have been made in numerous randomized trials, the summary of which showed an increased risk of fracture-healing complications (7.5 vs. 3.6%) and an increased reoperation rate (5.6 vs. 3.5%) for the nails (Parker and Handoll, 2004). The main problem with the nails was the occurrence of fractures at the tip of the intramedullary nails, and it may be that future modification to the design of these nails will reduce this complication.

Subtrochanteric Fractures

These fracture are less common accounting for about 5–10% of all hip fractures. They present a considerable challenge to the surgeon as the high mechanical forces in this area of bone leads to an increased risk of fixation failure. The SHS remains an acceptable method of treatment for this fracture, but is a technically difficult surgical procedure and requires an extensive surgical exposure. An alternative method of treatment is using an intramedullary nail (Figure 6). This method of treatment is currently becoming more extensively used as the design of these nails and instrumentation to accompany them continues to improve.

POSTOPERATIVE CARE

After surgery, it should be normal practice to sit the patient out of bed and begin to stand the patient on the day after surgery. After this, progress will vary considerably and will depend on each individual patient and the type of their fracture. Patients with an extracapsular fracture will tend to take longer to mobilize than those with intracapsular fractures.

Weight Bearing

With current surgical techniques and implants, there should be very few occasions in which weight bearing is restricted.

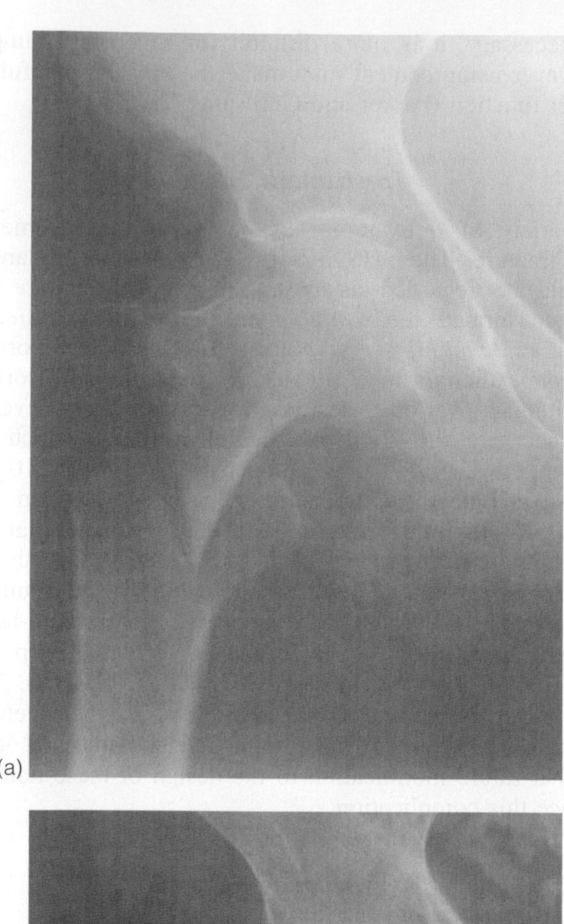

(a)

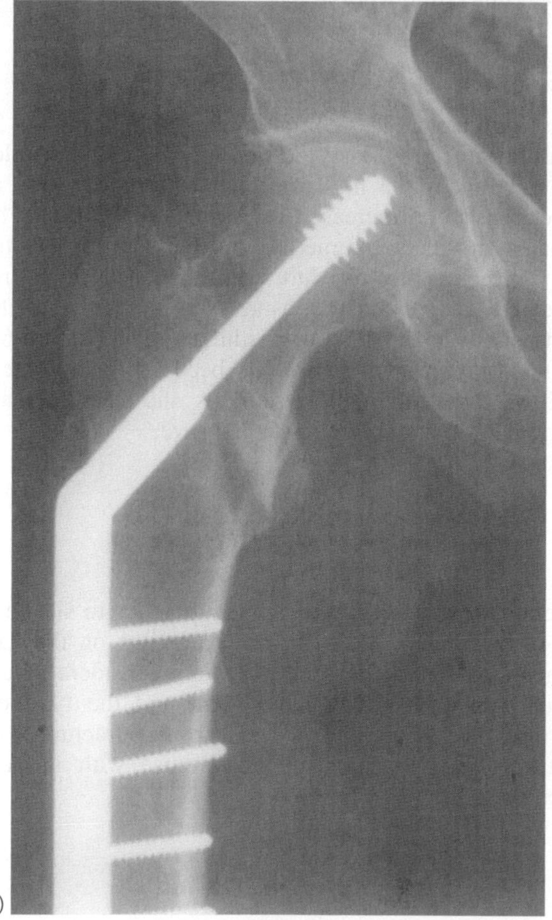

(b)

Figure 5 (a,b) A trochanteric fracture fixed with a sliding hip screw

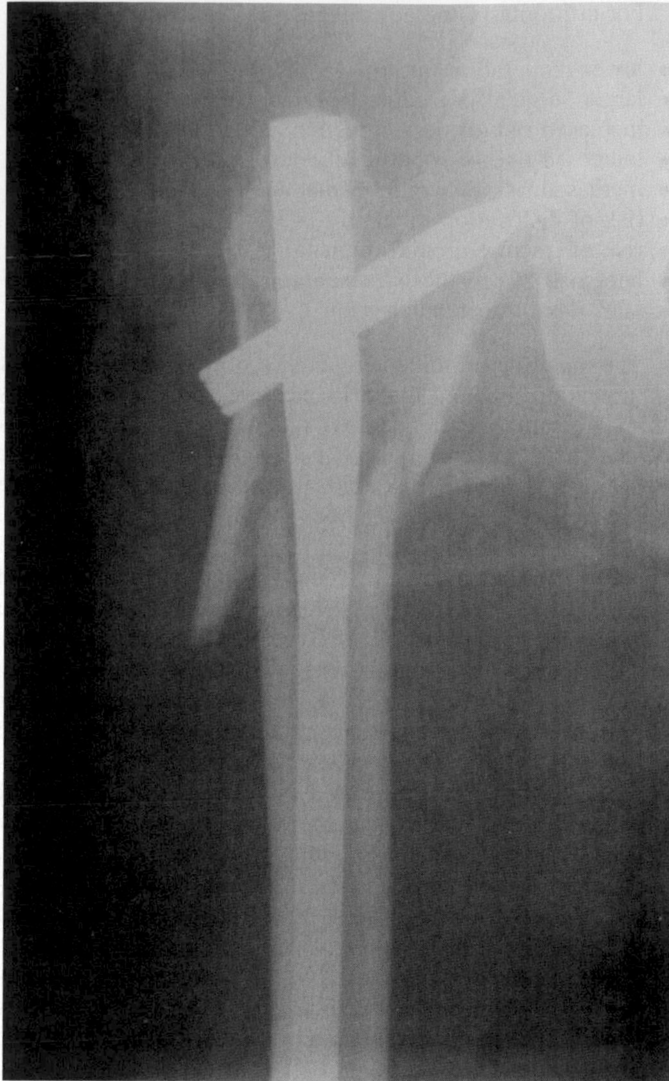

Figure 6 A subtrochanteric fracture fixed with an intramedullary nail

Most elderly patients who sustain a hip fracture will be unable to comply with any weight bearing restriction and certainly not the difficulties of walking "non-weight bearing". In practice, most patients will bear weight as pain tolerates, then become fully weight-bearing as the fracture heals.

Hip Movements

Traditional practice was to restrict hip flexion after an arthroplasty. This was to reduce the risk of prosthetic dislocation. This meant the patient required a raised bed and chairs, and was restricted from getting in and out of a car or bath. Such measures are still used for a total hip replacement, but for a hemiarthroplasty, should no longer be necessary. Refinements in surgical techniques with a more careful repair of the hip joint capsule reduce the risk of dislocation, and should make any restrictions on hip movements unnecessary.

Surgical Complications

Wound Healing Complications

Wound hematoma are the most common form of wound healing complication with an incidence of about 2–10%. Varying definitions of what constitutes a hematoma lead to differences in incidence, with some degree of bruising to be expected for all wounds. Small hematomas can be allowed to resolve spontaneously but larger collections will require surgical drainage.

Deep wound infection is the most devastating of complications that may occur after surgical treatment of a hip fracture, with a mortality approaching 50%. It is defined as infection of the wound below the level of the deep fascia and invariably involving the implant used. The incidence varies from about 1–5%, being somewhat higher after arthroplasty than after internal fixation of fracture. Treatment generally involves surgical debridement and often removal of the implant. This may mean that the patient is left with a "Girdlestone" hip – without a femoral head. A younger patient may be able to regain some degree of mobility with walking aids, but this is unlikely of older, frailer patients.

Superficial wound sepsis refers to infection of the wound that does not extend below the deep fascia layer. It is more common than deep sepsis but can be more effectively treated with antibiotics and, if indicated, with surgical debridement.

Internal Fixation of Intracapsular Fractures

The most common complication after this operation is failure of the fracture to heal (Figure 7). This may be seen as displacement of the fracture, which can occur within days or weeks of the fracture being treated. This is also termed *redisplacement of the fracture*. The terms *nonunion, pseudoarthrosis* or *delayed union* are generally used for those fractures that fail to heal after a period of a few months. Avascular necrosis or late segmental collapse refers to collapse of the femoral head due to insufficient blood supply (Figure 8). It normally occurs after 1 to 2 years of the fracture. Treatment of these complications is generally a replacement arthroplasty, although for a younger patient in whom there is a desire to retain the femoral head, various bone osteotomies or revascularization procedures may be used.

Other complications of internal fixation are irritations of the local tissues by the implant backing out into the local tissues. The patient may complain of pain around the implant and inability to lie on that side or of clicking around the hip. There will be local tenderness over the implant. Treatment is the removal of the implant.

Arthroplasty

Progressively increasing pain or reducing mobility after an arthroplasty may be due to one of a number of complications. Loosening of an arthroplasty is reported in about 2–30% of cases and is much more common after an uncemented

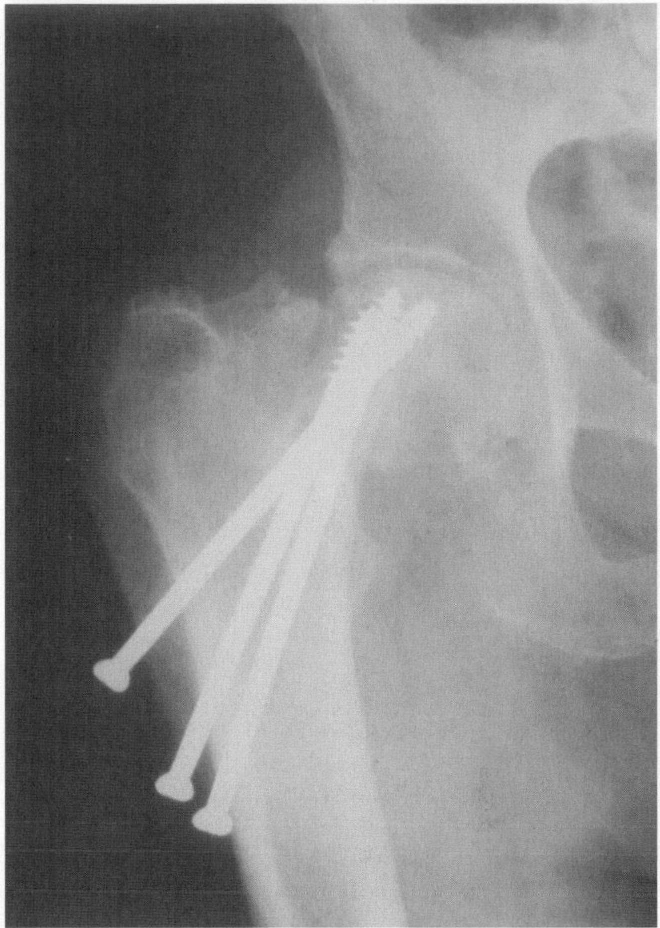

Figure 7 Redisplacement of a displaced intracapsular fracture that had been reduced and fixed with three screws

implant (Figure 9). The incidence is lower for cemented prosthesis and in those patients with limited functional demands or life expectancy. Treatment is by revision arthroplasty if symptoms are sufficiently severe. Acetabular wear can only occur after a hemiarthroplasty (Figure 10), as the acetabulum is resurfaced with a total hip replacement. Reported incidence varies from 5 to 50%, depending largely on the length of follow-up and is strongly related to the activities of the patient. Treatment is again by revision arthroplasty.

Other complications of arthroplasty are refracture around the implant which occurs in 1–5% of patients, generally after another fall. Treatment may be conservative with bed rest, bracing, traction, or alternatively operatively with either fixation of the fracture or replacement of the arthroplasty.

Sliding Hip Screw Fixation and Intramedullary Nail Fixation of Extracapsular Fractures

The most common surgical complication after this operation is cutout of the implant from the femoral head (Figure 11). The implant may protrude into the surrounding tissue or penetrate into the acetabulum. Symptoms will be increasing pain and impaired mobility. Treatment depends on the degree

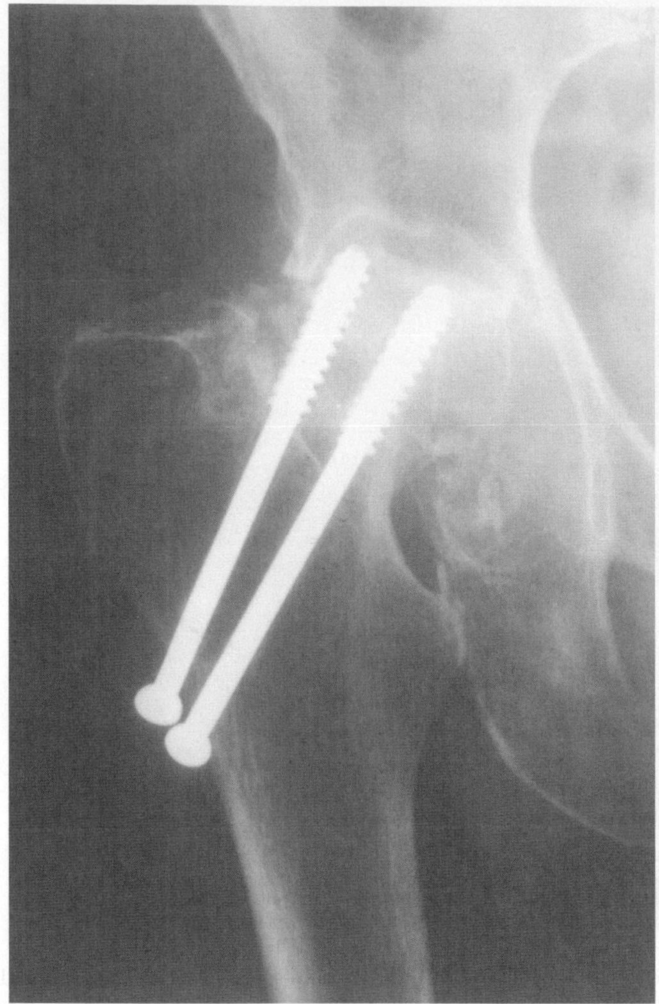

Figure 8 Avascular necrosis of the femoral head occurring after an intracapsular fracture

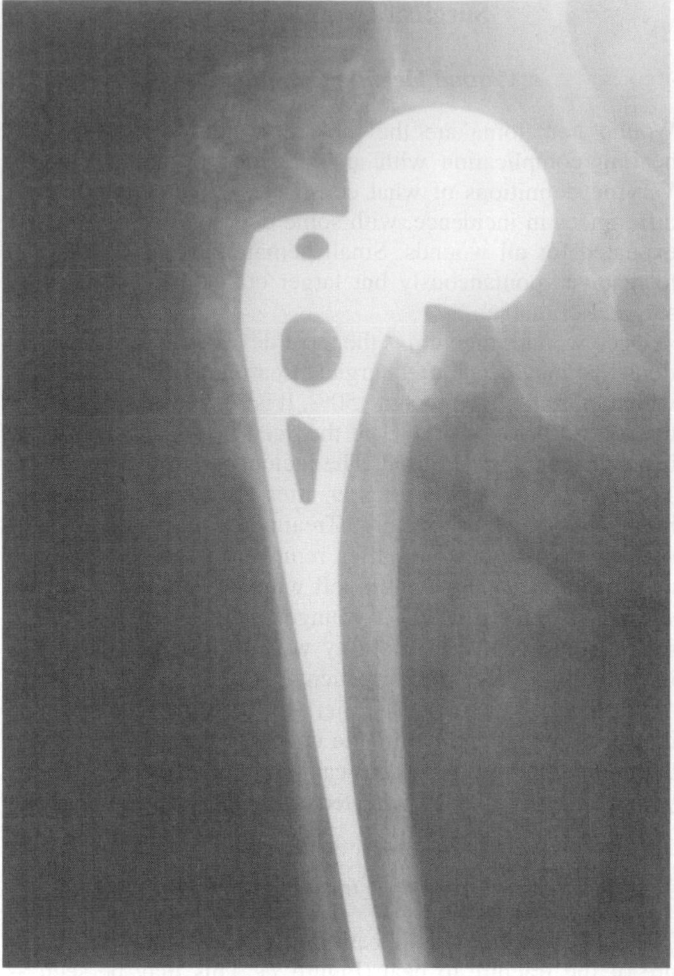

Figure 9 Loosening of an uncemented Austin Moore prosthesis. There is an area of radiolucency around the tip of the prosthesis. In addition, the prosthesis has sunk within the femur and there is ectopic calcification in the tissues around the hip joint

of the symptoms and fitness of the patient to undergo what may be a major revision surgery. Surgical treatment may be refixation of the fracture, replacement arthroplasty, or simple removal of the implant.

Other complications of SHS fixation are breakage of the implant, detachment of the plate from the femur, refracture around the implant, fracture below the implant, or nonunion of the fracture. All these complications may be treated by surgical methods. For subtrochanteric fractures, cutout of the implant is less common but for nonunion of the fracture, it is more common. The complications of intramedullary nail fixation are essentially the same as that of a SHS except that fracture around the tip of the nail is a specific complication related to nails, with an incidence of about 1–2%.

MEDICAL CARE

The management of older people with a fracture is increasingly recognized as an area requiring collaboration between the orthopedic surgeon, the geriatrician, and the multidisciplinary team on the trauma unit. The frailty of the elderly people who suffer a hip fracture means that their inpatient medical care is quite comparable to that of patients in a geriatric medical ward. There is a strong case for all patients admitted with this injury being assessed in respect of the four "giants of geriatrics" – falls, immobility, confusion, and incontinence. These commonly pose practical challenges to staff dealing with a patient with a hip fracture, and all four are recognized risk factors for poor outcome following this injury, as well as being risk factors for the development of the hip fracture, and for subsequent further fractures.

Apart from the ongoing surgical element of care described previously, the predominant way in which care differs from that on a geriatric medical ward is in patients' need for attention to secondary fracture prevention.

Secondary Fracture Prevention

The vast majority of older people admitted to a trauma ward, and nearly all of those admitted with hip fracture will have

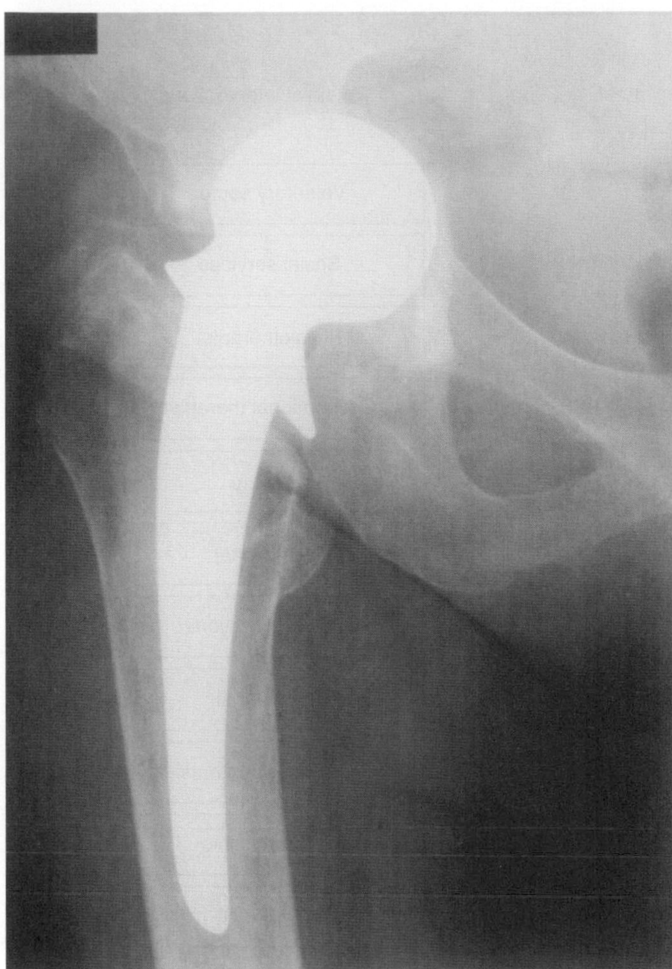

Figure 10 Acetabular wear of a cemented Thompson hemiarthroplasty. The prosthesis is eroding into the pelvis

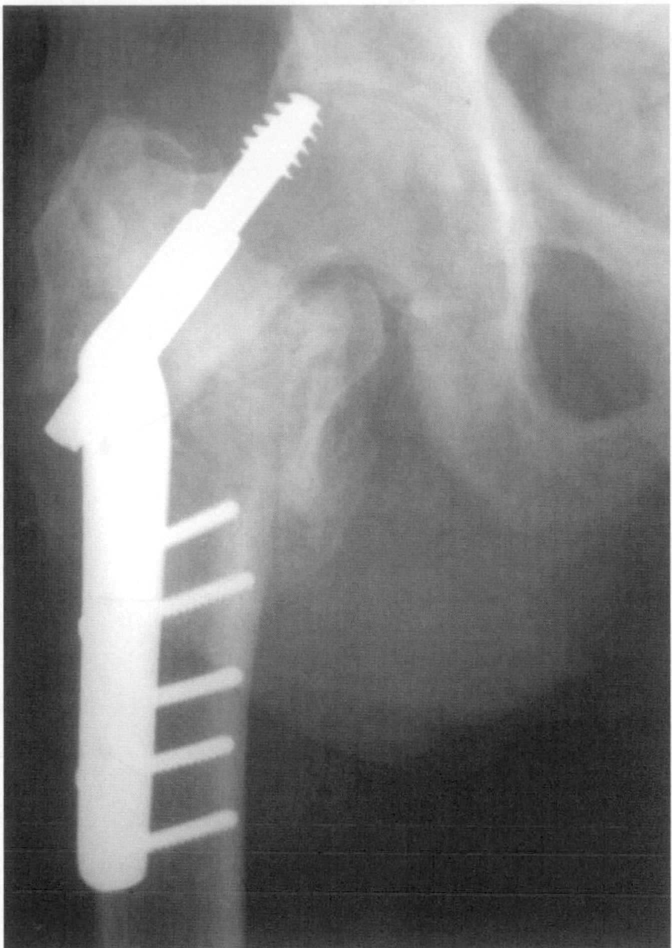

Figure 11 Cut-out of a sliding hip screw fixation of an unstable trochanteric fracture

sustained a "fragility" fracture (Johansen *et al.*, 1999) – a fracture resulting from only moderate trauma, usually a fall from standing height or less.

This implies that bone fragility and osteoporosis is contributing to the etiology of most hip fractures, and all people presenting with hip fracture in such circumstances need assessment of their risk of future fracture.

Hip fracture can be considered as the consequence of three factors:

- a fall leading to a fracture
- an impact that exerts stress on the hip
- a fragile bone.

The evidence for effective approaches to hip fracture prevention reflects this threefold causation with falls assessment, hip protection, and osteoporosis management each potentially playing a part.

Falls Assessment

It is beyond the scope of this article to try and look at falls assessment in depth. The complexity of the subject reflects its multifactorial nature, and the multidisciplinary approach necessary to its management (*see* **Chapter 112, Gait, Balance, and Falls**). However, optimal approaches to falls assessment are increasingly well defined, with international consensus as to the crucial elements of effective fall prevention (American Geriatrics Society, 2001). These guidelines argue for the assessment of all patients who have presented with a fall, or who exhibit gait and balance problems with a past history of falling (Figure 12). Nearly all patients with hip fracture will meet one or both of these indications, and so falls assessment should be made a routine part of their inpatient care.

A familiarity with this document is vital to any clinician involved in care of patients with hip fracture.

Many of the recommended elements of effective falls assessment will automatically form part of the rehabilitation process, with different members of the multidisciplinary team focusing attention on:

- gait and balance disorders
- optimization of mobility
- appropriate walking aids and footwear

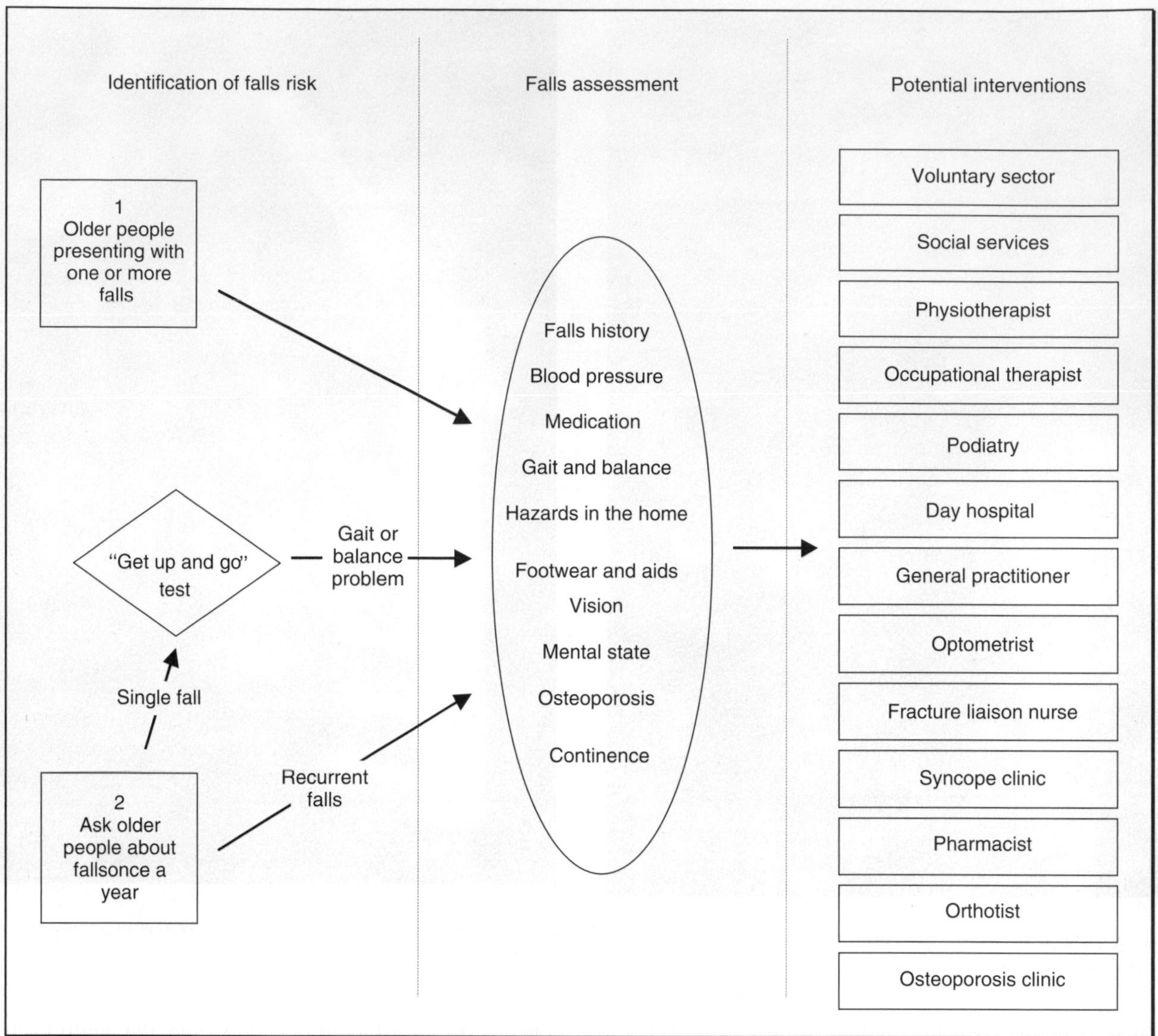

Figure 12 Falls assessment algorithm

- home environmental hazard modification
- assessment of vision, cognition, and continence.

A small proportion of patients will require specialist assessment, and the geriatrician is well placed to try and ensure that appropriate patients are triaged to specialist attention – for instance, in syncope and osteoporosis clinics.

A majority of patients will not need such specialist attention, but to complement the multidisciplinary issues listed, specific medical attention should be given to:

- assessment of the fall or falls that precipitated the fracture
- hip protection
- osteoporosis management
- medication review.

Most falls are simple accidents, with slips and trips resulting from gait and balance as the second commonest cause of hip fractures. Cardiovascular causes of falls are less frequent with hypotension, orthostatic hypotension, carotid sinus hypersensitivity, and vasovagal syncope predominating over cardiac arrhythmias (*see* **Chapter 83, Abnormalities of the Autonomic Nervous System**).

A detailed history of the circumstances leading to the fall including enquiry into previous falls is vital, as the description of the fall will allow examination and investigation to be most effective.

Where a medical cause of falls is suspected, the history is often suggestive of a specific diagnosis. Attention to medication history, examination including lying and standing blood pressure measurements (once the patient has recovered from postoperative hypovolemia), and a 12-lead ECG are most profitable. Such an approach will establish the cause for falls in a large proportion of patients presenting with hip fracture, so that more complex investigations such as 24-hour

ECG monitoring and echocardiography are relatively rarely needed.

Hip Protectors

It is recognized that a fall is less likely to lead to a fracture if it occurs on a carpeted surface, and it is possible that absorption of the force of impact may be effective in preventing a fracture.

Hip protectors are devices that are either based on a rigid exterior shell, or employing some form of foam laminate – integrated into underclothing so that they lie over the hip to protect the bone from the impact of a fall. There is no evidence of effectiveness of hip protectors from studies in which randomization was by individual patient within an institution, or for those living in their own homes.

Data from cluster randomized studies indicate that, for those living in institutional care with a high background incidence of hip fracture, a program of providing hip protectors appears to reduce the incidence of hip fractures. Acceptability by users of the protectors remains a problem due to discomfort and practicality. Cost-effectiveness remains unclear (Parker *et al.*, 2003).

These devices are of particular relevance to patients whose rehabilitation is impaired by anxiety over their risk of suffering a further fall and fracture and to patients who are at risk of repeated falls because of confusion and restlessness.

Osteoporosis Assessment

If a hip fracture results from "low trauma" (trauma no greater than a fall from a standing height), then this is suggestive of underlying bone fragility. Osteoporosis is by far the commonest underlying cause. Only 2–3% of hip fractures are "pathological", the majority of these reflecting metastatic disease, with only a very small proportion resulting from primary bone tumors, bone cysts, or Paget's disease.

Attention to the assessment and management of osteoporosis should be routine, following any low-trauma hip fracture. Strategies should be as inclusive as possible so that the frail and confused patients who are at highest risk of further falls and fractures are not excluded from receiving secondary prevention.

Results of trials specifically addressing the secondary treatment of osteoporosis after hip fracture are still awaited, but evidence from other clinical settings would support attention to the use of calcium and vitamin D status. Deficiency of sunlight exposure and dietary calcium is common among older people and can lead to secondary hyperparathyroidism, osteoporosis, and perhaps an increased risk of falls (Bischoff *et al.*, 2003). In a placebo-controlled study, the use of a daily supplement offering 1.2 g calcium and 800 IU vitamin D_3 led to a 28% reduction in hip fractures among elderly, mobile women living in residential care (Chapuy *et al.*, 1994).

Part of any approach to the secondary prevention of hip fracture should be to extrapolate these findings – and to offer calcium and vitamin D supplementation to frail older people who present with a low-trauma hip fracture, if they are expected to be house bound or institutionalized in the future.

These supplements are well tolerated, but should be avoided in patients known to have primary hyperparathyroidism, sarcoidosis, urinary calculi, and metastatic malignancy or myeloma. It is prudent to check that patients' serum calcium is not elevated before starting such supplementation to avoid precipitating hypercalcemia in patients with unrecognized hypercalcemia.

Calcium and vitamin D supplementation is unlikely to be effective in more younger and fitter patients who are not expected to be house bound and who already have an adequate calcium intake (broadly equating with consumption of a pint of milk a day). However, routine consideration of the need for supplementation is still important in these individuals, as correction of calcium and vitamin D deficiency is necessary before antiresorptive osteoporosis treatments are considered.

In the secondary prevention of low-trauma hip fracture, the first-line antiresorptive agent should be an oral bisphosphonate such as alendronate or risedronate (NICE, 2005). These agents are highly effective and have been shown to halve the risk of future fracture in patients with osteoporosis.

These drugs are usually taken as a single tablet once a week. Gastrointestinal intolerance is not uncommon, and the drugs should be taken first thing after getting up in the morning, washed down with a glass of tap water to minimize the risk of nausea, dyspepsia, and oesophageal pain or dysphagia. Effective absorption of the drug requires that no food, drink, or other medication is taken for at least half an hour after the tablet. Many patients with hip fracture will be unable to remember or cope with this prescription regime, unless appropriate supervision is available.

Consideration of bisphosphonate therapy usually requires assessment of bone mineral density to be undertaken (Royal College of Physicians, 1999; Eastell *et al.*, 2001). However, three-quarters of hip fracture patients are women, and their mean age is 83 years. An 83-year-old Caucasian woman with average bone density for her age would be expected to have a T-score of around -2.5, the WHO threshold for the diagnosis of osteoporosis. Thus, nearly half of this patient population would be predicted to have osteoporosis simply on the basis of their age, even before taking into account the additional risk demonstrated by the hip fracture itself.

The National Institute for Clinical Excellence has demonstrated that confirmation of osteoporosis is unnecessary in the over-75-year-old women who make up the majority of presentations with low-trauma hip fracture (NICE, 2005). These women should be offered a bisphosphonate without measuring their bone density. Bone densitometry should be performed in younger postmenopausal women and in men, as in these people bisphosphonate therapy is less cost-effective, unless a T-score of less than -2.5 has been confirmed.

Consideration should be given to the exclusion of other disease that will cause osteoporosis, especially if clinical assessment, operative findings, or a low Z-score on bone densitometry indicate greater bone fragility than would be expected for the patient's age. This is especially important in men where an underlying cause can be identified in half of the individuals. Clinical assessment might include questioning alcohol intake, breast examination, and screening investigations such as blood count, urea, electrolytes, liver and thyroid function tests, parathyroid hormone, serum and urine electrophoresis, with prostatic specific antigen and testosterone levels in men (*see* **Chapter 15, Alcohol Use and Abuse**).

Patients with moderate or severe renal impairment will not necessarily benefit from vitamin D supplementation and should not be given bisphosphonates. Activated vitamin D in the form of calcitriol (Tilyard *et al.*, 1992) or α-calcidol could be considered in these circumstances. Such drugs can be also used as second-line antiresorptive agents in patients who are unable to take a bisphosphonate for other reasons. Selective oestrogen receptor modulators (SERMs) are another form of second-line antiresorptive agent (NICE, 2005), but their use increases the risk of thromboembolism, making them unsuitable for use in the acute trauma setting.

One strategy for the secondary prevention of low-trauma fracture is the appointment of a specialist "fracture liaison" nurse. Though much of their work will be focused on the fracture clinic, they can also visit trauma wards to identify and assess low-trauma fracture patients, give advice, and arrange bone densitometry when appropriate. They will then follow up patients with the results of densitometry to advise on secondary prevention including the use of antiresorptive therapy where indicated. A clinician should report the scan, and availability of specialist clinic follow-up for more complex cases is clearly necessary to support such a nurse-led approach. Such an approach is superfluous if the geriatrician is routinely involved in hip fracture aftercare, as the management of osteoporosis will then be a routine part of comprehensive patient assessment.

Medication Review

Over a third of patients exhibit features of acute or chronic cognitive impairment and their medical history is often difficult to elicit. In such circumstances it is important to seek a collateral medical and medication history, and a phone call to the GP surgery will quickly elicit a drug list that can indicate relevant and unrecognized medical comorbidity. Many falls and fractures are a reflection of complex, often inappropriate polypharmacy, and a review of medication must be performed at an early stage of patient assessment.

The necessity for antipsychotic, sedative, hypnotic, and antidepressant therapy needs to be addressed alongside assessment of the patient's mental state. Such drugs may have been started during an acute upset in the past, and may have been continued unnecessarily. A period of observation in hospital offers the opportunity to assess the consequences of their withdrawal. Such drugs are associated with an increased risk of falls, and the inappropriate use of sedating medication will slow patients' rehabilitation and recovery.

Medical assessment should similarly include a review of the indication for vasodilator and diuretic therapy. Hypotension is common around the time of surgery, but persistent hypotension or postural hypotension in the postoperative period may necessitate a reduction in antihypertensive, antianginal or antifailure therapy.

Nonsteroidal therapy should be avoided in the perioperative period because of the increased risk of renal impairment and gastrointestinal bleeding during a period of stress and hypotension. Steroid therapy, anticonvulsant, and thyroid treatments can all be indicators of increased osteoporosis risk, and should be noted while previous and future osteoporosis treatment is being considered.

MODELS OF ORTHOGERIATRIC COLLABORATION

In addition to the medical aspects of hip fracture, many patients fear that the diagnosis of a hip fracture will lead to either death or loss of independence. Adequate information supported by a patient information booklet on the proposed treatment and outcome is useful to the patient. Planning for discharge of the patient back home should start from the time of admission.

Since the original descriptions of the benefits of collaboration between orthopedic surgeons and geriatricians in the 1960s (Irvine and Devas, 1963; Clarke and Wainwright, 1966), most trauma services in the United Kingdom have moved to develop at least some form of formal geriatrician input into the care of older inpatients recovering from fractures. A number of models of orthogeriatric care can be defined, but in general these are variations on the following four approaches.

Traditional Orthopedic Care

The elderly fracture patient is admitted to a trauma ward and the orthopedic surgical team manage their care and subsequent rehabilitation. Geriatrician input to such wards can take a variety of forms. In some units medical queries are dealt with by a consultative service, but in others there is regular input including weekly geriatrician visits.

Geriatric Orthopedic Rehabilitation Unit

Perioperative management by the orthopedic team is followed by early postoperative transfer to a geriatric rehabilitation unit, often between 5 and 10 days. The identification of appropriate patients may be left to orthopedic staff, or it may be led by specialist liaison nurses (Blacklock and Woodhouse, 1988), or be part of routine geriatrician rounds of the acute trauma wards.

The extent of orthopedic input to the rehabilitation ward also varies, depending on how early patients are moved from the acute trauma wards. Easy access to orthopedic surgical advice is necessary if momentum in rehabilitation is to be maintained. A weekly surgeon visit at a predictable time will allow all members of the multidisciplinary team to present concerns, problems, and x-rays.

Combined Orthogeriatric Care

The fracture patient is admitted to a specialized orthogeriatric ward under the care of both geriatricians and orthopedic surgeons. Surgical and geriatrician ward-rounds may happen independently, or be combined in weekly or twice-weekly multidisciplinary ward rounds. This degree of collaboration is central to the concept of a Geriatric Hip Fracture Service, with preoperative patient assessment by the geriatric medical team who will take the lead in postoperative multidisciplinary care. Rehabilitation may occur in this setting or in a separate rehabilitation unit.

Early Supported Discharge and Community Rehabilitation

Increasingly, community rehabilitation schemes are being implemented which help more able hip-fracture patients to be discharged directly home from the orthopedic ward. Earlier discharge may be facilitated by referral to a geriatric day hospital or a community rehabilitation team. Multidisciplinary assessment including contribution from the geriatrician is essential to ensure optimal patient selection for different forms of early supported discharge. Postdischarge rehabilitation will allow patients to maximize their independence, and graduate from a zimmer to a stick or no walking aid as appropriate. Practice walking out-of-door and advice about when to return to driving may also be given if appropriate.

Evidence for Effective Orthogeriatric Collaboration

The National Service Framework for Older People in England (Department of Health, 2001) states that "at least one general ward in an acute hospital should be developed as a center of excellence for orthogeriatric practice". However, evidence as to the effectiveness and cost-effectiveness of the different models is complex, and the National Service Framework does not recommend a particular type of orthogeriatric collaboration, but advocates that this should be agreed at local level.

A number of research trials have been published describing different models of care but only a few of these were of sufficient quality to allow their inclusion in the Cochrane review of Coordinated Multidisciplinary Hip Fracture Care (Cameron *et al.*, 2003). These studies consider different models of care, each adapted to local needs, and as a result it is difficult to draw clear conclusions from their findings. The Cochrane review concludes that there is "no conclusive evidence of the effectiveness of coordinated postsurgical care... but a trend towards effectiveness in all main outcomes".

The NHS Health Technology Assessment Programme has performed a systematic review of the evidence in respect of Geriatric Rehabilitation Following Fractures in Older People (Cameron *et al.*, 2000). This very comprehensive document considers four broad categories of approach that have been proposed as alternatives to traditional orthopedic care. The review is guarded in its conclusions about Geriatric Orthopedic Rehabilitation Units, and raises concern that the additional cost of such units does not appear to be justified by improvements in patient outcome. Pressures on acute hospital sites may encourage Trusts to consider such developments, but this may not be the most effective way for geriatricians to improve the outcome for older trauma inpatients.

Such concerns are supported by the results of the East Anglia Hip Fracture Audit (Parker *et al.*, 1998), which indicated increased length of stay in units that routinely transferred large proportions of trauma patients to rehabilitation in other wards. This is perhaps because the expectation of a move to a different unit for rehabilitation may encourage staff on the trauma ward to neglect discharge planning, as "rehabilitation is someone else's problem". Furthermore, momentum in rehabilitation can be lost at the time of the move while the patient settles in, and is reassessed by a new multidisciplinary team. Work in other countries has also shown that a focus on reduction of acute orthopedic length of stay and earlier transfer to other settings will tend to prejudice patients' rehabilitation, leading to increases in dependency and care costs in the long term (Fitzgerald *et al.*, 1988).

In contrast, the Cameron review concludes that there is good evidence to suggest that collaborative approaches in the acute setting such as the Geriatric Hip Fracture Service do appear effective in improving outcome. It also suggests a benefit from the use of intermediate care initiatives such as Early Supported Discharge schemes to expedite rehabilitation and discharge.

Thus, involvement of the geriatrician in the acute trauma wards is crucial. This will allow many aspects of high quality care to be built into the routine management of older trauma inpatients, perhaps through the development of evidence-based assessment and treatment protocols for patients with hip fracture (Johansen, 2004). It has been suggested that such protocols should be developed into formal Integrated Care Pathways for hip fracture (Cameron *et al.*, 2000), but our experience is that such pathways are often inconsistent with the needs of the heterogeneous population who present with this injury.

KEY POINTS

- Hip fracture is the most common cause of acute orthopedic admission in the elderly.

- Treatment is generally surgical – to fix the fracture or replace the femoral head.
- Perioperative mortality is about 5–10% with most patients having some loss of functional capacity.
- Multidisciplinary rehabilitation is necessary to optimize the chance of patients returning home.
- Interventions to reduce the risk of further fracture should routinely be considered.

KEY REFERENCES

- American Geriatrics Society, British Geriatrics Society, American Academy of Orthopaedic Surgeons. Guidelines for the prevention of falls in older persons. *Journal of American Geriatrics Society* 2001; **49**:664–72.
- Cameron ID, Handoll HHG & Finnegan TP *et al.* Co-ordinated multidisciplinary approaches for inpatient rehabilitation of older patients with proximal femoral fractures (Cochrane Methodology Review). *The Cochrane Library* 2003, Issue 4; John Wiley & Sons, Chichester.
- National Institute for Clinical Excellence. Secondary prevention of osteoporotic fragility fractures in post-menopausal women, *NICE*, 2005; www.nice.org.uk.
- Parker MJ, Pryor GA & Thorngren K-G. *Handbook of Hip Fracture Surgery*. 1997; Butterworth-Heinemann Publications, Oxford.
- Scottish Intercollegiate Guidelines Network (SIGN). *Prevention and Management of Hip Fractures in Older People* 2002; A National Guideline. Edinburgh SIGN No. 56 (www.sign.ac.uk).

REFERENCES

American Geriatrics Society, British Geriatrics Society, American Academy of Orthopaedic Surgeons. Guidelines for the prevention of falls in older persons. *Journal of American Geriatrics Society* 2001; **49**:664–72.

Avenell A & Handoll HHG. Nutritional supplementation for hip fracture aftercare in the elderly (Cochrane Review). *The Cochrane Library* 2004, Issue 2; John Wiley & Sons, Chichester.

Bischoff HA, Stahelin HB, Dick W *et al.* Effects of vitamin D and calcium on falls. *Journal of Bone and Mineral Research* 2003; **18**:343–51.

Blacklock C & Woodhouse KW. Correspondence. *Lancet* 1988; **i**:999.

Brennan J, Johansen A, Butler J *et al.* Place of residence and risk of fracture in older people: a population based study of over 65 year olds in Cardiff. *Osteoporosis International* 2003; **14**:515–9.

Burge RT, Worley D, Johansen A *et al.* The cost of osteoporotic fractures in the United Kingdom: projections for 2000–2020. *Journal of Medical Economics* 2001; **4**:51–62.

Cameron I, Crotty M, Currie C *et al.* Geriatric rehabilitation following fractures in older people: a systematic review. *Health Technology Assessment* 2000; **4**:2.

Cameron ID, Handoll HHG & Finnegan TP *et al.* Co-ordinated multidisciplinary approaches for inpatient rehabilitation of older patients with proximal femoral fractures (Cochrane Methodology Review). *The Cochrane Library* 2003, Issue 4; John Wiley & Sons, Chichester.

Chapuy MC, Arlot ME, Delmas PD & Meunier PJ. Effect of calcium and cholecalciferol treatment for 3 years on hip fractures in elderly women. *British Medical Journal* 1994; **308**:1081–2.

Clarke ANG & Wainwright D. Management of the fractured neck of femur in the elderly female: a joint approach of orthopaedic surgery and geriatric medicine. *Gerontology Clinics* 1966; **8**:321–6.

Department of Health. *National Service Framework for Older People* 2001; DoH, London, www.doh.gov.ulc/inst/olderpeople/index.htm.

Duncan DG, Beck SJ & Johansen A. Using dietetic assistants to improve the outcome of hip fracture – a randomised controlled trial of nutritional support in an acute trauma ward. *Journal of Human Nutrition and Dietetics* 2002; **15**:461.

Duncan D, Murison J, Martin R *et al.* Adequacy of oral feeding among elderly patients with hip fracture. *Age and Ageing* 2001; **30**(suppl 2):22.

Eastell R, Reid DM, Compston J *et al.* Secondary prevention of osteoporosis: when should a non-vertebral fracture be a trigger for action? *The Quarterly Journal of Medicine* 2001; **94**:575–97.

Fitzgerald JF, Moore PS & Dittus RS. The care of elderly patients with hip fracture: changes since implementation of the prospective payment system. *The New England Journal of Medicine* 1988; **319**:1392–7.

Handoll HHG, Farrar MJ, McBirnie J *et al.* Heparin, low molecular weight heparin and physical methods for preventing deep vein thrombosis and pulmonary embolism following surgery for hip fractures. *The Cochrane Library* 2004, Issue 3; John Wiley & Sons, Chichester.

Hay D & Parker MJ. Hip fracture in the immobile patient. *The Journal of Bone and Joint Surgery. British Volume* 2003; **85-B**:1037–9.

Hornby R, Grimley Evans J & Vardon V. Operative or conservative treatment for trochanteric fractures of the femur: a randomised epidemiological trial in elderly patients. *The Journal of Bone and Joint Surgery* 1989; **71-B**:619–23.

Irvine RE & Devas MB. The geriatric orthopaedic unit. *The Journal of Bone and Joint Surgery* 1963; **49-B**:186–7.

Johansen A. *Hip Fracture Assessment Care Pathway* 2004; www.eldermedcymru.com.

Johansen A, Evans R, Stone MD *et al.* The incidence of fracture in the United Kingdom: a study based on the population of Cardiff. *Injury* 1997; **28**:655–60.

Johansen A, Harding K, Evans R & Stone M. Trauma in elderly people: what proportion of fractures are a consequence of bone fragility? *Archives of Gerontology and Geriatrics* 1999; **29**:215–21.

Masson M, Parker MJ & Fleischer S Internal fixation versus arthroplasty for intracapsular proximal femoral fractures in adults (Cochrane Review). *The Cochrane Library* 2003, Issue 2; John Wiley & Sons, Chichester.

Melton LJ, Chrischilles EA, Cooper C *et al.* Perspective; how many women have osteoporosis? *Journal of Bone and Mineral Research* 1992; **7**:1005–10.

National Institute for Clinical Excellence. Secondary prevention of osteoporotic fragility fractures in post-menopausal women, *NICE*, 2005; www.nice.org.uk.

Parker MJ & Anand JK. What is the true mortality of hip fractures? *Public Health* 1991; **105**:443–6.

Parker MJ, Gillespie LD & Gillespie WJ Hip protectors for preventing hip fractures in the elderly (Cochrane Review). *The Cochrane Library* 2003, Issue 3; John Wiley & Sons, Chichester.

Parker MJ & Gurusamy K Arthroplasties (with and without bone cement) for proximal femoral fractures in adults (Cochrane Review). *The Cochrane Library* 2004, Issue 2; John Wiley & Sons, Chichester.

Parker MJ & Handoll HHG Gamma and other cephalocondylic intramedullary nails versus extramedullary implants for extracapsular hip fractures (Cochrane Review). *The Cochrane Library* 2004, Issue 1; John Wiley & sons, Chichester.

Parker MJ, Pryor GA & Thorngren K-G. *Handbook of Hip Fracture Surgery*. 1997; Butterworth-Heinemann Publications, Oxford.

Parker M, Todd C, Palmer C *et al.* Inter-hospital variations in length of hospital stay following hip fracture. *Age and Ageing* 1998; **27**:333–7.

Pathak G, Parker MJ & Pryor GA. Delayed diagnosis of femoral neck fractures. *Injury* 1997; **28**:299–301.

Pulmonary Embolism Prevention (PEP) Trial Collaborative Group. Prevention of pulmonary embolism and deep vein thrombosis with low dose aspirin: Pulmonary Embolism Prevention (PEP) trial. *Lancet* 2000; **355**:1295–302.

Royal College of Physicians. *Bone and Tooth Society of Great Britain. Osteoporosis Clinical Guidelines for Prevention and Treatment* 1999, Working party report on-line publication; Royal College of Physicians of London, www.rcplondon.ac.uk.

Salkeld G, Cameron ID, Cumming RG *et al.* Quality of life related to fear of falling and hip fracture in older women: a time trade off study. *British Medical Journal* 2000; **320**:341–6.

Scottish Intercollegiate Guidelines Network (SIGN). *Prevention and Management of Hip Fractures in Older People* 2002; A National Guideline. Edinburgh SIGN No. 56 (www.sign.ac.uk).

Tilyard MW, Spears GF, Thomson J & Dovey S. Treatment of post-menopausal osteoporosis with calcitriol or calcium. *The New England Journal of Medicine* 1992; **326**:357–62.

Torgerson DJ & Dolan P. The cost of treating osteoporotic fractures in the United Kingdom female population. *Osteoporosis International* 2000; **11**:551–2.

Versluysen M. Pressure sores in elderly patients: the epidemiology related to hip operations. *The Journal of Bone and Joint Surgery* 1985; **67-B**:10–3.

115

Diseases of the Joints

Terry L. Moore
Saint Louis University Health Sciences Center, St Louis, MO, USA

INTRODUCTION

The clinical presentation of arthritis is one of joint pain, swelling, morning stiffness, and limitation of motion (Nesher and Moore, 1994). These are symptoms common to all types of arthritis. Different diseases of the joint can present with signs and symptoms that appear quite similar. There are over a 100 types of arthritis that can affect the elderly (Table 1).

Nevertheless, a thorough medical history and physical examination, together with radiographic and laboratory testing, will identify the correct diagnosis in most cases of diseases of the joints (Table 2).

Arthritis has to be differentiated from periarticular or other musculoskeletal pain syndromes that commonly occur in the aged including fibromyalgia, rotator cuff tendinitis, trochanteric bursitis, polymyalgia rheumatica, and temporal arteritis.

OSTEOARTHRITIS

Osteoarthritis (OA) or degenerative joint disease is a chronic disorder characterized by softening and disintegration of articular cartilage with secondary changes in underlying bone, new growth of cartilage and bone (osteophytes) at the joint margins, and capsular fibrosis (Solomon, 2001). It is by far the most common form of chronic arthritis among the elderly. Its prevalence increases with age, occurring in greater than 50% of individuals older than 60 (Felson, 1990). Interphalangeal OA is particularly common in elderly people, affecting more than 70% of those older than 70 years (Solomon, 2001). Susceptibility to OA involves systemic factors affecting joint vulnerability including age, gender, genetic susceptibility, and nutritional factors; intrinsic joint vulnerabilities including previous damage, muscle weakness, malalignment, and so on; and extrinsic factors including obesity and physical activity (Felson, 2004) (Mankin and Brandt, 2001). The most common joints involved are those of weight bearing including the knees, hips, cervical and lumbosacral spine, proximal intraphalangeal (PIP) and distal intraphalangeal (DIP) joints of the hands, first carpometacarpal joints, and metatarsophalangeal (MTP) joints (Nesher and Moore, 1994; Solomon, 2001). Involvement is typically symmetric, although it can be unilateral at first depending on previous trauma or unusual stress. The pain may be insidious and relieved by rest initially, but as the disease progresses it becomes persistent and more severe with activity. Stiffness following periods of inactivity may also become common. The patient may complain of problems such as knee locking, unsteadiness, or giving away. Some patients, especially women, experience inflammatory OA or erosive OA, which particularly involves the PIPs and DIPs of the hands. These may exhibit inflammatory manifestations such as redness, tenderness, and local heat. Knees are often swollen with synovial fluid produced. Cervical and lumbosacral pain is a result of arthritis of hypophyseal joints, bony spur formation, pressure on ligaments or other surrounding tissues, or reactive muscle spasm. Impingement on nerve roots by osteophytes can cause radicular symptoms. Cord compression may result in spinal stenosis. In the cervical area, it causes localized pain and gait unsteadiness. At lumbar areas, it may result in spinal claudication, consisting of pain in the buttocks or legs while walking, which is relieved after 10 to 15 minutes of rest. Lumbar flexion and sitting usually relieve these symptoms, as opposed to aggravation of radicular disc symptoms by these positions.

Examination of the joints may detect crepitus, deformities, subluxation, swelling, bony overgrowths such as Heberden's nodes of the DIPs or Bouchard's nodes of the PIPs, and limitation of motion. Neurological evaluations may detect a radicular pattern of motor or sensory abnormalities, lower motor neuron or upper motor neuron signs in spinal stenosis, and sphincter abnormalities (Nesher and Moore, 1994).

No diagnostic laboratory tests are currently available. The synovial fluid, when present, is noninflammatory with a white count less than 1000 cells mm^{-3}. Radiological abnormalities may lag behind symptoms. Typical findings

Principles and Practice of Geriatric Medicine, 4th Edition. Edited by M.S. John Pathy, Alan J. Sinclair and John E. Morley.

Table 1 Common arthritides in the elderly

Osteoarthritis
Rheumatoid arthritis
Gout
Calcium pyrophosphate Deposition disease
Connective tissue diseases
Infectious arthritis

Table 2 Studies to screen for arthritis

Complete blood count (CBC)
Urinalysis
Erythrocyte sedimentation rate (ESR)
C-reactive protein (CRP)
Chemistry panel including studies for kidney, liver, muscle, and uric acid
Rheumatoid factor (RF)
Antinuclear antibody (ANA) and profile if indicated
Synovial fluid analysis if indicated (White count, crystal analysis, cultures)
X rays of appropriate joints or spinal areas

are joint space narrowing, subchondral sclerosis, osteophytes, and periarticular bone cysts. Oblique films of the spine must be obtained to evaluate the neuroforamina. Computerized tomography (CT) or magnetic resonance imaging (MRI) give better evaluation of the spine pathology and can differentiate OA changes from discopathy, another common problem in older persons (Solomon, 2001).

RHEUMATOID ARTHRITIS

Rheumatoid arthritis (RA) is a chronic inflammatory symmetrical disease of joints of unknown etiology, affecting about 1% of the general population worldwide and about 2% of persons 60 years and older in the United States (Firestein, 2001; Rasch *et al.*, 2003). Extraarticular manifestations may also contribute to disease symptomatology (Nesher *et al.*, 1991). Most elderly patients with RA have the disease onset before age 60 and commonly present with additional therapeutic problems when older because of the long duration of the disease and other illnesses. Older persons are more likely to develop joint deformities. Involvement of the cervical spine may result in pain, decreased range of motion, and neurological deficits. Extraarticular manifestations, such as rheumatoid nodules, secondary Sjögren's syndrome (SS), and vasculitis are more frequent in this group of patients (Nesher *et al.*, 1991).

Patients with elderly-onset rheumatoid arthritis (EORA) are those in whom RA develops after the age of 60. Most patients present with a gradual onset of pain, swelling, and stiffness in symmetrical joints, while in others, the onset may be more acute. Fatigue, malaise, and weight loss may be present. Joint symptoms are characteristically symmetric, although asymmetric presentation may occur. In the aged, asymmetric involvement may be seen in hemiplegic patients with sparing of the paralyzed side. All peripheral joints may be involved, but the most common are the PIPs and metacarpophalangeals (MCPs) of the hands involved in 90% as are the wrists, MTPs, and ankles. More centrally located joints, knees, hips, elbows, and shoulders are involved to a lesser extent. DIPs of the hands are usually spared. Large joints are commonly involved in EORA, the shoulders more often than in younger patients (Nesher *et al.*, 1991; Deal *et al.*, 1985).

The majority of patients experience intermittent periods of active disease alternating with periods of relative or complete remission. A minority will suffer no more than a few months of symptoms followed by complete remission, whereas a small group will have severe, progressive disease. EORA is considered by many to be milder than RA developing at a younger age, which may be related to the lower incidence of rheumatoid factor (RF) positivity in the elderly. RF-positive EORA patients are likely to have more severe disease (van der Heidje *et al.*, 1991). Most laboratory abnormalities are not specific for RA, with the possible exception of high-titer 19 seconds IgM RF. It should be noted that RF in low titers may occur in a small percentage of healthy older individuals, so a positive RF test by itself may not be diagnostic. The erythrocyte sedimentation rate (ESR) and C-reactive protein (CRP) are usually increased in RA, often correlating with disease activity. Radiological evaluation of involved joints in early stages is likely to show only soft tissue swelling. Later, the typical findings of symmetric joint space narrowing and erosions can support the clinical diagnosis (Nesher and Moore, 1994; Firestein, 2001; Nesher *et al.*, 1991).

GOUT

Gout is an inflammatory arthropathy caused by deposition of sodium monourate crystals in the joint (Wortman and Kelley, 2001). Its prevalence increases with age (Pascual and Pedraz, 2004). The typical presentation is that of an acute monoarthritis, most commonly occurring in the first MTP joint. The joint is usually extremely tender because it is associated with swelling and overlying erythema that sometimes mimics cellulitis or septic arthritis. Patients may be febrile and attacks can be precipitated by alcohol intake, use of diuretics, and stress, such as that occurring with surgical procedures or acute medical illness. Gout occurs more readily in joints damaged by other conditions such as OA. Polyarticular involvement of gout is not uncommon in older persons. It sometimes resembles RA. Such attacks tend to have a smoldering onset and longer course with a duration that is as long as 3 weeks. Chronic tophaceous gout is characterized by episodes of acute arthritis, chronic polyarthritis, joint deformities, and tophi. Radiographic findings are nonspecific in early stages. Punched out lesions or periarticular bone with overhanging borders are typically seen in chronic gout (Nesher and Moore, 1994; Wortman and Kelley, 2001; Pascual and Pedraz, 2004).

Laboratory findings include hyperuricemia in most cases (Wortman and Kelley, 2001). Most individuals with hyperuricemia never experience acute or chronic gout. About 10%

have normal serum levels during the attack. Therefore, the diagnosis should be established by the identification of typical sodium monourate crystals in synovial fluid, preferably with the use of a polarized microscope. This is accompanied by evaluating serum uric acid level and also performing a 24-hour urine for total serum urate spillage to define if the patient is an overproducer or undersecreter of uric acid.

CALCIUM PYROPHOSPHATE DEPOSITION DISEASE

Calcium pyrophosphate deposition disease (CPDD) is also a crystalline deposition arthropathy (Gohr, 2004). Its prevalence increases with age, being 10% in age 60 to 75 years and 30% in those 80 years or older (Reginato and Schumacher, 1988). Most cases are primary, but in some people it is associated with certain conditions such as hypothyroidism, hyperparathyroidism, and hemochromatosis. Many patients merely have asymptomatic chondrocalcinosis, commonly noted by X rays in the knees and wrists where linear punctate radiodensities are found within the cartilage (Gohr, 2004).

Typical presentation is usually of two types, that of chronic arthropathy that is sometimes polyarticular and presents with or without acute attacks with the knees most predominantly affected. Clinically, it may resemble OA or RA. Radiography may show features of both OA and CPDD, so it is not clear whether CPDD is primary or secondary. The second presentation is pseudogout, which is an acute monoarthritis, affecting mainly the knees and other large joints primarily and these resolve spontaneously within 3 weeks. It may infrequently affect a few articulations. Attack of pseudogout can be precipitated by stress or local trauma, and fever is common (Reginato and Reginato, 2001).

CONNECTIVE TISSUE DISEASE

Connective tissue disease, primary SS, and systemic lupus erythematosus (SLE), may present in the older population. Five percent of cases of SLE may begin after age 65 (Maddison, 1987). It may present with arthralgias or symmetric polyarthritis involving primarily finger joints, best resembling RA at this stage. Older onset SLE tends to be milder than the disease in younger patients with a lower incidence of nephropathy, neuropsychiatric manifestations, fever, and Raynaud's symptoms. There is an increased frequency of serositis, interstitial lung disease, and increase in sicca symptoms (Hahn, 2001). Primary SS, also, often presents in the aged (Thomas *et al.*, 1998). Patients complain of dryness of their eyes and also dryness in their mouth with swallowing difficulty. Nasal dryness, hoarseness, bronchitis, and skin and vaginal dryness may occur. The parotid glands may be swollen. Sicca symptoms (dry eyes and dry mouth) may be subtle and not obvious to the patients. Individual patients commonly have polyarthritis or arthralgias. Other features of the disease are myalgias, low-grade fever, and fatigue. Most have hypergammaglobulinemia and the frequency of developing lymphoproliferative disease is increased (Theander *et al.*, 2004).

Antinuclear antibodies are present in most SS and SLE patients, with antibodies to SS-A (Ro) and SS-B (La) occurring in the SS patients, and SLE patients having antibodies to double-stranded deoxyribonucleic acid (DNA), Sm, ribonucleoprotien (RNP), and SS-A/SS-B (von Mŭhlen and Tan, 1995). Other laboratory studies for evaluation include complement levels, antiphospholipid antibody studies, and other specific tests that may be helpful in diagnosing a particular connective tissue disease that is involved in the elderly patient (Illei *et al.*, 2004a,b).

Drug-induced lupus (DIL) is also a disease of older patients because inciting drugs are prescribed more frequently in the elderly. Symptoms are mild in most patients and resemble those of older onset SLE. The diagnosis is suggested by a history of administration of drugs like procainamide, hydralazine, α-methyldopa, propylthiouracil, or minocycline (Rubin, 1999). Most of these patients have positive ANA tests and antibodies to histones in 70 to 95% of the cases and occasional antibodies to myeloperoxidase. Other antibodies occur infrequently (Brogan and Olsen, 2003).

INFECTIOUS ARTHRITIS

Infectious arthritis typically presents as an acute monoarthritis of a large joint. It is associated with systemic signs of infection such as high fever, chills, and leukocytosis. Several factors predispose to an infected joint, including preexisting joint disease, a prosthetic joint, an infectious process elsewhere, or an immunocompromised state such as diabetes mellitus or treatment with corticosteroids (Vincent and Amirault, 1990). Infectious arthritis has to be entertained in all elderly patients with arthritis complaints. The presentation may be atypical in the aged because normal leukocyte counts and a normal temperature are not uncommon (Vincent and Amirault, 1990). In all cases of monoarthritis, synovial fluid should be aspirated, a Gram stain and culture performed, and a leukocyte count and differential determined. The leukocytes counts are usually $>50\,000$ cells mm^{-3}, primarily neutrophils; however, the initial count may be less than $10\,000$ cells mm^{-3} (Coutlakis *et al.*, 2002). The most common pathogen is *Staphylococcus aureus*, followed by streptococci and gram-negative bacilli (Ho, 2001). *Staphylococcus epidermidis* is common in a prosthetic joint infection. Early diagnosis is mandatory to prevent the high rate of complications; a 19% mortality rate has been reported, and 38% of patients may develop osteomyelitis (Vincent and Amirault, 1990). Treatment of infectious arthritis is determined by the type of organism that is isolated and then appropriate therapy is provided.

Table 3 Treatment modalities for arthritis in the aged

Physical therapy
Medications
(Noninflammatory arthritis)
Analgesics
Nonsteroidal antiinflammatories
(Inflammatory arthritis)
Nonsteroidal antiinflammatories
Disease-modifying agents
Biologics
Corticosteroids
Surgery

TREATMENT

Effective treatment of elderly arthritic patients combines physical therapy, medications, and in some cases, surgical intervention (Table 3).

PHYSICAL THERAPY

The value of physical therapy in improving the quality of life of the elderly patients with arthritis cannot be overemphasized. The main goals are pain relief, prevention of deformities, and maintaining mobility and independence (Nesher and Moore, 1994). Pain is relieved by periodic rest, splinting of affected joints, and locally applied heat. Although rest decreases joint pain and swelling, it may contribute to the development of contractures, disuse atrophy of muscles, and osteoporosis. In the aged, even brief periods of rest can result in loss of muscle strength and difficulty in resuming activities. An individual must maintain a certain level of activity even in the presence of active disease. Initial periods of relative rest should be followed by a program of passive and then active exercises designed to maintain range of motion and muscle strength. The patients should be encouraged to participate in body toning exercise programs such as regular swimming, walking, or water aerobics-type programs. Foot, hand, and cervical spine involvement can be helped with proper individualized footwear, paraffin baths, and cervical collars, respectively. Fabricated orthoses can help maintain alignment and support mechanically deranged joints. Assistive devices for walking, dressing, eating, and bathing can greatly improve the quality of life of these patients (Nesher and Moore, 1994; Calkins, 1991; Brandt *et al.*, 2003).

MEDICATIONS

Treatment decisions should consider several age-related changes that may affect drug absorption, distribution, metabolism, and elimination. The possibility exists that various treatments will have altered efficacy and be potentially more hazardous. Also, many elderly patients with arthritis have other diseases requiring other medications that could cause drug–drug interactions with the arthritis preparations.

Analgesic medications are given for mild arthralgias, especially for OA. Acetaminophen is commonly prescribed at a daily dose of 1 gm 3 to 4 times a day as needed. It has been shown to have equal efficacy to other anti-inflammatory agents for pain relief. It is a safe drug when used in therapeutic doses. It appears to be safe for patients with renal dysfunction or peptic ulcers; however, liver function studies must be followed to be sure there are no problems with hepatic toxicity (Brandt *et al.*, 2003). Other analgesics and opioid receptor agonists are effective in pain management, but their use should be limited to a short term, because abuse can lead to adverse effects, such as respiratory depression, drowsiness, constipation, and addiction. Propoxyphene is much safer than codeine for prolonged use and administration is much less addicting (Brandt *et al.*, 2003). The recent use of glucosamine and chondroitin sulfate for OA have been investigated and may be efficacious, especially glucosamine in some patients with OA of the hips and knees (Reginsten *et al.*, 2003). Diabetics and patients allergic to shellfish should not use these compounds. Also, the use of intra-articular injections of hyaluronic acid have been helpful to preserve knee cartilage and hip cartilage in some cases (Day *et al.*, 2004; Berg and Olsson, 2004).

Nonsteroid anti-inflammatory drugs (NSAIDs) are the most frequently prescribed medications for arthritis (Nesher and Moore, 1994). In many cases, they alone are sufficient to induce the desired effect. The use of NSAIDs as primary therapy for older patients with OA and RA is not without problems (Brandt *et al.*, 2003; Johnson and Day, 1991). Advanced age has been identified as a primary risk factor for adverse gastrointestinal (GI) events in users of NSAIDs (Willkens, 2004). Hospitalization for bleeding of the stomach or esophagus occurs far more frequently in older patients who use NSAIDs than those who do not. However, patients are often asymptomatic. The risk factors for such events are advanced age, a history of GI problems, and the simultaneous use of corticosteroids, anticoagulants, alcohol, or tobacco. These factors should be documented in individual patients and treated accordingly (Willkens, 2004). Adverse events such as epigastric pain, mental changes, fluid retention, changes in blood pressure, and occult or gross blood loss should be monitored closely. A complete blood count (CBC), urinalysis, and liver and kidney function tests should be attended initially and every 1 to 3 months thereafter to monitor toxicity in the elderly population. NSAIDs such as naproxen, fenoprofen, sulindac, and diclofenac have proved very effective in the treatment of OA or RA in patients. A concern about peptic ulcer disease has been relieved considerably by the availability of cyclooxygenase-2 (COX-2) inhibitors (Baigent and Patrono, 2003). However, caution is still needed in older patients who have a history of ulcer disease. Some physicians still add proton pump inhibitors to this therapy when it is used in high-risk patients. Also, the use of H2 blockers such as famotidine, and so on, can also be helpful. Both the older NSAIDs and COX-2 selective NSAIDs have the potential for decreasing renal blood flow causing fluid retention, creating abnormal salt and water metabolism, and interfering with drug excretion, so they are not without their toxicity in the elderly population (Perazella and Tray, 2001). The COX-2 antagonists celecoxib, rofecoxib, valdecoxib, and etoricoxib have been used extensively and have other advantages beyond decreased gastric acidity (Brune and Hinz, 2004). Clinical trials of these drugs have shown no effect on platelet aggregation or bleeding time at therapeutic doses and do not alter this anticoagulant effect of warfarin. However, the possibility of increased blood pressure, peripheral edema, or predisposal to myocardial infarctions or strokes because of their effect on thromboxane A_2 levels may be a contraindication to using some COX-2 inhibitors in the elderly population (Baigent and Patrono, 2003).

The nephrotoxic effect of NSAIDs is well documented. The most common mechanism leading to renal dysfunction is inhibition of renal prostaglandin synthesis, which may adversely affect renal blood flow in certain situations, leading to acute insufficiency (Perazella and Tray, 2001). At special risk are patients with preexisting changes in renal function, such as those changes related to aging, diabetes mellitus, hypertension, congestive heart failure, or use of concomitant diuretics. Preferably, NSAIDs should not be prescribed to patients with these conditions or anybody with a creatinine of 1.5 or higher. NSAID-related psychotic reactions and depression occur more commonly in the aged. Also, NSAIDs can interact with several medications commonly used in older persons, mainly anticoagulants, oral hypoglycemics, digoxin, seizure medications, and lithium (Johnson and Day, 1991). Combining NSAIDs with potassium-sparing diuretics increase the risk of hyperkalemia.

In RA, the baseline therapy is the use of NSAIDs and then the use of remittive agents very quickly to reduce erosions and joint space narrowing, which generally occur in the first 2 years (Johnson and Day, 1991). Disease-modifying agents (disease-modifying antirheumatic drugs or DMARDs) are second line agents in RA, but are used much more quickly today. The first that is usually prescribed is hydroxychloroquine in doses of 200 mg once to twice daily. It is considered effective in mild to moderate cases of RA. It is also effective in treating the arthritis and skin manifestations of SLE and SS (Nesher and Moore, 1996). The mainline therapy in RA now is usually triple therapy including an NSAID, hydroxychloroquine, and in the United States, methotrexate in doses of 10 to 25 mg weekly or in Europe sulfasalazine at doses of 2 to 3 g daily. These regimens appear to be effective for elderly patients with RA, as it is for younger ones. Methotrexate may have some toxicity in the elderly, but is limited mainly to hepatotoxicity and in those with abnormal renal function. The lowest reasonable dose should be used (Willkens, 2004; Nesher and Moore, 1996). CBC, urinalysis, and comprehensive metabolic panel every 6 to 8 weeks to monitor toxicity are recommended. Also, to reduce toxicity, the use of folic acid at 1 to 2 mg day^{-1} is very helpful. Sulfasalazine in 2 to 3 g daily dose should also be monitored every two months by CBC, urinalysis, and comprehensive metabolic panel to reduce toxicity. Other remittive agents such as azathioprine or leflunomide, may be used in RA with efficacy (Smolen, 2004). The recent advent of biologics including etanercept, infliximab, and adalimumab have been very helpful in bringing into remission elderly patients with RA (Calabrese, 2003). These biologics inhibit tumor necrosis factor (TNF). Etanercept, a TNF receptor antagonist, is given as 25 mg subcutaneous twice a week to 50 mg once a week. It has been shown to be very effective in decreasing sedimentation rate, joint activity, arthralgias, and reducing erosions and joint space narrowing. The same can also be said for the other new biologics, which are monoclonal antibodies directed toward TNF. The fully humanized antibody, adalimumab, is given as a 40 mg subcutaneous every 2 weeks, or the chimeric molecule, infliximab, an intravenous preparation, is given at dosages from 3 to 10 mg kg^{-1} at baseline, 2 to 6 weeks, and then every 4 to 8 weeks thereafter (Calabrese, 2003). All have been shown to have long-term efficacy and little toxicity (Cush, 2003). Injection site reactions may occur and are usually managed with antihistamines. The only other toxicity noted is the possible development of exacerbating an indolent tuberculosis infection. Therefore, a tuberculosis skin test and chest X-ray should be performed at baseline and yearly. Also, the possibility of aggravating any new infection has to be entertained. Therefore, a dose should be held if a viral or bacterial infection occurs. Also, the long-term effect of blocking TNF is not well understood (Ellerin *et al.*, 2003). They should not be used for any patient with a demyelinating disorder (Robinson *et al.*, 2001) and monitoring for any type of lymphoproliferative processes should occur (Brown *et al.*, 2002). However, early studies in the United States have shown no increase in lymphomas, tumors, or other side effects with these medications greater than is seen as a late outcome in RA.

Corticosteroids can be used in low doses of 5 to 10 mg of prednisone daily in some elderly seronegative RA patients or in patients with remittive seronegative symmetrical synovitis with pitting edema (RS3PE) (Nesher and Moore, 1996). However, higher doses predispose the patient to the multiple side effects of steroids in the elderly, including sodium and fluid retention, hypertension, hyperglycemia, osteoporosis, infections, and skin changes (Willkens, 2004; Nesher and Moore, 1996). With the advent of the new remittive agents and biologics, the use of steroids should be limited to only those who are unresponsive or cannot afford the other agents. If steroids are used, the use of calcium and vitamin D should be included with that therapy to prevent osteoporosis as much as possible. Intra-articular injections of steroid preparations are commonly employed in RA and OA in conjunction with other treatment modalities, especially when symptoms are limited to one or fewer joints (Nesher and Moore, 1996).

The treatment of acute gout in the elderly is still the use of colchicine, but at lower doses than in the past (Willkens, 2004). Generally, the dosage for long-term use of colchicine is one or two 0.6 mg tablets/day depending on the patient's renal function; however, only 0.3 mg in patients aged 70 years or older. When parental colchicine is used, the maximum dose used for an acute episode in or out of the hospital should be 1 mg day^{-1} intravenously. In renal compromised patients, the use of colchicine has resulted in neuromyopathy (Kuncl *et al.*, 1987). Allopurinol, a xanthine oxidase inhibitor, is another gout medication that can lower serum urate levels. It is best started slowly at 100 mg day^{-1}. If the hyperuricemia is not responding, the dosage should be advanced to 100 mg twice a day and then finally up to 300 mg day^{-1} (Nesher and Moore, 1994). Platelet counts and hypersensitivity reactions should be monitored. Anti-inflammatory agents such as naproxen or the COX-2 inhibitor, etoricoxib can also be used in acute gout (Rubin *et al.*, 2004). In general, uric acid lowering therapy should be administered when there are tophi, frequent attacks of gouty arthritis of over three per year, or evidence of uric acid overproduction is documented. Baseline 24-hour urine of uric acid spillage over 750 mg/24 hours or uric acid levels over 8 may indicate the need for therapy (Wortman and Kelley, 2001; Maddison, 1987).

In the treatment for pseudogout in adult patients, it has been shown that colchicine is less effective and is usually being managed by NSAIDs. The dosage of naproxen 500 mg twice a day, etoricoxib 60 mg once to twice a day, or diclofenac 50 mg 3 times a day can be very effective in the long-term management of patients with pseudogout (Reginato and Reginato, 2001).

SURGERY

The major goals of various orthopedic procedures are to relieve pain and to improve function (Nesher and Moore, 1994). Joint replacement, tendon repair, carpal tunnel release, and synovectomy are some of the frequently employed measures in RA (Sledge, 2001). In OA, treatments include bunion resection, decompression of spinal roots, and total knee and hip replacements. Arthroscopic lavage of knees has been reported to improve symptoms, but has not been widely employed as a therapeutic measure. Age itself is neither a contraindication to surgery nor a predictor of poor results. Rather, the presence of concurrent medical problems such as heart failure and pulmonary disease contribute more to perioperative morbidity and outcome. The goals, indications, and timing of surgery should be individualized depending on the patient's general health status, function impairment, degree of pain, and rehabilitation potential (Rosandrich *et al.*, 2004).

In summary, arthritis is a common condition among the aged. The most common type is OA and the most common inflammatory process is RA. Optimal management includes physical therapy and medication, possibly combined with surgery, if necessary. Treatment modalities should be offered sometimes to accommodate age-related changes and body mechanics and function. The long-term medical management of arthritis in the elderly requires close monitoring for potential adverse effects of medications.

KEY POINTS

- Arthritis is a common chronic condition among the aged.
- Osteoarthritis is the most common type.
- Rheumatoid arthritis is the most common inflammatory arthritis and can produce long-term morbidity if not treated aggressively.
- There are more than one hundred types of arthritis affecting the elderly.
- Gout, pseudogout, or infectious arthritis can present as red, hot, swollen joints, and only synovial fluid aspiration can differentiate.

KEY REFERENCES

- Cush JJ. Safety of new biologic therapies in rheumatoid arthritis. *Bulletin on the Rheumatic Diseases* 2003; **52**(8):1–6.
- Firestein GS. Etiology and pathogenesis of rheumatoid arthritis. In S Ruddy, ED Harris & CB Sledge (eds) *Kelley's Textbook of Rheumatology* 2001, p 921–66; W.B. Saunders Company, Philadelphia.
- Hahn BH. Systemic lupus erythematosus and related syndromes. In S Ruddy, ED Harris & CB Sledge (eds) *Kelley's Textbook of Rheumatology* 2001, pp 1089–103; W.B. Saunders Company, Philadelphia.
- Nesher G & Moorc TL. Recommendations for drug therapy of rheumatoid arthritis in the elderly patients. *Clinical Immunotherapeutics* 1996; **5**:341–50.
- Solomon L. Clinical features of osteoarthritis. In S Ruddy, ED Harris & CB Sledge (eds) *Kelley's Textbook of Rheumatology* 2001, pp 1409–18; W.B. Saunders Company, Philadelphia.

REFERENCES

Baigent C & Patrono C. Selective cyclooxygenase 2 inhibitors, aspirin, and cardiovascular disease. *Arthritis and Rheumatism* 2003; **48**:12–20.

Berg P & Olsson U. Intra-articular injection of hyaluronic acid of osteoarthritis of the hip: A pilot study. *Clinical and Experimental Rheumatology* 2004; **22**:300–6.

Brandt KD, Doherty M, Raffa BB *et al.* Controversies and practical issues in management of osteoarthritis. *Journal of Clinical Rheumatology* 2003; **9**(suppl 2):1–39.

Brogan BL & Olsen NJ. Drug-induced rheumatic syndromes. *Current Opinion in Rheumatology* 2003; **15**:76–80.

Brown SL, Green MH, Gershon SK *et al.* Tumor necrosis factor antagonist therapy and lymphoma development. *Arthritis and Rheumatism* 2002; **46**:3151–8.

Brune K & Hinz B. Selective cyclooxygenase-2 inhibitors: similarities and differences. *Scandinavian Journal of Rheumatology* 2004; **33**:1–6.

Calabrese LH. Molecular differences in anticytokine therapies. *Clinical and Experimental Rheumatology* 2003; **21**:241–8.

Calkins E. Arthritis in the elderly. *Bulletin on the Rheumatic Diseases* 1991; **40**:15–8.

Coutlakis PH, Roberts WN & Wise CM. Another look at synovial fluid leukocytosis and infection. *Journal of Clinical Rheumatology* 2002; **8**:67–71.

Cush JJ. Safety of new biologic therapies in rheumatoid arthritis. *Bulletin on the Rheumatic Diseases* 2003; **52**(8):1–6.

Day R, Brooks P, Conaghan PG & Peterson M. Double blind, randomized, multicenter, parallel group study of the effectiveness and tolerance of intraarticular hyaluronan in osteoarthritis of the knee. *Journal of Rheumatology* 2004; **31**:775–82.

Deal CL, Meenan RF & Goldenberg DL. The clinical features of elderly-onset rheumatoid arthritis: A comparison with younger-onset disease of similar duration. *Arthritis and Rheumatism* 1985; **28**:987–94.

Ellerin T, Rubin RH & Weinblatt ME. Infections and anti-tumor necrosis factor α therapy. *Arthritis and Rheumatism* 2003; **48**:3013–22.

Felson DT. The epidemiology of osteoarthritis: Results from the framingham osteoarthritis study. *Seminars in Arthritis and Rheumatism* 1990; **20**(suppl 1):42–9.

Felson DT. Obesity and vocational and avocational overload of the joint as risk factors for osteoarthritis. *Journal of Rheumatology* 2004; **31**(suppl 70):2–5.

Firestein GS. Etiology and pathogenesis of rheumatoid arthritis. In S Ruddy, ED Harris & CB Sledge (eds) *Kelley's Textbook of Rheumatology* 2001, p 921–66; W.B. Saunders Company, Philadelphia.

Gohr C. In vitro models of calcium crystal formation. *Current Opinion in Rheumatology* 2004; **16**:263–7.

Hahn BH. Systemic lupus erythematosus and related syndromes. In S Ruddy, ED Harris & CB Sledge (eds) *Kelley's Textbook of Rheumatology* 2001, pp 1089–103; W.B. Saunders Company, Philadelphia.

Ho G. Bacterial arthritis. *Current Opinion in Rheumatology* 2001; **13**:310–4.

Illei GG, Tackey E, Lapteva L & Lipsky PE. Biomarkers in systemic lupus erythematosus. I. General overview of biomarkers and their applicability. *Arthritis and Rheumatism* 2004a; **50**:1709–20.

Illei GG, Tackey E, Lapteva L & Lipsky PE. Biomarkers in systemic lupus erythematosus. II. Markers of disease activity. *Arthritis and Rheumatism* 2004b; **50**:2048–65.

Johnson AG & Day RO. The problems and pitfalls of NSAID therapy on the elderly. *Drugs & Aging* 1991; **1**:130–51.

Kuncl RW, Duncan G & Watson D. Colchicine myopathy and neuropathy. *New England Journal of Medicine* 1987; **316**:1562–8.

Maddison PJ. Systemic lupus erythematosus in the elderly. *Journal of Rheumatology* 1987; **14**(suppl 13):1892–6.

Mankin HJ & Brandt KD. Pathogenesis of osteoarthritis. In S Ruddy, ED Harris & CB Sledge (eds) *Kelley's Textbook of Rheumatology* 2001, pp 1391–407; W.B. Saunders Company, Philadelphia.

Nesher G & Moore TL. Clinical presentation and treatment of arthritis in the aged. *Clinics in Geriatric Medicine* 1994; **10**:659–75.

Nesher G & Moore TL. Recommendations for drug therapy of rheumatoid arthritis in the elderly patients. *Clinical Immunotherapeutics* 1996; **5**:341–50.

Nesher G, Moore TL & Zuckner J. Rheumatoid arthritis in the elderly. *Journal of the American Geriatrics Society* 1991; **39**:284–94.

Pascual E & Pedraz T. Gout. *Current Opinion in Rheumatology* 2004; **16**:282–6.

Perazella MA & Tray K. Selective cyclooxygenase-2 inhibitors: a pattern of nephrotoxicity similar to traditional non-steroidal anti-inflammatory drugs. *American Journal of Medicine* 2001; **111**:64–7.

Rasch EK, Hirsch R, Paulose-Ram R & Hochberg MC. Prevalence of rheumatoid arthritis in persons 60 years of age and older in the United States. *Arthritis and Rheumatism* 2003; **48**:917–26.

Reginato AJ & Reginato AM. Diseases associated with deposition of calcium pyrophosphate or hydroxyphosphate. In S Ruddy, ED Harris & CB Sledge (eds) *Kelley's Textbook of Rheumatology* 2001, pp 1377–90; W.B. Saunders Company, Philadelphia.

Reginato AJ & Schumacher HR. Crystal associated arthritis. *Clinics in Geriatric Medicine* 1988; **4**:295–301.

Reginsten J-Y, Bruyere O, Lecart M-P & Henrotin Y. Glucosamine and chondroitin sulfate compounds as structure-modifying drugs in the treatment of osteoarthritis. *Current Opinion in Rheumatology* 2003; **15**:651–5.

Robinson WH, Genovese MC & Moreland MW. Demyelinating and neurologic events reported in association with tumor necrosis factor α antagonism. *Arthritis and Rheumatism* 2001; **44**:1977–83.

Rosandrich PA, Kelley JT & Conn DL. Perioperative management of patients with rheumatoid arthritis in the era of biologic response modifiers. *Current Opinion in Rheumatology* 2004; **16**:192–8.

Rubin BR, Burton R, Navarra S *et al.* Efficacy and safety profile of treatment with etoricoxib 120 mg once daily in acute gout. *Arthritis and Rheumatism* 2004; **50**:598–606.

Rubin RL. Etiology and mechanisms of drug-induced lupus. *Current Opinion in Rheumatology* 1999; **11**:357–63.

Sledge CB. Principles of reconstructive surgery. In S Ruddy, ED Harris & CB Sledge (eds) *Kelley's Textbook of Rheumatology* 2001, pp 1699–788; W.B. Saunders Company, Philadelphia.

Smolen J. Practical management of rheumatoid arthritis patients treated with leflunomide. *Journal of Rheumatology* 2004; **31**(suppl 71):1–30.

Solomon L. Clinical features of osteoarthritis. In S Ruddy, ED Harris & CB Sledge (eds) *Kelley's Textbook of Rheumatology* 2001, pp 1409–18; W.B. Saunders Company, Philadelphia.

Theander E, Manthorpe R & Jacobsson LTH. Mortality and causes of death in primary Sjögren's syndrome. *Arthritis and Rheumatism* 2004; **50**:1262–9.

Thomas E, Hay EM, Hajeer A & Silman AJ. Sjögren's syndrome: a community-based study of the prevalence and impact. *British Journal of Rheumatology* 1998; **37**:1069–76.

van der Heidje DMFM, van Riel PLCM, van Leewen MA *et al.* Older versus younger onset RA: Results at onset and after 2 years of a prospective followup study of early RA. *Journal of Rheumatology* 1991; **18**:1285–9.

Vincent GM & Amirault JD. Septic arthritis in the elderly. *Clinical Orthopaedics and Related Research* 1990; **251**:241–60.

von Műhlen CA & Tan EM. Autoantibodies in the diagnosis of systemic rheumatic diseases. *Seminars in Arthritis and Rheumatism* 1995; **24**:323–58.

Willkens RF. Making the most of antirheumatic drugs in older patients. *Musculoskeletal Medicine* 2004; **21**:317–32.

Wortman RL & Kelley WN. Gout and hyperuricemia. In S Ruddy, ED Harris & CB Sledge (eds) *Kelley's Textbook of Rheumatology* 2001, pp 1339–76; W.B. Saunders Company, Philadelphia.

116

Back Pain

John V. Butler

Caerphilly District Miners Hospital, Caerphilly, UK

INTRODUCTION

Back pain is a very common complaint in both developed and developing countries, with a lifetime prevalence ranging from 11 to 84% (Walker, 2000). It has been traditionally perceived to be a problem affecting relatively younger adults where its major impact on the workplace, associated economic burdens and public health implications, have been well described. Both physicians and older patients have been guilty of regarding back pain as an inevitable part of aging, this despite the fact that prevalence of low back pain appears to decline with age, the majority of patients having their first presentation before the age of 65 years (Lavsky-Shulan *et al.*, 1985). The reasons for this decline are unclear but may partly be explained by a change in working life patterns and associated psychosocial adjustments that come with retirement.

While prevalence studies performed in older people are limited, a cohort of older American adults demonstrated that over one-fifth of patients age 68–100 years had back pain on most days, particularly in the lower back. Older people confined mostly to their homes were especially affected, while prevalence was demonstrably higher in women compared to men. This was notably more evident for mid or upper back pain (Edmond and Felson, 2000).

Back pain remains a very challenging assessment and diagnostic problem in elderly people. Its causes are often multiple, while the incidence of serious pathology is considerably higher than in younger people. Older patients commonly have pains that are of a different nature from those found in younger or middle-aged adults and often they show a marked discrepancy between imaging findings and demonstrable pain (Baumgartner, 1996). There is a large spectrum of presentations that range from acute and life-threatening, such as occurs with a leaking abdominal aortic aneurysm, to chronic persistent nonspecific back pain syndromes. While the majority of back pain presentations are self-limiting and will resolve within 6 weeks, identifying more serious causes requires a logical stepwise approach to establish the cause so that optimal treatment can be instigated. The physicians' dilemma is to differentiate between those back pains which may herald more sinister pathology from those of more benign disease. This is of particular importance in older people given the relatively higher proportion of identifiable secondary causes such as cancer, infection, and fracture in this group.

The health-care costs for the patient population suffering from back pain are very substantial. The total expenditure in the United States alone came to over $90 billion in 1998, which represented approximately 1% of its gross domestic product. It was also demonstrated that the elderly population, particularly females in this group, incurred higher costs on average when compared with younger individuals (Luo *et al.*, 2003). The human cost in terms of pain, depression, and disability as a result of back pain cannot be fully quantified but almost two-thirds of older people, again women more so than men, will experience functional limitations as a result of it (Edmond and Felson, 2003). Once back pain becomes chronic in older patients recovery is less effective compared to younger individuals, particularly in the context of an associated specific etiological diagnosis or psychosocial disorder (Van Doorn, 1995; Rossignol *et al.*, 1988).

DEFINITIONS

Back pain has many different phases that need to be defined in order to provide a clearer picture to the physician. This is particularly important for older people when multiple professional disciplines are usually involved in assessing and managing patients. Useful definitions that follow the natural history of back pain have been proposed using the following terms (VonKorff, 1994):

Transient back pain is an episode in which back pain is present on no more than 90 consecutive days and does not recur over a 12-month observation period.

Principles and Practice of Geriatric Medicine, 4th Edition. Edited by M.S. John Pathy, Alan J. Sinclair and John E. Morley.

Recurrent back pain is back pain present on less than half the days in a 12-month period, occurring in multiple episodes over the year.

Chronic back pain is back pain present on at least half the days in a 12-month period in a single or multiple episodes.

Acute back pain refers to pain that is not recurrent or chronic and whose onset is recent and sudden.

First onset refers to an episode of back pain that is its first occurrence in a person's lifetime.

A *flare-up* is a phase of back pain superimposed on a recurrent or chronic course when back pain is markedly more severe for the person.

An *episode of low back pain* is a period of pain in the lower back lasting for more than 24 hours, preceded and followed by at least 1 month without back pain (De Vet *et al.*, 2002).

NORMAL SPINE AGING

Back and neck pain may arise from several anatomical structures in the spine including intervertebral disks, facet joints, paravertebral musculature, spinal nerve roots as well as joint ligaments connecting vertebrae and spinal nerve roots. All of these structures are subjected to age-related degenerative changes and as such they play an important role in the etiology of back pain in older people. A wide range of genetic and environmental insults influence such changes. All parts of the spine undergo degenerative changes with aging (Andersson, 1998). Autopsy studies have shown that significant disk degeneration is evident in most spines by at least the fourth decade (Schmorl and Junghanns, 1971) and is ubiquitous by the sixth decade (Vernon-Roberts, 1988). This appears to occur earlier in men compared to women. The intervertebral disk is a cartilaginous structure but morphologically it is different to articular cartilage. It shows degenerative and aging changes earlier than does any other connective tissue in the body. These changes have frequently been cited as causing spine stiffness, neck and lower back pain which may be chronic or intermittent (Urban and Roberts, 2003).

Disk degeneration involves disruption of the normal annular fibers. Such degeneration occurs as a result of complex biochemical and biomechanical factors that the disk is subjected to throughout a lifetime. These include declining nutrition, loss of viable cells, cell senescence, reduced water content of the nucleus pulposus, accumulation of cell waste products such as proteoglycan fragments, and reduced ability to instigate repair of damaged tissues at a molecular level. Scoliosis for example is associated with decreased endplate permeability, which may reduce diffusion of nutrients leading to accelerated degenerative disease (Bibby *et al.*, 2001). Osteophyte growth from the margins of the vertebral bodies and facet joint osteoarthrosis are other characteristic features of the degenerative process but it remains unclear as to what triggers their progression. It is postulated that the latter occurs as a result of changing stresses on the facet joints with age. Environmental stresses to the spine, especially in those engaged in manual work, also appear to accelerate the development of degenerative changes, the disks being mostly affected. The relative risk ratio for disk degeneration with space narrowing was 1.8 in a comparison between concrete reinforcement workers compared to a matched group of house painters. Such disk narrowing and spondylotic changes occurred significantly earlier in the former group (Riihimaki *et al.*, 1989).

These degenerative changes especially when associated with disease processes in the back such as osteoarthritis, osteoporosis, and vertebral collapse are important contributory factors in causing impairment and resultant disability in older people.

CLINICAL EVALUATION

It has been suggested that instead of laboriously seeking an exact cause for a back pain presentation, the priority should be to answer three pertinent questions (Deyo, 1986). Is there a serious systemic disease causing the pain; is there neurological compromise requiring urgent intervention; and are psychosocial factors contributing to the pain syndrome?

The initial diagnostic evaluation of any back or neck pain presentation demands meticulous care in gathering a comprehensive history and performing a carefully structured examination. Appropriate investigations may then be pursued as guided by the clinical findings. If after the initial assessment no risk factors for a serious cause are evident, then no diagnostic tests are required but patients should be reassured, educated, and offered appropriate pain relief and early return to usual activity encouraged. Patients should be followed up at 2 weeks and if normal activity has not been reestablished a careful review of risk factors and response to initial treatment is recommended. If warning features suggesting serious pathology become apparent, then further investigation is mandatory (Rose-Innes and Engstrom, 1998).

Back pain may arise from several anatomical structures in the spine such as occurs in intervertebral disk herniation or spinal stenosis (*see* **Chapter 85, Cervical and Lumbar Spinal Canal Stenosis**). It may also be the presenting complaint in visceral diseases unrelated to the spine such as occurs in abdominal aortic aneurysm. Given the many demands on physician time, the need to be alert to worrying symptoms and signs, the so-called *red flags*, is of paramount importance in identifying serious disease. In a primary care setting of all patients presenting with back pain, 4% will have compression fractures, 3% will have spondylolisthesis, while a not insignificant 0.7% will have either primary or secondary cancers. One patient in 10 000 will have had spinal infections such as diskitis or osteomyelitis (Deyo *et al.*, 1992). A systematic assessment helps to separate the benign from serious pathology, and distinguishing spinal from nonspinal pain. Patients with a nonmechanical cause of pain such as cancer or those suitable for surgery may thus be identified and referred to the relevant specialist. The remainder may then be managed with appropriate analgesia and mobilization regimes.

History

A careful and thorough history of pain is essential in establishing the anatomical site of pain. All conventional aspects of pain should be assessed. The time of onset of pain is of particular importance, as well as the following questions: is it acute or insidious; what is the duration of pain, is it intermittent, persistent, or chronic in nature; what were the circumstances of how the pain developed; was there any associated trauma, however trivial; are there associated symptoms such as weight loss or rigors; does the pain radiate; are there any lower limb motor or sensory symptoms; what are the precipitating, aggravating, and relieving factors; what is the severity and intensity of the pain. Pain that is not relieved on lying down, while not specific, should increase suspicion of underlying infection or malignancy.

The past medical history should focus on clues such as a previous history of tuberculosis or trauma. Risk factors for osteoporosis should be sought after (*see* **Chapter 110, Epidemiology of Osteoporosis**). Careful attention to the drug history including over-the-counter and herbal medicines is required, particularly changes in medication that may correlate to the onset of pain. Patients who have received long-term corticosteroid medication should have a vertebral compression fracture assumed unless later excluded.

The family history should explore the possibility of conditions such as rheumatoid arthritis, which have a strong familial inheritance pattern. Points to be established in the social history include past and present smoking and alcohol intake, relevant occupations particularly where manual work or a more sedentary lifestyle was a strong feature. The review of systems should especially focus on symptoms that might point to more sinister pathology such as weight loss or a change in bowel habit. Symptoms of prostate disease in men and breast disease in women, even if deemed trivial by patients, should always be given serious attention.

Depression or anxiety states should also be sought, as these play an important role in the evolution of back pain syndromes.

Difficulties in history-taking may arise in some older patients who are reluctant to report pain or in cognitively impaired individuals. In these situations observation should be made for increased vocalizations such as moaning or crying or behavior changes such as grimacing or irritability, which may herald underlying pain. Caregivers may also be in a position to report any recent changes particularly in function that are not readily apparent. "Red flags" in the history in older patients include pain which is worse at rest or at night, a previous history of cancer or chronic infection, a trauma history, pain which has persisted for more than one month, prior corticosteroid or intravenous drug use, or a change in bladder habits (Rose-Innes and Engstrom, 1998).

Examination

A comprehensive physical examination should be performed when assessing older individuals with back or neck pain. This is important because the source of pain may not originate in the spine structures, or the pain may arise from more than one site. Patients should be examined in both the supine and standing positions with the spinal posture and range and symmetry of movements noted in the latter, while neurological assessment can be performed in the former. Leg length discrepancies, standing posture, as well as gait and postural sway disorders may also contribute to back pain; examination for these conditions should be made (Gurney, 2002).

Patients should also be sufficiently undressed so that the breasts in women and prostate gland in men can both be given careful attention. The genitalia should not be overlooked particularly in male patients as otherwise tumors or large hydroceles may be missed. Additional signs to be looked for in older women include the severity of flexed posture. This has been shown to correlate to the severity of vertebral pain, emotional status, muscular impairment, and motor function. It also has a measurable effect on resulting disability (Balzini *et al.*, 2003).

Alarming signs to be looked for include unexplained pyrexia or evidence of weight loss, a positive Lasegue (straight leg raising) test, percussion tenderness over the spine or costovertebral angles, the presence of an abdominal, rectal, or pelvic mass, or any focal neurological signs especially if these are progressive (Rose-Innes and Engstrom, 1998).

Trigger points may also provide useful diagnostic clues. These are discrete hyperirritable spots located in taut bands of skeletal muscle. In the back, these can manifest as low back pain or gait changes, while in the neck they may be important in the etiology of headache or temperomandibular joint pain. Palpation of the trigger point can elicit pain directly over the affected area or to a referred site (Alvarez and Rockwell, 2002).

Non-radiological Investigations

These will be guided by the clinical presentation. An elevated erythrocyte sedimentation rate (ESR), white blood cell count (WBC), alkaline phosphatase, prostate specific antigen or a monoclonal band on serum, or urine electrophoresis are all indications of serious disease. A septic screen to include urine, stool, and serial blood cultures should be performed wherever underlying sepsis is suspected. Cerebrospinal fluid should be examined and cultured where meningitis is a possibility and there are no contraindications to a lumbar puncture being performed.

It should be remembered that typical markers of infection are not always apparent in older people even in the face of overwhelming sepsis. Readers are referred to the appropriate chapters on metabolic bone disease (*see* **Chapter 109, Paget's Disease of Bone**; **Chapter 111, Osteoporosis and**

its Consequences: a Major Threat to the Quality of Life in the Elderly) and cancer (*see* **Chapter 128, Cancer and Aging**; **Chapter 129, Oncological Emergencies and Urgencies**; **Chapter 125, Prostate Diseases**; **Chapter 130, Breast Cancer in the Elderly**) for appropriate investigations where these are suspected.

Radiological Investigations

A high index of suspicion for most of the sinister causes of lower back pain can be arrived at through careful exploration of the history and examination. Routine imaging in older patients with acute low back pain should not be performed unless they present with suspected serious pathology such as trauma, acute vertebral collapse, a neurological deficit, or suspicion of infection or neoplasm is present.

There is a large spectrum of imaging studies that can be performed, but their use should be tailored to individual presentations. The potential benefits and limitations of such studies should always be borne in mind so as to avoid unnecessary and expensive investigations. Advanced imaging should be reserved for those in whom sinister disease is strongly suspected or those who would consider surgical intervention where appropriate. The simple question of how a patients' management to include diagnosis, treatment, and outcome will change on the basis of a positive or negative test result is a useful guide in determining the appropriateness of particular investigations. Readers are referred to **Chapter 144, Diagnostic Imaging and Interventional Radiology**, which further addresses these issues.

Plain Radiograph

In older adults with self-reported back pain, osteophytes are the most frequent radiographic feature. Together with endplate sclerosis they are found more frequently in men than in women. Disk space narrowing is usually the first indicator of degenerative disease on plain radiograph and appears to be more strongly associated with back pain than any other radiographic feature (Pye *et al.*, 2004). Even though the prevalence of degenerative change is high in older people, the therapeutic consequences of diagnosing this abnormality are minimal.

The diagnostic contribution of the frontal lumbar spine radiograph in community dwelling adults has been prospectively examined. In over 90% of cases the antero-posterior view was noncontributory, while a single lateral lumbar view can pick up important conditions such as infection, malignancy, or benign tumors (Khoo *et al.*, 2003). Plain film sensitivity is poor, however, as infections such as osteomyelitis tend to show up late, sometimes up to 8 weeks after symptoms begin (Smith and Blaser, 1991).

Ultrasound

There are several medical applications for diagnostic ultrasound. It is especially attractive in older people because of its ease of use, relative low cost, and noninvasive nature. It may identify intraabdominal causes of back pain such as abdominal aortic aneurysm, but it can also be used in assessing spine disorders. Such applications include measuring the spinal canal, detecting cord abnormalities, quantifying scoliotic curves, and examining soft tissue abnormalities. Ultrasound may also be used potentially as a preliminary diagnostic procedure for lumbar disk herniation, but it is distinctly inferior to magnetic resonance imaging (MRI) mainly due to lower diagnostic accuracy (Berth *et al.*, 2003).

Radioisotope Bone Scan

This is more sensitive at picking up metastatic disease than plain films and should be used where malignant disease is suspected clinically. It can also be used to identify infection in bone particularly where disease is occult. Degenerative disk disease, especially in its later stages, can also be identified in this way.

Computed Tomography

This is not as useful as MRI in viewing the spine. It is more helpful in diagnosing nonspinal sources of back pain such as abdominal aortic aneurysm.

Magnetic Resonance Imaging

This can be used where either neoplastic or infectious pathology are suspected. It may also be utilized in patients with radicular pain particularly those with a clear level of nerve root impingement or those with sciatica-type symptoms but where nerve root dysfunction is unclear. MRI scanning is often overutilized especially when compared to simple lumbar radiographs where no long-term benefit in terms of disability, pain, or general health status was identified (Jarvik *et al.*, 2003).

Bone Scintigraphy

This can be used to detect stress fractures and bone metastases. It may also be combined with nuclear medicine studies such as radio-labelled white blood cell scans in identifying and localizing occult infections particularly those deep seated in vertebral bone.

Specific Causes

The differential diagnosis of the many causes of back pain is presented in Table 1. It must be emphasized that the diagnostic probabilities in older patients are considerably different to younger people with a much higher prevalence of compression fractures, cancer, spinal stenosis, and abdominal aortic aneurysm. Readers are referred to the various chapters that address many of these individual causes in more detail.

Table 1 Differential diagnosis of low back pain

Mechanical low back or leg pain[a]	Nonmechanical spinal conditions	Visceral disease
Lumbar strain, sprain[b]	*Neoplasia*	*Disease of pelvic organs*
Degenerative processes of disks and facets	Multiple myeloma	Prostatitis
	Metastatic carcinoma	Endometriosis
Herniated disk	Lymphoma & Leukemia	Chronic pelvic
Spinal stenosis	Spinal cord tumors	Inflammatory disease
Osteoporotic compression	Retroperitoneal tumors	*Renal disease*
Fracture	Primary vertebral tumors	Nephrolithiasis
Spondylolisthesis	*Infection*	Pyelonephritis
Traumatic fracture	Osteomyelitis	Perinephric abscess
Severe kyphosis	Septic diskitis	*Aortic aneurysm*
Severe scoliosis	Paraspinous abscess	*Gastrointestinal disease*
Transitional vertebrae	Epidural abscess	Pancreatitis
Spondylolysis[c]	Shingles	Cholecystitis
Internal disk disruption or diskogenic low back pain[d]	*Inflammatory arthritis*	Penetrating ulcer
	Ankylosing spondylitis	
Presumed instability[e]	Psoriatic spondylitis	
	Reiter's syndrome	
	Inflammatory bowel disease	
	Paget's disease of bone	
	Osteochondrosis	

Adapted from NEJM by permission of Massachusetts Medical Society.
[a]The term "mechanical" is used here to designate an anatomical or functional abnormality without an underlying malignant, neoplastic, or inflammatory disease. [b]"Strain" and "sprain" are nonspecific terms with no pathoanatomical confirmation. "Idiopathic low back pain" may be a preferable term. [c]Spondylolysis is as common among asymptomatic persons as among those with low back pain, so its role in causing low back pain remains ambiguous. [d]Internal disk disruption is diagnosed by provocative diskography (injection of contrast material into a degenerated disk, with assessment of pain at the time of injection). However, it often causes pain in asymptomatic adults, and the condition of many patients with positive diskograms improves spontaneously. Thus, the clinical importance and appropriate management of this condition remain unclear. "Diskogenic low back pain" is used more or less synonymously with "internal disk disruption". [e]Presumed instability is loosely defined as greater than 10° of angulation or 4 mm of vertebral displacement on lateral flexion and extension radiograms. However, the diagnostic criteria, natural history, and surgical indications remain controversial.

Vertebral Fracture

On a plain x-ray if a fracture is confirmed, referral for specialist opinion should be done to address the underlying cause and to explore treatment options. If a fracture is not clearly evident but suspicions remain, then specialist referral and consideration for performing an isotope bone scan may be considered.

Neoplastic Disease

High suspicion for individual cancers warrants referral to the appropriate specialist. Multiple myeloma and metastatic disease, particularly prostate in men and breast in women, are much more common than primary spine tumors.

Infection

Infections can manifest in several spine structures including the bony vertebrae, the interstitial disks, paraspinal muscles, zygapophysial joints, and meninges. An elevated ESR or WBC supports the diagnosis, but once again it should be remembered that these are not always evident in older people.

The goals of management are early identification of causative organisms, preservation of neurological function, infection eradication with pain resolution, and spine stability. If serious infective pathology such as osteomyelitis, tuberculosis, or diskitis is suspected then appropriate specialist referral is warranted.

Osteomyelitis: The history is commonly of insidious onset over a period of weeks or months, and is usually localized in the thoracolumbar spine having been seeded via the haematogenous route (Lew and Waldvogel, 2004). Vertebral tenderness has sensitivity for underlying infection but lacks specificity. Pyrexia and raised white cell count may be absent in up to 50% of cases while blood cultures are commonly negative. Needle biopsy may be required to allow microbial and pathological examination so as to facilitate targeted and long lasting antimicrobial treatment. The ESR is commonly elevated and may be used as a marker to monitor response to treatment. A multidisciplinary approach involving expertise in orthopedics, radiology, and infectious disease is often required for optimal outcomes. The physiological and anatomical characteristics of bone often pose difficulty in eradicating infection. This is often compounded by the emergence of resistant organisms such as methicillin resistant *Staphloccocus aureus*.

Diskitis: This occurs when there is inflammation of the intervertebral disk space. This is frequently caused by an associated vertebral bone infection while endplate infection can also lead to vertebral osteomyelitis. Its incidence in Europe is approximately 1 in 50 000 inhabitants but is believed to be even higher in older people. Its onset is often insidious making diagnosis difficult. It commonly occurs secondary to a primary infective focus such as in the urinary tract. MRI is the preferred method of investigation, but biopsy may be required to confirm the diagnosis. Clinical symptoms, infective and inflammatory markers, temperature and interval radiological changes will guide antimicrobial treatment, the duration of which may be up to 12 weeks. Whilst epidural infection with neurological sequelae can occur, the prognosis is generally good (Lam and Webb, 2004).

Tuberculosis: Pott's disease is a common and serious form of tuberculous infection of the spine with potentially catastrophic sequelae including paraplegia. It commonly localizes to the thoracic spine involving the vertebral body. It too may have an insidious onset. Common presenting symptoms include leg weakness (69%), gibbus (46%), local pain (21%), and a palpable mass in 10% (Turget, 2001). Identification and sensitivity patterns of causative organisms, appropriate antituberculous chemotherapy with decompressive surgery when required are the mainstays of treatment.

Prolapsed Intervertebral Disc

Symptoms of prolapsed disk include backache that is commonly of abrupt onset, sciatica, or those suggestive of cauda equina syndrome (CES) as described later. Clinical signs will depend on the level of root involvement and are helpful in improving accuracy of the site of compression. A positive, straight leg-raising test is up to 80% accurate in diagnosing the condition. Pain on crossed straight leg-raising increases diagnostic accuracy even further. MRI should be considered as the gold standard for confirming clinical suspicion. Conservative treatments will incorporate many of the measures used for treating nonspecific low back pain including limited bed rest during the acute period with simple analgesia and controlled weight loss in obese patients. Both nonsteroidal anti-inflammatory drugs (NSAIDs) and muscle relaxants may have a role to play, but they should be used cautiously in older people given their significant adverse effect profile.

Epidural injections and traction under specialist supervision may be useful for pain that is difficult to control. Epidemiological studies suggest that pain will resolve in the majority of patients using conservative measures. Surgical decompression should be reserved for carefully selected individuals not responding to at least 1 month of conservative treatment and where the diagnosis is not disputed. The balance of potential risks and benefits, as always, needs to be carefully considered. There is considerable evidence that surgical diskectomy provides effective clinical relief for such patients. Chemonucleosis (injection of chymopapain into the disk space) is a less invasive, intermediate procedure between conservative and open surgery, which can be considered in less robust individuals, but it is less effective than open diskectomy.

Lumbar Spine Stenosis

This commonly affects older people and is often demonstrated incidentally on CT or MRI imaging (Hudgins, 1983). Disk degenerative disease, facet joint osteoarthritis, and ligamentum flavum hypertrophy are the commonest causes. It is often associated with incapacitating pain in the lower back and extremities, reduced mobility, lower limb paraesthesia, and weakness. In severe cases, bowel and bladder disturbance may become evident. Readers are referred to **Chapter 85, Cervical and Lumbar Spinal Canal Stenosis** for further details.

Cauda Equina Syndrome (CES)

Characteristics of CES include low back pain, sciatica, saddle anaesthesia, decreased rectal tone and perineal reflexes together with lower limb extremity and bowel or bladder dysfunction. There are many causes of this syndrome including infection, neoplasm, trauma (including iatrogenic procedures), and intervertebral disk herniation.

Decompression surgery is the treatment of choice but the optimal timing of this is unclear.

Emergency decompressive surgery compared to the "next available list" did not lead to significantly improved outcomes (Hussain *et al.*, 2003).

Abdominal Aortic Aneurysm

This is an important nonspinal cause of low back pain, which warrants special mention, as its incidence increases steeply with age. It is three times more common in men than women where it may affect up to 5% of individuals age 65–74 years. The only well established risk factor is cigarette smoking. Its natural history is highly variable, varying from an asymptomatic incidental clinical finding to abrupt rupture with presentations including acute severe back pain, an expanding pulsatile mass, as well as sudden death. Ultrasound or CT scanning help to confirm the diagnosis. Ruptured aneurysm is a surgical emergency, which carries a high perioperative mortality of up to 50%, while in untreated patients death is usually inevitable (Ernst, 1993). The UK Small Aneurysm trial suggests observing small aneurysms with transverse diameter between 4 and 5.5 cm with ultrasound surveillance every 6 months with elective surgical repair in suitable candidates if it grows at a rate of more than 1 cm per year. Once again the benefits and risks of major elective surgery must be carefully assessed for individual patients (UKSAT, 1998).

Nonspecific Low Back Pain

This is defined as pain between the costal margins and the inferior gluteal folds that is generally accompanied by painful limitation of movement. It remains the commonest cause of back pain in older people. It is affected by physical posture and activities and may be associated with referred pain. The diagnosis is made when no underlying disorder such as fracture or infection is evident. In the majority of patients no organic cause is identified although degenerative processes are often sited (Deyo and Weinstein, 2001). Many of the treatments used in its management have also been used for mechanical neck pains with varying degrees of success.

Nonpharmacological Interventions

Most patients including older people with acute back pain of a non-serious etiology will get better without any treatment or with simple analgesia alone. Nonspecific chronic low back pain, however, requires both a physical and psychosocial evaluation that may incorporate various nonpharmacological treatment measures. This is especially important in the context of multidisciplinary team management. Many older patients with lower back pain as well as their physicians are also interested in trying nonpharmacological therapies outside the conventional medical spectrum, particularly so as to avoid adverse drug effects of which older people are at high risk. Such measures have various degrees of benefit and are outlined below.

Bed Rest

There is limited quality research into bed rest as a treatment for lower back pain but current evidence suggests that bed rest should not be recommended for acute low back pain as this may delay recovery and potentially harm patients with complications such as deep vein thrombosis or pressure sores. Enforced bed rest should not be replaced, however, with enforced activity (Allen *et al.*, 1999).

Type of Mattress

Physicians are commonly asked by patients with lower back pain to advise on the type of bed or mattress that may relieve symptoms. In a randomized double-blinded controlled multicenter study which included patients up to 82 years, it was shown that a mattress of medium firmness improved pain and disability among patients with chronic nonspecific low back pain possibly by promoting sleeping in the fetal position or distributing body weight more evenly (Kovacs *et al.*, 2003).

Lumbar Supports

A restriction of trunk motion for flexion–extension and lateral bending as well as a reduction in required back muscle forces in lifting are proposed as mechanisms of action of lumbar supports. They have been used as both primary and secondary preventative measures for lower back pain. There is, however, no evidence that they are effective in the latter while there is moderate evidence that they are no more effective than no intervention, in the former (Jellema *et al.*, 2000).

There is still a requirement for high quality randomized controlled trials with inclusion of older people to address their value if any, while aid compliance will also need to be fully ascertained in such work. There are also valid concerns that prolonged use of such supports may lead to increased trunk muscle weakness and atrophy which may in turn exacerbate the underlying problem.

Massage

Advocates of massage therapy claim that it can minimize pain and disability, as well as speed up return to normal function. A systematic review of various massage treatments concluded that massage might be beneficial for patients with subacute and chronic nonspecific lower back pain, particularly when combined with exercise treatment and patient education. Patients included in the trials examined were predominantly a younger population. In this group acupuncture massage appears to be more effective than classic massage but more studies including older participants are required to confirm this as well as determining its cost-effectiveness (Furlan *et al.*, 2002). In elderly institutionalized individuals back massage has been shown to reduce anxiety levels but effects on pain control have not been examined(Fraser and Kerr, 1993). The effects of massage therapy for nonspecific neck pain are not clearly established yet.

Exercise Therapy

Exercise is a widely prescribed treatment for chronic low back pain aiming to improve performance in activities of daily living by improving impairments in back flexibility, strength, and endurance. Exercise also aims to reduce the intensity of back pain and associated disability by challenging established fears and attitudes patients might have. Tailored exercise programs addressing the specific needs and abilities of individual patients have been found to be a safe and effective way of reducing pain and functional dependency. In a systematic review there was strong evidence that exercise helps individuals with chronic low back pain to return to normal activities of daily living, but is not more effective for acute low back pain than inactive or other active treatments (Van Tulder *et al.*, 2000a).

Acupuncture

Both acupuncture and electroacupuncture are used worldwide as alternative medical therapies mainly for the treatment of acute and chronic pain. Endogenous opioid peptides in the central nervous system play an essential role in mediating their analgesic effect. In a systematic review acupuncture appears to be superior to various control interventions but there is insufficient evidence to establish its superiority to placebo (Tulder *et al.*, 2000). In a subsequent randomized controlled study, electroacupuncture was specifically examined in older patients over 60 years of age with chronic low back pain and was found to be a safe and effective adjunctive treatment in the intervention group (Ernst *et al.*, 2002).

Spinal Manipulation Therapy (SMT)

Spinal manipulation therapy (SMT) acts on the various components of the vertebral motion segment. It distracts the facet joints and with faster separation a cracking sound is heard. Relaxation of the paraspinal muscles occurs when they are forcibly stretched although the mechanisms of this are unclear. SMT is often used for both back and neck pain. In a systematic review incorporating 39 randomized controlled trials it was concluded that there is no evidence that SMT is superior to other treatments such as general practitioner care, analgesia, physiotherapy, exercise, or back schools for acute or chronic low back pain (Assendelft *et al.*, 2003). There is limited evidence that SMT is superior to general practitioner management for short-term pain reduction in chronic neck pain but no long-term benefit is gained. This is especially so when compared to more multidisciplinary rehabilitation exercise programs (Bronfort *et al.*, 2004). The safety profile of SMT in older patients has not been fully established particularly for the treatment of acute or chronic neck pain.

Transcutaneous Electrical Nerve Stimulation (TENS)

Transcutaneous electrical nerve stimulation (TENS) therapy was introduced in the 1970s as an alternative therapy to drug treatments for chronic pain. It is a noninvasive modality that is used for pain relief by electrically stimulating peripheral nerves via electrodes placed on the skin. Its mode of action is based on the gate-control theory of pain which proposes that the TENS mechanism generates neuroregulatory peripheral and central effects that modulate pain transmission. In a systematic review there was no evidence to support the use of TENS in the treatment of chronic low back pain although the meta-analysis lacked data on how TENS effectiveness is affected by the type and site of electrode applications or treatment durations, frequencies, and intensities (Milne *et al.*, 2004).

Behavioral Treatment

Behavioral interventions are commonly used in the treatment of disabling chronic low back pain. These are based on the rationale that psychosocial factors, patient attitudes and beliefs, as well as illness behavior are just as important in chronic low back pain syndromes as somatic disease (Waddell,1987).

Cognitive therapy aims to identify and modify patients' thoughts regarding their pain and disability. This can be done directly by cognitive restructuring techniques such as imagery or attention diversion, or indirectly by changing maladaptive beliefs and thoughts (Turner and Jensen, 1993).

A systematic review concluded that behavioral therapies appeared to be an effective treatment for patients with chronic low back pain, but it was unclear what type of patients would benefit while the reviewed trials predominantly examined younger populations (Van Tulder *et al.*, 2000b).

Biopsychosocial approaches have not been examined in older adults but in a working age population there is moderate evidence that multidisciplinary rehabilitation is effective for subacute low back pain (Karjalainen *et al.*, 2004a) but not for neck pain (Karjalainen *et al.*, 2004b). Routine physiotherapy for patients with mild to moderate low back pain may be no more effective in the long term than advice given by a physiotherapist (Frost *et al.*, 2004).

Back Schools

These have been predominantly studied in younger age-groups where a systematic review concluded that they may be effective for patients with recurrent and chronic low back pain in occupational settings. Their cost-effectiveness has not been established. The trials examined did not include older patients as participants (Van Tulder *et al.*, 2000c).

Neuroreflexology

Neuroreflexology is characterized by temporary implantation of a number of epidermal staples into trigger points in the back and into referred tender points in the ear. It is a separate entity to acupuncture as different zones of the skin are stimulated. It is performed without anaesthesia and takes about 60 minutes for the staples to be implanted. These remain in place for up to 90 days in the back and up to 20 days in the ear. A systematic review showed that it appears to be a safe and effective short-term treatment for chronic nonspecific low back pain, but further multinational randomized controlled trials are needed to confirm this (Kovacs *et al.*, 2002).

Radiofrequency Denervation

Radiofrequency current is a clinical tool used for creating discrete thermal lesions in neural pathways in order to interrupt transmission. Such currents can be used to block nociceptive pathways at various sites. It can be considered as a minimally invasive alternative to open surgery in suitably selected older patients. The technique was first developed in the 1970s and has been used as a palliative treatment in conditions such as trigeminal neuralgia and nerve root avulsion. It is a highly technical procedure, which requires a skilled operator and is not without its complications. In a systematic review, there was limited evidence that it provides short-term benefits in patients with lumbar zygapophysial joint pain and conflicting evidence in favor of a short-term benefit in cervical zygapophysial joint pain Niemisto *et al.* (2003).

Other Treatments

Other alternative treatments that have been tried for lower back pain include herbal medicines, homeopathy, balneotherapy, prolotherapy, heat and cold therapies, but evidence for their efficacy is limited.

Pharmacological Interventions

Readers are referred to **Chapter 84, Control of Chronic Pain** on pain management, particularly stepwise treatment of pain along the pathway of the standard analgesic ladder. A number of systematic reviews have addressed the benefits and problems of different category analgesics especially for nonspecific causes of back pain. Again it must be emphasized that pharmacological treatments beyond simple analgesia such as paracetamol, should be preferably avoided given the usually inevitable association with adverse effects in older people.

Nonsteroidal Anti-inflammatory Drugs (NSAIDs)

NSAIDs are the most frequently prescribed medications worldwide. Their potential for adverse effects including gastrointestinal, cardiovascular, and renal function, particularly in older people is well documented. It remains unclear whether or not they are more effective than simple analgesia such as paracetamol (Van Tulder *et al.*, 2000d).

Muscle Relaxants

Both benzodiazepines and nonbenzodiazepines have been evaluated in treating low back pain. The latter have greater efficacy than the former in treating acute pain, but the relatively high occurrence of adverse effects including gastrointestinal and central nervous system effects such as drowsiness and dizziness, of which older people may be more vulnerable to, suggests they should be used with great caution. Most studies have been performed in a relatively younger population where the nonbenzodiazepine drugs particularly carisoprodol have been shown to have most efficacy for acute lower back pain (Van Tulder *et al.*, 2004)

Antidepressants

Antidepressant drugs have been extensively used for chronic pain syndromes including chronic low back pain. Their efficacy has been postulated to be due to a combination of their antidepressant, sedative, and analgesic properties. Both tricyclic and tetracyclic antidepressants produce a moderate effect on symptom reduction in patients with chronic low back pain, independently of depression status. Selective serotonin reuptake inhibitors do not appear to have the same effect. It is unclear whether patient functional status improves though (Staiger *et al.*, 2003).

Neck Pain

Neck pain is second only to low back pain as the most common musculoskeletal disorder in population surveys and primary care with a point prevalence of 22% (Cote *et al.*, 2000). As such, it too represents a major cause of morbidity and health-care expenditure. Like low back pain it can be a difficult symptom to assess as often the pain is poorly localized and important symptoms and signs are often located peripherally. The aging neck is also prone to many of the degenerative processes described earlier, particularly as it is a relatively more mobile structure than the thoracic or lumbosacral spine. Cervical disk, vertebrae, as well as cord pathology can all produce symptoms and signs located elsewhere. Pain may be purely mechanical such as in spondylosis, myelopathy, or disk herniation, but other pathologies must also be considered, especially as these tend to occur more frequently in older people. These include:

rheumatological disorders such as rheumatoid and psoriatic arthritis, ankylosing spondylitis, fibromyalgia, polymyalgia rheumatica, and giant cell arthritis;
neurological disorders such as the neuropathies, brachial plexitis, and causes of meningeal irritation including subarachnoid hemorrhage;
neoplastic disease including primary and metastatic disease and multiple myeloma;
infective causes such as osteomyelits and diskitis as described previously. Herpes zoster infections may only become apparent with the appearance of the characteristic vesicular rash;
gastrointestinal disease including oesophageal spasm, gastro-oesophageal reflux disease, and pharyngeal pouch pathology;
trauma including both direct and indirect injuries;
referred pain including cardiovascular sources such as angina or arterial dissection.

Clinical Approach

A similar assessment process incorporating many of the features in assessing back pain will help guide appropriate investigations and treatment. Many of the specific causes of neck pain are addressed elsewhere in this textbook.

Cervical Spondylosis

This is usually caused by degenerative disk disease and is a very common cause of chronic neck pain in older people. Whiplash injuries in earlier adult life may also result in premature secondary cervical spondylosis. It can affect all levels of the cervical spine with degenerative disease evident in the intervertebral disks, vertebral body osteophytosis, and facet and laminal arch hypertrophy. Pain associated with cervical spondylosis may be local or referred elsewhere or both. Typical pain syndromes include that which develops at the back of the neck radiating to the occiput, shoulder, and upper limb if there is cervical root pressure from osteophytes or cervical disk disease. Pain responds variably to activity modification, neck immobilization, exercise programs, and appropriate analgesia.

Cervical spondylotic myelopathy is the most serious and disabling complication of the disease (*see* **Chapter 85, Cervical and Lumbar Spinal Canal Stenosis**). Simple neck immobilization can result in improvement in up to 50% of patients, while surgical intervention should be considered in patients presenting with severe or progressive neurological signs. However, there is no definite conclusion on the benefit/risk ratio of surgery (Fouyas *et al.*, 2002). Fortunately, neurological symptoms are uncommon, tending to occur more often in patients with associated congenital spinal stenosis.

KEY POINTS

- Back and neck pain are very common symptoms in older people.
- The incidence of serious pathology is much more common than in younger age-groups.
- "Red flag" symptoms and signs demand thorough investigation.
- Serious disease should be managed using the expertise of all appropriate specialists.
- Restoration of function and abolition of pain are the mainstays of management of nonspecific low back pain.

KEY REFERENCES

- Andersson GBJ. What are the age-related changes in the spine? *Bailliere's Clinical Rheumatology* 1998; **12**(1):161–73.
- Deyo R, Rainville J & Kent D. What can the history and physical examination tell us about low back pain. *The Journal of the American Medical Association* 1992; **268**(6):760–5.
- Deyo RA & Weinstein JN. Low back pain. *The New England Journal of Medicine* 2001; **344**:363–70.
- Lam SL & Webb JK. Discitis. *Hospital Medicine* 2004; **65**(5):280–6.
- Lew DP & Waldvogel FA. Osteomyelitis. *Lancet* 2004; **364**(9431): 369–79.
- Rose-Innes AP & Engstrom JW. Low back pain: an algorithmic approach to diagnosis and management. *Geriatrics* 1998; **53**(10):26–8, 33–6, 39–40.

REFERENCES

Allen C, Glasziou P & Del Mar C. Bed rest: a potentially harmful treatment needing more careful evaluation. *Lancet* 1999; **354**(9186):1229–33.

Alvarez DJ & Rockwell PG. Trigger points: diagnosis and management. *American Family Physician* 2002; **65**(4):653–60.

Andersson GBJ. What are the age-related changes in the spine? *Bailliere's Clinical Rheumatology* 1998; **12**(1):161–73.

Assendelft WJ, Morton SC, Yu EI *et al.* Spinal manipulative therapy for low back pain. A meta-analysis of effectiveness compared to other therapies. *Annals of Internal Medicine* 2003; **138**(11):871–81.

Balzini L, Vannucchi L, Benvenuti F *et al.* Clinical characteristics of flexed posture in elderly women. *Journal of the American Geriatrics Society* 2003; **51**(10):1419–26.

Baumgartner H. Lumbar pain in old age. *Schweizerische Rundschau Fur Medizine Praxis* 1996; **85**(43):1347–53.

Berth A, Mahlfeld K & Merk HR. Transabdominal ultrasonography in the diagnosis of lumbar disc herniation. *Ultraschall in der Medizin* 2003; **24**(6):383–7.

Bibby SR, Jones DA, Lee RB *et al.* The pathophysiology of the intervertabral disc. *Joint Bone Spine* 2001; **68**(6):537–42.

Bronfort G, Haas M, Evans RL *et al.* Efficacy of spinal manipulation and mobilisation for low back pain and neck pain: a systematic review and best evidence synthesis. *The Spine Journal* 2004; **4**(3):335–56.

Cote P, Cassidy JD & Carroll L. The factors associated with neck pain and its related disability in the Saskatchewan population. *Spine* 2000; **25**:1009–17.

De Vet HC, Heymans MW, Dunn KM *et al.* Episodes of low back pain: a proposal for uniform definitions to be used in research. *Spine* 2002; **27**(21):2409–16.

Deyo RA. Early diagnostic evaluation of low back pain. *Journal of General Internal Medicine* 1986; **3**:328–38.

Deyo R, Rainville J & Kent D. What can the history and physical examination tell us about low back pain. *The Journal of the American Medical Association* 1992; **268**(6):760–5.

Deyo RA & Weinstein JN. Low back pain. *The New England Journal of Medicine* 2001; **344**:363–70.

Edmond SL & Felson DT. Prevalence of back symptoms in elders. *The Journal of Rheumatology* 2000; **27**(1):220–5.

Edmond SL & Felson DT. Function and back symptoms in older adults. *Journal of the American Geriatrics Society* 2003; **51**(12):1702–9.

Ernst CB. Abdominal aortic aneurysm. *The New England Journal of Medicine* 1993; **328**:1167–72.

Ernst E, White AR & Wider B. Acupuncture for back pain: meta-analysis of randomised controlled trials and an update with data from the most recent studies. *Schmerz* 2002; **16**(2):129–39.

Fouyas IP, Statham PF & Sandercock PA. Cochrane review on the role of surgery in cervical spondylotic radiculomyelopathy. *Spine* 2002; **27**(7):736–47.

Fraser J & Kerr JR. Psychophysiological effects of back massage on the elderly. *Journal of Advanced Nursing* 1993; **18**(2):238–45.

Frost H, Lamb SE, Doll HA *et al.* Randomised controlled trial of physiotherapy compared with advice for low back pain. *British Medical Journal* 2004; **329**:708–11.

Furlan AD, Brosseau L, Imamura M *et al.* Massage for low-back pain: a systematic review within the framework of the Cochrane Collaboration Back Review Group. *Spine* 2002; **27**(17):1896–910.

Gurney B. Leg length discrepancy. *Gait & Posture* 2002; **15**(2):195–206.

Hudgins WR. Computer aided diagnosis of lumbar disc herniation. *Spine* 1983; **8**:604–15.

Hussain SA, Gullan RW & Chitnavis BP. Cauda equina syndrome: outcome and implications for management. *British Journal of Neurosurgery* 2003; **17**(2):164–7.

Jarvik JG, Hollingworth W, Martin B *et al.* Rapid magnetic resonance imaging vs radiographs for patients with low back pain: a randomised controlled trial. *The Journal of the American Medical Association* 2003; **289**(21):2810–8.

Jellema P, Van Tulder MW, Van Poppel MN *et al.* Lumbar supports for prevention and treatment of low back pain. *Spine* 2000; **26**(4):377–86.

Karjalainen K, Malmivaara A, van Tulder M *et al.* Multidisciplinary biopsychosocial rehabilitation for subacute low-back pain among working age adults (Cochrane Review). *The Cochrane Library* 2004a, Issue 3; John Wiley & Sons, Chichester.

Karjalainen K, Malmivaara A, van Tulder M *et al.* Multidisciplinary biopsychosocial rehabilitation for neck and shoulder pain among working age adults (Cochrane Review). *The Cochrane Library* 2004b, Issue 3; John Wiley & Sons, Chichester.

Khoo LA, Heron C, Patel U *et al.* The diagnostic contribution of the frontal lumbar spine radiograph in community referred low back pain – a prospective study of 1030 patients. *Clinical Radiology* 2003; **58**(8):606–9.

Kovacs FM, Abraira A, Pena A *et al.* Effect of firmness of mattress on chronic non-specific low-back pain: randomised, double-blind, controlled, multicentre trial. *Lancet* 2003; **362**:1599–604.

Kovacs FM, Llobera J, Abraira V *et al.* Effectiveness and cost-effectiveness analysis of neuroreflexotherapy for subacute and chronic low back pain in routine general practice. *Spine* 2002; **27**(11):1149–59.

Lam SL & Webb JK. Discitis. *Hospital Medicine* 2004; **65**(5):280–6.

Lavsky-Shulan M, Wallace RB, Kohout FJ *et al.* Prevalence and functional correlates of low back pain in the elderly: the Iowa 65+ Rural Health Study. *Journal of the American Geriatrics Society* 1985; **33**:23–8.

Lew DP & Waldvogel FA. Osteomyelitis. *Lancet* 2004; **364**(9431):369–79.

Luo X, Pietroban R, Sun S *et al.* Estimates and patterns of direct health care expenditures among individuals with back pain in the United States. *Spine* 2003; **29**(1):79–86.

Milne S, Welch V, Brosseau L *et al.* Transcutaneous electrical nerve stimulation (TENS) for chronic low-back pain (Cochrane Review). *The Cochrane Library* 2004, Issue 3; John Wiley & Sons, Chichester.

Niemisto L, Kalso E, Malmivaara A, Seitsalo S & Hurri H. Radiofrequency denervation for neck and back pain (Cochrane Review). *The Cochrane Library* 2003, Issue 3; John Wiley & Sons, Chichester.

Pye SR, Reid DM, Smith R *et al.* Radiographic features of lumbar disc degeneration and self-reported back pain. *The Journal of Rheumatology* 2004; **31**(4):753–8.

Riihimaki H, Wickstrom G, Hanninen K *et al.* Predictors of sciatic pain among concrete reinforcement workers and house painters. A five year follow-up. *Scandinavian Journal of Work, Environment and Health* 1989; **6**(15):415–23.

Rose-Innes AP & Engstrom JW. Low back pain: an algorithmic approach to diagnosis and management. *Geriatrics* 1998; **53**(10):26–8, 33–6, 39–40.

Rossignol M, Suissa S & Abenhaim L. Working disability due to occupational back pain: three year follow-up of 2300 compensated workers in Quebec. *Journal of Occupational Medicine* 1988; **30**:502–5.

Schmorl G & Junghanns H (Translated by EF Basemann) *The Human Spine in Health and Disease* 1971, Grune & Stratton, New York and London.

Smith AS & Blaser SI. Infections and inflammatory processes of the spine. *Radiologic Clinics of North America* 1991; **29**(4):809–27.

Staiger TO, Gaster B, Sullivan MD *et al.* Systematic review of antidepressants in the treatment of chronic low back pain. *Spine* 2003; **28**(22):2540–5.

Tulder MWVA, Cherkin DC, Berman B *et al. Cochrane Database of Systematic Reviews* 2000; **2**:CD001351.

Turget M. Spinal tuberculosis (Pott's disease): its clinical presentation, surgical management and outcome. A survey study on 694 patients. *Neurosurgical Review* 2001; **24**(1):8–13.

Turner JA & Jensen MP. Efficacy of cognitive therapy for chronic low back pain. *Pain* 1993; **52**:169–77.

UKSAT: The UK Small Aneurysm Trial Participants Mortality results for randomised controlled trial of early elective surgery or ultrasonographic surveillance for small abdominal aortic aneurysms. *Lancet* 1998; **352**:1649–55.

Urban JP & Roberts S. Degeneration of the intervertebral disc. *Arthritis Research & Therapy* 2003; **5**(3):120–30.

Van Doorn TWC. Low back disability among self-employed dentists, veterinarians, physicians and physical therapists in the Netherlands. *Acta Orthopaedica Scandinavica* 1995; **66**(suppl 263):1–64.

Van Tulder M, Malmivaara A, Esmail R *et al.* Exercise therapy for low back pain: a systematic review within the framework of the cochrane collaboration back review group. *Spine* 2000a; **25**(21):2784–96.

Van Tulder MW, Ostelo R, Vlaeyen JW *et al.* Behavioural treatment for chronic low-back pain. *Spine* 2000b; **25**(20):2688–99.

Van Tulder MW, Esmail R, Bombardier C *et al.* Back schools for non-specific low-back pain (Cochrane Review). *The Cochrane Library*, 2000c, Issue 3; John Wiley & Sons, Chichester.

Van Tulder MW, Scholten RJPM, Koes BW *et al.* Non-steroidal anti-inflammatory drugs for low back pain. (Cochrane review). *The Cochrane Library* 2000d, Issue 3; John Wiley & Sons, Chichester.

Van Tulder MW, Touray T, Furlan AD *et al.* Muscle relaxants for non-specific low-back pain (Cochrane Review). *The Cochrane Library* 2004, Issue 3; John Wiley & Sons, Chichester.

Vernon-Roberts B. Disc pathology and disease states. In P Ghosh (ed) *The Biology of the Intervertebral Disc* 1988, pp 73–120; CRC Press, Boca Raton.

VonKorff M. Studying the natural history of back pain. *Spine* 1994; **19**(18S):2041S–6S.

Waddell G. A new clinical model for the treatment of low back pain. *Spine* 1987; **12**:632–44.

Walker BF. The prevalence of low back pain: a systematic review of the literature from 1966 to 1998. *Journal of Spinal Disorders* 2000; **13**(3):205–17.

PART III

Medicine in Old Age

Section 10

Endocrine and Metabolic Disorders

117

Water and Electrolyte Balance in Health and Disease

Allen I. Arieff

University of California, San Francisco, CA, USA

INTRODUCTION

The major constituent of all body fluids is water and the major solutes are electrolytes. The body water is divided into major fluid compartments, which are the intracellular and extracellular spaces, and the extracellular space is further separated into plasma and interstitial components. Intracellular solutes are very different from those found in extracellular fluid. However, osmotic equilibrium dictates that the chemical potential of water must be the same in intra- and extracellular fluid. Since all cell membranes are readily permeable to water, osmolality throughout the body fluids is essentially the same, with only a few exceptions (renal medulla, CSF (cerebrospinal fluid)).

The volume and composition of both the intracellular and extracellular fluid may be altered by a variety of circumstances. In order for normal metabolic activity to be carried out, there must be maintenance of an optimal body fluid osmolality in both the extracellular and intracellular fluid. Homeostatic mechanisms are therefore constantly at work to maintain such an environment. Most major metabolic activities do not occur in the extracellular fluid, so there can be substantial alteration in its osmolality without causing any adverse effects.

Extracellular fluid serves to transmit substances (electrolytes, metabolites, nutrients) between cells and the various organ systems. It regulates both intracellular volume and ionic composition. Because of the requirement for osmotic equilibrium between the cells and the extracellular fluid, any alteration in extracellular fluid osmolality is accompanied by identical changes in intracellular osmolality, often with a concomitant change in cell volume. The brain, on the other hand, appears to regulate its osmolality primarily by alteration of intracellular solute content rather than by changes in cell volume (Ayus *et al.*, 1996; Arieff *et al.*, 1995). The ability of the extracellular fluid to transmit substances from plasma to organs and cells requires maintenance of a near-normal extracellular fluid volume. Maintenance of an intact plasma volume is also necessary to maintain cardiovascular stability and adequate tissue oxygen delivery. This chapter will describe the normal and abnormal regulation of body water, intracellular and extracellular volume, antidiuretic hormone (ADH), sodium, potassium, and osmolality. Abnormalities of sodium, osmolality, water, potassium, and ADH, as well as their management, will be described.

TOTAL BODY WATER AND PLASMA VOLUME

Total body water (TBW) varies as a function of age, sex, and weight. Body water in hospitalized adults who do not have abnormalities of fluid and electrolyte balance is about 43–54% of body weight. The relative water content of the body is highest in infants and children and decreases progressively with aging. The water content also depends on the percent of body fat, which is greater for women and obese individuals. The frequently quoted figure for TBW as 60% of body weight applies primarily to healthy young males. The percent of TBW varies widely as a function of age, sex, and body habitus, with a range of 42% (obese elderly women) to 75% (young children), while the mean figure for hospitalized adults is about 50% of body weight. The percent body water as a function of age, gender, and weight has recently been determined in a large number of subjects by radioisotope studies (Chumlea *et al.*, 2001). The intracellular volume is estimated from TBW and extracellular volume, but the extracellular volume can be measured directly by use of various chemical markers (insulin, sucrose, sulfate, Cl^-, CNS^-, Br^-). Measurement of TBW by various dilution techniques is relatively reproducible, but measurement of the extracellular volume is technically difficult, because there is no material that is known to distribute exclusively in

Principles and Practice of Geriatric Medicine, 4th Edition. Edited by M.S. John Pathy, Alan J. Sinclair and John E. Morley.

extracellular fluid. Thus, depending on the type of marker used, the extracellular volume will vary from 27–45% of TBW (Oh and Carroll, 1995).

Brain Cell Volume Regulation

Disorders of body water and electrolytes exert their most severe manifestations upon the brain. In general, hypoosmolar states tend to result in brain swelling, while hyperosmolar states lead to brain shrinkage. To understand how these conditions can affect the central nervous system, it is first necessary to understand how the brain can defend itself against alterations in body water and electrolytes. The principal osmotically active constituents of brain consist of both organic and inorganic solutes. Substantial evidence exists, both in humans and experimental animals, that there are several clinical situations where changes in plasma osmolality occur, but the apparent net loss or gain of cellular water and solute in brain does not account for the apparent change in tissue osmolality (McManus *et al.*, 1995). In these instances, there may be (1) inactivation of intracellular solute; (2) a gain in solute that is not the same as the usual commonly measured substances (urea, glucose, sodium, potassium, lactate). This undetermined solute has been called *idiogenic osmoles*. Furthermore, it is now known that the brain undergoes osmotic adaptation to hyperosmolar states in a manner that is distinctly different from that of most other mammalian tissues.

In clinical situations characterized by hypoosmolality, the brain minimizes swelling by lowering its intracellular osmolality with extrusion of sodium, potassium, chloride, and, possibly, amino acids (Arieff *et al.*, 1995; Vexler *et al.*, 1994a). The decrement of brain intracellular sodium and potassium is largely mediated by the effects of Na–K ATPase (Fraser and Arieff, 2001). The lowering of brain osmolality in this manner prevents the influx of water, which would lower brain osmolality at the expense of a gain in brain cell volume. In several different mammalian species, when hyponatremia is produced over periods of days to weeks, brain water content is normal to only slightly increased, and there is a markedly reduced cell content of both sodium and potassium (Arieff *et al.*, 1995).

Hyperosmolar States

The response of the brain to hyperosmolality has been extensively studied, with hyperosmolality produced using either NaCl, glucose, sodium, mannitol, glycerol, ethyl alcohol, or urea (Arieff *et al.*, 1977). It has been shown that the brain response depends on the type of solute accumulated. When hyperosmolality is caused by endogenous solutes, such as in hypernatremia or hyperglycemia, the increase in intracellular solute content necessary for osmotic equilibrium is largely accounted for by the osmoles of unknown nature (idiogenic osmoles) and, to a lesser extent, by increases in Na, K, and Cl, and amino acids (Ayus *et al.*, 1996). Other potential idiogenic osmoles present in the brain of animals with hypernatremia include myoinositol, betaine, phosphocreatine, and glycerophosphorylcholine (GPC), creatine, other methylamines, choline, sorbitol, and other polyols (Lien *et al.*, 1990). However, the osmotic contribution of any of these organic compounds has not been determined. It is possible that idiogenic osmoles arise from the osmotic activation of some solutes normally bound to polyvalent anions and released in response to the increase in ionic strength. The speed of brain volume regulation in hyperosmolality seems to vary with the type of solutes that cause the hyperosmolality. It appears that the speed of volume regulation is similar during hyperglycemia and hypernatremia. In glucose-induced hyperosmolality (in rabbits), the brain volume is restored to normal within 4 hours (Arieff *et al.*, 1977), similar to the findings after 4 hours of NaCl-induced hyperosmolality (Ayus *et al.*, 1996). Rapid infusion of urea can cause brain dehydration because the equilibration of urea in the brain is relatively slow. Although it takes less than 1 hour for urea to equilibrate in skeletal muscle, it takes 4–10 hours to reach equilibrium in the brain. In chronic uremia, despite the absence of a urea concentration gradient, there is substantial accumulation of idiogenic osmoles, suggesting that shrinkage of brain cells is not required for the formation of idiogenic osmoles. In contrast to chronic uremia, there is no accumulation of idiogenic osmoles in experimental acute uremia (Fraser and Arieff, 1997a).

HORMONAL AND PHYSICAL EFFECTS ON BRAIN ADAPTATION

The ability of the brain to adapt to either hyperosmolar or hypoosmolar states is markedly influenced by the effects of both hormones and physical factors (water content, ratio of brain size to skull size) (Fraser and Arieff, 2001). The most important of these hormones are vasopressin, estrogens, androgens, progesterone, and atriopeptin. The most important effects of physical factors on brain adaptation are the progressive alterations between the ratio of brain size to skull capacity, which occurs with the aging process (Gur *et al.*, 1991), and the gender differences between men and women (Arieff *et al.*, 1995). Recent studies demonstrate that physical factors are primarily responsible for the differences in brain adaptation between immature versus adult laboratory animals, as hormonal factors are not different (Fraser and Arieff, 2001).

VASOPRESSIN

Most studies of hyponatremia in both children and adults demonstrate that virtually all hyponatremic patients have increased blood levels of the hormone arginine vasopressin (Anderson *et al.*, 1985). There are multiple cerebral effects of vasopressin (Arieff *et al.*, 1993). Vasopressin administration in rodents, acting through cerebral V1 (Vasopressin 1) receptors, results in water movement into brain in the absence of hyponatremia, a significant decline in brain synthesis of ATP, decreased brain blood flow and CSF production, and impairment of several possible pathways for sodium efflux during hyponatremia (Kanda and Arieff, 1994; Kanda *et al.*, 1992). The decline of ATP synthesis in female rats after vasopressin administration may be related in part to brain ischemia from cerebral vasoconstriction. The vascular reactivity of vasopressin, a potent vasoconstrictive agent, is significantly greater in female rats than in males (Kozniewska *et al.*, 1995). Following blood loss, plasma vasopressin levels are significantly higher in female rats than in males. When hyponatremia is induced with either water alone or water plus a vasopressin analogue, desmopressin (DDAVP, which has no effect on the brain V1 receptor), the aforementioned cerebral effects of vasopressin are absent, demonstrating the importance of vasopressin in the pathogenesis of hyponatremic encephalopathy (Arieff *et al.*, 1995).

ESTROGEN, PROGESTERONE, AND ANDROGENS

The important mechanisms of early adaptation of brain to hyponatremia include extrusion of sodium from brain cells by several pathways (Fraser and Swanson, 1994; Vexler *et al.*, 1994b). Hyponatremic male laboratory animals are better able to extrude sodium to decrease brain cell osmolality than are females, resulting in significantly less brain swelling in males than in females both *in vivo* and *in vitro* (Fraser and Swanson, 1994). Following an initial fall in cerebral blood flow and loss of CSF via bulk flow, extrusion of sodium is the most important early defense of the brain against hyponatremia (Vexler *et al.*, 1994a). The major reasons for the increased morbidity and mortality in females compared to males include a diminished ability of the female brain to adapt to hyponatremia by limiting the amount of brain swelling. There is increasing evidence that these effects of gender may be mediated in part through the actions of certain steroid and peptide hormones, including estrogen, progesterone, and testosterone (Fraser and Swanson, 1994). In addition, there is substantial evidence that estrogen stimulates vasopressin release, whereas androgens suppress it (Arieff *et al.*, 1995). In addition to effects on vasopressin release, estrogen may antagonize brain adaptation via the Na^{+}-K^{+} ATPase system while androgens may enhance such adaptation (Fraser and Swanson, 1994).

Atrial Natriuretic Peptide (*see* Chapter 49, Mechanisms of Heart Failure)

Atrial natriuretic peptide (ANP) in the central nervous system appears to play an important role in the regulation of brain water content in several pathologic states characterized by cerebral edema. During the regulatory volume decrease observed with hyponatremia, an important initial response in the brain is a loss of sodium (Arieff *et al.*, 1995). ANP may act to decrease cell volume by effecting a net decrease of the intracellular sodium concentration in nerve cells (Kanda *et al.*, 1992). By decreasing sodium uptake in pathological states, the net effect of ANP would be a decrease in intracellular sodium, as it continues to be pumped out by Na^{+}-K^{+} ATPase. The effect of ANP in brain appears to be opposite to that of vasopressin (Del Bigio and Fedoroff, 1990). ANP also affects the regulation of CSF production and hence its pressure.

PHYSICAL FACTORS

There are two important factors that impact the physical elements of brain adaptation. The first is the aging process, which is marked by progressive alterations between the ratio of brain size to skull capacity. This ratio is highest at birth and progressively decreases with age. The second factor is gender. For reasons yet unknown, the ratio between skull size and brain size is different between adult men and women (Gur *et al.*, 1991). Other physical factors include CSF volume and brain water and electrolyte content. Physical factors may play an important role in adaptation to hyponatremia, particularly in small children and the elderly. In humans and laboratory animals, brain water content is more than 2.5 times higher in the young, decreasing progressively with advancing age (Gur *et al.*, 1991). In children, the ratio of brain to skull size is such that there is less room for expansion of the pediatric brain in the skull than there is in the adult (Gur *et al.*, 1991). Adult brain size is reached at about age six, while full skull size is not reached until about age 16. Additionally, the intracerebral volume of CSF is more than 10% greater in the adult than in the young (Gur *et al.*, 1991). When brain swelling occurs, the intracerebral loss of CSF increases the available volume in which the brain can expand. Since the percentage of CSF in the brain increases with age, adults have more room in the rigid skull for the brain to expand than do children (Gur *et al.*, 1991). In neonatal rats and dogs with hyponatremia, the ability of the brain to adapt to hyponatremia is impaired (Arieff *et al.*, 1995). The net result of the aforementioned physical factors is manifest in prepubescent children and menstruant women with hyponatremia (Arieff *et al.*, 1992). When symptomatic hyponatremia occurs in either group, the morbidity and mortality are very high, largely because of the effects of physical factors and decreased ability of the brain to adapt (Arieff *et al.*, 1992). In postoperative hyponatremia, a prospective study of 77 000 patients revealed that menstruant women are far more susceptible to brain damage from hyponatremia than are either men or postmenopausal women (Ayus *et al.*, 1992), a finding confirmed many times over (Steele *et al.*, 1997; Nzerue *et al.*, 2003).

Thirst and its Regulation

The sensation of thirst is an important general regulator of the body's water balance. The afferent stimuli for thirst sensation include both increases in plasma osmolality and decreases in extracellular volume. Increases in either plasma or CSF sodium concentration will also stimulate thirst and cause ADH to be released. At a normal plasma osmolality of approximately 285 mOsm/kg water, the circulating plasma ADH level is approximately $2\,\mathrm{pg\,ml^{-1}}$, which is the level needed to produce a half maximal urine concentration of approximately 600 mOsm/kg. Normal individuals do not usually experience thirst at this level of plasma osmolality. With dehydration, thirst is first expressed only when plasma osmolality reaches approximately 294 mOsm/kg water. This level of plasma osmolality represents a 2% increase above normal and is generally referred to as the *osmolar threshold* for thirst. At this level of plasma osmolality, ADH is maximally stimulated (usually above $5\,\mathrm{pg\,ml^{-1}}$) and is sufficient to achieve maximally concentrated urine (above 1000 mOsm/kg in young adults). A number of pharmacologic agents increase thirst, including tricyclic antidepressants and antihistamines. Certain hormones increase thirst, including ADH and angiotensin II.

A patient with defective thirst mechanism and intact osmolar regulatory center will appropriately release ADH in response to volume contraction and hypertonicity, but will become increasingly dehydrated because of the lack of thirst sensation. Such patients will not experience the desire to drink and have to be taught to drink water on a routine basis. They also have to learn to increase water intake with increased ambient temperature and physical activity. Such patients are classically described as having "essential hypernatremia" as their ability to normalize their serum sodium depends entirely on the ability to take in sufficient amounts of oral fluids. On the contrary, patients with intact thirst mechanism and decreased circulating ADH (diabetes insipidus) can often exist quite normally because of voluntary water intake stimulated by thirst. These patients may get into trouble only if access to water is prevented, as in the case of incapacity.

The afferent stimuli for the sensation of thirst include both osmolar and volume signals. However, it is not clear how these signals are transmitted to the thirst center. For example, increases in either plasma or CSF sodium concentrations can stimulate thirst (and ADH release); but it is not clear which is more important, or if changes in tonicity or sodium concentration are the primary stimuli. As is true for ADH release, it is clear that "effective" osmoles (those that are relatively restricted to the extracellular fluid, such as sodium salts or mannitol) are effective thirst stimuli. The cellular mechanisms by which changes in osmolality are translated into thirst are also unknown, although changes in brain cell volume have been proposed (McKinley *et al.*, 1988). Changes in intracellular volume seem more important in regulating thirst than changes in intracellular osmolality (without a change in intracellular volume), or changes in extracellular volume (without a change in intracellular volume) (McKinley *et al.*, 1988).

Complex roles for enkephalins and other opiate mediators in thirst regulation have recently been proposed, and the roles for prostaglandins and other neuroactive substances are also being explored. ADH may also have central dipsogenic effects (McKinley *et al.*, 1988). Thirst may also alter ADH distribution and metabolism, and substances such as isoproterenol may affect it by altering angiotensin II levels. Angiotensin II has substantial dipsogenic properties within the brain, but it does not cross the blood-brain barrier as does angiotensin I. Angiotensin I readily crosses the blood-brain barrier, and the brain has its own angiotensin converting enzyme (ACE) system, which converts angiotensin I to angiotensin II. The exact biochemical mechanism by which angiotensin II activates the cerebral thirst center is unknown. Such mechanisms are similar to those proposed for osmolar stimuli, suggesting that there may be a final common pathway for the two normal (physiologic) thirst stimuli (McKinley *et al.*, 1988).

Primary hypodipsia is a "pure" deficit in the thirst mechanism, requiring all other aspects of osmoregulation to be normal. The results of such a "pure" deficit in thirst may then be predicted as follows. The loss of thirst would result initially in decreased water intake and a tendency both to hyperosmolality and to effective arterial blood volume depletion. Both changes would stimulate ADH release and thereby increase renal water conservation. If water conservation is sufficient to offset the decrease in water intake (if plasma osmolality and blood volume are returned to near normal), the thirst deficit may go unrecognized by the patient. On the other hand, if renal water conservation is insufficient to compensate for the decreased water intake, symptoms of hyperosmolality and hypovolemia would supervene.

A meaningful evaluation of thirst deficits is difficult because drinking behavior is influenced by many stimuli that are unrelated to osmoregulation or volume regulation (Zerbe and Robertson, 1994). Definitive testing for thirst deficits should include both osmolar and volumetric stimuli, but only the former is usually evaluated. The test subject must be alert, oriented, and able to indicate whether or not thirst sensation is present. When studies of osmolar thirst stimuli are performed, the subject should be euvolemic (normal blood volume), and other dipsogenic stimuli (hyperthermia, exercise) should be minimized. A commonly used testing method is the administration of intravenous hypertonic NaCl (514 mM NaCl) solution at a rate sufficient to elevate the plasma osmolality from baseline to some arbitrary level that is at least 10% above baseline. The plasma osmolality should be determined at the baseline and at 30-minute intervals until the sensation of thirst is reported, or until the plasma osmolality has increased by at least 10% (Zerbe and Robertson, 1994). This technique will increase both blood volume and plasma osmolality, and the increased blood volume will tend to decrease hypovolemia-induced thirst. Moreover, the conclusion of the test is arbitrary if thirst is not elicited; thus, total absence of thirst (dipsia) can never be defined with certainty.

AGE-RELATED CHANGES IN SODIUM AND WATER HOMEOSTASIS

Hypernatremia is a frequent problem in older patients (Palevsky *et al.*, 1996). Thus, changes that may occur in the physiological responses of the elderly to hypernatremia may be of particular interest in understanding the pathogenesis of hypernatremia in the elderly. If healthy elderly men are compared to younger controls, there are differences in the response to 24 hours of water deprivation (Lindeman *et al.*, 1985). In the older men, there are deficits in both the intensity and threshold of the thirst response to specific stimuli, and in the subsequent water intake that follows the thirst. The ability to produce a concentrated urine during water deprivation also declines with advancing age. This may be related to a relative increase in renal medullary blood flow, which washes out medullary tonicity; increases in solute load per nephron (because of nephron dropout) resulting in an obligate osmotic diuresis; or impairment of renal tubular responsiveness to osmolality-mediated vasopressin release. Although there is an enhanced responsiveness to osmolality-mediated vasopressin release, there may be impaired responsiveness of vasopressin release to volume and pressure stimuli (Phillips *et al.*, 1984). In addition, there is a high prevalence of bacteriuria in elderly patients, which may impair urinary-concentrating ability. Finally, there is both a decline in glomerular filtration rate (GFR) and an increased incidence of renal disease with advancing age, both of which may contribute to impaired ability to conserve water (Lindeman *et al.*, 1985).

THIRST AND WATER METABOLISM IN THE ELDERLY

There are several alterations of water metabolism that have been described in elderly individuals. After 24 hours of water deprivation, elderly men (age above 67 years) exhibited greater increases in plasma osmolality, serum sodium and plasma vasopressin levels than did younger men (age below 31 years) (Phillips *et al.*, 1984). In addition, after 24 hours of water deprivation, elderly men were less thirsty, and their maximal urine osmolality was less, than observed in younger men (Phillips *et al.*, 1984). For a given serum osmolality, the plasma vasopressin levels are higher in older men than in their younger counterparts. Although there is thus an enhanced responsiveness to osmolality-mediated vasopressin release in older men, there may be impaired responsive volume stimuli. In addition, there is a high prevalence of bacteriuria in elderly patients, which may impair urinary-concentrating ability, and with increasing age, there is a decline of GFR, which may contribute to impaired ability to conserve water (Lindeman *et al.*, 1985; Palmer and Levi, 1997).

Despite the fact that maximal urine osmolality is less in elderly individuals, hyponatremia is the most common electrolyte abnormality encountered in the elderly, although hypernatremia is almost as frequent. Unlike the situation with hyponatremia, hypernatremia in the elderly carries a very poor prognosis, with a mortality in excess of 40%, seven times that observed in age-matched controls (Palevsky *et al.*, 1996; Snyder and Arieff, 1992). An important cause of hypernatremia is diabetes insipidus, which can be congenital (Bichet *et al.*, 1997), related to stroke, tumor, other causes of brain damage (Bichet, 1997), or as a complication of neurosurgery (Bichet, 1997; Arafah *et al.*, 1996a; Arafah *et al.*, 1996b).

REGULATION OF VASOPRESSIN

Arginine vasopressin (antidiuretic hormone, ADH) is the principal hormone responsible for the regulation of body water. ADH is synthesized in the hypothalamus and is carried in cortical CSF to portal blood flowing to the pituitary capillaries (Arieff *et al.*, 1993). The hormone is also secreted (from the hypothalamus) into the CSF of the third ventricle, where it binds to V1 receptor sites on neurons and blood vessels where its cerebral effects are mediated by intracellular second messengers (Faraci *et al.*, 1990). From the pituitary, vasopressin is then secreted into the bloodstream (Zerbe and Robertson, 1994). Neither ADH nor most other hormones that have effects on the brain have access to the brain parenchyma. These substances bind to brain cells and exert their effects inside the brain by means of second messengers. For ADH in brain, the second messengers include calcium, inositol triphosphate (IP3), and nitric oxide, and a linkage has been demonstrated between IP3 and vasopressin V1 receptors in the brain.

There are two primary stimuli for the release of ADH: (1) increased plasma osmolality; and (2) decreased intravascular volume (Share, 1996). Extracellular volume becomes important in the control of vasopressin elaboration only when there is a decrease of about 5%. With ADH release, ingested water is retained abnormally, which lowers plasma osmolality and repletes plasma volume. As these parameters are satisfied, ADH release is inhibited and any excess intake of water is eliminated in the urine. If a patient with normal kidneys takes in a normal daily solute load (1000 mosmoles), and is able to produce a maximally dilute urine (50 mOsm/kg), he will theoretically be able to ingest up to 20 l of water/day without becoming hyponatremic. However, in patients with poor nutrition (solute load of 250 mOsm/day), as in the case of beer potomania (Fenves *et al.*, 1996), water intake in excess of 5 l could lead to the development of hyponatremia. A similar situation would exist with a diet low in both NaCl and protein, combined with a water intake of less than 5 l per day, either as beer or other fluids (Goldman *et al.*, 1997). Similar cases have been reported after water intoxication associated with use of the recreational drug ecstasy (Balmelli *et al.*, 2001; Ben-Abraham *et al.*, 2003). A number of factors other than elevated plasma osmolality and hypovolemia can cause ADH release and override the effects of osmolality and volume. These include many medications, tumors, pulmonary lesions, intracranial processes, emesis, nausea, stress, hypoxia, and even anxiety and fear. Elevation in ADH levels secondary to these entities, along with a clinical syndrome consisting of a normal to increased intravascular volume, with hypoosmolality, urine osmolality above 100 mOsm/kg, and decreased plasma levels of sodium, urea, uric acid, and creatinine is known as the *syndrome of inappropriate secretion of antidiuretic hormone* (*SIADH*). The patient must have no other reason for increased ADH, such as volume depletion or hyperosmolality, or any of the nonosmotic stimuli for vasopressin release (Verbalis, 2001).

DIABETES INSIPIDUS

The absence of ADH effect upon the kidney results in diabetes insipidus. Diabetes insipidus is a clinical condition characterized by the decreased or absent renal effects of the hormone vasopressin, and it can be either nephrogenic or central in origin. Vasopressin is synthesized by the hypothalamus and is both stored and secreted by the posterior pituitary gland. In central diabetes insipidus, there is an impairment of either synthesis or release of vasopressin into the circulation. In nephrogenic diabetes insipidus, vasopressin is usually present in the circulation but the kidney response to the hormone is impaired or absent. Criteria for the diagnosis of diabetes insipidus include the presence of polyuria (urine output above 250 ml hour^{-1}) with hypotonic urine (urine osmolality below 100 mOsm/kg) in the absence of osmotic diuresis (plasma osmolality is below about 300 mOsm/kg without elevations in plasma levels of impermiant solutes, such as glucose, mannitol, urea). The diagnosis of central diabetes insipidus can be established by the above findings plus the following: (1) before the onset of polyuria, patients were able to excrete a hypertonic urine (urine osmolality above 300 mOsm/kg); (2) after several days of polyuria, when plasma is concentrated, the urine osmolality should remain below 100 mOsm/kg. At this time, vasopressin stimulation should be maximal and urine intensely concentrated; (3) no drugs have been administered, nor was there any medical condition present, which would predispose the patients to the development of nephrogenic diabetes insipidus; and (4) findings by radiologic evaluation or autopsy should demonstrate hypothalamic/pituitary damage but normal kidneys and renal tubular function. Both central and nephrogenic diabetes insipidus can lead to hypernatremia and permanent brain damage (Vin-Christian and Arieff, 1993).

In the syndrome of central diabetes insipidus, ADH is either not synthesized at all or not released into the circulation in quantities sufficient to maintain normal water balance. Complete diabetes insipidus is the inability to produce urine of greater osmotic concentration than that of plasma under an appropriate osmotic stimulus. Patients with partial diabetes insipidus include those who can produce a urine hypertonic to plasma but whose ADH production is below normal. Conscious patients with diabetes insipidus do not become dehydrated unless they also have a thirst defect, a combination that may occur with stroke, hypothalamic disease or after hypothalamic surgery. Renal function is normal in pituitary diabetes insipidus. Mild serum hyperosmolality and increased sodium concentration may be the only laboratory abnormalities detectable. Unconscious patients manifest polyuria and hypernatremia with worsening dehydration (Trivedi and Nolph, 1994).

If ADH is absent but thirst is normal, the patient will drink sufficient water to prevent the serum sodium from rising but will manifest polyuria and polydipsia as well. If ADH secretion is normal and thirst is absent, the patient will become progressively dehydrated with hypernatremia and small volumes of concentrated urine unless he drinks deliberately (primarily hyodipsia). If ADH and thirst are both absent, the patient will become very dehydrated and will manifest hypernatremia. The extreme dehydration will eventually lead to a reduction of GFR and the production of small volumes of concentrated urine. If ADH is partially deficient and thirst is normal, the patient will have a water diuresis with a normal plasma osmolality, leading to an eventual increase of plasma osmolality. This will provoke thirst and polydipsia (incomplete pituitary diabetes insipidus). If thirst is absent, the patient with partial diabetes insipidus will lose water and will not drink. The loss of water will raise serum sodium and osmolality to such a level that the quantity of ADH released is sufficient to permit the excretion of concentrated urine. This condition, sometimes described as "essential hypernatremia", is usually caused by a hypothalamic lesion (Zerbe and Robertson, 1994).

With nephrogenic diabetes insipidus, there is no impairment of the ability to secrete vasopressin, but there is rather an impairment of the ability of the hormone to affect the kidney. Arginine vasopressin binds to the vasopressin V2 receptor in the renal distal tubule (thick ascending limb of the loop of Henle) and collecting tubules. The V2 receptor is coupled to an adenylate cyclase, which generates cyclic AMP when stimulated. A number of pharmacological agents can lead to nephrogenic diabetes insipidus, and these include lithium, demethylchlortetracycline, methoxyflurane, and certain hypoglycemic agents such as glyburide (Morrison and Singer, 1994). Hyperparathyroidism with hypercalcemia can lead to nephrogenic diabetes insipidus, as can a number of renal interstitial disorders (Vin-Christian and Arieff, 1993).

Diabetes insipidus is most commonly of undetermined cause and is occasionally familial. The familial form, which is probably due to atrophy of the nerve cells in the area of the hypothalamus where ADH is synthesized, may present at any age. When the etiology is known, it most often results from metastatic tumors (breast or lung), granulomas (including sarcoidosis) in the areas of the sella or hypothalamus, surgical interruption of the hypothalamic-neurohypophyseal system, skull fractures, or cerebral vascular accidents. Among the most common causes of acute diabetes insipidus is head trauma associated with either falls or auto accidents (Trivedi and Nolph, 1994; White and Likavec, 1992). Cerebral hypoxema is another cause of diabetes insipidus, where patients have cerebral encephalomalacia associated with severe brain damage secondary to clinical circumstances as asphyxia, drug-induced respiratory failure, cardiac arrest, or shock. Diabetic insipidus has been infrequently reported after cerebral herniation complicating symptomatic hyponatremia (Fraser and Arieff, 1990), or cerebral edema associated with diabetic ketoacidosis or nonketotic hyperosmolar coma. In rare situations, clinical diabetes insipidus may not be apparent if both anterior and posterior pituitary cease to function, because glucocorticoid secretion may be impaired secondary to ACTH deficiency (Morrison and Singer, 1994). The diabetes insipidus will become apparent only when glucocorticoid replacement therapy is given (Arieff, 2003).

Diabetes insipidus is a well-recognized complication of blunt head trauma. Delay in diagnosis can occur when head trauma does not appear to be severe or when the patient is admitted to a service other than neurosurgery. Detailed assessment of anterior pituitary function in patients with traumatic diabetes insipidus usually requires a delay until the patient is medically stable. Generally, these patients are initially treated with adrenal steroid therapy for cerebral edema, and detailed evaluation of endocrine function is often difficult to obtain. The diabetes insipidus caused by head trauma may persist for several years, and may become permanent if the patient does not recover within 4–6 months (Arieff, 2003).

HYPONATREMIA

While diabetes insipidus generally occurs because of the absence of ADH effect upon the kidney, hyponatremia is usually associated with elevated plasma levels of ADH. Hyponatremia can be succinctly defined as an abnormally low plasma sodium concentration. Although the kidney is important in the pathogenesis of hyponatremia, the target organ for changes that produce morbidity and mortality is the brain. Hyponatremia has few important sequelae or clinical manifestations other than those associated with the central nervous system. Hyponatremia is the most common electrolyte abnormality seen in a general hospital population, with an incidence and prevalence of about 1.0 and 2.5%, respectively (Ayus *et al.*, 1992). The incidence of hyponatremia is similar among men and women, but brain damage occurs predominantly in young (menstruant) females and prepubertal individuals (Arieff *et al.*, 1992; Ayus *et al.*, 1992; Arieff, 1998). Brain damage from hyponatremia is generally uncommon in men but does occur in older (postmenopausal) women (Ayus and Arieff, 1999).

It is now clear that brain damage from hyponatremia can be associated with either hyponatremic encephalopathy or improper therapy of symptomatic hyponatremia. However, even with improper therapy of symptomatic hyponatremia, brain damage is exceedingly rare, occurring in less than 4% of such cases (Ayus and Arieff, 1996). More recent evidence strongly suggests that virtually all of the brain damage associated with hyponatremia is due to hypoxia (Nzerue *et al.*, 2003; Knochel, 1999). Clinical evidence suggests that the vast majority of brain damage from hyponatremia is associated with untreated hyponatremic encephalopathy, and occurs primarily in a limited number of clinical settings. These include (1) the postoperative state; (2) polydipsia-hyponatremia syndrome; (3) pharmacologic agents; (4) congestive heart failure; (5) acquired immunodeficiency syndrome (AIDS); hepatic insufficiency; and (6) malignancy (Figure 1).

Clinical Manifestations of Hyponatremia

The clinical signs and symptoms of hyponatremia are directly related to the development of cerebral edema, increased intracellular pressure, and cerebral hypoxia. Neurological manifestations of hyponatremia may be observed when the plasma sodium is below 130 mM. Early symptoms of hyponatremia from any cause may include apathy, weakness, muscular cramps, nausea, vomiting, and headache. The type of symptoms varies enormously among individuals, and no individual is likely to have any or all ascribed symptoms. More advanced clinical manifestations are shown in Table 1. In general, symptoms are more severe and occur at a higher level of serum sodium in younger women (age 16–49 years) than in either men or older women (Figure 2; Fraser and Arieff, 1997b).

Patients with chronic hyponatremia have been said to have less severe symptoms and a lower mortality. However, this has been shown to be incorrect, with the overall

Table 1 Objective and subjective manifestations of hyponatremic encephalopathy

Objective findings
Anorexia
Headache
Nausea
Emesis
Muscular cramps
Weakness
Subjective findings
Impaired response to verbal stimuli
Impaired response to painful stimuli
Bizarre (inappropriate) behavior
Hallucinations (auditory or visual)
Asterixis
Obtundation
Incontinence (urinary or fecal)
Respiratory insufficiency
Advanced subjective findings
Decorticate and/or decerebrate posturing
Bradycardia
Hypertension
Altered temperature regulation (hypo- or hyperthermia)
Hyperglycemia (secondary to central diabetes mellitus)
Dilated pupils
Seizure activity (usually grand mal)
Coma
Respiratory arrest
Cardiac arrest
Polyuria (secondary to central diabetes insipidus)

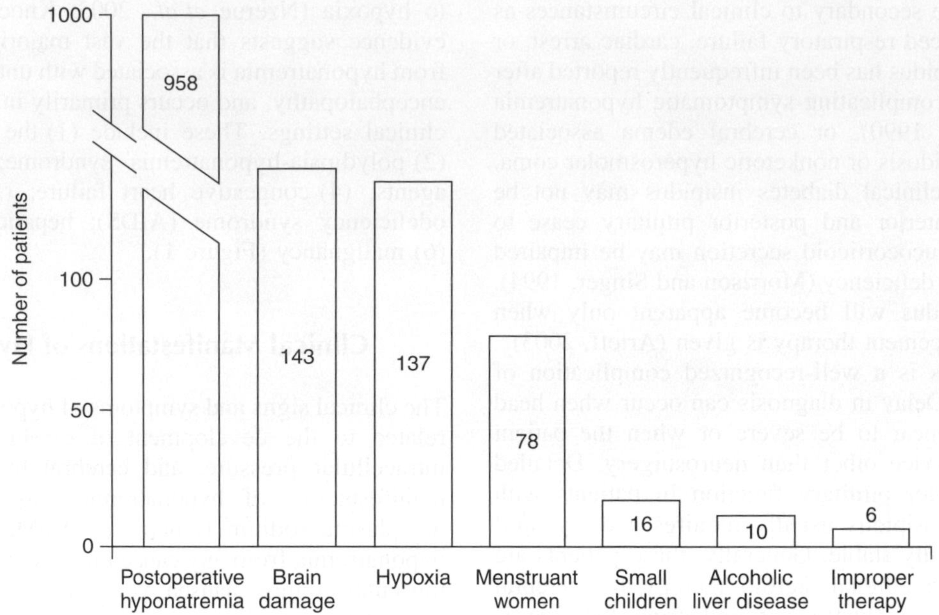

Figure 1 The major risk factors associated with permanent brain damage among hospitalized patients with hyponatremia (serum sodium below 128 mmol l^{-1}). Most patients (96%) suffered a hypoxic episode because of failure to initiate active therapy in a timely manner. In only 4% of patients suffering permanent brain damage could improper therapy for hyponatremia be implicated in the outcome. The incidence of hyponatremic encephalopathy in 11 published series from our laboratory comprising 958 hospitalized patients with hyponatremia was 23% (143/958). Among patients with hyponatremic encephalopathy, the overall morbidity was 15%

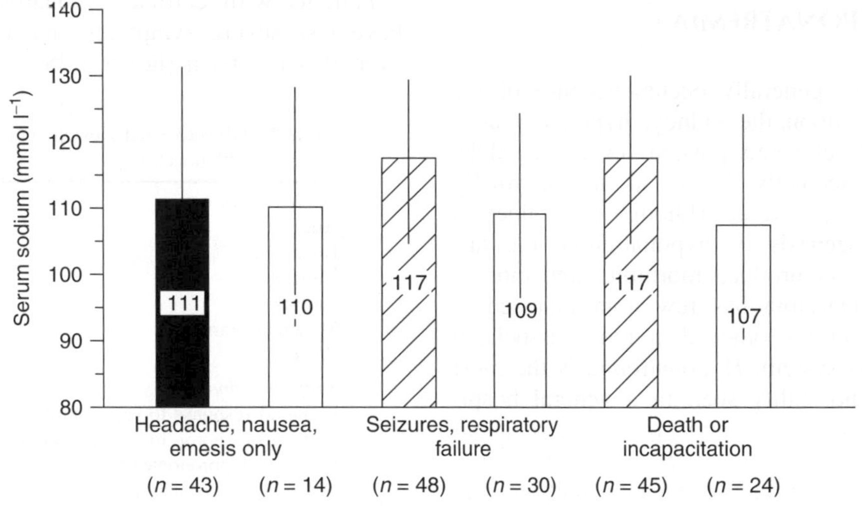

Figure 2 The plasma sodium in 136 patients with hyponatremic encephalopathy. The men and postmenopausal women with headache, nausea, and emesis only did not progress to respiratory failure. We have observed less than 10 menstruant women with headache, nausea, and emesis who did not progress to respiratory failure, and these are not included because of the small sample. The plasma sodium in menstruant women who progressed to respiratory failure or permanent brain damage was significantly higher ($p < 0.001$) than that of postmenopausal women who progressed to respiratory failure or permanent brain damage. The plasma sodium in menstruant women who progressed to respiratory failure or permanent brain damage was also significantly higher ($p < 0.001$) than that of either men or postmenopausal women who had headache, nausea, and emesis only ($p < 0.01$). We have observed less than 10 men (all age-groups) with headache, nausea, and emesis who progressed to either respiratory failure, death, or permanent brain damage, and these are not included because of the small sample size. The data is presented as the mean ±2 standard deviations (±2SD)

mortality from chronic hyponatremia being about 25% (Ayus and Arieff, 1999). However, in most clinical situations, it is very difficult to determine the duration of the hyponatremia, and the separation may in fact be largely artificial. Since chronic hyponatremia is more common in both men and elderly women, the less severe symptoms may be due not so much to the duration of hyponatremia as to the age, sex, and hormonal status of the patients. Young women are not prone to many of the disorders that may be associated with chronic hyponatremia, such as long-term diuretic use, congestive heart failure, and hepatic insufficiency. An important but poorly recognized cause of chronic hyponatremia is polydipsia in elderly women. The incidence is not known, but there have been many reported deaths (Ayus and Arieff, 1999; Posner *et al.*, 1967; Ashraf *et al.*, 1981).

Postoperative Hyponatremia (*see* Chapter 137, Perioperative and Postoperative Medical Assessment)

Postoperative hyponatremia is a common clinical problem in the United States and Western Europe, with an occurrence of about 1% (Ayus *et al.*, 1992; Ayus and Arieff, 1996), or about 250 000 cases per year, with an overall morbidity of approximately 5%. In the vast majority of cases, the patients tolerated the surgery without complications, being able to walk, talk, and eat after surgery before symptoms of encephalopathy developed. Initial symptoms are usually quite mild (Table 1). Because these symptoms are somewhat nonspecific, they are often mistakenly attributed to routine postoperative sequelae. However, if the symptoms are due to hyponatremia and left untreated, the patient may progress to more advanced manifestations (Table 1) (Fraser and Arieff, 1990; Arieff, 1986). Thus, symptomatic hyponatremia in postoperative patients is particularly dangerous and should be promptly treated. In this setting, premenopausal women are particularly at risk of developing hyponatremic encephalopathy and respiratory insufficiency when compared to men and postmenopausal women (Ayus *et al.*, 1992; Figure 3). Additionally, respiratory arrest occurs at a significantly higher plasma sodium (±SD) in menstruant women ($117 \pm 7\,\mathrm{mmol\,l^{-1}}$; range $104-130\,\mathrm{mmol\,l^{-1}}$) than in postmenopausal women ($107 \pm 8\,\mathrm{mmol\,l^{-1}}$; range $92-123\,\mathrm{mmol\,l^{-1}}$) (Figure 2). Although the frequency of permanent brain damage from hyponatremia following elective surgery is not known, recent studies suggest a morbidity of about 20% in patients with encephalopathy (Ayus *et al.*, 1992; Ayus and Arieff, 1996; Figure 3).

Polydipsia

Another common setting in which symptomatic hyponatremia can occur is with polydipsia. The polydipsia-hyponatremia syndrome (frequently known as *psychogenic polydipsia*) occurs primarily in individuals who have either schizophrenia, bipolar disorder, or certain eating disorders (Demitrack *et al.*, 1992; Vieweg, 1996). The average daily solute intake is about $1000\,\mathrm{mmol\,day^{-1}}$, and if the kidney can elaborate a maximally dilute urine (below 100 $\mathrm{mOsm\,kg^{-1}}$), the normal individual should theoretically be able to excrete in excess of $20\,\mathrm{l\,day^{-1}}$. To lower plasma sodium below $120\,\mathrm{mmol\,l^{-1}}$ requires retention of more than $80\,\mathrm{ml\,kg^{-1}}$ of water, so that to develop hyponatremia in the absence of elevated plasma levels of ADH requires ingestion of over $20\,\mathrm{l\,day^{-1}}$ in a 60-kg adult. Most patients with polydipsia-hyponatremia syndrome have actually ingested less water than that theoretically required. Instead, they have less fluid intake but both abnormal urinary diluting capacity and elevated plasma ADH levels (Vieweg, 1996; Goldman *et al.*, 1988). Beer potomania is a variation of polydipsia-hyponatremia syndrome, where the hyponatremia is associated with poor nutrition and massive ingestion of beer instead of water (Fenves *et al.*, 1996).

Primary polydipsia has been reported in almost all age-groups, from the very young to the elderly. Many such patients have histories of psychiatric disorders (usually schizophrenia, bipolar disorder, or bulimia nervosa) (Demitrack *et al.*, 1992; Vieweg, 1996). Symptoms of drug-induced primary polydipsia can often be mistaken for symptoms stemming from nonrelated psychiatric disorders (confusion, hallucinations, bizarre behavior). Accurate diagnosis

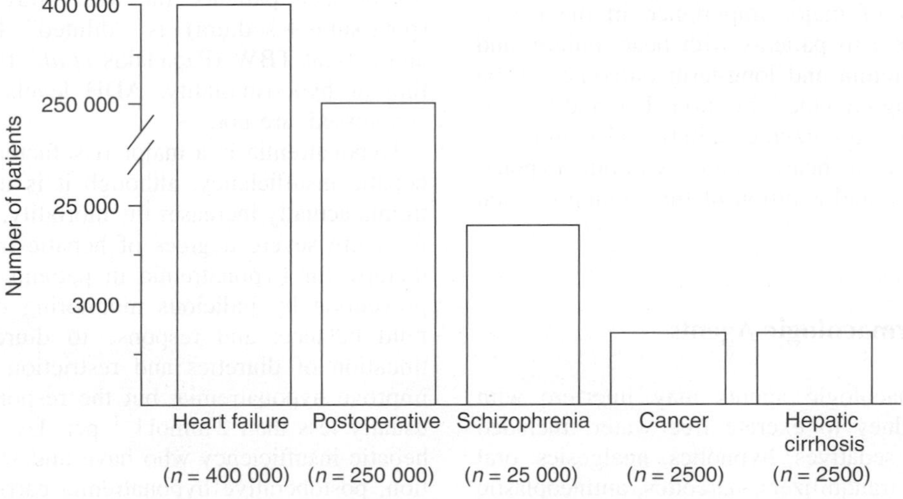

Figure 3 The clinical causes of hyponatremia that are likely to be associated with death or permanent brain damage. Of the five causes, only in the case of postoperative hyponatremia is there solid epidemiologic data. The other causes are estimated from the current literature. There is not enough data in the current literature to estimate the incidence of hyponatremia associated with AIDS, diuretic therapy, or hyponatremia-polydipsia syndrome

of symptoms stemming from drug-induced polydipsia and symptomatic hyponatremia may therefore be challenging. The clinical picture may be further complicated when the patient is taking phenothiazines or tricyclic antidepressants, which may increase ADH release, or diuretics, which can interfere with renal water excretion (Sandifer, 1983). Such patients may ingest excessive quantities of water, which can lead to symptomatic hyponatremia. Absent any medication, patients who are compulsive water drinkers disorders may also be at risk for both symptomatic hyponatremia and fatal water intoxication (Cheng *et al.*, 1990).

The mainstay of therapy of polydipsia is water restriction and treatment of underlying reversible causes of the disease. Such causes include drugs, certain psychiatric or neurologic disorders, hypercalcemia, and potassium depletion (resulting in nephrogenic diabetes insipidus). However, these patients are very adept at obtaining water, even under well-controlled circumstances, and their psychiatric disturbances may not easily be amenable to therapy.

Congestive Heart Failure (*see* Chapter 50, Heart Failure in the Elderly)

The most common cause of hyponatremia in the United States is congestive heart failure with an incidence of about 400 000 per year (Figure 1) (Lee and Packer, 1986). The pathogenesis of the hyponatremia is complex and may include activation of vasoconstrictor hormones, thirst stimulation, diuretic therapy, impaired renal water excretion, high plasma ADH levels, and elevated plasma renin activity. The one year mortality among patients with congestive heart failure exceeds 50%, although an undetermined number of these actually die from hyponatremia. Although the mortality from hyponatremia among patients with heart failure is thus difficult to estimate, there are many reported deaths and low plasma sodium is of major prognostic importance. Recent studies suggest that the renin-angiotensin system is of major importance in the pathogenesis of hyponatremia in patients with heart failure, and that both the hyponatremia and long-term outcome can be improved by converting-enzyme inhibition (Lee and Packer, 1986). However, converting-enzyme inhibition also improves survival in patients with heart failure without hyponatremia (SOLVD, 1991), and addition of furosemide is often required.

Pharmacologic Agents

A number of pharmacologic agents may interfere with the ability of the kidney to excrete free water. Included are large numbers of sedatives, hypnotics, analgesics, oral hypoglycemic agents, tranquilizers, narcotics, antineoplastic drugs, antidepressant agents, and diuretics (DeFronzo and Arieff, 1995). In most such instances, there is excessive net retention of ingested or infused free water. Those diuretics most commonly associated with hyponatremia are thiazides and "loop" diuretics (furosemide). In patients with thiazide-associated hyponatremia, there may be an idiosyncratic reaction to the drug, resulting in massive acute losses of sodium and potassium in the urine, often with associated polydipsia.

Acquired Immunodeficiency Syndrome (AIDS)

AIDS is a major cause of hyponatremia in the United States (Vitting *et al.*, 1990). The hyponatremia in patients with AIDS may be secondary to SIADH; volume deficiency with hypotonic replacement fluids; or adrenal insufficiency (Vitting *et al.*, 1990; Grinspoon and Bilezikian, 1992). Even in the presence of mineralocorticoid deficiency, glucocorticoid function may be intact, resulting in a normal ACTH stimulation test. Adrenal insufficiency is particularly suspect in hyponatremic AIDS patients who have disseminated cytomegalovirus or tuberculosis. Therapy with Florinef (fludrocortisone acetate) is indicated only if adrenal insufficiency is documented in hyponatremic patients with renal salt-wasting (Grinspoon and Bilezikian, 1992). Current data strongly suggest that patients who have AIDS and hyponatremia have both a higher mortality and longer duration of hospitalization than those who are normonatremic. However, with such a virulent disease as AIDS, it is difficult to determine the exact role of hyponatremia in the associated morbidity.

Hepatic Insufficiency (*see* Chapter 33, Liver and Gall Bladder)

Hyponatremia is a common disorder in patients with liver disease and it is almost always associated with excessive retention of free water. Regardless of the volume status in such patients, the total body exchangeable cation (potassium + sodium) is "diluted" by relatively greater amounts of TBW (Papadakis *et al.*, 1990). Even in the setting of hypoosmolality, ADH levels, which are normally suppressed, are not.

Hyponatremia is a major risk factor among patients with hepatic insufficiency, although it is unclear if the hyponatremia actually increases the mortality, or is merely a marker for more severe degrees of hepatic insufficiency. The best therapy for hyponatremia in patients with liver disease is prevention by judicious monitoring of serum electrolytes, fluid balance, and response to diuretic therapy. Discontinuation of diuretics and restriction of water intake will improve hyponatremia, but the response is generally slow, usually less than $2\,\mathrm{mmol\,l^{-1}}$ per day. Among patients with hepatic insufficiency who have undergone liver transplantation, postoperative hyponatremia carries a prohibitive mortality (Singh *et al.*, 1994). Cerebral demyelinative lesions are frequent in such patients, and appear to be related to upward changes in the plasma sodium concentration. Thus, patients with hepatic insufficiency, particularly those who have undergone liver transplantation, are at greatly increased risk for development of cerebral demyelinative lesions (Ayus *et al.*, 1987).

There is not a consensus of opinion regarding the optimal method or rate of correction of symptomatic hyponatremia in patients with liver disease. There is substantial clinical evidence that correction of severe symptomatic hyponatremia to mildly hyponatremic levels in nonalcoholic patients does not usually result in cerebral demyelinating lesions, such as central pontine myelinolysis. However, there is only limited data available in patients with liver disease, and data in patients who have undergone liver transplantation suggest that any increment of plasma sodium, whether such patients are hyponatremic or not, is potentially dangerous (Singh *et al.*, 1994). However, it has recently been shown that a substantial percent of patients with liver disease who have not been hyponatremic will have central pontine myelinolysis, which is asymptomatic (Sullivan and Pfefferbaum, 2001). Such data strongly support the concept that central pontine myelinolysis is common in alcoholic subjects and has nothing to do with hyponatremia.

Recent studies suggest that the major determinants of the occurrence of permanent brain damage in patients with liver disease and hyponatremia include at least four factors (Papadakis *et al.*, 1990; Ayus *et al.*, 1987): (1) the occurrence of a hypoxic episode (arterial pO_2 below 75 mmHg); (2) correction of serum sodium above 128–132 mmol l^{-1} within the initial 48 hours of therapy; (3) elevation of serum sodium by more than 25 mmol within the initial 24–48 hours of therapy; (4) the presence of hypernatremia (serum sodium above 145 mmol l^{-1}) in patients with liver disease receiving lactulose. The mortality in patients who have both liver disease and serum sodium below 120 mmol l^{-1} accompanied by central nervous symptoms is probably above 40% (Papadakis *et al.*, 1990). Therapy of the hyponatremia found in patients with liver disease should soon change. There are several vasopressin V2 receptor-blocking agents that are in various stages of clinical testing. These agents have proven effective in the therapy of hyponatremia associated with liver disease, and may soon be commercially available (Decaux, 2001; Gross *et al.*, 2001).

Malignancy-associated Hyponatremia (*see* Chapter 129, Oncological Emergencies and Urgencies)

A major group of patients with asymptomatic hyponatremia and normal to slightly expanded extracellular volume are those who have a malignancy that secretes a peptide having actions similar to antidiuretic hormone (arginine vasopressin, ADH), although some tumors actually secrete arginine vasopressin (Bartter and Schwartz, 1967). The most common of such malignancies associated with SIADH is lung cancer, particularly oat cell or bronchogenic carcinoma, although a large number of malignancies may be associated with elaboration of ADH. It is difficult to even estimate the mortality of hyponatremia associated with malignancy because most patients eventually die of the primary disease.

Management of Hyponatremia

The management of hyponatremia may be broadly divided into three groups: (1) active (usually hypertonic NaCl intravenously); (2) passive (usually water restriction); (3) supportive modalities (respiratory support, diuretics, intubation); (4) antagonism of effects of ADH on the kidney (declomycin, lithium); and (5) vasopressin V2 receptor antagonists. The most important decision is whether to treat a patient in a passive manner (water restriction being the cornerstone of such therapy) or if there is a need for active therapeutic intervention (infusion of hypertonic NaCl (500–850 mM NaCl), either with or without a loop diuretic). The decision should be primarily based upon the presence or absence of neurologic symptomatology.

In patients whose hyponatremia is asymptomatic, neither active therapy (with hypertonic NaCl) nor supportive measures are indicated. If the patient is volume-depleted, isotonic (154 mM) NaCl is usually the fluid of choice. If there is a hormone deficiency (adrenal, thyroid), appropriate replacement is indicated. If the patient has received a drug that may interfere with renal handling of sodium or water, the drug should be discontinued whenever possible. Although water restriction can theoretically be of benefit in some of these disorders, practical considerations diminish its usefulness. There are several medical regimens for the long-term management of patients with stable asymptomatic hyponatremia. Demeclocycline, a tetracycline antibiotic, in doses above 600 mg day^{-1} can be effectively used to produce a state of nephrogenic diabetes insipidus and has been successful in treating patients with SIADH (DeFronzo and Arieff, 1995).

The most important measures for the management of at-risk patients are prophylactic. Every hospitalized patient in the six groups discussed above should be considered at risk for the development of hyponatremia, and appropriate measures undertaken. The most important measure is the avoidance of intravenous hypotonic fluid to hospitalized patients. Other important procedures include monitoring of daily electrolytes, weight, and strict input and output. Symptomatic hyponatremia is a medical emergency, with a morbidity in excess of 15% (Ayus and Arieff, 1996). In patients with hyponatremic encephalopathy, the preponderance of clinical evidence demonstrates that correction by water restriction results in an unacceptable morbidity and mortality (Ayus and Arieff, 1999). Patients with hyponatremic encephalopathy should be constantly monitored, preferably in an intensive care unit. The first step in management of such patients is a secure airway with assisted ventilation if required. Therapy should be initiated with intravenous hypertonic sodium chloride (514 mmol l^{-1}) using an infusion pump, with the infusion designed to raise plasma sodium at a rate of about 1 mmol l^{-1} per hour. If the patient is actively seizing or has other clinical evidence of increased intracranial pressure, then the rate of hypertonic fluid administration should be adjusted to elevate plasma sodium by about 4–5 mmol l^{-1} $hour^{-1}$ over the first hour. Therapy with hypertonic NaCl should be discontinued when: (1) the patient becomes asymptomatic; (2) the patient's plasma sodium has increased by 20 mmol l^{-1}; or (3) the plasma sodium reaches a value in the range of 120 to 125 mmol l^{-1}. While active correction of symptomatic hyponatremia is in progress, monitoring of plasma electrolytes should be carried out every 2 hours, until the patient has become neurologically stable. In addition to hypertonic NaCl, therapy should include supportive measures when required. The plasma sodium should never be acutely elevated to hyper- or normonatremic levels, and should not be elevated by more than 25 mmol l^{-1} during the initial 48 hours of therapy (Ayus *et al.*, 1987). The technique has been described in detail elsewhere (DeFronzo and Arieff, 1995).

The patient's TBW, which varies as a function of age, sex, and body habitus, with a range of 42% (obese elderly women) to 75% (young children), should be estimated (Chumlea *et al.*, 2001). Correction of the plasma sodium should be initially planned using intravenous 514 mM NaCl, often combined with a loop diuretic (furosemide) (DeFronzo and Arieff, 1995) Infuse the 514 mM NaCl at a rate calculated to increase plasma sodium at a rate of 1 mmol l^{-1} per hour. The plasma sodium must be monitored at least every 2 hours, with appropriate adjustments in the infusion rate to reach the desired level.

There are possible complications of the therapy of hyponatremia. Therapy is usually not an important factor in the genesis of permanent brain damage in hyponatremic patients (Nzerue *et al.*, 2003; Ayus and Arieff, 1999; Figure 3). It had been suggested that the development of cerebral demyelinating lesions might somehow be related to the correction of hyponatremia (DeFronzo and Arieff, 1995). However, a number of studies have shown that cerebral demyelinating lesions develop only when patients with hyponatremia (1) are inadvertently made hypernatremic during treatment; (2) have an absolute increase in plasma sodium, which exceeds 25 mmol l^{-1} in the first 24–48 hours of therapy; (3) suffer an hypoxic event; (4) have severe liver disease (Singh *et al.*, 1994; Ayus *et al.*, 1987; Tien *et al.*, 1992). On the other hand, there is overwhelming evidence that treatment of symptomatic hyponatremia with hypertonic NaCl is associated with recovery and survival (Ayus and Arieff, 1999; DeFronzo and Arieff, 1995).

HYPERNATREMIC STATES

Hypernatremia is defined as an abnormally high concentration of plasma sodium. Because sodium with its accompanying anions comprises the great majority of osmoles in the plasma, hypertonicity always accompanies hypernatremia. However, a hyperosmolar state can exist in the absence of hypernatremia if another solute (such as glucose or urea) is present in excessive amounts. The subjects of uremia (Fraser and Arieff, 1997a) hyperglycemic nonketotic hyperosmolar coma and diabetic ketoacidosis are discussed in detail elsewhere and will not be covered here (Halperin *et al.*, 1995).

Brain Adaptation to Hypernatremia

Adaptation of the brain to hypernatremia determines survival, and a rapid increase of plasma sodium without the brain having an opportunity to adapt can lead to permanent brain damage. The response of excitable cells (central nervous system) to a hyperosmolar external fluid can be described as follows. Initially the cells shrink owing to osmotic water abstraction, but ultimately the cells nearly regain the water content they had in the control state by virtue of a combination of net solute uptake and generation of solute *de novo*. Several important differences exist in the response of brain cells versus those of other tissues, such as skeletal muscle and kidney. These are mainly in the types and quantity of solutes that accumulate within the cells as well as the mechanisms by which they accumulate (Strange and Morrison, 1992).

Previous studies have shown that there is some uptake of electrolytes (sodium and potassium) during adaptation of the brain to hypernatremia in rat brain (Ayus *et al.*, 1996). However, while regulatory increases in brain cell volume occur largely due to increases in brain cell content of monovalent cations, these are not the only solutes that accumulate during regulatory increases in brain cell volume. Recent studies have provided good support for the notion that a number of organic compounds account for some of the increase in total brain osmoles (Ayus *et al.*, 1996; Lien *et al.*, 1990). Studies of hypernatremia have shown that over the course of 7 days, water content of the brain decreases by approximately 10% but ultimately recovers to within 98–99% of control (Ayus *et al.*, 1996). This is largely accompanied by an increase in brain solute content. Most of this increase is accounted for by inorganic ions (Na^+, K^+, Cl), amino acids, and undetermined solute (idiogenic osmoles). The increase in undetermined solute (idiogenic osmoles) begins after only about 1 hour of hypernatremia and changes very little during 4 hours to 1 week of hypernatremia (Ayus *et al.*, 1996). The increase in undetermined solute serves to protect brain cell volume from further dehydration. However, this initial protective effect may eventually become deleterious during correction of hypernatremia if the plasma sodium is somehow decreased at a more rapid rate than the brain is able to dissipate the idiogenic osmoles. During treatment of experimental hypernatremia, brain edema may develop despite a significant decrease in brain content of (sodium + potassium), due to failure of amino acids and idiogenic osmoles to dissipate (Ayus *et al.*, 1996).

Causes of Hypernatremia

The causes of hypernatremia in children and adults have recently been reviewed (Arieff, 1995). There are a number of medical conditions that are commonly associated with hypernatremia, the etiology of which is quite different in children and adults. In infants, gastroenteritis with diarrhea is the most common cause while in elderly individuals, hypernatremia is often associated with infirmity and inability to freely obtain water, leading to gradual desiccation (Snyder and Arieff, 1992). Small children may also become hypernatremic after accidental administration of a high solute load, particularly accidental substitution of NaCl for sugar in preparation of formula or improper dilution of concentrated formulas (Finberg *et al.*, 1963). Children commonly develop hypernatremia after dehydration from diarrhea or emesis associated with common illnesses (Mocharla *et al.*, 1997; Moritz and Ayus, 1999).

In adults, causes of hypernatremia include nasogastric hyperalimentation, nonketotic hyperosmolar coma, acute renal failure, renal tubular damage, improper mixture of dialysis fluid, dehydration secondary to either fever or elevated ambient temperature, $NaHCO_3$ administration, and diabetes insipidus. Generally, diabetes insipidus is associated with hypernatremia only under circumstances where the patient is unable to freely obtain water or when the lesion responsible for the diabetes insipidus results in a decrease in thirst. Excessive administration of hypertonic solutions of $NaHCO_3$ to critically ill patients suffering cardiac arrest or lactic acidosis has been associated with a dangerously elevated plasma osmolality and infrequent survival. Severe hypernatremia has also been occasionally observed in patients inadvertently receiving intravenous hypertonic NaCl for therapeutic abortion.

Clinical Manifestations of Hypernatremia

The signs and symptoms of hypernatremia are variable. In experimental hyperosmolality, findings include nystagmus, myoclonic jerking of the extremities, severe weight loss, decreased food intake, and, ultimately, respiratory failure and death (Ayus *et al.*, 1996). In human subjects, preexisting abnormalities of mental status may make it difficult to detect any new neurological findings. In addition, since hypernatremia frequently occurs in the setting of a coexistent pathologic process, it may be difficult to ascribe any particular symptom or group of symptoms to hypertonicity *per se*. In children, there may be alternating periods of lethargy and irritability; tachypnea is frequently present. A history compatible with gastroenteritis is frequently obtained and may be the cause of the hypernatremia; conversely, nausea and vomiting are often seen even in the absence of diarrhea. Seizures are common and roughly correlate with the degree of hypernatremia. Associated abnormalities include metabolic acidosis, hyperglycemia, and weight loss (Moritz and Ayus, 1999).

In the elderly, some important differences exist (Snyder and Arieff, 1992). When considering only patients who were hypernatremic at the time of hospital admission, women were predominant. Although nearly half the hypernatremic patients had a febrile illness, other associated conditions assume more prominence than in infants. These include the postoperative state, diuretic administration, excessive intravenous solute administration (including nutritional supplements), and diabetes mellitus as the leading causes. Depression of the sensorium is frequently present and is highly correlated with the degree of hypernatremia. Altered mental status is also an independent predictor of subsequent mortality at any level of hypernatremia (Palevsky *et al.*, 1996; Snyder and Arieff, 1992).

Morbidity and Mortality of Hypernatremia

Hypernatremia is associated with considerable long-term morbidity and mortality both in children and adults. Most studies in children report morbidity and mortality figures of about 15%, with survivors of hypernatremia having a 10–15% likelihood of having permanent neurological deficits (Banister *et al.*, 1975) (Moritz and Ayus, 1999). In adults, the figures are similar. The mortality in elderly patients with hypernatremia was found to be 42% in one study, and neurological morbidity as assessed by changes in level of care was present in 38% of the survivors (Snyder and Arieff, 1992). One especially noteworthy finding in this series was the fact that mortality was higher in patients with hypernatremia developing in the hospital. These findings have recently been confirmed (Palevsky *et al.*, 1996; Long *et al.*, 1991). Authors have attributed this finding to a more complicated clinical setting and delayed recognition of hypertonicity in hospitalized subjects.

Essential Hypernatremia

The initial descriptions of the syndrome of essential hypernatremia included the following elements: (1) asymptomatic chronic hypernatremia, (2) clinical euvolemia, (3) hypodipsia, (4) partial central diabetes insipidus, and (5) absence of nephrogenic diabetes insipidus. In more physiologic terms, essential hypernatremia is a disorder of osmoregulation where the regulatory systems (ADH and thirst) are at least partially responsive to osmolar and volumetric stimuli. In the steady state, patients are hypernatremic, euvolemic (by the usual clinical evaluation), and asymptomatic (absence of thirst) (Goldberg *et al.*, 1967). By definition, if the plasma osmolality is substantially elevated, this steady state represents an upward resetting of the osmolar set point for ADH release and probably of the osmolar threshold for thirst perception (if the steady state plasma osmolality is above about 294 mOsm/kg H_2O). Volumetric stimuli for ADH release and for thirst perception must operate at normal or near-normal settings to maintain clinical euvolemia.

Thus, the syndrome of essential hypernatremia is the hyperosmolar counterpart of the syndrome of "reset osmostat". In the latter syndrome, asymptomatic euvolemic hyponatremia is maintained with a decreased osmolar set point for ADH release and a decreased osmolar threshold for thirst.

Hypernatremia and Liver Disease

A group of adult patients in whom the entity of hypernatremia with its attendant sequelae is not appreciated are chronic alcoholic subjects with end stage liver disease who present with fulminant liver failure and hepatic encephalopathy (Fraser and Arieff, 1985). Such patients are often treated with oral lactulose as therapy for their hepatic encephalopathy. Hypernatremia may complicate such therapy (Fraser and Arieff, 1985). Patients with lactulose-associated hypernatremia had a mortality of 87 versus 60% in those patients who did not develop hypernatremia.

Hypernatremia in patients with severe liver disease may be quite a common occurrence after therapy with intravenous osmotic diuretic agents and/or oral lactulose (Fraser and Arieff, 1985). The hypernatremia is associated with a high mortality and appears to be directly related to a negative free water balance (Arieff and Papadakis, 1988). Patients with liver disease who have undergone hepatic transplantation and then develop hypernatremia are particularly susceptible to the development of cerebral demyelinating lesions (Ayus *et al.*, 1987; Estol *et al.*, 1989; Wszolek *et al.*, 1989).

Treatment of Hypernatremia

The goal of therapy in hypernatremia is the reduction of plasma osmolality toward normal by the administration of free water in excess of solute. Hypernatremia is uncommonly associated with administration of excessive quantities of NaCl, but when such a situation is present, removal of solute must be considered. Removal of solute is usually accomplished by dialysis. When water administration is planned, the major therapeutic questions are the type and quantity of fluid to be given. In adult patients with hypernatremia, although 280 mM dextrose in water (5% dextrose in water, D5W) has commonly been utilized, this therapeutic modality has recently come into question.

Patients with hypernatremic dehydration should be treated with fluid that provides free water in excess of electrolytes. In both children and adults, fluid therapy is usually calculated so as to be administered over a period of about 48 hours. Despite such recommendations, little data in humans or animals is available as to the ideal rate of fluid administration. Fatal cases of cerebral edema, as well as permanent brain damage, have occurred when hypernatremia was completely corrected within 24 hours, while seizures with cerebral edema occur in more than 50% of hypernatremic rabbits when plasma sodium is reduced from 185 to 142 mmol l^{-1} in 4 hours. The pathophysiology of cerebral edema complicating rapid (less than 24 hours) correction of experimental hypernatremia (in rabbits) has recently been described (Ayus *et al.*, 1996). These studies highlight the dangers of overly rapid correction of hypernatremia. In addition, recent information suggests that therapy of hypernatremia with glucose-containing solutions (280 mM glucose/H_2O) may lead to cerebral intracellular lactic acidosis (Sheldon *et al.*, 1992), although this has not been confirmed in humans. Current recommendations for treatment of chronic hypernatremia in adults, when the hypernatremia is primarily due to water loss, are:

1. If there is evidence of circulatory collapse, the patient should receive initial resuscitation with colloid, such as plasma or a plasma substitute (such as isotonic NaCl), rapidly enough to correct shock and stabilize the circulatory system.
2. Fluid deficit should be estimated on the basis of serum sodium, body weight, and TBW. The deficit should be given over a 48-hour period, aiming for a decrement in serum osmolality of approximately 1–2 mOsm per liter per hour. Maintenance fluids, which include replacement of urine volume with hypotonic fluid, are given in addition to the deficit.
3. Hypotonic fluid should be administered. The usual replacement fluid will be 77 mmol l^{-1} NaCl. In general, solutions containing glucose should be avoided if possible.
4. Plasma electrolytes should be monitored at frequent intervals, usually about every 2 hours. It should be stressed that many adult patients with hypernatremia have serious underlying systemic illness, such as stroke, dementia, infection, or head trauma. Many such patients appear to die of their underlying illness rather than of hypernatremia *per se*. Close attention should be given to the treatment of associated medical conditions.
5. If the hypernatremia is secondary to excessive loss of other body fluids, the replacement fluid should be similar to the fluid actually lost.

The ideal treatment of hypernatremia represents a balance between free water administration and solute (sodium) excretion. Sodium removal can be accomplished with diuretics or dialysis. Infusion of glucose-containing fluids can be associated with intracellular lactic acidosis, and they should be avoided if possible. Overzealous correction can be accompanied by rehydration seizures that are probably due to acute cerebral edema from brain cellular water uptake.

DISORDERS OF POTASSIUM

Disorders of the plasma potassium concentration are almost as common as are those of sodium, but otherwise there are few similarities. Unlike sodium, most potassium is located intracellularly, primarily in skeletal muscle. Abnormalities of plasma or total body potassium do not affect the brain. The factors that regulate plasma potassium concentration consist primarily of the kidney and the hormones insulin, aldosterone, the renin-angiotensin system, and epinephrine (DeFronzo, 1994). Although the kidney is responsible for most abnormalities of plasma potassium, the primary target organs are the heart and skeletal muscle. Although a linear relationship was once suggested between plasma potassium and metabolic acidosis, such a causal relationship is now known not to exist, as in most conditions associated with metabolic acidosis, plasma potassium is not elevated. In the original study, virtually all of the patients with hyperkalemia had either diabetic ketoacidosis or acute renal failure (Burnell *et al.*, 1956). It is now known that patients with acute renal failure tend to have both metabolic acidosis and hyperkalemia independently. Among patients with diabetic ketoacidosis, breakdown of skeletal muscle as substrate for gluconeogenesis accounts for the hyperkalemia. Hyperkalemia is not generally present with other forms of metabolic acidosis.

Hyperkalemia

Hyperkalemia may develop from a shift of potassium from intracellular to extracellular compartments, from tissue (muscle) breakdown, or it can be secondary to decreased renal potassium excretion. An important cause of hyperkalemia has only been described in the past 5 years. ACE inhibitors have been prescribed in increasing quantities for the treatment of congestive heart failure (Juurlink *et al.*, 2004) and the prevention of diabetic nephropathy (Lewis *et al.*, 2001; Palmer, 2004). Among hospitalized patients, the major concerns relating to alterations of potassium homeostasis are effects on the heart, which is particularly vulnerable to increases in the serum potassium. The electrocardiographic (ECG) changes associated with hyperkalemia have previously been described (Altmann, 1995). In brief, the earliest change associated with hyperkalemia is a symmetrical increase in the amplitude or "tenting" of the T waves, which is best observed in the precordial leads. Such ECG changes usually cannot be appreciated on a "rhythm strip" generated from a cardiac monitor. These changes usually become manifest when the serum potassium reaches levels of 5.5–6.0 mmol l^{-1}. As the serum potassium concentration rises further (6.0–7.0 mmol l^{-1}), conduction through the conducting system and ventricles becomes delayed. This is reflected by a lengthening of the PR interval and widening of the QRS complex. With potassium concentrations of 7.0 to 7.5, atrial muscle conduction becomes impaired and there is a progressive flattening of the P wave; there is continued widening of the QRS complex and a further delay in A-V conduction. When the potassium concentration exceeds 8 mmol l^{-1}, atrial conduction ceases and the P waves disappear. As the QRS complex widens further, it merges with the T wave, producing a sine wave pattern. If these changes go unrecognized and appropriate therapy is not begun, ventricular fibrillation or asystole will follow. In addition to the classic sequence of events outlined above, virtually any type of arrhythmia or conduction disturbance may be seen in hyperkalemic patients. The first symptoms include paresthesias and weakness in the arms and legs. These may be followed by a symmetrical flaccid paralysis of the extremities that ascends toward the trunk and may involve the muscles of respiration, causing hypoxemia, and carbon dioxide retention.

Treatment of Hyperkalemia

Treatment of the hyperkalemic patient is dependent upon the severity and etiology of the hyperkalemia. Whether or not aggressive therapy should be instituted will depend both upon the degree of hyperkalemia and the presence of cardiac or neuromuscular manifestations. If a specific cause for the increase in serum potassium concentration can be identified, it should be eliminated. Regardless of etiology, there will be certain patients in whom the hyperkalemia is life threatening and rapid correction is indicated. If the serum potassium concentration has risen acutely to levels above 6.0 mmol l^{-1}, or if ECG changes of hyperkalemia are present, treatment should be initiated immediately. There are several possible therapeutic regimens for hyperkalemia, which are explained in detail elsewhere (Smith and DeFronzo, 1995).

Calcium has no effect on the serum potassium level, but its intravenous infusion will immediately antagonize the effects of hyperkalemia on the heart. Although calcium does not affect the resting membrane potential, it increases the threshold potential at which excitation occurs.

Sodium bicarbonate will increase plasma bicarbonate and arterial pH, shifting potassium into cells, thus lowering serum potassium. Sodium bicarbonate is administered intravenously as a 50 mmol bolus over 5 to 10 minutes. The onset of action is 5 to 10 minutes, with the effect lasting about 2 hours.

Insulin stimulates potassium uptake by extrarenal cells, primarily skeletal muscle. This is the result of a direct effect of insulin on the cell membrane and is independent of glucose transport or intracellular glucose metabolism. Glucose is administered only in order to prevent hypoglycemia. Ten units of insulin with 50 gm of glucose are administered over 1 hour. The onset of action occurs in about 30 minutes, with the effect lasting for 4 to 6 hours. The plasma potassium should decrease by 0.5–1.2 mmol l^{-1} within 1 to 2 hours.

None of the therapeutic maneuvers discussed above will result in a net removal of potassium from the body. These maneuvers serve as temporizing measures until more definitive therapy can be initiated. Hyperkalemia is frequently encountered in patients with renal failure, where little can be done to enhance renal potassium excretion. Nebulized albuterol may be effective in such patients (Allon *et al.*, 1989). However, in the patient with intact kidney function, measures that enhance urine flow and sodium delivery to the distal tubular sites of potassium secretion will augment renal potassium excretion. Such measures include diuretics, which act proximal to the potassium secretary sites, such as furosemide (40–80 mg intravenously).

Cation-exchange resins, such as sodium polystyrene sulfonate (Kayexalate), decrease the plasma potassium concentration by exchanging sodium for potassium in the gastrointestinal tract. Each gram of Kayexalate removes 0.5–1 mmol of potassium in exchange for 2–3 mmol of sodium. The usual dose of Kayexalate is 25 g either orally or as a retention enema. Since the resin is constipating, it should always be given with sorbitol or mannitol (15–30 ml of 70% sorbitol or mannitol every 30 minutes) to induce osmotic diarrhea, which can be sustained by administering additional doses every 6–8 hours. If the patient cannot tolerate oral administration, 50 g of Kayexalate with 50 g of sorbitol can be added to 200 ml of 10% dextrose in water and given per rectum.

Both peritoneal and hemodialysis are very effective in removing potassium from the body. If acute reduction of the serum potassium concentration is indicated, hemodialysis is the therapy of choice. Using a potassium-free dialysate, the plasma potassium begins to fall within minutes and one can remove about 30–40 mmol of potassium during the first hour, assuming an initial plasma potassium of 7 mmol l^{-1}. The hypokalemic effect persists as long as dialysis is continued. Peritoneal dialysis is also effective in removing potassium from the body but the rate of removal is much slower than can be accomplished with either hemodialysis or cation-exchange resins. Using standard 2 l exchanges with one exchange per hour will remove only about 5 mmol of potassium per hour.

HYPOKALEMIA

Hypokalemia is discussed in substantial detail elsewhere (Smith *et al.*, 1995) and can result from (1) redistribution of potassium from the extracellular to intracellular space, (2) dietary deficiency of potassium, (3) extrarenal (mainly gastrointestinal tract) losses, or (4) renal losses. The plasma potassium concentration has only an approximate relationship to total body potassium stores. In circumstances where there is movement of potassium out of cells (such as diabetic ketoacidosis), substantial potassium depletion can be masked by a relatively normal plasma concentration.

Alkalemia is a well-known cause of hypokalemia. The most important mechanism contributing to hypokalemia is enhanced urinary excretion of potassium. When alkalemia has been present for more than a few minutes, urinary excretion accounts for substantially more potassium loss than does sequestration within cells, a mechanism that has little effect upon serum potassium. Hypokalemia commonly accompanies gastrointestinal disease (when emesis is present). Since renal potassium conservation develops slowly when intake is reduced, a significant potassium loss may develop on this basis alone. The normal gastrointestinal tract secretes more than 6 l of fluid daily, which has an average potassium concentration of 5–10 mmol l^{-1}. Significant quantities of this gastrointestinal fluid may be lost owing to vomiting, nasogastric suctioning, diarrhea, external fistulae, or sequestration within an aperistaltic segment ("third spacing"). Depletion of hydrochloric acid by removal of gastric juices will result in metabolic alkalosis (for each H^+ ion lost from the GI tract, a bicarbonate has been generated and retained), sequestration of potassium within cells, and urinary potassium wasting. Similarly, when chronic metabolic acidosis develops due to diarrhea, loss of potassium in the urine is common. It should be emphasized that although gastrointestinal fluids contain significant quantities of potassium, the major route of potassium loss in patients with diarrhea or vomiting is often renal. The concentration of potassium in gastric juice is about 10–15 mmol l^{-1}. Hypokalemia in patients with vomiting or nasogastric suction could result directly from loss of potassium-rich gastric fluid. However, these factors tend to promote urinary potassium wasting to such an extent that this usually accounts for the majority of the total potassium deficit among patients with extensive emesis or nasogastric suction.

Since the concentration of potassium in bile and pancreatic juice is similar to that of plasma, external drainage of these secretions will not usually directly cause hypokalemia. However, any accompanying decrease in the extracellular volume will activate mechanisms for renal potassium excretion, such as secondary aldosteronism and metabolic alkalosis.

The potassium concentration in stool water is normally about 75 mmol l^{-1}. Since daily stool output contains only 100 ml of water, very little potassium is normally excreted by this route. However, stool volume in severe diarrheal illness can exceed 10 l per day. If the potassium concentration in these circumstances resembled basal values, the obligatory potassium wasting would rapidly deplete body stores. However, potassium concentration in diarrheal stool falls sharply in inverse proportion to daily stool volumes. With stool losses above 3 l day^{-1}, the stool potassium concentration is usually similar to that of plasma.

Treatment of Hypokalemia

Hypokalemia is usually defined by a serum potassium concentration below 3.5 mmol l^{-1}. Prior to initiation of therapy, one should estimate the potassium deficit. There is no exact relationship between serum potassium and intracellular potassium. In muscle tissue, which constitutes most of body bulk, the intracellular potassium is about 130 mmol kg^{-1} H_2O. A decrease in the serum potassium concentration of 1 mmol l^{-1}, from 4.0–3.0 mmol l^{-1}, corresponds to approximately a 10% reduction (about 300 mmol) in total body potassium content. Such deficits are not usually associated with clinical manifestations and can usually be corrected with oral potassium replacement. A decline in the serum potassium concentration from 4.0–2.0 mmol l^{-1} implies a 15–20% or greater decrease in total body potassium stores (about 600 mmol), and potassium may have to be replaced more rapidly, depending on the presence of clinical manifestations. When the serum potassium level drops to below about 2.0 mmol l^{-1}, it is difficult to estimate the true potassium deficit because the relationship between serum potassium concentration and total body potassium content becomes less linear. With serum potassium levels below 2.0 mmol l^{-1}, small additional decreases may be associated with huge deficits in total body potassium. The treatment for hypokalemia consists of potassium replacement, usually in the form of KCl. How rapidly potassium is replaced and whether the potassium is given intravenously or orally will depend upon both the absolute serum potassium concentration and attendant clinical manifestations.

In general, treatment of a low serum potassium concentration is not an emergency. Symptoms tend to be more severe in patients with acute hypokalemia than when the disorder is more protracted. Whenever possible, potassium replacement should be given orally. The best guide to the adequacy of potassium replacement is sequential monitoring of serum potassium. Although changes in total body potassium content are roughly reflected by changes in the serum potassium concentration, there is substantial variation among patients.

Potassium can be administered intravenously as chloride, phosphate, or bicarbonate salt, depending on the accompanying electrolyte and acid–base disturbance. Evidence of cardiac or neuromuscular dysfunction, the presence of severe hypokalemia (below 2.0–2.5 $mmol\,l^{-1}$), and the inability to administer potassium orally (postsurgery, emesis) are indications for intravenous potassium. In general, a maximum of 40 mmol of potassium chloride in 1 l of IV fluid should be administered per hour. Infusion of 0.75 mmol potassium/kg over 1–2 hours will increase plasma potassium from 3–4.5 $mmol\,l^{-1}$. Although this might lead to ECG changes, it would be unlikely to cause life-threatening arrhythmia. Furthermore, when potassium is given to patients with more profound hypokalemia (below 2.0–2.5 $mmol\,l^{-1}$ with body potassium deficits of 15–20%) a greater percent of the administered potassium will enter cells. Consequently, the increase of plasma potassium will be less than the 1–1.5 $mmol\,l^{-1}$ observed in normokalemic patients or mildly hypokalemic subjects. Thus, 0.75 $mmol\,kg^{-1}$ of body weight administered over 1–2 hours is a safe means of replacing potassium intravenously. If hypokalemia is severe (2.0 $mmol\,l^{-1}$ or less) and associated with cardiac arrhythmias such as premature ventricular contractions or ventricular tachycardia, potassium replacement must be more rapid, with as much as 80 mmol infused during the first hour.

KEY POINTS

- Hyponatremia is the most common electrolyte disorder in hospitalized patients; the symptoms are often dramatic, and if not managed properly, can lead to death or permanent brain damage.
- Hypernatremia affects about 3% of hospitalized elderly patients; the symptoms are very subtle, and the overall mortality when plasma sodium exceeds 150 mmol/l is in excess of 50%.
- The most common causes of hypernatremia in hospitalized elderly patients are administration of hypotonic intravenous fluids to hospitalized postoperative patients and inappropriate use of diuretics.
- Total body water varies as a function of age, gender, and body mass, with a range of 42% (elderly women) to 75% (young children) and an average of 50% in hospitalized adults.
- Hyperkalemia is most common in patients with renal insufficiency and in those taking aldactone plus ACE inhibitors for the treatment of heart failure. It can lead to fatal arrhythmia if not properly managed.

KEY REFERENCES

- Ayus JC, Wheeler JM & Arieff AI. Postoperative hyponatremic encephalopathy in menstruant women. *Annals of Internal Medicine* 1992; **117**:891–7.
- Chumlea WC, Guo SS, Zeller CM *et al.* Total body water reference values and prediction equations for adults. *Kidney International* 2001; **59**:2250–8.
- Fraser CL & Arieff AI. Epidemiology, pathophysiology and management of hyponatremic encephalopathy. *The American Journal of Medicine* 1997b; **102**:67–77.
- Juurlink DN, Mamdani MM, Lee DS & Redelmeier DA. Rates of hyperkalemia after publication of the randomized aldactone evaluation study. *The New England Journal of Medicine* 2004; **351**:543–51.
- Palevsky PM, Bhagrath R & Greenberg A. Hypernatremia in hospitalized patients. *Annals of Internal Medicine* 1996; **124**:197–203.

REFERENCES

Allon M, Dunlay R & Copkney C. Nebulized albuterol for acute hyperkalemia in patients on hemodialysis. *Annals of Internal Medicine* 1989; **110**:426–9.

Altmann P. Clinical manifestations of electrolyte disorders. In AI Arieff & RA DeFronzo (eds) *Fluid, Electrolyte and Acid – Base Disorders* 1995, 2nd edn, pp 527–72; Churchill Livingstone, New York & London.

Anderson RJ, Chung HM, Kluge R & Schrier RW. Hyponatremia: a prospective analysis of its epidemiology and the pathogenetic role of vasopressin. *Annals of Internal Medicine* 1985; **102**:164–8.

Arafah BM, Nekl K, Lechner R & Selman WR. Diabetes insipidus: endocrine and neuroendocrine abnormalities in the neurosurgical patient. In GT Tindall, PR Cooper & DL Barrow (eds) *The Practice of Neurosurgery* 1996a, pp 337–41; Williams & Wilkins, Baltimore.

Arafah BM, Nekl K, Lechner R & Selman WR. Neuroendocrine dysfunction following head trauma: endocrine and neuroendocrine abnormalities in the neurosurgical patient. In GT Tindall, PR Cooper & DL Barrow (eds) *The Practice of Neurosurgery* 1996b, pp 346–8; Williams & Wilkins, Baltimore.

Arieff AI. Hyponatremia, convulsions, respiratory arrest, and permanent brain damage after elective surgery in healthy women. *The New England Journal of Medicine* 1986; **314**:1529–35.

Arieff AI. Acid – base, electrolyte, and metabolic abnormalities. In JE Parrillo & RC Bone (eds) *Critical Care Medicine: Principles of Diagnosis and Management* 1995, pp 1071–105; Mosby – Year Book, Philadelphia.

Arieff AI. Postoperative hyponatraemic encephalopathy following elective surgery in children. *Paediatric Anaesthesia (London)* 1998; **8**:1–4.

Arieff AI. Neurologic aspects of endocrine disturbances. In RJ Joynt & RC Griggs (eds) *Clinical Neurology* 2003; Lippincott – Raven, Philadelphia.

Arieff AI, Ayus JC & Fraser CL. Hyponatraemia and death or permanent brain damage in healthy children. *British Medical Journal* 1992; **304**:1218–22.

Arieff AI, Guisado R & Lazarowitz VC. Pathophysiology of hyperosmolar states. In TE Andreoli, JJ Grantham & FC Rector Jr (eds) *Disturbances in Body Fluid Osmolality* 1977, pp 227–50; American Physiological Society, Bethesda.

Arieff AI, Kozniewska E & Roberts TPL. Role of vasopressin in brain damage from hyponatremic encephalopathy. In P Gross, D Richter & GL Robertson (eds) *Vasopressin* 1993, pp 243–57; John Libbey Eurotext, Montrouge.

Arieff AI, Kozniewska E, Roberts T *et al.* Age, gender and vasopressin affect survival and brain adaptation in rats with metabolic encephalopathy. *The American Journal of Physiology* 1995; **268**(5):R1143–52;(*Regulatory Integrative and Comparative Physiology* **337**).

Arieff AI & Papadakis MA. Hyponatremia and hypernatremia in liver disease. In M Epstein (ed) *The Kidney in Liver Disease* 1988, 3rd edn, pp 73–88; Williams & Wilkins, Baltimore.

Ashraf N, Locksley R & Arieff AI. Thiazide – induced hyponatremia associated with death or neurologic damage in outpatients. *American Journal of Medicine* 1981; **70**(6):1163–8.

Ayus JC & Arieff AI. Brain damage and postoperative hyponatremia: role of gender. *Neurology* 1996; **46**:323–8.

Ayus JC & Arieff AI. Chronic hyponatremic encephalopathy in postmenopausal women: association of therapies with morbidity and mortality. *The Journal of the American Medical Association* 1999; **281**:2299–304.

Ayus JC, Armstrong DL & Arieff AI. Effects of hypernatraemia in the central nervous system and its therapy in rats and rabbits. *Journal of Physiology (London)* 1996; **492**(Pt 1):243–55.

Ayus JC, Krothapalli RK & Arieff AI. Treatment of symptomatic hyponatremia and its relation to brain damage. A prospective study. *The New England Journal of Medicine* 1987; **317**:1190–5.

Ayus JC, Wheeler JM & Arieff AI. Postoperative hyponatremic encephalopathy in menstruant women. *Annals of Internal Medicine* 1992; **117**:891–7.

Balmelli C, Kupferschmidt H, Rentsch K & Schneemann M. Fatal brain edema after ingestion of ecstasy and benzylpiperazine. *Deutsche Medizinische Wochenschrift* 2001; **126**:809–11.

Banister A, Siddiqi S & Hatcher GW. Treatment of hypernatremia dehydration in infancy. *Archives of Disease in Childhood* 1975; **50**:179.

Bartter FE & Schwartz WB. The syndrome of inappropriate secretion of antidiuretic hormone. *The American Journal of Medicine* 1967; **42**:790–806.

Ben-Abraham R, Szold O, Rudick V & Weinbroum AA. 'Ecstasy' intoxication: life threatening manifestations and resuscitative measures in the intensive care setting. *European Journal of Emergency Medicine* 2003; **10**:309–13.

Bichet DG. Nephrogenic and central diabetes insipidus. In RW Schrier & CW Gottschalk (eds) *Diseases of the Kidney* 1997, 6th edn, pp 2429–49; Little, Brown & Company, Boston.

Bichet DG, Oksche A & Rosenthal W. Congenital diabetes insipidus. *Journal of the American Society of Nephrology* 1997; **8**:1951–8.

Burnell JM, Villamil M, Uyeno B & Scribner BH. The effect in humans of extracellular pH change on the relationship between serum potassium concentration and intracellular potassium. *The Journal of Clinical Investigation* 1956; **35**:935–9.

Cheng JC, Zikos D, Skopicki HA *et al.* Long term neurologic outcome in psychogenic water drinkers with severe symptomatic hyponatremia: the effect of rapid correction. *The American Journal of Medicine* 1990; **88**:561–6.

Chumlea WC, Guo SS, Zeller CM *et al.* Total body water reference values and prediction equations for adults. *Kidney International* 2001; **59**:2250–8.

Decaux G. Difference in solute excretion during correction of hyponatremic patients with cirrhosis or inappropriate secretion of ADH (SIADH) by oral vasopressin V2 receptor antagonist VPA-985. *The Journal of Laboratory and Clinical Medicine* 2001; **138**(1):18–21.

DeFronzo RA. Clinical disorders of hyperkalemia. In MH Maxwell, CR Kleeman & RG Narins (eds) *Clinical Disorders of Fluid and Electrolyte Metabolism* 1994, 4th edn, pp 697–754; McGraw – Hill Book Company, San Francisco.

DeFronzo RA & Arieff AI. Hyponatremia: pathophysiology and treatment. In AI Arieff & RA DeFronzo (eds) *Fluid, Electrolyte and Acid – Base Disorders* 1995, 2nd edn, pp 255–303; Churchill Livingstone, New York.

Del Bigio MR & Fedoroff S. Swelling of astroglia in vitro and the effect of arginine vasopressin and atrial natriuretic peptide. *Acta Neurochirurgica. Supplement* 1990; **51**:14–6.

Demitrack MA, Kalogeras KT, Altemus M *et al.* Plasma and cerebrospinal fluid measures of arginine vasopressin secretion in patients with bulimia nervosa and in healthy subjects. *The Journal of Clinical Endocrinology and Metabolism* 1992; **74**:1277–83.

Estol CJ, Faris AA, Martinez AJ & Barmada MA. Central pontine myelinolysis after liver transplantation. *Neurology* 1989; **39**:493–8.

Faraci FM, Mayhan WG & Heistad DD. Effect of vasopressin on production of cerebrospinal fluid: possible role of vasopressin (V1)-receptors. *The American Journal of Physiology* 1990; **258**:R94–8;(*Regulatory Integrative and Comparative Physiology* **27**).

Fenves AZ, Thomas S & Knochel JP. Beer potomania: two cases and review of the literature. *Clinical Nephrology* 1996; **45**:61–4.

Finberg L, Kiley J & Luttrell CN. Mass accidental salt poisoning in infancy: a study of a hospital disaster. *The Journal of the American Medical Association* 1963; **184**:187–90.

Fraser CL & Arieff AI. Hepatic encephalopathy. *The New England Journal of Medicine* 1985; **313**(14):865–73.

Fraser CL & Arieff AI. Fatal central diabetes mellitus and insipidus resulting from untreated hyponatremia: a new syndrome. *Annals of Internal Medicine* 1990; **112**:113–9.

Fraser CL & Arieff AI. Nervous system manifestations of renal failure. In RW Schrier & CW Gottschalk (eds) *Diseases of the Kidney* 1997a, 2625–46 6th edn; Little, Brown & Company, Boston.

Fraser CL & Arieff AI. Epidemiology, pathophysiology and management of hyponatremic encephalopathy. *The American Journal of Medicine* 1997b; **102**:67–77.

Fraser CL & Arieff AI. Na-K-APTase activity decreases with aging in female rat brain synaptosomes. *The American Journal of Physiology (Renal Physiology)* 2001; **281**:674–8.

Fraser CL & Swanson RA. Female sex hormones inhibit volume regulation in rat brain astrocyte culture. *The American Journal of Physiology* 1994; **267**:C909–14;(*Cell Physiology* **36**).

Goldberg M, Weinstein G, Adesman J & Bleicher SJ. Asymptomatic hypovolemic hypernatremia: a variant of essential hypernatremia. *The American Journal of Medicine* 1967; **43**:804–10.

Goldman MB, Luchins DJ & Robertson GL. Mechanisms of altered water metabolism in psychotic patients with polydipsia and hyponatremia. *The New England Journal of Medicine* 1988; **318**(7):397–403.

Goldman MB, Robertson GL, Luchins DJ *et al.* Psychotic exacerbations and enhanced vasopressin secretion in schizophrenic patients with hyponatremia and polydipsia. *Archives of General Psychiatry* 1997; **54**:443–9.

Grinspoon SK & Bilezikian JP. HIV disease and the endocrine system. *The New England Journal of Medicine* 1992; **327**:1360–5.

Gross P, Remann D, Henschkowski J & Damian M. Treatment of severe hyponatremia: conventional and novel aspects. *Journal of the American Society of Nephrology* 2001; **12**:S10–4.

Gur RC, Mozley PD, Resnick SM *et al.* Gender differences in age effect on brain atrophy measured by magnetic resonance imaging. *Proceedings of the National Academy of Sciences of the United States of America* 1991; **88**:2845–9.

Halperin ML, Goguen JM, Cheema-Dhadli S & Kamel KS. Diabetic emergencies. In AI Arieff & RA DeFronzo (eds) *Fluid, Electrolyte and Acid – Base Disorders* 1995, pp 741–75; Churchill Livingstone, New York.

Juurlink DN, Mamdani MM, Lee DS & Redelmeier DA. Rates of hyperkalemia after publication of the randomized aldactone evaluation study. *The New England Journal of Medicine* 2004; **351**:543–51.

Kanda F & Arieff AI. Vasopressin inhibits calcium-coupled sodium efflux system in rat brain synaptosomes. *The American Journal of Physiology* 1994; **266**:R1169–73;(*Regulatory Integrative and Comparative Physiology* **35**).

Kanda F, Sarnacki P & Arieff AI. Atrial natriuretic peptide inhibits the amelioride-sensitive sodium-hydrogen exchanger in rat brain.

The American Journal of Physiology 1992; **263**:R279–83;(*Regulatory Integrative and Comparative Physiology* **32**).

Knochel JP. Hypoxia is the cause of brain damage in hyponatremia. *The Journal of the American Medical Association* 1999; **281**:2342–3.

Kozniewska E, Roberts TPL, Vexler ZS *et al.* Hormonal dependence of the effects of metabolic encephalopathy on cerebral perfusion and oxygen utilization in the rat. *Circulation Research* 1995; **76**:551–8.

Lee WH & Packer M. Prognostic importance of serum sodium concentration and its modification by converting enzyme inhibition in patients with severe chronic heart failure. *Circulation* 1986; **73**:257–67.

Lewis EJ, Hunsicker LG, Clarke WR *et al.* Renoprotective effect of the angiotensin – receptor antagonist irbosartan in patients with Nephropathy due to type 2 diabetes. *The New England Journal of Medicine* 2001; **345**:851–60.

Lien YH, Shapiro JI & Chan L. Effects of hypernatremia on organic brain osmoles. *The Journal of Clinical Investigation* 1990; **85**(5):1427–35.

Lindeman RD, Tobin J & Shock NW. Longitudinal studies on the rate of decline in renal function with age. *Journal of the American Geriatrics Society* 1985; **33**(5):278–85.

Long CA, Marin P, Bayer AJ *et al.* Hypernatraemia in an adult in – patient population. *Postgraduate Medical Journal* 1991; **67**:643–5.

McKinley MJ, Allen A, Congiu M *et al.* Central integration of osmoregulatory vasopressin secretion, thirst and sodium excretion. In AW Crowley, JF Laird & DA Ausiello (eds) *Vasopressin: Cellular and Integrative Functions* 1988, pp 185–92; Raven Press, New York.

McManus ML, Churchwell KB & Strange K. Regulation of cell volume in health and disease. *The New England Journal of Medicine* 1995; **333**:1260–6.

Mocharla R, Schexnayder SM & Glasier CM. Fatal cerebral edema and intracranial hemorrhage associated with hypernatremic dehydration. *Pediatric Radiology* 1997; **27**:785–7.

Moritz ML & Ayus JC. The changing pattern of hypernatremia in hospitalized children. *Pediatrics* 1999; **103**:435–9.

Morrison G & Singer I. Hyperosmolal states. In Narins RG (ed) *Clinical Disorders of Fluid and Electrolyte Metabolism* 1994, 5th edn, pp 617–58; McGraw – Hill, New York.

Nzerue CM, Baffoe-Bonnie H, You W *et al.* Predictors of outcome in hospitalized patients with severe hyponatremia. *Journal of the National Medical Association* 2003; **95**:335–43.

Oh MS & Carroll HJ. Regulation of intracellular and extracellular volume. In AI Arieff & RA DeFronzo (eds) *Fluid, Electrolyte and Acid – Base Disorders* 1995, 2nd edn, pp 1–28; Churchill Livingstone, New York.

Palevsky PM, Bhagrath R & Greenberg A. Hypernatremia in hospitalized patients. *Annals of Internal Medicine* 1996; **124**:197–203.

Palmer BF. Managing hyperkalemia caused by inhibitors of the renin – angiotensin – aldosterone system. *The New England Journal of Medicine* 2004; **351**:585–92.

Palmer BF & Levi M. Renal function and disease in the aging kidney. In RW Schrier & CW Gottschalk (eds) *Diseases of the Kidney* 1997, 6th edn, pp 2293–317; Little, Brown & Company, Boston.

Papadakis MA, Fraser CL & Arieff AI. Hyponatraemia in patients with cirrhosis. *The Quarterly Journal of Medicine* 1990; **76**:675–88.

Phillips PA, Rolls BJ, Ledingham JGG *et al.* Reduced thirst after water deprivation in healthy elderly men. *The New England Journal of Medicine* 1984; **311**(12):753–9.

Posner JB, Ertel NH, Kossmann RJ & Scheinberg LC. Hyponatremia in acute polyneuropathy. *Archives of Neurology* 1967; **17**:530–41.

Sandifer MG. Hyponatremia due to psychotropic drugs. *The Journal of Clinical Psychiatry* 1983; **44**:301–3.

Share L. Control of vasopressin release: an old but continuing story. *News in Physiological Sciences* 1996; **11**:7–13.

Sheldon RA, Partridge JC & Ferriero DM. Postischemic hyperglycemia is not protective to the neonatal rat brain. *Pediatric Research* 1992; **32**:489–93.

Singh N, Yu VL & Gayowski T. Central nervous system lesions in adult liver transplant recipients. *Medicine (Baltimore)* 1994; **73**:110–8.

Smith JD & DeFronzo RA. Hyperkalemia. In AI Arieff & RA DeFronzo (eds) *Fluid, Electrolyte and Acid – Base Disorders* 1995, 2nd edn, pp 319–86; Churchill Livingstone, New York & London.

Smith JD, Perazella M & DeFronzo RA. Hypokalemia. In AI Arieff & RA DeFronzo (eds) *Fluid, Electrolyte and Acid – Base Disorders* 1995, 2nd edn, pp 387–426; Churchill Livingstone, New York & London.

Snyder NA & Arieff AI. Neurological manifestations of hypernatremia. In RA Griggs & AI Arieff (eds) *Metabolic Brain Dysfunction in Systemic Disorders* 1992, pp 87–106; Little, Brown & Company, Boston.

SOLVD. Effect of enalapril on survival in patients with reduced left ventricular ejection fractions and congestive heart failure. *The New England Journal of Medicine* 1991; **325**:293–302.

Steele A, Gowrishankar M, Abrahamson S *et al.* Postoperative hyponatremia despite near-isotonic saline infusion: a phenomenon of desalination. *Annals of Internal Medicine* 1997; **126**:20–5.

Strange K & Morrison R. Volume regulation during recovery from chronic hypertonicity in brain glial cells. *The American Journal of Physiology* 1992; **263**:C412–9;(*Cell Physiology* **32**).

Sullivan EV & Pfefferbaum A. Magnetic resonance relaxometry reveals central pontine myelinolysis in clinically asymptomatic alcoholic men. *Alcoholism, Clinical and Experimental Research* 2001; **25**:1206–12.

Tien R, Arieff AI, Kucharczyk W *et al.* Hyponatremic encephalopathy: is central pontine myelinolysis a component? *American Journal of Medicine* 1992; **92**:513–22.

Trivedi HS & Nolph KD. Nephrogenic diabetes insipidus presenting after head trauma. *American Journal of Nephrology* 1994; **14**:145–7.

Verbalis JG. The syndrome of inappropriate antidiuretic hormone secretion and other hypoosmolar disorders. In RW Schrier & CW Gottschalk (eds) *Diseases of the Kidney* 2001, 7th edn, pp 2511–48; Lippincott Williams & Wilkins, Philadelphia.

Vexler ZS, Ayus JC, Roberts TPL *et al.* Ischemic or hypoxic hypoxia exacerbates brain injury associated with metabolic encephalopathy in laboratory animals. *The Journal of Clinical Investigation* 1994a; **93**:256–64.

Vexler ZS, Roberts TPL, Kucharczyk J & Arieff AI. Severe brain edema associated with cumulative effects of hyponatremic encephalopathy and ischemic hypoxia. In U Ito, A Baethmann, KA Hossman *et al.* (eds) *Brain Edema IX* 1994b, pp 246–9; Springer – Verlag, Vienna.

Vieweg WVR. Special topics in water balance in schizophrenia. In DB Schnur & DG Kirch (eds) *Water Balance in Schizophrenia* 1996, pp 43–52; American Psychiatric Press, London.

Vin-Christian K & Arieff AI. Diabetes insipidus, massive polyuria and hypernatremia leading to permanent brain damage. *American Journal of Medicine* 1993; **94**:341–2.

Vitting KE, Gardenswartz MH, Zabetakis PM *et al.* Frequency of hyponatremia and nonosmolar vasopressin release in the acquired immunodeficiency syndrome. *The Journal of the American Medical Association* 1990; **263**:973–8.

White RJ & Likavec MJ. The diagnosis and initial management of head trauma. *The New England Journal of Medicine* 1992; **327**:1507–11.

Wszolek ZK, McComb RD, Pfeiffer RF *et al.* Pontine and extrapontine myelinolysis following liver transplantation. *Transplantation* 1989; **48**:1006–12.

Zerbe R & Robertson G. Osmotic and nonosmotic regulation of thirst and vasopressin secretion. In RG Narins (ed) *Clinical Disorders of Fluid and Electrolyte Metabolism* 1994, 5th edn, pp 81–100; McGraw – Hill, New York.

118

Endocrinology of Aging

John E. Morley *and* **Moon J. Kim**

Saint Louis University School of Medicine and Saint Louis Veterans' Affairs Medical Center, St Louis, MO, USA

INTRODUCTION

Hormones flow from the ductless glands into the circulation and regulate the metabolism of the body. With aging there is a decline in the circulating levels of a number of hormones. Deficiency of some of these hormones produces symptoms and signs similar to the changes seen with aging. This has led different authorities to suggest that aging is due to an endocrinopause, and that replacement of one or more hormones will result in a reversal of the aging process. Thus, it has been claimed that the aging process is due to the somatopause, adrenopause, menopause, or andropause. However, hormonal replacement has been as likely to produce negative effects as it has to lead to rejuvenation. Aging is also associated with changes at the receptor or postreceptor level that can alter hormonal responsiveness.

HORMONAL REGULATION AND AGING

Hormones are regulated by a classical negative feedback system. Each peripheral hormone is regulated by a central system consisting of the hypothalamic-pituitary unit. The hypothalamus produces releasing hormones (and occasionally inhibitory hormones) that create a feedforward system that regulates the pulsatility and the circadian rhythm of hormone release. These releasing hormones regulate the release of anterior pituitary hormones, which in return result in the release of endorgan hormones. The endorgan hormones then feed back at the pituitary and the hypothalamic level to inhibit further release of pituitary hormones (Figure 1). When disease occurs in the endorgan hormone, it leads to failure of the endorgan and, therefore, negative feedback with an increase in the pituitary hormone (HYPO-disease) or increased activity of the endorgan with suppression of pituitary hormone release (HYPER-disease). When this occurs, the disease is considered to be primary endorgan disease, for example, primary hypothyroidism. Alternatively, failure can occur in the hypothalamic-pituitary unit leading to a decrease in both the pituitary and the endorgan hormone and this is known as *secondary disease*, for example, secondary hypogonadism. Finally, excess production of either a hypothalamic releasing hormone or pituitary hormone can occur. An example of this central form of HYPER-disease would be Cushing's Syndrome.

Aging has effects on all levels of the hypothalamic-pituitary-gonadal axis. The circadian rhythm is controlled by the suprachiasmatic nucleus, which feeds information to the hypothalamus. The hypothalamic releasing hormones are responsible for maintaining the pulsatility of hormone release, which is essential for optimal hormonal action. With aging, the pulse generator leads not only to a decline in maximal hormone production, but also to an irregular or "chaotic" production of hypothalamic releasing hormones. This is amplified at the pituitary level where there is a decrease in the ability to respond to the hypothalamic signal. In addition, the endorgan itself has decreased responsiveness to the stimulus from the pituitary hormone (Veldhuis and Bowers, 2003; Veldhuis, 1999; Korenman *et al.*, 1990; Harman and Tsitouras, 1980; Matsumoto, 2002) (Figure 2).

In addition, with aging changes in hormonal binding to its receptor and postreceptor responsiveness can also occur. An example of this is the posterior pituitary hormone, arginine vasopressin (AVP) or antidiuretic hormone (ADH). There is a decline in the renal responsiveness to AVP with aging. This leads to an increase in basal secretion of AVP with aging. A small further increase in AVP then puts the older person at high risk of developing hyponatremia and syndrome of inappropriate ADH (Miller *et al.*, 1995). There is also an attenuation of the normal increase in AVP that occurs at night. This increase is important for reabsorption of fluid during sleep and, therefore, its attenuation with aging leads to increasing nocturia (Moon *et al.*, 2004).

Classically, endocrinologists have interpreted circulating hormone levels in the absence of an understanding of

Principles and Practice of Geriatric Medicine, 4th Edition. Edited by M.S. John Pathy, Alan J. Sinclair and John E. Morley.

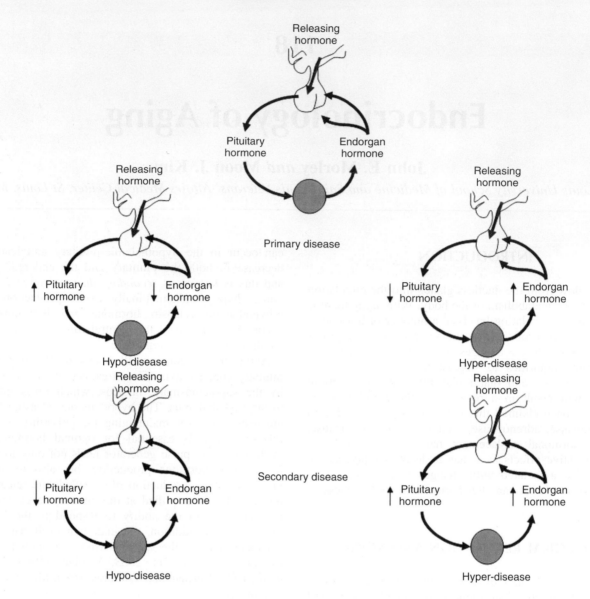

Figure 1 The normal hypothalamic-pituitary-endorgan and the effects of disease processes on it

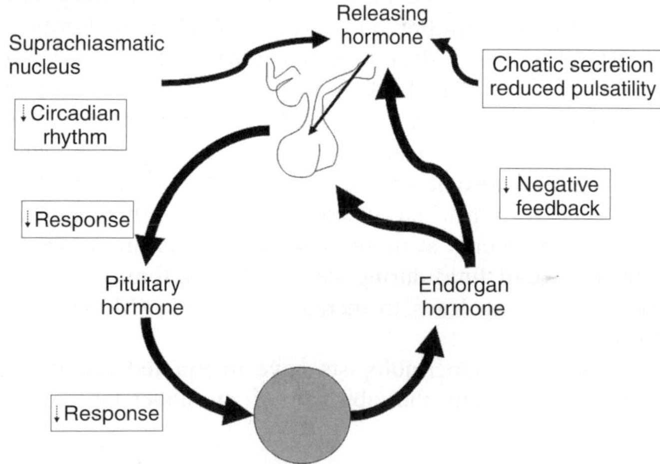

Figure 2 Effects of aging on the hypothalamic-pituitary-endorgan axis

the functioning of the receptor. This is becoming less acceptable as was shown recently by the example of the testosterone receptor and prostate cancer. The testosterone receptor contains a number of CAG repeats. The more the repeats, the less responsive the receptor is to testosterone. Prostate cancer occurs less often in males with a higher number of CAG repeats (Linja and Visakorpi, 2004).

Table 1 lists the hormonal changes seen with aging. The levels of circulating hormones are determined by their production and clearance rates. Thus, the level of thyroxine remains normal because both the production and clearance rates decrease equally. Cortisol levels are slightly increased as there is a greater decrease in clearance rates. Cholecystokinin levels increase markedly due to the decline in clearance rate (MacIntosh *et al.*, 2001).

It is generally believed that free hormone or tissue available hormone levels determine the effectiveness of the

Table 1 Hormonal changes associated with aging

Decreased	Normal	Increased
Growth hormone	Estrogen (men)	ACTH
Insulin Growth Factor-I	Luteinizing hormone (men)	Cholecystokinin
Testosterone	Thyroxine	Insulin
Estrogen (women)	Pancreatic polypeptide	Amylin
Dehydroepiandrosterone	Gastric inhibitory peptide	Luteinizing hormone (women)
Pregnenolone	TSH	FSH
Triaodothyronine	Glucagon-releasing peptide	Vasoactive intestinal peptide
25 $(OH)_2$ Vitamin D	Epinephrine	Cortisol
1,25(OH) Vitamin D	Prolactin	Parathyroid hormone
Aldosterone		Norepinephrine
Calcitonin		Glucagon

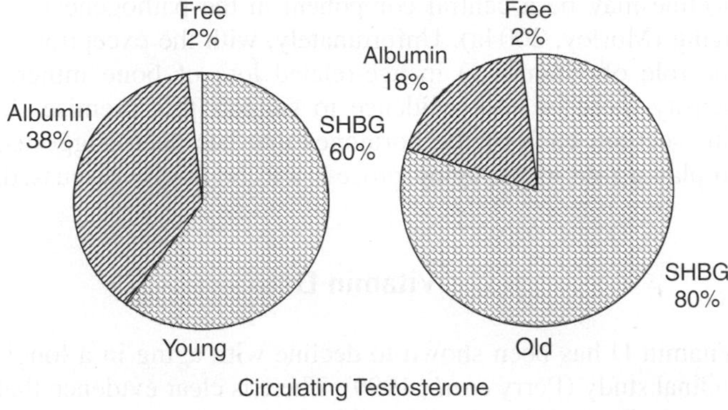

Figure 3 The effect of altered binding proteins with aging on the effect of tissue available hormones: the example of testosterone

hormone. Thus, in the case of testosterone in males there is a marked increase in sex hormone binding globulin (SHBG) with aging. The testosterone bound to SHBG is not thought to be available to tissues (Figure 3). The rest of the testosterone is free or bound to albumin, which is thought to be tissue available. Thus, measurement of the bioavailable testosterone gives a more accurate reflection of the true testosterone level than does a total testosterone measurement (Morley *et al.*, 2002). Similarly, a number of growth hormone binding proteins can produce marked changes in the ability of growth hormone to access its receptor.

EFFECTS OF AGING AND RELATED DISEASES ON ENDOCRINE DISEASES

With aging, there is a blurring of the boundaries between health and disease. The age-related decline in many hormone levels results in difficulties in making the biochemical diagnoses of endocrine disorders. The decreased functional reserve of endocrine organs that occurs with aging increases the propensity for older persons to develop endocrine deficiency disorders. With aging there is a decrease in T-suppressor lymphocytes and an increase in autoantibodies. Many endocrine disorders are due to autoimmune disease, and these changes amplify the possibility of an older person developing hypoendocrine disease in old age. There is also an increased likelihood of the development of polyglandular failure syndromes (Morley, 2001).

The decline in receptor and postreceptor responsiveness that occurs with aging often leads to atypical presentations. Apathetic thyrotoxicosis is, in part, due to the decreased postreceptor responsiveness for ß-adrenergic receptors that occurs with aging. The classical changes of apathetic thyrotoxicosis include depression, weight loss, atrial fibrillation, heart failure, blepharatosis, and proximal myopathy. Apathetic thyrotoxicosis occurs only in about 7% of older persons with hyperthyroidism. The presentations of endocrine disease in older persons are further confused by the fact that they often present with nonspecific symptoms, for example, delirium, fatigue, falls, weight loss, cognitive decline, or depression. These symptoms are common in older persons and can lead to delayed diagnosis. For example, Addison's disease can present with weight loss, fatigue, abdominal pain, diarrhea, and hyponatremia. The increase in cancer with aging can lead to ectopic hormone production with an increase in endocrine disorders such as the syndrome of inappropriate ADH.

Polypharmacy is common among older persons. This can lead to (1) interference with hormonal and metabolic measurements, for example, Vitamin C interferes with the measurement of glucose; (2) altered circulating hormone levels, for example, phenytoin and thyroxine; (3) decreased hormonal responsiveness, for example, spironolactone and aldosterone; (4) altered requirement for appropriate hormonal replacement dose, for example, rifampin increases the thyroxine replacement dose; (5) precipitation of latent disease, for example, thyrotoxicosis by iodine-containing medicines; (6) drug-hormone interaction, for example, coumadin and oral hypoglycemics to produce hypoglycemia; (7) production of metabolic abnormalities, for example, Vitamin A in megadoses produces hypercalcemia; (8) poor compliance with endocrine replacement therapies, and (9) adverse drug reactions.

Hypothyroidism represents a classical example of an endocrine condition that has major overlap with symptoms commonly seen in older persons. These include cold intolerance, slowed pulse, constipation, fatigue, cognitive changes, erectile dysfunction, dry skin, dry, brittle hair, and high blood pressure.

There are a number of endocrine disorders that occur virtually exclusively in older persons. These include osteoporosis, andropause, Paget's disease, and endothelioma-induced hypertension.

INSULIN RESISTANCE SYNDROME AND AGING

There is increasing awareness that insulin resistance syndrome is a cause of an accelerated aging process (Morley, 2004b). This condition is produced by a genetic propensity interacting with overeating and lack of exercise, that is, the couch potato syndrome (Figure 4). It is classically associated with visceral obesity, that is, an increase in intra-abdominal fat. This leads to an increased production of tumor necrosis factor α and leptin and a decrease in adiponectin (a hormone that decreases insulin resistance). The insulin resistance syndrome consists of hyperinsulinemia, diabetes mellitus, hypertension, hyperuricemia, hypertriglyceridemia, hypercholesterolemia, increased small, dense low-density lipoprotein (LDL) molecules, alterations in coagulation status, myosteatosis (fat infiltration into muscle), cognitive decline, and nonalcoholic steatohepatitis. Hypertriglyceridemia is a key in the development of the myosteatosis and the cognitive decline. Persons with insulin resistance have an increased incidence of myocardial infarction and stroke. The insulin resistance syndrome is associated with frailty, disability, and increased mortality.

Recent studies have suggested that a major component of the pathogenesis of the insulin resistance syndrome is accumulation of triglycerides and free fatty acids within muscle cells. This can occur either because of a failure of mitochondria leading to decreased utilization of intracellular fatty acids (primary syndrome) or because of excess circulating triglycerides and fatty acids (secondary syndrome). Accumulation of fatty acids within the cell leads to decreased activity of the insulin receptor substrate and therefore, a decrease in GLUT-transporter activity (Lowell and Shulman, 2005).

THE HORMONAL FOUNTAIN OF YOUTH

The parallel decline of many hormones with aging and age-related symptoms has led to the suggestion that the hormonal decline may be a central component in the pathogenesis of aging (Morley, 2004a). Unfortunately, with the exception of the role of vitamin D in age-related loss of bone mineral density there is little evidence to support this premise. In this section, each of the hormones that has been suggested to play a role in the aging process will be briefly discussed.

Vitamin D

Vitamin D has been shown to decline with aging in a longitudinal study (Perry *et al.*, 1999). There is clear evidence that vitamin D (800 IU) together with calcium decreases the rate of hip fracture in older persons (Chapuy *et al.*, 1994). This is associated with a decline in mortality. Vitamin D replacement in persons who have clear vitamin D deficiency improves muscle strength and decreases falls (Bischoff-Ferrari *et al.*, 2005; Bischoff-Ferrari *et al.*, 2004). Vitamin D deficiency should be suspected in any older person with a borderline low

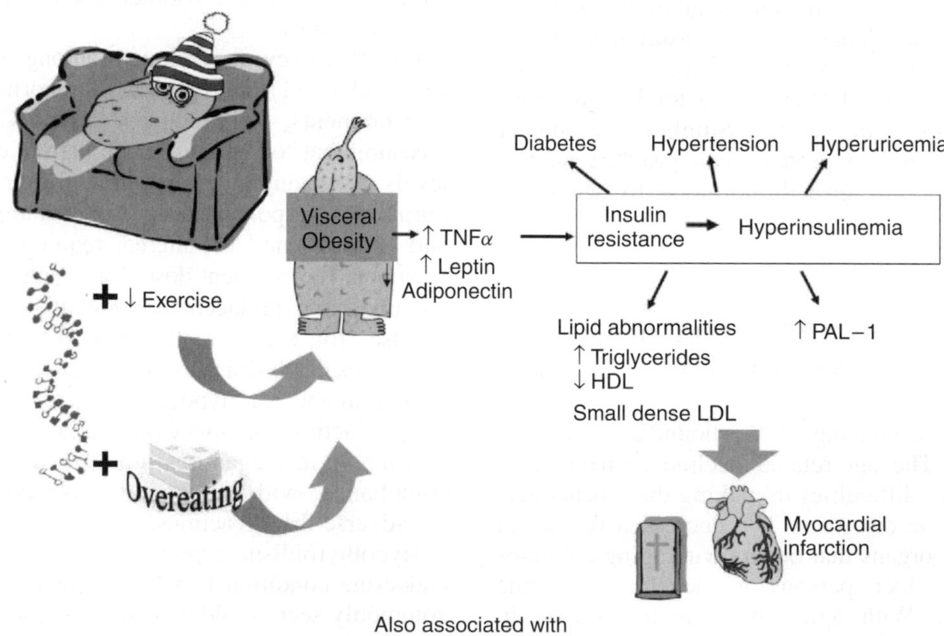

Figure 4 Metabolic syndrome: the deadly quintet (Camus, 1966; Reaven, 1993)

calcium level and an elevated alkaline phosphatase. Increased exposure to sunlight may be as efficacious in increasing Vitamin D levels as using Vitamin D replacement. However, there is some evidence that old skin when exposed to ultraviolet light is less effective than young skin, at manufacturing cholecalciferol.

Testosterone

Testosterone levels decline both in males and females with aging. The effects of testosterone replacement in males and females with aging is shown in Table 2. Testosterone replacement at relatively high doses in older males has been shown to increase muscle mass, strength, functional status, and bone mineral density (Page *et al.*, 2005; Matsumoto, 2002). Testosterone increases libido in both males and females. In males, testosterone increases erectile strength, volume of ejaculation and visuospatial cognition. The major side effect is an excessive increase in hematocrit. The effects of long-term testosterone replacement on benign prostate hypertrophy and prostate cancer are unclear at present. Testosterone can cause gynecomastia, produce water retention, and may worsen sleep apnea in a few individuals. The lack of long-term safety data for testosterone is a major concern. At present, testosterone should be considered a quality of life drug in both men and perhaps women (*see* **Chapter 11, Sexuality and Aging**; **Chapter 121, Ovarian and Testicular Function**). The development of selective androgen receptor modulators (SARMs) is under way in an attempt to avoid some of the potential side effects of testosterone. Nandrolone has been shown to be a potent anabolic agent in older persons.

Growth Hormone

The concept that growth hormone may be able to rejuvenate older men was given impetus by a publication of Rudman *et al.*, (1990) in the New England Journal of Medicine. Unfortunately, since this original publication, numerous studies have failed to demonstrate any major positive effects of growth hormone (Table 3; Morley, 1999). In addition, growth hormone has been shown to have a variety of side effects when administered for more than 3 months to older persons. There is some evidence that growth hormone may improve weight gain and function in malnourished older persons (Chu *et al.*, 2001; Kaiser *et al.*, 1991).

Studies in animals have suggested that growth hormone deficient animals live longer than growth hormone sufficient animals (Bartke, 2005). In addition, in a human study, persons with the highest levels of growth hormone had the highest mortality rate. At present, there is no evidence to support the use of growth hormone to slow aging or improve the quality of life of older persons.

Table 2 Effects of testosterone in older males and in postmenopausal females

Old males	Postmenopausal females
Increased muscle mass	Increased muscle mass
Increased strength	Increased bone mineral density
Increased function	Increased libido
Increased bone mineral density	Decreased mastalgia
Increased hematocrit	
Increased visuospatial cognition	
Increased libido	
Increased strength of erection	
Increased volume of ejaculation	

Table 3 Lesson from growth hormone studies in older persons

Growth hormone increases nitrogen retention
Growth hormone produces weight gain
Growth hormone increases muscle mass
Growth hormone possibly increases Type-II muscle fibers
Growth hormone does not increase strength
Growth hormone is associated with multiple side effects
Growth hormone may improve function in malnourished older persons

Insulin Growth Factor-1 (IGF-1)

Insulin Growth Factor-1 (IGF-1) is produced in peripheral tissues in response to growth hormone. In human studies, it has tended to produce hypoglycemia and minimal positive effects. In animals, it accelerates the growth of tumor cells. In muscle, three different forms of IGF are produced. One of these is mechanogrowth factor (MGF). MGF levels increase in response to resistance exercise. Stem cell replacement of MGF has reversed the muscle atrophy seen in older rats.

Ghrelin

Ghrelin is produced in the fundus of the stomach and released into the circulation. It causes the release of growth hormone and increases food intake (Table 4). MK-771, a ghrelin analog, while increasing growth hormone, has failed to produce major positive effects in older humans.

Dehydroepiandrosterone (DHEA)

Dehydroepiandrosterone (DHEA) is an adrenal hormone whose levels decline markedly with aging. It has been touted as the "mother hormone" by antiaging charlatans. DHEA has

Table 4 Ghrelin and aging

Ghrelin is produced in the fundus of the stomach
Ghrelin is slightly decreased with aging
Ghrelin increases food intake
Ghrelin releases growth hormone from pituitary
Ghrelin increases body mass
Ghrelin enhances memory
Ghrelin produces its food and growth hormone effects through nitric oxide synthase stimulation
MK-771 (a ghrelin agonist) had minimal effects in older humans

remarkable effects on the immune system and cognition in rodents. Unfortunately, a year long study of 50 mg, showed no effects on muscle mass or strength and only a small increase in libido in women over 70 years and some positive effects on the skin (Percheron *et al.*, 2003; Baulieu *et al.*, 2000; Berr *et al.*, 1996). It may have some small effects on insulin resistance. At doses of 100 mg, it has been reported to have effects on humans, but at this dose it is converted into substantial amounts of circulating testosterone.

Pregnenolone

Pregnenolone is produced by the adrenals from cholesterol. It is the true "mother hormone" as it is the precursor of DHEA. In mice, it is the most potent memory enhancer yet to be discovered (Flood *et al.*, 1992). Unfortunately, it has not been shown to have positive effects in humans.

Estrogen

Estrogens were originally touted as hormones that would make women "feminine forever". The Women's Health Initiative (WHI) has shown that premarin in older postmenopausal women increases breast cancer, pulmonary embolism, heart disease, and Alzheimer's disease while decreasing hip fracture and colon cancer (Sherwin, 2005; Goldzieher, 2004; Seelig *et al.*, 2004). While there are still scientists pursuing a better (safer) estrogen which will have the positive effects in women without the negative effects, estrogens should be avoided in women over the age of 60 at present. The use at the time of the menopause represents a quality of life decision.

Melatonin

Melatonin is synthesized from tryptophan in the pineal gland. Melatonin levels increase at night and fall to very low levels during the day. Melatonin has been used with minor success to enhance sleep in older persons. It does not alter the normal sleep structure. It may have a role in the treatment of seasonal affective disorder. Extravagant claims for the utility of melatonin have been based primarily on animal studies and include life extension, enhanced immune function and decreased tumor growth. Studies in humans to support these claims are virtually nonexistent. The rate of decline of melatonin with age is less than was originally thought.

KEY POINTS

- It has been suggested that multiple hormonal changes occur with aging which may play a role in the pathophysiological process associated with aging.
- Many hormones decline with aging but their replacement does not necessarily reverse aging effects.
- The role of melatonin and dehydroepiandrosterone in aging is unknown.
- The insulin resistance syndrome can be considered a cause of the accelerated aging process.
- Testosterone and other hormones may play a role in the treatment of sarcopenia, which is an important proximate occurrence in the development of functional decline in older persons.

KEY REFERENCES

- Matsumoto AM. Andropause: clinical implications of the decline in serum testosterone levels with aging in men. *The Journals of Gerontology. Series A, Biological Sciences and Medical Sciences* 2002; **57A**:M76–99.
- Morley JE. Hormones, aging, and endocrine disorders in the elderly. In PP Felig & LALA Frohman (eds) *Endocrinology and Metabolism* 2001, 4th edn, pp 1455–82; McGraw-Hill, New York.
- Morley JE. The metabolic syndrome and aging. *The Journals of Gerontology. Series A, Biological Sciences and Medical Sciences* 2004b; **59A**:139–42.
- Page ST, Amory JK, Bowman FD *et al.* Exogenous testosterone (T) alone or with finasteride increases physical performance, grip strength, and lean body mass in older men with low serum T. *The Journal of Clinical Endocrinology and Metabolism* 2005; **90**:1502–10.

REFERENCES

Bartke A. Insulin resistance and cognitive aging in long-lived and short-lived mice. *The Journals of Gerontology. Series A, Biological Sciences and Medical Sciences* 2005; **60A**:133–4.

Baulieu EE, Thomas G, Legrain S *et al.* Dehydroepiandrosterone (DHEA), DHEA sulfate, and aging: contribution of the DHEAge study to a sociobiomedical issue. *Proceedings of the National Academy of Sciences of the United States of America* 2000; **97**:4279–84.

Berr C, Lafont S, Debuire B *et al.* Relationships of dehydroepiandrosterone sulfate in the elderly with functional, psychological, and mental status, and short-term mortality: a French community-based study. *Proceedings of the National Academy of Sciences of the United States of America* 1996; **93**:13410–5.

Bischoff-Ferrari HA, Dawson-Hughes B, Willett WC *et al.* Effect of Vitamin D on falls: a meta-analysis. *The Journal of the American Medical Association* 2004; **291**:1999–2006.

Bischoff-Ferrari HA, Willett WC, Wong JB *et al.* Fracture preventions with vitamin D supplementation: a meta-analysis of randomized controlled trials. *The Journal of the American Medical Association* 2005; **293**:2257–64.

Camus JP. Gout, diabetes, hyperlipemia: a metabolic trisyndrome. *Revue du Rhumatisme et des Maldies Osteo-Articulaires* 1966; **33**:10–4.

Chapuy MC, Arlot ME, Delmas PD & Meunier PJ. Effect of calcium and cholecalciferol treatment for three years on hip fractures in elderly women. *British Medical Journal* 1994; **308**:1081–2.

Chu LW, Lam KS, Tam SC *et al.* A randomized controlled trial of low-dose recombinant human growth hormone in the treatment of malnourished elderly medical patients. *The Journal of Clinical Endocrinology and Metabolism* 2001; **86**:1913–20.

Flood JF, Morley JE, Roberts E *et al.* Memory-enhancing effects in male mice of pregnenolone and steroids metabolically derived from it.

Proceedings of the National Academy of Sciences of the United States of America 1992; **89**:1567–71.

Goldzieher JW. Hormone replacement therapy and the women's health initiative: the emperor has no clothes. *Endocrine Practice* 2004; **10**:448–9.

Harman SM & Tsitouras PD. Reproductive hormones in aging men. I. Measurement of sex steroids, basal luteinizing hormone, and Leydig cell response to human chorionic gonadotropin. *The Journal of Clinical Endocrinology and Metabolism* 1980; **51**:35–40.

Kaiser FE, Silver AJ & Morley JE. The effect of recombinant human growth hormone on malnourished older individuals. *Journal of the American Geriatrics Society* 1991; **39**:235–40.

Korenman SG, Morley JE, Mooradian AD *et al.* Secondary hypogonadism in older men: its relation to impotence. *The Journal of Clinical Endocrinology and Metabolism* 1990; **71**:963–9.

Linja MJ & Visakorpi T *et al.* Alterations of androgen receptor in prostate cancer. *The Journal of Steroid Biochemistry and Molecular Biology* 2004; **92**:255–64.

Lowell BB & Shulman GI. Mitochondrial dysfunction and type 2 diabetes. *Science* 2005; **307**:384–7.

MacIntosh CG, Morely JE, Wishart J *et al.* Effect of exogenous cholecystokinin (CCK)-8 on food intake and plasma CCK, leptin, and insulin concentrations in older and young adults: evidence for increased CCK activity as a cause of the anorexia of aging. *The Journal of Clinical Endocrinology and Metabolism* 2001; **86**:5830–7.

Matsumoto AM. Andropause: clinical implications of the decline in serum testosterone levels with aging in men. *The Journals of Gerontology. Series A, Biological Sciences and Medical Sciences* 2002; **57A**:M76–99.

Miller M, Morley JE & Rubenstein LZ. Hyponatremia in a nursing home population. *Journal of the American Geriatrics Society* 1995; **43**:1410–3.

Moon G, Jin MH, Lee JG *et al.* Antidiuretic hormone in elderly male patients with severe nocturia: a circadian study. *BJU International* 2004; **94**:571–5.

Morley JE. Growth hormone: fountain of youth or death hormone? *Journal of the American Geriatrics Society* 1999; **47**:1475–6.

Morley JE. Hormones, aging, and endocrine disorders in the elderly. In PP Felig & LALA Frohman (eds) *Endocrinology and Metabolism* 2001, 4th edn, pp 1455–82; McGraw-Hill, New York.

Morley JE. Is the hormonal fountain of youth drying up? *The Journals of Gerontology. Series A, Biological Sciences and Medical Sciences* 2004a; **59A**:458–60.

Morley JE. The metabolic syndrome and aging. *The Journals of Gerontology. Series A, Biological Sciences and Medical Sciences* 2004b; **59A**:139–42.

Morley JE, Patrick P & Perry HM III. Evaluation of assays available to measure free testosterone. *Metabolism: Clinical and Experimental* 2002; **51**:554–9.

Page ST, Amory JK, Bowman FD *et al.* Exogenous testosterone (T) alone or with finasteride increases physical performance, grip strength, and lean body mass in older men with low serum T. *The Journal of Clinical Endocrinology and Metabolism* 2005; **90**:1502–10.

Percheron G, Hogrel JY, Denot-Ledunois S *et al.* Double-blind placebo-controlled trial. Effect of 1-year oral administration of dehydroepiandrosterone to 60- to 8-year-old individuals on muscle function and cross-sectional area: a double-blind placebo-controlled trial. *Archives of Internal Medicine* 2003; **163**:720–7.

Perry HM III, Horowitz M, Morley JE *et al.* Longitudinal changes in serum 25-hydroxyvitamin D in older people. *Metabolism: Clinical and Experimental* 1999; **48**:1028–32.

Reaven GM. Role of insulin resistance in human disease (syndrome X): an expanded definition. *Annual Review of Medicine* 1993; **44**:121–31.

Rudman D, Feller Ag, Nagraj HS *et al.* Effects of human growth hormone in men over 60 years. *The New England Journal of Medicine* 1990; **323**:1–6.

Seelig MS, Altura BM & Altura BT. Benefits and risks of sex hormone replacement in postmenopausal women. *Journal of the American College of Nutrition* 2004; **23**:482S–96S.

Sherwin BB. Estrogen and memory in women: how can we reconcile the findings? *Hormones and Behavior* 2005; **47**:371–5.

Veldhuis JD. Recent insights into neuroendocrine mechanisms of aging of the human male hypothalamic-pituitary-gonadal axis. *Journal of Andrology* 1999; **20**:1–17.

Veldhuis JD & Bowers CY. Human GH pulsatility: an ensemble property regulated by age and gender. *Journal of Endocrinological Investigation* 2003; **26**:799–813.

119

The Pituitary Gland

James F. Lamb[1] ***and*** **John E. Morley**[2]

[1] Ohio State University College of Medicine and Public Health, Columbus, OH, USA, and [2] Saint Louis University School of Medicine and Saint Louis Veterans' Affairs Medical Center, St Louis, MO, USA

INTRODUCTION

The pituitary gland is the master endocrine gland as it detects and integrates multiple sources of information to regulate physiologic functions (Figure 1). The name pituitary originated from the Latin *pituita*, which means mucus. It was believed that the pituitary excreted mucus from the brain through the nose. Understanding age-related changes in this gland and the manifestations of pituitary disease in the elderly is becoming increasingly important as the population ages. The magnitude of these age-related changes is highly variable, and the confounding effect of illness on these changes must be appreciated. Interpreting age-associated changes in pituitary function must also take into account the rates and pulsatile secretion of hormones, the rapid changes in the levels of some hormones due to physiologic states such as stress, the binding of hormones to plasma proteins, the hormone clearance rates from the plasma, and the altered target tissue sensitivity to hormones. The comorbidity often seen in older persons can mask the usual presentation of pituitary disease and make the diagnosis and treatment of these disorders challenging.

This chapter will review the pertinent changes in the pituitary gland that occur with aging and the diseases that affect this gland and are relevant to the care of the older individual.

ANATOMY

The pituitary gland is functionally divided into an anterior lobe, a posterior lobe, and an intermediate lobe. It is located at the base of the brain within the sella turcica and is covered by the diaphragm sella. The pituitary stalk exits through the diaphragm sella to connect with the hypothalamus. The adult pituitary gland weighs 600 mg and measures 13 mm (transverse) ×6–9 mm (vertical) ×9 mm (anteroposteriorly) (Melmed and Kleinberg, 2003). The optic chiasm is located anterior to the pituitary stalk and is directly above the diaphragm sella, making the optic tracts vulnerable to compression by an expanding pituitary mass. The hypothalamus contains neurons that synthesize releasing and inhibiting hormones as well as the hormones arginine vasopressin and oxytocin of the posterior pituitary. The five cell types that secrete hormone in the anterior pituitary gland are listed in Table 1.

In the elderly, the pituitary gland is moderately decreased in size and contains areas of patchy fibrosis, local necrosis, vascular alterations, and cyst formation. Extensive cellular deposits of lipofuscin and regional deposits of amyloid are also seen. There are not any prominent age-associated alterations in the relative proportions of different types of pituitary secretory cells. The LH and FSH contents are somewhat increased in older people, but there are no age-related changes in the pituitary content of GH, PRL, and TSH (Blackman, 1987).

Blood Supply

The blood supply to the anterior pituitary is through a rich vascular network. The superior hypophyseal arteries (from the internal carotid arteries) supply the hypothalamus and form a capillary network and portal vessels from this network supply the anterior pituitary. These vessels form the conduit for the releasing and inhibiting hormones of the hypothalamus to the anterior pituitary cells. Inferior hypophyseal arteries from the posterior communicating and internal carotid arteries supply the posterior pituitary. Drainage is into the cavernous sinus and internal jugular veins.

Anterior Pituitary Disorders – Clinical Manifestations

Pituitary tumors are very common occurring at postmortem in 20–25% of persons (Costello, 1936). Microadenomas

Principles and Practice of Geriatric Medicine, 4th Edition. Edited by M.S. John Pathy, Alan J. Sinclair and John E. Morley.

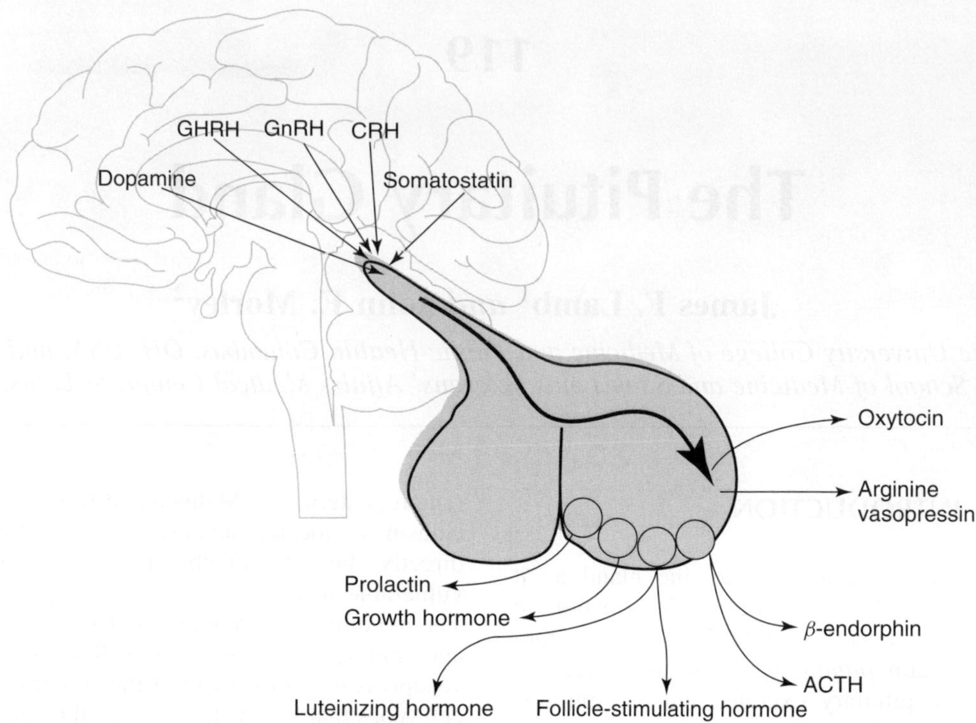

Figure 1 Hormones produced by the anterior pituitary and its hypothalamic controlling factors

Table 1 Pituitary cell type, their hormone, and their percentage

Cell type	Hormone	Stimulators	Inhibitors	Percentage of anterior pituitary cells
Corticotroph	POMC including ACTH	Corticotropin-releasing hormone, vasopressin, cytokines	Glucocorticoids	15–20
Somatotroph	GH	GH-releasing hormone, GH secretagogues	Somatostatin, IGF	50
Thyrotroph	Alpha subunit and beta subunit (thyrotropin)	TRH	T_3, T_4, dopamine, somatostatin, glucocorticoids	<10
Gonadotroph	FSH and LH	Gonadotropin-releasing hormone	Sex steroids, inhibin	10–15
Lactotroph	PRL	Estrogen, TRH	Dopamine	10–25

POMC, pro-opiomelanocortin peptides; ACTH, adrenocorticotrophic hormone; GH, growth hormone; FSH, follicle-stimulating hormone; LH, leuteinizing hormone; PRL, prolactin; TRH, thyrotropin-releasing hormone; IGF, insulin-like growth factor; T_3, triode thyronine; T_4, thyroxine.

are more common in men than in women and over half the tumors in older persons have immunoreactive prolactin staining in their cytoplasm. Despite the frequency of this occurrence, pituitary tumors in the elderly are a neglected subject in the literature. Outcome studies on the prevalence and treatment of the various types of pituitary adenomas are confounded by lack of long-term follow-up, comorbidity, and a referral bias toward younger patients (Turner and Wass, 1997). Pituitary tumors in persons over 60 years of age account for 3–13.4% of all brain tumors (Kleinschmidt-DeMasters *et al.*, 2003). Pituitary lesions present with a variety of manifestations, including pituitary hormone hypersecretion and hyposecretion, enlargement of the sella turcica, and visual loss. In the general adult population, hypersecreting pituitary adenomas are the most common cause of pituitary dysfunction, and the earliest symptoms are due to endocrinologic abnormalities. Visual loss and headache are later manifestations and are due to sellar enlargement. These later symptoms are seen only in patients with large tumors on extension above the sella (Aron *et al.*, 2004). Early visual symptoms include the hemifield slide phenomenon, that is, images floating apart from one another, and the inability to focus on two points at the same time, for example, the inability to do needlework. The classical visual sign of pituitary tumors is bitemporal hemianopsia. In older persons, this sign can be difficult to detect as some degree of bitemporal hemianopsia occurs as a normal part of the aging process.

In contrast, most clinically relevant pituitary tumors in the elderly are nonfunctioning and do not present with features of hormonal hypersecretion. Patients are more likely to be diagnosed with visual field deficits or as incidentalomas (Turner and Wass, 1997). In a study by Cohen *et al.* (1989) 73% of 22 pituitary tumors diagnosed in patients over 70 years of age were nonfunctioning. Cushing's disease was diagnosed in one, prolactinoma in one, and acromegaly in three. In the series by Kleinschmidt-DeMasters *et al.* (2003), of the 13 tumors one was a prolactinoma with subarachnoid hemorrhage and apoplexy and two secreted growth hormone. The other 10 were nonfunctioning.

Of the hormones hypersecreted by pituitary adenomas, prolactin (PRL) is the most common. Measuring PRL is an important part of the evaluation of patients with suspected pituitary disorders and should be performed in older patients presenting with gonadal dysfunction, secondary gonadotropin deficiency, or sella turcica enlargement. The characteristic syndromes of acromegaly and Cushing's disease are due to the hypersecretion of GH and ACTH, respectively, but are rare presentations of pituitary disease in the older population. The characteristic symptoms of acromegaly are given in Table 2. Even more rarely, ectopic GH-releasing hormone causing somatotroph hyperplasia leading to acromegaly and corticotropin-releasing hormone to Cushing's disease can be due to abdominal or chest tumors.

Hypopituitarism is another manifestation of a pituitary adenoma. The clinical presentation of hypopituitarism depends on which hormones are affected, the acuteness or chronicity of the disorder, and the severity of the hormone deficiencies (Table 3).

In adults, hypogonadism is the earliest clinical manifestation of an adenoma and is secondary to elevated PRL, ACTH and cortisol, or GH. The hypogonadism is due to impaired secretion of gonadotropin-releasing hormone rather than anterior pituitary distinction. Older persons with hypopituitarism may present with recurrent falls (Johnston *et al.*, 1996), hyponatremia (Mansell *et al.*, 1993), postural hypotension, and hypothyroidism with an inappropriately suppressed TSH (Belchetz, 1985). Tayal reported pituitary adenomas as the most common cause of hypopituitarism in 12 patients aged 63–89 years (Tayal *et al.*, 1994). The presenting features in this series were lethargy, hypotension, weakness, falls, weight loss, drowsiness, confusion, immobility, and urinary incontinence. Other symptoms of hypopituitarism in older adults include changes in body composition (abdominal obesity and loss of muscle leading to decreased exercise tolerance and fatigue – due to GH loss), decreased sexual function (owing to gonadotropin loss), hypoglycemia and hypocortisolism (caused by loss of ACTH), and polyuria and polydipsia (due to deficits in vasopressin). Other causes of hypopituitarism are given in Table 4.

Pituitary apoplexy, resulting from hemorrhage or infarction of the pituitary gland, usually occurs as a sudden crisis in a patient with a known or previously unrecognized pituitary tumor, but may occur in a normal gland. The risk factors for this condition are common in the elderly. Symptoms at presentation include the sudden onset of headache, stiff neck, oculomotor disturbances, and confusion (Turner and Wass, 1997).

An enlarged sella turcica is another presentation of pituitary disease. The enlargement is usually noted on X rays performed for other indications such as trauma, sinusitis, or mental status changes. Patients with an enlarged sella usually have a pituitary adenoma or empty sella syndrome as

Table 2 Symptoms of acromegaly in older persons with pituitary secreting tumors

Fatigue
Weakness
Swelling of hands and feet
Coarse facial features
Increased head size
Increased perspiration
Deepening of voice
Enlargement of lip, nose, and tongue
Joint pain
Snoring
Cardiomyopathy
Headaches
Visual loss

The diagnosis can often be made by looking at serial photos taken over the lifetime to detect the physical changes that occurred.

Table 3 Symptoms of hypopituitarism in older adults

Insufficient thyroid-stimulating hormone production
- Confusion
- Cold intolerance
- Weight gain
- Dry skin
- Constipation
- Hypertension
- Fatigue

Insufficient growth hormone production
- Fatigue
- Decreased strength

Insufficient gonadotropin production
- Fine wrinkled skin
- In males worsening libido

Insufficient corticotropin production (very rare)
- Fatigue
- Hypoglycemia
- Hypotension
- Intolerance of stress

Table 4 Causes of hypopituitarism

Primary hypopituitarism
- Pituitary tumors
- Hemosderosis
- Infections
- Sarcoidosis
- Radiation therapy
- Tuberculosis
- Hypophysitis (autoimmune disease)
- Surgery
- Impaired vascular supply

Secondary hypopituitarism
- Hypothalamic tumors
- Head injuries
- Multiple Sclerosis
- Inflammatory disease

the cause (Aron *et al.*, 2004). In the elderly, carotid artery aneurysms would also be in the differential diagnosis, while craniopharyngiomas and lymphocytic hypophysitis seen in younger populations would be less likely. Pituitary function in the empty sella syndrome is usually normal, although some patients have hyperprolactinemia. MRI confirms the diagnosis.

An increased suspicion of a pituitary/hypothalamic disorder should occur if patients present with unexplained unilateral or bilateral visual field deficits including bitemporal hemianopsia or visual loss. Vision changes were the most common presentation of pituitary adenomas in Cohen's series of 22 patients aged 70 years and over (Cohen *et al.*, 1989). These patients should have a neuro-ophthalmologic evaluation, MRI, and a serum prolactin as well as an assessment for hypopituitarism. Additional concerns of large pituitary lesions are that they may have lateral extension into the cavernous sinus leading to diplopia caused by dysfunction of the third, fourth, or sixth cranial nerve. These large tumors may also extend in an inferior direction through the sphenoid sinus and roof of the palate and lead to cerebrospinal fluid leakage. Seizures and personality changes can result from invasion of the temporal or frontal lobe. Hypothalamic encroachment can lead to hypogonadism, diabetes insipidus, and disorders of temperature regulation, appetite, and sleep. Headaches can be due to stretching of the dural plate and do not necessarily correlate with size or extension of the mass.

ANTERIOR PITUITARY DISORDERS – TREATMENT

Nonfunctioning Pituitary Tumors

The clinical features of these tumors are usually due to mass effects. Hypopituitary and hyperprolactinemia (caused by impingement on the pituitary stalk and interference with tonic inhibition of lactotroph cells by dopamine secreted by the hypothalamus) are usually present in varying degrees. Less than one-third of the time there is an elevation of follicle-stimulating hormone (FSH), LH, or their subunits.

There is no effective medical therapy. Nonfunctioning microadenomas (≤10 mm) have a benign natural history and can be followed with annual visual acuity and visual field testing and neuroimaging in the asymptomatic patient. Surgery and radiotherapy appear to be very effective in producing control of symptomatic nonfunctioning pituitary tumors. In Cohen's series (Cohen *et al.*, 1989), transsphenoidal surgery was performed in 64% of the 16 patients and was well tolerated with few postoperative complications. Vision was significantly improved in seven and unchanged in one. Temporary visual deterioration occurred in one patient and permanent deterioration occurred in another. In Brada's population aged 60 years and over, 79% of patients treated with radiotherapy had a diagnosis of nonfunctioning pituitary adenoma and, after 10 years of follow-up, only one showed evidence of tumor progression (Brada *et al.*, 1993). In the United States, 5497 pituitary surgery operations were performed between 1996 and 2000. There was a 0.6% death rate and a 3% discharge to long-term care. Age was a significant predictor of mortality and a worse outcome at hospital discharge (Barker *et al.*, 2003). Surgeons with a higher case load had much better outcomes.

Prolactinomas

In addition to symptoms caused by mass effects, postmenopausal women may present with galactorrhea and men can present with hypogonadism including decreased libido. Excluding medications, hypothyroidism, and other causes of hyperprolactinemia is an important step in the initial approach to this problem. In general, treatment consists of medical therapy with a dopamine agonist. The available dopamine agonists include bromocriptine, lisuride, pergolide, and cabergoline. Dopamine agonists can produce orthostans and delirium with hallucinations and delusions. Surgery is used for those intolerant or resistant to dopamine agonist therapy. Surgery is also indicated for those patients who require urgent decompression of the sella turcica for visual field deficits. Treatment is recommended for microprolactinoma (≤10 mm) to prevent osteoporosis, the infrequent occurrence of tumor progression, and the effects of prolonged hypogonadism.

The management of prolactinomas in the elderly is hindered by the lack of data. Several reviews include no elderly patients (Ciccarelli *et al.*, 1990; Soule *et al.*, 1996; Bevan *et al.*, 1992), so extrapolation from data in younger populations and individualizing treatment decisions is necessary.

Cushing's Disease

The diagnosis of Cushing's disease may be more challenging in the elderly because symptoms (weight gain, hypertension (HTN), diabetes mellitus (DM)) may be nonspecific and because elevated urinary cortisol exertion can be seen with Alzheimer's disease and multi-infarct dementia (Maeda *et al.*, 1991). Lack of cortisol suppression after low-dose dexamethasone is seen with depression and Alzheimer's disease as well as Cushing's disease and further complicates the diagnosis. In addition, up to 50% of ACTH tumors are not visible on MRI and require inferior petrosal sinus sampling and CRH-provocative testing.

Treatment of ACTH-producing tumors is by transsphenoidal resection. A higher relapse rate has been seen in younger patients versus older patients (Bochicchio *et al.*, 1995; Robert and Hardy, 1991). Metyrapone has also been used to treat Cushing's disease in the elderly (Donckier *et al.*, 1986).

Acromegaly

The predominant cause of acromegaly is GH-producing tumors, and the effects of GH are medicated by IGF-1 (produced by the liver). Symptoms are those of acromegaly as well as those caused by mass effects of the tumor. The best screening test for this disease is an IGF-1 level. Because the secretion of GH is pulsatile, random levels are not helpful with the diagnosis. The treatment of choice for a GH-secreting tumor is excision. Pharmacologic therapy with octreotide or radiotherapy can be considered if disease persists after excision.

Acromegaly in older patients appear to be a milder disease than in younger patients (Klijn *et al.*, 1980), and it has been suggested that treatment can be more conservative in this group (Clayton, 1993). It appears that elderly individuals respond well to both transsphenoidal surgery and medical treatment with somatostatin agonists (Turner and Wass, 1997).

Thyrotropin (TSH)-Secreting Tumors

About 2% of all pituitary tumors are TSH-secreting. They can present with symptoms of thyrotoxocosis. Among 25 patients with TSH-producing tumors, one was 60, one 63, and one 80 years old (Brucker-Davis *et al.*, 1999). There are few data for treatment in any age-groups for this rare tumor. Octreotide appears to be a safe and effective treatment (Charson *et al.*, 1993). However, in the older patients tumors tend to be large, requiring surgery and radiation. Often some tumor remnant remains in these patients.

Gamma-knife Radiosurgery

Gamma-knife radiosurgery is a new option for the management of pituitary tumors. The gamma-knife is a device that allows radiation to be delivered from outside the head to a precise position within the brain. It requires no incision. Multiple radiation beams are aimed at the pituitary. Each individual beam is too weak to damage the brain tissue it passes through, with the tissue destruction only happening at the place in the pituitary where the beams meet. Accuracy is to within a fraction of a millimeter: Occasionally, gamma-knife therapy can cause local swelling 2–12 months following the procedure. Otherwise, it is relatively side effect–free.

Empty Sella Turcica

Empty sella turcica has been diagnosed in men and women in their 60s and 70s. It is characterized by enlargement of the bony structure enclosing the pituitary together with loss of pituitary tissue. It occurs most commonly in overweight women with high blood pressure. Symptoms include cephalgia, hypopituitarism, or a runny nose. Most empty sellas are diagnosed incidentally during a radiological procedure of the head.

Table 5 Changes reported in hormones

Hormone	Increase	Decrease	None
Adrenocorticotrophin hormone	−	+	−
Follicle-stimulating hormone	+	+	−
Luteinizing hormone	+	+	−
Growth hormone	−	+	−
Thyroid-stimulating hormone	−	+	+
Prolactin	+	+	+

Anterior Pituitary Hormone Secretion – Functional Changes with Age

Functional changes in anterior pituitary hormone secretion occur with increasing age. Table 5 summarizes some of the changes that have been reported in these hormones (Rehman and Masson, 2001).

Gonadotropins (LH and FSH)

Blood concentrations of both LH and FSH abruptly and universally increase in about the sixth decade in women as ovarian secretion of estrogens decreases. These values gradually decline after age 75 years (Vaninetti *et al.*, 2000). Serum FSH and LH rise approximately twofold in men aged 75–85 years, and then decline gradually, as pituitary gonadotropic secretory capacity is reduced with advancing age. This is suggested by a decrease in the amplitude of LH and/or FSH responses to gonadotropin-releasing hormone (Harman *et al.*, 1982). There is a widespread of values at these ages, suggesting primary hypogonadism in some men and secondary (central) hypogonadism in others. Secondary hypogonadism may be the rule rather than the exception with aging (Kaiser and Morley, 1994). The mean LH pulse amplitude and the maximal pulse amplitude are lower in elderly than in younger males (Vermeulen, 1994).

The changes in the LH response to aging may be due to the effects of aging on the catecholamine responses in the hypothalamus. The estrous cycle in old female rats is reinstated by drugs that stimulate brain catecholamine neurotransmitters (Quadri *et al.*, 1973). Naloxone administered to old rats partially restores the LH surge. This suggests that opiates from the hypothalamus may be partly responsible for reduction in LH secretion (Allen and Kalra, 1986).

Prolactin (PRL)

Unlike other pituitary hormones, hypothalamic control of prolactin is mainly inhibitory through dopamine. Other than stimulating lactation in the post partum period, prolactin has no significant physiologic function. Hyperprolactinemia suppresses sex steroid production.

There is no consensus on the effects of aging on prolactin secretion. Investigators have reported decreases, increases, or no change in prolactin levels (Blackman, 1987). Sawin's analysis of prolactin levels from the Framingham cohort showed no significant difference in the prolactin levels between the age-matched sexes. The mean prolactin level in men for ages 40–49 years was $6.4 + 1-3.1\,\mathrm{mg\,ml^{-1}}$ compared with $8.4 \pm 3.8\,\mathrm{mg\,ml^{-1}}$ for ages 80–89 years. In age-matched women, the values of 6.9 ± 3.1 and $8.8 \pm 5.3\,\mathrm{mg\,ml^{-1}}$ corresponded to the same age groups as described for the men (Sawin *et al.*, 1989). Alterations of PRL in humans are probably of small magnitude and unlikely to affect sexual function in the older adult, but more likely the causes hyperprolactinemia in this population are medications and prolactinomas which should be evaluated (Harman and Blackman, 2000).

Growth Hormone

Both aging and sex effect growth hormone secretory dynamics. Young women have twice as high daily growth hormone production as young men. The fall in growth hormone over the life span is from $1200\,\mu\mathrm{g\,m^{-2}}$ in adolescents to $60\,\mu\mathrm{g\,m^{-2}}$ in older individuals (Veldhuis and Bowers, 2003). The fall in growth hormone secretion with aging is due both to a decrease in the orderly production of growth hormone releasing hormone from the hypothalamus and an increase in somatostatin production from the hypothalamus. The fall in growth hormone secretion leads to a decline in insulin-growth-factor-1.

Circulating growth hormone is bound to growth hormone binding proteins. With aging there is a decline in growth hormone binding proteins. The level of growth hormone binding proteins is approximately half that in nonagenarians compared to the 60-year-olds (Maheshwari *et al.*, 1996).

In older women, estrogen increases growth hormone secretion. In older men only high doses of aromatizable form of testosterone (200 mg) increased basal and the mytohemeral growth hormone production (Gentili *et al.*, 2002).

Overall aging is associated with multiple changes of the hypothalamic-growth hormone – insulin growth factor-1 axis and their binding proteins. Interactions with sex hormones further complicate these effects. However, studies with growth hormone or ghrelin analog replacement have failed to demonstrate physiologically important effects of these changes on the aging process.

POSTERIOR PITUITARY GLAND

The posterior pituitary gland is neural tissue and consists only of the distal axons of the hypothalamic magnocellular neurons. The cell bodies of these axons are located in the supraoptic and paraventricular nuclei of the hypothalamus. The axon terminals contain neurosecretory granules in which are stored the hormones oxytocin and vasopressin (antidiuretic hormone (ADH)). Diseases of the posterior pituitary (diabetes insipidus, syndrome of inappropriate ADH) modulate water homeostasis. Persons with diabetes insipidus (insufficient production of vasopressin) present with excessive thirst, polyuria, and dehydration. The major causes of diabetes insipidus are listed in Table 6.

Table 6 Causes of diabetes insipidus

- Hypothalamic malfunction or damage
- Brain injury including cerebrovascular accidents
- Tumors
- Meningitis and encephalitis
- Sarcoidosis
- Tuberculosis

Water excretion in the elderly is affected by physiologic changes of the aging process and leads to an increased risk of both hyponatremia and hypernatremia (Stout *et al.*, 1999; Davies, 1987). Multiple diseases common in elderly persons and the treatments for these diseases can further affect water balance. In addition, body water is reduced in the elderly. By age 75–80, total body water declines to 50% of the level in young adults and complicates studies of responses to dehydration, volume stimulation, and osmolar stimulation (Fulop *et al.*, 1985).

There is a reduced responsiveness of the renal collecting duct to vasopressin in older as compared with younger individuals, the consequences of which is an increased vulnerability to water deprivation (Davis and Davis, 1987). This decreased renal sensitivity to ADH is thought to be due to a decreased ability of vasopressin to stimulate aquaphorin-2 levels in the kidney, and results in a chronic increase in vasopressin secretion and an eventual depletion in posterior pituitary hormone stores. This may cause a decreased visualization of the bright spot on T-1 weighed MRI scans in elderly people (Terano *et al.*, 1996). The bright spot in the sella on MRI is due to stored hormone in neurosecretory granules in the posterior pituitary.

Vasopressin levels have a greater range of normal in older persons and do not correlate as directly with plasma osmolality (Johnson *et al.*, 1994; Favll *et al.*, 1993). Changes in vasopressin levels in response to osmotic stimulation are either normal (Stachenfeld *et al.*, 1996) or increased (Stachenfeld *et al.*, 1996; Ayos and Arieff, 1996), while the vasopressin response to volume depletion (mediated by baroreceptors) is increased (Phillips *et al.*, 1984).

Older persons also have a decrease in thirst in response to osmotic stimulation. As a result of the decrease in thirst and in the responsiveness of the kidney to vasopressin, it is easy for older patients to become dehydrated and hypernatremic despite an increase in vasopressin secretion (Weinberg and Minaker, 1995). Even when recovering from dehydration, older people drink less fluid to return their volume to normal (Phillips *et al.*, 1991).

Excreting a water load is also limited in the elderly. Decreases in glomerular filtration rate and a decreased suppression of vasopressin contribute to this phenomenon. Vasopressin is not shut off in the elderly as well as in the young in response to drinking and oral-pharyngeal receptor stimulation. Those older patients with increased levels of ADH secretion in response to a particular osmotic level have a downward alteration in their osmotic set point. This inability to execute a water load can lead to an increased tendency toward hyponatremia in the elderly. Almost 75% of patients with the syndrome of inappropriate ADH secretion are over 65 years of age (Harman and Blackman, 2000).

Given the issues raised above by numerous studies, healthy older adults probably exhibit normal secretion of vasopressin but do have a decreased thirst appreciation and a decreased ability to maximally concentrate the urine to retain water or to maximally dilute the urine to excrete water. Both hyponatremin (Roberts, 1993) and hypernatremia (Hoffman, 1991), to which older people are susceptible due to the physiologic changes noted above, can cause increased morbidity and mortality especially in the frail elderly and therefore warrant vigilance for their occurrence.

KEY POINTS

- Nonfunctioning pituitary tumors are extremely common in older persons.
- With aging there is a decline in anterior pituitary function.
- Diabetes insipidus is due to insufficient production of vasopressin and leads to excessive thirst and polyuria.
- Treatment for pituitary tumors includes medical, surgery and most recently gamma-knife radiation.

KEY REFERENCES

- Belchetz PE. Idiopathic hypopituitarism in the elderly. *British Medical Journal* 1985; **291**:247–8.
- Turner HE & Wass JAH. Pituitary tumors in the elderly. *Balliere's Clinical Endocrinology and Metabolism* 1997; **11**:407.
- Veldhuis JD & Bowers CY. Human GH pulsatility: an ensemble property regulated by age and gender. *Journal of Endocrinological Investigation* 2003; **26**:799–813.
- Vermeulen A. Clinical problems in reproductive neuroendocrinology of men. *Neurobiology of Aging* 1994; **15**:489–93.

REFERENCES

Allen LG & Kalra SP. Evidence that a decrease in opioid tone may evoke preovulatory leuteinizing hormone release in rats. *Endocrinology* 1986; **118**:2375–81.

Aron DC, Findling JW, Tyrrel JB. Hypothalamus and pituitary gland In *Basic and Clinical Endocrinology* 2004, 7th edn; Appleton and James.

Ayos JC & Arieff AI. Abnormalities of water metabolism in the elderly. *Seminars in Nephrology* 1996; **16**:277.

Barker FG II, Klibanski A & Swearingen B. Transsphenoidal surgery for pituitary tumors in the United States 1996–2000: mortality, morbidity, and the effects of hospital and surgeon volume. *Journal of Clinical Endocrinology and Metabolism* 2003; **88**:4709–19.

Belchetz PE. Idiopathic hypopituitarism in the elderly. *British Medical Journal* 1985; **291**:247–8.

Bevan JS, Webster J, Binke CW & Scanlon MF. Dopamine agonist and pituitary tumor shrinkage. *Endocrine Reviews* 1992; **13**:220–40.

Blackman MR. Pituitary hormones and aging. *Clinics in Endocrinology and Metabolism* 1987; **16**:981–94.

Bochicchio D, Losa M, Buchfelder M *et al.* Factors influencing the immediate and late outcome of Cushing's disease treated by transsphenoidal surgery. *Journal of Clinical Endocrinology and Metabolism* 1995; **80**:3114–20.

Brada M, Rajan B, Traish D *et al.* The long-term efficacy of conservative surgery and radiotherapy in the control of pituitary adenomas. *Clinical Endocrinology* 1993; **38**:571–8.

Brucker-Davis F, Oldfield EH, Skarulis MC *et al.* Thyrotropin-secreting pituitary tumors: diagnostic criteria, thyroid hormone sensitivity, and treatment outcome in 25 patients followed at the National Institutes of Health. *Journal of Clinical Endocrinology and Metabolism* 1999; **84**:476–87.

Charson P, Weintroub BD & Harrn AG. Octreotide therapy for thyroid-stimulating hormone-secreting pituitary adenomas. *Annals of Internal Medicine* 1993; **119**:236.

Ciccarelli E, Ghigo E, Miola C *et al.* Long-term follow-up of "cured" prolactinoma patients after successful adenomectomy. *Clinical Endocrinology* 1990; **32**:583–602.

Clayton RN. Modern management of acromegaly. *Quarterly Journal of Medicine* 1993; **86**:285–7.

Cohen DL, Bevan JS & Adams BT. The presentation and management of pituitary tumors of the elderly. *Age and Aging* 1989; **18**:247–52.

Costello RT. Subclinical adenoma of the pituitary gland. *American Journal of Pathology* 1936; **12**:205–14.

Davies I. Aging in the hypothalamo-neurohypophyseal-renal system. *Comprehensive Gerontology* 1987; **1**:12.

Davis PJ & Davis FB. Water excretion in the elderly. *Endocrinology and Metabolism Clinics of North America* 1987; **16**:867.

Donckier J, Borrin JM, Ramsey ID & Joplin GF. Successful control of Cushing's disease in the elderly with long term metyrapone. *Postgraduate Medical Journal* 1986; **62**:727–30.

Favll CM, Holmes C & Baylis PH. Water balance in elderly people. *Age Aging* 1993; **22**(2):114.

Fulop T, Worum I & Csogne J. Body composition in elderly people. *Gerontology* 1985; **31**:150.

Gentili A, Mulligan T, Godschalk M *et al.* Unequal impact of short-term testosterone repletion on the somatotropic axis of young and older men. *Journal of Clinical Endocrinology and Metabolism* 2002; **87**:825–34.

Harman SM & Blackman MR. The hypothalamic pituitary axes. In *Oxford Textbook of Geriatric Medicine* 2000, 2nd edn; Oxford University Press.

Harman SM, Tsitouras PD, Costa PT *et al.* Reproductive hormones in aging men. *Journal of Clinical Endocrinology and Metabolism* 1982; **54**:547–51.

Hoffman NB. Dehydration in the elderly. *Geriatrics* 1991; **46**(6):35.

Johnson AG, Grawford GA, Kelly D *et al.* Arginine vasopressin and osmolality in the elderly. *Journal of the American Geriatrics Society* 1994; **42**:399.

Johnston S, Hoult S & Chan CA. Falling again. *Lancet* 1996; **349**:26.

Kaiser FE & Morley JE. Gonadotropins, testosterone, and the aging male. *Neurobiology of Aging* 1994; **15**:559–63.

Kleinschmidt-DeMasters BK, Lillehei KO & Breeze RE. Neoplasms involving the central nervous system in the older old. *Human Pathology* 2003; **34**:1137–47.

Klijn JGM, Lamberts SWJ, de Jong FH *et al.* Interrelationships between tumor size, age, plasma growth hormone, and incidence of extra-sellar extension in acromegalic patients. *Acta Endocrinologica* 1980; **95**:289–97.

Maeda T, Tanimoto K, Terada T *et al.* Elevated urinary free cortisol in patients with dementia. *Neurobiology of Aging* 1991; **12**:161–71.

Maheshwari H, Sharma L & Baumann G. Decline of plasma growth hormone binding protein in old age. *Journal of Clinical Endocrinology and Metabolism* 1996; **81**:995–7.

Mansell P, Scott VL, Logan RF & Reckless JPD. Secondary adrenocortical insufficiency. *British Medical Journal* 1993; **307**:253–4.

Melmed S & Kleinberg D. The anterior pituitary. In: *Williams Textbook of Endocrinology* 2003, 10th edn; Saunders.

Phillips PA, Bretherton M, Johnston CI *et al.* Reduced osmotic thirst in healthy elderly men. *American Journal of Physiology* 1991; **261**:R166.

Phillips PA, Rolls BJ, Ledingham JG *et al.* Reduced thirst after water deprivation in healthy elderly men. *The New England Journal of Medicine* 1984; **311**:753.

Quadri SK, Kledzite GS & Meties J. Reinitiation of estrous cycles in old constant-estrous rats by central-acting drugs. *Neuroendocrinology* 1973; **11**:248–55.

Rehman HU & Masson EA. Neuroendocrinology of aging. *Age and Ageing* 2001; **30**:279–87.

Robert F & Hardy J. Cushing's disease: a correlation of radiological surgical and pathological findings with therapeutic results. *Pathology Research and Practice* 1991; **187**:617–21.

Roberts MM. Hyponatremia in the elderly. *Geriatric Nephrology and Urology* 1993; **3**:43.

Sawin CT, Carlson HE, Geller A *et al.* Serum prolactin and aging. *Journal of Gerontology* 1989; **44**:M131–5.

Soule SG, Farhi J, Conway GS *et al.* The outcome of hypophysectomy for prolactinomas in the era of dopamine agonist therapy. *Clinical Endocrinology* 1996; **44**:711–6.

Stachenfeld NS, Mack GW, Takamata A *et al.* Thirst and fluid regulatory responses to hypertonicity in older adults. *The American Journal of Physiology* 1996; **271**:R757.

Stout NR, Kenny RA & Baylis PH. A review of water balance in aging in health and disease. *Gerontology* 1999; **45**:61.

Tayal SC, Bansal SK & Chandra DK. Hypopituitarism. *Age and Ageing* 1994; **23**:320–2.

Terano T, Seya A, Tamura Y *et al.* Characteristics of the pituitary gland in elderly subjects from MRI. *Clinical Endocrinology* 1996; **45**:273.

Turner HE & Wass JAH. Pituitary tumors in the elderly. *Balliere's Clinical Endocrinology and Metabolism* 1997; **11**:407.

Vaninetti S, Baccarelli A, Romoli R *et al.* Effect of aging on serum gonadotropin levels in healthy subjects and patients with non-functioning pituitary adenomas. *European Journal of Endocrinology* 2000; **142**:144–9.

Veldhuis JD & Bowers CY. Human GH pulsatility: an ensemble property regulated by age and gender. *Journal of Endocrinological Investigation* 2003; **26**:799–813.

Vermeulen A. Clinical problems in reproductive neuroendocrinology of men. *Neurobiology of Aging* 1994; **15**:489–93.

Weinberg AD & Minaker KL. Dehydration. Evaluation and management in older adults. *Journal of the American Medical Association* 1995; **274**:1552.

120

Thyroid Disorders

Rachel F. Oiknine *and* Arshag D. Mooradian

Saint Louis University, St Louis, MO, USA

INTRODUCTION

Changes in thyroid gland anatomy and function occur with aging. However, distinguishing physiologic processes of normal aging from pathologic processes associated with disease is difficult. For example, clinical diagnosis of thyroid disease in the elderly is obscured by the presence of many signs and symptoms of hypothyroidism in euthyroid elderly persons, and the absence of many signs and symptoms that represent disease in hyperthyroid elderly persons. An understanding of the changes in thyroid gland anatomy, thyroid hormone economy, and thyroid hormone actions that occur with aging is important for accurate diagnosis and therapy.

CHANGES IN THYROID GLAND ANATOMY AND HISTOLOGY

Thyroid gland anatomy and histology change with aging. Grossly, thyroid weight may be increased, unchanged, or decreased (Denham and Wills, 1980; Mariotti *et al.*, 1995). Increased thyroid weight occurs with the development of a nodular goiter, which occurs more commonly in the elderly (Mariotti *et al.*, 1995). Thyroid nodularity may be related to iodine deficiency (Laurberg *et al.*, 1998), and so may not be attributed to the aging process alone. Microscopically, there is lymphocytic infiltration, fibrosis, reduction in follicle size, and flattening of follicular epithelium (Mariotti *et al.*, 1995). While the presence of thyroid nodules carries a risk for autonomous function and hyperthyroidism, and the presence of lymphocytic infiltrates in a patient with antithyroid antibodies suggests autoimmune thyroiditis and a risk for hypothyroidism, anatomic and histologic changes that occur with aging do not always correlate with abnormalities in thyroid function. Still, in one survey of thyroid glands from elderly patients obtained at postmortem examination, there was a statistically significant increased incidence of abnormal function in nodular versus normal thyroid glands. Microscopic changes, however, occurred in both nodular and normal thyroid glands (Denham and Wills, 1980).

CHANGES IN THYROID HORMONE ECONOMY

There are also changes in thyroid hormone economy with aging. These occur at various levels of the hypothalamus-pituitary-thyroid gland axis (Table 1). Beginning at the hypothalamus, there may be a reduction in thyrotropin-releasing hormone (TRH) concentration, as less TRH was released *in vitro* by hypothalamic tissue from older as compared to younger rats (Pekary *et al.*, 1987). There is no reduction in either the pituitary content of thyrotropin-stimulating hormone (TSH) or serum TSH concentration with aging. A comparison of serum TSH concentrations in a large group of older persons in the community-based Framingham Heart Study to their middle-aged offspring showed no significant difference in serum TSH concentrations among individuals without known thyroid disease (Hershman *et al.*, 1993). Although serum TSH concentration does not change with age, studies have demonstrated decreased pituitary sensitivity to TRH. The TSH response to TRH stimulation is proportional to the basal TSH concentration. Some, but not all studies have found that the peak TSH response to exogenous TRH is lower in the elderly. In one study, the TSH response was lower only in older women (Kaiser, 1987). In two other studies (Erfuth *et al.*, 1984; Snyder and Utiger, 1972), TSH response was lower in older men, while one study did not find any significant reduction in TSH response to TRH in older men (Harman *et al.*, 1984).

Another change in the hypothalamic-pituitary axis is demonstrated by a decrease in the pulse amplitude of nocturnal TSH secretions, although the pulse frequency is unchanged; the circadian variation of serum TSH concentrations in 78- to 83-year-old men was smaller compared with the TSH oscillation in younger subjects (Hermann *et al.*,

Principles and Practice of Geriatric Medicine, 4th Edition. Edited by M.S. John Pathy, Alan J. Sinclair and John E. Morley.

Table 1 Age-related changes in thyroid economy

No change	No change or ↓	↓	↑
TSH	Thyroid sensitivity to TSH	Production of T4, T3	Serum half-life of T4
Pituitary concentration of TSH	TSH response to exogenous TRH	Degradation of T4, T3	
T3	Diurnal variation in TSH secretion	Pulse amplitude of nocturnal TSH	
rT3			
TBG			
T4 and FT4		Thyroid gland uptake of iodine	
		TSH rise 2^0 to decreasing T4	

Source: Adapted from Mooradian, 1995 and Case and Mooradian, 2000.

1981). While the pituitary content of TSH and serum TSH concentrations may be unaltered, the reduced pituitary sensitivity to TRH and reduced pulse amplitude of TSH secretions could signal reduced biologic activity of TSH. Reduced biological activity of TSH may occur without a change in immunoreactive mass of TSH, since biologic activity is dependent on proper glycosylation of TSH, a process that is modulated by TRH.

Changes in the set point of pituitary-thyroid axis with aging are unclear. A cross-sectional study of euthyroid subjects showed that the slope of the curve correlating TSH and free thyroxine (FT4) is not altered in elderly subjects (Friedman *et al.*, 1992). However, a more direct estimate of pituitary sensitivity to thyroid hormone, measured by the pituitary response to thyroxine (T4) that is suppressed with exogenous iodide, shows a significant reduction in pituitary sensitivity to T4 in the elderly (Ordene *et al.*, 1983). In other words, the increase in TSH rise in the face of the decrease in T4 was blunted in elderly subjects. The latter observation can alternatively be interpreted as increased effectiveness of T4 in suppressing the TSH during hypothyroxinemia. Similar changes are seen in aging rat models (Mooradian, 1993; Mooradian and Wong, 1994). These changes could be partially attributed to either increased thyroid hormone receptors in the pituitary, or more importantly, increased conversion of T4 to triiodothyronine (T3) through increased activity of 5′ deiodinase type II (Donda *et al.*, 1987; Donda and Lemarchand-Beraud, 1989). Extrapolation of these results to humans is difficult, however, because of interspecies differences in thyroid hormone economy (Reymond *et al.*, 1992).

Finally, in humans, thyroid response to TSH may be reduced or remain unaltered. In one study, T3 responses to exogenous TSH in younger and older subjects were similar. However, these results are questioned because exogenous TSH was administered in very high doses (Van Coevorden *et al.*, 1989). There is also a decreased production of thyroid hormone with age such that T4 production decreases from 80 to 60 μg day^{-1}, and T3 production decreases from 30 to 20 μg day^{-1} (Mooradian, 1995; Case and Mooradian, 2000). While this appears to be a compensatory response to decreased thyroid hormone clearance, it may also be a function of reduced thyroidal sensitivity to TSH, as well as altered TSH secretory kinetics and TSH bioactivity (Choy *et al.*, 1982). Decreased T3 production also reflects decreased peripheral conversion of T4 to T3, as a result of decreased T4 production and possibly secondary to reduced activity of 5′ deiodinase type I. In general, thyroid hormone clearance is reduced in the elderly, with an increase in the half-life of T4 from 6.7 days in the third decade to 9.1 days in the seventh decade (Gregerman *et al.*, 1962). Finally, thyroidal uptake of iodine is reduced in the elderly (Gaffney *et al.*, 1982), reflecting decreased thyroid hormone production.

CHANGES IN THYROID HORMONE ACTION

Thyroid hormone acts by modulating gene expression, and specific gene products are positively or negatively regulated biomarkers of thyroid hormone action (Mooradian and Wong, 1994). Age-related changes in thyroid hormone action are reflected in changes in these gene products (Table 2). For example, there is a decrease in Na^+-K^+ ATPase activity in renal cortical and hepatic cells with age; this may be responsible for the decline in thyroid-induced thermogenesis (Mooradian *et al.*, 1994b). There is a decrease in malic enzyme activity; this may be responsible for a decline in thyroid-induced lipogenesis (Mooradian *et al.*, 1991; Mooradian and Albert, 1999). In addition to lipogenic enzymes, a

Table 2 Age-related changes: Thyroid hormone responsiveness of various markers of thyroid hormone action

Serum
Angiotensin-converting enzyme
Liver
ApoA1 Mrna
Malic enzyme activity
Malic enzyme mRNA
Fatty acid synthase
Spot14 (encodes liver protein which may be involved in lipogenesis)
Red blood cells
Na^+-K^+ ATPase
Ca^{++} ATPase
2-Deoxy-glucose transporter
Kidney
Na^+-K^+ ATPase
Thymocyte
2-Deoxy-glucose transporter
Heart
Isoproterenol-stimulated adenyl cyclase
Sarcoplasmic Ca-ATPase mRNA
α-Myosin heavy chain
β-Myosin heavy chain (negatively regulated biomarkers)
Pituitary
TSH sensitivity to T4 (negatively regulated biomarkers)
Cerebral cortex
Synaptosomal adrenergic transmission
THRP
NAT-1

Source: Adapted from Mooradian and Wong, 1994 and Case and Mooradian, 2000.

slue of biomarkers of thyroid hormone action in the liver, such as apoliprotein AI (Shah *et al.*, 1995; Mooradian *et al.*, 1996) and S14 (Mooradian *et al.*, 1994a), shows reduced responsiveness to thyroid hormones. The response of a serum marker of thyroid hormone action, namely angiotensin-converting enzyme, is also altered in aging (Mooradian and Lieberman, 1990). Similar alterations in thyroid hormone action have been observed in cardiac muscle. In this tissue, the response of myosin heave chain and calcium ATPase response to thyroid hormone is reduced in aged animals. There is also a decrease in isoproterenol-stimulated adenyl cyclase activity that may play a role in reduced thyroid-induced cardiac chronotropic activity (Mooradian and Scarpace, 1989). In addition, response of glucose transport isoforms (Mooradian *et al.*, 1999) and malondialdehyde modification of proteins (Chehade *et al.*, 1999) are altered in aged rats.

The effect of age on the thyroid hormone responsiveness of the cerebral cortex is not well studied as there are only few biomarkers of thyroid hormone action in the brain of mature animals (Haas *et al.*, 2004). The thyroid hormone responsiveness of adrenergic neurotransmission in synaptosomal membranes is reduced in aged rats (Mooradian and Scarpace, 1993). Two novel markers of thyroid hormone action in the brain, namely thyroid hormone responsive protein (THRP) (Shah *et al.*, 1997; Haas *et al.*, 2002; Mooradian *et al.*, 1998) and novel translational repressor (NAT-1) (Shah *et al.*, 1999), also show significant reduction to thyroid hormone responsiveness in senescent rats. The precise biological implications of these observations are not clear. However, THRP is identified as an important mediator of thyroid hormone–induced neurotoxicity in primary neauronal cultures (Haas *et al.*, 2005). Thus, an age-related decline in THRP responsiveness may have a neuroprotective role.

Possible mechanisms for changes in thyroid hormone action with age include impaired transport of T3 across plasma membranes, impaired tissue metabolism of thyroid hormone, and alterations in postreceptor processes modulating gene expression. Transport of T3 across plasma membranes is a carrier-mediated process that has been shown to be reduced by 50% in the liver of old rats, leading to a decrease in the number of nuclear receptors occupied by T3 while receptor affinity for T3 (Ka) measured *in vitro* is unchanged (Mooradian, 1990a,b). Second, tissue metabolism of the thyroid hormone is impaired as a result of a decrease in the deiodination rate of T4 to T3 (Gregerman *et al.*, 1962; Jang and Distefeno, 1985). Finally, there may be alterations in postreceptor processes that modulate gene expression; these could be related to alterations in transcription factors or secondary to structural changes of the gene. Changes in the activity of S14 gene expression in response to T3 reflect both age-related alterations in transcription factors and gene structure. A transcription factor P-1 binds S14 DNA and represses gene transcription, while another transcription factor, PS-1, binds S14 DNA and stimulates gene transcription. Aging is associated with decreased levels of P-1 (Mooradian *et al.*, 1994a), resulting in an age-related increase in basal expression of S14 gene. Also, there is an age-related demethylation of the S14 gene, reflecting structural changes that result in the increased expression of this gene with age (Wong *et al.*, 1989). Despite increased basal expression of this gene, its thyroid hormone responsiveness is reduced with age.

Overall, it appears that the thyroid hormone responsiveness of a host of biomarkers of the thyroid hormone action is blunted in aging. This age-related "relative" resistance to the thyroid hormone action may partly explain the myriad symptoms and signs of hypothyroidism that older subjects exhibit despite normal plasma levels of thyroid hormones. Alternatively, it can also account for the paucity of symptoms or signs of excess thyroid hormone in patients with apathetic hyperthyroidism.

CLINICAL IMPLICATIONS OF AGE-RELATED CHANGES IN THE THYROID

The clinical presentations of hypothyroidism and hyperthyroidism change in the elderly. In addition, because of age-related changes in thyroid hormone kinetics and alterations in drug effects and tolerability, the management of thyroid disease in the elderly can be challenging.

Hypothyroidism

Clinical diagnosis of hypothyroidism is difficult, as many signs and symptoms associated with hypothyroidism are present in euthyroid elderly individuals (Table 3). For example, slow mentation, fatigue, constipation, hair loss, dry skin, and delayed relaxation phase of deep tendon reflexes occur in both hypothyroid patients and euthyroid elderly individuals (Case and Mooradian, 2000) (Table 3). In healthy outpatient subjects followed in the Framingham Heart Study, the prevalence of clinically unrecognized hypothyroidism in subjects at the age of 60 and older was found to be approximately 2.5% (Sawin *et al.*, 1985). While hypothyroid patients and euthyroid elderly individuals may share

Table 3 Signs and symptoms of hypothyroidism commonly found in older euthyroid subjects

Signs	Dry skin
	Delayed deep tendon reflexes
	Gynecomastia
	Bradycardia
	Hypertension
Symptoms	Slow mentation
	Muscle fatigue
	Hair loss
	Decreased appetite
	Constipation
	Cold intolerance
	Decreased libido
	Depression

Source: Adapted from Case and Mooradian, 2000.

many of the same signs and symptoms, it is interesting that overall the elderly hypothyroid patient exhibits fewer number of signs and symptoms, and also fewer of the classical signs. In a study comparing clinical signs and symptoms of hypothyroidism between elderly patients and younger patients, indeed the most frequent clinical features in elderly patients were the nonspecific findings of fatigue and weakness. However, the mean number of clinical signs per patient was significantly smaller in the elderly patients, and also four classical signs of hypothyroidism, cold intolerance, paresthesias, weight gain, and cramps occurred significantly less frequently in elderly patients (Trivalle *et al.*, 1996).

Even more challenging is the diagnosis of secondary hypothyroidism. In these patients, serum TSH levels may be normal or subnormal and the free T4 levels are low. This condition is particularly common in people over the age of 85 (Sundbeck *et al.*, 1991). Many people with this set of thyroid function tests are also taking medications known to interfere with TSH and T4 levels, making the diagnosis of hypothyroidism particularly difficult.

Once hypothyroidism is diagnosed, treatment strategies must be tailored to the elderly patient. When initiating thyroid hormone replacement for hypothyroidism, dosages should be low (no more than $25\,\mu g\,day^{-1}$), and increased slowly, as the consequent increase in myocardial oxygen demand may precipitate coronary syndrome or congestive heart failure in patients with organic heart disease. The maintenance dose of thyroid hormone replacement will also be reduced in the elderly hypothyroid patient as compared to the younger patient; the mean daily dose of thyroid hormone replacement required to attain a euthyroid state in the elderly is $110\,\mu g\,day^{-1}$, while in younger subjects it is $130\,\mu g\,day^{-1}$ (Silverberg and Mooradian, 1998; Case and Mooradian, 2000). This is the result of alterations in thyroid hormone economy with aging, specifically, a decrease in the clearance rate of thyroid hormone. Should a hypothyroid elderly patient begin to require increasing doses of thyroid hormone replacement therapy, the possibility of decreased drug absorption should be considered. Several drugs including bile acid sequestrants (i.e. colestipol, cholestyramine), aluminum hydroxide, ferrous sulfate, calcium carbonate, and sucralfate can decrease absorption of exogenous oral thyroid hormone, rendering the patient hypothyroid again (Surks and Sievert, 1995). Finally, in any patient in whom secondary hypothyroidism is suspected, thyroid hormone replacement is withheld until adrenal insufficiency is excluded or glucocorticoid replacement therapy is initiated.

Treatment of subclinical hypothyroidism (isolated elevation of TSH levels) is generally recommended when the TSH is over $10\,mU\,ml^{-1}$, but may also be considered at TSH levels of $5-10\,mU\,ml^{-1}$ in the presence of antithyroid antibodies, as these patients are more likely to progress to overt hypothyroidism (2–3% vs. 4–5% annual rate) (Samuels, 1998). In addition to the development of overt hypothyroidism, subclinical hypothyroidism carries an increased risk of aortic atherosclerosis and myocardial infarction (Hak *et al.*, 2000), hyperlipidemia (Biondi *et al.*, 2002; Caraccio *et al.*, 2002; Danese *et al.*, 2000), left ventricular dysfunction (Biondi *et al.*, 2002), and nonspecific symptoms such as fatigue, dry skin, and cold intolerance (Cooper *et al.*, 1984). Treatment with thyroxine prevents overt hypothyroidism, reduces total cholesterol and low density lipoprotein (LDL) cholesterol (Biondi *et al.*, 2002; Caraccio *et al.*, 2002; Danese *et al.*, 2000), with a possible secondary reduction in the risk of atherosclerosis, normalizes left ventricular dysfunction (Biondi *et al.*, 2002), and alleviates nonspecific symptoms (Cooper *et al.*, 1984).

Finally, given the age-related decline in thyroid hormone responsiveness, the question remains whether supplementing euthyroid elderly patients with thyroid hormone would minimize some of the age-related changes that resemble hypothyroidism. Support of such a hypothesis would require safety and efficacy data from double-blind randomized studies with thyroid hormone replacement in elderly subjects with normal and increased TSH levels.

Hyperthyroidism

The clinical diagnosis of hyperthyroidism is difficult because many signs and symptoms of hyperthyroidism are absent in elderly patients. Apathetic thyrotoxicosis is an extreme example, in which apathy, lethargy, pseudodementia, weight loss, and depressed mood are the major findings. In one study, a comparison of clinical signs and symptoms of hyperthyroidism in older versus younger patients revealed the findings of hyperactive reflexes, increased sweating, polydipsia, heat intolerance, tremor, nervousness, and increased appetite occurred significantly less frequently in older hyperthyroid patients. Only the findings of atrial fibrillation and anorexia were significantly more frequent in older hyperthyroid patients (Trivalle *et al.*, 1996) (Table 4). Note that the increased incidence of cardiac complications in hyperthyroid elderly persons is attributed to the increased prevalence of organic heart disease in this population, as there is no increase in myocardial response to thyroid hormone in the elderly (Mooradian and Wong, 1994).

Table 4 Comparison between old and young patients with symptoms and clinical signs of hyperthyroidism

Symptoms and signs	Older patients incidence (%)	Younger patients incidence (%)
Tremor	44	84
Anorexia	32	4
Nervousness	31	84
Hyperactive reflexes	28	96
Increased sweating	24	95
Polydipsia	21	67
Heat intolerance	15	92
Increased appetite	0	57
Atrial fibrillation	35	2

Source: Reproduced from Trivalle *et al.*, 1996, by permission of Blackwell Publishing Ltd.
Note: $P < 0.001$ for all comparisons.

An age-related desensitization of β-adrenergic receptors may be responsible for the absence of other adrenergic-system related hyperthyroid symptoms (i.e. tremor) in the elderly hyperthyroid patient (Case and Mooradian, 2000).

The treatment strategy for hyperthyroidism does not change in the elderly. β-Blockers are used for symptom control, and antithyroid drugs are used to attain a euthyroid state. Once the patient becomes euthyroid, radioactive iodine ablation of the gland may be performed. Repeated treatments with radioactive iodine may be necessary to achieve remission in patients with toxic nodular goiters, a more common cause of hyperthyroidism in the elderly. In the elderly patient, there is no concern about potential adverse effects of radioactive iodine on the reproductive system, and the potential risks are minimal as compared to surgical thyroidectomy. A potential risk of radioactive iodine therapy is thyroid "storm"; however, this becomes less likely with antecedent use of an antithyroid drug. Another potential toxicity in those with bladder outlet obstruction or atonic bladders is the increased incidence of cystitis secondary to stasis of radioactive iodine in the bladder. These people will present with increased lower urinary tract symptoms (LUTS). Note that the possibility of agranulocytosis, which occurs in 0.3–0.6% of all patients who take antithyroid drugs, increases with age especially in those over 40 years old (Cooper *et al.*, 1983). Treatment for subclinical hyperthyroidism (low TSH and normal FT4 and FT3) is recommended if the TSH is $<0.1\,\mathrm{mU\,l^{-1}}$, in the presence of Graves' disease or nodular thyroid disease (Surks *et al.*, 2004). Note that single low TSH measurements often normalize upon retesting weeks to months later, so the decision to treat should be based on persistently low TSH levels (Parle *et al.*, 1991). The basis for treatment of subclinical hyperthyroidism is to prevent detrimental cardiac and skeletal effects that can result in substantial morbidity in the elderly. Cardiac effects include a threefold increase in the risk of atrial fibrillation (Sawin *et al.*, 1994), and an increase in left ventricular mass (Biondi *et al.*, 2002). The association of thromboembolic disease and atrial fibrillation makes subclinical hyperthyroidism a risk factor for thromboembolism in the elderly (Biondi *et al.*, 2002). The skeletal effect of subclinical hyperthyroidism is a decrease in bone mineral density (Foldes *et al.*, 1993) as thyroid hormone directly stimulates bone turnover (Foldes *et al.*, 1993). In postmenopausal women, subclinical hyperthyroidism is a risk factor for osteoporosis (Foldes *et al.*, 1993; AACE, 2002).

Occasionally, a diagnostic dilemma emerges when the signs and symptoms are nonspecific and the thyroid function tests cannot conclusively distinguish between secondary hypothyroidism and subclinical hyperthyroidism. In such instances, it is best if the patient is referred to an endocrinologist for reevaluation and if need be, a short course trial with antithyroid medicine to evaluate TSH secretory reserve. To differentiate between hypothalamic and pituitary causes of low TSH, the TRH stimulation test can be helpful. Unfortunately, at the present time, TRH is not available in the United States for clinical use.

THYROID NODULES AND CANCER

Aging is commonly associated with increased propensity for developing neoplasms (Mooradian, 1994). As such, the thyroid gland is not an exception. It has been estimated that the prevalence of thyroid nodules increases with age, especially in women. Although the prevalence of thyroid nodules in the general population is approximately 1–5%, in the elderly, 6–10% of the population may have solitary nodules (Gupta, 1995). The vast majority of these nodules are benign cysts or adenomatous changes. In perhaps 10% or less of the cases, cancer can be found. More than 60% of carcinomas are of papillary type, yet most benign adenomas are of follicular type. The most common causes of thyroid nodules are listed in Table 5. Some adenomas produce excessive amounts of thyroid hormone, typically T3, and present with hyperthyroidisms. These adenomas can be ablated with radioactive iodine therapy. Most patients with thyroid adenomas or carcinomas are euthyroid. Occasionally, hyperthyroidism and thyroid cancer may coexist and this combination may carry worse prognosis especially if the hyperthyroidism is secondary to Graves' disease. The increased risk in such patients is attributed to the presence of circulating thyroid-stimulating immunoglobulins that will promote thyroid cancer growth and unlike endogenous TSH cannot be suppressed with thyroid hormone therapy.

The etiology of thyroid adenomas and carcinomas are not completely understood. Endemic goiters secondary to iodine deficiency are associated with the increasing formation of hyperplastic nodules probably because of overstimulation with TSH. Follicular and anaplastic carcinomas have been associated with endemic goiters, while the papillary cancer is not associated with endemic goiters. It has been estimated that 4–17% of patients with nodular goiter may develop carcinomas, mostly of the papillary type (Gupta, 1995). In addition to overstimulation with TSH, another important risk factor is exposure to irradiation. Nevertheless, exposure to irradiation to the neck increases the risk of thyroid cancers, notably the differentiated variety such as follicular or papillary type. The medullary cancers and anaplastic cancers have not been associated with irradiation exposure.

Medullary carcinomas constitute 2–5% of all thyroid cancers and are rare in the elderly. In 20% of the cases, they are familial arising as a component of multiple endocrine

Table 5 Differential diagnoses of thyroid nodules

Benign thyroid nodules	Multinodular goiter Hashimoto's thyroiditis Cysts Follicular adenomas Hurthle-cell adenomas
Malignant thyroid nodules	Papillary carcinoma Follicular carcinoma Medullary carcinoma Anaplastic carcinoma Primary thyroid lymphoma Metastatic carcinoma

neoplasia (MEN). These tumors secrete calcitonin and carcinoembryonic antigen (CEA), and these are good markers for follow-up. If familial disease is suspected, genetic testing for Ret oncogene is now available commercially.

In general, well-differentiated thyroid cancers in the elderly carry poorer prognosis compared to younger middle-aged subjects. Thus, it is essential that elderly patients with thyroid cancer are given the full benefit of total thyroidectomy coupled with radioactive iodine ablation of the remnant.

An unusually aggressive form of thyroid cancer, namely anaplastic cancer of the thyroid is primarily a disease of the elderly. This rare disease should be considered in all patients who present with rapidly enlarging solid mass in the neck or are found to have widespread metastasis (Mooradian *et al.*, 1983).

The workup of a patient presenting with thyroid nodule is summarized in Figure 1. In general, if TSH is not suppressed, the first step is fine-needle aspiration biopsy (FNAB). The differential diagnosis includes adenomas, carcinomas, thyroiditis, and thyroid cysts. Solitary nodules or a predominant nodule within a multinodular goiter are candidates for biopsy. The clinical risk factors favoring cancer include age (less than 20 or more than 60), male gender, history of irradiation, history of thyroid cancer, rapid growth, fixation of the nodule to the surrounding tissue, hardness, cervical lymph node enlargement, and dysphagia or hoarseness (Gupta, 1995). If the biopsy reveals cystic nature of the nodule, every attempt should be made to biopsy the wall of the cyst to acquire enough cells for evaluation. Cysts that continue to grow will require reaspiration with possible ablation with alcohol or referral to surgery. If the biopsy shows cancerous cells or is equivocal, then the patient is referred for surgery. Under certain circumstances a second look rebiopsy may be helpful. The suppressive therapy for benign nodules is not recommended in the elderly with increased risk of underlying cardiovascular disease and dubious efficacy of therapy.

SCREENING FOR THYROID DISEASE

As the clinical presentation of thyroid disease is not reliable in the elderly population, the physician should consider periodic screening for biochemical abnormalities. Clinically relevant biochemical tests do not change physiologically with aging, and therefore can be used to diagnose or exclude disease. However, the physician should be aware of alterations in serum TSH levels that can occur as a result of nonthyroidal disease or medications, which may occur more commonly in elderly patients with multiple comorbidities. Serum TSH levels may be slightly increased or decreased as a result of illness (Wiersinga, 2000), and decreased as a result of medications such as dopamine or glucocorticoids (Scanlon and Toft, 2000). Recommendations for screening guidelines vary. While the American Thyroid Association (Ladenson *et al.*, 2000) recommends screening men and women aged 35 and older every 5 years, and more frequently in those at high risk, the American College of Physicians (Helfand and Redfern, 1998) recommends periodic screening of only women aged 50 and older. The US Preventive Services Task Force (USPSTF, 2004) has concluded that evidence is insufficient to recommend for or against routine screening for thyroid disease in adults, however, it recommends having a

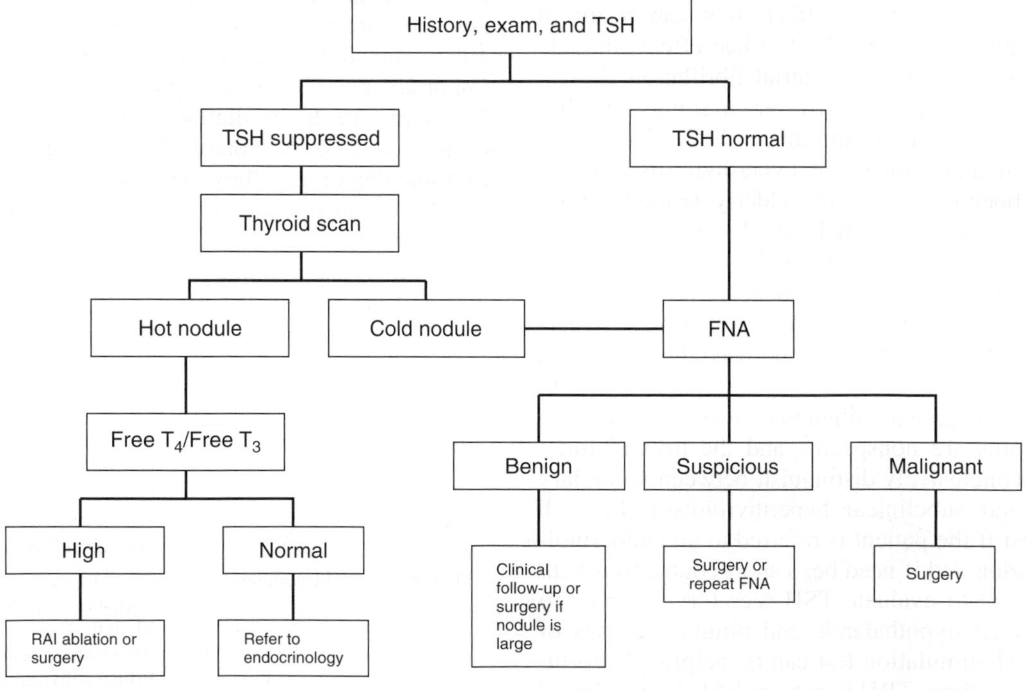

Figure 1 A suggested algorithm for workup of thyroid nodules. FNA: fine-needle aspiration biopsy

high index of suspicion in at-risk populations. Several studies including National Health & Nutrition Examination Survey (NHANES) III (Hollowell *et al.*, 2002) and The Colorado Thyroid Disease Prevalence Study (Canaris *et al.*, 2000) have shown an increased prevalence of elevated serum TSH in women and in the elderly. Thus, periodic screening with serum-sensitive TSH measurements in this at-risk population is recommended.

An understanding of the common etiologies of thyroid disease in the elderly would identify risk factors, the presence or absence of which would help determine screening frequency. The most common cause of hypothyroidism (Sawin, 2003) in the elderly is lymphocytic thyroiditis, which usually leads to an atrophic gland (as opposed to a goiter in younger persons). Elderly persons with other autoimmune diseases (i.e. type 1 diabetes mellitus, pernicious anemia) or a family history of thyroid disease are particularly at risk. Other causes of hypothyroidism in the elderly include head and neck radiation, a more common cause in elderly men with increased incidence of head and neck cancer, and medications (i.e. amiodarone, lithium). The most common cause of hyperthyroidism in the elderly is Graves' disease (Braverman, 1999), followed by an increased prevalence of toxic nodular goiter as compared to younger people. In addition, common iatrogenic causes of hyperthyroidism in the elderly include amiodarone therapy, use of iodinated contrast agents, iodine-containing expectorants, or supplements such as *kelp*.

The most effective way for screening for thyroid dysfunction is to order TSH with third-generation assays using one of the more recently developed immunoradiometric (IRMA) or immunochemilumenescence assays (IMCA). A suggested algorithm for evaluating thyroid dysfunction is shown in Figure 2. Generally, if serum TSH is normal, no further workup is needed. Increased TSH level over $10\,\mathrm{mU\,ml^{-1}}$ is usually diagnostic for primary thyroidal failure, unless there is a confounding variable such as interference with the assay, recovery from illness, or exposure to certain drugs, especially iodinated contrast agents. If free T4 is normal and TSH is less than $10\,\mathrm{mU\,ml^{-1}}$, subclinical hypothyroidism is suspected. For the latter, the presence of antithyroid peroxidase antibodies (anti-TPO) will help in the decision whether to initiate thyroid hormone replacement or to observe conservatively. If TSH is decreased and free T4 is low, evaluate the patient for pituitary hypothalamic dysfunction or surreptitious consumption of T3. If FT4 is elevated, then the diagnosis of hyperthyroidism is made, otherwise check for free T3 to exclude T3 toxicosis. If FT4 and FT3 are normal in the face of suppressed TSH, then the patient may either have subclinical hyperthyroidism or the set point of pituitary may be altered.

CONCLUSIONS

Thyroid gland anatomy and function change with age. Decreased thyroid hormone action, as evidenced by a decrease in gene products that are positively regulated by thyroid hormone, suggests that there may be an age-related resistance to thyroid hormone. Though an increase in serum thyroid hormone levels is expected in a resistance syndrome,

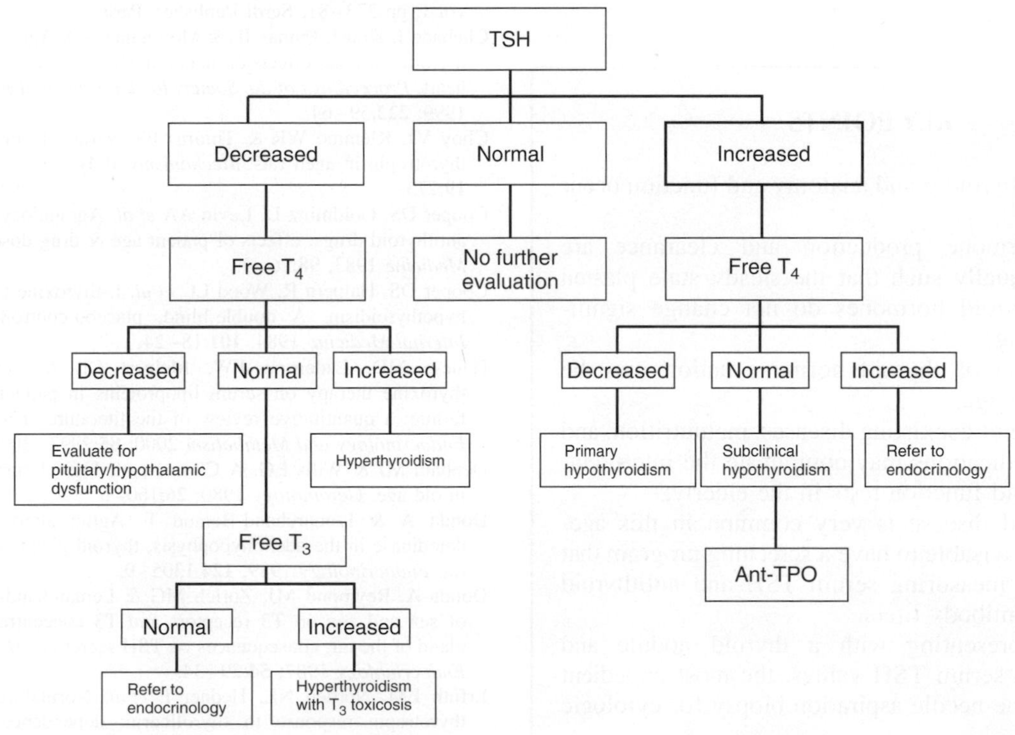

Figure 2 A suggested algorithm for diagnosing thyroid dysfunction

unchanged serum thyroid hormone levels in the euthyroid elderly person likely reflect additional changes in thyroid hormone economy that occur with aging. For example, increased suppressability of TSH, decreased conversion of T4 to T3, and decreased thyroidal sensitivity to TSH, may preclude expected increases in thyroid hormone concentrations (Case and Mooradian, 2000). While thyroid hormone resistance may account for clinical similarities among euthyroid elderly persons and hypothyroid subjects, and the lack of classical clinical findings in hyperthyroid elderly persons, it is unclear whether this actually reflects thyroid disease. Certainly, these clinical presentations are apparent in elderly persons with and without biochemical abnormalities. Therefore, the most important difference in the evaluation of thyroid disease in older versus younger persons lies in diagnosing the disease in the absence of clinical clues. In this case, the physician must rely on intermittent biochemical screening, as there are no age-related changes in the biochemical tests used in clinical practice to diagnosis thyroid disease. Once the disease is detected, there may be differences in treatment strategies as a result of age-related changes in thyroid hormone economy. Specifically, as thyroid hormone degradation decreases with age, the hypothyroid elderly patient will require a decreased dose of thyroid hormone replacement to avoid overreplacement. Finally, the physician must be aware of possible consequences of both untreated thyroid disease and overtreated thyroid disease, which may be exacerbated in the elderly patient based on the increased prevalence of underlying comorbidities in this population, for example, cognitive impairment, coronary artery syndrome, cardiac systolic dysfunction, atrial fibrillation, and metabolic bone disease.

KEY POINTS

- Changes in thyroid gland anatomy and function occur with aging.
- Thyroid hormone production and clearance are decreased equally such that the steady state plasma levels of thyroid hormones do not change significantly with age.
- Tissue effects of thyroid hormone action may be reduced with age.
- The presence of coexisting diseases, malnutrition, and a host of medications may complicate the interpretation of thyroid function tests in the elderly.
- Since thyroid disease is very common in this age-group, it is advisable to have a screening program that incorporates measuring serum TSH and antithyroid peroxidase antibody titers.
- For those presenting with a thyroid nodule and have normal serum TSH values, the most expedient workup is fine-needle aspiration biopsy for cytologic studies.

KEY REFERENCES

- Mariotti S, Franceschi C, Cosarizza A & Pinchera A. The aging thyroid. *Endocrine Reviews* 1995; **16**:686–715.
- Mooradian AD. Normal age-related changes in thyroid hormone economy. *Clinics in Geriatric Medicine* 1995; **11**:159–69.
- Mooradian AD & Wong NCW. Age-related changes in thyroid hormone action. *European Journal of Endocrinology* 1994; **131**:451–61.
- Samuels MH. Subclinical thyroid disease in the elderly. *Thyroid* 1998; **8**:803–13.
- Sawin CT. Thyroid disease in older persons. In LE Braverman (ed) *Diseases of the Thyroid* 2003, pp 85–105; Humana Press, Totowa.

REFERENCES

American Association of Clinical Endocrinologists. Medical guidelines for clinical practice for the evaluation and treatment of hyperthyroidism and hypothyroidism. *Endocrine Practice* 2002; **8**:457–67.

Biondi B, Palmieri EA, Lombardi G & Fazio S. Effects of subclinical thyroid dysfunction on the heart. *Annals of Internal Medicine* 2002; **137**:904–14.

Braverman LE. Subclinical hypothyroidism and hyperthyroidism in elderly subjects: should they be treated? *Journal of Endocrinological Investigation* 1999; **22**(suppl 10):1–3.

Canaris GJ, Manowitz NR, Mayor G & Ridgway EC. The Colorado thyroid disease prevalence study. *Archives of Internal Medicine* 2000; **160**:526–34.

Caraccio N, Ferrannini E & Monzani F. Lipoprotein profile in subclinical hypothyroidism: response to levothyroxine replacement, a randomized placebo-controlled study. *The Journal of Clinical Endocrinology and Metabolism* 2002; **87**:1533–8.

Case CC & Mooradian AD. Thyroid changes with aging. In JE Morley, HJ Armbrecht, RM Coe & B Vellas (eds) *The Science of Geriatrics. Facts, Research and Intervention in Geriatrics Series* 2000, vol 1, pp 273–81; Serdi Publisher, Paris.

Chehade J, Kim J, Pinnas JL & Mooradian AD. Age-related changes in the thyroid hormone effects on malondialdehyde modified proteins in the rat heart. *Proceedings of the Society for Experimental Biology and Medicine* 1999; **222**:59–64.

Choy VJ, Klemme WR & Timiras PS. Variant forms of immunoreactive thyrotropin in aged rats. *Mechanisms of Ageing and Development* 1982; **19**:273.

Cooper DS, Goldminz D, Levin AA *et al.* Agranulocytosis associated with antithyroid drugs: effects of patient age & drug dose. *Annals of Internal Medicine* 1983; **98**:26–9.

Cooper DS, Halpern R, Wood LC *et al.* L-thyroxine therapy in subclinical hypothyroidism. A double-blind, placebo-controlled trial. *Annals of Internal Medicine* 1984; **101**:18–24.

Danese MD, Ladenson PW, Meinert CL & Powe NR. Effect of thyroxine therapy on serum lipoproteins in patients with mild thyroid failure: a quantitative review of the literature. *The Journal of Clinical Endocrinology and Metabolism* 2000; **85**:2993–3001.

Denham MJ & Wills EG. A Clinico-pathological survey of thyroid gland in old age. *Gerontology* 1980; **26**:160–6.

Donda A & Lemarchand-Beraud T. Aging alters the activity of 5′-deiodinase in the adenohypophysis, thyroid gland, and liver of the male rat. *Endocrinology* 1989; **124**:1305–9.

Donda A, Reymond MJ, Zurich MG & Lemarchand-Beraud T. Influence of sex and age on T3 receptors and T3 concentration in the pituitary gland of the rat: consequences on TSH secretion. *Molecular and Cellular Endocrinology* 1987; **54**:29–34.

Erfuth EM, Norden NE, Hedner P *et al.* Normal reference interval for thyrotropin response to thyroliberin: dependence on age, sex, free thyroxine index, and basal concentrations of thyrotropin. *Clinical Chemistry* 1984; **30**:196.

Foldes J, Tarjan G, Szathmari M *et al.* BMD in patients with endogenous subclinical hyperthyroidism: is this thyroid status a risk factor for osteoporosis? *Clinical Endocrinology* 1993; **39**:521–7.

Friedman D, Reed RL & Mooradian AD. The prevalence of over medication with levothyroxine in ambulatory elderly patients. *Age* 1992; **15**:9–13.

Gaffney GW, Gregerman RI & Shock NW. Relationship of age to the thyroidal accumulation, renal excretion & distribution of radioiodine in euthyroid man. *The Journal of Clinical Endocrinology and Metabolism* 1982; **22**:784.

Gregerman RI, Gaffney GW, Shock NW & Crowder SB. Thyroxine turnover in euthyroid man with special reference to changes with age. *The Journal of Clinical Investigation* 1962; **41**:2065.

Gupta KL. Neoplasm of the thyroid gland. *Clinics in Geriatric Medicine* 1995; **11**:271–90.

Haas MJ, Li J-P, Pun K & Mooradian AD. Partial characterization of a cerebral thyroid hormone responsive protein (THRP). *Archives of Biochemistry and Biophysics* 2002; **399**:6–11.

Haas MJ, Mreyoud A, Fishman M & Mooradian AD. Microarray analysis of thyroid hormone induced changes in mRNA expression in the adult rat brain. *Neuroscience Letters* 2004; **365**(1):14–8.

Haas MJ, Fishman M, Mreyoud A & Mooradian AD. Thyroid hormone responsive protein (THRP) mediates thyroid hormone-induced cytotoxicity in primary neuronal cultures. *Experimental Brain Research* 2005; **160**(4):424–32.

Hak AE, Pols HP, Visser TJ *et al.* Subclinical hypothyroidism is an independent risk factor for atherosclerosis & myocardial infarction in elderly women: the Rotterdam Study. *Annals of Internal Medicine* 2000; **132**:270–8.

Harman SM, Wehmann RE & Blackman MC. Pituitary-thyroid hormone economy in healthy aging men: basal indices of thyroid function and thyrotropin responses to constant infusions of thyrotropin releasing hormone. *The Journal of Clinical Endocrinology and Metabolism* 1984; **58**:320.

Helfand M & Redfern CC. Screening for thyroid disease: an update. *Annals of Internal Medicine* 1998; **129**:144–58.

Hermann J, Heinen E, Kroll HJ *et al.* Thyroid function and thyroid hormone metabolism in elderly people. Low T3 syndrome in old age. *Klinische Wochenschrift* 1981; **59**:315–23.

Hershman JM, Pekary AE, Berg L *et al.* Serum thyrotropin and thyroid hormone levels in elderly and middle-aged euthyroid persons. *Journal of the American Geriatrics Society* 1993; **41**:823–8.

Hollowell JG, Staehling NW, Hannon WH *et al.* Serum TSH, T4, and thyroid antibodies in the United States population (1988 to 1994): National Health & Nutrition Examination Survey (NHANES III). *The Journal of Clinical Endocrinology and Metabolism* 2002; **87**:489–99.

Jang M & Distefeno JJ III. Same quantitative changes in iodothyroronine distribution and metabolism in mild obesity and aging. *Endocrinology* 1985; **116**:457–68.

Kaiser FE. Variability of response to thyrotropin-releasing hormone in normal elderly. *Age Ageing* 1987; **16**:345.

Ladenson PW, Singer PA, Ain KB *et al.* American thyroid association guidelines for detection of thyroid dysfunction. *Archives of Internal Medicine* 2000; **160**:1573–5.

Laurberg P, Pedersen KM, Hreidarsson A *et al.* Iodine intake and the pattern of thyroid disorders: a comparative epidemiological study of thyroid abnormalities in the elderly in Iceland and in Jutland Denmark. *The Journal of Clinical Endocrinology and Metabolism* 1998; **83**:765–9.

Mariotti S, Franceschi C, Cosarizza A & Pinchera A. The aging thyroid. *Endocrine Reviews* 1995; **16**:686–715.

Mooradian AD. Blood-brain transport of triiodothyronine is reduced in aged rats. *Mechanisms of Ageing and Development* 1990a; **52**:141–7.

Mooradian AD. The hepatic transcellular transport of 3, 5, 3′- triiodothyronine is reduced in aged rats. *Biochimica et Biophysica Acta* 1990b; **1054**:1–7.

Mooradian AD. Mechanisms of age-related endocrine alterations in mammals. *Drugs & Aging* 1993; **3**:81–97, 131–46.

Mooradian AD. Biology of aging. In G Felsenthal, SJ Garrison & FU Steinberg (eds) *Rehabilitation of the Aging and Elderly Patient* 1994, pp 3–10; Williams and Wilkins, Baltimore.

Mooradian AD. Normal age-related changes in thyroid hormone economy. *Clinics in Geriatric Medicine* 1995; **11**:159–69.

Mooradian AD & Albert SG. The age-related changes in lipogenic enzymes: the role of dietary factors and thyroid hormone responsiveness. *Mechanisms of Ageing and Development* 1999; **108**:139–49.

Mooradian AD & Lieberman J. Age-related decrease in serum angiotensin converting enzyme activity: the role of thyroidal status and food intake. *The Journals of Gerontology Biological Sciences* 1990; **45**:B24–7.

Mooradian AD & Scarpace PJ. The response of isoproterenol-stimulated adenylate cyclase activity after administration of L-triiodothyronine is reduced in aged rats. *Hormone and Metabolic Research* 1989; **21**:638–9.

Mooradian AD & Scarpace PJ. 3,5,3′-L-7triiodothyronine regulation of B-adrenergic receptor density and adenylyl cyclase activity in synaptosomal membranes of aged rats. *Neuroscience Letters* 1993; **161**:101–4.

Mooradian AD & Wong NCW. Age-related changes in thyroid hormone action. *European Journal of Endocrinology* 1994; **131**:451–61.

Mooradian AD, Allam CK, Khalil MF *et al.* Anaplastic transformation of thyroid cancer. *Journal of Surgical Oncology* 1983; **23**:95–8.

Mooradian AD, Chehade J & Kim J. Age-related changes in thyroid hormone effects on glucose transporter isoforms of rat heart. *Life Sciences* 1999; **65**:981–9.

Mooradian AD, Deebaj L & Wong NCW. Age-related alterations in the response of hepatic lipogenic enzymes to altered thyroid states in the rat. *The Journal of Endocrinology* 1991; **128**:79–84.

Mooradian AD, Fox-Robichaud A, Meijer ME & Wong NCW. Relationship between transcription factors and S_{14} gene expression in response to thyroid hormone and age. *Proceedings of the Society for Experimental Biology and Medicine* 1994a; **207**:97–101.

Mooradian AD, Habib MP, Dickerson F & Yetskievych T. The effect of age on L-3, 5, 3′, triiodothyronine induced ethane exhalation. *Journal of Applied Physiology* 1994b; **77**:160–4.

Mooradian AD, Li J & Shah GN. Age-related changes in thyroid hormone responsiveness protein (THRP) expression in cerebral tissue of rats. *Brain Research* 1998; **793**:302–4.

Mooradian AD, Wong NCW & Shah GN. Age-related changes in the responsiveness of apolipoprotein A_1 to thyroid hormone. *The American Journal of Physiology* 1996; **271**:R1602–7.

Ordene KW, Pan C, Barzel US & Surks MI. Variable thyrotropin response to thyrotropin-releasing hormone after small decreases in plasma thyroid hormone concentrations in patients of advanced age. *Metabolism* 1983; **32**:881–8.

Parle JV, Franklyn JA, Cross KW *et al.* Prevalence & follow-up of abnormal thyrotropin concentrations in the elderly in the United Kingdom. *Clinical Endocrinology* 1991; **34**:77–83.

Pekary AE, Mirell CJ, Turner LF Jr *et al.* Hypothalamic secretion of thyrotropin releasing hormone declines in aging rats. *Journal of Gerontology* 1987; **42**:447–50.

Reymond F, Denereaz N & Lemarchand-Beraud TL. Thyrotropin action is impaired in the thyroid gland of old rats. *Acta Endocrinologica* 1992; **126**:55.

Samuels MH. Subclinical thyroid disease in the elderly. *Thyroid* 1998; **8**:803–13.

Sawin CT. Thyroid disease in older persons. In LE Braverman (ed) *Diseases of the Thyroid* 2003, pp 85–105; Humana Press, Totowa.

Sawin CT Castelli WP, Hershman JM *et al.* The aging thyroid: thyroid deficiency in the Framingham study. *Archives of Internal Medicine* 1985; **145**:1386–8.

Sawin CT, Geller A, Wolf PA *et al.* Low serum thyrotropin concentrations as a risk factor for atrial fibrillation in older persons. *The New England Journal of Medicine* 1994; **331**:1249–52.

Scanlon MF & Toft AD. Regulation of thyrotropin secretion. In LE Braverman & RD Utiger (eds) *Werner & Ingbar's the Thyroid* 2000, pp 234–53; Lippincott Williams & Wilkins, Philadelphia.

Shah GN, Li J & Mooradian AD. Novel translational repressor (NAT-1) expression is modified by thyroid state and age in brain and liver. *European Journal of Endocrinology* 1999; **139**:649–53.

Shah GN, Li JP, Schneiderjohn P & Mooradian AD. Cloning and characterization of a complementary DNA for a thyroid hormone responsive protein in mature rat cerebral tissue. *The Biochemical Journal* 1997; **327**:617–23.

Shah NG, Wong NCW & Mooradian AD. Age-related changes in apolipoprotein A_1 expression. *Biochimica et Biophysica Acta* 1995; **1259**:277–82.

Silverberg AB & Mooradian AD. The thyroid and aging. Interdisciplinary topics in aging. *Functional Endocrinology of Ageing* 1998; **29**:27–43.

Snyder PH & Utiger RD. Response to thyrotropin releasing hormone (TRH) in normal man. *The Journal of Clinical Endocrinology and Metabolism* 1972; **34**:380.

Surks MI, Ortiz E, Daniels GH *et al.* Subclinical thyroid disease, U.S. Preventive Services Task Force (2004) screening for thyroid disease: recommendation statement. *Annals of Internal Medicine* 2004; **140**:125–7.

Surks MI & Sievert M. Drugs & thyroid function. *The New England Journal of Medicine* 1995; **333**:1688–94.

Sundbeck G, Eden S, Jagenburg R & Lindstedt G. Thyroid dysfunction in 85-year-old men and women. Influence of non-thyroidal illness and drug treatment. *Acta Endocrinologica* 1991; **125**:475–86.

Trivalle C, Doucet J, Chassagne P *et al.* Differences in the signs & symptoms of hyperthyroidism in older & younger patients. *Journal of the American Geriatrics Society* 1996; **44**:50–3.

U.S. Preventive Services Task Force. Scientific review & guidelines for diagnosis & management. *The Journal of the American Medical Association* 2004; **291**:228–38.

Van Coevorden A, Laurent E, Decoster C *et al.* Decreased basal and stimulated thyrotropin secretion in healthy elderly men. *The Journal of Clinical Endocrinology and Metabolism* 1989; **69**:177–85.

Wong NCW, Schwartz HL, Strait K & Oppenheimer JH. Thyroid hormone, carbohydrate and age-related regulation of a methylation site in the hepatic S14 gene. *Molecular Endocrinology* 1989; **3**:645–50.

Wiersinga WW. Nonthyroidal illness. In LE Braverman & RD Utiger (eds) *Werner & Ingbar's the Thyroid* 2000, pp 281–94; Lippincott Williams & Wilkins, Philadelphia.

121

Ovarian and Testicular Function

Syed H. Tariq

Saint Louis University School of Medicine, St Louis, MO, USA

MENOPAUSE

The word menopause originated from the Greek words "meno" meaning menses and "pause" meaning cessation. The diagnosis of menopause is made retrospectively and is clinically defined as *amenorrhea* for 12 months. Menopause can be "natural" or "induced". Induced menopause can result from bilateral oophorectomy. Premature ovarian failure is the onset of menopause before 40 years and is seen in some conditions like oophoritis. The average age at menopause is 51 years. Menopause is a normal event in a woman's life and is not considered as a disease. Menopause can be a positive and liberating experience for some women and negative for others.

In 2000, there were approximately 41.75 million women in the United States. The percentage of women over the age of 50 years has tripled in the last century. During this time, the mean life expectancy of women in the United States has increased from 50 years to 81.7 years, suggesting that menopause will occur at a time when women have yet to experience almost a third of their life span. In the next 20 years, about 40 million women will experience menopause. Early menopause occurs before the age of 46 and is seen in one-tenth of the women.

Menopause occurs in three stages: perimenopause, cessation of menses, and postmenopause. Perimenopause marks the beginning of the postmenopausal period; this transition is a slow process. During this time, the ovarian functions are changing and take between 2 and 8 years till the final menopausal period is reached. The majority of women experience menstrual irregularities during this time, followed by cessation of menses and then the postmenopausal stage. The Practice Committee of the American Society for Reproductive Medicine recommended using the term "menopausal transition" (MT) instead of using "perimenopause" or "climacteric" in scientific papers.

"The MT was defined by the Stages of Reproductive Aging Workshop (STRAW) held in 2001. It begins with variations in the length of menstrual cycle in a woman who has a rise in the monotropic follicle-stimulating hormone (FSH) and ends with the final menstrual period" (The Practice committee of the American Society for Reproductive Medicine, 2004).

RISK FACTORS OF EARLY MENOPAUSE

One-tenth of the women reach early menopause and the risk factors include:

1. smoking (appears to be dose and duration related) (Tauber, 1996; Olshansky *et al.*, 1990)
2. nulliparity
3. short menstrual cycles and
4. maternal history of early menopause.

Menopause offers the primary health-care provider an opportunity to assess a woman's health, her concerns, and her needs for health promotion and disease prevention measures.

HORMONAL CHANGE

During the perimenopause period, the ovarian follicles decrease in number through the process of apoptosis and the ovarian estrogen production also decreases (Driancourt and Thuel, 1998). Both luteinizing hormone (LH) and FSH rise, with the increase in FSH being more than the increase in LH (Santro *et al.*, 1997). FSH is responsible for the maturation of the follicles and ovulation, while LH provides the stimulus for ovulation and secretion of steroids from the corpus luteum. The rise in FSH is related to the loss of negative biofeedback by gonadal steroids and cessation of inhibin production by the ovarian follicles. Inhibin inhibits the secretion of FSH by acting on the pituitary gland, and increases cell proliferation and gonadotropin-dependent steroid production by its action on the gonads. Inhibin B levels fall before Inhibin A (Burger *et al.*, 1998). Androgen production by the ovaries continues under the

Principles and Practice of Geriatric Medicine, 4th Edition. Edited by M.S. John Pathy, Alan J. Sinclair and John E. Morley.

influence of elevated LH concentration. Activin functions as an autocrine/paracrine regulator and plays a role in the induction of FSH receptors and folliculogenesis (Li *et al.*, 1995). Since menopause is more than a state of estrogen deficiency, its replacement may not return the level of FSH to the premenopausal level. FSH is predominately under the control of inhibin. Inhibin remains low in menopause. FSH, therefore, will remain elevated even in the face of estrogen administration, and thus FSH may not be completely reliable as a measure of sufficient or reliable estrogen administration. There might be a further decline in the levels of gonadotropins with age and other comorbid conditions (Quint and Kaiser, 1985). During the transition to menopause, both estradiol and estrone concentrations fall, though the concentration of estradiol is much lower than the estrone, which is exactly opposite to that in the case of younger women. Estradiol in postmenopausal women comes from the peripheral aromatization of androgen from the ovarian and adrenal glands.

During menopause there is decrease in the production of the androgens, dehydroepiandrostenedione (DHEA) and dehydroepiandrostenedione sulphate (DHEAS), by the ovaries and adrenals (Longscope, 1978). There is a reduction of the total and bioavailable testosterone levels in postmenopausal women undergoing total abdominal hysterectomy with bilateral salpingo-oophorectomy compared to women undergoing hysterectomy alone with conservation of the ovary or ovaries (Meldrum *et al.*, 1981). Longitudinal hormonal studies have shown a decline in both testosterone and androstenedione approximately 3 years before the occurrence of menopause (Laughlin *et al.*, 2000).

CLINICAL FEATURES OF MENOPAUSE

Table 1 shows the changes associated with menopause (Tariq Syed and Morley, 2003).

Table 1 Changes with menopause

Skin	Dryness, loss of hair, atrophy, and loss of elasticity
Skeleton	Loss of teeth and development of osteoporosis
Breast	Softer consistency and smaller breast size
Endocrine	Hot flashes
	Flushing and sweating
	Palpitation
	Anxiety
	Sleep disruption
	Mood changes
	Decrease in libido
Neurological	Cognitive, sleep, and mood changes
Urogenital	Vaginal dryness
	Vaginal bleeding
	Itching/burning/irritation in the labial/mons
	Urge incontinence
	Dysuria
	Nocturia
	Dyspareunia
	Urinary tract infections

Hot Flashes

Hot flashes are one of the most common characteristic symptoms of menopause. Typically, a woman experiences intense heat (hot flashes) and subsequent cooling by cutaneous vasodilatation, perspiration, and chills (Overlie *et al.*, 1999; Bachmann, 1999). These symptoms last from a few seconds to several minutes and vary in intensity from being mild to intolerable. Hot flashes are more severe in women who have undergone oophorectomy (Shanafelt *et al.*, 2002). McKinlay *et al.* (1992) reported that 58% of the women experience hot flashes within 2 years of menopause. Hot flashes last for 1–5 years in two-thirds of women undergoing menopause, but in about 10–15% of the women it will last for more than 5 years (McKinlay *et al.*, 1992). Hot flashes are reported more in the western hemisphere (up to 80%) compared to as low as 10% in East Asia (Flint and Samil, 1999; Thompson *et al.*, 1973). Hot flashes vary in different cultures, with reports of fewer hot flashes in Chinese and Indonesian women. It is not clear whether these differences are related to the perception of menopause, use of herbs, genetic factors, or differences in the reporting of symptoms, or because of other factors (Beyene, 1986).

Kronberg (1990) reported that 87% of the women had current symptoms of hot flashes daily, 15% had more than 10 hot flashes lasting for 1–5 minutes daily, and 6% had hot flashes lasting more than 6 minutes. Hot flashes are reported when the cutaneous temperature exceeds 0.3 °C.

Hot flashes are associated with the disruption of sleep, work, and social relationships. At times hot flashes could be brought about by body contact, which could make relationships worse. The pathophysiology of hot flashes has not been fully elucidated. Hot flashes respond very well in a dose-response fashion to hormone replacement, but may take up to 12 weeks to see the improvement in symptoms (Kronberg, 1990). Human studies have failed to show any quantitative difference in estrogen levels and the occurrence of hot flashes (Steingold, 1985; Walsh and Schiff, 1990; Thompson *et al.*, 1973; Freedman, 2001). The abrupt drop in estrogen is more related to the symptoms of hot flashes rather than hypoestrogenemia (Silva and Boulant, 1986). LH pulses are temporally related to the occurrence of a hot flash but do not appear to be the cause of the flash. Other hormones that increase with a hot flash include adrenocorticotropic hormone (ACTH), cortisol, and neurotensin (Hammond, 1996; Lightman *et al.*, 1981). The active area of interest lies in the central adrenergic system. Clonidine, an α-2 adrenergic receptor agonist, has been shown to reduce vascular responsiveness to norepinephrine, epinephrine, and angiotensin (Freedman *et al.*, 1990). Clonidine is also effective in tamoxifen-induced hot flashes in women with breast cancer (Ginsburg *et al.*, 1985).

Sexual Dysfunction

The prevalence of sexual activity varies, 70% among those aged 45–54 (Pandya *et al.*, 2000) and 60% among those aged 55–64 (Fantl *et al.*, 1994). This prevalence is similar to that reported in community-based surveys from Europe and the United States (Greendale *et al.*, 1996; Dennerstein *et al.*, 2000; Diokno *et al.*, 1990). Hot flashes affect the quality of life markedly as well as adversely affect libido (Greendale *et al.*, 1996). It is not certain that reduced sexual activity is related to menopause *per se*, but may be related to some menopause-related symptoms that interfere with sexuality, for example, vaginal atrophy results in vaginal dryness and friability leading to dyspareunia and even reduced sexual arousal in some women (Fantl *et al.*, 1994; Lindgren *et al.*, 1993).

Estrogen is responsible for the development of primary and secondary sexual characteristics in women, although there is an increasing consensus regarding the role of androgens, as a major factor in enhancing libido. Lower testosterone levels in women have been found to be related to the reduction in the frequency of sexual intercourse, reduced sexual arousal, and a reduction in self-related sexual gratification scores (Osborn *et al.*, 1988; McCoy and Davidson, 1985). Free testosterone levels have a positive correlation with sexual desire (Osborn *et al.*, 1988). Testosterone replacement was shown to improve sexual desire in studies of women who have had oophorectomy and received higher doses of testosterone (Hutchinson, 1995; Sherwin and Gelfand, 1985). It is debatable if such a finding can be applied for similar testosterone replacement in women with natural occurring menopause. At the same time, the safety of the high dose of testosterone necessary for this effect is questioned (Sherwin *et al.*, 1985). It is unclear as to when and in whom androgen therapy should be utilized in women. The presence of depression and medications are major factors causing low libido. The risk and potential benefits of androgen remain to be elucidated. Doses for women can be individualized and the potential side effects monitored very closely, that is, hirsutism, lipid disorder, hepatic dysfunction, fluid retention, and potential polycythemia. A trial of low-dose oral methyltestosterone (1.25–5 mg daily) has been used for postmenopausal women who report low sexual desire. Myers *et al.* (1990) reported that a dose of 5 mg methyltestosterone showed an increase in self-stimulation, but not a self-reported arousal. In countries, where available, testosterone undecanoate can be used. Pharmacists have also compounded vaginal testosterone creams.

Urogenital Atrophy

Women with vaginal atrophy present with symptoms of dyspareunia, vaginal dryness, itching, and irritation frequently. At the onset of menopause, withdrawal of estrogen results in atrophic changes, that is, an increase in the friability of urogenital tissue and relevant pelvic organs. As a result, there is a decrease in the thickness and vascularity of the vulva and vaginal walls and a decrease in the size of the uterus. The secretion by the Bartholin's and cervical glands also decreases. In addition, the depleted lactobacillus from the vagina is replaced by normal flora. Normally, lactobacillus produces lactic acid to maintain a vaginal pH of 4.5, but with the loss of lactobacillus there is an increase in the vaginal pH (alkaline) resulting in an increase in urinary tract infections. Atrophic changes affecting the trigone, urethra, and bladder neck, acting in concert with postmenopausal reduction in α-adrenergic bladder neck receptors may result in urinary urgency and urge incontinence (Casson and Carson, 1996; Greendale *et al.*, 1999a; Rekers *et al.*, 1992). The prevalence of urogenital atrophy is estimated to be from 10 to 40% (Milsom *et al.*, 1993). Twenty-seven percent of the women reported vaginal dryness and dyspareunia and 36% complained of micturition symptoms, incontinence, or urinary tract infection at the time of menopause (Greendale and Judd, 1993). Symptoms of itching, burning, incontinence, and dyspareunia can be disabling (van Geelen *et al.*, 2000).

Depression

Several longitudinal population-based studies suggest no association between menopause transition and depression (Barlow *et al.*, 1997). Kaufert *et al.* (Pearlstein *et al.*, 1997) reported in a Canadian study that 51% of menopausal women had a positive depression screening (Center for Epidemiologic Studies Depression Scale) at least once during a 3 year period of observation, but these high scores were related to perceived poor health and not because of menopause. Two other studies have identified a higher incidence of depression in menopausal women with a preexisting history of depression (Kaufert *et al.*, 1992; Avis *et al.*, 1994). Although there is no scientific evidence associating menopause and the increase in the risk of depression, the failure of health professionals to differentiate without any doubt among transient periods of depressed mood, depressed mood due to adjustment disorder, and major depression has led to this myth in the mind of the layperson. Regardless of this, postmenopausal women complain of increased irritability, anxiety, and depressed mood.

Estrogen replacement appears to enhance mood and this could be the effect of β-endorphin, which increases with estrogen replacement. In postmenopausal women, the response of cortisol and prolactin to the antagonist (1-metchlorophenyl piperazine) was blunted as compared to younger women and those on estrogen replacement (Hunter, 1990). This diminished response to serotonin may explain some of the mood-altering effects of estrogen; however, it is not clear that these changes are persistent (Halbreich *et al.*, 1985). The combination of hormone replacement therapy (HRT) plus SSRIs (selective serotonin reuptake inhibitors) may confer benefit in treating depression (Oppenheim, 1984) compared to either one of the therapy alone. The impact of progesterone on mood is also unclear and studies exist showing conflicting results, as has been seen with estrogen (Schneider *et al.*, 1997; Sherwin, 1991).

Sleep

Sleep disruption is frequently perceived during the perimenopause period both by the subject and the health-care professional. Insomnia is not the immediate presenting issue in perimenopause, but its incidence is higher in women during this time in their life span (Greendale *et al.*, 1999b; Shaver and Zenk, 2000). Insomnia could present as difficulty in falling asleep, disruption of sleep by hot flashes, fragmented sleep, and early morning awakenings. Sleep studies had shown that the hot flashes and the rapid eye movement (REM) sleep tends to occur at the same time, thereby compromising the quality of sleep (Baker *et al.*, 1997). In asymptomatic women (without hot flashes), the higher prevalence of insomnia could be a result of obstructive sleep apnea. The prevalence of obstructive sleep apnea rises in women after menopause but remains stable with aging in men (Shaver *et al.*, 1988; Polo-Kantola *et al.*, 2001). There is poor correlation between estrogen levels and the level of insomnia. The etiology of insomnia is poorly explored at this time.

Cognition

Clinical studies have suggested the presence of estrogen receptors in the cerebral cortex, pituitary gland, limbic system, and hypothalamus. Until recently, the commonly held view was that estrogen/hormone therapy (ET/HT) helped prevent postmenopausal women from developing dementia, particularly Alzheimer's dementia (AD) because of the neuroprotective effect of estrogen on the brain (Lamberg, 1997). The Women Health Initiative Memory Study (WHIMS), a randomized, double-blind, placebo-controlled clinical trial, examined 93% of the postmenopausal women from Women Health Initiative (WHI) (Birge, 1997). The estrogen plus progestin segment of the study enrolled only women aged 65 and older, with an average age of 71 years. These patients were diagnosed with possible dementia. The results of the WHIMS were quite perplexing. Sixty-one women were diagnosed with possible dementia (most likely AD), and among these women 40 were on estrogen/progestin therapy, which is twice the number of women on placebo. A risk-benefit analysis suggested the discontinuation of estrogen/progestin therapy, as there were no significant differences in women 65 years and over. There was a higher incidence of diagnosing AD in the second year, which is very difficult to explain as it is a very slow and progressive disease. The causes of these findings need to be explored further. These findings do not apply to women in the menopausal transitional period. It should be remembered that women in this study received premarin and these findings may not apply to other forms of estrogen.

Coronary Heart Disease

Cardiovascular disease is the leading cause of death (43%) among women aged 50 and older (Shumaker *et al.*, 2003). Women have approximately 10 times the risk of heart disease in their lifetime than of breast cancer, reproductive cancer, or osteoporotic fracture. The HERS (Heart and Estrogen/Progestin Replacement Study) trial examined 2763 postmenopausal women with heart disease, suggesting no significant difference between ET/HT and placebo groups (Mosca *et al.*, 1997). However, there was an increase in the risk of cardiovascular events in the first year of hormone replacement, which decreased over time. HT is also associated with a significant risk in venous thromboembolism (VTE) and gall bladder disease; however, a significant improvement in lipid profile was observed in ET/HT users despite the lack of effect on cardiovascular disease, with a 11% lowering of low-density lipoprotein levels and a 10% increase in high-density lipoprotein (HDL) levels than in the placebo group despite the increase in events in the first year. The WHI Study also observed an increase in heart disease death, nonfatal myocardial infarction, pulmonary thromboembolic disease, and deep vein thrombosis. The findings from both HERS and WHI studies suggest not initiating HRT for the primary and/or secondary prevention of heart disease.

Stroke

The WHI study analyzed the risk of stroke among the 16 608 women enrolled in the study. The overall hazard ratio (HR) for stroke (fatal and nonfatal stroke) was 1.41 after an average of 5.2 years of follow-up (Hulley *et al.*, 1998). Those who used estrogen/progestin had a higher incidence of nonfatal stroke but not fatal stroke. A recent update of WHI confirms that there were 7 additional strokes per 10 000 women across all age-groups per year, representing a 31% increase in risk (Rossouw *et al.*, 2002). This increase is reported to exist from the second through the fifth year of estrogen/progestin usage.

Osteoporosis

The prevalence of low bone mineral density (BMD) in women 50 years and older is about 50–68% (Wassertheil-Smoller *et al.*, 2003; Looker *et al.*, 1998). Osteoporotic fracture accounts for 1.5 million low-impact fractures each year. The lifetime risk of hip, spine, and radial fracture is 40% for postmenopausal women, and most of these fractures are accounted for by white women. In the first year after hip fracture, the mortality rate is about 20%. Hip fracture results in a significant loss of function with about one-third requiring institutionalized care (Siris *et al.*, 2001). Loss of BMD begins in the fourth decade in both men and women at a rate of approximately 1% per year. Age-related bone loss results in about 25% of trabecular and cortical bone loss in women. Some women are predisposed to accelerated bone loss on entering menopause. During this time, the trabecular bone loss progresses at a rate of about 5% each year, and the etiology of accelerated bone loss during menopause is unclear.

PERIMENOPAUSAL EVALUATION

During the perimenopausal period, questions should be directed about vasomotor symptoms, menstrual irregularities, sexual dysfunction, prevention of osteoporosis, increased risk of cardiovascular events after menopause, and the exclusion of pregnancy to confirm menopause. Measuring hormonal levels to help diagnose menopause is not clear, but an FSH level of $40\,\mathrm{mIU\,L^{-1}}$ or greater is considered diagnostic of menopause. Several studies have shown wide fluctuations in the perimenopausal values for FSH, making it an unfavorable tool to be used for the diagnosis of menopause (Riggs and Melton, 1995; Santoro *et al.*, 1996).

MANAGEMENT OF PERIMENOPAUSAL SYNDROME

Hormone Replacement Therapy

Currently, 20–45% of the women in the United States between the ages of 50 and 75 take some form of HRT. About 8 million American women use estrogen alone and about 6 million American women use estrogen-progestin therapy. Approximately 20% of the women do so for more than 5 years. Earlier studies suggesting that HRT exerted a protective role against osteoporosis, cardiovascular disease, and dementia suggested that it could be the "fountain of youth" for women (Santoro *et al.*, 1996; Keating *et al.*, 1999). The HERS study (Mendelsohn and Karas, 1999) reported that the use of conjugated estrogen 0.625 mg and medroxyprogesterone acetate (MPA) did not reduce the risk of cardiovascular events in women with documented coronary artery disease. In fact, there was an increase in cardiovascular events in the group treated with HRT. The treatment also increased the rate of thromboembolic events and gallbladder disease. There was a pattern of early increase in the risk of coronary heart disease (CHD) events and no overall cardiovascular benefits; starting HRT treatment for the purpose of secondary prevention of CHD is not recommended. A follow-up study to the HERS II looked to determine whether the risk reduction observed in the later years of HERS persisted and resulted in an overall reduced risk of CHD events with additional years of follow-up. After 6.8 years, HT did not reduce the risk of cardiovascular events in women with CHD. HERS II recommends that postmenopausal HT should not be used to reduce the risk for CHD events in women with CHD (Hulley *et al.*, 1998).

The estrogen plus progestin component in the study by the WHI was a randomized controlled primary prevention trial (planned duration, 8.5 years) in which 16 608 postmenopausal women aged 50–79 years with an intact uterus were treated with HRT. The trial was stopped prematurely after a mean of 5.2 years of follow-up. The estimated HRs by the major clinical outcomes were as follows: CHD, 1.29 with 286 cases; breast cancer, 1.26 with 290 cases; stroke, 1.41 with 212 cases; pulmonary embolism (PE), 2.13 with 101 cases; colorectal cancer, 0.63 with 112 cases; endometrial cancer, 0.83 with 47 cases; hip fracture, 0.66 with 106 cases; and death due to other causes, 0.92 with 331 cases. The absolute increased risks per 10 000 person-years attributable to estrogen plus progestin were 7 more CHD events, 8 more strokes, 8 more PEs, and 8 more invasive breast cancers, while the absolute risk reductions per 10 000 person-years were 6 fewer colorectal cancers and 5 fewer hip fractures (Grady *et al.*, 2002).

Postmenopausal HT is known to increase the risk of venous thrombosis (VT). Cushman and colleagues reported (Writing Group for the Women's Health Initiative Investigators, 2002) the analyses of the data from the WHI Estrogen Plus Progestin trial, which included assessment of the interaction of HT with other demographic and clinical risk factors for VT. The authors found that HT increased the risks of VT associated with age, overweight or obesity, and factor V Leiden. In a second article, Smith and colleagues (Cushman *et al.*, 2004) compared the risk of first VT among women taking esterified estrogen or conjugated equine estrogen (CEE) with or without progestin, versus nonusers of HT. They found that the current use of conjugated equine estrogen, but not esterified estrogen, was associated with an increased risk of VT compared with nonuse, and the risk was increased with concomitant progestin use. With all this evidence, the use of HRT is not recommended as the risks outweigh the benefits.

Hot Flashes

The main triggers are spicy or hot food, caffeine, or alcohol, all of which should be avoided. Removing layers of clothing, drinking cold beverages, moving to an open window or cool place, putting ice on the forehead, or using a handheld fan are some ways to reduce the subjective effects of a flash. Even talking about a flash can help reduce the psychological effects it can produce.

Herbal Therapies

Many women in the United States use herbal therapies for menopausal symptoms (Smith *et al.*, 2004). The common herbs used in the United States include black cohosh (*Cimicifuga racemosa*), chaste tree berry (*Vitex agnus-castus*), dong quai (*Angelica sinensis*), Gingseng (*Panax gingseng*), evening primrose oil (*Oenethera biennis*), motherwort (*Leonurus cardiaca*), red clover (*Trifolium pratense*), and licorice (*Glycyrrhiza glabra*).

Black cohosh is the most popular herb used traditionally by Native Americans for gynecological conditions. There are four randomized controlled trials on black cohosh with 2–6 months follow-up in a total of 285 women. One of the four trials was placebo controlled (Beal, 1998), one used both treatment and placebo control (Jacobson *et al.*, 2001), and two were treatment controlled (Warnecke, 1985;

Stoll, 1987). Three studies showed no difference between black cohosh and the control and in the fourth trial, there was no difference between the treatment groups. All clinical studies of black cohosh have used the standardized product remifemin, however, the formulation and dosages were different. There is a concern for long-term use of these herbal products since there is no data available on its long-term safety, especially regarding endometrial or breast stimulation. Black cohosh may be useful for hot flashes but long-term use may not be safe as there is no data available regarding its safety.

Many foods contain phytoestrogens, primarily phenolic (rather than steroidal) compounds that include isoflavones, ligans, and coumestans. Isoflavones are found in soy. Lignan precursors are found in vegetables, rye, whole grain, seeds, and legumes.

Soy products are used in Japan, China, and Korea with a reported lower prevalence of menopausal symptoms in these countries (Lehmann-Willenbrock and Riedel, 1988; Lock *et al.*, 1988). Soy is also used in the United States, and currently there are 11 randomized controlled trials (RCT) with soy and soy extract in a total of 1172 women (Adlercreutz *et al.*, 1992; Van Patten *et al.*, 2002; Kronenberg and Fugh-Berman, 2002; Baber *et al.*, 1999; Knight *et al.*, 1999). The duration of these studies is from 1 to 4 months. Of these RCTs, six showed some difference in hot flashes such as severity, frequency, or symptoms score (Van Patten *et al.*, 2002). Comparisons are difficult because of variation in the dosage, menopausal symptoms of hot flashes, and menopausal status of patients. The products used in these studies ranged from soy foods to pure isoflavone products. Soy products have been used for years in Asian cuisines and are safe, but it is not wise to assume that products with high doses of isoflavones that are currently available in health stores are also safe. Studies of longer duration need to be conducted in order to ensure safety of these products and differentiate among whole foods, soy protein, and isoflavone.

Red clover is a Native American herb that is not traditionally used long term for hot flashes, and its effect on breast or endometrium stimulation is unknown. Red clover contains the phytoestrogens formononetin, biochanin A, daizein, and genistein. Two Australian RCTs of 3-month duration with 88 patients showed no significant difference of red clover extract compared to placebo for hot flashes (Kronenberg and Fugh-Berman, 2002; Baber *et al.*, 1999).

Dong quai, a Chinese herb is sold in the United States in the form of nontraditional herb combinations. Dong quai has been reported to produce no clinical benefit for hot flashes (Knight *et al.*, 1999). Dong quai contains coumarins and furocoumarins, which, if used with warfarin, can lead to an increase in bleeding tendencies and photosensitization respectively (Hirata *et al.*, 1997; Amato *et al.*, 2002). Dong quai does not contain the typically reported phytoestrogen and as such has a controversial effect on breast tissue stimulation (Fugh-Berman, 2000; Foster and Tyler, 1999).

Ginseng in one trial was shown to have a positive effect on mood but no benefit on menopausal symptoms and quality of life (Zava *et al.*, 1998). There are case reports linking both topical and ingestion of ginseng with postmenopausal bleeding (Wiklund *et al.*, 1999; Greenspan, 1983; Punnonen and Lukola, 1980). Ginseng also reduces the INR (international normalization ratio) in patients receiving coumadin.

Oil of evening primrose is being evaluated for hot flashes. In one trial, there was no benefit between evening primrose oil and placebo on hot flashes (Hopkins *et al.*, 1988).

In a recent literature review, postmenopausal vasomotor treatments that are safe in the short term are (Chenoy *et al.*, 1994): black cohosh, exercise, gabapentin, medroxyprogesterone acetate, paroxetine hydrochloride, and soy protein.

Initial small studies suggest the use of megestrol acetate and venlafaxine. One needs to be aware of the side effects of megestrol acetate such as thromboembolic disease and the rare Cushing's syndrome. The HOPE study, a randomized, double-blind, placebo-controlled trial (the Women's Health, Osteoporosis, Progestin, Estrogen study) examined 2673 healthy, postmenopausal women with an intact uterus. The reduction in vasomotor symptoms was similar with conjugated equine estrogen of $0.625\ \mathrm{mg\,d^{-1}}$ and medroxyprogesterone acetate of $2.5\ \mathrm{mg\,d^{-1}}$ (the most commonly prescribed doses) and all lower combination doses. CEE of $0.625\ \mathrm{mg\,d^{-1}}$ alleviated hot flashes more effectively than the lower doses of CEE alone. Vaginal maturation index improved in all active treatment groups. It was concluded that lower doses of CEE plus MPA relieve vasomotor symptoms and vaginal atrophy as effectively as commonly prescribed doses (Fugate and Church, 2004).

Atrophic Vaginitis

Both systemic and topical estrogen preparations are effective in treating the symptoms of atrophic vaginitis by reducing vaginal pH (Utian *et al.*, 2001) and restoring the premenopausal index. Some of the commonly used vaginal preparations are estrogen cream 0.625 mg, estriol cream, estradiol tablets, and estradiol rings. Nonhormonal preparations are also used and are effective such as polycarbophil or asroglide.

Sexual Dysfunction

Women with androgen deficiency due to chemotherapy and/or bilateral salpingo-oophorectomy have decreased libido and sexual responses. Sherwin *et al.* found that surgical menopausal women on estradiol and testosterone reported greater sexual desire, arousal, and more frequent fantasias than women on estradiol alone or placebo. These changes in behavior covaried with testosterone but not with estradiol serum concentration, which supports the hypothesis that testosterone, not estrogen, has a major role in female sexual interest (Stone *et al.*, 1975; Yu *et al.*, 1997).

Minimal data is available on the use of testosterone in older women. Testosterone, in addition to improving libido also decreases the hot flashes, improves the general well being, and decreases estrogen deficiency-related headaches and mastalgia. Testosterone has been demonstrated to increase BMD and lean body mass in postmenopausal women.

For women, oral testosterone (methyl testosterone) is available in combination with estrogen (Estratest), but may cause elevation of liver enzymes. Testosterone patches are also being developed for women. Testosterone gel can either be compounded by local pharmacist or obtained from androgel packets. Testosterone pellets can be implanted subcutaneously. Testosterone cream application can be utilized for treating atrophic vulvar dystrophy. It has been suggested that testosterone cream applied to the clitoris will increase orgasm in anorgasmic women. Tibolone is a unique agent that has mixed estrogenic-progestagenic-androgenic properties and as such appears to be an ideal replacement therapy. Effects of testosterone include hirsutism, deepening of voice, and an oily skin. DHEA has mixed androgenic-estrogenic properties in postmenopausal women. It has been shown to increase libido in women over 70 years of age. It is not recommended because of variable quality of DHEA and its potential carcinogenic effect on the postmenopausal breast.

Sildenafil was tried in postmenopausal women and it seems that it did not improve sexual function significantly, though it was well tolerated and improved lubrication and clitoral sensitivity (Cheng, 1999).

Finally, older women need to be educated about erectile dysfunction in the male partner along with female sexual aging. Women need to be educated that there is diminished erection and need for more genital stimulation, rather than assuming that the problem is her own inability to arouse her partner.

Postmenopausal Health Maintenance

Current evidence suggests that the use of HRT is no more justifiable, based on the increased adverse events related to its use. It is the responsibility of the physician and the women themselves to increase awareness of the important preventive component of women's health care. An increase in such awareness will result in a healthy lifestyle by bringing in a change in lifestyle.

Cardiovascular Disease

The results of HERS and HERS II study suggested that HRT is not beneficial in secondary prevention of cardiovascular disease but increases the risk of cardiovascular events in women with documented CHD. Lately, the WHI study also failed to demonstrate any benefit of HRT in the primary prevention of CHD or in the reduction of all-cause mortality. The WHI showed 29% increase in CHD event, 42% increase in stroke, a twofold increase in pulmonary embolism as well as an increase in deep vein thrombosis and a 26% increase in breast cancer. The WHI did show a 24% reduction in hip fracture and a 37% decrease in colorectal cancer, and there was no change in endometrial cancer, lung cancer, or the total incidence of cancer. It is important to recognize that the estrogen-only arm of the study in hysterectomized women was not stopped, suggesting progesterone was the main agent responsible for the adverse effects. Similarly, another study of hormone replacement in postmenopausal women reported a significant increase in the risk of ovarian cancer in women who received estrogen replacement for 10 or more years (Shaw *et al.*, 1997).

Postmenopausal Osteoporosis

The prevalence of low BMD in women over the age of 50 is 50–68% (Wassertheil-Smoller *et al.*, 2003; Looker *et al.*, 1998). The lifetime risk of hip, spine, and radial fracture is 40% for postmenopausal women. The mortality rate is 20% at 1 year after a fracture.

The National Osteoporosis Foundation supports the testing of BMD for all women over the age of 65, and women under the age of 65 with risk factors. Once osteoporosis is identified, the next step is to treat it appropriately.

SUMMARY

In summary, ovarian hypofunction results in menopause and at this stage using HRT is counterproductive. Cessation of menses, the hallmark of menopause is considered by many as the starting point for screening and treating chronic diseases. It is imperative to start educating women about the risks resulting from ovarian hypofunction and carry out discussions involving measures to modify risk factors of chronic diseases before the onset of menopause, and perform appropriate screening tests and implement preventive therapies (pharmacological or nonpharmacological) as indicated.

- Menopause is a normal rather than a disease process.
- Women in this age-group need education and understanding the process of menopause and while adapting to the new lifestyle.
- Emphasis needs to be placed on the preventive aspects of chronic diseases that occur during this time and to avoid HRT.

MALE HYPOGONADISM (ANDROPAUSE)

Hypogonadism is a clinical condition associated with testosterone deficiency with specific signs and symptoms, such as diminished libido and sense of energy, erectile dysfunction, decreased muscle mass and strength, decreased BMD, depression and anemia, increased fatigue, and impaired cognition (Matsumoto, 2002; Morley, 2001). When Hypogonadism occurs in the older men, the condition is called *andropause*, androgen deficiency of aging man (ADAM), and partial androgen deficiency of the aging male, male climacteric, male menopause, or even viropause.

Andropause is seen in men over 50 years of age. It has been described in the Chinese text of Internal Medicine in the sixteenth century. Testicular extract was used by Brown-Sequard for treating his menopausal symptoms. Testosterone was first isolated from the bull testes in the laboratory in 1930s. Werner described the symptoms of testosterone deficiency in the 1940s (Werner, 1946).

Hypogonadism affects an estimated 2–4 million men in the United States, and its prevalence increases with aging (Harman *et al.*, 2001; Morley *et al.*, 1997a). Currently, only 5% of the affected men are receiving treatment (Food and Drug Administration, 1996). Recent media attention to testosterone-replacement therapy has been fueled not only by the increased medical awareness of hypogonadism but also by the marketing of new topical testosterone formulations, and the desire of "baby boomers" to maintain vitality and health into their more mature years.

DECLINE IN TESTOSTERONE WITH AGING

Both cross-sectional and longitudinal studies have clearly shown that testosterone levels in men decrease with age at a rate of 1–2% per year (Korenman *et al.*, 1990; Kaiser *et al.*, 1998; Harman *et al.*, 2001; Haren *et al.*, 2001; Zmuda *et al.*, 1997). Circulating testosterone is mainly (60%) bound to sex hormone binding globulin (SHBG). About 38% is bound to albumin and 1–2% circulates freely in the blood. The SHBG increases with increase in age, which leads to an increase in bound testosterone; reflecting a total testosterone level higher than expected for the level of tissue available testosterone. The free and albumin-bound testosterone can enter the cell under physiological conditions and are available to activate the testosterone receptors. It is also believed that there is an alteration in the binding capacity of SHBG with aging (Haren *et al.*, 2001). Whatever the cause, there is a low amount of testosterone available to tissues in older adults. Total testosterone is an inappropriate measure of hypogonadism in older adults.

Both bioavailable testosterone and free androgen index (which can be calculated using the program at www.Issam.ch) are acceptable methods to measure testosterone levels in older adults. Using these measures, 2–30% of men between the ages of 40 and 59 years and 34–70% of men between the ages of 60 and 80 years are hypogonadal (Morley *et al.*, 1997a; Zmuda *et al.*, 1997; Khosala and Melton, 2001).

Reports indicate that testosterone-replacement therapy produces a wide range of benefits for men with hypogonadism, which includes libido (Tenover, 1998; Kim, 1999; Snyder *et al.*, 2000), bone density (Kenny *et al.*, 2001; Snyder *et al.*, 1999), muscle mass (Snyder *et al.*, 2000; Kenny *et al.*, 2001; Sih *et al.*, 1997), body composition (Snyder *et al.*, 2000; Sih *et al.*, 1997; Snyder *et al.*, 2001), mood (Snyder *et al.*, 2000; Dobs *et al.*, 1999), erythropoiesis (Snyder *et al.*, 2000; Dobs *et al.*, 1999), and cognition (Dobs *et al.*, 1999; Cherrier *et al.*, 2001; Moffat *et al.*, 2002).

Perhaps the most common controversial topic concerning the ongoing discussion of testosterone-replacement therapy is its long-term safety and risks. Recent reports from the HRT studies have aroused concerns that men receiving hormones may also be vulnerable to an increase in health risks.

PATHOPHYSIOLOGY OF HYPOGONADISM

The causes of hypogonadism in older adults seem to be multifactorial.

- Hypogonadism could be either primary or secondary, but in older adults it is mostly secondary in nature, that is, lower testosterone levels fail to elevate the LH outside the normal range (Korenman *et al.*, 1990; Leifke *et al.*, 2000).
- Decrease in Leydig cell function in the testes of older men (Mulligan *et al.*, 2001).
- Partial desensitization of Leydig cells to LH with aging (Mulligan *et al.*, 2001).
- Decrease in testosterone response to human chorionic gonadotropin (Harman and Tsitouras, 1980).
- Decrease in pituitary responsiveness to gonadotropin releasing hormone with aging (Winters and Atkinson, 1997).
- Testosterone replacement in older men is a more potent inhibitor of LH than in younger men (Winters and Atkinson, 1997).
- In healthy older men, there is a decrease in LH pulse amplitude and frequency and irregularity of the secretion of LH (Mulligan *et al.*, 2001; Pincus *et al.*, 1996).
- Increased aromatization of testosterone to estradiol and in 5α reductase activity to dihydrotestosterone (DHT). DHT levels stay stable, while testosterone decreases with aging (Ukkola *et al.*, 2001).
- There is a decrease in fertility and spermatogenesis with aging (Baccarelli *et al.*, 2001).
- Decrease in Inhibin B levels with aging (Baccarelli *et al.*, 2001).
- FSH levels increase more than LH with aging (Morley *et al.*, 1997a).

EFFECTS OF TESTOSTERONE REPLACEMENT IN OLDER ADULTS

Coronary Artery Disease

Testosterone was used successfully to treat angina. Studies have shown that low testosterone levels are associated with both coronary artery disease and the degree of atherosclerosis (Jaffe, 1997; English *et al.*, 2000a). Testosterone dilates the brachial artery and thereby increases the blood flow (Rosano *et al.*, 1999; Webb *et al.*, 1999) reduction in the ST depression during exercise stress test (Jaffe, 1997; Wu and Weng,

1993; English *et al.*, 2000b) reducing myocardial infarction (Anderson *et al.*, 1995) or causing no effect on myocardial infarction (Hajjar *et al.*, 1997). Anderson *et al.* (1995) reported that testosterone replacement decreases the prothrombotic factors and prothrombinase activity, and protein C and S appeared to be counterbalanced by an increase in antithrombin III activity and fibrinolytic activity. There was no effect on platelet activity. Testosterone-replacement therapies have not demonstrated an increase in the incidence of cardiovascular disease or events such as myocardial infarction, stroke, or angina (Hajjar *et al.*, 1997).

Lipid Profiles

Testosterone decreases cholesterol, low-density lipoprotein cholesterol levels, and HDL cholesterol levels (Sih *et al.*, 1997; Zgliczynski *et al.*, 1996; Anderson *et al.*, 1995; Wittert *et al.*, 2003; Tenover, 1992; Ferrando *et al.*, 2002; Morley *et al.*, 1993; Kang *et al.*, 2002). Whitsel *et al.* (2001) in their meta-analysis on the effect of intramuscular testosterone injection on serum lipid in hypogonadal men reported that HDL levels were reduced in three studies and remained unchanged in 15. Five studies showed reduction in total cholesterol, increase in 2, and unchanged in 12. Low-density cholesterol was either unchanged or reduced in 14 of the 15 studies.

Although the data appear reassuring, definitive assessment of long-term effects of testosterone-replacement therapy on cardiovascular health require prospective, large scale, placebo-controlled studies.

Libido and Erectile Dysfunction

Epidemiologic studies have shown that decreased sexual activity and libido are associated with a decrease in free or bioavailable testosterone levels (Davidson *et al.*, 1983; Schiavi *et al.*, 1991). These studies suggested that aging was a more important contributor than androgen levels in sexual behavior in healthy older men.

Testosterone replacement improves libido and quality of erection in hypogonadal men (Billingtom *et al.*, 1983; Nankin and Lin, 1986). Sildenafil is reported to improve erection in older men (Wagner *et al.*, 2001). It is reported that certain men with low testosterone do not respond to sildenafil alone unless their testosterone is replaced (Tariq *et al.*, 2003). This seems to be because testosterone is essential for the synthesis of nitric oxide synthase. DHT is also shown to be associated with the ability to maintain erection (Endo *et al.*, 2002).

Body Composition and Frailty

Aging is associated with a decrease in muscle mass and strength. Conservation of muscle mass and strength has been shown to be reversed with resistance training (Klein *et al.*, 2002; Evans, 2002; Trappe *et al.*, 2001). Excessive loss of muscle in a person results in sarcopenia and an increase in the risk of becoming frail (Gillick, 2001; Fried *et al.*, 2001; Lipsitz, 2002). Free testosterone index and bioavailable testosterone index are better predictors of muscle mass and strength (Baumgartner *et al.*, 1999a; Perry *et al.*, 2000).

Studies with testosterone replacement have clearly shown that it produces an increase in muscle mass, which is reported even in older men who are not hypogonadal (Wittert *et al.*, 2003; Tenover, 1992; Ferrando *et al.*, 2002; Morley *et al.*, 1993). Most of the studies have shown increased strength in the upper extremities in the case of hypogonadal men (Tenover, 1992; Bakhshi *et al.*, 2000; Morley, 1997), but failed to increase strength in men who were not hypogonadal (Kenny *et al.*, 2001; Snyder *et al.*, 1999). DHT is shown to increase knee flexion strength (Ly *et al.*, 2001). Testosterone replacement is also beneficial in improving the functional independence measure (FIM) during rehabilitation following hospitalization (Bakhshi *et al.*, 2000).

Leptin level increases with age in males and this has been shown to be associated with a decrease in testosterone (Morley, 1997; Baumgartner *et al.*, 1999b; Baumgartner *et al.*, 1999c; Munzer *et al.*, 2001; Morley *et al.*, 1997b).

Testosterone replacement decreases fat mass (Kenny *et al.*, 2001; Snyder *et al.*, 1999; Ferrando *et al.*, 2002) with subcutaneous adiposity being reduced to a greater extent than abdominal visceral fat (Munzer *et al.*, 2001).

Behavioral Effects

Epidemiologists have shown a strong correlation between low testosterone and cognitive decline with aging (Morley *et al.*, 1997b; Barrett-Connor *et al.*, 1999). Low testosterone in middle age is predictive of developing AD (Henderson and Hogervorst, 2004). Testosterone replacement improves working spatial memory and trail-making B (Kenny *et al.*, 2001; Janowsky *et al.*, 1994; Janowsky *et al.*, 2000; Cherrier *et al.*, 2001); effects on verbal memory are controversial (Janowsky *et al.*, 2000; Cherrier *et al.*, 2001) and in other studies it has shown failure to alter cognition (Kenny *et al.*, 2001; Sih *et al.*, 1997).

Dysphoria has been related to low levels of testosterone (Barrett-Connor *et al.*, 2000; Seidman *et al.*, 2002). Testosterone replacement did improve depression in one study (Giorgi *et al.*, 1992), but other studies have failed to show the same results (Sih *et al.*, 1997; Janowsky *et al.*, 2000; Seidman *et al.*, 2001; Reddy *et al.*, 2000).

Bone

Testosterone is converted by the process of aromatization to estradiol that acts on the bone. Testosterone increases BMD by acting on the osteoblasts. Testosterone increases BMD at the hip and lumbar spine (Katznelson *et al.*, 1996; Anderson *et al.*, 1996). There are no studies examining the effect of testosterone on hip fracture.

Polycythemia

Replacement of testosterone appears to stimulate erythropoiesis. Hemoglobin levels increase by 15–20% in boys at puberty, in parallel with serum testosterone levels. Lower testosterone levels are associated with anemia in men (Basaria and Dobs, 1999). A rise in hematocrit is generally beneficial in anemia; elevation above the normal range may have grave consequences for coronary, cerebrovascular, or peripheral vascular circulation (Basaria and Dobs, 1999; The Endocrine Society, 2002). Increase in hemoglobin is associated with the route of testosterone replacement. Injection increased hematocrit by 44%, transdermal nonscrotal patch by 15% (Dobs *et al.*, 1999), and scrotal patch by 5% (Leifke *et al.*, 2000). Wang *et al.* (2000) reported a direct relation between testosterone dosage and the incidence of erythrocytosis. Erythrocytosis was reported in 2.8% of men on 5 mg of nonscrotal patches, 11% with 50 mg day^{-1} and 18% with 100 mg day^{-1} gel respectively.

Benign Prostatic Hypertrophy

It is a well-established fact that androgens are required for the causation of benign prostatic hypertrophy (BPH) and that a decrease in serum testosterone causes a reduction in the size of the prostate (Huggins *et al.*, 1941). However, a number of studies have failed to show that testosterone replacement exacerbated the voiding symptoms of BPH or caused increased urinary retention compared to placebo (Kenny *et al.*, 2001; Sih *et al.*, 1997; Dobs *et al.*, 1999; Comhaire, 2000; Krieg *et al.*, 1993; Pechersky *et al.*, 2002; Marcelli and Cunningham, 1999; Slater and Oliver, 2000).

Prostate Cancer

Case reports have suggested that testosterone-replacement therapy may convert occult cancer into a clinically apparent lesion (Curran and Bihrle, 1999; Loughlin and Richie, 1997). To date, prospective studies have demonstrated a low frequency of prostate cancer in association with testosterone-replacement therapy. A compilation of published prospective trials of testosterone-replacement therapy followed for 6 to 36 months showed prostate cancer in 5 of 461 men (1.1%) (Zmuda *et al.*, 1997; Snyder *et al.*, 2000; Kenny *et al.*, 2001; Sih *et al.*, 1997; Dobs *et al.*, 1999; Wang *et al.*, 2000), a prevalence rate very similar to that in the general population. There is some concern that the underlying prevalence of occult prostate cancer in men with low testosterone levels appear to be substantial (Morgentaler *et al.*, 1996).

Despite decades of research, there is no compelling evidence to show that testosterone has a causative role in prostate cancer (Pechersky *et al.*, 2002; Marcelli and Cunningham, 1999; Carter *et al.*, 1995; Heikkila *et al.*, 1999; Hsing, 2001).

Other side effects include gynecomastia, water retention, hypertension, and sleep apnea.

Screening for Hypogonadism

Three screening questionnaires have been developed for hypogonadism. These tests are useful but not diagnostic. The Saint Louis University ADAM Questionnaire and the Aging Male Survey both have good specificity, but the Massachusetts Male Survey utilizes risk factors and has poor specificity.

TESTOSTERONE THERAPIES

Testosterone replacement can be achieved in several ways:

- Oral and injectable therapies.
- Transscrotal and transdermal patches.
- Subcutaneous gels.
- Buccal preparations.
- Selective androgen receptor molecule (no effects on prostate). These are under development.
- Sublingual and inhalation forms are under development.

CONCLUSION

Hypogonadism is a very common condition in older males. Appropriate screening is suggested to clinicians, and it is important to exclude the diagnosis of depression and hypothyroidism before initiating the laboratory work-up (bioavailable testosterone, etc.). Testosterone replacement is available in different forms with minimal side effects if closely monitored. From the current literature, there is no increase in the risk of prostate cancer in subjects with replacement therapy. A long-term study is required to answer the questions regarding the risks and benefits of testosterone therapy.

KEY POINTS

- Hypogonadism is very common in older males.
- Screening tools are available to screen high-risk patients.
- Bioavailable testosterone levels should be checked rather than total testosterone.
- Monitor therapy and watch for any side effects.

KEY REFERENCES

- Baumgartner RN, Waters DL, Morley JE *et al.* Age-related changes in sex hormones affect the sex difference in serum leptin independently of changes in body fat. *Metabolism – Clinical and Experimental* 1999c; **48**(3):378–84.

- Sih R, Morley JE, Kaiser FE *et al.* Testosterone replacement in older hypogonadal men: a 12-month randomized controlled trial. *Journal of Clinical Endocrinology and Metabolism* 1997; **82**:1661–7.
- Tariq Syed H & Morley JE. Maintaining sexual function in elderly women. *Women's Health in Primary Care* 2003; **6**(3):157–60.
- Morley JE. Andropause. Is it time for geriatrician to treat it? *Journals of Gerontology. Series A, Biological Sciences and Medical Sciences* 2001; **56**:M–263–5.
- Morley JE, Perry HM III, Kaiser FE *et al.* Effects of testosterone replacement therapy in old hypogonadal males: a preliminary study. *Journal of the American Geriatrics Society* 1993; **41**(2):149–52.

REFERENCES

Adlercreutz H, Hämäläinen E, Gorbach S & Goldin B. Dietary phyto-oestrogens and the menopause in Japan. *Lancet* 1992; **339**:1233.

Amato P, Christophe S & Mellon PL. Estrogenic activity of herbs commonly used as remedies for menopausal symptoms. *Menopause* 2002; **9**:145–50.

Anderson FH, Francis RM & Faulkner K. Androgen supplementation in eugonadal men with osteoporosis – effects of 6 months of treatment on bone mineral density and cardiovascular risk factors. *Bone* 1996; **18**(2):171–7.

Anderson RA, Ludlam CA & Wu FC. Haemostatic effects of supraphysiological levels of testosterone in normal men. *Thrombosis and Haemostasis* 1995; **74**:693–7.

Avis NE, Brambilla D, McKinlay SM & Vass K. A longitudinal analysis of the association between menopause and depression. Results from the Massachusetts Women's Health Study. *Annals of Epidemiology* 1994; **4**:214–20.

Baber RJ, Templeman C, Morton T *et al.* Randomized placebo-controlled trial of an isoflavone supplement and menopausal symptoms in women. *Climacteric* 1999; **2**:85–92.

Baccarelli A, Morpurgo PS & Corsi A. Activin A serum levels, and aging of the pituitary-gonadal axis: a cross sectional study in the middle-aged and elderly healthy subjects. *Experimental Gerontology* 2001; **36**:1403–12.

Bachmann GA. Vasomotor flushes in menopausal women. *American Journal of Obstetrics and Gynecology* 1999; **180**(3 Pt 2):S312–6.

Baker A, Simpson S & Dawson D. Sleep disruption and mood changes associated with menopause. *Journal of Psychosomatic Research* 1997; **43**(4):359–69.

Bakhshi V, Elliott M, Gentili A *et al.* Testosterone improves rehabilitation outcomes in ill older men. *Journal of the American Geriatrics Society* 2000; **48**(5):550–3.

Barlow DH, Cardozo LD, Francis RM *et al.* Urogenital ageing and its effect on sexual health in older British women. *British Journal of Obstetrics and Gynaecology* 1997; **104**(1):87–91.

Barrett-Connor E, Goodman-Gruen D & Patay B. Endogenous sex hormones and cognitive function in older men. *Journal of Clinical Endocrinology and Metabolism* 1999; **84**(10):3681–5.

Barrett-Connor E, Mueller JE, Von Muhlen DG *et al.* Low levels of estradiol are associated with vertebral fractures in older men, but not women: the Rancho Bernardo study. *Journal of Clinical Endocrinology and Metabolism* 2000; **85**(1):219–23.

Basaria S & Dobs AS. Risks versus benefits of testosterone therapy in elderly men. *Drugs & Aging* 1999; **15**:131–42.

Baumgartner RN, Waters DL, Gallagher D *et al.* Predictors of skeletal muscle mass in elderly men and women. *Mechanisms of Ageing and Development* 1999a; **107**(2):123–36.

Baumgartner RN, Ross RR, Waters DL *et al.* Serum leptin in elderly people: associations with sex hormones, insulin, and adipose tissue volumes. *Obesity Research* 1999b; **7**(2):141–9.

Baumgartner RN, Waters DL, Morley JE *et al.* Age-related changes in sex hormones affect the sex difference in serum leptin independently of changes in body fat. *Metabolism – Clinical and Experimental* 1999c; **48**(3):378–84.

Beal MW. Women's use of complementary and alternative therapies in reproductive health care. *Journal of Nurse-Midwifery* 1998; **43**:224–34.

Beyene Y. Cultural significance and physiological manifestations of menopause: a biocultural analysis. *Culture Medicine and Psychiatry* 1986; **10**:47–71.

Billingtom CJ, Mooradian AD & Morley JE. Testosterone therapy in impotent patients with normal testosterone. *Clinical Research* 1983; **31**:718A.

Birge SJ. The role of estrogen in the treatment and prevention of dementia: introduction. *American Journal of Medicine* 1997; **103**(3A):36S–45S.

Burger HG, Cahir N & Robertson DM. Serum inhibin A and B falls differentially as FSH rises in perimenopausal women. *Clinical Endocrinology* 1998; **48**:809–813.

Carter HB, Pearson JD, Metter EJ *et al.* Longitudinal evaluation of serum androgen levels in men with and without prostate cancer. *Prostate* 1995; **27**:25–31.

Casson PR & Carson SA. Androgen replacement therapy in women: myths and realities. *International Journal of Fertility* 1996; **41**:412–22.

Cheng TO. Warfarin danshen interaction. *Annals of Thoracic Surgery* 1999; **67**:892–6.

Chenoy R, Hussain S, Tayob Y *et al.* Effect of oral gamolenic acid from evening primrose oil on menopausal flushing. *British Medical Journal* 1994; **308**:501–3.

Cherrier MM, Asthana S, Plymate S *et al.* Testosterone supplementation improves spatial and verbal memory in healthy older men. *Neurology* 2001; **57**(1):80–8.

Comhaire FH. Andropause: hormone replacement therapy in the aging male. *European Urology* 2000; **38**:655–62.

Curran MJ & Bihrle W III. Dramatic rise in prostate-specific antigen after androgen replacement in a hypogonadal man with occult adenocarcinoma of the prostate. *Urology* 1999; **53**:423–4.

Cushman M, Kuller LH, Prentice R *et al.*, The Women's Health Initiative Investigators. Estrogen plus progestin and risk of venous thrombosis. *The Journal of the American Medical Association* 2004; **292**:1573–80.

Davidson JM, Chen JJ, Crapo L *et al.* Hormonal changes and sexual function in aging men. *Journal of Clinical Endocrinology and Metabolism* 1983; **57**(1):71–7.

Dennerstein L, Dudley EC, Hopper JL *et al.* A prospective population-based study of menopausal symptoms. *Obstetrics and Gynecology* 2000; **96**(3):351–8.

Diokno AC, Brown MB & Herzog AR. Sexual function in the elderly. *Archives of Internal Medicine* 1990; **150**:197–200.

Dobs AS, Meikle AW, Arver S *et al.* Pharmacokinetics, efficacy, and safety of a permeation-enhanced testosterone transdermal system in comparison with bi-weekly injections of testosterone enanthate for the treatment of hypogonadal men. *Journal of Clinical Endocrinology and Metabolism* 1999; **84**:3469–78.

Driancourt MA & Thuel B. Control of oocyte growth and maturation by follicular cells and molecules present in follicular fluid. A review. *Reproduction Nutrition Development* 1998; **38**:345–62.

Endo M, Ashton-Miller JA & Alexander NB. Effects of age and gender on toe flexor muscle strength. *Journals of Gerontology. Series A, Biological Sciences and Medical Sciences* 2002; **57**(6):M392–7.

English KM, Mandour O & Steeds RP. Men with coronary artery disease have lower levels of androgens than men with normal coronary angiograms. *European Heart Journal* 2000a; **21**:890–4.

English KM, Steeds RP, Jones TH *et al.* Low-dose transdermal testosterone therapy improves angina threshold in men with chronic stable angina: a randomized, double-blind, placebo-controlled study. *Circulation* 2000b; **102**:1906–11.

Evans WJ. Exercise as the standard of care for elderly people. *Journals of Gerontology. Series A, Biological Sciences and Medical Sciences* 2002; **57**(5):M260–1.

Fantl JA, Cardozo L & McClish DK. Estrogen therapy in the management of urinary incontinence in postmenopausal women: a meta-analysis. *Obstetrics and Gynecology* 1994; **83**:12–8.

Ferrando AA, Sheffield-Moore M, Yeckel CW *et al.* Testosterone administration to older men improves muscle function: molecular and physiological mechanisms. *American Journal of Physiology Endocrinology and Metabolism* 2002; **282**(3):E601–7.

Flint M & Samil RS. Culture and subcultural meanings of the menopause. *Annals of the New York Academy of Sciences* 1999; **592**:134–48.

Food and Drug Administration. Updates 1996, Rockville (Accessed January 6, 2004, at http://www.fda.gov/fdac/departs/196upd.html).

Foster S and Tyler VE. *Tyler's Honest Herbal* 1999, 4th edn; Haworth Pr, New York.

Freedman RR. Physiology of hot flashes. *American Journal of Human Biology* 2001; **13**(4):453–64.

Freedman RR, Woodward S & Sabharwal SC. Alpha 2-adrenergic mechanism in menopausal hot flushes. *Obstetrics and Gynecology* 1990; **76**(4):573–8.

Fried LP, Tangen CM, Walston J *et al.*, Cardiovascular Health Study Collaborative Research Group. Frailty in older adults: evidence for a phenotype. *Journals of Gerontology. Series A, Biological Sciences and Medical Sciences* 2001; **56**(3):M146–56.

Fugate SE & Church CO. Nonestrogen treatment modalities for vasomotor symptoms associated with menopause. *Annals of Pharmacotherapy* 2004; **38**:1482–99.

Fugh-Berman A. Herb-drug interactions. *Lancet* 2000; **355**:134–8.

Gillick M. Pinning down frailty. *Journals of Gerontology. Series A, Biological Sciences and Medical Sciences* 2001; **56**(3):M134–5.

Ginsburg J, O'Reilly B & Swinhoe J. Effect of oral clonidine on human cardiovascular responsiveness: a possible explanation of the therapeutic action of the drug in menopausal flushing and migraine. *British Journal of Obstetrics and Gynaecology* 1985; **92**(11):1169–75.

Giorgi A, Weatherby RP & Murphy PW. Muscular strength, body composition, and health responses to the use of testosterone enanthate: a double blind study. *Journal of Science and Medicine in Sport* 1992; **2**:341–55.

Grady D, Herrington D, Bittner V *et al.* Cardiovascular disease outcomes during 6.8 years of hormone therapy: Heart and Estrogen/progestin Replacement Study follow-up (HERS II) *The Journal of the American Medical Association* 2002; **288**(1):49–57.

Greendale GA & Judd HL. The menopause: health implications and clinical management. *Journal of the American Geriatrics Society* 1993; **41**(4):426–36.

Greendale GA, Hogan P & Shumaker S. Sexual functioning in post-menopausal women: the postmenopausal estrogen/progestin interventions trial. *Journal of Womens Health* 1996; **5**:445–58.

Greendale GA, Lee NP & Arriola ER. The menopause. *Lancet* 1999a; **353**(9152):571–80.

Greendale GA, Reboussin BA, Sie A *et al.* Effects of estrogen and estrogen-progestin on mammographic parenchymal density. Postmenopausal Estrogen/Progestin Interventions (PEPI) Investigators. *Annals of Internal Medicine* 1999b; **130**(4 Pt 1):262–9.

Greenspan EM. Ginseng and vaginal bleeding. *The Journal of the American Medical Association* 1983; **249**:2018.

Hajjar RR, Kasier FE & Morley JE. Outcomes of long-term testosterone replacement in older hypogonadal male: a retrospective analysis. *Journal of Clinical Endocrinology and Metabolism* 1997; **82**:3793–6.

Halbreich U, Asnis GM & Shindeldecker R. Cortisol secretion in endogenous depression. *Archives of General Psychiatry* 1985; **42**:904–8.

Hammond CB. Menopause and hormone replacement therapy: an overview. *Obstetrics and Gynecology* 1996; **87**(2 Suppl):2S–15S.

Haren M, Nordin BEC & Pearce CEM. The calculation of bioavailable testosterone. *Proceedings of the VII International Congress of Andrology* 2001, pp 209–21; Medimond, Englewood.

Harman SM, Metter EJ, Tobin JD *et al.* Longitudinal effects of aging on serum total and free testosterone levels in healthy men: Baltimore Longitudinal Study of Aging. *Journal of Clinical Endocrinology and Metabolism* 2001; **86**:724–31.

Harman SM & Tsitouras PD. Reproductive hormones in aging men. Measurement of sex steroids, basal luteinizing hormone, and Leydig's cell responsive to human chorionic gonadotropin. *Journal of Clinical Endocrinology and Metabolism* 1980; **51**:35–40.

Heikkila R, Aho K, Heliovaara M *et al.* Serum testosterone and sex hormone-binding globulin concentrations and the risk of prostate carcinoma: a longitudinal study. *Cancer* 1999; **86**:312–5.

Henderson VW & Hogervorst E. Testosterone and Alzheimer's disease – Is it men's turn now? *Neurology* 2004; **62**(2):170–1.

Hirata JD, Swiersz LM, Zell B *et al.* Does dong quai have estrogenic effects in postmenopausal women? A double blind, placebo-controlled trial. *Fertility and Sterility* 1997; **68**:981–6.

Hopkins MP, Androff L & Benninghoff AS. Ginseng face cream and unexplained vaginal bleeding. *American Journal of Obstetrics and Gynecology* 1988; **159**:1121–2.

Hsing AW. Hormones and prostate cancer: what's next? *Epidemiologic Reviews* 2001; **23**:42–58.

Huggins C, Stevens RE Jr & Hodges CV. Studies on prostatic cancer. II. The effects of castration on advanced carcinoma of the prostate gland. *Archives of Surgery* 1941; **43**:209–23.

Hulley S, Grady D, Bush T *et al.*, Heart and Estrogen/progestin Replacement Study (HERS) Research Group. Randomized trial of estrogen plus progestin for secondary prevention of coronary heart disease in postmenopausal women. *The Journal of the American Medical Association* 1998; **280**(7):605–13.

Hunter MS. Psychological and somatic experience of the menopause: a prospective study. *Psychosomatic Medicine* 1990; **52**:357–67.

Hutchinson KA. Androgens and sexuality. *American Journal of Medicine* 1995; **98**(1A):111S–115S.

Jacobson JS, Troxel AB, Evans J *et al.* Randomized trial of black cohosh for the treatment of hot flashes among women with a history of breast cancer. *Journal of Clinical Oncology* 2001; **19**:2739–45.

Jaffe MD. Effect of testosterone cypionate on post exercise ST segment depression. *British Heart Journal* 1997; **39**:1217–22.

Janowsky JS, Chavez B & Orwoll E. Sex steroids modify working memory. *Journal of Cognitive Neuroscience* 2000; **12**(3):407–14.

Janowsky JS, Oviatt SK & Orwoll ES. Testosterone influences spatial cognition in older men. *Behavioral Neuroscience* 1994; **108**(2):325–32.

Kaiser FE, Viosca SP & Morley JE. Impotence and aging: clinical and hormonal factors. *Journal of American Geriatric Society* 1998; **36**:511–9.

Kang SM, Jang Y, Kim JY *et al.* Effect of oral administration of testosterone on brachial arterial vasoreactivity in men with coronary artery disease. *American Journal of Cardiology* 2002; **89**(7):862–4.

Katznelson L, Finkelstein JS, Schoenfeld DA *et al.* Increase in bone density and lean body mass during testosterone administration in men with acquired hypogonadism. *Journal of Clinical Endocrinology and Metabolism* 1996; **81**(12):4358–65.

Kaufert PA, Gilbert P & Tate R. The Manitoba Project: a reexamination of the link between menopause and depression. *Maturitas* 1992; **14**:143–55.

Keating N, Cleary P, Aossi A & Zaslavsky A. Use of hormone replacement therapy by postmenopausal women in the United States. *Annals of Internal Medicine* 1999; **130**:545–53.

Kenny AM, Prestwood KM, Gruman CA *et al.* Effects of transdermal testosterone on bone and muscle in older men with low bioavailable testosterone levels. *Journals of Gerontology. Series A, Biological Sciences and Medical Sciences* 2001; **56**:M266–72.

Khosala S & Melton LJ III. Relationship of serum sex steroid levels to longitudinal changes in bone density in young verses old men. *Journal of Clinical Endocrinology and Metabolism* 2001; **86**:3555–61.

Kim YC. Testosterone supplementation in the aging male. *International Journal of Impotence Research* 1999; **11**:343–52.

Klein CS, Allman BL, Marsh GD & Rice CL. Muscle size, strength, and bone geometry in the upper limbs of young and old men. *Journals of Gerontology. Series A, Biological Sciences and Medical Sciences* 2002; **57**(7):M455–9.

Knight DC, Howes JB & Eden JA. The effect of Promensil, an isoflavone extract, on menopausal symptoms. *Climacteric* 1999; **2**:79–84.

Korenman SG, Morley JE, Mooradian AD *et al.* Secondary hypogonadism in older men: its relation to impotence. *Journal of Clinical Endocrinology and Metabolism* 1990; **71**:963–9.

Krieg M, Nass R & Tunn S. Effect of aging on endogenous level of 5(alpha)-dihydrotestosterone, testosterone, estradiol, and estrone in epithelium and stroma of normal and hyperplastic human prostate. *Journal of Clinical Endocrinology and Metabolism* 1993; **77**:375–81.

Kronberg F. Hot flashes: epidemiology and physiology. *Annals of the New York Academy of Sciences* 1990; **592**:52–86.

Kronenberg F & Fugh-Berman A. Complementary and alternative medicine for menopausal symptoms: a review of randomized, controlled trials. *Annals of Internal Medicine* 2002; **137**:805–13.

Lamberg L. 'Old and gray and full of sleep'? Not always. *The Journal of the American Medical Association* 1997; **278**(16):1302–4.

Laughlin GA, Barrett-Connor E, Kritz Silverstein D & Von Muhlen D. Hysterectomy, oophorectomy and endogenous sex hormone levels in older women: the Rancho Bernardo Study. *Journal of Clinical Endocrinology and Metabolism* 2000; **85**:645–51.

Lehmann-Willenbrock E & Riedel HH. Clinical and endocrinologic studies of the treatment of ovarian insufficiency manifestations following hysterectomy with intact adnexa. *Zentralblatt fur Gynakologie* 1988; **110**:611–8.

Leifke E, Gorenoi V & Wichers C. Age related changes in serum sex hormones, insulin-like growth factor and sex-hormone binding globulin levels in men; cross sectional data from a healthy male cohort. *Clinical Endocrinology* 2000; **53**:689–95.

Li R, Phillips DM & Mather JP. Activin promotes ovarian follicular development in vitro. *Endocrinology* 1995; **136**:849–56.

Lightman SL, Jacobs HS, Maguire AK *et al.* Climacteric flushing: clinical and endocrine response to infusion of naloxone. *British Journal of Obstetrics and Gynaecology* 1981; **88**(9):919–24.

Lindgren R, Berg G, Hammar M & Zuccon E. Hormonal replacement therapy and sexuality in a population of Swedish postmenopausal women. *Acta Obstetricia Et Gynecologica Scandinavica* 1993; **72**:292–7.

Lipsitz LA. Dynamics of stability: the physiologic basis of functional health and frailty. *Journals of Gerontology. Series A, Biological Sciences and Medical Sciences* 2002; **57**(3):B115–25.

Lock M, Kaufert P & Gilbert P. Cultural construction of the menopausal syndrome: the Japanese case. *Maturitas* 1988; **10**:317–32.

Longscope C. The differences of steroids production by peripheral tissues. In R Scholler (ed) *Endocrinology of the Ovary* 1978, pp 23–35; SEPE, Paris.

Looker AC, Wahner HW, Dunn WL *et al.* Updated data on proximal femur bone mineral levels of US adults. *Osteoporosis International* 1998; **8**(5):468–89.

Loughlin KR & Richie JP. Prostate cancer after exogenous testosterone treatment for impotence. *Journal of Urology* 1997; **157**:1845.

Ly LP, Jimenez M, Zhuang TN *et al.* A double-blind, placebo-controlled, randomized clinical trial of transdermal dihydrotestosterone gel on muscular strength, mobility, and quality of life in older men with partial androgen deficiency. *Journal of Clinical Endocrinology and Metabolism* 2001; **86**(9):4078–88.

Marcelli M & Cunningham GR. Hormonal signaling in prostatic hyperplasia and neoplasia. *Journal of Clinical Endocrinology and Metabolism* 1999; **84**:3463–8.

Matsumoto AM. Andropause: clinical implications of the decline in serum testosterone levels with aging men. *Journals of Gerontology. Series A, Biological Sciences and Medical Sciences* 2002; **57**:M76–99.

McCoy NL & Davidson JM. A longitudinal study of the effects of menopause on sexuality. *Maturitas* 1985; **7**(3):203–10.

McKinlay SM, Brambilla PJ & Posner JG. The normal menopause transition. *Maturitas* 1992; **14**:103–15.

Meldrum DR, Davidson BJ, Tatryn IV & Judd HL. Changes in circulating steroids with aging in postmenopausal women. *Obstetrics and Gynecology* 1981; **57**:624–8.

Mendelsohn M & Karas R. The protective effects of estrogen on the cardiovascular system. *New England Journal of Medicine* 1999; **340**:1801–11.

Milsom I, Ekelund P, Molander U *et al.* The influence of age, parity, oral contraception, hysterectomy and menopause on the prevalence of urinary incontinence in women. *Journal of Urology* 1993; **149**(6):1459–62.

Moffat SD, Zonderman AB, Metter EJ *et al.* Longitudinal assessment of serum free testosterone concentration predicts memory performance and cognitive status in elderly men. *Journal of Clinical Endocrinology and Metabolism* 2002; **87**:5001–7.

Morgentaler A, Bruning CO III & DeWolf WC. Occult prostate cancer in men with low serum testosterone levels. *The Journal of the American Medical Association* 1996; **276**:1904–6.

Morley JE. Anorexia of aging–physiologic and pathologic. *American Journal of Clinical Nutrition* 1997; **66**(4):760–73.

Morley JE. Andropause. Is it time for geriatrician to treat it? *Journals of Gerontology. Series A, Biological Sciences and Medical Sciences* 2001; **56**:M–263–5.

Morley JE, Kaiser FE, Perry HM III *et al.* Longitudinal changes in testosterone, luteinizing hormone and follicle-stimulating hormone in healthy older men. *Metabolism* 1997a; **46**:410–3.

Morley JE, Kaiser F, Raum WJ *et al.* Potentially predictive and manipulable blood serum correlates of aging in the healthy human male–progressive decreases in bioavailable testosterone, dehydroepiandrosterone sulfate, and the ratio of insulin-like growth factor 1 to growth hormone. *Proceedings of the National Academy of Sciences of the United States of America* 1997b; **94**(14):7537–42.

Morley JE, Perry HM III, Kaiser FE *et al.* Effects of testosterone replacement therapy in old hypogonadal males: a preliminary study. *Journal of the American Geriatrics Society* 1993; **41**(2):149–52.

Mosca L, Manson JE, Sutherland SE *et al.*, Writing Group. Cardiovascular disease in women: a statement for healthcare professionals from the American Heart Association. *Circulation* 1997; **96**(7):2468–82.

Mulligan T, Iranmanesh A, Gheorghiu S & Godschalk M. Amplified nocturnal luteinizing-hormone secretary burst frequency with selective attenuation of pulsatile testosterone secretion in healthy aged men-possible Leydig's cell desensitization to endogenous LH signaling-a clinical research–center study. *Journal of Clinical Endocrinology and Metabolism* 2001; **86**:5547–53.

Munzer T, Harman SM, Hees P *et al.* Effects of GH and/or sex steroid administration on abdominal subcutaneous and visceral fat in healthy aged women and men. *Journal of Clinical Endocrinology and Metabolism* 2001; **86**(8):3604–10.

Myers LS, Dixen J, Morrissette D *et al.* Effects of estrogen, androgen and progestin on sexual psychophysiology and behaviour in postmenopausal women. *Journal of Clinical Endocrinology and Metabolism* 1990; **70**:1124–31.

Nankin HR & Lin T. Chronic testosterone cypionate therapy in men with secondary impotence. *Fertility and Sterility* 1986; **40**:300–7.

Olshansky SJ, Carnes BA & Cassel C. In search of Methuselah: estimating the upper limits to human longevity. *Science* 1990; **250**:634–9.

Oppenheim G. A case of rapid mood cycling with estrogen: implications for therapy. *Journal of Clinical Psychiatry* 1984; **45**(1):34–5.

Osborn M, Hawton K & Gath D. Sexual dysfunction among middle aged women in the community. *British Medical Journal* 1988; **296**:259–62.

Overlie I, Moen MH, Morkrid L *et al.* The endocrine transition around menopause: five years prospective study with profiles of gonadotropins, estrogens, androgens, and SHBG among healthy women. *Acta Obstetricia Et Gynecologica Scandinavica* 1999; **10**:642–7.

Pandya KJ, Raubertas RF, Flynn PJ *et al.* Oral clonidine in postmenopausal patients with breast cancer experiencing tamoxifen-induced hot flashes: a University of Rochester Cancer Center Community Clinical Oncology Program study. *Annals of Internal Medicine* 2000; **132**(10):788–93.

Pearlstein T, Rosen K & Stone AB. Mood disorders and menopause. *Endocrinology and Metabolism Clinics of North America* 1997; **26**:279–94.

Pechersky AV, Mazurov VI, Semiglazov VF *et al.* Androgen administration in middle-aged and ageing men: effects of oral testosterone undecanoate on dihydrotestosterone, oestradiol and prostate volume. *International Journal of Andrology* 2002; **25**:119–25.

Perry HM, Miller DK, Patrick P & Morley JE. Testosterone and leptin in older African-American men: relationship to age, strength, function, and season. *Metabolism–Clinical and Experimental* 2000; **49**(8):1085–91.

Pincus SM, Mulligan T & Iranmanesh A. Older males secrete luteinizing hormone and testosterone more irregularly, and jointly more asynchronously, than younger males. *Proceedings of the National Academy of Sciences of the United States of America* 1996; **93**:14100–5.

Polo-Kantola P, Saaresranta T & Polo O. Aetiology and treatment of sleep disturbances during perimenopause and postmenopause. *CNS Drugs* 2001; **15**(6):445–52.

Punnonen R & Lukola A. Oestrogen-like effect of ginseng. *British Medical Journal* 1980; **281**:1110.

Quint AR & Kaiser FE. Gonadotropin determinations and thyrotropin releasing hormone and luteinizing hormone releasing in critically ill postmenopausal women with hypothroxinemia. *Journal of Clinical Endocrinology and Metabolism* 1985; **60**:464–71.

Reddy P, White CM, Dunn AB *et al.* The effect of testosterone on health-related quality of life in elderly males–a pilot study. *Journal of Clinical Pharmacy and Therapeutics* 2000; **25**(6):421–6.

Rekers H, Drogendijk AC, Valkenburg HA & Riphagen F. The menopause, urinary incontinence and other symptoms of the genito-urinary tract. *Maturitas* 1992; **15**(2):101–11.

Riggs BL & Melton LJ III. The worldwide problem of osteoporosis: insights afforded by epidemiology. *Bone* 1995; **17**(5 suppl):505S–11.

Rosano GMC, Leonardo F & Pagnotta P. Acute anti-ischemic effect of testosterone in men with coronary artery disease. *Circulation* 1999; **99**:1666–70.

Rossouw JD, Anderson GL, Prentice RL *et al.*, Writing Group for the Women's Health Initiative Investigators. Risks and benefits of estrogen plus progestin in healthy post-menopausal women: principal results from the Women's Health Initiative randomized controlled trial. *The Journal of the American Medical Association* 2002; **288**:321–33.

Santoro N, Brown JR, Adel T & Skurnick JH. Characterization of reproductive hormonal dynamics in the perimenopause. *Journal of Clinical Endocrinology and Metabolism* 1996; **81**(4):1495–501.

Santro N, Adel T & Skurnick J. Decreased inhibin tone and increase activan A secretion characterizes reproductive aging in women. *Fertility and Sterility* 1997; **71**:658–62.

Schiavi RC, Schreiner-Engel P, White D & Mandeli J. The relationship between pituitary-gonadal function and sexual behavior in healthy aging men. *Psychosomatic Medicine* 1991; **53**(4):363–74.

Schneider LS, Small GW, Hamilton SH *et al.*, Fluoxetine Collaborative Study Group. Estrogen replacement and response to fluoxetine in a multicenter geriatric depression trial. *American Journal of Geriatric Psychiatry* 1997; **5**(2):97–106.

Seidman SN, Araujo AB, Roose SP *et al.* Low testosterone levels in elderly men with dysthymic disorder. *American Journal of Psychiatry* 2002; **159**(3):456–9.

Seidman SN, Spatz E, Rizzo C & Roose SP. Testosterone replacement therapy for hypogonadal men with major depressive disorder: a randomized, placebo-controlled clinical trial. *Journal of Clinical Psychiatry* 2001; **62**(6):406–12.

Shanafelt TD, Barton DL, Adjei AA & Loprinzi CL. Pathophysiology and treatment of hot flashes. *Mayo Clinic Proceedings* 2002; **77**(11):1207–18.

Shaver J, Giblin E, Lentz M & Lee K. Sleep patterns and stability in perimenopausal women. *Sleep* 1988; **11**(6):556–61.

Shaver JL & Zenk SN. Sleep disturbance in menopause. *Journal of Women's Health & Gender-Based Medicine* 2000; **9**(2):109–18.

Shaw D, Leon C, Kolev S *et al.* Traditional remedies and food supplements: a five-year toxicological study (1991–1997). *Drug Safety* 1997; **17**:342–56.

Sherwin BB. The impact of different doses of estrogen and progestin on mood and sexual behavior in postmenopausal women. *Journal of Clinical Endocrinology and Metabolism* 1991; **72**(2):336–43.

Sherwin BB & Gelfand MM. Sex steroids and affect in the surgical menopause: a double-blind cross-over study. *Psychoneuroendocrinology* 1985; **10**:325–35.

Sherwin BB, Gelfand MM & Brender W. Androgen enhances sexual motivation in females: a prospective, crossover study of sex steroid administration in the surgical postmenopausal. *Psychosomatic Medicine* 1985; **47**:339–51.

Shumaker SA, Legault C, Rapp SR *et al.* Estrogen plus progestin and the incidence of dementia and mild cognitive impairment in postmenopausal women: the Women's Health Initiative Memory Study: a randomized controlled trial. *The Journal of the American Medical Association* 2003; **289**:2651–62.

Sih R, Morley JE, Kaiser FE *et al.* Testosterone replacement in older hypogonadal men: a 12-month randomized controlled trial. *Journal of Clinical Endocrinology and Metabolism* 1997; **82**:1661–7.

Silva NL & Boulant JA. Effects of testosterone, estradiol, and temperature on neurons in preoptic tissue slices. *American Journal of Physiology* 1986; **250**(4 Pt 2):R625–32.

Siris ES, Miller PD, Barrett-Connor E *et al.* Identification and fracture outcomes of undiagnosed low bone mineral density in postmenopausal women: results from the National Osteoporosis Risk Assessment. *The Journal of the American Medical Association* 2001; **286**(22):2815–22.

Slater S & Oliver RTD. Testosterone: its role in development of prostate cancer and potential risk from use as hormone replacement therapy. *Drugs & Aging* 2000; **17**:431–9.

Smith NL, Heckbert SR, Lemaitre RN *et al.* Esterified estrogens and conjugated equine estrogens and the risk of venous thrombosis. *The Journal of the American Medical Association* 2004; **292**:1581–7.

Snyder PJ, Peachey H, Berlin JA *et al.* Effects of testosterone replacement in hypogonadal men. *Journal of Clinical Endocrinology and Metabolism* 2000; **85**:2670–7.

Snyder PJ, Peachey H, Berlin JA *et al.* Effects of transdermal testosterone treatment on serum lipid and apolipoprotein levels in men more than 65 years of age. *American Journal of Medicine* 2001; **111**:255–60.

Snyder PJ, Peachey H, Hannoush P *et al.* Effect of testosterone treatment on bone mineral density in men over 65 years of age. *Journal of Clinical Endocrinology and Metabolism* 1999; **84**:1966–72.

Steingold KA. Treatment of hot flashes with transdermal estradiol administration. *Journal of Clinical Endocrinology and Metabolism* 1985; **61**:627–32.

Stoll W. Phytopharmacon influences atrophic vaginal epithelium – double-blind study – Cimicifuga vs. estrogenic substances [German]. *Therapeutikon* 1987; **1**:23–31.

Stone SC, Mickal A & Rye PH. Postmenopausal symptomatology, maturation index, and plasma estrogen levels. *Obstetrics and Gynecology* 1975; **45**(6):625–7.

Tariq SH, Haleem U, Omran ML *et al.* Erectile dysfunction: etiology and treatment in young and old patients. *Clinics in Geriatric Medicine* 2003; **19**(3):539–51.

Tariq Syed H & Morley JE. Maintaining sexual function in elderly women. *Women's Health in Primary Care* 2003; **6**(3):157–60.

Tauber CM (ed). *Statistical Handbook on Women in America* 1996, 2nd edn, pp 1–5; Oryx Press, Phoenix.

Tenover JL. Effects of androgen supplementation in ageing male. *Journal of Clinical Endocrinology and Metabolism* 1992; **75**:1092–8.

Tenover JL. Male hormone replacement therapy including "andropause". *Endocrinology and Metabolism Clinics of North America* 1998; **27**:969–87.

The Endocrine Society. Clinical bulletins in andropause: benefits and risks of treating hypogonadism in the aging male. *Endocrine Report* 2002; **2**:1–6.

The Practice committee of the American Society for Reproductive Medicine The menopausal transition. *Fertility and Sterility* 2004; **82**(1):S107–10.

Thompson B, Hart SA & Durno D. Menopausal age and symptomatology in a general practice. *Journal of Biosocial Science* 1973; **5**(1):71–82.

Trappe S, Godard M, Gallagher P *et al.* Resistance training improves single muscle fiber contractile function in older women. *American Journal of Physiology–Cell Physiology* 2001; **281**(2):C398–406.

Ukkola O, Gagnon J & Rankinen T. Age, body mass index, race and other determinants of steroid hormone variability: the Heritage Family Study. *European Journal of Endocrinology* 2001; **145**:1–9.

Utian WH, Shoupe D, Bachmann G *et al.* Relief of vasomotor symptoms and vaginal atrophy with lower doses of conjugated equine estrogens and medroxyprogesterone acetate. *Fertility and Sterility* 2001; **75**(6):1065–79.

van Geelen JM, van de Weijer PH & Arnolds HT. Urogenital symptoms and resulting discomfort in non-institutionalized Dutch women aged 50–75 years. *International Urogynecology Journal* 2000; **11**(1):9–14.

Van Patten CL, Olivotto IA, Chambers GK *et al.* Effect of soy phytoestrogens on hot flashes in postmenopausal women with breast cancer: a randomized, controlled clinical trial. *Journal of Clinical Oncology* 2002; **20**:1449–55.

Wagner G, Montorsi F, Auerbach S & Collins M. Sildenafil citrate (VIAGRA) improves erectile function in elderly patients with erectile dysfunction: a subgroup analysis. *Journals of Gerontology. Series A, Biological Sciences and Medical Sciences* 2001; **56**(2):M113–9.

Walsh B & Schiff I. Vasomotor flushes. *Annals of the New York Academy of Sciences* 1990; **592**:346–56.

Wang C, Swerdloff RS, Iranmanesh A *et al.* Transdermal testosterone gel improves sexual function, mood, muscle strength, and body composition parameters in hypogonadal men. *Journal of Clinical Endocrinology and Metabolism* 2000; **85**:2839–53.

Warnecke G. Beeinflussung klimakterischer beschwerden durch ein phytotherapeutikum: erfolgreiche therapie mit cimicifuga-monoextrakt. *Medizinische Welt* 1985; **36**:871–4.

Wassertheil-Smoller S, Hendrix S, Limacher M *et al.* Effect of estrogen plus progestin on stroke in postmenopausal women. The Women's Health Initiative: a randomized trial. *The Journal of the American Medical Association* 2003; **289**:2673–26.

Webb CM, Adamson DL, De Zeigler D & Collins P. Effect of acute testosterone on myocardial ischemia in men with coronary artery disease. *American Journal of Cardiology* 1999; **83**:437–9.

Werner AA. The male climacteric: report of two hundred and seventy-three cases. *The Journal of the American Medical Association* 1946; **132**:188–94.

Whitsel EA, Boyko EJ, Matsumoto AM *et al.* Intramuscular testosterone esters and plasma lipids in hypogonadal men: a meta-analysis. *American Journal of Medicine* 2001; **111**:261–9.

Wiklund IK, Mattsson LA, Lindgren R & Limoni C, Swedish Alternative Medicine Group. Effects of a standardized ginseng extract on quality of life and physiological parameters in symptomatic postmenopausal women: a double-blind, placebo-controlled trial. *International Journal of Clinical Pharmacology Research* 1999; **19**:89–99.

Winters SJ & Atkinson L, The Testoderm Study Group. Serum LH concentration in Hypogonadal men during transdermal testosterone replacement therapy through scrotal skin: further evidence that ageing enhances testosterone negative biofeedback. *Clinical Endocrinology* 1997; **26**:39–45.

Wittert GA, Chapman IM, Haren MT *et al.* Oral testosterone supplementation increases muscle and decreases fat mass in healthy elderly males with low-normal gonadal status. *Journals of Gerontology. Series A, Biological Sciences and Medical Sciences* 2003; **58**(7):618–25.

Writing Group for the Women's Health Initiative Investigators. Risks and benefits of estrogen plus progestin in healthy postmenopausal women. Principal results from the Women's Health Initiative randomized controlled trial *The Journal of the American Medical Association* 2002; **288**:321–33.

Wu SZ & Weng XZ. Therapeutic effects of an androgenic preparation on myocardial ischemia and cardiac function in 62 elderly male coronary heart disease patients. *Chinese Medical Journal* 1993; **106**:415–8.

Yu CM, Chan JCN & Sanderson JE. Chinese herbs and warfarin potentiation by 'danshen'. *Journal of Internal Medicine* 1997; **241**:337–9.

Zava DT, Dollbaum CM & Blen M. Estrogen and progestin bioactivity of foods, herbs, and spices. *Proceedings of the Society for Experimental Biology and Medicine* 1998; **217**:369–78.

Zgliczynski S, Ossowski M & Slowinska J. Effect of testosterone replacement on serum lipids and lipoproteins in hypogonadal and elderly men. *Atherosclerosis* 1996; **121**:35–43.

Zmuda JM, Cauley JA & Kriska A. Longitudinal relation between endogenous testosterone and cardiovascular disease risk factors in middle-aged men: a 13 year followup of former Multiple Risk Intervention Trial Participants. *American Journal of Epidemiology* 1997; **146**:609–17.

122

Type 2 Diabetes Mellitus in Senior Citizens

Alan J. Sinclair[1] ***and*** **Graydon S. Meneilly**[2]

[1] University of Warwick, Coventry, UK, and [2] University of British Columbia, Vancouver, BC, Canada

INTRODUCTION

Diabetes care systems for older people require an integrated multidimensional approach involving general practitioners, hospital specialists, and other members of the health-care team. There should be an emphasis on diabetes prevention and its complications, early treatment for vascular disease, and functional assessment of disability due to limb problems, eye disease, and stroke.

Inequalities of care are common in many health-care systems due to variations in clinical practice, particularly in relation to older people. This may be manifest as lack of access to services, inadequate specialist provision, poorer clinical outcomes, and patient and family dissatisfaction. The recent development of clinical guidelines that are responsive to the needs of older people with diabetes may be an important step to minimize deficits in care from country to country, worldwide.

Type 2 diabetes mellitus is a common disabling chronic cardiovascular and medical disorder that has a tremendous health, social, and economic burden, and has a high prevalence of 10–30% in subjects above 65 years of age across Europe. About 60% of total health-care expenditure on diabetes in this special group can be accounted for by acute-care hospitalizations and compared with nondiabetic counterparts, the relative risk for admission to hospital is 5.0. At any one time, about 1 in 12 district hospital beds are occupied by older people who have diabetes and their length of stay is double compared to nondiabetic inpatients. The introduction of insulin to their regimen results in expenditure quadrupling, presumably because of the additional resources required in both hospital and community settings to monitor and support the use of insulin.

A direct approach to the metabolic management of type 2 diabetes in older subjects is to concentrate on strategies designed to limit and ameliorate both defective insulin secretion and insulin resistance. Type 2 diabetes represents a cluster of cardiovascular-risk factors that represent a significant vascular threat, and in aging subjects, the added effects of aging and renal impairment increase the impact of this syndrome, while some of the features may be present up to 10 years before the onset of overt hyperglycemia, thus increasing the cardiovascular risk before the onset of diabetes. Since up to 50% of the variability in insulin action in insulin-resistant states may be associated with lifestyle differences: obesity, physical activity levels, and cigarette smoking, it becomes obvious that environmental, preventative, and health promotional strategies are of vital importance in limiting the impact of this epidemic.

Management of diabetes in older people can be relatively straightforward, especially when patients have no other comorbidities and when vascular complications are absent. In many cases, however, special issues arise that increase the complexity of management and lead to difficult clinical decision making. It is thus not surprising that the present state of diabetes care for older patients varies throughout Europe and North America. Although *geriatric diabetes* is developing as a subspeciality interest in the United Kingdom, there is little evidence of its presence in other national diabetes care systems and virtually no specific provision for those who are housebound or in institutional care.

Diabetes care for the old is, however, generally improving as more and more health-care systems are being audited, standards of care highlighted and deficiencies in care addressed. This chapter can be considered to be a learning program that aims to provide a succinct but comprehensive review of diabetes care for older people focusing on special areas of concern.

We have identified two principal aims: (1) To develop and enhance the knowledge and application of the principles of diabetes and diabetes care in older persons and (2) to provide clinicians with the knowledge and skills, and to influence attitudes to maximize their effectiveness in applying this learning within their own clinical setting. In addition, we have suggested that clinicians who study this chapter in depth should be able to demonstrate: (1) an in-depth understanding of diabetes in older people and to analyze their own organization's provision and care, with a view to enhancing

Principles and Practice of Geriatric Medicine, 4th Edition. Edited by M.S. John Pathy, Alan J. Sinclair and John E. Morley.

local care; (2) an understanding of the means by which the diabetes care team in their own organization and key players in their own community can be engaged in improving the quality of diabetes care for older people. Further goals might include the ability to (3) reflect on their personal learning and apply that learning to the approaches they take with team members, other care professionals, patients, and carers; and (4) analyze and evaluate outcomes in the delivery of care to older people who have diabetes, taking into account the roles of other care professionals and the beliefs of people from different ethnic and cultural backgrounds.

EPIDEMIOLOGY, PATHOGENESIS, AND MODES OF PRESENTATION

Within the next decade, it is projected that the number of diabetic individuals in the world will double to 221 million. Several important risk factors (Table 1) are likely to underpin this increase in prevalence such as advancing age of the population, greater numbers of people from ethnic minority backgrounds adopting a "transitional" lifestyle, greater levels of overweight and obesity, and more sedentary lifestyles. From an epidemiological perspective, aging is an important factor: in the United States, the number of people with diabetes aged 75 years and over doubled between 1980 and 1987. In most populations, peak rates are generally found in the sixth decade and, subsequently, although in Pima Indians, the peak rate is between the fourth and fifth decades.

Most developed countries have a prevalence rate of about 17% in white elderly subjects and 25% in nonwhite subjects. The prevalence of white British elderly is only around 9% although the prevalence in nonwhite British elderly is about 25% and the prevalence in British care homes is 25%.

There is an increasing view that diabetes in the elderly has a genetic basis (Meneilly, 2001). Older people with a family history are often more likely to develop this illness as they age. In genetically susceptible people, various factors may increase the likelihood of type 2 diabetes developing. Elderly patients with diabetes have normal hepatic production of glucose, which is in contrast to younger subjects (Meneilly and Ellitt, 1999). In lean elderly subjects, the principal defect appears to be impaired glucose-induced insulin release, while in the obese elderly, resistance to insulin-mediated glucose disposal is the major problem (Meneilly and Ellitt, 1999). Multiple drugs, reduced physical activity, and a diet with low intake of complex carbohydrates also contribute to this increasing prevalence. Further research into discovering the molecular abnormalities in older people with diabetes is warranted.

Table 1 Risk factors for diabetes mellitus in older subjects

- Aged 65 years and over
- People of Asian, Afro-Caribbean, or African origin
- BMI >27 kg m^{-2} and/or large waist circumference
- Those with manifest cardiovascular disease or hypertension with or without hyperlipidemia
- Presentation with a stroke
- Presentation with recurrent infections
- Use of diabetogenic drugs: for example, corticosteroids, estrogens
- A family history of diabetes mellitus
- Those with IGT/IFG

MODES OF PRESENTATION

Diabetes in older people has a varied presentation and may be insidious, which ultimately delays diagnosis (Sinclair, 2001) (Table 2). Detection of diabetes during hospital admissions for other comorbidities or acute illnesses is relatively common, although even when hyperglycemia has been recognized initially, about half the subjects receive no further evaluation for diabetes or treatment (Levetan *et al.*, 1998). Some patients do not have the classic features of either diabetic ketoacidosis or hyperosmolar nonketotic coma but present with a "mixed" disturbance of hyperglycemia (blood glucose levels 15–25 mM), arterial blood pH of 7.2 or 7.3 (not particularly acidotic), and without marked dehydration or change in level of consciousness.

IMPACT OF DIABETES MELLITUS

Older patients with diabetes appear to burden the hospital care system two to three times more than the general population (Damsgaard *et al.*, 1987a) and use primary care services two to three times more than nondiabetic controls (Damsgaard *et al.*, 1987b). This latter primary care study from Denmark indicated that insulin-treated patients accounted for more than half of the service provision, mainly due to chronic vascular disease, with a correspondingly high number of hospital clinic visits. Several UK-based studies

Table 2 Varying presentation of diabetes in older people

Asymptomatic (coincidental finding)	
Classical osmotic symptoms	
Metabolic disturbances	Diabetic ketoacidosis Hyperosmolar nonketotic coma "Mixed" metabolic disturbance
Spectrum of vague symptoms	Depressed mood Apathy Mental confusion
Development of "geriatric" syndromes	Falls or poor mobility: muscle weakness, poor vision, cognitive impairment Urinary incontinence Unexplained weight loss Memory disorder or cognitive impairment
Slow recovery from specific illnesses or increased vulnerability	Impaired recovery from stroke
	Repeated infections Poor wound healing

have defined the prevalence of elderly patients in hospital diabetic populations. This has ranged from 4.6% (Edinburgh (Harrower, 1980)) to 8.4% (Cardiff (Hudson *et al.*, 1995)).

Several important population-based and community studies have revealed that diabetes in older subjects is associated with considerable morbidity, mainly due to the long-term complications of diabetes. These include the Oxford Study (Cohen *et al.*, 1991), the Poole Study (Walters *et al.*, 1992), the Nottingham Community Study (Dornan *et al.*, 1992), and the Welsh Community Diabetes Study (Sinclair and Bayer, 1998). In the latter study, in subjects aged 65 years, one in three subjects with diabetes had been hospitalized in the previous 12 months (compared with one in six nondiabetic controls). One in four diabetic subjects required assistance with personal care and older people with diabetes had significantly lower levels of health status compared with nondiabetic counterparts. Visual acuity was impaired in 40% of diabetic subjects (compared with 31% controls) and diabetes was found to be associated with an increased risk of visual impairment (OR 1.50 (1.09–2.05)). Factors that were significantly associated with visual loss in diabetic subjects included advanced age, female sex, history of foot ulceration, duration of diabetes, and treatment with insulin.

Diabetic Foot Disease

A recent study from the Netherlands (Van Houtum *et al.*, 1995) identified increasing age and a higher level of amputation as important factors leading to increases in both the period of hospitalization and the associated costs. The 3-year survival following lower extremity amputation is about 50% (Palumbo and Melton, 1985), and in about 70% of cases, amputation is precipitated by foot ulceration (Larsson *et al.*, 1995). The principal antecedents include peripheral vascular disease, sensorimotor and autonomic neuropathy, limited joint mobility (which impairs the ability of older people to inspect their feet), and high foot pressures (Young and Boulton, 2001).

The majority of the elderly diabetic population is at increased risk of developing foot ulcers and various risk factors have been identified (Table 3). Peripheral sensorimotor neuropathy, which is the primary cause or contributory factor in the vast majority of cases, may cause common symptoms of numbness, lancinating and burning pain, "pins and needles", and hyperesthesia, which is typically worse at night, and evidence of high foot pressures leading to gait disturbances, falls, and other foot injuries. The presence of visual loss may exacerbate the consequences of this situation (Cavanagh *et al.*, 1993).

Table 3 Risk factors for foot ulceration in the elderly

Peripheral sensorimotor neuropathy
Automatic neuropathy
Peripheral vascular disease
Limited joint mobility
Foot pressure abnormalities, including deformity
Previous foot problems
Visual loss
History of alcohol abuse

Erectile Dysfunction

After the age of 60 years, erectile dysfunction (ED) may affect 55–95% of diabetic men, while the corresponding figure for nondiabetic counterparts is 50% (Vinik and Richardson, 2001). ED is defined as the inability to attain and maintain an erection satisfactory for sexual intercourse, and is a complex problem involving several mechanisms: vasculopathy, autonomic neuropathy, hormonal dysregulation, endothelia dysfunction, and psychogenic factors have all been implicated. Drug-related causes may be a particular problem in older patients, with thiazide diuretics, cimetidine, β-blockers and spironolactone especially being implicated. An alcohol history must be looked for. ED is evaluated initially with an interview with the patient and sexual partner where appropriate. A comprehensive history, full medical examination, blood testing for diabetes control, lipids, testosterone, and thyroid function tests are necessary. Other more sophisticated tests are available through diabetes ED clinics in most large centers and may involve testing for prolactin, other gonadotrophins, and for nocturnal penile tumescence. For many older patients, extensive testing is often avoided.

Metabolic Comas

Older subjects with diabetes may present with either diabetic ketoacidosis (DKA) and hyperglycemic hyperosmolar nonketotic (HONK) coma. HONK occurs predominantly in subjects aged over 50 years. Compared to the young, older subjects with hyperglycemic comas have a higher mortality, have a higher length of stay in hospital following admission, are less likely to have had diabetes diagnosed previously, are more likely to have renal impairment, and require a greater amount of insulin as treatment (Croxson, 2001).

The tendency to hyperosmolarity in HONK comas may be worsened in elderly people, who may not appreciate thirst well, may have difficulty drinking enough to compensate for their osmotic diuresis, and may also be on diuretics. It also appears that hyperosmolarity not only worsens insulin resistance but may also inhibit lipolysis.

Death may be due to the metabolic disturbance and to acute illnesses such as pneumonia and myocardial infarction. The cause of the hyperglycemia may be infection, infarction, inadequate hypoglycemic treatment or inappropriate drug treatment. Residents of care homes are also at increased risk of HONK coma associated with appreciable mortality (Wachtel *et al.*, 1991). Thiazide diuretics and steroids are known to increase blood glucose levels and may precipitate DKA; thiazide diuretics and frusemide may be particularly likely to precipitate HONK coma.

Diabetes-related Disability, Cognitive Dysfunction, and Depression

Diabetes is associated with both functional impairment and disability. The wide spectrum of vascular complications, acute metabolic decompensation, adverse effects of medication, and the effects of the condition on nutrition and lifestyle behavior may all create varying levels of impairment and/or disability. These changes may have adverse rebound effects on vulnerability to other comorbidities, independence, and quality of life.

In the *Health and Retirement Survey (1998)* (>6300 subjects aged 51–61 years at baseline), diabetes was identified as an important predictor of failing to recover from a mobility difficulty over a 2-year follow-up period (Clark *et al.*, 1998). In a systematic literature review of longitudinal studies examining the relationships between various risk factors and functional status outcomes (Stuck *et al.*, 1999), diabetes was one of five conditions (others were hypertension, stroke or TIA, arthritis), which reported 10 or more studies showing a significant association between the risk factor and subsequent functional decline.

In a study examining the relationship between various chronic disease states and disability, a survey from Madrid, Spain (Valderrama-Gama *et al.*, 2002), of 1001 subjects aged 65 years and over living at home showed that diabetes was one of four chronic diseases (the others were cerebrovascular disease, depression/anxiety disorders) that had a strong association with disability (OR, 2.18, 1.24–3.83).

The Welsh Community Diabetes Study (Sinclair and Bayer, 1998) revealed significant excesses in physical (Barthel ADL, $p < 0.0001$; Extended ADL, $p < 0.0001$), cognitive (Mini Mental State Examination (MMSE), $p < 0.001$; Clock Test, $p < 0.001$), mobility (use of walking aid, $p < 0.01$), and visual disabilities (Snellen VA chart, $p < 0.01$) in diabetic subjects assessed by objective measures.

In a cross-sectional survey of community-dwelling older Mexican Americans aged 65 years and over ($n = 2873$), the presence of diabetes predicted poorer performance on tests of lower limb function (Perkowski *et al.*, 1998).

The Third National Health and Nutrition Examination Survey (NHANES III) revealed that diabetes was a major cause of physical disability among subjects aged 60 years and over (Gregg *et al.*, 2000a). Disability in at least one of the physical tasks examined was reported in 63% of diabetic women (controls, 42%) and 39% of diabetic men (controls, 25%) with stronger associations between diabetes and more severe forms of disability. Diabetes was shown to have a two- to threefold increased likelihood of a mobility disorder, with coronary heart disease being a major contributor to this excess disability in both sexes, and stroke being an important contributor among men.

Other studies that have examined this relationship include the *Women's Health and Aging Study (2002)* (Volpato *et al.*, 2002) and the *Study of Osteoporotic Fractures (2002)* (Gregg *et al.*, 2002). In this latter study, in community-dwelling white women aged 65–99 (mean 71.7) years, diabetes was associated with a 42% increased risk of any incident disability and a 53–98% increased risk of disability for specific tasks, for example, walking two to three blocks on level ground, or doing housework.

Cognitive Dysfunction

A decline in cognitive function has been demonstrated in older subjects with type 2 diabetes (Strachan *et al.*, 1997). This can be demonstrated using relatively straightforward tests such as the Folstein MMSE (Folstein *et al.*, 1975) or the Clock Test (Shulman, 2000).

The Zutphen Study (1995) (Kalmijn *et al.*, 1995) and the Kuopio Study (1998) (Stolk *et al.*, 1997) showed that impaired glucose tolerance (IGT) is linked to cognitive dysfunction, and increased serum insulin may be associated with decreased cognitive function and dementia in women. The Rotterdam Study (1996) showed that type 2 diabetes may be associated with both Alzheimer's Disease and vascular dementia (Ott *et al.*, 1996), and the Rochester Study (1997) has demonstrated that the risk of dementia is significantly increased for both men and women with type 2 diabetes (Leibson *et al.*, 1997). In a 7-year follow-up study (The Hisayama Study, 1995), type 2 diabetes was associated with an increased risk of developing vascular dementia (Yoshitake *et al.*, 1995). Poor glucose control may be associated with cognitive impairment that recovers following improvement in glycemic control (Gradman *et al.*, 1993). A recent prospective cohort study involving 682 women with self-reported diabetes (mean age of population sample 72 years) followed up for 6 years indicated a twofold increased risk of cognitive impairment and a 74% increased risk of cognitive decline (Gregg *et al.*, 2000b). Women with diabetes for longer than 15 years had a threefold increase of having cognitive impairment at baseline and a doubling of the risk of decline.

In the Framingham Study (1997), type 2 diabetes and hypertension were found to be significant but independent risk factors for poor cognitive performance (on tests of visual organization and memory) in a large prospective cohort sample followed for over 20 years (Elias *et al.*, 1997). This relationship between cognitive decline and with the presence of either diabetes and hypertension was also observed in the Atherosclerosis Risk in Communities (ARIC) study (2001) in a 6-year follow-up of nearly 11 000 individuals aged 47–70 years at initial assessment (Knopman *et al.*, 2001). Hyperinsulinemia in hypertension has also been shown to be associated with poorer cognitive performance (Kuusisto *et al.*, 1993).

Various benefits may accrue from the early recognition of cognitive impairment in older people with diabetes (Table 4). Depending on its severity, cognitive dysfunction in older diabetic subjects may have considerable implications, which include increased hospitalization, less ability for self-care, less likelihood of specialist follow-up, and increased risk of institutionalization (Sinclair *et al.*, 2000).

Cognitive dysfunction may result in poorer adherence to treatment, worsen glycemic control due to erratic taking of

Table 4 Benefits of early recognition of cognitive impairment in diabetes

- Prompts the clinician to consider the presence of cerebrovascular disease and to review other vascular risk factors
- May be an early indicator of Alzheimer's Disease and provides early access to medication
- Allows patients and families to benefit early with social and financial planning and access to information about support groups and counseling
- Creates opportunities to consider interventions for diabetes-related cognitive impairment: optimizing glucose control; controlling blood pressure and lipids

diet and medication, and increase the risk of hypoglycemia if the patient forgets that he or she has taken the hypoglycemic medication and repeats the dose.

Type 2 Diabetes Mellitus and Depression

Diabetes was found to be significantly associated with depression, independent of age, gender, or presence of chronic disease in one study (Amato *et al.*, 1996), also, the presence of diabetes appears to double the odds of developing depression (Anderson *et al.*, 2001). The finding of depression was the single most important indicator of subsequent death in a group of diabetic patients admitted into hospital (Rosenthal *et al.*, 1998). Failure to recognize depression can be serious since it is a long-term, life-threatening, disabling illness, and has a significant impact on quality of life (Egede *et al.*, 2002). Depression may be associated with worsening diabetic control (Lustman *et al.*, 2000) and decreased treatment compliance. In the *Baltimore Epidemiological Project (1996),* a 13 year follow-up of more than 3400 household residents (about 1 in 7 was aged 65 years and over), major depressive disorder had an adjusted OR of 2.23 for predicting the onset of type 2 diabetes (Eaton *et al.*, 1996).

Importance of Functional Evaluation

Functional evaluation of older people with diabetes mellitus using well-validated assessment tools is an essential step in the initial assessment process. Evaluation of functional status should be a multidisciplinary approach and comprise at least three main areas for measurement: physical, mental, and social functioning. However, further evaluation with measures of self-care abilities and independent living skills (generally assessed by activities of daily living (ADL) tools) are also required. The benefits of functional assessment in the context of diabetes is indicated in Table 5.

Functional assessment is a primary component of Comprehensive Geriatric Assessment (CGA), which is an essential methodology for geriatric medical practice (Kane and Rubenstein, 1998). CGA is crucial at the initial assessment, and helpful in planning care and rehabilitation, and monitoring progress. CGA can be performed in many clinical and health-care locations, and not only involves a basic assessment of functional status but also includes various limited screening techniques, evaluation of social and medical problems, instigating initial treatment, and ensuring follow-up. CGA and its variants (including in-home assessment packages) have been demonstrated to reduce mortality (by 14% at 12 months), increase the chance of remaining at home after referral (26% at 12 months), reduce hospital admissions (12% at 12 months), with gains in cognition and physical function having also been observed (Stuck *et al.*, 1993). Not all patients gain from this approach, and targeting is required. Criteria for older subjects with type 2 diabetes who may derive benefit from comprehensive assessment methods with a measure of functional status are shown in Table 6. A summary of the various assessment methods in common use is given elsewhere in this textbook. The authors do not advocate that all practitioners in Europe should adopt CGA as a routine part of their assessment processes, but suggest that functional assessment become a routine measure in older people with type 2 diabetes at diagnosis and at regular intervals thereafter.

Table 5 Benefits of functional assessment: diabetes-related

- Measures ability to comply with treatment goals and adherence to nutritional advice
- Assesses self-care ability and ability to apply sick-day rules
- Assesses the impact of vascular complications of diabetes, for example, peripheral vascular disease, or neuropathy
- Assesses likely ability to gain from educational interventions
- Assesses need for carer support
- Identifies any quality-of-life issues related to the disease or its treatment

Table 6 Criteria for targeting patients with type 2 diabetes for comprehensive geriatric assessment

- Presence of a "geriatric syndrome": confusional state, depression, falls, incontinence, immobility, pressure sores
- Those with several coexisting morbidities apart from diabetes with complex drug regimens
- Those with disabilities due to lower limb vascular disease or neuropathy requiring a rehabilitation program
- Absence of a terminal illness or dementing syndrome

Treatment and Care Issues: Learning from Recent Literature

The major aims in the management of older people with type 2 diabetes involve both medical and patient-orientated factors (Table 7). An initial plan for the early evaluation of patients is reflected in Table 8, which should form a framework for instigating the appropriate treatment pathway. An important aim of risk assessment in the general population is to identify subclinical cardiovascular risk, which may be the principal cause of undetected functional impairment or frailty in older people. Coronary risk charts are often based on Framingham data (Wilson *et al.*, 1998; Menotti *et al.*, 2000) and can be used to identify either 5- or 10-year event rates, but it is important to note that cardiovascular-risk data are based generally on populations of individuals

Table 7 Major aims in managing older people with diabetes

Medical	Patient-orientated
Freedom from hyperglycemic symptoms	Maintain general well-being and good quality of life
Prevent undesirable weight loss	Acquire skills and knowledge to adapt to lifestyle changes
Avoid hypoglycemia and other adverse drug reactions	Encourage diabetes self-care
Estimate cardiovascular risk as part of screening for and preventing vascular complications	
Detect cognitive impairment and depression at an early stage	
Achieve a normal life expectancy for patients where possible	

Table 8 Care plan for initial management of diabetes in an elderly person

1. Establish realistic glycemic and blood pressure targets
2. Ensure consensus with patient, spouse or family, general practitioner, informal carer, community nurse, or hospital specialist
3. Define the frequency and nature of diabetes follow-up
4. Organize glycemic monitoring by patient or carer
5. Refer to social or community services as necessary
6. Provide advice on stopping smoking, increasing exercise, and decreasing alcohol intake

up to a maximum age of 74 years only. In a large proportion of older people with type 2 diabetes, excess cardiovascular risk is evident and active intervention should be considered.

A summary of the therapeutic areas for intervention and the relevant evidence base is provided in Table 9, and a table indicating the main types of insulin regimes employed is given in Table 10. The treatment algorithm that should be used as a framework for glucose regulation in older people with type 2 diabetes is shown in Appendix 1. In the United Kingdom, the license for thiazolinediones (TZD) (pioglitazone and rosiglitazones) has recently been modified to allow "triple" therapy (a TZD and both a sulphonylurea and metformin to be coprescribed).

Appendix 1: Algorithm for Glucose regulation based on reference – European Diabetes Working Party for Older People, 2001–2004

On the basis of these studies and interpretation of the likelihood that older people with type 2 diabetes may benefit (derived from the European Diabetes Working Party for Older People, 2001–2004), a number of major recommendations on therapy can be made.

Glucose Regulation

The management of blood glucose must form part of a multifaceted approach to dealing with the metabolic disorder of type 2 diabetes in older people since most patients have evidence of other cardiovascular-risk factors and at least half are likely to satisfy the criteria for the metabolic syndrome proposed by a WHO Expert Committee in 1998 (Alberti and Zimmet, 1998) and more recently by the International Diabetes Federation (Alberti and Zimmet, 2005).

While there is now overwhelming evidence that the level and duration of glycemia influences the development of diabetes-related complications, specific studies in older subjects (>70 years) with type 2 diabetes are lacking.

The majority of the studies conducted in older populations have involved patients of Caucasian ancestry affected by type 2 diabetes. The applicability of these results to the elderly type 1 diabetic patient or to the non-Caucasian type 2 diabetic patient remains to be assessed. However, no randomized controlled trials assessing the impact of achieving optimal glucose control on primary prevention of cardiovascular outcomes are available in the elderly diabetic patient.

Recommendations

The following represent some of the more important recommendations on glucose regulation taken from the European Guidelines (European Diabetes Working Party for Older People, 2001–2004):

1. At initial assessment and annually thereafter, older patients with type 2 diabetes should have a cardiovascular-risk assessment and evaluation of both microvascular and macrovascular complications. Evidence level 2++; Grade of recommendation C. *Evidence in subjects older than 75 years is lacking and a lower Grade of recommendation (D) may be applicable.*
2. For older patients with type 2 diabetes, with single system involvement (free of other major comorbidities), a target HbA1c (DCCT aligned) range of 6.5–7.5% and a fasting glucose range of 5–7.0 mmol l^{-1} should be aimed for. *The precise target agreed will depend on existing cardiovascular risk, presence of microvascular complications, and ability of individual to self-manage.*
3. For frail (dependent; multisystem disease; care home residency including those with dementia) patients where the hypoglycemia risk is high and symptom control and avoidance of metabolic decompensation is paramount, the target HbA1c range should be >7.5 to ≤8.5%, and the fasting glucose range >7 to ≤9.0.
4. Glibenclamide should not be prescribed for newly diagnosed cases of type 2 diabetes in older adults (>70 years) because of the marked risk of hypoglycemia.
5. In older adults with diabetes, the use of premixed insulin and prefilled insulin pens may lead to a reduction in dosage errors and an improvement in glycemic control.
6. Where the risk of hypoglycemia is considered moderate (renal impairment, recent hospital admission) to high (previous history, frail patient with multiple comorbidities, resident of a care home) and a sulphonylurea is considered, use an agent with a lower hypoglycemic

Table 9 Treatment targets and intervention studies for elderly diabetic patients

Blood glucose levels	Blood pressure	Blood lipid levels	Aspirin use
No specific studies in older people with diabetes	UKPDS: ≤140/80 mmHg (not based on older subjects)	Few studies in older people with diabetes	Antiplatelet Trialists Collaboration: 75–325 mg/day reduced major cardiovascular events in high-risk patients by 25%; NNT 26 (17–66)
	A 10 mmHg (systolic) and 5 mmHg (diastolic) fall in blood pressure in the intensive group resulted in a 24% decrease in risk of any diabetes-related endpoint, 44% reduction in risk of stroke, and 37% risk reduction in macrovascular disease	PROSPER: pravastatin for 3.2 years resulted in a 1.0 $mmol\,l^{-1}$ fall in LDL cholesterol and a modest RR of 15% for the primary composite outcome; no change in the decline of cognition was seen	
UKPDS: HbA1c <7%; fasting blood glucose <7 $mmol\,l^{-1}$	HOT Study: diastolic lowering to ≤83 mmHg	Heart Protection Study:	HOT Study: 75 mg/day reduced major cardiovascular events by 15% and myocardial infarction by 36%; stroke was unaffected
A reduction in HbA1c of 0.9% between the study groups resulted in a 12% reduction in risk of any diabetes-related endpoint, but no significant reduction in major cardiovascular events	A systolic BP less than 80 mmHg resulted in a 51% reduction in major cardiovascular events compared with the target group of equal to or less than 90 mmHg	Treatment with simvastatin for 5 years resulted in a fall of 1.0 $mmol\,l^{-1}$ of HDL cholesterol and a 25% RR in incidence of first nonfatal or fatal stroke	
	SHEP Study: systolic <150 mmHg	LIPID, CARE, 4S, VA-HIT studies: Total cholesterol <5 $mmol\,l^{-1}$ HDL cholesterol >1.0 $mmol\,l^{-1}$	
	A 34% reduction in risk of cardiovascular disease in the actively treated group was observed	Triglycerides <2.0 $mmol\,l^{-1}$	
	Syst-Eur Study: systolic BP <160 mmHg	ALLHAT-LLT : 4.9 years of pravastatin showed modest reductions in cholesterol only and did not reduce mortality or coronary heart disease	
	A fall of 23/7 mmHg in the actively treated group was associated with a 55% decrease in mortality, and a 69% reduction in cardiovascular end-points		
	MICRO-HOPE was not target driven but showed highly significant reductions in cardiovascular risk with ramipril for 4.5 years (22% RR in myocardial infarction; 33% RR in stroke). LIFE study: 24% RRR in primary composite endpoint of cardiovascular mortality, stroke, and all myocardial infarction after minimum 4 years of losartan treatment compared with atenolol. ALLHAT showed that after a mean of 4.9 years of follow-up, there were no significant differences in outcome between chlorthalidone, lisinopril, or amlodipine.	ASCOT-LLA: study stopped after 3.3 years showing highly significant benefits of atorvastatin; a fall of 1.0 $mmol\,l^{-1}$ of HDL cholesterol gave a 36% RR of primary end point but subgroup analysis of diabetic patients showed no benefit	

potential, for example, gliclazide, tolbutamide. *Risk of hypoglycemia: glibenclamide > glimepiride > gliclazide > tolbutamide* (Schernthaner *et al.*, 2004).

7. Optimal glucose regulation may help maintain cognitive performance, improve learning and memory, and may help to minimize symptoms of mood disorder in patients with depression.
8. Optimizing glucose control may help maintain functional status and may decrease the risk of falls.

Blood Pressure Regulation

Adverse cardiovascular outcomes (stroke and coronary heart disease) are clearly and directly related to increasing levels of blood pressure. In nondiabetic individuals, this is more pronounced in men than in women; antihypertensive treatment has been shown to produce worthwhile reductions in risk, especially in high-risk patients such as those with diabetes or the elderly, where the absolute benefit is greater.

Table 10 Practice orientated guidelines for insulin treatment in older people

	Indications	Advantages	Disadvantages
Once-daily insulin	Frail subjects Very old (>80 years) Symptomatic control	Single injection Can be given by carer or district nurse	Control usually poor Hypoglycemia common
Twice-daily insulin	Preferred if good glycemic control	Low risk of hypoglycemia	Normoglycaemia difficult to achieve
	Suitable for type 1 diabetes	Easily managed by most older diabetic people	Fixed meal times reduce flexibility Expensive
Basal/bolus insulin	Well-motivated individuals	Enables tight control	Frequent monitoring required to avoid hypoglycemia
	Can reduce microvascular complications	For acute illness in hospital Flexible meal times	
Insulin plus oral agents	If glycemic control is unsatisfactory with oral agents alone To limit weight gain in obese subjects	Limits weight gain by reducing total daily insulin Increased flexibility	May delay conversion to insulin in thin or type 1 patients

Increasing age is also an independent risk factor for cardiovascular disease even in low-risk individuals with normal blood pressure.

There is an age-related increase in systolic blood pressure but diastolic blood pressure tends to peak at 66–69 years of age and then falls. A large percentage of older patients will have isolated systolic hypertension where the diastolic blood pressure is not raised. Hypertension is also associated with the insulin resistance syndrome in older subjects, and in diabetic subjects who develop microalbuminuria, thus increasing the risk of nephropathy and end-stage renal failure.

Diagnosis of Hypertension in Diabetes

Established hypertension exists when blood pressure readings are persistently above 140/90 mmHg (Korotkov 1-V) over at least 1 month or when the diastolic blood pressure exceeds 110 mmHg, or when there is evidence of target organ damage. As the presence of diabetes imposes a greater cardiovascular risk, it is reasonable to have lower blood pressure thresholds for treatment in these subjects, but most guidelines indicate 140/90 mmHg as the treatment threshold with lower target values for those with diabetes. Four national/international sets of guidelines for hypertension have recently been published, and these can be downloaded from the relevant website or author address: for example, http://www.nhlbi.nih.gov/guidelines/hypertension/express.pdf

Each major guideline has a section on the management of hypertension in diabetes, but age-modification of targets and thresholds is not detailed. In addition, there have been no specific randomized controlled trials in older subjects with type 2 diabetes and hypertension that have directly investigated the benefits and outcomes of treating blood pressure to target.

On the basis of an analysis of these sets of guidelines and the relevant clinical evidence base, the European Diabetes Working Party for Older People, 2001–2004 have set targets described in the clinical recommendations below.

Recommendations

1. The threshold for treatment of high blood pressure in older subjects with type 2 diabetes should be 140/80 mmHg or higher present for more than 3 months and measured on at least three separate occasions during a period of lifestyle management advice (behavioral: exercise, weight reduction, smoking advice, nutrition/dietary advice).
   This decision is based on the likelihood of reducing cardiovascular risk in older subjects balanced with issues relating to tolerability, clinical factors, and disease severity, and targets likely to be achievable with monotherapy and/or combination therapy, and with agreement with primary care colleagues. As most subjects aged 70 years and over with type 2 diabetes and hypertension will already by definition have a high CV risk, no additional weighting for extent of CV risk has been applied. A lower value of blood pressure should be aimed for in those who are able to tolerate the therapy and self-manage, and/or those with concomitant renal disease.
2. For frail (dependent; multisystem disease; care home residency including those with dementia) patients, where avoidance of heart failure and stroke may be of greater relative importance than microvascular disease, an acceptable blood pressure is <150/<90 mmHg.
3. In patients with type 2 diabetes and a recent acute stroke (within 4 weeks), consideration should be given to an active treatment approach of raised blood pressure and lipids, vascular prophylaxis with antiplatelet therapy (aspirin), and optimizing blood glucose control to reduce the rate of recurrent stroke.
   The PROGRESS Study (2001) (PROGRESS Collaborative Group, 2001) *has shown large absolute risk reductions* ($NNT = 11$) with the ACE inhibitor, perindopril (in combination with the diuretic indapamide) in patients surviving from a stroke.
4. Optimal blood pressure regulation should be aimed for to help maintain cognitive performance and improve learning and memory.

Guidelines on Specific Treatment Strategy and Medication

5. In older patients with a sustained blood pressure (≥140/80 mmHg) and in whom diabetic renal disease is absent, first-line therapies can include: use of ACE inhibitors, angiotensin II receptor antagonists, long-acting calcium channel blockers, β-blockers, or thiazide diuretics. *In terms of comparable efficacy, safety, and cost-effectiveness, treatment with a thiazide diuretic may be preferred as the first-line therapy. Short-acting calcium channel blockers should not be used.*
   The choice of antihypertensive agent should take into account metabolic factors, the presence or not of renal impairment or cardiovascular disease, and the likelihood of causing postural hypotension, which may have particularly adverse consequences in older subjects. At the present time, α-adrenoreceptor blockers have no special indications in the treatment of hypertension in diabetes and may be harmful. The use of low-dose fixed combinations of two agents such as a thiazide diuretic plus an ACE inhibitor may also have additional advantages (*European Society of Cardiology, 2003*).
6. In older patients with a sustained blood pressure (≥140/80 mmHg) with microalbuminuria or proteinuria, treatment with an ACE inhibitor is recommended. *An angiotensin II receptor antagonist may be considered as an alternative to an ACE inhibitor where the latter class of drug is not tolerated or contraindicated.*

Lipid Regulation

Coronary heart disease (CHD) is the most common cause of mortality in type 2 diabetes and remains the principal challenge for older people with this metabolic disorder. Elevated levels of blood lipids is an independent risk factor for CHD, and there is published evidence of cardiovascular benefit using a lipid-lowering regimen, although this is limited in older subjects. As part of a multifaceted approach to the metabolic consequences of diabetes, effective management of blood lipids is essential to optimize vascular outcomes. Attention to risk factors such as smoking and other metabolic derangements such as blood pressure is also of paramount importance.

Cardiovascular Risk Assessment

Categories of risk based on lipoprotein levels in adults with diabetes mellitus according to most international recommendations are given without modification concerning age and duration of diabetes. Since general cardiovascular risk is increasing with both variables, especially age, cardiovascular risk in older diabetic patients is generally underestimated according to non-age-specific risk assessment. One approach is calculating global risk in individuals without overt cardiovascular disease (primary prevention) using the Framingham Heart Study equation or the WHO-ISH risk table (Kannel and McGee, 1979; Winocour and Fisher, 2003). Another method relies on a calculation of individual risk on the basis of epidemiological data. For the purposes of this chapter, "high" and "low" cardiovascular risks are described in Table 11.

Table 11 High and low 10-year cardiovascular risk definition

High risk
Has manifest cardiovascular disease (history of symptoms of coronary heart disease, stroke, or peripheral vascular disease) or a coronary (Risk Assessment Chart)[a] event risk of >15%;
Low risk
Does not manifest cardiovascular disease and whose coronary event risk[a] is ≤15%

Adapted from NICE (UK).
[a]On the basis of Joint British recommendations: (BMJ 2000; 320:705–708).

Several large-scale clinical trials have shown benefit with statin therapy of high-risk (cardiovascular-risk) individuals, and these included a proportion of older subjects. They have also demonstrated that these agents are well tolerated and safe, with no consistent additional risk of cancer or nonvascular morbidity or mortality. Previous statin trials indicate that the absolute reduction in LDL cholesterol produces similar proportional risk reductions in older and younger people.

Target Values for Total Cholesterol and LDL Cholesterol

Target values for treatment decisions based on total/LDL cholesterol level in adults with diabetes should be adopted without age limitation, especially in otherwise healthy and independent individuals ("single disease model"). Categories of risk are available depending on lipid levels (*American Diabetes Association criteria*), although treatment decisions based on an estimation of a 10-year cardiovascular (CV) risk may also be used (*National Institute for Clinical Excellence (NICE)* guidelines). Additional measurement of HDL cholesterol provides a more accurate assessment of CV risk because of the inverse relationship between CV risk and HDL cholesterol. These recommendations may not be directly applicable for old (>75 years) and very old (>85) patients because of the presence of multiple comorbidities, high dependency levels, care home residency and/or end-stage dementia ("frailty model") (Sinclair, 2000). In these situations, limited life expectancy or competing noncardiovascular causes for mortality (for example, cancer or infections), may mask or remove any benefit from lipid lowering and increase the likelihood of adverse drug reactions. Lipid regulation on an individual basis is required.

Initial Assessment of the Older Patient

Initial assessment should include enquiry about alcohol consumption, presence or not of renal, thyroid, or liver disease. An estimate of the level of physical activity is important, and overweight (and obese) subjects should be encouraged to lose weight and given exercise advice relative to their capability and overall functional status. Dietary modification may be of benefit as part of a revised lifestyle plan.

Assessments of total cholesterol, HDL-C, LDL-C, and triglycerides are usually required as part of the annual review process (Grade of recommendation C) and should preferably be fasting samples at the start of treatment for those with abnormal profiles.

For these *Guidelines*, an abnormal lipid profile in older subjects can be regarded as a total cholesterol of 5.0 mmol l^{-1} or higher, a LDL cholesterol of 3.0 mmol l^{-1} or higher, or triglycerides of 2.3 mmol l^{-1} or higher.

In general, pharmacological therapy of abnormal lipid levels should not be delayed or ignored because of the age of the individual and should be regarded as part of the routine interventions in managing older people with diabetes. In patients prescribed a statin, the clinician must always be alert to the potential side effects of treatment including reversible myositis and myopathy.

RECOMMENDATIONS

Some of the principal recommendations related to the use of statins and fibrates in older people with diabetes can be summarized as follows:

1. Statin therapy is well tolerated and can be safely used in older subjects with diabetes.
2. Primary Prevention: in subjects with no history of cardiovascular disease, a statin should be offered to patients with an abnormal lipid profile if their 10-year cardiovascular risk is >15%. *There is little evidence at the present time for primary preventative strategies for subjects aged greater than 80 years.*
3. Secondary Prevention: a statin should be offered to patients with an abnormal lipid profile who have proven cardiovascular disease.
4. A fibrate should be considered in patients with an abnormal lipid profile who have been treated with a statin for at least 6 months but in whom the triglyceride level remains elevated ($\geq$2.3 mmol l^{-1}).
5. A fibrate should be considered in patients with proven cardiovascular disease who have isolated high triglyceride levels ($\geq$2.3 mmol l^{-1}).
6. For patients with cardiovascular disease who have persistent raised fasting triglycerides above 10 mmol l^{-1}, referral to a specialist lipid or diabetes clinic is recommended.

CARE HOME DIABETES

Within the European Union, the structure and provision of diabetes care within residential care homes is highly variable. High-quality diabetes care is unlikely to be present in

Table 12 Concerns and deficiencies in diabetes care – institutional facilities

- Increasing number of institutionalized diabetic elderly
- Lack of specialist medical follow-up
- Inadequate dietary care and lack of structured health professional input
- Lack of individualized diabetes care plans
- Lack of educational and training programs for care home staff
- No major intervention studies assessing the benefits of metabolic control and/or educational strategies
- Few national standards of diabetes care

the majority of care homes with many underlying reasons accounting for this rather dismal situation. These include organizational difficulties within the institutions, lack of clarity relating to medical and nursing roles and responsibilities, funding issues, and a lack of a coherent professional framework for delivering diabetes care.

Several deficiencies of diabetes care within institutional settings have been identified (see Table 12). They represent a series of concerns that highlight the need for standards of diabetes care to be established.

A recent UK study highlighted problems in diabetes care delivery (Sinclair *et al.*, 1997). This study involved a medical examination of and semistructured interview with residents with diabetes of long-term care facilities in South Wales, which revealed a prevalence of known diabetes of 7.2%. A third of residents with diabetes tested had a HbA1c >11.0%, 40% of those on oral hypoglycemic agents were taking the long-acting sulphonylureas, chlorpropamide or glibenclamide, and none of the homes had a policy in place for recording hypoglycemic events. Only 8 out of 109 diabetic residents had a specialist follow-up arranged. Other health professional input was minimal.

More recently, a retrospective, cross-sectional study using the *SAGE* (Systematic Assessment of Geriatric Drug Use via Epidemiology) database reported that 47% of residents with diabetes were receiving no antidiabetic medication and that the presence of advanced age, being black, having a low ADL score, cognitive impairment, and a low body mass index (BMI) (<21) increased the likelihood of not receiving antidiabetic medication (Spooner *et al.*, 2001).

These and other studies indicate that diabetic residents of care homes appear to be a highly vulnerable and neglected group, characterized by a high prevalence of macrovascular complications, marked susceptibility to infections (especially skin and urinary tract), increased hospitalization rates, and high levels of physical and cognitive disability. Communication difficulties (because of dementia and/or stroke) lead to unmet care needs and lack of self-care abilities, and water and electrolyte disturbances increase the risk of metabolic decompensation.

PREVALENCE OF DIABETES MELLITUS IN CARE HOMES

A number of prevalence surveys of diabetes within care homes provide estimates of between 7.2 and 26.7%, depending on the method used for identifying those with diabetes.

Additional information from the population-based SAGE database in the United States (Spooner *et al.*, 2001), which involves five states and evaluation of all residents using the 350-item minimum data set (MDS), revealed a prevalence of diabetes of 18.1%, which decreased as age increased (e.g. 27% in those aged 65–74 years compared with 13% in those aged 85 years and over). The highest prevalence was recorded in Hispanics (28%) and black non-Hispanics (26%).

In a recent study of screening care home residents for diabetes using two-point (fasting and 2-hour postglucose challenge values) oral glucose tolerance tests, the overall prevalence rate (newly diagnosed + known diabetes) was calculated as 26.7%, with a rate of 30.2% for impaired glucose tolerance (Sinclair *et al.*, 2001). The majority of diagnoses were made according to the 2-hour values rather than the fasting glucose levels, but it may be argued that these residents are at greater cardiovascular risk and may benefit from an intervention.

Intervention Studies in Care Homes

Few intervention studies of diabetic residents of care homes have been reported. In Denver, Colorado, USA, an educationally based intervention study in 29 nursing homes consisted of providing workshops and follow-up consultations to administrative staff designed to assist in developing and implementing diabetes care policies and procedures (Hamman *et al.*, 1984). By 1 year, a significant increase in the adherence to previously published diabetes care plans was observed, and although hospital admission rates had not changed, total bed days were smaller. Affiliation to a university-based academic faculty may also lead to an improvement in outcomes for nursing home residents with diabetes. In a study from California, USA, significantly better glycemic control was observed in a small group ($n = 47$) of nursing home diabetic residents (mean age 81 years; HbA1 8.9% on oral agents) compared with a group of ambulatory diabetic residents (mean age 66 years; 11.8% on oral agents) with only a small number of associated hypoglycemic events (Mooradian *et al.*, 1988).

A small study (18 subjects) in Stanford, USA (Coulston *et al.*, 1990), demonstrated that residents of care homes who are in good health, and in good glycemic control (mean fasting glucose of 7 mmol l^{-1}), that the introduction of a "regular diet" compared with the standard "diabetes" diet had minimal effects on glucose control, lipid levels, and body weight over a 16-week period. In a small study of Italian nursing home residents with diabetes ($n = 30$; mean age 77 years), the substitution with insulin *lispro* treatment for 4 months as part of a series of treatment periods using regular insulin led to a significant decrease in mean daily blood glucose, HbA1c (7.6 vs 8.5% (regular), $p < 0.01$), and hypoglycemic episodes (Velussi, 2002).

More recently, in an academic nursing home facility, a 5-month educational program on dyslipidemia treatment aimed at physicians and nurse practitioners led to an improvement in the frequency of prescribing lipid-lowering therapy (Ghosh and Aronow, 2003). This New York–based study demonstrated an increase from 26 to 67% for diabetic residents.

Table 13 Importance of early detection of diabetes mellitus in care homes

- Improved metabolic control may improve cognition, decrease the risk of hyperosmolar coma, and lessen osmotic symptoms
- Earlier treatment may delay vascular complications and reduce disability
- Knowledge of diagnosis of diabetes prompts physician to be alert to diabetes-related complications, for example, hyperosmolar coma
- Earlier dietary intervention may delay treatment (and therefore limit adverse drug reactions) with oral agents
- Treatment can reduce symptoms and may increase quality of life and functional well-being

Rationale for Early Detection of Diabetes Mellitus in Care Homes

In view of the absence of clinical trial data, the rationale for early detection of diabetes mellitus has not been justified. However, each resident has a right to active investigation and intervention (where appropriate) and it is feasible that several benefits may accrue from such a policy (Table 13):

Aims of Care for Diabetic Residents

Residents with diabetes in care homes should receive a level of comprehensive diabetes care commensurate with their health and social needs. The two most important *aims of care according to the European Guidelines* (European Diabetes Working Party for Older People, 2001–2004) are as follows:

(1) To maintain the highest degree of quality of life and well-being without subjecting residents to unnecessary and inappropriate medical and therapeutic interventions.
(2) To provide support and opportunity to enable residents to manage their own diabetes condition where this is a feasible and worthwhile option.

Other crucial objectives of care include: (3) achieving a satisfactory (but optimal) level of metabolic control that reduces both hyperglycemic lethargy and hypoglycemia, and allows the greatest level of physical and cognitive function; (4) optimizing foot care and visual health that promotes an increased level of mobility, reduced risk of falls, and prevents unnecessary hospital admissions; (5) to provide a well-balanced nutritional and dietetic plan that prevents weight loss and maintains nutritional well-being; and (6) to effectively screen for diabetic complications regularly especially eye disease, peripheral neuropathy, and peripheral vascular disease that predispose to foot infection and ulceration.

Diabetes Care Home Provision – Modern Approaches

Several important strategies to improve the quality and outcomes of diabetes care within these settings have been proposed (BDA, 1999). A series of recommendations have been proposed by the European Diabetes Working Party on Older People:

Recommendations

1. At the time of admission to a care home, each resident requires to be screened for the presence of diabetes.
2. Each resident with diabetes should have an individualized diabetes care plan with the following minimum details: dietary plan, medication list, glycemic targets, weight, and nursing plan.
3. Each resident with diabetes should have an annual review where the medical component is undertaken either by a general practitioner, geriatrician, or hospital diabetes specialist.
4. If required, each resident with diabetes should have reasonable access to the following specialist services: podiatry, optometric services, hospital diabetes foot clinic, dietetic services, and diabetes specialist nurse.
5. Each care home with diabetes residents should have an agreed Diabetes Care Policy or Protocol that is regularly audited.

CONCLUSIONS

Diabetes mellitus in older subjects represents an often complex interplay between aging, functional loss, vascular disease, and the metabolic syndrome. Type 2 diabetes may be a potent cause of both premature and unsuccessful aging. Functional assessment and estimation of disability levels form part of the important screening process in older adults with diabetes. There is increasing evidence that improving metabolic control will have important benefits even in older subjects. The recently published European Guidelines on managing older people with type 2 diabetes represents an important step forward in the provision of clinical guidance of this often neglected but highly prevalent group. We should encourage more research by randomized controlled design studies that examine the benefits of metabolic intervention and explore the value and cost-effectiveness of different diabetes care models for managing the frail elderly diabetic subject.

KEY POINTS

- Diabetes mellitus has a high prevalence in aging populations and is associated with specific metabolic alterations.
- Cardiovascular disease is a major cause of morbidity and premature disability in older subjects with type 2 diabetes.
- Functional impairment remains a major challenge for clinicians managing older people with diabetes, and a working knowledge of assessment methodology is helpful in planning therapies.
- Cognitive dysfunction, depressive illness, and falls are important complications and strategies to prevent them require being included in the overall management plan.
- Further research (both basic science and clinical) into the pathogenesis and treatment of type 2 diabetes in senior citizens is urgently required.

KEY REFERENCES

- European Working Party for Older People. *Clinical Guidelines for Type 2 Diabetes Mellitus* 2001–2004, Website for downloading: www.eugms.org.
- Gregg EW, Beckles GL, Williamson DF *et al.* Diabetes and physical disability among older U.S. adults. *Diabetes Care* 2000a; **23**(9):1272–7.
- Meneilly GS & Ellitt T. Metabolic alterations in middle-aged and elderly obese patients with type 2 diabetes. *Diabetes Care* 1999; **22**:112–8.
- Rosenthal MJ, Fajardo M, Gilmore S *et al.* Hospitalization and mortality of diabetes in older adults. A 3-year prospective study. *Diabetes Care* 1998; **21**(2):231–5.
- Sinclair AJ & Bayer AJ. *All Wales Research in Elderly (AWARE) Diabetes Study* 1998; Department of Health, Report 121/3040, London: UK Government.
- Sinclair AJ. Diabetes in old age - changing concepts in the secondary care arena. *Journal of the Royal College of Physicians of London* 2000; **34**(3):240–4.

REFERENCES

Alberti KG & Zimmet PZ. Definition, diagnosis and classification of diabetes mellitus and its complications. Part 1: diagnosis and classification of diabetes mellitus provisional report of a WHO consultation. *Diabetic Medicine* 1998; **15**(7):539–53.

Alberti KG & Zimmet PZ. The IDF consensus worldwide definition of the metabolic syndrome 2005; available on: www.idf.org.

Amato L, Paolisso G, Cacciatore F *et al.*, The Osservatorio Geriatrico of Campania Region Group. Non-insulin-dependent diabetes mellitus is associated with a greater prevalence of depression in the elderly. *Diabetes & Metabolism* 1996; **22**(5):314–8.

Anderson RJ, Freedland KE, Clouse RE & Lustman PJ. The prevalence of comorbid depression in adults with diabetes: a meta-analysis. *Diabetes Care* 2001; **24**(6):1069–78.

BDA (British Diabetic Association). *Guidelines of Practice for Residents with Diabetes in Care Homes* 1999; BDA, London.

Cavanagh PR, Simoneau GG & Ulbrecht JS. Ulceration, unsteadiness and uncertainty: the biomechanical consequences of diabetes mellitus. *Journal of Biomechanics* 1993; **26**(suppl 1):23–40.

Clark DO, Stump TE & Wolinsky FD. Predictors of onset of and recovery from mobility difficulty among adults aged 51–61 years. *American Journal of Epidemiology* 1998; **148**(1):63–71.

Cohen DL, Neil HAW, Thorogood M *et al.* A population based study of the incidence of complications associated with type 2 diabetes in the elderly. *Diabetic Medicine* 1991; **8**:928–33.

Coulston AM, Mandelbaum D & Reaven GM. Dietary management of nursing home residents with non-insulin-dependent diabetes mellitus. *The American Journal of Clinical Nutrition* 1990; **51**(1):67–71.

Croxson SCM. Metabolic decompensation. In AJ Sinclair & P Finucane (eds) *Diabetes in Olde Age* 2001, 2nd edn, pp 53–66; John Wiley & Sons, Chichester.

Damsgaard EM, Froland A & Green A. Use of hospital services by elderly diabetics: the Frederica Study of diabetic and fasting hyperglycaemic patients aged 60–74 years. *Diabetic Medicine* 1987a; **4**:317–22.

Damsgaard EM, Froland A & Holm A. Ambulatory medical care for elderly diabetics: the Fredericia survey of diabetic and fasting hyperglycaemic subjects aged 60–74 years. *Diabetic Medicine* 1987b; **4**:534–8.

Dornan TL, Peck GM, Dow JDC *et al.* A community survey of diabetes in the elderly. *Diabetic Medicine* 1992; **9**:860–5.

Eaton WW, Armenian H, Gallo J *et al.* Depression and risk for onset of type II diabetes. A prospective population-based study. *Diabetes Care* 1996; **19**(10):1097–102.

Egede LE, Zheng D & Simpson K. Comorbid depression is associated with increased health care use and expenditures in individuals with diabetes. *Diabetes Care* 2002; **25**(3):464–70.

Elias PK, Elias MF, D'Agostino RB *et al.*, The Framingham Study. NIDDM and blood pressure as risk factors for poor cognitive performance. *Diabetes Care* 1997; **20**(9):1399–5.

European Working Party for Older People. *Clinical Guidelines for Type 2 Diabetes Mellitus* 2001–2004, Website for downloading: www.eugms.org.

Folstein MF, Folstein SE & McHugh PR. 'Mini-mental state'. A practical method for grading the cognitive state of patients for the clinician. *Journal of Psychiatric Research* 1975; **12**(3):189–98.

Ghosh S & Aronow WS. Utilization of lipid-lowering drugs in elderly persons with increased serum low-density lipoprotein cholesterol associated with coronary artery disease, symptomatic peripheral arterial disease, prior stroke, or diabetes mellitus before and after an educational program on dyslipidemia treatment. *The Journals of Gerontology. Series A, Biological Sciences and Medical Sciences* 2003; **58**(5):M432–5.

Gradman TJ, Laws A, Thompson LW & Reaven GM. Verbal learning and/or memory improves with glycemic control in older subjects with non-insulin-dependent diabetes mellitus. *Journal of the American Geriatrics Society* 1993; **41**(12):1305–12.

Gregg EW, Beckles GL, Williamson DF *et al.* Diabetes and physical disability among older U.S. adults. *Diabetes Care* 2000a; **23**(9):1272–7.

Gregg EW, Mangione CM, Cauley JA, *et al.*, Study of Osteoporotic Fractures Research Group. Diabetes and incidence of functional disability in older women. *Diabetes Care* 2002; **25**(1):61–7.

Gregg EW, Yaffe K, Cauley JA *et al.*, Study of Osteoporotic Fractures Research Group. Is diabetes associated with cognitive impairment and cognitive decline among older women? *Archives of Internal Medicine* 2000b; **160**(2):174–80.

Hamman RF, Michael SL, Keefer SM & Young WF. Impact of policy and procedure changes on hospital stays among diabetic nursing home residents – Colorado. *Morbidity and Mortality Weekly Report* 1984; **33**:621–9.

Harrower ADB. Prevalence of elderly patients in a hospital diabetic population. *The British Journal of Clinical Practice* 1980; **34**:131–3.

Hudson CN, Lazarus J, Peters J *et al.* An audit of diabetic care in three district general hospitals in Cardiff. *Practical Diabetes International* 1995; **13**(1):29–32.

Kalmijn S, Feskens EJ, Launer LJ *et al.* Glucose intolerance, hyperinsulinaemia and cognitive function in a general population of elderly men. *Diabetologia* 1995; **38**(9):1096–102.

Kane RA & Rubenstein LZ. Assessment of functional status. In MSJ Pathy (ed) *Principles and Practice of Geriatric Medicine* 1998, 3rd edn, pp 209–20; John Wiley & Sons, Chichester.

Kannel WB & McGee DL. Diabetes and cardiovascular disease: the Framingham Study. *The Journal of the American Medical Association* 1979; **241**:2035–8.

Knopman D, Boland LL, Mosley T, *et al.*, Atherosclerosis Risk in Communities (ARIC) Study Investigators. Cardiovascular risk factors and cognitive decline in middle-aged adults. *Neurology* 2001; **56**(1):42–8.

Kuusisto J, Koivisto K, Mykkanen L *et al.* Essential hypertension and cognitive function. The role of hyperinsulinemia. *Hypertension* 1993; **22**(5):771–9.

Larsson J, Apelqvist J, Agardh DD & Stenstrom A. Decreasing incidence of major amputation in diabetic patients: a consequence of a multidisciplinary footcare team approach? *Diabetic Medicine* 1995; **12**:770–6.

Leibson CL, Rocca WA, Hanson VA *et al.* Risk of dementia among persons with diabetes mellitus: a population-based cohort study. *American Journal of Epidemiology* 1997; **145**(4):301–8.

Levetan CS, Passaro M, Jablonski K *et al.* Unrecognised diabetes among hospital patients. *Diabetes Care* 1998; **21**:246–9.

Lustman PJ, Anderson RJ, Freedland KE *et al.* Depression and poor glycemic control: a meta-analytic review of the literature. *Diabetes Care* 2000; **23**(7):934–42.

Meneilly GS. Pathophysiology of diabetes in the elderly. In AJ Sinclair & P Finucane (eds) *Diabetes in Old Age* 2001, 2nd edn, pp 17–23; John Wiley & Sons, Chichester.

Meneilly GS & Ellitt T. Metabolic alterations in middle-aged and elderly obese patients with type 2 diabetes. *Diabetes Care* 1999; **22**:112–8.

Menotti A, Puddu PE & Lanti M. Comparison of the Framingham risk function-based coronary chart with risk function from an Italian population study. *European Heart Journal* 2000; **21**(5):365–70.

Mooradian AD, Osterweil D, Petrasek D & Morley JE. Diabetes mellitus in elderly nursing home patients. A survey of clinical characteristics and management. *Journal of the American Geriatrics Society* 1988; **36**(5):391–6.

Ott A, Stolk RP, Hofman A *et al.* Association of diabetes mellitus and dementia: the Rotterdam Study. *Diabetologia* 1996; **39**(11):1392–7.

Palumbo PJ & Melton LJ. Peripheral vascular disease and diabetes. *Diabetes in America, Diabetes Data* 1985; 15:1–21, NIH publication No 85–1468, US Government Printing Office, Washington.

Perkowski LC, Stroup-Benham CA, Markides KS *et al.* Lower-extremity functioning in older Mexican Americans and its association with medical problems. *Journal of the American Geriatrics Society* 1998; **46**(4):411–8.

PROGRESS Collaborative Group. Randomised trial of a perindopril-based blood-pressure-lowering regimen among 6,105 individuals with previous stroke or transient ischaemic attack. *Lancet* 2001; **358**(9287):1033–41.

Rosenthal MJ, Fajardo M, Gilmore S *et al.* Hospitalization and mortality of diabetes in older adults. A 3-year prospective study. *Diabetes Care* 1998; **21**(2):231–5.

Schernthaner G, Grimaldi A, Di Mario U *et al.* GUIDE study: double-blind comparison of once-daily gliclazide MR and glimepiride in type 2 diabetic patients. *European Journal of Clinical Investigation* 2004; **34**:535–42.

Shulman KI. Clock-drawing: is it the ideal cognitive screening test? *International Journal of Geriatric Psychiatry* 2000; **15**(6):548–61.

Sinclair AJ. Diabetes in old age – changing concepts in the secondary care arena. *Journal of the Royal College of Physicians of London* 2000; **34**(3):240–4.

Sinclair AJ. Issues in the initial management of type 2 diabetes. In AJ Sinclair & P Finucane (eds) *Diabetes in Old Age* 2001, 2nd edn, pp 155–64; John Wiley & Sons, Chichester.

Sinclair AJ, Allard I & Bayer A. Observations of diabetes care in long-term institutional settings with measures of cognitive function and dependency. *Diabetes Care* 1997; **20**(5):778–84.

Sinclair AJ & Bayer AJ. *All Wales Research in Elderly (AWARE) Diabetes Study* 1998; Department of Health, Report 121/3040, London.

Sinclair AJ, Gadsby R, Penfold S *et al.* Prevalence of diabetes in care home residents. *Diabetes Care* 2001; **24**(6):1066–8.

Sinclair AJ, Girling AJ & Bayer AJ, All Wales Research into Elderly (AWARE) Study. Cognitive dysfunction in older subjects with diabetes mellitus: impact on diabetes self-management and use of care services. *Diabetes Research and Clinical Practice* 2000; **50**(3):203–12.

Spooner JJ, Lapane KL, Hume AL *et al.* Pharmacologic treatment of diabetes in long-term care. *Journal of Clinical Epidemiology* 2001; **54**(5):525–30.

Stolk RP, Breteler MM, Ott A *et al.*, The Rotterdam Study. Insulin and cognitive function in an elderly population. *Diabetes Care* 1997; **20**(5):792–5.

Strachan MW, Deary IJ, Ewing FM & Frier BN. Is type II diabetes associated with an increased risk of cognitive dysfunction? A critical review of published studies. *Diabetes Care* 1997; **20**(3):438–45.

Stuck AE, Siu AL, Wieland GD *et al.* Comprehensive geriatric assessment: a meta-analysis of controlled trials. *Lancet* 1993; **342**(8878):1032–6.

Stuck AE, Walthert JM, Nikolaus T *et al.* Risk factors for functional status decline in community-living elderly people: a systematic literature review. *Social Science & Medicine* 1999; **48**(4):445–69.

Valderrama-Gama E, Damian J, Ruigomez A & Martin-Moreno JM. Chronic disease, functional status, and self-ascribed causes of disabilities among noninstitutionalized older people in Spain. *The Journals of Gerontology. Series A, Biological Sciences and Medical Sciences* 2002; **57**(11):M716–21.

Van Houtum WH, Lavery LA & Harkless LB. The costs of diabetes-related lower extremity amputations in the Netherlands. *Diabetic Medicine* 1995; **12**:777–81.

Velussi M. Lispro insulin treatment in comparison with regular human insulin in type 2 diabetic patients living in nursing homes. *Diabetes, Nutrition & Metabolism* 2002; **15**(2):96–100.

Vinik A & Richardson D. Erectile dysfunction. In AJ Sinclair & P Finucane (eds) *Diabetes in Old Age* 2001, 2nd edn, pp 89–102; John Wiley & Sons, Chichester.

Volpato S, Blaum C, Resnick H *et al.* Comorbidities and impairments explaining the association between diabetes and lower extremity disability: the Women's Health and Aging Study. *Diabetes Care* 2002; **25**(4):678–83.

Wachtel TJ, Tetu-Mouradjian LM, Goldman DL *et al.* Hyper-osmolarity and acidosis in diabetes mellitus: a three-year experience in Rhode Island. *Journal of General Internal Medicine* 1991; **6**:495–502.

Walters DP, Gatling W, Mullee MA *et al.* The prevalence of diabetic distal sensory neuropathy in an english community. *Diabetic Medicine* 1992; **9**:349–53.

Wilson PW, D'Agostino RB, Levy D *et al.* Prediction of coronary heart disease using risk factor categories. *Circulation* 1998; **97**(18):1837–47.

Winocour PH & Fisher M. Prediction of cardiovascular risk in people with diabetes. *Diabetic Medicine* 2003; **20**:515–27.

Yoshitake T, Kiyohara Y, Kato I *et al.* Incidence and risk factors of vascular dementia and Alzheimer's disease in a defined elderly Japanese population: the Hisayama Study. *Neurology* 1995; **45**(6):1161–8.

Young MJ & Boulton AJM. The diabetic foot. In AJ Sinclair & P Finucane (eds) *Diabetes in Old Age* 2001, 2nd edn, pp 67–88; John Wiley & Sons, Chichester.

APPENDIX

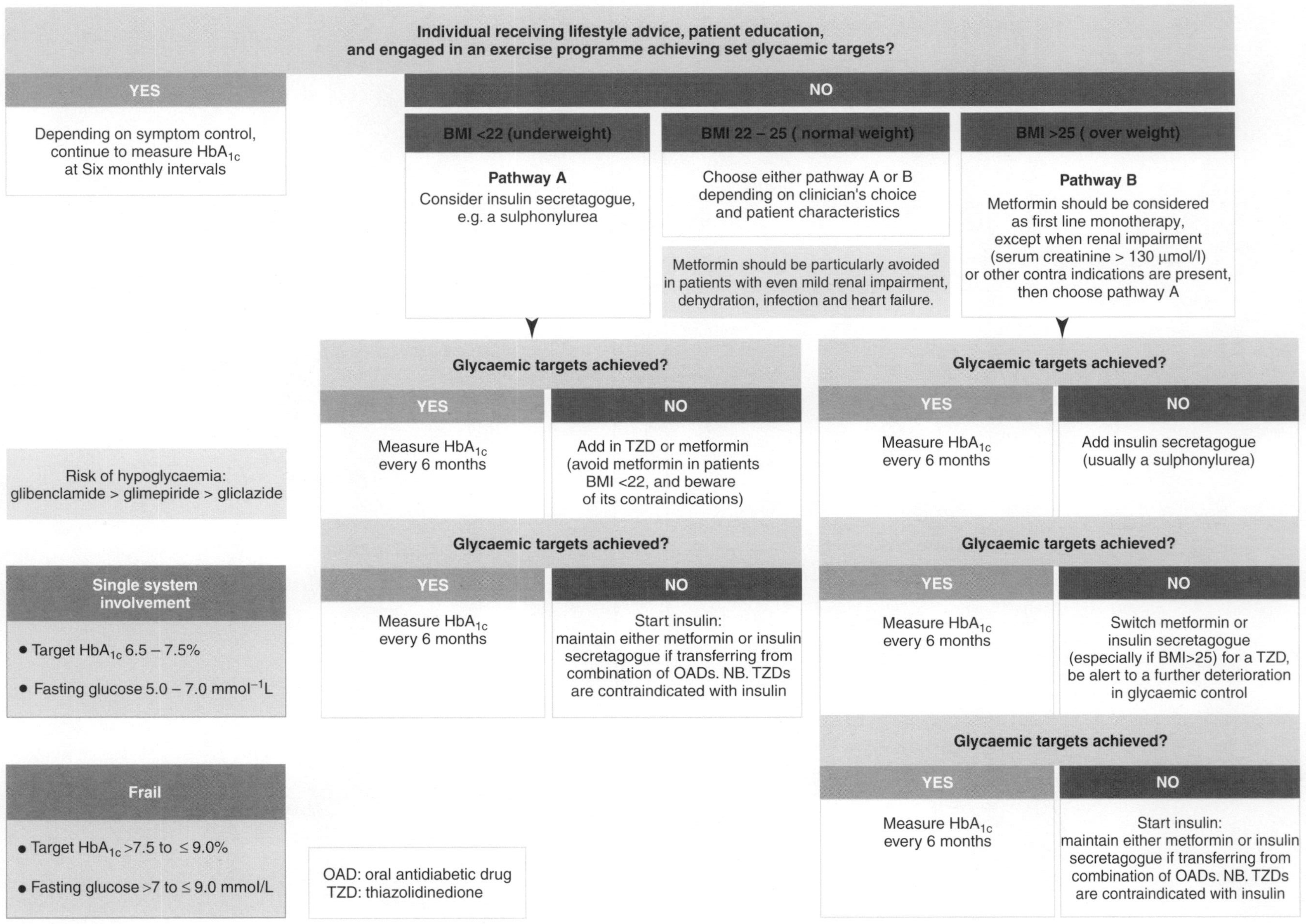

Individual receiving lifestyle advice, patient education, and engaged in an exercise programme achieving set glycaemic targets?

YES

Depending on symptom control, continue to measure HbA_{1c} at Six monthly intervals

NO

BMI <22 (underweight)

Pathway A
Consider insulin secretagogue, e.g. a sulphonylurea

BMI 22 – 25 (normal weight)

Choose either pathway A or B depending on clinician's choice and patient characteristics

Metformin should be particularly avoided in patients with even mild renal impairment, dehydration, infection and heart failure.

BMI >25 (over weight)

Pathway B
Metformin should be considered as first line monotherapy, except when renal impairment (serum creatinine > 130 μmol/l) or other contra indications are present, then choose pathway A

Pathway A:

Glycaemic targets achieved?

- **YES**: Measure HbA_{1c} every 6 months
- **NO**: Add in TZD or metformin (avoid metformin in patients BMI <22, and beware of its contraindications)

Glycaemic targets achieved?

- **YES**: Measure HbA_{1c} every 6 months
- **NO**: Start insulin: maintain either metformin or insulin secretagogue if transferring from combination of OADs. NB. TZDs are contraindicated with insulin

Pathway B:

Glycaemic targets achieved?

- **YES**: Measure HbA_{1c} every 6 months
- **NO**: Add insulin secretagogue (usually a sulphonylurea)

Glycaemic targets achieved?

- **YES**: Measure HbA_{1c} every 6 months
- **NO**: Switch metformin or insulin secretagogue (especially if BMI>25) for a TZD, be alert to a further deterioration in glycaemic control

Glycaemic targets achieved?

- **YES**: Measure HbA_{1c} every 6 months
- **NO**: Start insulin: maintain either metformin or insulin secretagogue if transferring from combination of OADs. NB. TZDs are contraindicated with insulin

Risk of hypoglycaemia: glibenclamide > glimepiride > gliclazide

Single system involvement

- Target HbA_{1c} 6.5 – 7.5%
- Fasting glucose 5.0 – 7.0 $mmol^{-1}L$

Frail

- Target HbA_{1c} >7.5 to ≤ 9.0%
- Fasting glucose >7 to ≤ 9.0 mmol/L

OAD: oral antidiabetic drug
TZD: thiazolidinedione

PART III

Medicine in Old Age

Section 11

Urogenital Disorders

123

Gynecology and the Older Patient

Radha Indusekhar, F. O'Mahony *and* P.M.S. O'Brien

University Hospital of North Staffordshire, Stoke-on-Trent, UK

Based in part on the chapter 'Gynaecology' by Jarmila Wiener and Joan Andrews, which appeared in *Principles and Practice of Geriatric Medicine*, 3rd Edition.

INTRODUCTION

The aging population presents a major challenge for the society and the health services worldwide. It is a reflection of longer life expectancy because of improvements in living standards and health care and falling mortality. In the United Kingdom, people aged 60 and above had outnumbered children under 16 (21 compared to 20%). By 2026, nearly 28% of the UK population will be over the age of 60 (Dening and Barapatre, 2004). Women constitute a majority of the elderly population as they outlive males by 5–7 years. Sixty-five years is the accepted starting point of old age, that is, the official retirement age in the western world. Female aging is unique in that it represents a combination of the aging processes and hormone deficiency. This chapter reviews the problems of the old-age gynecology patient with reference to the common symptomatology, the menopause, hormone replacement therapy, sexuality, and malignancies.

EFFECT OF AGING ON THE GENITAL TRACT

Vulva and Vagina

The lower genital tract undergoes atrophic changes with loss of connective tissue elasticity and thinning of the mucosa. There is a decline in intracellular glycogen production in the vagina, leading to a decrease in lactobacillae and lactic acid and an increase in the vaginal pH from acid to alkali. These changes lead to an increase in colonization by pathogenic bacteria and infective vaginitis. Senile or atrophic vaginitis is also common due to loss of vaginal tissue elasticity and shrinkage of the vagina. This can lead to postmenopausal bleeding and dyspareunia.

Cervix and Uterus

The cervix becomes atrophic and the ectocervix becomes flush with the vaginal vault. The squamocolumnar junction of the cervix recedes into the endocervical canal and it becomes difficult to obtain an accurate representative cervical smear. The uterus undergoes atrophy of myometrium and the uterine body becomes smaller. The endometrium becomes thinner and the glands become inactive.

Ovary and Fallopian Tube

In the perimenopausal years, the few remaining primordial follicles become unresponsive to the pituitary gonadotrophins and therefore the estrogen secretion falls. The ovaries become smaller and more wrinkled. The fallopian tubes become shorter with muscle replaced by fibrous tissue.

Pelvic Floor

Pelvic floor muscle weakness is due to the combined effects of estrogen withdrawal and age. This is compounded by the mechanical effects of previous childbirth. The endopelvic fascia surrounding both the genital tract and urinary tract atrophies. The fascial condensations of cardinal and uterosacral ligaments also atrophy, leading to an increased incidence of genital prolapse as age increases. In the elderly, chronic cough, constipation, and increased intra-abdominal pressure are other factors contributing to this.

Urethra and Bladder

Both the urethra and trigone of the bladder are sensitive to estrogen as they have estrogen receptors and there is deterioration in structure and function as a woman ages. The urethral

Principles and Practice of Geriatric Medicine, 4th Edition. Edited by M.S. John Pathy, Alan J. Sinclair and John E. Morley.

lumen becomes more slit shaped and the folds become coarser. The mucosal lining changes from transitional in the proximal two-thirds to nonkeratinizing squamous epithelium (Stanton, 1997). Urethral closure becomes less competent. There is a reduction in detrusor contraction power during voiding and the contractions fade shortly after initiation of voiding. The bladder capacity is also reduced in the elderly. All these features account for a greater prevalence of urinary incontinence in the elderly. Withdrawal of estrogen may lead to a high prevalence of urinary tract infection in the elderly, which is aggravated by voiding difficulty and may lead to stress incontinence, urge incontinence, frequency, urgency, and nocturia (Dantas *et al.*, 1981).

HORMONAL CHANGES

In premenopausal women, ovarian function is controlled by the two pituitary gonadotrophins, follicle stimulating hormone (FSH) and luteinising hormone (LH). These are controlled by the pulsastile secretion of gonadotrophin releasing hormone (GnRH) from the hypothalamus. The ovary has the maximum number of oocytes at 20–28 weeks of intrauterine life. There is a reduction in these cells from midgestation onwards and the oocyte stock becomes exhausted in the perimenopausal age-group. The ovary gradually becomes less responsive to gonadotrophins and this results in a gradual increase in FSH and LH levels, and a fall in estradiol concentration. As ovarian unresponsiveness becomes more marked, cycles tend to become anovulatory and complete failure of follicular development occurs. Estradiol production from the granulosa and theca cells of the ovary ceases and there is insufficient estradiol to stimulate the endometrium; amenorrhea ensues. FSH and LH levels are persistently elevated. FSH level >30 IU/l is generally considered to be the postmenopausal range.

THE MENOPAUSE AND THE HRT (HORMONE REPLACEMENT THERAPY)

Menopause is defined as the permanent cessation of menstruation. The word menopause is derived from the greek words *menos* (the month) and *pausos* (ending). It is a retrospective diagnosis since a woman is menopausal only after 12 months of amenorrhea. The average age of menopause is 51 years and the female life expectancy is now over 80 years. Postmenopausal women spend more than 30 years in a profound estrogen-deficient state. The early symptoms of menopause are vasomotor symptoms, mainly hot flushes, night sweats, insomnia, and so on. The long-term consequences are osteoporosis, urogenital atrophy, and connective tissue atrophy.

Vasomotor symptoms

There is good evidence from randomized placebo-controlled studies that estrogen is effective in treating hot flushes and improvement is noted within four weeks (MacLennan *et al.*, 2001). Relief of vasomotor symptoms is the commonest indication for HRT and is used for less than 5 years. It must be remembered that as old age approaches, the symptoms of the menopause appear to resolve spontaneously, though of course, the risk of osteoporosis increases.

Osteoporosis

Osteoporosis has been defined by WHO as a "disease characterized by low bone mass and micro-architectural deterioration of bone tissues, leading to enhanced bone fragility and a consequent increase in fracture risk". In postmenopausal women, there is an accelerated bone loss, so that by the age of 70 years, 50% of bone mass is lost. The risk factors for osteoporosis are family history, low body mass index (BMI), cigarette smoking, alcohol abuse, early menopause, sedentary lifestyle, corticosteroids, and so on. Fractures are the clinical consequences of osteoporosis. The most common sites of osteoporotic fractures are the distal forearm (wrist or Colles fracture), proximal femur and vertebrae. Vertebral fractures lead to loss of height and curvature of the spine with typical dorsal kyphosis ("Dowager's hump"). This can affect their quality of life and ultimately impair the respiratory function. There is evidence from randomized controlled trials that HRT reduces the risk of osteoporotic fractures (Cauley *et al.*, 2003; The Women's Health Initiative Steering Committee, 2004). But recent advice from regulatory authorities has been that HRT should not be used for osteoporosis prevention as the risks of such treatment outweigh the benefits (Managing the Menopause – British Menopause Society Council, 2004). After the publication of the Million Women study in 2003, the Committee on Safety of medicines (CSM) pronounced that HRT was no longer to be considered as first line therapy for the prevention of osteoporosis. Bisphosphonates are probably the best choice for the over 60s, though there is actually less data on long-term safety.

Urogenital symptoms

Symptoms such as vaginal dryness, soreness, superficial dyspareunia and urinary frequency and urgency respond well to local estrogen, in the form of pessaries, gel, and so on.

Risks of HRT

Breast Cancer

HRT appears to confer a similar degree of risk as that associated with late natural menopause. In absolute terms, the excess risk in the Womens Health Initiative (WHI) study with continuous combined HRT at 50–59 years was 5; 60–69 years, 8; and 70–79 years, 13 cases of breast cancer per 10 000 women per year (Chlebowski *et al.*, 2003). The unopposed estrogen only arm of this study did not show any evidence of an excess increase in breast cancer risk. The Million Women study found an increased risk with all HRT regimens, the greatest degree of risk was with combined HRT (Million Women Study Collaborators, 2003). So the addition of progestogen increases breast cancer risk compared with estrogen alone but this has to be balanced against the reduction in risk of endometrial cancer provided by combined therapy (Chlebowski *et al.*, 2003; Li *et al.*, 2003). Irrespective of the type of HRT prescribed, breast cancer risk falls after cessation of use, risk being no greater than that in women who have never been exposed to HRT by 5 years.

Endometrial Cancer

Unopposed estrogen replacement therapy increases endometrial cancer risk. Most studies have shown that this excess risk is not completely eliminated with monthly sequential progestogen addition especially when continued for more than 5 years. No increase has been found with continuous combined regimens (Anderson *et al.*, 2003).

Venous Thromboembolism

HRT increases risk of venous thromboembolism (VTE) twofold with the highest risk occurring in the first year of use. Advancing age and obesity significantly increase this risk. The absolute rate increase is 1.5 VTE events per 10 000 women in 1 year.

Cardiovascular Disease (Coronary Heart Disease and Stroke)

The role of HRT either in primary or secondary prevention remains uncertain and currently should not be used primarily for this indication. WHI study showed an early transient increase in coronary events. The excess absolute risk at 50–59 years was 4; 60–69 years, 9; and 70–79 years, 13 cases of stroke per 10 000 women per year. However, the timing, dose, and possibly, type of HRT may be crucial in determining cardiovascular effects. Therefore, HRT should currently not be prescribed solely for possible prevention of cardiovascular disease. The merits of long-term use of HRT need to be assessed for each woman at regular intervals. It should be targeted to the individual woman's needs.

Alzheimer's Disease

While estrogen may delay or reduce the risk of Alzheimer's disease, it does not seem to improve established disease. WHI study found a twofold increased risk of dementia in women receiving the particular combined estrogen and progestogen regimen. However, this risk was only significant in the group of women over the age of 75. More evidence is required before definitive advice can be given in relation to Alzheimer's disease.

Table 1 Common symptoms in the elderly

Postmenopausal bleeding
Discharge per vagina
Pelvic mass
Prolapse
Urinary incontinence
Vulval soreness or itching
Vulval pain

COMMON SYMPTOMS IN THE ELDERLY

Older women are usually reluctant to approach their practitioners due to embarassment when they suffer from the symptoms as in Table 1.

POSTMENOPAUSAL BLEEDING (PMB)

Postmenopausal bleeding is defined as bleeding from the genital tract after 1 year of amenorrhea. A woman not taking hormone replacement therapy who bleeds after the menopause has a 10% risk of having a genital cancer' (Gredmark *et al.*, 1995). In the vast majority of cases, the cause is benign, mainly atrophic vaginitis. The causes are as in Table 2.

Diagnosis

History should include the symptoms, drug history, and smear history. Examination may be difficult in an elderly patient and is further complicated by dementia, immobility, obesity, and arthritis. General examination including BMI, abdominal examination for masses, pelvic examination, both speculum and bimanual examination should be carried out.

Investigation

The principal aim of investigation is to exclude the possibility of cancer. Transvaginal ultrasound measurement

Table 2 Causes of postmenopausal bleeding

Atrophic	– Senile vaginitis Decubitus ulcer from a prolapse
Neoplasia	– Endometrial cancer Cervical cancer, vaginal cancer Vulval cancer, estrogen-secreting tumors, ovarian tumors Fallopian tube cancer, secondary deposits Endometrial polyps
Iatrogenic	– Bleeding on HRT Bleeding on tamoxifen Ring, shelf pessary
Infection	– Vaginal, endometrial
Others	– Hematuria, rectal bleeding, trauma, foreign body

of endometrial thickness will help in directing the need for an endometrial biopsy. An endometrial thickness of less than 5 mm is reassuring that the cavity is empty. The myometrium and ovaries can also be visualized for evidence of tumors. Investigation should also include a smear. Hysteroscopy is now the "gold standard" investigation for postmenopausal bleeding. The procedure can be carried out under general anesthetic or as an outpatient, although cervical stenosis associated with atrophic change may cause failures. It is mandatory for recurrent bleeding, and cystoscopy and sigmoidoscopy may be necessary if there is any doubt about the source of the bleeding.

Treatment

Treatment depends on the cause. If atrophic vaginitis, treatment is by local estrogen therapy. If any carcinoma, management is usually centralized in cancer units staffed by experienced gynecological oncologists.

DISCHARGE PER VAGINA

Vaginal discharge is a common gynecological complaint seen in the elderly. The causes are as in Table 3. Owing to the loss of vaginal tissue elasticity and shrinkage of the vagina, atrophic vaginitis is very common. Infective vaginitis is also common due to colonization by pathogenic bacteria when the vaginal pH shifts from acid to alkali.

UTEROVAGINAL PROLAPSE

Uterovaginal prolapse is a herniation of the female genital tract. It is extremely common with an estimated 11% of women undergoing at least one operation for this condition. The factors responsible for the development of prolapse are weakening of fascia and muscle support following the menopause and damage occurring during childbirth. Raised intra-abdominal pressure from an abdominal mass or cough is a contributory factor in some women as is congenital or postoperative weakness. Uterovaginal prolapse is commonly associated with urinary incontinence.

Table 3 Causes of discharge per vagina

Atrophic	– Postmenopausal vaginitis
Infective	– Bacterial vaginosis, candida, trichomoniasis.
Tumors	– Cervical polyp, intrauterine polyp Cervical cancer, endometrial cancer, Fallopian tube cancer – rare
Fistulae	– Vesicovaginal fistula, rectovaginal fistula
Pyometra	– associated with carcinoma of the endometrium
Others	– Foreign body, pessary

Classification

Anterior vaginal wall prolapse	
Urethrocele	– Urethral descent
Cystocele	– Bladder descent
Cystourethrocele	– Descent of bladder and urethra
Posterior vaginal wall prolapse	
Rectocele	– Rectal descent
Enterocele	– Small bowel
Apical vaginal prolapse	
Uterovaginal	– Uterine descent with inversion of vaginal apex
Vault	– Posthysterectomy inversion of vaginal apex

Diagnosis

Most commonly, the presenting symptom is a feeling of a lump coming down the vagina. They also present with a dragging or bearing down sensation of gradual onset which is worse with activity and settles with rest. A minor prolapse may become symptomatic in the presence of marked atrophic vaginitis. Trophic ulceration may occur with discharge and bleeding. Urinary symptoms such as frequency, urgency, incontinence, incomplete, or slow emptying result from distortion of the prolapsed bladder and urethra. Digital replacement of the anterior or posterior vaginal wall is sometimes necessary before micturition or defecation respectively.

A detailed obstetric history and sexual history to ascertain whether they are sexually active is important to decide the treatment. Also, a medical history like constipation, cough, and any major medical illness should be ruled out. A detailed social history is also important.

General examination: To assess if surgery is safe, to check BMI, and cardiorespiratory system examination.

Abdominal examination: Looking for pelvic masses.

Pelvic examination: Prolapse may be obvious when examining the patient in the dorsal position if it protrudes beyond the introitus, ulceration, and/or atrophy may be apparent. The anterior and posterior vaginal walls and cervical descent should be assessed with the patient in the left lateral position, using a firm Sims speculum. Combined rectal and vaginal digital examination can be an aid to differentiate rectocele from enterocele. Vaginal examination should be performed and pelvic mass excluded. Urine culture and sensitivity, cystometry, and cystoscopy to be considered when symptoms include both stress and urge incontinence and especially prior to consideration of surgery.

Management

The management of prolapse depends on the severity of symptoms, the degree of incapacity and the patient's operative fitness. Operative treatment by repair of prolapse with or without vaginal hysterectomy is most effective. Obesity, heavy smoking, and constipation require improvement before surgery. Most patients tolerate surgery very well because of improved anesthetics and minimal postoperative morbidity. When such surgery is undertaken in an older woman, it is important to ascertain the level of sexual activity as this will influence the degree of narrowing achieved by surgery. Age *per se* is not a contraindication to surgery. Medical disorders develop with advanced age and these dictate any reasons for avoiding anesthesia.

When surgery is contraindicated or declined, conservative methods may be used. A polyvinyl ring pessary will be successful, providing there is adequate perineum to retain the pessary. Some patients, particularly those with large prolapses and very little perineum, may do better with a shelf pessary. Either type needs changing at 4–6 months interval and the vagina should be inspected to ensure no ulceration has occurred. If ulceration occurs, the pessary should be removed for a few weeks and local estrogen used daily to allow epithelial healing.

Physiotherapy: Pelvic floor exercises are useful for the prevention and improvement of incontinence. But they require good patient motivation. Physiotherapy may improve symptoms from a small prolapse but it is unlikely to help with more degree of herniation.

URINARY INCONTINENCE

Urinary Incontinence is defined as the involuntary loss of urine that is objectively demonstrable and is a social or hygiene problem. The causes are as in Table 4. The prevalence increases with age, with approximately 10% of those aged between 45 and 64 years of age being affected, rising to 20% of those greater than 65 years. It is even higher in women who are institutionalized and may affect up to 40% of those in residential nursing homes. This places huge financial demands on health resources, with 2% of the total budget being spent on incontinence services alone. Many women will not seek advice because of embarrassment.

Uninhibited detrusor muscle contractions are usually the cause in geriatric patients owing to age-related changes in the central nervous system. Genuine stress incontinence (GSI) occurs when the bladder pressure exceeds the maximum urethral pressure in the absence of any detrusor contraction and this is common in the early postmenopausal years. In many women, the two conditions exist together.

Table 4 Causes of urinary incontinence

1. Genuine/urodynamic stress incontinence – Bladder neck hypermobility, urethral sphincter weakness
2. Detrusor instability – Idiopathic, secondary to neurological disease – hyperreflexia
3. Retention with overflow – motor neurone lesions, drugs, pelvic mass, severe prolapse
4. Fistulae – Ureteric, vesical, urethral
5. Miscellaneous – Urinary infection

Assessment

A good history will help to differentiate GSI from detrusor instability to some extent. Examination to rule out any associated prolapse or pelvic mass should be carried out in these patients. Urodynamic studies are necessary to confirm the diagnosis, especially prior to any surgical treatment.

Management

Simple measures like exclusion of urinary tract infection, restriction of fluid intake, modifying medication like diuretics when possible play an important role in the management of urinary incontinence.

Genuine Stress Incontinence (GSI)

Conservative management: The treatment of GSI should be nonoperative initially, and the best results for mild/ moderate leakage are with pelvic floor exercises. The rationale behind pelvic floor education is the reinforcement of cortical awareness of the levator ani muscle group, hypertrophy of existing fibers and a general increase in muscle tone and strength. Motivation and good compliance are the key factors associated with success. Local estrogen therapy may have a small effect by improving the urethral mucosa in women with estrogen deficiency.

Surgical Management – the Aims of Surgery:

- Restoration of the proximal urethra and bladder neck to the zone of intra-abdominal pressure transmission
- To increase urethral resistance.

The procedures are Burch's colposuspension, transvaginal tape (TVT), periurethral bulking using collagen, macroplastique.

Detrusor Instability (DI)

DI can be treated by bladder retraining and biofeedback, all of which tend to increase the interval between voids and inhibit the symptoms of urgency. Drug treatment is mainly by Anticholinergics like Oxybutynin, Tolteridine, Regurin combined with local estrogen.

SEXUALITY AND OLD AGE

In the past, it was mistakenly assumed that a woman well past the menopause will not be sexually active. In

1953, Kinsey *et al.* described reduced sexual activity in elderly women. In this group of women, orgasm was more likely to be achieved by masturbation than by coitus (Kinsey *et al.*, 1953). In fact, sexual drive is not exhausted with aging, and as life expectancy increases, it is necessary to recognize that continued sexual activity is an important requirement to promote satisfactory relationships, personal well-being and quality of life (Brown and Cooper, 2003). Many older people were grown up in sexually restricted times so that ignorance is widespread. The organization of institutions for elderly people does not recognize their sexuality, so their needs are ignored (White, 1982). It has been proved that sexual activity remains relatively constant within a stable relationship and declines only following death or illness of the partner (George and Weiler, 1981).

Sexual Response and Aging

In the elderly, the changes of vasocongestion, pudendal swelling, and vaginal lubrication are reduced and delayed, and resolution occurs more rapidly. Also, vaginal lubrication diminishes and there is less vaginal elasticity leading to shrinkage of the vagina. Coital trauma to the vagina and urethra causes dyspareunia, dysuria, and postmenopausal bleeding. Lesions of the vulva like lichen sclerosus (LS) and surgical scarring may make intercourse impossible for some older women.

Health Factors that Inhibit Sexual Activity in Elderly People

Physical factors

- Stress incontinence
- Diminishing mobility
- Decreasing muscle tone
- Uterine prolapse
- Skin tone and sensitivity
- Diseases like diabetes and cardiovascular problems
- Chronic conditions like arthritis.

Psychological factors

- Sense of unattractiveness
- Facing mortality; depression, bereavement, and grief reactions
- Loss of partner or friends
- Lack of contact with others and loneliness.

Effect of Chronic Illness and Surgery on Sexuality

Chronic urological and gynecological conditions causing pain on intercourse, chronic anxiety and stress, neurological disorders, depression and fatigue can result in loss of sexual desire. Disfiguring and mutilating operations, especially of the breasts, genitals and reproductive organs, often have a deleterious effect on a woman's self image and sexuality. Dyspareunia can be a major problem, not only because of lack of arousal or secondary vaginismus after surgery but also because of the amount of scar tissue within the pelvis. Women who have a stoma-like colostomy or ileostomy also experience psychological problems. Patients' greatest fears are loss of control, bad odor, noise, leaking bags, and their partner's feelings toward them. Healthy adaptation to a stoma depends on preoperative and postoperative counseling and understanding by stoma nurses.

Management

A detailed sexual history including the problem, the duration, the couple's past life together and emotional relationship should be taken. Early experiences, difficulties with previous partner and any episode of sexual assault is also important. Examination should aim to look for a physical cause of the sexual problem. Behavioral techniques play an important part in the management of sexual dysfunction. Ignorance about sexuality is common. Changing negative attitudes resulting from past experiences, parental or religious influences will help. Talking to each other about sexual anxieties or needs, and discussion with a therapist increases their mutual understanding and ability to communicate.

Psychological Therapy

The psychological approaches include giving accurate information, general counseling, psychosexual therapy, behavioral therapy, sexual and relationship therapy. Before any operation, it is essential to discuss with the woman, preferably with her partner, the full implications of the operation on their sexual life. This helps to minimize sexual dysfunction after the operation.

Pharmacological Therapy

There is now evidence from randomized controlled studies that testosterone therapy improves sexual satisfaction and mood in surgically menopausal women treated with concurrent estrogen (Burger *et al.*, 1987; Davis *et al.*, 2003). However, long-term safety data for combined estrogen-testosterone therapy are lacking, and the effects of testosterone-only therapy on such factors as plasma lipids in postmenopausal women are unknown.

The use of appropriate creams to help with vaginal soreness – such as estrogen cream, KY Jelly, or aromatic oils may enable a woman and her partner to enjoy sexual activity much more fully.

VULVAL DISORDERS

As the lower genital tract undergoes atrophic changes, the labia majora lose their fat and elastic tissue content and become smaller. The vulval epithelium becomes thin, leading to vulval irritation. Other symptoms are itching and soreness. The conditions affecting the vulva can be a part of a more widespread problem, such as psoriasis or conditions specific to the vulva. Vulval disorders are important because of the chronicity and severity of symptoms and the association with carcinoma. The common vulval disorders are as follows:

1. Lichen sclerosus
2. Squamous cell hyperplasia
3. Other dematoses
4. Vulvodynia or chronic vulval pain.

Lichen Sclerosus (LS)

LS is a chronic skin condition characterized by the thinning of the epithelium with loss of keratin which frequently extends around the anus. The etiology is uncertain, but there is an association with genetic and hormonal factors and autoimmune disease (Meyrick *et al.*, 1988). The clinical signs include pale ivory white plaques often with a crinkly atrophic surface, purpura, and scarring with gradual destruction of the normal vulval architecture. Complications include narrowing of the introitus and rarely squamous cell carcinoma. Punch biopsies should be taken of any suspicious areas. Squamous cell carcinoma is more likely when there is ulceration, raised lesions or lymph node involvement. The most effective treatment is to use topical steroid ointment clobetasol propionate 0.05% plus a soap substitute.

Squamous Cell Hyperplasia

The skin is usually reddened with exaggerated folds. In certain areas, after rubbing, lichenification can be seen. The term squamous cell hyperplasia is applied for those women who have histological evidence for the cause.

Other Dermatoses

The most common general diseases causing vulval itching or discomfort are diabetes, uraemia, and liver failure. Other causes are allergic dermatitis caused by irritants like perfumed soap, washing powder, and so on. General skin diseases like psoriasis, lichen planus, and scabies may also affect the vulva.

Vulvodynia (Vulval Pain)

Vulvodynia is defined as chronic pain, discomfort or burning in the absence of a relevant skin condition. This condition is common in elderly women. The etiology is uncertain but psychological and physical factors play a role. Depression is also a compounding factor. Treatment initially is empirical using topical steroids, anesthetic and estrogen cream. The use of antidepressants should be considered. A multidisciplinary approach involving specialists in dermatology, pain relief, psychiatry, and gynecology is essential for intractable cases.

GYNECOLOGICAL CANCER

The most common types of gynecological malignancies are cervical cancer, ovarian cancer, endometrial cancer, and vulval cancer. Occasionally, skin cancers or sarcomas can also be found in the female genitalia.

Cervical Cancer

Worldwide, cervical cancer is the most common gynecological malignancy. The etiological factors include multiple sexual partners, early age of coitus, human papilloma virus (HPV) 16 and 18 infection. In developed countries, there is an overall decline in incidence and mortality from cervical cancer as a result of the cervical screening program. There is a defined premalignant stage, namely, cervical intraepithelial neoplasia – CIN1, CIN2 and CIN3. Screening for cervical cancer is by cervical smear. Liquid-based cytology and HPV testing are new developments taking place in this field. Abnormal cytological findings are an indication for further investigation by colposcopy and if necessary, directed biopsies or excision biopsy.

Approximately 500 000 new cases of cervical cancer are diagnosed each year in the world with 80% of these occurring in the less developed world (Cancer Statistics, 2003). More than 80% of cervical cancers are squamous cell carcinomas. The presenting symptoms are postcoital bleeding, vaginal discharge, or postmenopausal bleeding. Pain is experienced late and is due to pelvic infiltration or bony metastases. The first sign of this cancer may be obstructive renal failure from hydronephrosis due to advanced disease. On inspection, cancer of the cervix presents as an ulcer, growth, or a friable warty looking mass which bleeds on touch. As the carcinoma progresses, the mobility of the cervix is affected and the cervix eventually becomes fixed. Diagnosis is by biopsy of suspicious areas, preferably under general anesthesia so that clinical staging can be done. Treatment for clinical invasive carcinoma of the cervix is by surgery, chemoradiotherapy or a combination of all three. The management of gynecological cancer patients is now mostly centralized in units staffed by gynecological oncologists, so that all the treatment modalities can be offered to patients. If the disease is in an early stage confined to the cervix, then either surgery or radiotherapy may be offered since the prognosis is equally good for both. Surgery is by radical hysterectomy and pelvic node dissection, that is, Wertheim's hysterectomy. In the elderly, radiotherapy is usually offered because of the fear of surgical complications. However, a fit patient will tolerate the procedure well and age by itself should be no bar to surgery. If the disease is in a late stage, then chemo-radiotherapy is the treatment of choice. In an unfit patient with advanced disease, palliative care may be the only option.

Endometrial Cancer

Carcinoma of the endometrium is considered as the gynecological cancer with a relatively favorable prognosis because of its early presentation with postmenopausal bleeding. The median age of patients with endometrial cancer is 61 years, with 80% of women being postmenopausal. The risk factors are obesity, diabetes mellitus, hypertension, nulliparity, late menopause, unopposed estrogen therapy and prior history of polycystic ovary syndrome. The presenting symptom in the elderly is almost always postmenopausal bleeding. Late diagnosis include pain and discharge from a pyometra. The diagnosis is by transvaginal ultrasound determination of endometrial thickness and outpatient endometrial biopsy. Outpatient hysteroscopy also may be undertaken, but if there is cervical stenosis, then hysteroscopy should be done under general anesthesia. Early disease is treated by total abdominal hysterectomy and bilateral salpingo-oophorectomy. In a poorly differentiated tumor or if the myometrium is involved beyond the inner third, postoperative radiotherapy is given. Advanced cancers are treated with radiotherapy. Progestational agents are used for recurrent disease to control vaginal bleeding and to reduce the pain from bony metastases.

Ovarian Cancer

Carcinoma of the ovary is common in developed countries. The peak incidence is in the 50–70 year age-group. Ovarian cancer remains the most lethal gynecological malignancy despite trials of many different treatment regimens to try to improve the poor prognosis. Most women present with advanced disease. There is no satisfactory screening method for ovarian neoplasia, but women with a family history of breast or ovarian cancer should be offered regular ultrasonic assessment and measurement of the tumor marker, Ca 125. This test is not sensitive or specific enough to be applied to the general population.

90% of ovarian carcinomas in older women are epithelial adenocarcinomas, but sex cord and germ cell tumors may also be seen in this age-group. Also, metastases may be seen from elsewhere, particularly colon and breast. Granulosa cell tumor is the most common sex cord tumor. This produces estrogen which can cause postmenopausal bleeding due to the resulting endometrial hyperplasia.

The presenting symptoms are often vague including abdominal discomfort, swelling, malaise, and weight loss. Later symptoms include abdominal pain and distension, ascites, and pleural effusion. Investigations include hematological, biochemical, imaging techniques like ultrasound and CT scan. Solid areas within an ovarian cyst and ascites are strongly suggestive of malignancy. The final diagnosis is by laparotomy.

Management

The mainstay of treatment is by debulking of the tumor with bilateral salpingo-oophorectomy, total hysterectomy, and omentectomy. Postoperative chemotherapy is used in all but early stages and indeed many patients will have residual disease after surgery. Taxol and Carboplatin are the chemotherapeutic agents of choice. Radiotherapy is limited to patients with symptomatic recurrence and is used only for palliation.

Vulval Cancer

Vulval cancer is a less common cancer and is most frequently seen in the 60–70 year age-group. The presenting symptoms are soreness, pruritus, irritation, ulceration, lump, or bleeding. Many women present very late because of embarrassment. Ninety-five percent of vulval carcinomas are squamous cell carcinomas, but basal cell carcinoma, malignant melanoma and adenocarcinoma of the Bartholin's gland may occur rarely. Diagnosis can be confirmed only by vulval biopsy.

Management

Radical vulvectomy with bilateral groin node dissection is the treatment of choice. The common complications are wound breakdown and infection. The primary tumor is resected and separate groin node dissections are performed to improve wound healing and reduce infection. The other complications are deep vein thrombosis, osteitis pubis, secondary hemorrhage, and so on. For patients unfit for surgery, wide excision of the lesion may be used as palliation. Pelvic irradiation is available for extensive nodal involvement.

HIV AND OLD AGE

The majority of those infected and affected by HIV are younger adults. The ability of highly active antiretroviral therapies (HAART) to extend survival means that those infected when younger may reach older age and so an increase in numbers of older individuals living with HIV is expected. There is evidence that older individuals engage in risky sexual behaviors and are drug users, suggesting potential for HIV transmission (Dougan *et al.*, 2004). For older women after menopause, condom use becomes unimportant, and normal aging changes such as a decrease in vaginal lubrication and thinning vaginal walls can put them at higher risk during unprotected sexual intercourse.

Doctors may not discuss with their older patients about HIV/AIDS because they do not think they are at risk or they presume symptoms to be age related. As a result, many older people are diagnosed at a later stage in their infection, and many have an AIDS diagnosis the first time they become aware of their HIV infection. Older people are more likely to be diagnosed with HIV at a generally higher viral load and lower CD4+ cell count, making them more susceptible to opportunistic infections. More aggressive therapy may be required to successfully suppress the virus.

Data from the Center for Disease Control (CDC) HIV/AIDS surveillance report showed that 11% of all AIDS cases reported in 1999 were among people aged 50 and above (Centre for Disease Control, 1998). This percentage has remained stable since 1991. However, the CDC notes an alarming trend in that older AIDS patients had a greater increase in opportunistic infections than did younger AIDS patients. The report also says a higher proportion of people aged 50 and above died within 1 month of AIDS diagnosis. These deaths can be attributed to original misdiagnosis and immune systems that naturally weaken with age. These statistics seem to confirm the idea that older adults are naive about their risk of contracting HIV and their providers aren't discussing that risk with them. A 1997 study of Texas doctors found that most physicians rarely or never discussed HIV and risk factors with their older patients (Skiest and Keiser, 1997). Compounding the problem, AIDS symptoms often are more difficult to diagnose in older people because they mimic some common diseases associated with old age. Because of the stigma, it can be difficult for women to disclose their HIV status to family, friends, and their community.

For these reasons, physicians should keep HIV in mind as a possibility, even with their older patients. HIV experts recommend that physicians routinely ask all patients about their sexual behaviors during the annual physical or gynecological examination. Providers should educate the population over 50 years about possible exposures to HIV and safer sex practices.

CONCLUSION

Gynecology for the elderly patient includes the whole spectrum of gynecological disorders of which cancer, prolapse, urinary incontinence, and the problems of late menopause are the most important ones. The advice given for such women changes with each decade. Of particular note is our increasing reluctance to give long-term HRT and our increasing likelihood of undertaking surgery in women who are healthy despite their age. Many women, through fear and embarrassment avoid telling their problems to general practitioners, geriatricians, or gynecologists and so present with long standing disease.

KEY POINTS

- The female aging process is unique in that it represents a combination of the aging processes and hormone deficiency.
- Managing the menopause should be targeted to individual women's needs. Hormone replacement still offers the potential for benefit to outweigh the harm, provided the appropriate regimen has been instigated in terms of dose, route, and combination.
- Age *per se* should not be a contraindication to surgical management for any gynecological problem.
- There is no age limit for the expression of sexuality. The management of sexual problems should be guided by the same principles irrespective of age and condition of the patient.
- Older women, out of fear and embarrassment neglect early symptoms of gynecological diseases, some of which are potentially lethal.

KEY REFERENCES

- Brown ADG & Cooper TK. *Gynaecological Disorders.* Geriatric Medicine: Women's health Section 2, chapter 90, 2003, pp 1135–44, Churchill Livingstone.
- Dening T & Barapatre C. Mental health and the ageing population. *The Journal of the British Menopause Society* 2004; **10**:49–53.
- Managing the Menopause – British Menopause Society Council. *Consensus Statement on Hormone Replacement Therapy*, June 2004.
- Million Women Study Collaborators. Breast cancer and hormone replacement therapy in the Million Women Study. *Lancet* 2003; **362**:419–27.
- Stanton SL. Gynaecology in the elderly. *Gynaecology* 1997, 2nd edn, pp 915–9; Churchill Livingstone.

REFERENCES

Anderson GL, Judd HL, Kaunitz AM *et al.*, Women's Health Initiative Investigators. Effects of estrogen plus progestin on gynaecologic cancer and associated diagnostic procedures: the Women's Health Initiative randomised trial. *The Journal of the American Medical Association* 2003; **290**:1739–48.

Brown ADG & Cooper TK. *Gynaecological Disorders.* Geriatric Medicine: Women's health Section 2, Chapter 90, 2003, pp 1135–44, Churchill Livingstone.

Burger HG, Hailes J, Nelson J & Menelaus M. Effect of combined implants of oestradiol and testosterone on libido in postmenopausal women. *British Medical Journal* 1987; **294**:936–7.

Cancer Statistics. *Cervical Cancer-UK* January 2003; Cancer Research UK, London.

Cauley JA, Robbins J, Chen Z *et al.*, Women's Health Initiative Investigators. Effects of estrogen plus progestin on risk of fracture and bone mineral density: the Women's Health Initiative randomised trial. *The Journal of the American Medical Association* 2003; **290**:1729–38.

Centre for Disease Control. AIDS among persons aged greater than or equal to 50 years- United States, 1991 – 1996. *Morbidity and Mortality Weekly Report* 1998; **47**:21–7.

Chlebowski RT, Hendrix SL, Langer RD *et al.* Influence of estrogen plus progestin on breast cancer and mammography in healthy postmenopausal women. The Women's Health Initiative randomised trial. *The Journal of the American Medical Association* 2003; **289**:3243–53.

Dantas A, Kasviki-Charvati P, Papanawiotou P & Marketos S. Bacteriuria and survival in old age. *The New England Journal of Medicine* 1981; **304**:939–43.

Davis S, Rees M, Ribot J & Moufarege A. Efficacy and safety of testosterone patches for the treatment of low sexual desire in surgically menopausal women. *59th Annual Meeting of the American Society for Reproductive Medicine*, San Antonio, 11–15th October 2003.

Dening T & Barapatre C. Mental health and the ageing population. *The Journal of the British Menopause Society* 2004; **10**:49–53.

Dougan S, Payne LJ, Brown AE *et al.* Past it? HIV and older people in England, Wales and Northern Ireland. *Epidemiology and Infection* 2004; **132**(6):1151–60.

George L & Weiler SJ. Sexuality in middle and late life. *Archives of General Psychiatry* 1981; **38**:919–23.

Gredmark T, Kvint S, Havel G & Mattsson L-A. Histopathological findings in women with postmenopausal bleeding. *British Journal of Obstetrics & Gynaecology* 1995; **102**:133–6.

Kinsey AC, Pomeroy WB, Martin CE & Gebhard PH. *Sexual Behaviour in the Human Female* 1953, WB Saunders, Philadelphia.

Li CI, Malone KE, Porter PL *et al.* Relationship between long durations and different regimens of hormone replacement therapy and risk of breast cancer. *The Journal of the American Medical Association* 2003; **289**:3254–63.

MacLennan A, Lester S & Moore V. Oral oestrogen replacement therapy versus placebo for hot flushes. *Cochrane Database of Systematic Reviews* 2001; **1**:CD002978.

Managing the Menopause – British Menopause Society Council. *Consensus Statement on Hormone Replacement Therapy*, June 2004.

Meyrick TRH, Ridley CM, McGibbon DH *et al.* Lichen sclerosis et atrophicus and autoimmunity; a study of 350 women. *The British Journal of Dermatology* 1988; **118**:41–6.

Million Women Study Collaborators. Breast cancer and hormone replacement therapy in the Million Women Study. *Lancet* 2003; **362**:419–27.

Skiest DJ & Keiser P. Human immunodeficiency virus infection in patients older than 50 years. A survey of primary care physicians' beliefs, practices, and knowledge. *Archives of Family Medicine* 1997; **6**:289–94.

Stanton SL. Gynaecology in the elderly. *Gynaecology* 1997, 2nd edn, pp 915–9; Churchill Livingstone.

The Women's Health Initiative Steering Committee. Effects of conjugated equine estrogen in postmenopausal women with hysterectomy: the Women's Health Initiative randomised controlled trial. *The Journal of the American Medical Association* 2004; **291**:1701–12.

White CB. Sexual interest, attitudes, knowledge and sexual history in relation to sexual behaviour in the institutionalised aged. *Archives of Sexual Behavior* 1982; **11**:11–22.

124

The Aging Bladder

James M. Cummings *and* **Kimberly C. Berni**
Saint Louis University, St Louis, MO, USA

INTRODUCTION

The increase in human life expectancy unmasked a variety of genitourinary complaints. Most physicians are familiar with lower urinary tract symptoms (LUTS) suffered by the aging male related to prostatic enlargement. Equally debilitating though are bladder symptoms found in both sexes totally unrelated to obstruction of any kind. Symptoms of frequency, urgency and urge incontinence, commonly lumped together under the term "overactive bladder" are very prevalent in the aging patient and confront the physicians who care for them on a daily basis.

A multitude of other influences on the bladder also exist that affect its performance over a lifetime. Certainly, injury from infection or surgery can affect vesical function over both long and short-term horizons. Changes in the bladder outlet via prostatic obstruction in males or overzealous surgery in women can have effects ranging from mild to devastating, on detrusor function. Alterations in the neurological milieu of the lower urinary tract can profoundly alter bladder function. These variations, when severe enough, can not only create difficult symptomatology for the patient but can also occasionally be detrimental to renal function.

In this chapter, we hope to examine the aging bladder from a number of angles. The alterations in vesical anatomy, both gross and microscopic, are important in dysfunctional voiding and incontinence associated with aging. Neuronal and hormonal changes influence the aging bladder. Pharmaceutical agents are under intense scrutiny as to their effect in the urinary tract as well as their side effects in the elderly patient. Finally, special disease states found mostly in the older population have specific effects on the urinary tract that must be considered in the overall therapy for those diseases.

ANATOMY OF THE AGING BLADDER

The normal bladder is characterized grossly by its pelvic position in the adult. In the older male, the macroscopic anatomy of the bladder is most commonly affected by the growth of the prostate gland. Although most commonly, benign prostate growth occurs in the transition zone surrounding the urethra, occasionally this growth becomes unrestrained in a cephalad manner and pushes the trigone superiorly to give the bladder an elevated appearance radiographically. Gross inspection of the bladder interior often demonstrates a trabeculated appearance (Cockett *et al.*, 1992). Trabeculations are often thought to be a sign of chronic obstruction in males, but have been observed in the female bladder as well (Groutz *et al.*, 2001).

In women, the anatomical position of the bladder is most often altered by defects in the pelvic floor musculature. This leads to the presentation of cystoceles, effectively a herniation of the bladder through the anterior vaginal muscle layers. This defect, as well as rectoceles and enteroceles are commonly noted in parous individuals, although the impact of aging, obesity, and possibly, neurological dysfunction can be substantial (Pinho *et al.*, 1990; Constantinou *et al.*, 2002; Cummings and Rodning, 2000; Bakas *et al.*, 2001). Perucchini has demonstrated localized striated urethral muscle loss with aging at the bladder neck and dorsal wall of the urethra (Perucchini *et al.*, 2002). Others have shown an increase in paraurethral connective tissue in elderly females with a reduction of blood vessels (Verelst *et al.*, 2002). Falconer has demonstrated altered collagen production in women with stress incontinence with poor quality collagen seen in postmenopausal women possibly contributing to disorders related to prolapse in the elderly (Falconer *et al.*, 1994, 1996).

The histologic appearance of the aging bladder can give clues about its ultimate ability to function as a storage facility for urine. Ultrastructural changes in the aging bladder include collagen deposition, muscle degeneration, and axonal degeneration (Elbadawi *et al.*, 1993). The degree of these changes may correlate with specific abnormalities in voiding and incontinence such as detrusor overactivity and impaired contractility (Elbadawi, 1995). Chronic ischemia of the bladder may play a large causative role in these changes (Azadzoi *et al.*, 1999a,b).

Principles and Practice of Geriatric Medicine, 4th Edition. Edited by M.S. John Pathy, Alan J. Sinclair and John E. Morley.

Table 1 Anatomical changes of the aging bladder

Gross anatomical changes
Trabeculations
Cystocele (females)
Muscle loss at bladder neck (females)
Histologic changes
Collagen deposition
Muscle degeneration
Axonal degeneration

Surgical procedures in both sexes can alter vesical anatomy. In females with pelvic prolapse and/or stress incontinence, certainly operations can successfully reposition the bladder and other pelvic organs toward normalcy. They also can cause difficulties if, for example, bladder neck prolapse is overcorrected and obstruction occurs. Certain women will suffer urgency and frequency symptoms even if no obstruction is present (Dunn *et al.*, 2004). In males, relief of obstruction at the level of the prostate may improve symptoms but changes in bladder configuration may not occur at the same rapid rate seen in symptom reduction. Furthermore, radical prostatectomy in the man with prostate cancer may alter bladder dynamics as well as cause sphincteric incontinence (Sebesta *et al.*, 2002). The anatomical changes of the aging bladder are summarized in Table 1.

BLADDER PHYSIOLOGY AND CORRELATION TO ANATOMY OF THE AGING BLADDER

Bladder function involves both the storage of urine and the expulsion of urine at a socially appropriate time. To maintain continence, the storage of urine must occur under low pressures and the bladder must empty adequately. Unfortunately, aging results in changes that occur intrinsically and extrinsically to the bladder that affect continence and emptying. Pathologic changes are seen in the bladder because of aging. In addition, nerve transmission can be altered because of age, disease states, surgical procedures, or drugs. Anatomic obstruction or lack of adequate support of the bladder neck also changes the ability of the bladder to empty and store urine.

The bladder consists of two parts: the body and the base or bladder neck. The smooth muscle fibers of the body are arranged randomly and those of the bladder neck are arranged in an inner longitudinal and outer circular layer. In the male urethra, the sphincter consists of both smooth muscles and striated muscles. The external sphincter consists of the periurethral striated muscle and the intramural striated muscle or rhabdosphincter. In the female, these muscles are attenuated. DeLancey proposes that female continence is created by a combination of muscular coaptation and passive compression of the urethra by the pubourethral hammock (DeLancey, 1989).

During urine storage, low level afferent bladder stimulation signals sympathetic contraction of the bladder neck and relaxation of the detrusor muscle or body of the bladder. This results in storage of urine under low pressure. The voiding reflex is initiated when afferent activity becomes intense. The pontine micturition center stimulates the parasympathetic pathway and inhibits the sympathetic pathway resulting in relaxation of the bladder outlet and contraction of the detrusor muscle and thus bladder emptying. The striated external sphincter, which has separate innervation from the bladder neck, is also influenced by the pontine micturition and storage centers. The voiding reflex results in inhibition of the external sphincter and the storage reflex results in activation of the pudendal nerve.

The bladder must be able to distend and contract adequately, for proper functioning. Structural changes in the tissues and abnormalities in bladder shape can alter urine storage and emptying. Bladder compliance is a measurable value defined as the change in volume divided by the change in intravesical pressure. A normally functioning bladder fills under a low pressure; therefore the bladder is compliant. Compliance is greatly affected by tissue composition, innervation, and vascular supply.

Histologic studies have shown that as collagen levels increase, compliance is lost (Macarak and Howard, 1999). Landau demonstrated that in bladders with poor compliance, the ratio of Type III to Type I collagen was significantly higher than that of normal bladders (Landau *et al.*, 1994). The aged bladder has a higher deposition of collagen; in addition, innervation of the detrusor smooth muscle changes with age. Neurochemical studies of human detrusor strips have shown an increase in purinergic neurotransmission and a decrease in cholinergic neurotransmission with age. It is felt that the shift in neurochemical transmission may change the resting tone of the bladder and contribute to the overactive bladder symptoms in aged bladders (Yoshida *et al.*, 2004).

Bladder wall blood flow is affected by intramural tension. A bladder with poor compliance has increased intravesical pressure and intramural tension, and therefore, a greater decrease in bladder blood flow (Ohnishi *et al.*, 1994). Ischemia can result in diminished contractility and patchy denervation (Van Arsdalen *et al.*, 1983). The end result is a bladder that empties inadequately and may have detrusor instability (Brading, 1997). Injured areas of the bladder can become weak and form diverticulum, resulting in ineffective bladder emptying.

The complexity of voiding dysfunction in the aged bladder makes it difficult to distinguish between the changes in the bladder that are secondary to the normal aging process and changes as a result of bladder outlet obstruction, or changes caused by diseases affecting the nervous system and/or vascular supply. Certainly, the LUTS of obstruction, instability, and impaired detrusor function often overlap. The changes seen in bladder function with aging must certainly overlap as well. A study by Homma found the symptoms of urgency, frequency, and nocturia increased with age in both men and women. The cystometric capacity declined with age in both sexes (Homma *et al.*, 1994).

Histologic changes in the aged bladder have been documented, including increased collagen deposition, widened spaces between muscle fibers, and ultrastructural changes of the smooth muscle cell membrane (Levy and Wight, 1990; Elbadawi *et al.*, 1993). Elbadawi *et al.* showed that aged bladders without urodynamic evidence of obstruction had muscle cell membranes with dominant dense bands and depleted caveolae (Elbadawi *et al.*, 1993). These findings were reproducible and different from the ultrastructural changes seen with obstructed, overactive or hypocontractile bladders (Hailemariam *et al.*, 1997). These findings are thought to represent dedifferentiation of the smooth muscle fibers.

Changes in bladder compliance, nerve transmission, and vascularity, occur as the bladder ages. Certainly, multiple disease processes may worsen these changes. With advanced age, the expected bladder symptoms might include increasing frequency and urgency with a decreased bladder capacity.

SPECIAL DISEASE STATES

Several disease states especially affect the bladder in the geriatric population. Irrespective of whether it is caused by neurological disease, endocrine problems, iatrogenic intervention, or the aging process itself, these problems exact a particular morbidity on the lower genitourinary tract. The following conditions are particularly important.

Parkinson's Disease

Parkinson's disease affects 1% of all patients over the age of 60 and is rarely seen in those under 40. In addition to the characteristic tremors and motion deficits, the loss of dopaminergic neurons in the substantia nigra of the basal ganglia affects voiding by reducing the inhibitory effect of the basal ganglia on the micturition reflex as demonstrated in several animal studies (Albanese *et al.*, 1988; Yoshimura *et al.*, 1992).

The voiding symptoms of Parkinson's disease are frequency, urgency, and urge incontinence. These irritative symptoms are present in well over half of all patients with the disorder (Pavlakis *et al.*, 1983). A significant problem from a diagnostic viewpoint is the presence of these symptoms in elderly males. These irritative voiding symptoms mimic the LUTS associated with bladder outlet obstruction related to Benign Prostatic Hyperplasia (BPH). Without urodynamic evaluation, the neurogenic component to the symptoms may be overlooked, or not quantified well, and inappropriate therapy instituted. Furthermore, men with multiple systems atrophy rather than true Parkinson's disease may actually have mild detrusor-sphincter dyssynergia, which again could mimic the obstructive symptoms of BPH (Stocchi *et al.*, 1997).

The typical urodynamic findings of Parkinson's are detrusor hyperreflexia on filling cystometry. As much as 79% of bladder dysfunction in these patients can be related to hyperreflexia (Araki *et al.*, 2000). Other findings are not uncommon though. Hyporeflexia is present in 16% of patients in Araki's study (Araki *et al.*, 2000). Obstruction can also be present particularly in the male with prostatic enlargement or stricture disease from previous interventions. Multichannel urodynamics is essential to the evaluation of voiding dysfunction in patients with Parkinson's Disease.

Cerebrovascular Accident (CVA)

Stroke can be considered a major health problem among elderly patients. Roughly three-fourths of the 400 000 stroke patients per year in the United States are over the age of 65. The impact of this disorder on voiding and continence can range from mild to profound. When occurring in the aged patient, its effects can magnify preexisting bladder conditions and cause great confusion as to what the proper therapy should be. Depending on the location of the ischemic event, the bladder may range from hyperreflexic to areflexic. One can therefore present with an entire range of symptoms anywhere from nocturia and urgency/urge incontinence to voiding difficulties and urinary retention (Sakakibara *et al.*, 1996). The presence of urinary incontinence in the acute phase of a Cerebrovascular Accident (CVA) is a powerful predictor of a negative outcome (Wade and Hewer, 1985).

The patient presenting with LUTS following a CVA can be a diagnostic dilemma. In one study, detrusor hyperreflexia was seen in 68% of patients, detrusor-sphincter dyssynergia in 14%, and uninhibited sphincter relaxation in 36% (Sakakibara *et al.*, 1996). In that same study, there were patients with retention who were noted to have detrusor areflexia with an unrelaxing sphincter. No correlation was seen between site of lesion and urodynamic findings. In the elderly post-CVA male, neurogenic bladder problems may coexist with obstruction from the prostate gland. Nitti found in a group of men with a mean age of 70 with voiding complaints following a stroke that detrusor hyperreflexia was present in 82% of the group, but pressure-flow characteristics of definite obstruction were present in 63% (Nitti *et al.*, 1996). Multichannel urodynamics can be an important adjunct in the urologic management of these patients.

Nocturia

Nocturia is commonly listed as a symptom by the older patients. In males, it is often perceived as related to prostate enlargement. But this symptom is also commonly noted among aging women (Lose *et al.*, 2001). Menopausal status may contribute to the presence of nocturia (Chen *et al.*, 2003). In all likelihood, nocturia is a manifestation of normal aging.

Other factors impacting the presence of nocturia in the aging individual include sleep difficulties and nocturnal polyuria. Sleep disturbances are common in the elderly population and nocturia may be more related to those problems, rather than to a urinary tract dysfunction. Furthermore, the patient with nocturia, whatever be its cause, will have poorer sleep (Middelkoop *et al.*, 1996). The problem of nocturnal polyuria in many of the elderly, which is reported as nocturia, can be difficult to manage. With lower renal concentrating ability, poorer conservation of sodium, loss of the circadian rhythm of antidiuretic hormone secretion, decreased production of renin-angiotensin-aldosterone, and increased release of atrial natriuretic hormone, there is an age-related alteration in the circadian rhythm of water excretion, leading to increased nighttime urine production in the older population. Exacerbated by age-related diminution in functional bladder volume and detrusor instability, nocturnal polyuria often leads to a dramatic version of nocturia (Miller, 2000).

Dementias

The elderly patient with dementia faces the dual difficulties of having to face the consequences of an aging bladder and in addition, the difficulties caused by an altered perception of his or her internal and external environments. This can lead to urinary incontinence or retention depending on what is influencing it, bladder factors or a central neurologic inability to properly perceive the urinary activity. The difficulties in the management of these patients' other significant conditions often pushes concerns about incontinence aside, but the fact remains that incontinence issues are the primary reason for institutionalization of the elderly patient.

Evidence of combined cerebral and urinary tract dysfunction comes from perfusion studies in elderly patients. From positron emission tomography (PET) scan studies, it has been demonstrated that the pontine micturition center in the dorsomedial pontine tegmentum, the periaqueductal gray matter and the pre-optic area of the hypothalamus are all active during various phases of micturition (Blok and Holstege, 1998). Furthermore, urge incontinence has been associated with underperfusion of the frontal areas of the brain (Griffiths, 1998). Clearly, cerebral atrophy, irrespective of the cause, can lead to disinhibition of the bladder and resulting incontinence. Treatment routines combining anticholinergic medications with prompted or timed voiding have been utilized to circumvent the loss of cerebral control over the micturition process in elderly patients afflicted with bladder dysfunction (Burgio *et al.*, 1998; Schnelle and Leung, 2004).

PHARMACOLOGY AS IT RELATES TO THE AGING BLADDER

With so many elderly at risk for bladder dysfunction, the use of medications among the elderly for urinary tract problems is rising almost exponentially. The number of prescriptions for one particular overactive bladder drug alone surpasses 50 000 per month, many presumably to older sufferers of the condition (Alza, 1999). Clearly, an understanding of how the common drugs for these urinary conditions work is essential for proper prescription and monitoring. Proper use of pharmaceuticals for urinary conditions can give maximum benefit to the patient's symptoms and pathology without engendering any undue risk in the aging population.

Receptors

The pharmacology of the bladder is primarily related to either the bladder itself or to the nervous innervation of the organ. At the level of the bladder itself, a number of receptor sites exist to varying degrees. These receptors govern to a great degree the function of the lower urinary tract and become more prominent in the elderly patient as various bladder conditions become more prevalent.

Among the adrenergic receptors, α- and β-receptors are found in the bladder although it has been thought that β-receptors predominate in the bladder body and α-receptors in the bladder base and bladder neck region. Urine storage is facilitated by relaxation caused by β-stimulation and tonic contraction in the area enriched by α-receptors (Khanna *et al.*, 1981). More recent work has elucidated (at least in the rabbit) that the division by receptors into bladder base and body may be overly simplistic and that further regionalization of the bladder based on differing mixes of α- and β-receptors might be more appropriate (Chou *et al.*, 2003). α-receptors are also well characterized in the prostatic urethra and stroma. Stimulation of these receptors causes contraction and thus possibly obstruction of the bladder neck (Caine, 1988).

Muscarinic receptors are the other major group of receptors influencing bladder behavior. These receptors, particularly the M2 and M3 subtypes are responsible for bladder contraction (Ehlert, 2003). The pharmacology of these receptors is influenced by their ubiquity. They are also found in gastrointestinal, airway, and salivary gland smooth muscle. Table 2 gives a summary of receptors located within the bladder and the effects of aging on these receptors.

Adrenergic Stimulation/blockade

α-stimulation in the elderly patient is most often a deleterious side effect from a pharmaceutical designed for action elsewhere. With the rich supply of α-receptors in the prostate, stimulation can cause contraction, and thus obstruction and

Table 2 Bladder receptors and aging

Receptor	Location	Action	Effect of aging
α-adrenergic	Prostate	Contraction smooth muscle	Stimulation-causes urinary retention Blockade-improves urine flow
α-adrenergic	Bladder base	Contraction smooth muscle	Shift in subtype may ameliorate bladder symptoms
β-adrenergic	Bladder body	Relaxation smooth muscle	Unknown at present
Muscarinic	Detrusor muscle (primarily M3)	Relaxation smooth muscle	Urinary retention Worsening of side effects at other locations

urinary retention (Beck *et al.*, 1992). α-blockade, although originally designed with hypertension in mind, has become a mainstay in the therapy of LUTS related to prostatic enlargement (Dunn *et al.*, 2002).

One effect of aging is the possible change in the type, sensitivity, and number of these receptors. With increasing age, α-adrenoceptor responsiveness either decreases or remains unchanged (Docherty and O'Malley, 1985). Furthermore, α-receptors in the aging bladder itself show a shift from the α-1a subtype to an α-1d predominance (Hampel *et al.*, 2004). If α-blockers have an effect in the bladder that aids in relief of LUTS as well as its effect on obstruction itself, then this change with aging could have implications for both short-term as well as long-term use in elderly men with prostate disease.

Antimuscarinics

Antimuscarinics are drugs that are utilized primarily in the therapy of symptoms of overactive bladder. Although the M2 subtype is the predominant population, it appears that the smaller population M3 subtype is the functionally important group (Fetscher *et al.*, 2002). Although several antimuscarinic agents exist in oral, intravesical, and transdermal forms, the lack of bladder M3 selectivity remains a problem.

In the elderly, antimuscarinic can be very effective for symptoms of frequency, urgency, and urge incontinence (Wein, 2003). Changes in the aging patient may, however, alter the pharmacology of these drugs in an adverse manner. Side effects such as dry mouth and constipation may be of more concern and less well tolerated in the elderly individual. Decreases in force of detrusor contraction in the aging male with an enlarged obstructing prostate gland may well push the patient into urinary retention. At least one of these agents crosses the blood-brain barrier and thus, particularly in the aging patient, could effect a higher incidence of confusion as a side effect (Todorova *et al.*, 2001). These effects could play a role in limiting the usefulness of the antimuscarinics in treating bladder dysfunction.

5-α Reductase Inhibitors

This group of drugs, although having therapeutic activity in the prostate gland, is known for their beneficial effect on bladder complaints caused by obstruction from the prostate gland. These agents inhibit the conversion of testosterone to dihydrotestosterone in the prostate gland and thus cause reduction in the size of the periurethral prostatic tissue (Tempany *et al.*, 1993). This leads to improvement in urinary flow and BPH related symptomatology. In the proscar long-term efficacy and safety study (PLESS), the main side effects in all age-groups are sexual side effects, particularly ejaculatory disturbances (Wessells *et al.*, 2003). This may be more profound in the elderly male with borderline sexual dysfunction although this was not borne out in the PLESS study.

SURGICAL DISEASE OF THE AGING BLADDER

Lower urinary tract surgery in the aged patient is common for two conditions having a large impact on the bladder – stress urinary incontinence in women and bladder outlet obstruction from prostatic enlargement in men. The elderly suffer disproportionately from these disorders but have benefited from advances in therapy for these conditions. With proper selection of treatment, this group of patients can enjoy great improvement in their quality of life related to their lower urinary tract.

Female Stress Urinary Incontinence

Stress incontinence occurs when abdominal pressure generated by such actions as coughing, sneezing, or other Valsalva maneuvers causes bladder pressure to exceed urethral pressure without a detrusor contraction and urine is expelled. Stress incontinence is associated with parturition, previous pelvic surgery and aging. Previously, major abdominal surgery was the only method considered for treatment and older age could be considered a relative contraindication. But with newer therapies, elderly women can be considered excellent candidates for realizing improvement in their condition.

Pelvic Floor Conditioning

Pelvic floor exercises have become a mainstay of conservative therapy for stress incontinence. They are absolutely safe and can be performed either alone or with biofeedback. Effectiveness as measured both subjectively by patient report as well as objectively with pad weights has been demonstrated in several studies (Bo *et al.*, 1999; Aksac *et al.*, 2003).

Some concern over the effectiveness in the elderly of pelvic floor rehabilitation can be raised. The reduction in estrogen effect on the vaginal tissues may reduce the benefit of these exercises in the elderly woman. Furthermore, the overall reduction of muscle tone with aging may also make these exercises less efficacious (Dimpfl *et al.*, 1998; Aukee *et al.*, 2003). Patients with significant intrinsic sphincter deficiency may not respond as well to pelvic floor conditioning. These exercises, however, are essentially risk-free, which makes them especially appealing as a first line effort for the elderly woman.

Pharmacologic Management

Stress urinary incontinence has been remarkably resistant to drug therapy in the past. Pharmacologic agents with α-adrenergic properties such as pseudoephedrine were occasionally utilized with moderate success in women with mild incontinence (Cummings, 1996). These medications were effective due to the presence of α-receptors in the bladder neck. These agents though, have recently been pulled out of use owing to adverse events and so are not readily available. Estrogen therapy may also play a role in the medical management of stress incontinence in the older, post-menopausal woman (Ishiko *et al.*, 2001) but its true benefit has been disputed in some studies (Jackson *et al.*, 1999).

Anticholinergic agents, although truly indicated for urgency and urge incontinence, are often prescribed for stress incontinence. These drugs may be helpful in women with mixed incontinence (urge and stress incontinence) by reduction of the urge component and thus improving overall continence. Patients with pure stress incontinence may perceive a worsening of the problem in that the bladder capacity will increase, and they will leak larger volumes of urine with stress maneuvers (Chutka and Takahashi, 1998).

Although it is appealing to consider these pharmaceuticals as first line therapy for stress incontinence in the aging woman, one must consider certain factors. α-adrenergic agents have been associated with CVAs and increases in blood pressure (Cantu *et al.*, 2003; Beck *et al.*, 1992). Certain anticholinergic medications cross the blood-brain barrier and can cause confusion and drowsiness in the older patient (Yarker *et al.*, 1995). These adverse effects may outweigh the usually small benefits these drugs provide for stress incontinence.

The serotonin-norepinephrine reuptake inhibitors (SNRI) are being shown to have a therapeutic effect in female stress incontinence. These drugs have been shown to facilitate urine storage and facilitate rhabdosphincter activity. Thus, a positive effect on stress incontinence could be expected and trials are under way to study this possibility (Thor and Donatucci, 2004). Safety in the geriatric population would also need evaluation.

Injection Therapy

The concept of injecting substances at the bladder neck to aid in coaptation and thus improve continence dates back to the use of sodium morrhuate by Murless in the 1930s (Murless, 1938). This led later to the use of Teflon popularized by Politano with good results (Lopez *et al.*, 1993). Concerns over the safety of Teflon injection led to the use of glutaraldehyde cross-linked bovine collagen and later development of other injectables such as carbon beads. Injection treatments have been shown to have an improvement rate of about 40% (Groutz *et al.*, 2000) with best results occurring in women without low leak point pressures or maximum urethral closure pressures (Gorton *et al.*, 1999).

This therapy may be a good alternative for the older female. It is minimally invasive with a low rate of complications. The anesthetic requirements are not significant, with some reporting use of local anesthetic only. The major downside, especially for the geriatric patient is the frequent need for multiple injections to achieve success. Still, this is an excellent option for the older woman desiring aggressive treatment, but reluctant to undergo major surgical procedures (Khullar *et al.*, 1997).

Operative Therapy

With multiple procedures described for female stress urinary incontinence, it is difficult to discern what the role of surgery might be for the aging female. Several factors are clear though. Older women are, as a rule, healthier now and thus better able to tolerate surgery. Surgery offers the best chance for successful resolution of stress incontinence. Finally, modifications of many procedures have allowed good results with less morbidity than was seen with earlier operations.

Sling procedures have evolved from being a procedure designed only for those with severe incontinence to a rational alternative for all women desiring operative therapy (Morgan *et al.*, 2000). The procedure is commonly done today with alternative materials for the sling such as cadaveric fascia or dermis as opposed to the classic descriptions of harvesting the patient's own fascia. Bone anchors are now commonly available for fixation of the sling, allowing for a lower degree of invasiveness via an exclusively transvaginal approach.

The taping procedures for stress incontinence have also shown good results with minimal morbidity and may be ideal alternatives for the elderly female. The tension-free vaginal tape procedure as popularized by Ulmsten (Ulmsten *et al.*, 1998) and its modifications (suprapubic tapes and transobturator tapes) place a sling-like material at the midurethra and are often done under local anesthetic with light sedation only (Tash and Staskin, 2003). These procedures have been shown to be safe enough and have quite good results to be a reasonable alternative for the more active older female who requires aggressive treatment, but desires minimal morbidity (Walsh *et al.*, 2004).

Benign Prostatic Hyperplasia (BPH) in the Older Male

Benign enlargement of the prostate gland in the human male is a condition inexorably linked with aging. When the vesicourethral junction becomes obstructed by the growing tissue, symptoms such as slowing of the urinary stream, hesitancy, straining to void and a sensation of incomplete emptying result. Furthermore, irritative symptoms such as urinary frequency, urgency, and nocturia may also become common. It is estimated that the prevalence of symptoms related to BPH may be as high as 50% in a multinational survey (Rosen *et al.*, 2003).

Medical Therapy

Two broad classes of drugs are utilized for therapy for BPH, α-receptor blockers and 5-α reductase inhibitors. The bladder neck region in males is rich in α-receptors and blockade of these causes relaxation of the smooth muscle in the prostatic urethra. This results in a decrease in the tonic luminal pressure in the prostatic fossa and allows for more efficient urine outflow from the bladder (Debruyne, 2000).

Early α-antagonists were designed primarily for use as antihypertensives and thus a major side effect when used for relief of voiding dysfunction from BPH was orthostasis. Normotensive men complained also of asthenia and fatigue (Lepor *et al.*, 2000). In older men with hypertension, attempted medical management of BPH along with hypertension became complex. Over the last several years, the introduction of α-adrenergic antagonists selective to the prostatic α-receptors has broadened the population that can be managed with these agents and includes many elderly men, ensuring also safe usage. (Dunn *et al.*, 2002).

The 5-α reductase inhibitors block the conversion of testosterone to dihydrotestosterone in the prostate gland, which is the active form stimulating prostate growth. With blockade, the prostate gland involutes and a reduction in prostate volume of up to 30% may be seen. This can result in an improvement in urinary flow and a decrease in symptomatology. The safety profile of these drugs is very good, making them a good choice in the older male, particularly those with very large prostate glands (Roehrborn *et al.*, 2004).

Combination therapy may also be of benefit in the elderly male. The recently completed Medical Therapy of Prostate Symptoms (MTOPS) study demonstrated a 66% decrease in acute urinary retention compared to placebo. α-blockade alone and 5-α reductase therapy alone showed 39% and 34% reductions respectively (McConnell *et al.*, 2003). Acute urinary retention in the elderly is a morbid event with an impact on quality of life similar to that of myocardial infarction; so prevention by means of a combined therapy may be worthwhile for the older population with LUTS related to BPH.

Minimally Invasive Therapy

A plethora of minimally invasive treatments for BPH now exist. Many are safe enough to be office-based and thus particularly applicable to the older male population. These therapies involve the delivery of energy to the prostate gland in order to heat the tissues to greater than 60 °C, which leads to protein denaturation and ultimately destruction of prostatic tissue and relief of obstruction. The differences in the methods lie in the type of heat delivery system; whether by externally generated microwaves (Osman *et al.*, 2003) or internally placed systems generating radiofrequency energy (Hill *et al.*, 2004) or laser energy (Costello *et al.*, 1999).

Safety makes these procedures particularly appealing for the older male (Berger *et al.*, 2003). Most of the complications center around irritative voiding symptoms. Bleeding essentially does not occur but postprocedure retention can be a problem. Furthermore, it takes several weeks before improvement in symptoms and flow occurs.

Transurethral Resection of the Prostate Gland (TURP)

The TURP procedure is still considered the "gold standard" of treatment for bladder outlet obstruction from BPH (Minardi *et al.*, 2004). It works quickly, since the obstructing tissue is removed immediately at the time of surgery. Symptom scores drop rapidly and flow rates are instantly improved. Although not without morbidity, improvements in instrumentation and optics have made this procedure much safer for the elderly patient, and in those with severe symptoms or retention, it is still the best choice for therapy, no matter what the age of the patient is, if he can reasonably tolerate anesthesia.

CONCLUSION

The effects of aging on lower urinary tract function can be profound. Anatomic variations, both at the macroscopic and ultrastructural levels occur frequently and induce functional changes. Disease states commonly seen in the older patient have significant impact on the bladder, which should be recognized as a major portion of the syndromes. Bladder changes from aging significantly impact on pharmaceutical effectiveness and alter the ability to manage many conditions. A multimodal approach including surgery to treat common geriatric disorders of the lower urinary tract can be both safe and very effective.

KEY POINTS

- Bladder anatomy changes with aging both macroscopically because of prostate enlargement in men and pelvic prolapse in women, as well as microscopically because of collagen deposition.
- Changes in anatomy lead to physiologic changes such as loss of compliance and variation in response to neurotransmitters and pharmaceuticals.
- Certain extravesical disease processes common in the older patient have a profound effect on the bladder.
- The common lower urinary tract symptom complexities of stress incontinence in women and obstructive voiding in women can be safely treated by a variety of means including surgery.

KEY REFERENCES

- Burgio KL, Locher JL, Goode PS *et al.* Behavioral vs drug treatment for urge urinary incontinence in older women: a randomized controlled trial. *The Journal of the American Medical Association* 1998; **280**:1995–2000.
- Elbadawi A, Yalla SV & Resnick NM. Structural basis of geriatric voiding dysfunction. II. Aging detrusor: normal versus impaired contractility. *The Journal of Urology* 1993; **150**:1657–67.
- Thor KB & Donatucci C. Central nervous system control of the lower urinary tract: new pharmacological approaches to stress urinary incontinence in women. *The Journal of Urology* 2004; **172**:27–33.
- Yoshida M, Miuamee K, Iwashita H *et al.* Management of detrusor dysfunction in the elderly: changes in acetylcholine and adenosine triphosphate release during aging. *Urology* 2004; **63**(3 suppl 1):117–23.

REFERENCES

Aksac B, Aki S, Karan A *et al.* Biofeedback and pelvic floor exercises for the rehabilitation of urinary stress incontinence. *Gynecologic and Obstetric Investigation* 2003; **56**:23–7.

Albanese A, Jenner P, Marsden CD & Stephenson JD. Bladder hyperreflexia induced in marmosets by 1-methyl-4phenyl-1,2,3,6-tetrahydropyridine. *Neuroscience Letters* 1988; **87**:46–50.

Alza Pharmaceuticals Press Release. *ALZA Corporation Announces Approval of Ditropan® XL 15 MG Tablets* 1999; June 24.

Araki I, Kitahara M, Oida T & Kuno S. Voiding dysfunction and Parkinson's disease: urodynamics abnormalities and urinary symptoms. *The Journal of Urology* 2000; **164**:1640–3.

Aukee P, Penttinen J & Airaksinen O. The effect of aging on the electromyographic activity of pelvic floor muscles. A comparative study among stress incontinent patients and asymptomatic women. *Maturitas* 2003; **44**:253–7.

Azadzoi KM, Tarcan T, Siroky MB & Krane RJ. Atherosclerosis-induced chronic ischemia causes bladder fibrosis and non-compliance in the rabbit. *The Journal of Urology* 1999a; **161**:1626–35.

Azadzoi KM, Tarcan T, Kozlowski R *et al.* Overactivity and structural changes in the chronically ischemic bladder. *The Journal of Urology* 1999b; **162**:1768–78.

Bakas P, Liapis A, Karandreas A & Creatsas G. Pudendal nerve terminal motor latency in women with genuine stress incontinence and prolapse. *Gynecologic and Obstetric Investigation* 2001; **51**:187–90.

Beck RA, Mercado DL, Seguin SM *et al.* Cardiovascular effects of pseudoephedrine in medically controlled hypertensive patients. *Archives of Internal Medicine* 1992; **152**:1242–5.

Berger AP, Niescher M, Spranger R *et al.* Transurethral microwave thermotherapy (TUMT) with the Targis system: a single-centre study on 78 patients with acute urinary retention and poor general health. *European Urology* 2003; **43**:176–80.

Blok BF & Holstege G. The central nervous system control of micturition in cats and humans. *Behavioural Brain Research* 1998; **92**:119–25.

Bo K, Talseth T & Holme I. Single blind, randomised controlled trial of pelvic floor exercises, electrical stimulation, vaginal cones, and no treatment in management of genuine stress incontinence in women. *British Medical Journal* 1999; **318**:487–93.

Brading AF. A myogenic basis for the overactive bladder. *Urology* 1997; **50**(suppl 6A):57–67.

Burgio KL, Locher JL, Goode PS *et al.* Behavioral vs drug treatment for urge urinary incontinence in older women: a randomized controlled trial. *The Journal of the American Medical Association* 1998; **280**:1995–2000.

Caine M. Alpha-adrenergic mechanisms in dynamics of benign prostatic hypertrophy. *Urology* 1988; **32**(6 suppl):16–20.

Cantu C, Arauz A, Murillo-Bonilla LM *et al.* Stroke associated with sympathomimetics contained in over-the-counter cough and cold drugs. *Stroke* 2003; **34**:1667–72.

Chen YC, Chen GD, Hu SW *et al.* Is the occurrence of storage and voiding dysfunction affected by menopausal transition or associated with the normal aging process? *Menopause* 2003; **10**:203–8.

Chou EC, Capello SA, Levin RM & Longhurst PA. Excitatory alpha1-adrenergic receptors predominate over inhibitory beta-receptors in rabbit dorsal detrusor. *The Journal of Urology* 2003; **170**:2503–7.

Chutka DS & Takahashi PY. Urinary incontinence in the elderly. Drug treatment options. *Drugs* 1998; **56**:587–95.

Cockett AT, Barry MJ, Holtgrewe HL *et al.* The American Urological Association Study. Indications for treatment of benign prostatic hyperplasia. *Cancer* 1992; **70**:280–3.

Constantinou CE, Hvistendahl G, Ryhammer A *et al.* Determining the displacement of the pelvic floor and pelvic organs during voluntary contractions using magnetic resonance imaging in younger and older women. *BJU International* 2002; **90**:408–14.

Costello AJ, Agarwal DK, Crowe HR & Lynch WJ. Evaluation of interstitial diode laser therapy for treatment of benign prostatic hyperplasia. *Techniques in Urology* 1999; **5**:202–6.

Cummings JM. Current concepts in the management of stress urinary incontinence. *Drugs of Today* 1996; **32**:609–14.

Cummings JM & Rodning CB. Urinary stress incontinence among obese women: review of pathophysiology and therapy. *International Urogynecology Journal & Pelvic Floor Dysfunction* 2000; **11**:41–4.

Debruyne FM. Alpha blockers: are all created equal? *Urology* 2000; **56**(5 suppl 1):20–2.

DeLancey JO. Anatomy and embryology of the lower urinary tract. *Obstetrics and Gynecology Clinics of North America* 1989; **16**:717–31.

Dimpfl T, Jaeger C, Mueller-Felber W *et al.* Myogenic changes of the levator ani muscle in premenopausal women: the impact of vaginal delivery and age. *Neurourology and Urodynamics* 1998; **17**:197–205.

Docherty JR & O'Malley K. Ageing and alpha-adrenoceptors. *Clinical Science (London)* 1985; **68**(suppl 10):133s–6s.

Dunn JS Jr, Bent AE, Ellerkman RM *et al.* Voiding dysfunction after surgery for stress incontinence: literature review and survey results. *International Urogynecology Journal and Pelvic Floor Dysfunction* 2004; **15**:25–31.

Dunn CJ, Matheson A & Faulds DM. Tamsulosin: a review of its pharmacology and therapeutic efficacy in the management of lower urinary tract symptoms. *Drugs & Aging* 2002; **19**:135–61.

Ehlert FJ. Contractile role of M2 and M3 muscarinic receptors in gastrointestinal, airway and urinary bladder smooth muscle. *Life Sciences* 2003; **74**:355–66.

Elbadawi A. Pathology and pathophysiology of detrusor in incontinence. *The Urologic Clinics of North America* 1995; **22**:499–512.

Elbadawi A, Yalla SV & Resnick NM. Structural basis of geriatric voiding dysfunction. II. Aging detrusor: normal versus impaired contractility. *The Journal of Urology* 1993; **150**:1657–67.

Falconer C, Ekman G, Malmstrom A & Ulmsten U. Decreased collagen synthesis in stress-incontinent women. *Obstetrics and Gynecology* 1994; **84**:583–6.

Falconer C, Ekman-Ordeberg G, Ulmsten U *et al.* Changes in paraurethral connective tissue at menopause are counteracted by estrogen. *Maturitas* 1996; **24**:197–204.

Fetscher C, Fleichman M, Schmidt M *et al.* M(3) muscarinic receptors mediate contraction of human urinary bladder. *British Journal of Pharmacology* 2002; **136**:641–3.

Gorton E, Stanton S, Monga A *et al.* Periurethral collagen injection: a long-term follow-up study. *BJU International* 1999; **84**:966–71.

Griffiths D. Clinical studies of cerebral and urinary tract function in elderly people with urinary incontinence. *Behavioural Brain Research* 1998; **92**:151–5.

Groutz A, Blaivas JG, Kesler SS *et al.* Outcome results of transurethral collagen injection for female stress incontinence: assessment by urinary incontinence score. *The Journal of Urology* 2000; **164**:2006–9.

Groutz A, Samandarov A, Gold R *et al.* Role of urethrocystoscopy in the evaluation of refractory idiopathic detrusor instability. *Urology* 2001; **58**:544–6.

Hailemariam S, Elbadawi A, Yalla SV & Resnick NM. Structural basis of geriatric voiding dysfunction. V. Standardized protocols for routine ultrastructural study and diagnosis of endoscopic detrusor biopsies. *The Journal of Urology* 1997; **157**:1783–801.

Hampel C, Gillitzer R, Pahernik S *et al.* Changes in the receptor profile of the aging bladder. *Der Urologe. Ausg. A* 2004; **43**:535–41.

Hill B, Belville W, Bruskewitz R *et al.* Transurethral needle ablation versus transurethral resection of the prostate for the treatment of symptomatic benign prostatic hyperplasia: 5-year results of a prospective, randomized, multicenter clinical trial. *The Journal of Urology* 2004; **171**:2336–40.

Homma Y, Imajo C, Takahashi S *et al.* Urinary symptoms and urodynamics in a normal elderly population. *Scandinavian Journal of Urology and Nephrology* 1994; **157**:27–30.

Ishiko O, Hirai K, Sumi T *et al.* Hormone replacement therapy plus pelvic floor muscle exercise for postmenopausal stress incontinence. A randomized, controlled trial. *The Journal of Reproductive Medicine* 2001; **46**:213–20.

Jackson S, Shepherd A, Brookes S & Abrams P. The effect of oestrogen supplementation on post-menopausal urinary stress incontinence: a double-blind placebo-controlled trial. *British Journal of Obstetrics and Gynaecology* 1999; **106**:711–8.

Khanna OP, Barbieri EJ & McMichael RF. The effects of adrenergic agonists and antagonists on vesicourethral smooth muscle of rabbits.

The Journal of Pharmacology and Experimental Therapeutics 1981; **216**:95–100.

Khullar V, Cardozo LD, Abbott D & Anders K. GAX collagen in the treatment of urinary incontinence in elderly women: a two year follow up. *British Journal of Obstetrics and Gynaecology* 1997; **104**:96–9.

Landau EH, Jayanthi VR, Churchill BM *et al.* Loss of elasticity in dysfunctional bladders: Urodynamic and histochemical correlation. *The Journal of Urology* 1994; **152**:702–5.

Lepor H, Jones K & Williford W. The mechanism of adverse events associated with terazosin: an analysis of the Veterans Affairs cooperative study. *The Journal of Urology* 2000; **163**:1134–7.

Levy BJ & Wight TN. Structural changes in the aging submucosa: new morphologic criteria for the evaluation of the unstable human bladder. *The Journal of Urology* 1990; **144**:1044–55.

Lopez AE, Padron OF, Patsias G & Politano VA. Transurethral polytetrafluoroethylene injection in female patients with urinary continence. *The Journal of Urology* 1993; **150**:856–8.

Lose G, Alling-Moller L & Jennum P. Nocturia in women. *American Journal of Obstetrics and Gynecology* 2001; **185**:514–21.

Macarak EJ & Howard PS. The role of collagen in bladder filling. *Advances in Experimental Medicine and Biology* 1999; **462**:215–23.

McConnell JD, Roehrborn CG, Bautista OM *et al.* Medical Therapy of Prostatic Symptoms (MTOPS) Research Group. The long-term effect of doxazosin, finasteride, and combination therapy on the clinical progression of benign prostatic hyperplasia. *The New England Journal of Medicine* 2003; **349**:2387–98.

Middelkoop HA, Smilde-van den Doel DA, Neven AK *et al.* Subjective sleep characteristics of 1,485 males and females aged 50–93: effects of sex and age, and factors related to self-evaluated quality of sleep. *The Journals of Gerontology. Series A, Biological Sciences and Medical Sciences* 1996; **51**:M108–15.

Miller M. Nocturnal polyuria in older people: pathophysiology and clinical implications. *Journal of the American Geriatrics Society* 2000; **48**:1321–9.

Minardi D, Galosi AB, Yehia M *et al.* Transurethral resection versus minimally invasive treatments of benign prostatic hyperplasia: results of treatments. Our experience. *Archivio Italiano Di Urologia, Andrologia* 2004; **76**:11–8.

Morgan TO Jr, Westney OL & McGuire EJ. Pubovaginal sling: 4-year outcome analysis and quality of life assessment. *The Journal of Urology* 2000; **163**:1845–8.

Murless BC. The injection treatment of stress incontinence. *The Journal of Obstetrics and Gynaecology of the British Empire* 1938; **45**:67–73.

Nitti VW, Adler H & Combs AJ. The role of urodynamics in the evaluation of voiding dysfunction in men after cerebrovascular accident. *The Journal of Urology* 1996; **155**:263–6.

Ohnishi N, Kishima Y, Hashimoto K *et al.* A new method of measurement of the urinary bladder blood flow in patients with low compliant bladder. *Hinyokika Kiyo. Acta Urologica Japonica* 1994; **40**:663–7.

Osman Y, Wadie B, El-Diasty T & Larson T. High-energy transurethral microwave thermotherapy: symptomatic vs urodynamic success. *BJU International* 2003; **91**:365–70.

Pavlakis AJ, Siroky MB, Goldstein I & Krane RJ. Neurourologic findings in Parkinson's disease. *The Journal of Urology* 1983; **129**:80–3.

Perucchini D, DeLancey JO, Ashton-Miller JA *et al.* Age effects on urethral striated muscle. II. Anatomic location of muscle loss. *American Journal of Obstetrics and Gynecology* 2002; **186**:356–60.

Pinho M, Yoshioka K, Ortiz J *et al.* The effect of age on pelvic floor dynamics. *International Journal of Colorectal Disease* 1990; **5**:207–8.

Rosen R, Altwein J, Boyle P *et al.* Lower urinary tract symptoms and male sexual dysfunction: the multinational survey of the aging male (MSAM-7). *European Urology* 2003; **44**:637–49.

Roehrborn CG, Bruskewitz R, Nickel JC *et al.* Proscar Long-Term Efficacy and Safety Study Group. Sustained decrease in incidence of acute urinary retention and surgery with finasteride for 6 years in men with benign prostatic hyperplasia. *The Journal of Urology* 2004; **171**:1194–8.

Sakakibara R, Hattori T, Yasuda K & Yamanishi T. Micturitional disturbance after acute hemispheric stroke: analysis of the lesion site by CT and MRI. *Journal of the Neurological Sciences* 1996; **137**:47–56.

Schnelle JF & Leung FW. Urinary and fecal incontinence in nursing homes. *Gastroenterology* 2004; **126**(1 suppl 1):S41–7.

Sebesta M, Cespedes RD, Luhman E *et al.* Questionnaire-based outcomes of urinary incontinence and satisfaction rates after radical prostatectomy in a national study population. *Urology* 2002; **60**:1055–8.

Stocchi F, Carbone A, Inghilleri M *et al.* Urodynamic and neurophysiological evaluation in Parkinson's disease and multiple system atrophy. *Journal of Neurology, Neurosurgery, and Psychiatry* 1997; **62**:507–11.

Tash J & Staskin DR. Artificial graft slings at the midurethra: physiology of continence. *Current Urology Reports* 2003; **4**:367–70.

Tempany CM, Partin AW, Zerhouni EA *et al.* The influence of finasteride on the volume of the peripheral and periurethral zones of the prostate in men with benign prostatic hyperplasia. *The Prostate* 1993; **22**:39–42.

Thor KB & Donatucci C. Central nervous system control of the lower urinary tract: new pharmacological approaches to stress urinary incontinence in women. *The Journal of Urology* 2004; **172**:27–33.

Todorova A, Vonderheid-Guth B & Dimpfel W. Effects of tolterodine, trospium chloride, and oxybutynin on the central nervous system. *Journal of Clinical Pharmacology* 2001; **41**:636–44.

Ulmsten U, Falconer C, Johnson P *et al.* A multicenter study of tension-free vaginal tape (TVT) for surgical treatment of stress urinary incontinence. *International Urogynecology Journal and Pelvic Floor Dysfunction* 1998; **9**:210–3.

Van Arsdalen KN, Wein AJ & Levin RM. The contractile and metabolic effects of acute ischemia on the rabbit urinary bladder. *The Journal of Urology* 1983; **130**:180–2.

Verelst M, Maltau JM & Orbo A. Computerised morphometric study of the paraurethral tissue in young and elderly women. *Neurourology and Urodynamics* 2002; **21**:529–33.

Wade DT & Hewer RL. Outlook after an acute stroke: urinary incontinence and loss of consciousness compared in 532 patients. *The Quarterly Journal of Medicine* 1985; **56**:601–8.

Walsh K, Generao SE, White MJ *et al.* The influence of age on quality of life outcome in women following a tension-free vaginal tape procedure. *The Journal of Urology* 2004; **171**:1185–8.

Wein AJ. Diagnosis and treatment of the overactive bladder. *Urology* 2003; **62**(5 suppl 2):20–7.

Wessells H, Roy J, Bannow J *et al.* PLESS Study Group. Incidence and severity of sexual adverse experiences in finasteride and placebo-treated men with benign prostatic hyperplasia. *Urology* 2003; **61**:579–84.

Yarker YE, Goa KL & Fitton A. Oxybutynin. A review of its pharmacodynamic and pharmacokinetic properties, and its therapeutic use in detrusor instability. *Drugs & Aging* 1995; **6**:243–62.

Yoshida M, Miuamee K, Iwashita H *et al.* Management of detrusor dysfunction in the elderly: changes in acetylcholine and adenosine triphosphate release during aging. *Urology* 2004; **63**(3 suppl 1):117–23.

Yoshimura N, Sasa M, Yoshida O & Takaori S. Dopamine D-1 receptor-mediated inhibition of the micturition reflex by central dopamine from the substantia nigra. *Neurourology and Urodynamics* 1992; **11**:535–45.

125

Prostate Diseases

Timothy D. Moon *and* Jennifer L. Maskel
University of Wisconsin and Veterans' Affairs Medical Center, Madison, WI, USA

INTRODUCTION

The prostate is perhaps the most diseased organ in the male body. The lifetime risk of being diagnosed with prostate cancer is approximately 16% while a 65-year-old male has about a 40% likelihood of having a focus of prostate cancer. Benign prostatic hyperplasia as an histological entity will affect almost all men if they live long enough and 25% will receive treatment during their lifetime. Prostatitis has a clinical prevalence of 16% in men over 65 while its histological prevalence is close to 100%.

The above perhaps underscores the importance of prostatic pathology upon the well being of older men. This chapter will review these basic diagnostic entities and the approach to treatment of the aging male.

BENIGN PROSTATIC HYPERPLASIA

Benign prostatic hyperplasia (BPH) has generally been used as a synonym for lower urinary tract symptoms (LUTS) (Abrams, 1994). While BPH is one cause of LUTS, age-related detrusor dysfunction, neurogenic disease, and diabetes are other major causes (Kelly and Zimmern, 2003). This chapter will address LUTS rather than BPH *per se*.

Anatomy

The prostate is a golf ball–sized organ, which lies between the bladder and the pelvic floor anterior to the rectum (Figure 1). The transition zone is situated around the urethra and is responsible for hyperplastic growth (benign prostatic hyperplasia). This may take the form of lateral lobes encroaching on the urethral lumen, or less frequently, a middle lobe of prostate, which may enlarge and develop like a tongue within the bladder (Figure 2). This may then act like a ball valve during urination.

The two major requirements for prostatic growth are androgens and aging. For a more detailed review of the molecular biology of prostatic growth this is reviewed in detail elsewhere (Roehrborn and McConnell, 2002).

Histologically prostatic growth is both epithelial and stromal (Roehrborn and McConnell, 2002). Most patients have varying degrees of stromal and glandular hyperplasia but with both elements usually being present.

Prevalence

BPH usually starts during the early 40s and increases thereafter. Several autopsy studies have been published demonstrating almost no existence before age 40, 50% prevalence by age 60, and with a peak of 90% by age 90 (Berry *et al.*, 1984). Clinically, the Baltimore longitudinal study of aging demonstrated a prevalence of 30% by the fifth decade, 50% in the sixth, and reaching 80% in the eighth decade of life (Arrighi *et al.*, 1991). The prevalence of moderate to severe symptoms for patients in various studies performed globally is enormous ranging from 10 to 60% for men in their sixth decade (Roehrborn and McConnell, 2002). A US study from Olmstead County demonstrated moderate to severe BPH symptoms in 31% of men in their sixth decade rising to 44% in their eighth decade (Chute *et al.*, 1993). Overall, from the patient perspective, the main criterion for initiating treatment is "bother"; how much do these symptoms intrude upon the patient's lifestyle? As patients react differently to the same set of symptoms, how the symptoms affect the patient is more important than an absolute count of the symptoms.

Natural History

The question, which most patients and physicians pose, is what will happen to my symptoms with time? Will I go into acute retention? One study evaluated LUTS in

Principles and Practice of Geriatric Medicine, 4th Edition. Edited by M.S. John Pathy, Alan J. Sinclair and John E. Morley.

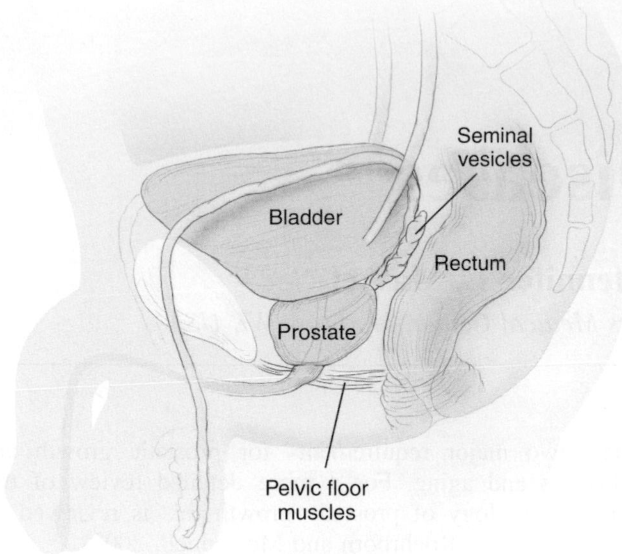

Figure 1 Sagitaal section of male pelvis

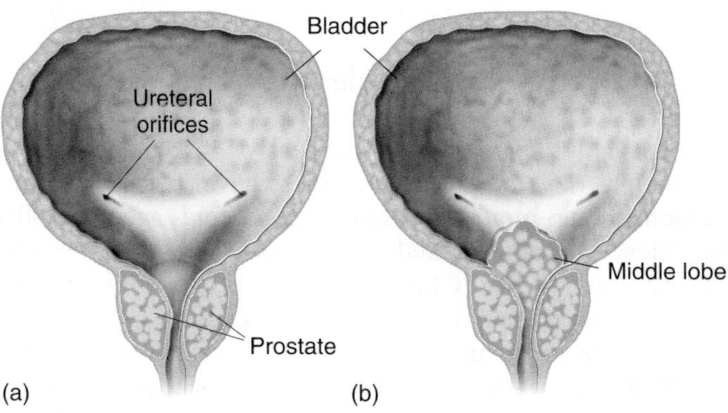

Figure 2 Coronal section of prostate and bladder (a) normal (b) with prostatic and middle lobe enlargement

community-dwelling men over age 60 years (Lee *et al.*, 1996). Of interest, 23% of men with severe symptoms at baseline were asymptomatic 1 year later. Most natural history data, however, comes from the placebo arms of randomized controlled trials for the treatment of LUTS (Flanigan *et al.*, 1998; McConnell *et al.*, 1998; McConnell *et al.*, 2003). The most significant of these is the recently published medical therapy of prostate symptoms (MTOPS) trial (McConnell *et al.*, 2003). Of the 737 men involved in the placebo arm only 18 men went into acute urinary retention during this study (5 years). This rate was 0.6 per hundred person years. The comparison rate in the best treatment arm (finasteride plus doxazosin) was 0.1 per hundred person years. These data demonstrate not only the natural history but also that while medical treatment decreased the acute urinary retention rate by a significant percentage (80%), the absolute risk is relatively small to begin with. Additionally, prostate size as measured by PSA, also correlates with acute urinary retention risk (McConnell *et al.*, 2003). Patients with a PSA less than $1.4\,\mathrm{mg\,ml^{-1}}$ had a very low risk of acute urinary retention.

Patient Evaluation

The key elements to patient evaluation are shown in Table 1. Urinary symptomatology may be evaluated using the international prostate symptoms score (Table 2). For an assessment of symptoms along with an impact score the BPH impact score can be used (Table 3) as an assessment of bother. For most patients, treatment is based upon the negative quality of life impact that they have (bother) rather than any absolute symptomatic criteria. Additionally, it is important to evaluate the rest of the patient's medical history to determine if other medical conditions may lead to bladder dysfunction, polyuria, and so on (Table 4).

A symptom score of 0–7 is considered mild while 8–19 is considered moderate, and 20–35, severe. The impact (Table 3) score should be used in conjunction with the International Prostate Symptom Score. For example, a patient with moderate symptoms but without any bother probably does not warrant treatment, while a patient who is bothered by his symptoms should at least have a discussion of treatment options along with their attendant risks and side effects.

Physical examination should include a rectal examination as well as a focused neurologic examination and evaluation of the patient's mental status. Clearly, dementia amongst many neurologic conditions will affect urinary symptomatology. Many demented patients are referred for incontinence while their bladder function is essentially normal for their age. Treatment of these patients will often be behavioral such as timed voiding (initiated by the caregiver), rather than interventional.

Laboratory Evaluation

Urinalysis is a specifically recommended test to rule out a urinary tract infection or bladder cancer (presence of hematuria). Additionally, the presence of glycosuria in diabetic patients may identify problems for management, not only of diabetes but secondarily, with associated lower urinary tract symptomatology. Patients with primarily irritative urinary symptoms (frequency, urgency, nocturia) should be considered for urinary cytology as well as all men with hematuria. Microscopic hematuria alone should lead to a formal urologic

Table 1 Patient evaluation (AUA Practice Guidelines Committee, 2003)

- Medical history of voiding dysfunction
  - Identify other etiologies and comorbidities for voiding dysfunction
  - Obtain international prostate symptom score
- Physical Examination
  - Include DRE, focused neurologic examination
- Urinalysis
- PSA for select patients
  - Life expectancy greater than 10 years or those for whom PSA measurement would change treatment options

Table 2 AUA BPH symptom score (AUA Practice Guidelines Committee, 2003)

	Not at all	Less than 1 time in 5	Less than half the time	About half the time	More than half the time	Almost always
1. Over the past month, how often have you had a sensation of not emptying your bladder completely after you finished urinating?	0	1	2	3	4	5
2. Over the past month, how often have you had to urinate again less than two hours after you finished urinating?	0	1	2	3	4	5
3. Over the past month, how often have you found you stopped and started again several times when you urinated?	0	1	2	3	4	5
4. Over the past month, how often have you found it difficult to postpone urination?	0	1	2	3	4	5
5. Over the past month, how often have you had a weak urinary stream?	0	1	2	3	4	5
6. Over the past month, how often have you had to push or strain to begin urination?	0	1	2	3	4	5
7. Over the past month, how many times did you most typically get up to urinate from the time you went to bed at night until the time you got up in the morning?	None	1 time	2 times	3 times	4 times	5 or more times

Total Symptom Score ______

Table 3 BPH impact index (AUA Practice Guidelines Committee, 2003)

1. Over the past month how much physical discomfort did any urinary problems cause you?	None ☐	Only a little ☐	Some ☐	A lot ☐
2. Over the past month, how much did you worry about your health because of any urinary problems?	None ☐	Only a little ☐	Some ☐	A lot ☐
3. Overall, how bothersome has any trouble with urination been during the past month?	Not at all bothersome ☐ Bothers me a little ☐	Bothers me some ☐ Bothers me a lot ☐		
4. Over the past month, how much of the time has any urinary problem kept you from doing the kind of things you would usually do?	None of the time ☐ A little of the time ☐ Some of the time ☐	Most of the time ☐ All of the time ☐		

Table 4 Medical diseases affecting urinary symptoms

Cardiac Disease	Especially CHF. Peripheral edema will revascularize at night adding to nocturia
Diabetes	Poorly controlled diabetes will act as osmotic diuretic
Neurologic disease	MS, SCI, PID with nerve compression
Mental disease	Dementia, Alzheimer's
Other urologic conditions	OAB, bladder cancer

CHF, Congestive Heart Failure; MS, Multiple Sclerosis; SCI, Cord Injury; PID, prolapsed intervertebral disc; OAB, overactive bladder.

workup generally consisting of a CT urogram, cystoscopy, and urinary cytology. These studies will evaluate the kidneys, ureters, bladder, and complete lower urinary tract for pathology.

Previously a serum creatinine was recommended, but studies have shown that in the absence of other medical issues this is not a helpful test (AUA Practice Guidelines Committee, 2003). European urologists (European Association of Urology, 2004), however, continue to recommend its collection as did the 4th International Consultation of Benign Prostatic Hyperplasia in 1997 (Koyanogi *et al.*, 1998).

The measurement of PSA remains controversial. In the BPH guidelines (AUA Practice Guidelines Committee, 2003), the general recommendations is for patients with a life expectancy of greater than 10 years or where measurement would make a difference to treatment. For example, in octogenarians, the diagnosis of prostate cancer is not usually a basis for treatment. However, if the patient had severe urinary tract symptomatology then it may be that treatment of the prostate cancer would be appropriate treatment for the LUTS. Patients whose symptoms are complex or who fail medical therapy may require further urodynamic evaluation. Either way this would require referral to an urologist. Measurement of urinary flow rates, post void residuals, ultrasounds, and other urodynamic studies are not generally considered routine.

Treatment

The treatment for LUTS may be separated into four groups: watchful waiting, medical therapy, minimally invasive treatment, and invasive surgical therapy (Table 5).

Watchful Waiting

For patients with mild symptoms and no complications (e.g. renal insufficiency, urinary tract infection) and who are not

Table 5 Treatment options for BPH

Watchful waiting	Symptoms minimal (IPSS < 8) and there is little bother. These are not mandatory indications for treatment
Medical therapy α blockers 5α reductase inhibitors Phytotherapy	Symptoms and/or bother are moderate but the patients wants treatment
Minimally invasive surgery Microwave Radiofrequency	Moderate to severe symptoms/bother Comorbid indications for surgery: Bleeding Renal failure Recurrent UTI Urinary retention
Invasive surgery TUIP TURP Open prostatectomy	Moderate to severe symptoms Indications for surgery Failure of other therapies

IPSS, International prostate symptom score; UTI, Urinary Tract infection; TURP, Transurethral Resection of Prostate; TUIP, transurethral incision of prostate.

bothered by their symptoms, monitoring of the symptoms without active intervention is appropriate. Generally, this would include all patients with symptom scores less than 8 and many with symptom scores between 8 and 19.

Medical Therapy (Lepor and Lowe, 2002)

Medical therapy consists of α-blockers, 5-α-reductase inhibitors, and phytotherapy.

α-blockers

The basis for this treatment utilizes the fact that the prostate and bladder neck are richly innervated by $\alpha 1_a$ receptors. The bladder body is primarily innervated with $\alpha 1_d$ receptors while $\alpha 1_b$ receptors are present on blood vessels throughout. By blocking the $\alpha 1_a$ and $\alpha 1_d$ receptors, the prostate and detrusor smooth muscle will relax, allowing for a better flow and reduced irritative urinary symptomatology. The effect on $\alpha 1_b$ receptors tends to cause vascular relaxation and potentially hypotension. Indeed, the earliest drugs (terazosin and doxazosin) were first approved by the FDA as hypotensive agents. Most of the α-blockers are non-subtype selective (alfuzosin, doxazosin, terazosin). Because of their effect upon blood vessels, the dose needs to be increased over several weeks. Even so, many patients, especially the elderly, may have problems with dizziness and postural hypotension. Alfuzosin (long acting) and tamsulosin, because of less effect upon blood pressure, do not require dose titration. Tamsulosin is a different class of drug and is primarily $\alpha\text{-}1_{a/d}$ specific. As such, it has less potential interaction with hypotensive agents than the other drugs. Overall, the efficacy of the drugs are similar, although the side effect profiles differ somewhat with perhaps tamsulosin having the best side effect profile.

Of special note is the interaction between α-blockers and the phospho-diesterase-5 inhibitors (Sildenofil, Tadalafil, and Vardenofil). Sildenofil (Viagara), tadalafil (cialis) and vardenafil (levitra) are contraindicated within 6 hours of taking α-blockers. Levitra is contraindicated with all α-blockers though work is underway to try and remove this FDA proscription. Tamsulosin is the only α-blocker approved by the FDA for use in combination with Cialis.

5-α-reductase Inhibitors

These drugs block the conversion of testosterone to dihydrotestosterone (the active metabolite). Two enzymes exist: type I in the skin and liver and type II in the reproductive organs. Dutasteride blocks both enzymes, while Finasteride blocks only the type II enzyme. Despite this difference, the overall suppression of testosterone is similar. Because of the mechanism of action, it takes 3–6 months for full clinical effect. Further, these drugs are most efficacious on large prostates (>50 g).

Combination Therapy

The recent MTOPS trial demonstrated maximal effect in reducing prostate size and improving symptoms by combining both an α-blocker (doxazosin) with a 5-α-reductase inhibitor (finasteride) (McConnell *et al.*, 2003). While the differences in risk for symptom progression and urinary retention were large (approximately 25% greater than single treatment alone (McConnell *et al.*, 2003)) the absolute reductions were relatively small: nine episodes to five episodes per 100 patient years for urinary retention and 25 per 100 patient years for symptom progression (>4 points on the symptom score). Two features of practical utility did stand out. Patients with small prostates had little risk of going into retention irrespective of treatment option. PSA has also been demonstrated to be a surrogate for prostate size. Patients with low PSA's (less than $1.4\,\mathrm{ng\,ml^{-1}}$) also have small prostates and minimal risk of retention. Conversely, patients with large prostates had a much greater risk of retention and therefore are likely to benefit more from this aspect of 5-α-reductase therapy.

Phytotherapy

A variety of plant extracts have been utilized for the treatment of LUTS. Unfortunately, because they are designated as food additives and not regulated by the Food and Drug Administration no good randomized prospective clinical trials have been performed. Despite this, several compounds do appear to have real activity. These are currently being studied in the Complimentary and Alternative Medicine (CAMUS) trial funded by the National Institutes of Health (NIH). This study will randomize patients to placebo, Saw Palmetto, Africanum Pygeum, or an α-blocker/5-α-reductase inhibitor combination. The results of this study will unfortunately not be available for several years.

Perhaps the most widely used plant is Seranoa Repens (Saw Palmetto). The extracts of this plant contain a mixture of fatty acids, sterols, flavenoids, and other compounds (Lowe and Fogelman, 2004). Its mechanism of action suggests 5-α-reductase inhibition, anti-inflammatory action and effects upon apoptosis.

One of the largest problems with these unregulated drugs is batch-to-batch variation and also manufacturer-to-manufacturer variation. Studies have been performed analyzing the active ingredients from multiple manufacturers demonstrating that the content varies between excess of that stated on the package to none at all.

Minimally Invasive Therapy

Surgical therapies are generally out with the scope of practice for gerontologists. For that reason, the following discussion will center on information, which will help the physician guide, the patient toward the best therapy for them. More detailed reviews of the subject have been published (Fitzpatrick and Mebust, 2002). The most commonly utilized methods for minimally invasive treatment are transurethral needle ablation (TUNA) and microwave thermotherapy. Both act by heating the prostatic tissue. The TUNA device is a rigid cystoscope like instrument passed transurethrally under vision. Two needles (which look a bit like snake fangs) can be extended from the instrument into the prostatic tissue. Utilizing a radiofrequency signal the tissue is heated between 46 and 100 °C. The microwave devices look like a urinary catheter with a normal balloon area (to seat it at the bladder neck) but with the microwave area distal to that. Using microwave energy the prostatic tissue is heated to 69 °C. Overall, tissue heated to greater than 45 °C will lead to hemorrhagic necrosis. These procedures are generally performed in the office or a surgicenter under local anesthetic or conscious sedation.

Overall, most studies show a marked reduction in Symptom Score (50% or more) and with improvement in peak flow from 30 to 100%. Comparative studies have not yet been performed, however, the NIH is sponsoring the trial of minimally invasive surgical therapy (MIST), which will compare TUNA with microwave thermotherapy with combined medical therapy (α-blocker plus 5-α-reductase inhibitor). The results of this trial however will again not be available for several years.

Given that most patients are treated for "bother" rather than absolute need the complication rates are extremely important. The complications of TUNA include postoperative urinary retention with rates of 13–42%. Forty percent will have retention for the first 24 hours. Likewise, 40% of patients will have irritative urinary symptoms early on after treatment. Up to 14% of patients will undergo another form of therapy within 2 years. To the extent that some patients without benefit will not undergo additional therapies this perhaps underscores the lack of efficacy rate.

The complications of microwave thermotherapy include 36% catheterization rate for 1 week postoperatively. Satisfaction rates have dropped off to 34% at 2 years. One recently reported study of microwave thermotherapy demonstrated that over a 5-year period, 29% underwent additional treatment while only 59 of 150 patients remained in the study (Miller *et al.*, 2003). While these dropout rates are similar to dropout rates for medical (drug) therapy the economic impact is greater. If drug therapy is stopped the cost (of the drug) also stops. Once a relatively expensive treatment is performed the total cost has already been incurred.

Despite all the cautionary notes mentioned earlier, Medicare has approved both TUNA and microwave thermotherapy for reimbursement. Because they are generally performed in the office/surgicenter setting, utilization has increased dramatically over the last few years.

Invasive Surgical Therapy

In today's society most patients with lower urinary tract symptomatology will first be tried on medical therapy. Depending upon the experience of the urologist, equipment availability, or the patient circumstances some patients may next be treated with minimally invasive therapy. If that fails or is not appropriate patients may proceed to invasive therapy namely transurethral incision of the prostate or transurethral resection of the prostate (TURP). Both of these procedures are performed in the hospital operating room under spinal or general anesthesia. The patients are generally admitted for at least one night postoperatively. If the prostate is small and especially if there is a high bladder neck (between the prostate prostatic urethra and bladder) then a transurethral incision of the prostate may be preferable. Not only is this a single cut from the bladder trigone to the verumontanum of the prostate simple, but there is much less blood loss than with a TURP. Additionally, because the whole bladder neck has not been resected the risk for bladder neck scarring and stricture formation is much less. In general, bladder neck contractures are seen more frequently after resections of small prostates rather than with large prostates. Additionally, men will usually have antegrade ejaculation afterwards, which is a major issue for many men of all ages (including octogenarians).

A transurethral resection of prostate entails resecting the tissue from the bladder neck to the prostatic apex. The "surgical capsule" represents the boundary between the transition and peripheral zones of the prostate. Most men have a catheter in for 1–2 days and take about 6 weeks to fully recover. Significant postoperative bleeding occurs in about 10% and may occur 10–14 days postoperatively. Because the lower urinary tract symptomatology is often associated with prostatic problems and bladder neck dysfunction the symptomatic improvement may not be as marked as urologists would like to think. Indeed, for the occasional patients with primarily irritative symptoms these may even become worse postoperatively. In general, however, the dysuria, frequency, and urgency routinely experienced postoperatively will resolve within 2 months.

More recently lasers have been used to resect the prostate. The technique entails resecting "the benign adenoma" and delivering it into the bladder where it is then morcellated and extracted. Overall, the surgical process is slower than traditional electrocautery but there is much less bleeding. For a detailed review of technical issues associated with these invasive surgical procedures this may be found elsewhere (Lepor and Lowe, 2002).

Open Prostatectomy

For patients with very large glands (>100 g), it is difficult to treat the adenoma within a reasonable time frame. For these patients an open suprapubic approach is best. A lower midline incision is made. Next a midline incision is made in the bladder, which may be extended into the prostatic capsule. The benign adenoma is then shelled out using finger disection. Major bleeders are oversewn and the bladder neck often reconstructed as part of oversewing of the bleeding vessels. A three-way irrigating catheter is inserted. There is often significant bleeding at the time of enucleation (≤500 ml). Otherwise the risks/complications are broadly the same as for a TURP.

PROSTATE CANCER

Prostate cancer is the most common cause of malignancy in men in the United States (Jenal *et al.*, 2003). The incidence of prostate cancer increases with age making this a pertinent topic in the geriatric population. Advances in diagnosis and treatment allow for earlier detection and improved treatment of the disease. The unique challenge in the geriatric population is patient selection for continued screening and choice of treatment modalities.

Epidemiology

Prostate cancer incidence in the United States has risen dramatically in the past three decades. The incidence of prostate cancer increased 2.7% annually from 1973 to 1988 (Jenal *et al.*, 2003). From 1988 to 1992 it increased 16.2% annually and then fell to 11.7% from 1992 to 1995. Since then data suggests that incidence rates may have leveled off and perhaps are following the curve established before the spike in 1992, which was almost certainly driven by the introduction of widespread use of PSA. African-American males have the highest rate of prostate cancer incidence in the United States (Jenal *et al.*, 2003).

Prostate cancer incidence is also age dependent. In men under 65 years the annual incidence is 58.8 cases per 100 000 men. In men over age 65, the incidence increases to 982.2 cases per 100 000 males per year (Jenal *et al.*, 2003). While screening and treatment advances have recently focused on the younger male, prostate cancer remains predominately a disease of the older male.

Screening and Detection

Early prostate cancer rarely causes symptoms as cancers generally arise in the peripheral portion of the gland. Symptoms from prostate cancer tend to arise with advanced or metatstatic disease. Often these take the form of urinary symptoms. Symptoms may include obstructive urinary symptoms, irritative urinary symptoms, hematuria, hematospermia, bone pain, weight loss, spinal cord compression, and fecal or urinary incontinence. Thus, screening for prostate cancer has become widespread and widely accepted. However, the method of screening and the population to be screened remain controversial. The challenge for the geriatric population is to define the population who will benefit from screening.

Prior to the widespread use of prostate-specific antigen (PSA) only individuals with palpable nodules, or symptoms resulting from prostate cancer underwent transrectal ultrasound guided biopsy (TRUS). Today, screening measurement of PSA often prompts the performance of prostate biopsies.

PSA, although widely utilized as a screening tool, is still controversial. The American Urological Association (AUA), American Cancer Society, and American College of Physicians all support the use of PSA as a screening modality as long as the patient has been given counseling regarding the use of PSA for early detection and treatment (Thompson *et al.*, 2000; Smith *et al.*, 2000; Coley *et al.*, 1997).

The AUA recommends screening only for men with a 10-year life expectancy. Using life assurance tables this approximates to age 74 years. The reason for 10 years is based upon the fact that for periods of less than 10 years it is difficult to show outcome differences for treated versus untreated patients. Thus, for the young geriatric population (65–75 years) recommendations are similar to those for younger men. For the true elderly (>75 years), the approach to screening needs to be individualized. Certainly, as population longevity increases it may be appropriate to screen, diagnose, and treat much older patients.

Prostate-specific Antigen

Prostate-specific-antigen (PSA) is a serine protease produced by both normal and malignant prostate cells. It functions in the liquefaction of the seminal coagulum (Han *et al.*, 2004). Approximately 90% of PSA exists bound to α-1-antichymotrypsin and α-2-macroglobulin. The remainder exists in the unbound or "free" form. Routine PSA assays detect all forms of PSA (Han *et al.*, 2004).

The normal range for PSA has generally been considered 0–4 ng ml^{-1}; however, age-specific cutoffs have been proposed (only for men <65 years) (Morgan *et al.*, 1996; Oesterling *et al.*, 1993). A comment should be made about the new data arising from the Prostate Cancer Prevention Trial. In this trial involving 18 882 men, patients were routinely biopsied at the end of the trial (Thompson *et al.*, 2004). It was found that men were diagnosed with high-grade cancers even with low PSA values (<1 ng ml^{-1}) raising questions about the validity of PSA screening in general. A number of refinements in PSA have been explored to increase its sensitivity as a screening tool.

PSA velocity – It has been shown that PSA increases more rapidly in men with prostate cancer than in men without the disease (Carter *et al.*, 1992). Normal PSA velocity should be less than $0.75\,\mathrm{ng\,ml^{-1}\,year^{-1}}$. In one series 72% of men with cancer had an increased PSA velocity compared with only 5% of men without cancer (Carter *et al.*, 1992). Other studies have supported this finding. Caution must be used with PSA velocity. The lab assays should be from the same laboratory over at least an 18-month period. In periods of less than 1 year, variations of up to 25% may occur in patients without prostate cancer (Riehmann *et al.*, 1993).

In addition to age-adjusted PSA (Table 6), physicians have also come to rely on free PSA and the ratio of free/total PSA to improve the specificity of PSA screening (Carter and Partin, 2002). Men with prostatic adenocarcinoma tend to have a larger percentage of PSA in the complexed or bound form and less in the unbound or free form when compared with men without prostate cancer (Carter and Partin, 2002).

The percentage of free PSA is only useful in men with a total PSA of $4-10\,\mathrm{ng\,ml^{-1}}$. A number of studies have looked at the optimal cutoff for free PSA. Using a cutoff free/total PSA a ratio of 25% was shown to detect 95% of cancers while preventing 20% of unnecessary biopsies (Catalona *et al.*, 1998). If the ratio is less than 20–25% a biopsy is indicated. As the percentage of free/total PSA decreases, the odds increase that there is prostate cancer within the gland. For example, with a free PSA >25% there is an 8% chance of prostate cancer, with a free PSA ratio <10, there is a 56% chance of cancer within the gland (Carter and Partin, 2002).

Additional studies have looked at the free/total PSA ratio in the black population and in men on finasteride. There appears to be no difference in detection using a free cutoff of 25% in black-and-white men (Catalona *et al.*, 2000). Finasteride has been found to decrease the PSA by approximately 50%. However, it decreases the free PSA by an equal amount and is thereby still an effective screening tool in men on this medication (Carter and Partin, 2002).

As longevity increases in men, so will the duration of PSA screening and thus presumably the detection of prostate cancer. This will inevitably lead to the detection of clinically insignificant cancers. Treatment decisions will need to be discussed with the patient and a plan initiated. No therapy for prostate cancer is without side effects. As such, care must be taken to screen only those men whose comorbidities will likely permit at least 10 years of additional life expectancy.

One possible exception to this rule is in an elderly man with severe LUTS that the clinician suspects could be related to prostate cancer. In that instance, PSA and TRUS to diagnose and treat the prostate cancer may alleviate symptoms and improve quality of life.

Once a palpable nodule is found on exam, or a patient has an elevated PSA on screening, a transrectal ultrasound guided biopsy (TRUS) is recommended. The optimal number of cores to perform has been widely studied and debated and is beyond the scope of this chapter. Depending upon the size of the prostate 6–12 cores are usual.

The biopsy is usually performed in the office setting. The patient lies on the side with the knees drawn up. An ultrasound probe is inserted via the rectum and images and measurements of the prostate are obtained. Then a series of needle biopsy samples are obtained transrectally using the ultrasound probe. Most men tolerate the biopsies with minimal discomfort. There is always a risk of continued bleeding from the biopsy sites and as such men should hold their aspirin, vitamin E, herbals, and anticoagulation medications for 5–7 days prior to the biopsy. The use of enemas and antibiotics (fluoroquinoline) prior to the biopsy is usual.

Tumor Grade

The most widely utilized pathologic grading system is the Gleason grading system (Gleason and Mellinger, 1974). The pathologist looks at the prostate cancer under relatively low magnification and assigns a score based on the glandular architecture. Two scores of 1–5 are assigned: the first number being the predominant pattern, and the second number being the secondary pattern. A Gleason grade of 1 being well differentiated and 5 being poorly differentiated, the scores are then added together for a sum of 2–10. For example, two areas of totally undifferentiated tumor would represent a Gleason $5 + 5 = 10$ and, thus, portend a very poor prognosis. Overall, a score of <4 is well differentiated, 5–6 (7) moderately differentiated, and (7) 8–10 poorly differentiated. Any element of a Gleason pattern 4 or a total score of 8 or higher indicate poorly differentiated disease and a worse long-term prognosis.

Table 6 PSA thresholds based on age and race

	"Normal" PSA ranges ($\mathrm{ng\,mL^{-1}}$)			
	Based on 95% specificity		Based on 95% sensitivity	
Age decade (Years)	White males	Black males	White males	Black males
40	0–2.5	0–2.4	0–2.5	0–2.0
50	0–3.5	0–6.5	0–3.5	0–4.0
60	0–4.5	0–11.3	0–3.5	0–4.5
70	0–6.5	0–12.5	0–3.5	0–5.5

Table 7 Prostate cancer staging

TNM	DESCRIPTION
TX	Primary tumor cannot be assessed
T0	No evidence of primary tumor
T1	Nonpalpable tumor not evident by imaging
T1A	Tumor found in tissue removed at TUR; 5% or less is cancerous with histological grade ≤7
T1B	Tumor found in tissue removed at TUR; >5% is cancerous or histological grade >7
T1C	Tumor identified by prostate needle biopsy owing to elevation in PSA
T2	Palpable tumor confined to the prostate
T2A	Tumor involves one lobe or less
T2B	Tumor involves more than one lobe
T3	Palpable tumor beyond prostate
T3A	Unilateral extracapsular extension
T3B	Bilateral extracapsular extension
T3C	Tumor invaded seminal vesicle(s)
T4	Tumor is fixed or invades adjacent structures (not seminal vesicles)
T4A	Tumor invades bladder neck, external sphincter, and/or rectum
T4B	Tumor invades levator muscle and/or is fixed to pelvic wall
N (+)	Involvement of regional lymph nodes
NX	Regional lymph nodes cannot be assessed
N0	No lymph node metastases
N1	Metastases in single regional lymph node, ≤2 cm in dimension
N2	Metastases in single (>2 but ≤5 cm) or multiople nodes with none <5 cm
N3	Metastases in regional lymph node >5 cm in dimension
M (+)	Distant metatstatic spread
MX	Distant metastases cannot be assessed
M0	No evidence of distant metastases
M1	Distant metastases
M1A	Involvement of nonregional lymph nodes
M1B	Involvement of bones
M1C	Involvement of other distant sites

Staging of Prostate Cancer

Stage is determined using the TNM staging system. This is shown in Table 7. Once biopsy confirms prostate cancer, the clinician's goal is to accurately assign a clinical stage, which will predict prognosis and aid in selection of appropriate therapy. The clinical stage is based on the digital rectal exam (DRE), PSA, and pathologic information as well as imaging modalities if indicated. For patients with a Gleason score of 7 or greater, we will obtain a bone scan. For PSA's in excess of 20–25 ng ml^{-1} a CT scan may help identify pathologic lymph nodes.

The PSA, Gleason grade, and TNM stage can be utilized to predict final pathologic stage. There are complex nomograms to help predict the probability of organ confinement, seminal vesical invasion, lymph node involvement (Partin *et al.*, 1997), and extracapsular spread (Partin *et al.*, 1997).

Natural History

In general, prostate cancer is considered to be a slow growing tumor. Indeed, the cliché that most people die with prostate cancer rather than from it holds true. The need for treatment is very much predicated upon life expectancy with 10 years being the threshold defining need for treatment. Two papers have been published demonstrating the relatively benign course with no treatment (Johansson *et al.*, 1997; Albertsen *et al.*, 1998).

Patients with Gleason 6 cancers have a <10% risk of dying of their cancer within 5 years. At the same time, their overall risk of dying is 10–20%. However, even for patients 70–74 years, the risk of dying from a Gleason 8–10 cancer is approximately 30% at 5 years. Thus even for older patients, the diagnosis of a high-grade cancer supports active intervention.

Treatment

There are a number of treatment modalities available for prostate cancer today (Table 8). Each case must be considered individually and each patient (and their family) involved in the decision-making process. Patients who are involved in their decision making and who are fully apprised of the risks, benefits, and possible complications are generally more satisfied despite side effects.

Watchful Waiting

As with any disease process, the first step is to decide to treat or not to treat. Watchful waiting is the conservative approach to prostate cancer. It means that the man makes the decision to monitor the PSA and treat only if the disease spreads or causes symptoms. This decision is based on the natural history of prostate cancer, the patient's age, their comorbidities, and their wishes.

It is imperative that the patient understands that with watchful waiting there is no plan to perform one of the

Table 8 Treatment options for prostate cancer

	Pro	Con
Watchful waiting	• Noninvasive • No immediate side effects of treatment • Disease may never impact quality of life • Treatment unlikely to impact survival in less than 10 years	• Quality of life impacted by worry about cancer • PSA will rise • Tumor may spread and cause local symptoms • Metastatic disease possible
Surgery	• Removal of cancer • Pathology available on whole gland	• Major operation • Impotence in 60–75% of men over age 70 • Some incontinence in 5–15% with higher rate in older men
Radiation	• Less invasive than surgery	• Additional pathology not available • Impotenence • Incontinence • Irritative GI and GU side effects both early and delayed possible • Bleeding

potentially curative therapies listed below if or when the disease progresses. It is to monitor for disease progression and intervene if and when the disease progresses. The intervention at that point is to slow progression, not to cure. If the intent is to cure the disease and the patient is an acceptable candidate, one of the curative modalities discussed below should be utilized.

While this concept is seemingly simple, it is not necessarily easily accepted by all patients. Some men worry constantly about their next PSA. Their quality of life suffers because of the stress. Other patients readily accept this. The patient must be involved in any therapy decision, including the decision to perform watchful waiting.

Radical Prostatectomy

Radical prostatectomy, or removal of the prostate gland, is a potentially curative therapy for prostate cancer. Like any therapy it carries risks. Utilizing a retropubic (lower midline incision), perineal, or laparoscopic approach, the prostate gland is removed in its entirety and the urethra and bladder are sutured together. Goals in performing prostate surgery in order of importance are cancer control, urinary continence, and preservation of sexual potency (Walsh, 2002).

Radical retropubic prostatectomy is the approach most commonly performed today. With refinements in surgical technique and better anesthetic agents morbidity and mortality have been greatly reduced.

There are several advantages of retropubic prostatectomy. It allows for removal of the entire prostate gland and pelvic lymph nodes with accurate pathologic staging. It is not uncommon for the final pathology to differ from that of the needle biopsy with upgrading in about 30%. Patients found on pathologic evaluation to have positive margins may be considered for adjuvant radiation or antiandrogen therapy.

Complications include hemorrhage, incontinence, and impotence. Blood loss can be quite variable but has generally been falling over the last decade. It was quite common for patients to donate autologous blood prior to surgery during the 1990s. This is becoming less common as average intraoperative blood losses fall and transfusion is less often necessary.

Incontinence is another complication. Refined surgical techniques and a better understanding of the anatomy make this complication less common in contemporary series. Total continence rates vary from 80 to 95%. Age does appear to influence continence with younger men fairing slightly better than older men (Catalona *et al.*, 1999). A study of Medicare patients revealed that about one-third of patients had at least some degree of stress incontinence. Severe incontinence, when consideration for an artificial sphincter is given, should occur in 1–2% and certainly less than 5%.

Erectile dysfunction is less common in contemporary series owing to the advent of a nerve-sparing prostatectomy. Potency in large series ranged from 63 to 68% with bilateral nerve sparing and from 41 to 50% with unilateral nerve sparing. Erectile function and dysfunction are graded phenomena. The patient's erectile function prior to surgery, age, and comorbidities all impact the postoperative state.

Potency rates are generally better in younger men and men without significant vascular disease or comorbidities that would predispose to vascular disease. Potency following radical bilateral nerve-sparing prostatectomy varied from 86 to 91% in men under the age of 50, to 25–40% in men older than age 70 (Catalona *et al.*, 1999; Walsh *et al.*, 1994). It has been stated that erectile preservation is rare in men over 70 years. Additional complications to discuss with a patient when contemplating prostatectomy include rectal injury (<1–3.6%), deep venous thrombosis or pulmonary embolism (2–3.1%), and bladder neck contracture (5–10%) (Taneja and deKernion, 2001).

Postoperatively, patients remain in the hospital for 1–2 days and have a urinary catheter for 1–2 weeks. Full recovery takes about 2 months. A surgical option becomes less common for patients over 70 and rare for patients over 75 years.

External Beam Radiation Therapy

Radiation therapy is another potentially curative therapy for prostate cancer. Linear accelerators and 3D conformational techniques have improved delivery of radiation to the prostate gland and decreased radiation exposure to adjacent organs. Radiation treatments are typically delivered daily, Monday–Friday. Treatment protocols vary, but patients usually receive 6–7 weeks of therapy.

Advantages of external beam radiation therapy are that it does not require a general anesthetic, it is noninvasive, does not require a prolonged postoperative recovery period, it is a potentially curative therapy, and has lower risks of incontinence or impotence than prostatectomy. If PSA begins to rise after radiation therapy, patients may still be candidates for other therapies.

Potential disadvantages also exist for external beam radiation therapy as with all the discussed modalities. As the prostate gland is treated *in situ*, there is no additional pathology available to the clinician and no information about margin or lymph node status.

Complications of external beam therapy may be divided into early and late. Early toxicity often occurs during the course of treatment. Gastro intestinal (GI) distress is common occurring in up to 33% of patients (Selch, 2001). GI symptoms include diarrhea, rectal pain, and bleeding. Genitourinary (GU) symptoms are also common during treatment. Urinary symptoms include dysuria, occurring in 12%, and hematuria, frequency, and urgency in 1–5% (Selch, 2001).

Late toxicities may occur immediately after treatment, but more commonly occur years after the completion of therapy. Impotence, GI, and GU morbidity are common. Impotence is often a delayed effect after conclusion of therapy. Potency is retained in 40–76% of men at a follow-up of 12–24 months. Conformational therapy has had minimal effect on potency (Roach *et al.*, 1996). Pretreatment level of function, as with prostatectomy is the most important determinant of posttreatment function.

The most complete analysis of late morbidity in radiation therapy was performed by RTOG (Pilepich *et al.*, 1984). Diarrhea ranged from 9–14%, proctitis 9–11%, and rectal bleeding from 8.7–13%. Additional late GI complications include rectal ulcer, anorectal stricture, and small bowel obstruction although these are much less common.

Delayed GU side effects from the RTOG study included cystitis 11–12%, hematuria 6–11%, and urethral stricture 3–7%. Ranges included are from three different protocols employed in the study.

Brachytherapy

Modern-day techniques have been refined significantly over those utilized in the 1970s. Improved imaging and delivery techniques have made the procedure safer and the disease free survival data more comparable to other techniques in properly selected patients with intermediate term results of nonrandomized trials (Blasko *et al.*, 1997).

Brachytherapy is the insertion of radioactive seeds into the prostate under general or spinal anesthesia. The prostate is imaged, usually by transrectal ultrasound. The prostate is mapped and a computer utilized to determine the dose and number of seeds needed to deliver optimal treatment to the prostate and minimal radiation to the adjacent tissues.

The advantages of brachytherapy include, rapid recovery period with the procedure performed as an outpatient or 23-hour observation, decreased erectile dysfunction and incontinence when compared with open surgery, and comparable results to external beam therapy in properly selected individuals (Jani and Hellman, 2003). Disadvantages include limitation of use to moderately differentiated tumors, lack of final pathologic specimen, erectile dysfunction, GU symptoms, and prostatitis (Jani and Hellman, 2003). Patients with anything but small low-grade tumors will be treated with additional external beam therapy to the pelvic nodes.

Irritative voiding symptoms are the most common side effects after implantation. Mild symptoms of urgency, frequency, dysuria, and hematuria occurred in up to 89% of patients in one large series in the first 4–8 months after the procedure. The symptoms continued after a year in 7% of that same group (Blasko *et al.*, 1993). Postprocedure urinary symptoms are related to the patient's pretreatment symptomatology.

Urinary retention occurs in 5–22% of patient's postimplant (Scherr *et al.*, 2001). Often the retention resolves with initiation of therapy and a temporary indwelling catheter; however, some patients will eventually require TURP. The degree of obstructive symptoms varies, but patients with preexisting obstructive symptoms are at higher risk for postprocedure complications. In fact, severe obstructive symptoms are a relative contraindication to brachytherapy.

A major problem exists for patients who remain in retention posttreatment. If this persists over several months it may be necessary to perform a TURP. When this is necessary, there is a significant risk for the patient having severe irritative LUTS, which can be quite debilitating (Scherr *et al.*, 2001).

Less than 1% of patients have postprocedure incontinence. The exception is in patients with a prior TURP whose risk in several large series was 11–17% (Scherr *et al.*, 2001). Erectile dysfunction after seed implantation was found to be 22% in one large series. Pretreatment potency was a predictor of posttreatment potency as was age. In men younger than 70, 85% were found to preserve potency compared with 50% of those older than 70 (Blasko *et al.*, 1997).

An additional phenomenon unique to brachytherapy is seed migration. One year after therapy, 18–20% of patients will have radiographic evidence of 1–3 seeds in the lungs (Scherr *et al.*, 2001). This is asymptomatic and does not cause clinical adverse outcomes. Additionally, seeds may migrate to the urethra and occasionally may require cystoscopic removal.

Cryotherapy

Cryotherapy of the prostate has been approved by the FDA for use in postradiation failures. Early use with the modality was hampered by problems with urethral and rectal injury. Efficacy in animal models has also been questioned. No good long-term trials are available.

Androgen Deprovation

For many elderly patients, watchful waiting will be the treatment of choice. Likewise, in this patient group (80+ years or younger with comorbidity) surgery and radiation carry greater risk for complications. Some patients will be diagnosed with high-grade tumors (≥Gleason 7). For those patients, primary treatment with hormonal therapy will be appropriate. This is generally achieved with one of the 3–12-month depot injections of the GnRH agonists (Leuprolide, Goserelin Acetate). Bilateral orchiectomy is equally effective, but has largely fallen out of favor for social reasons. Estrogen (Diethylstilbestrol) is rarely if ever used because of cardiovascular toxicity and feminization: GnRH antagonists have recently been introduced and their use may increase in the future.

Treatment of Disease Progression

If the prostate cancer progresses (locally or distant) then initial treatment is hormonal, utilizing the drugs mentioned in the preceding text. Patients receiving hormonal therapy may suffer from osteoporosis with attendant risks for fractures (Krupski *et al.*, 2004; Diamond *et al.*, 2004). Caucasian patients and those of lower BMI are at increased risk for fractures. For these patients, it makes sense to consider a baseline screening for bone density. For patients at risk for bone loss or when it is demonstrated, treatment with a bisphosphonate may be appropriate. At present these are not routinely indicated, but clearly the elderly (≥80 years) are at increased risk for osteoporosis and falls.

PROSTATITIS

Prostatitis is one of the most enigmatic disease labels in medicine. As a word, it implies inflammation of the prostate; yet in the current classification, one subcategory specifically excludes inflammation. The primary symptoms associated with this disease label are irritative LUTS and pelvic pain. It has often been associated with younger men (Moon *et al.*, 1997) though some recent data suggest increasing prevalence through old age (Roberts *et al.*, 1998; McNaughton Collins *et al.*, 2002).

Definition and Classification

The word prostatitis itself by traditional definition is one of inflammation (infection) of the prostate. The process has been subdivided into acute and chronic. Several decades ago it was recognized that not all patients had a bacterial infection and so the term nonbacterial prostatitis was coined. Next, there was a recognition that not all men with symptoms had either an infection or an inflammatory process and thus prostatodynia arose. Finally, in the current classification the recognition that men without symptoms often have histological prostatic inflammation led to the fourth category (Table 9). So what do these men have in common: essentially lower urinary tract symptomatology and pelvic pain. In the early 1990s, the National Institute of Diabetes and Digestive and Kidney Diseases brought together a group of experts and interested individuals to develop a consensus definition of prostatitis (Krieger *et al.*, 1999). This classification is now the basis for most research studies (Table 9). Categories 1 and 2 are fairly straightforward in that category 1 is acute bacterial prostatitis. Patients with this disease present with an acute urinary tract infection and frequently with systemic symptomatology. Patients with category 2 chronic bacterial prostatitis present with relapsing urinary tract infections. The primary requirement for category 3 prostatitis is pelvic pain. This is subdivided into 3a and 3b. 3a is inflammatory nonbacterial prostatitis for which expressed prostatic secretions demonstrate the presence of leukocytes. In category 3b, no leukocytes are present in the expressed prostatic secretions. Category 4 was introduced to cover the incidental finding of inflammation in the prostate in the absence of symptoms: for example, during a biopsy for possible prostate cancer.

Table 9 Classification of prostatitis

Category	Name	Factors
1	Acute Bacterial Prostatitis	Acute urinary tract Infection Systemic symptoms of fever, malaise, myalgia
2	Chronic Bacterial Prostatitis	Recurrent urinary tract infections Between symptomatic episodes cultures localize to prostate
3a	Inflammatory Chronic prostatitis/chronic pelvic pain syndrome	Pelvic Pain Leukocytes in expressed prostatic secretions usually with positive urinary symptomatology
3b	Noninflammatory CP/CPPS	Same as III a but no leukocytes in EPS
4	Asymptomatic inflammatory prostatitis	Incidental finding when prostate being evaluated for other reasons. For example, prostate cancer

Epidemiology

Until the last decade prostatitis was generally thought of as a young man's disease. Part of the reason for that belief occurs because there is significant overlap in the symptomatology between prostatitis symptoms and those of BPH/lower urinary tract symptomatology (Neal and Moon, 1994). However, various reviews of diagnostic coding and patient questionnaires have revealed an increasing incidence and prevalence with age (Roberts *et al.*, 1998; McNaughton Collins *et al.*, 2002). In one study reviewing physicians assigned prostatitis diagnoses in Olmsted County, MN, there were two age-associated peaks: patients aged 20–30 years had 4 cases per thousand person years and over 70 years at 5 cases per thousand person years (Roberts *et al.*, 1998). In another national health professional study, the overall prevalence was 16% with 75% of these patients being first treated before age 60 (McNaughton Collins *et al.*, 2002). Of interest, patients with a diagnosis of BPH had an eight-fold increased likelihood of being diagnosed with prostatitis suggesting either a causal association between the two diagnoses, or alternatively that there is much overlap between the two entities making separation more difficult (more likely). Indeed, in a population-based study from Canada evaluating prostatitis symptom scores, no difference was seen in the prevalence rates for patients less than or over 50 years of age (11.5 vs 8.5%, respectively) (Nickel *et al.*, 2001).

Etiology

The etiology of category 3 prostatitis is one of the least understood diagnoses in medicine. Category 1 (acute bacterial) prostatitis is a lower urinary tract infection. In addition to the usual lower urinary tract symptomatology (frequency, urgency, dysuria) the patient is usually constitutionally sick with hesitancy, poor flow, feeling of incomplete emptying, high fever, chills, nausea, and vomiting. In most cases, there are also obstructive voiding symptoms. The most common infectious agents are *Escherichia coli*, *Klebsiella*, *Proteus*, and *Pseudomonas*. The prevalence of gram-positive bacteria is a debated subject. Certainly, *Staphylococcus aureus*, and *Enterococci* may on occasion cause infection but infections with *Staphylococcus epidermis*, and *Corynebacterium* are debated (Nickel *et al.*, 2003). Of interest, the FDA has recently accepted more gram-positive cultures as evidence of chronic prostatitis than would earlier have been accepted (Bundrick *et al.*, 2003).

Category 2 (chronic bacterial) prostatitis presents as recurrent urinary tract infections where localization tests (performed between acute infections) would reveal prostatic infection. These patients account for only 5% of chronic prostatitis cases.

Category 3 chronic prostatitis (inflammatory 3a or noninflammatory 3b) represents the majority of patients. The etiology for these patients is unclear, but a variety of etiologic possibilities have been postulated (Nickel, 2002). These include dysfunctional voiding, immunologic factors, pelvic floor abnormalities, and psychological factors. Category 4 prostatitis reflects an incidental finding of prostatitis.

Diagnosis/Evaluation

The diagnosis of patients with prostatitis consists of taking a history and physical exam (Table 10). The primary area concerns urinary symptomatology. However, an evaluation of back problems (*referred* pain) and bowel function are important. In 1999, the NIH published a chronic prostatitis symptom index (Litwin *et al.*, 1999) (Table 11) which while not essential for individual practitioners allows researches to uniformally compare data and also monitor changes in patient symptoms.

The physical examination should include a rectal examination and focused neurological examination to rule out other causes of lower urinary tract symptomatology. At the time of rectal examination prostatic massage is performed to obtain an expressed prostatic secretion (EPS) or at least a VB3 (postmassage urine). The one exception to prostatic massage is in the patient with acute bacterial prostatitis where such an examination could lead to septicemia.

Laboratory Testing

Traditionally the urine specimen was divided into 4 specimens (4 glass test). These were the initial stream urine (VB1 – to evaluate for urethral organisms), midstream urine (VB2 – to evaluate for cystitis), EPS, and VB3 urines as a surrogate for EPS, which is not obtainable in all patients, and is intended to define a prostatic infection/inflammation.

If hematuria is noted on the VB1 or 2 specimens then the patient will need an evaluation for hematuria to rule out upper urinary tract abnormalities. Generally, this will consist of a CT urogram and cystoscopy. A urine cytology is also appropriate for patients with hematuria or severe irritative lower urinary tract symptomatology, which could be caused by transitional cell carcinoma or carcinoma *in situ*.

If patients fail initial therapy and where voiding dysfunction is a problem then formal pressure flow urodynamic evaluation may be necessary and appropriate. In either case, a referral to a urologist will be necessary.

Prostatic ultrasound is rarely helpful in this disease. Occasionally, it may identify rare abnormalities such as prostatic cysts, prostatic abscess, or an obstructed seminal vesicle.

Table 10 Evaluation of patients with prostatitis

History		
Symptom index		
Physical Exam		
Including renal scan		
Prostatic massage for collection of EPS/Postmassage Urine		
NOT ACUTE PROSTATITIS PATIENTS		
Laboratory Tests		
4 glass test	VB1	Initial stream urine
	VB2	Mid stream urine
	EPS	Expressed prostatic secretions
	VB3	Post massage urine
2 glass test – VB2, VB3		
Urine culture		
Urine cytology – If hematuria present		
Urodynamics – May be required to evaluate voiding dysfunction-if initial treatment fails		

Treatment

Despite the fact that most urologists, let alone primary physicians, don't evaluate prostatic fluid/VB3 for bacteria or other microorganisms the majority will initiate antibiotic therapy (McNaughton Collins *et al.*, 2002) (Table 12). Clearly, with chronic bacterial prostatitis being present in only 5% of patients this treatment will not be very effective. In the absence of prostatic cultures persistence with antibiotics, filling one after the other (an all too often seen occurrence) is futile. Fluoroquinolones have become the treatment of choice for chronic bacterial prostatitis. Drugs should be given for 2–4 weeks. If a true infection is found then therapy in some cases will be necessary for up to 12 weeks to eradicate it completely. Trimethopim and Sulfamethoxazole (Bactrim) have been used for many years. However, increasing bacterial resistance is reducing the appropriateness for this drug. Doxycycline is considered a second-line drug. The place of fungal infections in prostatitis is unclear, but occasionally some patients may benefit from a trial with an antifungal agent such as diflucan.

α-Blockers

The prostate is innervated with α-1 adrenergic receptors ($\alpha 1_a$ on the smooth muscles and $\alpha 1_b$ on the blood vessels). The bladder body also has adrenergic innervation but primarily with $\alpha 1_d$ receptors. Thus, a drug, which blocks $\alpha 1_{a/d}$ receptors, should lead to a reduction in irritative bladder symptoms ($\alpha 1_d$) and improvement in obstructive symptoms ($\alpha 1_a$). As many prostatitis patients are thought to have voiding dysfunction with reflux of urine into the prostatic ducts, resection of the prostate should reduce this problem and likely reduce chemical inflammation and symptoms. The use of α-blockers has recently been reviewed (Moon, 2004). No good large randomized clinical trials have been performed but the general sense is that they have a place in the

Table 11 NIH–Chronic Prostatitis Symptom Index (NIH–CPSI)

Pain or Discomfort

1. In the last week, have you experienced any pain or discomfort in the following areas?

	Yes	No
a. Area between rectum and testicles (perineum)	❑ 1	❑ 0
b. Testicles	❑ 1	❑ 0
c. Tip of the penis (not related to urination)	❑ 1	❑ 0
d. Below your waist, in your public or bladder area	❑ 1	❑ 0

2. In the last week, have you experienced:

	Yes	No
a. Pain or burning during urination?	❑ 1	❑ 0
b. Pain or discomfort during or after sexual climax (ejaculation)?	❑ 1	❑ 0

3. How often have you had pain or discomfort in any of these areas over the last week?

❑ 0 Never
❑ 1 Rarely
❑ 2 Sometimes
❑ 3 Often
❑ 4 Usually
❑ 5 Always

4. Which number best describes your AVERAGE pain or discomfort on the days that you had it, over the last week?

❑	❑	❑	❑	❑	❑	❑	❑	❑	❑	❑
0	1	2	3	4	5	6	7	8	9	10
NO PAIN									PAIN AS BAD AS YOU CAN IMAGINE	

Urination

5. How often have you had a sensation of not emptying your bladder completely after you finished urinating, over the last week?

❑ 0 Not at all
❑ 1 Less than 1 time in 5
❑ 2 Less than half the time
❑ 3 About half the time
❑ 4 More than half the time
❑ 5 Almost always

6. How often have you had to urinate again less than two hours after you finished urinating, over the last week?

❑ 0 Not at all
❑ 1 Less than 1 time in 5
❑ 2 Less than half the time
❑ 3 About half the time
❑ 4 More than half the time
❑ 5 Almost always

Impact of Symptoms

7. How much have your symptoms kept you from doing the kinds of things you would usually do, over the last week?

❑ 0 None
❑ 1 Only a little
❑ 2 Some
❑ 3 A lot

8. How much did you think about your symptoms, over the last week?

❑ 0 None
❑ 1 Only a little
❑ 2 Some
❑ 3 A lot

Quality of Life

9. If you were to spend the rest of your life with your symptoms just the way they have been during the last week, how would you feel about that?

❑ 0 Delighted
❑ 1 Pleased
❑ 2 Mostly satisfied
❑ 3 Mixed (about equally satisfied and dissatisfied)
❑ 4 Mostly dissatisfied
❑ 5 Unhappy
❑ 6 Terrible

therapeutic armamentarium. Unfortunately, the largest randomized clinical trials recently conducted by the NIDDK failed to define a drug effect (Alexander *et al.*, 2004). However, as the authors point out, the population was heavily pretreated and resistant to other treatments.

The use of α-blockers has also been tried in conjunction with antibiotics for patients with chronic bacterial prostatitis. The general conclusion is that combining the two drugs and continuing the α-blocker for 6 months will reduce the likelihood of recurrence (Barbalias *et al.*, 1998).

Table 12 Treatment of prostatitis

Antibiotics	Commentary
Fluoroquinolines	If culture negative, one therapeutic trial is sufficient
α-blockers	Studies mixed but efficacy predicated upon voiding dysfunction amenable to α blockade
Anti-inflammatory drugs	Nonsteroidal anti-inflammatory drugs should reduce inflammatory parameters
Physical therapy	Pelvic flow massage and myofascial release
Microwave therapy	Although approved for benign prostatic hypertrophy small scale studies suggest efficacy

Physical Therapy

Physical therapy covers two main entities: prostatic massage and pelvic floor massage/myofascial trigger point release. Prostatic massage has mixed reviews. A recent publication by a panel of North American "prostatitis experts" could not come to a concensus as potential benefits (Nickel *et al.*, 1999).

Pelvic Floor Massage

It has been suggested that some patients develop chronic tension in the pelvic floor muscles as a result of many factors (Anderson, 1999). These include dysfunctional voiding, sexual abuse, constipation, and even stress and anxiety. These abnormalities may lead to pelvic trigger points causing pain. Physical therapy to release these trigger points has been reported to improve symptoms in patients. However, these methods have not been studied in a randomized clinical trial.

Minimally Invasive Therapy

Microwave thermotherapy has been reported to alleviate symptoms in patients with category 3a chronic prostatitis. The hypothesized mechanism of action is by possible denervation of the prostate by heat therapy. However, no large long-term randomized clinical trials have been performed.

Other Therapies

Because prostatitis is in many reports a symptom complex rather than a disease process, many different interventions have been utilized. These include anti-inflammatory agents, muscle relaxants, hormone therapy, and phytotherapeutics. These have been reviewed elsewhere (Nickel, 2002).

KEY POINTS

- Benign prostatic hyperplasia (as an histologic entity) may or may not be the cause of lower urinary tract symptoms in older men.
- The key issue for whether or not to treat men with BPH/LUTS is BOTHER.
- Screening for prostate cancer is only appropriate for men with more than 10 years' life expectancy.
- Older (>70 yrs) patients with high-grade prostate cancer will still die from cancer as well as competing comorbidities.
- Most patients (>95%) with prostatitis do not have an infection.
- Prostatitis is probably a catchbag for multiple pathologic entities.

KEY REFERENCES

- Albertsen PC, Hanley JA, Gleason DF & Barry MJ. Competing risk analysis of men aged 55 to 74 years at diagnosis managed conservatively for clinically localized prostate cancer. *The Journal of the American Medical Association* 1998; **280**(11):975–80.
- AUA Practice Guidelines Committee. AUA Guideline on management of benign prostatic hyperplasia. Chapter 1: diagnosis and treatment recommendations. *The Journal of Urology* 2003; **170**:530–47.
- Krupski TL, Smith MR, Lee WC *et al.* Natural history of bone complications in men with prostate carcinoma initiating androgen deprivation therapy. *Cancer* 2004; **101**(3):541–9.
- McConnell JD, Roehrborn CG, Bautista OM *et al.* The long-term effect of Doxazosin, Finasteride, and combination therapy on the clinical progression of benign prostatic hyperplasia. *The New England Journal of Medicine* 2003; **349**:2387–98.
- Nickel JC. Prostatitis and related conditions. *Campbell's Urology* 2002, pp 603–30; W.B. Saunders.

REFERENCES

Abrams P. In support of pressure flow studies for evaluating men with lower urinary tract symptoms. *Urology* 1994; **44**:153–5.

Albertsen PC, Hanley JA, Gleason DF & Barry MJ. Competing risk analysis of men aged 55 to 74 years at diagnosis managed conservatively for clinically localized prostate cancer. *The Journal of the American Medical Association* 1998; **280**(11):975–80.

Alexander RB, Propert KJ, Schaeffer AJ *et al.* A randomized trial of Ciprofloxacin and tamsulosin in men with chronic prostatitis/chronic pelvic pain syndrome. *The Journal of Urology* 2004; **171**(4):232.

Anderson RU. Treatment of prostatodynia (pelvic floor myalgia or chronic non-inflammatory pelvic pain syndrome). In JC Nickel (ed) *Textbook of Prostatitis* 1999, pp 357–64; Isis Medical Media Limited, Oxford.

Arrighi HM, Metter EJ, Guess HA & Fozzard JL. Natural history of benign prostatic hyperplasia and risk of prostatectomy. The Baltimore longitudinal study of aging. *Urology* 1991; **38**(suppl 1):4–8.

AUA Practice Guidelines Committee. AUA Guideline on management of benign prostatic hyperplasia. Chapter 1: diagnosis and treatment recommendations. *The Journal of Urology* 2003; **170**:530–47.

Barbalias GA, Nikiforidis G & Liatsikos EN. α-Blockers for the treatment of chronic prostatitis in combination with antibiotics. *The Journal of Urology* 1998; **159**:883–7.

Berry SJ, Coffey DS, Walsh PC & Ewing LL. The development of human benign prostatic hyperplasia with age. *The Journal of Urology* 1984; **132**:474–9.

Blasko J, Grimm P & Ragde H. Brachytherapy and organ preservation in the management of carcinoma of the prostate. *Seminars in Radiation Oncology* 1993; **3**:240–9.

Blasko JC, Radge H & Grimm PD. Transperineal ultrasound-guided implantation of the prostate: morbidity and complications. *Scandinavian Journal of Urology and Nephrology. Supplementum* 1997; **137**:113–8.

Bundrick W, Heron SP, Ray P *et al.* Levofloxacin versus Ciprofloxacin in the treatment of chronic bacterial prostatitis: a randomized double-blind multicenter study. *Urology* 2003; **62**(3):537–41.

Carter HB & Partin AW. Diagnosis and staging of prostate cancer. In PC Walsh (ed) *Campbell's Urology* 2002, 8th edn, vol. 4, pp 3055–73; W.B. Saunders, Philadelphia.

Carter HB, Pearson JD, Metter JE *et al.* Longitudinal evaluation of prostate specific antigen levels in men with and without prostate disease. *The Journal of the American Medical Association* 1992; **267**:2215.

Catalona WJ, Carvalhal GF, Mager DE & Smith DS. Potency, continence, and complication rates in 1,870 consecutive radical retropubic prostatectomies. *The Journal of Urology* 1999; **162**(2):433–8.

Catalona WJ, Partin AW, Slawin KM *et al.* Use of the percentage free prostate-specific antigen to enhance differentiation of prostate cancer from benign prostatic disease: a prospective multicenter clinical trial. *The Journal of the American Medical Association* 1998; **279**:279–1542.

Catalona WJ, Partin AW, Slawin KM *et al.* Percentage of free PSA in black versus white men for detection and staging of prostate cancer: a prospective multicenter clinical trial. *Urology* 2000; **55**:372.

Chute CG, Panswer LA, Girman CJ *et al.* The prevalence of prostatism: a population-based survey of urinary symptoms. *The Journal of Urology* 1993; **150**:85–9.

Coley C, Barry MJ & Mulley AG. Clinical Guidelines: Part III: Screening for prostate cancer. *Annals of Internal Medicine* 1997; **126**:480.

Diamond TH, Bucci J, Kersley JH *et al.* Osteoporosis and spinal fractures in men with prostate cancer: risk factory and effects of androgen deprivation therapy. *The Journal of Urology* 2004; **172**(2):529–32.

European Association of Urology. 2004, Www.uroweb.org.

Fitzpatrick JM & Mebust WK. Minimally invasive and endoscopic management of benign prostatic hyperplasia. In PC Walsh (ed) *Campbell's Urology* 2002, 8th edn, Vol 2, chapter 40, pp 1379–422; W.B. Saunders, Philadelphia.

Flanigan RC, Reda DJ, Wasson JH *et al.* 5-year outcome of surgical resection and watchful waiting for men with moderately symptomatic benign prostatic hyperplasia: a department of veteran's affairs cooperative study. *The Journal of Urology* 1998; **160**:12–7.

Gleason DF, & Mellinger GT, Veterans Administration Cooperative Urological Research Group. Prediction of prognosis for prostatic adenocarcinoma by combined histologic grading and clinical staging. *The Journal of Urology* 1974; **111**:58–64.

Han M, Gann PH & Catalona WJ. Prostate-specific antigen and screening for prostate cancer. *The Medical Clinics of North America* 2004; **88**(2):245–65.

Jani AB & Hellman S. Early prostate cancer: clinical decision making. *The Lanet (London)* 2003; **361**(9362):1045.

Jenal A, Murray T, Samuels A, Cancer Statistics 2003. *CA: A Cancer Journal for Clinicians* 2003; **53**:5–26.

Johansson JE, Holmberg L, Johansson S *et al.* Fifteen-year survival in prostate cancer: a prospective, population-based study in Sweden. *The Journal of the American Medical Association* 1997; **277**(6):467–71.

Kelly CE, Zimmern PE. Clinical evaluation of lower urinary tract symptoms due to benign prostatic hyperplasia. *Atlas of the Prostate* 2003, 2nd edn, chapter 2, pp 11–23: Current Medicine Philadelphia PA, USA.

Koyanogi T, Artiboni W, Correa R *et al.* In L Denis, K Griffith, S Khoury *et al.* (eds) *Proceedings of the Fourth International Consultation of BPH, Paris, July 1997* 1998, pp 179–265; Health Publications, Plymouth.

Krieger JN, Nyberg L Jr & Nickel JC. NIH consensus definition and classification of prostatitis. *The Journal of the American Medical Association* 1999; **2841**(3):236–7.

Krupski TL, Smith MR, Lee WC *et al.* Natural history of bone complications in men with prostate carcinoma initiating androgen deprivation therapy. *Cancer* 2004, **101**(3):541–9.

Lee AJ, Russell EB, Garraway WM & Prescott RJ. Three-year follow-up of a community-based cohort of men with untreated benign prostatic hyperplasia. *European Urology* 1996; **30**:11–7.

Lepor H & Lowe FC. Evaluation and non-surgical management of benign prostatic hyperplasia. In PC Walsh (ed) *Campbell's Urology* 2002, 8th edn, vol 2, chapter 39, pp 1337–78; W.B. Saunders, Philadelphia.

Litwin MS, McNaughton Collins M, Fowler FJ Jr *et al.* The national institutes of health chronic prostatitis symptom index: development and validation of a new outcome measure. *The Journal of Urology* 1999; **162**:369–75.

Lowe FC & Fogelman F. Permixon: a review. *Current Prostate Reports* 2004; **2**:132–6.

McConnell JD, Bruskewitz RC, Walsh P *et al.* The effect of Finasteride on the risk of acute urinary retention and the need for surgical treatment among men with benign prostatic hyperplasia. *The New England Journal of Medicine* 1998; **338**:557–63.

McConnell JD, Roehrborn CG, Bautista OM *et al.* The long-term effect of Doxazosin, Finasteride, and combination therapy on the clinical progression of benign prostatic hyperplasia. *The New England Journal of Medicine* 2003; **349**:2387–98.

McNaughton Collins M, Meigs JB, Barry MJ *et al.* Prevalence and correlates of prostatitis in the health professionals follow-up study cohort. *The Journal of Urology* 2002; **167**:1363–6.

Miller PD, Kastner C, Ramsey EW & Parsons K. Cooled thermotherapy for the treatment of benign prostatic hyperplasia: durability of results obtained with the targis system. *Urology* 2003; **61**(6):1160–5.

Moon TD. Alpha-blockers in prostatitis. *Current Prostate Reports* 2004; **2**:143–7.

Moon TD, Hagen L & Heisey DM. Urinary symptomatology in younger men. *Urology* 1997; **50**(5):700–3.

Morgan TO, Jacobsen SJ, McCarthy WF *et al.* Age-specific reference ranges for prostate-specific antigen in black men. *The New England Journal of Medicine* 1996; **335**:304.

Neal DE Jr & Moon TD. Use of terazosin in prostatodynia and validation of a symptom score questionnaire. *Urology* 1994; **43**(4):460–5.

Nickel JC. Prostatitis and related conditions. *Campbell's Urology* 2002, pp 603–30; W.B. Saunders.

Nickel JC, Alexander R, Anderson R *et al.* Prostatitis unplugged? Prostate massage revisited. *Techniques in Urology* 1999; **5**(1):1–7.

Nickel JC, Alexander RB, Schaeffer AJ *et al.* Leukocytes and bacteria in men with chronic prostatitis/chronic pelvic pain syndrome compared to asymptomatic controls. *The Journal of Urology* 2003; **170**:818–22.

Nickel JC, Downey J, Hunter D & Clark J. Prevalence of prostatitis-like symptoms in a population-based study using the national institutes of health chronic prostatitis symptom index. *The Journal of Urology* 2001; **165**:842–5.

Oesterling JE, Jacobsen SJ, Chute CG *et al.* Serum prostate-specific antigen in a community-based population of healthy men: Establishment of age-specific reference ranges. *The Journal of the American Medical Association* 1993; **270**:860.

Partin AW, Kattan MW, Subong EN *et al.* Combination of prostate-specific antigen, clinical stage, and Gleason score to predict pathological stage of localized prostate cancer. A multi-institutional update. *The Journal of the American Medical Association* 1997; **277**:1445–51.

Pilepich MV, Krall J, George FW *et al.* Treatment-related morbidity in phase III RTOG studies of extended-field irradiation for carcinoma of the prostate [Clinical Trial Journal Article]. *International Journal of Radiation Oncology, Biology, Physics* 1984; **10**(10):1861–7.

Riehmann M, Rhodes PR, Cook TD, Analysis of variation in prostate-specific antigen values. *Urology* 1993; **42**(4):390–7.

Roach M, Chinn DM, Holland J *et al.* A pilot survey of sexual function and quality of life following 3D conformational radiotherapy for clinically localized prostate cancer. *International Journal of Radiation Oncology, Biology, Physics* 1996; **35**:869–74.

Roberts RO, Lieber MM, Rhodes T *et al.* Prevalence of a physician-assigned diagnosis of prostatis: the olmstead county study of urinary symptoms and health status among men. *Urology* 1998; **51**(4):578–84.

Roehrborn CG & McConnell JD. Etiology, pathopysiology, epidemiology, and natural history of benign prostatic hyperplasia. In PC Walsh (ed) *Campbell's Urology* 2002, 8th edn, vol 2, Chapter 38, pp 1297–336; W.B. Saunders, Philadelphia.

Scherr D, Bosworth J, Steckel J. Complications of brachytherapy in the treatment of localized prostate cancer. *Complications in Urologic Surgery: Prevention and Management* 2001, 3rd edn, pp 419–26; W.B. Saunders, Philadelphia.

Selch MT. Complications of radiation therapy for urologic cancer. *Complications of Urologic Surgery: Prevention and Management* 2001, 3rd edn, pp 133–41; W.B. Saunders, Philadelphia.

Smith RA, Mettlin CJ, Davis KJ *et al.* American Cancer Society guidelines for the early detection of cancer. *CA: A Cancer Journal for Clinicians* 2000; **50**:34.

Taneja SS, deKernion JB. Complications of radical retropubic prostatectomy. *Complications of Urologic Surgery: Prevention and Management* 2001, 3rd edn, pp 408–18; W.B. Saunders, Philadelphia.

Thompson I, Carroll P, Coley C *et al.* Prostate-specific antigen (PSA) best practice policy. American Urological Association. *Oncology* 2000; **14**:267.

Thompson IM, Pauler DK, Goodman PJ *et al.* *The New England Journal of Medicine* 2004; **350**:2239–46. Prevalence of prostate cancer among men with a prostate-specific antigen level $\leq$4.0 ng per milliliter.

Walsh PC. Anatomic radical retropubic prostatectomy. In PC Walsh (ed) *Campbell's Urology* 2002, 8th edn, vol 3, pp 3107–28; W.B. Saunders, Philadelphia.

Walsh PC, Partin AW & Epstein JI. Cancer control and quality of life following anatomical radical retropubic prostatectomy: results at 10 years. *The Journal of Urology* 1994; **152**:1831–6.

126

Urinary Incontinence

Margaret-Mary G. Wilson

Saint Louis University Health Sciences Center and Veterans' Affairs Medical Center, St Louis, MO, USA

Some men there are love not a gaping pig,
Some that are mad if they behold a cat,
And others when the bagpipe sings i'th' nose
Cannot contain their urine.

William Shakespeare (1564–1616),
Shylock, in The Merchant of Venice, act 4, sc. 1.

INTRODUCTION

Unlike other parameters of geriatric health, such as cognition, balance, and mood, continence is an attribute that is rarely appreciated until there is almost complete failure of the underlying physiological regulatory mechanisms. Additionally, despite the great strides that have been made in dissociating social stigma from a variety of diseases, including sexually transmitted diseases and acquired immune deficiency syndrome, urinary incontinence (UI) continues to suffer from the reluctance of both patient and provider to address the problem. Embarrassment, lack of awareness of the associated serious comorbidity and mortality, as well as ignorance regarding the availability and efficacy of several therapeutic options have been implicated as factors that deter due attention to this deadly disease (Dugan *et al.*, 2001; Horrocks *et al.*, 2004; Kinchen *et al.*, 2003; Shaw *et al.*, 2001). With the advent of the "baby boomers" and the projected increase in the proportion of older adults, UI and the attendant consequences will loom large on the horizon of geriatric disease. Thus, in this climate, health-care providers who fail to identify and adequately treat older adults with UI are delivering substandard care.

UI in older adults is a potentially devastating disease. Affected adults may exhibit significant functional decline and frailty, resulting in increased risk of institutionalization and death. Abundant data confirms the negative effect of UI on the quality of life of affected elders (Bradway, 2003; Johnson *et al.*, 2000).

Reported prevalence for UI varies from 15% among relatively healthy community-dwelling older adults to 65% among the frail elderly (Brandeis *et al.*, 1997; Holroyd-Leduc *et al.*, 2004; Landi *et al.*, 2003; Sgadari *et al.*, 1997). In the United States, more than 17 million adults suffer from UI (Hu *et al.*, 2004). However, available figures most likely underestimate the true prevalence of this syndrome for a variety of reasons. Major reasons identified for inaccurate reporting of the true prevalence of UI include failure to perceive the significance and ominous implications of UI by affected elders, and also the misconception that UI is an expected consequence of aging. Patient embarrassment, discomfort, and lack of awareness of effective treatment options are other barriers to self-reporting (Dugan *et al.*, 2001).

Annually, the direct cost of UI exceeds US $20 billion, with approximately 74% of this amount being spent on incontinence care in women. Two-thirds of the direct cost for UI care in women is spent on community-dwelling women (Hu *et al.*, 2004; Wilson *et al.*, 2001). Overall, the incremental lifetime medical cost of treating an older adult with UI approaches US $60 000 (Birnbaum *et al.*, 2003).

Indirect costs arising from factors such as reduced work productivity of the patient or the caregiver elevate the economic burden of UI even further. Of paramount importance in estimating the societal cost of UI is the recognition of associated intangible costs reflected in compromised quality of life, decreased feeling of well-being, psychological instability, and loss of self-esteem (Hu *et al.*, 2004).

RISK FACTORS

UI is less frequent in men. Zunzunegui Pastor *et al.* reported a prevalence of UI of 14% in older community-dwelling men compared to a prevalence of 30% among their female counterparts. Nevertheless, advancing age is associated with a higher frequency of UI in men, but not in women.

Principles and Practice of Geriatric Medicine, 4th Edition. Edited by M.S. John Pathy, Alan J. Sinclair and John E. Morley.

Additional associated factors include coexisting morbidity, cognitive dysfunction, functional impairment, gait abnormality, diuretic therapy, and obesity (Zunzunegui Pastor *et al.*, 2003). Notably, most independent risk factors for UI are potentially reversible (Landi *et al.*, 2003). The onus lies with providers to identify and treat such risk factors in all patients being evaluated for UI.

PATHOPHYSIOLOGY OF URINARY INCONTINENCE IN THE ELDERLY

Several age-related changes threaten lower urinary tract function in the elderly. These include an increase in the frequency of uninhibited detrusor contractions, impaired bladder contractility, abnormal detrusor relaxation patterns, and reduced bladder capacity. An increase in nocturnal urine production also occurs. Anatomically, prostatic size increases in men, while urethral shortening and urethral sphincter weakening occurs in women. In addition to these physiological and anatomical age-related changes, the increased frequency of lower urinary tract disease in older patients further increases the risk of UI (Enriquez, 2004; Kevorkian, 2004; Klauser *et al.*, 2004; Lluel *et al.*, 2003; Patel *et al.*, 2002; Tan, 2003; Whishaw, 1998; Yoshida *et al.*, 2004).

Although providers tend to defer screening for UI until later in life, the framework for UI is often laid much earlier in life. Predisposing factors for UI should be sought in all patients regardless of age. Female gender is an irreversible predisposing factor and mandates routine enquiry for UI in all women regardless of age. The presence of structural congenital abnormalities such as hypospadias, epispadias, and ambiguous genitalia may also compromise bladder continence. With aging and the increased likelihood of disease, inciting factors such as cerebrovascular disease, radical pelvic surgery and autonomic degeneration further increase the risk of UI (Allen *et al.*, 2004; Ayed *et al.*, 1995; McLoughlin & Chew, 2000; Mouriquand *et al.*, 2003). Available data indicates that the occurrence of cerebrovascular disease doubles the risk of UI in older females. Obesity, frailty, and diabetes are other strong predictors of the occurrence of UI (Enriquez, 2004; Klausner and Vapnek, 2003; Landi *et al.*, 2003; Namikawa, 1999; Ouslander, 2000). Additionally, older adults are more likely to become incontinent following the onset of UI-promoting factors such as constipation, obesity, and polyuria from uncontrolled hyperglycemia, hypercalcemia, or diuretic therapy. Traditional geriatric pathophysiological factors such as impaired cognitive function, functional impairment, and frailty may also precipitate incontinence as a manifestation of global decompensation.

CLASSIFICATION

Accurate classification of UI should include reference to both the temporal course and the mechanistics of involuntary urine

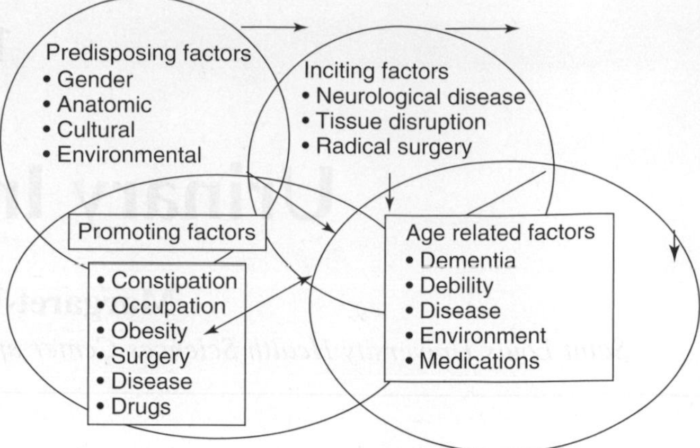

Figure 1 Risk factors for urinary incontinence

Table 1 Causes of reversible urinary incontinence

D Delirium	D Delirium
I Infection	R Restricted mobility, retention
A Atrophic vaginitis	I Infection, inflammation, impaction
P Pharmaceuticals	P Polyuria, pharmaceuticals
P Psychological disorders	
E Endocrine disorders	
R Restricted mobility	
S Stool impaction	

loss. Several mnemonics have been developed for the causes of transient or reversible incontinence (Figure 1; Table 1). Previously, continent patients who experience incontinence in the acute-care setting are likely to have underlying reversible causes of incontinence. Acute-care protocols that incorporate screening and detection of such risk factors are critical to reducing the incidence of incontinence in acutely hospitalized elders. Classification of UI in this manner also facilitates efficient and cost-effective intervention, as recognition and correction of causes of transient incontinence prevents unnecessary and expensive investigations and invasive studies.

Mechanistic classification of UI results in five major categories: UI associated with overactive bladder (OAB), stress incontinence, overflow incontinence, and functional incontinence. Combinations of these categories constitute the fifth category that is referred to as *mixed incontinence*. Bladder overactivity and impaired contractility frequently occur in conjunction in patients with diabetes mellitus. Similarly, benign prostatic enlargement often presents with symptoms of bladder overactivity as well as urinary retention (Johnson and Ouslander, 1999; Nasr and Ouslander, 1998; Ouslander, 2000; Ouslander and Schnelle, 1995).

Urinary Incontinence Associated with Overactive Bladder

Overactive bladder occurs in 1 of 4 adults over the age of 65, and is the most common cause of UI in the elderly, accounting for 40–70% of all cases. Characteristically, overactive bladder results from involuntary contractions of the detrusor muscle, resulting in a strong urge to pass urine in unusually low volumes. Clinically, OAB manifests with urgency, frequency, and nocturia with or without urge incontinence (Newman, 2004; Teleman *et al.*, 2004; Tubaro, 2004; Yoshida *et al.*, 2004). Persons with urge incontinence present with involuntary urine loss preceded by a sudden, urgent, and strong desire to void.

Electrical field stimulation studies have identified at least three different mechanisms of detrusor muscle contraction. The major mechanism is cholinergic, and is mediated through the effect of acetylcholine (Ach) on muscarinic bladder receptors. A second mechanism (purinergic) involves adenosine triphosphate (ATP)-mediated bladder contraction. A third and poorly defined mechanism is thought to be nonneuronal and attributed to local urothelial Ach production and a paracrine effect on local muscarinic receptors located in the bladder. Age-related reduction in cholinergic and purinergic bladder transmission has been identified. However, purinergic transmission appears to play a greater role in bladder contraction in older adults, indicating disproportionate age-related compromise in cholinergic function. Available data also indicates an age-related compromise of nonneuronal uroepithelial Ach production (Wuest *et al.*, 2005; Yoshida *et al.*, 2004).

Stress Incontinence

Stress incontinence is the underlying cause in 25% of women with UI, and results from anatomical or pathological disruption of the angle between the bladder neck and the urethra, thereby disrupting continence. Causes of stress incontinence include vaginal childbirth, and pelvic surgery such as hysterectomy or prostate surgery (Jackson *et al.*, 2004; Molander *et al.*, 2002; Van der Varrt *et al.*, 2002).

Characteristically, stress incontinence presents with involuntary urine loss resulting from increases in intra-abdominal pressure in the presence of a relatively incompetent urethral sphincter mechanism. Thus, involuntary urine loss may occur when the patient laughs, coughs, or sneezes. In severe cases, UI may occur with a change in posture from supine or sitting to standing.

Overflow Incontinence

Overflow incontinence results from bladder outlet obstruction, resulting in massive bladder distension. Consequently, involuntary urine loss results from a buildup of intravesical pressure until the mechanical outlet obstruction is overcome by sheer pressure. Persons with overflow incontinence complain of persistent trickling of urine in the presence of suprapubic distension. In men, prostatic enlargement is the most common cause of overflow incontinence. Pelvic masses, such as uterine fibroids, or cystoceles may cause similar obstructive symptoms in women (Borrie *et al.*, 2001; Chapple, 2001; Grosshans *et al.*, 1993).

Functional Incontinence

Functional incontinence refers to involuntary urine loss resulting from inability to gain access to toileting facilities for a variety reasons including limited mobility, impaired cognition, lack of motivation, environmental barriers, or restricted access. This is a common cause of incontinence in frail elders with dementia, cerebrovascular disease, Parkinson's disease, or delirium. Altered mental status from narcotics, sedatives, or narcoleptic agents are also frequently implicated (Chadwick, 2005; Vickerman, 2002). Inappropriate use of physical or chemical restraints, poor vision, depression, reduced exercise tolerance, gait abnormality, or fear of falling are other miscellaneous causes of functional incontinence.

COMPLICATIONS AND CONSEQUENCES OF URINARY INCONTINENCE

Deleterious effects of UI are far reaching and multidimensional. Various aspects of quality of life are affected. Older adults with UI frequently suffer from embarrassment and loss of self-confidence and self-esteem. Sixty percent of older adults with UI develop depressive symptoms. Unpredictable involuntary urine loss frequently results in the affected elders becoming increasingly isolated as a result of voluntary restriction of social interaction and travel. Limitation of physical activity in affected elders may compromise functional status and hasten progression to frailty. Intimate relationships may also be adversely affected by the onset of incontinence, as affected persons avoid sexual activity with partners for fear of involuntary urine loss during intercourse. Indeed, available data highlights an independent association between sexual dysfunction and UI in older men (Bradway, 2003; Hogan, 1997; Johansson *et al.*, 1996; Miner, 2004; Saltvedt *et al.*, 2002).

Financially, the economic costs of UI may be extremely burdensome. Protective garments and beddings are relatively expensive, and are often not covered by insurance plans. The productivity of older adults in the workforce may be negatively affected by the threat of frequent and unpredictable episodes of incontinence. Likewise, the productivity of caregivers of patients with UI may be compromised by their inability to cope with the demands of a relative with UI. Indeed, available data highlights UI as the most common cause of institutionalization of elders. Likewise, in long-term care facilities, the resident with UI imposes an additional annual financial burden of approximately $5000 to total health-care costs (Bradway, 2003; Hogan, 1997; Johansson *et al.*, 1996; Miner, 2004; Saltvedt *et al.*, 2002).

Table 2 Complications of urinary incontinence

- Recurrent urinary tract infections
- Skin infections
- Balanitis
- Pressure ulcers
- Falls
- Fractures
- Depression
- Decreased libido and sexual dysfunction
- Acute hospitalization
- Social isolation
- Caregiver stress
- Reduced feeling of well-being
- Institutionalization
- Increased health-care costs

Medical complications further compromise health-care related quality of life. In women with incontinence aged over 65, the incidence of falls and fractures increases significantly. Approximately, 20–40% of women with UI will fall within 12 months and of these about 10% will result in fractures, usually of the hip. Available data also indicates a strong association between UI, acute hospitalization, and institutionalization (Gray, 2003; Wilson, 2003, 2004). Thirty percent of women with UI over the age of 65 are likely to be hospitalized within 12 months. Older men are twice as likely to be hospitalized over a 12-month period (Saltvedt *et al.*, 2002). Of the myriad complications associated with UI, the most alarming is the independent association between UI and increased mortality (Table 2).

CLINICAL DETECTION OF UI

Older adults with UI rarely volunteer this information as a presenting complaint. The onus is therefore on the providers to screen for UI in all older adults. Several older patients labor under the misconception that UI is part of the normal aging process. Other patients may be embarrassed by the nature of the complaint, especially when interacting with a health-care provider of the opposite gender. Decreased awareness of available therapeutic options may also discourage the patient from complaining. As a result of these factors, delayed presentation is typical, with most patients with severe continence, manifesting with loss of large volumes of urine, present themselves after 2 years or more after the onset of symptoms (Miller *et al.*, 1999; Resnick *et al.*, 1994; Rodriguez *et al.*, 2003).

In most cases, a detailed history will enable accurate classification of UI (Table 3). Specific inquiry should be made regarding volume of urine lost, strength of urinary stream, position in which urine loss is most likely to occur, number of pads used, and associated fecal incontinence. Quality of life and caregiver burden should also be assessed. Additional information should be sought regarding risk factors, and predisposing factors (Figure 1). Enquiry should also be made as to a coexisting history of diabetes mellitus, hypercalcemia, impaired cognition, functional disability, or impaired sensory perception. Medication history is critical (Table 4). Diuretics and hyperosmolar agents such as mannitol may contribute to polyuria. Anticholinergic agents may cause obstruction and consequent overflow incontinence. Narcotics, sedative, and hypnotics may impair cognition or cloud consciousness.

An accurate voiding diary is an important tool that facilitates the quantification of severity and classification of UI. Serial diaries also facilitate assessment of response to intervention. Although 7-day diaries are still done, available evidence indicates that shorter voiding diaries (48 or 72 hours) are comparable in reliability and validity to the 7-day diaries and are perceived as less burdensome by patients (Ku *et al.*, 2004; Nygaard & Holcomb, 2000; Singh *et al.*, 2004).

Physical examination of the patient with UI must include a complete neurological, abdominal, urogenital, pelvic, and rectal examination. The integrity of relevant superficial spinal reflexes, the anal and bulbocavernosus reflexes, should be assessed. Response to the cough reflex can easily be evaluated during pelvic examination, facilitating exclusion of stress incontinence. Persons with stress incontinence may actually be observed to lose urine during coughing. Patients with intact perineal sensation and reflexes will exhibit reflex tightening of the anal sphincter during coughing.

Bedside measurement of postvoid residual (PVR) volumes is helpful in the diagnosis or exclusion of overflow

Table 4 Some common medications that may cause incontinence

- Diuretics
- Anticholinergics
- Antihistamines
- Antipsychotics
- Antidepressants
- Sedatives/hypnotics
- Alcohol
- Narcotics
- α-adrenergic agonists/antagonists
- Calcium channel blockers
- Hyperosmolar intravenous infusions

Table 3 Clinical differentiation of urinary incontinence

Symptoms	OAB/urge	Stress	Overflow	Functional
Urgency	Yes	No	No	Variable
Leakage during activity or cough	No	Yes	Variable	No
Volume leaked	Large	Small	Small/dribble	Large
Ability to reach toilet in time	Reduced	Normal	Normal	Reduced
Nocturia	Yes	No	Variable	Yes

incontinence due to bladder outlet obstruction. Postresidual volumes greater than 150 cc in older adults suggest inadequate bladder emptying. PVR volumes greater than 200 cc are highly indicative of urinary retention. Where available, ultrasound measurements of PVR volumes are preferred over direct measurement using a urethral catheter due to the less invasive nature of bladder scans and the consequent lower risk of urinary tract infection (Lehman and Owen, 2001; Sullivan and Yalla, 1996).

PRACTICAL APPROACH TO THE INVESTIGATION AND MANAGEMENT OF UI

Diagnostic Evaluation

Comprehensive physical examination should yield preliminary information relating to PVR volumes and urethral sphincter competence. The primary care provider should also remain alert to other specific indications for specialist urological evaluation and ensure prompt referral. Thus, urinary retention due to obstructive uropathy, hematuria, prostate disease, recent pelvic surgery, recurrent urinary tract infections, and stress incontinence should prompt early referral for urological examination. However, the majority of older patients with functional UI or urge incontinence associated with overactive bladder can be effectively managed by geriatric or primary care providers.

Although urodynamic studies in the assessment of patients with UI are routinely conducted by urologists, available data indicates that results of this test are unlikely to alter management in a significant proportion of older adults. In older adults with UI, urodynamic studies are likely to be most helpful in patients being considered for surgical intervention or in patients in whom the diagnosis remains unclear after a thorough history and physical examination (Lovatsis *et al.*, 2002; Thompson *et al.*, 2000). Guidelines issued by the Agency for Healthcare Policy and Research recommend limitation of initial diagnostic work-up to urinalysis and measurement of PVR volumes. The American Medical Director Association's guidelines (AMDA) for the management of UI are even more conservative in recommending urinalysis only in patients with suspected urinary tract infection and new or worsening UI. AMDA guidelines recommend PVR measurements only in men and female patients at risk of retention due to coexistent neurologic disorders or diabetes mellitus (AMDA, 2000; Resnick *et al.*, 2004). Bedside cystometric studies have fallen out of favor mainly due to poor diagnostic accuracy, as evidenced by lack of correlation with results of urodynamic studies and failure of cystometry results to alter management initiatives based exclusively on clinical criteria (Byun *et al.*, 2003; Resnick *et al.*, 1996). The associated increased risk of urinary tract infection associated with urethral catheterization is an additional disadvantage of bedside cystometry (Hung *et al.*, 2005; Ouslander *et al.*, 1987).

Management

Effective management incorporates both nonpharmacological and pharmacological strategies. Although, traditionally, pharmacological therapy was withheld until nonpharmacological strategies proved effective, there is emerging controversial evidence that suggests that the parallel institution of both strategies may yield better results (Goode, 2004; Ouslander *et al.*, 2001). Nevertheless, the increased risk of adverse drug effects and interactions in older adults justifies caution with this approach. Thus, an initial trial of nonpharmacological therapy alone remains the conventional approach to treatment. However, inadequate response to nonpharmacological management should prompt consideration of drug therapy. Invasive procedures or definitive surgical intervention are occasionally warranted in older adults who can tolerate such procedures.

Nonpharmacological Intervention

The nature of nonpharmacological intervention varies with the type of incontinence. In patients diagnosed with overactive bladder, the mainstay of nonpharmacological management is behavior modification, tailored to suit the individual patient. Mentally competent, functional and highly motivated persons are good candidates for patient-dependent intervention such as biofeedback therapy. In dependent or cognitively impaired patients, caregiver-dependent toileting protocols are more appropriate and likely to be more effective. Prompted voiding is a caregiver-dependent strategy that offers the patient a regular opportunity to use the toilet. The designated caregiver offers toileting assistance at scheduled intervals, usually starting with a short period of about 2 hours. Prompted voiding has the added advantage of providing the patient an opportunity for social interaction and positive reinforcement. Habit training is a more complex variant of this method, where persons with UI are encouraged to link voiding to specific activities, such as meals, drinks, or just before outings. Eventually, regular toileting becomes a "habit", and involuntary urine loss is preempted.

Older adults who are more severely cognitively impaired may be unable to respond appropriately to communication, and thus a simple timed toileting schedule may be more appropriate. In such cases, the caregiver toilets the patient consistently at predetermined intervals. Prompted voiding and habit training are also helpful in the management of older adults with functional incontinence. Environmental assessment, and modification if indicated, is a pivotal component of the management of functional incompetence. Adaptive equipment and assistive appliances may help facilitate efficient toileting and reduce incontinent episodes.

Rehabilitative exercises focusing on pelvic muscles and biofeedback therapy may be helpful in patients with stress incontinence or mixed incontinence. In patients with mixed incontinence, a combination of pelvic floor exercises and bladder sphincter biofeedback therapy has been shown to result in a reduction in episodes of involuntary loss (Teunissen *et al.*, 2004).

Pharmacological Therapy

Detrusor muscle contraction is dependent on the action of Ach on bladder muscarinic receptors. Thus, antimuscarinic drug treatment is appropriate for urge incontinence due to bladder overactivity being poorly responsive to nonpharmacological intervention. Traditionally, antimuscarinic drugs have formed the mainstay of management for this variant of UI. However, until recently, serious and prohibitive side effects such as delirium, cognitive impairment, orthostatic hypotension, falls, and cardiac arrhythmias have rendered this group of agents an unsafe choice to use in older adults. The emergence of selective antimuscarinic agents provides a safer alternative, although in older patients the occurrence of delirium, dry mouth, urinary retention, constipation, and blurring of vision are still troubling concerns.

Five different muscarinic receptor subtypes have been cloned (Table 5). M1, M4, and M5 receptor subtypes are found primarily, although not exclusively, in the nervous system. M2 and M3 receptors predominate in smooth muscle, although they are also present relatively small numbers in the brain and salivary glands. M2 and M3 receptors are also the major cholinergic receptors in the bladder. M3 receptors mediate direct detrusor muscle contraction, while M2 receptors appear to play a role in the inhibition of bladder relaxation and modulation of bladder contraction in pathological conditions, such as denervation injury or spinal cord disease. Differences in receptor subtype distribution are particularly important when considering adverse events associated with antimuscarinic agents in older adults.

Overall, oxybutynin and tolterodine are the two most commonly used antimuscarinic agents in the treatment of urge incontinence. Oxybutynin is a relatively nonselective antimuscarinic agent and acts primarily on M1, M2, and M3 receptor subtypes. Although oxybutynin has been shown to reduce episodes of UI by almost 50% in 60–80% of patients, there is a relatively high incidence of side effects, with approximately 75% of patients reporting discomfort arising from dry mouth. Tolerability is low, as evidenced by the high discontinuation rate (25%) due to peripheral anticholinergic side effects such as dry mouth, constipation, and blurred vision. Notably, central nervous system (CNS) side effects such as dizziness, cognitive dysfunction, delirium, and psychotic reactions have been reported in several studies, rendering oxybutynin a poor choice for the geriatric patient.

Table 5 Distribution of muscarinic receptors

- M1: Cortex, hippocampus, salivary glands
- M2: Hindbrain, heart, smooth muscle
- M3: Brain, salivary glands, heart, smooth muscle
- M4: Basal forebrain, striatum
- M5: Substantia nigra

Tolterodine is a more selective antimuscarinic agent that affects predominantly M2 and M3 receptor subtypes. Efficacy of tolterodine is comparable to oxybutynin. However, the incidence of peripheral anticholinergic side effects, such as dry mouth, is much lower. Additionally, only three case reports of cognitive dysfunction related to tolterodine use exist in the literature. Available data favor the use of the extended release formulations of tolterodine over the immediate release due to greater efficacy, higher tolerability, and higher adherence rates (Hartnett & Saver, 2001; Rovner and Wein, 2002).

More recently, two M3 selective inhibitors, darifenacin and solifenacin have emerged as viable pharmacological therapeutic options for overactive bladder. Available data suggests comparable efficacy with the older agents. However, adverse effects such as constipation and blurred vision, in conjunction with the notable paucity of safety and tolerability data in older adults preclude objective comment regarding prescription of these agents in geriatric practice (Jimenez Cidre, 2004; Robinson & Cardozo, 2004).

Trospium has recently been approved by the Federal Drug Administration in the United States for the treatment of overactive bladder in the elderly. However, this drug has been in use in Europe over the past three decades, and available literature indicates a relatively clean safety profile. Unlike the M2/M3 selective agents that are lipophilic, tertiary amines, trospium is a hydrophilic, quaternary amine. These unique biochemical properties render the blood-brain barrier relatively impermeable to trospium, thereby reducing the risk of unwanted CNS side effects. Additionally, available evidence indicates that trospium may exert a significant local effect on nonneuronal cholinergic receptors located in the detrusor muscle. Trospium is not metabolized by the cytochrome p450 system and, therefore, is less prone to drug interactions. Although available global data suggests that trospium is an effective agent and may be well suited for the treatment of urge incontinence in the elderly, further studies specifically relating to safety and tolerability in the frail elder are needed (Gaines, 2005; Rovner, 2004; Scheife and Takeda, 2005).

INVASIVE PROCEDURES AND SURGICAL MANAGEMENT

Periurethral sphincter collagen injections and vaginal pessaries are viable and reasonably effective options for older adults unable to tolerate surgery.

Sacral neuromodulation involves surgical implantation of a "bladder pacemaker" in the patient's hip attached to a lead wire that is threaded to a site within the sacral canal at the base of the spine. External programming results in the delivery of a painless electrical stimulus to the sacral nerves, which regulate bladder function. This allows patients to control urine storage and expulsion.

For some patients with stress or overflow incontinence, surgery may be the only effective treatment. Older men with overflow incontinence due to obstructive uropathy arising from prostatic enlargement may experience considerable relief following prostatectomy. Although several techniques have been described to treat stress incontinence, none of them is entirely satisfactory. The best long-term success rate has been documented following bladder neck slings. Prolene suburethral sling insertion is a new promising technique, with a documented cure rate of more than 80%. However, published follow-up does not exceed 3 years. Surgical complications of this procedure include retropubic hematoma, urinary tract infections and fibrosis, pubic osteomyelitis, urinary fistula, and transient postoperative urinary retention. Late complications include dysuria, urinary retention and detrusor instability, genital prolapse, sexual disorders, chronic pain, chronic urinary tract infections, and complications related to the use of biomaterials, including screws, synthetic tape, and artificial urinary sphincter. Nevertheless, quality of life studies after surgery for stress incontinence in younger patients shows consistent improvement. Data in older adults is lacking.

Tension-free vaginal tape (TVT) surgery, is a highly effective and minimally invasive alternative for treating patients with stress UI. Surgical complications include bladder perforation, urinary retention, pelvic hematoma suprapubic wound infection, persistent suprapubic discomfort, and intravaginal tape erosion (Abouassaly *et al.*, 2004; Ayoub *et al.*, 2004; Krissi *et al.*, 2004; Ouslander *et al.*, 1987).

KEY POINTS

- Urinary incontinence is a highly prevalent syndrome in older adults. Age-related physiological changes in bladder regulation and lower urinary tract dysfunction in the presence of coexisting morbidity increase the likelihood of urinary incontinence with aging.
- Urinary incontinence is classified into five major types: urge, stress, functional, overflow, and mixed incontinence. The most common type of incontinence in older adults is urge incontinence resulting from bladder overactivity.
- Routine screening for urinary incontinence is a critical component of routine geriatric evaluation. A comprehensive history and physical examination usually enables accurate diagnosis and classification. Initial diagnostic work-up should include urinalysis and postvoid residual measurements. Urodynamic studies are not indicated routinely and should be reserved for selected cases only.
- Treatment modalities comprise nonpharmacological, pharmacological, and surgical modalities. Selective antimuscarinic agents are the preferred pharmacological therapeutic option. Invasive modalities include periurethral collagen injections, vaginal pessary insertion, and sling procedures for stress incontinence.

KEY REFERENCES

- Klausner AP & Vapnek JM. Urinary incontinence in the geriatric population. *The Mount Sinai Journal of Medicine* 2003; **70**(1):54–61.
- Scheife R & Takeda M. Central nervous system safety of anticholinergic drugs for the treatment of overactive bladder in the elderly. *Clinical Therapeutics* 2005; **27**(2):144–53.
- Teunissen TA, de JA, van WC & Lagro-Janssen AL. Treating urinary incontinence in the elderly–conservative therapies that work: a systematic review. *The Journal of Family Practice* 2004; **53**(1):25–30, 32.
- Tubaro A. Defining overactive bladder: epidemiology and burden of disease. *Urology* 2004; **64**(6 suppl 1):2–6.
- Wilson MM. Urinary incontinence: bridging the gender gap. *The Journals of Gerontology. Series A, Biological Sciences and Medical Sciences* 2003; **58**(8):752–5.

REFERENCES

Abouassaly R, Steinberg JR, Lemieux M *et al.* Complications of tension-free vaginal tape surgery: a multi-institutional review. *BJU International* 2004; **94**(1):110–3.

Allen L, Rodjani A, Kelly J *et al.* Female epispadias: are we missing the diagnosis? *BJU International* 2004; **94**(4):613–5.

AMDA. American Medical Directors Association issues how-to guide for protocols on long-term care resident assessment. *LTC Regulatory Risk & Liability Advisor* 2000; **8**(25):7–8.

Ayed M, Ben AF, Loussaief H *et al.* Female hypospadias. Apropos of 3 cases. *Journal d'urologie* 1995; **101**(5–6):244–7.

Ayoub N, Chartier-Kastler E, Robain G *et al.* Functional consequences and complications of surgery for female stress urinary incontinence. *Progres en Urologie* 2004; **14**(3):360–73.

Birnbaum H, Leong S & Kabra A. Lifetime medical costs for women: cardiovascular disease, diabetes, and stress urinary incontinence. *Women's Health Issues* 2003; **13**(6):204–13.

Borrie MJ, Campbell K, Arcese ZA *et al.* Urinary retention in patients in a geriatric rehabilitation unit: prevalence, risk factors, and validity of bladder scan evaluation. *Rehabilitation Nursing* 2001; **26**(5):187–91.

Bradway C. Urinary incontinence among older women. Measurement of the effect on health-related quality of life. *Journal of Gerontological Nursing* 2003; **29**(7):13–9.

Brandeis GH, Baumann MM, Hossain M *et al.* The prevalence of potentially remediable urinary incontinence in frail older people: a study using the minimum data set. *Journal of the American Geriatrics Society* 1997; **45**(2):179–84.

Byun SS, Kim HH, Lee E *et al.* Accuracy of bladder volume determinations by ultrasonography: are they accurate over entire bladder volume range? *Urology* 2003; **62**(4):656–60.

Chadwick V. Assessment of functional incontinence in disabled living centres. *Nursing Times* 2005; **101**(2):65, 67.

Chapple CR. Lower urinary tract symptoms suggestive of benign prostatic obstruction–triumph: design and implementation. *European Urology* 2001; **39**(suppl 3):31–6.

Dugan E, Roberts CP, Cohen SJ *et al.* Why older community-dwelling adults do not discuss urinary incontinence with their primary care physicians. *Journal of the American Geriatrics Society* 2001; **49**(4):462–5.

Enriquez EL. A nursing analysis of the causes of and approaches for urinary incontinence among elderly women in nursing homes. *Ostomy/Wound Management* 2004; **50**(6):24–43.

Gaines KK. Trospium chloride (Sanctura)–new to the U.S. for overactive bladder. *Urologic Nursing* 2005; **25**(1):64–5, 52.

Goode PS. Behavioral and drug therapy for urinary incontinence. *Urology* 2004; **63**(3 suppl 1):58–64.

Gray ML. Gender, race, and culture in research on UI: sensitivity and screening are integral to adequate patient care. *The American Journal of Nursing* 2003; **103**(suppl):20–5.

Grosshans C, Passadori Y & Peter B. Urinary retention in the elderly: a study of 100 hospitalized patients. *Journal of the American Geriatrics Society* 1993; **41**(6):633–8.

Hartnett NM & Saver BG. Is extended-release oxybutynin (Ditropan XL) or tolterodine (Detrol) more effective in the treatment of an overactive bladder? *The Journal of Family Practice* 2001; **50**(7):571.

Hogan DB. Revisiting the O complex: urinary incontinence, delirium and polypharmacy in elderly patients. *Canadian Medical Association Journal* 1997; **157**(8):1071–7.

Holroyd-Leduc JM, Mehta KM & Covinsky KE. Urinary incontinence and its association with death, nursing home admission, and functional decline. *Journal of the American Geriatrics Society* 2004; **52**(5):712–8.

Horrocks S, Somerset M, Stoddart H & Peters TJ. What prevents older people from seeking treatment for urinary incontinence? A qualitative exploration of barriers to the use of community continence services. *Family Practice* 2004; **21**(6):689–96.

Hu TW, Wagner TH, Bentkover JD *et al.* Costs of urinary incontinence and overactive bladder in the United States: a comparative study. *Urology* 2004; **63**(3):461–5.

Hung JW, Tsay TH, Chang HW *et al.* Incidence and risk factors of medical complications during inpatient stroke rehabilitation. *Chang Gung Medical Journal* 2005; **28**(1):31–8.

Jackson RA, Vittinghoff E, Kanaya AM *et al.* Urinary incontinence in elderly women: findings from the Health, Aging, and Body Composition Study. *Obstetrics and Gynecology* 2004; **104**(2):301–7.

Jimenez Cidre MA. Urinary incontinence: anticholinergic treatment. *Revista de Medicina de la Universidad de Navarra* 2004; **48**(4):37–42.

Johansson C, Hellstrom L, Ekelund P & Milsom I. Urinary incontinence: a minor risk factor for hip fractures in elderly women. *Maturitas* 1996; **25**(1):21–8.

Johnson TM, Bernard SL, Kincade JE & Defriese GH. Urinary incontinence and risk of death among community-living elderly people: results from the National Survey on Self-Care and Aging. *Journal of Aging and Health* 2000; **12**(1):25–46.

Johnson TM & Ouslander JG. Urinary incontinence in the older man. *Medicine Clinics of North America* 1999; **83**(5):1247–66.

Kevorkian R. Physiology of incontinence. *Clinics in Geriatric Medicine* 2004; **20**(3):409–25.

Kinchen KS, Burgio K, Diokno AC *et al.* Factors associated with women's decisions to seek treatment for urinary incontinence. *Journal of Women's Health (Larchmt.)* 2003; **12**(7):687–98.

Klauser A, Frauscher F, Strasser H *et al.* Age-related rhabdosphincter function in female urinary stress incontinence: assessment of intraurethral sonography. *Journal of Ultrasound in Medicine* 2004; **23**(5):631–7.

Klausner AP & Vapnek JM. Urinary incontinence in the geriatric population. *The Mount Sinai Journal of Medicine* 2003; **70**(1):54–61.

Krissi H, Borkovski T, Feldberg D & Nitke S. Complications of surgery for stress incontinence in women. *Harefuah* 2004; **143**(7):516–9 548.

Ku JH, Jeong IG, Lim DJ *et al.* Voiding diary for the evaluation of urinary incontinence and lower urinary tract symptoms: prospective assessment of patient compliance and burden. *Neurourology and Urodynamics* 2004; **23**(4):331–5.

Landi F, Cesari M, Russo A *et al.* Potentially reversible risk factors and urinary incontinence in frail older people living in community. *Age and Ageing* 2003; **32**(2):194–9.

Lehman CA & Owen SV. Bladder scanner accuracy during everyday use on an acute rehabilitation unit. *SCI Nursing* 2001; **18**(2):87–92.

Lluel P, Deplanne V, Heudes D *et al.* Age-related changes in urethrovesical coordination in male rats: relationship with bladder instability? *American Journal of Physiology Regulatory, Integrative and Comparative Physiology* 2003; **284**(5):R1287–95.

Lovatsis D, Drutz HP, Wilson D & Duggan P. Utilization of preoperative urodynamic studies by Canadian gynaecologists. *Journal of Obstetrics and Gynaecology Canada* 2002; **24**(4):315–9.

McLoughlin MA & Chew DJ. Diagnosis and surgical management of ectopic ureters. *Clinical Techniques in Small Animal Practice* 2000; **15**(1):17–24.

Miller JM, Ashton-Miller JA, Carchidi LT & DeLancey JO. On the lack of correlation between self-report and urine loss measured with standing provocation test in older stress-incontinent women. *Journal of Women's Health* 1999; **8**(2):157–62.

Miner PB Jr. Economic and personal impact of fecal and urinary incontinence, *Gastroenterology* 2004; **126**(1 suppl 1):S8–13.

Molander U, Sundh V & Steen B. Urinary incontinence and related symptoms in older men and women studied longitudinally between 70 and 97 years of age. A population study. *Archives of Gerontology and Geriatrics* 2002; **35**(3):237–44.

Mouriquand PD, Bubanj T, Feyaerts A *et al.* Long-term results of bladder neck reconstruction for incontinence in children with classical bladder exstrophy or incontinent epispadias. *BJU International* 2003; **92**(9):997–1001.

Namikawa M. Pathophysiology of established urinary incontinence (UI) in the elderly and an ameliorative method for disuse syndrome including UI seen in the bed-ridden elderly–using prone position and its variations. *Nippon Ronen Igakkai Zasshi* 1999; **36**(6):381–8.

Nasr SZ & Ouslander JG. Urinary incontinence in the elderly. Causes and treatment options. *Drugs & Aging* 1998; **12**(5):349–60.

Newman DK. Report of a mail survey of women with bladder control disorders. *Urologic Nursing* 2004; **24**(6):499–507.

Nygaard I & Holcomb R. Reproducibility of the seven-day voiding diary in women with stress urinary incontinence. *International Urogynecology Journal and Pelvic Floor Dysfunction* 2000; **11**(1):15–7.

Ouslander JG. Intractable incontinence in the elderly. *BJU International* 2000; **85**(suppl 3):72–8.

Ouslander JG, Greengold B & Chen S. Complications of chronic indwelling urinary catheters among male nursing home patients: a prospective study. *The Journal of Urology* 1987; **138**(5):1191–5.

Ouslander JG, Maloney C, Grasela TH *et al.* Implementation of a nursing home urinary incontinence management program with and without tolterodine. *Journal of the American Medical Directors Association* 2001; **2**(5):207–14.

Ouslander JG & Schnelle JF. Incontinence ins the nursing home. *Annals of Internal Medicine* 1995; **122**(6):438–49.

Patel MD, Coshall C, Rudd AG & Wolfe CD. Cognitive impairment after stroke: clinical determinants and its associations with long-term stroke outcomes. *Journal of the American Geriatrics Society* 2002; **50**(4):700–6.

Resnick NM, Beckett LA, Branch LG *et al.* Short-term variability of self report of incontinence in older persons. *Journal of the American Geriatrics Society* 1994; **42**(2):202–7.

Resnick NM, Brandeis GH, Baumann MM *et al.* Misdiagnosis of urinary incontinence in nursing home women: prevalence and a proposed solution. *Neurourology and Urodynamics* 1996; **15**(6):599–613.

Resnick B, Quinn C & Baxter S. Testing the feasibility of implementation of clinical practice guidelines in long-term care facilities. *Journal of the American Medical Directors Association* 2004; **5**(1):1–8.

Robinson D & Cardozo L. The emerging role of solifenacin in the treatment of overactive bladder. *Expert Opinion on Investigational Drugs* 2004; **13**(10):1339–48.

Rodriguez LV, Blander DS, Dorey F *et al.* Discrepancy in patient and physician perception of patient's quality of life related to urinary symptoms. *Urology* 2003; **62**(1):49–53.

Rovner ES. Trospium chloride in the management of overactive bladder. *Drugs* 2004; **64**(21):2433–46.

Rovner ES & Wein AJ. Once-daily, extended-release formulations of antimuscarinic agents in the treatment of overactive bladder: a review. *European Urology* 2002; **41**(1):6–14.

Saltvedt I, Mo ES, Fayers P *et al.* Reduced mortality in treating acutely sick, frail older patients in a geriatric evaluation and management unit. A prospective randomized trial. *Journal of the American Geriatrics Society* 2002; **50**(5):792–8.

Scheife R & Takeda M. Central nervous system safety of anticholinergic drugs for the treatment of overactive bladder in the elderly. *Clinical Therapeutics* 2005; **27**(2):144–53.

Sgadari A, Topinkova E, Bjornson J & Bernabei R. Urinary incontinence in nursing home residents: a cross-national comparison. *Age and Ageing* 1997; **26**(suppl 2):49–54.

Shaw C, Tansey R, Jackson C *et al.* Barriers to help seeking in people with urinary symptoms. *Family Practice* 2001; **18**(1):48–52.

Singh M, Bushman W & Clemens JQ. Do pad tests and voiding diaries affect patient willingness to participate in studies of incontinence treatment outcomes? *The Journal of Urology* 2004; **171**(1):316–8.

Sullivan MP & Yalla SV. Detrusor contractility and compliance characteristics in adult male patients with obstructive and nonobstructive voiding dysfunction. *The Journal of Urology* 1996; **155**(6):1995–2000.

Tan TL. Urinary incontinence in older persons: a simple approach to a complex problem. *Annals of the Academy of Medicine, Singapore* 2003; **32**(6):731–9.

Teleman PM, Lidfeldt J, Nerbrand C *et al.* Overactive bladder: prevalence, risk factors and relation to stress incontinence in middle-aged women. *British Journal of Obstetrics and Gynaecology* 2004; **111**(6):600–4.

Teunissen TA, de JA, van WC & Lagro-Janssen AL. Treating urinary incontinence in the elderly–conservative therapies that work: a systematic review. *The Journal of Family Practice* 2004; **53**(1):25–30, 32.

Thompson PK, Duff DS & Thayer PS. Stress incontinence in women under 50: does urodynamics improve surgical outcome? *International Urogynecology Journal and Pelvic Floor Dysfunction* 2000; **11**(5):285–9.

Tubaro A. Defining overactive bladder: epidemiology and burden of disease. *Urology* 2004; **64**(6 suppl 1):2–6.

Van der Varrt C, Van der Bom JG, de L Jr, *et al.* The contribution of hysterectomy to the occurrence of urge and stress urinary incontinence symptoms. *British Journal of Obstetrics and Gynaecology* 2002; **109**(2):149–54.

Vickerman J. Thorough assessment of functional incontinence. *Nursing Times* 2002; **98**(28):58–9.

Whishaw M. Urinary incontinence in the elderly. Establishing a cause may allow a cure. *Australian Family Physician* 1998; **27**(12):1087–90.

Wilson MM. Urinary incontinence: bridging the gender gap. *The Journals of Gerontology. Series A, Biological Sciences and Medical Sciences* 2003; **58**(8):752–5.

Wilson MM. Urinary incontinence: a treatise on gender, sexuality, and culture. *Clinics in Geriatric Medicine* 2004; **20**(3):565–70.

Wilson L, Brown JS, Shin GP *et al.* Annual direct cost of urinary incontinence. *Obstetrics and Gynecology* 2001; **98**(3):398–406.

Wuest M, Morgenstern K, Graf EM *et al.* Cholinergic and purinergic responses in isolated human detrusor in relation to age. *The Journal of Urology* 2005; **173**(6):2182–9.

Yoshida M, Miyamae K, Iwashita H *et al.* Management of detrusor dysfunction in the elderly: changes in acetylcholine and adenosine triphosphate release during aging. *Urology* 2004; **63**(3 suppl 1):17–23.

Zunzunegui Pastor MV, Rodriguez-Laso A, Garcia de Yebenes MJ *et al.* Prevalence of urinary incontinence and linked factors in men and women over 65. *Atencion Primaria* 2003; **32**(6):337–42.

127

Renal Diseases

Carlos G. Musso[1] *and* Juan F. Macías-Núnez[2]

[1] Hospital Italiano de Buenos Aires, Buenos Aires, Argentina, and [2] University Hospital of Salamanca, Salamanca, Spain

INTRODUCTION

As the term 'Giants' in Geriatric Medicine has been coined to define the most frequent clinical conditions, there is also a group of renal conditions that we believe deserve the term "Nephrogeriatric Giants". For instance, although more than 50% of aged kidneys are normal in appearance, not all of them are actually normal because approximately 14% display cortical scars scattered across their surface (Griffiths *et al.*, 1976). Usually, if these scars are detected in a young person, they suggest pathology such as pyelonephritis, but in the aged kidney, in the absence of other abnormalities, these scars are a consequence of the normal aging process. Another aspect of the renal aging process is the change in kidney weight and size. The weight of the kidney slowly decreases to less than 300 g in the ninth decade of life. Renal length diminishes by 2 cm between the age of 50 and 80 years. The cortex is more affected than the medulla. In the latter, an increase is seen in the interstitial tissue; this is accompanied by fibrosis and increased fat content at the level of the renal sinus (McLachlan, 1987). A constant finding is the presence of cysts along the distal nephron (Baert and Steg, 1977).

After the age of 30, there is a gradual reduction in renal functional capacity. By the age of 60, these functions decrease to half the value they were at the age of 30 (Musso *et al.*, 2001). The deterioration of renal function with age can be explained in terms of either the progressive loss of functioning nephrons alone, or a decrease in the number of energy-producing mitochondria, lower concentration of adenosine triphosphatase activity and other enzyme levels, or decreased tubular cell transport capacity as observed in kidneys of old animals (Beauchene *et al.*, 1965). It is important to understand that these changes are not representative of any pathology, but only the normal aging process leading to a reduction in kidney function.

As has been previously stated, all the structural and functional changes of the aged kidney may be summarized under the heading of "Nephrogeriatric Giants"; six conditions that are so called because they are conditions in which there are profound modifications of renal physiology which occur in the majority of the elderly population (Musso, 2002):

1. Senile hypofiltration
2. Renal vascular alterations
3. Tubular dysfunction
4. Tubular frailty
5. Medullary hypotonicity
6. Obstructive uropathy.

NEPHROGERIATRIC GIANTS

Senile Hypofiltration

Glomerular sclerosis begins at approximately 30 years of age. The percentage of obsolete glomeruli varies between 1 and 30% in persons aged 50 years or more (McLachlan *et al.*, 1977). The glomerular tuft appears partially or totally hyalinized, and this is the basis of glomerulosclerosis which accompanies aging (Rosen, 1976). With age, there is a reduction in the length and surface of the glomerulus, which affects the effective filtration surface (Goyal, 1982). On microangiographic examination, there is obliteration, particularly of juxtamedullary nephrons, but not of those sited more peripherally, with the formation of a direct channel between afferent and efferent arterioles in this area of the kidney (Takazakura *et al.*, 1972). This presumably contributes to the maintenance of medullary blood flow. The mesangium, which accounts for 8% of glomerular volume at 45 years, increases to nearly 12% at the age of 70 (McLachlan, 1987).

Owing to the aforementioned changes, aging is accompanied by a decrease of glomerular filtration rate (GFR), renal plasma flow (RPF) and renal blood flow (RBF) (Cohen

Principles and Practice of Geriatric Medicine, 4th Edition. Edited by M.S. John Pathy, Alan J. Sinclair and John E. Morley.

and Ku, 1983). The GFR evaluation with ^{51}Cr EDTA confirms that the elderly have lower GFRs than the young. At the third decade of life, GFR reaches approximately 140 ml/minute/1.73 m^2, and from then on, GFR progressively declines at a rate of 8 ml/minute/1.73 m^2 per decade (Rowe *et al.*, 1976a). The fall in creatinine clearance (Ccr) is followed by a decrease in creatinine production, and the relationship between blood and urine creatinine levels changes with age (Swedko *et al.*, 2003). This may be the reason serum creatinine concentration of 1 mg dl^{-1} reflects a GFR of 120 ml/minute in a person 20 years old and 60 ml/minute at the age of 80. If an elderly person has a normal adult creatinine level, it should be remembered that the GFR is diminished and hence the dose of drugs metabolized/eliminated through the kidney should be corrected to the true GFR (Musso and Enz, 1996). To calculate the Ccr in the elderly, the nomogram of Cockcroft and Gault is quite useful in daily clinical practice (Cockcroft and Gault, 1976):

$$\text{Ccr} = \frac{(140 - \text{age}) \times (\text{body weight})}{72 \times \text{serum creatinine}}$$

In women, it is 15% lower. It is of paramount importance to know that although creatinine clearance diminishes with age, the value of plasma creatinine remains stable and comparable to young adults, ranging from 0.9 to 1.3 mg dl^{-1}. Therefore, if we only take into account plasma creatinine levels without calculating creatinine clearance, we may falsely interpret the GFR as normal, thereby failing to recognize reduced renal function. For patients with a normal plasma creatinine level, one simple way to calculate GFR is 130 – age in years, but for patients with plasma creatinine >1.5 mg dl^{-1}, it is mandatory to calculate GFR according to the nomograms or 24-hour urine collection.

Renal Vascular Alteration

In apparently normal elderly individuals, prearterioles, from which afferent arterioles arise, show subendothelial deposition of hyaline and collagen fibers resulting in an intimal thickening (McLachlan *et al.*, 1977). Small arteries exhibit a thickening of the intima due to proliferation of the elastic tissue. This is associated with atrophy of the media, which virtually disappears when intimal thickening is prominent. Afferent arterioles show reduplication of elastic tissue, with thickening of the intima preceding the subendothelial deposition of hyaline material. Another characteristic of the aging kidney is the formation of anastomoses among afferent and efferent arterioles of the capillary tuft (Darmady *et al.*, 1973).

Ischemic nephropathy from nonmalignant nephrosclerosis has emerged as an important cause of terminal renal failure in the elderly patient with essential hypertension (Ritz and Fliser, 1992). Antihypertensive agents may impair renal blood flow (through plasma volume contraction) and further aggravate the age-related decline in renal perfusion. A worsening of renal perfusion may activate counter-regulatory neurohormonal mechanisms, such as the renin-angiotensin-aldosterone system, which in turn may place the patient at increased risk for the development of glomerulosclerosis through promotion of vascular or mesangial hypertrophic changes or increased intraglomerular pressure, despite an associated reduction in systemic blood pressure (Weir, 1992).

Sometimes, renal function deteriorates suddenly and unexpectedly in hypertensive patients. This condition is commonly due to destruction of main renal arteries by atheroma, a cause of so-called *renovascular* renal failure. In hypertensive patients, poorly controlled blood pressure on several medications or rapid acceleration of hypertension can suggest renovascular disease. The classic association is a reversible renal failure after use of angiotensin-converting enzyme (ACE) inhibitors and unequal sized kidneys on echography. The importance of making the diagnosis is that it is often possible to regain some renal function, even in end-stage renal disease (ESRD), by intervention on the renal artery (Meyrier, 1996).

Tubular Dysfunction

Renal tubules undergo fatty degeneration with age, showing an irregular thickening of their basal membrane (McLachlan, 1987). By microdissection, the existence of diverticulae arising from the distal and convoluted tubules has been demonstrated, and this becomes more frequent with age. It has been suggested that these may serve as reservoirs for recurrent urinary tract infections in the elderly (Darmady *et al.*, 1973). There are also increasing zones of tubular atrophy and fibrosis, which may relate to the defects in concentration and dilution observed as part of the normal renal aging process (McLachlan, 1987).

Sodium (see Chapter 117, Water and Electrolyte Balance in Health and Disease)

Hypernatremia and hyponatremia are probably the commonest and most well known disturbances of the internal milieu in the elderly. In spite of the lower sodium tubular load, 24-hour urinary sodium output and fractional excretion of sodium are significantly greater in old and very old people (Macias *et al.*, 1987; Musso *et al.*, 2000). This suggests that the renal tubule of the elderly is unable to retain sodium adequately, either in absolute terms or when corrected to glomerular filtration. The mean half-time for a reduction of sodium excretion is 17.7 hours in persons under 30 years, reaching 30.9 hours in persons over 60, apparently mediated by the concomitant reduction in GFR (Meyer, 1989). As GFR declines with age and the amount of filtered sodium is lower than in young subjects; a salt load given to an elderly person takes longer to eliminate (Fish *et al.*, 1994). However, when sodium is restricted to 50 mmol/day, the period required to achieve equilibrium is 5 days in the young and 9 days in the elderly. As a result of these slow adaptations, both hypernatremia and hyponatremia are frequent findings in patients in geriatric wards (Solomon and Lye, 1990; Roberts and

Robinson, 1993). Under normal conditions, the elderly are not salt depleted because of replacement of renal sodium losses by salt contained in the diet. Problems may arise when patients are salt restricted for therapeutic reasons or when they become ill and lose their appetite. Both situations may easily lead to salt and volume depletion and even to acute renal failure (ARF). The incompetence of the aging kidney to conserve sodium may explain the facility with which the aged develop volume depletion (Macias *et al.*, 1980). The capacity of the aging kidney to adapt to a low salt intake (50 mmol/24 hour) is clearly blunted (Macias *et al.*, 1978). The proximal nephron behaves similarly in the young, old, and very old, whereas in the "distal nephron" (thick ascending limb of Henle's loop), a clear-cut difference in the handling of sodium in the elderly is evident, present in 85% of a study population of healthy elderly people (De Santo *et al.*, 1991; Musso *et al.*, 2004). The diminished capacity to reabsorb sodium by the ascending limb of Henle's loop in healthy elderly people has two direct important consequences. First, the amount of sodium arriving at more distal segments of the nephron (distal convoluted and collecting tubules) increases; and second, the capacity to concentrate in the medullary interstitium is also diminished, causing elderly subjects to exhibit both increased sodium excretion and an inability to maximally concentrate urine. Despite the elderly being more prone to an exaggerated natriuresis, total body sodium is not significantly decreased with age (Fulop *et al.*, 1985). Kirkland *et al.* (1983) found greater urinary elimination of water and electrolytes during the night in the elderly, which can, at least in part, explain the nocturia observed in 70% of elderly persons. Basal plasma concentrations of renin and aldosterone and the response to stimuli such as walking and salt restriction are also diminished in old age (Macias *et al.*, 1987). Thus, a dual effect of low aldosterone secretion and a relative insensitivity of the distal nephron to the hormone could account for diminished sodium reabsorption at this site. Atriopeptin in the elderly elicits a greater increase in natriuresis, calciuresis, diuresis, urinary, and plasma cyclic Guanydine monophosphate (cGMP) concentrations than in the young (Heim *et al.*, 1989).

Potassium (see Chapter 117, Water and Electrolyte Balance in Health and Disease)

Potassium content of the body is lower in the old than in the young and the correlation with age is linear (Cox and Shalaby, 1981). As 85% of potassium is deposited in muscle, and muscular mass diminishes with age, this may largely account for the fall in total body potassium, with other factors such as poor intake also playing some role (Lye, 1981). Under normal conditions, plasma potassium is normal in the elderly, but when diuretics are taken, they develop hypokalemia more rapidly than do the young (Kirkland *et al.*, 1983). The possible explanation for the tendency to develop potassium deficiency is an inability of the kidney to conserve potassium. On the other hand, it has been observed that the total renal excretion of potassium is significantly lower in the aged population than in the young. The clinical consequence of the tendency to excrete less potassium by the aging kidney, when total potassium urinary output is considered, is the vulnerability of elderly people to develop hyperkalemia (Lowental, 1994). This electrolyte disturbance is particularly frequent when elderly individuals are treated (either alone or in combination) with the following drugs: nonsteroidal antiinflammatory drugs (NSAIDs), ACE inhibitors, nonselective β-blockers (particularly during exercise) or potassium-sparing diuretics (especially in diabetics) (Andreucci *et al.*, 1996). Recently, a hyperfunction of the H+-K+ ATPase of the intercalar cells in the collecting tubules was described in old rats, generating a greater excretion of H+, and a greater reabsorption of potassium. This mechanism may also explain the trend in old people to develop hyperkalemia (Eiam-Ong and Sabatini, 2002).

Urinary Acidification

Macias *et al.* did not find differences in titratable acid, ammonia, or net acid excretion in response to an acute acid overload in old people, with respect to young controls. The maximal values of ammonia and titratable acid excretion, however, were reached four hours following the acid load in the young, and between six and eight hours in the old. The elderly subjects took longer to reach peak excretion, and experienced a greater fall in blood bicarbonate following the same dose of ammonium chloride (Macias *et al.*, 1983). Lindeman (1990) suggests that renal ammonium ion secretion in response to acid load is not different in healthy elderly subjects.

Calcium, Phosphate, and Magnesium

In general, it is a usual clinical finding to observe relatively low blood calcium and high phosphate levels in old age. In the urine, hyperphosphaturia is often found. Regarding calcium urinary output, some authors refer to the same range as for the young population, others have observed a tendency for it to be higher and other groups have found hypocalciuria (Galinsky *et al.*, 1987). These discrepancies may be explained by different calcium intake (dairy products) with or without the addition of vitamin D in these products. These changes in the metabolism of calcium and phosphate may be related to low levels of 1,25-dihydroxy-vitamin D found in the elderly, probably as a result of a deficit of renal 1-α-hydroxylase as an expression of the normal aging process. Serum levels of 24,25-dihydroxy-vitamin D are also low in the elderly. In addition, low plasma phosphate may lead to mild hyperparathyroidism, with further loss of bone mass (Perez del Molino and Alvarez, 2002; De Toro Casado and Macías Núñez, 1995). It is known that in old age, magnesium supplements are often required, probably because of a combination of diminished spontaneous intake of magnesium, poor intestinal absorption and increased urinary output. Approximately 80% of magnesium is filtered, 25% reabsorbed by proximal tubuli, and 65% by the thick ascending limb of Henle's loop, which is functionally altered in the elderly. Consequently, a diminution of the reabsorptive capacity of the ascending limb may account for the negative balance of magnesium if oral intake is lower than optimal (Seeling and Preuss, 1994).

Erythropoietin Hormone

Erythropoietin hormone is mainly produced by the peritubular interstitial cells near the proximal convoluted tubules. There is no difference in plasma erythropoietin levels among healthy young, old, and very old people (Musso *et al.*, 2004).

Urea

In healthy old and very old people, fractional excretion of urea (FEU) is increased in comparison to the younger population: 65 and 50% respectively. This phenomenon could be secondary to a senile alteration in the UT1 (urea channels) that perhaps produces an increase in urea permeability at the collecting tubules (Musso *et al.*, 2004).

Medullary Hypotonicity

Aging reduces the capacity of the kidney to concentrate the urine (Rowe *et al.*, 1976b). The maximum urinary concentration remains constant until about the third decade and then falls by about 30 mosmol/kg for each subsequent decade. The diminution of the concentrating ability has been related to the decrease in GFR that occurs with age. The relative increase in medullary blood flow could contribute to the impairment of renal concentration capacity. The defect in sodium chloride reabsorption in the ascending limb of Henle's loop, which is the basic mechanism for the adequate function of the countercurrent concentration mechanism, may be an important factor for the decrease in the capacity to concentrate urine, as seen in the aged. Moreover, the increased FEU in this group of people could contribute to their medullary hypotonicity, since normally urea accounts for 50% of the interstitial tonicity (Musso *et al.*, 2004). The decrease in responsiveness of collecting duct tubular epithelium to circulatory antidiuretic hormone (ADH), is another explanation for impairment of urine concentrating ability, and it may also explain why plasma vasopressin levels are higher in the elderly compared to the younger population (Bengele *et al.*, 1981; Andreucci *et al.*, 1996). When healthy active elderly volunteers are water restricted for 24 hours, the threshold for thirst is found to be increased and water intake reduced in comparison with a control group of younger subjects (Phillips *et al.*, 1984). Dryness of the mouth, a decrease of taste, alteration in mental capacity or cortical cerebral dysfunction, and a reduction in the sensitivity of both osmoreceptors and baroreceptors may all contribute to the increased threshold for thirst. Finally, angiotensin concentration, a powerful generator of thirst, is lower in the elderly (Andreucci *et al.*, 1996). Total body water is slightly diminished with age, so that it comprises only 54% of total body weight, probably because old people have a greater proportion of body fat than the young. The diminution seems to be predominantly intracellular. Males have a higher volume than females, regardless of age (Macias *et al.*, 1987; Andreucci *et al.*, 1996; Shannon *et al.*, 1984). Thus, a low plasma volume in an elderly subject is almost always the result of disease (Macias *et al.*, 1987). Urinary dilution has not been extensively investigated in the old, but it has been found to be decreased. There is a minimum urine concentration of only 92 mosmol kg^{-1} in the elderly compared with 52 mosmol kg^{-1} in the young (Dontas *et al.*, 1972). Maximum free water clearance was also reduced in the elderly from 16.2 ml/minute to 5.9 ml/minute. Again, the functional impairment of the diluting segment of the thick ascending limb described above seems to account for the remainder of the diminution in the capacity to dilute urine as observed in the aged (Macias *et al.*, 1978).

Tubular Frailty

Tubular cells are frail in the elderly, and because of that they progress easily to acute tubular necrosis (ATN), and they also recover slowly from this histological alteration. Owing to these reasons, ARF is a frequent disturbance in the elderly (Musso, 2002; Macías Núñez *et al.*, 1996). The commonest causes of ARF in the old population are (Macías Núñez *et al.*, 1996; Musso and Macías Núñez, 2002):

1. *Prerenal causes*: loss of fluids (vomiting and diarrhea, diuretics); inadequate fluid intake; loss of plasma (burns); loss of blood (hemorrhage); shock (cardiogenic and septicemic).

2. *Renal causes*: ATN due to the persistence of the state of prerenal uremia and/or to nephrotoxins; rapidly progressive damage due to collagen disorders, Goodpasture's syndrome, Henoch-Schonlein purpura; arterial or venous thrombosis; acute interstitial nephritis (toxicity with drugs).

3. *Postrenal (obstructive) causes*: stones, clot, tumor, stricture, prostatic hypertrophy.

Prerenal and postrenal causes of ARF are of particular importance since their early identification and treatment may prevent the development of established ATN (Musso and Macías Núñez, 2002). The incidence of ARF in the elderly is higher than in the young, because of the frequency of systemic illnesses, poly pharmacy, and because of the renal aging process itself (Kafetz, 1983). There is also the intriguing role played by accumulation of superoxide radicals with aging. Some illnesses may predispose the aged kidney to develop ARF: cardiac insufficiency, diabetes mellitus, myeloma, prostatic enlargement, vasculitis, rapidly progressive idiopathic glomerulonephritis (GN), mesangiocapillary GN, and the proliferative variety of systemic lupus erythematosus (Frocht and Fillit, 1984). Other etiological agents are septic shock, postsurgical ARF and cardiogenic shock. Poly pharmacy includes the use of diuretics, laxatives, analgesics, NSAIDs, and ACE inhibitors, which are all frequently taken by the elderly. The cause of ARF in a particular individual is often multifactorial, that is, inadequate fluid replacement before surgery, followed by dehydration, hypotension, infection, or inappropriate antibiotics (particularly aminoglycosides).

In the old, the renal indices for diagnosing ARF may be slightly different from those accepted for younger populations. For instance, in the elderly, a urinary sodium output lower than 70 mmol l^{-1} in a patient with clinical and biochemical findings of ARF suggest a prerenal cause or acute reversible renal hypoperfusion. When urinary sodium output is higher than 70 mmol l^{-1} one should think in terms of ATN (Macías Núñez *et al.*, 1996; Musso and Macías Núñez, 2002; Musso *et al.*, 1996). Initial treatment involves rapid correction of fluid and electrolyte balance. If diuresis is not restored with volume expansion, frusemide can be administered. Other measures, such as administration of low dose dopamine infusion (2–7 μg/kg/minute), may be employed to increase renal tubular flow and promote glomerular vasodilation (Musso and Macías Núñez, 2002). Sometimes renal replacement therapy is needed. A greater than 40% survival was achieved in critically ill elderly patients with severe ARF by the use of continuous hemodiafiltration (Bellomo *et al.*, 1994). These findings support an aggressive renal replacement approach in such patients and suggest that continuous hemodiafiltration may be ideally suited to their management. Age *per se* is not an important determinant of survival in patients with ARF (Druml *et al.*, 1994). Prophylaxis is of paramount importance: maintenance of an adequate extracellular volume and drug dosage regimen tailored to the patient's GFR are essential (Macías Núñez *et al.*, 1996; Musso and Macías Núñez, 2002).

Obstructive Uropathy (*see* Chapter 125, Prostate Diseases)

Prostatic hypertrophy occurs to some extent in almost all aging males, but in a proportion it provides a slow obstruction to urinary outflow, with entry into uremia. It is often not recognized until it is too late, largely because the patient becomes polyuric rather than oliguric (Sacks *et al.*, 1989). By the time it is diagnosed, irreversible damage may have taken place, so that even with the relief of obstruction, renal function recovers only partially. The use of α-blockers may help to relieve bladder outlet obstruction and reduce the need for catheterization. Other causes of urinary tract obstruction include uterine prolapse, stones, strictures, and neurogenic bladder due to diabetes mellitus and posterior column dysfunction (Klahr, 1987).

Urinary Tract Infection in the Elderly

Urinary tract infection is the most common infectious disease of the elderly and is especially prevalent in debilitated, institutionalized old individuals. The pathogenesis is strongly related to obstructive uropathy or its treatment: abnormal bladder function, bladder outlet obstruction, urolithiasis, tumors, use of long-term indwelling catheters. Moreover, the incidence of bacteriuria increases with advancing age since there are nonobstructive mechanisms that predispose aged people to urinary infection such as: vaginal and urethral atrophy and puddling related to bed rest. Infection is usually asymptomatic, and there is currently no indication for the treatment of usually asymptomatic bacteriuria except before invasive genitourinary procedures. Catheter-acquired bacteriuria should probably be treated following catheter removal. These individuals are always bacteriuric, usually with a complex polymicrobial flora. For symptomatic infection, the goal of treatment is relief of symptoms and not sterilization of the urine. Treatment has not been shown to prevent subsequent symptomatic episodes, is associated with antimicrobial adverse effects, and promotes the emergence of resistant organisms. Overuse of antimicrobials should be avoided (Rodríguez Pascual and Olcoz Chiva, 2002; Nicolle, 1994).

CHRONIC RENAL FAILURE (CRF)

Introduction

CRF is a syndrome characterized by progressive and generally irreversible deterioration of renal competence due to destruction of nephronal mass. CRF is predominantly a disease of the elderly, because the population incidence of CRF rises steadily with age, being at least 10 times more common at the age of 75 than at 15–45 years (Feest *et al.*, 1990). The causes of ESRD in the elderly differ substantially from those in younger populations (Verbeelen *et al.*, 1993). The most common disorders that lead to renal failure in old age are hypertension, diabetes mellitus, nephrosclerosis, and obstructive uropathy although in as many as one-third of cases it proves impossible to identify any specific cause. Two common causes of ESRD in the elderly are vascular disease of the main renal arteries and prostatic. A further problem worth noting is that of amyloidosis (Labeeuw *et al.*, 1996). Pathogenic mechanisms by which the failing kidney may produce specific clinical features are as follows:

(1) As the sclerosis of the glomeruli advances, glomerular hyperfiltration appears in the remaining nephrons. In this manner, it is possible to eliminate more intoxicating products per functioning nephron. This mechanism appears beneficial in the first instance, but the price paid for hyperfiltrating is an acceleration of glomerular sclerosis (Anderson and Brenner, 1987).
(2) Retention of uremic toxins (polyamines, guanidines, middle molecules, and hormonal peptides).
(3) High levels of parathormone (PTH) is currently accepted as the major uremic toxin-Erythropoietin and 1,25-dihydroxycholecalciferol deficiencies result in anemia and low calcium, respectively.

(4) Phosphate retention leads to secondary hyperparathyroidism and renal osteodystrophy. Clinically, it is convenient to divide CRF into three phases. In the early phase, until GFR reaches 50 ml/minute, there are no clear clinical symptoms. The reduction of creatinine clearance is a laboratory finding. As CRF progresses and creatinine clearance falls to about 25 ml/minute, the clinical picture of CRF appears. During this period, polyuria with clear urines and nocturia are present in nearly all patients. With GFR lower than 15 ml/minute, the full clinical picture becomes evident. The skin acquires a characteristic yellow–brown pallor and pruritus is frequent. Soft-tissue calcifications due to high calcium phosphate production are very common. In the eyes, conjunctival and corneal calcifications occur when the calcium phosphate product is raised, producing the "red eye of renal failure". Patients complain of asthenia, anorexia, and vomiting. In the cardiorespiratory system, pulmonary edema, hypertension, heart failure, coronary disease, and arrhythmia may be seen. The nervous system shows polyneuropathy, clonus, and even uremic coma in the most advanced period of the disease. Secondary hyperparathyroidism, carbohydrate intolerance, hypothyroidism, hyperprolactinemia, and hypogonadism are frequent endocrinological disturbances. A deficit of cellular immunity, polynuclear dysfunction, and clotting alterations are also present. In the late phase, all the above problems increase and when creatinine clearance is lower than 10 ml/minute, it is necessary to start replacement therapy (Musso and Macías Núñez, 2002; Glickman *et al.*, 1987).

Management

A low protein diet, proposed to relieve uremic symptoms, has shown little effect, and protein restriction in the elderly is associated with a high risk of malnutrition; as a result, we should provide a diet with a protein content between 0.6–1 $g\,kg^{-1}$ body weight.

Concerning secondary hyperparathyroidism, it remains necessary to suppress PTH secretion with calcitriol, a low-phosphate diet, and phosphate binders. Calcium acetate is preferable as a phosphate binder, because calcium carbonate needs hydrochloric acid to get converted into active calcium chloride, so there is a risk that this drug will remain ineffective in the elderly, who are frequently affected by low gastric acid secretion. The new calci-mimetic drugs should also be of value, although at the moment there is no clinical experience in aged patients. When urinary output falls below 2 l/day, sodium and potassium intake must be restricted, adding loop diuretics. Calcium blockers and ACE inhibitors are recommended to lower high blood pressure and to slow down the progression of renal disease (Vendemia and D'Amico, 1995).

Dialysis

During the 1970s, older patients with ESRD were almost never considered as candidates for renal replacement therapy (RRT), due to limited resources, whereas during the last decade, patients aged 75 and over with ESRD have been accepted routinely on to dialysis programs. Up to one-third of new patients entering dialysis throughout the world are now older than 65 years (D'Amico, 1995). Today, almost all clinicians believe that the majority of elderly uremics can be rehabilitated satisfactorily, and that age by itself does not constitute a major impediment to dialysis and/or transplantation (Piccoli *et al.*, 1993). Elderly patients on dialysis are prone to develop more serious forms of bone disease than the young, because of osteopenia, unbalanced diet, reduced physical activity and lack of exposure to sunlight. Malnutrition is frequently present and cachexia may contribute to death. Of routine laboratory tests, a low serum albumin is the most powerful independent risk factor for mortality. To prevent this, it is advisable to provide more than 1 $g\,kg^{-1}$ body weight of proteins for patients on hemodialysis (HD), and more than 1.2 g for those on chronic ambulatory peritoneal dialysis (CAPD), with a diet containing more than 6.3 g/day of essential amino acids(Musso and Macías Núñez, 2002).

The most common practical problems during treatment by HD of people aged 65 or more are (Ismail *et al.*, 1993; Lerma *et al.*, 1995; Vandelli *et al.*, 1996):

1. Difficulty in surgical fashioning of the arteriovenous fistula due to concomitant arteriosclerosis or insufficient venous dilatation. As a general rule, it is wise to plan surgery for fistula early, when the creatinine clearance is around 20–15 ml/minute. If all local access fails, transposition of a saphenous vein graft to the radial or cubital artery in a loop may allow hemodialysis, and seems to give better results than other artificial grafts.
2. Some 50–60% of elderly patients complain of weakness, hypotension, headaches and vomiting, cramps, and cardiovascular instability in the first two hours of HD. Such episodes can be alleviated by maintenance of a hemoglobin level over 10 $g\,dl^{-1}$ and an albumin level about 4 $g\,dl^{-1}$, careful titration of "dry weight", gentle and slow ultrafiltration, avoidance of vasodilator drugs in the predialysis period, and of course, the use of bicarbonate instead of acetate will also help.
3. Angina is frequent in older patients with coronary artery disease, and this may be facilitated by anemia, left ventricular hypertrophy and perhaps the higher free radical production exhibited by the elderly treated by hemodialysis. To prevent these episodes, it may be useful to maintain a high hematocrit above 30% by transfusion, intravenous iron, androgens, and/or administration of erythropoietin hormone.
4. Arrhythmias are very frequent in the elderly during dialysis because metastatic calcification, amyloid infiltration, cardiac hypertrophy and hypertension are more frequent than in younger patients. Hypokalemia and acidosis are contributory factors to the development of supraventricular and ventricular rhythm disturbances.

5. The commonest causes of gastrointestinal bleeding in elderly patients are angiodysplasia and gastritis provoked by uremia and worsened by intake of NSAID.
6. Impaired cellular immunity may lead to a higher incidence of viral infections and malignant tumors.

CAPD is also not without complications in the aged (Ismail *et al.*, 1993; Grapsa *et al.*, 2000):

1. dialysate leakage and formation of hernias;
2. peritonitis is the most common complication, but its incidence is not significantly different in elderly and young patients. The use of a Y-connector reduces the risk of infection, even in handicapped elderly patients;
3. exit site and tunnel infections requiring antibiotic treatment occur with the same frequency in young and in elderly patients, and catheter survival is also similar in both groups;
4. diverticulitis due to the frequency of intestinal diverticulosis in the elderly. Constipation is common, and is almost invariable in the elderly on dialysis;
5. backache, probably related to increased lordosis, secondary to carrying 2 l of dialysate fluid in the peritoneal cavity;
6. hypotension and worsening of peripheral vascular disease, particularly in those with preexisting ischemia of the lower limbs;
7. peritoneal dialysis imposes a nutritional stress in that from 8 to 15 g of first-class protein, mainly albumin, are lost each day in dialysate, and this amount increases during and following episodes of peritonitis.

CAPD is better for patients with residual diuresis, severe hypotension, complicated and/or short-lived vascular access, intradialytic arrhythmias, angina, or cardiovascular instability. CAPD is a satisfactory alternative treatment for elderly ESRD patients. Most studies confirm that survival of elderly patients on CAPD and HD is similar. Other forms of peritoneal dialysis include chronic cycling peritoneal dialysis (CCPD) and nightly automated peritoneal dialysis (APD); the latter can be an alternative treatment for more vulnerable elderly patients (Grapsa and Oreopoulos, 2000; Carrasco *et al.*, 1999).

Transplantation

Renal transplantation in the elderly remains controversial, despite being recognized as the most successful and cheapest treatment for patients with ESRD. Until the beginning of the 1980s, patients as young as 45 years were considered to be a "high-risk" group: allograft survival in this age-group was only 20% at 1 year, due to a high incidence of infections and cardiovascular complications (Simmonds *et al.*, 1971). These ideas are no longer present due to improved care of transplant recipients and the introduction of cyclosporin. However, the reality is that only 4% of patients aged 65–74 under treatment for ESRD receive a renal transplant. The USRDS report for 1991 notes that the actual 10-year survival for transplant recipients aged 55–59 was only 22%, only 10.5% for those aged 60–64, and 8% for those aged 65–69 years (Cameron *et al.*, 1994; USRDS, 1991). Triple therapy regimen (prednisolone, azathioprine, and cyclosporin A, all in relatively low doses) used in most European transplant units can be used in the elderly almost without modification. It is prudent to lower the dose of both cyclosporin, to avoid toxicity, and prednisolone, to avoid the many side effects of these drugs, especially on skin and bone. Elderly patients have decreased hepatic enzyme activity, especially the P450 system, and therefore require a lower cyclosporin dose. Because of that, other new drugs such as mycofenolate or rapamycine may be of help although clinical trials of the effect of these drugs in renal transplant in persons aged over 65 are lacking. It is unclear whether antilymphocyte globulin or monoclonal antibodies such as OKT3 should be used in the elderly. The success of transplantation in geriatric ESRD patients over the last decade is due to improved patient selection as well as the use of cyclosporin A and lower doses of corticosteroids, with achievement of 1-year patient and graft survival rates of 85 and 75%, respectively. For patients older than 60 or 65 years, the 5-year "functional" graft survival is 55–60%. Although overall results are excellent, the management of transplantation in the elderly requires an understanding of pharmacology, immunology and physiology peculiar to this age-group. Although elderly patients experience fewer rejection episodes than younger patients, graft loss in the elderly transplant recipient is due mainly to patient death. Most common causes of death in the elderly transplant recipient are cardiovascular disease and infection related to peaks of immunosuppression (Morris *et al.*, 1991; Ismail *et al.*, 1994).

AGED KIDNEY ALTERATIONS

Secondary to Systemic Diseases

Many features of common renal syndromes are different in elderly subjects. In a comparison of the elderly with patients of younger age-groups, it appeared that amyloidosis, MN, vasculitis, hypertension, and diabetes mellitus had a significantly higher incidence in the elderly. However, apart from greater critical water and electrolyte balance and tendency to develop cardiac failure, the causes, symptomatology, and investigations are largely the same as in the young.

Hypertension (see Chapter 48, Hypertension)

Renal diseases, including acute and chronic failure, may cause hypertension but on the other hand, hypertension itself can result in renal damage (Parfrey *et al.*, 1981). It accounts for 33% of ESRD in the elderly (Labeeuw *et al.*, 1996). A pathological rise in arterial pressure with age in Western society may result from an increase in dietary sodium or decreased dietary potassium, or both. A renal lesion develops later, possibly as a consequence of this primary increase in blood pressure. This is associated with resetting of pressure natriuresis, so that higher blood pressure is needed to maintain a given sodium excretion. It seems that renal hemodynamics in essential hypertension are adjusted mainly to ensure a consistent GFR. Albuminuria and renal dysfunction have recently been recognized as important complications in the patient with essential hypertension. Albuminuria is associated with more severe hypertension, with evidence of more advanced target organ damage (e.g. left ventricular hypertrophy), and is more prevalent in high-risk groups (e.g. older people). Ischemic nephropathy from nonmalignant nephrosclerosis has emerged as an important cause of terminal renal failure in the elderly patient with essential hypertension (Ritz and Fliser, 1992). Antihypertensive agents may impair renal blood flow (through plasma volume contraction or reduction) and further aggravate the age-related decline in renal perfusion. An understanding of the antihypertensive actions in an elderly patient may have a significant influence on renal function. A worsening of renal perfusion may activate counterregulatory neurohormonal mechanisms, such as the renin-angiotensin-aldosterone system, which in turn may place the patient at increased risk for the development of glomerulosclerosis through promotion of vascular or mesangial hypertrophic changes or increased intraglomerular pressure, despite an associated reduction in systemic blood pressure (Weir, 1992).

Atheroembolic Disease of the Elderly

Atheroembolism of the kidney occurs when plaque material breaks free from the diseased vessel and enters the distal microcirculation. Cholesterol crystals are the most easily recognizable of the embolic material, and usually vessels of about 80 mm diameter are affected. Diagnosis is made in a vasculopathic patient aged over 60 years, who has undergone an angiographic procedure or vascular surgery, and fever, muscle pain, weight loss, leucocytosis with eosinophilia, consumption of platelets, hypocomplementemia, and appearance of autoantibodies. Livedo reticularis and digital infarcts occurred in more than 30% of patients. Skin, muscle, and kidney biopsies remain the main tools for diagnosis. Confusion with vasculitis is not rare. Recovery of renal function rarely occurs and the mortality is very high (Cameron, 1995).

Diabetic Nephropathy (see Chapter 122, Type 2 Diabetes Mellitus in Senior Citizens)

Renal disease is now one of the commonest fatal complications of diabetes, especially in the elderly, where it causes about 22% of the ESRD cases (Labeeuw *et al.*, 1996). The condition of intercapillary glomerulosclerosis was first described by Kimmelstein and Wilson. Clinically, longstanding proteinuria with gradual decline in renal function leads to development of nephrotic syndrome, hypertension, and heart failure (Airoldi and Campanini, 1993). Results of treatment of ESRD in patients with non-insulin-dependent diabetes mellitus (type 2) showed a survival rate of 58% at 1 year and 14% at 5 years, independent of treatment modality. Patients who received a renal allograft had a higher survival rate as compared with patients on HD treatment (5-year survival, 59 vs 2%, $P < 0.005$). Renal transplantation improved survival of elderly diabetic patients without vascular complications and should be the treatment of choice in this specific group of patients (Hirschl *et al.*, 1992).

Collagen Disorders

These are chronic multisystem inflammatory diseases that commonly involve the kidney. The lesion is always some form of vasculitis. In systemic lupus erythematosus, necrosis and thrombosis of small vessels lead to ischemic changes. In progressive systemic sclerosis, there is obliterative thickening of the interior of small arteries and thickening of basement membrane due to fibroblastic proliferation and deposition of collagen. Rheumatoid arthritis commonly affects the kidney with proteinuria and renal impairment. In systemic vasculitis in elderly patients, it is not uncommon that kidney involvement, glomerulitis or necrotizing vasculitis, and circulating antineutrophil cytoplasm activity (ANCA), is what leads to diagnosis of the disease. Hematuria is almost a constant in vasculitis nephropathy. ANCA-related renal disease can be treated successfully with cyclophosphamide and steroids, and elderly patients should not be excluded from treatment, including dialysis if necessary (Musso and Macías Núñez, 2002; Garrett *et al.*, 1992).

Primary Glomerulopathies and Nephrotic Syndrome

During the past decade, controversy has raged about the necessity of renal biopsy for the management of the idiopathic nephrotic syndrome. The debate has centered on whether a precise diagnosis is imperative for steroid treatment or whether such therapy can be given blindly. There is a positive approach to the performance of a renal biopsy in the management of the nephrotic syndrome in the elderly (Moran *et al.*, 1993). Firstly, because at present it is known that the indications for renal biopsy, and the incidence of biopsy complications are the same for elderly and young adults. Secondly, because steroid therapy is not free of complications in the old population, it is therefore better to use this medication with histological support. Consequently, renal biopsy and histological observations are useful aids in estimating the prognosis and therapy selection for renal disorders even in elderly patients (Labeeuw *et al.*, 1996; Moulin *et al.*, 1991). When the number of glomerulopathy cases are properly related to the size of the general population of corresponding age-group, primary GN in the elderly was found to be the most diffuse biopsy-proven renal disease, even more frequent than primary GN in the adult (Vendemia *et al.*, 2001). Incidence of immunoglobulin A (IgA) nephropathy is three- to fourfold higher in patients aged 20–60 years than in the elderly. In contrast, membranous nephropathy (MN) is 3 times more frequent in the elderly than in young people (Simon *et al.*, 1995). Nephrotic syndrome accounts for 50% of renal biopsy indications in elderly patients, with its most frequent causes being: MN, minimal change disease and amyloidosis (Labeeuw *et al.*, 1996). MN in some patients is related to drugs or an underlying malignancy (20%). Usually the tumor, most commonly adenocarcinoma of the lung or colon, is obvious at the time of presentation (Labeeuw *et al.*, 1996; Vendemia *et al.*, 2001). Regarding minimal changes disease, it has some particular characteristics when it appears in the elderly: senile structural renal changes make its histological diagnosis difficult; its clinical presentation is usually "atypical", that means in the context of hypertension, microhematuria and/or renal failure; it may be associated with drugs (NSAID) or malignancies (lymphoma) (Labeeuw *et al.*, 1996). Crescentic GN reaches its greatest incidence in older people aged 60–79 years, and its typical clinical presentation is an ARF of rapid evolution. Steroids and other immunosuppressive drugs (cyclophosphamide, etc.) can be used in the old as in the young, though paying special attention to its side effects (Labeeuw *et al.*, 1996; Vendemia *et al.*, 2001).

Plasma Cell Dyscrasias and Primary Amyloidosis

Myeloma has been recognized for many years as a cause of renal disease in the elderly, usually ARF or CRF accompanied by proteinuria. Recovery from ARF is common in myeloma, perhaps because dehydration and desalination plays a role, itself the result of mobilization hypercalcemia. However, once ESRD has been reached, return of renal function is rare. Other types associated with abnormal plasma cell products are light chain nephropathy and fibrillary or immunotactoid nephropathy. In both conditions, the marrow is usually of normal to ordinary cytology, but there are often paraprotein spikes in serum or light chains in the urine. Finally, in primary amyloidosis patients are nephrotic and often develop renal failure (Musso and Macías Núñez, 2002; Kafetz, 1983; Frocht and Fillit, 1984; Musso *et al.*, 1996; Bellomo *et al.*, 1994; Druml *et al.*, 1994; Sacks *et al.*, 1989; Klahr, 1987; Rodríguez Pascual and Olcoz Chiva, 2002; Nicolle, 1994; Feest *et al.*, 1990; Verbeelen *et al.*, 1993; Labeeuw *et al.*, 1996; Anderson and Brenner, 1987; Glickman *et al.*, 1987; Vendemia and D'Amico, 1995; D'Amico, 1995; Piccoli *et al.*, 1993; Ismail *et al.*, 1993; Lerma *et al.*, 1995; Vandelli *et al.*, 1996; Grapsa and Oreopoulos 2000; Carrasco *et al.*, 1999; Simmonds *et al.*, 1971; Cameron *et al.*, 1994; USRDS, 1991; Morris *et al.*, 1991; Ismail *et al.*, 1994; Parfrey *et al.*, 1981; Cameron, 1995).

DRUGS AND THE KIDNEY

The kidneys in elderly subjects are particularly susceptible to the toxic effect of drugs and other chemical agent for the following reasons: (1) there is a rich blood supply; (2) drugs are concentrated in the hypertonic medulla; (3) drug accumulation is associated with impaired renal function; (4) hypersensitivity reaction with vasculitis is common in the kidney; (5) concomitant inhibition of hepatic enzymes increases drug toxicity. There is evidence that metabolic activation of some drugs within the kidney is responsible for nephrotoxicity while other drug reactions seem to be immunologically mediated (Evans, 1980).

The high rates of drug-induced ARF, worsening chronic renal dysfunction and systemic toxicity of renal excreted drugs can be minimized by carefully assessing renal function, avoiding potentially nephrotoxic drugs as much as possible and closely monitoring drug concentrations and renal function when drugs must be used (Thomson, 1995). NSAIDs may induce a variety of acute and chronic renal lesions. Acute interstitial nephritis can follow the use of nearly all NSAIDs, but the number of reported cases is low. Most of these patients are elderly and develop a nephrotic syndrome with ARF while taking NSAIDs for months. Renal biopsy shows acute tubulo-interstitial lesions with minimal changes in the glomeruli. The renal signs usually improve after discontinuing the drug, with or without steroid therapy, but chronic renal insufficiency or even ESRD are possible hazards. Interstitial nephritis results mainly from a delayed hypersensitivity response to NSAID, and nephrotic syndrome results from changes in glomerular permeability mediated by prostaglandins and other hormones. Patients taking NSAIDs for months or years may develop papillary necrosis, chronic interstitial nephritis, or even ESRD (Kleinknecht, 1995). The use of ACE inhibitors has increased greatly during recent years, and they are used in the treatment of elderly patients who often have generalized atherosclerosis. During treatment with ACE inhibitors, kidney function must be controlled before and following 1 to 2 weeks of treatment, since treatment with ACE inhibitors can cause pronounced changes in renal hemodynamics and kidney function (Rasmussen *et al.*, 1995). ACE inhibitors reduce angiotensin II production, with a decrease in total renal vascular resistance. The mechanism of ARF involves two major factors: sodium depletion and reduction in renal perfusion pressure. ARF is usually asymptomatic, nonoliguric, associated with hyperkalemia, and in nearly every case, completely reversible after discontinuation of the ACE inhibitors. The use of ACE inhibitors in the elderly should be practised with caution (Toto, 1994).

Toxicity of Drugs Administered to Patients with Renal Impairment

This depends on multiple factors, particularly the proportion of the drug normally excreted by the kidneys and the likely toxic effect of drugs. Thus the elderly are more susceptible to ototoxicity and nephrotoxicity with aminoglycosides, neuropathy with nitrofurantoin, and hypoglycemia with chlorpropamide (Castleden, 1978). Digoxin is mainly excreted by the kidney and, consequently, the same dose of digoxin produces higher blood levels and a longer blood half-life in old subjects than in the young. Its cardiac toxicity is enhanced by hypokalemia, a very common association due to the concomitant use of diuretics and the known tendency of the elderly to take a diet deficient in potassium. Dose adjustment may be achieved by reducing the amount given at the same intervals or by giving the same dose at longer intervals (Musso and Enz, 1996).

CONCLUSIONS

The aging kidney becomes less efficient in coping with stressful situations such as overload or deprivation. If attention is not paid to this decrease in functional capacity, it is possible to predispose elderly patients to situations such as ARF or congestive cardiac failure. In elderly patients, drug abuse is frequent, dehydration is very common, and renal artery stenosis and urinary outflow obstruction are important but often symptomless. With clinical experience, it is possible to overcome these difficulties and prevent renal failure. Kidney transplantation in elderly patients shows that long-term survival is at least as good, quality of life is improved and treatment is cheaper than HD or CAPD.

Acknowledgment

The authors are very grateful for the assistance of Sarah Dunt, Anna-Louise Nichols, and Tom Wingfield in the preparation of this chapter, enabled by the successful Erasmus-Socrates Exchange Program between The University of Salamanca, Spain, and The University of Liverpool, UK.

KEY POINTS

- The "Nephrogeriatric Giants" are six conditions that represent profound structural and physiological renal modifications which occur in the majority of the elderly population. These conditions are senile hypofiltration, renal vascular alteration, medullary hypotonicity, obstructive uropathy, tubular dysfunction, and frailty.
- Indications for renal biopsy, and the incidence of biopsy complications are the same for elderly and young adults.
- Main causes of renal failure in the old population are hypertension, atheroembolic disease, diabetes mellitus, vasculitis, plasma cell dyscrasias, and nephrotoxic drugs.
- CRF is predominantly a disease of the elderly and age by itself does not constitute a major impediment to dialysis and/or transplantation.

KEY REFERENCES

- Macias JF, Garcia-Iglesias C, Bondia A *et al.* Renal handling of sodium in old people: a functional study. *Age and Ageing* 1978; **7**:178–81.
- Macías Núñez JF, López Novoa JM & Martínez Maldonado M. Acute renal failure in the aged. *Seminars in Nephrology* 1996; **16**:330–8.
- Musso CG. Geriatric nephrology and the "nephrogeriatric giants". *International Urology and Nephrology* 2002; **34**:255–6.
- Musso CG, Fainstein I, Kaplan R & Macías Núñez JF. Tubular renal function in the oldest old. *Revista Espanola de Geriatria y Gerontologia* 2004; **39**(5):314–9.
- Vendemia F, Gesualdo L, Schena FP & D'amico G. Epidemiology of primary glomerulonephritis in the elderly. Report from the Italian registry of renal biopsy. *Journal of Nephrology* 2001; **14**:340–52.

REFERENCES

Airoldi G & Campanini M. Microalbuminuria: theoretical bases and new applications. *Recenti Progressi in Medicina* 1993; **84**:210–24.

Anderson S & Brenner BM. The aging kidney: structure, function, mechanisms, and therapeutic implication. *Journal of the American Geriatrics Society* 1987; **35**:590–3.

Andreucci V, Russo D, Cianciaruso B & Andreucci M. Some sodium, potassium and water changes in the elderly and their treatment. *Nephrology, Dialysis, Transplantation* 1996; **11**(suppl 9):9–17.

Baert L & Steg A. Is the diverticulum of the distal and collecting tubules a preliminary stage of the simple cyst in the adult? *The Journal of Urology* 1977; **118**:707–10.

Beauchene RE, Fanestil DD & Barrows CH. The effect of age on active transport and sodium-potassium-activated ATPase activity in renal tissue of rats. *Journal of Gerontology* 1965; **20**:306–10.

Bellomo R, Farmer M & Boyce N. The outcome of critically ill elderly patients with severe acute renal failure treated by continuous hemodiafiltration. *The International Journal of Artificial Organs* 1994; **17**:466–72.

Bengele HH, Mathias RS, Perkins JH & Alexander EA. Urinary concentrating defect in the aged rat. *The American Journal of Physiology* 1981; **240**:147–50.

Cameron JS. Renal disease in the elderly: particular problems. In G D'Amico & G Colasanti (eds) *Issues in Nephrosciences* 1995, pp 111–7; Wichting, Milano.

Cameron JS, Compton F, Koffman G & Bewick M. Transplantation in elderly recipients. *Geriatric Nephrology and Urology* 1994; **4**:93–9.

Carrasco M, García Ramón R & Gonzalez Rico M. Diálisis peritoneal en el anciano. In J Montenegro & J Olivares (eds) *La Diálisis Peritoneal* 1999, pp 479–90; Dibe, Spain.

Castleden CM. Prescribing for the elderly. *Prescribers' Journal* 1978; **18**:90.

Cockcroft DW & Gault MH. Prediction of creatinine clearance from serum creatinine. *Nephron* 1976; **16**:31–41.

Cohen MP & Ku L. Age-related changes in sulfation of basement membrane glycosaminoglycans. *Experimental Gerontology* 1983; **18**:447–50.

Cox JR & Shalaby WA. Potassium change with age. *Gerontologie* 1981; **27**:340–4.

D'Amico G. Comparability of the different registries on renal replacement therapy. *American Journal of Kidney Diseases* 1995; **25**:113–8.

Darmady EM, Offer J & Woodhouse MA. The parameters of the ageing kidney. *The Journal of Pathology* 1973; **109**:195–207.

De Santo N, Anastasio P, Coppola S *et al.* Age-related changes in renal reserve and renal tubular function in healthy humans. *Child Nephrology and Urology* 1991; **11**:33–40.

De Toro Casado R & Macías Núñez JF. Physiologic characteristics of the renal ageing: clinical consequences. *Anales de Medicina Interna* 1995; **12**:157–9.

Dontas AS, Marketos S & Papanayioutou P. Mechanisms of renal tubular defects in old age. *Postgraduate Medical Journal* 1972; **48**:295–303.

Druml W, Lax F, Grim G *et al.* Acute renal failure in the elderly 1975-1990. *Clinical Nephrology* 1994; **41**:342–9.

Eiam-Ong S & Sabatini S. Effect of ageing and potassium depletion on renal collecting tubule k-controlling ATPases. *Nephrologie* 2002; **7**:87–91.

Evans DB. Drugs and the kidney. *British Journal of Hospital Medicine* 1980; **24**:244–51.

Feest TG, Mistry CD, Grimes DS & Mallick NP. Incidence of advanced chronic renal failure and the need for end-stage renal replacement treatment. *British Medical Journal* 1990; **301**:897–903.

Fish LC, Murphy DJ, Elahi D & Minaker KL. Renal sodium excretion in normal aging: decreased excretion rates lead to delayed sodium excretion in normal aging. *Journal of Geriatric Nephrology and Urology* 1994; **4**:145–51.

Frocht A & Fillit H. Renal disease in the geriatric patient. *Journal of the American Geriatrics Society* 1984; **32**:28–43.

Fulop T, Worum I, Csongor J *et al.* Body composition in elderly people. *Gerontology* 1985; **31**:6–14.

Galinsky D, Meller Y & Shany S. The aging kidney and calcium regulating hormones: vitamin D metabolites, parathyroid hormone and calcitonin. In JF Macias & JS Cameron (eds) *Renal Function and Disease in the Elderly* 1987, p 121; Butterworths, London.

Garrett PJ, Dewhurst AG, Morgan LS *et al.* Renal disease associated with circulating antineutrophil cytoplasm activity. *The Quarterly Journal of Medicine* 1992; **85**:731–49.

Glickman JL, Kaiser D & Bolton K. Aetiology and diagnosis of chronic renal insufficiency in the aged: the role of the renal biopsy. In JF Macias & JS Cameron (eds) *Renal Function and Disease in the Elderly* 1987, pp 485–508; Butterworths, London.

Goyal VK. Changes with age in the human kidney. *Experimental Gerontology* 1982; **17**:321–31.

Grapsa E & Oreopoulos DG. Continuous ambulatory peritoneal dialysis in the elderly. In R Gokal & K Nolph (eds) *The Textbook of Peritoneal Dialysis* 2000, pp 419–33; Kluwer Academic Publishers, Dordrecht.

Griffiths GJ, Robinson KB, Cartwright GO & McLachlan MSF. Loss of renal tissue in the elderly. *The British Journal of Radiology* 1976; **49**:111–7.

Heim JM, Gottmann K, Weil J *et al.* Effects of a bolus of atrial natriuretic factor in young and elderly volunteers. *European Journal of Clinical Investigation* 1989; **19**:265–71.

Hirschl MM, Heinz G, Sunder-Plassmann G & Derfle K. Renal replacement therapy in type 2 diabetic patients: 10 years. *American Journal of Kidney Diseases* 1992; **20**:564–8.

Ismail N, Hakim RM & Helderman JH. Renal replacement therapies in the elderly: Part II. Renal transplantation. *American Journal of Kidney Diseases* 1994; **23**:1–15.

Ismail N, Hakim RM, Oreopoulos DG & Patrikaerea A. Renal replacement therapies on the elderly: Part I. Hemodialysis and chronic peritoneal dialysis. *American Journal of Kidney Diseases* 1993; **22**:759–82.

Kafetz K. Renal impairment in the elderly: a review. *Journal of the Royal Society of Medicine* 1983; **76**:398–401.

Kirkland JL, Lye M, Levy DW & Banerjee AK. Patterns of urine flow and electrolyte secretion in healthy elderly people. *British Medical Journal* 1983; **285**:1665–7.

Klahr S. Obstructive uropathy in the elderly. In JF Macias & JS Cameron (eds) *Renal Function and Disease in the Elderly* 1987, pp 432–55; Butterworths, London.

Kleinknecht D. Interstitial nephritis, the nephrotic syndrome, and chronic renal failure secondary to nonsteroidal anti-inflammatory drugs. *Seminars in Nephrology* 1995; **15**:228–35.

Labeeuw W, Caillette A & Dijoud F. La biopsie rénal chez le sujet âgé. *La Presse Médicale* 1996; **25**:611–4.

Lerma JL, Tabernero JM, Gascon A *et al.* Influence of age and hemodialysis on the production of free radicals. *Geriatric Nephrology and Urology* 1995; **5**:93–6.

Lindeman RD. Overview: renal physiology and pathophysiology of ageing. *American Journal of Kidney Diseases* 1990; **16**:275–82.

Lowental DT. Vulnerability to hyperkalemia. *Journal of Geriatric Nephrology and Urology* 1994; **4**:121–5.

Lye M. Distribution of body potassium in healthy elderly subjects. *Gerontologie* 1981; **27**:286–92.

Macias JF, Bondia A & Rodriguez Commes JL. Physiology and disorders of water balance and electrolytes in the elderly. In JF Macias & JS Cameron (eds) *Renal Function and Disease in the Elderly* 1987, pp 67–93; Butterworths, London.

Macias JF, Garcia-Iglesias C, Bondia A *et al.* Renal handling of sodium in old people: a functional study. *Age and Ageing* 1978; **7**:178–81.

Macias JF, Garcia-Iglesias C, Tabernero JM *et al.* Renal management of sodium under indomethacin and aldosterone in the elderly. *Age and Ageing* 1980; **9**:165–72.

Macias JF, Garcia-Iglesias C, Tabernero JM *et al.* Behaviour of the ageing kidney under acute acid overload. *Nefrologia* 1983; **3**:11–6.

Macías Núñez JF, López Novoa JM & Martínez Maldonado M. Acute renal failure in the aged. *Seminars in Nephrology* 1996; **16**:330–8.

McLachlan MSF. Anatomic structural and vascular changes in the ageing kidney. In JF Macias & JS Cameron (eds) *Renal Function and Disease in the Elderly* 1987, pp 3–26; Butterworths, London.

McLachlan MSF, Guthrie JC, Anderson CK & Fulker MJ. Vascular and glomerular changes in the ageing kidney. *The Journal of Pathology* 1977; **121**:65–77.

Meyer BR. Renal function in ageing. *Journal of the American Geriatrics Society* 1989; **37**:791–800.

Meyrier A. Renal vascular lesions in the elderly: nephrosclerosis or atheromatous renal disease? *Nephrology, Dialysis, Transplantation* 1996; **11**(suppl 9):45–52.

Moran D, Korzets Z, Bernheim J *et al.* Is renal biopsy justified for the diagnosis and management of the nephrotic syndrome in the elderly? *Gerontology* 1993; **39**:49–54.

Morris GE, Jamieson NV, Small J *et al.* Cadaveric renal transplantation in elderly recipients: is it worthwhile? *Nephrology, Dialysis, Transplantation* 1991; **6**:887–92.

Moulin B, Dhib M, Sommervogel C *et al.* Intérêt de la biopsie rénal chez le vieillard. *La Presse Médicale* 1991; **20**:1881–5.

Musso C & Enz P. Pharmacokinetics in the elderly. *Revista Argentina de Farmacología Clínica* 1996; **3**:101–5.

Musso C, Fainstein I & Kaplan R. The patient with acid-base and electrolytes disorders. In JF Macias, F Guillén Llera & JM Rivera Casado (eds) *Geriatrics Since the Beginning* 2001, pp 245–52; Glosa, Barcelone.

Musso CG, Fainstein I, Kaplan R & Macías Núñez JF. Tubular renal function in the oldest old. *Revista Espanola de Geriatria y Gerontologia* 2004; **39**(5):314–9.

Musso CG. Geriatric nephrology and the "nephrogeriatric giants". *International Urology and Nephrology* 2002; **34**:255–6.

Musso CG & Macías Núñez JF. The aged kidney: morphology and function. Main nephropathies. In A Salgado, F Guillén & I Ruipérez (eds) *Geriatrics Handbook* 2002, pp 399–412; Masson, Barcelone.

Musso CG, Macías Núñez JF & Mayorga M. Worth of the urinary sodium in the differential diagnosis between renal and pre-renal acute renal failure in the elderly. *Revista Argentinade Geriatría y Gerontología* 1996; **16**:129–36.

Musso CG, Macías Núñez JF, Musso CAF *et al.* Fractional Excretion of sodium in old old people on a low sodium diet. *Federation of American Societies for Experimental Biology* 2000; **14**:A659.

Nicolle LE. Urinary tract infection in the elderly. *The Journal of Antimicrobial Chemotherapy* 1994; **33**:99–109.

Parfrey PS, Markandu ND, Roulston JE *et al.* Relation between arterial blood pressure, dietary sodium intake and renin system in essential hypertension. *British Medical Journal* 1981; **283**:94.

Perez del Molino P & Alvarez L. Metabolic bonne diseases in the elderly. In A Salgado, F Guillén & I Ruipérez (eds) *Geriatrics Handbook* 2002, pp 447–58; Masson, Barcelone.

Phillips PA, Rolls BJ, Ledingham DM *et al.* Reduced thirst after water deprivation in healthy elderly men. *The New England Journal of Medicine* 1984; **311**:753–9.

Piccoli G, Bonello F, Massara C *et al.* Death in conditions of cachexia: the price for the dialysis treatment of the elderly? *Kidney International* 1993; **43**:282–6.

Rasmussen K, Heitmann M, Nielsen JI & Mogelvang JC. Renal function during treatment with angiotensin converting enzyme inhibitors. *Ugeskrift for Laeger* 1995; **157**:5377–81.

Ritz E & Fliser D. Clinical relevance of albuminuria in hypertensive patients. *Clinical and Investigative* 1992; **70**:s114–9.

Roberts MM & Robinson AG. Hyponatremia in the elderly: diagnosis and management. *Geriatric Nephrology and Urology* 1993; **3**:43–50.

Rodríguez Pascual C & Olcoz Chiva M. Infectious diseases in geriatric patients. In A Salgado, F Guillén & I Ruipérez (eds) *Geriatrics Handbook* 2002, pp 542–8; Masson, Barcelone.

Rosen H. Renal disease of the elderly. *The Medical Clinics of North America* 1976; **60**:1105.

Rowe JW, Andres R, Tobin JD *et al.* The effect of age on creatinine clearance in man: a cross-sectional and longitudinal study. *Journal of Gerontology* 1976a; **31**:155–63.

Rowe JW, Shock NW & De Fronzo RA. The influence of age on the renal response to water deprivation in man. *Nephron* 1976b; **17**:270–8.

Sacks SH, Aparicio SAJR, Bevan A *et al.* Late renal failure due to prostatic out flow obstruction: a preventable disease. *British Medical Journal* 1989; **298**:180–9.

Seeling MS & Preuss HG. Magnesium metabolism and perturbation in the elderly. *Geriatric Nephrology and Urology* 1994; **4**:101–11.

Shannon RP, Minaker KL & Rowe JW. Aging and water balance in humans. *Seminars in Nephrology* 1984; **4**:346–53.

Simmonds RL, Kjellstrand CM, Buselmeier TS *et al.* Renal transplantation in high risk patients. *Archives of Surgery* 1971; **103**:290–8.

Simon P, Ramee MP, Autuly V *et al.* Epidemiology of primary glomerulopathies in a French region. Variations as a function of age in patients. *Nephrologie* 1995; **16**:191–201.

Solomon LR & Lye M. Hypernatremia in the elderly patient. *Gerontology* 1990; **36**:171–9.

Swedko P, Clark H, Paramsothy K & Akbari A. Serum creatinine is an inadequate screening test for renal failure in the elderly patients. *Archives of Internal Medicine* 2003; **163**:356–60.

Takazakura E, Sawabu N, Handa A *et al.* Intrarenal vascular changes with age and disease. *Kidney International* 1972; **2**:224–30.

Thomson NM. Drugs and the kidney in the elderly. *The Medical Journal of Australia* 1995; **162**:543–7.

Toto RD. Renal insufficiency due to angiotensin-converting enzyme inhibitors. *Mineral and Electrolyte Metabolism* 1994; **20**:193–200.

USRDS (United States Renal Data System). Annual data report. *American Journal of Kidney Diseases* 1991; **18**(suppl 2):38–48.

Vandelli L, Medici G, Perrone S & Lusvarghi E. Haemodialysis in the elderly. *Nephrology, Dialysis, Transplantation* 1996; **11**(suppl 9):89–94.

Vendemia F & D'Amico G. Management of chronic renal failure in the elderly. In G D'Amico & G Colasanti (eds) *Issues in Nephrosciences* 1995, pp 119–26; Wichting, Milano.

Vendemia F, Gesualdo L, Schena FP & D'amico G. Epidemiology of primary glomerulonephritis in the elderly. Report from the Italian registry of renal biopsy. *Journal of Nephrology* 2001; **14**:340–52.

Verbeelen D, de Neve W, van der Niepen P & Sennessael J. Dialysis in patients over 65 years of age. *Kidney International* 1993; **43**:s27–30.

Weir MR. Hypertensive nephropathy: is a more physiologic approach to blood pressure control an important concern for the preservation of renal function? *The American Journal of Medicine* 1992; **93**:s27–37.

PART III

Medicine in Old Age

Section 12

Cancer

128

Cancer and Aging

Claudia Beghe[1,2] *and* Lodovico Balducci[1,3]

[1] University of South Florida College of Medicine, Tampa, FL, USA, [2] James A. Haley Veterans' Hospital, Tampa, FL, USA, and [3] H. Lee Moffitt Cancer Center and Research Institute, Tampa, FL, USA

Cancer is the second most common cause of death and a major cause of disability for individuals aged 65 and older (Yancik and Ries, 2004). Cancer control is a key to a more prolonged and more active survival. After reviewing the epidemiology of cancer in the elderly and the biologic interactions of cancer and age, we will examine effectiveness and safety of cancer prevention and treatment in the older aged person.

EPIDEMIOLOGY

The incidence of most common cancers increases with age (Figure 1) up to age 80–85 and plateaus thereafter (Yancik and Ries, 2004). Autopsy studies suggest that after age 95 cancer ceases to be a major cause of morbidity and mortality, and even the incidence of occult malignancies may decrease (Stanta *et al.*, 1997). Seemingly, the prevalence of common cancers increases also with age, as early diagnosis and new forms of treatment have transformed many neoplasms into chronic diseases that may influence the function and the quality of life of older individuals. This area deserves more investigation (Caranasos, 1997).

Four epidemiological facts may have clinical implications. First, while cancer incidence has increased both among people younger than 65 and those 65 and older since 1950, cancer-related mortality has decreased for the young but increased for the old ones (Wingo *et al.*, 2003). This may be due in part to remediable causes, including the fact that older individuals are less likely to undergo cancer screening and to receive aggressive antineoplastic treatment. For example, breast cancer is diagnosed at a more advanced stage in women over 70 despite the fact that this neoplasm becomes more indolent with age (Randolph *et al.*, 2002).

Second, the incidence of some neoplasms, including non-Hodgkin's lymphomas and malignant brain tumors, has increased since 1970 mainly in older individuals (Yancik and Ries, 2004; Wingo *et al.*, 2003). This phenomenon, that so far is unexplained, should alert the practitioner that with the aging of the population certain diseases may become more common and that age may be associated with increased susceptibility to certain neoplasias.

Third, an age-related shift in incidence and mortality has been seen for some cancers. For example, lung cancer–related mortality has declined by more than 10% in individuals 50 and younger, but has increased around 20% for those 70 and older (Wingo *et al.*, 2003). Nowadays, lung cancer in elderly ex-smokers is becoming progressively more common. Smoking cessation has likely resulted in reduced death rate from cardiovascular and chronic obstructive lung diseases, and in reduced growth rate of occult cancer. In support of this hypothesis, lung cancer may be more indolent in older individuals. The emergence of more indolent lung cancer with a prolonged preclinical phase justifies new studies of early detection of lung cancer in ex-smokers.

Fourth, cancer may affect preferentially older individuals in good general condition. In Italy, Ferrucci *et al.*, (2003) and Repetto *et al.*, (1998) demonstrated that cancer patients aged 70 and older were less likely to present functional dependence or comorbidity than age-matched individuals without cancer. The Surveillance, Epidemiology and End Result study (SEER) showed that women aged 80 and older with breast cancer had a more prolonged survival than women of the same age without breast cancer (Diab *et al.*, 2000). These findings support cancer prevention and treatment in older individuals as they indicate that cancer is indeed a cause of death and morbidity for the elderly.

BIOLOGICAL INTERACTIONS OF CANCER AND AGING

These interactions may occur in two areas: carcinogenesis, and tumor biology.

Principles and Practice of Geriatric Medicine, 4th Edition. Edited by M.S. John Pathy, Alan J. Sinclair and John E. Morley.

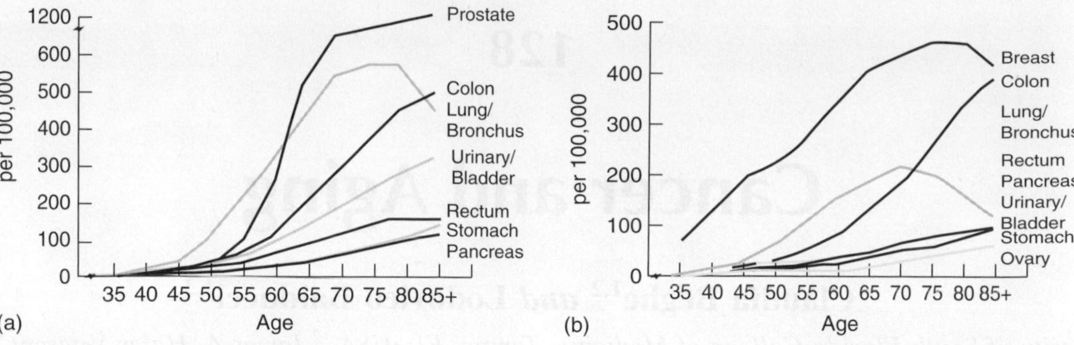

Figure 1 (a) Cancer incidence rates in men. (b) Cancer incidence rates in women

Aging and Carcinogenesis

Carcinogenesis is a stepwise process that involves a number of serial genomic changes, including activation of cellular oncogenes and inhibition of antiproliferative genes (antioncogenes) (Anisimov, 2005). These changes are effected by substances called *carcinogens* that in experimental models have been distinguished into early- and late-stage carcinogens. The action of the latter is reversible and is the focus of a modern strategy of cancer control, chemoprevention.

The association of aging and cancer may be explained by three, nonmutually exclusive mechanisms. First, as carcinogenesis is time consuming, cancer is more likely to become manifest late in life. Second, aging is associated with molecular changes similar to those of carcinogenesis, including formation of DNA adducts and DNA hypermethylation. Older individuals harbor a larger concentration of cells primed to the action of late-phase environmental carcinogens. Both experimental and clinical data support this hypothesis (Anisimov, 2005). A possible explanation for the increased incidence of lymphoma and malignant brain tumors recently observed in older individuals is that these individuals are a natural monitoring system for new environmental carcinogens, that is, in the presence of new carcinogens older individuals develop cancer at an earlier time. Third, paradoxically, proliferative senescence, that is the loss of self-replicative ability of the aging cells, may predispose to cancer, as senescent cells may become immortalized (Hornsby, 2004). The pathogenesis of slowly growing neoplasms, such as follicular lymphoma, may be traced to the loss of programmed cell death (apoptosis) by the aging lymphocytes (Balducci and Aapro, 2004).

Age and Tumor Biology

The clinical behavior of some neoplasms may change with the age of the patient (Table 1) (Balducci and Aapro, 2004). At least two mechanisms may explain these changes. If one thinks of a tumor as a plant, the growth of the plant may be determined by the nature of the seed (the tumor cell), and of the soil (the tumor host). In the case of acute myelogenous leukemia (AML), the prevalence of resistance to cytotoxic chemotherapy increases after age 60, which may explain the poor outcome of AML in the elderly (Lancet *et al.*, 2000). The prognosis of NHL (Non Hodgkin's Lymphoma) may worsen through a "soil" mechanism: age is associated with increased circulating concentrations of interleukin-6 (IL-6), an independent poor prognostic factor (The International Non-Hodgkin's Lymphoma Prognostic Factors Project 1993; Preti *et al.*, 1997), as IL-6 stimulates lymphoid proliferation. In the case of breast cancer, both a "seed" and a "soil" mechanism may conspire to

Table 1 Example of neoplasms whose biology may change with aging

Cancer	Change in prognosis	Mechanism
Acute myelogenous leukemia	Worse, increased resistance to chemotherapy	Seed: 1. Increased prevalence of MDR1 2. Increased prevalence of stem-cell leukemia
Non-Hodgkin's lymphoma	Worse, decreased response rate to chemotherapy, decreased disease-free survival	Soil: Increased circulating concentration of IL-6
Breast	Better: More indolent disease	Seed: 1. Higher prevalence of hormone-responsive tumors 2. Lower proliferation rate 3. Higher prevalence of well-differentiated tumors Soil: 1. Endocrine senescence 2. Immune senescence
Ovary	Worse: reduced response to chemotherapy and disease-free survival	Unknown
Lung, nonsmall cell	Better, presentation at earlier stages, more indolent disease	Seed: More differentiated, slowly growing tumor

Note: MDR, multi drug resistance.

generate a more indolent tumor (Balducci *et al.*, 2004): the prevalence of well-differentiated-hormone-receptor-rich tumors increases with age, and at the same time endocrine senescence may disfavor the growth of hormone-responsive neoplasms. As already mentioned, lung cancer is more likely to affect elderly ex-smokers, whose tumor has undergone a lower number of mutations and is less aggressive.

A major breakthrough in tumor biology has been the development of microarray techniques, able to reveal the full genetic profile of a tumor. The overexpression of certain genes has been associated with different biologic behaviors, including growth rate and susceptibility to cytotoxic chemotherapy (Sikic, 1999). Microarrays may allow identification of biologic differences between the tumor cells of younger and older patients.

Little is known about the host-related changes that may influence tumor growth. In addition to endocrine senescence, immune senescence and proliferative senescence of the stromal cells may play a role. Immune senescence may favor the growth of highly immunogenic tumors, while proliferative senescence of fibroblasts is associated with increased production of tumor growth factors (Hornsby, 2004). It is also worthwhile remembering that frailty is associated with increased concentration of catabolic cytokines in the circulation (Cohen *et al.*, 2003) and with sarcopenia (Stanta *et al.*, 1997) that may inhibit tumor growth.

The mechanisms by which age may influence tumor aggressiveness represent a widely open research area.

Two considerations are clinically pertinent: (i) Aging may be associated with more indolent as well as more aggressive tumors. (ii) Age itself is a poor predictor of tumor behavior and each cancer should be managed according to the individual characteristics of the tumor and of the patient. If it is true that 67% of AML in individuals aged 60 and older present MDR (Multi Drug resistance), it is also true that 33% of these patients have a neoplasm sensitive to chemotherapy. If 80% of breast cancer patients aged 65 and older have a hormone-receptor-rich tumor for which cytotoxic chemotherapy produces limited benefits, 20% of these women have aggressive hormone-receptor-poor tumors that may need front-line cytotoxic chemotherapy.

CANCER PREVENTION

Cancer prevention represents the most obvious way to reduce the impact of cancer on mortality, disability, and quality of life. Primary prevention involves elimination of environmental carcinogens or block and reversal of carcinogenesis with chemoprevention. Secondary prevention involves early detection of cancer at a curable stage by screening asymptomatic individuals at risk.

Chemoprevention of Cancer

Chemoprevention appears the most practical form of primary cancer prevention (Beghe' and Balducci, 2004). Potential drawbacks include cost and toxicity of treatment. Figure 2 illustrates the possible mechanisms of action of chemopreventative agents. Chemoprevention may inhibit the reactions that activate procarciongens into carcinogens and facilitate those that catabolize carcinogens. The crossroad of chemical, radiation, and light-induced carcinogenesis, electrophylic DNA adducts, may be reversed by DNA repairing enzymes, whose activity is enhanced by selenium, calorie restriction, and epigallocatechin galate (Hursting *et al.*, 1999). Endogenous substances that influence carcinogenesis, such as reactive oxygen species, hormones, growth factors, and eicosenoids, represent another target of chemoprevention.

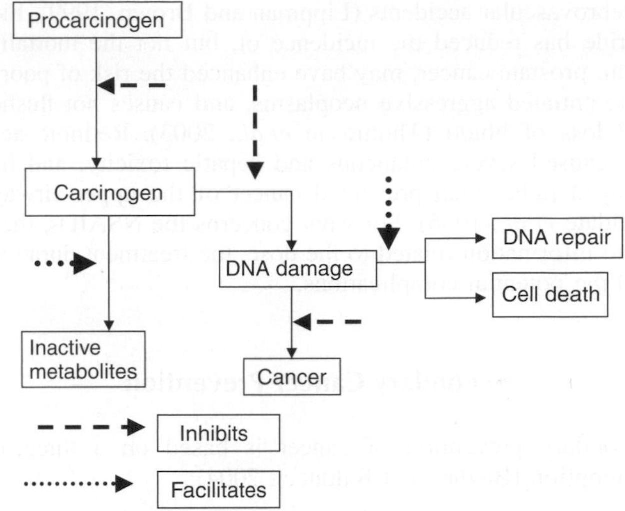

Figure 2 Mechanism of action of chemoprevention

Three groups of agents were proven to prevent cancer in humans: hormonal agents, retinoids, and NSAIDs. In randomized controlled studies, the SERM tamoxifen (Lippman and Brown, 1999) has prevented breast cancer, and the reductase inhibitor finasteride prostate cancer (Thompson *et al.*, 2003). Other hormonal agents of interest for the prevention of breast cancer include the SERM raloxifen that unlike tamoxifen does not cause endometrial cancer, and the aromatase inhibitors. In randomized controlled studies, retinoic acid has reversed preneoplastic lesions and delayed the occurrence of secondary cancers in the upper airways (Oridate *et al.*, 1986). In a prospective study, the COX-2 inhibitor rofecoxib has caused regression of preneoplastic polyps (Steinbach *et al.*, 2000); two large retrospective studies suggest that aspirin may prevent death from cancer of the large bowel (Thun *et al.*, 1991; Chemoprevention Working Group, 1999) and another retrospective study that it may reduce the risk of breast cancer (Terry *et al.*, 2004). Furthermore, NSAIDs and aromatase inhibitors appear synergistic *in vitro*.

These encouraging results cannot be translated as yet into clinical indications. Tamoxifen prevents only indolent well-differentiated hormone-responsive tumors and has not reduced breast cancer-related mortality. Though rare, the complications of tamoxifen have been potentially serious, including endometrial cancer, deep vein thrombosis, and cerebrovascular accidents (Lippman and Brown, 1999). Finsteride has reduced the incidence of, but not the mortality from, prostate cancer, may have enhanced the risk of poorly differentiated aggressive neoplasms, and causes hot flushes and loss of libido (Thompson *et al.*, 2003). Retinoic acid has caused severe cutaneous and hepatic toxicity, and has delayed rather than prevented cancer of the upper airways (Oridate *et al.*, 1986). For what concerns the NSAIDs, there is no information related to the dose, the treatment duration, and the potential complications.

Secondary Cancer Prevention

Secondary prevention of cancer is based on a threefold assumption (Beghe' and Balducci, 2004):

- Clinical manifestations of cancer are preceded by a prolonged preclinical phase, including invasive cancer and premalignant lesions.
- Screening tests may diagnose cancer in the preclinical and even the premalignant phase.
- Early diagnosis of cancer is associated with improved chances of surgical curability.

A reduction in cancer-related deaths in randomized clinical trials is considered the definitive proof that secondary prevention is effective. This end point has been criticized for two reasons. First, it may take several years and result in unnecessary loss of lives and the conclusions of the trial may be obsolete, because by the time of completion new and more sensitive screening techniques might have been developed. Second, one may wonder how meaningful a reduction of cancer-related mortality is in elderly individuals when overall mortality is unaffected. This issue is exemplified by a randomized study of radical prostatectomy versus observation in men up to age 75 in Sweden that demonstrated radical prostatectomy is associated with a reduction in cancer-related but not overall mortality (Holmberg *et al.*, 2002). For a number of older men with prostate cancer, maybe the majority, prostatectomy is costly, dangerous, and without appreciable benefit. At the same time, however, screening may improve patient quality of life even when it does not seem to affect mortality. It is possible that early detection of some cancers, such as breast cancer, might reduce the risk of cancer-related complications.

Age itself has diverging effects on the outcome of screening (Beghe' and Balducci, 2004). On one hand, the positive predictive value of screening tests may increase with age, owing to increased prevalence of common cancers. On the other hand, reduced life expectancy and development of more indolent tumors may lessen the benefits of screening. Also, the yield of screening tests decreases with the number of times they have been performed, as the initial tests have eliminated most prevalence cases.

Two combined approaches may help identify asymptomatic older individuals for whom cancer screening is indicated. The first involves an estimate of the effects of screening on quality of life. Chen *et al.* have identified a profile of older patients for whom the benefits of screening may overwhelm the risk of complications (Chen *et al.*, 2003). These are the so-called risk takers, who are willing to undergo dangerous forms of cancer treatment even when the benefits are minimal. The second approach identifies patients at higher risk of development of a certain type of cancer. In a decision analysis, Kerlikowske *et al.* demonstrated that mammography is most beneficial for women in the upper quintile of bone density, who are those at higher breast cancer risk (Kerlikowske *et al.*, 1999).

Randomized and controlled clinical trials have demonstrated that screening mammography reduces the mortality of breast cancer in women aged 50–70 (Kerlikowske *et al.*, 1995) and screening for colorectal cancer with fecal occult blood reduces the mortality for individuals aged 50–80 (Frazier *et al.*, 2000). Presumably, serial endoscopies may be at least as effective as examination of stools for occult blood, and are the preferred form of screening in many centers (Frazier *et al.*, 2000). In the absence of data, it appears prudent to screen persons with a life expectancy of five years or longer for breast and colorectal cancer, as the earliest benefits of screening have been observed five years after the institution of the screening program (Walter *et al.*, 2004). Controversy lingers on the benefits of screening asymptomatic men for prostate cancer: in any case it is unlikely that this intervention may reduce cancer-related mortality in men over 70. Screening for cervical cancer after age 60 is another area of controversy. It is recommended in women at risk, because they are sexually active, especially if they have multiple partners, and for those who have never been screened before age 60. No proof exists of the value of screening for lung, ovarian, or endometrial cancer. In these cases, screening is justified only in the context of clinical trials.

CANCER TREATMENT

Local treatment of cancer involves surgery and radiation therapy; systemic treatment involves cytotoxic chemotherapy, and hormonal, biological, and targeted therapy. Cancer therapy may have different goals including curative, adjuvant, and palliative. Adjuvant treatment is administered to prevent recurrence of cancer in patients at high risk of recurrence after definitive therapy: Palliative treatment is aimed at relieving symptoms and prolonging the survival of patients with incurable cancer.

Two new treatment approaches deserve mention: neoadjuvant and combined modality treatment. Neoadjuvant treatment mainly involves chemo and hormonal therapy and is administered prior to definitive therapy, with the goal of making this more effective and less radical. Neoadjuvant chemotherapy of breast cancer has allowed breast preservation in the majority of patients. Combined modality treatment that generally involves a combination of cytotoxic chemotherapy and radiation therapy has been used to allow organ preservation and to obtain better outcome than with either individual forms of treatment. Combined modality treatment has allowed organ preservation in patients with resectable cancer of the head and neck area, of the esophagus, and of the anus, and has prolonged the survival of patients with locally advanced cancer of the lung and of the head and neck.

Surgery

The incidence of surgical complications, including mortality, increases after age 70, according to Medicare data (Berger and Roslyn, 1997). The majority of these complications should be ascribed to emergency surgery, however, mainly related to large bowel obstruction and resulting Gram-negative sepsis (Berger and Roslyn, 1997). With the exception of pneumonectomy, most elective surgical procedures appear well tolerated by older individuals (Berger and Roslyn, 1997; Kemeny *et al.*, 2000). Unfortunately, the risk of emergency abdominal surgery increases with age, which underlines the importance of regular screening for colorectal cancer, as early detection would minimize the risk of colonic obstruction.

Recent advances in anesthesia and in surgical techniques have reduced the risk of postoperative complications in the elderly. The addition of amnesic drugs to the anesthetic cocktail has allowed reducing the dose of traditional anesthetics and opioids, and has minimized the risk of respiratory and cardiovascular complications of anesthesia even in centenarians (Miguel and Vila, 2004). Furthermore, a number of procedures, including mastectomy, may be performed under local anesthesia and are accessible also to patients with severe respiratory diseases. The advent of sentinel lymph-node mapping to recognize patients at risk for lymph-node metastases has allowed the foregoing of full lymph-node dissection in patients with cancer of the breast and melanoma (Singletary *et al.*, 2004). The value of this approach is being explored also in cancer of the head and neck areas and in gynecological cancer. The extent of surgery has become more limited for several cancers, including rectal cancer that seldom requires nowadays an abdominal-perineal resection. Laser endoscopic surgery may be curative in early stages of esophageal and bronchial cancer and may maintain the patency of these organs through the latest stages of the disease. Radiosurgery (γ knife) proved as effective as standard surgery for small brain tumors and is investigated in other malignancies (Hevezi, 2003). Radio-frequency ablation (RFA) that may be performed in many patients without general anesthesia and under CT guidance was proven effective in the management of primary and secondary liver tumors, and may be utilized also for small kidney cancers (Tranberg, 2004).

Radiation Therapy

A number of retrospective studies in Europe and in the United States have shown that external beam irradiation is well tolerated even in individuals over 80, more than three-quarters of whom are able to receive full doses of radiation (Zachariah and Balducci, 2000). The risk of mucositis may increase with age during radiation of the chest, involving the esophagus, and of the pelvis. In these cases it is extremely important to assure hydration and nutrition. Prophylactic peg tubes are recommended in patients undergoing treatment of the upper digestive tract and of the esophagus.

The advent of conformational radiation therapy has minimized toxicity of normal tissues and maximized therapeutic efficacy. Brachytherapy, that is delivering of radiation by implant of radioactive material, is another safe and effective form of treatment. Of special interest for older men is brachytherapy of prostate cancer (Zachariah and Balducci, 2000).

New forms of radiation therapy include hyper fractionated radiation therapy that may improve therapeutic efficacy by reducing the time intervals between treatments, and also lead to reduced treatment duration. The safety of this form of treatment in elderly patients is being explored.

Together with radiation therapy one should mention *radioisotopes* that have gained new momentum in the last few years. Radioactive strontium and sumerium relieve pain from multiple bone metastases and are generally well tolerated, though they may cause myelosuppression and limit the use of cytotoxic chemotherapy (Roque *et al.*, 2003). In addition, monoclonal antibodies targeted to the CD20 antigens, in combination with radioactive yttrium (Zevelin) or Iodine (Bexaar), induce remission in 40% of patients with low-grade lymphomas resistant to cytotoxic chemotherapy (Harris, 2004). The use of these agents as front-line treatment is being explored. These compounds may cause prolonged and substantial myelodepression.

Hormonal Therapy

Breast, prostate, and endometrial cancer may respond to hormonal therapy.

Estrogen deprivation is the mainstay breast cancer treatment. For almost 30 years this has been achieved with SERM, tamoxifen, and toremifene. These compounds have reduced the recurrence rate of breast cancer after surgery and the development of contralateral breast cancer by almost 50%, and have relieved the symptoms and prolonged the survival of 50–60% of patients with metastatic breast cancer (Buluwela *et al.*, 2004). SERMs still represent the preferred form of hormonal treatment of breast cancer in men. Tamoxifen and toremifene prevent bone loss, but cause hot flushes and vaginal discharge in the majority of patients. In addition, they increase the risk of endometrial cancer, deep vein thrombosis and ischemic strokes, especially in presence of obesity, but these complications are rare. In postmenopausal women, the aromatase inhibitors that prevent the transformation of androgen into estrogen were proven superior to tamoxifen both in the adjuvant and the metastatic setting (Arora and Potter, 2004). These compounds appear better tolerated than the SERMs in terms of vasomotor and genitourinary complications, and have not been associated with endometrial cancer, thrombosis, or stroke. The nonsteroidal aromatase inhibitors anastrozole and letrozol increase the rate of bone loss and bone fracture, while examestane, which has a steroidal configuration, may delay bone loss. A new SERM, faslodex, is also available. Unlike tamoxifen and toremifene, faslodex is a complete estrogen antagonist and does not cause endometrial cancer or hypercoagulability, and is effective in about a fourth of the patients whose disease has progressed while taking tamoxifen (Buluwela *et al.*, 2004). Though the role of this compound vis-a-vis the aromatase inhibitors is not clear, parenteral (intramuscular) administration every 4 weeks makes faslodex particularly suitable for older women with poor compliance for oral medications. Progestins are still used as third line treatment of metastatic breast cancer, while the role of estrogen at high doses and androgen has become extremely limited.

The mainstay treatment of prostate cancer is androgen deprivation that may be effected by orchiectomy, oral estrogen, LH-RH (luteinizing hormone-releasing hormone) analogs, LH-RH antagonists (abarelix), and ketoconazol in high doses (Hellerstedt and Pienta, 2003). Currently, the LH-RH analogs are almost universally used as front-line treatment of metastatic prostate cancer, whereas ketoconazol is indicated for patients whose disease has progressed with LH-RH analogs. The only current indication for the use of abarelix is metastasis causing impending urinary obstruction or epidural compression. In these cases, the LH-RH analogs, which cause initially a spate in testosterone concentration, may stimulate tumor growth and precipitate a life-threatening complication. Long-term complications of androgen deprivation including osteoporosis, fatigue, and hot flushes (Holzbeierlein *et al.*, 2003) are seen with increased frequency as androgen deprivation is initiated in patients experiencing a PSA recurrence of prostate cancer whose life expectancy is in excess of 10 years (Han *et al.*, 2001).

Cytotoxic Chemotherapy

Cytotoxic chemotherapy destroys preferentially tissues with high concentration of proliferating cells (Cova and Balducci, 2004). While preferentially harmful to neoplastic tissues, chemotherapy may also affect a number of normal tissues.

Age is associated with a number of pharmacologic changes affecting effectiveness and toxicity of chemotherapy. These include pharmacokinetics, pharmacodynamics, and susceptibility of normal tissues to antineoplastic drugs (Table 2). Biological availability of oral drugs does not appear to change at least up to age 80 (Carreca and Balducci, 2002). Oral formulation of antineoplastic agents is becoming increasingly common, and appears particularly suitable for older individuals, thanks to home administration and more flexible dose titration. As the GFR declines almost universally with age, it is recommended to adjust the doses of medication to renal function, with the provision to increase the dose in subsequent treatment cycles in absence of toxicity, to avoid the risk of undertreatment (Balducci, in press). The volume of

Table 2 Pharmacologic changes of age

Pharmacokinetics	1. Reduced intestinal absorption 2. Reduced renal excretion 3. Reduced volume of distribution of hydrosoluble drugs 4. Reduced hepatic uptake and reduced activity of cytochrome p450 reactions
Pharmacodynamics	1. Reduced rate of DNA repair 2. Reduced intracellular catabolism of drugs
Susceptibility of normal tissues	1. Increased duration and severity of myelotoxicity 2. Increased risk of cardiomyopathy from anthracyclines 3. Increased risk of peripheral (platinol, alkaloids, taxanes, epipodophyllotoxins), and central nervous toxicity (cytarabine in high doses) 4. Increased risk of mucositis (fluorouracil, fluorouridine, anthracyclines)

distribution of hydrosoluble agents declines owing to reduced water content; consequently, the shape of the AUC (Area Under Curve) is changed with higher peak concentrations of free drug. Anemia may exacerbate this problem, as many agents are bound to red blood cells. For this reason, it is recommended that the hemoglobin of older patients receiving chemotherapy be maintained at 12 gm dl^{-1} or higher (Balducci, in press).

Myelosuppression, mucositis, peripheral neuropathy, and cardiomyopathy are the complications of chemotherapy that become more common with age. The risk of neutropenic infections as well as the duration and complications of hospitalization from neutropenic infections increase after age 65. Fortunately, hemopoietic growth factors and, in particular, filgrastim are effective also in older individuals. A pegylated form of filgrastim, peg-filgrastim, is particularly suitable for older individuals, as it requires a single administration per cycle of chemotherapy (Balducci, in press). Anemia is also a common manifestation of myelosuppression that is associated with fatigue and functional dependence (Balducci, 2003; Knight *et al.*, 2004), and may enhance the risk of chemotherapy related toxicity. Epoietin or darbepoietin ameliorate anemia in 60–70% of the patient. Mucositis may lead to dehydration from lack of fluid intake and diarrhea, with serious and even lethal consequences (Stein *et al.*, 1995). Prevention of mucositis may involve the use of oral capecitabine in lieu of intravenous fluorouracil and management with an oral solution of lysine. A keratynocute growth factor is undergoing clinical trials with promising results. In any case, an older person presenting with dehydration should be immediately admitted to the hospital for aggressive fluid resuscitation. No antidotes to neurotoxicity are available. Precautions include avoidance of combination of neurotoxic drugs (e.g. cisplatin and paclitaxel), and timely discontinuance of a neurotoxic drug in the presence of weakness. Age is a risk factor for anthracycline induced cardiomyopathy (Hequet *et al.*, 2004). Though this complication is rare for total doses of doxorubicin lower than $300\,\mathrm{mg\,m^{-2}}$, it increases steeply with higher doses. Furthermore, a recent study in patients with lymphoma revealed that asymptomatic myocardial dysfunction may affect up to one-fourth of patients treated with doxorubicin. Cardiomyopathy may be prevented by infusional doxorubicin (which is cumbersome), by concomitant administration of the antidote desrazoxane, which may increase the risk of myelodepression and mucositis, and by substitution of doxorubicin by pegylated liposomal doxorubicin (doxil) with a much more favorable toxicity profile (Theodoulou and Hudis, 2004).

Finally, it should be underlined that a number of new cytotoxic agents are particularly suitable for older individuals, even for frail individuals. These include capecitabine, vinorelbine, gemcitabine, weekly taxanes, and pegylated liposomal doxorubicin (doxil).

Most of these medications do not cause alopecia or severe nausea and vomiting or myelotoxicity.

Targeted Therapy

These agents target specific components or processes of the neoplastic cells, leading to their destruction or to inhibition of their proliferation. As the targets are specific to or overexpressed in neoplastic cells, these compounds promise to spare normal tissues. For practical purposes, we may distinguish monoclonal antibodies and small molecules antagonizing specific processes (Table 3).

Monoclonal antibodies may be naked or tagged (Harris, 2004). Naked antibodies may cause immune destruction of the cells or antagonize growth factor receptors. Tagged antibodies are used as carriers of toxins, cytotoxic agents, and radioisotopes. Rituximab targets the CD20 antigen, mainly expressed on B-lymphocytes. As single agent, rituximab induces a response rate of approximately 40% in low-grade lymphoma; in combination with chemotherapy, it improves the response rate in virtually all forms of B-cell lymphomas Alemtuzumab is directed against the CD52 antigen, overexpressed on B-lymphocytes, but also in normal hemopoietic precursors. This drug has an approximately 30% response rate in patients with CLL (Chronic Lymphocytic Leukemia) refractory to chemotherapy, but is associated with significant myelotoxicity. Tositumomab (Bexaar) and Ibitumomab tiuxetan (Zevalin) are also monoclonal antibodies targeting CD20 and they are bound respectively to radioactive iodine and Yttrium. They have produced prolonged remissions in patients with low-grade lymphomas, refractory to other forms of treatment, including rituximab, but their use has been complicated by substantial myelotoxicity. Mylotarg targets the CD33 antigen of myelopoietic cells and is active in patients with AML refractory to chemotherapy, but induces substantial myelosuppression

Cell proliferation may be inhibited by targeting the growth factor receptors (Trastuzumab, Herceptin), the activation of these receptors (cetuximab, erbitux), the intracellular signal transduction (gefitinib, Iressa, farnesyl transferase inhibitors), and the surface tyrosine phosphokinase (Imanitib) (Herbst, 2004; Ravandi *et al.*, 2004).

Imanitib, an inhibitor of the tyrosine phosphokinase encoded by the hybrid Bcr/abl oncogene, has resulted in higher rate of hematological remission and improved survival in patients with chronic myelogenous leukemia (CML) (Sledge, 2004). Trastuzumab has shown significant activity in those 30% of women with breast cancer that overexpress the growth factor receptor, genfitinib is indicated in a small group of patients with adenocarcinoma of the lung (Murray *et al.*, 2004), and cetuximab is indicated in carcinoma of colon and rectum (Folprecht and Kohne, 2004).

Proteosome inhibition may also lead through cell destruction through apoptosis (Adams, 2004) or programmed cell death. Bortezomib (velcade) produces a response in approximately 40% of multiple myeloma patients refractory to other forms of treatment.

Another important target of antineoplastic therapy is angiogenesis, as tumor cells cannot survive without the production of new vessels (Drevs *et al.*, 2002). Thalidomide, an inhibitor of angiogenesis, proved effective in patients with multiple myeloma and those with myelodysplasia, whereas bevacizumab (Avastin), a monoclonal antibody directed against the vascular endothelial growth factor (VEGF), in combination with chemotherapy, has prolonged the survival of patients with colorectal cancer (Hurwitz *et al.*, 2004).

Table 3 Targeted therapies

Group of compounds	Target	Indication(s)
Monoclonal antibodies		
a. Naked		
Rituximab	CD20	B-cell lymphoma
Trastuzumab (Herceptin)	HER-2 neu	Breast cancer
Alemtuzumab (CamPath)	CD52	CLL; low-grade lymphoma
Cetuximab	EGFR	Colorectal cancer
Bevacizumab	VEGF	Colorectal cancer
b. Tagged		
Gemtuzumab ozogamicin (Mylotarg)	CD33	Acute myelogenous leukemia
I-131 tositumomab (Bexaar)	CD20	Low-grade lymphoma
Ibitumomab tiuxetan (Zevalin)	CD20	Low-grade lymphoma
Small molecules		
Imanitib mesylate (Gleevec)	Tyrosine kinase	CML, Gastric stromal cell tumors
Gefitinib (Iressa)	EGFR-TK	Lung cancer
Bortezomib (Velcade)	26-S proteasome	Multiple myeloma
Thalidomide (Talidomid)	Angiogenesis	Multiple myeloma, myelodysplasia, malignant gliomas

Note: EGFR-TL, epithelial growth factor receptor–associated tyrosine kinase.

CONCLUSIONS

Cancer in the older person is an increasingly common problem, to the point that it has been proposed to consider cancer a geriatric syndrome. Preventative and treatment strategies should be tailored to the situation of each patient, based on life expectancy and treatment tolerance.

Chemoprevention is a promising cancer prevention strategy that may benefit older individuals, but its clinical use at present is limited. Screening for breast and colorectal cancer appear beneficial for people with a life expectancy of 5 years and longer; screening for other common cancers (prostate, lung, cervix, ovary) is the object of ongoing studies.

Elective surgery, with the possible exception of pneumonectomy, and radiotherapy appear well tolerated by persons of any age, while the risks of emergency surgery increase with age. Early detection of colorectal cancer may minimize the need of emergency surgery.

A number of advances have improved the tolerance of cytotoxic chemotherapy by older individuals: these include myelopoietic growth factors, that minimize neutroopenia and neutropenic infections, recombinant epoietin and darbepoietin for the treatment of anemia and the prevention of functional dependence, and the development of newer and safer drugs. In particular, capecitabine should be used in lieu of fluorouracil in older individuals and pegylated liposomal doxorubicin "in lieu" of other anthracyclines, when indicated.

Targeted therapy represents a very promising and novel approach to the treatment of cancer that may be particularly beneficial to older individuals.

With proper patient selection and adequate support, antineoplastic treatment may be as effective in older patients as it is in younger patients and age should not be considered a contraindication.

KEY POINTS

- The biologic interactions of cancer and age include carcinogenesis and tumor biology. Older individuals may be more susceptible to environmental carcinogens as they harbor a higher concentration of cells in advanced carcinogenetic stages than younger individuals. Breast and lung cancer are more indolent; AML, B-cell lymphoma and ovarian cancer are less responsive to treatment.
- Chemoprevention is promising, but clinical indications are wanted. Screening for breast and colorectal cancer is indicated for persons with a life expectancy of 5 and more years.
- New surgical techniques (radiosurgery, RFA) and radiation therapy techniques (brachytherapy) are minimally invasive and may prove particularly beneficial for older patients.
- Patients aged 65 and older receiving moderately cytotoxic chemotherapy should receive support with hemopoietic growth factors (filgrastim, pegfilgrastim, epoietin α, darbepoietin).
- New chemotherapy drugs, including capecitabine, pegylated liposomal doxorubicin, weekly taxanes, vinorelbine, and gemcitabine, may be safely used even in frail individuals.

KEY REFERENCES

- Anisimov VV. Biologic interactions of aging and cancer. In L Balducci & M Extermann (eds) *Biological Basis of Geriatric Oncology* 2005, pp 17–50 Springer New york.
- Balducci L. Guidelines for the management of the older cancer patient. *Journal of the National Comprehensive Cancer Network* (in press).
- Beghe' C & Balducci L. Biological basis of cancer prevention in the older adult. In L Balducci & M Extermann (eds) *Biological Basis of Geriatric Oncology* 2004; Kluwer.

REFERENCES

Adams J. The proteasome: a suitable antineoplastic target. *Nature Reviews Cancer* 2004; **4**:349–60.

Anisimov VV. Biologic interactions of aging and cancer. In L Balducci & M Extermann (eds) *Biological Basis of Geriatric Oncology* 2005, pp 17–50 Springer New york.

Arora A & Potter JF. Aromatase inhibitors: current indications and future prospects for treatment of post-menopausal breast cancer. *Journal of the American Geriatrics Society* 2004; **52**:611–16.

Balducci L. Anemia, cancer and aging. *Cancer Control: Journal of the Moffitt Cancer Center* 2003; **10**:478–86.

Balducci L. Guidelines for the management of the older cancer patient. *Journal of the National Comprehensive Cancer Network* (in press).

Balducci L & Aapro M Epidemiology of cancer and aging. In L Balducci & M Extermann (eds) *Biological Basis of Geriatric Oncology* 2004; Kluwer.

Balducci L, Silliman RA & Diaz N. Breast cancer in the older woman: the oncologist viewpoint. In L Balducci, GH Lyman, WB Ershler & M Extermann (eds) *Comprehensive Geriatric Oncology* 2004, 2nd edn; Harwood Academic Publishers, Amsterdam.

Beghe' C & Balducci L. Biological basis of cancer prevention in the older adult. In L Balducci & M Extermann (eds) *Biological Basis of Geriatric Oncology* 2004; Kluwer.

Berger DH & Roslyn JJ. Cancer surgery in the elderly. *Clinics in Geriatric Medicine* 1997; **13**:119–42.

Buluwela L, Constantinidou D, Pike J *et al.* Estrogen receptors and anti-estrogen therapy. *Cancer Treatment Research* 2004; **119**:271–92.

Caranasos GJ. Prevalence of cancer in older persons living at home and in institutions. *Clinics in Geriatric Medicine* 1997; **13**:15–32.

Carreca I & Balducci L. Oral chemotherapy for the older patient with cancer. *American Journal of Cancer* 2002; **1**:101–8.

Chemoprevention Working Group. Prevention in the next millenium: report of the Chemoprevention Working Group to the American Association for Cancer Research. *Cancer Research* 1999; **59**:4743–58.

Chen H, Cantor A, Meyer J *et al.* Can older cancer patients tolerate chemotherapy? *Cancer* 2003; **97**:1107–1114.

Cohen HJ, Harris F & Pieper CF. Coagulation and activation of inflammatory pathways in the development of functional decline and mortality in the elderly. *American Journal of Medicine* 2003; **114**:180–87.

Cova D & Balducci L. Cytotoxic chemotherapy in the older patient. In L Balducci, GH Lyman, WB. Ershler & M Extermann (eds)

Comprehensive Geriatric Oncology, 2004, pp 463–488 2nd edn; Taylor & Francis.

Diab SG, Elledge R & Clark GM. Tumor characteristics and clinical outcome of elderly women with breast cancer. *Journal of the National Cancer Institute* 2000; **92**:550–6.

Drevs J, Laus C, Mendinger M *et al.* Antiangiogenesis: current clinical data and future perspectives. *Onkologie* 2002; **25**:520–27.

Ferrucci L, Guralnik GM, Cavazzini C *et al.* The frailty syndrome: a critical issue in geriatric oncology. *Critical Reviews in Oncology Hematology* 2003; **46**:127–137.

Folprecht G & Kohne CH. The role of new agents in the treatment of colorectal cancer. *Oncology* 2004; **66**:1–7.

Frazier AL, Colditz GA & Fuchs CS. Cost-effectiveness of screening for colorectal cancer in the general population. *Journal of the American Medical Association* 2000; **284**:1954–59.

Han M, Partin AW, Pound CR *et al.* Long term biochemical disease-free and cancer-specific survival following anatomic radical retropubic prostatectomy. The 15-year Johns Hopkins experience. *Urology Clinics of North America* 2001; **28**:555–65.

Harris M. Monoclonal antibodies as therapeutic agents for cancer. *Lancet Oncology* 2004; **5**:292–302.

Hellerstedt BA & Pienta KJ. The truth is out there: an overall perspective on androgen deprivation. *Urology Oncology* 2003; **21**:272–81.

Hequet O, Le QH, Moullet I *et al.* Subclinical late cardiomyopathy after doxorubicin therapy for lymphoma in adults. *Journal of Clinical Oncology* 2004; **22**:1864–71.

Herbst RS Review of epidermal growth factor receptor biology. *International Journal of Radiation Oncology Biology Physics* 2004; **59**(2 suppl):21–6.

Holmberg L, Bill-Axelson A, Hegelsen F *et al.* A randomized trial comparing radical prostatectomy with watchful waiting in early prostate cancer. *New England Journal of Medicine* 2002; **347**:781–9.

Holzbeierlein JM, Castle EP & Thrasher JB. Complications of androgen deprivation therapy for prostate cancer. *Clinics in Prostate Cancer* 2003; **2**:147–52.

Hornsby PJ. Replicative senescence and cancer. In L Balducci & M Extermann (eds) *Biological Basis of Geriatric Oncology* 2004; Kluwer.

Hevezi JM. Emerging technology in cancer treatment: radiotherapy modalities. *Oncology (Huntington)* 2003; **17**:1445–56.

Hursting SD, Slaga TJ, Fisher SM *et al.* Mechanism-based cancer prevention approaches: targets, examples, and the use of transgenic mice. *Journal of the National Cancer Institute* 1999; **91**:215–25.

Hurwitz H, Fehrenbacher L, Novotny W *et al.* Bevacizumab plus irinotecan, fluorouracil and leucovorin for metastatic colorectal cancer. *New England Journal of Medicine* 2004; **350**:2335–42.

Kemeny MM, Busch-Devereaux E, Merriam LT *et al.* Cancer surgery in the elderly. *Hematology Oncology Clinics of North America* 2000; **14**:193–212.

Kerlikowske K, Grady D, Rubin SM *et al.* Efficacy of screening mammography. A meta-analysis. *Journal of the American Medical Association* 1995; **273**:149–54.

Kerlikowske K, Salzman P, Phillips KA *et al.* Continuing screening mammography in women aged 70 to 79 years. *Journal of the American Medical Association* 1999; **282**:2156–63.

Knight K, Wade S & Balducci L. Prevalence and outcomes of anemia in cancer: a systematic review of the literature. *American Journal of Medicine* 2004; **116**(suppl 7A):11s.

Lancet JE, Willman CL & Bennett JM. Acute myelogenous leukemia and aging. *Hematology Oncology Clinics of North America* 2000; **14**:251–67.

Lippman SM & Brown PH. Tamoxifen prevention of breast cancer: an instance of the fingerpost. *Journal of the National Cancer Institute* 1999; **91**:1809–19.

Miguel R & Vila H. Anesthesia in older cancer patients. In L Balducci, GH Lyman, WB Ershler & M Extermann (eds) *Comprehensive Geriatric Oncology* 2004, 2nd edn; Harwood Academic Publishers.

Murray N, Salgia R & Fossella FV. Targeted molecules in small cell lung cancer. *Seminars in Oncology* 2004; **33**(Suppl 1):106–11.

Oridate N, Lotan D, Xu XC *et al.* Differential induction of apoptosis by all-trans-retinoic acid and N-(4-Hydroxiphenyl)retinamide in human head and neck squamous cell carcinoma cell lines. *Clinical Cancer Research* 1986; **2**:855–63.

Preti HA, Cabanillas F, Talpaz M *et al.* Prognostic value of serum interleukin 6 in diffuse large-cell lymphoma. *Annals of Internal Medicine* 1997; **1127**:186–94.

Randolph WM, Mahnken JD, Goodwin JS *et al.* Using Medicare data to estimate the prevalence of breast cancer screening in older women: comparison of different methods to identify screening mammograms. *Health Services Research* 2002; **37**:1643–57.

Ravandi F, Kantarjian H, Giles F *et al.* New agents in acute myeloid leukemia and other myeloid disorders. *Cancer* 2004; **100**:441–54.

Repetto L, Granetto C, Venturino A *et al.* Prognostic evaluation of the older cancer patient. In L Balducci, GH Lyman & WB Ershler (eds) *Comprehensive Geriatric Oncology* 1998, pp 281–6; Harwood Academic Publishers, Amsterdam.

Roque M, Martinez MJ, Alonso P *et al.* Radioisotopes for metastatic bone pain. *Cochrane Database System Review* 2003; 4CDOO3347.

Sikic BI. New approaches in cancer treatment. *Annals of Oncology* 1999; **10**(suppl 6):149–53.

Singletary SE, Dowlatshahi K, Dooley W *et al.* Minimally invasive operation for breast cancer. *Current Problems in Surgery* 2004; **41**:394–447.

Sledge JW. HERe-2 stay: the continuing importance of translational research in breast cancer. *Journal of the National Cancer Institute* 2004; **19**(96):725–7.

Stanta G, Campagner L, Cavallieri F *et al.* Cancer of the oldest old: what we have learned from autopsy studies. *Clinics in Geriatric Medicine* 1997; **13**:55–68.

Stein BN, Petrelli NJ, Douglass HO *et al.* Age and sex are independent predictors of 5-fluorouracil toxicity. *Cancer* 1995; **75**:11–17.

Steinbach G, Phillips R.KS & Lynch PM. The effect of Celecoxib, a cyclooxygenase 2 inhibitor in familial adenomatous polyposis. *New England Journal of Medicine* 2000; **342**:1996–52.

Terry MB, Gammon MD, Zhang FF *et al.* Association of frequency and duration of aspirin use and hormone receptor status with breast cancer risk. *Journal of the American Medical Association* 2004; **291**:2433–40.

The International Non-Hodgkin's Lymphoma Prognostic Factors Project. A predictive model for aggressive non-Hodgkin's lymphoma. *New England Journal of Medicine* 1993; **329**:987–94.

Theodoulou M & Hudis C. Cardiac profiles of liposomal anthracyclines: greater cardiac safety versus conventional doxorubicin? *Cancer* 2004; **100**:2052–63.

Thompson IM, Goodman DJ, Tanger CM *et al.* The influence of finasteride on the development of prostate cancer. *New England Journal of Medicine* 2003; **349**:215–24.

Thun MJ, Namboodiri MM, Heath CW Jr *et al.* Aspirin use and reduced risk of fatal colon cancer. *New England Journal of Medicine* 1991; **325**:1593–96.

Tranberg KG. Percutaneous ablation of liver tumours. *Best Practices Research Clin Gastroenterol* 2004; **18**:125–45.

Walter LC, Linquist K, Covinsky KE *et al.* Relationship between health status and use of screening mammography and papanicolau smears among women older than 70 years of age. *Annals of Internal Medicine* 2004; **140**:681–8.

Wingo PA, Cardinez CJ, Landis SH *et al.* Long term trends in cancer mortality in the United States, 1930–1998. *Cancer* 2003; **97**(S21):3133–3275.

Yancik R & Ries L. Cancer in the older person: an international issue in an aging world. *Seminars in Oncology* 2004; **31**:128–136.

Zachariah B & Balducci L. Radiation therapy of the older patient. *Hematology Oncology Clinics of North America* 2000; **14**:131–67.

129

Oncological Emergencies and Urgencies

Samuel Spence McCachren
Thompson Cancer Survival Center, Knoxville, TN, USA

INTRODUCTION

Studies of cancer in the "very old" (older than 80 years) have been hampered by several factors including inaccuracies in death certificates, failure to diagnose malignancy in the setting of multiple illnesses, and a reduction in frequency of seeking medical attention in this age-group. It is known that nearly half of all cancers and almost two-thirds of all cancer deaths in the United States occur in people more than 65 years old (Yancik, 1983). Moreover, the incidence appears to be increasing with age.

During the past three decades there has been a noteworthy increase in our desire as well as the technology to treat some cancers (Bailar and Smith, 1986). Extrapolating from therapeutic progress in the 1980s and 1990s, we should anticipate further enhancement in our capacity to treat an even larger number of individuals with malignant disease, especially those with somewhat more resistant solid tumors, which are most common at older ages. These facts, coupled with steady growth in the size of the elderly population, indicate a need to prepare for more oncological crises. Moreover, a predominance of certain neoplasms, particularly solid tumors of breast, lung, colon, and prostate, with their particular attendant acute complications, could swell the number of emergencies even further.

Simultaneously, physicians have witnessed a remarkable gain in the ability to deal with and effectively manage the intensive care needs of patients with any disease. Early on, as intensive care units (ICU) attempted to cope with unmanageable numbers of referrals, there developed an unwritten and sometimes unspoken attitude about rationing beds, a policy which not infrequently precluded individuals with incurable forms of malignancy, especially if the patient was "old". With enlightenment and an increase in the numbers of ICU beds, this obstacle to heroic clinical management in the setting of cancer has begun to disappear (Pontoppidin *et al.*, 1976), especially for young patients who have leukemia or lymphoma.

Neoplastic diseases can bring about both acute and chronic complications either by their natural progression or by our treatment of them. They have the capacity to invade contiguous structures, such as blood vessels or viscus organs; cause a host of mechanical events by obstruction or compression; secrete a variety of ectopic hormones, some resulting in severe metabolic effects; and proliferate so extensively that vital organs are literally replaced. In addition, we have a therapeutic armamentarium that can irreversibly damage any of the vital organs or severely compromise the host's defenses. These statements prevail no matter what age-group one is discussing. There appears to be nothing particularly different in this regard about elderly patients. Although older patients may have more obvious cerebral dysfunction in the setting of fever, sepsis, hypotension, or hypercalcemia, and their marrow reserve may be less robust, there is no valid evidence that age alone is a criterion for withholding intensive life support or for that matter withholding treatment of the basic disease process (Cohen *et al.*, 1983; Peterson, 1982; Kennedy, 1985).

A growing volume of literature (Vaeth and Meyer, 1985) discusses cancer and its management in the elderly. There is also literature now written specifically about the concept of malignant disease in the emergency department (Brown *et al.*, 1983) but few publications specifically address the management of medical or surgical emergencies that occur in people over 65 as a consequence of a malignancy.

From experience in our own emergency departments, it is possible to list in order of decreasing frequency the more common reasons for attendance by adult patients with a known neoplasm. There is first fever and a close second is fever with granulocytopenia already defined by their referring physician; inability to eat or drink; pain; dyspnea from advancing cancer in the lung, nausea and/or vomiting following recent chemotherapy; general decline in performance status due to several factors ("failure to thrive"); weakness associated with severe anemia in need of blood transfusion; demonstrated thrombocytopenia in need of platelet transfusion; hypercalcemia; intestinal dysfunction

Principles and Practice of Geriatric Medicine, 4th Edition. Edited by M.S. John Pathy, Alan J. Sinclair and John E. Morley.

(including gastric outlet obstruction and partial or complete obstruction of small more often than large bowel); request by the family that the patient be allowed to die in the hospital; gastrointestinal bleeding from various sites and for several different reasons; altered mental status; spinal cord compression; and hemoptysis. Some, of course, come for a second opinion about their diagnosis of cancer and are already under therapy by a physician at another university or community hospital.

In this chapter, we discuss the life-threatening complications associated with cancer in the elderly and how to manage such events. Both the reader and the author must be mindful of those potentially fatal intercurrent problems that are independent of neoplasia and that occur more frequently in the old than in the young. Urosepsis with shock, myocardial infarction, pulmonary embolism, rupture of an abdominal or thoracic aortic aneurysm, upper gastrointestinal hemorrhage, perforation of large bowel, cardiac arrhythmias, and massive stroke with aspiration are specific examples. They require consideration in differential diagnosis far more often than in the young.

From a review of several major treatises on the subject of oncological emergencies (Yarboro and Bornstein, 1981; Yarboro *et al.*, 1978), it is clear that urgencies, true emergencies, and various serious problems are usually extensively intermixed. Although there is room for debate about the definition of the term medical emergency, most can agree about what items should be included in that category. For example, ventricular fibrillation, respiratory arrest, status epilepticus, intracranial (transtentorial) herniation, tension pneumothorax, septic shock, hemorrhagic shock, advanced pulmonary edema, pericardial tamponade, and massive hemoptysis all demand therapeutic action within seconds to minutes. We think about malignant tumors being capable of occasionally producing many of these events, but certain ones in particular are more commonly associated. Cancers erode into a carotid artery with exsanguination or into a pulmonary artery with death by asphyxiation. Intracranial metastases have been relatively silent until their size produces intractable seizures or uncal herniation. Pericardial involvement can cause a gradual filling of the pericardial space by fluid with modest symptoms until a critical volume rapidly results in total compromise of cardiac dynamics. And severe granulocytopenia, especially during cytotoxic chemotherapy, may lead to sepsis with profound hypotension. Only a few entities in emergency medicine are unique to malignancy: cerebral and pulmonary leukostasis (McKee and Collins, 1974), tumor lysis syndrome (Kalemkerian *et al.*, 1997; Zusman *et al.*, 1973) and, usually, superior vena cava (SVC) syndrome (Bell *et al.*, 1986).

The situations selected for inclusion are not unique to the older population, although some are more commonly seen in the later years of life. Disseminated intravascular coagulation (DIC) is frequently associated with advanced carcinoma of the prostate, clearly an older man's affliction. Hyperviscosity syndrome, with its attendant cerebral and cardiac consequences, generally is less well tolerated in the elderly patient.

It should be pointed out that there are two distinct settings in which one of these acute changes in clinical course might occur. The ideal would be for the patient to appear first in his/her personal physician's office. That doctor, thoroughly familiar with the clinical course to date, is quite prepared to decide about the appropriate intensity of investigation and support for the patient, and dispatches the patient to the hospital, calling ahead with orders and a plan of action. The second common scenario takes place in an emergency department and is more difficult for the patient and the physician, who has neither knowledge about this person's course to date nor about the many other factors that might bear on a decision to intervene in heroic ways. Because the latter setting is a more typical arena for the suddenness that characterizes emergencies and because of the extra challenge created by seeing a new physician, we have elected to discuss recognition and management of many oncological emergencies as though the reader is a physician in an emergency room (ER) seeing each patient for the first time.

FIRST TIME PRESENTATION BECAUSE OF ACUTE SYMPTOMS

Even though it is much less common that patients present with an urgent manifestation of a heretofore undiagnosed neoplasm, it certainly can and still does happen. In that situation it is always best to treat aggressively since critical questions about the quality of life or the reversibility of the acute process usually cannot be answered quickly in the emergency setting (Kalia and Tintinalli, 1984). Such is clearly the case for acute cecal dilatation as occurs in patients with a competent ileocecal valve and distal colonic occlusion by an adenocarcinoma. This is not an insignificant matter when one considers that the incidence of colorectal cancer is highest in the elderly; that the disease can be relatively "silent", especially if one ignores constipation; and that localized "potentially curable disease" is found in nearly two-thirds of patients presenting as emergencies although the perioperative mortality is twice as high as in those who undergo elective operation (Waldron *et al.*, 1986).

There are other instances wherein a combination of denial and minimal morbidity during early stages of a primary malignancy has resulted in presentation of an acute manifestation due to advanced disease before patient or clinician is aware of the diagnosis. This certainly happens with breast cancer, which, for example, can metastasize to pericardium causing tamponade. Another example of an unusual first time presentation of acute symptoms has been reported for previously undetected laryngeal carcinoma that declared itself by impending obstruction of the airway that was successfully managed by an "emergency" laryngectomy (Griebie and Adams, 1987). Fortunately, physicians who work principally or only in large and busy accident rooms have a practiced, sensible approach to these types of unusual presentations, that is, rapid formulation of a differential diagnosis while quickly mobilizing urgent procedures and consultations.

SPINAL CORD COMPRESSION

A diagnosis of this catastrophe is an easy matter by the time paraplegia and loss of sphincter control have occurred, but an optimal outcome requires much earlier recognition. In the face of vague or isolated symptoms, one must have much more clinical acumen in order to prevent one of the worst disasters that can befall a patient with cancer, namely, loss of locomotion and continence. Such deficits could be even more devastating for the widow or widower who had until that moment been able to manage an independent existence despite having a malignant disease.

Presenting symptoms of metastatic cord compression are generally shared by all primary tumors (Mullins *et al.*, 1971; Torma, 1957). A prodromal phase, present in almost every case, is characterized by pain somewhere along the spinal axis, with or without an accompanying radicular pattern. More importantly, many patients have a sense of dysfunction in their lower extremities even when there are no definite neurological findings. This subtle awareness by the patient may not be volunteered, or worse, if reported may be discounted as an acceleration in a natural process of aging because of the general systemic effects by a tumor with attendant weight loss and decrease in activity. Pain can antedate rapid deterioration of spinal cord function by days, weeks, and even months while other symptoms typically occur days to weeks before the critical sign that brings the patient to an ER. If these early subtle warnings were recognized it could turn emergency medicine into elective medicine.

Once clinical suspicions are aroused, one must follow through the appropriate diagnostic pathway. Although at least two-thirds of plain radiographs of the spine will show bony abnormalities, such as erosion of pedicles, partial to complete vertebral collapse, or a paraspinous soft-tissue abnormality, they do not establish the exact boundaries of cord compression. For appropriate neurosurgery or irradiation treatment, the exact boundaries of the compression must be known. This is easily determined by magnetic resonance imaging (MRI) when it is available. If MRI is unavailable, then myelography (either routine or with computed tomography) is needed.

Selection of the appropriate treatment depends upon the rapidity of onset, the severity as well as the duration of neurological deficit, the level of block, and the primary tumor. A first step in therapy of every case is relief of probable edema with corticosteroids. Dexamethasone, 100 mg intravenously as an initial "bolus" is probably excessive and unproved in any scientific study but has become accepted as standard in many places. That large dose is followed by 20 mg every six hours (by mouth or intravenously). A radioresponsive tumor detected early on predicts for excellent outcome using radiation therapy plus corticosteroids (Gilbert *et al.*, 1978; Ushio *et al.*, 1977). More importantly, that approach avoids surgery with risk of mortality ranging between 6 and 13% and the prolonged debility or lengthy incapacitation that often characterizes the postoperative course of elderly individuals who undergo laminectomy. Chemotherapy is often useful in cases due to lymphomas or other chemotherapy responsive malignancies.

Obviously, laminectomy should be performed in four situations: malignancy is suspected but the tumor type is unknown (needle biopsy may suffice for diagnosis); prior high dose radiation at that level of the cord; individuals with rapidly progressing or acute as well as severe neurological deficits found to have a complete block at myelography; and patients who fail to show a rapid response to radiation. Because laminectomy rarely results in complete removal of tumor, postoperative irradiation should be considered in all cases (Wild and Porter, 1963; Wright, 1963).

MASSIVE HEMOPTYSIS

Infectious disorders have dominated any listing by etiology for causes of massive hemoptysis, but the oncological category is becoming more important along with pulmonary tuberculosis, bronchiectasis, and chronic necrotizing pneumonia (Conlan *et al.*, 1983). Emergency physicians readily consider tuberculosis when confronted with hemoptysis, particularly in older patients and especially in residents of or refugees from underdeveloped countries. However, the elderly represent that fraction of the world's population which is enlarging the fastest; and they are the most likely to get cancer. At the current time, they may (hopefully they do) represent the last male generation of heavy smokers but it is recognized that a history of smoking combined with advanced age increases the incidence of lung cancer.

It is noteworthy that the definition used to quantify serious hemoptysis by such terms as significant or massive varies from 2 dl (Yoh *et al.*, 1967) to more than 3 dl or up to 5–6 dl (Crocco *et al.*, 1968). Clearly some patients can survive quite striking episodes of expectoration of blood, up to 600 ml in 12 hours, while others have instantaneous death with sudden first hemoptysis even when the cause is not neoplastic (Bobrowitz *et al.*, 1983). Regardless of the definition used for massive, the danger is asphyxiation due to obstruction of the tracheobronchial tree rather than exsanguination, although that too can occur. Finally, any amount of hemoptysis can be excessive to the patient with underlying lung disease who has also sustained loss of parenchyma by tumor, surgery, and/or irradiation. In that setting, even as little as 150 ml can lead to a clot capable of occluding a mainstem bronchus with resultant lethal pulmonary insufficiency.

In rare cases, a patient may present with life-threatening bronchial hemorrhage that is due to previously undiagnosed pulmonary neoplasms. However, the probable etiologic diagnosis should be obvious in almost all patients with profuse hemoptysis due to lung cancer because bleeding directly from bronchogenic carcinoma early on is rarely brisk and tumor erosion into a major blood vessel is usually a late sign. In any event, except in the unusual situation where a patient has a living will or durable power of attorney and can express or has previously expressed wishes that no further intervention take place, emergency management should proceed as for any critical patient: the ABCs (airway, breathing, circulation) must be secured. Whereas in an elective surgical situation an experienced anesthetist may selectively intubate each lung with a double lumen Carlen's or Robertshaw tube, in the most urgent setting with severe respiratory distress, intubation of the mainstem bronchus of the nonbleeding lung must be achieved as rapidly as possible. The patient is then positioned with the "suspected" side dependent. That, combined with suctioning, affords the only opportunity to prevent further drowning of the normal lung. Next, large bore intravenous catheters are inserted for resuscitation by crystalloid followed by blood products. Then and only then can one be more deliberate about further studies.

There are differences of opinion in the literature about surgical versus medical approaches to treatment even when the etiology of pulmonary hemorrhage is infectious (Bobrowitz *et al.*, 1983). However, even for the most aggressive thoracic surgeon there are some contraindications to resection including inadequate pulmonary reserves and very late stage disease, while cancer itself poses special problems, especially if it was deemed irresectable at the time of initial diagnosis and there has been subsequent radiation. All of these compromising descriptors are frequently the rule for lung cancer patients over age 70. So, after resuscitation with both the patient and the situation under control, there may be time for more definitive study of the site that is hemorrhaging and time to consider a nonsurgical therapeutic intervention such as bronchial artery embolization or laser bronchoscopy if the endobronchial growth itself is bleeding.

The expectoration of huge quantities of blood is usually much more frightening than hematemesis or copious hematochezia for both the patient and family, but also for the physician. There is nothing more distressing or taxing than trying to have a meaningful dialogue in an ER about a patient's wishes when that person is repeatedly coughing up large amounts of blood. Yet, our staff has had to do just that on several occasions in order to help the individual and/or family sort out whether they wanted heroic measures including intubation or merely sedation because it was clear that the malignancy was very advanced and no longer amenable to standard modalities of therapy.

In general, both geriatricians and oncologists should be urging upon almost all patients the concept and the execution of two legal instruments, a living will and a durable power of attorney. Hopefully, one or both would be in place when and if this cataclysmic event of massive hemoptysis occurs in any patient with advanced lung cancer.

HYPERCALCEMIA (*see* Chapter 108, Age-related Changes in Calcium Homeostasis and Bone Loss)

Hypercalcemia is a common complication of a number of neoplasms, whether associated with skeletal metastases, ectopic parathyroid hormone (PTH), PTH-like substances, interleukin-1 (as in adult T-cell leukemia/lymphoma), other humoral factors, or coincidental hyperparathyroidism. Although hypercalcemia occurring during the course of malignancy is usually attributable to the neoplasm, one must not forget to consider benign causes such as primary hyperparathyroidism, vitamin D intoxication and sarcoidosis. In any case, treatment in an emergency is similar, with definitive management requiring a later diagnosis.

Once a clinician considers hypercalcemia in the differential diagnosis of apathy, depression, malaise, somnolence, confusion, personality change, new polyuria–polydipsia, or rapidly evolving anorexia with nausea plus constipation, it is easy to establish the presence of a significant elevation in serum calcium. Changes in mental faculties and strength are more easily recognized in younger individuals, whereas in the elderly such events can be too easily blamed on many things including their poor tolerance of analgesics, anxiolytics, hypnotics, and antiemetics. This is especially true when symptoms occur very gradually. On rare occasion, elevations in serum calcium can appear with such rapidity that the event can be fatal within a few days (Cornbleet *et al.*, 1977).

Because normal serum calcium is maintained with 95% confidence limits of 2.24 to 2.58 $\mathrm{mmol\,l^{-1}}$ (9.0–10.5 $\mathrm{mg\,dl^{-1}}$) for men and 2.22 to 2.57 (8.9–10.4 $\mathrm{mg\,dl^{-1}}$) for women, it is important to consider a level of 2.64 $\mathrm{mmol\,l^{-1}}$ (10.6 $\mathrm{mg\,dl^{-1}}$) as a signal of abnormal calcium homeostasis. Values above 2.74 mmol l (11.0 $\mathrm{mg\,dl^{-1}}$) should be considered an indication to initiate treatment. (Each local laboratory confirms its own range of normal values, so that the above should be taken only as a guideline.) Although the hypercalcemic crisis is still reversible, it is easier to treat earlier before renal effects, with azotemia, or cardiovascular effects, with Mobitz II and other arrhythmias, have developed. It should be remembered that both the inotropic and toxic effects of digitalis preparations are potentiated by calcium and that digitalis preparations are commonly prescribed for elderly patients.

Essentially all patients will have become dehydrated and benefit from intravenous saline to restore vascular volume, with a consequent improvement in calcium excretion. Unless clearly contraindicated, this approach should be initiated immediately. Since large volumes of saline may be required and are usually administered rapidly, there is a need for careful monitoring of cardiac status. Potassium balance must be observed carefully. Once adequate hydration is assured, frusemide (furosemide) augments the calciuresis by decreasing renal tubular resorption of sodium and calcium. Thiazides should not be used since they inhibit calciuresis. Before the availability of potent antiresorptive agents it was common to suggest a fluid intake and output of 4–6 l daily. We now aim to maintain normovolemia and a more modest fluid flux. This minimizes the risk of volume overload in the debilitated patient and edema in the hypoalbuminemic patient.

Glucocorticoids can be helpful in the management of hypercalcemia caused by lymphoma, myeloma, and sometimes breast cancer. It is usual to prescribe prednisone in a dose of 60 mg daily, but the response is slower than with saline and diuretics, occurring over several days, so that this agent should be started promptly along with rehydration. We are less dependent on glucocorticoids since the advent of potent antiresorptive agents.

Salmon calcitonin in a dose of $8\,\text{IU}\,\text{kg}^{-1}$ body weight, by intramuscular injection every six hours for several days, has been useful in controlling hypercalcemia in some patients. Intramuscular administration gives more reliable absorption than the subcutaneous route. Tachyphylaxis may occur, limiting the effectiveness of this treatment. However, the efficacy of calcitonin in managing hypercalcemia due to epidermoid carcinoma has been questioned (Warrell *et al.*, 1988).

The use of bisphosphonates such as pamidronate and zolendronate has been a major advance in management of hypercalcemia of malignancy (Harvey, 1995). These agents very effectively reduce bone resorption. Increases in serum phosphate may occur during treatment, a potentially useful side effect in those patients with hypophosphatemia. Pamidronate 60–90 mg is administered intravenously over 2–4 hours, after rehydration. Zolendronate 4 mg iv may be administered over 15 minutes. Adequate saline should be used to ensure continued calciuresis. The dose can be repeated if required. Bisphosphonates are now our first line of therapy after rehydration.

The most recent addition to our armamentarium is gallium nitrate, administered at a dose of $200\,\text{mg}\,\text{m}^{-2}\,\text{day}^{-1}$ over 24 hours for five consecutive days. Its use is contraindicated in patients with significant renal insufficiency. Although some combination of the measures discussed will generally control the excessive serum calcium, occasionally for prolonged periods of time, ultimately the underlying disease must be managed. One must consider early administration of specific treatment for the malignant tumor.

Following the early clinical recognition of its ability to lower serum calcium in most patients with hypercalcemia caused by malignancy, plicamycin (mithramycin) became a standard therapy. The availability of bisphosphonates has greatly reduced its use. Whereas most texts recommend a dose of $25\,\mu\text{g}\,\text{kg}^{-1}$ body weight by intravenous "push" every 24 hours for two to three doses, often we find a lower dose of $15\,\mu\text{g}\,\text{kg}^{-1}$ body weight will suffice. It can be useful in older patients in whom fluid balance is precarious. Plicamycin may be difficult to obtain, and is myelosuppressive. It is no longer a part of our armamentarium.

For patients in the truly terminal stage of a tumor refractory to standard therapy, especially if complicated by skeletal pain, hypercalcemia may contribute to analgesia and on occasion may allow a more comfortable, dignified demise. Knowledge of a patient's wishes and clinical course to date therefore assumes critical importance.

HYPONATREMIA (*see* Chapter 117, Water and Electrolyte Balance in Health and Disease)

At serum sodium levels below $115\,\text{mmol}\,\text{l}^{-1}$ ($115\,\text{mEq}\,\text{l}^{-1}$), especially when the fall is rapid, brain edema can occur. Hyponatremia of this severity leads to alteration in mental status with lethargy and, in severe cases, coma, seizures, and death. The elderly are more susceptible to the effects of hyponatremia, and may manifest mental status impairment at higher levels of serum sodium. Other physical findings are generally unhelpful in the diagnosis, and routine evaluation of serum electrolytes is mandatory in patients with otherwise unexplained alterations of mental status.

Hyponatremia may be seen in several situations: water redistribution associated with mannitol infusions; pseudohyponatremia due to hyperparaproteinemia or hyperlipidemia; and acute water intoxication. More common causes are renal sodium loss due to diuretic therapy, extrarenal sodium loss during vomiting/diarrhea, and sudden withdrawal of glucocorticoid therapy. The hyponatremia in these situations is usually not life threatening.

The syndrome of inappropriate antidiuretic hormone (SIADH) secretion can cause a severe decrease in sodium that may be life threatening. Diagnostic features include (i) hypo-osmolality of serum; (ii) inappropriately high osmolality of urine for the concomitant plasma hypo-osmolality; (iii) normal renal function; (iv) continued renal excretion of sodium; (v) clinical normovolemia; and (vi) normal adrenal function. SIADH is most frequently seen with small cell undifferentiated carcinoma of the lung, but abnormalities in water homeostasis have been reported with many neoplasms, and especially in association with pulmonary or central nervous system metastases.

Optimal therapy is to correct the underlying disease by chemotherapy and/or radiotherapy while restricting "free water" intake to $500–1000\,\text{ml}\,\text{day}^{-1}$. Correction by this method may take 7 to 10 days. More serious hyponatremia can be reversed in an average of three to four days with the addition of demeclocycline, an antidiuretic hormone (ADH) antagonist (Trump, 1981). For potentially fatal hyponatremia, such as in patients with seizures, coma, or other neurological abnormalities, more rapid correction is required. We utilize infusions of 3% saline combined with frusemide $0.5–1.0\,\text{mg}\,\text{kg}^{-1}$ intravenously, with careful attention to intravascular volume, until the serum sodium is above a critical level (Hantman *et al.*, 1973).

SUPERIOR VENA CAVA (SVC) SYNDROME

Although SVC obstruction was seen with benign disease (such as tuberculosis and aneurysms) in the past, most cases in the developed world are now due to malignancy. Most neoplastic SVC obstruction is due to bronchogenic carcinoma, but Hodgkin's disease, non-Hodgkin's lymphoma, and other malignancies may be associated. Benign causes include thrombosis complicating central venous catheters (becoming more common as permanently implanted catheter use is increasing), and mediastinal fibrosis (primary, or secondary to radiation or surgery). The SVC and tributaries are easily compressed by expanding masses, causing impaired venous return and eventually tracheal, facial, and arm edema. Cerebral edema may occur in severe cases. With gradual obstruction a rich collateral circulation develops, and signs and symptoms may be subtle. With more rapid obstruction, the patient may present as a true emergency. Signs and their frequency of appearance at presentation include: thoracic vein distention (67%), neck vein distention (59%), facial edema (56%), tachypnea (40%), facial plethora (19%), cyanosis (15%), upper extremity edema (10%), vocal cord paralysis (4%), and Horner's syndrome (2%). Vocal cord paralysis and Horner's syndrome usually imply involvement of adjacent structures.

The syndrome is rarely so severe that immediate definitive treatment is necessary. For patients who initially present with SVC obstruction, there is usually time to search for a diagnosis. Sputum cytology and bronchoscopy usually provide a diagnosis. Often easily biopsied masses are found elsewhere in the body. In patients without tracheal edema, mediastinoscopy or even thoracotomy may be performed safely, notwithstanding older literature which suggests that an unacceptable risk of bleeding accompanies these procedures. "Blind" supraclavicular node biopsies may afford a diagnosis in up to 60% of cases.

Emergency treatment, without awaiting a diagnosis, is indicated when there is cerebral dysfunction, symptomatic impairment of cardiac output or upper airway edema. Adequate oxygenation and circulation should be obtained. If intubation of the edematous trachea is required, it should be performed by an experienced anesthetist under controlled conditions to avoid trauma. For patients known to have small cell carcinoma of the lung or lymphoma, chemotherapy is the treatment of choice (unless the tumor is known to be resistant). When the history is unknown, radiation therapy is promptly administered. We proceed with diagnostic maneuvers during the initial stages of radiation. Responses are usually seen within seven days, and are obtained in 70% of patients with bronchogenic carcinoma and 95% of patients with lymphoma. Lack of improvement in spite of tumor regression on radiographic studies suggests that thrombosis of the SVC may have developed. The usefulness of prophylactic anticoagulation in preventing SVC thrombosis must be weighed against the risk of hemorrhage in a venous system under increased pressure. We do not routinely anticoagulate patients with SVC obstruction. Corticosteroids have been recommended to reduce accompanying inflammation and edema, but there are no controlled trials to support their use.

A recent advance has been the development of intravascular SVC stents to relieve obstruction (Stock *et al.*, 1995). Relief is typically rapid. We have found this approach useful in patients who have previously received mediastinal radiation, and who lack other life-threatening comorbid conditions. Catheter-associated SVC thrombosis is best treated by immediate thrombolytic therapy, administered when possible directly to the thrombus to minimize systemic fibrinolysis. An alternative is anticoagulation and catheter removal.

MALIGNANT PERICARDIAL EFFUSIONS AND CARDIAC TAMPONADE

Although many patients with metastatic cancer are found to have cardiac or pericardial metastases at autopsy, only about 30% of these patients had symptoms attributable to this involvement, and in less than 10% was the diagnosis of malignant pericardial effusion made before death. The most common tumors associated with tamponade are bronchogenic carcinoma, breast cancer, lymphoma, leukemia, melanoma, gastrointestinal malignancy, and sarcomas. Occasionally tamponade may be due to cardiac encasement by tumor or to postirradiation pericarditis.

Eventually there is interference with diastolic filling and the stroke volume decreases, with subsequent fall in blood pressure and compensatory tachycardia. As ventricular pressure rises, the mean pressures rise and eventually equalize in the left atrium, the pulmonary circulation, and the vena cava. The major complaint of patients is typically dyspnea, often with cough, or retrosternal chest pain. Hiccups, hoarseness, nausea, vomiting, and epigastric pain are occasional complaints. Eventually there is a decrease in cerebral blood flow which may result in seizures or altered mental status. There is often peripheral cyanosis, engorged neck veins, pulsus paradoxus, facial plethora, low systemic and pulse pressures, and distant heart sounds. With persistent increases in venous pressure, edema, ascites, and hepatosplenomegaly may occur. A chest radiograph is abnormal in most patients, showing either an enlarged cardiac shadow, mediastinal widening, or hilar adenopathy. The electrocardiogram may be normal or show sinus tachycardia, low QRS voltage, ST segment elevation, T wave changes, or electrical alternans. If any suspicion of tamponade arises, an echocardiogram is the test of choice. With optimal techniques of echocardiography, right heart catheterization is rarely necessary to differentiate tamponade or constriction from cardiomyopathy.

Immediate removal of pericardial fluid should be performed as an emergency if there is cyanosis, shock, dyspnea, a pulse pressure less than 20 mm Hg, a paradox greater than 50% of pulse pressure, or peripheral venous pressure greater than 13 mm Hg (Spodick, 1967). Typically, this has been performed by pericardiocentesis using a subxiphoid approach and insertion of a Silastic catheter over a guide wire (Davis *et al.*, 1984). This is a temporary measure, but may allow stabilization of a patient, as well as a diagnosis by pericardial fluid cytology.

Pericardiectomy with creation of a pericardial window, generally utilizing a subxiphoid approach, provides long-term control of the tamponade, and provides diagnostic material in cases in which tumor cells are not shed into the pericardial fluid (Osuch *et al.*, 1985). In our center, this is also the preferred method for emergency management of tamponade, since an experienced surgical team is immediately available. Pericardiocentesis remains a viable temporary measure for situations in which access to pericardiectomy is not immediately available.

HYPERVISCOSITY SYNDROME

Emergency department visits because of altered mental status, visual disturbance, ischemic neurological symptoms, purpura, ecchymoses, epistaxis, or gastrointestinal bleeding are common for older patients. One cause to be considered, especially in elderly patients, is hyperviscosity syndrome due to high serum levels of an abnormal monoclonal immunoglobulin (McGrath and Penny, 1976). Plasma cell neoplasms, multiple myeloma, and Waldenström's macroglobulinemia occur predominantly in the elderly. In these patients, there is frequently expansion of plasma volume, which can create an appearance of congestive heart failure. There is also renal dysfunction in many individuals.

Usually plasma viscosity must be increased to four times normal before disturbances in hemostasis or circulation becomes evident (Crawford *et al.*, 1985). Ancillary laboratory abnormalities often include varying degrees of cytopenia with the expanded plasma volume contributing to the reduction in packed red cell volume. Examination of a blood film always demonstrates rouleaux formation; and the sedimentation rate is elevated. Diagnosis is completed by examination of the bone marrow aspirate and by serum protein electrophoresis and immunofixation electrophoresis. One should not delay treatment while waiting for results of laboratory studies. Physical examination is usually unhelpful in diagnosis, since the classic "boxcar" pattern of circulation in the retinal vessels is seen only in the most severe forms of hyperviscosity syndrome. Plasma viscosity may be rapidly and acutely reduced by plasmapheresis. Despite anemia, patients with hyperviscosity syndrome must undergo plasmapheresis before transfusion since red cell infusions will increase viscosity and may aggravate disturbances in perfusion.

PATHOLOGICAL FRACTURES

Fractures of weight-bearing bones are common in the elderly due to osteopenia. This tendency is enhanced in patients with cancer due to local metastatic disease or to tumor enhanced osteopenia. In pathological fractures of the axial skeleton, there is danger of neurological damage due to bony instability, and patients should be immobilized until surgical consultation is obtained. Pain control with rapidly acting narcotic analgesics is usually required. In these situations, particularly with vertebral pedicle involvement, surgical stabilization may be required (Drew and Dickson, 1980).

Long bone lesions often cause pain with weight bearing on use of that extremity and there is always a risk of pathological fracture. In the lower extremity, we consider prophylactic internal fixation and/or radiation therapy for areas of destruction more than 3 cm in length or when involvement exceeds 30% of the thickness of the cortex. (For the upper extremity, the corresponding dimensions are 5 cm and 50%.) Once a pathological fracture occurs, internal fixation is usually necessary for adequate healing and pain relief. In patients who present with pathological fractures, one immobilizes the affected extremity, provides adequate analgesia, establishes an intravenous line to ensure adequate hydration, estimates blood loss around the fracture site, and prepares for internal fixation as soon as practical if the patient's general condition is stable. Rapid fixation permits rapid mobilization. Radiation therapy to the involved site is begun as soon as feasible.

HEMATOLOGICAL EMERGENCIES

Leukostasis

This is an uncommon problem in a general medical setting, essentially occurs primarily in the situation of previously undiagnosed acute leukemia, and must be recognized rapidly for appropriate therapy. Patients present with varying degrees of mental confusion, and are sometimes even comatose; they may have respiratory insufficiency and often demonstrate evidence of inadequate peripheral perfusion. White blood cell counts are greater than 100×10^9/l and composed predominantly of blasts indicative of acute leukemia. This syndrome is rarely if ever a problem in chronic leukemia with similar leukocyte counts, since cells are smaller and possibly have greater deformability.

Therapy is directed toward reduction of circulating blasts and maintenance of perfusion. Patients should not be transfused initially, even if profound anemia is present. It is better to wait until leukocyte counts are falling and the clinical condition is improving, since early red cell transfusions can increase blood viscosity at presentation and even be fatal. While maintaining careful fluid balance, arrangements should be made for urgent therapeutic leukopheresis under the care of an oncologist or hematologist. Chemotherapy should be instituted promptly after diagnosis, to help prevent the progression of leukostasis after leukopheresis. In the case of acute promyelocytic leukemia, chemotherapy may induce a coagulopathy, and the combination of leukopheresis and retinoid therapy may be appropriate as well.

Thrombocytopenia (*see* Chapter 38, Disorders of Hemostasis)

There is no consensus regarding precise platelet counts below which transfusion of platelets is mandatory. Thrombocytopenia predisposes to bleeding at platelet counts less than 50×10^9/l but especially below 20×10^9/l if the level has fallen rapidly. If platelet function is abnormal, bleeding is frequently seen in this range, and is an indication for platelet transfusion. If platelet function is normal, then lower counts may be tolerated. Thrombocytopenia may occur because of marrow suppression by drugs, other marrow dysfunction or peripheral platelet destruction. When uncertain, a bone marrow aspirate is required for evaluation. Acutely, one transfuses platelets immediately for any bleeding or significant headache (which may be due to an early intracranial hemorrhage) and avoids salicylates or nonsteroidal anti-inflammatory agents that interfere with platelet function. Six pooled platelet concentrates or a single donor platelet aphereis collection will usually raise the platelet count some $40-60 \times 10^9$/l in an average sized adult (Kruskall *et al.*, 1988). Definitive therapy then is directed toward the cause of the thrombocytopenia.

Neutropenia

This is relatively uncommon except in acute leukemia or a setting of cytotoxic drug therapy, although extensive marrow involvement with tumor may also be a cause. Bone marrow failure in the elderly may also present in this manner. Definitive diagnosis and treatment of the underlying cause may require specialty consultation. Once the granulocyte count falls below 1×10^9/l, risk of infection increases dramatically. Therefore, any fever should prompt immediate examination; culture of blood, urine, and sputum; a chest radiograph; and prompt empiric broad-spectrum antibiotic therapy. Evaluation of the cerebrospinal fluid may be advisable in selected cases.

DISSEMINATED INTRAVASCULAR COAGULATION (DIC)

DIC crosses several clinical boundaries including infection, obstetrical catastrophes, neoplasia, shock, acidosis, and even heat stroke. DIC is certainly a well-recognized complication of malignant neoplasm. Cancer of the lung, pancreas, breast, prostate, stomach, and colon are particularly likely to precipitate a disturbance of coagulation by release of thromboplastic material from tumor tissue (Levi, 2004). The one hematological malignancy most likely to trigger DIC is acute promyelocytic leukemia and of all the neoplastic processes, it should be the most easily recognized.

Between 13 and 25% of patients with chronic DIC have underlying prostate carcinoma (Sack *et al.*, 1977). Moreover, prostate cancer is the second most common form of malignancy in American males over the age of 50 years and the incidence increases each decade thereafter. Therefore, since prostate cancer increases with age, and because DIC is a frequent complication of that malignancy, physicians in ERs should expect occasionally to see an elderly man with a life-threatening bleeding disorder or thrombotic disorder that is clearly related to cancer only.

Inclusion of this topic in a chapter devoted to oncological emergencies is appropriate but much more difficult to discuss than other problems because its clinical presentation can be variable and quite enigmatic; well-defined criteria for the diagnosis of acute and chronic DIC do not exist; coagulation tests are not infrequently deranged in random studies of patients with a broad spectrum of cancers (Peck and Reizuam, 1973); and treatment of this intricate coagulopathy remains controversial. Either thrombotic or fibrinolytic events may predominate in a patient with DIC, resulting in a picture of either thrombosis or of bleeding. The balance may shift from time to time, and, not infrequently, sites of thrombosis and of bleeding exist simultaneously.

Clinically significant expressions of the syndrome are usually manifest by bleeding, often from a combination of sites. Systemic signs of consumption coagulopathy can be quite inconstant since they reflect both the cause of the disordered clotting scheme and the organ dysfunctions that are secondary to defibrination as well as thrombosis. In a patient with cancer, one should evaluate primary roles for sepsis, shock, hemorrhage, venous thrombosis, embolism, thromboembolism, or the tumor itself, not to mention potential intra-abdominal disasters such as a perforated viscus of more rarely acute pancreatitis.

This disorder is an extremely complex disarray of the hemostatic mechanisms, in which there can be evidence of accelerated coagulation without overt bleeding such that the formation of microthrombi overshadows activation of fibrinolysis. Although criteria for diagnosis vary, basic tests for DIC center around three areas: assays for clotting factors, studies of cellular elements, and determination of fibrinolysis. We initially evaluate the prothrombin time, activated partial thromboplastin time, thrombin clot time, and serum fibrinogen level. These may be abnormal in DIC and the degree of abnormality is a clue to the severity of the condition. Fibrin D-dimer measurement detects the lysis of cross-linked fibrin, and if elevated confirms the presence of a fibrinolytic component in the clinical situation. Inspection of the blood film is mandatory to evaluate the presence of schistocytes, which connote microvascular thrombosis with intravascular red cell fragmentation. The platelet count is also often depressed due to consumption in the coagulation process. These studies do not usually define the exact pathophysiologic processes underway in the patient, but provide a "snapshot" of the situation at a single moment. Observation of changes in these tests over several hours or days is necessary to appropriately treat the hemostatic abnormalities.

Aggressive effort to trace and treat the underlying precipitating disorder is the best method to initiate therapy. Septicemia and shock may be difficult to treat but disseminated cancer is even less easily ablated. We strive to maintain reasonably normal levels of clotting factors, by transfusions if necessary, but also by anticoagulation if it appears that factors are being consumed due to extensive intravascular thrombosis. For situations in which excessive fibrinolysis plays a role, antifibrinolytic agents might be appropriate. The target is a moving one, and expert hematological consultation and access to a capable coagulation laboratory greatly facilitate managing patients with clinically significant DIC.

CENTRAL NERVOUS SYSTEM EVENTS

Mass lesions of the brain in patients with cancer may be due to a primary brain tumor, metastatic disease, postirradiation brain necrosis, hemorrhage, or abscess. Lung and breast primaries account for most metastases and symptoms are related to location of masses and the rate of increase in intracranial pressure.

Headache is often throbbing and present on awakening, clearing in hours but recurring periodically during the day. It is exacerbated by cough, Valsalva, or sudden movements. Headaches of a fleeting or stabbing nature, or those that increase in severity throughout the day, are unusual for tumor.

Any new onset of seizures (usually focal) without obvious cause in a patient over 30 years of age suggests tumor, especially in an individual known to have malignant disease. Other more classical findings in brain metastasis are focal neurological deficits or papilledema.

Computed tomography (CT) of the brain is generally the initial test. MRI scans are less readily available, and more expensive, although more sensitive. MRI scans may be most helpful in determining the exact number of lesions in patients being considered for excision of brain metastases or for stereotactic radiation. Once a mass lesion is identified, its origin must still be determined. At 6–12 months posttherapy, postirradiation brain necrosis can mimic a return of the original tumor but papilledema is not present. A biopsy may be required to distinguish between them. Positron-emission tomography is helpful in this situation but its availability is limited. In the setting of long-term steroid therapy or recurrent neutropenia, an abscess may present merely as a mass lesion without fever. A variety of disorders can mimic potential brain metastasis upon presentation, including: other kinds of headaches; ethanol withdrawal seizures; cerebrovascular accidents; pseudotumor cerebri; subdural hematomia; encephalitis and arachnoiditis. All should be evaluated appropriately.

If a mass lesion felt to be a tumor is demonstrated, initial therapy with dexamethasone is begun as for spinal cord compression. If herniation is imminent, then mannitol 12.5–25 g is given intravenously along with dexamethasone and neurosurgery and radiation oncology are consulted immediately.

Cerebrovascular complications in patients with cancer originate from several different causes, have been well described, and will be overlooked if not considered in the appropriate setting (Graus *et al.*, 1985). Nonbacterial thrombotic endocarditis and attendant cerebral infarction should not have any age dependence but atherosclerosis is the most frequent cause of cerebral infarction found at autopsy and certainly is more age related. Usual risk factors for cerebrovascular disease are often overshadowed in a patient with malignancy because frequently there are several other things going on. There are perhaps two clues in the approach to the diagnosis of cerebrovascular disease in patients with cancer: first, the clinical presentation is often a diffuse encephalopathy rather than an acute focal deficit and secondly, the type of event is related sometimes to the primary tumor, but also to the extent of cancer, evidence of central nervous system infiltration, or the presence of superimposed complications such as immunosuppression, infection, coagulopathy, and any recent invasive procedures (Graus *et al.*, 1985).

GASTROINTESTINAL EMERGENCIES

Major gastrointestinal calamities in the setting of cancer are related to obstruction, perforation, hemorrhage, and inflammation. These may be due to effects of tumor or therapy. Obstruction of the bowel may result from primary tumor, recurrent or metastatic tumor, adhesions, or scarring from radiation. Patients present with combinations of pain, nausea, vomiting, constipation, and distention. The greatest threat is in those individuals with a competent ileocecal valve and a distal obstruction wherein cecal perforation may occur. Immediate surgical decompression is indicated should cecal dilatation to 12–14 cm be seen on a plain film of the abdomen. When the ileocecal valve is not competent, large bowel obstruction as well as small bowel dilatation respond well to suction, along with fluid and electrolyte replacement, such that surgery can be delayed or sometimes avoided.

In patients presenting to an ER with abdominal pain, 2% were discovered to have cancer (usually of the colon) and there was rarely obstruction or perforation (DeDombal *et al.*, 1980). Of patients older than 50 years presenting with abdominal pain, 7% developed cancer. Data from a cooperative study in Scotland, England, and Denmark suggest that 10% of all patients with gastrointestinal malignancies present to an ER and 3% do so with an intra-abdominal catastrophe. The remainder present as acute "unexplained" abdominal pain. Characteristics more common in those found to have cancer were pain lasting longer than 48 hours, intermittent pain, worsening pain, constipation, abdominal distention, and an abdominal mass (DeDombal *et al.*, 1980). Surgery, when performed as an emergency in the elderly, especially for gastrointestinal malignancies, was believed to carry a higher risk. However, recent studies have shown no change in morbidity or mortality by decade if patients of similar nutritional status without coexisting organ system disease are compared (Boyd *et al.*, 1980). Complications are less related to age than to preoperative nutritional status and preoperative impairment of other organ systems. However, emergent surgery overall does have a higher risk than for similar procedures performed electively. The lesson here is that with proper attention, the elderly can undergo appropriate procedures with similar morbidity and mortality as patients who are younger but with similar coexisting conditions. Conditions that adversely affect risk include pulmonary insufficiency, cardiac dysfunction, hypertension, renal insufficiency, hepatic disease, diabetes, or previous major surgery (Boyd *et al.*, 1980).

VENOUS THROMBOSIS AND EMBOLISM (*see* Chapter 55, Venous Thromboembolism)

Thromboembolic events are common in patients with malignancies and can be attributed to a lack of activity and to a hypercoagulable state which characterizes some neoplasms (Di Nisio *et al.*, 2004). It is important to realize that a predisposition to thrombosis may be present and that the presentation may be gradual. For instance, multiple small pulmonary emboli may be responsible for worsening pulmonary insufficiency. Yet in patients with malignancies one sometimes avoids thrombolytic therapy since many patients have had surgery, have structural lesions, or have coexisting cytopenias, and often life expectancy as well as mobility are greatly limited such that prevention of a postphlebitic syndrome is of less concern than in other patients.

Age alone is not a contraindication to appropriate thrombolytic therapy or anticoagulation, although it may complicate management. The elderly patient is more likely to fall, complicating anticoagulation. The appetite and diet may be variable, complicating control of oral anticoagulation. There may also be an increased risk of gastrointestinal bleeding in these patients. If anticoagulation is contraindicated or unsuccessful, then insertion of a caval filter may at least prevent subsequent pulmonary embolism.

EMERGENCIES DUE TO NEOPLASMS OF THE HEAD AND NECK

Squamous cell carcinomas of the floor of the mouth, the tongue, the tonsils, and the larynx essentially occur during middle and older life. Therefore, two disasters, upper airway obstruction and external massive hemorrhage from the carotid system, are not unusual in the elderly. However, the usually slow growth of epidermoid carcinoma in the head and neck region provides ample warning of such complications, and more than enough time to decide how or whether to treat it. Unfortunately, a specific plan for such an exigency is uncommon or rarely transcribed.

Tracheostomy is indicated in every patient in whom there is or it is expected that there will be airway compromise. By following this principle, it should be possible to perform tracheostomy under controlled circumstances in the operating room, thereby avoiding having to do it under emergency and uncontrolled circumstances. There are rare exceptions, such as patients with bilateral thyroid cancer and primary or metastatic pulmonary neoplasms that might be seen with airway obstruction at the glottic level due to bilateral vocal cord paralysis in the adducted position. In that setting, it is possible to have more subtle signs and the etiology of the recurrent laryngeal nerve dysfunction might not be immediately apparent.

For the patient with a tracheostomy tube already in place, there are still two more threats. Rarely a life is lost because of the inability to reinsert tubes during the changing of them before the tract is well defined or when there is high-grade airway obstruction. Finally, dislodgement of a tube can be catastrophic and has characteristic signs including recurrent airway obstruction, despite an earlier tracheostomy; absence of airflow via the tube during attempts at deep respiration; inability to suction pulmonary secretions from it; and a normal voice. A proper instruction sheet warns of these signs and advises the patient and/or family to alert their physician promptly or to call for help through a number for emergency medical services.

Hemorrhage may ensue from extensive cancers that erode major vessels or because of necrosis of vessel walls subsequent to injury by some combination of exposure, radiation, surgery, cytotoxic chemotherapy, and oral cutaneous fistula formation. Attempts at local control or grafting of the vessel are of no avail. Carotid artery hemorrhage by tumor erosion is the most life-threatening emergency seen in oncological disorders. However, it rarely occurs de novo, being heralded by a small transient bleed prior to the final disruption. Certainly there is more than enough time for the physician of a patient with head and neck cancer to decide whether hemorrhage from the carotid system is going to be accepted as the terminal event should it occur. Unfortunately, decisions like that are both painful and distasteful, resulting in heroic attempts by emergency teams in the absence of such decision making and in the absence of written orders.

A deeply invasive tumor at the base of the tongue, with erosion of branches of the external carotid system, is one of the most common causes of major arterial hemorrhage from the mouth. This type of hemorrhage may require ligation of both external carotid arteries in order to stop the bleeding, since there is such extensive cross circulation.

UTILIZATION OF INTENSIVE CARE UNITS (ICUs)

Early in the course of neoplastic disease, when expectations of a successful outcome are real, there is almost never any reason to withhold supportive measures, including an ICU, in order to overcome an early complication of the disease *per se* or its treatment. On the other hand, it is legitimate to ask what to do about that patient with advanced cancer who is in the third trimester of the illness and whose intercurrent problems suddenly escalate. There appears to be no simple stopping point in the progression of attempts at diagnostic or therapeutic intervention. Often there is a clinical temptation to believe that just a bit more intervention, such as endotracheal intubation, open lung biopsy and aggressive support on an ICU, will surmount the complication. This is a scene played out frequently, leading to marginally useful results and extraordinarily high costs. Of the many controversies that attend this highly charged decision about admitting cancer patients to intensive care wards is one still incompletely resolved even by the courts: which patient has the right to refuse life-saving extraordinary therapy (Emanuel, 1988). Another challenge faced by critical care specialists who often control access to these units is the matter of unattainable certainty in formulating prognosis upon which life-and-death decisions should be based (Reuben *et al.*, 1988). It is impossible to give specific advice in this area of the practice of medicine since physicians are waiting for a societal commitment to the solution of certain problems (Bayer *et al.*, 1983). Nevertheless, physicians should not practice emergency medicine in the field of oncology without first carefully reflecting about the issues involved in the use of ICUs, and without examining/understanding the policies for control of the ICUs at their own hospital.

EMERGENCY MEDICAL SERVICES AND CANCER

The interface between emergency medical services and the dying patient is both complex and difficult. It ranges from the extreme, where an ambulance delivers paramedical staff to the bedside of a patient experiencing dyspnea, coma, or shock, to the appearance of a patient in an ER with varied or several complaints (usually reported by a relative or caregiver rather than the individual who has the malignancy). In the first scenario, the paramedical staff may be told about a living will, but the existence of such cannot be immediately documented. Sometimes a family member might just report that this individual patient would not want to be resuscitated. At such times, there is not comfortable agreement about what to do and in many states living wills were designed for use in hospital rather than as instruments to instruct medical technicians after a request for emergency care has already been initiated. Today general legal and ethical standards offer these paramedical personnel no truly safe alternative than to initiate life-saving techniques upon encountering an unresponsive patient or one in severe physiological distress. In the second setting, a visit to an ER, the reason for attendance may turn out to be plural, something we call a multifactorial presentation. Everything seems to be going a little bit wrong and actually it is a matter of family or caregivers wearing out or refusing to cope any longer. The problem then becomes one of dealing with a chronic disease in an inappropriate setting, by a busy physician who has limited knowledge about the patient's previous course.

Our capabilities for intervening are great and increase steadily with each decade. One challenge is to intervene appropriately and not let a potentially reversible crisis progress to irreversibility. We also must be wise enough not to make a bad situation worse. All of this requires an intense effort toward preventing individual pieces of the medical care system from becoming disconnected. Physicians can do that by remaining aware of their responsibilities especially in the area of communication. Certainly patients having an acute event during a chronic illness should rarely turn up in an ER unannounced. Finally, in the realm of therapy, we should all do well to remember the words of Max Born (Born, 1968): "intellect distinguishes between the possible and the impossible; reason distinguishes between the sensible and the senseless; even the possible can be senseless". There should be no real doubt about some of the sensible goals of treatment in patients with cancer whether they are in the first or the tenth decade of life. They are: activate every important modality of treatment in an attempt at cure; preserve locomotion and continence; protect the ability to think; relieve pain or suffering; and support dignity (Silberman, 1986).

KEY POINTS

- The presentation of cancer in the elderly may be as a urgent problem with either an anatomic or metabolic cause.
- Hypercalcemia may have subtle symptoms in the elderly, and requires a high index of suspicion.
- Weakness may be a result of spinal cord compression, central nervous system metastases, metabolic derangements due to cancer, or be unrelated to a patient's malignancy.
- Cancer is associated with a pronounced tendency towards thrombosis.
- Encourage patients and families to formally make known their wishes regarding end of life care, before an urgent situation arises.

KEY REFERENCES

- Di Nisio M, Squizzato A, Klerk CPW *et al.* Antithrombotic therapy and cancer. *Current Opinion in Hematology* 2004; **11**:187–91.
- Graus F, Rogers LR & Posner JB. Cerebrovascular complications in patients with cancer. *Medicine* 1985; **64**:16–35.
- Harvey HA. The management of hypercalcemia of malignancy. *Support Care Cancer* 1995; **3**:123–9.
- Stock KW, Jacob AL, Proske M *et al.* Treatment of malignant obstruction of the superior vena cava with the self-expanding Wallstent. *Thorax* 1995; **50**:1151–6.
- Yarboro JW & Bornstein RS. *Oncologic Emergencies* 1981; Grune and Stratton, New York.

REFERENCES

Bailar JC & Smith EM. Progress against cancer? *The New England Journal of Medicine* 1986; **314**:1226–32.

Bayer R, Callahan D, Fletcher J *et al.* The care of the terminally ill: morality and economics. *The New England Journal of Medicine* 1983; **309**:1490–94.

Bell DR, Woods RL & Levi JA. Superior vena caval obstruction: a 10-year experience. *The Medical Journal of Australia* 1986; **145**:566–568.

Bobrowitz ID, Ramakrishna S & Shim Y-S. Comparison of medical v surgical treatment of major hemoptysis. *Archives of Internal Medicine* 1983; **143**:1343–6.

Born M. *My Life and My Views* 1968; Charles Scribner and Son, New York.

Boyd JB, Bradford B & Watne AL. Operative risk factors of colon resection in the elderly. *Annals of Surgery* 1980; **192**:743–46.

Brown MW, Bradley JA & Calman KC. Malignant disease in the accident and emergency department. *The British Journal of Clinical Practice* 1983; **37**:205–8.

Cohen HJ, Silberman HR, Forman W *et al.* Effect of age on response to treatment and survival in multiple myeloma. *Journal of the American Geriatrics Society* 1983; **31**:272–7.

Conlan AA, Hurwitz SS, Krige L *et al.* Massive hemoptysis. *The Journal of Thoracic and Cardiovascular Surgery* 1983; **85**:120–4.

Cornbleet M, Bondy PK & Powels TJ. Fatal irreversible hypercalcemia in breast cancer. *British Medical Journal* 1977; **i**:145–9.

Crawford J, Cox EB & Cohen HJ. Evaluation of hyperviscosity in monoclonal gammopathies. *The American Journal of Medicine* 1985; **79**:13–22.

Crocco JA, Rooney JJ, Fankushen DS *et al.* Massive hemoptysis. *Archives of Internal Medicine* 1968; **121**:495–8.

Davis S, Rambotti P & Grignani F. Intrapericardial tetracycline sclerosis in the treatment of malignant pericardial effusion. An analysis of 35 cases. *Journal of Clinical Oncology* 1984; **2**:631–6.

DeDombal FT, Matharu SS, Stuniland JR *et al.* Presentation of cancer to hospital as 'acute abdominal pain'. *The British Journal of Surgery* 1980; **69**:413–16.

Di Nisio M, Squizzato A, Klerk CPW *et al.* Antithrombotic therapy and cancer. *Current Opinion in Hematology* 2004; **11**:187–91.

Drew M & Dickson RB. Osseous complications of malignancy. In J Lohick (ed) *Clinical Cancer Management* 1980, p 18; GR Hall, Boston.

Emanuel EJ. A review of the ethical and legal aspects of terminating medical care. *The American Journal of Medicine* 1988; **84**:291–301.

Gilbert RW, Kim JH & Posner JB. Epidural spinal cord compression from metastatic tumour: diagnosis and treatment. *Annals of Neurology* 1978; **3**:40–51.

Graus F, Rogers LR & Posner JB. Cerebrovascular complications in patients with cancer. *Medicine* 1985; **64**:16–35.

Griebie MS & Adams BL. 'Emergency' laryngectomy and stomal recurrence. *The Laryngoscope* 1987; **97**:1020–4.

Hantman D, Rossier B, Zohlman R *et al.* Rapid correction of hyponatremia in the syndrome of inappropriate secretion of antidiuretic hormone – an alternative treatment to hypertonic saline. *Annals of Internal Medicine* 1973; **78**:870–5.

Harvey HA. The management of hypercalcemia of malignancy. *Support Care Cancer* 1995; **3**:123–9.

Kalemkerian GP, Darwish B & Varterasian ML. Tumor lysis syndrome in small cell carcinoma and other solid tumors. *American Journal of Medicine* 1997; **103**:363–8.

Kalia S & Tintinalli J. Emergency evaluation of the cancer patient. *Annals of Emergency Medicine* 1984; **13**:723–30.

Kennedy BJ. Specific considerations for the geriatric patient with cancer. In P Calabresi, P Schein & S Rosenberg (eds) *Medical Oncology* 1985, pp 1433–45; Macmillan, New York.

Kruskall MS, Mintz PD, Bergin JJ *et al.* Transfusion therapy in emergency medicine. *Annals of Emergency Medicine* 1988; **17**:327–35.

Levi M. Current understanding of disseminated intravascular coagulation. *British Journal of Haematology* 2004; **124**:567–76.

McGrath MA & Penny R. Paraproteinemia: blood hyperviscosity and clinical manifestations. *The Journal of Clinical Investigation* 1976; **58**:1155–9.

McKee LC & Collins RD. Intravascular leukocyte thrombi and aggregates as a cause of morbidity and mortality in leukemia. *Medicine* 1974; **53**:463–78.

Mullins GM, Glynn MB, El-Mahdi AM *et al.* Malignant lymphoma of the spinal epidural space. *Annals of Internal Medicine* 1971; **74**:416–23.

Osuch JR, Khandehar JN & Fry WA. Emergency subxyphoid pericardial decompression for malignant pericardial effusion. *The American Surgeon* 1985; **51**:298–303.

Peck SD & Reizuam CW. Disseminated intravascular coagulation in cancer patients: supportive evidence. *Cancer* 1973; **31**:1114–19.

Peterson BA. Acute non-lymphocytic leukemia in the elderly. In CD Bloomfield (ed) *Biology and Treatment in Adult Leukemias* 1982, pp 199–235; Martinus Nijhoff, The Hague.

Pontoppidin H, Abbott W, Brewster D *et al.* Optimum care for hopelessly ill patients. In Report of the Clinical Care Committee of the Massachusetts General Hospital. *The New England Journal of Medicine* 1976; **295**:362.

Reuben DB, Mor V & Hiris J. Clinical symptoms and length of survival in patients with terminal cancer. *Archives of Internal Medicine* 1988; **148**:1586–91.

Sack GH, Levin J & Bell WR. Trousseau's syndrome and other manifestations of chronic disseminated coagulopathy in patients with neoplasms: clinical pathologic and therapeutic features. *Medicine* 1977; **56**:1–37.

Silberman HR. Minimizing the economic hardships of diagnosis and treatment. In J Laszlo (ed) *Physician's Guide to Cancer Care Complications* 1986; Marcel Dekker, New York.

Spodick DH. Acute cardiac tamponade pathologic physiology diagnosis and management. *Progress in Cardiovascular Diseases* 1967; **10**:64–96.

Stock KW, Jacob AL, Proske M *et al.* Treatment of malignant obstruction of the superior vena cava with the self-expanding Wallstent. *Thorax* 1995; **50**:1151–6.

Torma T. Malignant tumours of the spine and spinal extradural space: a study based on 250 histologically verified cases. *Acta Chirurgica Scandinavica* 1957; **225**:1–138.

Trump DL. Serious hyponatremia in patients with cancer: management with demeclocycline. *Cancer* 1981; **47**:2908–12.

Ushio Y, Posner T, Kim JH *et al.* Treatment of experimental spinal cord compression caused by extradural neoplasms. *Journal of Neurosurgery* 1977; **47**:380–90.

Vaeth JM & Meyer J. Cancer and the elderly. In JM Vaeth & J Meyer (eds) *Frontiers of Radiation Therapy in Oncology* 1985, vol 20; Karger, Basel, New York.

Waldron RP, Donova IA, Drumm J *et al.* Emergency presentation and mortality from colorectal cancer in the elderly. *The British Journal of Surgery* 1986; **73**:214–16.

Warrell TP, Israel R, Frisone M *et al.* Gallium nitrate for accurate treatment of cancer-related hypercalcemia. *Annals of Internal Medicine* 1988; **108**:669–74.

Wild WO & Porter RW. Metastatic epidural tumor of the spine: a study of 45 cases. *Archives of Surgery* 1963; **87**:137–42.

Wright RL. Malignant tumors of the spinal extradural space: results of surgical treatment. *Annals of Surgery* 1963; **157**:227–31.

Yancik R. Old age as the context for the presentation and treatment of cancer. In R Yancik & PP Carbone (eds) *Perspectives on Prevention and Treatment of Cancer in the Elderly* 1983, p 95; Raven Press, New York.

Yarboro JW & Bornstein RS. *Oncologic Emergencies* 1981; Grune and Stratton, New York.

Yarboro JW, Bornstein RS & Mastrangelo MJ. *Oncologic emergencies*. *Seminars in Oncology* 1978; **5**:123–231.

Yoh CB, Hubaytar RT, Ford JM *et al.* Treatment of massive hemorrhage in pulmonary tuberculosis. *The Journal of Thoracic and Cardiovascular Surgery* 1967; **54**:503–10.

Zusman J, Brown BM & Nesbit ME. Hyperphosphatemia, hyperphosphaturia, and hypocalcemia in acute lymphoblastic leukemia. *The New England Journal of Medicine* 1973; **289**:1135–40.

Breast Cancer in the Elderly

Robert E. Mansel *and* **Anurag Srivastava**
Wales College of Medicine, Cardiff University, Cardiff, UK

THE PRESENTATION

Diagnosis of breast cancer in the elderly is made by the discovery of a lump in 60–80% women. Since screening is applied less rigorously to elderly patients, the majority of women present with a palpable lump. Some studies reveal that the stage at presentation is more advanced in the elderly women (Goodwin *et al.*, 1986; Homes and Hearne, 1981). A patient care evaluation survey was conducted by Commission on Cancer of the American College of Surgeons for 1983 and 1990 (Busch *et al.*, 1996). They surveyed all states of United States including Puerto Rico and Canada and studied 17 029 women in 1983 and 24 004 women in 1990. Twenty percent of women in 1983 and 23% in 1990 were 75 years of age or older. The survey included 2000 hospitals (25 patients from each). The percentage of cancers detected by physicians' examination decreased in the younger group from 27% in 1983 to 21% in 1990, whereas in the elderly, the corresponding figures were 41% and 34% respectively.

Veronesi's group from Milan reported various features of presentation and choice of therapy in the elderly (Gennari *et al.*, 2004). They studied 2999 postmenopausal patients referred for surgery at the European Institute of Oncology, Milan, Italy, from 1997 to 2002. The patients were grouped according to age: young postmenopausal (YPM age 50–64 years, $n = 2052$), older postmenopausal (OPM age 65–74, $n = 801$), and elderly postmenopausal (EPM age ≥ 75, $n = 146$). EPM patients had larger tumors compared with YPM patients (pT4: 6.7 vs 2.4%) and more nodal involvement (lymph node positivity: 62.5 vs 51.3%). EPM patients showed a higher degree of estrogen and progesterone receptor expression, less peritumoral vascular invasion and less human epidermal growth factor receptor-2 (HER-2)/*neu* expression than YPM patients. Although, comorbidities were more often recorded for elderly patients (72% EPM vs 45% YPM), it did not influence surgical choices which were similar across groups (breast conservation: 73.9, 76.9, and 72.9%, respectively). No systemic therapy was recommended for 19.1% of the EPM compared with 5.4 and 4.7% of the two other groups.

In women over 70 years, estrogen receptor positive tumors are more common, range 69 to 95% compared with all tumors, range 53 to 72% (Busch *et al.*, 1996).

Pathologically infiltrating ductal carcinoma accounts for 77 to 85% of all tumors in the elderly women as compared to 68% in younger women. There is an increase in the proportion of papillary and mucinous carcinoma with advancing age. Whereas the number of lobular carcinoma *in situ*, comedo, medullary, and inflammatory carcinoma decreases with advancing age, the prevalence of ductal carcinoma *in situ* (DCIS) increases until 75 years, after which it declines (Rosen *et al.*, 1985; Law *et al.*, 1996).

In summary, elderly women generally present with large palpable estrogen receptor positive, infiltrating ductal carcinoma with a positive lymph node (Law *et al.*, 1996).

STAGE OF PRESENTATION

Age and delay – there is generally a delay in the diagnosis of breast cancer in elderly women. In a study by Berg and Robbins (1961), the diagnosis was delayed by more than 6 months in 28% of women under 70 years of age compared to 42% delay in women above the age of 70. Similarly, Devitt (1970) observed a delay of more than 6 months in diagnosis in 35% of women above the age of 70, compared to 28% below the age of 70. The tumor is generally advanced in elderly group as shown in Table 1.

COMORBIDITY: THE MAIN REASON TO JUSTIFY UNDERTREATMENT

Women suffering from heart disease, obstructive airway disease, stroke, or other major incapacitating illnesses receive inadequate diagnostic and therapeutic attention.

Principles and Practice of Geriatric Medicine, 4th Edition. Edited by M.S. John Pathy, Alan J. Sinclair and John E. Morley.

Table 1 TNM Stage with age at presentation

Age(yrs)	I	II	III	IV	Reference
>80	52%	18%	6%	24%	Robin and Lee (1985)
>80	25%	49%	15%	10%	Davis *et al.* (1985)
>75	53%	22%	12%	13%	Host (1986)

TNM, tumor nodes metastases.

Nicolucci *et al.* (1993) analyzed the data on 1724 women treated in 63 general hospitals in Italy. A comorbidity index was computed from individual disease value (IDV) and functional status (FS). IDV summates the severity and presence of specific complications for each disease suffered on a scale of 0–3, with 0 = full recovery and 3 = life-threatening disease. FS from signs and symptoms of 12 system categories evaluated the impact of all conditions, whether diagnosed or not, on patients' health status. The study showed higher proportions of inadequate diagnosis and therapy in the elderly group. The quality of care was assessed by a score based on observed degree of compliance with standard care. The median value of overall diagnostic and staging score was 60%. About one-third of surgical operations were inappropriate; 24% of cases with stage I-II disease had unnecessary Halsted mastectomy, and breast conservation in smaller tumors of ≤2 cm was underutilized. The presence of one or more coexistent diseases was associated with failure to undergo axillary dissection and lower utilization of conservative surgery.

Newschaffer *et al.*, 1996 from the Virginia Cancer Centre evaluated 2252 women with breast cancer (without metastasis). In the group of women above 85 years, the odds of being treated surgically were one-third of those women in 66–74 years age-group. The odds of getting breast-conserving surgery with radiotherapy (RT) were 0.55. Even after adjusting for comorbidity, the odds ratio remained the same.

Ganz *et al.* (2003) examined health-related quality of life (QoL) of a cohort of older women with breast cancer. They used standardized QoL measures in a group of 691 women of 65 and above who were interviewed 3 months after surgery and twice in the following year. Physical and mental health scores declined significantly in the follow-up year, independent of age. However, a cancer-specific psychosocial instrument showed improvement in the scores. Better 3-month physical and mental scores and better emotional support predicted more favorable self-perceived health, 15 months after surgery. The authors concluded that significant decline occurs in the physical and mental health of older women in 15 months after surgery, whereas cancer-specific QoL measure improved over time.

Alvan Feinstein, a famous clinical epidemiologist from Yale, has said that the failure to classify and analyze comorbid disease has led to many difficulties in medical statistics (Feinstein, 1970). There are four reasons for measuring comorbidity correctly: (1) to be able to correct for confounding thus improving internal validity of the study, (2) to be able to identify effect modification, (3) the desire to use comorbidity as a predictor of outcome, and (4) to construct a comprehensive single comorbid scale that is valid, to improve the statistical efficiency. de Groot *et al.* (2003) have recently reviewed various comorbidity indices. The following indices have been applied for patients with breast cancer: "Charlson Index" – this is the most extensively studied method and includes 19 diseases which are weighted on the basis of strength of association with mortality. The "disease count index" simply counts the coexisting diseases but lacks a consistent definition and weighting for different diseases. The "Kaplan index" uses the type and severity of comorbid condition, for example, types are classified vascular (hypertension, cardiac disease, peripheral vascular disease) and nonvascular (lung, liver, bone, and renal disease). It has good predictive validity for mortality. It may be worthwhile for all the agencies involved in breast cancer research to adopt one of the above indices and record it prospectively.

SCREENING IN THE ELDERLY

Presently, all women in the United Kingdom between age 50 and 65 are being offered breast cancer screening. Although those above 65 are eligible, they have not been called *routinely*. Till recently, those already on the regular screening were not recalled after they reached the age of 65.

The NHS Breast Cancer screening Programme in the UK, 2005 has screened more than 14 million women and has detected over 80 000 cancers. The NHS Breast Screening Programme is saving at least 300 lives per year. This figure is set to rise to 1250 by 2010. By 2010, the effect of the screening program, combined with improvements in treatment and other factors (including cohort effects), could result in up to a halving of the breast cancer death rate in women aged 55–69 from that seen in 1990. The program has now expanded to invite women between 65 and 70.

Thus, from Table 2 it can be seen that with increasing age the number of cancers detected goes up.

In order to enhance the rate of breast examination by doctors in women above 65 years and to increase compliance with mammography, Herman *et al.* (1995) conducted a randomized clinical trials (RCT) at the Metro Health Medical Center Cleveland, Ohio. All house staff in Internal Medicine were asked to fill a questionnaire about their attitude toward prevention of breast cancer in elderly people after providing some basic information (Monograph and a lecture).

In one arm (controls), no specific interventions were offered. In the next group (education), nurses provided educational leaflets to patients attending the clinics. In the third group (prevention), nurses filled the request forms and

Table 2 Result of UK breast cancer screening – 2004 review NHS Breast Cancer screening Programme in the UK, 2005

Age	Cancer detected per 1000 women screened
50–64	7.6
65–69	20.6

Table 3 Rates of examination and mammography by intervention

Group	Breast exam (%)	Mammography (%)
Control ($n = 192$)	18	18
Education ($n = 183$)	22	31
Prevention ($n = 165$)	32	36

facilitated women to undergo mammography. Their results are given in the Table 3:

The study suggests that encouragement and education of older women by motivated doctors and nurses improves compliance. Chen *et al.* (1995) reported the mortality rate of women aged 65–74 screened in the Swedish 2-county trial – 77 080 women were randomized to undergo screening every 33 months and 55 985 women served as controls. Of the screened group, 21 925 were in the age-group 65–74. In the control arm, 15 344 women belonged to the age-group 65–74 years. The relative breast cancer mortality in the screened group was 0.68, demonstrating a survival advantage in the elderly population.

RISK FACTORS IN ELDERLY

Age: With advancing age, the risk of developing breast cancer rises.

In a cohort of National Surgical Adjuvant Breast and Bowel Project's Breast cancer prevention trial of USA, the presence of nonproliferative lower category benign breast disease (LCBBD) has been found to increase the risk of invasive breast cancer. The overall relative risk (RR) of breast cancer was 1.6 for LCBBD, compared to women without any LCBBD. This risk increased to 1.95 (95% confidence interval (CI) 1.29–2.93) among women aged 50 and over (Wang *et al.*, 2004).

Hormone replacement therapy (HRT) has been identified as a *risk factor for breast cancer.* The impact of HRT on the incidence and death due to breast cancer in the United Kingdom was assessed through a study on 1 million women (Million Women Study Collaborators, 2003). In this prospective cohort of 1 084 110 women aged 50–64, current users of HRT were found to have a higher risk of developing breast cancer than nonusers (RR = 1.66; 95% CI 1.58–1.75). The risk was highest for combined estrogen-progestogen (RR = 2; 95% CI 1.88–2.12) than for estrogen alone (RR = 1.3; 95% CI 1.2–1.4) and for tibolone (RR = 1.45; 95% CI 1.25–1.68) compared to those who never used. There was a dose response relationship of increasing risk of cancer, with increasing duration of HRT usage, the highest being with combined estrogen + progestogen used for 10 years or more (RR = 2.31; 95% CI 2.08–2.56).

The Danish Nurses Cohort study (Stahlberg *et al.*, 2004) provided data on 10 874 nurses (aged 45 years and above). Of these, 244 women developed breast cancer. After adjusting for confounding, increased risk was found with current use of estrogens (RR = 1.96; 95% CI 1.16–3.35), for combined use of estrogen + progesterone (RR = 2.7; 95% CI 1.96–3.73), for current use of Tibolone (RR = 4.27; 95% CI 1.74–10.51), compared to never ever use of HRT. In current users of combined HRT with progestins, continuous combined use has higher risk (RR = 4.16; 95% CI 2.56–6.75) than cyclical combined use (RR = 1.94; 95% CI 1.26–3).

Natural History of Breast Cancer in the Elderly

It has long since been thought that breast cancer in the elderly is rather indolent and a biologically less aggressive disease. Singh *et al.* (2004) studied the *metastatic proclivity* as indicated by the virulence (defined as the rate of appearance of distant metastasis) and *metastagenecity* (defined as the ultimate likelihood of developing distant metastasis). These authors examined 2136 women who underwent mastectomy without systemic adjuvant therapy at the University of Chicago Hospitals between 1927 and 1987. The median follow-up period was 12 years. Distant disease-free survival(DDFS) was determined and virulence (V) and *metastagenecity* (M) were obtained from log linear plots of DDFS. No significant difference was observed between size of primary tumor in age-group <40 years, 40–70 years and >70 years. Significantly, fewer women above 70 years presented with positive nodes. In women with negative nodes, the DDFS was higher among age 40–70 years, compared with those among age over 70. However, no significant difference was observed in the DDFS in the node positive group in any of the age categories. The 10-year DDFS for age 40–70 was 33% and for women >70 it was 38%. Among the node negative women, V was 3% per year for age 40–70 years, as well as for age >70 years and M was 0.2 for age 40–70 years and 0.35 for age >70 years. In women with positive nodes, both V (11% per year vs 10% per year) and M (0.7 vs 0.65) were similar in both age-groups. These authors concluded that there was no evidence that breast cancer was more indolent in the elderly. Therefore, similar diagnostic and therapeutic efforts should be made in the elderly as in the younger women, the only modification made on the basis of comorbidity.

TREATMENT OF OPERABLE DISEASE

The optimum treatment of breast cancer in the elderly is not yet well established. It is reasonable to apply the principles of therapy largely learned from studies in the younger cohort of women, viz. breast-conserving wide tumor excision and axillary dissection for smaller lesions, mastectomy for the larger tumors, tamoxifen for estrogen receptor (ER)-positive lesions and chemotherapy for node positive or >1 cm tumors and radiotherapy for locally advanced lesions. Unlike the treatment of younger women, which is based on sound high-level evidence from meta-analyses of large RCTs, the therapy for the elderly is not evidence based, as there is paucity of large RCTs. The women over 65 years have been excluded from many trials. In order to fill up this lacuna in knowledge, two European Organization for Research and Treatment of Cancer (EORTC) trials were set up. In Britain, a CRC trial and a trial at Nottingham were conducted to answer the question of what would be the best therapy for the elderly. The results of these trials are summarized below. Moreover, a decision analysis has also been performed by (Punglia *et al.*, 2003). Truong *et al.* (2004) have reported an overview of literature on breast-conserving therapy (BCT) in elderly women with early breast cancer. They found a paucity of prospective data and numerous retrospective series of diverse treatments with conflicting results. Their observation supports BCT + postoperative RT as the standard of care for the elderly.

Crowe *et al.* (1994) reported the outcome of modified radical mastectomy (MRM) in a group of 1353 women (age range 22–75). The hazard ratio for death were similar in all the three age-groups (<45, 46–65and >65). This data demonstrates that older women achieve similar results as younger ones, provided they are treated adequately.

Among cooperative group clinical trials sponsored by the National Cancer Institute for early-stage breast cancer, women of 65 years and above constitute only 18% of participants, although they constitute 49% of eligible pool of all newly diagnosed cases. Physicians have been incriminated as the key barrier to enrolling older women in trials (Kemeny *et al.*, 2003).

The Cancer Research UK Breast Cancer Trial Group (Fennessy *et al.*, 2004) conducted a RCT for women over 70 years of age with operable breast cancer. Of 455 patients, from 27 hospitals in the United Kingdom, 225 were randomized to surgery + tamoxifen and 230 to receive tamoxifen alone. The analysis was based on a median follow-up of 12 years. The local control was better achieved when surgery was combined with tamoxifen. Fifty-seven patients randomized to surgery and 141 to tamoxifen alone progressed. The hazard ratio (HR) for local progression for tamoxifen as compared to mastectomy was 17.24; 95% CI 6.4–47.6 and for tamoxifen compared to BCT, 5.99; 95% CI 4.12–8.7. The risk of local progression was greater in the BCT arm compared to mastectomy (HR = 2.98; 95% CI 1.06–8.39). The 5 year risk of local progression was 8% after mastectomy, 18% after breast conservation and 64% in women who had tamoxifen alone.

The 10 year survival was 37.7% for surgery + tamoxifen and 28.8% for tamoxifen alone. Primary tamoxifen therapy is inferior to mastectomy and breast-conserving surgery in achieving local control. Among patients randomized to surgery + tamoxifen, the risk of local progression was greater in those who had breast conservation than in those who had a mastectomy (Fennessy *et al.*, 2004).

A strong consensus prevails that by the time the breast tumor is palpable, dissemination has already occurred and local treatment can only provide local control. Surgery cannot influence development of metastases. Data from mature randomized trials challenges this belief. Thus, local treatment offers more than local control and may prevent the spread of breast cancer from residual cancer left behind after surgery.

ROLE OF RADIOTHERAPY

In a study of 558 women aged ≥50 years, by the University of Pennsylvania, who had been treated with breast conservation and RT, for stage I and II breast cancer, there were 173 women who were aged ≥65years. Treatment included complete gross excision of tumor, pathological axillary lymph node staging and breast irradiation. Women ≥65 years and those between 50–64 years, were found to have large T2 lesions (43% vs 34%; p = 0.05), ER negativity (9% vs 16%; p = 0.13). The proportion of axillary node positivity (24%) as well as the mortality rates due to breast cancer at 10 years (13%) was similar in elderly patients and those in the 50–64 age-group. The overall survival at 10 years (77% vs 85%; p = 0.14), local failure (13% vs 12%; p = 0.6) and freedom from distant metastasis (83% vs 78%; p = 0.45) were similar. The study revealed that breast cancer in the elderly is not an indolent disease and has many aggressive prognostic factors. Moreover, breast-conserving surgery and RT achieves good local control and a survival comparable to women below 65 years (Solin *et al.*, 1995).

In a decision analysis of a hypothetical cohort, by a Markov model including postmenopausal women with ER-positive T1 tumors (≤2 cm), Punglia *et al.* (2003) from Harvard Medical School, computed the benefits of adding RT to conservative breast surgery and tamoxifen versus BCT + tamoxifen (tam.) alone. The modeled recurrence free survival benefit of radiation was 3.35 years for women of 50 years and 0.61 years for women at 80. A 50 year old was less likely to die from breast cancer when treated with RT + tam. than with tam. alone (relative risk reduction, RRR = 54%). An 80 year old had a RRR = 42% when RT was added to tamoxifen. Compared with the untreated group, the adjusted hazard ratio of breast cancer mortality was 0.4 for tamoxifen alone (95%CI 0.2–0.7), 0.4 for BCT alone (95%CI 0.1–1.4), 0.2 for mastectomy alone (95% CI 0.1–0.7) and 0.1 for BCT + adjuvant therapy (95%CI 0.03–0.4).

It is thought by some that in a selected group of elderly women, radiation could be avoided. Gruenberger *et al.* (1998) from University of Vienna evaluated the need of RT in a retrospective review of 356 women above 60 years, treated by quadrantectomy + axillary dissection followed or not followed by adjuvant radiation. Among node negative, ER-positive cases, there was no benefit of RT as locoregional recurrence rate was 3% with or without radiation. In this subgroup (ER positive, node negative women), adjuvant tamoxifen reduced LR to 2% with or without radiation. These authors suggest that elderly women aged 60 or above with a T1, ER positive, node negative tumor, may be spared the toxicity of RT when treated by conservation surgery, axillary dissection, and tamoxifen.

Milan Trials of Breast conservation: Prof. Veronesi of Milan Institute has been a great proponent of breast conservation. He initially developed the technique of quadrantectomy plus radiotherapy (QUART) and later reduced the extent of resection to only lumpectomy. The results of the Milan trials were published in a meta-analysis of data from 1973 patients treated in three consecutive randomized trials by four different radiosurgical procedures: Halsted mastectomy, QUART, lumpectomy plus RT, and quadrantectomy without RT (Veronesi *et al.*, 1995). Median follow-up for all patients was 82 months. The annual rates of local recurrence was 0.2 for patients treated with Halsted mastectomy and 0.46 for QUART, 2.45 for lumpectomy plus radiotherapy and 3.28 for quadrantectomy without RT. The local recurrences were much higher in patients under 45 years of age as compared to women over 55 years. Overall survival was identical in the four groups of patients. This study indicated that in elderly patients, lumpectomy and RT is a satisfactory option.

ADJUVANT ENDOCRINE THERAPY

Since the majority of tumors in the postmenopausal women are ER positive, hormonal manipulation by antiestrogen molecules or aromatase inhibitors is used with advantage in over 60% of cases.

Crivellari *et al.* (2003) reported the results of International Breast Cancer Study Group Trial IV conducted in many centers from the United States, Australia, Sweden, Switzerland, Italy, and Slovenia. From 1978 to 1981, 349 women 66 to 80 years of age with pathologically involved nodes after total mastectomy and axillary clearance were randomly assigned to receive 12 months of tamoxifen (20 mg daily) plus prednisolone (7.5 mg daily) (T + P) or no adjuvant therapy. At 21 years, median follow-up T + P prolonged the disease-free survival and overall survival – 15-year DFS 10 versus 19% in control; hazard ratio 0.71; 95% CI 0.58–0.86. The therapy was also superior in controlling breast cancer recurrences.

The long-term use of tamoxifen is associated with increased hazard of thrombotic episodes and endometrial proliferation. In an RCT (Rutqvist and Mattsson, 1993) of adjuvant tamoxifen (tamoxifen 40 mg daily for 2–5 years) versus no adjuvant therapy among 2365 postmenopausal women with early breast cancer in Stockholm, there was significantly reduced hospital admission due to cardiac disease. The relative hazard (tam. vs control) was 0.68 (95% CI 0.48–0.97; $p = 0.03$). Comparing 5- versus 2-year therapy, there was grater protection from cardiac disease with longer use of tamoxifen (relative hazard = 0.37, 95% CI 0.15–0.92, $p = 0.03$).

The results from meta-analysis of RCTs on early breast cancer have been published by the (Early Breast Cancer Trialists' Collaborative Group (EBCTCG), 2005).

For ER-positive disease only, allocation to about 5 years of adjuvant tamoxifen reduces the annual breast cancer death rate by 31% (SE 3), largely irrespective of the use of chemotherapy and of age (<50, 50–69, ≥70 years), progesterone receptor status, or other tumor characteristics.

Mastectomy or Tamoxifen?

Professor RW Blamey and his group reported the results of a trial comparing tamoxifen alone with wedge mastectomy for women above age 70. They randomized 135 women with operable, <5 cm tumors –68 to tamoxifen (20 mg b.d.) group and 67 to mastectomy arm. Those women developing local recurrence or progression in the tamoxifen arm underwent wedge mastectomy later. In the wedge mastectomy group, local recurrences were treated with further excision or RT, and if tumor recurred again, patients were given tamoxifen. The mortality from metastatic breast cancer was 10% in the tamoxifen group and 15% in the mastectomy group. In the mastectomy group, 70% remained alive and free of recurrence at 24 months, compared with 47% in the tamoxifen group. Authors concluded that since many patients in the tamoxifen arm eventually required surgery, optimum treatment should include surgery and tamoxifen (Robertson *et al.*, 1988).

This issue was also evaluated by EORTC 10 851 multicenter trial (Fentiman *et al.*, 2003a). Women above 70 years with operable breast cancer were randomized to either MRM (82 cases) or tamoxifen – 20 mg daily (82 cases). The tamoxifen was given till death or relapse. The median follow-up was for 11.7 years for MRM and 10.2 years in the tam. group. Eleven percent of women in the MRM arm and 62% in the tam. group developed locoregional progression, the difference being highly significant ($p < 0.001$). The risk of distant progression was noted in 20% of MRM and 23% of those getting tam. alone ($p = 0.654$). For overall survival, the modified logrank test gave a $p = 0.001$, rejecting the null hypothesis of nonequivalence, thus indicating that the two groups are similar in terms of overall survival.

The GRETA trial: Mustacchi *et al.* (2003) reported the results of a multicenter RCT on tamoxifen alone versus surgery followed by adjuvant tamoxifen in elderly women. Between 1987 and 1992, women above 70 with operable breast cancer were randomized – 239 to surgery + tamoxifen (20 mg/day) and 235 to tamoxifen alone. The tamoxifen was given for 5 years. At a median follow-up of 80 months, 274 patients had died, there was no difference between the two groups as regards the overall and breast cancer survival. Local progression was noted in 27 cases in surgery group and 106 in the tam. alone group. They concluded that minimal surgery followed by tam. appears to be appropriate therapy for older women as compared to tamoxifen alone.

EORTC 10 850 study (Fentiman *et al.*, 2003b): In this multicenter study, 236 women above 70 years with operable breast cancer were randomized to either modified radical mastectomy (MRM; $n = 120$) or wide excision + tamoxifen (WLE + tam.; $n = 116$). No other adjuvant therapy was given. The tamoxifen group received 20 mg daily till death or relapse. The median follow-up period was 10.9 years for the mastectomy and 10.4 years for the WLE + tam. group. Women experienced locoregional recurrences in 16% in MRM arm versus 26% in the WLE + tam. group. Distant relapse was observed in 28% in MRM and only 13% in WLE + tam. group. There was a higher risk of local relapse and a significantly reduced risk of distant relapse in the WLE + tam. arm. The multivariate Cox's modeling revealed no treatment effect according to time to progression (Hazard ratio = 0.89; $p = 0.06$). In terms of overall survival, all predictors except for age were removed. A model with age showed that the patients in the most elderly group had the highest mortality hazard.

Newer forms of hormone therapy have now been tried in the elderly group. A RCT using exemestane (Coombes *et al.*, 2004) has been reported. After 2–3 years of tamoxifen, 2362 patients were switched to exemestane and 2380 continued on tamoxifen. After a median follow-up of 30 months, the first recurrence (local or systemic) was noted. There were 183 recurrences in the exemestane arm and 266 in the tamoxifen arm. This represents a 32% risk reduction with exemestane. The overall survival was similar – 93 deaths in exemestane and 106 in tamoxifen. Contralateral cancer occurred in nine in exemestane and 20 in tamoxifen group.

The duration and type of hormone therapy in the elderly is a matter of debate. The benefits of tamoxifen for 2 years are not very much different from tamoxifen given for 5 years. In an RCT of 2 versus 5 years of tamoxifen for women above 50 years, no difference in overall survival was observed even in ER-positive patients (hazard ratio = 0.98; 95% CI 0.72–1.32). Prolonging the therapy from 2 to 5 years doubled the risk of thromboembolic events (absolute excess number of thromboembolic events in 5-year arm as opposed to 2-year arm was 2.48 of 1000 women years for age 50–55, 2.96 of 1000 women years for women 56 to 65, and 2.75 of 1000 women years for women 66 to 70 years at diagnosis) and this excess risk was counterbalanced by the benefit derived from protection from contralateral breast cancer (Sacco *et al.*, 2003). Recently, aromatase inhibitors have been recommended in place of tamoxifen as endocrine therapy for ER positive tumors. The aromatase inhibitor anastrozole was compared with tamoxifen for 5 years in 9366 postmenopausal women with localized breast cancer. After a median follow-up of 68 months, anastrozole prolonged disease-free survival with a hazard ratio 0.87, 95% CI 0.78–0.97 and time to recurrence and reduced distant metastases (HR 0.86, 95% CI 0.74–0.99) and contralateral breast cancer (42% reduction, 95% CI 12–62). Anastrozole was associated with fewer side effects than tamoxifen, especially gynecological and vascular events, but fractures were increased (Howell *et al.*, 2005).

Ragaz and Coldman (1998), calculated the relative risk of mortality from thromboembolic events with tamoxifen use at age 50 to be 1.5. At age 80, it rose to 17.5.

The duration of tamoxifen use in women above 70 is an open question as there is no good data about long-term morbidity in this age-group. Newer aromatase inhibitors like anastrozole seem to carry a reduced risk of thrombotic episodes and need further evaluation in the elderly who are more prone to arterial and venous thrombosis.

CHEMOTHERAPY

Owing to concerns of excessive toxicity, there is a defeatist attitude toward chemotherapy in the elderly. Hence, women above 65 are not included in chemotherapy trials. In the National Institute of Health (NIH) consensus, chemotherapy is recommended only for women below 70 years of age.

Allocation to about 6 months of anthracycline-based poly-chemotherapy (e.g. with 5 flourouracil, adiamycin and cytoxan (FAC) or 5 flourouracil, epirubicin and cyclophosphamide (FEC)) reduces the annual breast cancer death rate by about 38% (SE 5) for women younger than 50 years of age when diagnosed and by about 20% (SE 4) for those of age 50–69 years when diagnosed, largely irrespective of the use of tamoxifen and of ER status, nodal status, or other tumor characteristics. Such regimens are significantly ($2p = 0.0001$ for recurrence, $2p < 0.00001$ for breast cancer mortality) more effective than cyclophosphamide, methrotraxate and 5 flourouracil (CMF) chemotherapy. Few women of age 70 years or older entered these chemotherapy trials (Early Breast Cancer Trialists' Collaborative Group (EBCTCG), 2005).

Recently, Taxanes have been tried in older women with good tolerance. Taxanes are considered a most effective drug in breast cancer, and have been tried on weekly regimens. The toxicity of weekly therapy is much lower than 3 weekly courses. Since there is decreased clearance of both paclitaxel and docetaxel in elderly, it seems safer to use lower doses of weekly regimens. A dose of paclitaxel 80 mg m^{-2} per week and docetaxel 36 mg m^{-2} per week is usually well tolerated with impressive response. Severe neutropenia, the dose limiting toxicity of 3 weekly regimen, is rare in weekly therapy (Wildiers and Paridaens, 2004).

In a phase II study of weekly docetaxel 36 mg m^{-2} among 47 frail or elderly patients with metastatic breast cancer, a response rate of 30% with low toxicity was achieved (D'hondt *et al.*, 2004).

TREATMENT OF ADVANCED DISEASE

Patients with locally advanced disease need evaluation by a combined breast care team and should be offered good local control by limited surgery and radiation followed by tamoxifen and chemotherapy (preferably Taxanes). Women presenting with a fungating or bleeding ulcer should not be denied the benefit of limited surgical ablation and coverage of the defect with a myocutaneous flap. Palliative hemostatic fractions of radiation may help arrest bleeding. Women with dissemination of cancer need systemic chemoendocrine administration till the level of tolerance and, later, tender loving care for the debility.

PROGNOSTIC FACTORS IN ELDERLY BREAST CANCER

Ian Fentimen, in an editorial in a recent issue of British Journal of Surgery (1), pointed out that 60% of deaths from breast cancer occurred in women of age 65 and above because of late diagnosis and treatment.

The outcome of the elderly patients and the posttreatment QoL has been studied by a number of authors.

Age has been considered an important determinant of the type of treatment and hence the outcome. In the CRUK, trial age and tumor size were found to predict mortality independently (Fennessy *et al.*, 2004).

Data from six regional National Cancer Institute Surveillance Epidemiology End Result Cancer registries evaluated a population-based random sample of 1800 patients in the age-group of 55 and above. Seventy-three percent of the women presented with stage I and II breast cancer, 10% with III and IV, and 17% did not have stage assignment. Of the 1017 cases with stage I and II, node negative disease, 95% of women received therapy in agreement with NIH consensus. Patients in older age-group were less likely to receive therapy according to the consensus statement. Women aged 70 years and above were significantly less likely to receive axillary lymph node dissection. Diabetes, renal failure, stroke, liver disease, and history of smoking were significant predictors of early mortality in a statistical logistic regression model that included age and disease stage. These authors concluded that patient care decision making occurs in the context of age and other comorbid conditions. Comorbidity in older patients results in less number of axillary dissections. As a result, information on axillary node is not available in many elderly patients. Breast cancer was the underlying cause of death in 51% and heart disease in 17%. The number of women getting breast conservation therapy is also reduced and comorbidity also increases the risk of death from breast cancer (Yancik *et al.*, 2001).

QUALITY-OF-LIFE ISSUES

The impact of the diagnosis of breast cancer and the effect of different therapeutic modalities has been addressed by a number of authors. Kroenke *et al.* (2004) from Harvard School of Medicine and Harvard school of Public Health reported changes in physical and psychological functions before and after breast cancer by age at diagnosis. From 122 969 women from the Nurses' Health Study (NHS) and NHS2 of age 29 to 71 years, who responded to a pre- and postfunctional status assessment, who were included, 1082 women were diagnosed with breast cancer between 1992 and 1997. FS was assessed using Short form SF-36. Mean changes in health-related quality of life (HRQoL) scores was computed. Compared with women ≤40 years without breast cancer, women with breast cancer experienced a functional decline. Young women who developed breast cancer experienced the largest decline in HRQoL as compared with older women in multiple domains such as physical roles, bodily pain, social functioning, and mental health. Much of the decline in HRQoL was age related (age ≥65 years).

A telephone survey was conducted from a random cross-sectional sample of 1812 medicare beneficiaries of 67 years and above treated for breast cancer 3–5 years earlier. The QoL and satisfaction with treatment were evaluated. The use of axillary dissection was the only surgical treatment that affected outcome, increasing the risk of arm problems fourfold (95% confidence interval 1.56–10.51). Having arm problems exerted a negative independent effect on all outcomes. Processes of care were also associated with QoL and satisfaction. Women who perceived high levels of agism or felt that they had no choice of treatment reported more bodily pain, lower mental health scores and less general satisfaction. These same factors as well as high perceived racism were significantly associated with diminished satisfaction with the medical care system. The authors concluded that with the exception of axillary dissection, the process of care and not the therapy itself are the most important determinants of long-term QoL in older women (Mandelblatt *et al.*, 2003).

VARIATION IN CARE OF ELDERLY

Monica Morrow in a review on treatment in the elderly noted that screening by physical exam and mammography is underutilized for the older women. Since mastectomy offers excellent local control and has only less than 1% operative mortality in women above 65, it should be offered to more (suitable) patients. She further points that failure to use adjuvant therapy when indicated is one of the most frequent problems in management of elderly (Morrow, 1994).

Pattern of care of elderly women is different from that offered to younger patients. In the study by Commission on Cancer of the American College of Surgeons for 1983 and 1990 (Busch *et al.*, 1996) in 1983, 23% of older women received total or partial mastectomy without axillary dissection compared with 8% of younger females. In 1990, the rate of total or partial mastectomy without nodal dissection was 20.6% in older women and 10% in younger women. The use of reconstruction was limited in the older women. The percentage of elderly females receiving reconstruction was 1.2% in 1983 and 1.3% in 1990. The operative mortality rates were higher in the older age-group (2.9% in 1983 and 1.5% in 1990). RT was used less frequently in the older group in both study years.

Gold and Dick (2004) reported the variation in the care of women with DCIS across the registries of the Surveillance, Epidemiology, and End Result (SEER) program in the United States. They studied 2701 women from SEER database from 1991 to 1996 aged 65 or over, diagnosed with unilateral DCIS. The results indicated significant geographic and temporal variations in treatment with increasing use of breast conservation alone. The treatment choice is explained by the particular SEER registry, diagnosis year, marital status, race, age, urban/rural status, educational attainment, and number of radiation oncologists. Increasing variability in treatment implies continued uncertainty about optimal therapy of DCIS.

In another retrospective review study from Italy on 1724 cases (median age 61, range 17–89) treated in 63 hospitals, 541 (38%) were inappropriately treated. More than two-thirds of these inappropriate surgical procedures were unnecessary Halsted Mastectomy. There was considerable geographical variation in the rate of appropriateness (range 52–88%). The authors suggested an urgent need of technology transfer to promote more appropriate surgical care and increased patient participation (Scorpiglione *et al.*, 1995). The same authors in another report on the same subjects (1724 cases) showed that elderly patients were less likely to have intensive diagnostic work-up, greater use of radical surgery and less use of limited surgery, independently of their overall health status. The presence of one or more coexistent diseases was associated with a failure to undergo axillary clearance and a lower utilization of conservative surgery, independent of age. The authors recommend the development of practice guidelines and their implementation to improve the quality of care (Nicolucci *et al.*, 1993).

In an editorial in Journal of Clinical Oncology, Rebecca A. Silliman (2003) chided clinicians for not offering definitive treatment to elderly women with breast cancer. Although breast cancer-specific mortality has declined among women younger than 70 years, they are either stable in 70–79 years or increased in women above 65 years of age. This proportion is likely to grow as older age is the most important risk factor for breast cancer and gains in life expectancy will result in more women being at risk for longer periods. Currently, the average life expectancy of a 75 year old is 12 years (17 years if she is healthy) and that of 85 years is 6 years (9 years if she is healthy). Owing to paucity of good evidence-based data, there is considerable controversy about what constitutes appropriate care for older women. More than one-fourth (27%) of breast cancer deaths in 2001 in the United States were in the age-group of 80 years and older. Although the patient's health status, patient and family preferences and support, and patient–physician interactions explain in part, age-related treatment variations, age alone remains an independent risk factor for less than definitive breast cancer care.

In a cohort of 407 octogenarian women from Canton province of Geneva, Switzerland, Bouchardy *et al.* (2003) addressed the relationship between undertreatment and breast cancer mortality. They used tumor registry data including sociodemographic data, comorbidity, tumor, and treatment characteristics, and the cause of death. The main problem they noted in analyzing this data was the issue of missing information – 20% for comorbidity, 49% for tumor grade, 74% for ER status. Because of loss of data on these important prognostic factors, there was a problem in multivariate analysis and incomplete control of confounding, decreasing the statistical power and precision. Both mastectomy plus adjuvant therapy and breast-conserving surgery plus adjuvant therapy appear to protect against death from causes other than breast cancer, suggesting residual confounding either because comorbidity was not well measured or because undertreatment of breast cancer is associated with undertreatment of other medical conditions. This cohort of Swiss women differed from women presenting elsewhere. The average tumor size in this group was 30 mm, only 22% presented in stage I, 22% received no therapy, 32% got tamoxifen alone. Despite the limitations of this study, it highlights the link between undertreatment and high rate of breast cancer recurrence and mortality.

A similar study from Quebec, Canada, assessed the variation in care with age. Herbert-Croteau *et al.* (1999) selected a stratified random sample of 1174 women from new cases of node negative breast cancer of age 50 and above. Women over 70 were less likely to receive definitive locoregional treatment than younger women (48 vs 83%; $p < 0.0001$). Older women were less likely to receive breast-conserving surgery (76 vs 86%; $p < 0.0001$) and RT (54 vs 90%; $p < 0.0001$), axillary dissection (55 vs 86%; $p < 0.0001$), or receive chemotherapy (1.2 vs 13%; $p < 0.0001$). Tamoxifen was given equally to both the groups (66 vs 64%; $p = 0.41$). Adjusting for comorbidity and other disease characteristics, age remained the strong determinant of definitive therapy (odds ratio 0.14; 95% CI 0.12–0.18 for age ≥70 vs age 50–69 years). The authors lamented that elderly women receive less aggressive therapy independent of comorbidity.

CONCLUSIONS

Breast Cancer in the elderly is inadequately diagnosed with a significant delay. Many women are improperly treated, as there is a lack of practice guidelines for women above 65 years of age. Screening and prevention strategies need to be applied more rigorously to older women. The same therapeutic principles and selection criteria should be utilized as established for the younger women. Breast care providers need to be cognizant of the associated illnesses and tailor therapy to suit the tolerance of the individual case.

GUIDELINES FOR THERAPY

The present knowledge base supports the following general guideline for the elderly:

<4 cm tumor, ER+ve → BCT + axillary dissection + RT + Tamoxifen

<4 cm tumor, ER+ve on warfarin/ Stroke /Deep vein thrombosis

→ BCT + axillary dissection + RT + Anastrozole

<4 cm tumor, ER−ve → BCT + axillary dissection + RT + Chemotherapy with weekly Taxanes if patient is rich, otherwise CMF; Consider Herceptin

>4 cm tumor, ER+ve → MRM + RT + Tamoxifen

>4 cm tumor, ER−ve → MRM + RT + Chemotherapy; Consider Herceptin. Consider downstaging for large tumors by neoadjuvant Anastrozole/Tamoxifen with or without chemotherapy prior to operation.

More elderly patients should be recruited in trials to expand the evidence base not confounded by ageist bias. Oncologists ought to explore newer modes of delivering less toxic chemotherapy, intraoperative radiotherapy and biological response modifiers. Interventions to address the physical and emotional needs of older women with breast cancer should be developed.

KEY POINTS

- Improve awareness among the geriatric care providers for early diagnosis.
- Apply screening and prevention strategies similar to younger women to reduce the burden of disease and morbidity of therapy.
- Apply same therapeutic principles as in younger women.
- Recruit more elder women in therapeutic trials and develop practice guidelines.
- Be cognizant of comorbidity and tailor therapy accordingly.

KEY REFERENCES

- Early Breast Cancer Trialists' Collaborative Group (EBCTCG). Effects of chemotherapy and hormonal therapy for early breast cancer on recurrence and 15-year survival: an overview of the randomised trials. *Lancet* 2005; **365**:1687–717.
- Howell A, Cuzick J, Baum M *et al.*, ATAC Trialists' Group. Results of the ATAC (Arimidex, Tamoxifen, alone or in combination) trial after completion of 5 years' adjuvant treatment for breast cancer. *Lancet* 2005; **365**(9453):60–2.
- Million Women Study Collaborators. Breast cancer and hormone-replacement therapy in the million women study. *Lancet* 2003; **362**:419–27.
- Solin LJ, Schultz DJ & Fowble BL. Ten year results of the treatment of early stage breast carcinoma in elderly women using breast-conserving surgery and definitive breast irradiation. *International Journal of Radiation Oncology, Biology, Physics* 1995; **33**(1):45–51.
- Veronesi U, Salvadori B, Luini A *et al.* Breast conservation is a safe method in patients with small cancer of the breast. Long-term results of three randomised trials on 1,973 patients. *European Journal of Cancer* 1995; **31A**(10):1574–9.

REFERENCES

Berg JW & Robbins GF. Modified mastectomy for older, poor risk patients. *Surgery, Gynecology & Obstetrics* 1961; **113**:631–4.

Bouchardy C, Rapiti E, Fioretta G *et al.* Undertreatment strongly decreases prognosis of breast cancer in elderly women. *Journal of Clinical Oncology* 2003; **21**:3580–7.

Busch E, Kemeny M, Fremgen A *et al.* Patterns of breast cancer care in the elderly. *Cancer* 1996; **78**:101–11.

Chen H-H, Tabar L, Faggerberg G & Duffy SW. Effect of breast screening after age 65. *Journal of Medical Screening* 1995; **2**:10–4.

Coombes RC, Hall E, Gibson LJ *et al.*, Intergroup Exemestane Study. A randomized trial of exemestane after two to three years of tamoxifen therapy in postmenopausal women with primary breast cancer. *The New England Journal of Medicine* 2004; **350**(11):1081–92.

Crivellari D, Price K, Gelber RD *et al.* Adjuvant endocrine therapy compared with no systemic therapy for elderly women with early breast cancer: 21-year results of international breast cancer study group trial IV. *Journal of Clinical Oncology* 2003; **21**(24):4517–23.

Crowe JP, Gordon NH, Shenk RR *et al.* Age does not predict breast cancer outcome. *Archives of Surgery* 1994; **129**:483–8.

Davis SJ, Karrer FW, Moose BJ *et al.* Characteristics of breast cancer in women over 80 years of age. *American Journal of Surgery* 1985; **150**:655–8.

de Groot V, Beckerman H, Lankhorst GJ & Bouter LM. How to measure comorbidity: a critical review of available methods. *Journal of Clinical Epidemiology* 2003; **56**:221–9.

Devitt JE. The influence of age on the behaviour of carcinoma of the breast. *Canadian Medical Association Journal* 1970; **103**:923–6.

D'hondt R, Paridaens R, Wildiers H *et al.* Safety and efficacy of weekly docetaxel in frail and/or elderly patients with metastatic breast cancer: a phase II study. *Anti-cancer Drugs* 2004; **15**(4):341–6.

Early Breast Cancer Trialists' Collaborative Group (EBCTCG). Effects of chemotherapy and hormonal therapy for early breast cancer on recurrence and 15-year survival: an overview of the randomised trials. *Lancet* 2005; **365**:1687–717.

Feinstein AR. The pre-therapeutic classification of co-morbidity in chronic disease. *Journal of Chronic Diseases* 1970; **23**:455–68.

Fennessy M, Bates T, MacRae K *et al.* Late follow-up of a randomized trial of surgery plus tamoxifen versus tamoxifen alone in women aged over 70 years with operable breast cancer. *The British Journal of Surgery* 2004; **91**:699–704.

Fentiman IS. Improving the outcome for older women with breast cancer. *The British Journal of Surgery* 2004; **91**:655–6.

Fentiman IS, Christiaens MR, Paridaens R *et al.* Treatment of operable breast cancer in the elderly: a randomized clinical trial EORTC 10851 comparing tamoxifen alone with modified radical mastectomy. *European Journal of Cancer* 2003a; **39**:309–16.

Fentiman IS, Van Zijl J, Karydas I *et al.* Treatment of operable breast cancer in the elderly: a randomized trial EORTC 10850 comparing modified radical mastectomy with tumorectomy plus tamoxifen. *European Journal of Cancer* 2003b; **39**:300–8.

Ganz PA, Guadagnoli E, Landrum MB *et al.* Breast cancer in older women: quality of life and psychosocial adjustment in the 15 months after diagnosis. *Journal of Clinical Oncology* 2003; **21**(21):4027–33.

Gennari R, Curigliano G, Rotmensz N *et al.* Breast carcinoma in elderly women: features of disease presentation, choice of local and systemic treatments compared with younger postmenopausal patients. *Cancer* 2004; **101**(6):1302–10.

Gold HT & Dick AW. Variations in treatment for Ductal Carcinoma in situ in elderly women. *Medical Care* 2004; **42**(3):267–75.

Goodwin JS, Samet JM, Key CR *et al.* Stage at diagnosis of cancer varies with the age of the patient. *Journal of the American Geriatrics Society* 1986; **34**:20.

Gruenberger T, Gorlitzer M, Soliman T *et al.* It is possible to omit postoperative irradiation in a highly selected group of elderly breast cancer patients. *Breast Cancer Research and Treatment* 1998; **50**(1):37–46.

Herbert-Croteau N, Brisson J, Latreille J *et al.* Compliance with consensus recommendations for the treatment of early stage breast carcinoma in elderly women. *Cancer* 1999; **85**(5):1104–13.

Herman CJ, Speroff T & Cebul RD. Improving compliance with breast cancer screening in older women. *Archives of Internal Medicine* 1995; **155**:717–22.

Homes FF & Hearne E. Cancer stage-to-age relationship: implication for cancer screening in the elderly. *Journal of the American Geriatrics Society* 1981; **29**:55.

Host H. Age as a prognostic factor in breast cancer. *Cancer* 1986; **57**:2217–21.

Howell A, Cuzick J, Baum M *et al.*, ATAC Trialists' Group. Results of the ATAC (Arimidex, Tamoxifen, alone or in combination) trial after completion of 5 years' adjuvant treatment for breast cancer. *Lancet* 2005; **365**(9453):60–2.

Kemeny MM, Peterson BL, Kornblith AB *et al.* Barriers to clinical trial participation by older women with breast cancer. *Journal of Clinical Oncology* 2003; **21**:2268–75.

Kroenke CH, Rosner B, Chen WY *et al.* Functional impact of breast cancer by age at diagnosis. *Journal of Clinical Oncology* 2004; **22**(10):1849–56.

Law TM, Hesketh PJ, Porter KA *et al.* Breast cancer in elderly women. *The Surgical Clinics of North America* 1996; **76**(2):289–308.

Mandelblatt JS, Edge SB, Meropol NJ *et al.* Predictor of long – term outcomes in older breast cancer survivors: perceptions versus patterns of care. *Journal of Clinical Oncology* 2003; **21**(5):855–63.

Million Women Study Collaborators. Breast cancer and hormone-replacement therapy in the million women study. *Lancet* 2003; **362**:419–27.

Morrow M. Breast disease in elderly women. *The Surgical Clinics of North America* 1994; **74**(1):145–61.

Mustacchi G, Ceccherini R, Milani S *et al.*, Italian Cooperative Group GRETA. Tamoxifen alone versus adjuvant tamoxifen for operable breast cancer of the elderly: long-term results of the phaseIII randomized controlled multicenter GRETA trial. *Annals of Oncology* 2003; **14**(3):414–20.

Newschaffer CJ, Penberthy L, Desch CE *et al.* The effect of age and comorbidity in the treatment of elderly women with non metastatic breast cancer. *Archives of Internal Medicine* 1996; **156**:85–90.

NHS Breast Cancer screening Programme in the UK. 2005, www.cancer-screening.nhs.uk/breastscreen/publications/nhsbsp_annualreview2004; http://www.cancerscreening.nhs.uk/breastscreen/ - footnote5#footnote5.

Nicolucci A, Mainini F, Penna A *et al.* The influence of patient characteristics on the appropriateness of surgical treatment for breast cancer patients. progetto oncologia femminile. *Annals of Oncology* 1993; **4**(2):133–40.

Punglia RS, Kuntz KM, Lee JH & Recht A. Radiation therapy plus tamoxifen versus tamoxifen alone after breast-conserving surgery in postmenopausal women with stage I breast cancer: a decision analysis. *Journal of Clinical Oncology* 2003; **21**(12):2260–7.

Ragaz J & Coldman A. Survival impact of adjuvant tamoxifen on competing causes of mortality in breast cancer survivors, with analysis of mortality from contralateral breast cancer, cardiovascular events, endometrial cancer and thromboembolic episodes. *Journal of Clinical Oncology* 1998; **16**:2018–24.

Robertson JF, Todd JH, Ellis IO *et al.* Comparison of mastectomy with tamoxifen for treating elderly patients with operable breast cancer. *British Medical Journal* 1988; **297**(6647):511–4.

Robin RE & Lee D. Carcinoma of the breast in women 80 years of age and older: still a lethal disease. *American Journal of Surgery* 1985; **140**:606–9.

Rosen P, Lesser M & Linne D. Breast carcinoma at the extremes of age: a comparison of patients younger than 35 years and older than 75 years. *Journal of Surgical Oncology* 1985; **28**:90.

Rutqvist LE & Mattsson A, The Stockholm Breast Cancer Study Group. Cardiac and thromboembolic morbidity among postmenopausal women with early stage breast cancer in a randomized trial of adjuvant tamoxifen. *Journal of the National Cancer Institute* 1993; **85**(17):1398–406.

Sacco M, Valentini M, Belfiglio M *et al.* Randomized trial of 2 versus 5 years of adjuvant tamoxifen for women aged 50 years or older with early breast cancer: Italian interdisciplinary group for cancer evaluation study of adjuvant treatment in breast cancer. *Journal of Clinical Oncology* 2003; **21**:2276–81.

Scorpiglione N, Nicolucci A, Grill R *et al.* Appropriateness and variation of surgical treatment of breast cancer in Italy: when excellence in clinical research does not match with generalized good quality care. *Journal of Clinical Epidemiology* 1995; **48**(3):345–52.

Silliman RA. What constitutes optimal care for older women with breast cancer? *Journal of Clinical Oncology* 2003; **21**(19):3554–6.

Singh R, Hellman S & Heimann R. The natural history of breast carcinoma in the elderly, implications for screening and treatment. *Cancer* 2004; **100**(9):1807–13.

Solin LJ, Schultz DJ & Fowble BL. Ten year results of the treatment of early stage breast carcinoma in elderly women using breast-conserving surgery and definitive breast irradiation. *International Journal of Radiation Oncology, Biology, Physics* 1995; **33**(1):45–51.

Stahlberg C, Pedersen AT, Lynge E *et al.* Increased risk of breast cancer following different regimens of hormone replacement therapy frequently used in Europe. *International Journal of Cancer* 2004; **109**(5):721–7.

Truong PT, Wong E, Bernstein V *et al.* Adjuvant radiation therapy after breast-conserving surgery in elderly women with early-stage breast cancer: controversy or consensus? *Clinical Breast Cancer* 2004; **4**(6):407–14.

Veronesi U, Salvadori B, Luini A *et al.* Breast conservation is a safe method in patients with small cancer of the breast. Long-term results of three randomised trials on 1,973 patients. *European Journal of Cancer* 1995; **31A**(10):1574–9.

Wang J, Costanino JP, Tan-Chiu E *et al.* Lower-category benign breast disease and the risk of invasive breast cancer. *Journal of the National Cancer Institute* 2004; **96**(8):616–20.

Wildiers H & Paridaens R. Taxanes in elderly breast cancer patients. *Cancer Treatment Reviews* 2004; **30**(4):333–42.

Yancik R, Wesley MN, Ries LAG *et al.* Effect of age and comorbidity in postmenopausal breast cancer patients aged 55 years and older. *The Journal of the American Medical Association* 2001; **285**:885–92.

PART III

Medicine in Old Age

Section 13

Functional Disorders and Rehabilitation

131

Multidimensional Geriatric Assessment

Laurence Z. Rubenstein[1] *and* **Andreas E. Stuck**[2]

[1] Geriatric Research Education and Clinical Center, UCLA – Greater Los Angeles Veterans' Affairs Medical Center, CA, USA, and [2] Department of Geriatric Medicine, Spital Bern Ziegler, Bern, Switzerland

INTRODUCTION

The essence of a good geriatric practice is the expert management of the medical, psychological, and social needs of elderly patients and their family caregivers. In order to accomplish this, the members of the interdisciplinary geriatric team – whether based in a hospital geriatric unit, an outpatient clinic, a nursing home, or a home-care program – must work closely together to carefully assess the patient's risks and problems and translate the knowledge into care plans that will have far-reaching effects on both the patient's and the caregiver's lives.

Such multidimensional assessment implies the detailed investigation of the elderly individual's total situation in terms of physical and mental state, functional status, formal and informal social support and network, and physical environment. This requires the clinician to become involved in collecting, interpreting, synthesizing, and weighing a formidable amount of patient-specific information. Much of this differs in kind from the physical symptoms and signs, laboratory values, radiology results, and other data that are traditionally combined to reach a medical diagnosis.

Definition

Multidimensional geriatric assessment is a diagnostic process, usually interdisciplinary, intended to determine an elderly person's medical, psychosocial, functional, and environmental resources and problems, with the objective of developing an overall plan for treatment and long-term follow-up. The process differs from the standard medical evaluation in its concentration on elderly people with their often complex problems, its emphasis on functional status and quality of life, and its frequent use of interdisciplinary teams and quantitative assessment scales.

As described in this chapter, multidimensional geriatric assessment can vary in its level of detail, its purpose, and other aspects depending on the clinical circumstances. Therefore, multidimensional assessment denotes both the relatively brief multidimensional screening assessment for preventive purpose in a patient's home as well as the interdisciplinary work-up of a newly hospitalized patient. Despite this broad definition, the term must meet the primary criteria above. For example, a multidimensional evaluation of an elderly person without any link to the overall plan for treatment and follow-up does not meet these criteria. Similarly, a home visit emphasizing psychosocial and environmental factors, but not including a medical evaluation of the elderly person, is not a multidimensional assessment, since one of the key components of the multidimensionality is not included.

Rationale

While the principles of geriatric assessment may be valid in the treatment of younger persons as well, since biopsychosocial factors play an important role in medicine for patients of all age-groups, there is additional justification for using this multidimensional approach in elderly people for various reasons:

- *Multimorbidity and complexity*: Many elderly people suffer from multiple conditions, and multidimensional assessment helps to deal with these complex situations through its systematic approaches and its setting of priorities.
- *Unrecognized problems*: Many elderly people suffer from problems that have not been reported to the physician or may not even be known to the elderly person. One of the reasons problems may go undetected is that they may be falsely considered as nonmodifiable consequences of aging. Multidimensional geriatric assessment is a method for identifying previously unknown problems.
- *Chronic conditions*: Many elderly people suffer from chronic conditions. Diagnostic information without information on functional relevance of the underlying condition

Principles and Practice of Geriatric Medicine, 4th Edition. Edited by M.S. John Pathy, Alan J. Sinclair and John E. Morley.

is often of limited value for therapeutic decisions or for monitoring follow-up.

- *Interaction with social and environmental factors*: Once functional impairments or dependencies arise, the elderly person's condition is strongly influenced by his or her social and physical environment. For example, the arrangement of the elderly person's in-home environment and the availability of his or her social network might determine whether a person can continue to live in his or her home.
- *Functional status*: One of the main objectives of medicine for elderly people is to prevent or delay the onset of functional status decline. Epidemiological research has shown that functional status decline is related to medical, functional, psychological, social, and environmental risk factors. Therefore, for both rehabilitation as well as prevention, the approach of multidimensional assessment helps to take into account potentially modifiable factors in all relevant domains.
- *Intervention studies*: Multiple intervention studies that compared the effects of programs on the basis of the concept of multidimensional geriatric assessment with usual care did show benefits of geriatric assessment, including better patient outcomes and more efficient health-care use.

Brief History of Geriatric Assessment

The basic concepts of geriatric assessment have evolved over the past 70 years by combining elements of the traditional medical history and physical examination, the social worker assessment, functional evaluation and treatment methods derived from rehabilitation medicine, and psychometric methods derived from the social sciences.

The first published reports of geriatric assessment programs (GAPs) came from the British geriatrician Marjory Warren, who initiated the concept of specialized geriatric assessment units during the late 1930s while in charge of a large London infirmary. This infirmary was filled primarily with chronically ill, bedfast, and largely neglected elderly patients who had not received proper medical diagnosis or rehabilitation and who were thought to be in need of lifelong institutionalization. Good nursing care kept the patients alive, but the lack of diagnostic assessment and rehabilitation kept them disabled. Through evaluation, mobilization, and rehabilitation, Warren was able to get most of the long bedfast patients out of bed and often discharged home. As a result of her experiences, Warren advocated that every elderly patient receive comprehensive assessment and an attempt at rehabilitation before being admitted to a long-term care hospital or nursing home (Matthews, 1984).

Since Warren's work, geriatric assessment has evolved. As geriatric care systems have been developed throughout the world, GAPs have been assigned central roles, usually as focal points for entry into the care systems (Brocklehurst, 1975). Geared to differing local needs and populations, GAPs vary in intensity, structure, and function. They can be located in different settings, including acute hospital inpatient units and consultation teams, chronic and rehabilitation hospital units, outpatient and office-based programs, and home-visit outreach programs. Despite diversity, they share many characteristics. Virtually all programs provide multidimensional assessment, utilizing specific measurement instruments to quantify functional, psychological, and social parameters. Most use interdisciplinary teams to pool expertise and enthusiasm in working toward common goals. Additionally, most programs attempt to couple their assessments with an intervention, such as rehabilitation, counseling, or placement.

Today, geriatric assessment continues to evolve in response to increased pressures for cost containment, avoidance of institutional stays, and consumer demands for better care. Geriatric assessment can help achieve improved quality of care and plan cost-effective care. This has generally meant more emphasis on noninstitutional programs and shorter hospital stays. Geriatric assessment teams are well positioned to deliver effective care for elderly persons with limited resources. Geriatricians have long emphasized judicious use of technology, systematic preventive medicine activities, and less institutionalization and hospitalization.

COMPONENTS OF GERIATRIC ASSESSMENT

A typical geriatric assessment begins with a functional status "review of systems" that inventories the major domains of functioning. The major elements of this review of systems are captured in two commonly used functional status measures – basic activities of daily living (ADL) and instrumental activities of daily living (IADL). Several reliable and valid versions of these measures have been developed (Rubenstein *et al.*, 1987a; Rubenstein *et al.*, 1995a; Kane and Kane, 2000; Osterweil *et al.*, 2000; Gallo *et al.*, 2000), perhaps the most widely used being those by Katz *et al.* (1963), Lawton and Brody (1969), and Barthel (Mahoney and Barthel, 1965; Wade and Colin, 1988). These scales are used by clinicians to detect whether the patient has problems performing activities that people must be able to accomplish to survive without help in the community. Basic ADL include self-care activities such as eating, dressing, bathing, transferring, and toileting. Patients unable to perform these activities will generally require 12–24-hour support by caregivers. Instrumental activities of daily living include heavier housework, going on errands, managing finances, and telephoning – activities that are required if the individual is to remain independent in a house or an apartment.

In order to interpret the results of impairments in ADL and IADL, physicians will usually need additional information about the patient's environment and social situation. For example, the amount and type of caregiver support available, the strength of the patient's social network, and the level of social activities in which the patient participates will all influence the clinical approach taken in managing the detected deficits. This information could be obtained by an experienced nurse or a social worker. A screen for mobility and fall risk is also extremely helpful in quantifying function and disability, and several observational scales are available (Tinetti, 1986; Mathias *et al.*, 1986). An assessment of nutritional status and risk for undernutrition is also important in understanding the extent of impairment and for planning care (Vellas and Guigoz, 1995). Likewise, a screening assessment of vision and hearing will often detect crucial deficits that need to be treated or compensated for.

There are two other key pieces of information that must always be gathered in the face of functional disability in an elderly person. These are a screen for mental status (cognitive) impairment and a screen for depression (Rubenstein *et al.*, 1987a; Rubenstein *et al.*, 1995a; Gallo *et al.*, 2000). Among the several validated screening tests for cognitive function, the Folstein Mini-mental State is one of the best tests because of its efficiency to test the major aspects of cognitive functioning (Folstein *et al.*, 1975). Among the various screening tests for geriatric depression, the Yesavage Geriatric Depression Scale (Yesavage *et al.*, 1983), and the Zung Self-rating Depression Scale (Zung, 1965) are in wide use, and even shorter screening versions are available without significant loss of accuracy (Hoyl *et al.*, 1999).

The major measurable dimensions of geriatric assessment, together with examples of commonly used health status screening scales, are listed in Table 1 (Rubenstein *et al.*, 1987a; Rubenstein *et al.*, 1995a; Kane and Kane, 2000; Osterweil *et al.*, 2000; Gallo *et al.*, 2000; Katz *et al.*, 1963; Lawton and Brody, 1969; Mahoney and Barthel, 1965; Wade and Colin, 1988; Tinetti, 1986; Mathias *et al.*, 1986; Vellas and Guigoz, 1995; Folstein *et al.*, 1975; Yesavage *et al.*, 1983; Zung, 1965; Hoyl *et al.*, 1999; Rubenstein, 1996; Hedrick, 1995; Kane, 1995; Rubenstein *et al.*, 2001; Gurland and Wilder, 1995; Duke University Center for the Study of Aging and Human Development, 1978; Lubben, 1988; Kahn *et al.*, 1960; Chambers *et al.*, 1982; Reisberg *et al.*, 1982; Hoehn and Yahr, 1967; Stewart *et al.*, 1988; Nelson *et al.*, 1987; Bergner *et al.*, 1981; Jette *et al.*, 1986). The instruments listed are short, have been carefully tested for reliability and validity, and can be easily administered by virtually any staff person involved with the assessment process. Both observational instruments (e.g. physical examination) and self-report (completed by patient or proxy) are available. Components of them – such as watching a patient walk, turn around, and sit down – are routine parts of the geriatric physical examination. Many other kinds of assessment measures exist and can be useful in certain situations. For example, there are several disease-specific measures for stages and levels of dysfunction for patients with specific diseases such as arthritis (Chambers *et al.*, 1982), dementia (Reisberg *et al.*, 1982), and parkinsonism (Hoehn and Yahr, 1967). There are also several brief global assessment instruments that attempt to quantify all dimensions of the assessment in a single form (Stewart *et al.*, 1988; Nelson *et al.*, 1987; Bergner *et al.*, 1981; Jette *et al.*, 1986). These latter instruments can be useful in community surveys and some research settings but are not detailed enough to be useful in most clinical settings. More comprehensive lists of available instruments can be found by consulting published reviews of health status assessment (Rubenstein *et al.*, 1987a; Rubenstein *et al.*, 1995a; Kane and Kane, 2000; Osterweil *et al.*, 2000; VanSwearington and Brach, 2001).

SETTINGS OF GERIATRIC ASSESSMENT

A number of factors must be taken into account in deciding where an assessment should take place – whether it should be done in the hospital, in an outpatient setting, or in

Table 1 Measurable dimensions of geriatric assessment with examples of specific measures

Dimension	Basic context	Specific examples
Basic ADL (Hoyl *et al.*, 1999; Hedrick, 1995)	Strengths and limitations in self-care, basic mobility, and incontinence	Katz (ADL) (Katz *et al.*, 1963), Lawton personal self-maintenance scale (Lawton and Brody, 1969) Barthel index (Mahoney and Barthel, 1965; Wade and Colin, 1988)
IADL (Hedrick, 1995)	Strengths and limitations in shopping, cooking, household activities, and finances	Lawton (IADL) (Lawton and Brody, 1969) OARS, IADL section (Duke University Center for the Study of Aging and Human Development, 1978)
Social activities and supports (Kane, 1995)	Strengths and limitations in social network and community activities	Lubben social network scale (Lubben, 1988) OARS, Social resources section (Duke University Center for the Study of Aging and Human Development, 1978)
Mental health Affective (Gurland and Wilder, 1995)	Degree of anxiety, depression, and happiness	Geriatric depression scale (Yesavage *et al.*, 1983; Hoyl *et al.*, 1999) Zung depression scale (Zung, 1965)
Mental health Cognitive (Gurland and Wilder, 1995) Questionnaire (Kahn *et al.*, 1960)	Degree of alertness, orientation, concentration, and mental task capacity	Folstein mini-mental state (Folstein *et al.*, 1975) Kahn mental status
Mobility, gait, and balance (Lawton and Brody, 1969; Wade and Colin, 1988)	Quantification of gait, balance, and risk of falls	Tinetti mobility assessment (Tinetti, 1986) Get-up-and-go test (Mathias *et al.*, 1986)
Nutritional checklist (Vellas and Guigoz, 1995) Adequacy (Vellas and Guigoz, 1995)	Current nutritional status and risk of malnutrition	Nutritional screening Mini-nutritional assessment (Rubenstein *et al.*, 2001)

ADL, Activities of Daily Living; IADL, Instrumental Activities of Daily Living.

the patient's home. Mental and physical impairment make it difficult for patients to comply with recommendations and to navigate multiple appointments in multiple locations. Functionally impaired elders must depend on families and friends, who risk losing their jobs because of chronic and relentless demands on time and energy and in their roles as caregivers, and who may be elderly themselves. Each separate medical appointment or intervention has a high time-cost to these caregivers. Patient fatigue during periods of increased illness may require the availability of a bed during the assessment process. Finally, enough physician time and expertise must be available to complete the assessment within the constraints of the setting.

Most geriatric assessments neither require the full range of technology nor the intense monitoring found in the acute-care inpatient setting. Yet, hospitalization becomes unavoidable if no outpatient setting provides sufficient resources to accomplish the assessment fast enough. A specialized geriatric setting outside an acute hospital ward, such as a day hospital or subacute inpatient geriatric evaluation unit, will provide the easy availability of an interdisciplinary team with the time and expertise to provide needed services efficiently, an adequate level of monitoring, and beds for patients unable to sit or stand for prolonged periods. Inpatient and day hospital assessment programs have the advantages of intensity, rapidity, and ability to care for particularly frail or acutely ill patients. Outpatient programs are generally cheaper and avoid the necessity of an inpatient stay.

Assessment in the Office Practice Setting

A streamlined approach is usually necessary in the office setting. An important first step is setting priorities among problems for initial evaluation and treatment. The "best" problem to work on primarily might be the problem that most bothers a patient or, alternatively, the problem upon which resolution of other problems depends (alcoholism or depression often fall into this category).

The second step in performing a geriatric assessment is to understand the exact nature of the disability by performing a task or a symptom analysis. In a nonspecialized setting, or when the disability is mild or clear cut, this may involve taking only a careful history. When the disability is more severe, more detailed assessments by a multidisciplinary or interdisciplinary team may be necessary. For example, a patient may present with difficulty in dressing. There are multiple tasks associated with dressing, any one of which might be the stumbling block (e.g. buying clothes, choosing appropriate clothes to put on, remembering to complete the task, buttoning, stretching to put on shirts, or reaching downward to put on shoes). By identifying the exact areas of difficulty, further evaluation can be targeted toward solving the problem.

Once the history reveals the nature of the disability, a systematic physical examination and ancillary laboratory tests are needed to clarify the cause of the problem. For example, difficulty in dressing could be caused by mental status impairment, poor finger mobility, or dysfunction of shoulders, back, or hips. An evaluation by a physical or occupational therapist may be necessary to pinpoint the problem adequately, and evaluation by a social worker may be required to determine the extent of family dysfunction engendered by or contributing to the dependency. Radiologic and other laboratory tests may also be necessary.

Each abnormality that could cause difficulty in dressing suggests different treatments. By understanding the abnormalities that contribute the most to the functional disability, the best treatment strategy can be undertaken. Often one disability leads to another – impaired gait may lead to depression or decreased social functioning; and immobility of any cause, even after the cause has been removed, can lead to secondary impairments in performance of daily activities due to deconditioning and loss of musculoskeletal flexibility.

Almost any acute or chronic disease can reduce functioning. Some common but easily overlooked causes of dysfunction in elderly people include impaired cognition, impaired special senses (vision, hearing, balance), unstable gait and mobility, poor health habits (alcohol, smoking, lack of exercise), poor nutrition, polypharmacy, incontinence, psychosocial stress, and depression. In order to identify the contributing causes of the disability, the physician must look for worsening of the patient's chronic diseases, occurrence of a new acute disease, or appearance of one of the common occult diseases listed above. The physician does this through a refocused history guided by the functional disabilities detected and their differential diagnoses, and a focused physical examination. The physical examination always includes, in addition to usual evaluations of the heart, lungs, extremities, and neurologic function, postural blood pressure, vision and hearing screening, and a careful observation of the patient's gait. The mini-mental state examination, already recommended as part of the initial functional status screen, may also determine the parts of the physical examination that require particular attention as part of the evaluation of dementia or acute confusion. Finally, basic laboratory testing including a complete blood count and a blood chemistry panel, as well as tests indicated on the basis of specific findings from the history and physical examination, will generally be necessary.

Once the disability and its causes are understood, the best treatments or management strategies for it are often clear. When a reversible cause for the impairment is found, a simple treatment may eliminate or ameliorate the functional disability. When the disability is complex, the physician may need the support of a variety of community or hospital-based resources. In most cases, a strategy for long-term follow-up and often, formal case management should be developed to ensure that needs and services are appropriately matched up and followed through.

Preventive Home Visits

Preventive home visitation programs in elderly people are part of a national policy in several countries. The rationale is to delay or prevent functional impairment and subsequent nursing home admissions by primary prevention (e.g. immunization and exercise), secondary prevention (e.g. detection of untreated problems), and tertiary prevention (e.g. improvement of medication use).

This is a typical description of a preventive home visitation program (Stuck *et al.*, 1995a). "The assessment included a medical history taking, a physical examination, hematocrit and glucose measurements in blood samples obtained by finger stick, a dipstick urinalysis, and a mail-in fecal occult-blood test. The subjects were also evaluated for functional status, oral health, mental status (presence or absence of depression and cognitive status), gait and balance, medications, percentage of ideal body weight, vision, hearing, extensiveness of social network, quality of social support, and safety in the home and ease of access to the external environment. The nurse practitioners discussed each case with the project geriatricians, developed rank-ordered recommendations, and conducted in-home follow-up visits every three months to monitor the implementation of the recommendations, make additional recommendations if new problems were detected, and facilitate compliance. If additional contact was considered necessary, the nurse practitioner telephoned the participant or was available by telephone. All the participants were encouraged to take an active role in their care and to improve their ability to discuss problems with their physicians. Only in complex situations did the nurse practitioners or study physicians contact the patients' physicians directly".

A variety of studies have shown the advantage of the home environment in conducting a multidimensional assessment. The yield of a home visit does not seem to be limited to the preventive application; home visits can also play an important role as part of outpatient or inpatient programs.

Inpatient Geriatric Assessment

If a referral to a specialized geriatric setting has been chosen, the process of assessment will probably be similar to that described above, except that the greater intensity of resources and the special training of all the members of the multidisciplinary team in dealing with geriatric patients and their problems will facilitate carrying out the proposed assessment and the plan more quickly, and in greater breadth and detail. In the usual geriatric assessment setting, the key disciplines involved include, at a minimum, physicians, social workers, nurses, and physical and occupational therapists, and optimally may also include other disciplines such as dieticians, pharmacists, ethicists, and home-care specialists. A special geriatric expertise among the interdisciplinary team members is crucial.

The interdisciplinary team conference, which takes place after most team members have completed their individual assessments, is critical. Most of the successful trials of geriatric assessment have included such a team conference. By bringing the perspectives of all disciplines together, the team conference generates new ideas, sets priorities, disseminates the full results of the assessment to all those involved in treating the patient, and avoids duplication or incongruity. The development of fully effective teams requires commitment, skill, and time as the interdisciplinary team evolves through the "forming, storming, and norming" phases to reach the fully developed "performing" stage (Campbell and Cole, 1987). The involvement of the patient (and carer if appropriate) at some stage is important in maintaining the principle of choice (Campbell and Cole, 1987; Wieland *et al.*, 1996).

Hospital-home Assessment Programs

A number of additional published reports have described another multidimensional assessment model in which hospitalized elderly patients in need of comprehensive assessment are referred to an in-home assessment program that occurs in their homes following the hospital discharge. The advantages of this approach include shortening the hospital stay, providing the assessment in the home environment that allows evaluation of the home itself and how the patient functions therein, and allowing careful targeting of the in-home assessment to individuals who can derive maximal benefit.

A special approach has been tested in elderly patients with cardiac risk. In these patients, geriatric assessment in the hospital was combined with a systematic ambulatory follow-up. An early detection of heart failure and optimizing patient adherence with medication prescriptions were the key ingredients of these programs (Gwadry-Sridhar *et al.*, 2004). Several studies have confirmed that geriatric assessment also reduces unnecessary or inappropriate medications use.

EFFECTIVENESS OF GERIATRIC ASSESSMENT PROGRAMS

A large and still growing literature supports the effectiveness of GAPs in a variety of settings. Early descriptive studies indicated a number of benefits from GAPs such as improved diagnostic accuracy, reduced discharges to nursing homes, increased functional status, and more appropriate medication prescribing. Since they were descriptive studies, without concurrent control patients, they were neither able to distinguish the effects of the programs from simple improvement over time nor did these studies look at long-term, or many short-term outcome benefits. Nonetheless, many of these early studies provided promising results (William *et al.*, 1964; Lowther *et al.*, 1970; Brocklehurst *et al.*, 1978; Applegate *et al.*, 1983; Rubenstein *et al.*, 1987b).

Improved diagnostic accuracy was the most widely described effect of geriatric assessment, most often indicated by substantial numbers of important problems that were uncovered. Frequencies of the new diagnoses that were found ranged from almost 1 to more than 4 per patient. The factors contributing to the improvement of diagnosis in GAPs include the validity of the assessment itself (the capability of a structured search for "geriatric problems" to find them), the extra measure of time and care taken in the evaluation of the patient (independent of the formal elements of "the assessment"), and a probable lack of diagnostic attention on the part of referring professionals.

Improved living location on discharge from health-care setting was demonstrated in several early studies, beginning with T. F. Williams' classic descriptive prepost study of an outpatient assessment program in New York (Williams *et al.*, 1973). Among the patients referred for nursing home placement in the county, the assessment program found that only 38% actually needed skilled nursing care, while 23% could return home, and 39% were appropriate for board and care or retirement facilities. Numerous subsequent studies have shown similar improvements in living locations (Rubenstein *et al.*, 1984; Hendriksen *et al.*, 1984; Thomas *et al.*, 1993; Vetter *et al.*, 1984; Vetter *et al.*, 1992; Winograd *et al.*, 1993; Collard *et al.*, 1985; Allen *et al.*, 1986; Hogan *et al.*, 1987; Hogan and Fox, 1990; Williams *et al.*, 1987; Gilchrist *et al.*, 1988; Reid and Kennie, 1989; Pathy *et al.*, 1992; Hansen *et al.*, 1992; Gayton *et al.*, 1987). Several studies that examined mental or physical functional status of patients before and after comprehensive geriatric assessment coupled with treatment and rehabilitation showed patient improvement on measures of function (Rubenstein *et al.*, 1984; Hendriksen *et al.*, 1984; Thomas *et al.*, 1993; Vetter *et al.*, 1984; Vetter *et al.*, 1992; Hogan *et al.*, 1987; Reid and Kennie, 1989).

The Pioneering Studies of Geriatric Assessment

Beginning in the 1980s, controlled studies appeared that corroborated some of the earlier studies and documented additional benefits such as improved survival, reduced hospital and nursing home utilization, and in some cases, reduced costs (Rubenstein *et al.*, 1984; Hendriksen *et al.*, 1984; Thomas *et al.*, 1993; Vetter *et al.*, 1984; Vetter *et al.*, 1992; Winograd *et al.*, 1993; Collard *et al.*, 1985; Allen *et al.*, 1986; Hogan *et al.*, 1987; Hogan and Fox, 1990; Williams *et al.*, 1987; Gilchrist *et al.*, 1988; Reid and Kennie, 1989; Pathy *et al.*, 1992; Hansen *et al.*, 1992; Gayton *et al.*, 1987; Rubenstein *et al.*, 1995b; Rubenstein *et al.*, 1988; Schuman *et al.*, 1978; Lefton *et al.*, 1983; Berkman *et al.*, 1983; Lichtenstein and Winogard, 1984; Burley *et al.*, 1979; Tulloch and Moore, 1979; Rubenstein *et al.*, 1995c). These studies were by no means uniform in their results. Some showed a whole series of dramatic positive effects on function, survival, living location, and costs, while others showed relatively few, if any, benefits. However, the GAPs being studied were also very different from each other in terms of the process of care offered and patient populations accepted. To this day, controlled trials of GAPs continue, and as results accumulate, we are able to understand the aspects that contribute to their effectiveness and the ones that do not.

One striking effect confirmed for many GAPs has been a positive impact on survival. Several controlled studies of different basic GAP models demonstrated significantly increased survival, reported in different ways and with varying periods of follow-up. Mortality was reduced for Sepulveda geriatric evaluation unit patients by 50% at 1 year, and the survival curves of the experimental and control groups still significantly favored the assessed group at 2 years (Rubenstein *et al.*, 1984; Rubenstein *et al.*, 1995b; Rubenstein *et al.*, 1988). Survival was improved by 21% at 1 year in a Scottish trial of geriatric rehabilitation consultation (Reid and Kennie, 1989). Two Canadian consultation trials demonstrated a significantly improved 6-month survival (Hogan *et al.*, 1987; Hogan and Fox, 1990). Two Danish community-based trials of in-home geriatric assessment and follow-up demonstrated reduction in mortality (Hendriksen *et al.*, 1984; Hansen *et al.*, 1992), and 2 Welsh studies of in-home GAPs had beneficial survival effects among patients assessed at home and followed for 2 years (Vetter *et al.*, 1984; Vetter *et al.*, 1992). On the other hand, several other studies of geriatric assessment found no statistically significant survival benefits (Winograd *et al.*, 1993; Allen *et al.*, 1986; Gilchrist *et al.*, 1988; Reid and Kennie, 1989).

Multiple studies followed patients longitudinally after the initial assessment and thus were able to examine the longer-term utilization and cost impacts of assessment and treatment. Some studies found an overall reduction in nursing home days (Rubenstein *et al.*, 1984; Reid and Kennie, 1989; Schuman *et al.*, 1978; Lefton *et al.*, 1983). Hospital utilization was examined in several reports. For hospital-based GAPs, the length of hospitalization was obviously affected by the length of the assessment itself. Thus, some programs appear to prolong the initial length of stay (Rubenstein *et al.*, 1987b; Berkman *et al.*, 1983; Lichtenstein and Winogard, 1984), while others reduce initial stay (Collard *et al.*, 1985; Reid and Kennie, 1989; Pathy *et al.*, 1992; Hansen *et al.*, 1992; Burley *et al.*, 1979). However, studies following patients for at least 1 year have usually shown a reduction in use of acute-care hospital services, even in those programs with initially prolonged hospital stays (William *et al.*, 1964; Hendriksen *et al.*, 1984; Williams *et al.*, 1987).

Compensatory increases in use of community-based services or home-care agencies might be expected with declines in nursing home placements and use of other institutional services. These increases have been detected in several studies (Hendriksen *et al.*, 1984; Vetter *et al.*, 1984; Hogan *et al.*, 1987; Tulloch and Moore, 1979) but not in others (Rubenstein *et al.*, 1984; Williams *et al.*, 1987; Gayton *et al.*, 1987). Although increased use of formal community services may not always be indicated, it usually is a desirable goal. The fact that several studies did not detect increases in use of home and community services probably reflects the unavailability of community service or referral networks rather than that more of such services were not needed.

The effects of these programs on costs and utilization parameters have only seldom been examined comprehensively, because of methodologic difficulties in gathering comprehensive utilization and cost data, as well as statistical limitations in comparing highly skewed distributions. The Sepulveda study found that the total first-year direct health-care costs had been reduced because of overall reductions in nursing home and rehospitalization days, despite significantly longer initial hospital stays in the geriatric unit (Rubenstein *et al.*, 1984). These savings continued through 3 years of follow-up (Rubenstein *et al.*, 1995b). Hendriksen's in-home program (Hendriksen *et al.*, 1984) reduced the costs of medical care, apparently through successful early case-finding and referral for preventive intervention. Williams' outpatient GAPs (Williams *et al.*, 1987) detected reductions in medical care costs primarily because of the reductions in hospitalization. Although it would be reasonable to worry that prolonged survival of frail patients would lead to increased service use and charges, or, of perhaps greater concern, to worry about the quality of the prolonged life, these concerns may be without substance. Indeed, the Sepulveda study demonstrated that GAPs could improve not only survival but can also prolong high-function survival (Rubenstein *et al.*, 1984; Rubenstein *et al.*, 1995b) while at the same time reduce the use of institutional services and costs.

Meta-analyses of Controlled Studies

A 1993 meta-analysis attempted to resolve some of the discrepancies between study results, and tried to identify whether particular program elements were associated with particular benefits (Stuck *et al.*, 1993; Stuck *et al.*, 1995b). This meta-analysis included published data from the 28 controlled trials completed as of that date, involving nearly 10 000 patients, and was also able to include substantial amounts of unpublished data systematically retrieved from many of the studies. The meta-analysis identified five GAP types: hospital units (six studies), hospital consultation teams (eight studies), in-home assessment services (seven studies), outpatient assessment services (4 studies), and hospital-home assessment programs (three studies). The meta-analysis confirmed many of the major reported benefits for many of the individual program types. These statistically and clinically significant benefits included reduced risk of mortality (by 22% for hospital-based programs at 12 months, and by 14% for all programs combined at 12 months), improved likelihood of living at home (by 47% for hospital-based programs and by 26% for all programs combined at 12 months), reduced risk of hospital (re)admissions (by 12% for all programs at study end), greater chance of cognitive improvement (by 47% for all programs at study end), and greater chance of physical function improvement for patients in hospital units (by 72% for hospital units).

Clearly, not all studies showed equivalent effects, and the meta-analysis was able to indicate a number of variables at both the program and patient levels that tended to distinguish trials with large effects from ones with more limited ones. When examined on the program level, hospital units and home-visit assessment teams produced the most dramatic benefits, while no major significant benefits in office-based programs could be confirmed. Programs that provided hands-on clinical care and/or long-term follow-up were generally able to produce greater positive effects than purely consultative programs or ones that lacked follow-up. Another factor associated with greater demonstrated benefits, at least in hospital-based programs, was patient targeting; programs that selected patients who were at high risk for deterioration yet still had "rehabilitation potential" generally had stronger results than less selective programs.

The 1993 meta-analysis confirmed the importance of targeting criteria in producing beneficial outcomes. In particular, when use of explicit targeting criteria for patient selection was included as a covariate, increases in some program benefits were often found. For example, among the hospital-based GAPs studies, positive effects on physical function and likelihood of living at home at 12 months were associated with studies that excluded patients who were relatively "too healthy". A similar effect on physical function was seen in the institutional studies that excluded persons with relatively poor prognoses. The reason for this effect of targeting on effect size no doubt lies in the ability of careful targeting to concentrate the intervention on patients who can benefit, without diluting the effect with persons too ill or too well to show a measurable improvement.

Recent Studies of Geriatric Assessment

Studies performed after the 1993 meta-analysis have been largely corroborative. A recent meta-analysis confirmed that inpatient comprehensive assessment programs for elderly hospital patients may reduce mortality, increase the chances of living at home at 1 year, and improve physical and cognitive function (Ellis and Langhorne, 2005). However, with principles of geriatric medicine becoming more diffused into usual care, particularly at places where controlled trials are being undertaken, differences between GAPs and control groups seem to be narrowing (Reuben *et al.*, 1995; Burns *et al.*, 2000; Stuck *et al.*, 2000; Boult *et al.*, 2001; Elkan *et al.*, 2000; Rubenstein and Stuck, 2001). For example, a recent study of inpatient and outpatient geriatric assessment and management has failed to demonstrate substantial benefits in elderly patients (Cohen *et al.*, 2002). Other studies however continue to reveal major benefits of inpatient programs (Saltvedt *et al.*, 2004). Effects of outpatient GAPs have been less impressive, with a recent meta-analysis showing no favorable effects on mortality outcome (Kuo *et al.*, 2004). For cost reasons, growth of inpatient units has been slow, despite their proven effectiveness, while outpatient programs have increased, despite their less impressive effect size in controlled trials. However, some newer trials of outpatient programs have shown significant benefits in areas not found in earlier outpatient studies, such as functional status, psychological parameters, and wellbeing, which may indicate improvement in the outpatient care models being tested (Burns *et al.*, 2000; Stuck *et al.*, 2000; Boult *et al.*, 2001; Elkan *et al.*, 2000; Rubenstein and Stuck, 2001).

A recent meta-analysis of preventive home visits revealed that home visitation programs are effective if based on multidimensional geriatric assessments with extended follow-up, and if offered to elderly persons with relatively good function at baseline (Stuck *et al.*, 2002). On the basis of a large number of trials, the findings from this meta-analysis indicate that preventive home visitation programs are effective only if interventions are based on multidimensional geriatric assessment, include multiple follow-up home visits, and target persons with relatively good function at baseline. The NNV (number needed to visit) to prevent one admission in programs with frequent follow-up visits is around 40. Recently, it has been confirmed that a key component of successful programs is a systematic approach for teaching primary care professionals. These results have important policy implications. In countries with existing national programs of preventive home visits, the process and organization of these visits should be reconsidered on the basis of the criteria identified in this meta-analysis. In the United States, a system for functional impairment risk identification and appropriate intervention to prevent or delay functional impairment seems promising. There are a variety of chronic disease management programs specifically addressing the care needs of the elderly (Vass *et al.*, 2005). Engrafting the key concepts of home-based preventive care programs into these programs should be feasible, as they continue to evolve, and are cost-effective. Identifying risks and dealing with them as an essential component of the care of elderly persons is central to reducing the emerging burden of disability and improving the quality of life in the elderly.

CONCLUSION

Published studies of multidimensional geriatric assessment have confirmed its efficacy in many settings. A continuing challenge has been obtaining adequate financing to support adding geriatric assessment services to existing medical care. Despite GAPs' many proven benefits, and their ability to reduce costs documented in controlled trials, health-care financers have been reluctant to fund GAPs – presumably out of concern that the programs might be expanded too fast and that costs for extra diagnostic and therapeutic services might increase out of control. Many practitioners have found ways to "unbundle" the geriatric assessment process into component services and receive adequate support to fund the entire process. In this continuing time of fiscal restraint, geriatric practitioners must remain constantly creative in order to reach the goal of optimal patient care.

While there is no single optimal blueprint for geriatric assessment, the participation of the multidisciplinary team and the focus on functional status and quality of life as major clinical goals are common to all settings. Although the greatest benefits have been found in programs targeted to the frail subgroup of elderly persons, a strong case can be made for a continuum of GAPs – screening assessments performed periodically for all elderly persons and comprehensive assessment targeted to frail and high-risk patients. Clinicians interested in developing these services will do well to heed the experiences of the programs reviewed here in adapting the principles of geriatric assessment to local resources. Future research is still needed to determine the most effective and efficient methods for performing geriatric assessment and on developing strategies for best matching needs with services.

KEY POINTS

- Multidimensional geriatric assessment is an efficient and effective way for evaluating complex elderly patients and planning improved care.
- The process of multidimensional geriatric assessment usually involves the systematic evaluation of function, medical conditions, psychological parameters, and social networks through use of an interdisciplinary team and validated assessment measures.
- Multidimensional geriatric assessment has been shown to improve function and survival while reducing health-care utilization and costs.

KEY REFERENCES

- Kane RL & Kane RA. *Assessing Older Persons* 2000; Oxford University Press, New York.
- Rubenstein LZ, Josephson KR, Wieland GD *et al.* Effectiveness of a geriatric evaluation unit: a randomized clinical trial. *The New England Journal of Medicine* 1984; **311**:1664–70.
- Rubenstein LZ, Wieland D & Bernabei R. *Geriatric Assessment Technology: The State of the Art* 1995a; Kurtis Publishers, Milan.
- Stuck AE, Egger M, Hammer A *et al.* Home visits to prevent nursing home admission and functional decline in the elderly: systematic review and meta-regression analysis. *The Journal of the American Medical Association* 2002; **287**:1022–8.
- Stuck AE, Siu AL, Wieland GD *et al.* Comprehensive geriatric assessment: a meta-analysis of controlled trials. *Lancet* 1993; **342**:1032–6.

REFERENCES

Allen CM, Becker PM, McVey LJ *et al.* A randomized controlled clinical trial of a geriatric consultation team: compliance with recommendations. *The Journal of the American Medical Association* 1986; **255**:2617–21.

Applegate WB, Akins D, Vander Zwaag R *et al.* A geriatric rehabilitation and assessment unit in a community hospital. *Journal of the American Geriatrics Society* 1983; **31**:206–10.

Bergner M, Bobbit R & Carter WB. The sickness impact profile: validation of a health status measure. *Medical Care* 1981; **19**:787–805.

Berkman B, Campion E, Swagerty E & Goldman M. Geriatric consultation teams: alternative approach to social work discharge planning. *Journal of Gerontological Social Work* 1983; **5**:77–88.

Boult C, Boult LB, Morishita L *et al.* A randomized clinical trial of outpatient geriatric evaluation and management. *Journal of the American Geriatrics Society* 2001; **49**:351–9.

Brocklehurst JC. *Geriatric Care in Advanced Societies* 1975; MTP, Lancaster University Park Press, Baltimore.

Brocklehurst JC, Carty MH, Leeming JT & Robinson JH. Medical screening of old people accepted for residential care. *Lancet* 1978; **ii**:141–3.

Burley LE, Currie CT, Smith RG & Williamson J. Contribution from geriatric medicine within acute medical wards. *British Medical Journal* 1979; **263**:90–2.

Burns R, Nichols LO, Martindale-Adams J *et al.* Interdisciplinary geriatric primary care evaluation and management: two-year outcomes. *Journal of the American Geriatrics Society* 2000; **48**:8–13.

Campbell LJ & Cole KD. Geriatric assessment teams. *Clinics in Geriatric Medicine* 1987; **3**:99–110.

Chambers LW, MacDonald LA, Tugwell P *et al.* The McMaster health index questionnaire as a measure of quality of life for patients with rheumatoid disease. *The Journal of Rheumatology* 1982; **9**:780–4.

Cohen HJ, Feussner JR, Weinberger M *et al.* A controlled trial of inpatient and outpatient geriatric evaluation and management. *The New England Journal of Medicine* 2002; **346**:905–12.

Collard AF, Bachman SS & Beatrice DF. Acute care delivery for the geriatric patient: an innovative approach. *Quality Review Bulletin* 1985; **2**:180–5.

Duke University Center for the Study of Aging and Human Development. *The OARS Methodology* 1978; Duke University Press, Durham.

Elkan R, Kendrick D, Dewey M *et al.* Effectiveness of home based support for older people: systematic review and meta-analysis. *British Medical Journal* 2000; **323**:1–9.

Ellis G & Langhorne P. Comprehensive geriatric assessment for older hospital patients. *British Medical Bulletin* 2005; **71**:43–57.

Folstein M, Folstein S & McHugh P. Mini-mental state: a practical method for grading the cognitive state of patients for the clinician. *Journal of Psychiatric Research* 1975; **12**:189–98.

Gallo JJ, Fulmer T, Paveza GJ & Reichel W. *Handbook of Geriatric Assessment* 2000, 3rd edn; Aspen Publishers, Rockville.

Gayton D, Wood-Dauphine S, de Lorimer M *et al.* Trial of a geriatric consultation team in an acute care hospital. *Journal of the American Geriatrics Society* 1987; **35**:726–36.

Gilchrist WJ, Newman RH, Hamblen DL & Williams BO. Prospective randomized study of an orthopaedic geriatric inpatient service. *British Medical Journal* 1988; **297**:1116–8.

Gurland BH & Wilder D. Detection and assessment of cognitive impairment and depressed mood in older adults. In LZ Rubenstein, D Wieland & R Bernabei (eds) *Geriatric Assessment Technology: The State of the Art* 1995; Kurtis Publishers, Milan.

Gwadry-Sridhar FH, Flintoft V, Lee DS *et al.* A systematic review and meta analysis of studies comparing readmission rates and mortality rates in patients with heart failure. *Archives of Internal Medicine* 2004; **164**:2315–20.

Hansen FR, Spedtsberg K & Schroll M. Geriatric follow-up by home visits after discharge from hospital: a randomized controlled trial. *Age and Ageing* 1992; **21**:445–50.

Hedrick SC. Assessment of functional status: activities of daily living. In LZ Rubenstein, D Wieland & R Bernabei (eds) *Geriatric Assessment Technology: The State of the Art* 1995; Kurtis Publishers, Milan.

Hendriksen C, Lund E & Stromgard E. Consequences of assessment and intervention among elderly people: three-year randomized controlled trial. *British Medical Journal* 1984; **289**:1522–4.

Hoehn MM & Yahr MD. Parkinsonism: onset, progression, and mortality. *Neurology* 1967; **17**:427–42.

Hogan DB & Fox RA. A prospective controlled trial of a geriatric consultation team in an acute care hospital. *Age and Ageing* 1990; **19**:107–13.

Hogan DB, Fox RA, Badley BWD & Mann OE. Effect of a geriatric consultation service on management of patients in an acute care hospital. *Canadian Medical Association Journal* 1987; **136**:713–7.

Hoyl T, Alessi CA, Harker JO *et al.* Development and testing of a 5-item version of the geriatric depression scale. *Journal of the American Geriatrics Society* 1999; **47**:873–8.

Jette AM, Davies AR, Calkins DR *et al.* The functional status questionnaire: reliability and validity when used in primary care. *Journal of General Internal Medicine* 1986; **1**:143.

Kahn R, Goldfarb A, Pollack M *et al.* Brief objective measures of mental status in the aged. *American Journal of Psychiatry* 1960; **117**:326–8.

Kane RA. Assessment of social function: recommendations for comprehensive geriatric assessment. In LZ Rubenstein, D Wieland & R Bernabei. (eds) *Geriatric Assessment Technology: The State of the Art* 1995; Kurtis Publishers, Milan.

Kane RL & Kane RA. *Assessing Older Persons* 2000; Oxford University Press, New York.

Katz S, Ford AB, Moskowitz RW *et al.* Studies of illness in the aged. The index of ADL: a standardized measure of biological psychosocial function. *The Journal of the American Medical Association* 1963; **185**:914–9.

Kuo HK, Scandrett KG, Dave J & Mitchell SL. The influence of outpatient comprehensive geriatric assessment on survival: a meta-analysis. *Archives of Gerontology and Geriatrics* 2004; **39**:245–54.

Lawton MP & Brody EM. Assessment of older people: self-maintaining and instrumental activities of daily living. *The Gerontologist* 1969; **9**:179–86.

Lefton E, Bonstelle S & Frengley JD. Success with an inpatient geriatric unit: a controlled study. *Journal of the American Geriatrics Society* 1983; **31**:149–55.

Lichtenstein H & Winogard CH. Geriatric consultation: a functional approach. *Journal of the American Geriatrics Society* 1984; **32**:356–61.

Lowther CP, MacLeod RDM & Williamson J. Evaluation of early diagnostic services for the elderly. *British Medical Journal* 1970; **3**:275–7.

Lubben JE. Assessing social networks among elderly populations. *Family and Community Health* 1988; **8**:42–52.

Mahoney FI & Barthel DW. Functional evaluation – the Barthel Index. *Maryland State Medical Journal* 1965; **14**:61–5.

Mathias S, Nayak USL & Isaacs B. Balance in elderly patients: the "get up and go" test. *Archives of Physical Medicine and Rehabilitation* 1986; **67**:387–9.

Matthews DA. Dr. Marjory Warren and the origin of British geriatrics. *Journal of the American Geriatrics Society* 1984; **32**:253–8.

Nelson E, Wasson J, Kirk J *et al.* Assessment of function in routine clinical practice: description of the Coop chart method and preliminary findings. *Journal of Chronic Diseases* 1987; **40**:55S.

Osterweil D, Brummel-Smith K & Beck JC. *Comprehensive Geriatric Assessment* 2000; McGraw-Hill, New York.

Pathy MSJ, Bayer A, Harding K & Dibble A. Randomized trial of casefinding and surveillance of elderly people at home. *Lancet* 1992; **340**:890–3.

Reid J & Kennie DC. Geriatric rehabilitative care after fractures of the proximal femur: one-year follow-up of a randomized clinical trial. *British Medical Journal* 1989; **299**:25–6.

Reisberg B, Ferris SH, DeLeon MJ *et al.* The global deterioration scale for assessment of primary degenerative dementia. *American Journal of Psychiatry* 1982; **139**:1136–9.

Reuben DB, Borok GM, Wolde GT *et al.* A randomized clinical trial of comprehensive geriatric assessment consultation for hospitalized HMO patients. *The New England Journal of Medicine* 1995; **332**:1345–50.

Rubenstein LV. Using quality of life tests for patient diagnosis or screening. In B Spilker (ed) *Quality of Life and Pharmacoeconomics in Clinical Trials* 1996, 2nd edn; JB Lippincott, Philadelphia.

Rubenstein LZ, Campbell LJ & Kane RL. *Geriatric Assessment* 1987a; W. B. Saunders, Philadelphia.

Rubenstein LZ, Josephson KR, Wieland GD *et al.* Geriatric assessment on a subacute hospital ward. *Clinics in Geriatric Medicine* 1987b; **3**:131–43.

Rubenstein LZ, Harker JO, Salva A *et al.* Screening for undernutrition in geriatric practice: developing the short-form Mini-nutritional Assessment (MNA-SF). *Journals of Gerontology. Series A, Biological Sciences and Medical Sciences* 2001; **56**:M366–72.

Rubenstein LZ, Josephson KR, Wieland GD *et al.* Effectiveness of a geriatric evaluation unit: a randomized clinical trial. *The New England Journal of Medicine* 1984; **311**:1664–70.

Rubenstein LZ & Stuck AE. Preventive home visits for older people: defining criteria for success. *Age and Ageing* 2001; **30**:107–9.

Rubenstein LZ, Wieland D & Bernabei R. *Geriatric Assessment Technology: The State of the Art* 1995a; Kurtis Publishers, Milan.

Rubenstein LZ, Josephson KR, Harker JO & Wieland D. The Sepulveda GEU study revisited: long-term outcomes, use of services, and costs. *Aging Clinical and Experimental Research* 1995b; **7**:212–7.

Rubenstein LZ, Wieland D & Bernabei R. Geriatric assessment: international research perspective. *Aging Clinical and Experimental Research* 1995c; **7**:157–260.

Rubenstein LZ, Wieland D, Josephson KR *et al.* Improved survival for frail elderly inpatients on a geriatric evaluation unit (GEU): who benefits? *Journal of Clinical Epidemiology* 1988; **41**:441–9.

Saltvedt I, Saltnes T, Mo ES *et al.* Acute geriatric intervention increases the number of patients able to live at home. A prospective randomized study. *Aging Clinical and Experimental Research* 2004; **16**:300–6.

Schuman JE, Beattie EJ, Steed DA *et al.* The impact of a new geriatric program in a hospital for the chronically ill. *Canadian Medical Association Journal* 1978; **118**:639–45.

Stewart AL, Hays RD & Ware JE. Communication: the MOS short-form general health survey: reliability and validity in a patient population. *Medical Care* 1988; **26**:724–35.

Stuck AE, Aronow HU, Steiner A *et al.* A trial of annual comprehensive geriatric assessments for elderly people living in the community. *The New England Journal of Medicine* 1995a; **333**:1184–9.

Stuck AE, Wieland D, Rubenstein LZ *et al.* Comprehensive geriatric assessment: meta-analysis of main effects and elements enhancing effectiveness. In LZ Rubenstein, D Wieland & R Bernabei (eds) *Geriatric Assessment Technology: The State of the Art* 1995b; Kurtis Publishers, Milan.

Stuck AE, Egger M, Hammer A *et al.* Home visits to prevent nursing home admission and functional decline in the elderly: systematic review and meta-regression analysis. *The Journal of the American Medical Association* 2002; **287**:1022–8.

Stuck AE, Minder CE, Peter-Wuest I *et al.* A randomized trial of in-home visits for disability prevention in community-drelling older people at low and high risk for nursing home admission. *Archives of Internal Medicine* 2000; **160**:977–86.

Stuck AE, Siu AL, Wieland GD *et al.* Comprehensive geriatric assessment: a meta-analysis of controlled trials. *Lancet* 1993; **342**:1032–6.

Thomas DR, Brahan R & Haywood BP. Inpatient community-based geriatric assessment reduces subsequent mortality. *Journal of the American Geriatrics Society* 1993; **41**:101–4.

Tinetti ME. Performance oriented assessment of mobility problems in elderly patients. *Journal of the American Geriatrics Society* 1986; **34**:119–26.

Tulloch AH & Moore V. A randomized controlled trial of geriatric screening and surveillance in general practice. *The Journal of the College of General Practitioners* 1979; **29**:733–42.

VanSwearington JM & Brach JS. Making geriatric assessment work: selecting useful measures. *Physical Therapy* 2001; **81**:1233–52.

Vass M, Avlund K, Lauridsen J & Hendriksen C. Feasible model for prevention of functional decline in older people: municipality-randomized, controlled trial. *Journal of the American Geriatrics Society* 2005; **53**(4):563–8.

Vellas B & Guigoz Y. Nutritional assessment as part of the geriatric evaluation. *Geriatric Assessment Technology: The State of the Art* 1995; Kurtis Publishers, Milan.

Vetter NJ, Jones DA & Victor CR. Effects of health visitors working with elderly patients in general practice: a randomized controlled trial. *British Medical Journal* 1984; **288**:369–72.

Vetter NJ, Lewis PA & Ford D. Can health visitors prevent fractures in elderly people? *British Medical Journal* 1992; **304**:888–90.

Wade DT & Colin C. The Barthel ADL Index – a standard measure of physical disability. *International Disability Studies* 1988; **10**:64–7.

Wieland D, Kramer BJ, Waite MS & Rubenstein LZ. The interdisciplinary team in geriatric care. *The American Behavioral Scientist* 1996; **39**:655–64.

William J, Stokoe IH, Gray S *et al.* Old people at home: their unreported needs. *Lancet* 1964; **i**:1117–20.

Williams TF, Hill JH, Fairbank ME & Knox KG. Appropriate placement of the chronically ill and aged: a successful approach by evaluation. *The Journal of the American Medical Association* 1973; **266**:1332–5.

Williams ME, Williams TF, Zimmer JG *et al.* How does the team approach to outpatient geriatric evaluation compare with traditional care: a report of a randomized controlled trial. *Journal of the American Geriatrics Society* 1987; **35**:1071–8.

Winograd CH, Gerety M & Lai N. A negative trial of inpatient geriatric consultation: lessons learned. *Archives of Internal Medicine* 1993; **153**:2017–23.

Yesavage J, Brink T, Rose T *et al.* Development and validation of a geriatric screening scale: a preliminary report. *Journal of Psychiatric Research* 1983; **17**:37–49.

Zung WWK. A self rating depression scale. *Archives of General Psychiatry* 1965; **12**:63–70.

132

Function Assessment Scales

Fredric D. Wolinsky

The University of Iowa, Iowa City, IA, USA and Center for Research in the Implementation of Innovative Strategies and Practices, Iowa City Veterans' Affairs Medical Center, Iowa City, IA, USA

THEORETICAL FRAMEWORK

The functional assessment literature may be somewhat crudely characterized by two statements. On the one hand, functional assessment is critically important in gerontology and geriatrics. On the other hand, there is little agreement on how to do it right. How can there be so much confusion about such an important area? Jette *et al.* suggest that the confusion stems from:

"... similar terms used to describe outcomes that are operationalized in myriad ways. Lack of sensitivity of existing outcome instruments to detect important changes in disability status hinders the evaluation of interventions. Use of disability or health status measures not designed for evaluative purposes frequently results in ceiling or floor effects, if the content of the measures lacks sufficient breadth or if the increments in the ratings are too global."

(Jette *et al.*, 2002:M209)

Therefore, in order to understand functional assessment, it would seem most helpful to start with a conceptual framework. The model that is most appropriate to functional assessment was first proposed by Nagi (1965, 1969, 1976, 1991). A simplistic rendering of Nagi's conceptual model is shown in Figure 1. The four core components of the disablement process are: *active pathology, impairment, functional limitations*, and *disability*. The arrows reflect the principal pathway: a progressive stream in which active pathology may result in impairment, impairment may result in functional limitation, and functional limitation may result in disability.

To fully understand Nagi's model, it is essential to know exactly how he defined each of the four core components, and the best way to do this is to rely on the definitions provided in his reflective chapter included in the 1991 IOM report. In Nagi's own words, the four concepts are defined as follows:

"1. The state of *active pathology* may result from infection, trauma, metabolic imbalance, degenerative disease processes, or other etiology. Such a condition involves (a) interruption of or interference with normal processes and (b) the simultaneous efforts of the organism to regain a normal state." (pp. 313–314)

"2. The concept of *impairment* indicates a loss or abnormality of an anatomical, physiological, mental, or emotional nature. The concept comprises three distinct categories: (1) all conditions of pathology, which are by definition impairments because such conditions involve anatomical, physiological, mental, or emotional deviation; (2) residual losses or abnormalities that remain after the active state of pathology has been controlled or eliminated (e.g. healed amputations, residual paralysis); and (3) abnormalities not associated with pathology (e.g. congenital formations)." (p. 314)

"3. *Functional limitations* and impairments both involve function. The difference, however, is in the level at which the limitations are manifested. Functional limitation refers to manifestations at the level of the organism as a whole.... Although limitations at a lower level of organization may not be reflected at higher levels, the reverse is not true.... Functional limitations are the most direct way through which impairments contribute to disability." (pp. 314–315)

"4. *Disability* refers to social rather than to organismic functioning. It is an inability or limitation in performing socially defined roles and tasks.... Not all impairments or functional limitations precipitate disability, and similar patterns of disability may result from different types of impairments and limitations in function. Furthermore, identical types of impairments and similar functional limitations may result in different patterns of disability." (p. 315).

Disease histories are the principal measure of *active pathology*. Although clinical examination and laboratory testing represent the gold standard, self-reported disease histories are generally used to minimize the costs of data collection. Study subjects are typically asked to report whether a physician has ever told them that they have a particular disease, such as angina, arthritis, asthma, cancer, coronary artery disease (CAD), congestive heart failure, chronic obstructive pulmonary disease, diabetes, a heart attack, hypertension, kidney disease, or a stroke. Either a series of individual binary markers are then used for each disease, or a simple summary score is calculated.

Essentially, *impairments* are decrements to normal functional abilities that have not progressed far enough to affect

Principles and Practice of Geriatric Medicine, 4th Edition. Edited by M.S. John Pathy, Alan J. Sinclair and John E. Morley.

Active pathology ➛ Impairment ➛ Functional limitation ➛ Disability

Figure 1 A simplistic representation of the main pathway in Nagi's (1965, 1969, 1976, 1991) conceptual scheme for the epidemiology of disability

an individual's ability to perform a given task, even though she/he may recognize that the deficit exists. That is, study subjects may have statistically significantly less balance, quadriceps strength, and digital dexterity than extant age and sex norms would suggest, but these impairments do not yet pose difficulties in terms of her/his ability to perform routine functions such as bending over to pull on socks and tie one's shoes. As with disease histories, impairments can be assessed in multiple ways, including self-reported symptoms (e.g. dizziness or shortness of breath), examinations by a physician or other clinician, or epidemiologic field testing (e.g. gait speed, balance, or strength evaluations).

When impairments progress to the point where they inhibit the individual's ability to perform routine sensory motor or cognitive functions, such as walking, stair-climbing, reaching out to grab an object, vision, hearing, memory or processing speed, they are considered to have become *functional limitations*. The measurement of functional limitations can involve either self-report or observed performance. Self-report measures ask study subjects if they have no, some, or great difficulty in standing for long periods, lifting or carrying weights of approximately ten pounds, going up and down stairs, walking, stooping-bending-kneeling, using hands and fingers, and reaching out with either or both arms. Alternatively, performance evaluations involve observation of the study subject as she/he simulates the sensory motor functions involved in such tasks.

Disability involves difficulties in the performance of work and independent living. The work dimension has received relatively little attention in gerontology and geriatrics given the thorny problems of status determination among older adults, many of whom are either fully or partially retired. Independent living, however, has received considerable attention, and has given rise to variously named measures of activities of daily living (ADLs). The more basic ADLs involve personal care activities and are typically measured by asking study subjects if they have difficulty (yes/no), *due to health reasons*, in performing activities such as bathing or showering, dressing, eating, getting in or out of a bed or a chair, walking across a room, getting outside, or using the toilet. When study subjects indicate difficulty with a particular task, the follow-on question is how much – some difficulty, a lot of difficulty, or are they unable to perform the task at all. Higher level or instrumental ADLs (IADLs) involve activities like meal preparation, shopping for groceries or personal items, keeping track of expenses and paying bills, using the telephone, doing light housework, doing heavy housework, or managing medications. As with ADLs, study subjects expressing difficulty with IADL tasks are asked about the degree of difficulty. Performance-based (observed) measures have been developed for both ADLs and IADLs, although their associated time and prop demands have limited their practicality.

What sets disability apart, conceptually, is that it is essentially a social (i.e. relational) phenomenon involving the performance of task and role assignments. That is, it goes beyond the individual and involves the social role and task expectations that society places on the individual in the context of her/his environment. In contrast, active pathology, impairment, and functional limitations can be measured within the individual, inasmuch as these concepts are all attributes or properties of the individual.

Although Figure 1 implies that the disablement process is linear, fixed, and unrecoverable, this is not so. To underscore this point, Figure 2 contains Verbrugge and Jette's (1994) clarification and elaboration of the model. It contains the four core components: active pathology, impairment, functional limitation, and disability. What makes Figure 2 different is that risk factors, extra-individual factors, and intra-individual factors have been added because these moderate the rate of progression and flow through the main pathway.

Risk factors include long-term or permanent behaviors and attributes of the study subjects and the places where they live, which increase the incidence of functional limitations and/or disabilities. The position of risk factors on the far left side of the model indicates that they exist prior to or at the onset of the disablement process. In contrast, the extra-individual and intra-individual factors appear where functional limitations are manifest, and are shown as moderators whose function is to buffer progression along the main disablement pathway. Buffering interventions involve avoiding disability onset, slowing down its progression, or returning the study subject to the prior functional ability. Such interventions can reside within the study subject (e.g. personal activity accommodation), or come from extra-individual sources (e.g. standby assistance/help or environmental modifications). To be sure, some intra- and extra-individual factors have negative effects, and exacerbate the disablement process. This happens when therapeutic side effects do more harm than good, when the atrophic response of study subjects initiates downward spirals, or when inflexible role obligations are faced.

Figure 2 provides further clarifications. One involves the distinction between "intrinsic" versus "actual" disability. The former taps the study subject's abilities without the use of aids (devices) or aides (people), whereas the latter taps abilities when assistive devices or personnel are available. In this sense, actual disability reflects person-environmental-fit failure, and can be seen as an indicator of unmet need. Feedback loops resulting in secondary conditions or dysfunctions are also explicitly recognized. Finally, it is clear that disability has important consequences, such as reduced quality of life and increased odds of depression, hospitalization, nursing home placement, and death. These outcomes would be placed after an arrow flowing out of disability.

PRINCIPLES OF PSYCHOMETRIC ASSESSMENT

Psychometrics is another word for measurement science. When constructing scales to measure functional assessment,

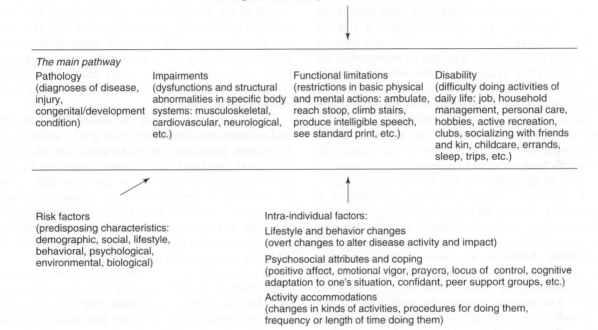

Extra-individual factors:

Medical care and rehabilitation
(surgery, physical therapy, speech therapy, counseling, health education, job retraining, etc.)

Medications and other therapeutic regimens
(drugs, recreational therapy/aquatic exercise, biofeedback/meditation, rest/energy conservation, etc.)

External supports (personal assistance, special equipment and devices, standby assistance/supervision, day care, respite care, meals-on-wheels)

Built, physical, and social environments (structural modifications at job/home, access to buildings and to public transportation, improvement of air quality, reduction of noise and glare, health insurance and access to medical care, laws and regulations, employment discrimination, etc.)

The main pathway

Pathology	Impairments	Functional limitations	Disability
(diagnoses of disease, injury, congenital/development condition)	(dysfunctions and structural abnormalities in specific body systems: musculoskeletal, cardiovascular, neurological, etc.)	(restrictions in basic physical and mental actions: ambulate, reach stoop, climb stairs, produce intelligible speech, see standard print, etc.)	(difficulty doing activities of daily life: job, household management, personal care, hobbies, active recreation, clubs, socializing with friends and kin, childcare, errands, sleep, trips, etc.)

Risk factors
(predisposing characteristics: demographic, social, lifestyle, behavioral, psychological, environmental, biological)

Intra-individual factors:

Lifestyle and behavior changes
(overt changes to alter disease activity and impact)

Psychosocial attributes and coping
(positive affect, emotional vigor, prayers, locus of control, cognitive adaptation to one's situation, confidant, peer support groups, etc.)

Activity accommodations
(changes in kinds of activities, procedures for doing them, frequency or length of time doing them)

Figure 2 Verbrugge and Jette's (1994) conceptual scheme for the disablement process

or any other construct, there are four key principles to consider: reliability, validity, responsiveness, and clinically important change (DeVellis, 2003; Trochim, 2004). These principles can be intuitively understood by considering a repeated target shooting scenario. The target consists of a series of concentric circles, with the innermost being the bull's-eye. When shooting at the target, the marksperson is trying to do two things. One is to hit the bull's-eye. The other is to have a tight cluster of shots in the target. After the marksperson fires all of his/her bullets, the target is repositioned (usually further away) and the process is repeated. Hitting the bull's-eye is analogous to validity. Having a tight cluster is analogous to reliability. Proper adjustment (resighting) after the target has been moved is analogous to responsiveness. Clinically important change is analogous to whether the target has been repositioned in a trivial (i.e. lateral movement that maintains the same distance from the marksperson), or a meaningful (i.e. greater distance) manner.

The bullet holes from each round represent the scale items. As with sampling principles, the larger the sample, the more representative and stable the obtained estimate. The best estimate of the actual value is the centroid (average) from that round of bullets. Reliability coefficients essentially gauge the magnitude of the average distance from each bullet hole to the centroid. Classical test theory dictates that:

$$X = t + e$$

where X represents the bullet holes (items), t represents the bull's-eye (true score), and e represents the distance to the centroid (amount of error). Because t is a latent value (never observed), the average of the Xs is considered the best estimate when five assumptions hold: (1) the expected value of the error score is zero (random error distribution); (2) the true score and error score are uncorrelated (homoscedasticity), (3) the true score for one marksperson is uncorrelated with the error score of another (independent observations); (4) the error scores for different markspersons are uncorrelated (no omitted confounders); and, (5) the amount of error for each bullet hole is equal (common factor loadings). Reliability problems involve random error, whereas validity problems involve systematic error. That is, reliability gauges the dispersal around the centroid (size of the cluster), whereas validity indicates whether the centroid is properly positioned in the bull's-eye. Thus, it is possible for a scale to be very reliable but invalid because it is consistently missing the mark.

There are four major ways to assess reliability: (1) test–retest; (2) alternative forms; (3) split halves; and (4) internal consistency. Test–retest reliability involves the correlation between scores on the same scale administered at two different points in time, and makes two strong assumptions. The first assumption is that the construct being measured does not change between the two administrations (i.e. the bull's-eye is not moved), and the second is that the two observations are independent. An issue here is the length of the interval between administrations – if it is too short, reproducibility will be biased upwards because subjects may try to remember their prior answers or interviewers try to remember their prior readings. If the interval between administrations is too long, reliability is attenuated because there is greater opportunity for change in the true score. To some extent, alternative forms reliability overcomes the memory and reactivity problems that limit test–retest reliability by using two different forms of the same test. The new problem here, however, is how do you construct alternative forms of the same test that are truly equivalent?

These difficulties give rise to assessing reliability at a single point in time. Split half reliability accomplishes this by dividing the set of scale items into two subscales and then using the correlation between those subscales as the reliability estimate. Although this resolves the assumption that the true score has not changed over time (because both subscales are administered at the same time), it poses a new problem – how do you separate the items into the two subscales? This is not a trivial issue, inasmuch as there are 125 unique ways to divide 10 items into two five-item subscales. Internal consistency reliability overcomes this problem by focusing on the average interitem correlation among items in the scale, where the reliability estimate is defined as:

$$r_{tt} = \frac{k^* \bar{r}_{ij}}{[1 + (k - 1)\bar{r}_{ij}]}$$

where r_{tt} is coefficient alpha (the t subscripts represent the true score), k is the number of items in the scale, and $\bar{r}_{ij}$ is the average interitem correlation coefficient. Coefficient alpha ranges between zero (unreliability, or when the variance in the errors is equal to the variance in X) and one (perfect reliability), and is a lower bound estimate or conservative measure of the scale's reliability. Current reliability standards require a minimum reliability coefficient of 0.70 for basic science and a minimum reliability coefficient of 0.90 when diagnostic and treatment decisions are being made.

Compared to evaluating the reliability of a scale, assessing its validity is more difficult. After all, reliability assessments involve correlations between observed scores at two different points in time (test–retest or alternative forms), or between components of the same score at the same time (split halves or internal consistency). In contrast, validity assessments involve a greater leap of faith inasmuch as the correlations between observables must be linked to the latent constructs. There are three main methods for evaluating validity: (1) content; (2) criterion; and (3) construct. Content validity is the most primitive approach, and is basically concerned with face and sampling validity. Face validity is simply whether items look like they are measuring what they are supposed to be, a rather subjective process. Some objectivity can be had by having an expert panel review the items and reach consensus about their face validity. The problems here lie in the picking of the experts, and whether these experts really know what the items will mean to the intended population. Sampling validity involves conceptually identifying all of the domains of the construct, and then developing multiple measures of each domain. It is akin to assuming that the population pool of potential items is known, and that stratified sampling of items within domains has occurred. Even when used in combination, face and sampling validity approaches cannot be said to make a strong case for the validity of the scale.

Criterion-related validity is reasonably straightforward, and assumes that some criterion or gold standard is available. It involves correlating the scale score with the known criterion (gold standard). The criterion value can be ascertained retrospectively (postdictive), at the same time (concurrent), or in the future (predictive). Thus, neither the timing of the criterion assessment nor the theoretical relationship between the gold standard and the latent construct is important. All that matters is that there is a known gold standard (criterion) with which to correlate the scale score.

Construct validity is a theory-driven approach that involves embedding the latent construct in a conceptual model that includes other latent constructs that are also measurable. Expected relationships between the construct measured by the scale score and the other constructs in the model are specified (positive or negative, strong or weak, null), and then these latent construct level correlations are estimated using the observable data (scale scores). The closer that the observed correlations conform to the theoretical expectations, then the greater the degree of construct validity. The main limitation here involves knowing how strong or weak the various correlations should be. The multitrait, multimethod matrix approach is the underlying framework for such determinations, and a good grasp of its principles leads directly to both exploratory and confirmatory factor analyses, which are the common approaches to construct validation.

Determining the responsiveness of a scale score generally involves known-group comparisons. Sometimes known-group comparisons are used in criterion validity, such as when a depression scale is administered to patients who have been diagnosed with depression, and to the general public. It is assumed that the diagnosed patients will register more depressive symptoms on the scale score than the community sample. Similarly, if study subjects are being followed over the course of a year to evaluate the responsiveness of an ADL scale, one would expect the change in the ADL scale score to be greatest among those who reported having an acute event like a heart attack, stroke, or hip fracture than among those not reporting having had such events. That is, the assumption would be made that those suffering such an acute event would have diminished ADL abilities (their bull's-eye should have moved, because this is a known effect of such acute events), and that this should be reflected in greater baseline-to-follow-up differences in their scale scores. A more subjective approach is to ask the study subjects at the posttest assessment whether their ability to perform ADLs has diminished since the pretest. If the ADL scale is responsive, then the change in scores among those who answered in the affirmative should be greater than those who did not.

Determining whether the difference between pretest and posttest scale score assessments is clinically meaningful is less straightforward. The issue is whether the observed change in scale scores represents movement of the bull's-eye versus random measurement error. The most widely used approach relies on Cohen's (1969) effect-size measures. Cohen suggested that the magnitude of group-level differences (as in intervention versus control) could best be gauged by (1) obtaining the average change from baseline to the end of the study in each group, (2) subtracting the average change in the control group from the average change in the intervention group, and (3) dividing the result by the pooled standard deviation obtained from both groups at baseline. The result (effect size) is a measure of the average change attributable to the intervention expressed relative to the amount of variation in the population.

Cohen (1969) further suggested that effect sizes ≥ 0.20 were small, effect sizes ≥ 0.50 were medium, and effect sizes ≥ 0.80 were large. The main problem with Cohen's effect-size approach is that the categorization of levels is arbitrary and atheoretical. Nonetheless, a recent meta-analysis (Norman *et al.*, 2003) of 38 studies containing 68 effect-size estimates found that the mean estimated meaningfully important difference was equivalent to an effect size of 0.50. Furthermore, if seven response options exist for each question in the scale, an effect size of 0.50 is remarkably close to estimates of human abilities to discriminate between two feeling states (Miller, 1956). Thus, in the absence of known-groups or criterion guidelines for how much change in scale scores is clinically relevant, an effect-size difference of 0.50 is a plausible rule of thumb.

IMPAIRMENTS

It is well established that the assessment of physical impairments in older adults is crucial, and there is growing con*sensus* that performance-based estimates in this area have distinct advantages over self-reports, especially with respect to sensitivity and responsiveness (Avlund, 1997; Berg and Norman, 1996; Gross, 2004; Guralnik, 1997; Ostir *et al.*, 2002; Reuben and Siu, 1990; Reuben *et al.*, 1995). Building upon initial work conducted as part of the EPESE (Established Populations for the Epidemiologic Study of the Elderly; Guralnik *et al.*, 1994, 1995), Guralnik and colleagues have developed, refined, and provided considerable psychometric evidence for a standardized physical performance measure of lower body function using data from the 1002 moderately to severely disabled women participating in the Women's Health and Aging Study (WHAS), a 3-year prospective community-based cohort study. The focus on lower body function derives from the substantial evidence that mobility-related dysfunction is the most detrimental, and that such limitations drive the disablement process.

The standardized, lower body physical performance measure was designed to be administered by a single lay interviewer within the spatial limitations typically encountered in the study subject's home. It consists of a hierarchical balance test, a 4-m walk, and repetitive chair stands. A summary score (0–5) is determined for each component, with those unable to perform the task scored as a zero. The hierarchical balance test involves tandem, semi-tandem, and side-by-side stands:

> "For each stand, the interviewer first demonstrated the task, then supported one arm while participants positioned their feet, asked if they were ready, then released the support and began timing. The timing was stopped when participants moved their feet or grasped the interviewer for support, or when 10 seconds had elapsed. Each participant began with the semi-tandem stand, in which the heel of one foot was placed to the side of the first toe of the other foot, with the participant choosing which foot to place forward. Those unable to hold the semi-tandem position for 10 seconds were evaluated with the feet in the side-by-side position [for a maximum of 10 seconds]. Those able to maintain the semi-tandem position for 10 seconds were further evaluated with the feet in full-tandem position, with the heel of one foot directly in front of the toes of the other foot [for a maximum of 10 seconds]."
>
> (Guralnik *et al.*, 1994, p. M86)

The summary balance scale score was determined as follows. Subjects who could not hold the side-by-side stand for a full 10 seconds, who tried but were unable to hold this stand at all, or who did not attempt any of the three stands either based on their concerns or those of the interviewer (for safety reasons) were scored as a zero. Subjects who were able to hold the side-by-side stand for a full 10 seconds, but who could not hold the semi-tandem stand for a full 10 seconds were scored as a one. Subjects who held the semi-tandem stand for a full 10 seconds but could not hold the tandem stand for at least two seconds were scored as a two. Subjects who were able to hold the tandem stand for 3 to 9 seconds were scored as a three, and subjects who could hold the tandem stand for the full 10 seconds were scored as a four.

The 4-m walk was performed at the study subject's normal pace, with a 3-m course substituted when necessary given unobstructed spatial constraints in the home (which occurred 9% of the time; Ostir *et al.*, 2002). A premeasured flat cord was used to layout the walking course, with the starting line, end of course line (for the interviewer's benefit), and stopping line (for the study subject's benefit) appropriately indicated. Subjects were instructed to "...walk to the other end of the course at your usual speed, just as if you were walking down the street to go to the store" (Guralnik *et al.*, 1994, p. M86). Each study subject was asked to perform this gait speed test twice, with the faster timing of their two trials (expressed in meters/second to adjust for two course lengths) used in the analyses. Scores were categorized into approximate quartiles with cut-points at ≤0.43, ≤0.60, ≤0.77, and ≥0.78 m second, with these quartiles assigned scores of one to four, respectively, and those unable to perform the test scored as a zero.

The repetitive chair stand test was performed as follows. Interviewers demonstrated the chair stand protocol using a straight-backed chair without arms, and having the arms folded across their chests. After the study subject demonstrated that she/he could perform a single chair stand safely, interviewers then asked them to perform five repetitive chair stands as quickly as possible. Timings from the start of the test to the peak of the fifth rise were categorized into approximate quartiles, with cut-points at ≥16.7, ≥13.7, ≥11.2, and ≤11.1 seconds assigned scores of one to four, respectively, with those unable to perform the test scored as a zero.

The overall score for the standardized lower body functional performance measure is the simple sum of the three categorical component scores, and thus ranges from 0 to 12. In general, the distribution of WHAS study subjects across the overall score range approximates the intended uniform function, with the notable exception of relatively few subjects in the best performing category (Guralnik *et al.*, 1995; Onder *et al.*, 2002). The short-term (weekly) test–retest reliability of the overall score has been shown to be excellent in multiple comparisons (≥0.88), and the long-term (six-month) test–retest reliability is very good (0.72 to 0.79; Ostir *et al.*, 2002). Furthermore, the overall score has been shown to be highly predictive of subsequent disability (ADL limitations) over both 2- and 4-year follow-ups (Guralnik *et al.*, 1995; Ostir *et al.*, 1998), and lower values on the overall score have been highly associated with increased risk of nursing home admission, health services use, and death (Ferrucci *et al.*, 2000; Guralnik *et al.*, 1994; Penninx *et al.*, 2000). Finally, the responsiveness of the overall score has been well established in that study subjects experiencing any of four incident medical events (heart attack, stroke, hip fracture, or congestive heart failure) had substantially poorer lower body function performance scores at their follow-up assessment (Ostir *et al.*, 2002). Thus, the standardized lower body functional performance measure has excellent psychometric properties and should be considered the test of choice for future epidemiologic and/or office-based clinical assessments.

FUNCTIONAL LIMITATIONS

Functional capacity refers to the ability to perform specific tasks that require fine and/or gross motor skills and actions (Nagi, 1991; Verbrugge and Jette, 1994). As indicated earlier, the items originally used by Nagi (1976) to measure functional limitations included standing for long periods, lifting or carrying weights of approximately ten pounds, going up and down stairs, walking, stooping-bending-kneeling, using hands and fingers, and reaching out with either or both arms. Subjects were simply asked whether they had no, some, or great difficulty in performing these tasks. Because functional limitations affect the organism as a whole, self-reports can provide reliable and valid measures (Avlund *et al.*, 1996; Siu *et al.*, 1990; Wolinsky and Miller, 2005). The problems with extant functional limitation scales, however, are that they have seldom covered the full spectrum of gross and fine motor scales, and their reproducibility and responsiveness have been inadequate (Linn and Linn, 1980; Reuben, 1995).

Recently, Jette and colleagues (Jette *et al.*, 2002; Haley *et al.*, 2002) have developed the Late-Life Function and Disability Instrument (Late-Life FDI) to overcome these problems. Building on Nagi's (1976, 1991) conceptual framework for the epidemiology of disability, the Late-Life FDI focuses on discrete activities and expands the range of actions under study beyond basic physical skills, which have been shown to be rather ineffective measures for capturing the variation in functional abilities found in the general population of community-dwelling older adults. After an extensive review of the literature, focus groups with older adults, and consultation with measurement experts, 54 items were initially developed to tap the full range of functional limitations, and after initial pilot testing, 48 of these were retained. A convenience sample of 150 older community-dwelling adults aged 60 years old and older from central and eastern Massachusetts was empanelled for further development and evaluation purposes.

Exploratory factor analyses were used to identify the 32 items that formed the most reliable and valid scales tapping three domains – basic lower extremity functions, advanced lower extremity functions, and upper extremity functions – that satisfied established criteria for simple structure (unidimensional scales, unipolar principal factor loadings ≥0.40, and no factorial complexity; DeVellis, 2003). Table 1 contains the final items for each scale and lists the items in ascending order of the degree of item difficulty. That is, the items are ordered from the easiest to accomplish functions to the most difficult to accomplish functions. Item difficulty calibrations were determined using Item Response Theory (IRT; Wright and Masters, 1982) methods. Scale scores are transformed to range between 0 (worst function) and 100 (best function).

Cronbach's alphas were 0.96 for the basic lower extremity scale, 0.96 for the advanced lower extremity scale, and 0.86 for the upper extremity scale. Test–retest reliability coefficients obtained on a small subset at approximately 2 weeks were ≥0.91. Responsiveness was evaluated using known-groups comparisons, with four groups (no functional limitations, slight, moderate, or severe functional limitations) determined based on scores from the SF-36 physical function scale. For each of the functional limitations domains, a monotonic and statistically significant decline in scale scores was observed progressing from the no functional limitations group to the severe functional limitations group. Although further research is needed on a nationally representative sample in order to establish population-based norms, the Late-Life FDI functional limitations scales are extremely promising and their use is epidemiologic and office-based clinical settings is strongly encouraged.

Table 1 The functional status items of the late-life function and disability instrument, by domain and in ascending order of difficulty (Haley *et al.*, 2002)

How much difficulty do you have ...without the help of someone else and without the use of assistive devices? (Responses: none, a little, some, quite a lot, or cannot do)

The 14 basic lower extremity items
Wash dishes while standing
Put on and take off coat
Walk around one floor of home
Pick up a kitchen chair
Get in and out of a car
Make bed
Reach overhead while standing
Go up and down a flight of stairs
Bend over from standing position
Up and down from a curb
Open heavy outside door
On and off a step stool
On and off bus
Stand up from a low soft couch

The 11 advanced lower extremity items
Walk several blocks
Walk 1 mile with rests
Get up from floor
Go up and down 1 flight, no rails
Go up and down 3 flights, inside
Carry while climb stairs
Run to catch bus
Walk a brisk mile
Walk on slippery surface
Hike a few miles including hills
Run one-half mile

The 7 upper extremity items
Hold full glass of water in one hand
Put on and take of pants
Use common utensils
Reach behind back
Pour from a large pitcher
Remove wrapping with hands only
Unscrew lid without assistive device

Source: From *J Gerontol A Biol Sci Med Sci*, 2002; **57**:M217–M222.

DISABILITY

Disability refers to the ability to perform ADLs and IADLs (Nagi, 1991; Verbrugge and Jette, 1994). Despite considerable work on the development and evaluation of ADL and IADL scales, however, a number of problems remain (Avlund *et al.*, 1993; Fitzgerald *et al.*, 1993; Katz *et al.*, 1963; Kempen and Suurmeijer, 1990; Thomas *et al.*, 1998; Wolinsky and Johnson, 1991; Wolinsky and Miller, 2005). As with functional limitations, the principal problems with disability scales involve the lack of conceptual clarity, the limited spectrum of activities that are tapped, and limited responsiveness for the detection of change (Jette, 1994, 2003; Jette and Keysor, 2003). Thus, Jette and colleagues (2002) set out to develop a more comprehensive, reliable, valid, and responsive disability measure.

Using the same approach and sample as in the development of the Late-Life FDI, functional limitations scales (Haley *et al.*, 2002), Jette *et al.* (2002) developed the Late-Life FDI disability scales. A refined list of 25 life tasks were administered to the 150 community-dwelling adults aged 60 years old or older in central and eastern Massachusetts. Unlike the functional limitations items, the disability questions are asked twice, once to determine how often the study subject does the life task, and once to determine the extent of their limitations in performing the life task.

Exploratory factor analyses were used to identify the 16 items that formed the most reliable and valid scales tapping the two domains – frequency of performance, and limitation in capability – that satisfied established criteria for simple structure (unidimensional scales, unipolar principal factors loadings ≥0.40, and no factorial complexity; DeVellis, 2003). Table 2 contains the final items and lists the items in ascending order of the degree of item difficulty, with item difficulty calibrations again determined using IRT methods (Wright and Masters, 1982). Scale scores are transformed to range between 0 (worst function) and 100 (best function).

Table 2 The 16 disability items of the late-life function and disability instrument, by domain and in ascending order of difficulty (Jette *et al.*, 2002)

Frequency items
How often do you
(Responses: very often, often, once in a while, almost never, never)
- take care of your own personal care needs?
- take care of your own health?
- keep in touch with others?
- provide meals for yourself and family?
- take care of household business and finances?
- take care of local errands?
- take care of inside of home?
- go out with others in public places?
- visit friends in their homes?
- provide care or assistance to others?
- take part in regular exercise program?
- invite people into your home?
- take part in organized social activities?
- travel out of town?
- work at a volunteer job?
- take part in active recreation?

Limitation items
To what extent do you feel limited in
(Responses: not at all, a little, somewhat, a lot, completely)
- taking care of your own health?
- taking care of your own personal care needs?
- taking care of household business and finances?
- providing meals for yourself and family?
- keeping in touch with others?
- taking care of local errands?
- taking part in organized social activities?
- going out with others in public places?
- inviting people into your home?
- providing care or assistance to others?
- visiting friends in their homes?
- taking care of inside of home?
- taking part in regular exercise program?
- working at a volunteer job?
- traveling out of town?
- taking part in active recreation?

Source: From *J Gerontol A Biol Sci Med Sci*, 2002; **57**:M209–M216.

Cronbach's alphas were 0.82 for the frequency of performance scale and 0.92 for the limitation in capability scale, and test–retest reliability coefficients were 0.68 and 0.82, respectively. Responsiveness was evaluated using known-groups comparisons, again with four groups (no functional limitations, slight, moderate, or severe functional limitations) based on scores from the SF-36 physical function scale. For each of the disability domains, a monotonic and statistically significant decline in scale scores was observed progressing from the no functional limitations group to the severe functional limitations group. Thus, the Late-Life FDI disability scales are also extremely promising and their use is strongly encouraged in epidemiologic and office-based settings. Taken together, it takes less than 25 minutes to administer all of the Late-Life FDI scales.

HEALTH-RELATED QUALITY OF LIFE

Health-related quality of life (HRQoL) is an important consequence of the disablement process for older adults. The most widely used HRQoL instrument in the world, regardless of study subject age, is the SF-36, which comprehensively addresses all facets of the classic WHO (1947) definition. A detailed description of the SF-36 developmental process and procedures is readily available elsewhere (Ware, 1996), and the exact wording of the items for both the original version and the second version (SF-36 V2) can be found in the SF-36 web page (www.sf-36.org). Thirty-five of the 36 items make up eight scales: physical functioning (10 items), role limitations due to physical functioning (4 items), bodily pain (2 items), general health perceptions (5 items), vitality (4 items), social functioning (2 items), role limitations due to emotional problems (3 items), and mental health (5 items). The remaining item asks respondents about any health changes over the past year, but is not used in any of the scales. Within scales, a proration imputation method is used for missing data. That is, as long as the subject answers at least half of the items within a scale, the average of those items is imputed for any items not answered in that scale. Because of the different number of items and response options in each scale, raw scores are transformed to range from 0 (worst health) to 100 (best health).

The original version of the SF-36 was selected in 1998 by the Centers for Medicare and Medicaid Services (CMS) as the core instrument for monitoring the quality of care proved by managed care organizations (MCOs). To evaluate MCOs, CMS requires each Medicare + Choice plan, Social HMO (SHMOs), and Section 1876 risk and cost contract plan to participate in the Health Outcomes Survey (HOS). Each HOS-participating plan annually identifies a random sample of 1000 beneficiaries for the National Center for Quality Assurance (NCQA). NCQA and its approved subcontractors then mail out the HOS protocol to the samples during the baseline line year and during the follow-up survey 2 years later. Plans are evaluated based on a trichotomous classification of the obtained change scores as better, the same, or worse HRQoL. The HOS calls for five successive cohorts (samples) starting in 1998 and 2000 for cohort one, and finishing in 2002 and 2004 for cohort five. Baseline response rates have been in the upper 60% range, and retention rates among survivors who remained in the health plans have been in the lower 80% range.

Deidentified data files from the HOS are now available (www.ncqa.org) for public use. The 1998 baseline data are used here to demonstrate the reliability, validity, and responsiveness of the SF-36 for older adults. As reported by Gandek *et al.* (2004), the reliability and validity of the SF-36 based on these data is good. Item analyses indicated that 95% or more of the respondents completed all of the items within any given scale. Floor and ceiling effects were modest for physical function and pain scales, low for the general health, vitality and mental health scales, substantial for the role physical and role emotional scales, and notable for the social function scale. Internal consistency reliability coefficients (Cronbach's alpha) for the eight SF-36 scales exceeded 0.80 and were greater than 0.90 for the physical and mental component summary scales. Indeed, the only unexpected results involved the exploratory factor analyses. In contrast to the hypothesized model of separate physical and mental composites, a unidimensional second-order factor structure was identified based on eigenvalue and scree criteria. When a two-factor solution was forced, however, the role emotional and mental health scales did load principally on the second factor, with near zero loadings on the first factor. Thus, overall, the 1998 HOS baseline data provide considerable support for the SF-36's underlying conceptual model.

To address the responsiveness of the SF-36, additional analyses were conducted for this chapter using the 1998 baseline HOS data for subjects aged 65 years old or older. Table 3

Table 3 Mean scores for each of the eight SF-36 scales by the number of diseases for subjects 65 years old or older in the baseline (1998) Center for Medicaid and Medicare Services (CMS) Health Outcomes Study (HOS)[a]

Number of diseases (*N*)	Physical function	Role-physical	Bodily pain	General health	Vitality	Social function	Role-emotional	Mental health
None (47 345)	74.2	71.8	71.2	73.5	64.7	86.9	84.5	81.5
1 (51 193)	67.6	63.1	65.9	67.3	59.5	83.0	80.0	79.0
2 (25 650)	59.6	51.6	60.4	59.7	53.4	77.2	73.4	76.4
3 (10 755)	53.1	42.3	56.2	53.3	48.7	72.2	68.9	74.3
4 (4744)	47.6	35.3	51.9	47.8	44.1	67.5	63.7	72.1
≥5 (2128)	38.6	25.0	45.7	40.2	36.1	58.4	55.2	67.3

[a]Where 0 = worst possible health, and 100 = best possible health. *p*-values obtained from global analysis of variance tests within columns were all <0.001. Shaded cells reflect deviations from expected monotonic decline within columns.

Table 4 Mean scores for each of the eight SF-36 scales by the number of activities of daily living (ADLs) for which subjects 65 years old or older in the baseline (1998) Center for Medicaid and Medicare Services (CMS) Health Outcomes Study (HOS) Reported Difficulty[a]

Number of six ADLs(N)	Physical function	Role-physical	Bodily pain	General health	Vitality	Social function	Role-emotional	Mental health
None (88 171)	79.8	78.3	75.7	73.8	66.9	90.3	87.5	82.6
1(20 253)	54.2	43.6	55.3	59.1	50.7	76.8	72.5	76.0
2(15 207)	41.4	27.6	45.5	52.5	42.9	67.7	64.4	72.7
3(5643)	31.7	17.3	40.0	45.4	37.4	56.7	54.1	68.0
4(3906)	25.0	11.8	34.6	41.2	33.2	48.9	47.5	65.0
5(2636)	20.2	9.33	1.03	7.13	0.84	1.54	0.86	1.0
6(1841)	33.7	25.5	42.0	42.5	38.0	48.9	44.2	60.0

[a]Where 0 = worst possible health, and 100 = best possible health. P-values obtained from global analysis of variance tests within columns were all <0.001. Shaded cells reflect deviations from expected monotonic decline within columns.

Table 5 Unstandardized partial regression coefficients obtained from multivariable linear regression of the eight SF-36 scales on demographics, ADLs, and diseases for subjects 65-years old or older in the baseline (1998) Center for Medicaid and Medicare Services (CMS) Health Outcomes Study (HOS)[a]

Independent variables	Physical function	Role-physical	Bodily pain	General health	Vitality	Social function	Role-emotional	Mental health
Demographics								
Age ≥ 75	−5.36	−8.02	−0.05	−0.50	−1.67	−1.37	−5.61	−0.57
Male	4.94	2.18	3.35	−0.38	2.08	1.55	2.32	2.18
Black	−1.89	0.08	0.99	−2.72	3.36	−1.48	−4.09	0.91
Other race	−0.55*	0.31	1.02	−1.51	1.89	−2.79	−2.43	−0.78
Education	2.85	3.35	1.52	2.73	1.67	1.44	4.87	2.49
ADLs								
Bathing	−12.59	−11.18	−4.93	−7.78	−6.51	−12.28	−11.06	−5.18
Dressing	−5.44	−5.65	−4.67	−3.58	−3.22	−6.80	−4.34	−2.28
Eating	1.82	−2.58	−0.76*	−5.29	−3.72	−6.64	−10.26	−7.43
Chair/bed transfer	−9.03	−15.33	−12.15	−5.21	−7.91	−6.82	−7.17	−3.26
Walking	−26.91	−31.22	−18.36	−12.48	−13.91	−13.02	−11.31	−4.70
Toileting	0.33	1.29*	−1.14	−0.43	0.42	−3.26	3.36	−2.00
Diseases								
Hypertension	−2.27	−2.65	−2.07	−3.19	−2.31	−1.06	−1.19	−1.43
Angina/CAD	−3.48	−7.65	−5.07	−6.03	−4.31	−3.39	−3.49	−2.23
CHF	−7.43	−8.20	−1.85	−7.69	−5.09	−5.36	−4.74	−1.67
AMI	−1.48	−2.50	−0.51*	−2.50	−1.58	−1.09	−0.83*	−0.54**
Stroke	−3.60	−5.31	0.27	−3.25	−3.03	−3.27	−4.31	−1.90
Diabetes	−2.56	−2.81	−1.22	−4.93	−2.64	−1.84	−3.66	−0.98
Cancer	−2.86	−5.77	−2.28	−4.65	−3.46	−3.10	−2.44	−1.01
Intercept	86.36	91.71	72.50	73.01	68.32	91.66	91.25	76.08
R-Squared	0.52	0.34	0.33	0.35	0.31	0.31	0.16	0.15
Number of cases	126,102	123,242	124,655	125,044	124,595	124,753	122,821	124,552

[a]Where 0 = worst possible health, and 100 = best possible health. Shaded cells reflect p-values > 0.05; p-values < 0.05 indicated by one asterisk (*), p-values < 0.01 indicated by two asterisks (**), with all other p-values < 0.001.

contains the mean scores for each of the eight SF-36 scales by the number of self-reported diseases (hypertension, angina or CAD, congestive heart failure, heart attack, stroke, diabetes, and cancer). As shown, the progressive decline in scale scores with increasing comorbidity holds for each scale. As expected, the extent of the decline is greatest for those scales tapping the physical health components of HRQoL than for those tapping the mental health components. Table 4 contains similar data based on the number of ADL limitations (bathing, dressing, eating, getting out of a chair, walking across a room, and toileting). In general, the same pattern holds, with the exception of those who were limited in all six ADLs, which is likely an artifact of the relatively small sample in that group.

Although the data shown in Tables 3 and 4 provide rather convincing known-groups evidence of the responsiveness of the SF-36 scales, those differences are crude (one-way analyses of variance) and aggregated. To estimate the net effects of each ADL and disease on the eight SF-36 scales, multiple linear regression analyses were conducted, adjusting for age, gender, race, and education. Table 5 contains the intercepts, unstandardized regression coefficients, and R-squared values obtained from these analyses. The unstandardized regression coefficients can be interpreted as the attributable change in the SF-36 scale score for older adults having that ADL limitation or disease, adjusted for the other ADLs and diseases, as well as the sociodemographic factors. As shown, although nearly all effects are statistically significant given the very large sample sizes, the dominant effect for all scales is associated with the walking ADL item, followed by the bathing ADL item. This is as expected and is consistent with the remarkable predictive power of lower body impairments on subsequent health outcomes. Somewhat less expected is the more modest effect of the individual diseases on HRQoL, although this may be reflective of their mediation through the ADLs. It is also worth noting that the R-squared value is greatest (0.52) for the physical function scale and smallest for the role emotional and mental health scales. This is consistent with the results of the exploratory factor analysis and supports the general notion that the mental health component of the SF-36 is not as responsive to disease and disability as the physical health component.

Acknowledgment

Supported by NIH grant R01 AG-022913 to Fredric D. Wolinsky. The opinions expressed here are those of the authors and do not necessarily reflect those of the NIH or any of the academic or governmental institutions involved. Address all correspondence to Fredric D. Wolinsky, the John W. Colloton Chair in Health Management and Policy, College of Public Health, the University of Iowa, 200 Hawkins Drive, E-205 General Hospital, Iowa City, Iowa 52242. Internet: fredric-wolinsky@uiowa.edu

KEY POINTS

- Despite the clinical and pragmatic importance of functional assessment, this area of geriatrics suffers from conceptual confusion and methodological limitations.
- Functional assessment scales should be based on established theoretical models of the disablement process and traditional psychometric principles.
- On the basis of the theoretical and methodological considerations, the following state-of-the-art measures were selected and are recommended for each of the principal components of the disablement process:
  - for *impairments*: the standardized lower body physical performance measure
  - for *functional limitations*: the functional component of the Late-Life Functional Disability Instrument (Late-Life FDI)
  - for *disability*: the disability component of the Late-Life Functional Disability Instrument (Late-Life FDI)
  - for *health-related quality of life*: the SF-36.

KEY REFERENCES

- Nagi SZ. An epidemiology of disability among adults in the United States. *Milbank Memorial Fund Quarterly. Health and Society* 1976; **54**:439–67.
- Nagi SZ. Disability concepts revisited: implications for prevention. In AM Pope & AR Tarlov (eds) *Disability in America: Toward a National Agenda for Prevention* 1991, pp 309–27; National Academy Press, Washington.
- Verbrugge LK & Jette AM. The disablement process. *Social Science & Medicine* 1994; **38**:1–14.
- Haley SM, Jette AM, Coster WJ *et al.* Late life function and disability instrument: II. Development and evaluation of the function component. *Journal of Gerontology: Medical Sciences* 2002; **57A**:M217–22.
- Jette AM, Haley SM, Coster WJ *et al.* Late life function and disability instrument: I. Development and evaluation of the disability component. *Journal of Gerontology: Medical Sciences* 2002; **57A**:M209–16.

REFERENCES

Avlund K. Methodological challenges in measurements of functional ability in gerontological research: a review. *Aging Clinical and Experimental Research* 1997; **9**:164–74.

Avlund K, Kreiner S & Schultz-Larsen K. Functional ability scales for the elderly: a validation study. *European Journal of Public Health* 1996; **6**:35–42.

Avlund K, Schultz-Larsen K & Kreiner S. The measurement of instrumental ADL: content validity and construct validity. *Aging* 1993; **5**:371–83.

Berg K & Norman KE. Functional assessment of balance and gait. *Clinics in Geriatric Medicine* 1996; **12**:705–23.

Cohen J. *Statistical Power Analysis for the Behavioural Sciences* 1969; Academic Press, London.

DeVellis RF. *Scale Development: Theory and Applications* 2003; Sage Publications, Thousand Oaks.

Ferrucci L, Penninx BWJH, Leveille SG *et al.* Characteristics of nondisabled older adults who perform poorly in objective test of lower extremity function. *Journal of the American Geriatrics Society* 2000; **48**:1102–10.

Fitzgerald JF, Smith DM, Martin D *et al.* Replication of the multidimensionality of activities of daily living. *Journal of Gerontology: Social Sciences* 1993; **48**:S28–31.

Gandek B, Sinclair SJ, Kosinski M & Ware JE. Psychometric evaluation of the SF-36 health survey in medicare managed care. *Health Care Financing Review* 2004; **25**(4):5–25.

Gross DP. Measurement properties of performance-based assessment of functional capacity. *Journal of Occupational Rehabilitation* 2004; **14**:165–74.

Guralnik JM. Assessment of physical performance and disability in older persons. *Muscle & Nerve* 1997; **5**:S14–6.

Guralnik JM, Ferrucci L, Simonsick EM *et al.* Lower-extremity function in persons over the age of 70 years as a predictor of subsequent disability. *The New England Journal of Medicine* 1995; **332**:556–61.

Guralnik JM, Simonsick EM, Ferrucci L *et al.* A short physical performance battery assessing lower extremity function: association with self-reported disability and prediction of mortality and nursing home admission. *Journal of Gerontology: Medical Sciences* 1994; **49A**:M85–94.

Haley SM, Jette AM, Coster WJ *et al.* Late life function and disability instrument: II. Development and evaluation of the function component. *Journal of Gerontology: Medical Sciences* 2002; **57A**:M217–22.

Jette AM. How measurement techniques influence estimates of disability in older populations. *Social Science & Medicine* 1994; **38**:937–42.

Jette AM. Assessing disability in studies on physical activity. *American Journal of Preventive Medicine* 2003; **25**:122–8.

Jette AM, Haley SM, Coster WJ *et al.* Late life function and disability instrument: I. Development and evaluation of the disability component. *Journal of Gerontology: Medical Sciences* 2002; **57A**:M209–16.

Jette AM & Keysor JJ. Disability models: implications for arthritis exercise and physical activity interventions. *Arthritis and Rheumatism* 2003; **49**:114–20.

Katz S, Ford A, Moskowitz R *et al.* Studies of illness in the aged. The index of ADL: a standardized measure of biological and psychological function. *Journal of the American Medical Association* 1963; **185**:914–9.

Kempen GI & Suurmeijer TP. The development of a hierarchical polychotomous ADL-IADL scale for noninstitutionalized elders. *The Gerontologist* 1990; **30**:497–502.

Linn BS & Linn MW. Objective and self-assessed health in the old and very old. *Social Science & Medicine* 1980; **14A**:311–5.

Miller GA. The magic number seven plus or minus two: some limits on our capacity for processing information. *Psychological Review* 1956; **63**:81–97.

Nagi SZ. Some conceptual issues in disability and rehabilitation. In MB Sussman (ed) *Sociology and Rehabilitation* 1965, pp 100–13; American Sociological Association, Washington.

Nagi SZ. *Disability and Rehabilitation: Legal, Clinical, and Self Concepts and Measurement* 1969; Ohio State University Press, Columbus.

Nagi SZ. An epidemiology of disability among adults in the United States. *Milbank Memorial Fund Quarterly. Health and Society* 1976; **54**:439–67.

Nagi SZ. Disability concepts revisited: implications for prevention. In AM Pope & AR Tarlov (eds) *Disability in America: Toward a National Agenda for Prevention* 1991, pp 309–27; National Academy Press, Washington.

Norman GR, Sloan JA & Wyrwich KW. Interpretation of changes in health related quality of life: the remarkable universality of half a standard deviation. *Medical Care* 2003; **41**:582–92.

Onder G, Penninx BWJH, Lapuerta P *et al.* Change in physical performance over time in older women: the Women's Health and Aging Study. *Journal of Gerontology: Medical Sciences* 2002; **57A**:M289–93.

Ostir GV, Markides KS, Black SA & Goodwin JS. Lower body functioning as a predictor of subsequent disability among older Mexican Americans. *Journal of Gerontology: Medical Sciences* 1998; **53**:M491–5.

Ostir GV, Volpato S, Fried LP *et al.* Reliability and sensitivity to change assessed for a summary measure of lower body function: results from the Women's Health and Aging Study. *Journal of Clinical Epidemiology* 2002; **55**:916–21.

Penninx BWJH, Ferrucci L, Leveille SG *et al.* Lower extremity performance in nondisabled older persons as a predictor of subsequent hospitalization. *Journal of Gerontology: Medical Sciences* 2000; **55**:M691–7.

Reuben DB. What's wrong with ADLs? *Journal of the American Geriatrics Society* 1995; **43**:936–7.

Reuben DB & Siu AI. An objective measure of physical function of elderly outpatients: the physical performance test. *Journal of the American Geriatrics Society* 1990; **38**:1105–12.

Reuben DB, Valle LA, Hays RD & Siu AL. Measuring physical function in community-dwelling older persons: a comparison of self-administered, interviewer-administered, and performance-based measures. *Journal of the American Geriatrics Society* 1995; **43**:17–23.

Siu A, Reuben D & Hays R. Hierarchical measures of physical function in ambulatory geriatrics. *Journal of the American Geriatrics Society* 1990; **38**:1113–9.

Thomas VS, Rockwood K & McDowell I. Multidimensionality in instrumental and basic activities of daily living. *Journal of Clinical Epidemiology* 1998; **51**:315–21.

Trochim W. *Social Research Methods* 2004; Atomic Dog Press, Philadelphia, and http://www.socialresearchmethods.net.

Verbrugge LK & Jette AM. The disablement process. *Social Science & Medicine* 1994; **38**:1–14.

Ware JE. The SF-36 health survey. In B Spilker (ed) *Quality of Life and Pharmacoeconomics in Clinical Trials* 1996, 2nd edn, pp 337–45; Lippincott-Raven Publishers, Philadelphia.

Wolinsky FD & Johnson RJ. The use of health services by older adults. *Journal of Gerontology: Social Sciences* 1991; **46**:S345–57.

Wolinsky, FD & Miller DK. Revisiting the disablement process. In JM Wilmoth & KF Ferraro (eds) *Gerontology: Perspectives and Issues* 2005, 3rd edn; Springer Publishing, New York.

World Health Organization. *Constitution of the World Health Organization* 1947; World Health Organization, New York.

Wright B & Masters G. *Rating Scale Analysis* 1982; MESA Press, Chicago.

133

Frailty

John E. Morley

Saint Louis University School of Medicine and Saint Louis Veterans' Affairs Medical Center, St Louis, MO, USA

INTRODUCTION

Frailty can be defined as that condition when a person loses the ability to carry out important, practiced social activities of daily living when exposed to either psychological or stressful conditions (Morley *et al.*, 2005). It should be distinguished from disability. Frailty represents a form of predisability.

Frailty has been objectively defined by Linda Fried and her colleagues at John's Hopkins University (Table 1) (Fried *et al.*, 2004, 2001). Their definition includes weight loss, exhaustion, weakness, walking speed, and low physical activity. By this definition, approximately 6.9% of the older population are frail. Females are more often classified as frail than are males of the same age. Frailty is the beginning of a cascade that leads to functional deterioration, hospitalization, institutionalization, and death (Figure 1). Over our lifetime, there is a peak in vitality between 20 and 30 years of age, after which there is a gradual physiological decline in performance (Figure 2). This decline can be delayed by positive behaviors, such as exercise, or accelerated by negative factors such as disease. However, eventually all individuals, if they live long enough, will cross the frailty threshold. This chapter will discuss the factors involved in the acceleration of the life slope toward the frailty threshold.

PATHOPHYSIOLOGY OF FRAILTY

The causes of frailty are multifactorial. The backdrop for the development of frailty is the physiological changes of aging. The interaction of normal physiology with genes, lifestyle, environment, and disease determines which individuals will become frail. In most individuals, frailty is caused by the failure to generate adequate muscle power and/or the failure to have sufficient executive function to appropriately utilize the available executive function. The major causes of frailty are illustrated in Figure 3.

Disease

Numerous disease processes can directly or indirectly result in frailty. Many diseases produce an excess of cytokines that can lead to a decrease in muscle mass, food intake, and cognitive function. Diseases also lead to a decline in levels of the anabolic hormone, testosterone.

Congestive heart failure (CHF) is a condition that is classically associated with frailty. Persons with CHF have a marked decline in their VO_{2max}, leading to an inability to perform endurance or resistance tasks. Left-sided heart failure leads to intestinal wall edema. This results in bacterial translocation into the lymphatic and systemic circulation. The bacterial endotoxins (lipopolysaccharides) result in the activation of the immune system and release of cytokines, such as TNFα. This results in anorexia, loss of muscle mass, weight loss, hypoalbuminemia, and hypocholesterolemia (Figure 4). In CHF, the best predictors of poor outcome are weight loss and hypocholesterolemia (Von Haehling *et al.*, 2004). Activation of the angiotensin II system that leads to cleaving of actomyosin and subsequent clearance of muscle protein by the ubiquitin-proteasome system may also play a role. Angiotensin-converting enzyme inhibitors reverse weight loss and frailty in some persons with CHF.

Persons with chronic obstructive pulmonary disease have a decrease in endurance, weight loss due to poor food intake, and increased resting metabolic rate and thermic energy of eating. They lose muscle because of low testosterone levels and increased circulating cytokine levels.

Diabetes mellitus is classically associated with an increase in frailty, injurious falls, disability, and premature death (Figure 5). Again, the causes are multifactorial, and include low testosterone, increased angiotensin II, increased cytokines, peripheral neuropathy, reduced executive function, and accelerated atherosclerosis (Maty *et al.*, 2004; Rodriguez-Saldana *et al.*, 2002; Miller *et al.*, 1999; Sinclair, 1999).

Persons with anemia have reduced endurance, decreased muscle strength, orthostasis, increased falls, increased frailty,

Principles and Practice of Geriatric Medicine, 4th Edition. Edited by M.S. John Pathy, Alan J. Sinclair and John E. Morley.

Table 1 Objective definition of frailty

- Weight loss (10 lbs in 1 year)
- Exhaustion (self-report)
- Weakness (grip strength: lowest 20%)
- Walking speed (15 feet; slowest 20%)
- Low physical activity (Kcals/week: lowest 20%)

Source: From J Gerontol A Biol Sci Med Sci, 2001; **56**:M146 M156. Copyright 2001 The Gerontological Society of America. Reproduced by permission of the publisher.

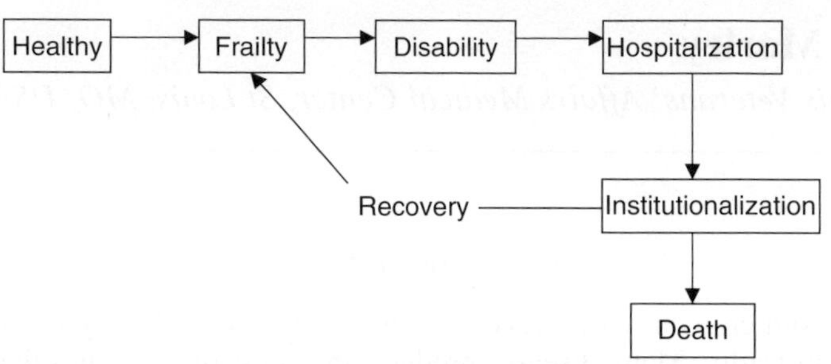

Figure 1 The pathway from frailty to death

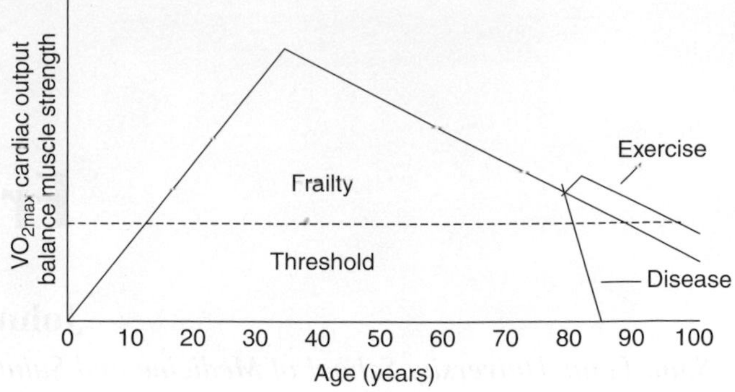

Figure 2 The frailty threshold

decreased mobility, increased disability, and increased mortality (Figure 6). Both erythropoietin and darbopoetin-α can reverse the anemia and many of these changes (Cesari *et al.*, 2004a; Thomas, 2004). The use of these agents has led to a marked increase in the quality of life of patients with chronic kidney failure, anemia of chronic disease, and myelofibrosis.

Polymalgia rheumatica results in painful muscles with proximal myopathy. The diagnosis is confirmed by finding an elevated erythrocyte sedimentation rate. Treatment of this condition with corticosteroids reverses the frailty it produces. Unfortunately, this totally reversible condition is often misdiagnosed by clinicians.

Endocrine disorders, such as hyperthyroidism, hypothyroidism, and hypoadrenalism, can have insidious onset in older persons. When this occurs, they are the classical causes of the frailty syndrome.

Pain

Joint pain, that is, the arthritides, is classically associated with immobility. Immobility, over time, leads to loss of muscle mass and power and to a decline in endurance, the hallmarks of frailty. Pain can further induce frailty secondarily to increasing depression in older persons.

Decreased Food Intake

Older persons develop a physiological anorexia of aging that is associated with a loss of weight. The causes of the anorexia of aging are multifactorial (Morley, 1997). Social causes, such as isolation and dysphoria, and the decline in smell and increase in taste threshold are obvious causes. Recently, there have been a number of studies that demonstrated

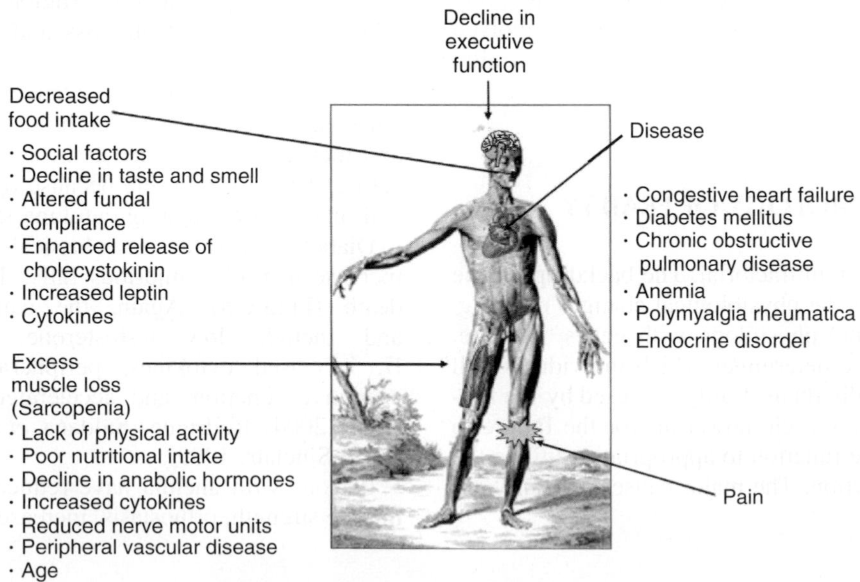

Figure 3 The major causes of frailty

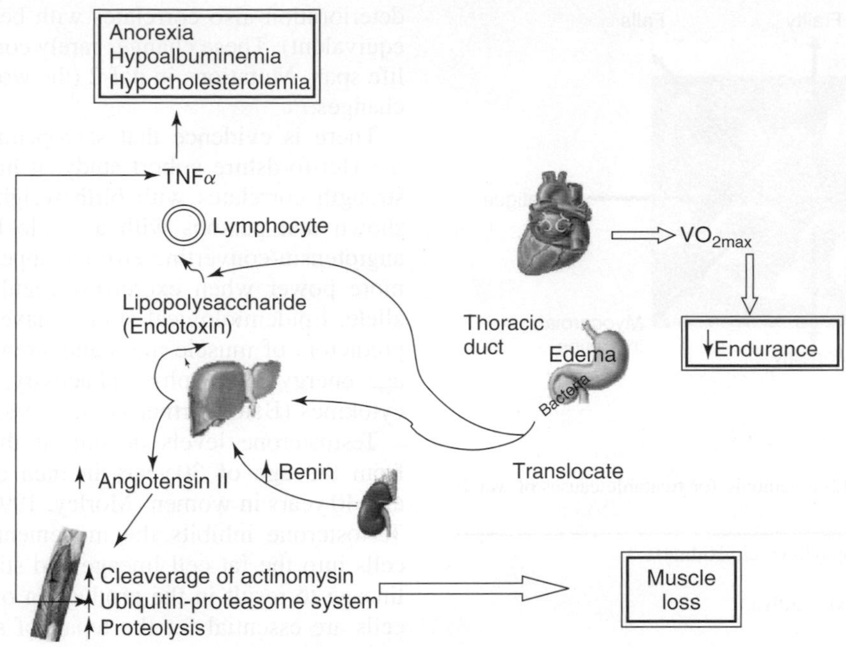

Figure 4 The pathogenesis of frailty in congestive heart failure

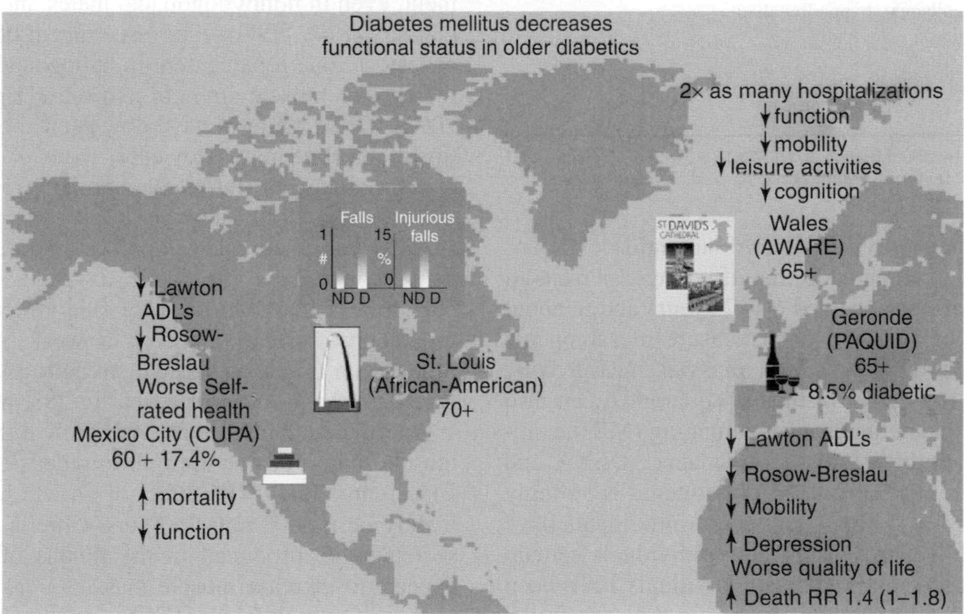

Figure 5 Frailty and diabetes mellitus

that decreased compliance and adaptive relaxation of the stomach results in a more rapid antral filling and early satiety. Excess production of cholecystokinen from the duodenum in response to a fatty meal is another cause of anorexia in older persons. High circulating cytokine levels in older persons have been associated with anorexia. Males have a greater decrease in both absolute and relative amounts of food intake over the life span. This appears to be due to the fall in testosterone, which results in an increase in leptin levels and, therefore, a greater anorexia.

In addition to the physiological anorexia of aging, many reversible causes of anorexia occur in older persons. These are easily remembered by the mnemonic, MEALS-ON-WHEELS (Table 2).

Sarcopenia

Sarcopenia is the excessive loss of muscle mass that occurs in older persons (Morley *et al.*, 2001; Roubenoff, 2003). It

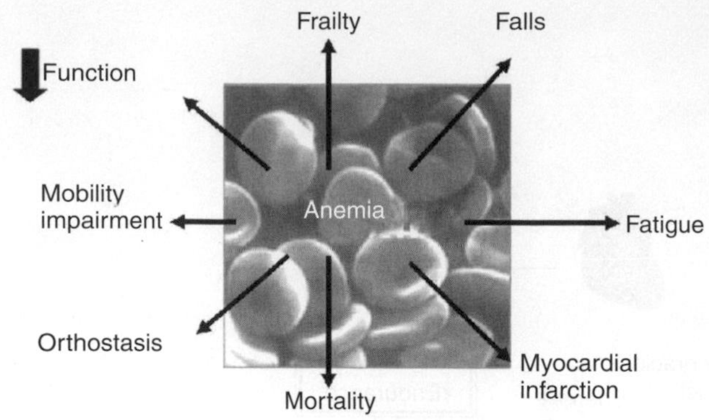

Figure 6 Frailty and anemia

Table 2 MEALS-ON-WHEELS mnemonic for treatable causes of weight loss

Medications (e.g. digoxin, theophylline, cimetidine)
Emotional (e.g. depression)
Alcoholism, elder abuse, anorexia tardive
Late-life paranoia
Swallowing problems
Oral factors
Nosocomial infections (e.g. tuberculosis)
Wandering and other dementia related factors
Hyperthyroidism, hypercalcemia, hypoadrenalism
Enteral problems (e.g. gluten enteropathy)
Eating problems
Low salt, low cholesterol, and other therapeutic diets
Stones (cholecystitis)

Source: From J Gerontol A Biol Sci Med Sci, 2002; **57**:M209–M216. Copyright 2002 The Gerontological Society of America. Reproduced by permission of the publisher.

is usually defined as a greater than two standard deviations amount of lean tissue compared to that of younger persons. It occurs in 13–24% of persons aged 60–70 years and in about 50% over 80 years of age. The best measure of sarcopenia is based on the appendicular skeletal mass as measured by DEXA, divided by the height in meters squared. It can also be calculated using magnetic resonance imaging (MRI), computed tomography, or bioelectrical impedance. DEXA and MRI measures are highly correlated. Sarcopenia is strongly correlated with disability. Most sarcopenic individuals have lost fat as well. However, a subset of individuals remain fat while losing muscle mass. These individuals have been characterized as the "sarcopenic obese" or the "fat frail". Longitudinally, those with obese sarcopenia have been found to be the most likely to develop future disability and mortality (Baumgartner *et al.*, 2004). Myosteatosis – the infiltration of fat into muscle – appears to be a separate condition related to insulin resistance. Mitochondrial failure or elevated circulating triglycerides lead to accumulation of triglycerides within the cell. This alters the function of the insulin receptor substrate and, therefore, the GLUT transporter, leading to insulin resistance.

The development of sarcopenia and its effect on frailty have been characterized in the worm *Caenorhabditis elegans*. In *C. elegans*, muscle deterioration (sarcopenia) with aging leads to a decline in body movement. The muscle deterioration also correlates with behavior deficits (a frailty equivalent). These changes rarely correlated with a decreased life span. Mutations in daf-2 (the worm's IGF-1) delay these changes.

There is evidence that sarcopenia originates at birth. In the Hertfordshire cohort study, it has been shown that grip strength correlates with birth weight. Genetic studies have shown that persons with a single I or double I allele for angiotensin-converting enzyme appear to be able to generate more power when exercising regularly than those with D allele. Epidemiological studies have suggested that the best predictors of muscle mass and strength in older persons are age, energy intake, physical activity, IGF-1, testosterone, and cytokines (Baumgartner *et al.*, 1999).

Testosterone levels decline at the rate of 1% per year from the age of 30 years in men and rapidly between 20 and 40 years in women (Morley, 1997; Harman *et al.*, 2001). Testosterone inhibits the movement of pluripotential stem cells into the fat cell lineage and stimulates the muscle cell lineage to result in the production of satellite cells. Satellite cells are essential for the repair of skeletal muscle (Bhasin, 2003). Testosterone also stimulates muscle protein synthesis and inhibits the ubiquitin-proteasome pathway, resulting in a decrease in muscle protein turnover. Testosterone replacement, even in nonhypogonadal males, increases muscle mass (Wittert *et al.*, 2003). Pharmacological doses of testosterone or testosterone replacement in hypogonadal males lead to an increase in muscle strength and muscle power (Matsumoto, 2002). These changes have now been shown to lead to functional improvement. However, there is a small amount of evidence that testosterone has similar effects in older women.

A number of selective androgen receptor molecules (SARMs) are being developed, in an attempt to find androgenic compounds that have a specific effect on muscle but are less likely to produce side effects (Table 3). Dehydroepiandrosterone (DHEA), a weak androgen, failed to produce an effect on muscle strength or muscle mass when given at 50 mg daily for a year to 288 men and women.

Another anabolic hormone, growth hormone, increases muscle mass but not strength in older persons (Harman and Blackman, 2004). The effect of growth hormone is predominantly on type-II muscle fibers. Ghrelin, a growth hormone secretagogue produced in the fundus of the stomach, also appears to increase muscle mass.

Insulin growth factor (IGF) is produced in three alternative forms in muscle. One of these forms, a mechanogrowth

Table 3 Selective androgen receptor molecules

Steroids
Nandrolone
Oxymethalone
Oxandrolone
Nonsteroidal
2-Quinoline
Coumarin
Phthalimide
Bicalcutamide
Acetothiolutamide

factor (MGF) is produced in response to mechanical overload (McKoy *et al.*, 1999). The ability of MGF to be produced in response to mechanical overload declines with aging. Resistance exercise increases MGF in human quadriceps, and this increase is greater when growth hormone is also given. IGF enhances satellite cell production. Localized IGF transgene expression sustains hypertrophy and regeneration of senescent skeletal muscle (Musaro *et al.*, 2001).

Myostatin D inhibits muscle growth. A double deletion of myostatin D in mice leads to muscle hypertrophy, a veritable "mighty mouse". Double deletions of myostatin D in cows and in a single human result in marked muscle hypertrophy (Schuelke *et al.*, 2004).

Motor unit functioning is essential for the maintenance of muscle function. Motor unit firing rate is significantly decreased in the old-old, that is, those over 80 years of age. Ciliary neurotrophic factor (CNTF) levels decline with age and this decline correlates with the decrease in muscle strength with aging. Administration of CNTF leads to twofold increase in soleus muscle size.

Cytokines are soluble peptide messengers that are synthesized by white cells, neuronal cells, and adipocytes. Excess of tumor necrosis-α and interleukin-6 leads to loss of muscle strength. High levels of C-reactive protein and interleukin-6 are associated with a decrease in handgrip strength and in physical performance (Cesari *et al.*, 2004b).

Elevated homocysteine levels and peripheral vascular disease lead to poor blood flow to muscles, with muscle atrophy and decreased function. Creatine is an essential amino acid for muscle. Creatine, together with exercise, may improve muscle performance in older persons.

In the end, the development of sarcopenia depends on an imbalance of the normal everyday renewal cycle of muscle. There is either an excess of atrophy and apoptosis or a diminution of hypertrophy and satellite cell production. Figure 7 provides a schematic view of the biochemistry of sarcopenia.

CONCLUSION

Frailty is a predisability state. It is best defined objectively by the criteria developed by Linda Fried and her colleagues at John's Hopkins University. The causes of frailty are multifactorial. Frailty can have a single cause, such as anemia. Reversal of the anemia with iron, folate, vitamin B12 or erythopoetin will, in this case, reverse frailty. In

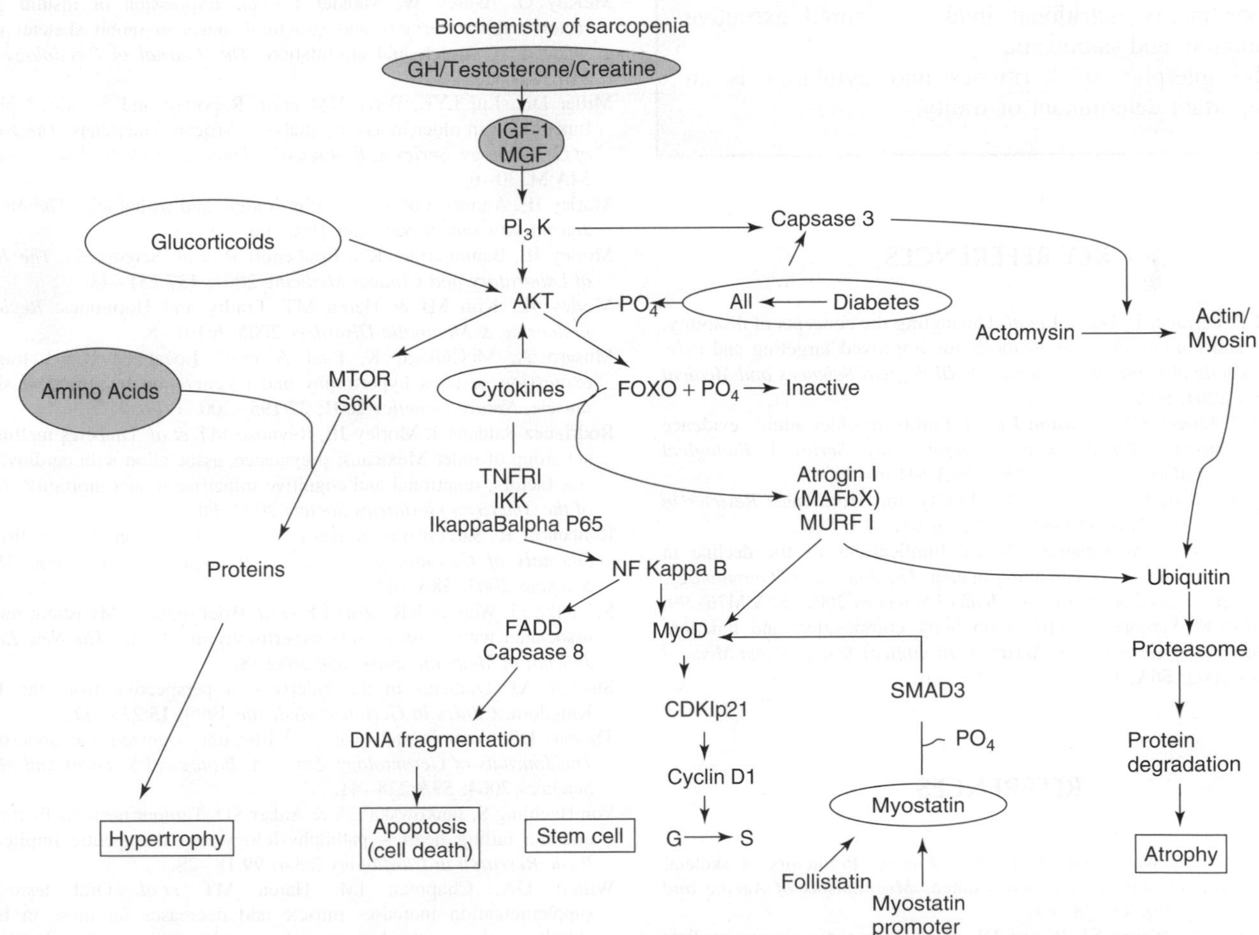

Figure 7 Schematic view of the biochemistry of sarcopenia

Table 4 Preventive strategies to slow the onset of frailty

Food intake maintained
Resistance exercises
Atherosclerosis prevention
Isolation avoidance
Limit pain
Tai Chi or other balance exercises
Yearly check for testosterone deficiency

other cases, frailty is due to the interplay of hormones and cytokines with disease processes and poor-quality nutritional intake. In these cases, the management of frailty requires a careful assessment of the causative factors and a multifaceted treatment regimen. One approach to the preventive strategies necessary to slow the onset of frailty is given in Table 4.

KEY POINTS

- Frailty is predisability and can be objectively defined by the Fried criteria.
- Frail persons are precipitated into disability by experiencing a stressful event.
- Causes of frailty include chronic diseases, pain, poor-quality nutritional intake, impaired executive function, and sarcopenia.
- The interplay of hormones and cytokines is an important determinant of frailty.

KEY REFERENCES

- Fried LP, Ferrucci L, Darer J *et al.* Untangling the concepts of disability, frailty, and comorbidity: implications for improved targeting and care. *The Journals of Gerontology. Series A, Biological Sciences and Medical Sciences* 2004; **59A**:255–63.
- Fried LP, Tangen CM, Walston J *et al.* Frailty in older adults: evidence for a phenotype. *The Journals of Gerontology. Series A, Biological Sciences and Medical Sciences* 2001; **56A**:M146–56.
- Morley JE, Kim MJ & Haren MT. Frailty and Hormones. *Reviews in Endocrine & Metabolic Disorders* 2005; **6**:101–8.
- Matsumoto AM. Andropause: clinical implications of the decline in serum testosterone levels with aging in men. *The Journals of Gerontology. Series A, Biological Sciences and Medical Sciences* 2002; **57A**:M76–99.
- Roubenoff R. Sarcopenia: effects on body composition and function. *The Journals of Gerontology. Series A, Biological Sciences and Medical Sciences* 2003; **58A**:1012–7.

REFERENCES

Baumgartner RN, Waters DL, Gallagher D *et al.* Predictors of skeletal muscle mass in elderly men and women. *Mechanisms of Ageing and Development* 1999; **48**:378–84.

Baumgartner RN, Wayne SJ, Waters DL *et al.* Sarcopenic obesity predicts instrumental activities of daily living disability in the elderly. *Obesity Research* 2004; **12**:1995–2004.

Bhasin S. Testosterone supplementation for aging-associate sarcopenia. *The Journals of Gerontology. Series A, Biological Sciences and Medical Sciences* 2003; **58A**:1002–8.

Cesari M, Penninx BW, Lauretani F *et al.* Hemoglobin levels and skeletal muscle: results from the InCHIANTI study. *The Journals of Gerontology. Series A, Biological Sciences and Medical Sciences* 2004a; **59A**:249–54.

Cesari M, Penninx BWJH, Pahor M *et al.* Inflammatory markers and physical performance in older persons: the InCHIANTI study. *The Journals of Gerontology. Series A, Biological Sciences and Medical Sciences* 2004b; **59A**:242–8.

Fried LP, Ferrucci L, Darer J *et al.* Untangling the concepts of disability, frailty, and comorbidity: implications for improved targeting and care. *The Journals of Gerontology. Series A, Biological Sciences and Medical Sciences* 2004; **59A**:255–63.

Fried LP, Tangen CM, Walston J *et al.* Frailty in older adults: evidence for a phenotype. *The Journals of Gerontology. Series A, Biological Sciences and Medical Sciences* 2001; **56A**:M146–56.

Harman SM & Blackman MR. Use of growth hormone for prevention or treatment of effects of aging. *The Journals of Gerontology. Series A, Biological Sciences and Medical Sciences* 2004; **59A**:652–8.

Harman SM, Metter JE, Tobin JD *et al.* Longitudinal effects of aging on serum total and free testosterone levels in healthy men. *The Journal of Clinical Endocrinology and Metabolism* 2001; **86**:724–31.

Matsumoto AM. Andropause: clinical implications of the decline in serum testosterone levels with aging in men. *The Journals of Gerontology. Series A, Biological Sciences and Medical Sciences* 2002; **57A**:M76–99.

Maty SC, Fried LP, Volpato S *et al.* Patterns of disability related to diabetes mellitus in older women. *The Journals of Gerontology. Series A, Biological Sciences and Medical Sciences* 2004; **59A**:148–53.

McKoy G, Ashley W, Mander J *et al.* Expression of insulin growth factor-1 splice variants and structural genes in rabbit skeletal muscle induced by stretch and stimulation. *The Journal of Physiology* 1999; **516**:583–92.

Miller DK, Lui LYL, Perry HM *et al.* Reported and measured physical functioning in older inner-city diabetic African Americans. *The Journals of Gerontology. Series A, Biological Sciences and Medical Sciences* 1999; **54A**:M230–6.

Morley JE. Anorexia of aging – physiologic and pathologic. *The American Journal of Clinical Nutrition* 1997; **66**:760–73.

Morley JE, Baumgartner RN, Roubenoff R *et al.* Sarcopenia. *The Journal of Laboratory and Clinical Medicine* 2001; **137**:231–43.

Morley JE, Kim MJ & Haren MT. Frailty and Hormones. *Reviews in Endocrine & Metabolic Disorders* 2005; **6**:101–8.

Musaro A, McCullagh K, Paul A *et al.* Localized IGF-1 transgene expression sustains hypertrophy and regeneration in senescent skeletal muscle. *Nature Genetics* 2001; **27**:195–200.

Rodriguez-Saldana J, Morley JE, Reynoso MT *et al.* Diabetes mellitus is a subgroup of older Mexicans: prevalence, association with cardiovascular risk factors, functional and cognitive impairment, and mortality. *Journal of the American Geriatrics Society* 2002; **50**:111–6.

Roubenoff R. Sarcopenia: effects on body composition and function. *The Journals of Gerontology. Series A, Biological Sciences and Medical Sciences* 2003; **58A**:1012–7.

Schuelke M, Wagner KR, Stolz LE *et al.* Brief report – Myostatin mutation associated with gross muscle hypertrophy in a child. *The New England Journal of Medicine* 2004; **350**:2682–8.

Sinclair AJ. Diabetes in the elderly – a perspective from the United Kingdom. *Clinics in Geriatric Medicine* 1999; **15**:225–37.

Thomas DR. Anemia and quality of life: unrecognized and undertreated. *The Journals of Gerontology. Series A, Biological Sciences and Medical Sciences* 2004; **59A**:238–41.

Von Haehling S, Jankowska EA & Anker SD. Tumour necrosis factor-alpha and the failing heart – pathophysiology and therapeutic implications. *Basic Research in Cardiology* 2004; **99**:18–28.

Wittert GA, Chapman IM, Haren MT *et al.* Oral testosterone supplementation increases muscle and decreases fat mass in healthy elderly males with low-normal gonadal status. *The Journals of Gerontology. Series A, Biological Sciences and Medical Sciences* 2003; **58A**:618–25.

134

Rehabilitation

Paul M. Finucane[1] *and* Philip J. Henschke[2]

[1] University of Limerick, Limerick, Ireland, and [2] Repatriation General Hospital, Daw Park, South Australia, Australia

INTRODUCTION

The human and economic consequences of avoidable dependency in older people are indeed great. Sixty years ago, Marjorie Warren identified this reality in her short but powerful paper describing the "proper care and rehabilitation of older persons" (Warren, 1946). She emphasized the need to help elderly people regain their best possible functional independence, the primary elements of which are mobility and self-care without assistance.

Older people who typically benefit from rehabilitation will have had a disabling event of recent onset. This is commonly an age-related event such as a stroke, hip fracture, other fall-related injury or deconditioning, following a major medical or surgical illness. Many elderly people will have ongoing limitations from other diseases such as osteoarthritis or Parkinson's disease.

Rehabilitation of older persons differs from that in the young. There is less physiological reserve with which to combat a disabling insult, so that recovery is typically prolonged and, at its conclusion, the previous state of function and health is often not fully regained. The specific diseases to which elderly people are susceptible are extensively described throughout this textbook. This chapter focuses on the process of optimizing recovery from the major disabling diseases of old age and on strategies for adaptation to their long-term sequelae.

TERMINOLOGY AND CLASSIFICATIONS

For many years, the World Health Organization (WHO) has sought to apply various classification systems to aspects of health and disease, most notably through its International Classification of Disease, now in its tenth revision (ICD-10) (World Health Organization, 1992–1994). Such systems provide a unified and standard language and framework for the description of health and health-related states across geographical boundaries, disciplines, and sciences.

To complement the ICD, WHO introduced its International Classification of Impairments, Disabilities, and Handicaps (ICIDH) in 1980 (World Health Organization, 1980). This stated that any illness could be considered at three levels: impairment, disability, and handicap. In simple terms, *impairment* refers to the pathological process affecting the person, *disability* to the resulting loss of function, and *handicap* to any consequent reduction in that individual's role in society.

The ICIDH had significant limitations, including the use of pejorative terms that emphasized the negative consequences of ill health and also insufficiently recognized its social and societal dimensions. Consequently, in 2001, WHO produced a revised classification known as the *International Classification of Functioning, Disability and Health* (ICF), which challenged traditional views on health and disability and allowed positive experiences to be described (World Health Organization, 2001). The ICF provides a mechanism to document the impact of the social and physical environment on a person's functioning.

The International Classification of Functioning, Disability and Health has the following two *parts*, each with two *components*:

Part 1. Functioning and Disability
- (a) Body Functions and Structures
- (b) Activities and Participation

Part 2. Contextual Factors
- (c) Environmental Factors
- (d) Personal Factors

The classification structure further divides each component into various *domains* and each domain into a number of *categories*, which form the units of classification.

The ICF provides the following definitions:

Impairment: problems in body function or structure such as a significant deviation or loss.

Principles and Practice of Geriatric Medicine, 4th Edition. Edited by M.S. John Pathy, Alan J. Sinclair and John E. Morley.

Activity: the execution of a task or action by an individual.

Activity limitations: difficulties an individual might have in executing activities.

Participation: involvement in a life situation.

Participation restrictions: problems an individual may experience in involvement in life situations.

Environmental factors: the physical, social, and attitudinal environment in which people live and conduct their lives.

Components of the ICF can be expressed in both positive and negative terms. Thus, *functioning* is an umbrella term for all body functions, activities, and participation, while *disability* is a collective term for impairments, activity limitations, or participation restrictions.

As illustrated by Figure 1, an individual's functioning is a result of a complex interaction between the health condition and contextual factors (i.e. environmental and personal factors). The interaction between these is highly dynamic such that any intervention in one area is likely to impact the other, perhaps in ways that are not easily predictable.

As an example, consider an individual with Parkinson's disease. The impairment (problems in body function or structure) is described elsewhere in this text. As a consequence, the person may have a number of activity limitations such as difficulty with personal care and mobility. In turn, the person cannot pursue former hobbies and interests (participation restriction). These restrictions are exacerbated by the fact that the person is widowed and lives alone in a first floor apartment. Now, suppose that she falls on the stairs and fractures her hip. This new impairment causes her to lose confidence and further restrictions in activity and participation result. She becomes even more isolated, withdrawn, and depressed; the feedback loops illustrated in Figure 1 indicate how vicious circles can develop with the person's level of activity and participation continuously deteriorating.

Simply stated, rehabilitation is a process that seeks to minimize activity and participation restrictions resulting from impairment. Many and more comprehensive definitions exist; perhaps the most widely accepted is the UN definition (United Nations, 2003):

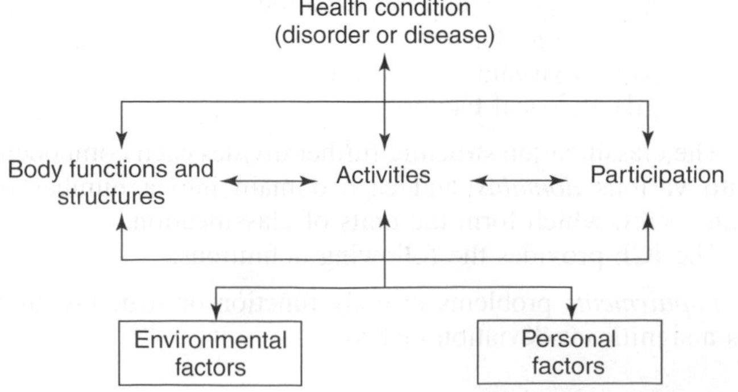

Figure 1 The complex interaction between health status, activity, and participation

> Rehabilitation means a goal-orientated and time-limited process aimed at enabling an impaired person to reach an optimum mental, physical and/or social functional level, thus providing him or her with the tools to change his or her own life. It can involve measures intended to compensate for a loss of function or a functional limitation (for example the use of technical aids) and other measures intended to facilitate social adjustment or readjustment.

Figure 1 also illustrates how rehabilitation programs can impact at various points in the impairment-activity-participation cycle. Not only can they prevent the progression of impairment to activity restriction and of activity restriction to participation restriction, they can also prevent further impairments and the development of vicious circles.

The Determinants of Activity and Participation Restrictions

As summarized in Table 1, a number of factors determine the extent to which activity and participation restrictions result from a given impairment. The type of impairment is clearly of paramount importance, with some diseases being inherently more likely to cause restrictions than others. The site of the lesion is also important as is well illustrated by stroke disease, where relatively large lesions in some parts of the brain may be relatively asymptomatic while much smaller lesions in strategic areas may cause major problems.

Elderly patients often have a number of coexisting impairments contributing to activity and participation restrictions (Figure 2). The rehabilitation program can be influenced as much by the existing as by the new impairments.

Elderly people have less physiological reserves. The aging process is characterized by a gradual functional decline in most bodily systems – a phenomenon that is relatively unimportant when organs and physiological systems are "at rest" but is most relevant when they are placed under stress by a disabling illness or event.

It must be emphasized that even very old people have the capacity to recover from such major events, and failure to make progress at rehabilitation can seldom be attributed to a lack of physiological reserve alone. Of far greater

Table 1 Determinants of activity and participation restrictions

Determinants
Determinants of activity restriction
Type of impairment (nature and severity of the disease process)
Presence of associated impairments
Degree of physiological reserve
Level of physical fitness
Determinants of participation restriction
Intrinsic factors
Attitude
Personality
Ability to adjust
Cultural issues
Extrinsic factors
Financial resources
Housing
Other resources
Social supports (spouse, family, neighbors, friends, pets)

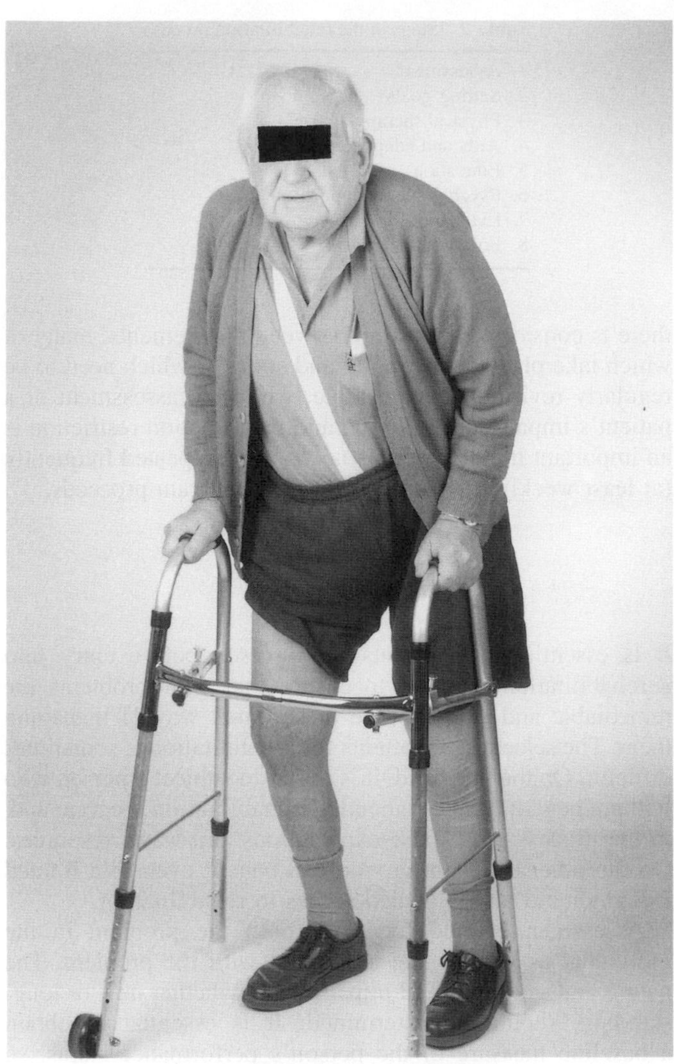

Figure 2 A 76-year old man with osteoarthritis who is undergoing rehabilitation following a right total knee replacement. He had a left above-knee amputation some years previously because of peripheral vascular disease, and this greatly impacts on the rehabilitation process

importance is the lack of activity and physical fitness that typifies elderly people in modern societies (Finucane *et al.*, 1997). Many of today's older people grew up in an era when exercise was not encouraged and sports and recreation facilities were relatively inaccessible. An age-related decline in muscle mass (sarcopenia) and strength is aggravated by physical inactivity (Castille *et al.*, 2003), and numerous studies have shown an association between sarcopenia and activity restriction (Janssen *et al.*, 2002). Weight training increases muscle strength in older people and has a positive effect on some functional limitations (Lathan *et al.*, 2004). Although little research has been done on the relationship between physical fitness and the ability to overcome impairment, it is probable that those who are unfit have a worse outcome from rehabilitation.

The degree of participation restriction resulting from activity restriction is influenced by a variety of intrinsic and extrinsic factors (Table 1). Intrinsic factors include the person's attitude in adjusting to activity restriction. A person who suffers a functional loss typically goes through a grief reaction similar to that seen following bereavement. Some people demonstrate better coping strategies than others. They are more positive in their approach, assume greater control of their situation, and find adaptive solutions to problems more readily. The psychological aspects of rehabilitation are discussed in more detail later in this chapter.

Extrinsic factors that impact participation include the resources and supports at one's disposal in dealing with activity restriction. In societies where public health care and welfare systems are poorly developed, personal finance is required for the many components of a rehabilitation program. These include the provision of physical therapy, prosthetic devices, home modification, and ongoing care. Of even greater importance are the social supports on which the person can rely on at all stages of the rehabilitation program, and particularly upon returning to their usual environment. In this regard, elderly people are often disadvantaged, with many females in particular, being widowed and living alone. In Australia, for example, 20% of people aged 65 years and over and 27% of elderly people with activity restriction live alone (Australian Bureau of Statistics, 1998). In recent decades, other demographic trends, such as the disappearance of the nuclear family and recruitment of the traditional informal carers, especially women, into paid employment have increased the social isolation and reduced the supports available to elderly people.

Psychological Aspects of Rehabilitation

The onset of impairment, particularly if unexpected or catastrophic, is generally associated with some emotional disturbance. Expected feelings include a sense of loss with regard to one's physical or mental faculties, to relationships with others or to inanimate objects such as one's home or other possessions. Normally, a grief reaction occurs with phases of denial, anger, and depression leading to a degree of acceptance sufficient to allow a relatively normal life to be resumed. However, adjustment to impairment is sometimes abnormal. For example, over 40% of older people with acute myocardial infarction have depressive symptoms, and this adversely affects the prognosis (Shiotani *et al.*, 2002). High levels of depression have also been found following stroke (Burvill *et al.*, 1995; Mast *et al.*, 2004), despite participation in a rehabilitation program (Young and Forster, 1992).

The manner in which people adapt to impairment greatly influences the development of activity and participation restriction. Some people appear inherently more adaptable and optimistic than others when faced with a potentially adverse situation. At one end of the spectrum are "highly motivated" people who set ambitious goals and work hard at achieving them. At the other end are those who appear to submit to their impairment, disengage, surrender power and autonomy, and adopt a "sick role".

Psychological theories exist to explain such different responses. An excellent model based on behaviorist concepts has been proposed by Kemp (1988), who contends that motivation is a dynamic process driven by four elements: the individual's wants; beliefs; the rewards to achievement; and the cost to the patient. The first three elements drive motivation in one direction, and this is counteracted by the cost of the behavior in terms of pain and effort. Thus, if a person really wants something, believes it to be attainable and potentially rewarding, he will strive to achieve it, provided the cost is acceptable. On the other hand, a goal is unlikely to be achieved if it is not strongly desired, if the person believes that it cannot be attained, if there is little reward for achieving it or if the actual or perceived cost of striving for the goal is too great. Using this framework, the rehabilitation specialist can help individuals in a number of ways, including setting goals, challenging incorrect beliefs, establishing rewards, and minimizing the physical and mental cost of the rehabilitation process (cf. section on Psychosocial Support).

THE PRINCIPLES OF REHABILITATION

The principles of rehabilitation are broadly similar irrespective of the problem with which one is dealing and the environment in which one is working. *Early intervention* is crucial, as much avoidable activity and participation restriction can occur soon after the onset of impairment. Certain problems should be anticipated and avoided, as once they have occurred, they may be irremediable. For example, a person with a flaccid hemiplegia is at risk of shoulder subluxation and its long-term sequelae. Proper handling and limb positioning in the immediate post-stroke period can minimize this risk.

Another key principle is the need for a *team approach*. A properly resourced team will include input from medical and nursing staff, physiotherapists, occupational therapists, speech pathologists, clinical psychologists, dietitians, and social workers. The particular expertise of different team members is complementary. Medical staff are primarily concerned with the assessment and management of impairment. Remedial therapists have particular skills in dealing with activity restriction. Social workers are best equipped to deal with participation restriction. Nursing staff in particular have a holistic brief with areas of expertise capable of influencing both activity and participation restriction.

To function effectively, team members need to communicate. When they are colocated (e.g. in a designated rehabilitation unit), exchange of information tends to occur regularly and informally. Most teams also have regular formal meetings to discuss the progress of individual patients, to revise goals, plan discharge, and organize follow-up in the community.

THE REHABILITATION PROCESS

A number of steps (see Table 2) are identifiable. While these steps are presented in chronological sequence, in practice, there is considerable overlap between the elements, many of which take place concurrently and some of which need to be regularly revisited. For example, while the assessment of a patient's impairment, activity, and participation restriction is an important initial step, this needs to be repeated frequently (at least weekly) as the rehabilitation program proceeds.

Table 2 Steps in the rehabilitation process

1. Assessment
2. Setting goals
3. Physical therapy
4. Aids and adaptations
5. Education
6. Psychological support
7. Evaluation
8. Follow-up

Assessment

It is essential that patients be assessed before entry into a rehabilitation program to ensure that their problems are remediable and to determine the optimal way of managing them. The selection of patients for rehabilitation is sometimes difficult. On the one hand, it is unfair to subject a person who will not benefit from a demanding rehabilitation program and, in the process, raise false expectations and waste resources. On the other hand, those who can benefit even to a limited extent should not be denied access to rehabilitation.

Assessment should focus on both the problem in the individual as well as the individual with the problem. The nature and severity of all impairments, whether new or longstanding, should be determined. It is essential to obtain a baseline measure of the person's performance status, so that subsequent progress can be monitored and the efficacy of rehabilitation reviewed. A variety of assessment tools are available, ranging from simple subjective measures to objective measures that tend to be more complex and time consuming. The choice of the measure to use will depend on the clinical context. Busy clinicians can usually acquire a reasonable understanding of the extent of activity and participation restriction by asking a few simple questions and by making some equally simple observations. Detailed assessment of activity restriction using standardized scales is generally left to remedial therapists, while social workers have the necessary knowledge and expertise to optimally assess participation restriction.

Assessment of Activity and Activity Restriction

Assessment begins with the clinical history. For the person who has suffered a recent impairment, it is important to determine the premorbid as well as the current functional status. A common approach is to focus on activities of daily living (ADLs). These are classified as items of personal care (e.g. washing, grooming, dressing, using toilet, eating, etc.) and those involving the use of "instruments" – hence known as *instrumental ADLs* (IADLs). The latter include such tasks as preparing meals, using the telephone, doing laundry and other housework, gardening, shopping, and using public transport. If difficulty is reported with any of these tasks, it is important to determine how the person manages. Are these tasks neglected or do others provide help?

A more formal, objective, and standardized assessment of activity restriction is generally required, particularly when patients are entering a rehabilitation program. A plethora of assessment scales and measures exist and the strengths and weaknesses of the major ones have been described (Barer, 1993). As yet, there is no consensus on the best assessment scales to use, and this lack of uniformity inhibits comparative research. A model drawn from the education literature explains the difficulty in reaching such a consensus (van der Vluten, 1996).

The model in question contends that the utility (U) of any assessment tool is governed by the formula:

$$U = V \times R \times A \times C$$

where V = validity; R = reliability; A = acceptability; and C = cost. While the ideal tool will score highly in the first three areas and be low on cost, in practice, assessment tools with high validity and reliability tend to be costly (i.e. resource intensive) and to have low acceptability (e.g. due to their intrusive nature). The converse is equally true; tools that are acceptable and easy to administer tend to have low validity and reliability. The multiplication factor in the equation is important, because if any one element of the equation measures zero or close to zero, then the overall utility of the assessment tool will also be zero or close to it. As a rule, therefore, the utility of any assessment tool is a trade-off between these elements.

Despite these considerations, the United Kingdom's Royal College of Physicians and British Geriatrics Society jointly endorse a number of standardized functional assessment scales for elderly patients, all of which have stood the test of time (Table 3). Collectively, these assess the following domains: ADLs, vision, hearing, communication, cognitive function and memory, depression, and quality of life (Royal College of Physicians and British Geriatrics Society Joint Workshops, 1992).

The use of assessment scales such as these facilitates the exchange of information between acute-care facilities, rehabilitation units, and community-based health-care teams. Standardized functional assessments also allow the effectiveness of rehabilitation to be measured. This is an essential preliminary step in allowing comparisons of different approaches to treatment in large randomized multicenter trials. Standardized assessment can also help to minimize the repeated questioning and examination that tends to characterize the multidisciplinary approach to rehabilitation.

Other assessment scales deserve special consideration. Neurodegenerative disorders are common in older patients, and Wade has provided a valuable reference for commonly used assessment measures in neurological rehabilitation (Wade, 1992). The drive toward output-driven health

Table 3 Standardized functional assessment scales for elderly patients

Domain assessed	Recommended scale	Comments
Basic ADL	Barthel Index (Mahoney and Barthel, 1965; Collin *et al.*, 1988)	Observation of what the patient *does*. Maximum of 20 points (Royal College of Physicians and British Geriatrics Society Joint Workshops, 1992). Ceiling effect in ambulatory patients.
Vision, hearing, communication	Lambeth Disability Screening Questionnaire (Peach *et al.*, 1980)	Postal questionnaire
Memory and cognitive function	AMT (Hodkinson, 1972)	10 questions from longer Roth-Hopkins test. Can be shortened by dropping some time-related questions (Jitapunkul *et al.*, 1991)
Depression	Geriatric Depression Scale (Yesavage *et al.*, 1983)	Screening test with 30 questions; 15 questions in short form (Yesavage, 1988)
Subjective morale	Philadelphia Geriatric Center Morale Scale (Davies and Challis, 1986)	Distinct from depression, although some overlap

ADL, activities of daily living; AMT, Abbreviated Mental Test.
Reproduced from Royal College of Physicians and British Geriatrics Society Joint Workshops, 1992. Copyright British Geriatrics Society.

funding in many countries has stimulated the development of outcome measures in medical rehabilitation. The Functional Independence Measure (FIM) is used in many countries, most notably the United States, to rate patient progress in a rehabilitation setting against 18 common functions concerning self-care, sphincter control, mobility, locomotion, communication, and social cognition (Keith *et al.*, 1987). The Uniform Data System for Medical Rehabilitation (UDSMR) was established to implement the FIM and to evaluate those centers that use it. Attempts have been made to use the aggregated data to identify the most effective and efficient aspects of rehabilitation programs (Johnston *et al.*, 2003). A useful review of the value of output-based research in medical rehabilitation is available (Wilkerson and Johnston, 1997).

Assessment of Participation and Participation Restriction

As individuals uniquely interact with their environment, any reduced role in society (participation restriction) that results from activity restriction will be unique to the individual. Furthermore, it is possible for somebody to develop major participation restriction in one area and have little or no restriction in another. Thus, the person who loses mobility following a lower limb amputation may have to give up playing golf but can continue to drive a car. As explained earlier, the level of participation restriction is mainly determined by one's ability to adapt to activity restriction. Some people largely fail to adapt, while in others the onset of activity restriction prompts a redefinition rather than loss of their social role. Potential losses in one area may be offset by gains elsewhere and, thereby, participation restriction may be minimal. Some people even claim that their lives have been enriched as a consequence of impairment and activity restriction.

It follows that an assessment of participation restriction can only be obtained from gaining an in-depth understanding of the individual and the manner in which he or she has come to terms with activity restriction. Such measurements are always subjective. They are also unstable over time and can be influenced by psychobehavioral variables such as mood. For these reasons, the assessment of participation restriction is largely neglected in both clinical and research settings.

Goal Setting

Assessment should culminate in the setting of rehabilitation goals. To avoid frustration and disappointment, goals should be realistic and take account of the individual's impairment and premorbid functional status. It is sometimes appropriate to set modest goals, such as helping an amputee patient to become wheelchair-independent rather than to walk. It is essential that all multidisciplinary team members, and particularly the patient, are involved in setting goals and that there is general agreement on the targets set (Wade, 1998). A rehabilitation program can be doomed from the outset if key people differ on what each is trying to achieve. Significant areas of conflict should therefore be identified, analyzed, and resolved at this early stage. In our experience, conflict in this situation usually arises when the patient's targets are considered to be unrealistically high by health professionals. However, there is some evidence to suggest that patients with ambitious goals make greater progress than those with more modest targets (Guthrie and Harvey, 1994). The pragmatic approach therefore is to set goals that are ambitious but achievable.

Short-term (intermediate) as well as long-term (final) goals should be identified. In the context of rehabilitation, as elsewhere in life, achieving a succession of intermediate goals is often the best way to arrive at the final goal. Setting realistic time frames within which to achieve goals is part of the process. The rate of progress at rehabilitation is often difficult to predict, particularly at the time of entry to a program. The goals to be achieved and the time frame within which to achieve them should therefore be flexible, regularly reviewed, and modified if necessary. Again, it is essential that all concerned be involved in the revision of goals and that consensus be reached.

Physical Therapy

A detailed description of the role of the various multidisciplinary rehabilitation team members is outside the scope of this chapter. In brief, medical staff concentrate on the identification and management of the presenting problem and any coexisting impairments. Underlying risk factors should be identified and minimized; potential complications should be anticipated and prevented. Thus, in an arteriopath who has had an embolic stroke, doctors have a role in monitoring anticoagulation, controlling hypertension, and managing coexisting angina pectoris and diabetes mellitus. Occupational therapists assess ability to manage ADLs and to devise strategies to overcome any identified problems. Physiotherapists plan and implement therapies that target specific problems and enhance cardiorespiratory, neuromuscular, and locomotor functions. Speech pathologists have skills in dealing with communication problems and swallowing disorders. In specific situations, input from other health professionals (e.g. podiatrists, dietitians) may be invaluable.

Aids and Adaptations

The use of aids has the potential to reduce activity and participation restriction for many impaired people. Devices range from the simple and inexpensive to the technologically advanced. They help people in diverse ways, from carrying out ADLs to the maintenance of mobility and the management of incontinence. The appropriate use of the most commonly used aids has been well described by Mulley (1989). It should be emphasized that the provision of an aid is not always the correct option for a restricted elderly person as its inappropriate use can cause dependence rather than promote independence. However, those in genuine need often do not avail of even basic and relatively inexpensive aids and appliances (Edwards and Jones, 1998).

Advice on the suitability of aids is best left to occupational therapists or others with particular expertise. Physiotherapists can advise on the selection of mobility aids, speech therapists on communication aids, audiologists on hearing aids, and continence advisors on continence aids. Such people can also provide follow-up and ensure that aids are properly used and maintained and continue to serve their purpose.

Special mention should be made of prostheses (devices that replace body parts) and orthoses (devices applied to the external surface of the body to provide support, improve function, or restrict or promote movement). Their design and construction require particular skill and access to increasingly sophisticated technology. Well-resourced rehabilitation centers will either employ or have access to prosthetists and orthotists who form part of the multidisciplinary team.

Adapting to the environment in which the person normally functions also promotes activity and participation. Home modifications include the installation of simple handrails or ramps, or improving access to shower and toilet areas. Early input from an occupational therapist, often including a home visit, ensures that modifications are appropriate and available at the time of discharge from hospital.

Education and Secondary Prevention

Education is a vital component of rehabilitation, as through it the patient acquires the knowledge, skills, and attitudes to minimize the activity and participation restrictions that can result from impairment. Modern concepts of adult learning emphasize the central role of the student in any learning situation and the need for active (rather than passive) participation. When applying such principles to the rehabilitation setting, the unique educational needs (in terms of knowledge, skills, and attitudes) of the individual must first be determined. The central role of the patient in setting the educational agenda needs to be acknowledged. If there is a discrepancy between the person's perceived needs and his or her actual needs as determined by health professionals, a compromise needs to be reached.

Generally, patients will require knowledge about their impairment, its etiology, underlying risk factors, management strategies, and prognosis. Such knowledge helps to foster compliance with treatment regimens and has a beneficial effect on attitudes. The skills that people require will also be highly specific and can range from cognitive skills to the more practical. Educated patients are empowered to take charge of their health and to institute life changes to maintain it and thus facilitate secondary prevention.

Education should be integrated into all stages of the rehabilitation program. Ideally, it occurs informally and each and every contact with a health professional affords an opportunity for education. It is important that rehabilitation team members acknowledge their role as educators, even to the extent of acquiring formal educational skills. Formal educational activities can complement the more informal. These can occur on a one-to-one basis or in a group setting. The format can vary from the distribution of educational literature to didactic presentations and small group discussions. Small group discussions have the added advantage of allowing patients to learn from one another and provide mutual support and encouragement so that the rehabilitation unit functions as a "therapeutic community".

Psychosocial Support

It is important that rehabilitation team members have at least a basic understanding of those common psychological issues that impact the rehabilitation process. These include the physiology of grief and loss and the psychology of motivation. Practical skills are also required in helping patients adjust to their loss, mentally as well as physically. The first step is to get to know and understand the patient, and especially his or her beliefs, goals, and fears. This calls for good communication skills and particularly good listening skills. Many people fear the unknown, and informing them about their condition and the rehabilitation process helps to reduce anxiety. Some people will be as concerned about potential future problems (e.g. the risk of a further stroke) as about the immediate one. If such concerns do not surface spontaneously, they should be sought and dealt with.

Psychological support can be provided simply and effectively through reassurance and positive feedback. Patients may need reassurance regularly and from different team members. There is also a need to maintain a consistently positive approach both to patients and to their progress at rehabilitation; there is much anecdotal evidence on the way in which a careless negative remark from a health professional can profoundly demoralize a patient. Demonstrating respect for a patient as an individual fosters feelings of self-worth and enhances motivation. However, attempts at providing positive feedback should never lead to dishonesty or insincerity and care must be taken not to generate false expectations.

The need for psychological support in the patient's spouse and other relatives should not be forgotten. Usually, such people will also be powerful providers of support. In a hospital-based rehabilitation setting, patients can offer each other support and encouragement – the so-called "therapeutic community". The formation of self-help groups is particularly useful in providing ongoing psychological and practical support once the patient is discharged from the rehabilitation program.

Discharge Planning and Follow-up

Discharge from an in-hospital rehabilitation program should signal a transition in the process rather than its conclusion. Many patients will benefit from continuing outpatient rehabilitation aimed at either achieving further gains or preventing the loss of those gains already made. Arrangements for aftercare will vary according to the needs of the individual and the availability of services. At the very least, it is important that the patient be followed up so that any exacerbation of activity or participation restriction can be evaluated and, if possible, remedied.

Evaluation

Rehabilitation programs are costly in terms of both money and manpower resources. Efforts should therefore be made to demonstrate their effectiveness. This involves the collection of data that compares people on entry to and discharge from the program. Data collection is becoming increasingly standardized and this allows comparison to be made between facilities and between different treatment strategies. Such research, which has formerly been relatively neglected, is now coming of age. It holds promise that we will not only be able to prove the overall efficacy of rehabilitation programs but also to demonstrate the elements of programs that contribute to their success (Johnston *et al.*, 2003).

THE REHABILITATION SETTING

Rehabilitation can be provided in various settings, including stand-alone rehabilitation hospitals, designated rehabilitation units in general hospitals, undifferentiated hospital wards, nursing homes, and residential care center, day hospitals, community day centers, outpatient rehabilitation centers, and the patient's own home. Each of these settings has specific advantages and disadvantages, detailed discussion of which is outside the scope of this chapter. Ideally, a range of options should be available to meet the specific needs of the individual patient at a given time.

In larger hospitals, it is usual to colocate patients with similar rehabilitation needs, often resulting from a specific impairment. Thus, for example, Stroke Units and Ortho-geriatric Units have long been in fashion. Such units foster staff expertise and facilitate research, education, and training. Though Stroke Units have been shown to improve survival and functional outcomes (Stroke Unit Trialists' Collaboration, 2001), evidence on the efficacy of Ortho-geriatric Units is less convincing (Cameron *et al.*, 2001).

Community-based rehabilitation has come of age in recent decades as a complement to hospital-based rehabilitation. In practice, community-based rehabilitation only suits a narrow range of patients, generally those from the least disabled end of the spectrum and who are otherwise well supported in the community. "Intermediate care" is a term to describe intensive, short-term, community or home-based rehabilitation that aims to prevent hospitalization, to facilitate early discharge from hospital and/or to maximize independent living (Stevenson and Spencer, 2002).

SPECIFIC REHABILITATION PROBLEMS

Cardiac Rehabilitation

Cardiac rehabilitation is defined as:

> The process by which patients with cardiac disease, in partnership with a multidisciplinary team of health professionals, are encouraged and supported to achieve and maintain optimal physical and psychological health.
>
> (Scottish Intercollegiate Guidelines Network, 2002)

It has evolved over the past 50 years, since Levine and Lown first recommended early mobilization rather than prolonged bed-rest following myocardial infarction (Levine and Lown, 1952). Initial cardiac rehabilitation programs were exercise-based and aimed at reducing morbidity and mortality following myocardial infarction. Such programs are effective, resulting in a 27% reduction in all-cause mortality (Jolliffe *et al.*, 2001).

Since its inception, the scope of cardiac rehabilitation has expanded to include such problems as ischemic heart disease, cardiac failure, coronary revascularization, and valve replacement surgery. The nature of the intervention has also expanded to include education, psychological support, lifestyle advice, risk factor reduction, and drug therapy (Dalal *et al.*, 2004). Home-based programs now complement those that are hospital-based, and these may particularly suit some elderly people. Outcomes increasingly focus on improved exercise tolerance and quality of life in addition to reduced mortality (Marchionni *et al.*, 2003).

The Scottish Intercollegiate Guidelines Network (SIGN) have produced comprehensive guidelines on cardiac rehabilitation (Scottish Intercollegiate Guidelines Network, 2002), which have been endorsed by the British Association for Cardiac Rehabilitation. These recognize the four phases of rehabilitation outlined in Table 4.

In Phase 1, early mobilization reduces the risk of thromboembolic disease and other problems associated with immobility. Low-level self-care activities can begin shortly after the acute event and then gradually accelerate. Thus, people with an uncomplicated infarct might feed themselves from the outset, sit out of bed within 24 hours and walk to the toilet within 48 hours. Spouses, partners, and other family members are ideally involved from this initial stage and should also be offered reassurance and information.

The early post-discharge period (Phase 2) is a time when many patients and their families are apprehensive and require particular support. Relevant written information and a telephone "help line" are among the strategies used to provide this.

Though Phase 3 revolves around a structured exercise program, this is just one of its elements (Table 4). This phase is increasingly offered in the community rather than in the traditional hospital setting. As described later, the exercise regimen must be adapted to the individual.

Physical activity and lifestyle changes need to be maintained (Phase 4) if the initial benefits of cardiac rehabilitation are to be sustained. In this regard, many people find that involvement in a local cardiac support group and participation in group activities to be invaluable.

A detailed description of the exercise programs suitable for people with cardiac disease is outside the scope of this chapter and is available elsewhere (Scottish Intercollegiate Guidelines Network, 2002). An initial assessment is essential to identify high-risk patients who either need a modified exercise program and/or who need to be carefully monitored. Ideally, this will include a simple test of functional capacity such as a shuttle walking test (Tobin and Thow, 1999) or a six-minute walking test (Demers *et al.*, 2001). Those identified as high-risk need more careful evaluation, perhaps including a comprehensive exercise stress test.

Aerobic, low to moderate intensity exercise is likely to suit the majority of elderly patients in a cardiac rehabilitation program. This is generally undertaken in a group setting and at least twice weekly for a minimum of eight weeks.

Table 4 The four phases of cardiac rehabilitation

1. The inpatient stage, following an acute cardiac event, includes medical evaluation, reassurance, education and correction of misconceptions, risk factor assessment, mobilization, and discharge planning.
2. Following hospital discharge, when patients may need physical and psychological support.
3. Structured exercise training, together with continuing educational and psychological support and advice on risk factor reduction.
4. Long-term maintenance of physical activity and lifestyle change.

However, weekly hospital-based group exercise, together with a home-based exercise program, can be just as effective.

The intensity of exercise can be monitored either by perceived exertion or by heart rate, as measured with a simple pulse monitor. With the former, the aim is to achieve "comfortable breathlessness". The target heart rate is derived from the maximal heart rate, which, in turn, can be estimated at 220 minus age (in years). A training effect is best seen at 65–80% of maximal heart rate (Kavanagh, 1995). Thus, an 80-year old person would have a target heart rate of 90–110 b.p.m when exercising.

Patients with unstable angina, cardiac valve stenosis or cardiac failure, or with a history of cardiac arrhythmia, are most at risk of an exercise-induced cardiac event. Such patients require a particularly careful evaluation prior to entry into a rehabilitation program and close medical supervision is then essential. For all who exercise, warm-up and cool-down exercises minimize the risk of musculoskeletal injury and cardiac arrhythmia. Extremes of temperature and overexertion should be avoided and exercise should cease immediately if the person feels unwell. All symptoms should be reported and medically assessed.

Access to a formal cardiac rehabilitation program is not always possible and these are particularly unsuited to elderly people with coincidental respiratory, neurological, or musculoskeletal disorders. However, even chair-bound elderly people can benefit from some form of low-intensity exercise following a cardiac event.

As psychosocial factors predispose to heart disease (Hemingway and Marmont, 1999), it is not surprising that they are particularly prevalent following an acute cardiac event. Thus, over 40% of elderly patients have some depressive symptoms following acute myocardial infarction (Shiotani *et al.*, 2002). Psychological distress in the early post-infarction period predicts a subsequent reduction in quality of life (Mayou *et al.*, 2000). Though psychological rehabilitation aims to reduce such distress, evidence of its efficacy is conflicting (Jones and West, 1996; Milani and Lavie, 1998). The key components of psychological rehabilitation are relaxation, stress management, and counseling. The formats for delivery range from individual to group therapy sessions.

The final important element of cardiac rehabilitation is patient education. This should span the entire program and activities can range from the highly structured and formal to the informal and opportunistic. Patients need to understand their disease, its implications, and the prospect of recovery. They also need to know about underlying risk factors and how these can be minimized in the future – that is, secondary prevention. Lifestyle modification should be recommended for those who smoke, are obese, hypertensive, or with lipid abnormalities. As such modifications impact the spouse and other family members, they should be involved in educational activities. The range of educational material and its manner of delivery (e.g. written material, audiotapes, videotapes, Internet material) continue to expand.

Pulmonary Rehabilitation

Pulmonary rehabilitation is defined as:

> An art of medical practice wherein an individually tailored, multidisciplinary program is formulated which through accurate diagnosis, therapy, emotional support and education, stabilizes or reverses both the physio- and psycho pathology of pulmonary disease and attempts to return the patient to the highest possible functional capacity allowed by his pulmonary handicap and overall life situation.
>
> (American College of Chest Physicians and American Association of Cardiovascular and Pulmonary Rehabilitation Guidelines Panel, 1997)

For people with chronic obstructive pulmonary disease (COPD), there is now good evidence that pulmonary rehabilitation substantially reduces dyspnoea and fatigue, enhances patient control of the disease, and modestly increases exercise capacity (Lacasse *et al.*, 2001). Pulmonary rehabilitation also improves health-related quality of life (American College of Chest Physicians and American Association of Cardiovascular and Pulmonary Rehabilitation Guidelines Panel, 1997) and may reduce hospital admissions (Calverley and Walker, 2003). Similar levels of benefit are seen in all adults, including the "old-old" (Katsura *et al.*, 2004), who should therefore be considered for pulmonary rehabilitation (Couser *et al.*, 1995). People with significant chronic lung disease other than COPD (e.g. asthma, interstitial/restrictive lung disease) also benefit from rehabilitation (Foster and Thomas, 1990).

The key elements of pulmonary rehabilitation are summarized in Table 5. An initial assessment allows the rehabilitation program to be tailored to the individual. While clinical and laboratory tests (e.g. radiology, pulmonary function tests) help to define the nature and severity of lung disease, these are unlikely to improve with rehabilitation. Formal exercise testing, together with blood gas analysis (or oximetry)

Table 5 Elements of pulmonary rehabilitation

Assessment
Define the nature and severity of lung disease
Identify continuing risk factors
Identify comorbidities
Assess nutritional status
Check immunization status (especially against *Pneumococcus* and influenza)
Assess lifestyle factors contributing to activity and participation restriction
Exercise test ± blood gas analysis/oximetry ± ECG monitoring
Intervention
Optimize medical management
Exercise program
Breathing exercises
Patient education
Lifestyle and dietary modification
Psychosocial support
Follow-up
Establish benefits of rehabilitation
Assess need for continued rehabilitation

and cardiac monitoring, should be performed at this stage to determine exercise tolerance, the tendency to hypoxia, and the risk of cardiac dysrhythmia. For those who are hypoxic at rest or who desaturate with exertion, a modified exercise program with supplementary oxygen and appropriate monitoring might still be feasible (Roig *et al.*, 2004).

Exercise training is the cornerstone of the rehabilitation process, and both upper and lower limb exercise improve limb strength and exercise tolerance (American College of Chest Physicians and American Association of Cardiovascular and Pulmonary Rehabilitation Guidelines Panel, 1997). Ventilatory muscle training only benefits a minority of patients with COPD. Ideally, exercise should be undertaken three times weekly, should last a minimum of 20 minutes, should induce a heart rate of not less than two-thirds of the maximum expected in the absence of lung disease, and should last at least 6 weeks and preferably 3 months (Clark, 1994).

In most centers, group exercise programs are conducted in outpatient settings. On the basis of the initial assessment already described, a program of graded exercises is provided for each individual, leading to a gradual increase in exercise capacity and tolerance. Exercise protocols for people with mild, moderate, and severe chest disease are available (American Association of Cardiovascular and Pulmonary Rehabilitation, 2004).

Pulmonary rehabilitation includes education to help patients reach a greater understanding of their disease and the factors that may contribute to its progression and retardation (American Association of Cardiovascular and Pulmonary Rehabilitation, 2004). Lifestyle and dietary modifications may be appropriate and people may need practical help to achieve these. Those who smoke, for example, not only need to understand the consequences of this habit and the advisability of stopping, but may also need access to smoking cessation programs. Psychosocial support of the elderly patient with chronic chest disease involves techniques to reduce anxiety and depression. While such techniques are often used, there is no clear evidence of their efficacy (Milani and Lavie, 1998). Participation in a rehabilitation program alone often provides a degree of psychosocial support, especially when this is undertaken in a group setting and where support is maintained following discharge from the rehabilitation program.

The gains achieved through pulmonary rehabilitation are often lost over time unless specific strategies to maintain them are put in place (Spruit *et al.*, 2004). While some form of follow-up is always required, a continuous maintenance program is ideal. In this regard, self-help groups who encourage and support one another have a particularly valuable role to play.

Musculoskeletal Disorders

This is a collective term for a number of heterogeneous conditions that differ in their duration (i.e. acute, subacute or chronic), their etiology (e.g. traumatic, inflammatory, degenerative) and the tissues involved (e.g. bone, joint, muscle). They are the commonest cause of disability in old people, such that in the United States, almost 60% of people aged 65 years and over report arthritis or chronic joint symptoms (Centers for Disease Control, 2002). Such problems will affect over 21 million older Americans in 2005 and over 41 million by 2030 (Centers for Disease Control, 2003).

Despite their heterogeneity, musculoskeletal disorders tend to result in similar restrictions in activity and participation. Pain, reduced mobility, and other functional losses are prominent features, which are interlinked and tend to reinforce one another. For example, people with arthritis may avoid those activities that exacerbate joint pain. As a result, muscles are weakened and joints become unstable and easily injured. This leads to more pain and further avoidance of exercise. Cardiorespiratory fitness may then become critically reduced, particularly in the very old in whom ADLs require oxygen uptakes close to the age-associated maximum. The net result is an unfit, inactive, arthritic person whose independence is compromised.

Detailed discussion of the management of pain of musculoskeletal origin is beyond the scope of this chapter and is dealt with elsewhere. However, it should be emphasized that appropriate treatment depends on an accurate diagnosis. For example, corticosteroids are the agents of choice in polymyalgia rheumatica but must be avoided when pain is from an osteoporotic vertebral crush fracture. The timing of analgesic use is also important. For example, pain in osteoarthritis is often exacerbated by exercise, so that it may be better to take medication before a particular activity rather than to continuously use potentially toxic analgesics. Non-pharmacological approaches to pain management should also be considered. For example, protecting arthritic hand joints with moulded splints can allow pain-free function with minimal loss of dexterity. A cane held in the contralateral hand reduces weight on an arthritic hip and thereby limits pain. For knee pain, the patient should experiment with holding a cane in either hand. Cane length is important to avoid secondary problems with other joints. Length should equal the distance from the wrist crease to the floor. Stick rubbers should be regularly checked and replaced when worn, to reduce the risk of falls. Resistant pain is best managed by a multidisciplinary team approach, and nowadays, most large centers have access to a pain management team and, with it, the expertise of anesthetists, psychiatrists, and others.

Daily range-of-motion exercises are particularly important in attempting to restore function in arthritic joints. However, compliance with such measures is low for people of all ages. The additional stimulus of joining others in a group activity with an added social component increases compliance. It is essential that footwear be appropriate. Patients with painful knees will benefit from wearing soft-soled shoes with cushioned heels (e.g. jogging shoes). A rocker bottom shoe (Figure 3) can reduce pain from rigid toes by assisting in weight transfer from posterior to anterior. This reduces the force needed to propel the body over the metatarsophalangeal (MTP) joints. Metatarsalgia can be reduced by

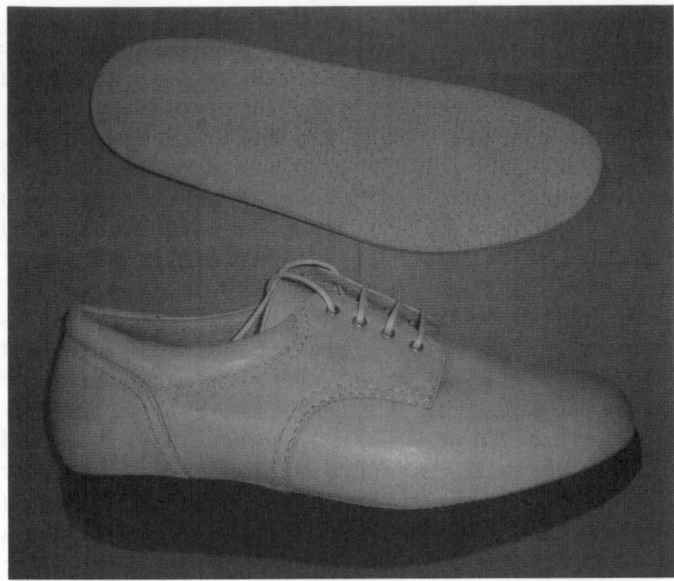

Figure 3 Rockerbottom shoe with an insole

an internal pad placed proximal to the MTP joints. When the hind foot is involved through medial arch collapse, an orthosis designed to support the medial arch often helps. Heat, including baths and spas, has been traditionally used for arthritic joints. There is no evidence that hydrotherapy causes measurable functional improvement in arthritic joints, although it does lead to greater self-confidence (Ahern *et al.*, 1995).

With regard to loss of function, a home-based assessment by an occupational therapist is often invaluable. Simple ergonomic measures and aids (e.g. tap turners, zipper pulls, sock pulls, stretch laces, long-handled shoehorns, and Velcro fasteners) can notably reduce joint strain and consequent pain.

In the context of the arthritic patient, the importance of secondary prevention should not be forgotten. Pathological changes occur against a backdrop of age-related changes in joints and soft tissues, which themselves limit flexibility. However, these age-related changes are reversible and exercise will increase joint flexibility (Raab *et al.*, 1988) and improve the strength, size, and resilience of cartilage, ligaments, and muscles. The arthritic patient should be encouraged to seek physical fitness and set him/herself realistic goals.

In the context of musculoskeletal disorders, evidence for the efficacy of structured rehabilitation programs is lacking, perhaps because research of sufficient rigor has yet to be undertaken. Multidisciplinary rehabilitation, based on time-limited and goal-directed interventions, is only of proven benefit in the management of chronic back pain, other types of chronic pain, and following hip fracture in frail elderly people (Cameron, 2004). The prevalence and impact of musculoskeletal disorders on elderly people means that further research to identify the effective elements of rehabilitation should become an even greater priority.

The Elderly Amputee Patient

The majority of lower limb amputations in elderly patients occur as a consequence of peripheral vascular disease (Ephraim *et al.*, 2003). While limb-threatening ischemia is occasionally due to a sudden embolic event, most patients have a long period of worsening ischemia prior to amputation. Many people are diabetic and have concurrent cardiac and other vascular disease, while others have smoking-induced chronic lung disease. Despite this, rehabilitation has much to offer older people following a lower limb amputation (Esquenazi, 2004) and many rise to the challenge of walking even with bilateral below-knee prostheses.

This stated, elderly people who require a lower limb amputation are a high-risk group. Perioperative mortality is in the range of 10–30%, two-year survival is 40–50%, and five-year survival is 30–40%. These survival rates have not changed significantly in the past 50 years, even with better anesthetic and surgical techniques (Cutson and Bongiorni, 1996).

When faced with an ischemic limb that cannot be salvaged by vascular reconstruction, the surgeon often has to choose between a transfemoral (i.e. above-knee) or transtibial (i.e. below-knee) amputation. Preservation of the knee is critical for the elderly amputee so that proprioceptive and neuromuscular control can be maintained and particularly so that energy expenditure can be minimized. It takes 40% more energy to walk with an above-knee than with a below-knee prosthesis (James, 1973). However, injudicious efforts to salvage a knee joint can result in an ischemic stump, which fails to heal and later necessitates a more proximal amputation. The need for a second surgical procedure is potentially disastrous as it increases the anesthetic risk, prolongs the period of immobility, increases the risk of deconditioning, and delays entry into rehabilitation.

Following limb amputation, stump management for early prosthetic intervention should commence by the use of rigid removable dressings to reduce edema, promote healing, and protect against incidental trauma. It is important that early physical therapy be directed at strengthening the arms, the abdominal muscles, the lower back, and the remaining leg. Prescription of a lower limb prosthesis is almost always indicated, even in the presence of other major medical problems. The prosthesis helps to facilitate transfers, standing and walking, and has added cosmetic value. It used to be argued that an older amputee should have crutch-walking capacity before a prosthesis should be offered. However, as walking without bearing weight on the amputated side has a higher energy cost than walking on the prosthesis, this criterion is neither valid nor fair. While some decline the offer of a prosthesis and accept wheelchair mobility, most elderly people, and particularly those with few comorbidities, are happy with their prosthesis and use it well (Pezzin *et al.*, 2004). As with any other medical intervention, a prosthesis should never be prescribed without considering the unique needs and wishes of each patient. The demands of using a prosthesis should be fully explained. For a below-knee amputee, the full range of knee extension should be maintained. It is therefore important to avoid prolonged periods of sitting in a chair without corrective exercises and a minimum of 20–30 minutes of prone lying should occur twice daily to promote full extension. The skin coming into contact with the prosthesis needs to be durable and toughened; this is best achieved by graded use of the prosthesis. Massaging the stump improves circulation and prevents adhesions during the healing process, and patients should be encouraged to do this.

Modern transtibial prostheses consist of a socket, a shank, and an ankle and foot mechanism (Figure 4). The socket is the major determinant of the comfort and stability of the prosthesis. In general, it is designed to transfer most of the weight onto the patellar tendon and a good fit is critical for achieving this. The stump is edematous in the early postoperative period and then shrinks over time. Temporary sockets are therefore required until this process is complete and a permanent socket is cast. The most commonly used socket materials are plastic laminate. The socket may incorporate a suction device to suspend the limb. When a nonsuction socket is used, an interface material (stump socks or other plastic resilient material) is needed. Stump socks should be washed daily with mild soap and warm water, rinsed thoroughly, and allowed to dry flat. The inner surface of the socket should be cleaned each evening with a warm soapy cloth.

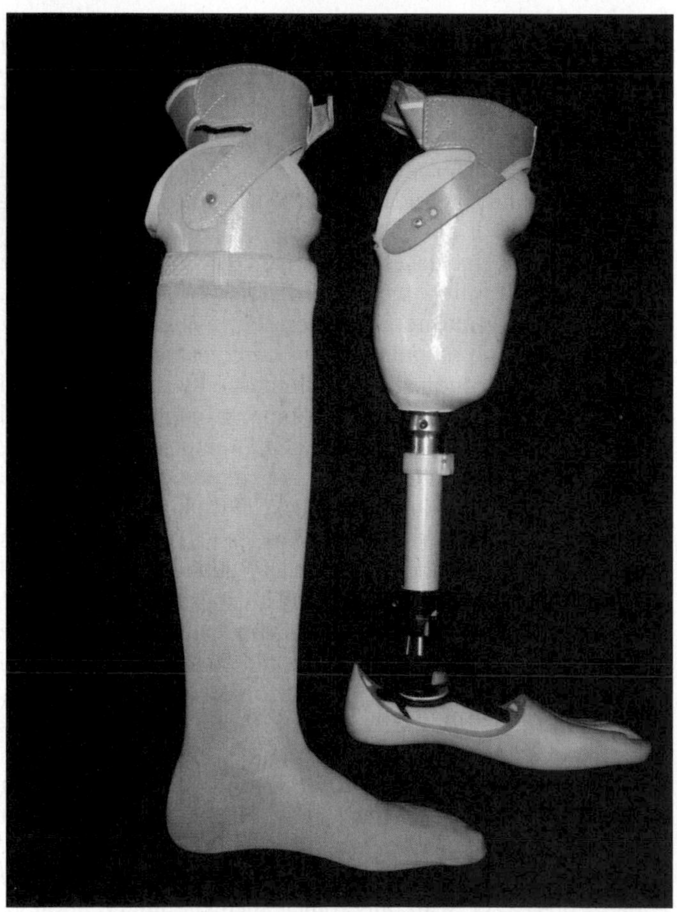

Figure 4 Two types of lower limb prostheses are shown with a solid ankle-cushion heel (SACH) foot on the left and an articulated flexible ankle mechanism fitted on the right prosthesis, which additionally shows the central pylon before final covering

Shanks have traditionally had an "exoskeletal" design, using willow or lightweight balsa wood covered with laminated plastic. A more modern "endoskeletal" limb (Figure 4) has a central pillar, made of carbon-fiber or lightweight metal to support the body weight, and is surrounded by a soft cover approximating the feel of a normal limb.

An artificial foot may be rigid or have an ankle that allows movement in one or more planes. Prescription is dependent on the level of client activity and on the condition of the stump. There is no evidence that any one design is inherently superior (Hofstad *et al.*, 2002). The advantages of a rigid ankle are lightness, low initial and maintenance cost, easy fitting, and good appearance. The solid ankle-cushion heel (SACH) foot has a rigid ankle, a compressible heel, and a light foot. It is particularly suited to the frail, less active patient who does not take long steps. SACH feet provide long service and are now almost always used for below-knee limbs.

Once a comfortable, stable, and functional limb has been provided, the next stage of training is to help the patient to walk on it properly. Gait retraining and the provision of additional mobility aids are complex subjects, discussion of which is outside the scope of this chapter.

When peripheral vascular disease leads to limb amputation, the remaining limb is often significantly ischemic so that 15–20% of people undergo a contralateral amputation within 2 years and some 40% within 4 years (Weiss *et al.*, 1990). The viability of the remaining leg can often be enhanced by surgery and by minimizing risk factors for vascular disease (e.g. poor diabetic control, cigarette smoking, etc.). Foot hygiene should be promoted and trauma to the leg should be avoided, particularly by wearing appropriate footwear.

Comprehensive rehabilitation of the elderly amputee involves more than the provision of a prosthesis. Comorbidity, prosthetic component selection and resettlement with tenuous or absent social supports all present formidable challenges. A more comprehensive review of this area, including the care of the bilateral amputee, is available (Esquenazi, 1993). The elderly amputee may draw encouragement from the life of the famed actress Sarah Bernhardt, who had an above-knee amputation at the age of 71 and thereafter continued her acting career until her death 8 years later.

The nonpainful sensation of a phantom limb is normal after amputation. Initially, this can be so deceptive that a patient inadvertently attempts to walk or reaches to scratch the missing limb. Over time, patients sense the limb retracting or "telescoping" into the stump. Phantom pain is a separate, though perhaps related phenomenon, which affects some 50–80% of people following a limb amputation (Flor, 2002).

The pathophysiology of phantom pain is poorly understood, though central and peripheral nervous system factors together with psychological factors are implicated (Halbert *et al.*, 2002). It can usually be differentiated from stump pain, as it is localized in the phantom and is variously described as burning, crushing, or lancinating. Phantom pains may be continuous or intermittent. The limb may be perceived as twisted or deformed. Management includes explaining to the patient that such bizarre sensations are commonplace and do not indicate mental instability or illness. While patients with chronic pain before amputation have a higher incidence of phantom pain, attempts to control pain before and during surgery do not consistently reduce the subsequent development of phantom pain.

The management of phantom pain is challenging, particularly on the rare occasion when it is very debilitating. There is little evidence from randomized controlled trials to guide clinicians and, when reported, improvement rates are a little better than with placebo (Halbert *et al.*, 2002). Anesthetic and surgical techniques (e.g. local anesthesia, sympathectomy, cordotomy) are as disappointing as pharmacological approaches. Tricyclic antidepressants and sodium-channel blocks are often used because of their efficacy in neuropathic pain, but are of no proven benefit. Transcutaneous electrical nerve stimulation (TENS) seems to provide modest relief at best (Katz and Melzack, 1991). However, patients do need ongoing psychological support and help to develop coping with strategies (Hill *et al.*, 1995).

Neurological Rehabilitation

The array of pathological processes that involve the brain and other parts of the nervous system tend to divide into those that are acute and nonprogressive on the one hand and those that are chronic and progressive on the other. Examples of the former include stroke, acquired brain injury, and spinal cord injury, while examples of the latter include Parkinson's disease, Motor Neuron Disease, and the dementing illnesses. Collectively, they present an array of rehabilitation challenges, particularly relating to mobility, balance and stability, communication and swallowing, and cognition. A multidisciplinary team approach to the management of chronic pain in older people is also starting to emerge (Helme, 2001).

This brief section deals only with the rehabilitation of some common chronic progressive neurological disorders of old age. The complex area of rehabilitation following stroke is addressed elsewhere in this text (*see* **Chapter 74, Stroke Rehabilitation**), while acquired brain injury and spinal cord injury are so uncommon in elderly people as to not warrant discussion here.

Perhaps the first matter to consider is the rationale for rehabilitation in people with progressive neurological disorders as it could be argued that their relentless nature makes resource-intensive approaches to rehabilitation inappropriate. This also raises complex ethical and practical issues regarding the overlap between rehabilitation and palliative care. In the context of a progressive dementing illness, particular challenges arise when, for example, patients lack both the intellectual capacity to fully engage in rehabilitation and to provide informed consent to participate. However, the loss of intellectual capacity cannot alone justify a decision to deny a person access to therapy that can improve his or her quality of life.

With progressive neurological disorders such as Parkinson's disease, rehabilitation has tended to focus on gait and speech problems (Montgomery, 2004). While these are the most distressing aspects of the disease for many patients, they are also the most difficult to modify. This may partly explain why randomized controlled trials have failed to demonstrate a benefit from physiotherapy or occupational therapy in Parkinson's disease (Deane *et al.*, 2003a,b). However, a lack of proof of efficacy is not proof of inefficacy and all experienced clinicians will have encountered very many patients with Parkinson's disease in whom rehabilitation made a significant contribution to improved functional status and quality of life.

Dementia is by far the commonest progressive neurological disorder in older people. With dementia, two particular considerations arise: the impact of rehabilitation on the dementing process *per se* and the impact of a coincidental dementia on rehabilitation for another disorder (e.g. hip fracture or stroke). With regard to the former, most research to date has focused on the potential benefits of exercise; a recent meta-analysis of 30 trials involving over 2000 patients concluded that exercise training increases fitness, physical function, cognitive function, and positive behavior in people with dementia (Heyn *et al.*, 2004). There is also accumulating evidence that those with mild to moderate dementia at least benefit from rehabilitation for such problems as hip fracture (Huusko *et al.*, 2000).

Future Challenges

The principles and practice of rehabilitation have evolved considerably since Marjorie Warren first highlighted its potential role in geriatric medicine some 60 years ago. However, progress has been slow in at least two areas. The first concerns access to rehabilitation for elderly people even in countries with well-developed health services. For example, it is estimated that only 2% of Canadians who might benefit access pulmonary rehabilitation and only 1% of those in need access musculoskeletal rehabilitation (Brooks *et al.*, 1999; Arthritis Foundation, Association of State and Territorial Health Officers, CDC, 1999). The mismatch between resources and demand is an even greater problem in developing countries.

The second area where progress has been slow is in identifying the most cost-effective elements of the rehabilitation process in different clinical situations. Further research in this area is essential for resources to be optimally targeted, for funding to be secured, and for geriatric rehabilitation to advance as a discipline. Many health-care systems are struggling with demographic change and a consequent increased demand for hospital resources at a time when acute hospital beds are being reduced. As acute hospital care and long-term residential care tend to be separately funded and poorly coordinated, pressures to reduce lengths of acute hospital stay tend to erode rehabilitation services in the acute hospital. Community-based rehabilitation services are not expanding to fill the gap and are anyway unsuited to many elderly people who lack the live-in support of a carer.

A lack of investment in rehabilitation is also a false economy measure as it leads to avoidable and costly institutional care (Young *et al.*, 1998). Sixty years ago, Marjorie Warren highlighted the social injustice of failing to optimally meet the rehabilitation needs of elderly people and their families. Such concerns are still relevant today.

KEY POINTS

- In 2001, the WHO introduced its International Classification of Functioning, Disability and Health (ICF). This challenges traditional views on health and disability, while providing a mechanism to document the impact of the social and physical environment on a person's functioning.
- Rehabilitation is a stepwise process where the various stages often overlap, may occur concurrently, and may need to be regularly revisited.
- Education is a vital component of rehabilitation, as through it, the patient acquires the knowledge, skills, and attitudes to minimize the activity and participation restrictions that can result from impairment.
- A failure to optimally meet the rehabilitation needs of older people and their families is socially unjust, just as a lack of investment in rehabilitation is a false economy measure, leading to avoidable and costly institutional care.

KEY REFERENCES

- Cameron ID, Handoll HHG, Finnegan TP *et al.* Co-ordinated multidisciplinary approaches for inpatient rehabilitation of older persons with proximal femoral fractures. *Cochrane Database of Systematic Reviews* 2001; (3):CD000106.
- Jolliffe JA, Rees K, Taylor RS *et al.* Exercise-based rehabilitation for coronary heart disease. *Cochrane Database of Systematic Reviews* 2001; (1):CD001800.
- Lacasse Y, Brosseau L, Milne S *et al.* Pulmonary rehabilitation for chronic obstructive pulmonary disease. *Cochrane Database of Systematic Reviews* 2001; (4):CD003793.
- Royal College of Physicians and British Geriatrics Society Joint Workshops. *Standardised Assessment Scales for Elderly People* 1992; The Royal College of Physicians of London and the British Geriatrics Society, London.
- World Health Organization. *International Classification of Functioning, Disability and Health: ICF* 2001; World Health Organization, Geneva.

REFERENCES

Ahern M, Nicholls E, Siminiato E *et al.* Clinical and psychological effects of hydrotherapy in rheumatic diseases. *Clinical Rehabilitation* 1995; **9**:204–12.

American Association of Cardiovascular and Pulmonary Rehabilitation. *Guidelines for Pulmonary Rehabilitation Programs* 2004, 3rd edn; AACVPR.

American College of Chest Physicians and American Association of Cardiovascular and Pulmonary Rehabilitation Guidelines Panel. Pulmonary rehabilitation: joint AACP/AACVPR evidence-based guidelines. *Chest* 1997; **112**:1363–96.

Arthritis Foundation, Association of State and Territorial Health Officers, CDC. *National Arthritis Plan: A Public Health Strategy* 1999; Arthritis Foundation, Atlanta.

Australian Bureau of Statistics. *Disability, Ageing and Carers Australia* 1998; ABS Catalogue No 4430.0, Australian Bureau of Statistics, Belconnen.

Barer D. Assessment in rehabilitation. *Reviews in Clinical Gerontology* 1993; **3**:169–86.

Brooks D, Lacasse Y & Goldstein RS. Pulmonary rehabilitation programs in Canada: national survey. *Canadian Respiratory Journal* 1999; **6**:55–63.

Burvill PW, Johnson GA, Jamrozik KD *et al.* Prevalence of depression after stroke: the Perth Community Stroke Study. *The British Journal of Psychiatry* 1995; **166**:320–7.

Calverley PMA & Walker P. Chronic obstructive pulmonary disease. *Lancet* 2003; **362**:1053–61.

Cameron ID. How to manage musculoskeletal conditions: when is 'Rehabilitation' appropriate? *Best Practice & Research. Clinical Rheumatology* 2004; **18**:573–86.

Cameron ID, Handoll HHG, Finnegan TP *et al.* Co-ordinated multidisciplinary approaches for inpatient rehabilitation of older persons with proximal femoral fractures. *Cochrane Database of Systematic Reviews* 2001; (3):CD000106.

Castille EM, Goodman-Gruen D, Kritz-Silverstein D *et al.*, The Rancho Bernardo Study. Sarcopenia in elderly men and women. *American Journal of Preventive Medicine* 2003; **25**:226–31.

Centers for Disease Control. Prevalence of self-reported arthritis or chronic joint symptoms among adults – United States, 2001. *Morbidity and Mortality Weekly Report* 2002; **51**:948–50.

Centers for Disease Control. Projected prevalence of self-reported arthritis or chronic joint symptoms among persons aged $\geq$ 65 years – United States, 2005–2030. *Morbidity and Mortality Weekly Report* 2003; **52**:489–91.

Clark CJ. Setting up a pulmonary rehabilitation programme. *Thorax* 1994; **49**:270–8.

Collin C, Wade DT, Davies S & Horne V. The Barthel ADL index: a reliability study. *International Disability Studies* 1988; **10**:61–3.

Couser JI, Guthmann R, Hamadeh MA & Kane CS. Pulmonary rehabilitation improves exercise capacity in older elderly patients with COPD. *Chest* 1995; **107**:730–4.

Cutson TM & Bongiorni DR. Rehabilitation of the older lower limb amputee: a brief review. *Journal of the American Geriatrics Society* 1996; **44**:1388–93.

Dalal H, Evans PH & Campbell JL. Recent developments in secondary prevention and cardiac rehabilitation after acute myocardial infarction. *British Medical Journal* 2004; **328**:693–7.

Davies B & Challis D. *Matching Resources to Needs in Community Care* 1986; Personal Social Services Research Unit, University of Kent, Canterbury.

Deane KOH, Ellis-Hill C, Playford ED *et al.*, Cochrane Movement Disorders Group. Occupational therapy for Parkinson's disease. *Cochrane Database of Systematic Reviews* 2003a; (3).

Deane KHO, Jones D, Ellis-Hill C *et al.*, Cochrane Movement Disorders Group. Physiotherapy for Parkinson's disease. *Cochrane Database of Systematic Reviews* 2003b; (3).

Demers C, McKelvie RS, Negassa A & Yusuf S. Reliability, validity, and responsiveness of the six-minute walk test in patients with heart failure. *American Heart Journal* 2001; **142**:698–703.

Edwards NI & Jones DA. Ownership and use of assistive devices among older people in the community. *Age and Ageing* 1998; **27**:463–8.

Ephraim PL, Dillingham TR, Sector M *et al.* Epidemiology of limb loss and congenital limb deficiency: a review of the literature. *Archives of Physical Medicine and Rehabilitation* 2003; **84**:747–61.

Esquenazi A. Geriatric amputee rehabilitation. *Clinics in Geriatric Medicine* 1993; **9**:731–43.

Esquenazi A. Amputation rehabilitation and prosthetic restoration: from surgery to community reintegration. *Disability and Rehabilitation* 2004; **26**:831–6.

Finucane P, Giles L, Withers RT *et al.* Exercise profile and subsequent mortality in an elderly Australian population. *Australian and New Zealand Journal of Public Health* 1997; **21**:155–8.

Flor H. Phantom-limb pain: characteristics, causes, and treatment. *Lancet. Neurology* 2002; **1**:182–9.

Foster S & Thomas HM. Pulmonary rehabilitation in lung disease other than chronic obstructive pulmonary disease. *The American Review of Respiratory Disease* 1990; **141**:601–4.

Guthrie S & Harvey A. Motivation and its influence on outcome in rehabilitation. *Reviews in Clinical Gerontology* 1994; **4**:235–43.

Halbert J, Crotty M & Cameron ID. Evidence for the optimal management of acute and chronic phantom pain: a systematic review. *The Clinical Journal of Pain* 2002; **18**:84–92.

Helme RD. Chronic pain management in older people. *European Journal of Pain* 2001; **5**:31–6.

Hemingway H & Marmont M. Psychological factors in the aetiology and prognosis of coronary heart disease: systematic review of prospective cohort studies. *British Medical Journal* 1999; **318**:1460–7.

Heyn P, Abreu BC & Ottenbacher KJ. The effects of exercise training on elderly persons with cognitive impairment and dementia: a meta-analysis. *Archives of Physical Medicine and Rehabilitation* 2004; **85**:1694–704.

Hill A, Niven CA & Knussen C. The role of coping in adjustment to phantom limb pain. *Pain* 1995; **62**:79–86.

Hodkinson HM. Evaluation of a mental test score for assessment of mental impairment in the elderly. *Age and Ageing* 1972; **1**:233–8.

Hofstad C, Van der Linde H, Van Limbeek J & Postema K. Prescription of prosthetic ankle-foot mechanisms after lower limb amputation. *Cochrane Database of Systematic Reviews* 2002; (4):CD003978.

Huusko TM, Karppi P, Avikainen V *et al.* Randomized, clinically controlled trial of intensive geriatric rehabilitation in patients with hip fracture: subgroup analysis of patients with dementia. *British Medical Journal* 2000; **321**:1107–11.

James U. Oxygen uptake and heart rate during prosthetic walking in the healthy male unilateral above-knee amputee. *Scandinavian Journal of Rehabilitation Medicine* 1973; **5**:71–80.

Janssen I, Heymsfield SB & Ross R. Low relative skeletal muscle mass (sarcopenia) in older people is associated with functional impairment and physical disability. *Journal of the American Geriatrics Society* 2002; **50**:889–96.

Jitapunkul S, Pillay I & Ebrahim SB. The abbreviated mental test: its use and validity. *Age and Ageing* 1991; **20**:332–6.

Johnston MV, Wood KD & Fiedler R. Characteristics of effective and efficient rehabilitation programs. *Archives of Physical Medicine and Rehabilitation* 2003; **84**:410–8.

Jolliffe JA, Rees K, Taylor RS *et al.* Exercise-based rehabilitation for coronary heart disease. *Cochrane Database of Systematic Reviews* 2001; (1):CD001800.

Jones DA & West RR. Psychological rehabilitation after myocardial infarction: multicentre randomised controlled trail. *British Medical Journal* 1996; **313**:1517–21.

Katsura H, Kanemaru A, Yamada K *et al.* Long-term effectiveness of an inpatient pulmonary rehabilitation program for elderly COPD patients: comparison between young-elderly and old-elderly groups. *Respirology* 2004; **9**:230–6.

Katz J & Melzack RA. Auricular transcutaneous electrical nerve stimulation (TENS) reduces phantom limb pain. *Journal of Pain and Symptom Management* 1991; **6**:77–83.

Kavanagh T. The role of exercise training in cardiac rehabilitation. In D Jones & R West (eds) *Cardiac Rehabilitation* 1995, pp 54–82; Br Med J Books, London.

Keith RA, Granger CV, Hamilton BB & Sherwin FS. The functional independence measure: a new tool for rehabilitation. *Advances in Clinical Rehabilitation* 1987; **1**:6–18.

Kemp BJ. Motivation, rehabilitation and aging: a conceptual model. *Topics in Geriatric Rehabilitation* 1988; **3**:41–51.

Lacasse Y, Brosseau L, Milne S *et al.* Pulmonary rehabilitation for chronic obstructive pulmonary disease. *Cochrane Database of Systematic Reviews* 2001; (4):CD003793.

Lathan N, Anderson C, Bennett D & Stretton C. Progressive resistance strength training for physical disability in older people (Cochrane review). In *The Cochrane Library* 2004, issue 3; John Wiley & Sons, Chichester.

Levine SA & Lown B. Armchair treatment of acute coronary thrombosis. *The Journal of the American Medical Association* 1952; **148**:1365–9.

Mahoney FJ & Barthel DW. Functional evaluation: the Barthel index. *Maryland State Medical Journal* 1965; **14**:61–5.

Marchionni N, Fattirolli F, Fumagalli S *et al.* Improved exercise tolerance and quality of life with cardiac rehabilitation of older patients after myocardial infarction. *Circulation* 2003; **107**:2201–6.

Mast BT, MacNeill SE & Lichtenberg PA. Post-stroke and clinically defined vascular depression in geriatric rehabilitation patients. *The American Journal of Psychiatry* 2004; **12**:84–92.

Mayou RA, Gill D, Thompson DR *et al.* Depression and anxiety as predictors of outcome after myocardial infarction. *Psychosomatic Medicine* 2000; **62**:212–9.

Milani RV & Lavie CJ. Prevalence and effects of cardiac rehabilitation on depression in the elderly with coronary heart disease. *The American Journal of Cardiology* 1998; **81**:1233–6.

Montgomery EB. Rehabilitative approaches to Parkinson's disease. *Parkinsonism and Related Disorders* 2004; **10**:S43–7.

Mulley GP. *Everyday Aids and Appliances* 1989; Br Med J Publications, London.

Peach H, Green S, Locker D *et al.* Evaluation of a postal screening questionnaire to identify the disabled. *International Rehabilitation Medicine* 1980; **2**:189–93.

Pezzin LE, Dillingham TR, MacKenzie EJ *et al.* Use and satisfaction with prosthetic limb devices and related services. *Archives of Physical Medicine and Rehabilitation* 2004; **85**:723–9.

Raab DM, Agre JC, McAdam M & Smith EL. Light resistance and stretching exercise in elderly women: effect on flexibility. *Archives of Physical Medicine and Rehabilitation* 1988; **69**:268–72.

Roig RL, Worsowicz GM, Stewart DG & Cifu DX. Geriatric rehabilitation. 3. Physical medicine and rehabilitation interventions for common disabling disorders. *Archives of Physical Medicine and Rehabilitation* 2004; **85**:S12–7.

Royal College of Physicians and British Geriatrics Society Joint Workshops. *Standardised Assessment Scales for Elderly People* 1992; The Royal College of Physicians of London and the British Geriatrics Society, London.

Scottish Intercollegiate Guidelines Network. *Cardiac Rehabilitation: A National Clinical Guideline* 2002; SIGN Publication No 57, SIGN, Edinburgh.

Shiotani I, Sato H, Kinjo K *et al.* Depressive symptoms predict 12-month prognosis in elderly patients with acute myocardial infarction. *Journal of Cardiovascular Risk* 2002; **9**:153–60.

Spruit MA, Troosters T, Trappenburg JCA *et al.* Exercise training during rehabilitation of patients with COPD: a current perspective. *Patient Education and Counseling* 2004; **52**:243–8.

Stevenson J & Spencer L. *Developing Intermediate Care: A Guide for Health and Social Service Professionals* 2002; Kings Fund, London.

Stroke Unit Trialists' Collaboration. Organised inpatient (stroke unit) care for stroke. *Cochrane Database of Systematic Reviews* 2001; (3):CD000197.

Tobin D & Thow MK. The 10m shuttle walk test with Holter monitoring: an objective outcome measure for cardiac rehabilitation. *Coronary Health Care* 1999; **3**:3–17.

United Nations. *World Programme of Action Concerning Disabled Persons* 2003; Division for Social and Policy Development, United Nations, http://www.un.org/esa/socdev/enable/diswpa01.htm.

van der Vluten CPM. The assessment of professional competence: developments, research and practical implications. *Advances in Health Sciences Education* 1996; **1**:41–67.

Wade DT. Evidence relating to goal planning in rehabilitation. *Clinical Rehabilitation* 1998; **12**:273–5.

Wade DT. *Measurements in Neurological Rehabilitation* 1992; Oxford University Press, Oxford.

Warren M. Care of the chronic aged sick. *Lancet* 1946; **I**:841–3.

Weiss GN, Gorton TA, Read RC & Neal LA. Outcomes of lower extremity amputations. *Journal of the American Geriatrics Society* 1990; **38**:877–83.

Wilkerson DL & Johnston MV. Outcomes research and clinical program monitoring systems: current capability and future directions. In M Fuhrer (ed) *Medical Rehabilitation Outcomes Research* 1997; PH Brookes, Baltimore.

World Health Organization. *International Classification of Impairments, Disabilities and Handicaps* 1980; World Health Organization, Geneva.

World Health Organization. *International Statistical Classification of Diseases and Related Health Problems* 1992–1994, Tenth Revision, vols 1–3; World Health Organization, Geneva.

World Health Organization. *International Classification of Functioning, Disability and Health: ICF* 2001; World Health Organization, Geneva.

Yesavage JA. Geriatric Depression Scale. *Psychopharmacology Bulletin* 1988; **24**:709–11.

Yesavage JA, Brink TL, Rose TL *et al.* Development and validation of a geriatric depression screening scale – a preliminary report. *Journal of Psychiatric Research* 1983; **17**:37–49.

Young JB & Forster A. The Bradford community stroke trial: results at six months. *British Medical Journal* 1992; **304**:1085–9.

Young J, Robinson J & Dickinson E. Rehabilitation for older persons. *British Medical Journal* 1998; **316**:1109–10.

PART III

Medicine in Old Age

Section 14

Special Issues

135

Skin Disorders in the Elderly

Daniel S. Loo, Mina Yaar *and* Barbara A. Gilchrest
Boston University School of Medicine, Boston, MA, USA

INTRODUCTION

Changing population demographics around the world, resulting in an increasing elderly population, lead to heightened awareness of health issues in this portion of the population. Among these, prevention and treatment of the highly prevalent skin disorders constitute a major concern. Approximately one in five Americans, 55 years or older, sees a physician each year for dermatologic diagnosis (Smith *et al.*, 2001): the most prevalent in both men and women is actinic keratosis, and nonmelanoma skin cancer is in the top four most common dermatologic conditions (Smith *et al.*, 2001). Moreover, fatal skin diseases like blistering disorders, malignant melanoma, and cutaneous T-cell lymphoma are disproportionately common in the elderly. A better understanding of the pathophysiology of aging processes in the skin would help prevent and treat dermatoses in the geriatric population, but much can be done even with therapies now available.

The following sections briefly outline current theories of skin aging and their implications on skin problems in the elderly, then discuss individual dermatoses and practical considerations for therapy.

MECHANISMS OF AGING

Aging is a complex process that affects the individual at different levels. At the cellular level, aging culminates in senescence (permanent loss of proliferative capacity) or apoptosis (death), leading to functional deficits as a result of cell loss, failure to replace lost cells, and compromised differentiated function of remaining cells. This continuous functional attrition, is unquestionably injurious to the individual, but appears to provide "secondary gain" as a cancer preventive mechanism (Campisi, 1996). Over time, genomic DNA is continuously exposed to damaging agents such as reactive oxygen species generated as a result of oxidative cellular metabolism and environmental carcinogens including solar irradiation, air pollution, and cigarette smoke. Cumulative DNA damage, particularly when affecting oncogenes and tumor suppressor genes, may lead to malignant transformation, but only in cells still capable of proliferation. Thus, it appears overall beneficial for the individual to lose such damaged cells and bear the resulting functional losses (*see also* **Chapter 2, A Biological Perspective on Aging**, **Chapter 3, Immunity and Aging** and **Chapter 4, Physiology of Aging**).

Telomeres and DNA Damage

Existing data suggest that aging is influenced both by inherent, genetic, as well as environmental factors. At the DNA level, telomeres, the terminal portion of eukaryotic chromosomes consisting of thousands of repeats of a tandem sequence TTAGGG, appear to govern the number of cellular divisions through progressive shortening, thus serving as the "biologic clock." (Ahmed and Tollefsbol, 2001).

It is interesting that the 3′ telomere strand is composed of DNA bases that constitute the target for DNA damaging agents such as UV irradiation, reactive oxygen species and benzo(a)pyrene, the carcinogen in cigarette smoke and automobile exhaust. UV irradiation leads to the formation of pyrimidine dimers, most commonly between adjacent thymidines (Patrick, 1977); reactive oxygen species primarily cause 8-oxo-guanine (Oikawa and Kawanishi, 1999); and benzo(a)pyrene forms adducts at guanine nucleotides (Jack and Brookes, 1980). Indeed, one-third of the 3′ strand (TTAGGG) is dithymidines (TT) and half is guanine (G) residues. This suggests a mechanism by which repeated UV irradiation or exposure to other environmental carcinogens might accelerate cellular aging through preferential telomere damage.

Indeed, human syndromes that display premature aging like Cockayne, Werner's and ataxia telangiectasia display mutations in genes that participate in DNA damage repair. In Cockayne syndrome, which is characterized by increased sensitivity to UV irradiation, developmental abnormalities,

Principles and Practice of Geriatric Medicine, 4th Edition. Edited by M.S. John Pathy, Alan J. Sinclair and John E. Morley.

and premature aging (Kraemer, 2003), a DNA helicase is mutated (Troelstra *et al.*, 1992) and the patients display increased sensitivity to oxidative and UV-induced DNA lesions. In ataxia telangiectasia, progeric skin changes including xerosis, develop at a young age in the majority of patients (Paller, 2003). The ATM gene mutated in ataxia telangiectasia encodes a kinase that mediates DNA damage responses (Savitsky *et al.*, 1995). In Werner's syndrome, patients display growth arrest, senile cataracts, premature balding and graying of hair, sclerodermoid appearance of the skin, loss of subcutaneous fat, and wasting of muscles at a young age (Nehlin *et al.*, 2000). A DNA helicase is mutated in Werner's syndrome, (Yu *et al.*, 1996) associated with rapid telomere shortening and decreased telomere repair as well as hair graying, atrophic and sclerotic skin and loss of subcutaneous fat, atherosclerotic heart disease, and death in early middle age. Together, these syndromes strongly support the role of DNA damage in the aging process.

The Immune System

The immune system has a role in controlling infections and also in surveillance against cancer development. With increasing age, infections become more prevalent and constitute one of the principal causes for mortality in people 65 years or older (Mouton *et al.*, 2001). In addition, the elderly display an increased incidence of cancer and inflammatory diseases, suggesting dysregulation of the immune system. With aging, both the cell-mediated and humoral immunity deteriorate. T-cells display reduced proliferation and cytokine production in response to specific triggers (Jankovic *et al.*, 2003). Recent studies based on murine data suggest that T-cell dysfunction and impaired age-associated response to pathogens and vaccines may be the result of decreased apoptosis of naive T cells early during infection/vaccination, compromising the ability of memory T cells to proliferate and expand (Jiang *et al.*, 2003). Similarly, with regard to humoral immunity, vaccination studies show that older individuals fail to select antigen activated B cells in the germinal centers of the lymph nodes, a process that may adversely affect humoral immunity (Dunn-Walters *et al.*, 2003). These decrements in immune response render the elderly more susceptible to infections and, possibly, to cancer development.

SKIN AGING

Skin aging can be divided into intrinsic or chronologic aging, those changes in the skin that are the result of passage of time alone; and photoaging, those changes in the skin that are the result of chronic sun exposure which are compounded by chronologic aging.

Intrinsic Aging

Clinical and Histological Changes

Intrinsically, aged skin appears pale, dry, lax, displaying gravitational and expression wrinkles, and a variety of benign neoplasms. Histological modifications present in chronologically aged skin are summarized in Table 1. These include flattening of the dermal–epidermal junction with decreased contact between the epidermis and the dermis and as a result, decreased exchange of molecules between the two compartments (Kurban and Bhawan, 1990). Also, this dermal–epidermal effacement leads to easier separation of the epidermis from the dermis upon minor trauma, rendering the elderly more prone to superficial erosions. Other changes include increased variability in epidermal thickness and in individual keratinocyte size as well as widening of the spaces between the keratinocytes (Yaar and Gilchrest, 2003). Also, there is a decreased number of enzymatically active melanocytes, the neural crest derived cells that reside in the basal layer of the epidermis and produce the pigment melanin that is protective against UV irradiation. Langerhans cells, the skin immune effector cells responsible for antigen presentation also decrease with age (Yaar and Gilchrest, 2003).

In the dermis, there is loss of volume, with cell depletion and decreased vascularity. Dermal changes in collagen, elastin, and glycosaminoglycans, the latter composing the ground substance of the dermis that occupies the spaces between the fibrous components of the dermis, occur. Both collagen and elastic fibers appear more compact as a result of decreased ground substance. In addition, the number of collagen bundles and the amount of elastic fibers decrease in part because of decreased synthesis and in part because of increased degradation (Yaar and Gilchrest, 2003; Tzaphlidou, 2004). Also, there is a decrease in the number of superficial dermal capillary loops that supply the epidermis, perhaps

Table 1 Histologic features of aging human skin[a]

Epidermis	Dermis	Appendages
Flattened dermal–epidermal junction	Atrophy (loss of dermal volume)	Depigmented hair
Variable thickness	Fewer fibroblasts	Loss of hair
Variable cell size and shape	Fewer mast cells	Conversion of terminal to vellus hair
Occasional nuclear atypia	Fewer blood vessels	Atrophy of glands
Fewer melanocytes	Fewer capillary loops	
Fewer Langerhans cells	Lymphatic involution	

[a]Modified from Yaar M and Gilchrest BA, Aging of the skin, Dermatology in General Medicine (Eds Freedberg IM *et al.*), 2003, p 1386, with permission of the McGraw-Hill Companies.

in part due to decreased epidermal angiogenic cytokines like vascular endothelial growth factor, decreased receptors on blood vessels, or both (Ryan, 2004). Similarly, lymphatic involution occurs and the walls of both the vascular and lymphatic vessels show replacement of elastic fibers by more rigid collagen (Ryan, 2004). In addition, skin appendages including hair follicles, eccrine and apocrine sweat glands, and sebaceous glands, display gradual age-associated atrophy.

Physiologic Functions

Physiologic functions that decline with age are summarized in Table 2. Although barrier function is mostly retained with age, there is a significant delay in barrier recovery after trauma. Decreased wound healing in the elderly is a result of decreased cell proliferation, decreased angiogenesis, as well as decreased collagen synthesis (Yaar and Gilchrest, 2003).

Owing to changes in their structure and perhaps also as a result of decreased epidermal or dermal stimuli, aged vessels display decreased ability to constrict or dilate upon temperature change. The lymphatics which, similar to blood vessels, are already compromised, are often overloaded by a deteriorating venous system, particularly in dependent areas, leading to lymphatic malfunction. With aging, there is decreased immune responsiveness in large part because of decreased and malfunctioning Langerhans cells, but other contributing factors include decreased access of Langerhans cells to capillary loops and lymphatics as well as decreased white cell reactivity in response to antigenic stimulus. An endocrine function of human skin that declines with age, in part because of decreased epidermal 7-dehydrocholesterol, is vitamin D production (MacLaughlin and Holick, 1985). Age-associated atrophy of cutaneous appendages result in decreased sweat and sebum production. Finally, there is an age-associated decrease in DNA damage repair capacity (Goukassian *et al.*, 2000).

Photoaging

UV Effect on Cellular Membranes

In addition to UV effects on DNA, UV irradiation also directly affects cellular membranes and their components (Fisher *et al.*, 2002). UV irradiation activates cell surface receptors including epidermal growth factor, interleukin 1 and tumor necrosis factor-α receptors, leading to intracellular signaling and synthesis of transcription factors, nuclear proteins that bind the DNA to enhance or repress gene transcription. One transcription factor that is quickly and prominently induced by UV irradiation is AP-1. AP-1 interferes with collagen gene transcription in fibroblasts, decreasing the levels of the major procollagens I and III. In addition, AP-1 stimulates the transcription of genes that encode matrix degrading enzymes such as metalloproteinases which degrade collagen.

Table 2 Functions of human skin that decline with age[a]

Barrier recovery	Wound healing
Cell proliferation	Vitamin D production
Thermoregulation	Sweat production
Lymphatic drainage	Sebum production
Immune responsiveness	DNA repair

[a]Modified from Yaar M and Gilchrest BA, Aging of the skin, Dermatology in General Medicine (Eds Freedberg IM *et al.*), 2003, p 1386, with permission of the McGraw-Hill Companies.

Clinical and Histological Changes

Photodamaged skin is dry and sallow displaying coarse and fine wrinkles, irregular pigmentation in the form of lentigines, lesions that are referred to by the layperson as "liver spots", which are small macules displaying variegated light to dark brown color and slight border irregularity; gutate hypomelanosis, multiple punctate hypopigmented spots; and persistent hyperpigmentation, or permanent bronzing of the skin (Yaar and Gilchrest, 2003). It frequently displays multiple premalignant lesions (actinic keratosis) and occasionally displays malignant lesions primarily, basal cell and SCCs. At times, facial skin may display a pattern of papular, yellowish aggregations with open comedones (Favre–Racouchot disease) and telangiectasis.

The histologic characteristics that correlate with these clinical changes are listed in Table 3. The epidermis of photodamaged skin is frequently acanthotic. There is loss of keratinocyte polarity, and there are many atypical keratinocytes (Yaar and Gilchrest, 2003). Melanocyte distribution is uneven, with areas of increased density of hypertrophic dopa-positive melanocytes and areas with reduced melanocyte numbers. Generally, elastosis, which is the overgrowth of abnormal elastic fibers, is the major histologic sign of photodamaged skin (Yaar and Gilchrest, 2003). Also, collagen fibrils appear fragmented and disorganized (Fisher *et al.*, 2002). In contrast, with sun-protected skin, photodamaged skin displays increased cellularity with abundant mast cells, histiocytes, other mononuclear cells, lymphocytic infiltrate, and numerous fibroblasts. Also, in contrast with sun-protected skin, the few remaining dermal blood vessels appear dilated and tortuous.

Physiologic functions that decline with chronologic skin aging appear to be more severe in sun-exposed skin, particularly compromised wound healing capacity and decreased immune responsiveness (Yaar and Gilchrest, 2003).

INFECTIONS/INFESTATIONS

Tinea Pedis

"Athlete's foot" or tinea pedis is the most common fungal infection in the elderly. Long-standing infections are

Table 3 Features of actinically damaged skin[a,b]

Clinical abnormality	Histologic abnormality
Dryness (roughness)	Increased compaction of stratum corneum, increased thickness of granular cell layer, reduced epidermal thickness, reduced epidermal mucin content
Actinic keratoses	Nuclear atypia, loss of orderly, progressive keratinocyte maturation; irregular epidermal hyperplasia, and/or hypoplasia; occasional dermal inflammation
Irregular pigmentation	
Freckling	Reduced or increased number of hypertrophic, strongly dopa-positive melanocytes
Lentigines	Elongation of epidermal rete ridges; increases in number and melanization of melanocytes
Guttate hypomelanosis	Reduced number of atypical melanocytes
Persistent hyperpigmentation (bronzing)	Increased number of dopa-positive melanocytes, and increased melanin content per unit area, and increased number of dermal melanophages
Wrinkling	
Fine surface lines	None detected
Deep furrows	Contraction of septae in the subcutaneous fat
Stellate pseudoscars	Absence of epidermal pigmentation, altered fragmented dermal collagen
Elastosis (fine nodularity and/or coarseness)	Nodular aggregations of fibrous to amorphous material in the papillary dermis
Inelasticity	Elastotic dermis
Telangiectasia	Ectatic vessels often with atrophic walls
Venous lakes	Ectatic vessels often with atrophic walls
Purpura (easy bruising)	Extravasated erythrocytes and increased perivascular inflammation
Comedones (maladie de Favre et Racouchot)	Ectatic superficial portion of the pilosebaceous follicle
Sebaceous hyperplasia	Concentric hyperplasia of sebaceous glands

[a]Basal cell carcinoma, squamous cell carcinoma and melanoma also occur in otherwise normal actinically damaged skin but, unlike the table entries, affect only a small minority of individuals with photoaging. [b]Modified from Yaar M and Gilchrest BA, Aging of the skin, Dermatology in General Medicine (Eds Freedberg IM *et al.*), 2003, p 1386, with permission of the McGraw-Hill Companies.

frequently associated with involvement of the toenail (onychomycosis). Tinea pedis usually begins in the interdigital web spaces as erythema and scale, sometimes spreading to involve the lateral, medial, and plantar surfaces of the foot (moccasin distribution) (Figure 1). Pruritus is a frequent complaint. The differential diagnosis of interdigital tinea pedis includes erythrasma (Corynebacterium) and gram-negative toe web infection (Pseudomonas). The potassium hydroxide (KOH) preparation is a simple and quick bedside test that can help confirm the diagnosis. Dry scale is removed with a 15 blade and placed on a glass slide. One drop of KOH with 20% dimethyl sulfoxide is added before the cover slip is placed on top. Direct microscopy with the 10 × magnification reveals branching hyphae (Figure 2). Topical azole cream (ketoconazole, spectazole) applied twice daily, or terbinafine 1% cream applied once daily for 3–4 weeks is effective. Patients should be instructed to apply the cream in the toe web spaces and to the lateral, medial, and plantar surfaces of the foot. Reinfection is a common problem. Prophylactic measures include complete drying of the feet after bathing and wearing cotton socks to eliminate the moist environment in which tinea proliferates, avoiding going barefoot in public places, and once weekly application of antifungal cream to the feet.

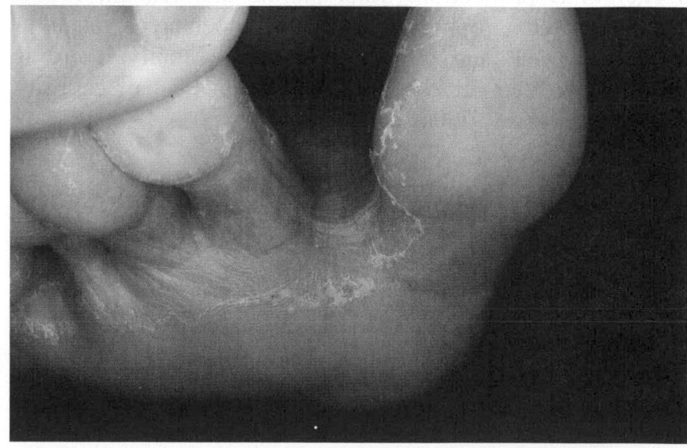

Figure 1 Interdigital tinea pedis with dry white scale

Onychomycosis

Onychomycosis is fungal infection of the nail bed with subsequent involvement of the nail plate, usually caused by contiguous spread from tinea pedis. Thus, most patients will also have clinical findings of interdigital or moccasin-type tinea pedis. Toenails are more often involved than finger nails.

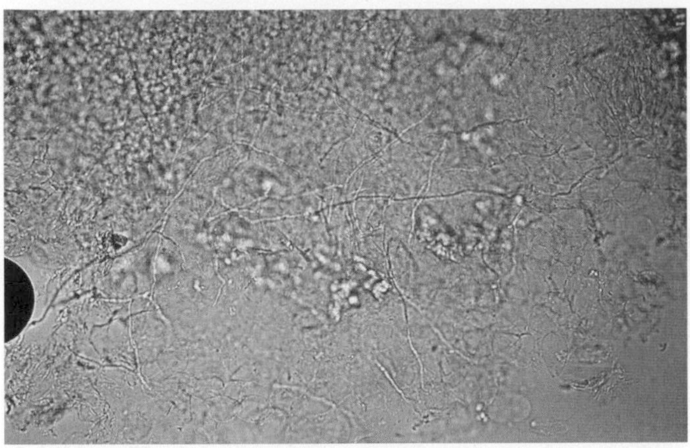

Figure 2 KOH preparation demonstrates long branching hyphae

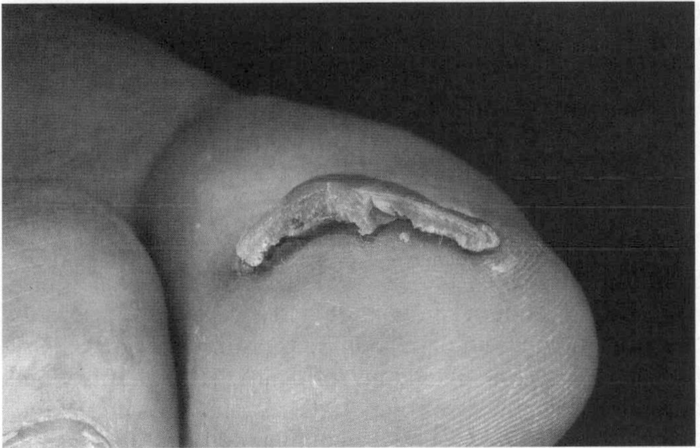

Figure 3 Onychomycosis. The nail demonstrates subungual hyperkeratosis and onycholysis

The characteristic clinical features are yellow discoloration, thickening of the nail bed (subungual hyperkeratosis) and separation of the nail bed from the nail plate (onycholysis) (Figure 3). The differential diagnosis includes pincer nail deformity, onychogryphosis, psoriasis, and lichen planus. Because only 50% of dystrophic toenails are caused by fungal infections, and systemic antifungal therapy is expensive ($400–$600), confirmatory testing is highly recommended. Sensitivity of KOH preparation and culture is highly dependent on proper specimen collection. A nail clipper is used to remove the nail proximally to the point where the nail plate meets the nail bed. This area is cleaned with an alcohol towelette and a small curette or 15 blade used to remove the soft yellow subungual debris. This specimen is placed on a glass slide for KOH preparation (as previously described) or plated on a dermatophyte test medium (DTM), which contains a pH indicator that turns the agar from yellow to red in the presence of dermatophyte. Color change is usually apparent within 2 weeks. (Elewski *et al.*, 2002) Recent studies support histologic examination of a nail clipping with periodic acid-Schiff stain (PAS) to be the most sensitive test (92%), compared to KOH preparation (80%) and fungal culture (59%) (Weinberg *et al.*, 2003).

Onychomycosis is usually asymptomatic and does not affect activities of daily living. Not all patients will require treatment, nor are all patients interested in therapy. However, onychomycosis may cause pain and limited mobility, and in diabetic patients, it can serve as a portal of entry for secondary bacterial infections. Topical antifungals are not effective because they cannot penetrate the nail bed or nail plate, and thus systemic therapy is required. Terbinafine 250 mg daily for 3–4 months is the treatment of choice for dermatophyte onychomycosis. (Sigurgeirsson *et al.*, 2002) For onychomycosis caused by yeast (Candida), the azoles must be selected (itraconazole 200 mg daily for 3–4 months, fluconazole 150 mg weekly for 6 months). Active hepatitis is a contraindication to taking these systemic therapies. For those patients at risk for liver disease, baseline liver function tests (AST, ALT) are recommended. Before the initiation of therapy, review of the patient's medication list is crucial to prevent potential drug interactions. Itraconazole is contraindicated in patients taking astemizole, terfenadine, triazolam, midazolam, cisapride, lovastatin, and simvastatin.

Herpes Zoster

Herpes zoster, commonly known as "shingles", is caused by reactivation of varicella–zoster virus in the dorsal root ganglion. Immunosuppressed individuals, particularly those with hematological malignancy and human immunodeficiency virus (HIV) infection, are at increased risk. The distribution is unilateral and dermatomal (Figure 4). The primary lesions are grouped vesicles on an erythematous base (Figure 5). Over time, the vesicles become pustules and form dried yellow or hemorrhagic crusts. The differential diagnosis includes herpes simplex, varicella, and acute contact dermatitis. Pain precedes the eruption in more than 90% of cases. Rarely, neuralgia is the only manifestation (zoster sine herpete). The classic clinical findings are usually adequate to

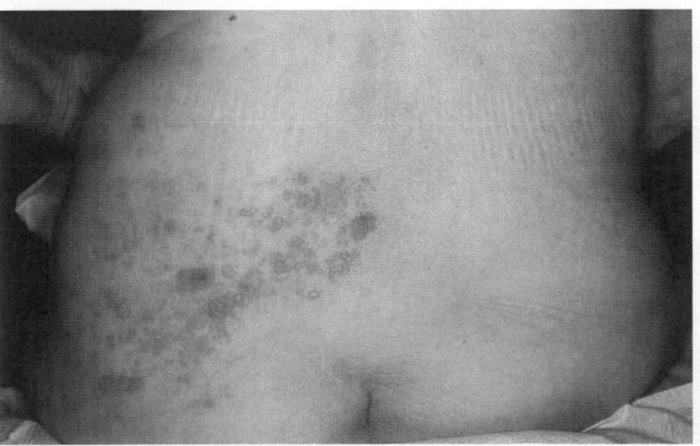

Figure 4 Herpes zoster in the classic dermatomal distribution

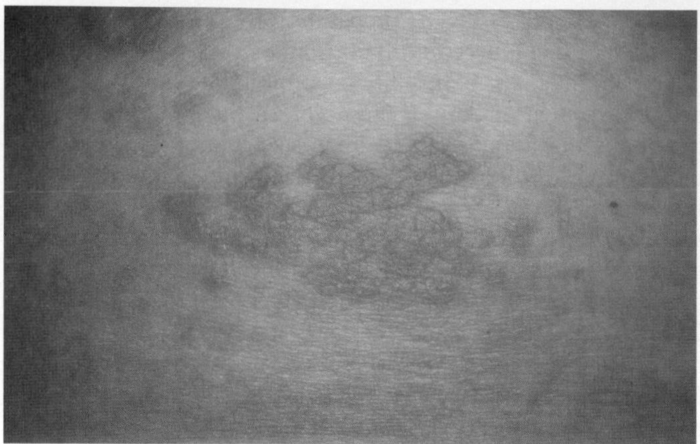

Figure 5 Herpes zoster with grouped vesicles on an erythematous base

make the diagnosis. The Tzanck smear and viral cultures are simple bedside confirmatory tests with variable sensitivity and specificity, dependent upon technique and timing of specimen collection. The Tzanck smear is performed by using iris scissors to unroof fresh vesicles and then a 15 blade is used to scrape the base of the subsequent erosion. This is smeared into a thin layer on a glass slide and briefly heated. Wright or Giemsa stain is applied for about 30 seconds and then rinsed off with water. The specimen is viewed with direct microscopy under 40 × magnification. Demonstration of multinucleated giant cells can be seen in herpes simplex and varicella–zoster infection (Figure 6). For viral cultures, the appropriate specimen is fluid from a vesicle, not dried crusts. Varicella–zoster cultures can take 1–2 weeks with frequent false-negative results. Direct fluorescent antibody is a specific and rapid test (1–2 hours), but not available in most outpatient settings.

Complications include ophthalmic involvement, dissemination, and postherpetic neuralgia. Patients with involvement of the V1 branch of the trigeminal nerve, particularly the side and tip of the nose (Hutchinson's sign), require immediate ophthalmologic consultation to rule out ocular involvement including keratitis and acute retinal necrosis. Immunocompromised patients are at risk for dissemination, defined as more than 20 vesicles outside the primary and immediately adjacent dermatomes. Rarely, this can be followed by visceral involvement (lung, liver, brain). The most common complication is postherpetic neuralgia, pain that persists after resolution of the cutaneous eruption. This affects at least half of the patients older than 60 and most frequently follows facial dermatome involvement.

Systemic antiviral therapy (acyclovir 800 mg po 5 times/day for 7–10 days, famciclovir 500 mg po 3 times/day for 7 days, valacyclovir 1 g po 3 times/day for 7 days) is effective if begun within 48–72 hours of rash onset. These drugs reduce acute pain, accelerate healing, and reduce the incidence and severity of postherpetic neuralgia. The addition of systemic corticosteroids can further reduce acute pain, but has questionable effects on the incidence and severity of postherpetic neuralgia. In immunocompromised patients and those with complications, intravenous acyclovir should be used. Postherpetic neuralgia can be treated with amitriptyline (25–75 mg po qHS) or gabapentin (900–3200 mg day^{-1}) in divided doses.

Scabies

Scabies is caused by the *Sarcoptes scabiei* mite, which burrows into the stratum corneum. It is transmitted by close body contact with other humans. Fomite transmission is rare. Risk factors include nursing home residence, HIV and acquired immunodeficiency syndrome (AIDS), and crowded living conditions. Affected patients complain of severe generalized pruritus for weeks and may report close contacts with similar symptoms. The best locations to find the mite are the interdigital web spaces between the fingers, volar wrists, penis, and areola. The primary lesions are 5–10 mm linear or serpiginous burrows, often with a gray dot at one end representing the mite (Figure 7). A generalized hypersensitivity reaction to the mite results in erythematous papules, diffuse eczematous dermatitis, lichenified plaques, and excoriations.

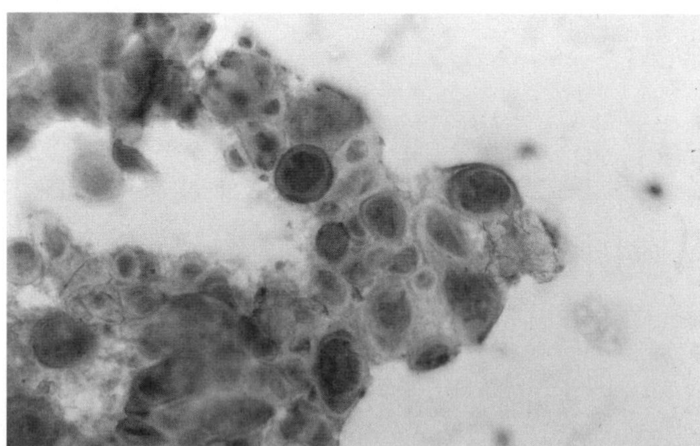

Figure 6 Tzanck smear with multinucleated giant cells

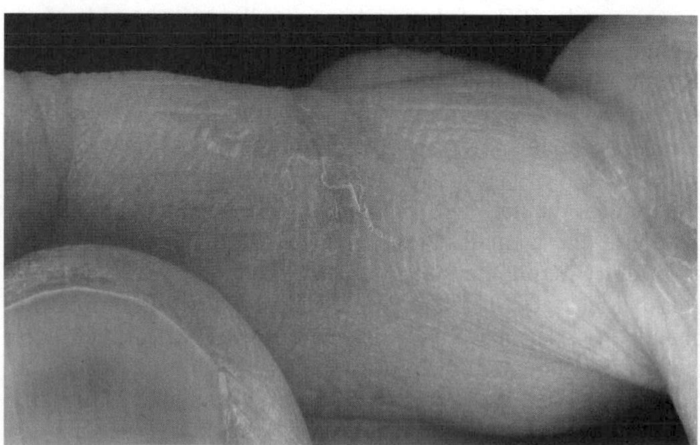

Figure 7 Serpiginous scabies burrow of the medial index finger

The differential diagnosis includes atopic dermatitis, contact dermatitis, drug eruption, and the urticarial phase of bullous pemphigoid. Less common presentations include nodules (nodular scabies), thick hyperkeratotic crusted plaques (Norwegian or crusted scabies), and vesicles or bullae (bullous scabies). Diagnosis is confirmed using direct microscopy, but proper specimen collection is essential for demonstrating the mite. Place one drop of mineral oil on the center of a glass slide. Touch this oil with the belly of a 15 blade (such that skin scrapings will adhere to the blade). Hold the blade perpendicular to the skin and scrape an epidermal burrow to remove the stratum corneum. Pinpoint bleeding occurs at the correct depth. Wipe the scrapings onto the center of the glass slide and repeat for two more burrows to increase the yield. Place a cover slip on top and view under scanning magnification (×4). Presence of the mite, mite parts, eggs or feces confirms the diagnosis (Figure 8). However, because a typical patient harbors very few mites even when severely symptomatic, a classical presentation even in the absence of a positive scraping may be adequate justification for treatment.

Nodular scabies is a prolonged hypersensitivity reaction to remnants of the mite. The lesions are pruritic firm erythematous to brown nodules often occurring on the genitals and intertriginous sites. Immunocompromised patients may develop severe thick hyperkeratotic crusts (Norwegian scabies). Compared to other scabies patients, they are extremely contagious as each crust contains hundreds of mites.

Comprehensive management includes mite eradication, alleviation of pruritus, and prevention of transmission. The patient and all close contacts should be treated simultaneously, as infected individuals may remain asymptomatic for 2 weeks or longer, until they mount a delayed hypersensitivity reaction to the mites. Topical treatments include permethrin 5% cream or lindane 1% lotion. Detailed instructions are required for proper application. A 60-g tube is prescribed for whole body application. Patients should take a bath or shower and completely dry before application. The topical agent should be applied to the entire skin surface (from the neck down), with particular attention to finger web spaces, feet, genitals, buttocks, and intertriginous sites. It should be washed off in 8 hours. This regimen should

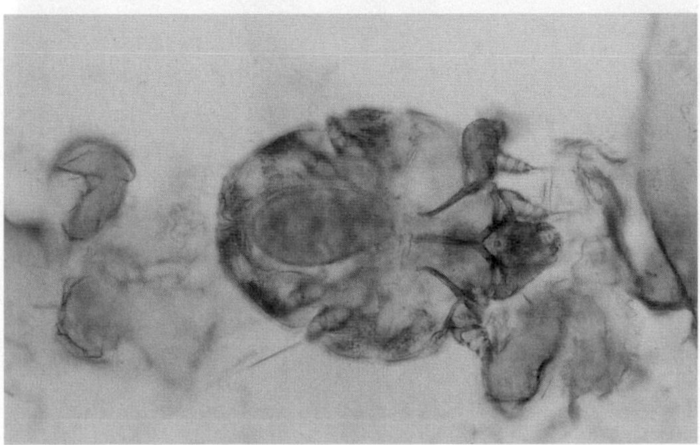

Figure 8 Scabies scrapings demonstrate gravid female mite

Table 4 Steroid compound potency rating

Class[a]	Compound
1	Clobetasol proprionate 0.05% Halobetasol proprionate 0.05%
2	Fluocinonide 0.05% Diflorasone diacetate 0.05%
3	Triamcinolone acetonide 0.5% Desoximetasone 0.05%
4	Mometasone furoate 0.1% Triamcinolone acetonide 0.1%
5	Hydrocortisone valerate 0.2% Prednicarbate 0.1%
6	Desonide 0.05% Triamcinolone acetonide 0.025%
7	Hydrocortisone 1% Hydrocortisone 2.5%

[a]Class 1 (strongest) → Class 7 (weakest).
Most steroids are available both as a cream and ointment. For the same concentration, the ointment is slightly more potent than the cream and more soothing to inflamed skin, although often less cosmetically acceptable than cream formulations. Most topical steroids are most effective if applied twice daily initially and then tapered as improvement occurs. Class 1 steroids should be used only in severe inflammatory or pruritic skin conditions.
Atrophy, telangiectasias, and striae may occur with prolonged use of potent topical steroids (class 1 & 2). The Food and Drug Administration (FDA) has approved use of all class 1 steroids for only 2 weeks (package insert). *The face, genitals, intertriginous areas, and mucosal surfaces* absorb steroids more readily and are more prone to these side effects. *Potent topical steroids should not be used >2 weeks on the face, genitals, intertriginous areas, or on mucosal surfaces.* Potent topical steroids applied to >50% total body surface area may be absorbed sufficiently to have systemic effects such as adrenal axis suppression.

be repeated for 1 week to eradicate newly hatched mites that may have survived treatment in the egg form. For asymptomatic contacts, one application may be adequate. Overexposure to lindane has been reported to cause central nervous system (CNS) toxicity and thus small children and patients with extensively eroded skin or crusted scabies, expected to have enhanced percutaneous absorption, should not be treated with this agent. For cases resistant to topical treatment, or in the immunocompromised host (such as AIDS patients), ivermectin $0.2\,\mathrm{mg\,kg^{-1}}$ as an oral dose repeated at 10–14 days should be considered. This is a practical option for nursing home epidemics when proper application of topical agents is difficult to achieve.

Although scabicides are very effective at mite eradication, they have little short-term effect on the severe pruritus that patients experience. Class I steroid ointments (clobetasol, halobetasol) applied twice to three times daily or a systemic corticosteroid taper over 2–3 weeks will help alleviate the itching while the hypersensitivity reaction abates (Table 4). To prevent fomite transmission, all clothes worn within 2 days of treatment, towels, and bed sheets should be machine washed in hot water or dry cleaned.

INFLAMMATORY DISORDERS

Dry Skin, Pruritus, and Asteatotic Dermatitis

Dry skin or xerosis is a common problem and manifests as pruritus. This is often exacerbated by hot showers and overuse of soaps, as well as high indoor heat and low humidity. Symptoms are more common in the winter. Extremities are more affected than the face or trunk. Erythematous patches and slightly raised plaques with fine dry scale and subsequent superficial cracking may be seen (asteatotic dermatitis) (Figure 9). The differential diagnosis includes atopic dermatitis, contact dermatitis, or a systemic cause of generalized pruritus (hepatobiliary obstruction, chronic renal failure, hypo or hyperthyroidism, Hodgkin's lymphoma). Detailed history taking and subsequent laboratory workup will help exclude internal causes of pruritus.

Patient education is the key to management of xerosis and asteatotic dermatitis. Limit application of soaps to intertriginous sites. Moisturizers containing lactic acid or urea should be applied daily to the trunk and extremities immediately after bathing or showering, to retain water in the stratum corneum. During winter months, a humidifier in the bedroom is helpful. For asteatotic patches, application of a class 3 topical steroid ointment to affected areas twice daily for 2–3 weeks is effective (Table 4).

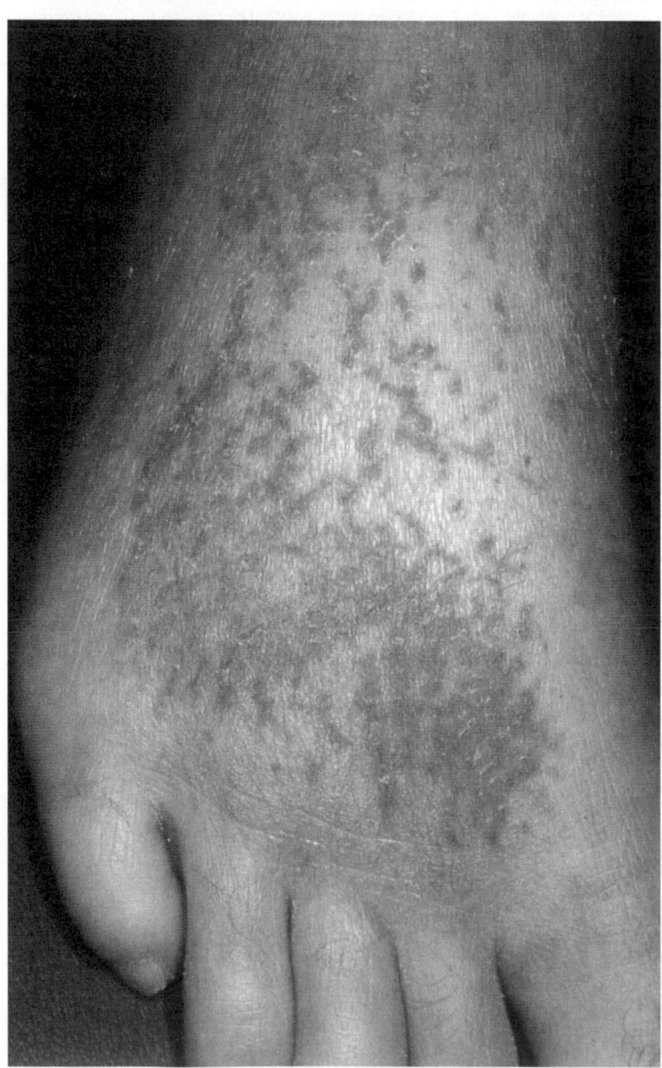

Figure 9 Asteatotic dermatitis with fine cracking of the skin surface

Seborrheic Dermatitis

Seborrheic dermatitis is strongly associated with overgrowth of a commensal yeast of the *Malassezia* species. The scalp, face, and chest are involved, particularly around the ears, eyebrows, nasolabial folds, and beard areas. The primary lesion is an erythematous patch or slightly raised plaque with greasy yellow scale (Figure 10). The differential diagnosis includes scalp psoriasis, rosacea, eczema, photosensitivity disorders, or airborne allergic reaction. Anti-dandruff shampoos containing zinc pyrithione 1%, selenium sulfide 1%, or ketoconazole 1% are effective for patients with scalp and facial involvement. They should be applied daily for 1 week and then tapered to 2–3 times per week to prevent recurrences. Patients should be instructed to massage the lather into the face for a few minutes before rinsing. Ketoconazole 2% shampoo may be more effective. For facial involvement, apply ketoconazole 2% cream or a class 6 steroid cream applied twice daily for 2–3 weeks (Table 1). For scalp pruritus, a class 2 steroid solution can be applied as needed.

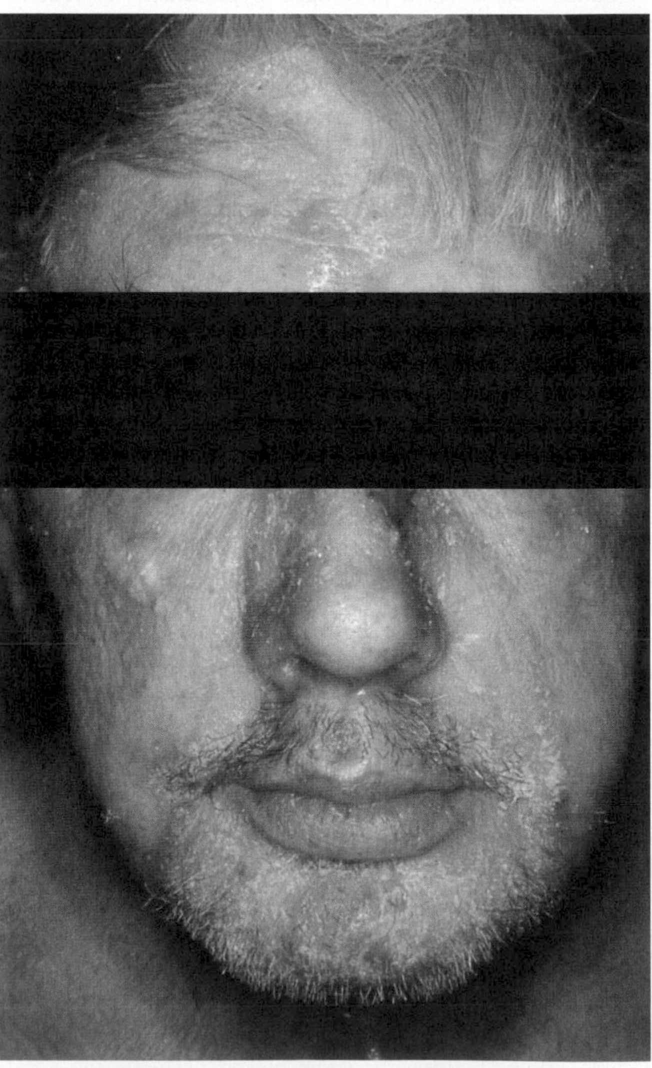

Figure 10 Seborrheic dermatitis. Erythema and scale involving the eyebrows and nasolabial creases

Psoriasis

Psoriasis is a hereditable T-cell-mediated inflammatory dermatosis; one-third of patients have a positive family history. Occasionally, it may be precipitated by an episode of streptococcal pharyngitis, classically as guttate psoriasis with many small plaques widely distributed over the body. Otherwise, psoriasis most often symmetrically affects extensor surfaces (elbows, knees, lumbosacral area), and scalp. The flexures and genital area may also be involved (inverse psoriasis). The primary lesion is an erythematous papule or plaque with thick, layered, silvery scale (Figure 11). The nails may demonstrate yellow–brown oil spots, pitting, and onycholysis (Figure 12). The differential diagnosis includes eczema, seborrheic dermatitis, and lichen planus. The diagnosis is usually made clinically, although in uncertain cases a biopsy will reveal characteristic changes. Five to thirty percent of patients with cutaneous psoriasis may also present with arthritis of the small and large joints. Rare presentations of generalized pustular psoriasis (von Zumbusch) or erythroderma (greater than 90% total body surface area involvement) may be life threatening and require hospitalization.

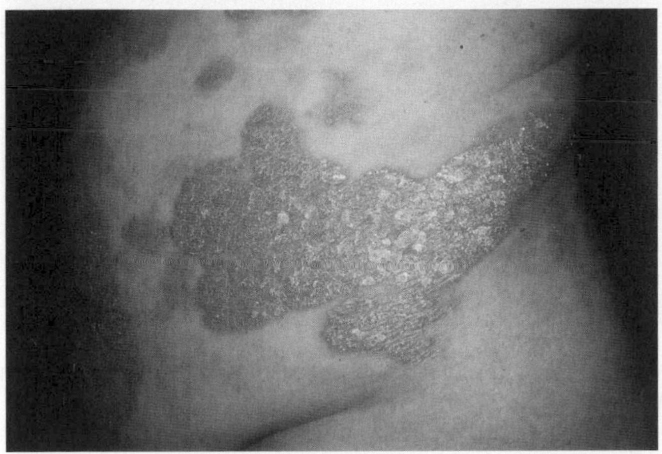

Figure 11 Plaque psoriasis. Erythematous plaque with thick, silvery scale

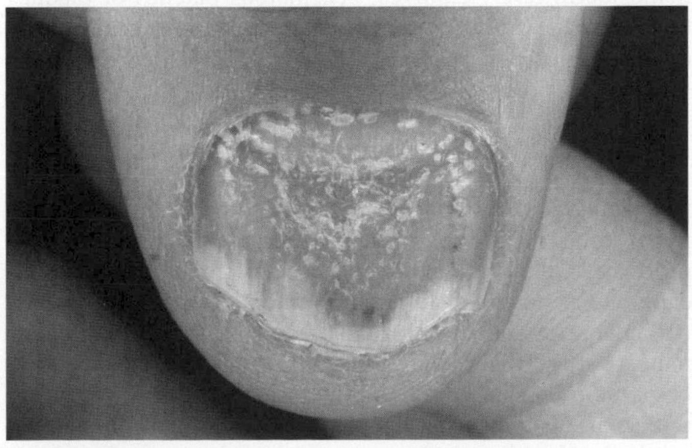

Figure 12 Nail psoriasis demonstrates pitting and onycholysis

The broad range of therapeutic options for psoriasis includes topical creams and ointments, ultraviolet light, traditional systemic agents (methotrexate, acitretin, cyclosporine) and most recently, biologic immunomodulators. Appropriate choice of therapy is largely dependent on disease severity, as determined primarily by total body surface area involvement. For patients with less than 25% involvement, topical therapies are generally effective (Lebwohl and Ali, 2001). Class 1 or 2 corticosteroid ointments are applied to affected areas of the trunk and extremities twice daily, whereas class 4 or 5 corticosteroid creams are preferred for the face or intertriginous sites to avoid steroid side effects (Table 1). Previously untreated patients usually respond best, allowing treatments to be tapered or even discontinued after a few weeks, but long-standing disease may require near-constant steroid use for good control. Calcipotriene 0.005% cream or ointment, and tazarotene 0.05/0.1% cream or ointment have a different mechanism of action and work synergistically when used in combination with topical steroids. They should be applied at different times, as simultaneous application may compromise efficacy of one or both agents. Monotherapy with calcipotriene or tazarotene is not as effective as use of a class 1 steroid. Cutaneous irritation is a common side effect of both of these steroid-sparing agents.

For patients with greater than 25% involvement and/or minimal improvement with topical treatment, ultraviolet light is an effective alternative. Oral psoralen and UVA (PUVA) or narrow band UVA (311 nm) treatments are administered 2–3 times per week, usually with substantial improvement in 1 month. For some patients, systemic therapies may be more appropriate or convenient than phototherapy or topical treatment (Lebwohl and Ali, 2001). Methotrexate, acitretin, and cyclosporine may result in adverse effects of hepatic fibrosis, hypertriglyceridemia, and renal failure, respectively. Thus, each of these medications requires appropriate monthly lab monitoring. The newest biologic agents (etanercept, alefacept, efalizumab) target specific T-cell interactions including antigen presentation, leukocyte trafficking, and cytokine production (Singri *et al.*, 2002). These agents demonstrate rapid improvement with comparable efficacy to traditional systemic therapies, without damage to internal organs. However, they are also immunosuppressive and very expensive, \$12 000 to \$20 000 per year per patient (Craze and Young, 2003).

Rosacea

"Adult acne" is characterized by vascular hyperreactivity and inflammatory papules and pustules. It occurs most commonly in women aged 40 to 50. The central face is predominantly involved (forehead, nose, cheeks, chin). The primary lesions are erythematous papules and pustules (Figure 13). Many patients present only with erythema, telangiectasias, and a history of flushing. Secondary bulbous deformity of the nose occurs rarely (rhinophyma). Ocular involvement with scleral injection and discomfort may occur in up to 50% of patients.

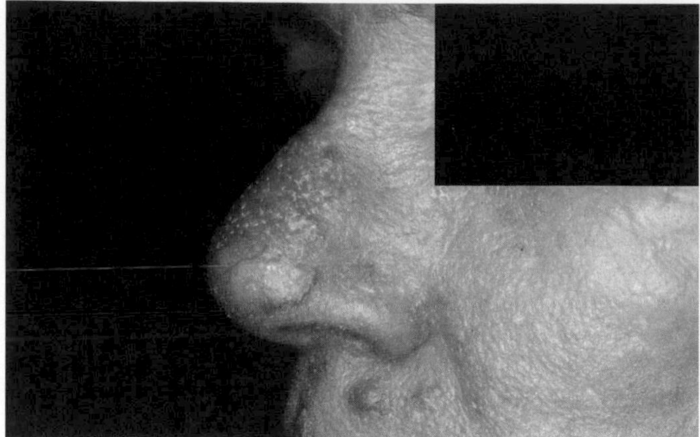

Figure 13 Rosacea. Papules and pustules of the central face and cheeks

A standard clinical classification system into erythematotelangiectatic, papulopustular, phymatous, and ocular subtypes has been suggested (Wilkin *et al.*, 2002).

Flushing is known to be triggered by any environmental stimulus that increases skin temperature of the head and neck including sunlight, hot showers, exercise, alcohol, hot beverages, and spicy food. All patients should be advised to apply daily sunscreen with a sun protection factor of 15 or greater. Physical blockers that contain titanium dioxide and zinc oxide are well tolerated. Topical antibiotics including metronidazole 0.75% cream or gel and sodium sulfacetamide 10%/sulfur 5% lotion applied twice daily are first line therapies that can reduce the number of inflammatory lesions and also the erythema (Pelle, 2003). Systemic antibiotics (tetracycline 500 mg po twice daily on an empty stomach, doxycycline 100 mg twice daily) work well for patients with more severe or extensive papules and pustules. Pulsed-dye laser treatments are very effective for the telangiectasias of rosacea, although it will not prevent development of new telangiectasias.

Stasis Dermatitis

This inflammation and discoloration of the lower extremities results from chronic venous insufficiency. Pooling of fluid in the lower extremities increases capillary pressure, causing extravasation of red blood cells and hemosiderin deposition in the dermis. The anterior shins are most commonly affected, followed by the calves, dorsal feet, and ankles. Primary lesions are red to brown hyperpigmented macules coalescing into larger patches (Figure 14). Varicosities and pedal edema are often present. Secondary changes include erythema, fine cracking, and scales. Ulceration may occur in up to 30% of patients. The differential diagnosis includes pigmented purpuric dermatosis, minocycline induced hyperpigmentation, and contact dermatitis.

Compression and leg elevation are mainstays in the management of chronic venous insufficiency and may help reduce development of ulcers. Open toe, below the knee compression stockings at 20–30 mm Hg should be worn daily. Elevation of the legs above the level of the heart when the patient is sitting or lying down will reduce venous pooling. Although the brown discoloration from hemosiderin rarely resolves, eczematous patches or plaques can be successfully treated with a class 4 topical steroid cream applied twice daily.

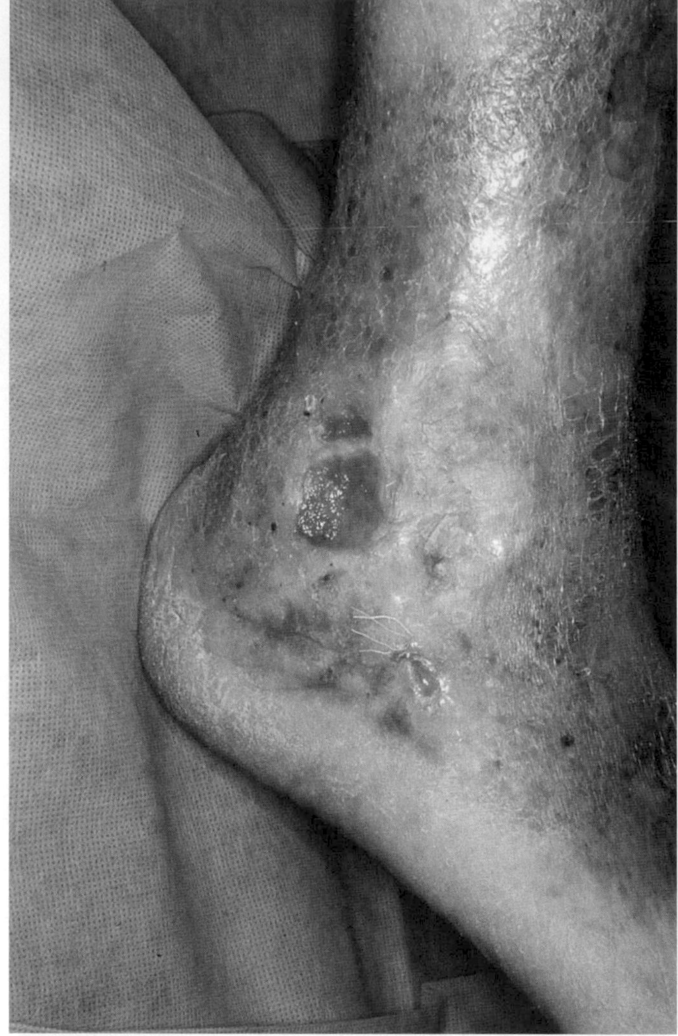

Figure 14 Stasis dermatitis. Brown discoloration with ulcer of the lateral malleolus

Drug Eruption (Morbilliform)

Maculopapular eruptions are the most common types of cutaneous drug reactions, occurring during the first 2 weeks of a new medication. The most common drugs implicated are penicillins (ampicillin, amoxicillin), sulfonamides (trimethoprim–sulfamethoxazole), nonsteroidal antiinflammatory drugs (naproxen, piroxicam), anticonvulsants (carbamazepine, phenytoin), and antihypertensives (captopril, diltiazem). The distribution is symmetric, usually beginning on the head and neck or upper trunk and progressing down the limbs. Primary lesions are erythematous macules and

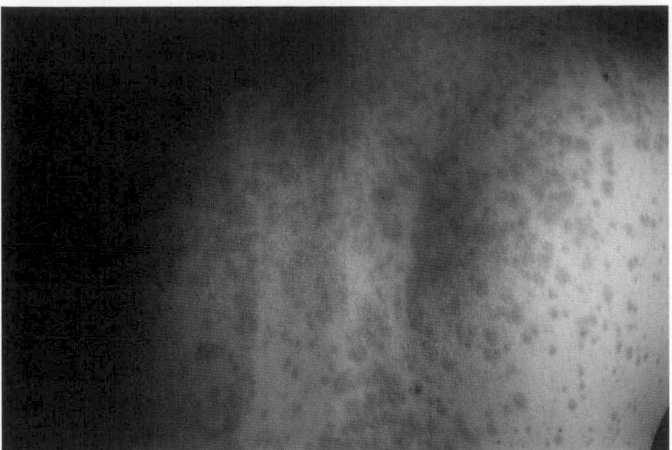

Figure 15 Morbilliform drug eruption from trimethoprim–sulfamethoxazole

papules forming areas of confluence (Figure 15). Pruritus is often present. The differential diagnosis includes viral exanthem.

Drug hypersensitivity syndrome is a potentially life threatening complication and presents as a triad of fever, cutaneous eruption (80% morbilliform), and internal organ involvement (hepatitis, nephritis, lymphadenopathy). This occurs on first exposure to the drug, with symptoms starting 1–6 weeks after exposure. In suspected cases, laboratory tests to evaluate potential asymptomatic internal organ involvement include transaminases, complete blood cell count, urinalysis, creatinine. The first step in managing a suspected drug reaction is to immediately discontinue the most likely culprit along with any unnecessary medications. Application of cool compresses or, in severe cases, a class I steroid cream applied twice daily or a predisone taper for 2–3 weeks may provide symptomatic relief of accompanying pruritus.

Bullous Pemphigoid

Bullous pemphigoid is an autoimmune blistering disease resulting from IgG autoantibodies and C3 binding to specific antigens at the dermal–epidermal junction (BP180, BP230) with subsequent inflammatory response and bulla formation. It predominantly affects individuals over the age of 60. The distribution favors the flexures including the medial thighs, groin, axilla, abdominal folds, neck, antecubital, and popliteal fossa. Pruritus is a common symptom. The blisters are often preceded by an "urticarial phase" of erythematous and edematous papules and plaques. The primary lesions are tense bullae, ranging from 0.5 to 3 cm in size, in contrast to the smaller flaccid blisters of pemphigus vulgaris (Figure 16). After the blisters rupture, secondary changes of erosions and dried yellow to hemorrhagic crust may also be observed. These lesions heal with dyspigmentation, but rarely scarring. The differential diagnosis includes porphyria cutanea tarda, arthropod bite reaction, acute contact dermatitis, scabies (urticarial phase), and epidermolysis bullosa.

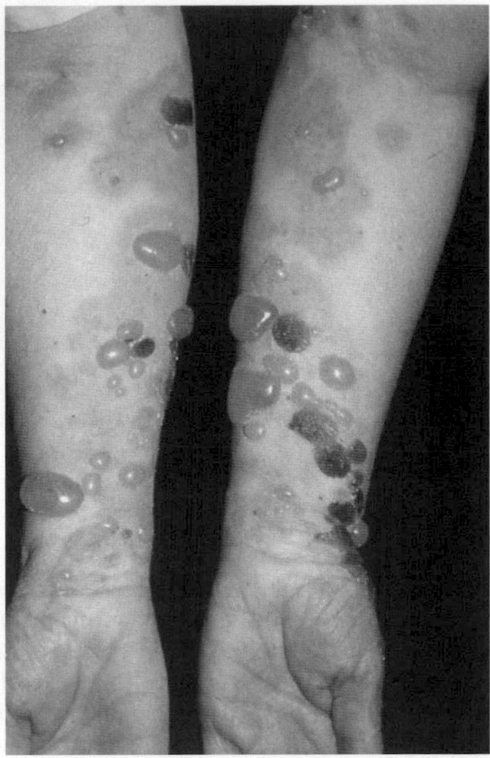

Figure 16 Volar forearms of a patient with bullous pemphigoid demonstrating tense blisters, ruptured bullae, and hemorrhagic crusts

Two biopsies are required to confirm the diagnosis. One biopsy of the blister for H&E (hematoxylin and eosin) demonstrates the subepidermal split and the eosinophil-rich infiltrate. Another biopsy of perilesional skin for immunofluorescence demonstrates linear deposition of IgG and C3 along the basement membrane zone.

Suppression of the immune system is the cornerstone of therapy. Prednisone at 0.5 to 1.0 mg kg^{-1} day^{-1} gradually tapered over 3 to 6 months is the first choice. For patients not responding rapidly, or requiring a high maintenance dose of predisone, a steroid-sparing agent such as mycophenolate mofetil or azathioprine should be given in combination with prednisone to allow a reduction in dose, and eventual discontinuation of the steroid. Tetracycline (500 mg 4 times/day) with nicotinamide (500 mg 3 times/day) may be effective in patients with limited disease.

BENIGN NEOPLASMS

Seborrheic Keratosis

This common growth of adulthood occurs after the age of thirty on face and trunk. The primary lesion is a 5–15 mm brown papule or plaque with a warty surface and a greasy feel on palpation. There is often a variety of colors in a single lesion ranging from beige to dark brown to black. On closer inspection, small 1 mm horn cysts may be apparent

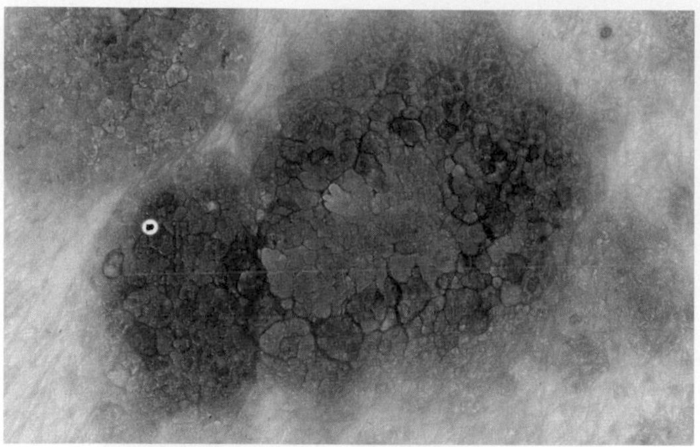

Figure 17 Seborrheic keratosis with horn cysts

(Figure 17). The pathogenesis of seborrheic keratosis is not well established, although the lesions occur more commonly on sun-exposed sites. The differential diagnosis includes pigmented basal cell carcinoma (BCC), melanoma, and warts (verruca vulgaris). Diagnosis is usually made clinically. However, if pigmented BCC or melanoma is highly suspected, a biopsy is recommended. Seborrheic keratoses are usually asymptomatic and require no treatment. If the lesions are inflamed, irritated, or cosmetically undesirable, they can easily be removed by cryotherapy, curettage, or shave excision.

Epidermoid Cyst

Synonyms for epidermoid cyst include wen, sebaceous cyst, or epidermal inclusion cyst. This common cutaneous cyst is usually located on the face, scalp, or trunk. The primary lesion is 5–30 mm flesh-colored to yellow, dermal to subcutaneous nodule (Figure 18). It often has a central punctum that may express foul smelling cheese-like keratin when pressure is applied. Epidermoid cysts are freely mobile over the underlying tissues. They can arise primarily from sebaceous follicles or from traumatically implanted epithelium. Although these cysts are usually asymptomatic and require no treatment, they can be cosmetically annoying or rupture from pressure. Ruptured cysts extrude keratin into the dermis and the resulting foreign body reaction leads to erythema, swelling, and pain. Incision and drainage followed by tetracycline 500 mg po twice daily for 2 weeks or intralesional triamcinolone acetonide 5 mg ml^{-1} will relieve the acute inflammation. Definitive treatment requires excision with removal of the entire cyst wall.

PREMALIGNANT AND MALIGNANT NEOPLASMS

Actinic Keratosis

Actinic keratosis is a precursor lesion to SCC. Actinic keratoses are seen commonly in middle-aged, fair-skinned Caucasians in a photo-distribution including the face, lips, ears, dorsal hands, and forearms, the result of cumulative lifetime of sun exposure. The primary lesion is a 5–10-mm rough, adherent, white scaly papule or plaque, often on an erythematous base (Figure 19). On palpation, it feels gritty, with a sandpaper-like texture. Early lesions are often more readily detected by palpation than visual inspection. The differential diagnosis includes seborrheic keratosis. Immunosuppressed patients, particularly transplant recipients, are at higher risk for actinic keratoses. There is a low risk of progression to invasive carcinoma for an individual lesion, estimated at far less than 1% per year by most authorities, but individuals with multiple actinic keratoses are at high risk of skin cancer by virtue of their diffused photodamage.

Regular sun avoidance prevents progression of actinic keratoses and allows regression of many. Daily application of sunscreen with sun protective factor 15 or greater, long-sleeve shirts, and broad-brimmed hats are recommended. Isolated lesions are often frozen with liquid nitrogen in the office setting. Liquid nitrogen can be applied with a

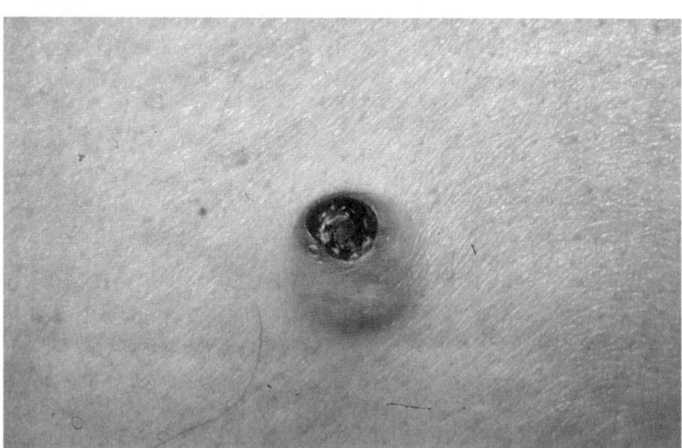

Figure 18 Epidermoid cyst with central punctum

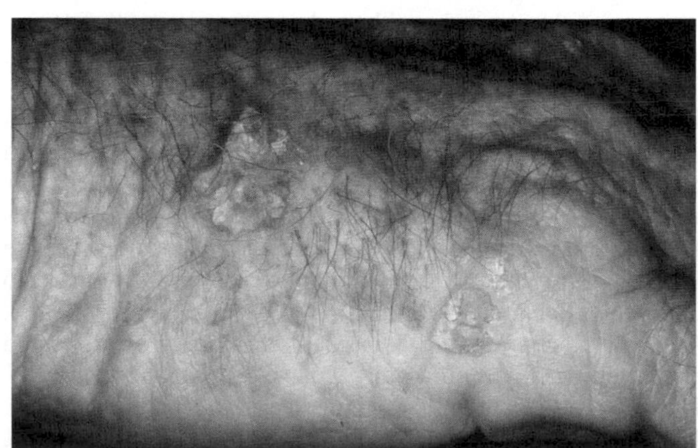

Figure 19 Hypertrophic actinic keratoses of the dorsal hand

cotton-tipped applicator or an open-spray technique with a handheld nitrogen unit, until the lesion turns white. This is repeated for a second cycle. Patients will experience stinging or burning during the treatment followed by erythema and sometimes blistering of the treated lesion. Other treatments include 5-fluorouracil 5% cream, imiquimod 5% cream, chemical peels, and photodynamic therapy. 5-fluorouracil 5% cream is applied twice daily for 3 weeks. Patients must be informed that treated areas will become progressively and often severely inflamed and eroded. A return visit scheduled in 1–2 weeks for patient assessment and reassurance is recommended. Compliance can be improved by dividing the affected area into smaller subunits and treating one subunit at a time to minimize the inflammatory reaction. Imiquimod 5% cream, recently approved in the United States for the treatment of actinic keratoses, is applied to the entire treatment area before bedtime and left on for 8 hours, twice weekly for 16 weeks (Lebwohl *et al.*, 2004). Side effects are similar to 5-fluorouracil. Recent studies with photodynamic therapy (application of a photosensitizing drug with exposure to its activating wavelength of light to achieve destruction of target tissue) demonstrate efficacy comparable to topical therapies and cryotherapy, with approximately 90% disappearance of lesions (Touma *et al.*, 2004; Piacquadio *et al.*, 2004). Advantages of this procedure include rapid healing and disappearance of treated lesions within 1 month, physician-controlled delivery allowing complete and homogeneous treatment of the face and/or scalp, eliminating the need for patient compliance. Because patients with actinic keratoses are also at risk for skin cancer, including melanoma, they should be examined annually.

Basal Cell Carcinoma (BCC)

BCC accounts for approximately 75% of all skin cancer, more than 1 million cases per year in the United States. It is also related to chronic ultraviolet light exposure, affecting predominantly fair-skinned Caucasians and involving the head and neck more often than the trunk and extremities. The nose is the most common site. The primary lesion is a translucent or pearly papule with visible telangiectasias (Figure 20). Late changes include central crusting or ulceration. Patients often complain that these lesions "do not heal" and they may break down or bleed. Histologic confirmation by shave or punch biopsy techniques is required to confirm the diagnosis. The differential diagnosis includes SCC, keratoacanthoma, and sebaceous hyperplasia. BCC is a very slow growing tumor that rarely metastasizes. However, if left untreated, significant morbidity can result from local invasion and extension to underlying cartilage, fascia, muscle, and bone.

Appropriate choice of therapy is dependent on the risk for recurrence and metastasis (Miller, 2000). Low risk tumors are defined as primary tumors measuring up to 2 cm on the trunk and extremities or up to 1 cm on the head and neck, with well-defined clinical borders, and occurring in an immunocompetent patient. Excision with 4-mm margins and electrodesiccation, and curettage (ED&C) have comparable cure rates of 90%. High-risk tumors have one or more of the following characteristics: recurrent tumor; size greater then 2 cm on the trunk and extremities or greater than 1 cm on the head and neck; poorly defined clinical borders; occurring in an immunosuppressed patient. These are best excised with concurrent histologic confirmation of clear margins before closure (Mohs surgery). Cure rates at 5 years are then 98–100%. For patients with a prior BCC, the 3-year cumulative risk for recurrence is 44% (Marcil and Stern, 2000). An annual skin examination is sufficient for detecting new BCCs. The number of prior skin cancers is a strong risk factor for development of subsequent skin cancers; thus patients with multiple BCCs should be examined more frequently.

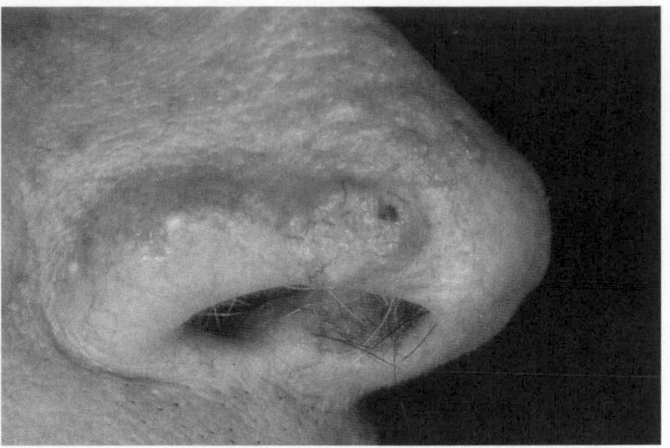

Figure 20 Nodular basal cell carcinoma with telangiectasias

Squamous Cell Carcinoma (SCC)

SCC is the second most common skin cancer, approximately 20% of the total, and derives from keratinocytes above the basal layer of the epidermis, often with actinic keratoses as precursor lesions. It predominantly affects the habitually sun-exposed head, neck, and dorsal hands, although SCC can also arise at sites of chronic inflammation, in areas of prior radiation or old burn scars, or on the genitals. The primary lesion is a firm indurated papule, plaque, or nodule (Figure 21). Secondary changes include hyperkeratotic scale or central ulceration with crust. These lesions do not heal and often break down and bleed. Biopsy with shave or punch technique is required to confirm the diagnosis. The differential diagnosis includes BCC and keratoacanthoma. SCC on the lips or ears has a 10–15% risk of spread to cervical nodes. SCC should be suspected in any persistent nodule, plaque or ulcer, especially when occurring in sun-damaged skin or on the lower lip. Immunosuppressed patients (transplant recipients) are at higher risk for SCC due to impaired cell-mediated immunity.

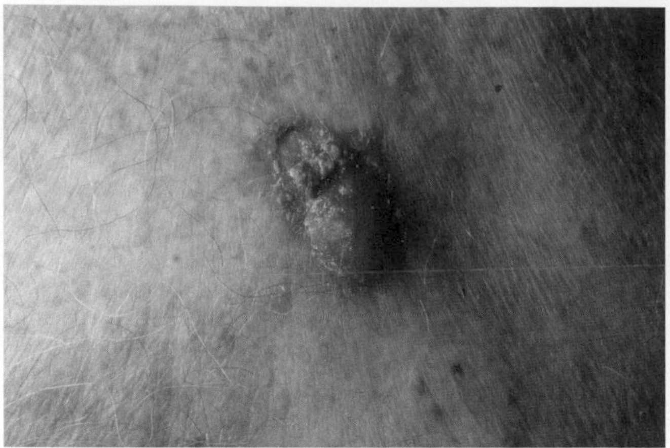

Figure 21 Squamous cell carcinoma of central chest

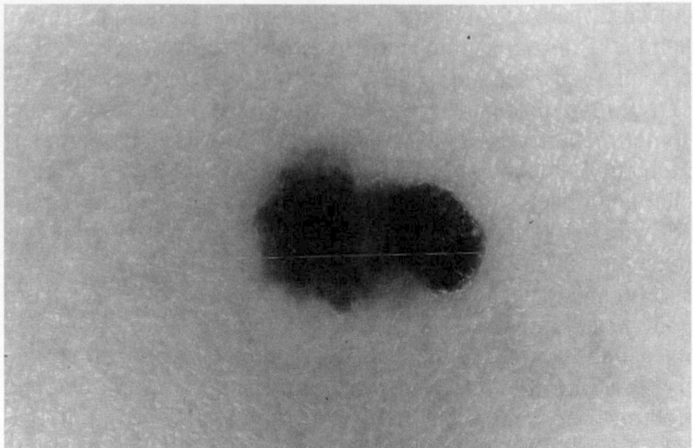

Figure 22 Superficial spreading melanoma demonstrating a nodular area likely to represent deep invasion

ED&C and excision have comparable cure rates of 90% for low risk tumors (defined for BCC). Mohs surgery is suggested for high-risk tumors defined as having one or more of the following: recurrent tumor; tumor measuring >2 cm on the trunk and extremities, or >1 cm on the head and neck; location on the genitals, lips, ears, site of prior radiation or scar; tumor with poorly defined clinical borders; and tumor occurring in an immunosuppresed host (Miller, 2000). For patients with a prior SCC, the 3-year cumulative risk for another SCC is 18% (Marcil and Stern, 2000). Annual follow-up examinations for at least 3 years are recommended. Patients with multiple SCCs should be seen more frequently.

Melanoma

Melanoma comprises 5% of all skin cancers. It is derived from melanocytes and has the greatest potential for metastasis. The incidence of melanoma is increasing faster than any other cancer. The lifetime risk of melanoma in an individual in the United States born in 2004 is estimated at greater than 1 in 70. Older men have the highest incidence of melanoma and the highest mortality rates from melanoma. In the United States, the incidence of thick tumors (>4 mm) has continued to increase in men 60 years and older (Jemal *et al.*, 2001). Nearly 50% of all melanoma deaths involve white men 50 years and older. Risk factors include light complexion (red-blonde hair), blistering sunburns during childhood, tendency to tan poorly and sunburn easily, and a positive family history. Additional risk factors in the middle-aged population include age greater than 50 years, male sex, and history of actinic keratoses or nonmelanoma skin cancer.

There are three clinical and histologic subtypes of melanoma: nodular (15%), superficial spreading (70%), and lentigo maligna melanoma (15%). The latter usually evolve after many years from a variegate, gradually enlarging macule on the face and neck of the elderly. The other types arise most commonly on the trunk or legs. The primary lesion is a brown to black macule, papule, plaque, or nodule with one or more of the following features: asymmetry, border irregularity, color variegation, and diameter greater than 6 mm (Figure 22). Patients may notice an increase in size of a pigmented lesion and bleeding. The differential diagnosis includes solar lentigo, seborrheic keratosis, dysplastic nevus, and pigmented BCC. If possible, suspected lesions should be excised with 1–2 mm margin of normal skin down to the subcutaneous fat.

Melanoma is treated by surgical excision with margins determined by histological tumor thickness (Breslow depth). (Balch *et al.*, 2001) Tumor thickness and presence or absence of histologic ulceration are the most important prognostic factors (Balch *et al.*, 2001). Patients with thin melanomas (<1.0 mm) have the best prognosis (>90% five-year survival rate), whereas those with thick tumors (>4 mm) have a 50% five-year survival rate. Evaluation of nodal involvement with sentinel lymph node biopsy provides regional lymph node staging information for patients at high risk for metastatic melanoma (primary melanomas >1.0 mm in depth, and for tumors ≤1 mm when histological ulceration is present) (Perrott *et al.*, 2003). Newly diagnosed and established melanoma patients require periodic complete skin examinations including mucosal sites, genitals, buttocks, palms and soles, lymph nodes, and palpation for hepatosplenomegaly. They should also be instructed on how to perform monthly self-skin exams. Frequency of follow-up, laboratory tests, and imaging studies depend on the stage of disease.

CUTANEOUS MANIFESTATIONS OF INTERNAL MALIGNANCY

There is a variety of skin signs associated with internal malignancy. Although uncommon, these findings with subsequent diagnostic testing may help one to discover an otherwise occult malignancy. Some cutaneous markers for malignancy are listed in Table 5.

Table 5 Cutaneous manifestations of internal malignancy

Skin sign	Physical findings	Associated malignancies
Metastases	≥1 cm firm nodule(s) on the scalp, flesh-colored to pink to black	Breast, lung, genitourinary
Bazex syndrome	Erythematous scaly plaques on the ears, nose, cheeks, hand, feet and knees. Hyperkeratosis of the palms & soles	Upper respiratory & digestive tracts
Paget's disease	Unilateral erythematous sharply defined plaque of the nipple and areola. Unresponsive to potent topical steroids	Breast
Generalized pruritus	Unexplained itching not associated with dry skin	Hodgkin's disease Leukemia/ lymphoma Mycosis fungoides
Dermatomyositis	Swelling of the face & eyelids with a pink to violaceous hue. Flat-topped violaceous papules over the PIP and DIP joints. Proximal muscle weakness	Lungs Gastrointestinal Breast
Erythema gyratum repens	Wavy erythematous plaques with fine peripheral scale in a concentric pattern (wood grain appearance). Lesions migrate over the skin surface	Lung, breast, stomach, other
Erythroderma	Erythematous patches or plaques with exfoliative scale covering ≥90% of total body surface area	Lymphoma, leukemia, Sezary syndrome
Acquired ichthyosis	Dry fish-like scale involving the extremities	Lymphoma, multiple myeloma, Lung, breast, cervical cancer
Acanthosis nigricans	Hyperpigmented velvety plaques involving the flexures (axilla, groin, neck)	Stomach Other gastrointestinal or genitourinary

KEY POINTS

- Successful management of dermatophyte infections (tinea pedis, onychomycosis) requires adequate patient education, correction of underlying predisposing factors, and prophylactic measures against recurrence.
- Inflammatory disorders are chronic, but can be effectively controlled with a routine skin care regimen (application of moisturizer, sunscreen) and topical therapies.
- Benign lesions may be biopsied or removed if they become irritated or cosmetically undesirable.
- Recommendations for skin cancer prevention include regular sun avoidance, daily application of sunscreen, long-sleeve shirts, and broad-brimmed hats.
- Patient education, early detection, and adequate monitoring are the keys to timely diagnosis of skin cancer.

KEY REFERENCES

- Elewski BE, Leyden J, Rinaldi MG & Atillasoy E. *Archives of Internal Medicine* 2002; **162**:2133–8.
- Jemal A, Devesa SS, Hartge P & Tucker MA. *Journal of the National Cancer Institute* 2001; **93**:678–83.
- Marcil I & Stern RS. *Archives of Dermatology* 2000; **136**:1524–30.
- Yaar M & Gilchrest BA. In IM Freedberg, AZ Eisen, K Wolff *et al.* (eds) *Fitzpatrick's Dermatology in General Medicine* 2003, vol 2 pp 1386–98; McGraw-Hill, New York.

REFERENCES

Ahmed A & Tollefsbol T. *Journal of the American Geriatrics Society* 2001; **49**:1105–9.

Balch CM, Buzaid AC, Soong SJ *et al. Journal of Clinical Oncology* 2001; **19**:3635–48.

Campisi J. *Cell* 1996; **84**:497–500.

Craze M & Young M. *Journal of the American Academy of Dermatology* 2003; **49**:S139–42.

Dunn-Walters DK, Banerjee M & Mehr R. *Biochemical Society Transactions* 2003; **31**:447–8.

Elewski BE, Leyden J, Rinaldi MG & Atillasoy E. *Archives of Internal Medicine* 2002; **162**:2133–8.

Fisher GJ, Kang S, Varani J *et al. Archives of Dermatology* 2002; **138**:1462–70.

Goukassian D, Gad F, Yaar M *et al. FASEB Journal* 2000; **14**:1325–34.

Jack P & Brookes P. *International Journal of Cancer* 1980; **25**:789–95.

Jankovic V, Messaoudi I & Nikolich-Zugich J. *Blood* 2003; **102**:3244–51.

Jemal A, Devesa SS, Hartge P & Tucker MA. *Journal of the National Cancer Institute* 2001; **93**:678–83.

Jiang J, Anaraki F, Blank KJ & Murasko DM. *Journal of Immunology* 2003; **171**:3353–7.

Kraemer KH. In IM Freedberg AZ Eisen, K Wolff *et al.* (eds) *Fitzpatrick's Dermatology in General Medicine* 2003, vol 2, pp 1508–21; McGraw-Hill, New York.

Kurban RS & Bhawan J. *The Journal of Dermatologic Surgery and Oncology* 1990; **16**:908–14.

Lebwohl M & Ali S. *Journal of the American Academy of Dermatology* 2001; **45**:649–61, quiz 662-4.

Lebwohl M, Dinehart S, Whiting D *et al. Journal of the American Academy of Dermatology* 2004; **50**:714–21.

MacLaughlin J & Holick MF. *The Journal of Clinical Investigation* 1985; **76**:1536–8.

Marcil I & Stern RS. *Archives of Dermatology* 2000; **136**:1524–30.

Miller SJ. *Dermatologic Surgery* 2000; **26**:289–92.

Mouton CP, Bazaldua OV, Pierce B & Espino DV. *American Family Physician* 2001; **63**:257–68.

Nehlin JO, Skovgaard GL & Bohr VA. *Annals of the New York Academy of Sciences* 2000; **908**:167–79.

Oikawa S & Kawanishi S. *FEBS Letters* 1999; **453**:365–8.

Paller AS. In IM Freedberg, AZ Eisen, K Wolff *et al.* (eds) *Fitzpatrick's Dermatology in General Medicine*, 2003, vol 2, pp 1833–6; McGraw-Hill, New York.

Patrick MH. *Photochemistry and Photobiology* 1977; **25**:357–72.

Pelle MT. *Advances in Dermatology* 2003; **19**:139–70.

Perrott RE, Glass LF, Reintgen DS & Fenske NA. *Journal of the American Academy of Dermatology* 2003; **49**:567–88, quiz 589-92.

Piacquadio DJ, Chen DM, Farber HF *et al. Archives of Dermatology* 2004; **140**:41–6.

Ryan T. *Micron* 2004; **35**:161–71.

Savitsky K, Bar-Shira A, Gilad S *et al. Science* 1995; **268**:1749–53.

Sigurgeirsson B, Olafsson JH, Steinsson JB *et al. Archives of Dermatology* 2002; **138**:353–7.

Singri P, West DP & Gordon KB. *Archives of Dermatology* 2002; **138**:657–63.

Smith ES, Fleischer AB Jr, & Feldman SR In BA Gilchrest (ed) *Clinics in Geriatric Medicine* 2001, vol 17, pp 631–41; W.B. Saunders, Philadelphia.

Touma D, Yaar M, Whitehead S *et al. Archives of Dermatology* 2004; **140**:33–40.

Troelstra C, van Gool A, de Wit J *et al. Cell* 1992; **71**:939–53.

Tzaphlidou M. *Micron* 2004; **35**:173–7.

Weinberg JM, Koestenblatt EK, Tutrone WD *et al. Journal of the American Academy of Dermatology* 2003; **49**:193–7.

Wilkin J, Dahl M, Detmar M *et al. Journal of the American Academy of Dermatology* 2002; **46**:584–7.

Yaar M & Gilchrest BA. In IM Freedberg, AZ Eisen, K Wolff *et al.* (eds) *Fitzpatrick's Dermatology in General Medicine* 2003, vol 2 pp 1386–98; McGraw-Hill, New York.

Yu CE, Oshima J, Fu YH *et al. Science* 1996; **272**:258–62.

136

Pressure Ulceration

Joseph E. Grey *and* **Keith G. Harding**
University of Wales College of Medicine, Cardiff, UK

INTRODUCTION

A pressure ulcer may be defined as an area of localized damage to the skin and underlying tissue caused by pressure, shear, friction or a combination of these (European Pressure Ulcer Advisory Panel). Pressure Ulcers are known by a variety of other terms including bed sore, decubitus ulcer, pressure sore, and dermal ulcer. However, these terms do not accurately reflect the nature or etiology of the wound and are thus best avoided. Pressure ulcers arise as a local breakdown of soft tissue as a result of compression between a bony prominence and an external surface. The majority of pressure ulcers develop on the lower half of the body: two-thirds of these occur around the pelvis and one-third on the lower limbs. Common sites of pressure ulceration are shown in Figure 1. Pressure ulcers are most common in the elderly population, especially those older than 70 years, up to one-third of whom will have undergone surgery for a hip fracture. A second distinct population are those with spinal cord injuries with a reported prevalence of 20–30% 1–5 years after injury.

Over four hundred thousand people develop a pressure ulcer annually in the United Kingdom. Pressure ulcers most commonly arise in the hospital setting with a prevalence ranging from 3 to 14% in the acute setting. This rate varies between specialties; 2% in general surgical patients and 10% in orthopedic patients, reflecting, in part, the age differences of the two groups (Clark and Watts, 1994). The incidence in the acute setting is between 1 and 5%, though in patients who are bed- or chair-bound for more than 1 week, the incidence rises to almost 8%. Development of a new pressure ulcer is associated with a fivefold increase in length of hospital stay (Lazarus *et al.*, 1994).

In long-term facilities, the prevalence ranges from 1.5 to 25%. The prevalence of pressure ulceration in nursing homes is not appreciably higher than in the acute hospital setting. Around 20% of pressure ulcers develop at home and a further 20% in nursing homes. Pressure ulceration in an elderly person carries a fivefold increase in mortality, with the in-hospital mortality rate of 25 to 33%. By 2020, the number of people aged over 65 years in the United Kingdom will rise by 20%: The incidence of pressure ulceration will rise concomitantly.

Pressure ulcers are responsible for a significant degree of morbidity, both physical and psychological. Moreover, they represent a huge financial burden, both to the individual and to society as a whole. In 1993, the cost of pressure ulcers to the NHS was estimated at between £180 and £321 million (Touche, 1993). More recent studies have shown that this cost has escalated to between £1.4 and £2.1 billion annually, equivalent to 4% of the total NHS expenditure (Bennett *et al.*, 2004): This was believed to be a conservative estimate as the figures did not reflect the cost of associated problems such as methicillin resistant staphylococcus aureus (MRSA) infection, heel pressure ulcers associated with peripheral vascular disease and pressure ulcers in diabetics.

The cost of healing a grade IV pressure ulcer was found to be ten times that of healing a grade I pressure ulcer (Bennett *et al.*, 2004). Osteomyelitis complicating pressure ulceration significantly increases the need for hospital admission with a lengthy in-patient course and increased financial cost, mostly reflecting nursing time. Most pressure ulcers are avoidable, with the cost of preventing pressure ulceration representing a significant potential cost saving to the patient and to the health-care system. The cost to society of pressure ulceration continues to increase as a result of increased litigation. In the United States, development of a pressure ulcer in a care home or hospital may be regarded in a court of law as evidence of clinical negligence.

PATHOGENESIS

The four main extrinsic factors implicated in the etiology of pressure ulceration include interface pressure (the load perpendicular to the tissue surface), shear (the load parallel

Principles and Practice of Geriatric Medicine, 4th Edition. Edited by M.S. John Pathy, Alan J. Sinclair and John E. Morley.

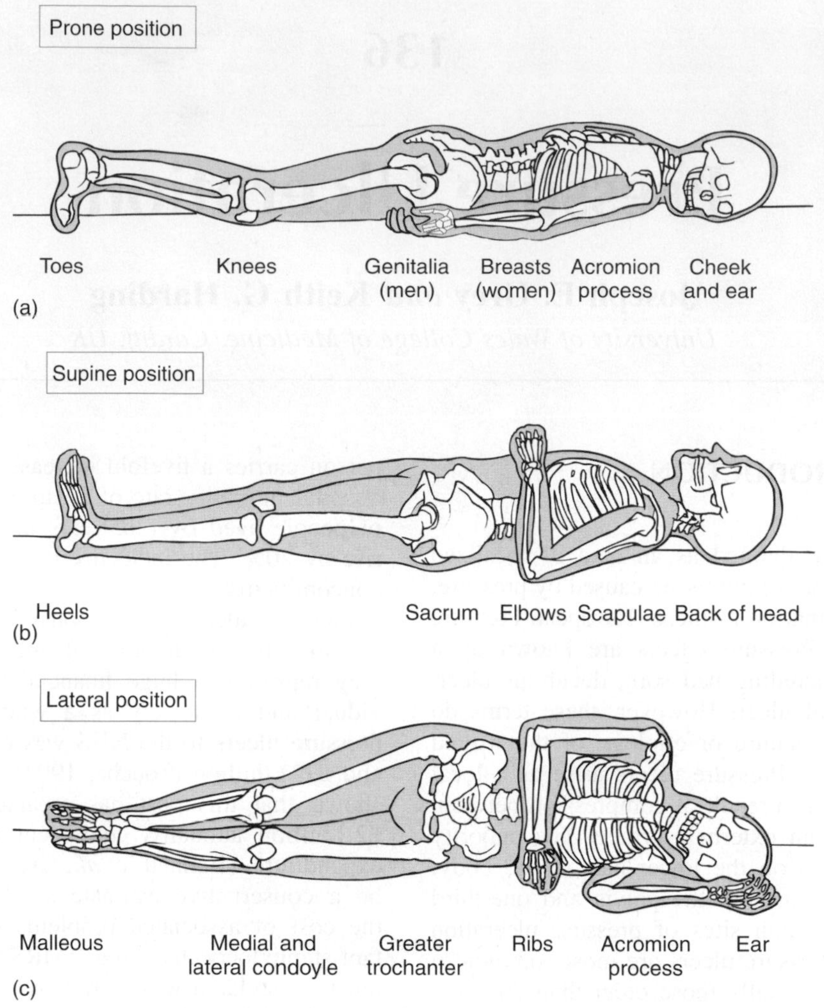

Figure 1 Common sites of pressure ulceration in the at-risk individual in (a) the prone position, (b) the supine position, (c) the lateral position

to the tissue surface), friction (the load acting tangentially to the tissue surface), and moisture. While direct (interface) pressure is the most important etiological factor, all four are closely interrelated.

In the 1930s, Landis estimated, in healthy volunteers, that normal capillary pressure ranged from 32 mm of mercury (mmHg) on the arterial side of the circulation to 12 mmHg on the venous side (Landis, 1930). When pressure of short duration is relieved, the tissue demonstrates reactive hyperemia, reflecting increased blood flow to the area. A sustained high closing pressure in excess of 32 mmHg was postulated to lead to decreased capillary blood flow, occlusion of blood vessels and lymphatics and tissue ischemia (Figure 2). The closing pressure was revised in later work by Landis to between 45 and 50 mmHg. Pressure as low as 40 mmHg has, however, been found to cause tissue anoxia in some elderly patients (Bader and Gant, 1988).

Dermal capillaries are coiled at their bases and are thus more resistant to occlusion by pressure. The subcutaneous vessels run parallel to the deep fascial planes and are more likely to be occluded by external pressure leading to tissue damage (Bliss, 1993). Prolonged pressure may, therefore, lead to ischemic changes and pressure ulceration due to perfusion/reperfusion injury from build up of inflammatory molecules.

The highest pressures occur over bony prominences at the bone/muscle interface (Figure 3). Thus, an external pressure of 50 mmHg may rise to over 200 mmHg at a bony prominence, leading, with time, to deep tissue destruction, which may not be evident on the surface of the skin. Such pressures may decrease transcutaneous oxygen tensions to almost zero. Pressures as high as 150 mmHg have been recorded from patients lying on ordinary mattresses (Lindan, 1961; Houle, 1969); regular relief from high pressures in the at-risk patient is, therefore, essential to prevent pressure ulceration.

Such changes are ultimately responsible for necrosis of muscle, subcutaneous tissue, dermis and epidermis and consequent pressure ulcer formation. It will be apparent though, that high pressure of short duration will lead to more rapid tissue damage while low pressure leads to a more insidious onset of tissue damage and ulceration

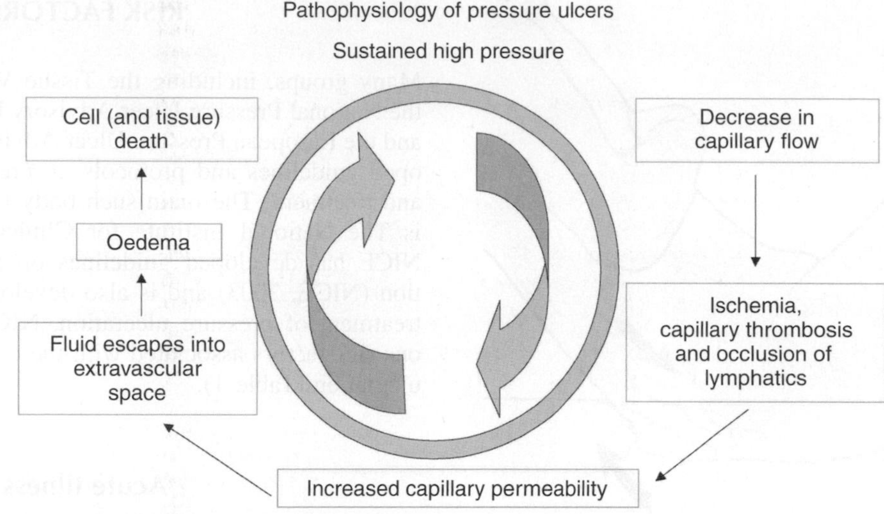

Figure 2 Schematic representation of the mechanism of pressure-induced tissue damage

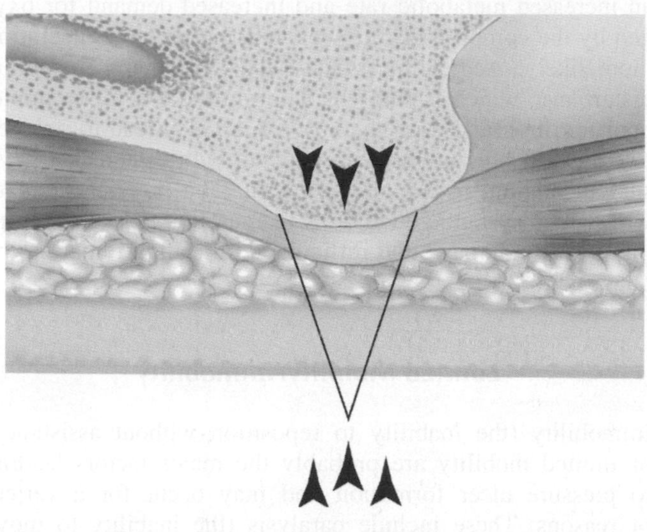

Figure 3 Conical pattern of pressure distribution over a bony prominence, illustrating the fact that seemingly low external pressure rises to a much higher pressure at the bone/muscle interface. Thus, tissue damage may be unrecognized as the skin may still be intact

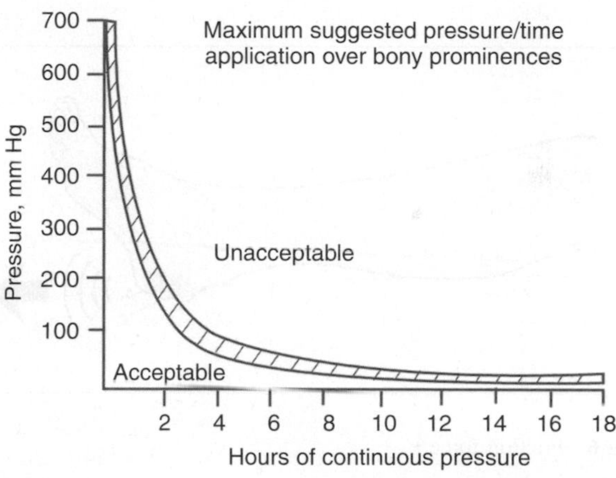

Figure 4 Guidelines on sitting tolerance based on the magnitude of localised pressure (From Reswick J and Rogers J. Experiences at Rancho Los Amigos Hospital with Devices and Techniques to Prevent Pressure Sores. Bedsore Biomechanics. Baltimore: University Park Press)

(Figure 4). However, duration of pressure is also important and tissue damage may be avoided in the face of sustained pressure, which is relieved intermittently. This forms the basis of the rationale of regular turning of patients at risk of pressure ulceration, though the minimum frequency is still a matter of debate. Clinically, pressures of 70–100 mmHg have been recorded over bony prominences supported by standard NHS mattresses (Collier, 2004). Pressure-reducing mattresses reduce this pressure to between 30 and 40 mmHg (Collier, 1996).

Shear force (the load parallel to the tissue surface) is generated owing to the motion of bone and subcutaneous tissue relative to the skin, which is restrained from moving due to frictional forces (Figure 5). For example, when a seated patient slides down the chair or when the head of a bed is elevated to greater than 30°, the sacral skin remains fixed with respect to the support surface while the sacrum moves, and the deep fascial blood vessels are stretched and distorted. In such circumstances, the pressure required to occlude the blood vessels is greatly reduced, which reduces the rate of recovery from tissue anoxia (Schubert and Héraudj, 1994). In the elderly individual, reduced skin elastin content predisposes to the adverse effects of shear. While interface pressure is of more importance in generating tissue damage, the concomitant presence of shear increases the risk of ischemic damage. The effect of shear may be reduced through the use of vapor-permeable mattress covers, which reduce the amount of moisture.

Friction, acting tangentially to the tissue surface, opposes the movement of one surface against another (Figure 6). Frictional forces may lead to the formation of intraepidermal

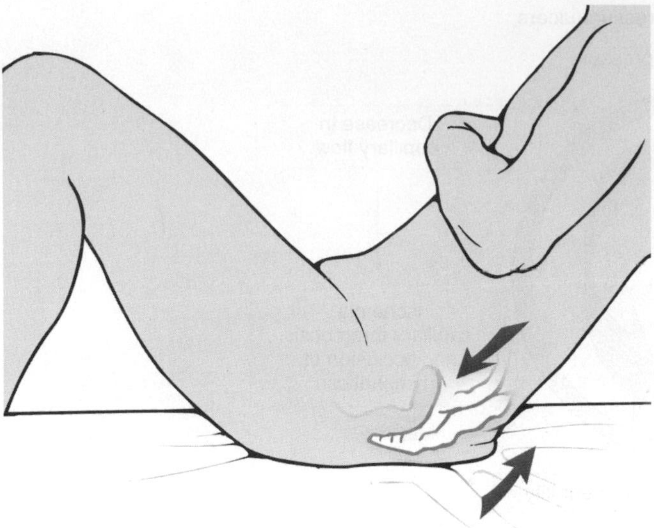

Figure 5 Shear force

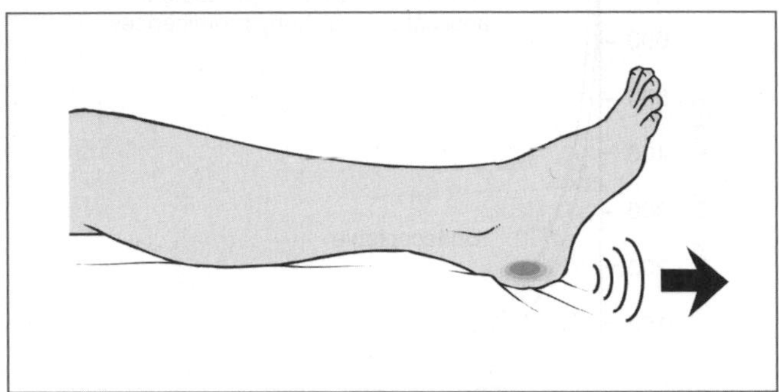

Figure 6 Friction force

blisters, which in turn lead to superficial skin erosions, initiating or accelerating pressure ulceration. Such forces occur, for example, when a patient is dragged across a bedsheet, pulling the sheet under the patient, sliding transfer from bed to chair, or as a result of ill-fitting prosthetic devices or footwear. Friction reduces the amount of pressure required for ulceration to occur.

It must be emphasized that pressure damage reflects a complex interplay of these three forces, each playing a greater or lesser role depending on the situation pertaining at that time and also affected by the presence of moisture.

While moisture, by itself, does not cause pressure ulceration, an excessively moist environment caused by, for example, perspiration, urinary or fecal incontinence or excessive wound drainage enhances the deleterious effects of pressure, friction, and shear. It also causes maceration of the skin, which compounds these factors. Friction and moisture are important factors leading to superficial skin breakdown and produce the greatest effects in areas of high pressure: The effects of friction are increased up to fivefold in the presence of moisture. Pressure and shear forces exert their effects on deeper structures (Hall, 1984; Herman and Rothman, 1989).

RISK FACTORS

Many groups, including the Tissue Viability Society (UK), the National Pressure Ulcer Advisory Panel (NPUAP) (USA) and the European Pressure Ulcer Advisory Panel, have developed guidelines and protocols on pressure ulcer prevention and treatment. The main such body in the United Kingdom is The National Institute for Clinical Excellence (NICE). NICE has developed guidelines on pressure ulcer prevention (NICE, 2003) and is also developing guidelines on the treatment of pressure ulceration. NICE has identified various risk factors associated with the development of pressure ulceration (Table 1).

Acute Illness

Pressure Ulceration is more common in immobile patients who develop pyrexia (Bar and Pathy, 1998). This leads to an increased metabolic rate and increased demand for oxygen by the compromised tissues, making pressure ulceration more likely. Acute illness also leads to general metabolic disturbance which is further compromised by, for example, poor nutrition and drug therapy, which may lead to reduced tolerance of pressure and, in patients with established pressure ulceration, to impaired healing. The precise extent to which such systemic conditions increase the risk of developing pressure damage and difficulties in healing remain to be quantified.

Limited Mobility/Immobility

Immobility (the inability to reposition without assistance) or limited mobility are probably the major factors leading to pressure ulcer formation and may occur for a variety of reasons. These include paralysis (the inability to move due to loss of motor nerve function) due to neurological problems such as stroke and spinal cord injury, which lead to hemi-, para- or quadriplegia. Paralysis also leads to decreased muscle bulk and reduction of subcutaneous tissue, which, in turn, predisposes to pressure ulceration. Physical illness, including arthritis and orthopedic problems, leads to difficulty in changing position due, for example, to pain as well as joint deformity and lack of strength. The elderly are

Table 1 Risk factors for pressure ulceration

Acute illness
Extremes of age
Level of consciousness
Malnutrition/dehydration
Limited mobility/immobility
History of pressure damage
Sensory impairment
Severe chronic or terminal disease
Vascular disease

particularly prone to such problems. Obesity may lead to reduced mobility.

One of the commonest reasons for immobility in the elderly is fracture of the neck of femur. Fractured neck of femur has been shown in a cross-sectional study to be a risk factor for the development of a pressure ulcer (Scheckler and Peterson, 1986). Between 50 and 60% of patients with fracture of the femur develop a pressure ulcer, most of which develop within five days to two weeks of admission and occupying 20% of orthopedic beds (Versluysen, 1985, 1986).

Being bed- or chair-bound significantly increases the risk of pressure ulceration; appropriate pressure-relieving surfaces should be provided. Individuals with increased limb tone (spasticity) may benefit from interventions such as physiotherapy, muscle relaxants, nerve block, or surgery.

The number of nocturnal movements is correlated with development of pressure ulcers. One study has shown that 90% of ulceration in older patients occurred in those who have less than 20 spontaneous movements per night: No pressure ulcers were recorded in those patients with more than 50 movements per night (Exton-Smith and Sherwin, 1961). Reduced nocturnal mobility is associated with use of sedative medication and a high-pressure ulcer risk score (Barbenel *et al.*, 1986).

Other risk factors, which have been found to increase the incidence of pressure ulceration in the immobile patient, include dry skin, a preexisting grade I pressure ulcer (non-blanchable erythema of intact skin) and fecal incontinence (Allman *et al.*, 1995). In patients with spinal cord injuries who develop pressure ulcers, the serum albumin, prealbumin and cellular adhesion molecules (which have a role in immunity and wound healing) have been shown to be lower than those without injuries (Cruse *et al.*, 2000).

Impact of Age

Age alone is not an independent risk factor for pressure ulcer development. The fact that the frequency of pressure ulcer rises with age is a consequence of the comorbidities associated with advancing age (Allman *et al.*, 1995). The effects of all such risk factors should be minimized through their optimal management. The elderly are more likely to have underlying chronic disease, which may be severe, contribute to immobility, increase the risk of pressure ulceration and may impair healing. As many as 70% of patients with pressure ulcers are over 70 years of age (Barbenel *et al.*, 1977). Individuals between 70 and 75 years of age have double the incidence of pressure ulcers compared with 55–69 year-olds. The greatest incidence of pressure ulcers occurs in the 80–84-year age-group (Ek and Bowman, 1982). More than two-thirds of the elderly with pressure ulcers are female (Nyquist and Hawthorn, 1987).

Age-related susceptibility to skin breakdown in the face of other comorbidities may occur owing to loss of dermal vessels, thinned epidermis, flattening of the dermo-epidermal junction, decreased elastin content and increased skin permeability (Carter and Balin, 1983). Significant risk factors for the development of pressure ulcers in the chronically sick patient include cerebrovascular accident (CVA), impaired nutritional intake, being bed- or chair-bound and having fecal incontinence (Berlowitz and Wilking, 1989). The incidence of fracture of the neck of femur increases with age and is a significant risk factor for pressure ulcer development.

Severe Chronic or Terminal Illness

Chronic and terminal illnesses are, by nature, more common with increasing age. In hospitals, the main focus of treatment is the underlying illness, and the prevention and treatment of pressure ulcers may be seen as a lower priority. Caution should be exercised in the use of drugs used in such diseases: Drugs such as sedatives and analgesics may lead to immobility, while antihypertensives may cause alteration of skin blood flow (Kanj *et al.*, 1998).

Diabetes is a major cause of morbidity and may be associated with pressure ulcer formation. Diabetics are at risk of vascular disease, which may lead to reduced tissue perfusion. Diabetic sensory neuropathy impairs the ability to sense and react to pressure, pain, and temperature. Autonomic and motor neuropathy lead to dry skin, which cracks easily, and to altered foot architecture, which itself predisposes to diabetic foot ulceration as a result of altered foot pressure.

Chronic respiratory disease such as chronic obstructive pulmonary disease (COPD) may lead to decreased tissue oxygenation and thus tissue that is more prone to pressure damage. Chronic cardiovascular disease and peripheral edema may also predispose to pressure ulceration. Inadequate circulation due, for example, to cardiovascular or peripheral vascular disease will lead to poor tissue oxygenation and may predispose to pressure ulcer formation. Anemia, similarly, leads to reduced oxygenation and increased susceptibility to pressure damage: Pragmatically, the hemoglobin should, if possible, be maintained above $10\,\mathrm{g\,dl^{-1}}$.

Individuals with terminal illness are at high risk of pressure ulceration. Prevalence of pressure ulcers in such patients ranges from 37 to 50% (Hatcliffe and Dawe, 1996) and reflect the severity of the underlying disease. While most pressure ulcers are avoidable, they may reflect the multisystem failure that often accompanies terminal illness. In these cases, aggressive preventative measures may be inappropriate; patient comfort and dignity should be of prime concern.

Vascular Disease

Peripheral vascular disease is particularly associated with smoking and diabetes. It leads to reduced blood perfusion and increased risk of pressure ulceration: The heels, feet, and toes are at particular risk (Figure 7).

Malnutrition and Dehydration

Attention to nutrition is critical in the prevention and management of pressure ulcers. There is a correlation between

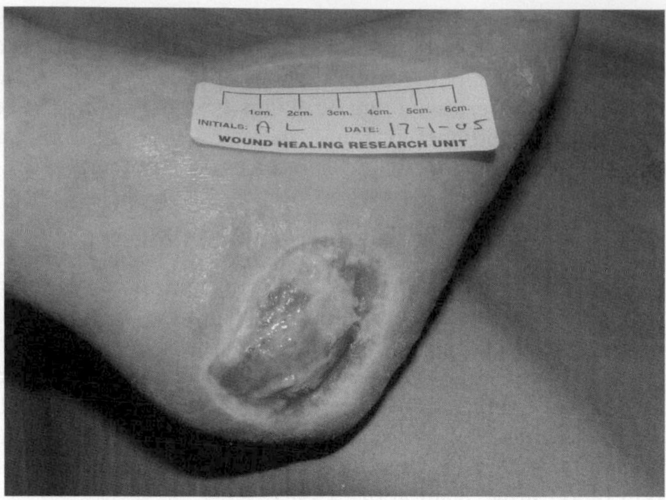

Figure 7 Heel pressure ulcer

the degree of malnutrition and the extent and severity of pressure ulceration (Allman *et al.*, 1986). In addition, malnutrition retards the healing of established pressure ulcers (Herman and Rothman, 1989). Malnutrition (protein-energy), impaired oral intake, and the development of pressure ulceration are closely interrelated. The relative risk of pressure ulcer development in high-risk malnourished patients is more than double that of patients with normal nutritional status (Thomas *et al.*, 1996). Two-thirds of severely malnourished nursing home residents were found in one study to have pressure ulcers, compared with none in mild to moderately malnourished residents (Pinchcofsky-Devin and Kaminski, 1986). Furthermore, malnutrition is associated with increased mortality in nursing home residents (Bourdel-Marchasson *et al.*, 2000).

Studies on the prevention of pressure ulceration through nutritional intervention are inconclusive (Mathus-Vliegen, 2004). However, it is generally accepted that, in order to prevent pressure ulceration in undernourished and malnourished patients, an energy intake of 35 kcal per kg body weight is required. 1.5 g kg^{-1} of protein and 1 ml per kcal per day fluid intake with the addition of the recommended daily allowance of micronutrient should be provided (though there are no good data on the amount or type) (EPUAP; Chernoff *et al.*, 1990; Breslow *et al.*, 1993; Mathus-Vliegen, 2004). In individuals with established pressure ulceration, the nutritional demands may be greater.

Patients at high risk and those with established pressure ulceration should be assessed and reviewed by a dietician. Provision of adequate nutrition may involve supplementary feeding, either assisted or enteral (via a nasogastric or PEG tube), though there may be a degree of morbidity associated, including diarrhea, incontinence, and limited mobility while attached to the feed – in themselves risk factors for pressure ulcer formation. Supplementation with high protein dietary supplements for 15 days to older, critically ill patients has shown a reduction in pressure ulcer development (Bourdel-Marchasson *et al.*, 2000). Practically, however, this may prove difficult to maintain in many patients.

Serum Albumin concentration is often used to assess the degree of nutrition. A concentration of less than 35 g l^{-1} is generally taken as a reflection of poor nutrition and a risk factor for the development of pressure ulcers. It should be remembered that this is at best a crude surrogate for degree of nutrition as the half-life of albumin is relatively long (of the order of 21 days) and hypoalbuminemia may be encountered in a variety of acute illnesses. Serum prealbumin, transferrin and lymphocyte count may be better markers of (mal) nutrition. Other measures of nutritional status predictive of pressure ulcer formation include decreased body weight, reduced triceps, skin-fold thickness, and lymphocytopenia (Allman *et al.*, 1995).

Sensory Problems

Sensory deficits give rise to altered ability to perceive the pain and discomfort associated with persistent local pressure, leading to reduced repositioning. Such deficits occur in individuals with neurological problems such as neuropathies (e.g. diabetic), which especially predispose to heel ulceration. Medical or psychological conditions may lead to altered conscious levels with resultant decrease in mobility. Medication is an especially common cause of altered conscious levels; these include sedatives, analgesics, and anesthetics. The effects of sensory loss in patients with stroke or spinal cord injury may be compounded by motor deficits or increased tone (spasticity), which limit mobility and the ability to reposition.

RISK ASSESSMENT

There are a plethora of pressure ulcer risk assessment scales in use, though there is little evidence that any one is superior to another or that their use has led to a reduction in pressure ulcer incidence (Whitfield *et al.*, 2000). The scales attempt to stratify the risk according to the number of known risk factors present, in order that preventive measures are instituted. They are designed for use in individuals who are bed- or chair-bound or who have limited ability to reposition themselves. Some are more comprehensive than others. They all contain a core of basic components (Table 2).

Table 2 Components of risk assessment scales

Age
Mobility
Activity
Level of consciousness
Nutrition
Continence
Skin status
Illness severity

However, some of the grading of the risk factors is subjective and observer dependent (Healey, 1996). This may be reflected in the low sensitivity (ability of the tool to correctly identify those patients who will develop a pressure ulcer) and specificity (ability of the tool to correctly identify those patients who will not develop a pressure ulcer) that the assessment scales exhibit. When using a risk assessment scale, it is judicious to consider whether it is valid, reliable, applicable to the patient group being assessed, subjective or objective, user friendly, and useful (Collier, 2004). It should be self evident that risk assessment scales are of use only if the at-risk patient identified receives appropriate intervention.

NICE has, echoing advice from the Department of Health (Essence of Care) in the United Kingdom, made suggestions on the use of pressure ulcer assessment scales (Table 3).

In Europe, the commonest scales used are Waterlow, Norton, and Braden. Others used include Gosnell and Knoll. The Waterlow scale is commonly used in the United Kingdom (Table 4).

Table 3 Points to be considered when choosing support surface

Identified level of risk
Skin assessment
Comfort
General health state
Lifestyle and abilities
Critical care needs
Acceptability of the pressure-relieving equipment to patient and/or carer

Prevention of Pressure Ulcers

Since direct pressure, shear forces, friction, and moisture are prerequisites for the development of pressure ulceration, pressure relief or redistribution should be the mainstay of any preventive strategy. Prevention may reduce the incidence of pressure ulceration by up to 50% (Anderson *et al.*, 1983; Seiler, 1985). Pressure ulcer prevention is further aided by the recognition that patients with limited or no mobility are at risk. Patients, carers, and health-care workers should be educated in this respect and also in recognizing early signs of pressure damage. While risk assessment tools will aid in this respect, they are no substitute for good clinical care and observation.

At-risk patients should have daily evaluations of the skin, concentrating particularly on the common at-risk areas, especially the bony prominences, including the sacral, ischial, trochanteric, and heel areas (Ayello, 1992). The skin should be kept clean and well hydrated (DeLisa and Mikulic 1985). Excess moisture should be minimized and may require the use of barrier creams or sprays and the use of absorbent pads for fecal and/or urinary incontinence. The skin over bony

Table 4 Waterlow risk assessment scale

WATERLOW PRESSURE SORE PREVENTION/TREATMENT POLICY

RING SCORES IN TABLE, ADD TOTAL. SEVERAL SCORES PER CATEGORY CAN BE USED

BUILD/WEIGHT FOR HEIGHT	★
AVERAGE	0
ABOVE AVERAGE	1
OBESE	2
BELOW AVERAGE	3

CONTINENCE	★
COMPLETE/ CATHETERISED	0
OCCASION INCONT	1
CATH/INCONTINENT OF FAECES	2
DOUBLY INCONT	3

SKIN TYPE VISUAL RISK AREAS	★
HEALTHY	0
TISSUE PAPER	1
DRY	1
OEDEMATOUS	1
CLAMMY (TEMP↑)	1
DISCOLOURED	2
BROKEN/SPOT	3

MOBILITY	★
FULLY	0
RESTLESS/FIDGETY	1
APATHETIC	2
RESTRICTED	3
INERT/TRACTION	4
CHAIRBOUND	5

SEX AGE	★
MALE	1
FEMALE	2
14 - 49	1
50 - 64	2
65 - 74	3
75 - 80	4
81+	5

APPETITE	★
AVERAGE	0
POOR	1
N.G. TUBE/ FLUIDS ONLY	2
NBM/ANOREXIC	3

SPECIAL RISKS	★
TISSUE MALNUTRITION	★
e.g.: TERMINAL CACHEXIA	8
CARDIAC FAILURE	5
PERIPHERAL VASCULAR DISEASE	5
ANAEMIA	2
SMOKING	1
NEUROLOGICAL DEFICIT	★
eg: DIABETES, M.S, CVA, MOTOR/SENSORY PARAPLEGIA	4 - 6
MAJOR SURGERY/TRAUMA	★
ORTHOPAEDIC - BELOW WAIST, SPINAL	5
ON TABLE > 2 HOURS	5
MEDICATION	★
CYTOTOXICS, HIGH DOSE STEROIDS ANTI-INFLAMMATORY	4

SCORE	10+ AT RISK	15+ HIGH RISK	20+VERY HIGH RISK

OBTAINABLE FROM: NEWTONS, CURLAND, TAUNTON, TA3 5SG

prominences should not be massaged deeply, as this may cause, rather than prevent, damage (Ek *et al.*, 1985, 1987).

In individuals not at risk of pressure ulceration, pressure relief or redistribution is an automatic, frequent, and usually reflex reaction to pressure, while in bed or seated. Individuals who are unwell or immobile turn much less frequently. These at-risk individuals should be repositioned regularly. While there are no firm data on frequency of repositioning, current practice suggests that a minimum 2-hourly repositioning schedule should be instituted, alternating the individual between lying on their back and then alternate sides (Knox *et al.*, 1994).

When positioned on the side, the individual's back should be angled at 30° with respect to the support surface in order to minimize pressure over the greater trochanter and lateral malleolus (Seiler and Stahelin, 1985). Direct ("kissing") contact of the bony prominences such as knees and ankles should be avoided through judicious use of cushions and foam wedges. "Doughnut" cushions should be avoided as they may lead to, rather than prevent, ulceration, possibly as a result of reduction of blood flow to the area of tissue which herniates through the center of the "doughnut" (Allman, 1989a,b).

Friction and shear forces should be minimized; abolition of these forces is neither possible nor desirable, else the patient would slip off the support surface! While repositioning, the individual should be lifted, rather than dragged across the bed or out of a wheelchair. The support surface should be kept clean and free of any debris (e.g. food), which may exacerbate any pressure damage. Shear damage may be diminished by keeping the head of the bed at 30° or less, thus preventing undue pressure on the sacrum, ischial tuberosities, and heels. A variety of heel (Figure 8) and elbow protectors are in use (e.g. sheepskin) but evidence on their efficacy is lacking.

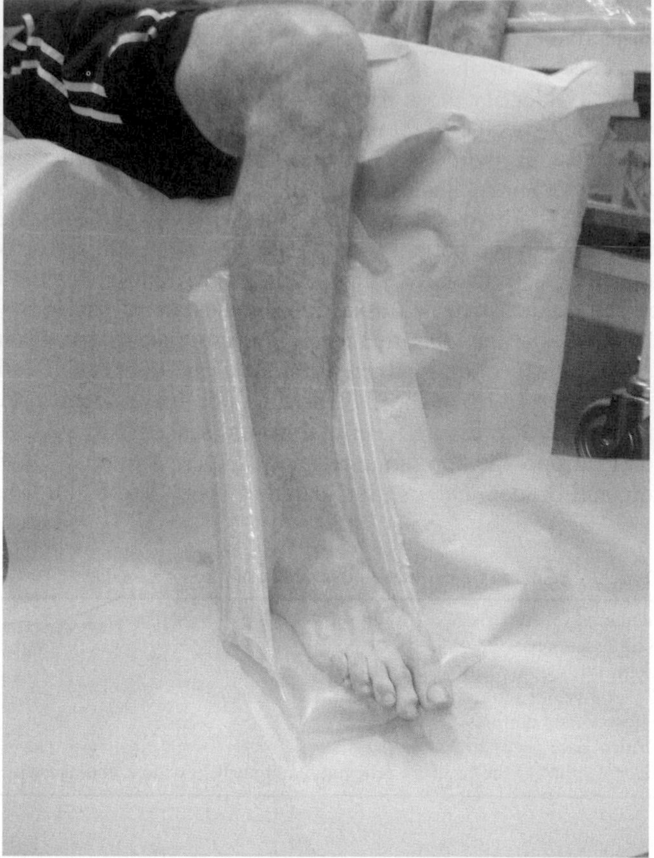

(a)

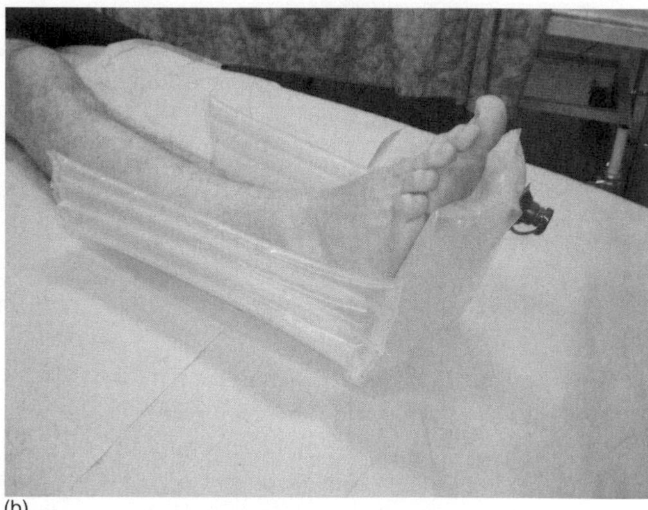

(b)

Figure 8 Repose Bootee, heel protector

Pressure-relieving Devices

There is a bewildering array of pressure-relieving and pressure-reducing support surfaces available. These include beds, mattresses, mattress overlays, cushions, chairs, and wheelchairs. There is, however, very little good-quality data supporting the use of particular pieces of equipment (Rycroft-Malone and Duff, 2000; Rithalia, 2004a). Furthermore, there appears to be a deal of uncertainty as to what the equipment actually achieves (Collins, 2004). There is also potential conflict in trying to combine a piece of equipment that is liked by the patient, meets the treatment objective, and is suitable for a particular care setting (Fletcher, 1995).

NICE in the United Kingdom has, in its guidelines, stated that pressure-relieving devices should be based on cost considerations as well as an overall assessment of the individual. They further state that holistic assessment should include the points listed in Table 3 and should not be based solely on scores derived from risk assessment scales (NICE).

However, much clinical practice in identifying the patient at risk of pressure ulcers and provision of the appropriate pressure-relieving surface continues to be dependent on the risk assessment scales. Indeed, the Waterlow scale, for example, links a risk score to a particular intervention (Watts and Clark, 1993; Winman and Clark, 1997). Moreover, many pressure ulcer prevention protocols and manufacturers of pressure-relieving surfaces imply that there are reliable cut-off points for identifying appropriate surfaces dependent on the degree of risk determined by the risk assessment scale.

NICE guidelines advocate the use of the terms "vulnerable to pressure ulcers" and "at elevated risk of pressure ulcers" in recognition of the limitations of risk assessment scales (NICE).

The implementation of holistic prevention programs, including provision of support surfaces, use of risk assessment tools, repositioning schedules, nutrition, and education programs have all resulted in reductions in pressure ulcer incidence (Xakellis *et al.*, 1998; Lyder *et al.*, 2002). This highlights the fact that good care is essential in both prevention and treatment of pressure ulcers. All prevention strategies require staff education. There should be a written pressure ulcer prevention and treatment policy. There should also be a multidisciplinary approach to prevention and treatment strategies including doctors, nurses, dieticians, physiotherapists, occupational therapists, speech and language therapists, housekeeping staff, catering, and supplies officers.

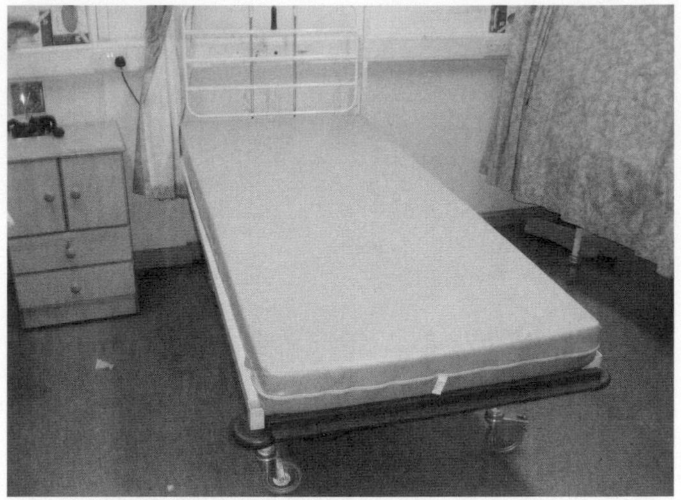

Figure 9 Standard hospital mattress

Mattresses

NICE guidelines recognize that there is little good-quality data on what support surface should be used in a particular circumstance. They suggest, as a minimum provision, that those individuals vulnerable to pressure ulcers should be placed on a high-specification (though low-tech) foam mattress with pressure-relieving properties. The guidelines further advise that alternating pressure or other high pressure-relieving systems should be considered in the following circumstances:

1. as a first-line preventive strategy for people at elevated risk (based on holistic assessment);
2. when the individual's previous history of pressure ulcer prevention and/or clinical condition indicates that they are best cared for on a high-tech device;
3. when a low-tech device has failed.

Support surfaces may be broadly divided into those that provide pressure reduction and those that provide pressure relief. Pressure-reducing systems produce the effect by increasing the surface area in contact with the support surface brackets (pressure = force/area). This is often the reason cited for nursing the patients in bed rather than in a chair, sitting for long periods (Gebhardt and Bliss, 1994). Pressure-relieving systems sequentially remove the source of pressure from parts of the body, usually by alternately inflating and deflating cells within mattress or mattress overlays.

Support systems are more commonly classified as static or dynamic systems. Static systems are generally, but not exclusively, nonpowered, low-tech devices of which the hospital mattress is the most basic example (Figure 9). They commonly comprise a sandwich of different densities of foam or other surfaces which are profiled (Collins, 2004). Other examples of static, pressure-reducing services include foam overlays and water-, gel- and air-filled devices designed to be placed over a standard mattress.

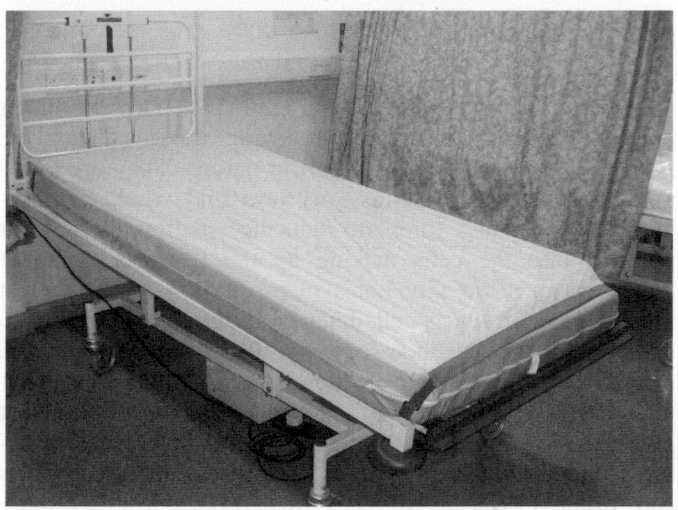

Figure 10 "Repose" mattress overlay

Comparative studies of some overlays have shown that they are no better than good-quality foam mattresses (Medical Devices Agency, 1994). However, a randomized, controlled, prospective trial comparing a low cost, low-pressure inflatable mattress ("Repose", Figure 10) designed to be placed on a standard hospital mattress showed no difference when compared to a high-tech dynamic support mattress and patients at high risk of pressure ulceration indicating that certain low-tech static pressure-relieving systems can be as effective as high-tech pressure-relieving systems in treating certain patient groups (Price *et al.*, 1999).

Static systems (Figure 11) are generally suitable for those individuals able to adopt a variety of positions. The system should not be able to "bottom out", that is, the mattress (or overlay) or any part of it providing less than 2.5 cm of support. The surfaces are appropriate for patients at low risk of pressure ulcer development.

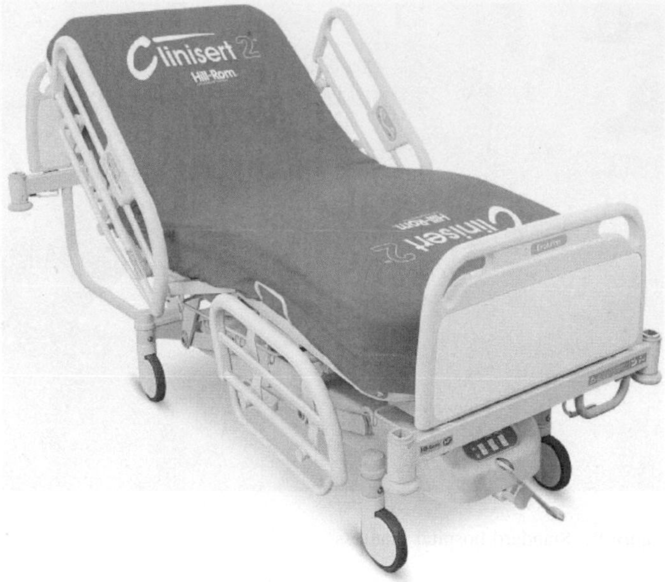

Figure 11 Static mattress

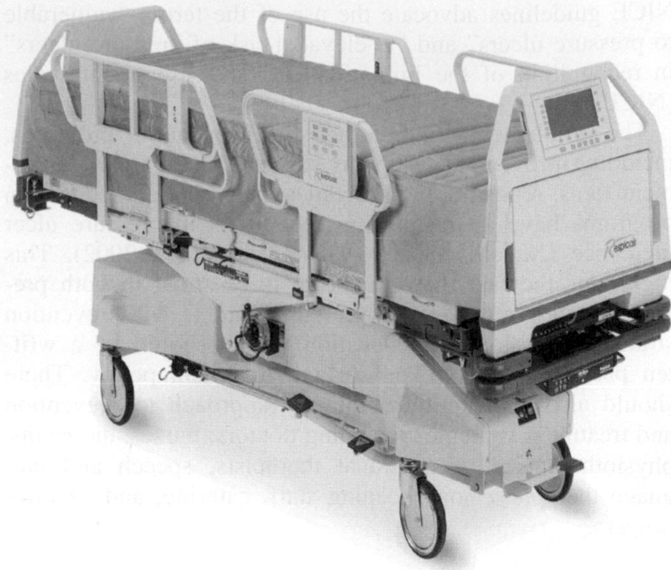

Figure 12 Dynamic mattress

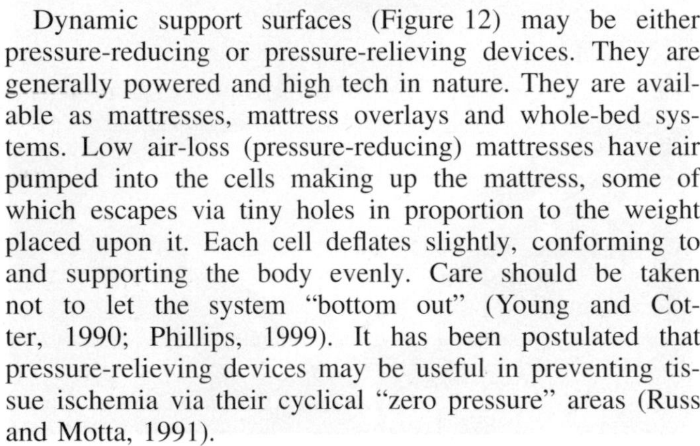

Dynamic support surfaces (Figure 12) may be either pressure-reducing or pressure-relieving devices. They are generally powered and high tech in nature. They are available as mattresses, mattress overlays and whole-bed systems. Low air-loss (pressure-reducing) mattresses have air pumped into the cells making up the mattress, some of which escapes via tiny holes in proportion to the weight placed upon it. Each cell deflates slightly, conforming to and supporting the body evenly. Care should be taken not to let the system "bottom out" (Young and Cotter, 1990; Phillips, 1999). It has been postulated that pressure-relieving devices may be useful in preventing tissue ischemia via their cyclical "zero pressure" areas (Russ and Motta, 1991).

Dynamic pressure-relieving surfaces are also powered high-tech devices. The pressure relief is generally facilitated by alternately inflating and deflating cells, so that one set of cells cyclically supports the body. The body is, therefore, relieved of pressure when a set of cells deflates. Usually, the two or three cells under the head of the patient are static, thus promoting patient comfort. Cell layers, sizes, shapes, and cell cycles vary between mattresses, depending on the manufacturer. Some dynamic systems adopt a static mode which is useful when carrying out certain procedures, for example, in the event of power failure or when transferring the patient from area to area. Table 5 lists the characteristics of different types of mattresses (Kanj *et al.*, 1998; Lyder, 2003).

Air-fluidized systems (pressure reducing) are filled with small silicone-coated beads through which air is pumped on a continuous basis, providing a dynamic surface (Figure 13). The patient's pressure points are, therefore, constantly moving. The dry particles are able to absorb fluid, which are then removed from the system, thus helping to prevent maceration and decrease the effect of moisture on the various forms of pressure.

Dynamic support surfaces are indicated for patients at elevated risk of developing a pressure ulcer, those patients with pressure ulcers who are unable to be nursed completely off the pressure ulcers, those with very large or multiple ulcers, and those with ulcers which are not healing.

In the United States, the center for Medicare and Medicaid to services has divided support services into three categories based upon reimbursement costs (Lyder, 2003).

Table 5 Selected characteristics for classes of support surfaces

Performance characteristics	Air-fluidized (high air loss)	Low-air loss	Alternating air (dynamic)	Static flotation (air or water)	Foam	Standard hospital mattress
Increased support area	Yes	Yes	Yes	Yes	Yes	No
Low moisture retention	Yes	Yes	No	No	No	No
Reduced heat accumulation	Yes	Yes	No	No	No	No
Shear reduction	Yes	?	Yes	Yes	No	No
Pressure reduction	Yes	Yes	Yes	Yes	Yes	No
Dynamic	Yes	Yes	Yes	No	No	No
Cost per day	High	High	Moderate	Low	Low	Low

From Bergstrom *et al.*, 1994.

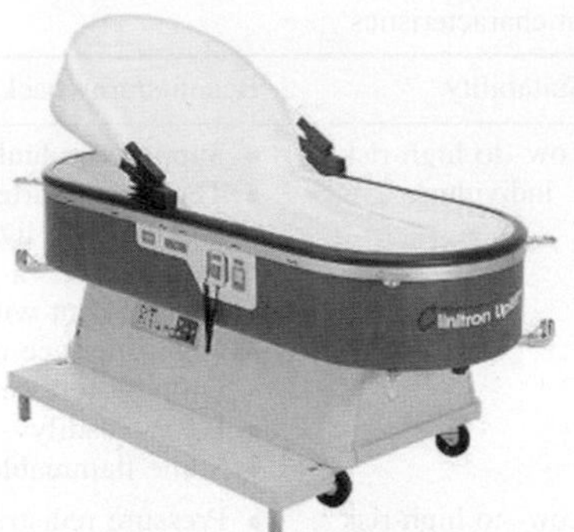

Figure 13 Air-fluidized mattress

Group 1 – Static support surfaces not requiring electricity.
Group 2 – Dynamic surfaces powered by electricity or pump including alternating and low air-loss mattresses.
Group 3 – Air-fluidized beds.

While such devices have been shown to reduce the incidence of pressure ulceration, there is no data to show that one particular type is better than another (Rithalia, 2004b). Furthermore, there is no evidence that high-tech pressure-relieving mattresses and overlays are more effective than high specification (low-tech) mattresses and overlays (NICE; Price *et al.*, 1999).

Seating

An often-neglected area of pressure-relieving support surfaces is seating, including both chairs and cushions. Again, however, there is a paucity of clinical evidence that one seat or cushion (from the enormous array of both that are available) is better than another. Suitable seating is essential to prevent pressure damage and to maintain a balanced, symmetrical seating posture (Collins, 2004). The provision of adequate seating in an acute hospital is generally very poor. A "one size fits all" approach seems to have been adopted with little thought given to providing pressure relief or reduction. All too often the seating is in poor condition (Versluysen, 1986). There is very little access to pressure-relieving cushions. In the person's own home and care homes, the elderly and disabled are often expected to sit for long periods in unsuitable chairs.

Ideally, provision of seating, including pressure-relieving cushions, should promote good sitting balance (Figure 14) and provide comfort by taking into account the individual's postural alignment, weight distribution, balance and stability and pressure relief or redistribution factors. The pelvis provides the interface between the seat and or cushion and the rest of the body. The main points of contact between the pelvis and seat are the ischial tuberosities, the tissue over which, not surprisingly, is the area particularly prone to pressure ulceration. In people without mobility problems, sitting is a dynamic process, the individuals changing their

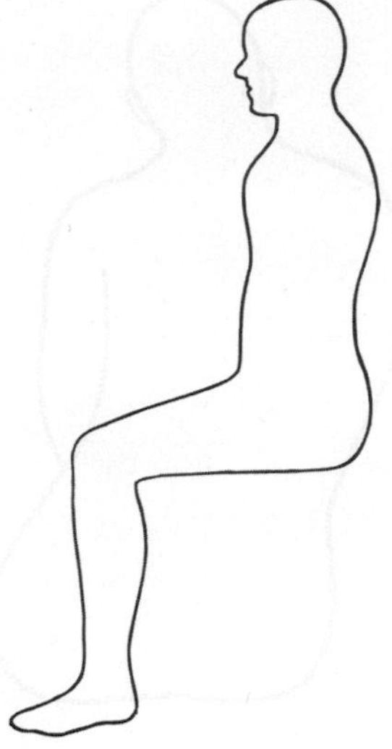

Figure 14 Ideal sitting position

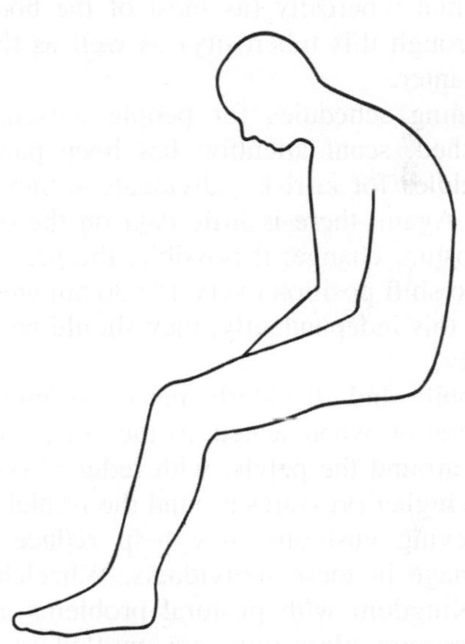

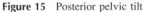

Figure 15 Posterior pelvic tilt

position when they become uncomfortable and thus relieving pressure, particularly over the ischial tuberosities.

Elderly, immobile, and disabled individuals often have a poor sitting posture, leading to what is known as *posterior pelvic tilt* (Figure 15). This may arise as a result of gravity, an unsupportive or inappropriate chair or wheelchair and poor trunk control, amongst other factors. Since the pelvis rotates posteriorly, the sacrum becomes more at risk of pressure damage. In addition, the ischial tuberosities slide forward, increasing shear and friction forces with a concomitant increase in the risk of pressure ulceration. A further consequence of the body slipping forward is that the heels become prone to further shear and frictional pressure, increasing the risk of pressure ulceration.

If the seat of the chair sags, the pelvis may tilt laterally (Figure 16), leading to increased risk of pressure ulceration

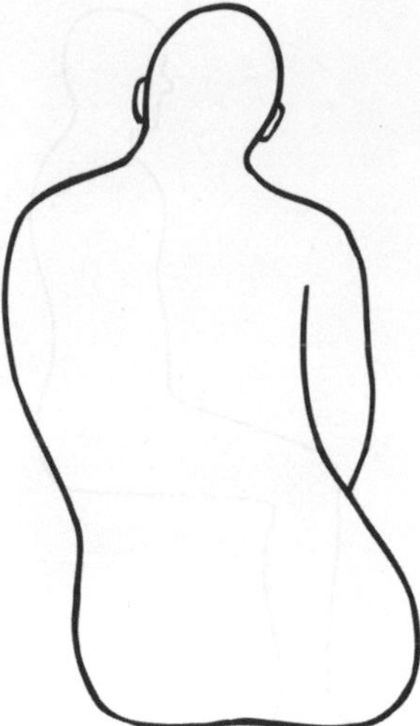

Figure 16 Lateral pelvic tilt

over one ischial tuberosity (as most of the body weight is supported through this tuberosity) as well as the ipsilateral greater trochanter.

While turning schedules for people nursed in bed are well established, scant attention has been paid to repositioning schedules for at-risk individuals sitting in chairs or wheelchairs. Again, there is little data on the optimum frequency of posture change: if possible, the person should be encouraged to shift position every 15–30 minutes. If they are unable to do this independently, they should be repositioned at least hourly.

The immobile and ill elderly person is more at risk of pressure ulceration when seated, as they often have reduced muscle bulk around the pelvis, with reduced skin elasticity. This leads to higher pressures around the ischial tuberosities. Pressure-relieving cushions may help reduce the risk of pressure damage in these individuals. Wheelchair users in the United Kingdom with postural problems and who are at risk of pressure ulceration, are entitled to be assessed for and provided with a suitable cushion or seating system (Collins, 2004).

The wide range pressure-relieving cushions available reflects, in part, a degree of lack of evidence of efficacy (Bar and Pathy, 1998). However, studies have shown that cushions markedly reduce interface pressure, shear and friction forces (Palmieri *et al.*, 1984). In addition, cushions provide support and stability for the pelvis and enable the individuals to maintain their balance when reaching for things (Fletcher, 1995). Cushions should enhance the ability to transfer either independently or with assistance and should be comfortable (Bennett *et al.*, 1981). The cushion choice is dependent on the degree of pressure relief needed, lifestyle factors, postural stability, continence (bladder and/or bowel) and cost. The cushion should also be compatible with the chair or wheelchair (Garber *et al.*, 1996, 2000). When choosing an armchair, attention should be paid to the seat base, cushion, backrest (with or without recline) and armrests.

Table 6 Cushion characteristics

Cushion type	Suitability	Benefits/drawbacks
Static	Low- to high-risk individuals	• Supports ischial tuberosities • Thighs supported and isolated • Inexpensive, lightweight, many variations • Bottoms out with time • High interface pressures • Difficult to clean • Wears readily • Some flammable
Air filled Gel filled Fluid filled	Low- to high-risk individuals	• Pressure redistribution and reduction • Good stability • Absorbs dynamic movements • Good for wheelchairs • Air filled – lightweight and cleanable • Dependent on correct inflation • Liable to puncture • More difficult transfers • Fluid filled – heavy
Dynamic	High-risk individuals Individuals with pressure ulcers	• Pressure relieving • Increase sitting tolerance • Varying inflation • Mechanical breakdown • Leaks • Regular battery charging

Cushions, like mattresses and mattress overlays, may be classified as either static or dynamic (Figure 17). The static cushions are used mainly for pressure ulcer prevention, while dynamic cushions are used for individuals at elevated risk of pressure ulceration and those with established pressure ulcers. Table 6 illustrates the advantages and disadvantages of a range of cushions.

MANAGEMENT OF ESTABLISHED PRESSURE ULCERATION

The management of established pressure ulcers has much in common with their prevention. The aim of treatment of pressure ulceration is to provide adequate pressure relief and further protection of vulnerable areas, prevent progression, and facilitate rapid healing within a multidisciplinary, holistic approach to the individual. Apart from treating the pressure ulcer, attention should focus on treatment of any underlying diseases, especially those that may adversely affect wound healing and mobility. Review of medication should ensure that there is no inappropriate sedation (which could lead to immobility). Similar nutritional regimes should be instituted in patients with pressure ulcers as for those at risk of pressure ulceration.

Pressure Relief

The type of pressure relief for individuals with pressure ulcers is dependent on their needs. If the individual is

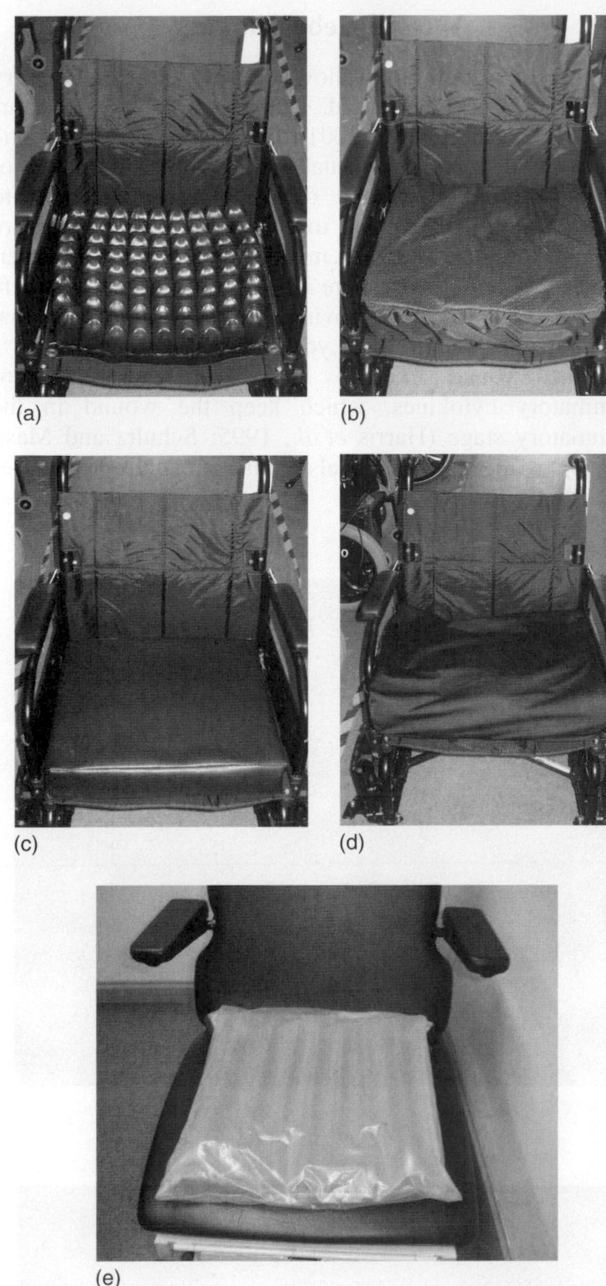

Figure 17 Pressure-relieving cushions

able to be nursed off the pressure ulcer, a static support surface accompanied by a regular turning schedule may be appropriate (Hanan and Scheele, 1991). Should it not be possible to nurse the patient off the ulcer and if the pressure ulcer demonstrates no evidence of healing or deteriorates on a static surface, a dynamic support system should be employed (Table 5).

Some studies in both long- and short-term care settings have demonstrated that dynamic mattresses promote healing of pressure ulcers compared to static foam mattresses, regardless of the size and depth of pressure ulcer (Allman *et al.*, 1987; Ferrell *et al.*, 1993). The major drawback of many dynamic mattresses is their expense, which is felt by some to be excessive compared to their benefits (Lubin and Powell, 1991; Kanj *et al.*, 1998).

Pressure Ulcer Classification

There are several classification schemes for established pressure ulceration. The European Pressure Ulcer Advisory Panel (EPUAP) has developed a simple to use, four-grade classification of pressure ulcers, reflecting increasing severity of pressure damage (Table 7, Figure 18). There is no "ideal" classification system; for example, grade 1 ulceration may go unnoticed in people with darkly pigmented skin. Clinicians should also beware the pressure ulcer covered with eschar: Such wounds cannot be accurately graded until the eschar has been removed. Undermining and sinuses commonly occur and affect grading as well as healing potential.

With moist wound healing techniques and optimal management of other medical conditions and nutrition, most grade 2 ulcers will heal after two weeks' treatment: Grades 3 and 4 ulcers take an average of 6 weeks to 3 months to heal (65% grade 2, 14% grade 3 and 0% grade 4 over a 6-week follow-up period) (Xakellis and Chrischilles, 1992; Xakellis and Frantz, 1996, Xakellis *et al.*, 1998). Generally, grades 1, 2, and 3 pressure ulcers are most amenable to local therapy, whereas grade 4 ulcers may require surgical repair (Kanj *et al.*, 1998). It has been suggested, however, that if there is not a 30% reduction in the area of a deep pressure ulcer after 2 weeks of treatment, the wound will be unlikely to heal in any reasonable period of time without reevaluation of treatment modalities (van Rijswijk, 1993).

Tools have been developed in an attempt to assess the healing of pressure ulcers. Two that have been evaluated include (1) the pressure sore status tool (PSST) (r 17 lyder) which is made up of 13 wound characteristics (e.g. edema, depth, size, exudate, etc.) and can be used to assess any chronic wound and (2) the pressure ulcer scale for healing (PUSH) tool (Stotts *et al.*, 2001) which is similar to the PSST, comprising only three wound characteristics (length and width of the ulcer, exudate amount, and tissue type); it also takes less time to complete than the PSST. These tools, however, are not widely used.

Photography of the pressure ulcer, made much easier with the advent of digital technology, is a key part of

Table 7 Pressure Ulcer Classification

Grade 1:	Nonblanchable erythema of intact skin. Discoloration of the skin, warmth, induration or hardness may also be used as indicators, particularly on individuals with darker skin
Grade 2:	Partial-thickness skin loss involving epidermis, dermis, or both. The ulcer is superficial and presents clinically as an abrasion or blister
Grade 3:	Full-thickness skin loss involving damage to or necrosis of subcutaneous tissue that may extend down to, but not through, underlying fascia
Grade 4:	Extensive destruction, tissue necrosis, or damage to muscle, bone or supporting structures with or without full thickness skin loss.

the assessment process. However, consistent methodology is essential. Documenting the distance from which the photo was taken is important in order to obtain an accurate representation of the actual size of the ulcer (Lyder, 2003). Patient identification, date, and location should be recorded on the photo.

Local Wound Management

A key measure in effective management of pressure ulcers is comprehensive evaluation of the wound and surrounding skin (Table 8). Other causes of skin ulceration should be excluded, including ischemia, vasculitis, radiation injury, and pyoderma gangrenosum: A detailed history and careful examination should help distinguish these.

Wound Debridement

Moist necrotic tissue is yellow or gray (Figure 19): dry necrotic tissue is thick, hard, leathery and black (eschar) (Maklebust and Sieggreen, 2001). In the presence of necrotic tissue, wound healing is usually impossible. Removal of necrotic tissue, eschar, and debris is essential, both to facilitate wound healing and to accurately stage a pressure ulcer. While the use of debridement is largely based on expert opinion (Vowden, 2004), there is evidence that debridement stimulates healing by removing the necrotic tissue that impedes healing (Brem and Lyder, 2004).

Chronic wound exudate has high levels of pro-inflammatory cytokines, which keep the wound in the inflammatory stage (Harris *et al.*, 1995; Schultz and Mast, 1998). There are also high levels of matrix metalloproteinases

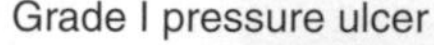

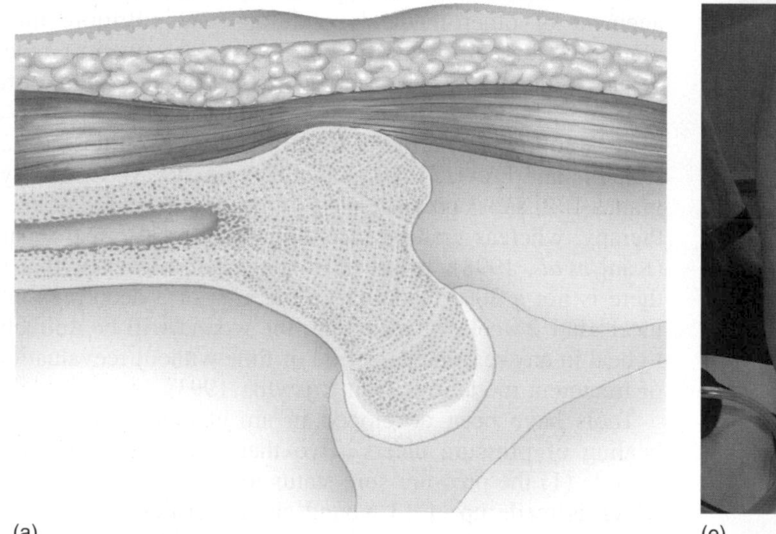
(a)

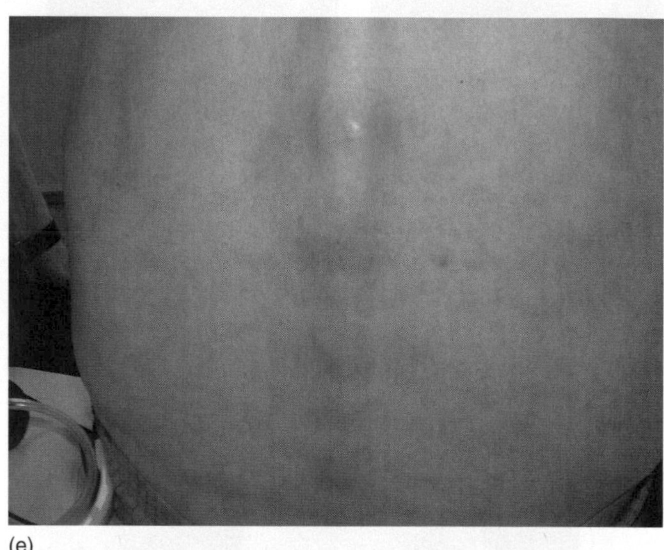
(e)

Grade II pressure ulcer

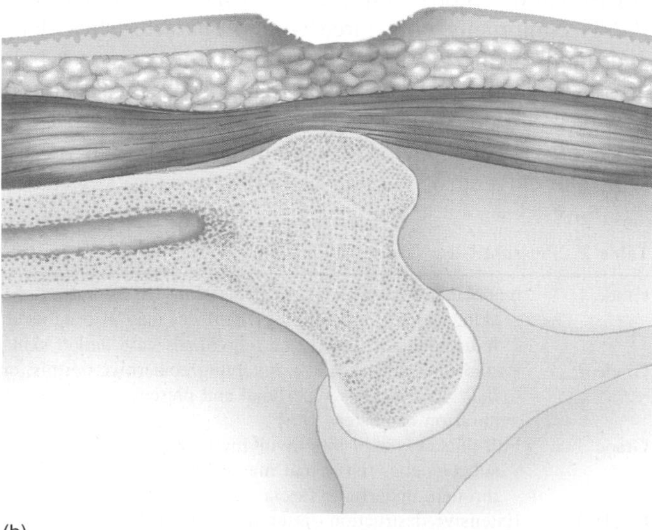
(b)

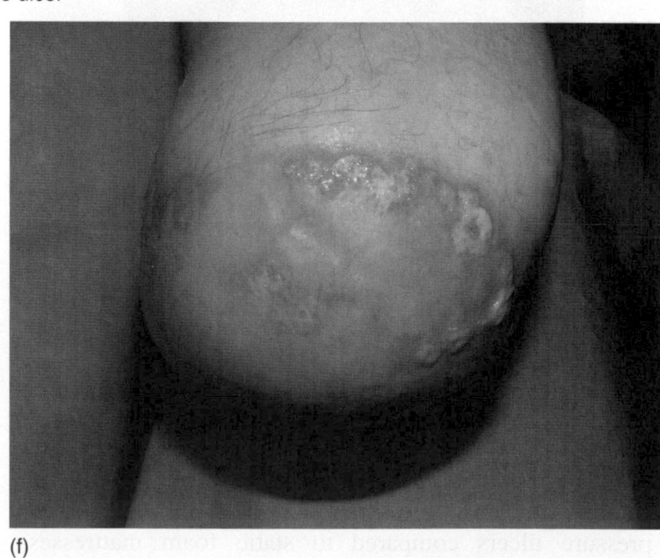
(f)

Figure 18 (a–h) Diagrammatic representations and pictures of the four grades of pressure ulcers

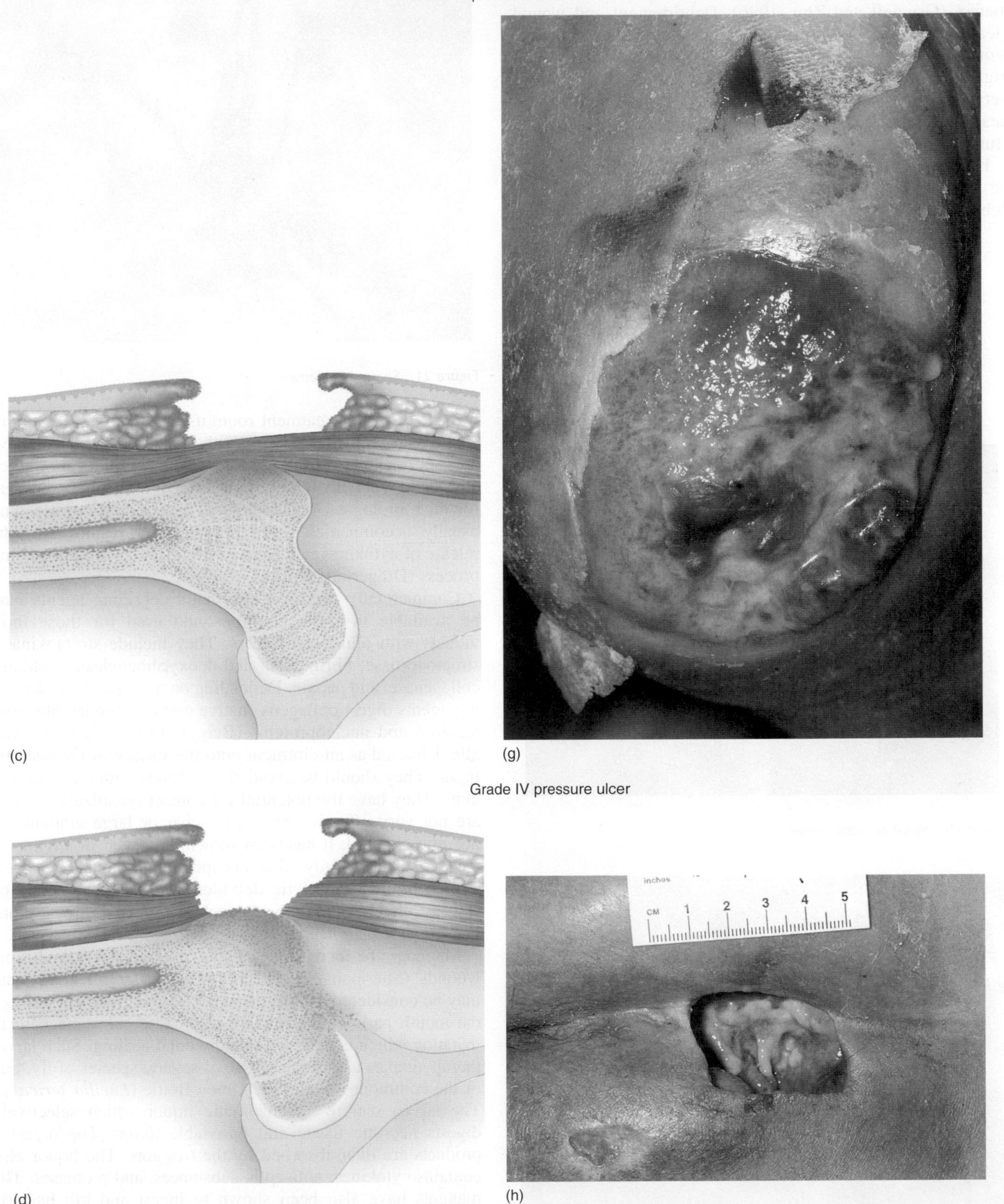

Figure 18 (*Continued*)

(MMPs), which destroy or alter the newly formed wound matrix (Grinnell and Zhu, 1996). Debridement and wound cleansing helps to remove the exudate and stimulate wound healing. Necrotic wounds are also associated with high levels of bacterial contamination. A direct correlation between high bacterial levels in wound tissues and delay in healing has been documented in pressure ulcers (Stotts and Hunt, 1997).

Eschar (Figure 20), devitalized and infected tissue may be removed by sharp, autolytic, enzymatic, or surgical debridement. Simple sharp debridement (Figure 21) at the bedside or in the treatment room using a scalpel, scissors or curette is useful when dealing with thick eschar and extensive areas of devitalized tissue. Prior treatment with local or block anesthetic may be required. Debrided tissue may be sent for microbiological or histological analysis. Minor bleeding usually accompanies sharp debridement, resulting in the release of cytokines, which may stimulate the wound healing process (Dräger and Winter, 1999).

Table 8 Wound characteristics

Size
Depth
Wound bed
Undermining
Amount and type of exudates
Surrounding skin

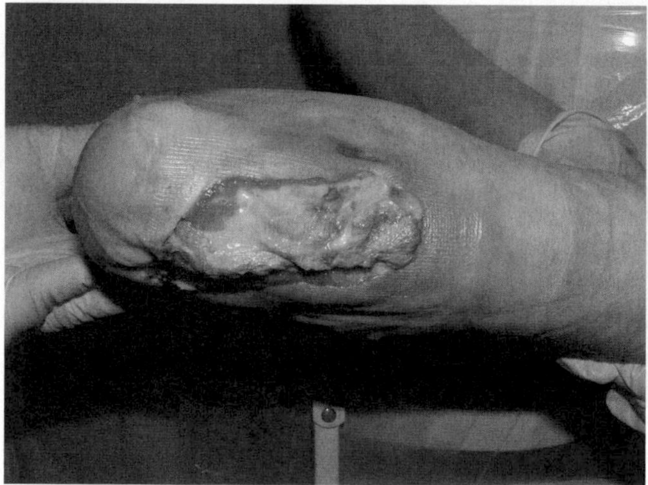

Figure 19 Moist necrotic tissue

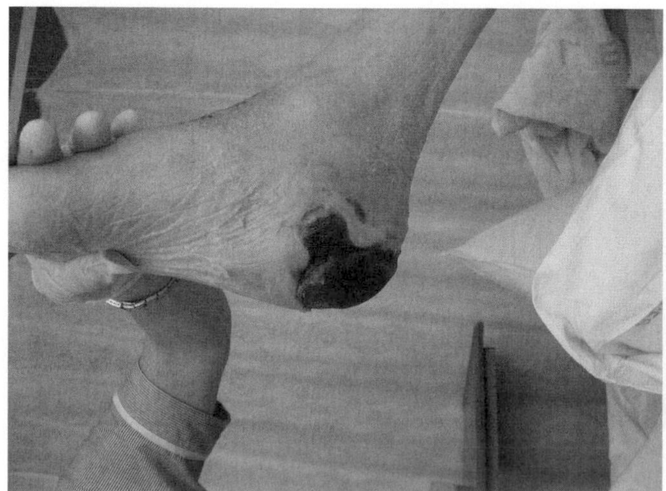

Figure 20 Wound covered with eschar

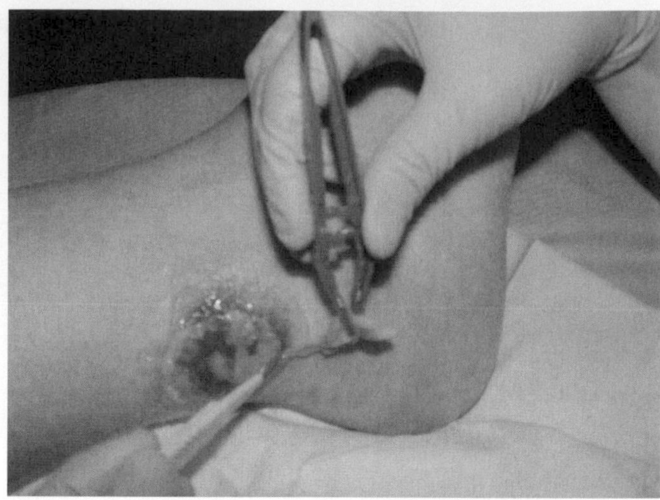

Figure 21 Sharp debridement

Commercially prepared enzymatic debriding agents may be available in some countries and used for those individuals with uninfected ulcers. They include streptokinase, streptodornase, fibrinolysin and deoxyribonuclease, sutilans, collagenase, and papain. Depending on the type, these debriding agents digest collagens (native and denatured), fibrinous material and nucleoproteins (Berger, 1993). They are usually delivered as an ointment onto the surface of the necrotic tissue. They should be avoided in wounds with exposed tendons. They have the potential for contact sensitization. They are not very effective on hard eschar or large amounts of necrotic material. It has been shown, however, in a randomized controlled study, that cheaper, amorphous Hydrogels (which promote autolytic debridement; see below) may be just as effective in debridement as enzyme preparations (Martin *et al.*, 1996).

Maggots are increasingly being used to debride chronic wounds (Sherman *et al.*, 2000; Thomas *et al.*, 1998) and may be considered a form of enzymatic debridement, though the mouth parts of the maggot also cause some mechanical irritation which is believed to aid wound healing. Such larval therapy makes use of the larvae of several species of fly, one of the commonest being the Green Bottle (*Lucilia sericata*). The larvae secrete an enzymatic liquor which selectively digests necrotic tissue and nonviable tissue: The digested products are then absorbed by the maggots. The liquor also contains cytokines, antiseptic substances, and proteases. The maggots have also been shown to ingest and kill bacteria (Fleischmann, 2004). Between 100 and 200 sterile maggots are used to debride wounds and are left in place for two to three days.

Mechanical debridement is still commonly used in some countries. The most common method is the wet to dry technique, usually using woven cotton gauze. This is soaked in saline and allowed to dry out and become adherent to the wound surface. However, this method can lead to damage of healthy viable tissue when the dressing is removed and should be avoided (Kanj *et al.*, 1998). Hydrotherapy and wound irrigation have been used to debride wounds, but evidence is limited (Palmier and Trial, 2004).

Autolytic debridement occurs in all wounds and is the body's own way of clearing necrotic tissue and debris from the area by the activity of the native enzymes within the ulcer (Thomas *et al.*, 1999). The process relies on leucocytic activity and endogenous proteolytic enzymes. Bacterial proteases also contribute to the process (Baharestani, 1999). The intrinsic process is slow and further delayed by aging, malnutrition, and chronic disease (Himel 1995).

Autolytic debridement may be promoted through the maintenance of a moist wound environment and is enhanced by the use of modern dressings, which are either moisture retentive or which hydrate the devitalized tissue. Frequent wound cleansing to eliminate the partially degraded tissue fragments is a necessary part of effective autolytic debridement. Several studies have shown that autolytic debridement is effective in digesting nonmobile tissue and more selective and less traumatic than mechanical techniques (Mulder *et al.*, 1993; Flanagan, 1995, Bale *et al.*, 1998, Colin *et al.*, 1996). Autolytic debridement is painless; easy to use; able to be combined with other forms of debridement; suitable for most wounds and patients; cost-effective; and widely available (Vowden, 2004; Mulder, 1995).

Wound Cleansing

This has been defined as "a process, which removes less adherent inflammatory molecules (such as cytokines and MMPs) from the wound surfaces and renders the wound less conducive to microbial growth" (Gardner and Frantz, 2004). The EPUAP in Europe and the American NPUAP have developed guidelines for cleansing pressure ulcers (Table 9).

Although not isotonic, and since contact with the wound is brief, tap water suitable for drinking may be used to cleanse pressure ulcers. While sterile saline (0.91% sodium chloride) is more commonly used, it is more expensive and some studies have shown that there is a lower wound infection rate in wounds irrigated with tap water compared with wounds irrigated with sterile saline (Angeras *et al.*, 1992).

Antiseptics have long been used in an attempt to kill bacteria within a wound. However, they are also toxic to nonbacterial cells found in the wound such as fibroblasts and macrophages. In addition, they may have limited effect on bacteria within wound tissue (Ayello, 2004). In general, antiseptics should not be routinely used and when they are, it should be for a limited period only. Systemic antibiotics should be used if the wound is infected.

Topical antimicrobial treatments demonstrated to enhance wound bed preparation without inhibiting the wound healing process include iodine-based dressings (e.g. Iodosorb) and noncrystalline silver-based dressings (for example, Acticoat (Smith and nephew); Actisorb 220 (Johnson and Johnson) and Aquacel Ag (Convatec)): the latter reported to minimize the potential of fungal infection (Johnson, 1991; Wright *et al.*, 1999; Thomas and McCubbin, 2003). Silver compounds may be of use to treat wounds that have developed a bio-film, which is produced by some bacteria (Ziegler *et al.*, 2004). Cadexomer iodine and silver compounds have been shown to reduce the bacterial burden.

Table 9 EPUAP and AHCPR guidelines for cleansing pressure ulcers (Bergstrom *et al.*, 1994; Fletcher, 2001)

European Pressure Ulcers Advisory Panel:

1. Cleanse wounds as necessary with tap water or with water, which is suitable for drinking, or with saline (strength of evidence = C).
2. Use minimal mechanical force when cleansing or irrigating the ulcer. Showering is appropriate. Irrigation can be useful for cleaning a cavity ulcer (C).
3. Antiseptics should not routinely be used to clean wounds but may be considered when bacterial load needs to be controlled after clinical assessment. Ideally, antiseptics should only be used for a limited period of time until the wound is clean and surrounding inflammation reduced (C).

Agency for Health Care Policy and Research (AHCPR):

1. Cleanse wounds initially and at each dressing change (strength of evidence = C).
2. Use minimal mechanical force when cleansing the ulcer with gauze, cloth or sponges (C).
3. Do not clean ulcer wounds with skin cleansers or antiseptic agents (e.g. povidone iodine, iodophor, sodium hypochlorite solution (Dakin's solution), hydrogen peroxide, acetic acid) (B).
4. Use normal saline for cleansing most pressure ulcers (C).

Wound irrigation is sometimes employed to help cleanse and debride a pressure ulcer. This ranges from use of saline filled syringes to pulsatile, battery-operated irrigation systems. The EPUAP and American Agency for Health Care Policy and Research, AHCPR (Bergstrom *et al.*, 1994; Fletcher, 2001), recommend 4–50 psi as safe and effective irrigation pressures (the health-care professional carrying out wound irrigation should ensure that they and the patient are protected from splashback and splatter).

Frequent showering with large amounts of water helps reduce the bacterial burden on the wound surface and provides psychological benefits to the patient (Bauer *et al.*, 2000). The shower should not be aimed directly at the wound, rather directed above it, so that the water irrigates the wound without too much force (Ayello, 2004).

Dressings

Dressings play a major role in the treatment of pressure ulcers. The occlusion that dressings provide promotes moist wound healing, facilitates re-epithelialization, reduces associated pain, enhances autolytic debridement and provides a barrier to bacteria (Leipziger *et al.*, 1985; Alvarez *et al.*, 1989; Friedman and Su, 1984, Mertz *et al.*, 1985). There are estimated to be more than 300 different dressings marketed for pressure ulcer care (Lyder, 2003). The major dressing classification and their uses are identified in Table 10.

Table 10 Dressings suitable for pressure ulcers

Dressing type	Pressure ulcer grade	Advantages/disadvantages
Semipermeable film	1 Minimally exuding 2	Promote moist environment Adheres to healthy skin but not to wound Allows visual checks May be left in place for several days No cushioning Not for infected or heavily exuding wounds
Foams	Low to moderately exuding, noninfected 2–3	Degree of cushioning May be left in place 2–3 days Needs secondary dressing
Hydrogels	Low to moderately exuding 2–4	Supplies moisture to low exuding wounds Useful for cavities and sinuses May be left in place for several days Needs secondary dressing May cause maceration
Hydrocolloids	Low to moderately exuding 3–4	Absorbable Conformable Good in "difficult areas" – heel, elbow, sacrum May be left in place for several days May cause maceration
Hydrofibres	Moderate to Highly exuding 2–4	Useful in cavities, sinuses, undermining wounds Highly absorbent Nonadherent May be left in place for several days Needs secondary dressing
Alginates	Moderate to Highly exuding 2–4	Useful in cavities, sinuses, undermining wounds Highly absorbent Needs secondary dressing Needs to be changed daily

Semipermeable (polyurethane) films are thin, transparent, nonabsorbent and coated on one side with hypoallergenic adhesive. They are suitable for grade 1 and minimally exuding grade 2 pressure ulcers. They are applied directly to the wound.

Hydrogels are insoluble polymers with hydrophilic sites containing more than 80% water and are available as an amorphous gel or translucent sheet. They are semitransparent and absorbent. They are nonadherent and dry out easily. They require a secondary dressing. They feel cool and soothing when applied to the wound. They are suitable for low to moderately exuding grades 2–4 ulcers. They are also suitable for wounds not spontaneously exuding, providing a moist environment.

Hydrocolloids are adherent, conformable, absorbent dressings: pastes and granules are also available and are especially suited to deeper wounds. Their conformability makes them suitable for use on "difficult" areas of the body including the sacrum, heels, and elbows. They can be left in place for several days. They are suitable for low to moderately exuding grades 3 and 4 ulcers. As they liquefy, Hydrocolloids form a yellowish gel-like material with a characteristic odor, which may, in the unwary, be mistaken for infection. They may stimulate excess granulation. They should be used with care if muscle, tendon, or bone is exposed. Hydrocolloids may be used on a range of wound beds, from ulcers that are infected to those that are epithelialising.

Alginates are polymers, which are derived from seaweed, either as calcium or sodium alginate. They are particularly useful in cavities, sinuses, and undermining grade 4 ulcers and moderately to highly exuding grades 2–4 ulcers. They are also suitable for sloughy and granulating wounds. They require a secondary dressing. They are hemostatic and useful for wounds that bleed.

Hydrofibre dressings are a form of hydrocolloid. They are highly absorbent and form a cohesive gel through interaction with wound exudates, thereby also maintaining a moist wound environment. They may be used on sloughy to granulating wounds. Hydrofibres are nonadherent and may be left in place for several days. They require a secondary dressing. They are used in similar situations as alginate dressings.

There are a plethora of other wounds dressings available. Their use should be guided by the characteristics of the wound, for example, site, size, depth, undermining, stage, drainage, surrounding skin involvement, wound infection, sinuses, underlying osteomyelitis, and so no. Dressing availability, cost, and ease of application may also need to be considered (Mulder and LaPan 1988; Eaglstein, 2001).

Infection

It is important to realize that all pressure ulcers will be colonized with bacteria. This does not, however, equate with infection. Wound cultures from pressure ulcer swabs are polymicrobial. Aerobic bacteria include, *Staphylococcus aureus*, *Staphylococcus epidermis*, β-hemolytic streptococcus Group A, *Escherichia coli*, *Pseudomonas aeruginosa*, *Proteus mirabilis*, *Providentia stuartii*, *Serratia marcescens*, *Enterococcus species*, *Enterobacter species*, and *Acenetobacter species* (Parish and Witkowski, 1989; Witkowski and Parish, 2000). Anaerobic organisms may also be present. Even when heavily colonized, most pressure ulcers eventually go on to heal (Mertz and Eaglestein, 1984; Dagher *et al.*, 1987; Hutchinson, 1989). Colonized wounds lack the signs of infection, which may include all or any of the features listed in Table 11.

Table 11 Signs of pressure ulcer infection

Warmth
Redness
Pain
Swelling
Odor
Increased wound exudate – serous, sero-sanguinous, purulent
Contact bleeding

When a pressure sore is infected, there is invasion of previously healthy tissue by microorganisms. A bacterial load of greater than 10^6 bacteria per gram of tissue has been found to impair wound healing (Sapico *et al.*, 1986; Parish and Witkowski, 1989; Witkowski and Parish, 2000). Infection is usually accompanied by at least some of the signs listed in Table 11. However, some of the signs may be attenuated or absent in patients with, for example, decreased sensation, abnormal neurological function or disturbed immunological response such as may occur in an elderly patient or patient with spinal cord injury. Cellulitis may complicate pressure ulcer infection as a result of spread of infection to surrounding tissue.

Bacteremia is a further serious complication of infected pressure ulcers. Bacteremia may lead to sepsis, endocarditis and death, with mortality rates between 50 and 70% (Sugarman *et al.*, 1982). Approximately one-quarter to one-third of nonhealing pressure ulcers are associated with underlying osteomyelitis arising through direct extension from an infected pressure ulcer or blood dissemination (Sugarman, 1987; Allman, 1989a,b).

Systemic treatment of an infected pressure ulcer and/or accompanying cellulitis, bacteremia, or osteomyelitis should be guided by culture and sensitivity of the organism(s). It may be prudent to start broad-spectrum antibiotic therapy while awaiting the results of tissue culture and sensitivity or blood cultures. However, swab results may not accurately reflect deep tissue cultures, which themselves may vary from one part of the ulcer to another (Kanj *et al.*, 1998). Curettage of the ulcer base following debridement is more reliable than swab samples (Sapico *et al.*, 1984; Lipsky *et al.*, 1990). Ulcer biopsy, if possible, will yield better tissue cultures (Daltrey *et al.*, 1981). Common pathogenic organisms include *S. aureus*, Bacteroides species, and gram-negative rods (Brown and Smith, 1999). A malodorous wound may be a sign of infection with anaerobes or *Bacteroides fragilis* (a facultative anaerobe). Gross tissue necrosis is usually caused by a combination of aerobic and anaerobic bacteria (Kanj *et al.*, 1998). Treatment should initially be with parenteral antibiotics.

Diagnosis of osteomyelitis and identification of the responsible pathogen is similarly fraught with difficulty. The traditional investigation of X-ray changes, elevated erythrocyte sedimentation rate and leucocytosis has a specificity of 33% and sensitivity of 60% (Darouiche *et al.*, 1994; Brown and Smith, 1999). More sensitive investigations include bone scans and MRI or CT scanning (Figure 22). Bone scans may be difficult to interpret, as the soft tissue inflammation from an infected wound is associated with a high false-positive rate. If the bone scan is abnormal, bone biopsy and culture may be necessary to determine infection and to identify the causative organism. A negative bone scan, however, makes osteomyelitis unlikely (Sugarman, 1987). MRI is now considered the investigation of choice for osteomyelitis (Sugarman, 1985). There is no consensus as to the duration of antibiotic treatment of osteomyelitis. Initial parenteral administration of antibiotics followed by oral antibiotics for a minimum of four to eight weeks is usual. Treatment may be monitored by measuring inflammatory markers such as ESR and CRP. Surgical debridement of the bone may be necessary.

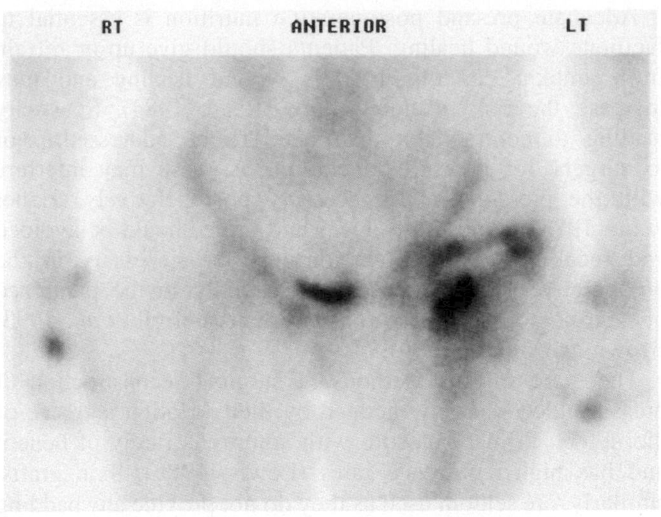

Figure 22 Bone scan of osteomyelitis underlying pressure ulcer of left hip

Sinus tracks may occur as a result of pressure ulceration. They occur in both superficial and deep ulcers and may extend to joint space and cause osteomyelitis. The sinuses may communicate with other structures including viscera (e.g. bowel and bladder). A sinogram or MRI may be necessary to delineate the extent and communication of these sinuses.

Other complications of pressure ulcers include squamous cell carcinoma (which may metastasize), with an estimated incident of 0.5%. Septic arthritis, amyloidosis, endocarditis, meningitis, and pseudoaneurysm formation may occur rarely.

Surgical Treatment of Pressure Ulcers

Surgical reconstruction may be appropriate treatment for some grade 3 and 4 pressure ulcers and may reduce healing times. An average healing time of 13 weeks has been demonstrated for grade 3 pressure ulcers if treated by skin grafting, and five weeks for those treated with musculocutaneous flaps (Brandeis *et al.*, 1990). It has been suggested that surgery is the preferred method of treatment when the rate of healing with conservative management is less than 40% (Siegler and Lavisso-Mourey, 1991).

Surgical treatment of pressure ulcers is usually reserved for those patients whose health outcomes and quality of life would significantly be improved by such intervention. There is, by extension, a definite place for palliative care for some patients with pressure ulcers whose medical and nutritional status is severely compromised, with control of symptoms rather than healing being the priority.

Successful reconstructive surgery is predicated on the optimization of the individual's medical and nutritional status. Surgery to close the defects is of long duration, with a potential for significant blood loss: postoperative immobilization is also protracted.

Adequate pre-and postoperative nutrition is essential to facilitate wound healing. Patients should give up or refrain from smoking as this hinders wound healing and may increase the risk of flap failure (Read, 1984). Spasticity leading to contractions may need to be addressed prior to surgery for pressure ulceration, as these may interfere with the pressure relief necessary postoperatively (Haher *et al.*, 1983). Exposure to feces and urine should be avoided and fecal or urinary diversion may be necessary in the preoperative planning process, especially in the paralyzed or neurologically compromised patient (Ferrell *et al.*, 1993; Brown and Smith, 1999).

There are various methods of surgical reconstruction of pressure ulcers largely dictated by their location and size of the defect. Primary closure with sutures is rarely of benefit and has high recurrence rates (Lewis, 1989). Skin grafts, similarly, are seldom used as they do not provide any padding and only provide a superficial barrier. Additionally, they exhibit "poor take" over exposed bone (Granick *et al.*, 1994).

Musculocutaneous and fasciocutaneous flaps are the most widely used method for reconstructing pressure ulcers. A fascial or muscular unit, the overlying skin and their blood supply, in a pedicle of tissue, is used to fill the defect made by the pressure ulcer (after debridement of devitalized tissue). Such flaps are, as a consequence of their preserved blood supply, able to withstand pressure and shear trauma. They are also particularly useful when treating pressure ulcers complicated by osteomyelitis by bringing highly vascularized muscle into the area of infection, which has been removed at the time of surgery (Daniel *et al.*, 1979; Mathes *et al.*, 1993; Bruck *et al.*, 1991; Anthony *et al.*, 1992).

Other flaps used include axial flaps – a vascularized segment of skin and subcutaneous tissue is raised and rotated into the defect; microvascular flaps – tissue with a single arteriovenous pedicle is raised, the vessels transected, and anastamosed to recipient vessels adjacent to the pressure ulcer defect; free flaps – muscle flaps where the original blood supply is disconnected and reconnected to vessels at the tissue defect site – rarely used, chiefly since less complicated options are usually available (Kostako-glu *et al.*, 1993).

Postoperatively, patients require immobilization, remaining in bed with vigilant pressure relief. A low air-loss mattress or an air-fluidized bed may be necessary. Immobilization for 2 to 4 weeks is usual. Flap viability must closely be monitored. Postoperative complications include hematoma (most common, therefore, meticulous intraoperative hemostasis is necessary), wound infection, flap necrosis, dehiscence, seroma, and infection.

Adjunctive Therapies

Adjunctive therapies are increasingly being employed in an attempt to heal pressure ulcers. Some of these are very effective and are becoming part of the armoury of standard treatment. Yet others are experimental or in the research stage.

VAC Therapy

Vacuum assisted closure (VAC) therapy is one of many synonyms in use for topical negative pressure therapy (TNP); though the term VAC is widely used in the United Kingdom (Figure 23). The technique has found an increasing role in the treatment of chronic wounds with large amounts of exudates, such as pressure ulcers (Philbeck *et al.*, 1999). The VAC dressing is open pored (polyurethane or polyvinyl chloride), shaped to fit the wound and sealed within it using a semiocclusive dressing. A negative pressure is delivered across the wound bed via a drainage tube embedded within the foam and connected to a negative pressure device (Banwell, 1999).

The negative pressure promotes granulation tissue formation (Morykwas *et al.*, 1997). This may be facilitated by reducing tissue edema directly, by removing fluid, or indirectly by eliminating factors that promote edema, thus preventing microvascular compromise (Morykwas *et al.*, 1997, 1999). Reduced edema may, however, reflect increase in local blood flow (Thomas and Banwell, 2004). Removal of fluid has also been postulated to remove factors inhibitory to wound healing (Banwell, 1999). Furthermore, TNP has been shown to reduce bacterial colonization of wounds both experimentally and clinically (Mullner *et al.*, 1997; Morykwas *et al.*, 1997; Obdeijn *et al.*, 1999; Giovanni *et al.*, 2001), which may further enhance wound healing.

Several studies have demonstrated the efficacy of VAC therapy in the treatment of pressure ulcers (Baynham *et al.*, 1999; Azad and Nishikawa, 2002; Coggrave *et al.*, 2002). Dressings may only need to be changed twice weekly, thus reducing patient discomfort and cost (Schneider *et al.*, 1998). The duration of VAC therapy depends on clinical improvement, patient compliance, and resources. VAC therapy has been advocated by some in the treatment of pressure ulcers complicated by underlying osteomyelitis (Ford *et al.*, 2002), while others feel that osteomyelitis is a contraindication to its use (Lyder, 2003); other relative contraindications

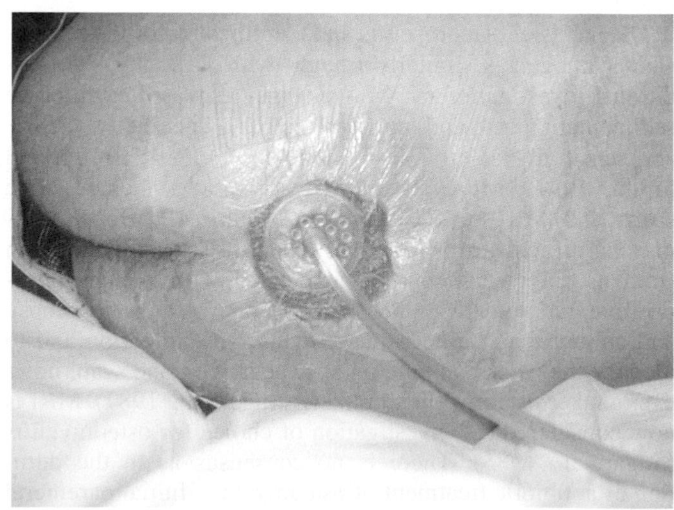

Figure 23 VAC therapy on sacral pressure ulcer

include application over an open joint; peritoneal or pleural space; in patients with a coagulopathy; over a tumor, though it may be considered as part of palliative wound control (Banwell, 1999).

Physical Modalities

Many physical therapies have been used to treat pressure ulcers. However, the therapeutic efficacy of hyperbaric oxygen, infrared, UV, low energy and laser irradiation, and ultrasonography has little evidence to support their use in the treatment of pressure ulceration (Bello and Phillips, 2000). Radiant heat (Normotherapy) is thought to increase blood flow and promote fibroblast and other factors associated with pressure ulcer healing (Xia *et al.*, 2000; Kloth *et al.*, 2000): Further evaluation with controlled trials is required.

Electrical stimulation has been recommended by the Agency for Health Care Research (USA) for stages 2 to 4 pressure ulcers which have not responded to conventional therapy (Ovington, 1999). The basis of the therapy is founded on the observation that when tissue is damaged, a current of injury is generated that may trigger biological repair (Weiss *et al.*, 1990). Electrical stimulation has been shown to enhance wound healing in human and animal models: This is thought to affect the migration, proliferation, and functional capacity of fibroblasts, neutrophils, and macrophages; promote collagen and DNA synthesis and increase the number of receptor sites for specific growth factors (Falanga *et al.*, 1997; Gentzkow *et al.*, 1993; Kloth and McCulloch, 1996; Baker *et al.*, 1996). However, it has been postulated that it is in fact the occlusive dressing used which may enhance wound healing by providing the moist environment necessary to maintain endogenous current flow (Jaffe and Vanable, 1984).

Larval Therapy

Sterile larvae (maggots, Figure 24) were first used as a treatment for infected or chronic wounds in the early twentieth century. Over recent years, there has been a resurgence of interest in their use for the debridement of a variety of infected or necrotic acute and chronic wounds including pressure ulcers. Two species of larvae are commonly used: *Lucilia species* and *Phaenicia species*.

While they often have a significant effect on sloughy and infected wounds, their exact mechanism of action is not fully understood. Maggots have been shown to ingest and kill some bacteria and studies have also shown that larval secretions kill or inhibit the growth of a number of bacterial species including *S. aureus* (including MRSA) and *Streptococcus*. Furthermore, the metabolic activity of the maggots increases wound pH, preventing the growth of such bacteria (Thomas and Jones, 1998).

The digestive juices of the larvae contain growth factors, antiseptic substances, and enzymes such as proteases (Fleischmann, 2004). Fibroblast growth stimulating factor has been demonstrated in the hemolymph and alimentary secretions of larvae (Prete, 1997). The presence of larvae or their metabolites may stimulate cytokine production by wound macrophages, thus stimulating the wound-healing process (Thomas and Jones, 1998). Larvae secrete powerful proteases, mainly of the serine class, which break down dead tissue, which is used for sustenance by the larvae (Young *et al.*, 1996).

Despite promising reports and widespread use, there are as yet, no large randomized, controlled trials to support the use of larvae in the treatment of pressure ulcers.

Growth Factors

Growth factors are secreted regulatory proteins that control survival, growth, differentiation, and effector function of tissue cells. They require a receptor, which may not be constitutive, to exert their effect. A large number of growth factors have been described and characterized. Since wound healing is an inflammatory process, much research has been carried out to determine whether they may be useful clinically in the treatment of chronic wounds including pressure ulcers. Initial promise, however, has not translated into clinical reality to any great extent.

Platelet-derived growth factor (PDGF) is one of the first growth factors released in acute wounds and as such has been investigated as a potential therapy to promote healing of chronic wounds. PDGF is a dimeric glycoprotein, released predominantly by platelet alpha granules. Topically applied recombinant PDGF-BB (rh PDGF-BB) has been shown in various small trials to produce a statistically significant reduction in pressure ulcer volume in the treatment group (Mustoe *et al.*, 1994). Other trials have shown an improvement in the rate of re-epithelialization of pressure ulcers with exogenously applied PDGF-BB (Robson, 1991; Cox, 1993). The trials highlighted the importance of simple good basic care in the treatment of pressure ulcers.

A further small, placebo controlled, double-blind study using recombinant basic fibroblast growth factor (rh b-FGF) in patients with chronic grades 3 and 4 pressure ulcers demonstrated no difference in the percentage volume reduction between different arms of the study. The volume reduction compared to baseline in the actively treated group was, however, significant (Robson *et al.*, 1992a,b).

Drawbacks of such trials are that they tend to be small and of short duration; large randomized, controlled trials are needed.

It is perhaps not surprising that growth factors have not proved the panacea in the healing of chronic wounds. Growth factors are present at different stages of healing and exert their effects depending on the wound microenvironment at a particular time and presence, or absence, of other growth factors. In addition, there is a balance between growth factors and enzymes responsible for their activation and degradation, which also vary at different stages in the wound healing cascade. Ideally, a diagnostic test to ascertain which of the wounds are deficient in specific growth factors is needed:

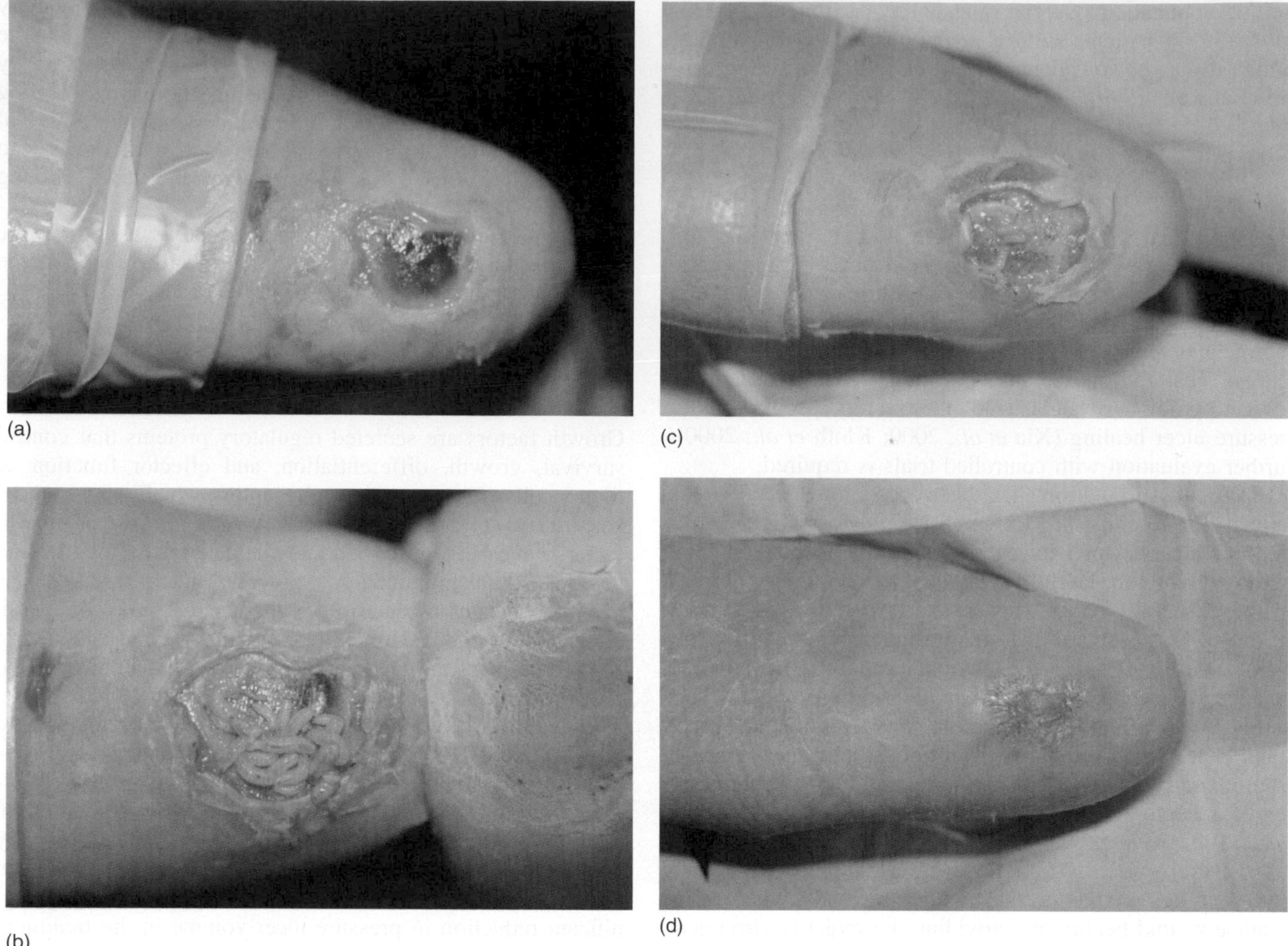

Figure 24 Debridement of heel pressure ulcer with Larval therapy (a) Pre-treatment, (b) 3 days post larval therapy, (c) 7 days post larval therapy, (d) Healed pressure ulcer (Pictures courtesy of Dr S Thomas, Zoobiotic Ltd.)

Then, perhaps, the promise of exogenously applied growth factors will be fulfilled.

Tissue Engineering

Tissue engineered "skin equivalents" have been developed to treat both acute and chronic wounds: They are formed by growing allogeneic cells in a synthetic matrix *in vitro*. The "skin equivalents" may be categorized as (1) those containing epidermal elements alone; (2) those comprising dermal elements, and (3) composite grafts containing both epidermal and dermal elements (Phillips, 1998). Most of the allogeneic cells are derived from neonatal foreskins and are seeded into a variety of collagen gels or bioabsorbable meshes. Much work has been carried out into their use on chronic wounds such as venous leg ulcers and diabetic foot ulcers with good effect. There have been some promising small trials using "skin equivalents" to treat pressure ulcers, but no large trials have been undertaken. It is an area that merits further study.

Other Therapies

Many other therapies for the treatment of pressure ulcers have been investigated. Topical agents include honey, sugar, vitamins, zinc, magnesium, gold, phenytoin, yeast extract, insulin, and aloe vera gel. Light therapy and ultrasound have also been tried (Kanj *et al.*, 1998). All require further evaluation and large-scale trials to establish their efficacy.

KEY POINTS

- Pressure ulcers are common, especially in the elderly patient.

- Pressure ulcers are caused by direct pressure, friction and shear forces, individually or often acting in concert with each other: Moisture exacerbates the effects of pressure, friction and shear.
- At-risk individuals should have regular risk assessments: Risk assessment scales are not a substitute for clinical judgment.
- The effects of risk factors should be minimized through optimal management.
- Adequate pressure relief is essential in the prevention and treatment of pressure ulcers.
- Accurate pressure ulcer grading assists in the choice of treatment, dressings, and adjunctive therapies.

KEY REFERENCES

- European Pressure Ulcer Advisory Panel (EPUAP). *Pressure Ulcer Prevention and Treatment Guidelines*, www.epuap.org.
- National Institute for Clinical Excellence. *Pressure Ulcer Risk Management and Prevention (Guideline B)* 2003; NICE, London, www.nice.org.uk.
- National Pressure Ulcer Advisory Panel (NPUAP, USA). *Pressure Ulcer Prevention and Treatment Guidelines*, www.npuap.org.

REFERENCES

Allman RM. Pressure ulcers among the elderly. *The New England Journal of Medicine* 1989a; **320**:850–3.

Allman RM. Epidemiology of pressure sore in different populations. *Decubitus* 1989b; **2**:30–3.

Allman RM, Goode PS, Patrick MM *et al.* Pressure ulcer risk factors among hospitalized patients with activity limitation. *The Journal of the American Medical* 1995; **273**(11):865–70.

Allman RM, Laprade CA, Noel LB *et al.* Pressure sores among hospitalized patients. *Annals of Internal Medicine* 1986; **105**(3):337–42.

Allman RM, Walker JM, Hart MK *et al.* Air-fluidized beds or conventional therapy for pressure sores. A randomized trial. *Annals of Internal Medicine* 1987; **107**:641–8.

Alvarez O, Rozint J & Wiseman D. Moist environment for healing; matching the dressing to wounds. *Wounds* 1989; **1**:35–51.

Anderson KE, Jensen O, Kvorning SA *et al.* Decubitus prophylaxis: a prospective trial of the efficiency of alternating pressure air mattresses and water mattresses. *Acta Dermato-venereologica. Supplementum (Stockh)* 1983; **63**:227–30.

Angeras MH, Brandberg A, Falk A & Seeman T. Comparison between sterile saline and tap water for the cleaning of acute traumatic soft tissue wounds. *The European Journal of Surgery* 1992; **158**:347–50.

Anthony JP, Huntsman WT & Mathes SJ. Changing trends in the management of pelvic pressure on ulcers: a 12 year review. *Decubitus* 1992; **5**:44–7, 50–1.

Ayello E. Teaching the assessment of patients with pressure ulcers. *Decubitus* 1992; **5**(7):53–4.

Ayello EA. Cleansing and cleaners. In L Teot, PE Banwell & UE Ziegler (eds) *Surgery in Wounds* 2004; Springer, Berlin.

Azad S & Nishikawa H. Topical negative pressure may help chronic wound healing. *British Medical Journal* 2002; **324**:1100.

Bader DL & Gant CA. Changes in transcutaneous oxygen tension as a result of prolonged pressures at the sacrum. *Clinical Physics and Physiological Measurement* 1988; **9**:33–40.

Baharestani M. The clinical relevance of debridement. In Baharestani M, Goltrup F, Holstein P *et al.* (eds) *The Clinical Relevance of Debridement* 1999; Springer, Berlin.

Baker L, Rubayi S, Villar F & DeMuth SK. Effects of electric stimulation wave form on healing of ulcers in human beings with spinal cord injury. *Wound Repair and Regeneration* 1996; **4**:21–8.

Bale S, Banks V, Haglestein S & Harding KG. A comparison of two amorphous hydrogels in the debridement of pressure sores. *Journal of Wound Care* 1998; **7**:65–8.

Banwell PE. Topical negative pressure therapy in wound care. *Journal of Wound Care* 1999; **8**:79–84.

Bar CA & Pathy MSJ. Pressure ulcers. In MSJ Pathy (ed) *Principles and Practice of Geriatric Medicine* 1998, 3rd edn; Wiley, London.

Barbenel JC, Ferguson-Pell MW & Kennedy R. Mobility of elderly patients in bed. Measurement and association with patient condition. *Journal of the American Geriatrics Society* 1986; **34**(9):633–6.

Barbenel JC, Jordan MM, Nicol SM & Clark MO. Incidence of pressure sores in the greater glasgow health board area. *Lancet* 1977; **2**:548–50.

Bauer C, Geriach MA & Doughty D. Care of metastatic skin lesions. *Journal of Wound, Ostomy, and Continence Nursing* 2000; **27**:247–51.

Baynham SA, Kohlman P & Katmer HP. Treating stage IV pressure ulcers with negative pressure therapy: a case report. *Ostomy/Wound Management* 1999; **45**:28–32, 34–35.

Bello YM & Phillips TJ. Recent advances in wound healing. *The Journal of the American Medical* 2000; **283**:716–8.

Bennett G, Dealey C & Posnett J. The cost of pressure ulcers in the U.K. *Age and Ageing* 2004; **33**:230–5.

Bennett L, Kavner D, Lee BY *et al.* Skin blood flow in seated geriatric patients. *Archives of Physical Medicine and Rehabilitation* 1981; **62**(8):392–8.

Berger MM. Enzymatic debriding preparations. *Ostomy/Wound Management* 1993; **39**:61–9.

Berlowitz DR & Wilking SV. Risk factors for pressure sores. A comparison of cross-sectional and cohort-derived data. *Journal of the American Geriatrics Society* 1989; **37**(11):1043–50.

Bliss M. Aetiology of pressure sores. *Clinical Gerontologist* 1993; **3**:379–97.

Bourdel-Marchasson I, Barateau M, Rondeau V *et al.* A multi-center trial of the effects of oral nutritional supplementation in critically ill older inpatients. GAGE Group. Groupe Aquitain Geriatrique d'Evaluation. *Nutrition* 2000; **16**(1):1–5.

Brandeis GH, Morris JN, Nash DJ & Lipsitz LA. The epidemiology and natural history of pressure ulcers in elderly nursing home residents. *The Journal of the American Medical* 1990; **264**:2905–9.

Brem H & Lyder RN. Protocol for the successful treatment of pressure ulcers. *American Journal of Surgery* 2004; **188**:9S–17S.

Bergstrom N, Bennett MA, Carlson CE *et al. Clinical Practice Guideline Number 15; Treatment of Pressure Ulcers* 1994; AHCPR publication 95–0652, US department of health and human services. Public health service, agency for health care policy and research, Rockville.

Breslow RA, Hallfrisch J, Guy DG *et al.* The importance of dietary protein in healing pressure ulcers. *Journal of the American Geriatrics Society* 1993; **41**(4):357–62.

Brown DL & Smith DJ. Bacterial colonization/infection and the surgical management of pressure ulcers. *Ostomy/Wound Management* 1999; **45**(suppl 1A):109S–18S.

Bruck JC, Butlemyer R, Grabosch A & Gruhl L. More arguments in favour of myocutaneous flaps for the treatment of pressure sores. *Annals of Plastic Surgery* 1991; **26**:85–8.

Carter DM & Balin AK. Dermatological aspects of aging. *The Medical Clinics of North America* 1983; **67**:531–43.

Chernoff RS, Milton KY & Lipschitz DA. The effect of a very high protein liquid formula on decubitus ulcer healing in long-term tube-fed institutionalised patients. *Journal of the American Dietetic Association* 1990; **90**:A130–9.

Clark M & Watts S. The incidence of pressure sores within a national health service trust hospital during 1991. *Journal of Advanced Nursing* 1994; **20**:33–6.

Coggrave M, West H & Leonard B. Topical negative pressure for pressure ulcer management. *British Journal of Nursing* 2002; **11**:S29–36.

Colin D, Kurring PA & Yvon C. Managing sloughy pressure sores. *Journal of Wound Care* 1996; **5**:444–6.

Collier M. Pressure reducing mattresses. *Journal of Wound Care* 1996; **5**:207–11.

Collier M. Effective prevention requires accurate risk assessment. *Journal of Wound Care/Therapy Weekly* 2004; **13**:3–7.

Collins F. A guide to the selection of specialist beds and mattresses. *Journal of Wound Care/Therapy Weekly* 2004; **13**:14–8.

Cox DA. Growth factors in wound healing. *Journal of Wound Care* 1993; **6**:339–42.

Cruse JM, Lewis RE, Roe DL *et al.* Facilitation of immune function, healing of pressure ulcers, and nutritional status in spinal cord injury patients. *Experimental and Molecular Pathology* 2000; **68**(1):38–54.

Dagher FJ, Algoni SV & Smith A. Bacterial studies of leg ulcers. *Angiology* 1987; **29**:641–53.

Daltrey DC, Rhodes B & Chattwood JG. Investigation into the microbial flora of healing and non-healing decubitus ulcers. *Journal of Clinical Pathology* 1981; **34**:701–5.

Daniel RK, Hall EJ & Macleod MK. Pressure sores: a reappraisal. *Annals of Plastic Surgery* 1979; **3**:53–63.

Darouiche RO, Landon GC, Klima M *et al.* Osteomyelitis associated with pressure sores. *Archives of Internal Medicine* 1994; **154**:753–8.

DeLisa JA & Mikulic MA. Pressure ulcers. What to do if preventive management fails. *Postgraduate Medicine* 1985; **77**(6):209–12, 218–20.

Dräger E & Winter H. Surgical debridement versus enzymatic debridement – benefits and drawbacks. In Baharestani M, Goltrup F, Holstein P *et al.* (eds) *The Clinical Relevance of Debridement* 1999; Springer, Berlin.

Eaglstein WH. Moist wound healing with occlusive dressings: a clinical focus. *Dermatologic Surgery* 2001; **27**:175–81.

Ek AC & Bowman GA. A descriptive study of pressure sores: the prevalence of pressure sores and the characteristics of patients. *Journal of Advanced Nursing* 1982; **7**:51–7.

Ek AC, Gustavsson G & Lewis DH. The local skin blood flow in areas at risk for pressure sores treated with massage. *Scandinavian Journal of Rehabilitation Medicine* 1985; **17**(2):81–6.

Ek AC, Gustavsson G & Lewis DH. Skin blood flow in relation to external pressure and temperature in the supine position on a standard hospital mattress. *Scandinavian Journal of Rehabilitation Medicine* 1987; **19**(3):121–6.

Exton-Smith AN & Sherwin RW. The prevention of pressure sores. Significance of spontaneous bodily movements. *Lancet* 1961; **2**:1124–6.

Falanga V, Bourguignon GL & Bourguignon LY. Electrical stimulation increases the expression of fibroblast receptors for transforming growth factor-beta. *The Journal of Investigative Dermatology* 1997; **88**:488–A.

Ferrell BA, Osterweil D & Christenson P. A randomized trial of low-air-loss beds for treatment of pressure ulcers. *The Journal of the American Medical* 1993; **269**:494–7.

Flanagan M. The efficacy of a hydrogel in the treatment of wounds with non-viable tissue. *Journal of Wound Care* 1995; **4**:264–7.

Fleischmann W. Maggot debridement. In L Teot, PE Banwell & UE Ziegler (eds) *Surgery in Wounds* 2004; Springer, Berlin.

Fletcher J. Selecting pressure relieving equipment. *Journal of Wound Care* 1995; **4**:254.

Fletcher J. Updating the EPUAP pressure ulcer prevention and treatment guideline. *European Pressure Ulcer Advisory Panel Review* 2001; **3**:78–82.

Ford CN, Reinhard ER & Yeh D. Interim analysis of a prospective, randomized trial of vacuum-assisted closure versus the healthpoint system in the management of pressure ulcers. *Annals of Plastic Surgery* 2002; **49**:55–61.

Friedman SJ & Su WP. Management of leg ulcers with hydrocolloid occlusive dressing. *Archives of Dermatology* 1984; **120**:1329–36.

Garber SL, Rintala DH, Hart KA & Fuhrer MJ. Pressure ulcer risk in spinal cord injury: predictors of ulcer status over 3 years. *Archives of Physical Medicine and Rehabilitation* 2000; **81**:465–71.

Garber SL, Rintala DH, Rossi CD *et al.* Reported pressure ulcer prevention and management techniques by persons with spinal cord injury. *Archives of Physical Medicine and Rehabilitation* 1996; **77**:744–9.

Gardner SE & Frantz RA. Wound bioburden. In S Baranoski & EA Ayello (eds) *Wound Care Essentials: Practice Principles* 2004, pp 91–116; Lippinkott Williams & Wilkins, Springhouse.

Gebhardt KS & Bliss MR. Preventing pressure ulcers in orthopaedic patients – s prolonged chair nursing detrimental? *Journal of Tissue Viability* 1994; **4**:51–4.

Gentzkow GD, Alon G, Taler GA *et al.* Healing of refractory stage III and IV pressure ulcers by a new electrical stimulation device. *Wounds* 1993; **5**:160–72.

Giovanni UM, Demaria R & Teot L. Benefits of negative pressure therapy in infected surgical wounds after cardiovascular surgery. *Wounds* 2001; **132**:82–7.

Granick MS, Eisner AN & Solomon MK. Surgical management of decubitus ulcers. *Clinics in Dermatology* 1994; **12**:71–9.

Grinnell F & Zhu M. Fibronectin degradation in chronic wounds depends on the relative levels of elastase, alpha1-proteinase inhibitor, and alpha2-macroglobulin. *The Journal of Investigative Dermatology* 1996; **106**:335–41.

Haher JN, Haher TR, Devlin VJ *et al.* The release of flexure contractures as a prerequisite for the treatment of pressure sores in multiple sclerosis: a report of 10 cases. *Annals of Plastic Surgery* 1983; **11**:246–9.

Hall DA. *The Biomedical Basis of Gerontology* 1984; John Wright, Guildford.

Hanan K & Scheele L. Albumin vs. weight as a predictor of nutritional status and pressure ulcer development. *Ostomy/Wound Management* 1991; **33**:22–7.

Harris IR, Yee KC, Walters CE *et al.* Cytokine and protease levels in healing and non-healing chronic venous leg ulcers. *Experimental Dermatology* 1995; **4**:342–9.

Hatcliffe S & Dawe R. Monitoring pressure sores in a palliative care setting. *International Journal of Palliative Nursing* 1996; **2**:182–6.

Healey F. Classification of pressure sores: 2. *British Journal of Nursing* 1996; **5**(9):567–8, 570, 572–4.

Herman LE & Rothman KF. Prevention, care and treatment of pressure (decubitus) ulcers in intensive care unit patients. *Journal of Intensive Care Medicine* 1989; **4**:117–23.

Himel H. Wound healing: focus on the chronic wound. *Wounds* 1995; **7**:70A–7A.

Houle RJ. Evaluation of seat devices designed to prevent ischaemic ulcers in paraplegic patients. *Archives of Physical Medicine and Rehabilitation* 1969; **50**:587–94.

Hutchinson JJ. Prevalence of wound infection and occlusive dressings; a collective survey of reported research. *Wounds* 1989; **1**:124–33.

Jaffe LF & Vanable JW Jr. Electric fields and wound healing. *Clinics in Dermatology* 1984; **2**:34–44.

Johnson A. A combative healer with no ill-effect. Iodosorb in the treatment of infected wounds. *Professional Nurse* 1991; **7**:60, 62, 64.

Kanj LF, Wilking SV & Phillips TJ. Pressure ulcers. *Journal of the American Academy of Dermatology* 1998; **38**:517–36.

Kloth LC, Berman JE, Dumit-Minkel S *et al.* Effects of a normal normothermic dressing on pressure ulcer healing. *Advances in Skin and Wound Care* 2000; **13**:69–74.

Kloth LC & McCulloch JM. Promotion of wound healing with electrical stimulation. *Advances in Wound Care* 1996; **9**:42–5.

Knox DM, Anderson TM & Anderson PS. Effects of different turn intervals on skin of healthy older adults. *Advances in Wound Care* 1994; **7**(1):48–52, 54–6.

Kostako-glu N, Keocik A, Ozymilaz F & Safak T. Expansion of fascial flaps: histopathologic changes and clinical benefits. *Plastic and Reconstructive Surgery* 1993; **91**:72–9.

Landis T. Micro-injection studies of blood pressure in human skin. *Heart* 1930; **15**:209–28.

Lazarus GS, Cooper DM, Knighton DR *et al.* Definitions and guidelines for assessment of wounds and evaluation of healing. *Archives of Dermatology* 1994; **130**:489–93.

Leipziger LS, Glushko V, DiBernardo B *et al.* Dermal wound repair: role of collagen matrix implants and synthetic polymer dressings. *Journal of the American Academy of Dermatology* 1985; **12**:409–19.

Lewis VL Jr. Tensor fasciae latae VY retroposition flap. *Plastic and Reconstructive Surgery* 1989; **84**:1016–7.

Lindan O. Etiology of decubitus ulcers; an experimental study. *Archives of Physical Medicine and Rehabilitation* 1961; **42**:774–83.

Lipsky BA, Percoraro RE & Wheat LS. The diabetic foot: soft tissue and bone infection. *Infectious Disease Clinics of North America* 1990; **4**:409–39.

Lubin BS & Powell T. Pressure sores and specialty beds: cost containment and ensurance of quality care. *Journal of ET Nursing* 1991; **18**:190–7.

Lyder CH. Pressure ulcer prevention and management. *The Journal of the American Medical* 2003; **289**:223–6.

Lyder CH, Shannon R, Empleo-Frazier O *et al.* A comprehensive program to prevent pressure ulcers in long-term care: exploring costs and outcomes. *Ostomy/Wound Management* 2002; **48**:52–62.

Maklebust J, Sieggreen M. *Pressure Ulcer: Guidelines for Prevention and Management* 2001, 3rd edn, Springhouse.

Martin SJ, Corrado OJ & Kay EA. Enzymatic debridement for necrotic wounds. *Journal of Wound Care* 1996; **5**:310–1.

Mathes SJ, Feng LJ & Hunk TK. Coverage of the infected wound. *Annals of Surgery* 1993; **198**:420–9.

Mathus-Vliegen EM. Old age, malnutrition, and pressure sores: an ill-fated alliance. *The Journals of Gerontology. Series A, Biological Sciences and Medical Sciences* 2004; **59**(4):355–60.

Medical Devices Agency. *Static Mattress Overlays: Evaluation P52* 1994; DoH.

Mertz PM & Eaglestein WH. The effect of semi-occlusive dressing on the microbial population in superficial wounds. *Archives of Surgery* 1984; **119**:287–9.

Mertz PM, Marshall DA & Eaglestein WH. Occlusive wound dressings to prevent bacterial invasion and wound infection. *Journal of the American Academy of Dermatology* 1985; **12**:662–8.

Morykwas MJ, Argenta LC, Shelton–rown EI & McGuirt W. Vacuum–assisted closure: a new method for wound control and treatment: animal studies and basic foundation. *Annals of Plastic Surgery* 1997; **38**:553–62.

Morykwas MJ, David LR, Schneider AM *et al.* Use of sub-atmospheric pressure to prevent progression of partial–thickness burns in a swine model. *The Journal of Burn Care and Rehabilitation* 1999; **201**:15–21.

Mulder GD. Cost-effective managed care: gel versus wet-to-dry for debridement. *Ostomy/Wound Management* 1995; **41**:68 70, 72, 74 passim.

Mulder GD & LaPan M. Decubitus ulcers: update on new approaches to treatment. *Geriatrics* 1988; **43**:37–9, 44–5, 49–50.

Mulder GD, Romanko KP, Sealey J & Andrews K. Controlled randomised study of a hypertonic gel for the debridement of dry eschar in chronic wounds. *Wounds* 1993; **5**:112–5.

Mullner T, Mrkonjic L, Kwasny O & Vecsei V. The use of negative pressure to promote the healing of tissue defects: a clinical trial using the vacuum sealing technique. *British Journal of Plastic Surgery* 1997; **50**:194–9.

Mustoe TA, Cutler NR, Allman RM *et al.* A phase II study to evaluate recombinant platelet-derived growth factor-BB in the treatment of stage 3 and 4 pressure ulcers. *Archives of Surgery* 1994; **129**:213–9.

National Institute for Clinical Excellence. *Pressure Ulcer Risk Management and Prevention (Guideline B)* 2003; NICE, London, www.nice.org.uk.

Nyquist R & Hawthorn PJ. The prevalence of pressure sores within an area health authority. *Journal of Advanced Nursing* 1987; **12**(2):183–7.

Obdeijn MC, de-Lange MY, Lichtendahl DH & de Boer WJ. Vacuum-assisted closure in the treatment of poststernotomy mediastinitis post op. *The Annals of Thoracic Surgery* 1999; **686**:2358–60.

Ovington LG. Dressings and adjunctive therapies: AHCPR guidelines revisited. *Ostomy/Wound Manage* 1999; **45**(suppl 1A):94–106.

Palmier S & Trial C. Uses of high-pressure water jets in wound debridement. In L Teot, PE Banwell & UE Ziegler (eds) *Surgery in Wounds* 2004; Springer, Berlin.

Palmieri l, Haelen T & Cochran GVB. A comparison of sitting pressures on wheelchair cushions measured by air cell transducers and miniature electronic transducers. *Bulletin of Prosthetics Research* 1984; **17**:5–8.

Parish LC & Witkowski JA. The infected decubitus ulcer. *International Journal of Dermatology* 1989; **28**:643–7.

Philbeck TE Jr, Whittington KT, Millsap MH *et al.* The clinical and cost – effectiveness of externally applied negative pressure wound therapy in the treatment of wounds in home health care medicare patients. *Ostomy/Wound Manage* 1999; **45**:41–50.

Phillips TJ. New skin for old. Developments in biological skin substitutes. *Archives of Dermatology* 1998; **134**:344–9.

Phillips L. Providing correct pressure-relieving devices for optimum outcome. *British Journal of Nursing* 1999; **8**(21):1447–52.

Pinchcofsky-Devin GD & Kaminski MV Jr. Correlation of pressure sores and nutritional status. *Journal of the American Geriatrics Society* 1986; **34**(6):435–40.

Prete P. Growth effects of *Phaenicia sericata* larval extracts on fibroblasts: mechanism for wound healing by maggot therapy. *Life Sciences* 1997; **60**:505–10.

Price P, Bale S, Newcombe R & Harding K. Challenging the pressure sore paradigm. *Journal of Wound Care* 1999; **8**(4):187–90.

Read RC. Presidential address: systemic effects on smoking. *American Journal of Surgery* 1984; **148**:706–11.

Rithalia SV. Evaluation of alternating pressure air mattresses: one laboratory-based strategy. *Journal of Tissue Viability* 2004a; **14**(2):51–8.

Rithalia SV. Evaluation of alternating-pressure air mattresses: How to do it. In M Clark (ed) *Pressure Ulcers: Recent Advances in Tissue Viability* 2004b; Quay books, Salisbury.

Robson MC. Growth factors and wound healing: part 2. Role in normal and chronic would healing. *American Journal of Surgery* 1991; **166**:74–81.

Robson MC, Phillips LG, Lawrence WT *et al.* The safety and effect of topically applied recombinant basic fibroblast growth factor on healing of chronic pressure sores. *Annals of Surgery* 1992a; **216**:401–6.

Robson MC, Phillips LG, Thomason A *et al.* Platelet-derived growth factor BB for the treatment of chronic pressure ulcers. *Lancet* 1992b; **339**:23–5.

Russ GH & Motta GJ. Eliminating pressure: is less than 32 mmHg enough for wound healing? *Ostomy/Wound Management* 1991; **34**:60–3.

Rycroft-Malone J & Duff L. Pressure ulcer guidelines. *Nursing Standard* 2000; **14**(40):31.

Sapico FL, Ginunas VJ, Thornhill–Joynes M *et al.* Quantitative microbiology of pressure sores in different stages of healing. *Diagnostic Microbiology and Infectious Disease* 1986; **5**:31–8.

Sapico FL, Witter JL, Canawati HN *et al.* The infected foot of the diabetic patient: quantitative microbiology and analysis of clinical features. *Reviews of Infectious Diseases* 1984; **6**:S171–S6.

Schneider AM, Morykwas MJ & Argenta LC. A new and reliable method of securing skin graph to the difficult recipient bed. *Plastic and Reconstructive Surgery* 1998; **1024**:1195–8.

Schubert V & Héraudj J. The effects or pressure and shear on skin micro-circulation in elderly stroke patients lying in supine or semi-recumbent positions. *Age and Ageing* 1994; **23**:405–50.

Schultz GS & Mast BA. Molecular analysis of the environment of healing and chronic wounds: cytokines, proteases and growth factors. *Wounds* 1998; **10**(suppl F):1F–11F.

Seiler WO. Decubitus ulcers: preventive techniques for the elderly patient. *Geriatrics* 1985; **40**:53–60.

Seiler WO & Stahelin HB. Decubitus ulcers: preventive techniques for the elderly patient. *Geriatrics* 1985; **40**(7):53–60.

Scheckler WE & Peterson PJ. Infections and infection control among residents of eight rural Wisconsin nursing homes. *Archives of Internal Medicine* 1986; **146**(10):1981–4.

Sherman RA, Hall MJ & Thomas S. Medicinal maggots: an ancient remedy for some contemporary afflictions. *Annual Review of Entomology* 2000; **45**:55–81.

Siegler EL & Lavisso-Mourey R. Management of stage III pressure ulcers in moderately demented nursing home residents. *Journal of General Internal Medicine* 1991; **6**:507–13.

Stotts NA & Hunt TK. Pressure ulcers. Managing bacterial colonization and infection. *Clinics in Geriatric Medicine* 1997; **13**:565–73.

Stotts NA, Rodeheaver GT, Thomas DR *et al.* An instrument to measure healing in pressure ulcers: development and validation of the pressure ulcer scale for healing (PUSH). *The Journals of Gerontology. Series A, Biological Sciences and Medical Sciences* 2001; **56**:M795–9.

Sugarman B. Infection and pressure sores. *Archives of Physical Medicine and Rehabilitation* 1985; **66**:177–9.

Sugarman B. Pressure sore and underlying bone infection. *Archives of Internal Medicine* 1987; **147**:553–5.

Sugarman B, Brown D & Musher D. Fever and infection in spinal cord injury patients. *The Journal of the American Medical* 1982; **248**:66–70.

Thomas S, Andrews A & Jones M. The use of larval therapy in wound management. *Journal of Wound Care* 1998; **7**:521–4.

Thomas GPL & Banwell PE. Topical negative–pressure therapy in wound management. In L Teot, TE Banwell & UE Ziegler (eds) *Surgery in Wounds* 2004; Springer, Berlin.

Thomas DR, Goode PS, Tarquine PH & Allman RM. Hospital-acquired pressure ulcers and risk of death. *Journal of the American Geriatrics Society* 1996; **44**(12):1435–40.

Thomas AM, Harding KG & Moore K. The structure and composition of chronic wound eschar. *Journal of Wound Care* 1999; **8**:285–7.

Thomas S & Jones M. The use of larval therapy in wound management. *Journal of Wound Care* 1998; **7**:521–4.

Thomas S & McCubbin P. A comparison of the antimicrobial effects of four silver-containing dressings on three organisms. *Journal of Wound Care* 2003; **12**:101–7.

Touche R. *The Cost of Pressure Sores. Report to Department of Health* 1993; Department of Health, London.

van Rijswijk L. Full-thickness pressure ulcers: patient and wound healing characteristics. *Decubitus* 1993; **6**:16–21.

Versluysen M. Pressure sores in elderly patients. The epidemiology related to hip operations. *The Journal of Bone and Joint Surgery* 1985; **67**:10–3.

Versluysen M. How elderly patients with femoral fracture develop pressure sores in hospital. *British Medical Journal* 1986; **292**:1311–3.

Vowden P. Autolytic debridement. In L Teot, PE Banwell & UE Ziegler (eds) *Surgery in Wounds* 2004; Springer, Berlin.

Watts S & Clark M. *Pressure Ulcer Prevention: A Review of Policy Documents. Final Report to the Department of Health* 1993; University of Surrey.

Weiss DS, Kirsner R & Eaglstein WH. Electrical stimulation and wound healing. *Archives of Dermatology* 1990; **126**:222–5.

Whitfield MD, Kaltenthaler EC, Akehurst RL *et al.* How effective are prevention strategies in reducing the prevalence of pressure ulcers? *Journal of Wound Care* 2000; **9**(6):261–6.

Winman G & Clark MA. A randomised, stratified survey of the current use of an alternating pressure air mattress within the national health service. *Journal of Tissue Viability* 1997; **7**:84–90.

Witkowski JA & Parish LC. The decubitus ulcer: skin failure and destructive behavior. *International Journal of Dermatology* 2000; **39**:894–6.

Wright JB, Lam K, Hansen D & Burrell RE. Efficacy of topical silver against fungal burn wound pathogens. *American Journal of Infection Control* 1999; **27**:344–50.

Xakellis GC & Chrischilles EA. Hydrocolloid versus saline-gauze dressings in treating pressure ulcers: a cost-effectiveness analysis. *Archives of Physical Medicine and Rehabilitation* 1992; **73**:463–9.

Xakellis GC & Frantz R. The cost of healing pressure ulcers across multiple health care settings. *Advances in Wound Care* 1996; **9**:18–22.

Xakellis GC Jr, Frantz RA, Lewis A & Harvey P. Cost-effectiveness of an intensive pressure ulcer prevention protocol in long-term care. *Advances in Wound Care* 1998; **11**(1):22–9.

Xia Z, Sato A, Hughes MA & Cherry GW. Stimulation of fibroblast growth in vitro by intermittent radiant warming. *Wound Repair and Regeneration* 2000; **8**:138–44.

Young J & Cotter D. Pressure sores: do mattresses work? *Lancet* 1990; **336**:182–3.

Young AR, Mesusen MT & Bowles VM. Characterisation of ES products involved in wound initiation by *Lucilia cuprina* larvae. *International Journal for Parasitology* 1996; **26**:254–2.

Ziegler UE, Dietz UA & Schmidt K. Wound-bed preparation – promotion of granulation tissue. In L Teot, PE Banwell & UE Ziegler (eds) *Surgery in Wounds* 2004; Springer, Berlin.

FURTHER READING

Ayello EA, Mezey M & Amella EJ. Educational assessment and teaching of older clients with pressure ulcers. *Clinics in Geriatric Medicine* 1997; **13**(3):483–96.

Bates-Jensen BM. The pressure sore status tool a few thousand assessments later. *Advances in Wound Care* 1997; **10**:65–73.

Daechsel D & Conine TA. Special mattresses: effectiveness in preventing decubitus ulcers in chronic neurologic patients. *Archives of Physical Medicine and Rehabilitation* 1985; **66**(4):246–8.

Galpin JE, Chow AW, Bever AS *et al.* Sepsis associated with decubitus ulcers. *The American Journal of Medicine* 1976; **61**:346–50.

Gorse GJ & Messner RL. Improved pressure sore healing with hydrocolloid dressings. *Archives of Dermatology* 1987; **123**:766–71.

Graham A. The use of growth factors in clinical practice. *Journal of Wound Care* 1998; **7**:464–466.

Leigh IH & Bennett G. Pressure ulcers: prevalence, etiology, and treatment modalities. A review. *American Journal of Surgery* 1994; **167**:25S–30S.

Pearson A, Francis K, Hodgkinson B & Curry G. Prevalence and treatment of pressure ulcers in northern New South Wales. *The Australian Journal of Rural Health* 2000; **8**:103–10.

Pressure ulcers: The management of pressure ulcers in primary and secondary care, *NICE*, 2005; www.NICE.org.uk.

Sugarman M, Hawes M, Musher DM *et al.* Osteomyelitis beneath pressure sore. *Archives of Internal Medicine* 1983; **143**:683–8.

137

Perioperative and Postoperative Medical Assessment

D. Gwyn Seymour
University of Aberdeen, Aberdeen, UK

INTRODUCTION

Over the past 25 years, almost all surgical specialities have seen a dramatic increase in admissions of elderly and very elderly patients. The numbers being referred have been over and above that which would have been expected from demographic change alone and the rate of increase has usually been faster than the rise in surgical activity seen in younger adults, particularly in regard to elective procedures. Trends for two operations having a major effect on quality of life are shown in Figures 1 and 2. It seems that old people themselves, and their lay and professional advisers, are increasingly willing to consider surgery in old age. On the other hand, the idea that there are individuals who are "too old for surgery" is still very pervasive. There is concern that rates of surgery may be suboptimal, especially for higher technology interventions such as coronary surgery (Wood and Bain, 2001), and there is also evidence that elderly patients in lower socioeconomic groups have lower rates of surgery than their contemporaries in higher socioeconomic groups (Seymour and Garthwaite, 1999).

This chapter discusses the approach that needs to be taken in elderly patients in the immediate preoperative and postoperative period, concentrating on the medical aspects of assessment. However, it must not be forgotten that the fundamental aim of a preoperative assessment is the same whatever the patient's age: there is a need to estimate whether the likely benefits of the surgical procedure in that particular individual will outweigh the likely risks.

The chapter begins with a discussion of the relationship between old age and postoperative morbidity and mortality. This is followed by a brief discussion of the causes and consequences of emergency surgery in older people. Consideration is then given to the major organ systems that are of particular relevance in the medical assessment of the older surgical patient, and pointers are given to active research areas that are likely to affect practice in the near future. The problems of surgical diagnosis, strategies for the management of individual surgical conditions, and details of the technical aspects of surgery and anesthesia are not considered here, but have been reviewed by Crosby *et al.* (1992) and in a recent multiauthor book by Rosenthal *et al.* (2001). Additionally, a policy document on "Anaesthesia and Peri-operative Care of the Elderly" has been produced by a Working Party of the Association of Anaesthetists of Great Britain and Ireland (2001). Finally, the recent (Scottish Intercollegiate Guidelines Network, 2004) Guideline on Postoperative Management in Adults, while not confined to the older surgical patient, is of considerable relevance to older people as they make up a major proportion of patients who develop problems following surgery. The SIGN (Scottish Intercollegiate Guidelines Network) Guidelines are intended for use by nonspecialists in the early postoperative period, giving advice on early detection and management of common problems, and, equally importantly, indicating when more specialist help should be sought.

AGE AND POSTOPERATIVE OUTCOME

Where age is the only risk factor studied, most statistical analyses in adult patients show a positive correlation between age and the rate of adverse postoperative outcome, and a simple interpretation would be that surgery should be discouraged in extreme old age. However, there are a number of flaws in this simplistic analysis. Firstly, there is the assumption that the outcome in an elderly individual can be predicted with accuracy from the "average" outcome of patients of the same age. As shown in the following, age as a risk factor for predicting adverse outcome in *individual* surgical patients lacks both sensitivity and specificity. Secondly, mortality figures do not tell us about the balance of risk and

Principles and Practice of Geriatric Medicine, 4th Edition. Edited by M.S. John Pathy, Alan J. Sinclair and John E. Morley.

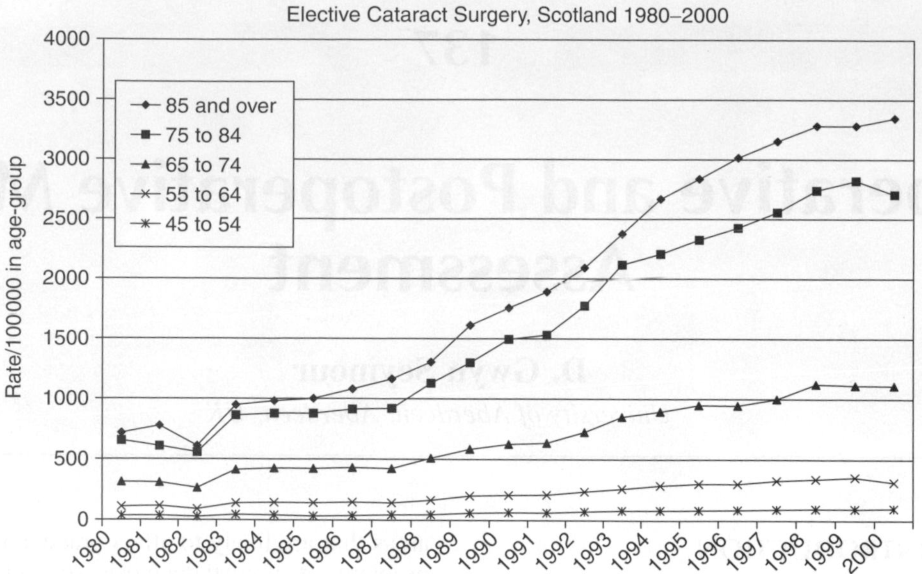

Figure 1 Elective Cataract Surgery, Scotland 1980–2000. On the basis of data supplied by the Information and Statistics Division of NHS Scotland

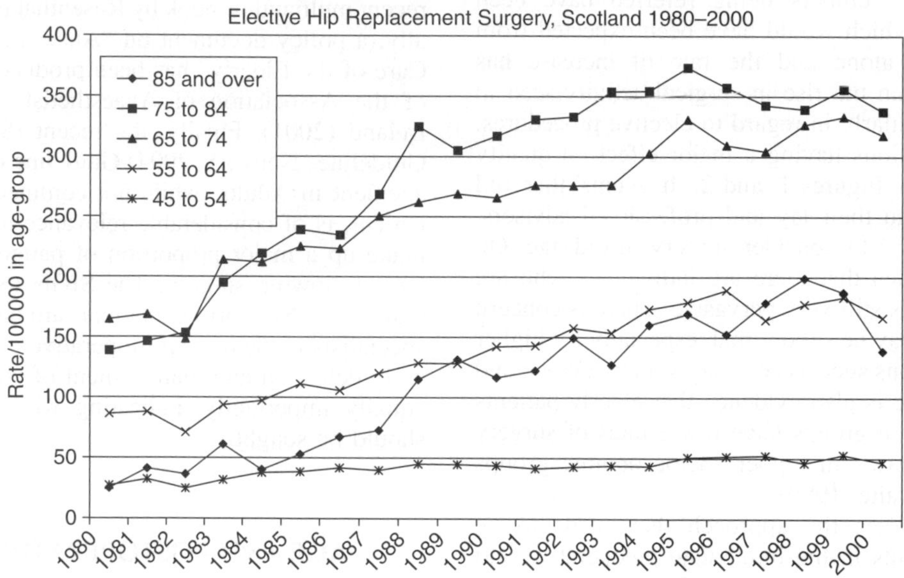

Figure 2 Elective Hip Replacement Surgery, Scotland 1980–2000. On the basis of data supplied by the Information and Statistics Division of NHS Scotland

benefits in individual patients. For example, in extreme circumstances, such as a ruptured aortic aneurysm, the mortality rate for nonoperative therapy is nearly 100% and so a postoperative mortality rate of 25–40% might be highly acceptable. Thirdly, outcome data related to broad surgical categories of disease do not take into account the tendency for more serious pathology to occur with advancing age. For example, young adults admitted urgently with abdominal pain tend to have conditions such as uncomplicated appendicitis or nonspecific abdominal pain, where mortality rates are low. As patients get older, an "acute abdomen" often turns out to be because of a perforated viscus, carcinoma, vascular events, or other major pathology which have a much higher rate of mortality and morbidity (de Dombal, 1991).

It is also wrong to assume that a positive correlation between age and postoperative adverse outcome indicates that the adverse outcome is a direct result of the aging process. In fact, there is little evidence that age *in the absence of disease* is a major risk factor for postoperative morbidity and mortality. This assertion is supported by several lines of evidence. For instance, a study from the United States, which used the Medisgroups system to grade the severity of preoperative medical problems of general surgical patients aged 65 years and over, found no relationship between age and outcome, once the preoperative status had been taken into account (Dunlop *et al.*, 1993). Similarly, the APACHE III (Acure Physiology and Chronic Health Evaluation) prognostic system, which has been applied widely in intensive care units, indicated that around 47% of the variability in mortality was associated with the severity of illness, 6% with a type of disease, while only 3% appeared to be attributable to age (Knaus *et al.*, 1991).

Thus, the great body of evidence suggests that the major factor in the association between age and adverse postoperative outcome comes about *not as a result of aging itself, but through a secondary association with age-associated disease* (Lubin, 1993; Seymour, 1999).

AGE, EMERGENCY SURGERY, AND POSTOPERATIVE OUTCOME

It has been known for many years that nonelective surgery is associated with a higher rate of postoperative problems than is elective surgery. Survival curves from a study of elderly general surgical patients in North Wales (Edwards *et al.*, 1996) have suggested that, while both age and nonelective surgery were associated with postoperative mortality, nonelective surgery had a strong association with short- and medium-term survival, while age had a major effect on long-term postoperative survival. However, the interpretation of the association between nonelective surgery and adverse outcome in older patients is complicated by the fact that there is also a positive correlation between increasing age and the tendency to be admitted nonelectively.

An excellent series of reports produced in England and Wales by the National Confidential Enquiry into Perioperative Deaths (NCEPOD) have focused attention on postoperative deaths which might have been preventable. They have pointed to deaths following emergency surgery (often carried out out-of-hours by less experienced staff on medically unstable patients) as a continuing cause for concern. The reports also show that over two-thirds of postoperative deaths occur in patients aged 71 years and over. Within Scotland, the SASM (Scottish Audit of Surgical Mortality) audits all postoperative deaths and has come to similar conclusions.

CARDIAC PROBLEMS

Cardiac Surgery (*see* Chapter 52, Cardiac Surgery in the Elderly)

In patients who are undergoing cardiac operations such as coronary artery bypass grafts or valve replacement, surgery is usually carried out under elective conditions and detailed information about cardiac status is available preoperatively. Furthermore, such patients tend to be treated postoperatively in intensive care units. Under such circumstances postoperative mortality rates tend to be gratifyingly low even in older patients. In the previous edition of this textbook, reference was made to a survey of patients undergoing cardiac operations in Washington DC. Even at that time, a quarter of patients were aged 70 years and over and they had a 30-day mortality of 5.3%, compared with a 2.7% 30-day mortality in patients aged 69 years or under (Katz *et al.*, 1995). Around the same time, Unsworth-White and colleagues from St George's Hospital in London concluded that while the risks of cardiac surgery "above 70 years of age, and certainly above 80 years of age, are appreciably higher... they are not prohibitive" (Unsworth-White *et al.*, 1993), and, in common with the Washington unit, about a quarter of their cardiac patients were aged 70 and over. In the last 10 years, there have been several hundred publications on cardiac surgery in old age, and in many areas, particularly North America, it is becoming almost routine. Alexander *et al.* (2000), from North Carolina, reviewed hospital outcome in 67 764 patients (4743 aged 80 years and over) undergoing cardiac surgery in 22 centers involved in the National Cardiovascular Network. The overall incidence of morbidity and mortality in the octogenarians was lower than that previously reported, but remained higher than the rates encountered in younger patients. However, in octogenarians without significant comorbidity, mortality rates approached those of younger patients.

While these results are encouraging, the elderly individual opting for open-heart surgery needs to be aware of the risks as well as the benefits. In an editorial giving a "cardiologist's perspective", Sprigings (1999) points out that the reported rate of postoperative stroke in some series of octogenarians undergoing aortic valve surgery is above 10%. As the nonsurgical treatment of severe aortic stenosis is unsatisfactory, Sprigings accepts that the decision to recommend surgery in those with severe symptoms and no other medical problems is not difficult, but there remain many other elderly cardiac patients in whom there is true uncertainty as to the right course of action. In all cardiac surgery, but particularly in conditions other than aortic stenosis, there is a widespread appreciation that the quality of life and the functional capacity as well as survival need to be taken into consideration, and cardiac surgery in old age can have major impact on the first two of these factors (Jaeger *et al.*, 1994; Walter and Mohan, 1995; Awad *et al.*, 1995; Olsson *et al.*, 1996).

Noncardiac Surgery

The major postoperative cardiac complications are myocardial infarction (MI) and acute heart failure. The former may be difficult to diagnose in the early postoperative period as pain can be masked by anesthesia and analgesia, and surgical trauma to muscles may make interpretation of cardiac enzyme changes difficult, although newer enzyme tests such as troponin-I and troponin-T offer the potential for enhanced specificity (Surveillance for perioperative MI, 2002). Using traditional clinical criteria, postoperative MI has been estimated to occur following 1–4% of general surgical operations in the over-65s and cardiac failure has been reported in 4–10%, with the mortality rate associated with postoperative myocardial infarction being around 50% (Seymour *et al.*, 1992). The rate of postoperative cardiac complications in patients aged 75 and over is 2–3 times that of those aged 65–74 (Seymour *et al.*, 1992). Depending on the definitions and diagnostic tests used, much higher estimates of perioperative MI rates have been reported. Thus, Badner *et al.* (1998) in a group of 323 patients aged 50 or over undergoing noncardiac surgery reported a 5.3% incidence of postoperative MI when the criteria were based on autopsy data, new Q waves on ECG, and creatine kinase (CK-2) levels. However, when cardiac troponin-T levels greater than 0.2 mcg l^{-1} were incorporated into the diagnostic criteria, the estimated rate of perioperative MI rose to 11.2% and further relaxation of ECG criteria led to an estimate of 20.7%.

In day-to-day medical practice, the main need for preoperative cardiac assessment arises in the elderly patient who is undergoing *noncardiac* surgery. Thus, Mangano (1990) estimated that, for each patient undergoing cardiac surgery in the United States, there are up to 10 other "cardiac" patients (i.e. patients with known heart disease or two or more major cardiac risk factors) undergoing noncardiac surgery. Mangano estimates that a third of all patients aged 65 and over fall into this "cardiac" category, and a proportion of the remaining two-thirds will have occult ischemic heart disease which may reveal itself only during the perioperative period.

The "cardiac assessment of the noncardiac surgical patient" has accordingly become a major focus of research in recent years. The earliest reports in this field identified a number of individual risk factors which were correlated with an increase in adverse postoperative cardiac outcomes. These included previous myocardial infarction, congestive heart failure, angina, age, hypertension, diabetes, arrhythmias, peripheral vascular disease, valvular heart disease, smoking, and previous cardiac surgery (Badner *et al.*, 1998). Later, researchers attempted to construct multifactorial indices of cardiac risk from these individual risk factors (Goldman *et al.*, 1977; Detsky *et al.*, 1986), but, as recognized by their originators, there are limitations in applying these indices to individual patients (Mangano & Goldman, 1995; Mangano, 1995). A major milestone in this field was the appearance of the 1996 guidelines on perioperative cardiovascular evaluation for noncardiac surgery, issued jointly by the American College of Cardiology and the American Heart Association (AAC/AHA) (Eagle *et al.*, 1996). These were subsequently updated in 2002 taking account of 400 or so references that had appeared between 1995 and 2000 (Eagle *et al.*, 2002). The first point to make of both of the AAC/AHA reports is that they found relatively few randomized control trials (RCTs) on which to base their recommendations. Part of the problem is that most of the studies quantifying postoperative risks are necessarily of an observational or cohort design, although RCTs may be feasible at a later stage. Another problem with RCT studies in the field of perioperative risk reduction is that the interventions may be complex and consist of changes in practice and organization rather than simple drug interventions. However, as in most cases the field of cardiology lends itself to drug interventions, an important development between the 1996 and 2002 AAC/AHA reports was the appearance of trials showing short- and long-term cardiac benefits of β-blockade in surgical patients (see pages 32–35 of the 2002 report), with the two publications by Poldermans *et al.* (1999) and Boersma *et al.* (2001) being particularly influential. Other important additions to be found in the 2002 AAC/AHA update are discussions of renal insufficiency, better quantification of the predictive role of preoperative functional capacity, more detailed guidance on preoperative cardiac assessment, and an assessment of the role of percutaneous coronary intervention.

The fundamental three-part strategy of risk prediction used in the 1996 ACC/AHA report remained unchanged in the 2002 version. Indeed, a similar strategy is likely to be a suitable model for use in risk prediction outside the cardiovascular field. The three separate areas of risk considered are:

(a) major clinical predictors of risk
(b) functional capacity
(c) surgery-specific risk.

Within category (a), "major" clinical predictors are identified as *unstable coronary syndromes*, decompensated heart failure, congestive heart failure, significant arrhythmias, and severe valvular disease. In the "intermediate" clinical predictor group are found mild angina, previous myocardial infarction, compensated or stable congestive cardiac failure, diabetes, and renal insufficiency. The "minor" clinical predictors are advanced age, abnormal ECG, non-sinus rhythm, history of stroke, and uncontrolled hypertension.

In respect to category (b), specialists in geriatric medicine will readily identify with the concept that age by itself in the absence of disease is not a major predictor of an adverse outcome. Similarly, they will concur with the importance of functional capacity in determining the outcome. The 1996 ACC/AHA report introduced the concept of defining functional capacity in terms of metabolic equivalents (MET levels) and this approach deserves to be more widely known both in medicine and surgery. Perioperative cardiac problems are much increased when a patient is unable to meet a four MET level of activity: this is roughly equivalent to climbing a flight of stairs, walking up a hill or walking on level ground at a speed of 4 mph or 6.4 kmph. The 2002 report has continued to champion the MET concept, and was able to incorporate a publication by Reilly *et al.* (1999) relating self-reported exercise tolerance to the risk of serious perioperative complications.

Category (c), the third element of the ACC/AHA risk assessment, classifies surgical procedures into high, intermediate and low risk. Examples of "high" risk (cardiac risk often >5%) include emergency major operations particularly in the elderly, aortic and other major vascular surgery, peripheral vascular surgery, and procedures likely to be associated with large fluid shifts or blood loss. "Intermediate" (cardiac risk generally <5%) procedures include carotid endarterectomy, head and neck surgery, interperitoneal and intrathoracic surgery, orthopedic surgery, and prostate surgery. “Low” risk procedures (cardiac risk generally <1%) include endoscopic procedures, superficial procedures, cataract surgery, and brain surgery.

The final part of the ACC/AHA risk assessment strategy is to weigh up the relative importance of categories (a), (b), and (c) in an individual patient, recognizing, for example, that adverse clinical predictors and functional impairment are much more to be feared in a patient undergoing intermediate or major surgery than they are in a patient undergoing minor surgery. As in 1996, an algorithm is provided for this purpose in the ACC/AHA 2002 report. The ACC/AHA guidelines will be reviewed annually from now on, and revisions will be published on the Internet (www.acc.org and www.americanheart.org). In addition, a recent paper by Mukherjee and Eagle (2003) provides a readily accessible summary of the current approach to perioperative cardiac assessment, illustrating the application of the ACC/AHA guidelines to a 68 year old patient with a cardiac history in whom elective surgery is being considered.

RESPIRATORY PROBLEMS (*see* Chapter 61, Respiratory Disease in the Elderly)

As Pulford and Connolly have pointed out (Pulford and Connolly, 1996), attempts to make a precise distinction between those changes in the lung that are caused by aging and those that are caused by accumulated damage from pollutants and lung disease are “doomed to failure”. However in general, we can say that the aging lung undergoes (a) *structural changes*, with increased rigidity of the chest wall, reduced alveolar area, and increases in lung compliance, functional residual capacity and residual volume; and (b) *physiological changes*, with a reduction in exercise capacity and impaired control of ventilation (from a mixture of central and peripheral changes including reduced sensitivity to hypoxia). Pulford and Connolly identify an increase in closing volume (i.e. small airways collapse at higher lung volumes during expiration), as the single most clinically important result of all these changes in the aging lung, and increased closing volumes probably have a significant role in causing postoperative atelectasis.

Respiratory complications remain a significant cause of postoperative morbidity and potentially preventable postoperative mortality (Seymour and Vaz, 1989; Williams Russo *et al.*, 1992). In a recent review of factors influencing a range of postoperative complications in older people, Jin and Chung (2001) quote estimated incidences of 2–10% for postoperative respiratory complications in elderly people. They identify the site of surgery as being the best single predictor of postoperative respiratory complications, with incisions near the diaphragm having the highest rate of complications. Other clinical risk factors identified are duration and type of anesthesia, chronic obstructive lung disease, asthma, preoperative hypersecretion of mucus, chest deformation, and smoking within the month prior to surgery. Research into perioperative respiratory risk reduction has been less extensive than in the field of cardiac risk, but research themes have included the ability of preoperative symptoms, signs, and pulmonary function testing to predict postoperative outcome, and on the preventive methods, including physiotherapy, which can be applied in patients shown to be at risk (ACP, 1990; Zibrak *et al.*, 1990; Celli, 1993). A further important discovery has been the recognition that postoperative hypoxemia is common, and that it may occur several days after anesthesia.

A series of three publications from Lawrence (Lawrence *et al.*, 1995; Lawrence *et al.*, 1996; De Nino *et al.*, 1997) and his colleagues in Texas has reexamined the factors associated with perioperative respiratory complications and the efficacy of attempts to reduce respiratory morbidity and mortality. The first of these publications showed that, in terms of cost and morbidity, respiratory complications were as important as cardiac complications. The second publication found that postoperative respiratory complications were statistically associated with abnormal preoperative lung signs, abnormal chest radiology, overall morbidity, and the Goldman Cardiac index. However, when combined with these clinical predictors, spirometry did not improve risk prediction. A formal cost-effective analysis contained in the third publication led to the conclusion that, at the time of the study, preoperative spirometry in the United States was “blowing away” $8 million to $20 million Medicare dollars each year. An earlier systematic review of the role of preoperative spirometry in non-thoracic surgery had similarly found it difficult to demonstrate a clear-cut benefit of spirometry over and above that of preoperative clinical assessment (Thomas and McIntosh, 1994). A more recent report by Smetana (1999) has indicated that obesity and age may be less important predictors of respiratory risk than they were reported to be in earlier studies.

In the absence of definitive evidence in many areas, what should be our preoperative strategy in attempting to minimize postoperative respiratory complications in older patients? Many of the recommendations in this area are based on clinical experience or extrapolation from what is known about respiratory risk, rather than on randomized intervention trials. They include (Seymour, 1999) cessation of smoking 6 to 8 weeks before surgery, “pulmonary toilet” combined with physiotherapy for those at highest risk, care with the temperature and humidification of anesthetic gases, adequate analgesia, early removal of nasogastric tubes, and early mobilization.

How much technology should we use when assessing preoperative respiratory risk in older patients? Jin and Chung (2001) recommend obtaining a preoperative chest X ray in all patients aged 60 and over, but particularly in patients with respiratory symptoms, smoking, obesity, and cardiopulmonary disease. In those with an abnormal chest X ray, basic pulmonary function tests are recommended. If these are abnormal, they trigger pre- and postoperative prophylaxis in patients undergoing nonresective or upper abdominal surgery. Patients in whom pulmonary resection is being considered require more intensive evaluation.

Postoperative Hypoxemia

A major discovery in the postoperative care of middle-aged and elderly patients in recent years has been that profound postoperative hypoxemia can occur many days after surgery (Catley *et al.*, 1985; Knill *et al.*, 1990). It used to be assumed that once the immediate sedative affects of general anesthesia had disappeared, that is, within a few hours of surgery, then the main risk period for hypoxemia had passed. However, with the discovery of pulse oximeters, which provided a noninvasive means of monitoring oxygen desaturation, it became clear that many patients were undergoing profound but clinically silent desaturations at night, sometimes up to a week after surgery. It is plausible that some of the arrhythmias and episodes of sudden death occurring several days after surgery which were previously attributed solely to cardiac causes were in fact the result of hypoxemia. However, while some authors claim that there is a close relationship between hypoxemia and cardiac disturbances such as ischemia or arrhythmias (Pateman and Hanning, 1989; Reeder *et al.*, 1991; Gill *et al.*, 1992; Stausholm *et al.*, 1995), others are not so convinced (Smith *et al.*, 1996).

The nocturnal desaturations can be reduced by giving continuous intranasal oxygen (McBrien and Sellers, 1995) for several days after surgery ("3 days and 5 nights" is a common regimen) and so these findings have considerable practical importance. Research efforts in the 1990s have been directed at explaining the mechanism of nocturnal desaturation in more detail, and trying to predict which patients are most at risk, so that this oxygen therapy can be better targeted. However, a final consensus has yet to emerge. If it is currently difficult to predict which elderly postoperative patients will develop postoperative hypoxemia, and if there is *prima facie* evidence that hypoxemia is harmful, it might appear logical to use oximetry to monitor the great majority of older people in the perioperative period, despite the costs in time, money, and inconvenience. However, scientific doubts about the efficacy of an "oximetry for all" approach have been raised by a large randomized study that was able to demonstrate that pulse oximetry reduced the *incidence* of postoperative hypoxemia, but which failed to demonstrate the expected *benefits* in postoperative complications (Moller *et al.*, 1993a; Moller *et al.*, 1993b).

Further, research is clearly warranted in this area. It seems likely that the final explanation of the variation in individual adverse effects of hypoxemia will be complex, and might, for instance, depend not only on the absolute level of oxygen, but also on the presence of hypocarbia, and/or the patient's previous level of hypoxemia. Research is also needed into the potential for hypoxemia to cause delirium and impair wound healing (Rosenberg, 1994).

RENAL FUNCTION AND FLUID STATUS

Postoperative Renal Failure and Renal Dysfunction

Deaths as the sole result of acute renal failure in the postoperative period are relatively rare after general surgery in older patients. Out of a total of 546 patients aged 65 years and over, undergoing general surgery in two prospective studies (Seymour and Vaz, 1989; Seymour and Pringle, 1982), the number of potentially preventable postoperative deaths was 26 but in only one was acute renal failure judged to be the *sole* cause of death. However, renal failure may also contribute to death in patients with multiple problems such as postoperative sepsis and cardiac failure.

Major vascular or cardiac operations are associated with an increased risk of renal failure when compared with general surgery. In a prospective study of 734 predominantly middle-aged cardiac surgery patients with normal preoperative renal function, Zanardo *et al.* (1994) recorded postoperative renal dysfunction in 11.4% and acute renal failure in 3.7%. Mortality rates were 0.8% for those with normal postoperative renal function, 9.5% for those with renal dysfunction, and 44.4% for those with acute renal failure.

Transient postoperative renal impairment is much more common than acute renal failure. Because the acute stress response results in difficulty in excreting a water load, it has been argued that a degree of postoperative oliguria is inevitable. However, careful fluid replacement, good analgesia, and controlled anesthesia can usually minimize this effect (Sweny, 1991; Burchardi and Kacmarczyk, 1994). Transient postoperative hyponatraemia is also a common phenomenon. Some episodes are related to difficulties in excreting a water load, but in urological practice the infusion of large amounts of hypotonic fluid into the bladder can also lead to significant retention of water and subsequent hyponatraemia. In the first few days following surgery or trauma, isotonic fluid sequestration in wound sites (the "third space") may also lead to subtle volume deficiencies (Van Zee and Lowry, 1995).

While anesthesia can have direct pharmacological effects on renal function and body fluid regulation, and while direct toxic effects have been reported with methoxyflurane, it appears that, in the majority of patients with postoperative renal impairment, nonanesthetic factors (such as volume impairment, sepsis, cardiovascular complications, the acute stress response, and the effects of mechanical ventilation) are more important (Sweny, 1991; Burchardi and Kacmarczyk, 1994)

Novis *et al.* (1994) have reviewed 28 studies of the preoperative risk factors associated with postoperative acute renal failure in patients undergoing general, biliary, vascular, and cardiac surgery. Preoperative renal impairment emerged as the most consistent predictor of postoperative impairment, and cardiac risk factors such as left ventricular dysfunction were better predictors than chronological age. In the search for potentially preventable risk factors for postoperative renal failure, patients with unrelieved obstructive jaundice deserve particular mention, as up to 10% will develop postoperative renal failure, and they may require specific prophylactic measures (Parks *et al.*, 1994; Fogarty *et al.*, 1995; Green and Better, 1995).

Assessment and Treatment of Fluid–electrolyte Imbalance (*see* Chapter 117, Water and Electrolyte Balance in Health and Disease)

Because the aging kidney and cardiovascular system often have limited homeostatic ability (Phillips *et al.*, 1993), particular care needs to be taken not to deplete or overload the older patient with fluids during the perioperative period. Preoperative water and/or salt depletion are particularly likely in patients with vomiting, diarrhea, pyrexia, or anorexia. Volume deficits may not be apparent in a patient who is lying quietly in bed and may only be revealed at the time of anesthetic induction, when blunting of the normal regulatory mechanisms may result in profound hypotension in a patient who has a deficiency of water and/or salt.

A careful preoperative assessment of elderly patients looking for evidence of water or salt depletion is, therefore important, although such an assessment is more difficult in the older patient than it is in the younger adult for a number of reasons (Gross *et al.*, 1992). For instance, skin turgor is often reduced in normal elderly people, especially on sun-exposed areas. Longitudinal tongue furrows are probably a better indicator of cell shrinkage (Gross *et al.*, 1992) but are difficult to quantify. A dry tongue may be a sign of water loss, but is more commonly associated with mouth breathing. Absence of sweating in the axillae has also been suggested as a sign of water loss, with a reported sensitivity of 50%, a specificity of 82%, a positive predictive value of 45%, and a negative predictive value of 84% in a group of elderly medical patients (Eaton *et al.*, 1994).

In trying to assess the individual patient, it is important to realize that the clinical and pathological effects of water depletion on the one hand and salt depletion on the other are quite different (Van Zee & Lowry, 1995). Levinsky (1994) has argued that the word "dehydration" should strictly be applied to pure water depletion, but the term is often used more generally to encompass combined deficits of salt and water (Weinberg and Minaker, 1995).

Water depletion tends to have its initial effect on the intracellular rather than the extracellular space. The early physical *signs* of pure water depletion are subtle and include drowsiness, mental confusion, and a low-grade fever (Van Zee and Lowry, 1995). The major *symptom* associated with water depletion is thirst. However, patients with serious surgical or medical illnesses may be too ill or too sedated to experience this otherwise powerful sensation, or there may be preexisting communication difficulties such as dysphasia. In addition, in a proportion of older patients, the thirst mechanism seems to be impaired (Phillips *et al.*, 1993; Weinberg and Minaker, 1995).

As signs and symptoms are an unreliable way of diagnosing water depletion, it is fortunate that a high serum sodium can be used as a diagnostic aid. It has been estimated that 90% of cases of hypernatraemia encountered in elderly hospitalized patients are due to water depletion (Lye, 1984). In patients relying on nasogastric feeding, it is also very important to make sure that adequate amounts of water are given, as standard regimens may contain very little free water (Weinberg and Minaker, 1995).

In a retrospective series of adult hospital patients with serum sodium of over $150\,\mathrm{mmol\,l^{-1}}$, mortality rates were over 54% (Long *et al.*, 1991), probably reflecting the severity of the underlying illness. However, care should be taken not to replace the deficit too quickly, as cerebral edema may result. Van Zee and Lowry (1995) recommend that only half of the calculated water deficit should be administered within the first 24 hours, with the remainder being replaced over the next 1–2 days. Water repletion can be achieved by 5% dextrose infusions intravenously or subcutaneously, or by providing water by mouth or through a nasogastric tube.

In the presence of hypernatraemia, the water deficit can be estimated as follows (Van Zee and Lowry, 1995)

1. Estimate the normal body water. The normal body water (liters) is usually estimated as being 60% of the body weight (kg) (*see* **Chapter 117, Water and Electrolyte Balance in Health and Disease**), but in older patients, a multiplication by 0.55 may be more accurate because of age changes in body composition.
2. Estimate the actual body water, using the formula: Actual total body water (l) = normal total body water (l)

$$\times \frac{\text{normal serum sodium}(\mathrm{mmol\ l^{-1}})}{\text{actual serum sodium}(\mathrm{mmol\ l^{-1}})}$$

3. Estimate the water deficit by subtracting (2) from (1).

Salt depletion (sometimes referred to as volume depletion, as salt loss is usually associated with a corresponding loss of water) can occur in the elderly preoperative patient through mechanisms such as vomiting and diarrhea. In addition, many elderly patients are on diuretics, often for dubious reasons. Whereas, water depletion tends to have its main impact intracellularly, salt depletion primarily causes shrinkage of the extracellular compartment. The extracellular compartment includes the intravascular space and so salt depletion tends to lead to hypotension (particularly postural hypotension) and tachycardia.

While salt depletion produces more definite physical signs than does water depletion, these signs may be less obvious in elderly people than in the young (Seymour *et al.*, 1992; Gross *et al.*, 1992). For example, if there is a preexisting degree of systolic hypertension, a subsequent fall in resting systolic blood pressure may go unnoticed. Standing the patient up will help to bring out postural hypotension, but postural hypotension may also be present in a quarter of apparently fit elderly people who are not volume depleted (Weinberg and

Minaker, 1995). The development of tachycardia in response to volume depletion is an autonomic reflex and such reflexes may be blunted in some elderly people and/or the ability of the heart to develop a tachycardia may be impaired in old age.

A bedside estimation of volume depletion which is underused in clinical practice is to look for a *low* jugular venous pressure by lying patients flat or even in a head-down position (Seymour *et al.*, 1992). In doubtful cases, a direct measurement of central venous pressure or even pulmonary artery pressure may be necessary, with or without a fluid challenge, but in the future noninvasive techniques should become available (McIntyre *et al.*, 1992; Vanoverschelde *et al.*, 1995). While a high serum sodium is an indicator of water depletion, the same is unfortunately not true of a low serum sodium as an indicator of salt depletion (Van Zee and Lowry, 1995).

In prescribing fluids in elderly patients over the perioperative period, there is unfortunately no magic formula that will allow an exact assessment of need to be made, and it is not possible to write prescriptions for days on end without further reference to the patient (Scottish Intercollegiate Guidelines Network, 2004). Some broad rules for quantifying the loss may be helpful, however.

1. A water loss of 2 kg or more is probably significant in an older patient (Lye, 1984).
2. In regard to younger adults, a saline loss of 4% of the body weight is "mild", 6–8% is "moderate", and 10% is "severe" (Shires and Canizaro, 1986). Because of their limited homeostatic reserve, elderly patients are likely to be even more at risk from a given percentage of saline loss.
3. In the younger surgical patient, Tweedle (1984) has estimated that 4 l of saline are lost before signs of depletion appear, and 4 l of saline are gained before edema develops. Again, the older patient is probably operating within narrower margins.

Some of the special problems in prescribing fluids in the elderly patient are discussed in Seymour *et al.* (1992). However, the basic approach, in surgical patients of all ages (Scottish Intercollegiate Guidelines Network, 2004; Van Zee and Lowry, 1995), is to assess the likely *preexisting* fluid losses, using a mixture of the clinical and biochemical methods already described, and to prescribe fluids that will both replace *preexisting* losses and keep up with *ongoing* losses as they occur. There is also a need to *adjust for baseline needs*, especially in patients who are taking nothing by mouth.

There are no simple guidelines on the rate of fluid administration. In young patients with a severe volume deficiency (as defined above), Shires and Canizaro 1986) recommend an initial infusion rate of $2\,\mathrm{l\,h^{-1}}$, with a halving of this rate as soon as signs of improvement appear. When rates of infusion are above $1\,\mathrm{l\,h^{-1}}$, however, they recommend that a physician be in constant attendance. For older patients, they point out that rapid repletion may be needed, but they advocate a more cautious approach, together with close monitoring via a central venous line or a pulmonary artery catheter.

Postoperative fluid, electrolyte and renal management of adults of all ages was an aspect of postoperative care that was considered by a recent SIGN Guideline (Scottish Intercollegiate Guidelines Network, 2004), but it was stated that there were very few relevant randomized controlled trials in the field, and that the recommendations relied heavily on clinical consensus.

NUTRITIONAL ASSESSMENT (*see* Chapter 24, Epidemiology of Nutrition and Aging; Chapter 25, Absorption of Nutrients)

Nutrition and Surgical Outcome

The two key questions in this area are, firstly, the degree to which under-nutrition affects surgical outcome and secondly, whether nutritional therapy is effective in reducing postoperative morbidity and mortality. The clinical assessment of malnutrition presents several problems, as recently discussed by Allison (2000). For example, there is no generally accepted definition of malnutrition to act as the basis for assessment, and even when a patient is severely underweight there is evidence that recent loss of weight is more important than the absolute level of weight achieved. Furthermore, while a low or falling body weight is reasonable evidence that energy intake is deficient (except perhaps in oedematous patients treated with large dose of diuretics), it is a poorer guide to protein deficiency and an even more indirect guide of micronutrient levels. The recent ESPEN (European Society for Parenteral and Enteral Nutrition) Guidelines for Nutrition Screening point out that different screening tools are required in different settings (community, hospital, and elderly) and propose a range of tools for further use in evaluation studies (Kondrup *et al.*, 2003).

A number of biochemical indicators have been identified as *metabolic markers of protein-calorie malnutrition* and may have a role in clinical assessment, but they can also be misleading. For instance, while a low albumin may be a marker of protein malnutrition, hypoalbuminaemia is also a common finding in chronic disease in old age or as an accompaniment of acute sepsis (Milne *et al.*, 2004; Avenell and Handoll, 2004). Patients with a low albumin from acute or chronic disease also tend to have a poorer postoperative outcome but it does not necessarily follow that the poor outcome arises directly from poor nutrition. More importantly, it does not follow that pre- and/or postoperative nutritional supplementation will reduce postoperative complications.

The assessment of malnutrition in elderly patients presents additional problems, and it is often difficult to tell whether a patient is "lean and fit" or "thin and frail". Measurement of Body Mass Index (BMI) classically depends on

surgical situations. However, withdrawal delirium tends to cause more diagnostic confusion in the latter situation, as a history of preoperative alcohol abuse or regular tranquilizer use may not have been elicited and so the occurrence of delirium in the first or second postoperative day may be falsely attributed to postoperative causes. Prospective studies of risk factors are difficult to carry out and so the large-scale investigation by Marcantonio and colleagues is particularly welcome (Marcantonio *et al.*, 1994). Independent correlates of postoperative delirium in this study included: age 70 or over; self-reported alcohol abuse; poor cognitive status; poor functional status; markedly abnormal preoperative sodium, potassium or glucose; noncardiac thoracic surgery; and aortic aneurysm surgery. In a large randomized controlled study of patients undergoing elective total knee replacement, Williams Russo *et al.* (1995) found no statistical difference between the incidence of postoperative delirium in patients following general anesthesia (12/128 or 9.4%) and that following epidural anesthesia (16/134 or 12%).

A useful general concept introduced by Inouye, and applicable to both medical and surgical patients, is that there should be an attempt to identify separate "predisposing" and "precipitating" factors for delirium (Inouye and Charpentier, 1996; Inouye, 1999). These two factors interact: for example, patients with a large number of predisposing factors require only a small precipitant to tip them into a delirious state. While there have been advances in multivariate risk scores to predict the risk of delirium both in surgical and medical situations (Marcantonio *et al.*, 1994; Inouye *et al.*, 1993), perhaps the biggest practical development has been the concept of adopting a series of preventative measures in *all* patients undergoing medical and surgical treatment to minimize the risk of delirium developing. These appear to be able to reduce delirium in the short-term in medical (Inouye *et al.*, 1999; Rizzo *et al.*, 2001) and surgical patients (Marcantonio *et al.*, 2001), although long-term benefits still need to be proven (Bogardus *et al.*, 2003).

As in acute delirium in nonsurgical situations, the postoperative patient who is delirious needs an urgent physical diagnosis (Scottish Intercollegiate Guidelines Network, 2004) as the delirium is usually due to treatable but potentially serious medical problems.

Postoperative Dementia

Can dementia appear for the first time purely as the result of a general anesthetic? In an often-quoted 5-year retrospective study, Bedford (1955) found 18 people in the Oxfordshire area in whom there was reasonable evidence that dementia had occurred for the first time after an apparently uneventful anesthetic, but in a subsequent prospective study of 678 elderly surgical patients (Simpson *et al.*, 1961) only one such patient was found. These two reports stimulated many more studies of long-term cognitive function after surgery. Some of these studies have randomized elective orthopedic patients to regional and general anesthetic treatment and have compared values on psychometric tests 3–6 months after surgery with preoperative values. Williams Russo *et al.* (1995) confirmed the results of previous studies in finding no long-term difference in mental functioning between elderly patients undergoing elective orthopedic surgery under regional anesthesia and those undergoing a general anesthetic. However, while there was no difference between the two types of anesthetic group, the cognitive function of 12 out of the 231 (7/114 epidural and 5/117 general anesthesia) patients examined at 6 months was worse than it had been preoperatively. The authors point out that this decline might have occurred in a similar elderly group of patients not having surgery, but long-term follow-ups of nonoperative patients using the same cognitive assessment protocol were not carried out as part of that study.

The study by Jones *et al.* (1990) also failed to find any objective differences in cognitive and functional competence between general and regional anesthetic groups 3 months after elective knee or hip replacement. However, 11 out of 64 general anesthesia patients and 10 out of 65 regional anesthesia patients considered that their memory and concentration were worse than they were preoperatively. Jones *et al.* commented that these subjective changes might have been too subtle to pickup on formal testing, or might represent mild depression or the state of postoperative fatigue that has also been reported in younger patients. Their overall conclusion, however, was that "modern anesthesia, either general or regional, seemed to have no significant long-term effects on mental function in elderly patients".

A potential criticism of all the earlier studies was that pre- and postoperative cognitive state was not measured in a standardized way. Because of this, the ISPOCD (International Study of Post Operative Cognitive Dysfunction) investigators set out to perform a definitive study of cognitive impairment after general surgery in older patients. They used a standardized battery of cognitive tests before and after elective surgery and looked at changes 1 week and 3 months after the surgery took place. In addition, a range of predictive factors including hypoxemia was investigated in the anticipation that these would be correlated with postoperative cognitive change. The main ISPOCD1 study was published in 1998 (Moller *et al.*, 1998) but unfortunately did not provide the reassurance for older people that had been anticipated. Perioperative hypoxemia and hypotension appear to have no relationship to postoperative cognitive dysfunction, but nevertheless, in around 16% of patients, careful psychological testing revealed cognitive deficits at 3 months which had not been present prior to elective surgery. Statistically, the only risk factor which was correlated with an adverse cognitive outcome, despite a series of multivariable analyses, was age.

The ISPOCD investigators have therefore embarked on a series of investigations under the broad heading of ISPOCD2 to examine further hypotheses about the causes of postoperative cognitive impairment. In addition, a sample of the original ISPOCD1 patients has now been followed for two years postoperatively (Abildstrom *et al.*, 2000). The cognitive performance of these ISPOCD1 patients at two years was compared with that of patients of similar age who had not undergone surgery and it appeared that the prevalence of cognitive dysfunction was similar in both populations. In other words, the events around surgery and anesthesia appeared to have led to a degree of cognitive loss which lasted at least 3 months (i.e. was more prolonged than simple postoperative delirium), but by 2 years the nonoperated population had "caught up".

PROPHYLAXIS AGAINST THROMBOEMBOLISM

The concept underlying the commonest form of prophylaxis against thromboembolism is that doses of heparin that would be insufficient to *treat* thromboembolism are often sufficient to *prevent* venous thrombosis, provided that they are given prior to surgery. The decision whether to give prophylaxis or not, and whether to use heparin and/or another approach such as graded pressure stockings, depends on patient factors (e.g. age, malignancy, obesity, immobility, and many other factors increase the risk of thromboembolism) and the nature of the surgical procedure (e.g. prolonged operations involving the hip or pelvis provide a greater thrombotic stimulus than shorter operations involving the periphery)(Seymour *et al.*, 1992). There is also need to balance the risks of bleeding against the risks of thromboembolism, and some of the newer forms of heparin may be used in selected conditions such as total hip replacement. Published guidelines of preoperative protocols for prophylaxis against thromboembolism are widely available (see, for example, SIGN Guideline 62, 2002), but in practice it is best to harmonize procedures with local guidelines.

PROPHYLAXIS AGAINST SEPSIS

Using antibiotics for prophylaxis against postoperative sepsis should not be confused with the use of full therapeutic courses of antibiotics once sepsis has occurred. In the former situation, the aim is to achieve high blood levels of an antibiotic at the time of the initial surgical incision and during the surgical procedure. Typically, this is achieved by giving an intravenous cephalosporin 30 minutes before surgery, followed by up to two further doses if the operative procedure is prolonged. While general reviews can set the scene (Scottish Intercollegiate Guidelines Network, 2000), local guidelines need to be followed, particularly as the sensitivity of bacteria to antibiotics varies from area to area. Guidelines also deal with the selection of patients for prophylaxis against sepsis. For instance, surgery on the gut has a much higher rate of postoperative sepsis than does a more peripheral procedure. However, risks and benefits also need to be balanced. For example, in elective joint surgery the risk of infection is low, but the consequences of infection are very serious and so there is a lower threshold for giving prophylactic antibiotics. Different preventive strategies need to be adopted when a patient has a preexisting heart valve lesion. Here, a surgical operation, a surgical procedure such as cystoscopy, or even a diagnostic procedure such as a barium enema, has the potential to provide a bacteremia that may lead to subsequent endocarditis.

CONCLUDING REMARKS

This chapter has been able to give only a brief introduction to the care of the elderly surgical patient, a subject on which whole textbooks are now being written. It is hoped that the conceptual framework of the chapter will allow the reader to pursue individual aspects of the subject in more detail, by reading some of the references, but more importantly by carrying out specific literature searches in response to the problems of individual elderly surgical patients. The optimal care of an elderly surgical patient requires an interdisciplinary approach from surgeons, anesthetists, physicians, nurses, and professions allied to medicine and many others and, for this reason, interdisciplinary organizations are now starting to emerge. These include the Age Anaesthesia Association founded several years ago by members of the Association of Anaesthetists of Great Britain and Ireland, but which also includes members from within surgical and medical specialties.

KEY POINTS

- The absolute and relative rates of surgery in old age are increasing year by year, but referral rates for elective surgery in very elderly patients may still be suboptimal.
- The major part of the statistical association between age and adverse postoperative outcome arises not as a result of aging itself, but through a secondary association with age-association disease.
- There is a growing body of evidence relating to the assessment, monitoring, and treatment of preoperative comorbidity and postoperative complications, but further targeted research work is needed in these areas.
- The American College of Cardiology/American Heart Association guidelines on perioperative evaluation for noncardiac surgery are of relevance in the cardiovascular assessment of older patients.
- In caring for older surgical patients in hospital, in addition to careful preoperative assessment, there is need for close scrutiny in the early postoperative period, particularly at the time when the older patient is transferred back to the general ward.

KEY REFERENCES

- Eagle KA, Berger PB, Calkins H *et al.* ACC/AHA guideline update for perioperative cardiovascular evaluation for noncardiac surgery – executive summary a report of the American College of Cardiology/American

Heart Association Task Force on Practice Guidelines. *Circulation* 2002; **105**:1257–67;OR *Journal of the American College of Cardiology* 2002; **39**:542–53, Available on www.acc.org or www.americanheart.org.

- Jin F & Chung F. Minimising perioperative adverse events in the elderly. *British Journal of Anaesthesia* 2001; **87**:608–24.
- Moller JT, Cluitmans P, Rasmussen LS *et al.* Long-term postoperative cognitive dysfunction in the elderly ISPOCD1 study. ISPOCD investigators. International Study of Post-Operative Cognitive Dysfunction. *Lancet* 1998; **351**:857–61.
- Rosenthal RA, Zenilman ME & Katlic MR (eds). *Principles and Practice of Geriatric Surgery* 2001; Springer, New York.
- The Association of Anaesthetists of Great Britain and Ireland. *Anaesthesia and Peri-operative Care of the Elderly* 2001; London, (available on www.aagbi.org).

REFERENCES

Abildstrom H, Rasmussen LS, Rentowl P *et al.* Cognitive dysfunction 1–2 years after non-cardiac surgery in the elderly. ISPOCD group. International Study of Post-Operative Cognitive Dysfunction. *Acta Anaesthesiologica Scandinavica* 2000; **44**:1246–51.

Alexander KP, Anstrom KJ, Muhlbaier LH *et al.* Outcomes of cardiac surgery in patients ≥80 years: results from the National Cardiovascular Network. *Journal of the American College of Cardiology* 2000; **35**:731–8.

Allison SP. Malnutrition, disease, and outcome. *Nutrition* 2000; **16**:590–3.

American College of Physicians. Preoperative pulmonary function testing. *Annals of Internal Medicine* 1990; **112**:793–4.

Avenell A & Handoll HHG. *Nutritional Supplementation for Hip Fracture Aftercare in the Elderly* Cochrane Database of Systematic Reviews 2004.

Awad W, Cooper G & Blauth C. Cardiac surgery in the elderly. *Journal of the Royal College of Physicians of London* 1995; **29**:252.

Badner NH, Knill RL, Brown FE *et al.* Myocardial infarction after noncardiac surgery. *Anesthesiology* 1998; **88**:572–8.

Bedford PD. Adverse cerebral effects of anaesthesia on old people. *Lancet* 1955; **2**:259–63.

Boersma E, Poldermans D, Bax JJ *et al.* for the DECREASE (Dutch Echocardiographic Cardiac Risk Evaluation Applying Stress Echocardiography) Study Group. Predictors of cardiac events after major vascular surgery: Role of clinical characteristics, dobutamine echocardiography, and beta-blocker therapy. *JAMA* 2001; **285**:1865–73.

Bogardus ST Jr, Desai M, Williams CS *et al.* The effects of a targeted multicomponent delirium intervention on postdischarge outcomes for hospitalized older adults. *American Journal of Medicine*. 2003; **114**:383–90.

Burchardi H & Kacmarczyk G. The effect of anaesthesia on renal function. *European Journal of Anaesthesiology* 1994; **11**:163–8.

Catley DM, Thornton C, Jordan C *et al.* Pronounced, episodic oxygen desaturation in the postoperative period: its association with ventilatory pattern and analgesic regimen. *Anesthesiology* 1985; **63**:20–8.

Celli BR. What is the value of preoperative pulmonary function testing? *The Medical Clinics of North America* 1993; **77**:309–25.

Crosby DL, Rees GAD & Seymour DG (eds). *The Ageing Surgical Patient: Anaesthetic, Operative and Medical Management* 1992; Wiley, Chichester.

de Dombal FT. Acute abdominal pain in the elderly patient. *Diagnosis of Acute Abdominal Pain* 1991, 2nd edn, pp 161–71; Churchill Livingstone, Edinburgh.

De Nino LA, Lawrence VA, Averyt EC *et al.* Preoperative spirometry and laparotomy: blowing away dollars. *Chest* 1997; **111**:1536–41.

Detsky AS, Abrams HB, McLaughlin JR *et al.* Predicting cardiac complications in patients undergoing non-cardiac surgery. *Journal of General Internal Medicine* 1986; **1**:211–9.

Dunlop WE, Rosenblood L, Lawrason L *et al.* Effects of age and severity of illness on outcome and length of stay in geriatric surgical patients. *American Journal of Surgery* 1993; **165**:577–80.

Dyer CB, Ashton CM & Teasdale TA. Postoperative delirium. A review of 80 primary data-collection studies. *Archives of Internal Medicine* 1995; **155**:461–5.

Eagle KA, Berger PB, Calkins H *et al.* ACC/AHA guideline update for perioperative cardiovascular evaluation for noncardiac surgery – executive summary a report of the American College of Cardiology/American Heart Association Task Force on Practice Guidelines. *Circulation* 2002; **105**:1257–67;OR *Journal of the American College of Cardiology* 2002; **39**:542–53, Available on www.acc.org or www.americanheart.org.

Eagle KA, Brundage BH, Chaitman BR *et al.* ACC/AHA Task Force Report. Guidelines for perioperative cardiovascular evaluation for noncardiac surgery. *Journal of the American College of Cardiology* 1996; **27**:910–48;OR *Circulation* 1996; **93**:1278–317.

Easton JD & Wilterdink JL. Carotid endarterectomy: trials and tribulations. *Annals of Neurology* 1994; **35**:5–17.

Eaton D, Bannister P, Mulley GP *et al.* Axillary sweating in clinical assessment of dehydration in ill elderly patients. *BMJ* 1994; **308**:1271.

Edwards AE, Seymour DG, McCarthy JM *et al.* A five year survival study of general surgical patients aged 65 years and over. *Anaesthesia* 1996; **51**:3–10.

Fogarty BJ, Parks RW, Rowlands BJ *et al.* Renal dysfunction in obstructive jaundice. *The British Journal of Surgery* 1995; **82**:877–84.

Gill NP, Wright B & Reilly CS. Relationship between hypoxaemic and cardiac ischaemic events in the perioperative period. *British Journal of Anaesthesia* 1992; **68**:471–3.

Goldman L, Caldera DL, Nussbaum SR *et al.* Multifactorial index of cardiac risk in noncardiac surgical procedures. *The New England Journal of Medicine* 1977; **297**:845–50.

Green J & Better OS. Systemic hypotension and renal failure in obstructive jaundice – mechanistic and therapeutic aspects. *Journal of the American Society of Nephrology* 1995; **5**:1853–71.

Gross CR, Lindquist RD, Woolley AC *et al.* Clinical indicators of dehydration severity in elderly patients. *The Journal of Emergency Medicine* 1992; **10**:267–74.

Hill GL. Surgical nutrition: time for some clinical common sense. *The British Journal of Surgery* 1988; **75**:729–30.

Howard L & Ashley C. Nutrition in the perioperative patient. *Annual Review of Nutrition* 2003; **23**:263–82.

Inouye SK. Predisposing and precipitating factors for delirium in hospitalized older patients. *Dementia and Geriatric Cognitive Disorders* 1999; **10**:393–400.

Inouye SK, Bogardus ST Jr, Charpentier PA *et al.* A multicomponent intervention to prevent delirium in hospitalized older patients. *The New England Journal of Medicine* 1999; **340**:669–76.

Inouye SK & Charpentier PA. Precipitating factors for delirium in hospitalized elderly persons. Predictive model and interrelationship with baseline vulnerability. *JAMA* 1996; **275**:852–7.

Inouye SK, Viscoli CM, Horwitz RI *et al.* A predictive model for delirium in hospitalized elderly medical patients based on admission characteristics. *Annals of Internal Medicine* 1993; **119**:474–81.

Jaeger AA, Hlatky MA, Paul SM *et al.* Functional capacity after surgery in elderly patients. *Journal of the American College of Cardiology* 1994; **24**:104–8.

Jensen MB & Hessov I. Randomization to nutritional intervention at home did not improve postoperative function fatigue or well being. *British Journal of Surgery* 1997; **84**:113–8.

Jin F & Chung F. Minimising perioperative adverse events in the elderly. *British Journal of Anaesthesia* 2001; **87**:608–24.

Jones MJT, Piggott SE, Vaughan RS *et al.* Cognitive and functional competence after anaesthesia in patients aged over 60: controlled trial of general and regional anaesthesia for elective hip or knee replacement. *BMJ* 1990; **300**:1683–7.

Katz NM, Hannan RL, Hopkins RA *et al.* Cardiac operations in patients aged 70 years and over: mortality, length of stay, and hospital charge. *The Annals of Thoracic Surgery* 1995; **60**:96–101.

Knaus WA, Wagner DP, Draper EA *et al.* The APACHE III prognostic system. Risk prediction of hospital mortality for critically ill hospitalized adults. *Chest* 1991; **100**:1619–36.

Knill RL, Moote CA, Skinner MI *et al.* Anesthesia with abdominal surgery lead to intense REM sleep during the first postoperative week. *Anesthesiology* 1990; **73**:52–61.

Kondrup J, Allison SP, Elia M *et al.* ESPEN guidelines for nutrition screening 2002. *Clinical Nutrition* 2003; **23**:415–21.

Lawrence VA, Dhanda R, Hilsenbeck SG & Page CP. Risk of pulmonary complications after elective abdominal surgery. *Chest* 1996; **110**:744–50.

Lawrence VA, Hilsenbeck SG, Mulrow CD *et al.* Incidence and hospital stay for cardiac and pulmonary complications after abdominal surgery. *Journal of General Internal Medicine* 1995; **10**:671–8.

Levinsky NG. Fluids and electrolytes. In KJ Isselbacher, E Braunwald, JD Wilson *et al.* (eds) *Harrison's Principles and Practice of Internal Medicine* 1994, 13th edn, pp 242–53; McGraw-Hill, New York.

Long CA, Marin P, Bayer AJ *et al.* Hypernatraemia in an adult in-patient population. *Postgraduate Medical Journal* 1991; **67**:643–5.

Lubin MF. Is age a risk factor for surgery? *The Medical Clinics of North America* 1993; **77**:327–35.

Lye M. Electrolyte disorders in the elderly. *Clinics in Endocrinology and Metabolism* 1984; **13**:377–98.

MacFie J, Woodcock NP, Palmer MD *et al.* Oral dietary supplements in pre- and post-operative surgical patients; a prospective and randomised clinical trial. *Nutrition* 2000; **16**:723–8.

Mangano DT. Perioperative cardiac morbidity. *Anesthesiology* 1990; **72**:153–84.

Mangano DT. Preoperative risk assessment: many studies, few solutions. Is a cardiac risk assessment paradigm possible? *Anaesthesiology* 1995; **83**:897–901.

Mangano DT & Goldman L. Preoperative assessment of patients with known or suspected coronary disease. *The New England Journal of Medicine* 1995; **333**:1750–6.

Marcantonio ER, Flacker JM, Wright RJ & Resnick NM. Reducing delirium after hip fracture: a randomised trial. *Journal of the American Geriatrics Society* 2001; **49**:516–22.

Marcantonio ER, Goldman L, Mangione CM *et al.* A clinical prediction rule for delirium after elective noncardiac surgery. *JAMA* 1994; **271**:134–9.

McBrien ME & Sellers WFS. A comparison of three variable performance devices for postoperative oxygen therapy. *Anaesthesia* 1995; **50**:136–8.

McIntyre KM, Vita JA, Lambrew CT *et al.* A noninvasive method of predicting pulmonary-capillary wedge pressure. *The New England Journal of Medicine* 1992; **327**:1715–20.

Mills SA. Cerebral injury and cardiac operations. *The Annals of Thoracic Surgery* 1993; **56**(suppl 5):S86–91.

Milne AC, Potter J & Avenell A. *Protein and Energy Supplementation in Elderly People at Risk from Malnutrition* Cochrane Database of Systematic Reviews 2004.

Moller JT, Cluitmans P, Rasmussen LS *et al.* Long-term postoperative cognitive dysfunction in the elderly ISPOCD1 study. ISPOCD investigators. International Study of Post-Operative Cognitive Dysfunction. *Lancet* 1998; **351**:857–61.

Moller JT, Johannessen NW, Espersen K *et al.* Randomized evaluation of pulse oximetry in 20,802 patients: II. Perioperative events and postoperative complications. *Anesthesiology* 1993b; **78**:445–53.

Moller JT, Pedersen T, Rasmussen LS *et al.* Randomized evaluation of pulse oximetry in 20,802 patients: I. Design, demography, pulse oximetry failure rate, and overall complication rate. *Anesthesiology* 1993a; **78**:436–44.

Mukherjee D & Eagle KA. Perioperative cardiac assessment for noncardiac surgery. Eight steps to the best possible outcome. *Circulation* 2003; **107**:2771–4.

National Confidential Enquiry into Peri-Operative Deaths (NCEPOD). *Recently Renamed National Confidential Enquiry into Patient Outcome and Death* Reports available from www.ncepod.org.uk.

Novis BK, Roizen MF, Aronson S *et al.* Association of preoperative risk factors with postoperative acute renal failure. *Anesthesia and Analgesia* 1994; **78**:143–9.

Olsson M, Janfjall H, Orth-Gomer K *et al.* Quality of life in octogenarians after valve replacement due to aortic stenosis. A prospective comparison with younger patients. *European Heart Journal* 1996; **17**:583–9.

Parks RW, Diamond T, McCrory DC *et al.* Prospective study of postoperative renal function in obstructive jaundice and the effect of perioperative dopamine. *The British Journal of Surgery* 1994; **81**:437–9.

Pateman JA & Hanning CD. Postoperative myocardial infarction and episodic hypoxaemia. *British Journal of Anaesthesia* 1989; **63**:648–50.

Phillips PA, Johnston CI & Gray L. Disturbed fluid and electrolyte homeostasis following dehydration in elderly people. *Age and Ageing* 1993; **22**:S26–33.

Poldermans D, Boersma E, Bax JJ *et al.* for the DECREASE (Dutch Echocardiographic Cardiac Risk Evaluation Applying Stress Echocardiography) Study Group. The effect of bisoprolol on perioperative mortality and myocardial infarction in high-risk patients undergoing vascular surgery. *The New England Journal of Medicine* 1999; **34**:1789–94.

Pulford EC & Connolly MJ. Respiratory disease in old age. *Reviews in Clinical Gerontology* 1996; **6**:21–39.

Redmond JM, Greene PS, Goldsborough MA *et al.* Neurologic injury in cardiac surgical patients with a history of stroke. *The Annals of Thoracic Surgery* 1996; **61**:42–7.

Reeder MK, Muir AD, Foex P *et al.* Postoperative myocardial ischaemia: temporal association with nocturnal hypoxaemia. *British Journal of Anaesthesia* 1991; **67**:626–31.

Reilly DF, McNeely MJ, Doerner D *et al.* Self-reported exercise tolerance and the risk of serious perioperative complications. *Archives of Internal Medicine* 1999; **116**:355–62.

Ricotta JJ, Faggioli GL, Castilone A *et al.* Risk factors for stroke after cardiac surgery: Buffalo Cardiac-Cerebral Study Group. *Journal of Vascular Surgery* 1995; **21**:359–64.

Rizzo JA, Bogardus ST Jr, Leo-Summers L *et al.* Multicomponent targeted intervention to prevent delirium in hospitalized older patients: what is the economic value? *Medical Care* 2001; **39**:740–52.

Rosenberg J. Hypoxaemia in the general surgical ward – a potential risk factor? *The European Journal of Surgery* 1994; **160**:657–61.

Rosenthal RA, Zenilman ME & Katlic MR (eds). *Principles and Practice of Geriatric Surgery* 2001; Springer, New York.

Rothwell PM, Slattery J & Warlow CP. A systematic review of the risks of stroke and death due to endarterectomy for symptomatic carotid stenosis. *Stroke* 1996a; **27**:260–5.

Rothwell PM, Slattery J & Warlow CP. A systematic comparison of the risks of stroke and death due to carotid endarterectomy for symptomatic and asymptomatic stenosis. *Stroke* 1996b; **27**:266–9.

Schor JD, Levkoff SE, Lipsitz LA *et al.* Risk factors for delirium in hospitalized elderly. *JAMA* 1992; **267**:827–31.

Scottish Audit of Surgical Mortality (SASM). Reports available from www.sasm.org.uk.

Scottish Intercollegiate Guidelines Network. *SIGN Guideline 45. Antibiotic Prophylaxis in Surgery* 2000; July, Available at www.sign.ac.uk.

Scottish Intercollegiate Guidelines Network. *SIGN Guideline 62. Prophylaxis of Venous Thromboembolism* 2002; October, Available at www.sign.ac.uk.

Scottish Intercollegiate Guidelines Network. *SIGN Guideline 77. Postoperative Management in Adults. A Practical Guide to Postoperative Care for Clinical Staff* 2004; August, (available on www.sign.ac.uk).

Seymour DG. The aging surgical patient – an update. *Reviews in Clinical Gerontology* 1999; **9**:221–44.

Seymour DG & Garthwaite PH. Age, deprivation category and rates of inguinal hernia surgery in men. Is there evidence of inequity of access to healthcare? *Age and Ageing* 1999; **28**:485–90.

Seymour DG & Pringle R. A new method of auditing surgical mortality rates: application to a group of elderly general surgical patients. *BMJ* 1982; **284**:1539–42.

Seymour DG, Rees GAD & Crosby DL. Introduction and general principles. In DL Crosby, GAD Rees & DG Seymour (eds) *The Ageing Surgical Patient: Anaesthetic, Operative and Medical Management* 1992, pp 1–90; Wiley, Chichester.

Seymour DG & Vaz FG. A prospective study of elderly surgical patients II. Post-operative complications. *Age and Ageing* 1989; **18**:316–26.

Shires GT & Canizaro PC. Fluid and electrolyte management of the surgical patient. In DC Sabiston (ed) *Textbook of Surgery. The Biological Basis of Modern Surgical Practice* 1986, 13th edn, pp 64–86; WB Saunders, Philadelphia.

Simpson BR, Williams M, Scott JF *et al.* The effects of anaesthesia on old people. *Lancet* 1961; **2**:887–93.

Sizer T, Russell CA, Wood S *et al.* Standards and Guidelines for Nutritional Support of Patients in Hospital. *A Report by a Working Party of the British Association for Parenteral and Enteral Nutrition* 1996; British Association for Parenteral and Enteral Nutrition (BAPEN), Maidenhead.

Smetana GW. Preoperative pulmonary evaluation. *The New England Journal of Medicine* 1999; **340**:937–44.

Smith HL, Sapsford DJ, Delaney ME *et al.* The effect on the heart of hypoxaemia in patients with severe coronary artery disease. *Anaesthesia* 1996; **51**:211–8.

Sotaniemi KA. Long-term neurologic outcome after cardiac operation. *The Annals of Thoracic Surgery* 1995; **59**:1336–9.

Sprigings DC. Cardiac surgery in the elderly: a cardiologist's perspective. *Heart* 1999; **82**:121–2.

Stausholm K, Kehlet H & Rosenberg J. Oxygen therapy reduces post-operative tachycardia. *Anaesthesia* 1995; **50**:737–9.

Surveillance for perioperative MI. *ACC/AHA Guideline Update on Peri-operative Cardiovascular Evaluation for Noncardiac Surgery* 2002, pp 41–2, Available on www.acc.org or www.americanheart.org.

Sweny P. Is postoperative oliguria avoidable? *British Journal of Anaesthesia* 1991; **67**:137–45.

The Association of Anaesthetists of Great Britain and Ireland. *Anaesthesia and Peri-operative Care of the Elderly* 2001; London, (available on www.aagbi.org).

Thomas JA & McIntosh JM. Are incentive spirometry, intermittent positive pressure breathing, and deep breathing exercises effective in the prevention of pulmonary complications after upper abdominal surgery? A systematic overview and meta-analysis. *Physical Therapy* 1994; **74**:3–16.

Tweedle DEF. Electrolyte disorders in the surgical patient. *Clinics in Endocrinology and Metabolism* 1984; **13**:351–76.

Unsworth-White MJ, Holmes L & Treasure T. Cardiac surgery in older people. *British Journal of Hospital Medicine* 1993; **49**:457.

Van Zee KJ & Lowry SF. *American College of Surgeons, Surgery vol 1* 1995; Section on Emergency Care, Chapter 11, pp 1–16; Scientific American, New York.

Vanoverschelde JL, Robert AR, Gerbaux A *et al.* Noninvasive estimation of pulmonary arterial wedge pressure with Doppler transmittal flow velocity pattern in patients with known heart disease. *The American Journal of Cardiology* 1995; **75**:383–9.

Walter PJ & Mohan R. Coronary bypass surgery in the elderly – a multi-disciplinary opinion. Summary of proceedings of an international symposium held at Antwerp, Belgium, March 9–11, 1994. *Quality of Life Research* 1995; **4**:279–87.

Weinberg AD, Minaker KL and The Council on Scientific Affairs, American Medical Association. Dehydration. Evaluation and management in older adults. *JAMA* 1995; **274**:1552–5.

Williams Russo P, Charlson ME, MacKenzie R *et al.* Predicting post-operative pulmonary complications. Is it a real problem? *Archives of Internal Medicine* 1992; **152**:1209–13.

Williams Russo P, Sharrock NE, Mattis S *et al.* Cognitive effects after epidural vs general anesthesia in older adults. A randomized trial. *JAMA* 1995; **274**:44–50.

Windsor JA. Underweight patients and the risks of surgery. *World Journal of Surgery* 1993; **17**:165–72.

Windsor JA & Hill GL. Weight loss with physiological impairment. A basic indicator of surgical risk. *Annals of Surgery* 1988; **207**:290–6.

Wood R & Bain M. Equity and healthy ageing. In R Wood & M Bain (eds) *The Health and Well-being of Older People in Scotland. Insights from National Data* 2001, pp 66–79; Information and Statistics Division, Common Services Agency for NHSScotland, Edinburgh, http://www.isdscotland.org/isd/files/older.pdf.

Zanardo G, Michielon P, Paccagnella A *et al.* Acute renal failure in the patient undergoing cardiac operation. Prevalence, mortality rate, and main risk factors. *The Journal of Thoracic and Cardiovascular Surgery* 1994; **107**:1489–95.

Zibrak JD, O'Donnell CR & Marton K. Indications for pulmonary function testing. *Annals of Internal Medicine* 1990; **112**:763–71.

138

Anesthesia in Older People

Suzanne Crowe

Adelaide & Meath Hospital incorporating the National Children's Hospital, Dublin, Ireland

INTRODUCTION

Elderly surgical patients present a specific challenge to anesthesiologists and may be at greater risk of an adverse outcome (Kazmers *et al.*, 1998). This is accounted for by a reduced ability to maintain or restore physiological homeostasis in the face of surgical and medical disease (Miller, 1998). This is exacerbated further by the presence of medical comorbidity such as cardiac or pulmonary disease or diabetes mellitus (Committee on Perioperative Cardiovascular Evaluation for Noncardiac Surgery, 1996). The statistical likelihood of having a coincident medical pathology increases with advancing years. The elderly have a higher rate of mortality associated with anesthesia and surgery than their younger counterparts. Postoperative adverse events on the cardiac, pulmonary, renal, and cerebral systems are the main concerns for older surgical patients at high risk. The very fact that the patient requires hospital admission for their surgery exposes them to risk, with familiar hazards including nosocomial infection, administration of the wrong drug, and side effects of certain procedures and investigations. Elderly patients are more likely to experience an adverse event during their hospital stay.

The elderly, and in particular those older than 85 years, are the fastest growing segment of the European and North American populations (Hall, 1997). Accordingly, overall life expectancy and active life expectancy have increased (General Office for Statistics, 1995). The number of older patients presenting for surgery and anesthesia is increasing and should not be a bar to surgery (Crosby *et al.*, 1992). The complexity of surgical procedures is also expanding. In 2001, The Association of Anaesthetists of Great Britain and Ireland called for this expansion to be recognized and incorporated into service provision. They also called for greater availability of 24-hour recovery facilities, High Dependency Unit (HDU), and Intensive Therapy Unit (ITU) bed for these patients. The National Confidential Enquiry into Perioperative Deaths (NCEPOD, 1999) has highlighted the importance of availability of high dependency and intensive care facilities for the safe care of older patients: "the decision to operate includes the commitment to provide appropriate supportive care".

This chapter elaborates on some of the risks to the elderly patient during the perioperative period and how they may be managed in order to minimize postoperative morbidity and mortality in this vulnerable patient group.

THE OUTCOME OF SURGERY AND ANESTHESIA IN THE ELDERLY

Mortality after surgery and anesthesia is defined as the death rate within 30 days (NCEPOD, 1999). The outcome of older patients from surgery, in general terms, has been studied by several authors in the past two decades (Chelluri *et al.*, 1992; Hosking *et al.*, 1989; Djokovic and Hedley-Whyte, 1979), suggesting that health-care practitioners have anecdotally identified areas for potential clinical improvement for many years. However, there are no recent surgical outcome studies for older patients. These early studies suggest that older patients have acceptable rates of perioperative mortality. There have been many advances in surgery and anesthesia, such as laparoscopic surgery, ultrashort-acting anesthetic medications, and regional pain management over the past two decades, reducing mortality rates (Table 1, Figure 1). Higher mortality rates are associated with higher American Association of Anesthesiologists (ASA) grade of physical status grade and emergency procedures (ASA, 1963). ASA is an independent predictor of mortality (Table 2). The highest risk surgical procedure in older patients is an exploratory laparotomy, because of the high risk of bowel infarction and disseminated carcinomatosis. The presence of preoperative renal, liver, and central nervous system impairment were predictors of poorer outcome.

Principles and Practice of Geriatric Medicine, 4th Edition. Edited by M.S. John Pathy, Alan J. Sinclair and John E. Morley.

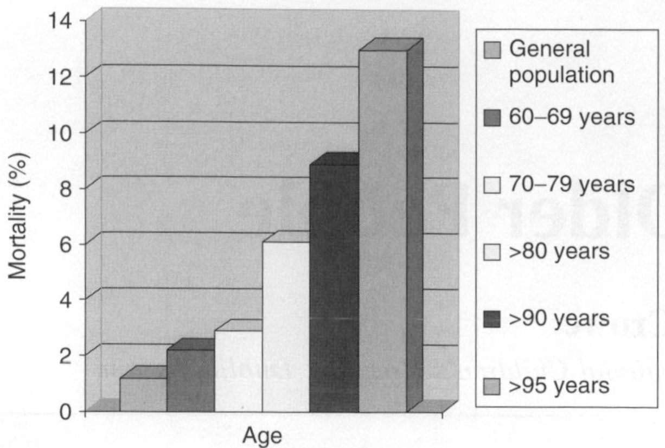

Figure 1 Mortality associated with surgery and anesthesia

Table 1 Mortality associated with surgery and anesthesia

Age (years)	Mortality rate
General population	1.2% (Pedersen *et al.*, 1990)
60–69	2.2% (Pedersen *et al.*, 1990)
70–79	2.9% (Pedersen *et al.*, 1990)
>80	5.8–6.2% (Djokovic and Hedley-Whyte, 1979)
>90	8.4% (Hosking *et al.*, 1989)
>95	13% (Djokovic and Hedley-Whyte, 1979)

Table 2 ASA grading of physical status (American Society of Anesthesiologists 1963)

Grade	
I	Normal healthy patient
II	Patient with mild systemic disease
III	Patient with severe systemic disease
IV	Patient with severe systemic disease which presents a constant threat to life
V	Moribund patient not expected to survive without operation

Source: Reproduced by permission of American Society of Anesthesiologists, Inc.

CARDIOVASCULAR MORBIDITY ASSOCIATED WITH SURGERY AND ANESTHESIA

The age-related changes that occur within the cardiovascular system are responsible for the higher incidence of perioperative myocardial infarction, cardiac failure, and arrhythmias in this age-group. There is a reduction in the sensitivity of the parasympathetic system to changes in baroreceptor stretch, blood pressure, and heart rate. The sensitivity of the sympathetic system also declines. This diminishes the body's ability to compensate for sudden change. There is a progressive stiffening of both the arterial and venous vessels, again reducing capacity for vasoconstriction or dilatation in the face of loss of intravascular volume. Stiffening of the myocardium occurs also, affecting diastolic relaxation and filling pressures. This may lead onto diastolic dysfunction with an increase in left atrial pressure and pulmonary congestion. Superimposed on physiological change, anesthetic agents cause peripheral vasodilatation, with a decrease in systemic vascular resistance. As many elderly patients have a contracted intravascular volume secondary to diuretic therapy, this can mean a sudden fall in tissue perfusion pressure. Anesthetic agents are myocardial depressants, particularly in higher doses, and have the capacity to adversely affect cardiac output.

Preoperative assessment is focused on identifying those risk factors that have been identified in studies as being predictive of adverse postoperative outcome (Table 3) (Goldman *et al.*, 1977; Eagle *et al.*, 1996). Following the initial interview, the patient's baseline level of function is assessed. If there are no significant predictors in the history, evaluation may be safely confined to detailed physical examination and a 12-lead electrocardiogram (ECG). ECG will identify patients with left ventricular hypertrophy or ST segment depression. These patients may require further investigation with an exercise ECG, depending on the surgical procedure planned. Patients who cannot exercise because of claudication or arthritis may be assessed with a dobutamine stress echocardiograph. Coronary angiography is reserved for patients with angina at rest or unstable angina. On the basis of the results, preoperative revascularization may be warranted. Clinically detected cardiac murmurs and features of congestive cardiac failure are further evaluated using echocardiography. Preoperative valve replacement is indicated for patients with severe disease. Less severe valve lesions or those following valve surgery require prophylactic antibiotic administration.

Arrhythmia detected at rest or during exercise should be treated if possible before surgery. If sinus rhythm is not achieved, rate control with anticoagulation is acceptable. Type II or type III heart block requires insertion of a temporary or permanent pacemaker.

Using the information gained from the history, examination, and further investigations, the anesthetic management is aimed at maximizing myocardial perfusion through maintenance of tissue perfusion pressure and oxygenation throughout the intraoperative and postoperative period. Postoperative admission to the HDU or intensive care unit should be anticipated for elderly patients with significant cardiac symptoms, especially those undergoing abdominal or thoracic procedures. Invasive monitoring of blood pressure and central venous pressure is commenced early and continued throughout the perioperative period. Regional anesthesia provides superior analgesia postoperatively and may reduce the

Table 3 Predictive factors for postoperative cardiovascular morbidity

Myocardial infarction within previous 3 months
Decompensated congestive cardiac failure
Arrhythmia (except premature atrial contractions)
Unstable angina or angina at rest (New York Heart Association Grade IV)
Uncontrolled hypertension
Severe valvular disease
Poor general medical condition
Poor exercise capacity
Diabetes mellitus
History of stroke

incidence of adverse cardiac events in certain patients, such as vascular and abdominal surgery. The institution of perioperative β-receptor blockade has been shown to reduce the risk of myocardial ischemia and is generally well tolerated by older patients (Poldermans *et al.*, 1999). β-blockade is thought to increase the time spent in diastole, increasing filling, and increasing time for coronary artery perfusion.

A combination of intravenous fluid infusion and vasopressor agents are used to maintain mean arterial blood pressure within 20% of the patient's baseline, awake blood pressure. Episodes of hypotension must be managed promptly and oxygenation increased during the period of reduced flow.

Postoperatively, the patient requires a similar level of care and monitoring. Supplemental oxygen therapy, optimum analgesia, rate control, and judicious blood transfusion will assist in maximizing myocardial oxygen supply.

Particular attention should focus on the first 3 days, when myocardial infarction is most likely to occur. Many episodes of ischemia in this age-group may be silent and may not be associated with the development of Q waves on the ECG. A low index of suspicion, the presence of new ST changes, in combination with serial estimations of serum troponin T and I concentrations will assist in early diagnosis.

RESPIRATORY MORBIDITY ASSOCIATED WITH SURGERY AND ANESTHESIA

The physiological changes associated with aging predispose the older patient to respiratory complications after surgery and anesthesia. A mixed obstructive/restrictive pattern develops from the decrease in total lung capacity, elastic recoil of the thorax, pulmonary parenchymal compliance, and vital capacity. Decreased compliance and muscle power mean a fall in forced expiration and reduced capacity to cough and clear secretions. Closing capacity, dead space, and residual volume increase so that the lungs of the supine patient become atelectatic. These changes do not occur in a uniform manner throughout the lungs, resulting in areas of good ventilation in combination with underventilated segments. A decrease in pulmonary blood flow combined with progressive loss of alveolar surface area diminishes the resting arterial oxygen tension from 95 ± 2 mmHg at age 20 to 73 ± 5 mmHg at 75 years. Occurring in tandem, there is an age-associated loss of central nervous system sensitivity to changes in arterial oxygen and carbon dioxide tensions. The physiological and structural changes cause an increase in ventilation/perfusion mismatch. This is exacerbated by the effect of anesthesia, in particular, general anesthesia. In addition, general anesthesia reduces reflex pulmonary hypoxic vasoconstriction. Regional anesthesia impacts less on the respiratory system as it does not necessitate intubation of the trachea, avoids the effect of intermittent positive pressure ventilation, and provides highly effective postoperative pain relief.

Preoperative preparation of the patient involves a detailed history and examination in combination with functional assessment. Taking the patient for a walk, including two flights of stairs, during the preoperative visit provides a useful measure of the patient's baseline physiological status. Smoking cessation for at least 8 weeks is to be recommended (Smetana, 1999). Chest physiotherapy in the 24 hours preceding surgery provides some physical benefit and facilitates instruction for deep breathing and coughing postoperatively. Patients with active pulmonary infection require more postponement of surgery and more aggressive medical treatment.

The anesthetic technique should employ regional analgesia/anesthesia where possible. Short-agents such as propofol, remifentanil, sevoflurane, and atracurium are most suitable for general anesthesia. Muscle relaxants should always be reversed at the end of the procedure. Invasive monitoring may be used to advantage to guide fluid therapy as the older patient will tolerate rapid expansion of intravascular and extravascular volumes poorly due to the changes in pulmonary compliance, perfusion, and renal function. This may be continued into the postoperative period in the context of intensive care or HDU admission. Postoperatively, oxygen supplementation and chest physiotherapy should be continued for a minimum of 5 days as this is the greatest period of risk of nocturnal hypoxia and the onset of pneumonia.

CENTRAL NERVOUS SYSTEM MORBIDITY ASSOCIATED WITH SURGERY AND ANESTHESIA

Elderly patients are at risk of serious central nervous system morbidity and mortality due to neuronal loss associated with aging, the presence of coincident pathology such as cerebrovascular atherosclerosis, and a reduction in neurotransmitter concentrations. This makes them less able to adapt successfully to the challenges imposed by surgery and anesthesia. The morbidity associated with anesthesia and surgery in the older patient most commonly takes the form of postoperative confusion (POC) or stroke.

Postoperative Confusion

The risk factors for the development of POC are listed in Table 4. POC is associated with an increased rate of morbidity, delayed return to baseline function, and delayed discharge home from hospital. To date, there is little evidence for an overall strategy to reduce the incidence in surgical patients, but some general recommendations may be made. Consideration should be given to admitting the patient as a daycase, as elderly patients become less disorientated when in familiar surroundings with familiar carers. The preoperative assessment should highlight particular issues that could be modified or preempted, such as alcohol withdrawal depression. Hearing aids and spectacles should be left with the patient until induction of anesthesia and returned to the patient a soon as possible. Medications listed

Table 4 Risk factors for the development of postoperative confusion

Preoperative factors
Older age
Depression/Anxiety
Dementia
Preoperative sensory deficit in hearing or vision
Alcohol withdrawal/Sedative withdrawal
Preoperative use of multiple medications
Intraoperative factors
Hypoxia
Hypocarbia
Hypotension
Postoperative factors
Inadequate analgesia
Perioperative factors
Sepsis
Surgical procedure
Cardiac surgery
Orthopedic surgery especially joint replacement
Perioperative medications
Anticholinergics: Atropine, scopolamine. Glycopyrrolate to a lesser extent
Barbiturates
Benzodiazepines
Antihistamines

in Table 3 should be avoided. Intraoperative monitoring of blood pressure, ventilation, and oxygenation requires a meticulous approach. Regional analgesic techniques should be employed where possible to reduce the use of sedating narcotics in the postoperative period. There is no difference in the incidence of POC between the intraoperative use of general anesthesia and spinal or epidural anesthesia (Chung *et al.*, 1997). Postoperatively, if the patient is confused, they should be nursed in a quiet, dark room. Organic causes should be treated promptly. Haloperidol 0.25–2 mg orally at night may be useful. Low doses of diazepam or chlorpromazine may be used as adjuncts if the patient does not respond to simple measures. Physical restraints usually serve to antagonize the patient further and should not be used. Referral to the occupational therapy and social work departments will be necessary to assist with cognitive assessment, follow-up, and discharge planning.

Long-term cognitive impairment has been documented by the International Study of Postoperative Cognitive Dysfunction (ISPOCD) (Moller *et al.*, 1998). Ten per cent of patients were found to have cognitive deficits 3 months after surgery, with age as the only significant predictive factor.

Postoperative Stroke

There have been few studies to determine the incidence of stroke occurring after surgery and anesthesia. The incidence from small retrospective studies would seem to suggest that the incidence is low–; in the order of 0.25% when a patient is undergoing noncarotid vascular surgery (Larsen *et al.*, 1988; Sultana *et al.*, 1997). Stroke most commonly occurs between the 5th and 26th day postoperatively. Risk factors for postoperative stroke are in Table 5 (Jin and Chung, 2001).

Table 5 Risk factors for postoperative stroke in the elderly

Preoperative factors:	Preexisting cerebrovascular disease
	Ischemic cardiac disease
	Atherosclerosis
	Carotid occlusion
	Preoperative vascular disease
	Hypertension
	Diabetes mellitus
	Physical inactivity
Intraoperative and postoperative factors:	Hemodynamic instability
	Hypoxemia

Source: From Jin and Chung (2001) Copyright The Board of Management and Trustees of the British Journal of Anaesthesia. Reproduced by permission of Oxford University Press/British Journal of Anaesthesia.

Patients with poorly controlled preoperative hypertension should have their surgery postponed to allow time to institute adequate pharmacological control. Patients with clinically detected carotid bruits should have further investigations and, if necessary, referral to a vascular surgeon before their intended procedure. The severity of the neurological deficit and the potential for rehabilitation after perioperative stroke varies enormously, and therapy must be directed at the individual patient.

RENAL MORBIDITY ASSOCIATED WITH SURGERY AND ANESTHESIA

Renal function is known to deteriorate with age, and, therefore, greater care will be needed to maintain renal function perioperatively. Decline in numbers of the functional unit, the glomerulus with age, means that glomerular filtration rate falls from 125 ml minute^{-1} in the young adult to 80 ml minute^{-1} in the older individual. As this fall in glomerular filtration rate (GFR) is usually accompanied by a decrease in muscle mass, there is rarely an increase in serum creatinine. During the perioperative period, the kidney will be exposed to many challenges: rapid fluid shifts in the intravascular and extravascular compartments, numerous medications administered simultaneously, electrolyte changes, and acid–base abnormalities (Epstein, 1996). In the face of these challenges, the underlying loss of function becomes exposed, leading to the development of postoperative renal failure. Atherosclerosis of the vascular supply of the kidney and coincident disease due to diabetes mellitus or hypertension further complicates the situation. In addition, the elderly patient tends to be taking a greater number of prescribed medications that have the potential to interact with anesthetic agents and conditions arising during surgery, such as hypotension.

Anesthetic drugs have little direct effect on renal function. Anesthetic agents reduce cardiac output with subsequent renal vasoconstriction, which may cause a fall in renal perfusion. Enflurane and isoflurane produce fluoride when metabolized, which may cause renal injury if the anesthesia is very prolonged. Sevoflurane produces a substance known as *compound A* at low fresh gas flows, which is nephrotoxic if not removed by effective scavenging of waste anesthetic gases (Conzen *et al.*, 2002). It is unusual for either of these chemical entities to present a problem in the clinical context.

Management of the patient starts with a high index of suspicion. Following a detailed preoperative review, fluid and electrolyte status should be closely monitored in the pre-, intra- and postoperative periods. Nephrotoxic medications should be stopped preoperatively if possible. Medications that deplete the intravascular volume and lead to electrolyte loss should be reviewed in the context of the patient's state of hydration and the planned surgical procedure. For example, a patient taking a loop diuretic scheduled for elective inguinal hernia repair should probably continue taking the medication, while a patient with low urinary output scheduled for emergency laparotomy for bowel obstruction should have the loop diuretic reviewed by the anesthesiologist. The dosing intervals of medications excreted by the kidney such as aminoglycosides may need to change and doses titrated to plasma levels. The development of perioperative renal failure increases the requirement for renal replacement, intensive care admission, and mortality. Acute tubular necrosis accounts for the majority of cases of renal failure. Prevention is based on optimizing the circulation preoperatively, close hemodynamic monitoring perioperatively, and maintenance of adequate perfusion pressures, including the judicious use of inotropes. Intraoperative low-dose dopamine infusion promoting renal vasodilatation and the use of mannitol as a free radical scavenger have been advocated (Kellum and Decker, 2001; Lameire *et al.*, 2003).

PERIOPERATIVE HYPOTHERMIA

Elderly patients are at a greater risk of developing perioperative hypothermia than younger patients owing to a number of factors. They have a reduced muscle mass, with a lower basal metabolic rate. This is often accompanied by reduced fat stores secondary to malnutrition. The shivering mechanism occurs later in response to cooling. In young patients, shivering begins peripherally at 1 °C less the normal core temperature of 36.5 °C. As patients age, this may not occur until their core temperature has fallen by 2 °C. Shivering increases cellular oxygen demands by 20–30%, increasing myocardial oxygen consumption, which may be deleterious for the older patient with cardiovascular pathology. Less vasoconstriction occurs in the older patient for a given fall in temperature, meaning that more heat is lost to the environment.

Surgery and anesthesia have a detrimental effect on thermoregulation. Anesthetic agents cause peripheral vasodilatation with abolition of the shivering mechanism so that patients lose the ability to compensate for cooling. The opening of major cavities such as the abdomen and thorax increases the amount of heat lost to the environment. The effect of perioperative hypothermia are listed in Table 6.

Prevention of hypothermia is more efficient and cost effective than warming the patient postoperatively. Patients should be kept in a warm room with blankets during their admission to the operating department. Induction of anesthesia should take place in a similar environment. Anesthetic gases should be warmed and humidified. Intravenous fluids should be warmed. Sterile preparation of the operative site should take place using warmed sterile solutions. A warm ambient temperature of the operating room should be maintained until the patient is draped. Forced air warming blankets may be placed under the drapes. At the end of the procedure, warm blankets should be placed over the patient during their transfer to the postanesthetic care unit.

Table 6 The effect of perioperative hypothermia

- Increased cardiac morbidity
- Increased incidence of cardiac arrhythmias
- Altered platelet function
- Increased blood loss
- Increased blood viscosity – combined with vasoconstriction may cause higher incidence of deep venous thrombosis
- Shift of oxygen dissociation curve to left with less oxygen released by hemoglobin to the tissues
- Inhalation of cold gases causes reduction in protective reflexes in respiratory tract through effects on cilia motility
- Increased incidence of postoperative wound infection
- Increased incidence of postoperative decubitus ulcers
- Decreased drug metabolism, resulting in longer recovery times
- Prolonged hospitalization

PREOPERATIVE ASSESSMENT

When carrying out a preoperative assessment of the older patient, it is important to place the function of the cardiovascular and respiratory systems into the context of the whole patient. It must be remembered that patients may have mild cognitive impairment affecting their memory, or they may be embarrassed and unwilling to admit disability. Answers may be slow as information is recalled. The history may be extensive and complicated and so sufficient time should be allotted to the interview. The clinical presentation of disease may differ greatly from that in younger patients. Conditions such as hyper and hypothyroidism are notoriously difficult to diagnose in the older patient. It is best if the assessment takes place several days before the planned surgery to allow enough time for further investigations if necessary. Attendance at a preanesthetic outpatient clinic will mean the patient can meet all of the multidisciplinary team members together, providing enhanced perioperative and discharge planning.

Following the interview, the anesthesiologist must review the patient's medical chart and carry out a comprehensive physical examination. Keeping in mind the demands and implications of each surgical procedure, the anesthetic plan will then be made and discussed with the patient. The anesthesiologist should expect much variation between each elderly patient. Routine investigations based on age alone are not warranted and should be directed by the clinical evaluation (Fleisher, 2001).

Particular issues to be addressed over the course of the assessment are:

1. The planned surgery. The surgical procedures most frequently carried out in the elderly are listed in Table 7.
2. The cognitive status of the patient. Does the patient answer questions in a coherent manner? Will they be suitable for ambulatory admission or a regional anesthetic technique?
3. The baseline function of the patient. Can they dress themselves; do the shopping, walk up a short flight of stairs?
4. Does the patient have symptoms suggestive of cardiac disease? Remember, patients may not report symptoms because of reduced mobility.
5. Does the patient have signs or symptoms of respiratory disease? Shortness of breath at rest is an important prognostic sign.
6. What are the patient's current medications and their compliance with them?
7. Previous anesthetic experiences.
8. Vital signs on examination especially blood pressure, pulse rate, and rhythm.

Meticulous attention to detail when planning the perioperative care of the patient can reduce the incidence of minor morbidity. Reduction of minor incidents may prevent escalation into life-threatening events.

Table 7 Pharmacological analgesic options

Agent	Advantages	Side effects
Acetaminophen (Paracetamol)	Oral and rectal route Opioid sparing	Hepatotoxicity, do not exceed 4 g/24 hours
NSAID	Oral, rectal, and parenteral route Opioid sparing	Gastric irritation Renal toxicity Antiplatelet effects
COX-II Inhibitors	Oral and parenteral route Opioid sparing Less severe gastric irritation and renal toxicity than NSAIDs	Gastric irritation Renal toxicity
Opioids	Oral, rectal, parenteral, spinal, epidural route Profound analgesia available as short-acting and long-acting preparations	Sedation/Confusion/Dysphoria Respiratory depression Metabolites may be toxic, for example, normeperidine Nausea/Vomiting Ileus Pruritus Urinary retention when administered into CSF/epidural space Bradycardia Hypotension especially if patient is dehydrated

NSAID, Non-steroidal Anti-Inflammatory; COX-II, Cyclo-oxygenase-II.

PAIN ASSESSMENT AND MANAGEMENT IN THE ELDERLY

Pain Assessment

Effective pain management in the elderly is subject to all of the usual barriers to pain management, such as fear of addiction. With the older surgical patient, there are additional problems to be overcome.

The assessment of pain forms the basis of successful pain relief. It is necessary to obtain a baseline measure of pain before instituting pharmacological measures to reduce that pain. Assessment allows the treatment to be evaluated and the need for further pain relief established (Katz and Melzack, 1999).

The needs of the older patient in assessing pain have not yet been fully met (Cook *et al.*, 1999). Conventional pain scores such as the visual analogue score (VAS) have limited application in this age-group due to the prevalence of mild/moderate cognitive impairment, hearing difficulties, and poor eyesight. The older patient may differ significantly in their cultural interpretation of pain and pain relief (Severn and Dodds, 1997).

Reporting of pain may be altered in this age-group because of the misperception among older patients that it is necessary for pain to follow surgery and that staff are doing all that they can to relieve it. They may also fear reporting that they have pain in case this means something has gone wrong, or that they may be seen as being "difficult". Health-care staff may mistake patients who do not report pain for patients who do not *have* pain. Attempts have been made to validate other scores such as the Faces Pain Score in older adults, but at present, there is no single system suitable for all elderly patients (Wong and Baker, 1988; Herr *et al.*, 1998). The accuracy of pain assessments may be increased by making the assessment more frequently, particularly following the administration of each analgesic dose.

Another hurdle to achieving adequate pain relief is the assumption that elderly patients do not experience pain to the same extent as younger patients. There is very little evidence for this misperception (Oberle *et al.*, 1990).

The Effect of Pain in Older Surgical Patients

The consequences of pain in surgical patients include (Ballantyne *et al.*, 1998; Rodgers *et al.*, 2000):

- sympathetic hyperactivity, producing tachycardia, myocardial ischemia, hypertension via the adrenal hormonal axis;
- decreased pulmonary function with atelectasis and hypoxemia, as a result of poor cough and reduced mobility;
- increased risk of deep venous thrombosis (DVT), as a result of reduced mobility;
- potential development of a chronic pain state through sensitization of pain pathways;

- postoperative delirium. This is particularly the case in patients who have predisposing risk factors for delirium such as visual, hearing, or cognitive deficit;
- increased length of stay.

Adequate pain relief in all patients may reduce postoperative morbidity (Ballantyne *et al.*, 1998).

The preoperative assessment visit should be used as an opportunity to discuss with the patient the postoperative analgesia pertinent for their procedure, particularly when regional analgesic techniques are planned. Education and reassurance may be provided to the patient and their family, diminishing their concerns regarding addiction and side effects. Instruction may be given on the use of equipment for patient controlled analgesia (PCA), which may be reinforced later by a visit from the acute pain team.

Pharmacological Management of Pain

A continuous, multimodal approach to postoperative pain management is indicated for elderly patients because it minimizes potential adverse effects from high doses of any single agent. Changes in drug absorption, distribution, metabolism, and elimination may affect the eventual plasma level and effect of a given analgesic drug. Increased gastric pH and decreased gastric motility reduce or delay drug absorption. The volume of distribution of drugs changes because of an increase in total body fat and a decrease in body water. Water-soluble opiates such as morphine have a smaller volume of distribution and therefore can produce higher plasma levels. Lipid-soluble drugs, such as fentanyl, have a larger volume of distribution and can produce a prolonged duration of action in older patients (Dodds, 1995). Reduced serum albumin concentrations and other plasma proteins from chronic illness or poor nutrition will reduce drug distribution, increasing the potential for adverse affects. Concurrent medical conditions, for example, renal impairment, may reduce excretion of the drug from the body. Liver disease may reduce drug metabolism and lead to accumulation of active drug and active drug metabolites. Reduced muscle mass leads to unpredictable absorption of drugs administered by the intramuscular route (Dodds, 1995).

The pharmacological analgesic options available are listed in Table 7. The key to effective pain management in patients of all ages is regular and appropriate assessment, combined with regular administration of multimodal analgesic agents.

The Role of Regional Analgesia

The intraoperative use of regional anesthetic techniques either in combination with general anesthesia or alone has been shown to reduce short- and long-term cardiac and mortality in the elderly following total hip arthroplasty, vascular surgery, and abdominal surgery. It is thought to do this by sympatholysis, attenuating the stress response and improving myocardial oxygenation. Regional analgesia continued into the postoperative phase provides more profound analgesia with lower doses of narcotics than intravenous opioid administration, thus minimizing the potential for sedation, respiratory depression, and ileus. It decreases the incidence of respiratory complications in patients undergoing abdominal and thoracic procedures and decreases admission rates to the intensive care unit and overall length of stay (Rodgers *et al.*, 2000). Regional analgesia decreases the rate of postoperative deep venous thrombosis due to relative vasodilatation of the venous plexus in the lower limbs and by decreasing the time to mobilization. Continuous epidural analgesia postoperatively can cause hypotension and lower extremity motor and sensory deficits. For this reason, nursing and medical staff require training on the recognition and management of potential complications of regional analgesic techniques.

The Role of Patient Controlled Analgesia (PCA) in the Elderly

Intravenous PCA has been shown to be safe in elderly patients (Egbert *et al.*, 1990), but health-care staff frequently hesitate to prescribe it because of the concern that it may cause confusion or inadequate analgesia in the older patient. Older patients should not be automatically excluded from using PCA, either via the intravenous or the epidural route. The cognitive state and physical abilities of each patient should be assessed on an individual basis.

ETHICAL CONSIDERATIONS FOR PERIOPERATIVE CARE OF THE ELDERLY

Decisions regarding surgery and anesthesia become more complicated in the older patient particularly when their ability to make a competent decision is compromised through cognitive impairment or illness. *Paternalism* on the part of the physician does not respect the patient's fundamental right to autonomy. Patients must be provided with the information they require, in a suitable format, to empower them with decision-making capacity. Informed consent leading to the choice of a treatment option or informed refusal of a treatment option must be respected by all professionals. If there is concern regarding the older patient's ability to assimilate information and decide, then further advice should be taken before deeming the patient "incompetent". Formal assessment of mental state may be necessary. If legal incompetence is concluded, decisions about the cessation or instigation of treatment may be taken by a proxy. This is often a family member. However, it may not be valid to assume that the proxy knows the wishes of a patient as they may never have discussed issues such as withdrawal of treatment. The proxy may be appointed on a formal basis through enduring power of attorney, or the patient may make their wishes known through an advanced directive. The legal standing of advanced directives varies across legal jurisdictions. If there is no proxy available, doctors may make decisions about care "in the best interests" of the patient. Efforts should be made early in the patient's admission to anticipate important decisions about medical care so that the patient may be involved as much as possible and proxy decision making is avoided. The patient's current and potential quality of life may impact on the decision to proceed to surgery or not.

Previously made decisions concerning resuscitation, often referred to as do-not-resuscitate (DNR) orders, should be revised before a patient is admitted to the operating department for surgery. The outcome of cardiac arrest differs greatly from that on the general ward, with 60% of patients surviving to hospital discharge compared with 7–17% of patients who sustain cardiopulmonary arrest on the ward (Martin *et al.*, 1991). This because cardiac arrest in the operating theater is monitored and witnessed, whereas a patient may be arrested on the ward for a variable length of time before resuscitation efforts begin. In addition, cardiac arrest in the operating theater is often due to reversible causes such as arrhythmia, medication administration or hypovolemia, which when promptly managed, restore adequate circulation to the patient. In the light of this, a patient with a terminal process such as pancreatic cancer, with a DNR order on the ward, may have this decision reversed during the period he is in the operating theater for palliative ileostomy, if that is what the patient wishes following informed consent.

Table 8 Summary of the anesthetic management of elderly patients

Preoperative assessment for identifying high-risk patients
Careful history
Physical examination
Twelve-lead ECG
Functional status assessment
Nutrition assessment
Preoperative preparation
Effective control of coexisting disease
Stopped smoking for 8 weeks
Training in cough and lung expansion techniques
Chest physiotherapy for elderly at risk of pulmonary complications
Correction of malnutrition
Routine precautions for major surgery
Temperature monitor and control
Ripple mattress
DVT prophylaxis
Intra-arterial pressure monitoring
Hemodynamic stability
Combination of anesthetic and vasopressor, β-blockers and vasodilatation
Avoid fluid overload
Quick recovery from anesthesia
Use short-acting anesthetic agents
Combine epidural anesthesia with GA for major abdominal and thoracic surgery
Antagonize neuromuscular blocking drugs
Postoperative period
Prevent hypoxemia: supplemental oxygen, reversal of neuromuscular drugs
Prevent hypothermia: keep warm perioperatively
Effective postoperative pain control: regular multimodal analgesia

Source: From Jin and Chung (2001) Copyright The Board of Management and Trustees of the British Journal of Anaesthesia. Reproduced by permission of Oxford University Press/British Journal of Anaesthesia.

STRATEGY TO REDUCE POSTOPERATIVE MORBIDITY AND MORTALITY IN THE ELDERLY

Reduction in anesthesia- and surgery-related morbidity and mortality involves a strategy that encompasses both individual organ systems and a wider view of the perioperative process (Table 8).

Preoperative Nutritional Supplementation

Up to 40% of older patients admitted to hospital are malnourished (McWhirter and Pennington, 1994).

Elderly patients with malnutrition are poor candidates for surgery and anesthesia, as it places them at particular risk from hypothermia, decubitus ulcers, drug overdose, local and systemic infection, anemia, and wound breakdown. The most common form of malnutrition in this age-group is protein-calorie malnutrition (Bonjour *et al.*, 1996). Low protein intake is associated with low intakes of calcium and vitamin D, both of which are necessary in the formation of callus after fracture. Loss of muscle secondary to malnutrition increases fatigability, decreases strength, and reduces the ability to maintain adequate ventilation.

The evidence from recent studies, including a Cochrane review, suggests that nutritional supplementation should be confined to those patients who are malnourished, in order to achieve an acceptable risk-benefit ratio, where side effects to the patient are balanced against a demonstrable clinical effect (Avenell and Handoll, 2000). The evidence to date suggests that simple oral supplements are the optimum method of supplementation as oral supplementation is more cost effective, more tolerable, and psychologically more acceptable to patients than nasogastric or parenteral nutrition. It has not been extensively studied however.

Simple qualitative assessment of nutritional status on admission to hospital may be carried out as part of the routine nursing assessment (Allison, 1995). Because of the prevalence of poor nutrition in older patients presenting for surgery, prompt preoperative referral to a dietician of all patients who are deemed malnourished on nursing assessment should take place. This will facilitate early institution of simple oral supplementation in the postoperative phase, with nasogastric supplementation in patients who are severely malnourished. The emphasis should be on restoring function and decreasing perioperative morbidity rather than rapid weight gain.

Prevention of Perioperative Decubitus Ulcers

The older surgical patient presents a unique challenge to the perioperative care team in the prevention of pressure ulcers. It is suggested that 25% of pressure ulcers are acquired intraoperatively (Aronovitch, 1999). For many patients, pressure ulcers mean increased pain, longer hospital stays, and reduced quality of life. A pressure ulcer can be defined as an area of localized damage to the skin and underlying tissue, caused by a disruption in the blood supply, preventing oxygen and vital nutrients from reaching the cells (EPUAP, 1998). Schultz *et al.* (1999) suggested that a pressure sore beginning in the operating theater develops initially in muscle and the subcutaneous tissues before progressing outwards to the dermis and epidermis. This causes an erythematous area, which may be mistaken for a burn. This may go on to become an established pressure sore. Pressure sores occurring in surgical patients are often not attributed to their time spent in theater, as the initial damage may not be apparent until several hours or days have passed (Vermillion, 1990).

The development of a pressure ulcer is considered to be largely preventable with the implementation of an effective preventive strategy (EPUAP, 1998), and the occurrence of pressure ulcers has been used as a proxy measurement of quality care.

Anesthetized patients are subjected to prolonged pressure on dependent body parts as neither the position or duration of surgery can be altered. Duration of surgery is a major risk factor in pressure ulcer formation, in conjunction with the patient's level of tissue tolerance and the support surface. Other risk factors for pressure ulcer formation have been well established (Table 9). A constellation of these features is frequently found in the older patient presenting for surgery.

On the basis of the literature to date, prevention of decubitus ulcers in the perioperative period should concentrate on the following points:

Table 9 Risk factors for the development of perioperative decubitus ulcers

Extrinsic
Pressure
Shear
Friction
Moisture
Intrinsic
Age (>40 years)
Nutritional status
Body mass index
Comorbidity
Core temperature
Low diastolic pressure
Low serum albumin
Immobility prior to surgery
Operating room factors
Duration of surgery
Surgical position
Type of mattress
Positioning devices
Warming devices
Epidural anesthesia/analgesia
Anesthetic agents
Type of surgery
Extracorporeal circulation
Inappropriate manual handling

- early assessment of risk factors, combined with full history and clinical examination;
- meticulous attention during manual handling, particularly after the patient has been anesthetized;
- caution during positioning for surgery;
- specialized table mattresses such as alternating air devices or gel overlays should be used for patients at particular risk;
- maintain normothermia;
- maintain diastolic blood pressure above 35 mmHg;
- low-dose local anesthetic infusions for regional analgesic techniques;
- frequent reevaluation.

The Role of Daycase Admission

There is no upper age limit for daycase admission, and older patients may benefit cognitively from reduced disruption to their daily environment and routine. Prior consultation at the preoperative assessment clinic should screen patients for suitability. Patients should be medically stable and able to understand simple instructions with regard to medications and fasting. A reminder telephone call the evening before surgery is useful in encouraging compliance. Patients require a responsible companion to accompany them home and to stay overnight. It is this issue that most often causes difficulty. Community services and follow-up need to be in place before the patient leaves the hospital.

Choice of Surgical Approach

The appropriateness of the surgery may need to be reviewed in older patients who, because of their preoperative baseline, are at particular risk of a poor outcome. Unnecessary surgery that exposes the patient to a high risk/low benefit ratio should not be undertaken without expert opinion and full informed consent from the patient. If possible, a less invasive surgical approach may be utilized, for example, thoracoscopic evacuation of hemothorax or laparoscopic-assisted colonic resection. These techniques result in less pain, a quicker recovery, and a shorter hospital stay.

Perioperative Audit

There is an important role for perioperative audit in the care of the older surgical patient. Attendance at preoperative assessment clinics, proportion of patients cancelled for medical reasons on the morning of surgery, unplanned admission to the intensive care unit, incidence of postoperative myocardial infarction, patient satisfaction, and 30-day mortality are just a few examples of outcome measures that may provide scope for audit and implementation of change in individual surgical units.

CONCLUSIONS

Good anesthetic care of the older person involves an assiduous approach to both minor and major elements of the perioperative process. The preparation of the patient begins early and is best carried out in a multidisciplinary unit that is focused on the needs of the elderly. Most information required to plan the anesthetic may be gained from a detailed history and clinical examination of the patient. Occasionally, special investigations or preparatory procedures are required.

Short-acting agents and/or regional anesthesia are recommended, providing there are no special indications for general anesthesia or contraindications to regional techniques. Provision of adequate pain relief with regular assessment and formal charting of pain scores should be adopted as routine practice. Fluid and electrolyte management should not be left to the most junior member of the team – consideration of the fluid, electrolyte, and nutritional needs of the patient should be a priority throughout the perioperative course. Oxygen supplementation should be continued routinely to reduce the incidence of hypoxemia preoperatively and postoperatively.

KEY POINTS

- Advanced age is not a barrier to anesthesia and surgery.
- Anesthesia should be carried out, or closely supervised, by an anesthesiologist with sufficient experience of anesthesia in elderly patients.
- Adequate time must be allocated for a detailed preoperative assessment.
- Invasive monitoring and regional anesthesia should be utilized liberally.
- The intraoperative anesthesia care should be viewed as part of a continuum, with therapy such as oxygen supplementation, analgesia, and fluid management continued into the postoperative period.

KEY REFERENCES

- Ballantyne JC, Carr DB, deFerranti S *et al.* The comparative effects of postoperative analgesic therapies on pulmonary outcome: cumulative meta-analyses of randomized, controlled trials. *Anesthesia and Analgesia* 1998; **86**:598–612.
- Jin F & Chung F. Minimizing perioperative adverse event in the elderly. *British Journal of Anaesthesia* 2001; **87**(4):608–24.
- Lameire NH, De Vriese AS & Vanholder R. Prevention and nondialytic treatment of acute renal failure. *Current Opinion in Critical Care* 2003; **9**(6):481–90.
- McWhirter JP & Pennington CR. Incidence and recognition of malnutrition in hospital. *British Medical Journal* 1994; **308**:945–8.
- Moller JT, Cluitmans P, Rasmussen LS *et al.* Long-term postoperative cognitive dysfunction in the elderly ISPOCD1 study. ISPOCD Investigators. International Study of Postoperative Cognitive Dysfunction. *Lancet* 1998; **351**:357–61.

REFERENCES

Allison SP. Cost-effectiveness of nutritional support in the elderly. *The Proceedings of the Nutrition Society* 1995; **54**(3):693–9.

American Society of Anesthesiologists. New classification of physical status. *Anesthesiology* 1963; **24**:11.

Aronovitch SA. Intraoperatively acquired pressure ulcer prevalence: a national study. *Journal of Wound, Ostomy and Continence Nursing* 1999; **26**(3):130–6.

Avenell A & Handoll HH. Nutritional supplementation for hip fracture aftercare in the elderly. *Cochrane Database Systematic Review* 2000; **4**:CD001880.

Ballantyne JC, Carr DB, deFerranti S *et al.* The comparative effects of postoperative analgesic therapies on pulmonary outcome: cumulative meta-analyses of randomized, controlled trials. *Anesthesia and Analgesia* 1998; **86**:598–612.

Bonjour JP, Schurch MA & Rizzoli R. Nutritional aspects of hip fractures. *Bone* 1996; **20**:79–82.

Chelluri L, Pinsky MR & Grenvik AN. Outcome of intensive care of the 'oldest old' critically ill patients. *Critical Care Medicine* 1992; **20**:757–61.

Chung F, Meier R, Lautenschlager E *et al.* General or spinal anesthesia: which is better in the elderly? *Anesthesiology* 1997; **67**:422–7.

Conzen PF, Kharash ED, Czerner SF *et al.* Low flow sevoflurane compared with low flow isoflurane anesthesia in patients with stable renal insufficiency. *Anesthesiology* 2002; **97**(3):578–84.

Cook AKR, Niven CA & Downs MG. Assessing the pain of people with cognitive impairment. *International Journal of Geriatric Psychiatry* 1999; **14**:421–5.

Crosby DL, Rees GAD & Seymour DG (eds) *The Ageing Surgical Patient: Anaesthetic, Operative and Medical Management* 1992; Wiley, London.

Djokovic JL & Hedley-Whyte J. Prediction of outcome of surgery and anesthesia in patients over 80. *Journal of the American Medical Association* 1979; **242**:2301–6.

Dodds C. Anaesthetic drugs in the elderly. *Pharmacology & Therapeutics* 1995; **66**:369–86.

Eagle KA, Brundage BH, Chaitman BR *et al.*, Report of the American College of Cardiology/American Heart Association Task Force on Practice Guidelines. Committee on Perioperative Cardiovascular Evaluation for Noncardiac Surgery. Guidelines for perioperative cardiovascular evaluation for noncardiac surgery. *Circulation* 1996; **93**:1278–317.

Egbert AM, Parks LH, Short LM & Burnett ML. Randomized trial of postoperative patient-controlled analgesia vs. intramuscular narcotics in frail elderly men. *Archives of Internal Medicine* 1990; **150**:1897–903.

Epstein M. Aging and the kidney. *Journal of the American Society of Nephrology* 1996; **7**:1106–22.

European Pressure Ulcer Advisory Panel. A policy statement on prevention of pressure ulcers. *British Journal of Nursing* 1998; **7**(15):888–90.

Fleisher LA. Routine laboratory testing in the elderly: is it indicated? *Anesthesia and Analgesia* 2001; **93**:249–50.

General Office for National Statistics. *Life Tables and Mortality Statistics* 1995; Her Majesty's Stationary Office, London.

Goldman L, Calderal DL & Nussbaum SR. Multifactorial index of cardiac risk in non-cardiac surgical procedures. *The New England Journal of Medicine* 1977; **297**:845–50.

Hall WJ. Update in geriatrics. *Annals of Internal Medicine* 1997; **127**:557–64.

Herr KA, Mobilly PR, Kohout FJ & Wagenaar D. Evaluation of the faces pain scale for use with the elderly. *The Clinical Journal of Pain* 1998; **14**(1):29–38.

Hosking MP, Lobdell CM, Warner MA *et al.* Anaesthesia for patients over 90 years of age. Outcomes after regional and general anaesthetic techniques for two common surgical procedures. *Anaesthesia* 1989; **44**:142–7.

Jin F & Chung F. Minimizing perioperative adverse event in the elderly. *British Journal of Anaesthesia* 2001; **87**(4):608–24.

Katz J & Melzack R. Measurement of pain. *Surgical Clinics of North America* 1999; **79**:231–52.

Kazmers A, Perkins AJ & Jacobs LA. Outcomes after abdominal aortic aneurysm repair in those >80 years of age: recent veterans affairs experience. *Annals of Vascular Surgery* 1998; **12**:106–12.

Kellum JA & Decker JM. Use of dopamine in acute renal failure: a meta-analysis. *Critical Care Medicine* 2001; **29**(8):1526–31.

Lameire NH, De Vriese AS & Vanholder R. Prevention and nondialytic treatment of acute renal failure. *Current Opinion in Critical Care* 2003; **9**(6):481–90.

Larsen SF, Zaric D & Boysen G. Postoperative cerebrovascular accidents in general surgery. *Acta Anaesthesiologica Scandinavica* 1988; **32**:698–701.

Martin RL, Soifer BE & Stevens WC. Ethical issues in anesthesia. Management of the do-not-resuscitate patient. *Anesthesia and Analgesia* 1991; **73**:221–5.

McWhirter JP & Pennington CR. Incidence and recognition of malnutrition in hospital. *British Medical Journal* 1994; **308**:945–8.

Miller R. The biology of aging and longevity. In WR Hazzard & JP Blass (eds) *Principles of Geriatric Medicine and Gerontology* 1998; McGraw-Hill, New York.

Moller JT, Cluitmans P, Rasmussen LS *et al.* Long-term postoperative cognitive dysfunction in the elderly ISPOCD1 study. ISPOCD Investigators. International Study of Postoperative Cognitive Dysfunction. *Lancet* 1998; **351**:357–61.

National Confidential Enquiry into Peri-Operative Deaths. Department of Health, London, November 1999.

Oberle K, Paul P & Wry J. Pain, anxiety and analgesics: a comparative study of elderly and younger surgical patients. *Canadian Journal on Aging* 1990; **91**:13–22.

Pedersen T, Eliasen K & Henriksen E. A prospective study of mortality associated with anaesthesia and surgery: risk indicators of mortality in hospital. *Acta Anaesthesiologica Scandinavica* 1990; **34**:176–82.

Poldermans D, Boersma E, Bax JJ *et al.*, Dutch Echocardiographic Cardiac Risk Evaluation Applying Stress Echocardiography Study Group. The effect of bisoprolol on perioperative mortality and myocardial infarction in high-risk patients undergoing vascular surgery. *The New England Journal of Medicine* 1999; **341**(24):1789–94.

Rodgers A, Walker N, Schug S *et al.* Reduction of postoperative mortality and morbidity with spinal and epidural anaesthesia: results from overview of randomized trials. *British Medical Journal* 2000; **321**:1493, www.bmj.org.

Schultz A, Bein M, Dumond K *et al.* Aetiology and incidence of pressure ulcers in surgical patients. *AORN* 1999; **70**(3):434–9.

Severn AM & Dodds C. Cognitive dysfunction may complicate assessment of pain in elderly patients. *British Medical Journal* 1997; **315**:551.

Smetana GW. Preoperative pulmonary evaluation. *The New England Journal Medicine* 1999; **340**:937–44.

Sultana CJ, Campbell JW, Pisanelli WS *et al.* Morbidity and mortality of incontinence surgery in elderly women: an analysis of medicare data. *American Journal of Obstetrics and Gynecology* 1997; **176**:344–8.

The Association of Anaesthetists of Great Britain and Ireland. *Anaesthesia and Peri-Operative Care of the Elderly* 2001; AAGBI, London.

Vermillion C. OR acquired pressure sores. *Decubitus* 1990; **3**(1):26–30.

Wong D & Baker C. Pain in children: comparison of assessment scales. *Pediatric Nursing* 1988; **14**(1):9–17.

FURTHER READING

Howell SJ, Sear YM, Yeates DM *et al.* Risk factors for cardiovascular death after elective surgery under general anesthesia. *Brit Journal of Anesthesia* 1998; **80**:14–9.

139

Health Issues in the Aging Female

Carolyn D. Philpot
Saint Louis University School of Medicine, St Louis, MO, USA

CANCER

Cancer is one of the leading causes of death in women (Levi *et al.*, 2001). The aging female is at risk for endometrial, ovarian, breast, cervical, vulvar, and vaginal cancer. Since there is risk with increasing age, reviewing the risk factors are important to help promote a good quality of life. Proper screening, early detection, treatment, and management of comorbidities are essential.

Endometrial Cancer

Endometrial cancer is the fourth most common malignancy in women after breast, colorectal, and lung cancer. Peak incidence occurs in women between 50 and 60 years of age, and the incidence appears to be climbing. The 5-year survival rate for all stages of endometrial cancer has been estimated at 65%.

Risk factors include nulliparity, obesity, and prolonged use of unopposed exogenous estrogen. The most common symptom is postmenopausal vaginal bleeding.

Besides a physical examination and pap smear, a pelvic ultrasonography and either a endometrial biopsy or dilation and curettage is required for diagnosis or exclusion of diagnosis of endometrial cancer. (A positive Pap test for endometrial cancer will only show in 35–50% of the cases and should not be the only determinant in diagnosis.) Optimal treatment is a hysterectomy with bilateral oophorectomy, and dissection of the retroperitoneal lymph nodes in the pelvic and para-aortic region (Geisler and Geisler, 2001). Additional treatment, such as chemotherapy, radiation or both may also be indicated for advanced stages of cancer and discussion is needed with the patient's oncologist and geriatrician to weigh the risks with the benefits.

Ovarian Cancer

After endometrial cancer, ovarian cancer is the second most common gynecological malignancy. Peak incidence occurs in women aged between 50 and 60. Risk factors include uninterrupted ovulation (nulliparity or contraceptive usage) and inherited genetic mutations.

Symptoms usually are nonspecific. Abdominal pain, abdominal distention, and gastrointestinal disturbances are complaints sometimes voiced from women with ovarian cancers, but symptoms may not develop until late in the disease process. Screening, except for high-risk patients, may include ultrasonography and tumor markers; however, it is thought to be of limited value.

Ovaries are generally small and not palpable in the postmenopausal woman and if, upon physical exam, an ovary is able to be palpated, immediate evaluation is warranted since it is suggestive of ovarian cancer. Initial treatment involves surgical removal of the tumor. Chemotherapy may be considered depending on the tumor stage, the patient's comorbidities, and benefits versus risks. Since most ovarian cancers are detected when the tumor is advanced, long-term prognosis is usually poor.

Breast Cancer

Approximately 50% of all new breast cancer cases occur in women over the age of 65. The incidence of breast cancer increases up to the age of 80, levels out between the ages of 80 and 85, and then is thought to decline. It is difficult to evaluate those over 85 years owing to limited data.

Risk factors for developing breast cancer may include personal or family history of breast cancer and/or colon or endometrial cancer in first-degree relatives, nulliparity or late first pregnancy at 31 years of age or older, late menopause, early menarche, abdominal obesity, estrogen replacement therapy, history of atypical hyperplasia on biopsy for benign breast disease (Chlebowski *et al.*, 2003).

Screening for breast cancer in a postmenopausal woman includes monthly self–breast examinations, an annual physical exam by a physician or other health-care provider, and a yearly, or every 2 years, mammogram. Research has shown that screening for breast cancer in women aged 50 to 70

Principles and Practice of Geriatric Medicine, 4th Edition. Edited by M.S. John Pathy, Alan J. Sinclair and John E. Morley.

has improved survival by early detection. There are many doctors that feel that mortality could be reduced 25–30% if all women received proper mammographic screening. There is limited data on breast screening in woman over 70 years, but it is thought that mammography is of benefit. Since 10–20% of all breast cancers are not picked up on mammography, physical examination is also important.

Less than 50% of all women 65 years or older have ever had a mammogram, and those who have had a mammogram, have obtained one on a routine basis. There has been argument among physicians against instituting routine screening for breast cancer in the elderly woman, stating that disability and shorter life expectancy may have a direct effect on the desirability and cost-effectiveness of screening. On the other hand, the life expectancy of a healthy woman in her mid-to-late 70s is approximately 10 more years, and for a healthy woman aged 85, 7 more years. Thus, screening appears to be warranted.

The clinical characteristics of breast cancer are the same, despite the age of the individual. Cancer is generally suspected when breast lesions palpated feel firm or abnormalities are detected on mammography. A palpable breast mass in a postmenopausal woman requires immediate attention since most palpable masses are malignant. All breast masses in this age-group should have a biopsy whether the mass was palpated and/or detected on mammography.

Prognosis is determined by the stage of the disease. Owing to lack of clinical studies, it is unclear if women over the age of 65 have the same clinical course as compared to that of younger women. The course of treatment is prompted by the stage of the disease. Until recently, many elderly women with breast cancer were not aggressively treated; however, today many older women with breast cancer are working with their oncologists and geriatricians discussing various treatment options.

Cervical Cancer

Cervical cancer occurs in women of all ages but its incidence peaks in women aged 40 to 50 years (Benedet *et al.*, 2001). Symptoms vary and hinge on the stage of the tumor. Some women may be asymptomatic, while others may show clinical signs of postmenopausal or postcoital bleeding. Routine Pap testing is the best method of screening. If the Pap test results are positive, colposcopy-directed biopsies and endocervical curettage are used to establish diagnosis.

Radical hysterectomy is the recommended treatment for cervical cancer. Adjuvant radiation or chemotherapy may also be used. The combined cure rate for all cervical cancers is 50–60%.

Vulvar Cancer

Vulvar cancer accounts for approximately 3–4% of all gynecological malignancies in the United States (Beller *et al.*, 2001a). The average age at diagnosis is 70 years, and the incidence increases with age. The most common symptoms exhibited in vulvar cancer are vulvar pruritus, pain, and a palpable vulvar lesion; however, many women are asymptomatic (Hyde *et al.*, 2002). A discharge may be present. Histology generally reveals squamous cell carcinoma. Biopsy may be indicated for diagnosis. Treatment is generally surgical and for extensive lesions, a radical vulvectomy with unilateral or bilateral inguinal lymphadenectomy is recommended. Radiation and chemotherapy may also be considered adjuvant therapy. Prognosis for early-staged lesion are generally favorable. The 5-year survival rate is 80–90% if there is no metastasis to the lymph node and 16–30% if lymph node metastasis is present.

Vaginal Cancer

Vaginal cancer is relatively rare (Beller *et al.*, 2001b). The average age at diagnosis is 60 to 65 years. It is estimated that 95% of these lesions are squamous cell carcinomas. Vaginal bleeding or discharge is an early symptom. Pain or postcoital bleeding may be exhibited in sexually active women. Where the tumor involves the anterior vaginal wall, it may cause dysfunction with voiding, since the vaginal wall may invade into the urethra. Biopsy is indicated for diagnosis. Radiation therapy is the main choice of treatment; however, surgery and chemotherapy may be utilized in specific cases. Prognosis is dependant upon the size and location of the tumor. The 5-year survival rate for all types is estimated to be from 25–48%.

MENOPAUSE

Menopause is the permanent cessation of menses as a result of ovarian aging. It is clinically diagnosed after 12 months of amenorrhea. The perimenopausal transition is defined as the time prior to the permanent cessation of menses and is identified with irregular menstrual cycles. Transitional time has been shown to vary in length from 2 to 8 years.

The average age, in the United States, at which menopause occurs is 51.

Early symptoms of menopause include irregular menstrual cycles, headache, fatigue, changes in mood and cognition, insomnia, and hot flashes (Table 1). Some women may experience vertigo, heart palpitations, and tachycardia. A later clinical presentation may include urinary incontinence, dry skin, breast changes, genital atrophy with dyspareunia, vaginitis, and cystitis.

Early symptoms of menopause is often irregular menstrual periods. They may vary in frequency, duration, and blood flow amount. Menstrual bleeding that is unusually heavy, lasts more than 10 days, or that occurs more often than once every 3 weeks should be clinically evaluated for possible neoplasms.

Another early symptom of menopause is hot flashes. About 80% of perimenopausal women report hot flashes

Table 1 Signs and symptoms of menopause

Irregular menstrual cycle
Insomnia
Hot flashes
Mood swings
Cognitive changes
Skin changes
Genitourinary atrophy
Headache
Fatigue
Vertigo
Heart palpitations/tachycardia

and up to 50% of these women may continue to have symptoms for up to 5 years. Hot flashes may also occur after surgical menopause. Research shows that short-term use of hormone replacement therapy (HRT) will help relieve severe vasomotor symptoms, but will not abolish symptoms.

Women who have had bilateral salpingo oophorectomy are at high risk for cardiovascular disease. This is especially true if HRT was not initiated. Early natural menopause is also at high risk.

Diagnosing menopause may be determined by elevated serum levels of follicle-stimulating hormone. Estrogen replacement therapy is the best treatment for symptoms of menopause. Duration of estrogen replacement therapy is controversial and each case should be reviewed for risk versus benefit.

Postmenopausal Vaginal Bleeding

About 20–30% of postmenopausal vaginal bleeding is due to atypical adenomatous endometrial hyperplasia or endometrial cancer. It may also be caused by the use of estrogen or progesterone or by genital atrophy resulting from low estrogen levels.

History taking should include past and present gynecological problems. A drug history should indicate whether any exogenous estrogens were used. A pelvic and bimanual exam should be performed to rule out any trauma, tumors, or bleeding from atrophic sites. A Pap test should also be performed to aid in diagnosis. Transvaginal ultrasonography may be useful for diagnosis. If the endometrial thickness is less than 5 mm, cancer or endometrial hyperplasia is doubtful. Endometrial thickness over 5 mm is suspicious for malignancy and further work-up is promptly warranted. Endometrial biopsy may then be indicated as well as a full fractional dilatation and curettage (D & C).

If postmenopausal bleeding is found to be cancerous, then treatment should be tumor specific. If cancer is nondetected, estrogen is initiated because it may be secondary to atrophy. For those women taking exogenous hormones, the estrogen dosage may need to be decreased and progesterone increased. If bleeding continues, a more aggressive work-up is needed.

Postmenopausal Hormone Replacement Therapy

Approximately 6 million women in the United States are taking HRT. The use of estrogen ranges from relief of postmenopausal symptoms to what was assumed, until recently, long-term health benefits. Until recently, it was felt that estrogen replacement had a protective effect against cardiovascular disease. From the data collected by the Heart and Estrogen/Progestin Replacement Study Follow-up (HERS II) trial and other recent secondary prevention studies, the new recommendations are against initiating or continuing its use for the primary prevention of cardiovascular disease. The Women's Health Initiative (WHI) study stated that estrogen and progestin therapy should not be initiated or continued for the primary prevention of coronary heart disease and was suggestive that it may stimulate breast cancer growth and hinder breast cancer diagnosis. This combination of hormone replacement also showed an increase in pulmonary embolus.

Sexual Dysfunction in the Menopausal Woman

Many women have experienced a lack of interest (decreased libido) or arousal in sexual activity (sexual arousal disorder), achieving orgasm (female orgasmic disorder), or have had pain prior or during sexual activity (dyspareunia) (Gutmann, 2005; Kingsburg, 2004). When one or more of these symptoms occur, causing anguish and interference with interpersonal relationships, it is diagnosed as female sexual dysfunction (FSD). The exact prevalence is unknown; however, one survey found that more than 40% of women aged 18 to 59 alluded to having sexual dysfunction. It has also been suggested that the prevalence of FSD increases while women are going through menopause transition.

Perimenopausal and postmenopausal women have repeatedly reported that they have lost an interest in sex and do not find sex "pleasurable". Studies have shown that there is a decline in sexual functioning from early to late perimenopause. In late perimenopausal to postmenopausal women, studies reveal that there is a decrease in libido and sexual responsitivity, an increase in dyspareunia, and a decline in sexual activity. Screening questions that are useful for FSD are given in Table 2.

The causes of FSD are multifactorial. Hormonal, physical, and psychosocial changes are key components of FSD.

Table 2 Screening questions for female sexual dysfunction

1. Are you currently involved in a sexual relationship? With men? With women? Both? Multiple partners?
2. How often do you engage in sexual activity? Intercourse? Masturbation?
3. Do you feel that your sex drive has changed? Less? Same? Increased?
4. Do you have difficulty in obtaining an orgasm? Inability? Pain with?
5. Are you satisfied with your current sexual relations?
6. Do you have any sexual concerns that you would like to discuss?

Hormonal Changes

There is a decline of circulating androgens during the late reproductive years. Androgen deficiency is associated with a decline in libido, decline in sensitivity to sexual stimulation, and arousability.

Estrogen deficiency can cause changes in the genitourinary system. Estrogen therapy, both topical and systemic, has been shown to improve vaginal atrophy, increase blood flow to the vagina and increase lubrication.

Physical Changes

In addition to the hormonal changes that occur in the genitourinary system, other conditions can contribute to FDS. Limited movement or pain from arthritis may be a factor. Recent pelvic surgery or trauma is another. Some medications, such as, antihistamines, antidepressants, and blood pressure medication can lead to a decreased libido and inability to achieve orgasm.

Psychosocial Changes

A woman may have concerns over the well being of her sexual partner. If she or her sexual partner is ill, or have a debilitating disease, it can have a direct impact on sexual function. Women, who live longer than men, often are without a sex partner. Not having a partner does not mean they are no longer in need of nurturing, affection, and physical contact. Depression and anxiety can contribute to FDS.

Research has shown that only 14% of Americans aged 40 to 80 have been asked by their doctor if they had any sexual problems within the past 3 years. Since this number is relatively small, the physician or health-care provider needs to remember to inquire about the patient's sexual health along with the history taking during physical exam.

Data from a large survey has indicated that 68% of men and women thought their physician would be uncomfortable talking about sex, and 71% thought that if sexual problems were disclosed, nothing would be done about the problem. Only 14% out of 1384 women ever reported sexual problems to their health-care provider in a study conducted by the American Association of Retired Persons. Of those women discussing sexual problems, most confer with their gynecologist rather than their private medical doctor (PCP). It is felt that physicians do not talk about sex because of a lack of education, comfort and confidence, and lack of time and treatment options (Table 2).

OSTEOPOROSIS

Osteoporosis is a major risk factor for fractures in the older population and is estimated to account for approximately 1.5 million low trauma fractures yearly (Ribeiro *et al.*, 2000). The lifetime risk of sustaining a fracture to the spine (symptomatic), hip or distal radius in white women is approximately 40% (while only 13% in white men) aged 50 years and older. The 6-month mortality rate from a hip fracture is approximately 10–20%. Of the survivors, about 25% will require assisted or nursing home care and approximately 50% will require an assistive device to aid in their ambulation. Osteoporotic fractures are associated with annual costs in the United States ranging between 7 and 20 billion dollars. One to one-and-a-half percent of all hospital beds in Europe are occupied by patients with osteoporosis. This European figure is expected to more than double in the next 50 years. In the United States, the estimated prevalence of osteoporosis is 8 million in women and 2 million in men and the estimated related health costs exceed 14 billion dollars annually. Primary osteoporosis occurs mainly in older people aged 51 to 75 years, and can be arranged in two groups: postmenopausal osteoporosis and age-related bone loss (senescence). The incidence of primary osteoporosis is six times more common in women than in men. Women are at higher risk because they have a lower peak bone mass compared to men and have an acceleration of bone loss during menopause.

Primary osteoporosis is thought to be atypical in premenopausal women, while secondary osteoporosis composes only a small amount of elderly women. (Elderly women may have a combination of both primary and secondary osteoporosis.)

Age-related bone loss is complex and multifactorial. As one ages, changes occur in cortical bone, trabecular bone, and bone marrow. Studies show that there is a decline in bone mineral density after the third decade of life and continues to decline at a rate of approximately 0.5% per year. During menopause, women, however, have an accelerated bone mineral density loss at an estimated rate of 3–5%.

Hormonal changes of vitamin D and reduction of calcium absorption also have an impact on aging bone. Vitamin D levels decrease with age and vitamin D deficiency in elderly people is common. Absorption rates also decline by 40%. Aging changes in skin reduce the amount of 7-dehydrocholesterol, the precursor and rate of conversion of vitamin D_3. Declining renal function leads to a drop of activity of 1-α-hydroxylase, which is responsible for the activation of vitamin D_3. Lower calcium levels then occur from these changes causing activation of the calcium sensor receptor in the parathyroid gland. Parathyroid hormone is secreted, stimulating osteoclast activity, which keeps serum calcium levels in homeostasis at the price of bone mineralization. Secondary osteoporosis may also have many other conditions causing bone loss such as various endocrine and neoplastic abnormalities, gastrointestinal disease, and drug usage (Table 3).

Osteoporosis has no symptoms; therefore, a thorough evaluation is critical for detection of osteoporosis. Assessment begins with a complete history alluding to its risk factors as stated in Table 4. Major risk factors for osteoporosis

Table 3 Secondary causes of osteoporosis

Endocrine
Hyperthyroidism
Cushing's syndrome
Osteomalacia
Paget's disease
Primary hyperparathyroidism
Gastrointestinal
Malabsorption syndromes
Alcoholism
Neoplastic states
Bone Metastases
Multiple myeloma
Medication
Glucocorticoids
Anticonvulsants
Excessive thyroid hormone replacement

Table 4 Risk factors for osteoporosis

Advanced age
Female gender
Race (more prevalent among white, Asian, and Hispanic decent)
Heredity (approximately 50–80% of peak bone mass is genetically determined)
Small body size/weight (<127 pounds)
Smoking
Alcoholism
Sedentary lifestyle/immobility
Low dietary calcium/vitamin D intake
History of previous fractures/falls
Decrease long life exposure to estrogen
Certain medication (anticonvulsants, gluccocorticoids, thyroid hormone, barbiturates)
Caffeine use
Early menopause or oophorectomy

are increased age, female, ethnicity, and thin body habitus. History of previous fracture(s) needs further assessment, focusing on whether the fracture occurred with only minimal trauma (suggestive of low bone density). Physical examination for osteoporosis should look for secondary causes. For example, an ill, cachectic woman may need assessment for malnutrition, malignancy, or malabsorption syndrome. A loss of body height may indicate vertebral compression fracture(s), or dorsal kyphosis from osteoporosis may be seen on clinical exam.

Laboratory evaluation should reflect clinical findings. All women with osteoporosis should receive a chemistry profile including electrolytes, kidney and liver function, glucose, calcium, phosphorus, and albumin. They should also have a complete blood count to rule out anemia and malignancy. Thyroid function should be assessed in women over 50 years. Other lab tests should be ordered as individually warranted such as 25(OH)-vitamin D and parathyroid hormone for those with low serum calcium to look for vitamin D deficiency and secondary hyperparathyroidism.

The combination of history taking, physical examination, and lab tests will help in diagnosing osteoporosis or other secondary causes.

Bone densitometry is the only test which confirms diagnosis of osteoporosis in the absence of fracture. To confirm diagnosis of primary osteoporosis, one needs to rule out secondary osteoporosis, malignancy, and osteomalacia. Although many women have some type of knowledge about osteoporosis, health-care providers need to educate the general population about the importance of taking certain steps to aid in its prevention. Treatment includes providing calcium and vitamin D supplementation, which can reduce the risk of fracture up to 30%. Estrogen therapy can prevent bone loss in menopausal women and is the treatment of choice in postmenopausal women. The second best choice in the treatment of osteoporosis is the use of biphosphonates. This group of drugs increases bone mass, thus decreasing the risk for fractures. Other medications used include selective estrogen receptor modulators and calcitonin. Other treatment modalities include exercise with a focus on muscle strengthening, weight bearing, and balance. Direct effects on bone may be relatively small but will aid in decreasing the incidence of falls which may lead to fractures (Messinger-Rapport and Thacker, 2002).

KEY POINTS

- The Women's Health Initiative has decreased the enthusiasm for hormone replacement therapy in older women.
- Screening for cancer remains important in older women.
- Female sexual dysfunction is a relatively common problem in older women.
- Osteoporotic fractures are a major cause of disability and mortality in older women.

KEY REFERENCES

- Blair KA & White N. Are older women offered adequate health care? *Journal of Gerontological Nursing* 1998; **24**(10):39–44.
- Chlebowski RT, Hendrix SL, Langer RD *et al.* Influence of estrogen plus progestin on breast cancer and mammography in healthy postmenopausal women. *The Journal of the American Medical Association* 2003; **289**:3243–53.
- Kingsburg S. Just ask! talk to patients about sexual function. *Sexuality, Reproduction and Menopause* 2004; **2**(4):199–203.
- Messinger-Rapport BJ & Thacker HL. Prevention for the older woman: a practical guide to prevention and treatment of osteoporosis. *Geriatrics* 2002; **57**(4):16–27.

REFERENCES

Blair KA & White N. Are older women offered adequate health care? *Journal of Gerontological Nursing* 1998; **24**(10):39–44.

Beller U Sideri M, Maisonneuve P *et al.* Carcinoma of the vulva. FIGO annual report. *Journal of Epidemiology and Biostatistics* 2001a; **6**:153.

Beller U Sideri M, Maisonneuve P *et al.* Carcinoma of the vagina. FIGO annual report. *Journal of Epidemiology and Biostatistics* 2001b; **6**:141.

Benedet JI Odicino F, Maisonneuve P *et al.* Carcinoma of the cervix. FIGO annual report. *Journal of Epidemiology and Biostatistics* 2001; **6**:5.

Chlebowski RT, Hendrix SL, Langer RD *et al.* Influence of estrogen plus progestin on breast cancer and mammography in healthy postmenopausal women. *The Journal of the American Medical Association* 2003; **289**:3243–53.

Geisler JP & Geisler HE. Radical hysterectomy in the elderly female: a comparison to patients age 50 or younger. *Gynecologic Oncology* 2001; **80**:258.

Gutmann JN. Exploring sexual dysfunction in the menopausal woman. *Sexuality, Reproduction, and Menopause* 2005; **3**(1):8–11.

Hyde SE, Ansink AC, Burger MP *et al.* The impact of performance status on survival in patients 80 years and older with vulvar cancer. *Gynecologic Oncology* 2002; **84**:388.

Kingsburg S. Just ask! talk to patients about sexual function. *Sexuality, Reproduction, and Menopause* 2004; **2**(4):199–203.

Levi F, Lucchini F, Negri E *et al.* Changed trends of cancer mortality in the elderly. *Annals of Oncology* 2001; **12**(10):1467–77.

Messinger-Rapport BJ & Thacker HL. Prevention for the older woman: a practical guide to prevention and treatment of osteoporosis. *Geriatrics* 2002; **57**(4):16–27.

Ribeiro V, Blakeley J & Laryea M. Women's knowledge and practices regarding the prevention and treatment of osteoporosis. *Health Care for Women International* 2000; **21**(4):347–53.

140

Antiaging

Alfred L. Fisher
University of California, San Francisco, CA, USA

INTRODUCTION: WHAT IS ANTIAGING MEDICINE AND WHY IS IT APPEALING?

Antiaging medicine involves the use of treatments specifically designed to slow, prevent, or reverse the effects of aging on people, which is in contrast to medical treatments that prevent or treat specific diseases. While proponents describe this approach as "the future of medicine", in fact, the search for the "fountain of youth" is hardly a new endeavor (Gammack and Morley, 2004). For example, stories about specific plants or bodies of water that convey eternal youth are common in ancient mythology, and the Bible contains references to a River of Immortality that flowed from the Garden of Eden. More recently in the thirteenth century, Roger Bacon suggested that a balanced diet, exercise, rest, and the "breath of a virgin" would extend life span. Ponce de Leon, the colonial governor of Puerto Rico, discovered Florida while searching for Bimini, where the Fountain of Youth was reportedly located. Even Nobel laureates were not immune to the seduction of antiaging therapies. Elie Metchnikoff believed aging was due to toxins released by the gut, and ate yogurt in an attempt to ward off the effects of these toxins. Linus Pauling took mega doses of vitamin C as an antiaging treatment. While many of these early stories are amusing, the rapid increase in knowledge about the biologic mechanisms involved in aging and the physiologic changes associated with aging have made the quest for antiaging therapies more rational, and due to the establishment of companies dedicated to developing antiaging therapies, more serious than ever.

The current plausibility of antiaging therapies combined with two other powerful social forces has fueled the explosion in interest and spending on antiaging therapies. These two forces are the growth of the Internet and the graying of many Western countries. First, the Internet now provides anyone the opportunity to exchange information or opinion about any topic on websites with little to no supervision. As health is an important topic to most people, an internet search on any health related topic will literally yield thousands to hundreds of thousands of "hits", each linked to a unique website. Some websites provide accurate and helpful information while others provide incorrect information and yet others provide information intended to sell a product that is also available on the same website. Along with being a source of information, the Internet has also developed into a virtual shopping mall for thousands of small businesses to sell wares around the globe. Second, the populations of the United States, Western Europe, and Japan are aging with a significant increase in the numbers of individuals older than 50 years. This "newly old" population is in better physical health than prior generations and often has had the experience of watching their parents age and cope with the consequences. Consequently, there has been a rise in interest in holistic approaches and disease prevention. These two forces have created a ready marketplace of interested consumers who are interested in and willing to purchase antiaging treatments.

The growth of the antiaging medicine movement and the progress of biogerontologists in unraveling basic mechanisms involved in aging have also had impacts upon the geriatrics community. Some in the geriatrics community have been drawn into the battle between antiaging medicine providers and biogerontologists about the relative lack of safety or effectiveness data for any of the currently touted antiaging therapies (Olshansky *et al.*, 2002). Antiaging medicine providers have also attacked the field of geriatrics as being unnecessary because of the dramatic effects that antiaging treatments will have on human aging. Often it seems that the discussion of antiaging treatments has become so overtaken with hyperbole that rational discussion has fallen by the wayside (Turner, 2004). This has left many in the geriatrics community skeptical about the claims of either antiaging medicine providers or biogerontologists, while at the same time uneasy about the social and health effects of success emanating from either camp.

This chapter will explore the topic of antiaging therapies on multiple levels. First, the idea of an antiaging treatment will be defined and the rationale for thinking why such a treatment could ever be developed will be discussed.

Principles and Practice of Geriatric Medicine, 4th Edition. Edited by M.S. John Pathy, Alan J. Sinclair and John E. Morley.

Second, some currently touted antiaging therapies along with the data, or the lack of data, supporting their use will be presented. Finally, the ethical issues behind the development and the use of antiaging treatments and the potential effects of a successful treatment in the field of geriatrics will be discussed.

WHAT IS AN ANTIAGING THERAPY?

Aging has multiple effects on people. The aging phenotype involves cosmetic changes like gray hair and wrinkles, physiologic changes like decreases in cardiovascular or pulmonary function and physiologic reserves, psychological changes like declines in short-term memory, and medical changes such as a marked increase in susceptibility to a large number of diseases as well as an increased risk for functional decline. An antiaging therapy could similarly act in one or more ways to counteract the aging process or its direct effects (Fisher and Hill, 2004). Specifically, an antiaging treatment could modify the biochemical and molecular events involved in aging and hence directly address the aging process. Alternately, an antiaging therapy could act more indirectly to either lessen the susceptibility to age-associated diseases or to correct physiologic changes associated with aging that result in aspects of the aging phenotype. Obviously, an intervention could work in multiple ways as exercise, for example, both corrects physiologic changes associated with aging by correcting declines in physical strength and stamina in part due to sarcopenia and also decreases the susceptibility to disease by raising HDL (high-density lipoprotein) cholesterol and preventing osteoporosis. Interestingly, therapies that act to lessen the susceptibility to age-associated disease are already commonly used in conventional medicine practice as preventive care practices, such as mammography, immunizations, colonoscopy, hypertension treatment, and cholesterol screening, and have as an expressed goal the prevention of diseases that increase in prevalence along with age. While these preventative care practices would never have been considered antiaging therapies, their goals do overlap with those of antiaging medicine. Consistent with this, most guidelines for preventive care include recommended ages for when to start screening and treatment. As preventive medicine is well known among physicians and discussed in detail both in the other chapters of this text and elsewhere, this chapter will instead focus on "antiaging" therapies that are intended to directly modify the aging process or its direct consequences.

The terms "antiaging medicine" or "antiaging therapy" are applied rather broadly in popular culture. Often, magazine articles or television programs will refer to cosmetic procedures like face-lifts, the use of botulinum toxin (Botox) to minimize wrinkles, or teeth whitening as "antiaging medicine". However, these treatments do not have any real effect on the aging process or its direct effects on individual health and functioning, and hence for the purposes of this chapter do not represent "antiaging" therapies. Furthermore, the providers of plastic surgery, Botox, or teeth whitening neither intend or claim to alter the effects of aging at a biochemical level or to improve the health or functioning of any organ systems. Instead, these procedures simply represent temporary measures to address specific cosmetic aspects of the aging phenotype.

Consequently, an antiaging therapy should have three features: (1) the medication or treatment acts by modifying the aging process or its direct effects; (2) it should promote continued good health or reduce disability; and (3) it should not simply be targeted to symptoms associated with normal aging (Fisher and Hill, 2004). First, an antiaging medicine or therapy by definition should act to address either the aging process or its direct effects on molecules, cells, tissues, or organs. An antiaging therapy needs to alter causal mechanisms related to aging such as oxidative stress, unfolded proteins, cell senescence, or hormone changes. Prolonging life by itself is not a true measure of a therapy, as immunization, proper sanitation, use of seat belts, and specific disease treatments, such as the use of aspirin in patients with coronary artery disease, can all produce increased longevity without being an antiaging therapy. A therapy can either act in a specific tissue or can act systemically.

Second, the use of an antiaging therapy should promote continued good health or reduce disability. An important goal of antiaging medicine is to address two major failings of treatments focused on specific diseases, which are the decline of overall patient health and functioning over time due to aging, and the related increase in disability. An antiaging therapy should address the causative role that aging plays in future disease and disability. A true failure, both from the societal and individual perspective, would be a treatment that simply results in the prolongation of poor health and functional disability, such as prolonging time in a nursing home.

Third, an antiaging therapy should not simply target symptoms associated with the aging phenotype, like gray hair, wrinkled skin, or normal short-term memory loss, without having some effect on the underlying aging process and altering its role in health and disease. Symptomatic treatment is an important part of geriatric medical care, and it is common in geriatrics to use treatments that mask symptoms, such as the use of pain control medications, or to minimize the functional effects of symptoms, for example, through the prescription of adaptive devices. Furthermore, cosmetics, hair dye, aesthetic dentistry, or cosmetic surgery procedures can be a useful way for patients to cope with aging. However, none of these treatments can rightly be thought of as providing benefit beyond altering temporarily the experience of aging.

ARE PATIENTS USING ANTIAGING THERAPIES?

While there is little information about the exact number of antiaging medicine providers, the number of patients using treatments, and the amount of money spent yearly on antiaging treatments, the use of antiaging treatments clearly do contribute to the $4 billion spent annually on alternative and complementary treatments (Butler, 2000). The American Academy of Anti-Aging Medicine ("A4M") reports having 12 500 members on their official website (http://www.worldhealth.net/, accessed June 30, 2004). Furthermore, the Internet contains literally millions of websites dedicated to providing information on, and selling, antiaging therapies as a Yahoo search done on June 30, 2004 with the search term "antiaging" yielded 3 490 000 hits. Additionally, a Harris Interactive poll conducted in October 2002 found that while the majority of those surveyed were skeptical of antiaging therapies and providers, 7% of those surveyed had either personally used or knew someone who used an antiaging therapy (Harris Interactive Inc., 2003). Over half of this group felt that the therapy was either very beneficial or somewhat beneficial while only 27% felt it was harmful. Hence, while the number of antiaging treatment users is small at this time, there are enough current users to support a fairly significant number of providers and vendors of products. These antiaging medicine users seem to be satisfied overall with the products and services and probably have become loyal repeat patients.

IS THERE A SCIENTIFIC BASIS FOR ANTIAGING THERAPIES? (*see* Chapter 2, A Biological Perspective on Aging)

During the last 10–15 years, knowledge about the aging process in humans and lower animals has greatly expanded. Both genetic and drug interventions have produced significant increases in longevity in model animals and have helped elucidate biologic mechanisms involved in the normal aging of these animal species (Guarente and Kenyon, 2000). While a complete understanding of the aging process is still far off, some basic principles about aging have emerged. Though no current product has been conclusively shown to alter one of these mechanisms and alter human aging, it is reasonable to assume that future drugs will be designed and tested, with a few, perhaps, being effective. The next section will briefly discuss some of the biologic mechanisms involved in aging in lower animals and presumably in humans, which represent potential targets for current and future aging therapies.

OXIDATIVE STRESS

As early as the 1950s, aging was proposed to be, at least in part, due to the collective damage to proteins, lipids, and nucleic acids from oxidative stress (Harman, 2003). The generation of chemical energy by mitochondria, destruction of pathogens by immune cells, and many other catabolic and anabolic biochemical reactions produce reactive oxygen or reactive nitrogen species. These species can then chemically modify and consequently damage proteins, DNA, or lipids either in cells or in tissues (Table 1). With sufficient damage to cellular proteins and DNA, cell and organ dysfunction could occur and result in aging of the animal. Study of aged model animals has shown the accumulation of oxidative damage with markers of oxidative damage being elevated two to three fold between reproductive maturity and death.

Consistent with the hypothesis, the scavenging of reactive oxygen species either by antioxidants or proteins with antioxidant actions results in increased longevity of experimental animals (Table 1). Additionally, many of the genetic

Table 1 Antiaging therapies

Aging mechanism	Effects	Treatment strategy	Treatment	Evidence of benefit from human studies
Oxidative stress	Damage to lipids, proteins, and DNA	Antioxidants	Vitamin A	−−¶
			β-carotene	+/−
			Vitamin C	+/−¶
			Vitamin E	+/−¶
			α-Lipoic acid	+/−
Hormone changes	(1) Production of symptoms associated with aging through reductions in hormone levels from young adulthood.	(1) Hormone replacement	(1) Growth hormone	−−
			Estrogen	−−
			Testosterone	+/−
			DHEA	+/−
	(2) Regulation of organismal aging by hormones	(2) Hormone Manipulation or Inhibition.	(2) ? IGF-1 Antagonists	?
Cell senescence	Loss of dividing cells and possible effects of dysfunctional senescent cells	? Inhibition of cell senescence, destruction of senescent cells	?	?
Caloric restriction	Increases lifespan by 30–50%, slows morphologic changes, and delays development of age-related disease	? Activation of *sir2* proteins	Resveratrol	+ (Observational studies of red wine consumption)

Improvements in scientific understanding of the biology of aging has allowed the rational development of antiaging therapies designed to address specific mechanisms. While no treatment has been tested in clinical studies for specific effects on aging, clinical studies of age-related diseases have allowed examination of potential benefits and side effects of treatments. Key to symbols: ?, unknown; ++, clear evidence of benefit; +, evidence of benefit; +/−, inconsistent evidence of benefit; −, lack of benefit; −−, evidence of harm that outweighs benefit; ¶, evidence of harm for specific subsets of patients (see text for details).

mutations identified, which extend lifespan have as one of their actions the induction of antioxidant proteins, for example, the *daf-2* gene in the worm, *Caenorhabditis elegans*, which doubles the worm lifespan, acts in part through the induction of catalase and superoxide dismutase through a downstream signaling cascade. So, far the effects of long-term treatment of humans with antioxidants on aging are not known. A diet favoring the intake of fruits and vegetables rich in antioxidants appears to protect against several age-related diseases, but whether this ultimately translates into retarded aging or increased longevity is unknown (Thomas, 2004). Furthermore, it is not clear if the dietary benefits are due to antioxidants, as multiple clinical trials studying the effects of antioxidant vitamin supplements on specific age-related diseases have yielded largely negative results.

MODULATION OF AGING BY HORMONES

There has been great interest in the role of hormones in causing or preventing aging (Table 1). In humans, it is clear that many hormones, such as growth hormone, dehydroepiandrosterone (DHEA), and sex hormones among others, change during aging, with this change usually representing a significant decline in hormone levels by old age (Horani and Morley, 2004). For some of these hormones, deficiency in younger people produces some of the symptoms felt to be associated with aging in older persons, such as fatigue, muscular weakness, decline in lean body mass, difficulty concentrating, and decrease in the sense of well-being (Morley, 2004). With regard to geriatric patients, these symptoms often reflect more of a caricature of aging than the reality of day-to-day life, are largely nonspecific with regard to any single hormone, and have a multitude of potential causes beyond hormone deficiencies. However, these observations have led to significant interest in the role that single or multiple relative hormone deficiencies may play in the aging phenotype. Effects of hormone supplements on geriatric patients will be discussed in a later section.

Interestingly, genetic experiments in lower animals have demonstrated hormones as also being important modulators of the aging process (Guarente and Kenyon, 2000). In these animals, the levels of these hormones in early to mid-adulthood can have dramatic effects on the rate of aging during adulthood and the ultimate lifespan of the animal (Table 1). For example, in the worm, *C. elegans*, the *daf-2* gene encodes a receptor in the insulin/insulin-like growth factor-1 (IGF-1) family. Ordinarily, *daf-2* signals in early adulthood to curtail maximal longevity. Animals lacking this receptor are unable to receive the signal and age at a much slower rate than normal animals. Many of the target genes induced in the absence of the *daf-2* have recently been described and include multiple heat shock proteins, catalase, superoxide dismutase, and proteins involved in immune defense, like antimicrobial peptides. Interestingly, no single target gene mediates all of the lifespan increases, but instead, each gene has a relatively small but additive effect.

Genes analogous to *daf-2* have been identified in other animals including mice and humans (Tatar *et al.*, 2003). In mammals, *daf-2* is felt to be more homologous to the IGF-1 receptor than the insulin receptor. IGF-1 is made by the liver and muscles in response to growth hormone. Work with mouse mutants have suggested that signaling by growth hormone and IGF-1 shortens lifespan in the same way as in the worm. Two types of mouse mutants, Ames and Snell dwarf mice, lack the somatotropes in the pituitary gland responsible for making growth hormone and are dwarves and long-lived. Laron dwarf mice lack the growth-hormone receptor and are also long-lived. Knockout mice lacking the IGF-1 receptor have been generated. These mice are normal in size, but are also long-lived. Additionally, in mice, as in humans, the levels of growth hormone decline with age. If adult mice are given exogenous growth hormone to increase the serum levels, these mice demonstrate accelerated aging. Together, this suggests that the *daf-2*/IGF-1 signaling pathways play a conserved role in lifespan determination.

If hormones can regulate aging, then why are the levels not set to maximize lifespan? The answer is that most of these hormones have multiple physiologic roles beyond the control of aging. The levels of hormones that maximize lifespan often have negative consequences too, such as impacts on fertility or survival when food is limiting. For example, competition experiments have found that *daf-2* mutant worms quickly disappear from a mixed population under lab conditions designed to mimic the worm's harsh native environment. These hormones act to manage the trade-offs needed for growth, survival, and reproduction. Since energy is usually a limited resource, energy spent on reproduction, growth, or daily activity is not being spent on the self-maintenance needed to minimize the impacts of aging. As environmental conditions are variable, the levels of these hormones can be adjusted to maximize the ability to cope with the conditions. These findings suggest that hormonal manipulation could have dramatic effects on aging though important trade-offs may be involved (Table 1).

CELL SENESCENCE

Leonard Hayflick noted in the 1960s that primary cell lines divided a limited number of times before cell senescence or cell death results. It is thought that the Hayflick limit reflects the loss of telomeres and activation of p53 (Campisi, 2003). Telomeres are repetitive sequences found at the end of chromosomes that are needed to prevent shortening of chromosomes during DNA replication. An enzyme known as *telomerase* is able to maintain telomeres after cell division by synthesizing and adding these repeats to the end of the chromosome. Mice express telomerase in all tissues, but in humans, the expression is much more limited, with expression in germ cells and a limited number of stem cells.

One function of telomeres is to protect the ends of chromosomes through the recruitment of telomere-binding proteins that prevent the end from triggering the double strand break–repair mechanism, producing the activation of p53 and break–repair enzymes. p53 either halts cell division to allow repair before DNA replication or can result in cell death via apoptosis. In cells that have lost telomeres due to multiple rounds of DNA replication without repair by telomerase, the chromosomal ends now behave as a bare DNA end and activate p53. In contrast to double strand DNA breaks, the chromosome end without telomeres cannot be repaired. Hence, p53 activation becomes permanent and results in permanent cell senescence or in some cases in cell death. In older people, it is likely that in tissues, like skin, that have frequent cell division but no telomerase, some of the cells have lost enough telomeres to become senescent (Table 1). Besides being unable to divide, senescent cells often show changes in gene expression resulting in alterations in the secretion of growth factors and synthesis of extracellular matrix, which can have harmful effects on other nonsenescent cells in a tissue.

Finding ways to prevent or reverse cell senescence could be an attractive target for antiaging therapies (Table 1). For example, the activation of telomerase in tissue culture cells that usually lack the enzyme has been shown to prevent cellular senescence. However, cancer cells also activate telomerase during oncogenesis, and telomerase inhibitors are being studied as an anticancer therapy (Campisi, 2003). Hence, alterations in cellular senescence pathways would have to be carried out selectively as the senescence pathways also represent cellular mechanisms to prevent the development of cancer.

CALORIC RESTRICTION

Caloric restriction is an almost uniformly effective means of increasing lifespan of animal species (Koubova and Guarente, 2003). This manipulation involves decreasing the calorie intake by 40–60% compared with *ad lib* fed animals while providing adequate calories and nutrients to prevent malnutrition (Table 1). Animals treated with caloric restriction show an average increase in lifespan of 30–40% compared with control animals and a slowing of the phenotypic changes of aging. Additionally, restricted animals develop age-associated disease and disability at later ages relative to *ad lib* fed animals. The presumed effectiveness and simplicity of caloric restriction make it an attractive antiaging approach for humans. However, caloric restriction also likely results in significant feelings of hunger, which ultimately limits the applicability and desirability of this approach. Consequently, there is intense interest in understanding the mechanisms underlying the caloric restriction response as a means to develop ways to uncouple caloric restriction from the beneficial effects.

While the exact mechanism of action of caloric restriction is unknown, there is evidence to support the presence of several mechanisms (Koubova and Guarente, 2003). It is also definitely possible that the currently identified mechanisms are all secondary to an unknown process. Animals undergoing caloric restriction show changes in metabolism resulting in declines in the production of reactive oxygen species. This decline along with increases in protein turnover results in decreases in the levels of proteins showing oxidative damage. Additionally, changes in metabolism accompany a change in energy utilization from glucose to fatty acid-derived ketone bodies. Several prominent hormonal changes that accompany this switch in mammals are significant reductions in insulin, growth hormone, and IGF-1 production. Prolonged caloric restriction also produces a reduction in fat mass due to the consumption of fat calories. The reduced fat mass probably also causes a dramatic change in the production of a variety of known and unknown fat-derived hormones. Future experiments with lower animals should help determine whether the hormonal and metabolic changes accompanying caloric restriction play a cause or effect role.

An important clue in the study of caloric restriction came from work with the *sir2* gene in yeast (Koubova and Guarente, 2003). This gene was originally identified as a mutation that increases the reproductive lifespan of yeast. The *sir2* gene encodes a (nicotinamide adenosine dinucleotide) NAD-dependent histone and protein de-acetylase, which is able to remove acetyl groups from specific lysine residues in the presence of the co-factor NAD+. At least in yeast, *sir2* appears to play a role in mediating the antiaging effects of caloric restriction. Caloric restriction results in the induction of enzymes that convert nicotinamide to NAD. Nicotinamide is generated by the de-acetylation reaction when the acetyl group is transferred from lysine to NAD. Nicotinamide is also a potent noncompetitive inhibitor of *sir2*. Hence, the conversion of nicotinamide to NAD removes an inhibitor of *sir2* and increases the available substrate for the reaction. Interestingly, resveratrol, which is a plant polyphenol found in red wine, was identified as a potent *in vitro* activator of *sir2*, and was subsequently shown to greatly increase the yeast lifespan (Howitz *et al.*, 2003). For yeast, resveratrol is able to mediate these effects independent of caloric restriction, suggesting that it acts like a caloric restriction mimetic (Table 1). It will be interesting to determine if *sir2* homologs in people and mammals play similar roles in the responses to caloric restriction. If so, there is the exciting possibility that the effects of red wine in people, like the prevention of cardiovascular and neurologic disease or cancer prevention, are due to caloric restriction mimetic effects mediated through mammalian *sir2* proteins.

DATA FOR CURRENT THERAPIES

No current antiaging therapy has been shown to either slow aging or reverse the effects of aging in people (Olshansky *et al.*, 2002). However, even this statement has some significant limitations as none of the currently touted antiaging therapies have been tested in clinical studies, such as a randomized controlled trial, specifically designed to address whether these drugs act as antiaging therapies. These conclusions have been largely based upon the lack of effectiveness of antiaging therapies in trials often designed for purposes only peripherally related to antiaging. For example, antioxidant vitamins have been tested in large long-term studies designed to address whether these vitamins can be used to prevent diseases such as cardiovascular disease or specific types of cancer (Thomas, 2004). While both cardiovascular disease and cancer are both aging-associated diseases, neither of these diseases is synonymous with aging, as some people will live an entire life without developing either disease. Growth hormone comes closest to being studied in human clinical trials designed to test its effect on aging (Vance, 2003). Several trials have given growth hormone to older subjects to assess the effects of the drug on strength, stamina, and body composition. These studies have been limited by small study sizes and a short duration of treatment. Plus, questions can be asked about whether assessing strength, stamina, and body composition are appropriate or the best measures of the aging phenotype.

This discussion illustrates a major stumbling block that scientists, physicians, antiaging medicine practitioners, and pharmaceutical companies interested in developing antiaging therapies will need to contend with, which is the lack of a convenient and widely accepted means of testing candidate therapies. It is unrealistic to expect that candidate therapies will undergo the long-term trials lasting for several decades to definitively prove effects on aging or its direct effects on people. These trials need large sample sizes, likely needing to be multicenter to exclude geographic and lifestyle effects, and extended trial times to conclusively show differences between control and treated groups. However, the cost of starting such a trial would likely be prohibitive, and the danger is that sufficient patients would drop out, relocate, or develop medical conditions violating inclusion criteria so that in the end the data could be useless. An important research goal in the near future is to develop widely accepted surrogate markers for aging that would allow the testing of antiaging therapies in a more rapid fashion, looking for changes in surrogate markers as opposed to long-term effects on aging (Baker and Sprott, 1988). While this means of testing would be less satisfying, it would ultimately be much more practical.

The remainder of this section will review the data for several types of currently touted antiaging therapies: antioxidants, growth hormone, and several types of steroid hormones such as testosterone and DHEA.

ANTIOXIDANTS

As discussed earlier, there is significant evidence from experimental animals that oxidative stress contributes to organismal aging (Harman, 2003). Besides aging, there is evidence that oxidative damage is involved in age-associated diseases such as atherosclerosis, cancer, Parkinson's disease, and Alzheimer's disease (Harman, 2003). Observational studies have consistently shown that increased dietary consumption of fruits and vegetables rich in antioxidant compounds protect against the development of these age-associated diseases (Lawlor *et al.*, 2004; Thomas, 2004). However, observational studies suffer from the potential bias that changes in consumption of specific fruits and vegetables could represent a marker for an unmeasured variable that actually accounts for the observed differences (Lawlor *et al.*, 2004). Consequently, prospective clinical studies have been conducted to test whether the use of antioxidants alone alter the development or progression of specific age-related diseases (Table 1). On the basis of wide availability, low cost, and safety concerns, human studies have used pharmacologic doses of antioxidant vitamins, specifically vitamin A, the vitamin A precursor β-carotene, vitamin C, and vitamin E. An important caution is that the observational (National Health and Nutrition Examination Survey) NHANES studies have failed to demonstrate any major increase in lifespan in persons taking vitamin supplements compared to nonusers.

VITAMIN E (*see* Chapter 29, Vitamins and Minerals in the Elderly)

Vitamin E is a lipid-soluble vitamin, which is thought to act biologically as an antioxidant (Table 1). Vitamin E is most commonly given as α-tocopherol, though three other tocopherols and four tocotrienols are chemically related but have lesser biologic activity (Thomas, 2004). The dosages of vitamin E used in clinical studies have ranged from 150 IU per day to 2000 IU per day. Vitamin E is the safest of the lipid-soluble vitamins, and with high doses of vitamin E, nausea, flatulence, and diarrhea have been commonly reported. Vitamin E also raises the vitamin K requirement and can cause bleeding in patients on oral anticoagulants. The only other side effects noted have been an increase in falls in a study using demented patients and an increase in hemorrhagic stroke in older male smokers.

Prospective observational studies have found that the use of vitamin E supplements for two or more years is associated with a reduction in the risk of coronary artery disease by 20–40% in patients without preexisting coronary artery disease. However, subsequent randomized studies have produced largely negative results (Eidelman *et al.*, 2004). The Primary Prevention project, which studied patients with cardiovascular risk factors, but no history of cardiovascular disease, found no effect of vitamin E during 3.6 years of follow-up, though a beneficial effect of low-dose aspirin was seen in a separate treatment arm. Also, the α-tocopherol and β-carotene Cancer Prevention Study (ATBC), which studied male smokers in southwestern Finland, showed little to no effect of vitamin E in patients without coronary artery disease either in the development of angina or myocardial infarction. With regard to secondary prevention in patients with coronary artery disease, a subgroup analysis of the ATBC study, the Heart Outcomes Prevention Evaluation study, the HDL-Atherosclerosis Treatment study, the MRC/BHF Heart Protection Study, the Women's Angiographic Vitamin and Estrogen Study (WAVES), and the Italian GISSI study showed no effect of vitamin E supplementation on cardiac outcomes. In contrast, the smaller Cambridge Heart Antioxidant Study showed a roughly 50% reduction in recurrent myocardial infarction. Also, patients on chronic hemodialysis are felt to be exposed to additional oxidative stress due to dialysis, and the Secondary Prevention with Antioxidants of Cardiovascular Disease in End-stage Renal Disease (SPACE) study, which included a majority of patients with coronary artery disease, showed a roughly 50% reduction in all cardiovascular endpoints and a greater reduction in myocardial infarction. A smaller number of studies have evaluated the effects of vitamin E on atherosclerosis at other sites and with most finding no evidence for benefit. Two studies evaluating the progression of carotid atherosclerosis via ultrasound over 3 to 4.5 years found no effect of vitamin E on intimal thickening, though the Antioxidant Supplementation in Atherosclerosis Prevention (ASAP) study found a reduction in thickening in men treated with a combination of vitamin E and vitamin C. Subgroup analyses from the ATBC study found no protective benefit for vitamin E on the development of abdominal aortic aneurysm or peripheral vascular disease. Finally, results from the HDL-Atherosclerosis study suggests that the use of an antioxidant cocktail including vitamin E could be harmful in patients with normal low-density lipoprotein (LDL) and low HDL levels treated with niacin and simvastatin, as the use of the antioxidants blunted the effects of niacin and simvastatin on raising HDL, reducing progression of atherosclerosis, and reducing cardiovascular events (Brown *et al.*, 2001). Similarly, the Women's Angiographic Vitamin and Estrogen study found that the use of vitamin E and C supplements had no effect on the progression of coronary artery narrowing, but significantly increased the chances of death from cardiovascular causes. In summary, there is little evidence for a benefit of vitamin E in the primary or secondary prevention of cardiovascular disease (Eidelman *et al.*, 2004). However, on the basis of current evidence, it may be reasonable to use vitamin E in patients receiving chronic hemodialysis.

Vitamin E has also been studied with regard to stroke, cancer, Alzheimer's disease, cataracts, and age-related macular degeneration. The effects of vitamin E supplementation on stroke were studied using data from the ATBC study. While vitamin E was associated with an overall higher risk of hemorrhagic stroke, both hypertensive patients and hypertensive patients with diabetes had a decreased risk of cerebral infarction. However, the hypertensive patients without diabetes had an elevated risk of subarachnoid hemorrhage that was not seen in diabetic patients. It is not clear at this time if these data represent a protective effect of vitamin E for hypertensive and diabetic patients. Several studies have examined the effects of vitamin E on the development of cancer with largely negative results. In smokers, the ATBC study found no effect on the development of lung cancer, an increase in the incidence of stomach cancer, and fewer cases of prostate and colorectal cancer (The α-Tocopherol β-Carotene Cancer Prevention Study Group, 1994). Follow-up studies of vitamin E in the prevention of colorectal cancer have produced mixed results. One study found no effect of vitamin E on the development of bladder cancer. One study has found no effect of vitamin E on the development of breast cancer. The decrease in prostate cancer seen in the ATBC study has been suggested to be due in part to lowered serum androgen levels as patients receiving vitamin E had significantly lower serum levels of testosterone and androstenedione. There is weak data supporting the use of vitamin E for delaying the progression of Alzheimer's disease as one study evaluated the effectiveness of vitamin E in patients with Alzheimer's disease of moderate severity (Sano *et al.*, 1997). The raw data showed no benefit from the use of vitamin E; however, the placebo group scored significantly higher on the entry mini-mental state examination (MMSE), making comparison difficult. When the baseline MMSE score was used as a covariate in interpreting the data, a significant delay was observed in the composite end point of time to death, institutionalization, loss of ability to perform two of three basic activities of daily living (ADL's), or development of severe dementia (670 days versus 440 days). Treatment of smokers as part of the ATBC trial with vitamin E for 6 years had no effect on the incidence of age-related macular degeneration at the end of the study. However, the Age-related Eye Disease study found that treatment of patients with preexisting age-related macular degeneration, with a combination of antioxidants including vitamin E resulted in a decrease in the progression to advanced macular degeneration (AREDSRG, 2001). However, another study found no effect on the progression of age-related macular degeneration with the use of a vitamin E supplement alone. With regard to cataract formation, one study found no effect of an antioxidant regimen including vitamin E, and another study found no effect of vitamin E alone on the development of cataracts. The Roche European American Cataract Trial, which used an antioxidant mixture including vitamin E, found a small decrease in the growth rate of cataracts, though this was more pronounced with patients enrolled at the US site and not with patients enrolled at the UK site. In conclusion, there is little evidence that the use of vitamin E has a protective effect in the development of cancer and little evidence that vitamin E is useful in slowing the progression of Alzheimer's disease. The use of vitamin E as part of a combination of antioxidants appears promising for slowing the progression of age-related macular degeneration, but not for the prevention of cataract.

The effect of vitamin E on respiratory infections has also been investigated. In a post-hoc analysis of the ATBC study, the use of vitamin E was found to have no effect on the development of pneumonia requiring hospitalization. A small study found that the use of a multivitamin supplement including vitamin E might improve the response to influenza vaccination. However, in a community-based study, the use of a vitamin E supplement had no effect on the incidence of upper respiratory tract infections (URI) and actually seemed to increase the severity and duration of symptoms during a URI (Graat *et al.*, 2002).

VITAMIN A (*see* Chapter 29, Vitamins and Minerals in the Elderly)

Vitamin A belongs to a group of over 600 naturally occurring compounds known as *carotenoids*. All of the carotenoids have antioxidant activity (Table 1), but only around 50 of the carotenoids have provitamin A activity, which means that they can be converted in the body to vitamin A (Thomas, 2004). The main dietary carotenoids are β-carotene, which is a vitamin A precursor, and lycopene, which has potent antioxidant properties but does not have provitamin A activity. Vitamin A also has additional biologic roles. Specifically, vitamin A is metabolized to retinol and plays a key role in vision as part of the rhodopsin protein that converts light to electrical signals in photoreceptor cells. Additionally, several vitamin A metabolites act as hormones and play important roles in the development as well as the regulation of cell growth and differentiation. These metabolites, known as *retinoids,* act as hormones via interactions with several retinoic acid receptors, which bind DNA and alter gene expression in response to hormone binding in a manner similar to thyroid hormone receptors.

The recommended daily allowance (RDA) for vitamin A is 5000 IU (1.5 mg) per day, with an intake of 10 000 IU per day that was felt to be safe. Several recent studies have raised concerns that chronic vitamin A consumption in the 10 000 IU range per day can worsen osteoporosis and result in an elevated risk of hip fracture in postmenopausal women (Feskanich *et al.*, 2002). This may be due in part to an increased production of parathyroid hormone (PTH) with resultant hypercalcemia. In addition to concerns about the effects on osteoporosis, it is seen that vitamin A is the most toxic of the lipid-soluble vitamins with both acute toxicity and chronic toxicity. Acute toxicity requires the ingestion of more than 200 000 IU per day as could be seen in a drug overdose. Chronic toxicity occurs following the ingestion of 50 000 IU per day for over 3 months. Symptoms of chronic toxicity include hair loss, mouth sores, nausea and vomiting, dry skin, hepatomegaly, and increased intracranial pressure, which can result in headaches and altered mental status. In contrast, since the conversion of β-carotene is highly regulated, the consumption of the provitamin β-carotene is felt to be safe with the main adverse event being yellowing of the skin. As a result of these safety issues, most studies use β-carotene instead of vitamin A.

Observational studies showed that a higher intake of fruits and vegetables containing both β-carotene and other carotenoids is associated with lower risks of cancer and cardiovascular disease with risk reductions of up to 30% being observed (Thomas, 2004). However, randomized studies designed to test for protective effects of supplements containing β-carotene with respect to cancer and cardiovascular disease have been very disappointing.

With regard to cancer, the ATBC study found that a group of Finnish male smokers treated with β-carotene had no decrease in cancer at the major sites and instead showed increases in the incidence of lung, prostate, and stomach cancer (The α-Tocopherol β-carotene Cancer Prevention Study Group, 1994). Additionally, the β-carotene and Retinol Efficacy trial (CARET), which treated smokers, former smokers, and workers exposed to asbestosis with vitamin A and β-carotene for 4 years, was stopped prematurely partly because of a 59% increase in lung cancer mortality in the treatment arm (Omenn *et al.*, 1996). The CARET study additionally found no change in the incidence of cancer at other sites. It is especially concerning that a later study using the CARET data found that the use of the β-carotene and vitamin A supplement actually blocked the protective effects of dietary carotenoids. The Physician's Health study found no impact of β-carotene on the incidence of cancer including lung cancer during 12 years of treatment. However, this study, in contrast to ATBC and CARET, had few smokers and former smokers. Women treated with β-carotene in the Women's Health study for roughly 2 years, then followed for 2 years more, demonstrated no change in the incidence of cancer.

The effects of β-carotene supplements on cardiovascular disease have also been tested in clinical trials with the ATBC study, the Physician's Health study, the MRC/BHF Heart Protection study, the CARET study, and the Women's Health study showing no positive effect of β-carotene on cardiovascular outcomes such as myocardial infarction or stoke (Hasnain and Mooradian, 2004). Additionally, two studies using the ATBC cohort looked at the effect of β-carotene on the risk of abdominal aortic aneurysm (AAA) formation and the progression of intermittent claudication due to peripheral vascular disease and did not see benefit from supplement use. Also, results from the HDL-Atherosclerosis study suggests that the use of an antioxidant cocktail including β-carotene could be harmful in patients with normal LDL and low HDL levels treated with niacin and simvastatin, as the use of the antioxidants blunted the effects of niacin and simvastatin on raising the HDL, reducing progression of atherosclerosis, and reducing cardiovascular events (Brown *et al.*, 2001). The ATBC study also examined the effect of β-carotene use on the development of both cataracts and age-related macular degeneration and failed to find evidence of benefit. In contrast, the Age-Related Eye Disease study has found that the use of β-carotene as part of an antioxidant mixture reduced the development of advanced age-related macular degeneration in patients with preexisting disease (AREDSRG, 2001).

Hence, despite benefits seen in observational studies of a diet rich in carotenoids, there is no evidence from randomized studies for the benefits of vitamin A or β-carotene supplements with regard to cancer, cardiovascular disease, or eye disease. Additionally, there is significant evidence for potential harm with the use of supplements for smokers and former smokers with regard to lung cancer and for postmenopausal women with regard to osteoporosis.

VITAMIN C (*see* Chapter 29, Vitamins and Minerals in the Elderly)

Vitamin C is a water-soluble vitamin that is found in citrus fruits, melons, strawberries, tomatoes, peppers, leafy vegetables, and broccoli (Thomas, 2004). In the body, vitamin C is involved in multiple oxidation-reduction reactions including the cross-linking between protein strands involved in the synthesis of collagen. Vitamin C also has antioxidant properties, and the use of vitamin C as an antiaging therapy, among other uses, was actively promoted by Nobel laureate Linus Pauling (Table 1). The RDA for vitamin C is 90 mg per day for men and 75 mg per day for women. Oral supplementation beyond these levels has progressively less effect upon the serum vitamin C levels as both the absorption from the GI tract and excretion via the urine is tightly regulated. Vitamin C has low toxicity even in large doses with the most common side effects consisting of GI upset, flatulence, and diarrhea. As vitamin C is metabolized to oxalate, there is also the possibility that high-dose supplementation could lead to oxalate kidney stones. Vitamin C supplementation, along with vitamin E supplements, may reduce the rate of *Helicobacter pylori* eradication in patients being treated with lansoprazole-amoxicillin-metronidazole triple treatment. Additionally, the use of vitamin C supplements can also be problematic in patients with diabetes, as vitamin C impairs tests measuring glucose in blood and urine. There is also a theoretical concern that supplementation with 500 mg per day of vitamin C could lead to oxidative damage to DNA as levels of 8-oxoadenine, a form of adenine produced by oxidative damage, are increased in patients taking vitamin C daily for 6 weeks (Podmore *et al.*, 1998).

Compared with vitamin A and vitamin E, few studies have evaluated vitamin C alone on the incidence of cardiovascular disease or cancer. Both the MRC/BHF Heart Protection Study and the WAVE study showed no benefit in cardiovascular outcomes with the use of an antioxidant supplement containing vitamin C (Hasnain and Mooradian, 2004). In addition, similar to vitamin E and vitamin A, the HDL-Atherosclerosis study suggested that the use of an antioxidant cocktail including vitamin C could be harmful in patients with normal LDL and low HDL levels, who are treated with niacin and simvastatin (Brown *et al.*, 2001). Preclinical studies have suggested that vitamin C supplementation may have a positive effect on vascular endothelial function and vascular tone. Hence, three studies have examined the effects of vitamin C supplementation on hypertension in patients with mixed results. A 1-month trial of vitamin C in diabetic patients showed a significant decrease in blood pressure, but an 8-month study in nondiabetic elderly patients saw a significant decline in blood pressure with supplementation only for the first month with nonsignificant effects for the remainder of the study. Additionally, a 5-year study found no effect of vitamin C on blood pressure. However, the ASAP study found that the use of a vitamin E and vitamin C supplement decreased the progression of atherosclerosis in patients with elevated serum cholesterol. Also in post-hoc analysis, a study treating patients with a multivitamin containing vitamin C found that elevation of plasma vitamin C levels correlated with reduction in C-reactive protein levels. There is little benefit observed for vitamin C in the prevention of cancer. One exception is stomach cancer where patients with preexisting precancerous lesions of the stomach had a significantly decreased rate of progression to stomach cancer when given vitamin C. Vitamin C has also been tested for age-related macular degeneration, as part of an antioxidant mixture, and shown to decrease the rate of progression to advanced macular degeneration. The Roche European American Cataract Trial, which used an antioxidant mixture including vitamin E, found a small decrease in the growth rate of cataracts, though this was more pronounced with patients enrolled at the US site and not with patients enrolled at the UK site. Vitamin C has recently been tried as a topical therapy in patients with photodamage with positive results in terms of appearance and the synthesis of new collagen. Also, the oral use of an antioxidant mixture including vitamin C may help prevent the development of photodamage. In conclusion, vitamin C has potential benefits in patients at high risk for stomach cancer, in patients with early age-related macular degeneration, and in patients with photodamage when given topically. Otherwise, there is no evidence of benefit and concerns about use related to DNA damage, kidney stones, and inhibition of lipid modifying therapy.

α-LIPOIC ACID

α-Lipoic acid is considered to be one of the most potent antioxidants, as it is able to reduce and hence regenerate other antioxidants such as vitamin E and glutathione (Table 1). Clinical studies testing α-lipoic acid are rather limited. Small studies have suggested that it may be helpful in treating diabetic neuropathy, improving diabetic control, treating photodamage of the facial skin, and retarding the progression of neurodegenerative diseases, but there is a need for further studies before this agent can be recommended.

WHAT DO THE NEGATIVE RESULTS IN CLINICAL TRIALS OF ANTIOXIDANTS MEAN?

How should the largely negative results of randomized studies of the antioxidant vitamins be interpreted? Some have suggested that these data draw into question the oxidative damage theory of aging and age-related disease while others have pointed out that the negative results could be due to reasons other than oxidative damage not being involved (Shishehbor and Hazen, 2004). For example, no dose finding studies have been carried out to determine the optimal dosages of antioxidants in people. Also, the levels of these antioxidant vitamins are regulated both in plasma and in tissues via regulation of absorption, excretion, transport, and metabolism. Hence, studies may have used inadequate doses of antioxidants, or more importantly the antioxidants studied may be unable to reach adequate levels in the proper anatomic or cellular locations. For example, a study of carotid endarterectomy patients found that use of vitamin E supplements lead to increased plasma vitamin E levels, but no increases in levels in the atheroma. An additional limitation of the current studies is that the effectiveness of the antioxidant supplements in actually lowering markers of oxidative stress was not demonstrated. Moreover, the antioxidant vitamins chosen on the basis of dietary epidemiologic studies may not represent the antioxidants responsible for the clinical effect and in fact may not even act in patients as antioxidants. For example, a study examining the effects of vitamin E supplements on serum vitamin E levels and oxidative stress found increased serum levels of serum vitamin E in patients taking increasing doses of the vitamin, but that the increased serum levels did not translate into changes in measures of lipid peroxidation as a measure of membrane oxidative damage (Meagher *et al.*, 2001). This study calls into question both the dosages of vitamin E used in existing studies and the appropriateness of using vitamin E as an antioxidant in patients eating a standard American diet. There are also concerns about the duration of therapy, as it is unclear when antioxidants would be most effective. Most animal studies treated animals for their entire lives, whereas clinical studies have started much later, treating adult patients, often for secondary prevention. Interest in newer antioxidants, such as the catalase/superoxide dismutase mimetics, will hopefully lead to future studies designed to address both clinical concerns as well as these more practical concerns.

HORMONES AS ANTIAGING THERAPIES

As discussed earlier, it is clear that many hormones, such as growth hormone, DHEA, and sex hormones among others, change during aging, with this change usually representing a significant decline in hormone levels by old age. For some of these hormones, deficiency in younger people produces some of the symptoms felt to be associated with aging in older persons, which has lead to significant interest in the role that single or multiple relative hormone deficiencies may play in the aging phenotype (Horani and Morley, 2004).

Clinical studies have examined the effects of growth hormone, testosterone, DHEA, and estrogen/progesterone supplementation on patients (Table 1). However, many of these studies have been of short duration and used clinical end points, such as change in lean body mass instead of physical strength, gait, or ADL function, which may have questionable relevance (Horani and Morley, 2004). Furthermore, none of the hormone-replacement therapies have undergone the long-term clinical testing needed to determine if they do represent an antiaging therapy that can slow, reverse, or ameliorate the effects of aging.

GROWTH HORMONE (*see* Chapter 118, Endocrinology of Aging)

Growth hormone is a polypeptide hormone that is made by the pituitary gland and acts primarily on liver and muscle to result in the production of IGF-1, which then acts on the ultimate target tissues (Horani and Morley, 2004). Growth-hormone secretion reaches its maximum during the growth spurt accompanying puberty before beginning a steady decline of approximately 14% per decade in both men and women. Much of this decline is due to a selective reduction in the nocturnal pulsatile secretion of growth hormone, with declines in both pulse height and pulse frequency seen. Some of the changes associated with aging are reminiscent of those seen in adult patients with frank growth-hormone deficiency, such as reduction in lean body mass, increase in body fat especially abdominal obesity, decrease in muscular strength, and difficulty with cognitive functioning. These observations led Dr Daniel Rudman to suggest in the mid-1980s that during aging a growth-hormone somatopause occurs, which may contribute to the aging phenotype (Rudman, 1985). In support of this hypothesis, Rudman observed a decrease in IGF-1 levels between healthy older patients in the community and frail patients living in a nursing home setting. However, other studies have failed to find a correlation between IGF-1 levels and physical or cognitive functioning.

There has been much interest in testing the effects of supplementing growth hormone in the elderly (Table 1). Trials with patients have shown that responses to growth hormone or growth hormone secretagogues, as measured by serum IGF-1 levels, persist in the elderly. Most studies have enrolled relatively healthy patients with low baseline IGF-1 levels and have treated the patients with doses of growth hormone adjusted to produce IGF levels in patients that fall in the low to mid-normal range seen in young adults. Few long-term growth-hormone trials have been conducted with most trials ending after a few months. Treatment with growth hormone has shown increases in lean body mass, increases in skin thickness, and decreases in fat mass (Rudman *et al.*, 1990). These changes were more pronounced in elderly men than in postmenopausal women. Interestingly, the increases in muscle mass have not been accompanied by significant increases in physical strength or stamina. A recent study conducted at the national institute of health (NIH) demonstrated that there are small but synergistic increases in strength and stamina when growth hormone was combined with testosterone in men (Blackman *et al.*, 2002). Effects of growth hormone on cognition and memory have not been well studied but so far the results are mixed. Growth-hormone treatment has been shown in several studies to improve bone mineral density both with respect to total body and to the lumbar spine, but whether these increases impact on fracture risk is not known.

Growth hormone has also been tested for benefits in patients with specific acute or chronic diseases due to its anabolic actions (Ruokonen and Takala, 2002). Trials with growth hormone have suggested that it might be beneficial in burn and postoperative patients to reverse catabolism. However, trials in intensive care unit (ICU) patients have shown mixed results with a large multicenter study demonstrating a dramatic increase in mortality among treated patients. A small study suggested that treatment of patients with dilated cardiomyopathy with growth hormone lowers circulating levels of inflammatory cytokines and improves left ventricular contractile function. This result is promising but will need to be replicated in a larger study and be linked to improvements in cardiac outcomes like functional class, hospitalization, and mortality.

Growth-hormone treatment has shown side effects of lower extremity edema, gynecomastia, carpal tunnel syndrome, arthralgias, and headache (Horani and Morley, 2004). These side effects are common and reversible with lowering of the growth-hormone dose by 25–50%. More concerning is the increase in glucose intolerance and frank diabetes seen in clinical trials with growth-hormone treatment which is due to decreases in peripheral uptake of glucose (Blackman *et al.*, 2002). Given the strong associations between insulin resistance and diabetes and cardiovascular disease, this finding may make long-term growth hormone use risky.

Growth hormone also carries two potential risks, which are: a possible increase in cancer risk given the cell growth stimulant properties of IGF-1, and a possible acceleration of aging caused by growth-hormone supplementation. With regard to cancer, several epidemiologic studies have found associations between IGF-1 levels and the risk of colon, breast, lung, and prostate cancer (Horani and Morley, 2004). With regard to aging, studies in mice suggest that increases in growth hormone and IGF-1 signaling may lead to lifespan shortening instead of prolongation. Mice deficient in growth hormone live longer than those with normal growth-hormone levels (Tatar *et al.*, 2003). Additionally, treatment of mice with supplemental growth hormone in adulthood is also associated with premature aging.

At this time, the modest benefits of growth hormone, high cost, and potential long-term risks weigh against the use of growth hormone in the elderly. Longer-term studies of growth hormone are needed to determine if the increases in muscle mass prevent decline or improve function long term, to determine the possible dangers associated with long-term use, and to compare growth hormone with less costly interventions.

TESTOSTERONE (*see* Chapter 118, Endocrinology of Aging; Chapter 121, Ovarian and Testicular Function)

Testosterone replacement for men has been advocated by some endocrinologists as well as by many in the antiaging field (Table 1). In men, testosterone levels peak during late adolescence, then decrease at a rate of roughly $100\,\mathrm{ng\,dL^{-1}}$ per decade afterwards because of decreases in testosterone production (Horani and Morley, 2004; Yialamas and Hayes, 2003). Additionally, most circulating testosterone is not bioavailable as it is bound by sex hormone-binding globulin, and the levels of sex hormone-binding globulin also increase with age. Hence, depending upon whether total or bioavailable testosterone is measured and the specific definition of hypogonadism, 10–49% of men in their fifties to sixties, 30 to 70% of men in their seventies, and 35–70% of men in their eighties have hypogonadism. Along with declines in testosterone levels, aging men experience decreases in muscle mass and strength, decreases in bone mass, increases in fat mass, decreases in sexual interest and potency, and decreases in cognitive function, which mimic similar symptoms seen in younger hypogonadal men (Horani and Morley, 2004).

Several studies have studied the supplementation of testosterone in men with low testosterone levels either via injections or via a scrotal patch, but no long-term studies have been conducted (Horani and Morley, 2004; Yialamas and Hayes, 2003). Most studies have treated older men with low testosterone levels and have shown an increase in lean body mass accompanied by a decrease in fat mass. The increase in muscle mass has usually not been accompanied by an increase in strength with the possible exception of men with very low testosterone levels, that is, less than $200\,\mathrm{ng\,dL^{-1}}$. Additionally, the increases in muscle mass have not led to improvements in frailty or functioning. Testosterone has also been found to have positive effects on markers of bone turnover, though this has not consistently led to increases in bone mineral density. This may be due to the effects of testosterone on bone being predominantly mediated through aromatization to estradiol. Sexual function has shown mixed results with supplementation, with men with lower initial testosterone levels tending to have the most significant improvements. With respect to sexual function, testosterone supplementation has shown benefit for improving libido, while for potency, conflicting results have been seen. The effects of testosterone supplementation on memory and cognitive function have also been tested with mixed results. Additionally, testosterone supplementation has not been beneficial in patients with mild cognitive impairment. There is data to suggest that testosterone replacement can improve mood, sense of well-being, and concentration, but testosterone does not improve symptoms of major depression.

Concerns have been raised regarding potential effects of supplementation on prostate and cardiovascular disease (Rhoden and Morgentaler, 2004). Studies have consistently found no connection between supplementation and the development of benign prostate hyperplasia (BPH) symptoms. A few studies have found small increases in prostate specific antigen (PSA) in elderly men receiving exogenous testosterone, though these studies have not lasted long enough and enrolled sufficient numbers to determine if this translates to an increased risk of prostate cancer. While hormone ablation has proven to be a successful treatment for prostate cancer, epidemiologic studies have not found a relationship between testosterone levels and the subsequent development of prostate cancer (Horani and Morley, 2004; Yialamas and Hayes, 2003). However, given the theoretical concern for increased development of prostate cancer or increased growth of subclinical tumors with supplementation, most advocate digital rectal examination and PSA testing prior to beginning testosterone treatment, with follow-up every 6 months (Rhoden and Morgentaler, 2004). At follow-up testing, an increase in PSA of $2\,\mathrm{ng\,ml^{-1}}$ over baseline or an increase of $0.75\,\mathrm{ng\,ml^{-1}\,year^{-1}}$ or greater should trigger the stopping of testosterone and prostate biopsy to exclude cancer. With regard to cardiovascular disease, most studies have found that administration of testosterone leads to no change or slight decreases in the HDL cholesterol which are counterbalanced with no change or slight decreases in total cholesterol and LDL cholesterol. Additionally, testosterone causes coronary artery dilatation and has been shown to decrease angina in patients with symptomatic coronary artery disease. Other side effects include worsening of sleep apnea and erythrocytosis, which can be seen in up to 25% of patients receiving treatment. This can be easily managed either by decreasing the dose of testosterone given or by using phlebotomy or blood donation.

Despite the lack of long-term trials showing safety and effectiveness, several professional societies have recommended that men with testosterone deficiency, diagnosed by free or total testosterone, and symptoms of androgen deficiency be offered testosterone replacement after initial prostate cancer screening (Rhoden and Morgentaler, 2004). While testosterone may address some of the symptoms of aging in men, the data to support the claims made for testosterone replacement, especially for non-deficient men by some in the antiaging field, appears to be lacking.

ESTROGEN (*see* Chapter 118, Endocrinology of Aging; Chapter 121, Ovarian and Testicular Function)

The hormonal changes accompanying menopause are among the most pronounced hormone changes during aging and are frequently accompanied by prominent symptoms (Horani and Morley, 2004). Consequently, estrogen or estrogen/progesterone hormone-replacement therapy (HRT) has been available for sometime. Observational studies consistently indicated benefits for HRT beyond the treatment of menopause with a possible role in the prevention of cardiovascular disease, colorectal cancer, dementia, and osteoporosis. As a result, most physicians advocated the use of HRT, and many women opted for it, which resulted in 38% of postmenopausal women in the United States using HRT as of just a few years ago. However, the results of randomized studies did not show evidence of benefits, and in contrast, demonstrated evidence of harm with the use of HRT (Table 1). Consequently, HRT is no longer recommended for use other than for short-term treatment of menopausal symptoms, and the number of HRT users has plummeted (Grady, 2003).

Clinical studies have shown HRT to be beneficial for treating the symptoms of menopause, including hot flashes, night sweats, insomnia, vaginal dryness, and mood swings, and preventing osteoporosis (Grady, 2003). The symptoms of menopause can be treated in other ways, such as using clonidine or selective-serotonin reuptake inhibitors, but these approaches are not as effective as HRT. Osteoporosis is also effectively treated with HRT with increases in bone mineral density and decreases in fractures observed. However, osteoporosis can also be treated with either bisphosphonates or raloxifene, which is a selective modulator of estrogen receptors, with roughly equivalent effectiveness. Hence, the clearest indication for HRT would be to manage menopausal symptoms.

Much of the interest in HRT was generated by benefits with regard to the prevention of cardiovascular disease, colorectal cancer, and dementia seen in earlier observational trials. However, the randomized Heart and Estrogen/Progestin Replacement Study (HERS) and Women's Health Initiative (WHI) study have failed to demonstrate these benefits. The only possible exception is colorectal cancer, where the WHI did show a slight decrease in cases of colorectal cancer suggesting a possible benefit. In contrast, for cardiovascular disease data from HERS, WHI, the Estrogen Replacement and Atherosclerosis trial, and HERS II demonstrated that HRT could be harmful in both women with preexisting coronary artery disease and even in women without a history of cardiovascular disease, as increases in myocardial infarctions were seen during the early study years. Initially, it appeared that the increase in cardiovascular events seen in the first 1–2 years of use would be then offset by a subsequent decrease in cardiovascular events. However, data from the HERS follow-up study, HERS II, demonstrated that there was no decrease in cardiovascular events with continued use (Grady *et al.*, 2002). For dementia, the randomized Women's Health Initiative Memory Study (WHIMS) showed an increased risk of dementia with HRT use during almost 5 years of follow-up (Shumaker *et al.*, 2003). This increase in dementia could perhaps be due to an increase in vascular dementia, given the increase in stroke observed. The impact of HRT on the quality of life and mental health was also explored by using the HERS cohort. This study found that the use of HRT had no impact upon physical function, depressive symptoms, overall mental health, or measures of energy or fatigue. Only women with flushing related to menopause at the start of the study showed any improvement in mental health and depressive symptoms from the use of HRT. Overall, the physical function, depressive symptoms, overall mental health, and measures of energy or fatigue were impacted more by co-morbid illnesses and disease severity than the use of HRT. As this study occurred as part of the HERS study, which enrolled only women with documented coronary artery disease, the results may not be easily generalized to other groups of patients.

HRT users have an increased risk of endometrial cancer, venous thromboembolism, breast cancer, and gallbladder disease (Manson and Martin, 2001). The risk of endometrial cancer is limited to women taking estrogen-only HRT, as women taking estrogen and progestin combination therapy have no increase in risk. Hence, women without a history of hysterectomy should only be given combination therapy. The risk of thromboembolism is elevated by a factor of roughly 2, but since thromboembolism is rare in otherwise healthy postmenopausal women, the absolute increase in risk is still rather small. For breast cancer, the overall risk appears to be increased by 35% compared to nonusers at 5 years, and the increase in risk increases with continued use. The use of HRT also appears to increase the risk of gallbladder disease by 40–50%.

DHEA (*see* Chapter 118, Endocrinology of Aging)

Dehydroepiandrosterone or DHEA appears to be used rather widely as an antiaging treatment especially since it is widely available over the counter as a non-FDA regulated nutritional supplement (Horani and Morley, 2004). DHEA and its sulfated derivative, DHEAS, are synthesized by the adrenal cortex and at the time of maximum production represent the most abundant steroids in the body. Levels of these hormones peak in the 20s then begin a 2% per year decline such that in 80-year-old patients the levels are only 10–20% of the earlier levels (Arlt, 2004; Horani and Morley, 2004). While the functions of DHEA and DHEAS are not completely understood, it appears that these steroids have functions in both peripheral tissues and the central nervous system (CNS). In peripheral tissues, DHEA serves as a precursor for sex steroid generation and is converted to androstenedione, testosterone, and estradiol. In contrast, in the CNS, DHEA appears to have direct effects on gamma-aminobutryic acid (GABA) and *N*-methyl-D-asparate (NMDA) receptors on neurons (Arlt, 2004).

Low levels of DHEA have been correlated with an increased risk of breast cancer in premenopausal women, an increase in cardiovascular disease and mortality in elderly men in several studies, a lower bone mineral density in perimenopausal women, and a higher likelihood of depressed mood in elderly women. DHEA levels have shown no consistent relationship with cognitive decline in either sex. Hence, there is significant interest in determining whether these observations represent a correlation with aging or, alternately, are caused by lower DHEA levels (Arlt, 2004; Horani and Morley, 2004).

Several studies have supplemented DHEA levels to those seen in young adults often with 50–100 mg doses per day (Table 1). Effects of DHEA supplementation on mood and sense of well-being have been assessed in several studies with mixed but generally positive results. However, some of the studies have used nonvalidated questionnaires for patient evaluation, making comparison difficult. The effects of DHEA on bone mineral density have also been assessed with mixed results, and additionally, a small study found no effect of DHEA on markers of bone turnover. DHEA has been found to have positive effects on skin thickness and indicators such as hydration, sebum production, and pigment, though there were sex differences observed. Women had more improvement in pigmentation and sebum production, while men had more improvement in hydration and thickness. Analysis of body composition with use has found mixed results, with some studies showing increases in muscle mass and decreases in fat mass and with other studies showing no effect. The observed increases in muscle mass did not seem to translate into increases in strength except in one study. In studies, adverse effects on lipid profile, except for small decreases in HDL levels, and glycemic control were generally not seen. In fact, one study suggested that DHEA could improve insulin sensitivity in postmenopausal women. A study treating women with adrenal insufficiency with DHEA saw hepatitis as an adverse effect, but this was reversible after DHEA was discontinued. Concerns have also been raised about the use of DHEA leading to prostate cancer in men or breast or ovarian cancer in women, though no clinical studies have demonstrated an increased risk of cancer with use. In conclusion, at least in the short-term, DHEA supplementation appears safe but there is little evidence that supplementation is beneficial in older patients (Arlt, 2004; Horani and Morley, 2004). Long-term studies to establish the benefits of supplementation, assess safety, and determine the durability of benefits will be needed before routine supplementation can be recommended. Also, patients and practitioners should be aware that many of the DHEA products on the market do not contain bioavailable DHEA.

IS MANIPULATING AGING A GOOD THING TO DO?

It is rather interesting to note the amount of debate surrounding this issue in the absence of any proven means to alter human aging. However, aging is ultimately a normal part of the human life cycle, so a major issue underlying the entire antiaging field is whether treating aging itself as opposed to illness or disability linked to aging is appropriate or desirable (Fisher and Hill, 2004; Miller, 2002; President's Council on Bioethics, 2003; Turner, 2004). Plus, there is likely to never be a treatment that postpones aging indefinitely, so unlike a cure for acquired immune deficiency syndrome (AIDS) or specific cancers that would end that illness for the rest of life, an antiaging treatment would likely be only temporary in effect. Despite this, the desire to escape aging and achieve enhanced longevity seems almost innate in people, given the frequency with which this theme has appeared in literature and history. While the personal value of retarding or reversing either aging or its effects is very individual, much of its value relates back to wanting to maintain hope for the future and prolong a life that is seen as active, full, and rewarding.

Proponents of antiaging medicine put forth several arguments as to why treatments should be aggressively developed (Miller, 2002; Turner, 2004). Some point to the multitude of health benefits experienced by experimental animals treated with caloric restriction or genetic manipulations, such as reductions in age-related diseases and disability. An effective antiaging therapy offers the promise of addressing geriatric syndromes like frailty, which have proven difficult to diagnose and manage via conventional medical treatment. Alternatively, treatment started in middle age could prevent the development of neurodegenerative diseases, such as Alzheimer's disease, that are a major source of anxiety. Furthermore, a treatment that could ensure the long, active, and healthy "golden years" that working adults daydream about would have tremendous individual value. Finally, actuarial estimates show that developing "cures" for all of the major causes of death would add only a few years to the current life expectancy (Fisher and Hill, 2004). Current disease-focused medical research and practice hence could involve significant investments of time and resources with a smaller benefit than a modestly effective antiaging therapy.

Opponents of antiaging medicine also have strong arguments (President's Council on Bioethics, 2003). While many people would like a longer and healthier life, how will the additional time be spent? People envision this time to be spent in leisure activities funded by working adults through pensions or Social Security. However, this is not financially viable and for the vast majority of people would entail working years longer than prior generations. Will a treatment that provides more time for work instead of play still be as attractive? Others worry about the shift in resources from younger people to older people that would accompany the development and use of a successful antiaging therapy. Would education and children's health still be important? Will a world with a perpetually healthy, productive, and increasingly well-trained workforce still welcome children and have a place for them as they grow up? Additionally, during the last decade, concerns have been raised about the appropriate as opposed to inappropriate use of treatments such as cancer screening, automatic implantable cardiac defibrillators, and artificial nutrition in frail, older patients. Will an antiaging therapy be used appropriately or will it add to the treatment burden placed on patients at the end of life with the accompanying human and financial costs? Finally, in a world that is increasingly populated by humans, will there be sufficient space, water, and food for everyone?

It is difficult to reconcile the two sides at this point without more information about the antiaging treatment under debate. Consequently, much of the debate has focused on conceptions of what might exist in the future, sometimes with this conception being probably unrealistic, such as lifespan gains of hundreds of years (Turner, 2004). Being concerned about the social effects of a treatment that extends lifespan to 200 years or more is very reasonable, while a treatment that extends lifespan by 5–10 years but reduces the incidence of Alzheimer's disease by 75% carries fewer ethical concerns. Clearly, the future development of the antiaging medicine field needs to be shaped by public debate, but the current climate which is clouded by hyperbole and unrealistic expectations will make this difficult.

POSSIBLE IMPACTS OF ANTIAGING THERAPIES ON GERIATRIC PRACTICE

Many wonder about the future role of geriatrics, given patient interest in antiaging therapies and the scientific breakthroughs that offer the potential to fuel the development of effective treatments. Some in the antiaging medicine field have tried to paint a dim picture for the future of geriatrics by calling the specialty "dead" because of the gains in health and longevity they feel their therapies will offer. Some in the geriatrics field have joined with biogerontology scientists to attack the safety and effectiveness of currently touted antiaging therapies. Others in the geriatrics field have questioned the wisdom of developing antiaging therapies and worry whether this would become another expensive therapy forced upon frail seniors as being "standard of care". The aura of hyperbole that surrounds some claims for current antiaging therapies and scientific breakthroughs has only further escalated the war of words and has led some to fear for the future of society were an antiaging therapy to be developed.

Clearly, the development of an effective antiaging therapy would have a profound effect on society, the practice of medicine in general, and the specialty of geriatrics, in particular. However, it is unlikely that any antiaging therapy would end the practice of geriatrics. The chances of the development of a 100% effective antiaging therapy that completely halts aging, let alone reverses aging, is rather unlikely. Instead, the antiaging therapies that will emerge are likely to face many of the same issues as therapies for heart disease, stroke, cancer, and other chronic medical conditions, namely, that the treatment will be less than 100% effective, will require continuous use, and will involve trade-offs between benefits and side effects. For example, in many experimental animals there are distinct trade-offs between longevity and fertility. Additionally, since aging involves multiple mechanisms occurring simultaneously to varying degrees in all tissues and organs, probably the best that can be expected is an antiaging therapy that slows or reverses some but not all aspects of aging. Consistent with this, even experimental animals treated with combinations of powerful genetic or drug manipulations to slow aging fail to become immortal and instead eventually age and die. As a result, geriatric patients will still exist in a world with antiaging therapies, and apart from being perhaps older and having more tales to tell, may still face many of the medical, social, and functional problems of today's patients.

Instead of ending the field of geriatrics, the development of effective antiaging therapies might very well open new opportunities to intervene in the chronic medical problems and geriatric syndromes that plague many older patients. Potentially, the treatment of older people with an antiaging treatment could be very different in terms of the dosing, routes, indications, and goals of treatment. For example, an antiaging treatment that benefits middle-aged patients might have no benefit for an old patient in terms of longevity, but short-term intensive use might be an important adjunct during peri-operative care to prevent specific complications or to assist rehabilitation. Alternately, treatments such as hormonal manipulations may emerge, which offer the potential to maximize health and vitality today at the expense of future longevity. This would obviously be a treatment only for frail, older patients as a way to finish life's final tasks or opt for continued independence instead of prolonged dependence. Finally, decisions about selecting a treatment, whether to start a treatment, and when to stop therapy will almost certainly rely upon the key principles in geriatrics of focusing on maximizing function and elucidating a patient's goals of care to help patients choose treatments consistent with these goals.

KEY POINTS

- Patients are interested in antiaging treatments, but few are currently using them. New discoveries by researchers studying aging have made the development of an effective antiaging treatment in the future a reasonable possibility.
- There is little evidence from randomized controlled trials that antioxidant vitamins prevent age-related diseases such as cardiovascular disease or cancer.
- DHEA and testosterone might be beneficial for older patients but data from long-term clinical studies to prove benefits and safety are lacking.
- Clinical studies have shown postmenopausal HRT to only be beneficial for the treatment of menopausal symptoms and osteoporosis. However, the use of HRT carries many risks, such as increased risk of breast cancer, heart attack, and dementia, which outweigh these small benefits.
- The ethical debate about the development and use of antiaging treatments is still in its early phases. A major hurdle for this area is the currently vague ideas about what an antiaging therapy might realistically do.

KEY REFERENCES

- Harris Interactive Inc. Anti-aging medicine, vitamins, minerals and food supplements: a public opinion survey conducted for the International Longevity Center. *Journal of Anti-Aging Medicine* 2003; **6**:83–90.
- Horani MH & Morley JE. Hormonal fountains of youth. *Clinics in Geriatric Medicine* 2004; **20**:275–92.
- President's Council on Bioethics. *Age Retardation: Scientific Possibilities and Moral Challenges* 2003; http://bioethicsprint.bioethics.gov/background/age_retardation.html.
- Rudman D. Growth hormone, body composition, and aging. *Journal of the American Geriatrics Society* 1985; **33**:800–7.
- Shishehbor MH & Hazen SL. Antioxidant studies need a change of direction. *Cleveland Clinic Journal of Medicine* 2004; **71**:285–8.

REFERENCES

Age-Related Eye Disease Study Research Group. A randomized, placebo-controlled, clinical trial of high-dose supplementation with vitamins C and E, beta carotene, and zinc for age-related macular degeneration and vision loss: AREDS report no. 8. *Archives of Ophthalmology* 2001; **119**:1417–36.

Arlt W. Dehydroepiandrosterone and aging. *Best Practice & Research Clinical Endocrinology & Metabolism* 2004; **18**:363–80.

Baker GT III & Sprott RL. Biomarkers of aging. *Experimental Gerontology* 1988; **23**:223–39.

Blackman MR, Sorkin JD, Munzer T *et al.* Growth hormone and sex steroid administration in healthy aged women and men: a randomized controlled trial. *JAMA* 2002; **288**:2282–92.

Brown BG, Zhao XQ, Chait A *et al.* Simvastatin and niacin, antioxidant vitamins, or the combination for the prevention of coronary disease. *New England Journal of Medicine* 2001; **345**:1583–92.

Butler RN. 'Anti-aging' elixirs. *Geriatrics* 2000; **55**:3–4.

Campisi J. Cancer and ageing: rival demons? *Nature Reviews Cancer* 2003; **3**:339–49.

Eidelman RS, Hollar D, Hebert PR *et al.* Randomized trials of vitamin E in the treatment and prevention of cardiovascular disease. *Archives of Internal Medicine* 2004; **164**:1552–6.

Feskanich D, Singh V, Willett WC & Colditz GA Vitamin A intake and hip fractures among postmenopausal women. *JAMA* 2002; **287**:47–54.

Fisher AL & Hill R. Ethical and legal issues in antiaging medicine. *Clinics in Geriatric Medicine* 2004; **20**:361–82.

Gammack JK & Morley JE. Anti-aging medicine-the good, the bad, and the ugly. *Clinics in Geriatric Medicine* 2004; **20**:157–77.

Graat JM, Schouten EG & Kok FJ. Effect of daily vitamin E and multivitamin-mineral supplementation on acute respiratory tract infections in elderly persons: a randomized controlled trial. *JAMA* 2002; **288**:715–21.

Grady D. Postmenopausal hormones–therapy for symptoms only. *New England Journal of Medicine* 2003; **348**:1835–7.

Grady D, Herrington D, Bittner V *et al.* Cardiovascular disease outcomes during 6.8 years of hormone therapy: Heart and Estrogen/progestin Replacement Study follow-up (HERS II). *JAMA* 2002; **288**:49–57.

Guarente L & Kenyon C. Genetic pathways that regulate ageing in model organisms. *Nature* 2000; **408**:255–62.

Harman D. The free radical theory of aging. *Antioxidants and Redox Signaling* 2003; **5**:557–61.

Harris Interactive Inc. Anti-aging medicine, vitamins, minerals and food supplements: a public opinion survey conducted for the International Longevity Center. *Journal of Anti-Aging Medicine* 2003; **6**:83–90.

Hasnain BI & Mooradian AD. Recent trials of antioxidant therapy: what should we be telling our patients? *Cleveland Clinic Journal of Medicine* 2004; **71**:327–34.

Horani MH & Morley JE. Hormonal fountains of youth. *Clinics in Geriatric Medicine* 2004; **20**:275–92.

Howitz KT, Bitterman KJ, Cohen HY *et al.* Small molecule activators of sirtuins extend Saccharomyces cerevisiae lifespan. *Nature* 2003; **425**:191–6.

Koubova J & Guarente L. How does calorie restriction work? *Genes & Development* 2003; **17**:313–21.

Lawlor DA, Davey SG, Kundu D *et al.* Those confounded vitamins: what can we learn from the differences between observational versus randomised trial evidence? *Lancet* 2004; **363**:1724–7.

Manson JE & Martin KA. Clinical practice. Postmenopausal hormone-replacement therapy. *New England Journal of Medicine* 2001; **345**:34–40.

Meagher EA, Barry OP, Lawson JA *et al.* Effects of vitamin E on lipid peroxidation in healthy persons. *JAMA* 2001; **285**:1178–82.

Miller RA. Extending life: scientific prospects and political obstacles. *Milbank Quarterly* 2002; **80**:155–74.

Morley JE. Is the hormonal fountain of youth drying up? *The Journals of Gerontology. Series A, Biological Sciences and Medical Sciences* 2004; **59**:458–60.

Olshansky SJ, Hayflick L & Carnes BA. Position statement on human aging. *The Journals of Gerontology. Series A, Biological Sciences and Medical Sciences* 2002; **57**:B292–7.

Omenn GS, Goodman GE, Thornquist MD *et al.* Risk factors for lung cancer and for intervention effects in CARET, the Beta-Carotene and Retinol Efficacy Trial. *Journal of the National Cancer Institute* 1996; **88**:1550–9.

Podmore ID, Griffiths HR, Herbert KE *et al.* Vitamin C exhibits pro-oxidant properties. *Nature* 1998; **392**:559.

President's Council on Bioethics. *Age Retardation: Scientific Possibilities and Moral Challenges* 2003; http://bioethicsprint.bioethics.gov/background/age_retardation.html.

Rhoden EL & Morgentaler A. Risks of testosterone-replacement therapy and recommendations for monitoring. *New England Journal of Medicine* 2004; **350**:482–92.

Rudman D. Growth hormone, body composition, and aging. *Journal of the American Geriatrics Society* 1985; **33**:800–7.

Rudman D, Feller AG, Nagraj HS *et al.* Effects of human growth hormone in men over 60 years old. *New England Journal of Medicine* 1990; **323**:1–6.

Ruokonen E & Takala J. Dangers of growth hormone therapy in critically ill patients. *Current Opinion in Clinical Nutrition and Metabolic Care* 2002; **5**:199–209.

Sano M, Ernesto C, Thomas RG *et al.*, The Alzheimer's Disease Cooperative Study. A controlled trial of selegiline, alpha-tocopherol, or both as treatment for Alzheimer's disease. *New England Journal of Medicine* 1997; **336**:1216–22.

Shishehbor MH & Hazen SL. Antioxidant studies need a change of direction. *Cleveland Clinic Journal of Medicine* 2004; **71**:285–8.

Shumaker SA, Legault C, Rapp SR *et al.* Estrogen plus progestin and the incidence of dementia and mild cognitive impairment in postmenopausal women: the Women's Health Initiative Memory Study: a randomized controlled trial. *JAMA* 2003; **289**:2651–62.

Tatar M, Bartke A & Antebi A. The endocrine regulation of aging by insulin-like signals. *Science* 2003; **299**:1346–51.

The Alpha-Tocopherol Beta Carotene Cancer Prevention Study Group. The effect of vitamin E and beta carotene on the incidence of lung cancer and other cancers in male smokers. *New England Journal of Medicine* 1994; **330**:1029–35.

Thomas DR. Vitamins in health and aging. *Clinics in Geriatric Medicine* 2004; **20**:259–74.

Turner L. Biotechnology, bioethics and anti-aging interventions. *Trends in Biotechnology* 2004; **22**:219–21.

Vance ML. Can growth hormone prevent aging? *New England Journal of Medicine* 2003; **348**:779–80.

Yialamas MA and Hayes FJ. Androgens and the ageing male and female. *Best Practice & Research Clinical Endocrinology & Metabolism* 2003; **17**:223–36.

Ethical Issues

Maureen Junker-Kenny *and* Davis Coakley

Trinity College, Dublin, Ireland

INTRODUCTION

In the past, diseases that presented in old age were seen as part of the aging process. The advent of geriatric medicine changed this, and physicians began to understand the importance of identifying pathology in old age and of treating it. All students are now taught to look for multiple pathology when assessing elderly patients. Such is the enthusiasm for this approach that the impression is sometimes given that if all the elements giving rise to multiple pathology in an old person could be successfully treated, old age itself would disappear. Similarly, the obsession of modern society with maintaining youth through such measures as creams, vitamins, exercise, and surgery may also result in a denial of aging. In view of this, we begin this chapter with a philosophical reflection on old age. Moreover, an integral vision of old age can serve as a criterion for practical judgments. Old age is an authentic period of a person's life, not simply a process of decay. It is therefore necessary to establish the general grounds of this specific phase of human life to discover the ethical task that it poses before treating problems of applied ethics which present in old age.

OLD AGE AS AN AUTHENTIC PERIOD OF HUMAN LIFE

How can the process of aging be seen as a period of growth and fulfillment rather than a period of decay and degeneration? In many traditions from ancient China to Greece, in the Hebrew and Christian Bibles, to reach old age has been regarded as a divine blessing. In contrast to the high cultures of antiquity that were based on tradition, modern society, with its ever-increasing speed of change, does not show a similar veneration of old age. Yet, because of greater affluence and medical advances, the ancient wish for a long life has come to be true for the majority of the population in the industrialized countries. The average span of life has been lengthened by up to a third, and yet there is a lack of a definite place in the structures of society for the citizens who reach this phase. Is there a solution to this dilemma? What cultural wisdom needs to be redeveloped under the changed conditions of the modern world? In order to answer these questions, the intrinsic values of an age that has matured beyond the mid-life concerns of building a career and raising a family need to be identified. These values are based on the general traits that mark human existence (Auer, 1995a).

PRINCIPLES OF HUMAN PERSONHOOD

Human personhood can be characterized by three elements: autonomy, finitude, and historicity. While all three are present in each stage of human existence, they acquire a new edge in the final stage of life.

Autonomy

Autonomy can be defined as self-government by reason. It is closely linked to the "Categorical Imperative", which, in its humanistic formulation demands to "always treat humanity, whether in your own person or in the person of any other, never simply as a means, but always at the same time as an end" (Kant, 1964a). This principle underlines both the dignity of each person, and their mutual obligation to recognize the equal value of the other. Autonomy, according to Kant, is a mandate to direct oneself by the law of reason in one's life, not simply a "freedom to choose". It cannot be used to defend individualism free of obligations to others, and it includes duties toward oneself. (For a critical discussion of the difference between Kant's original concept of autonomy and current biomedical and consumerist understandings which owe more to JS Mill's emphasis on individuality that civil liberty has to protect against "the tyranny of the majority", (see O'Neill, 2002)). However,

Principles and Practice of Geriatric Medicine, 4th Edition. Edited by M.S. John Pathy, Alan J. Sinclair and John E. Morley.

one problem remains with regard to the ethics of aging. If the unconditional recognition of the other is based on the dignity of each person's freedom, how can this prerequisite be verified? What about fellow human beings whose mental condition undermines their autonomy? It is important to examine the precise wording of Kant's foundation of dignity and understand its implications. (In the kingdom of ends, everything has either a price or a dignity. If it has a price, something else can be put in its place as an equivalent; if it is exalted above all price and so admits of no equivalent, then it has a dignity... that which constitutes the sole condition under which anything can be an end in itself has not merely a relative value – that is, a price – but has intrinsic value – that is, dignity (Kant 1964b)).

(1) It is a transcendental definition of dignity that refers to "conditions of the possibility", as opposed to an empirical one, such as being free of pain. But what is "that which constitutes the sole condition under which anything can be an end in itself"? It is not rationality as such, but in its moral orientation. "Morality is the only condition under which a rational being can be an end in himself... Therefore morality and humanity insofar as it is capable of morality, is the only ground of the dignity of human nature and of every rational nature". The decisive factor for being able to call human beings autonomous is their *capability* for morality, a faculty that can, but does not need to be actualized. It is crucial for the ethics of the end as well as of the beginning of human life that here, quite a different criterion for personhood is established than, for example, consciousness, agency, or the ability to have and voice interests. (2) Kant's understanding of dignity makes it clear that dignity is not at our disposal. Concretely, the specific difference between "having dignity" and "having a price" means that we cannot take stock of our own or anybody else's life. Kant's prohibition of suicide as irreconcilable with autonomy shows the distance between the concept he inaugurated and its current biomedical and cultural use. (3) It contradicts "teleological" arguments for which the empirical capacity to pursue the "goals and purposes of life" is the decisive criterion. Here, the gulf that separates Kant's arguments from some natural law positions becomes visible.

We will return to some practical consequences of Kant's ethics of dignity in the sections on euthanasia.

Finitude

It was the Danish religious philosopher Soren Kierkegaard who made the precarious position of human freedom the basis of his philosophical anthropology. In his *Sickness unto Death* (1849), the human self is portrayed as a "synthesis of the infinite and the finite, of the temporal and the eternal, of freedom and necessity" (Kierkegaard, 1968). The infinity of our intentions contrasts sharply with the finitude of our span of life which cuts short our ability to realize these intentions. Cultural tendencies toward maximizing instant gratification collude with the individual's desire to avoid the unwelcome perspective of death rather than take a reflective stance. The alternative then for a person who has reached this final phase of life lies between affirming and denying his or her own life history.

Historicity

Historicity is the third characteristic of human personhood. Humanity and each individual member spell out their essence only through the course of history and whilst the historical constellations are shared, a person's uniqueness can only be appraised through his response to these conditions. Each phase of life has its own criteria of fulfillment. The task posed for the older person by the historicity of human life is to welcome the opportunity to be accountable both to oneself and to younger generations by being a living link with the past.

THE ETHICAL TASK OF OLD AGE

The demand of choosing for oneself accompanies human existence in all the turns of a person's life. This task may be evaded in middle age by absorbing one's energies totally in a career or in other activities but in old age this cannot be done as easily. The choice at this age then is to either affirm or deny the way one's life has been shaped by oneself and others (Auer, 1995b). If this striving for the unity of one's life is accepted as the genuine task of old age, then the reminiscing of older people should not be discounted as merely a peculiar trait of the aged. Their challenge is to confront the choices they made and that were made for them and to appropriate them.

Attempts to concentrate solely on the present can even be seen as a move to escape from the task of integrating one's life, as one form of denial of a personal journey inevitably marked by disadvantages, wrong turns, and losses. It is a sign of mental health and moral courage to face up to these aspects of one's past and to be reconciled to them. Reconciliation and appropriation do not denote passive and resigned acceptance. They can refer to the ability or wisdom to sustain the tension of opposing poles in one's personality (Erikson *et al.*, 1986). The way in which a person meets the challenges of this phase is crucial for the fulfillment or failure of the whole of his or her life. Currently, many physicians in geriatric medicine see their role purely in terms of treating illness in old age. However, there is also a deeper role and this is the task of accompanying an aging person in a manner that allows him or her to accept and shape the final phase of life in a conscious and personal way (Schockenhoff, 1993).

AGEISM AND RESOURCE ALLOCATION

If one accepts that old age has its own task as outlined above, then one must reject philosophies which value only that period of life when one can take advantage of what have been described as "the prime benefits of life" (Callahan, 1987). The American ethicist Daniel Callahan has been a particular advocate of the concept of a natural lifespan beyond which life-extending treatment would automatically be excluded (Callahan, 1987; Homet and Holstein, 1990). According to Callahan, the natural lifespan ends in most people by the late 70s or early 80s. This attitude of ascribing little or no value to the final years of life has been driven largely by a desire to ration health care resources in this age-group. Over the last decade, a great emphasis has been placed on the need to find morally acceptable criteria on which finite resources can be distributed in the face of infinite needs (Elford, 1987). However, it is a task that should apply to resources not just for the elderly but for all citizens. One of the more sophisticated approaches was developed by Daniels's application of Rawls's theory of justice to resource allocation for the elderly which argues for rationing on the basis of lifetime fair shares of health care (Daniels, 1985). The "prudential lifespan" argument allows for factors such as the redistribution of funds from life-extending measures to nursing home care and domiciliary support for disabled elderly persons. Although this model cannot be accused of ageism, neither can it be declared as just, as it does not address the larger frame of resource decisions made in the political system. In other words, any proposal on rationing can be just only if it forms part of an overall system that is just and when adequate resources are provided in the first place (Wicclair, 1993). The advantage of the Rawlsian approach is that it demands fair access for rich and poor alike to the basic goods of health care. However, in the absence of any just and fair scheme of resource distribution, steps must be taken to safeguard a certain level of resource for the needs of the elderly so that a generation in society that has contributed its share to the political economy will not be short changed.

The issue of resource allocation is not just one of finance. It is also a question of the social imagination being prepared to envisage structures which do justice to the fact that medicine is now more than ever dealing with an aging population. It is a challenge for modern society that is weak on prevention and strong on repair to redirect its health care structures toward a more community-based approach. If the ethical debate on resource allocation is constructed in terms of justified interests of different groups, the starting point is already biased (Mieth, 1993). What is needed is a step back from the financial constraints and a critical analysis of the prevailing priorities. The proper use of resources may then be achieved by adapting the health care system to take into account the needs of an aging society.

It could be argued that too much attention has been paid to the whole subject of rationing health care in the elderly, whereas the real debate should focus on the adequate provision of health care in this age-group. It is still the case that many elderly people who suffer from stroke are deprived of full access to multidisciplinary rehabilitation. In other instances, rehabilitation has to be truncated after an inadequate period because of pressure on resources. Older patients may have to opt for long-term institutional care as they never reach their full potential for recovery. The amount of waste and unnecessary spending in some areas of health is also a matter for ethical consideration, particularly when there is a question of further rationing in an already deprived area. The growth of evidence-based medicine and surgery should be of considerable assistance in addressing these very important issues.

Age has been described as a risk factor for inadequate treatment (Wetle, 1987). Greenfield *et al.* demonstrated that the elderly are more likely to be given inadequate therapy for breast cancer even when controlling for stage of disease, functional status, and comorbidity (Greenfield *et al.*, 1987). It cannot be ethical to make decisions on treatment purely on the basis of chronological age. Frequently, negative characteristics are attributed to older people and this stereotyping is allowed to cloud decisions on individual patients. Negative imagery is also often used when describing elderly patients in ethical debates. Overemphasis on the extremes of disability and incompetence in discussions on issues relating to the elderly can be prejudicial to the majority of elderly people when decisions are made on resource allocation and also prejudicial to the individual when decisions are being made on treatment options. The majority of the elderly reside at home, with only 5% in institutional care (National Council on Ageing & Older People, 2000) (*see* **Chapter 161, Health and Care for Older People in the United Kingdom**). Case histories often describe 75-year-olds with various problems as if this was the extreme of life. Yet, the average life expectancy of a woman of this age is now well over a decade – a very significant length of life at any age.

The physician has an ethical responsibility to defend the best interests of the patient at all times and to act as advocate when required. This may mean, for instance, resisting pressure to discharge patients prematurely because the length of stay has exceeded a figure dictated by the DRGs (diagnostic related groups), or some other system. It must be emphasized that DRG lengths of stay are only mean figures and that the needs of the individual patient must always be paramount. The ethic of patient advocacy is perceived to be under threat in Western society where physicians are increasingly expected to assume the role of a gatekeeper. Under these circumstances, and in view of the demographic shifts in Western societies to low birth rates and greater longevity, there is a real danger that an ethic of cost-effectiveness could assume an unhealthy dominance in many areas of medicine relating to older people (Jecker, 1994).

QUALITY OF LIFE

Clinical decisions in the older age-group are increasingly influenced by perceptions of the individual's quality of life (QoL) either before treatment or as anticipated after treatment. Yet assessments of QoL have been shown to be very subjective. The work of Pearlman *et al.* has demonstrated that physicians who decided to intubate and physicians who decided not to intubate the same hypothetical individual both used assessment of the QoL as the major factor in making their decision (Pearlman *et al.*, 1982). The use of QoL assessment in decision making is ethically justifiable provided that the assessor does not inject a negative bias on the basis of the patient's age. QoL assessments interface with ethical considerations on many issues relating to the elderly and it has been the subject of substantial research. When physicians make judgments on the quality of life of their patients they do so usually on the basis of their qualifications as human beings rather than on their scientific knowledge. When they do make judgments from a professional perspective the criteria are often heavily influenced by a disease-related focus which concentrates on symptoms and limitations. Moreover, there are many papers in the literature which demonstrate major disagreements in many areas of medicine between assessments of patients, QoL provided by patients themselves and those provided by their doctors (Slevin *et al.*, 1988). Some more recently developed QoL measures seek to incorporate the individual perspective on QoL in the overall evaluation. For instance, in the Schedule for the Evaluation of Individual Quality of Life (SEIQoL), it is the individual him/herself who decides what QoL means, thus avoiding the problem of a professionally defined QoL (McGee, 1996).

EUTHANASIA

It is claimed that a natural consequence of the principle of autonomy, as outlined, is to be in control of the time and conditions of one's own death. It is up to the individuals concerned to decide on the value of their own existence to themselves. It can be argued that it is equally reprehensible to force a person who is willing to die to continue to live as it would be to condemn someone to die although he or she wants to live. Ethically, the question is whether these two options are as symmetrical as they are presented. The presupposition of this interpretation of the autonomy argument is that a person's life only needs to be protected as long as the individual deems it valuable. However, this position has been challenged on a number of grounds.

It is debatable whether the concept of autonomy can be stretched to include the ability to control one's own death. In its classical formulation, human finitude was the frame in which every act of autonomous self-determination was set. Both the beginning and the end of one's life were seen as a matter of contingency over which one had no choice. The question is which view is more in keeping with human freedom: to anticipate and "overtake" one's death by administering it oneself, or to accept one's death as one of the conditions of human freedom and make it one's own. The first view identifies the concept of human dignity with one's scope of power, whereas the second insists that dignity reaches beyond it since it also consists in taking a stance toward what happens to oneself. In the latter perspective, it is argued, the ultimate loss of power experienced in dying cannot negate dignity since this concept refers exactly to what is not at our disposal. A similar point is made when life itself is seen as something that has its own ethically relevant value quite apart from the value that the individual might ascribe to it. There is an ongoing debate on how its value relates to other values such as freedom, truth, or solidarity. The question as to whether there is true "symmetry" between forcing someone either to live or to die against his or her will has also been debated on temporal grounds. Even if forced, life is only for a definite period, whereas death is indefinite and irrevocable (Lamb, 1988).

In recent years, there has been much debate on the possible broader social consequences of legalizing voluntary euthanasia. Many fears have been articulated, including the fear that respect for human life in its ailing and dying forms will be eroded, and that the solidarity between generations, which is expressed in caring for the elderly, may be sacrificed for the demands of the healthy active members of society (*see* **Chapter 152, Carers and the Role of the Family**). It has also been suggested that the introduction of voluntary euthanasia may shift the burden of proof toward having to make a case for one's continuing interest in life in order to achieve medical treatment. It is claimed that an older person may feel obliged to calculate the value of his or her life against the costs to the family and to the state for maintaining it (Randall, 1993). In this latter situation, the decision to opt for euthanasia may not have been arrived at autonomously but be driven by the assumed expectations of others (Jecker, 1994).

Another controversial area relates to any implied obligation of medical personnel to assist patients who wish to die. It is argued that this would conflict with generally accepted statements of professional ethics and, in particular, with the principle of nonmaleficence. It is also claimed that making it legal for doctors to assist voluntary euthanasia could undermine the general attitude of trust the public has in their physicians who are expected to act in favor of life (Randall, 1993). The advocates of voluntary euthanasia see these fears as being greatly exaggerated by its opponents. However, others argue that even if the consequences are only feared their gravity is such that it should counsel against embarking on this course (Beauchamp and Childress, 1994). There are also reports in the literature of significant abuses of legal and professional standards regarding physician-assisted deaths in the Netherlands. These reports appear to substantiate the concerns of those physicians and ethicists who worry about the possibility of a "slippery slope" phenomenon if Western societies move to legalize physician-assisted death even under very restricted circumstances (Jecker, 1994; Pijnenborg *et al.*, 1993; Biggar, 2004).

Euthanasia has been legalized in the Netherlands and Belgium. The fear has been expressed that popular acclaim for euthanasia as a solution to suffering may divert attention from the development of palliative care services. According to surveys among oncologists, requests for euthanasia are very rare. They usually stem from poor pain control, and the patients almost invariably change their minds when their physical symptoms are controlled and when they are placed in a supportive environment (Cundiff, 1992). Heintz refutes assertions that adequate palliative care renders euthanasia redundant and he suggests that requests for euthanasia reflect people's needs to maintain a sense of "intactness" and to retain control over events (Heintz, 1994).

NONVOLUNTARY EUTHANASIA

The ethical debate with regard to the extent of medical obligations toward incompetent patients has centered on people in a persistent vegetative state (PVS). Yet the positions formulated in this context on continuing or withholding treatment or care would also be relevant for old and terminally ill patients who are comatose or confused and cannot make their preferences known. Under these conditions decisions must be made for another person on the basis of his or her own best interests. It is therefore a paternalistic or vicarious decision. The person in question lacks the very attributes of autonomy, the abilities for self-reflection, rational decision making and communication. However, the concept of autonomy might inform the quality of life judgments of the person authorized to decide on behalf of the patient. The proxy might evaluate the other's quality of life as lacking the fundamental trait that gives it value, namely, freedom. It would be in keeping with some understandings of autonomy to restrict the obligations toward the reciprocal recognition of persons to free agents. Yet it is equally possible to encompass within the demand for recognition those fellow humans who do not yet or no longer share the rationality, consciousness, and reflexivity of the fully autonomous subject. With this anticipatory, asymmetric, innovative understanding of recognition, comatose and PVS patients would enjoy equal rights to care and treatment on the basis of their being members of the human species. This approach, which gives respect and protection to human life also in its incompetent stages, has been dismissed by some as "speciesism", whereas its advocates describe it as the highest ethical principle (Meilaender, 1987). A transcendental concept of dignity is the basis of this latter argument. (In her "Explanatory Memorandum" to the "Report on the Protection of the Human Rights and Dignity of the Terminally Ill or Dying" (Council of Europe), the Austrian Rapporteur Edeltraut Gatterer specifies: "(3)... Dignity is a consequence of being human. Thus, a condition of being can by no means afford a human being its dignity nor can it ever deprive him or her of it. (4)... Pain, suffering, or weakness do not deprive a human being of his or her dignity. (5)... One possesses dignity and its subsequent rights not due to the recognition of other human beings, but due to one's descent from them ... (6) An individual's dignity can be respected or violated, yet it can neither be granted nor lost. Respect for human dignity is independent of factual reciprocity. Respect for human dignity is also due where reciprocity is not, not yet, or no longer possible (i.e. toward patients in a coma). To believe that human dignity may be divided or limited to certain stages or conditions of life is a form of disregard for human dignity.")

The position espoused by Meilaender (1987) of unconditional respect and the continuance of care for the embodied other has been criticized as "vitalism" as it seems to accord the highest value to biological human life irrespective of its possibilities of expression. Critics of this approach offer an alternative one and that is to respect physical life as a condition for the values and goals of life such as communication that transcend the biological level. From this teleological view that derives the value of life from its ability to attain its purposes and ends, they would argue that hydration and nutrition for PVS patients who can no longer "pursue life's goals" can be withdrawn (Shannon and Walter, 1993). The best interests of the patient should be the only consideration taken into account, and the only burden considered should be the burden of treatment on the patient and not the burden on the family, clinical staff, or society. This reasoning avoids the danger of social Darwinism, of sacrificing the weaker members of the community to the interests of the more powerful ones. It is thus based on a position that acknowledges the basic rights of individuals, competent or incompetent, as a limit which cannot be overridden in favor of the presumed needs of a collectivity. It is articulated in the face of a perceived danger that the aggressive use of medical technology may fail to accept the limits of human finitude.

The care of patients with no detectable mental capacity is an extreme example of the ethical principles at stake in situations of asymmetric communication where the competence to decide on further treatment has to be *referred* to a proxy. Much more frequent in geriatric medical practice would be situations where the patient's autonomy is not totally lacking, but where its degree is in doubt. Then, the principle of autonomy can conflict with the principles of beneficence and nonmaleficence. Here, apart from the assessment of the patient's competence to make decisions, difficult judgments on the quality of life also come into consideration. It is in this latter situation that differences of perspective may play a critical role. For instance, the value placed on a patient's life by a professional staff member may differ quite considerably from that of family and life-long friends who will have empathy and insights from sharing life's experiences with the person.

ADVANCE DIRECTIVES

There has been a growing interest in many countries in the concept of advance directives. In the United States, the Patient Self Determination Act (1991) requires all health care institutions to advise patients of their rights to accept or refuse medical care and to execute an advance directive. Legal frameworks for advanced directives are also in existence in Belgium, Germany, Holland, and Switzerland. Directives can take the form of a written instruction or be expressed by the appointment of a proxy to make decisions on behalf of the patient under certain circumstances. Directives of this nature have been generally well received by physicians as they decrease the possibility of legal actions over decisions made in good faith, and they extend patient autonomy (Editorial, 1992). However, reservations have been expressed about the meaning and durability of advance directives (Emanuel and Emanuel, 1990). Advance directives are based on the assumption that patients can anticipate their choice under future circumstances when death is imminent. Danis *et al.* in a prospective study found that some patients' wishes were unstable and suggested that the advance directive should be looked upon as an instruction for future care rather than a prediction of future wishes (Danis *et al.*, 1994). Preferences for life sustaining treatments appear only to be moderately stable, and the likelihood of choosing such treatments increases with worsening health (Emanuel *et al.*, 1994; Danis *et al.*, 1994). Under these circumstances it would be important to ask patients routinely how closely they wish their health care provider to adhere to their advance directives. There may also be problems both in providing and in eliciting the necessary information to make a properly informed advance directive. The patient will be required to make decisions about potential quality of life and a range of complex possible medical interventions. The listing of potential procedures may divert attention from the overall treatment goals and may give rise to inappropriate care (Brett, 1991).

Decisions about level of care are based on a complex interaction of the benefits and burdens of different therapies with individual patient goals. Fried and Gillick have shown that there are multiple points in the course of a community-dwelling patient's final illness at which choices about level of care can be made (Fried and Gillick, 1995). During this process, a significant number of elderly patients or their surrogates choose less intensive therapy. Many of these choices relate to diagnostic procedures and therapies whose relative benefits and burdens change depending upon the patient's condition, the aims of treatment, and the availability of different options. Decisions such as these, which are intimately dependent on specific circumstances, cannot easily be made by reference to advance directives. Moreover, Fried and Gillick point out that if alternatives are consistently explained during the course of an illness, the pattern of decisions made by a previously competent patient can provide guidance for both the physician and family when the patient can no longer take part in the discussions (Fried and Gillick, 1995). Dresser and Robertson have also pointed out that it is difficult, if not impossible, for competent individuals to predict their interests in future treatment situations when they are incompetent because their needs and interests will have changed radically (Dresser and Robertson, 1989). Research has shown that directives that are overly medicalized in format are largely ineffective in practice. In view of the complexity of advance decision making, a statutory basis for advance directives may, in fact, be contrary to the purpose of exercising autonomy.

BENEFICENCE AND PATERNALISM

Health care professionals need to be aware of the danger of regarding patients and family members who challenge their opinion as incompetent, and they must question the extent to which their own values may color their professional judgments (Finucane *et al.*, 1993). The frequency of end-of-life decisions that are most strongly determined by cultural factors, such as patients' autonomy, criteria for medical futility, or legal status (euthanasia, nontreatment decisions), varies much between countries (van der Heide *et al.*, 2003). The communication framework of Charles *et al.* which defines three distinct components of decision making – information exchange, deliberation about treatment options, and responsibility for the choice – may help model the physician–patient encounter (Charles *et al.*, 1999). There is also the danger that the principle of beneficence can lead to a paternalistic attitude. Data from the SUPPORT (Study to Understand Prognosis and Preferences for Outcomes and Risks of Treatment) project canvassed about 1000 seriously ill elderly patients and found that only approximately one-quarter had ever discussed cardiopulmonary resuscitation (CPR) with a physician (Krumholz *et al.*, 1998). Beneficence must be balanced against a patient's right to take risks. There should always be respect for the personhood of others and patients must not be seen as problems but as persons with problems. The dignity of the individual is promoted through informed consent and opportunities for choice and risk taking (Everett, 1993). For instance, an elderly person considered to be at risk may wish to keep on living unsupervised and less protected in his or her own home instead of moving to a nursing home.

However, despite its potential abuse in situations of unequal power the principle of beneficence testifies to a society's concern for the elderly. Beneficence as an ethical principle is being eroded in a number of Western countries where doctors are being encouraged to regard their patients as customers (Randall, 1993). Under these circumstances it should not be surprising if the ethics of the market place begin to find a place at the patient's bedside.

MEDICAL FUTILITY

Most physicians accept that it is reasonable to withhold therapy when treatment offers potentially little benefit but might impose great burdens on a patient (Luchins and Hanrahan, 1993). This acceptance is borne out by the widespread introduction of "do not resuscitate" (DNR) policies in hospitals and nursing homes. However, it needs to be kept in mind that the presence of a DNR order may affect physicians' willingness to order a variety of treatments not related to CPR, and physicians should elicit additional information about patients' treatment goals to inform these decisions (Beach and Morrison, 2002; Zweig *et al.*, 2004). The pre-eminence given to autonomy in modern society as an ethical principle can sometimes lead physicians to disregard other moral considerations and common sense when making clinical decisions. The employment of futile treatments cannot be demanded in law or by ethics and it serves no purpose to discuss in detail with dying patients treatment propositions that are unrealistic (Finucane and Harper, 1996). The discussion of medical futility has contributed an important dimension to the ethics of decision making near the end of life by focusing attention on the questions "what are we trying to achieve?" and "are we able to do it?" (Weber and Campbell, 1996) Doctors rarely receive training on how to deal with these complex ethical issues and there is a great need for educational programs which would foster the development of appropriate skills in this area (Husebo *et al.*, 2004; Hinka *et al.*, 2002).

Some physicians appear to believe that it is obligatory to use every available medical measure, no matter how futile, in order to prolong the life of a patient unless he or she is given or has been given directions to the contrary. Other physicians allow their own judgments to be overridden by acceding to the requests of patients (or their surrogates), who demand treatment which offers no benefit (Schneiderman *et al.*, 1990). Fried and Gillick have highlighted the conflicts which arise in long-term care when surrogates demand treatments which are viewed by the clinical staff as being excessively burdensome on the patients and technically futile (Kant, 1964a). They argue that the solution to the problem is to develop institutional policies within long-term care facilities that would restrict the scope of treatment facilities that could be made by surrogates. These policies would be derived from the experiences of the multidisciplinary team and would help construct a care plan for individual patients within which the proxy would be consulted on the implementation of specific therapies.

ETHICS AND GENETIC INFORMATION

The issue of freedom comes up again with regard to genetic information. The ethical problems of predictive genetic testing for incurable disease have become more of a concern for physicians in geriatric medicine in recent years. For instance, the relatives of patients suffering from Alzheimer's disease may be faced with the choice of discovering or ignoring their own genetic status (Post, 1994). The advantages of knowing lie in the possibility of relief from fear after a negative test result or in the ability to plan one's life and one's own reproductive choices after a positive test result. Yet, even here research on sufferers from Huntington's chorea and their families has shown that the relief of those family members who find out that they have been spared the defective gene is overshadowed by a sense of loss which has been compared to survivor's guilt (Burgess, 1994). The dangers of reducing persons to the sum of their genes or even further to their own one defective gene, of social discrimination, and of workplace and insurance disadvantages are equally present. The right to privacy opposes any obligation for genetic screening. The principle of equality is also endangered when data banks display genetic risk factors of affected citizens, thus enabling staff to predict the likely course of other people's lives. What is most at risk, however, when genetic screening is prescribed rather than being left to an individual's own initiative, is the realization of freedom as spontaneity. This means being able to embark on life's journey without knowing the outcome and being able to choose courses of action like everyone else without having to grieve in advance about future loss of self in a genetically predicted dementia.

KEY POINTS

- Integrating the unity of one's life is proposed as the genuine task of old age.
- Ageism should not be a factor in determining resource allocation, and when attempting to evaluate the quality of life of an older individual one must be aware of the limitations of purely professional assessments.
- Reports appear to substantiate the concerns of physicians and ethicists about the possibility of a 'slippery slope' phenomenon following legalization for physician-assisted death even under very restricted conditions. Research has shown that advanced directives, which are overtly medicalized, are usually ineffective in practice.
- The employment of futile treatments cannot be demanded in law or by ethics, and it serves no purpose to discuss in detail treatment possibilities with dying patients, which are unrealistic.
- Genetic testing may result in positive or negative consequences for an individual and these should be explained fully when counselling with regard to genetic testing.

KEY REFERENCES

- Biggar N. *Aiming to Kill. The Ethics of Suicide and Euthanasia* 2004, pp 120–51; Darton, Longman and Todd, London.
- Danis M, Garrett J, Harris R & Patrick D. Stability of choices about life-sustaining treatments. *Annals of Internal Medicine* 1994; **120**:567–73.
- Everett G. Autonomy and paternalism: an ethical dilemma in caring for the elderly. *Perspectives* 1993; **17**:2–5.
- O'Neill O. *Autonomy and Trust in Bioethics*, 2002, pp 28–48; Cambridge University Press, Cambridge.
- Wicclair MR. *Age-rationing, Ageism and Justice. Ethics and the Elderly* 1993, p 102; Oxford University Press, Oxford.

REFERENCES

Auer A. Das angereicherte Sinngefuge des Alterns im Horizont der erhöhten Lebenserwartung. *Geglucktes Altern* 1995a, pp 73–84; Herder, Freiburg.

Auer A. Die individual-ethische Perspektive: Altern als persönliche Herausforderung des einzelnen. *Geglücktes Altern* 1995b, pp 159–76; Herder, Freiburg.

Beach MC & Morrison RS. The effect of do-not-resuscitate order on physician decision-making. *Journal of the American Geriatrics Society* 2002; **50**(12):2057.

Beauchamp TL & Childress JF. Respect for autonomy. *Principles of Biomedical Ethics* 1994, 4th edn, p 141; Oxford University Press, Oxford.

Biggar N. *Aiming to Kill. The Ethics of Suicide and Euthanasia* 2004, pp 120–51; Darton, Longman and Todd, London.

Brett AS. Limitations of listings specific medical interventions in advance directives. *The Journal of the American Medical Association* 1991; **266**:825–8.

Burgess MM. Ethical issues in genetic testing for Alzheimer's disease: lessons from Huntington's disease. *Alzheimer Disease and Associated Disorders* 1994; **8**:71–8.

Callahan D. *Setting Limits. Medical Goals in an Aging Society* 1987; Simon and Schuster, New York.

Charles C, Gafni A & Whelan T. Decision-making in the physician-patient encounter: revisiting the shared treatment decision- making model. *Social Science & Medicine* 1999; **49**:651–61.

Cundiff D. *Euthanasia is Not the Answer: A Hospice Physician's View* 1992, p 24; Humana Press, Totowa.

Daniels N. *Just Healthcare* 1985; Cambridge University Press, Cambridge.

Danis M, Garrett J, Harris R & Patrick D. Stability of choices about life-sustaining treatments. *Annals of Internal Medicine* 1994; **120**:567–73.

Dresser RS & Robertson JA. Quality of life and non-treatment decisions for incompetent patients: a critique of the orthodox approach. *Law, Medicine and Health Care* 1989; **17**:234–44.

Editorial. Advance directives. *Lancet* 1992; **340**:1321–2.

Elford RJ. A response (cf. to Grimley Evans, the Sanctity of Life). In RJ Elford (ed) *Medical Ethics and Elderly People* 1987, pp 93–105; Churchill Livingstone, Edinburgh.

Emanuel EJ & Emanuel LL. Living wills: past present and future. *The Journal of Clinical Ethics* 1990; **1**:9–19.

Emanuel LL, Emanuel EJ, Stoeckle JD *et al.* Advance directives: stability of patient treatment choices. *Annals of Internal Medicine* 1994; **154**:209–17.

Erikson EH, Erikson JM & Kivnick HQ. Ages and stages. *Vital Involvement in Old Age* 1986, pp 32–8; Norton, London.

Everett G. Autonomy and paternalism: an ethical dilemma in caring for the elderly. *Perspectives* 1993; **17**:2–5.

Finucane TE & Harper M. Ethical decision-making near the end of life. *Clinics Geriatric Medicine* 1996; **12**:369–77.

Finucane P, Myser C & Ticehurst S. Is she fit to sign, doctor? practical ethical issues in assessing the competence of elderly patients. *The Medical Journal of Australia* 1993; **159**:400–3.

Fried TR & Gillick MR. The limits of proxy decision making: overtreatment. *Cambridge Quarterly of Healthcare Ethics* 1995; **4**:524–9.

Greenfield S, Blanco DM & Elashoff RM. Patterns of care related to age of breast cancer patients. *The Journal of the American Medical Association* 1987; **257**:2766–70.

Heintz APM. Euthanasia: can be part of good terminal care. *British Medical Journal* 1994; **308**:1656.

Hinka H, Kosunen E & Lammi EK. Treatment decision in end-of-life scenarios involving terminal cancer and terminal dementia. *Palliative Medicine* 2002; **16**(3):195–204.

Homet P & Holstein M (eds). *A Good Old Age? The Paradox of Setting Limits* 1990; Simon and Schuster, New York.

Husebo BS, Husebo S & Hysing-Dahl B. Old and given up for dying? palliative care in Nursing Homes. *Illness, Loss and Crisis* 2004; **1**:52–9.

Jecker NS. Physician-assisted death in the Netherlands and the United States: ethical and cultural aspects of health policy development. *Journal of the American Geriatrics Society* 1994; **42**:672–8.

Kant I. *Groundwork of the Metaphysic of Morals (1787)* translated and analysed by HJ Paton, 1964a, p 97; Harper and Row, New York.

Kant I. *Groundwork of the Metaphysic of Morals*, trans. HJ Paton, 1964b, pp 102–3; Harper & Row.

Kierkegaard S. *Fear and Trembling and The Sickness unto Death*, translated by WLowrie, 1968; Princeton University Press, Princeton.

Krumholz H, Philips R, Hemel M *et al.* Resuscitation preference among patients with severe congestive heart failure. *Circulation* 1998; **21**: 77–81.

Lamb D. The contagiousness of killing. *Down the Slippery Slope. Arguing in Applied Ethics* 1988, p 48; Croom Helm, London.

Luchins DJ & Hanrahan P. What is appropriate health care for end-stage dementia? *Journal of the American Geriatrics Society* 1993; **41**:25–30.

McGee HM. Ethics and the assessment of quality of life. *Irish Journal of Psychological* 1996; **17**:156–77.

Meilaender G. On removing food and water: against the stream. In T Shannon (ed) *Bioethics* 1987, 3rd edn, pp 215–22; Paulist Press, Mahwah.

Mieth D. The problem of 'justified interests' in genome analysis. A socioethical approach. In H Haker *et al.* (eds) *The Ethics of Human Genome Analysis. European Perspectives* 1993, pp 272–89; Attempto Verlag, Tübingen.

National Council on Ageing & Older People, *A Framework for Quality in Long Term Residential Care for Older People in Ireland* 2000; National Council on Ageing and Older People, Dublin.

O'Neill O. *Autonomy and Trust in Bioethics*, 2002, pp 28–48; Cambridge University Press, Cambridge.

Pearlman RA, Inui TS & Carter WB. Variability in physician bioethical decision making: a case study of euthanasia. *Annals of Internal Medicine* 1982; **97**:420–5.

Pijnenborg L, van der Maas PJ, van Delden JJM & Looman CWN. Life-terminating acts without explicit request of patient. *Lancet* 1993; **341**:1196–9. For a review of ethical debates and legal decisions on the Dutch law up to 2003, see Biggar 2004.

Post SG. Ethical commentary: genetic testing for Alzheimer disease. *Alzheimer Disease and Associated Disorders* 1994; **8**:66–7.

Randall F. Two lawyers and a technician. *Palliative Medicine* 1993; **7**:193–8.

Schneiderman LJ, Jecker NS & Jonsen AR. Medical futility: its meaning and ethical implications. *Annals of Internal Medicine* 1990; **112**:949–54.

Schockenhoff E. Die Verantwortung fur das fremde Leben: Abtreibung und Euthanasie. *Ethik des Lebens. Ein Theologischer Grundriss* 1993, p 329; Grunewald, Mainz.

Shannon T & Walter JJ. The PVS patient and the forgoing/withdrawing of nutrition and hydration. In T Shannon (ed) *Bioethics* 1993, 4th edn, pp 173–98; Paulist Press, Mahwah.

Slevin ML, Plant H, Lynch D *et al.* Who should measure quality of life, the doctor or the patient? *British Journal of Cancer* 1988; **57**:109–12.

van der Heide A, Deliens L, Faisst K *et al.*, EURELD consortium. End-of life decision making in six European countries: descriptive study. *The Lancet* 2003; **362**:345–50.

Weber LJ & Campbell ML. Medical futility and life sustaining treatment decisions. *The Journal of Neuroscience Nursing* 1996; **28**:56–60.

Wetle T. Age as a risk factor for inadequate treatment. *The Journal of the American Medical Association* 1987; **258**:516.

Wicclair MR. *Age-rationing, Ageism and Justice. Ethics and the Elderly* 1993, p 102; Oxford University Press, Oxford.

Zweig SC, Kruse RL & Binder EF. Effect of do-not-resuscitate orders on hospitalization of nursing home residents evaluated for lower respiratory infections. *Journal of the American Geriatrics Society* 2004; **52**:51–8.

142

Restraints and Immobility

Elizabeth A. Capezuti[1] ***and*** **Laura M. Wagner**[2]

[1]*New York University, New York, NY, USA, and* [2]*Baycrest Centre for Geriatric Care, Toronto, ON, Canada*

INTRODUCTION

Immobility is strongly associated with functional decline among older adults. Restrictive devices such as physical restraints and siderails deter mobility. Despite a growing body of literature documenting the negative consequences associated with immobilizing older adults with restrictive devices, the practice persists in both acute and long-term health care settings, where most health care providers continue to believe that restraints are an effective strategy in keeping older adults safe. This chapter provides an overview of the effects of immobility, with an emphasis on the consequences of prolonged physical restraint and restrictive siderail usage. Finally, clinical strategies and organizational approaches to replace restraints and restrictive siderails, and the evidence to support their use are presented.

IMMOBILITY

Immobility is the restriction of time spent out of bed (or chair) by medical orders, restrictive devices, chemical restraints, lack of mobility aids, human assistance, or encouragement. Immobility has been correlated with muscle atrophy, loss of muscle strength and endurance, bone loss, joint contractures, and problems with balance and coordination that lead to increased incidence of falls (Bloomfield, 1997; Covertino *et al.*, 1997; Allen *et al.*, 1999). Moreover, reduced bone mass, which is a consequence of decreased weight-bearing and physical activity, can contribute to the increased likelihood that falls will result in serious injury (Grisso *et al.*, 1991). Other secondary effects of immobility include increased risk of infection, new pressure sores, contractures, and functional incontinence. Table 1 lists the effects of immobility (Lofgren *et al.*, 1989; Frengley and Mion, 1986; Robbins *et al.*, 1987).

It is well documented that functional decline, including new walking dependence occurs in one-third to one-half of older hospitalized patients (Fortinsky *et al.*, 1999; Hirsch *et al.*, 1990; Mahoney, 1998; Mahoney *et al.*, 1998; McCusker *et al.*, 2002). Functional decline or "deconditioning" refers to the loss of the ability to perform basic activities of daily living. Attributed primarily to the effects of immobilization by "forced bed rest, immobilizing devices (e.g. catheters), restraint use, and lack of encouragement of independence in self-care", (Inouye *et al.*, 1993; p., 1353) functional decline has been correlated with numerous negative consequences. A systematic review of thirty studies examining correlates of functional decline found that between 15 and 76% of hospitalized elders experience diminished performance in at least one activity of daily living at discharge. Of those with decline at discharge, only half will recover function at three months postdischarge, and, for many, this decline will result in permanent loss of independent living (McCusker *et al.*, 2002; Fortinsky *et al.*, 1999; Sager *et al.*, 1996; Covinsky *et al.*, 1997). Functional decline is considered a profound marker of morbidity and mortality (Thomas, 2002; Walter *et al.*, 2001) resulting in longer lengths of stay, greater costs, and increased rate of nursing home (NH) placement (Fortinsky *et al.*, 1999; Inouye *et al.*, 1993; Janelli, 1995; McCusker *et al.*, 2002).

There is strong support in the literature linking prolonged physical restraint use with the consequences of immobility (Inouye *et al.*, 2000; Inouye *et al.*, 1999; Selikson *et al.*, 1988; Mahoney, 1998). This process, labeled "spiraling immobility" by Tinetti and Ginter (1988), creates a "catch-22" situation in which an older person, perceived to be at risk of falling, is restrained to prevent falling and is then unable to ambulate again, independently or safely, due to the immobilizing consequences of physical restraint. Other restrictive devices (e.g. full enclosure siderails) or practices (e.g. lack of assistance out of bed) also contribute to immobilization. Table 2 summarizes the effects of physical restraints and siderails.

Principles and Practice of Geriatric Medicine, 4th Edition. Edited by M.S. John Pathy, Alan J. Sinclair and John E. Morley.

Table 1 Effects of immobility

Musculoskeletal
Muscle atrophy
Loss of muscle strength and endurance
Osteoporosis
Joint contractures
Problems with balance and coordination
Gastrointestinal
Constipation
Impaction
Integumentary
Pressure Ulcers
Respiratory
Pneumonia
Atelectasis
Cardiovascular
Deep Vein Thrombosis
Pulmonary Embolism
Orthostasis

Table 2 Negative effects of physical restraints and siderails

Musculoskeletal
Immobility
Contractures
Falls
Decreased muscle mass, tone, strength
Osteoporosis
Fractures
Rhabdomyolysis
Neurological
Brachial plexus injury
Axillary vein thrombosis
Compressive neuropathy
Cardiovascular
Stress-induced cardiac arrhythmias
Orthostasis
Dependent edema
Psychological
Depression
Agitation
Increased Confusion
Integumentary
Pressure ulcers
Skin tears, bruises, abrasions
Cellulitis
Gastrointestinal/Genitourinary
Incontinence
Constipation
Infectious Disease
Nosocomial infections
Miscellaneous
Strangulation/Death
Entrapment
Asphyxiation
Hyperthermia

PHYSICAL RESTRAINTS

Physical restraints are defined as "any manual method or physical or mechanical device, material, or equipment attached or adjacent to the individual's body that the individual cannot remove easily which restricts freedom of movement or normal access to one's body" (Centers for Medicare and Medicaid Services, 1999). Examples of physical restraints include chest/vest, pelvic, combination of wrist, mitt or ankle, as well as geriatric chairs with fixed tray tables, and cushion tables in wheelchairs. These devices are generally not easily removed by the older adult (Braun and Capezuti, 2000).

Restraint use in NHs varies among countries and institutions as demonstrated in a study comparing restraint practices in NHs in Denmark, France, Ireland, Italy, Japan, Spain, Sweden, and the United States. A chair that prevents rising was the most common form of restraint while limb restraints were the least commonly used (CMS, 2004). Trunk restraints were more prevalent in Sweden and the United States than other restraint types (Ljunggren *et al.*, 1997). In general, the study found a very low prevalence of restraint use in Denmark, Iceland, and Japan with less than 9% of NH residents restrained at any time (Ljunggren *et al.*, 1997). Between 15 and 17% of the residents were restrained in France, Italy, Sweden, and the United States. Spain demonstrated the highest usage with almost 40% of residents restrained. Restraint practice patterns were attributed to cultural backgrounds and ethical views (Ljunggren *et al.*, 1997). Another study found that 24% of older adults are restrained in Sweden (Karlsson *et al.*, 1996), and at least 49% of residents in Dutch NHs are restrained (Hamers *et al.*, 2004).

In the United States, approximately 40% of NH residents were restrained in the 1980s (Evans and Strumpf, 1989). Combined with the research and heavy regulatory oversight in the United States, the prevalence of restraint use among NH residents dropped to 13% by 1998 and almost 9% in 2003 (Health Care Financing Administration, 1998; Zinn, 1994). In addition to diminished usage, restraints employed in NHs are "less restrictive" compared to the previous decade; wheelchair cushions and seat belts are more often used than the more restrictive vest restraints. Restraint use continues to vary widely throughout the United States (Phillips *et al.*, 1996), with some regions reporting almost 20% usage (Capezuti and Talerico, 1999) while others continue with even higher usage (Castle, 2002).

Spurred by the practice shift in the NH setting, reduction in hospital physical restraint use began in the early 1990s (Frengley and Mion, 1998; Sullivan-Marx and Strumpf, 1996). In the United States, the Joint Commission on Accreditation of Healthcare Organizations (JCAHO) developed standards to help reduce physical restraints (Capezuti *et al.*, 2000; Joint Commission on Accreditation of Healthcare Organizations, 1996; Bryant and Fernald, 1997). In American hospitals, the prevalence varies from 3.4 to 24.3% in nonintensive and intensive care settings, respectively (Minnick *et al.*, 1998). Restraint use is more often employed to prevent treatment interference than to avert falls, thus arm/limb restraints prevail over chest/vest restraints (Frengley and Mion, 1998; Mion, 1996; Mion *et al.*, 1996).

SIDERAILS

Siderails, also *referred* to as bed rails, cotsides, guardrails, safety rails, or sideboards, are adjustable metal or rigid plastic bars that attach to the bed and come in a variety of sizes (e.g. full-length, 1/2 length, split rails) (Braun and Capezuti, 2000). Many NH beds include bilateral, full-length siderails, while hospital beds generally have four "half" or "split" siderails, allowing diverse combinations of rails from one upper rail to both upper and lower rails (Levine *et al.*, 2000). Siderails are defined as restraints or "restrictive" devices when used to impede a patient's ability to voluntarily get out of bed (Capezuti, 2000). Since the use of restraints in bed have been drastically reduced in both NHs and hospitals, siderails have become the most frequently used restraint to prevent older adults from independent or accidental egress from bed (O'Keefe *et al.*, 1996; Capezuti *et al.*, 2002; van Leeuwen *et al.*, 2001).

In 1992, the United States Centers for Medicare and Medicaid Services (CMS; formerly the Health Care Financing Administration, 1992) issued guidelines to NHs that classified siderails as restraints when they prevent voluntary egress (Health Care Financing Administration, 1992). These guidelines were updated in both 1997 and 1999 to emphasize that restraints are defined according to their functional application as any device, material, or equipment that inhibits mobility or change in position, and are not easily removed by the person (Department of Health and Human Services, 1997; 1999). Similarly, the 1999 CMS Hospital Conditions of Participation and 2001 JCAHO standards redefined siderail use as restraints for hospitals using this functional definition (Capezuti and Braun, 2001).

Similar to physical restraints, siderail use varies among countries and institutions. Several surveys conducted in four areas of Australia described restraint prevalence among a sample of 36 000 NH residents as ranging from 15.3 to 26% (Retsas and Crabbe, 1997). Of those restrained, the most frequently used restraints were siderails. Australian nurses, like their American counterparts, frequently restrained residents due to fear of legal retribution. Interestingly, such fears are not raised in the British literature. A study conducted in a British hospital reported that 8.4% of patients had full-length siderails raised. Despite such low usage compared to American hospitals, the researchers questioned the appropriateness of bedrails (O'Keefe *et al.*, 1996). A British medical journal editorial described the "absurd" and "distasteful" use of siderails in the United States (Anonymous, 1984). The British aversion toward siderails is traced to a 1975 policy established by the Joint Working Party of the British Geriatrics Society and the Royal College of Nursing that clearly discourages routine bedrail use (Everitt and Bridel-Nixon, 1997). In 1999, the Royal College of Nursing issued guidelines aimed at further reduction of restraints; bedrails are listed as the most likely form of restraint.

There are no national statistics available for siderail prevalence in American NHs (Braun and Capezuti, 2000), however, several studies report rates of restrictive siderail use in NHs ranging from 18 to 64% (Tinetti *et al.*, 1991; Capezuti *et al.*, 2002; Wagner *et al.*, 2003). There are also no national figures or large multisite studies that quantify current siderail usage in American hospitals, though one study reports 20% usage following siderail reduction efforts (Si and Neufeld, 1999), and another reports a prevalence rate of 30% of nighttime use among patients in medical surgical units and 67% in the critical care setting (Capezuti *et al.*, 2000). The continued use of both restraint and siderail usage is based on embedded practices of health care providers who for decades have linked these devices to patient safety and protection (Brush and Capezuti, 2001; Strumpf and Tomes, 1993).

RISK FACTORS AND JUSTIFICATION

Use of restrictive devices depends on three factors: patient characteristics, organizational attributes, and health care providers' justification. Prevalence of restrictive devices varies with age, functional status, and cognition (Strumpf *et al.*, 1998). Greater age, worsened physical health, a previous fall, and the presence of depression or other psychiatric disorders have been associated with restraint use (Frengley and Mion, 1986; Tinetti *et al.*, 1991; Berland *et al.*, 1990).

Impaired cognition is the most significant patient factor associated with restraint and siderail use (Capezuti and Talerico, 1999; Strumpf and Tomes, 1993; Castle and Mor, 1998; O'Keefe *et al.*, 1996; Capezuti *et al.*, 1996). Among ambulatory NH residents, a restraint prevalence of 37% was reported in confused residents, while nonconfused residents were virtually never restrained (Capezuti *et al.*, 1996). In one study examining continued use of physical restraints following a restraint reduction intervention, patient factors such as physical dependency, lower cognitive status, behavior, presence of treatment devices, presence of psychiatric disorders, and perceived fall risk were all significantly associated with continued restraint use. Confused older adults and elders are also the most likely to be restrained in hospitals (Sullivan-Marx *et al.*, 1999; Bourbonniere *et al.*, 2003).

Castle and colleagues reported that organizational attributes, rather than patient factors, was more predictive of restraint use after the implementation of American federal regulations for NHs. These include high nursing aide–patient ratios, reduced occupancy rates, and prospective Medicaid reimbursement (Castle *et al.*, 1997). Similarly, in hospitals, high utilization of licensed practical nurses rather than registered nurses and nurse staffing patterns on weekend shifts are strongly associated with restraint use (Bourbonniere *et al.*, 2003).

Justification for restraints is also based on the health care providers' view that these devices prevent vulnerable older adults from injury secondary to falls, behavioral symptoms, or treatment interference. The most common reason cited for restraint and siderail use is prevention of falls (Braun and Capezuti, 2000). Among the cognitively impaired who demonstrate impaired gait and diminished safety awareness, restraints, and siderails are used to prevent independent transfer from chairs or bed. There is no empirical evidence, however, to support the use of these devices to prevent falls.

Numerous studies demonstrate a significant incidence of falls and injury among restrained confused patients in both NH and hospital settings (Capezuti *et al.*, 1996; Neufeld *et al.*, 1999; Capezuti *et al.*, 1999a; Shorr *et al.*, 2002; Tinetti *et al.*, 1992). One study prospectively observed fall-related incidents and injuries after the initiation of physical restraints among previously unrestrained ambulatory NH residents. After adjusting for confounding factors such as disorientation, physical restraint was associated with continued fall-related incidents and, most importantly, serious injury. They also found that intermittent restraint use in ambulatory residents led to increased fall-related serious injuries. The researchers concluded that the immobilizing effect of intermittent restraint use on muscle and bone strength was responsible for these results. Another study examining the relationship between restraint use and falls among 332 NH residents found that restraints were not associated with a significantly lower risk of falls or fall-related injuries (Capezuti *et al.*, 1996).

There is also no evidence to support the use of restrictive siderails to prevent falls. One NH study examined resident outcomes associated with consistent restrictive siderail status when compared to residents with no or nonrestrictive siderail use for one year (Capezuti *et al.*, 2002). Controlling for cognition, functional and behavioral status, the study found no indication of a decreased risk of falls or recurrent falls with restrictive siderail use. Similarly, a retrospective hospital-based study found that the incidence of falls from bed with siderails elevated was equal to, or higher, compared to the outcome when siderails were not elevated. Those patients with impaired cognition status were found to be the most likely to fall from bed when the siderails were elevated (van Leeuwen *et al.*, 2001). The evidence to date demonstrates the ineffectiveness of restrictive devices in prevention of falls and fall-related injuries (American Geriatrics Society, The British Geriatrics Society and The American Academy of Orthopaedic Surgeons, 2001).

Another major reason that health care providers choose restrictive devices is to reduce or control behavioral symptoms. Interestingly, although restraints are employed to "treat" these symptoms, the use of these devices is strongly correlated with physical or verbal aggression, especially among those with dementia (Talerico and Evans, 2001; Talerico *et al.*, 2002; Kolanowski *et al.*, 1994; Cohen-Mansfield and Werner, 1995). Delirium has also been found to be highly correlated with restraint use in several large-scale studies (Inouye and Charpentier, 1996; McCusker *et al.*, 2001; Morrison and Sadler, 2001). Federal regulations and JCAHO standards in the United States prohibit usage of restrictive devices to manage behavioral symptoms in NHs or medical/surgical (nonpsychiatric) care settings.

Behavioral symptoms, such as anxiety, agitation, physical aggression, and delirium, may result in patient interference with medical treatments. Treatment interference refers to both removal and manipulation of a monitoring or treatment device (e.g. feeding tubes, urinary catheters, intravenous lines, oxygen therapy) (Bryant and Fernald, 1997; Werner and Mendelson, 2001; Matthiesen *et al.*, 1996; Sullivan-Marx and Strumpf, 1996). This can be especially dangerous when the treatment or device fulfills a life-saving or life-maintaining function such as mechanical ventilatory support. Hand restraints may not prevent unplanned extubations in agitated patients (Chevron *et al.*, 1998). Some suggest that since many of those with unplanned extubations do not require reintubation, the problem lies primarily with poor adjustment of sedation (Chevron *et al.*, 1998; Tung *et al.*, 2001). Thus, restraints may be a marker of insufficient sedation that requires more attention to implementation of evidence-based guidelines for sedation of intubated patients (Slomka *et al.*, 2000; Bair *et al.*, 2000). The lack of evidence to support routine restrictive device usage to prevent falls or reduce behavioral symptoms is thus compounded by the numerous complications associated with use of these devices.

COMPLICATIONS

Use of restrictive devices is not without risk. In the 1980s and 1990s, research describing the negative physical and psychological sequelae associated with restrictive devices was the major impetus for changing the practice in hospitals and NHs (Evans and Strumpf, 1989). Psychologically, restrained older adults experience anger, humiliation, depression, and low self-esteem (Strumpf and Evans, 1988; Mion *et al.*, 1989; Happ *et al.*, 2001).

As described earlier in this chapter, the most common physical consequence of prolonged restraint or siderail use is immobility (Selikson *et al.*, 1988; Capezuti and Talerico, 1999; Inouye *et al.*, 2000; Inouye *et al.*, 1999; Mahoney, 1998). Other harmful medical outcomes associated with restraint include hyperthermia (Greenland and Southwick, 1978), rhabdomyolysis (Lahmeyer and Stock, 1983), brachial plexus injury (Scott and Gross, 1989), axillary vein thrombosis (Skeen *et al.*, 1993), compressive neuropathy (Vogel and Bromberg, 1990), Hess' sign (O'Connor *et al.*, 2003) and stress-induced cardiac arrhythmias (Robinson *et al.*, 1993). Siderails have been identified as a vector for nosocomial infections. Microbes cultured from siderails have been associated with subsequent integumentary and respiratory ailments (Mayer *et al.*, 2003; Noskin *et al.*, 1995; Bonten *et al.*, 1996; Podnos *et al.*, 2001; Slaughter *et al.*, 1996; Catalano *et al.*, 1999).

Although less common, restrictive devices have also been associated with fatal outcomes such as strangulation and asphyxiation (Robinson *et al.*, 1993; Katz, 1987; Miles and Irvine, 1992). Strangulation can occur due to improper application of a vest restraint or when an older adult with a vest restraint slips between two half rails. Asphyxiation results from gravitational chest compression when an older adult is suspended by a vest or belt restraint in a bed or chair (Joint Commission on Accreditation of Healthcare Organizations, 1998; Miles and Irvine, 1991). Asphyxiation can also occur if a person is entrapped within siderails. Between 1995 and 2001, the United States Food and Drug Administration (FDA) received 381 reports of siderail entrapment cases. Of these, 237 were deaths, 73 were injuries, and 71 cases were of near misses (Joint Commission on Accreditation of Healthcare Organizations, 2002).

Entrapments occur through the siderail bars; through the space between split siderails; between the siderail and mattress; or between the head or footboard, siderail, and mattress (Parker and Miles, 1997; Miles, 2002). All deaths involved entrapment of the head, neck, or thorax, while most injuries involved fractures, cuts, and abrasions. Persons at high risk for entrapment include older adults with preexisting conditions such as altered mental status (dementia or delirium), restlessness, lack of muscle control, or a combination of these factors (Parker and Miles, 1997; Todd, 1997). More recently, cases of asphyxiation deaths due to patients becoming trapped between therapeutic overlay air mattresses and siderails have been reported (Miles, 2002). These negative consequences associated with restraint use have served as an impetus for research aimed at identifying alternative "best-practices" to restrictive devices.

OUTCOMES OF RESTRICTIVE DEVICE REDUCTION

In the last decade, several studies have described the relationship between restraint reduction and fall/ injury rates. In a longitudinal prospective study comparing NH residents in one facility before and after a restraint reduction intervention, physical restraint use was reduced from 31.2 to 1.6%; however, no major differences were found in the number of residents falling before and after the reduction of physical restraint use (Werner *et al.*, 1994). Evans *et al.* (1997) and reported the results of the first controlled clinical trial testing the effectiveness of two interventions designed to reduce restraint use (a six-month education program and the educational program combined with unit-based, individualized consultation by a gerontologic advanced practice nurse compared to a control NH). All three NHs reduced restraint use; however, only the education plus consultation NH significantly reduced their usage. Secondary analyses of this dataset demonstrated that there was no statistically significant correlation between restraint removal/reduction and increases in falls or fall-related minor injuries (Capezuti *et al.*, 1998a). Another secondary analysis of the Evans *et al.* data set also found no increase in falls following nighttime restraint removal among a subsample of confused NH residents (Capezuti *et al.*, 1999a).

Fall-related injuries are rarely examined statistically, since the number of subjects required is often cost-prohibitive for most research studies. Fall-related minor injury in older persons, however, has significant implications for morbidity and mortality (Grisso *et al.*, 1992). Capezuti and colleagues reported that continued restraint use (versus restraint removal) was the only characteristic to significantly increase risk of fall-related minor injury (bruises, abrasions, certain sprains, and other soft tissue injuries that do not result in hospitalization or bed rest) (Capezuti *et al.*, 1998a). A two-year prospective project of 2075 patients residing in sixteen diverse NHs in California, Michigan, New York, and North Carolina evaluated the effect of an educational intervention for physical restraint reduction. The 90% reduction in restraint use (from 41% to 4%) resulted in an increase in minor injuries and falls; however, there was significant decrease in the percentage of injuries of moderate to serious severity (Neufeld *et al.*, 1999).

The only published studies of fall outcomes following siderail reduction have been conducted in rehabilitation settings (Hanger *et al.*, 1999; Si and Neufeld, 1999). One study conducted in a 25-bed rehabilitation unit within a NH found that the reduction in restrictive siderails resulted in no significant increase in fall rates and there were fewer injuries in those without siderails (Hanger *et al.*, 1999). A second study was conducted in several rehabilitation units of a New Zealand hospital, where the researchers evaluated fall outcomes following a policy change and educational effort aimed at siderail reduction (Si and Neufeld, 1999). There was a significant decrease in siderail usage and yet the bed-related fall rate did not significantly change. In summary, results from studies of restrictive device reduction efforts have demonstrated that they can be removed without negative consequences.

Although none of the studies represent a randomized clinical trial, no significant differences were found in the number of patients falling prior to or following the reduction of physical restraint use. Further, the studies demonstrate no statistically significant difference in falls compared with historical controls when restrictive siderails are removed (Agostini *et al.*, 2001). The positive outcomes associated with restrictive device reduction may represent not only the safe removal of these devices, but also the effectiveness of interventions aimed at decreasing the likelihood of falling. Both individual alternatives and the most effective strategies used to implement these interventions have been evaluated in the NH and hospital settings.

APPROACHES TO REDUCE RESTRICTIVE DEVICE USAGE

Restrictive devices are used to reduce injury risk from falls or treatment interferences that are often due to multiple causative factors. Optimal resolution also requires multiple interventions that rely on coordination via interdisciplinary dialogue and action (Tinetti *et al.*, 1995). Comprehensive assessment, coordinated care management and individualized intervention plans targeting identified risk factors have been found to be the most successful strategies to reduce restrictive devices.

"Best practice" approaches to restrictive device reduction are described in the literature or by professional associations as clinical practice guidelines for use in the NH and acute-care hospital (Joint Commission on Accreditation of

Healthcare Organizations, 1998; van Leeuwen *et al.*, 2001; American Geriatrics Society, 1991; Happ, 2000b; Maccioli *et al.*, 2003; Hospital Bed Safety Workgroup, 2003). Professional standards as well as governmental and accreditation regulations emphasize that a decision to use physical restraints and/or siderails should only be made after clinical evaluation and interdisciplinary care planning determines the purpose for the intervention. Further, alternatives to restrictive devices should be implemented and evaluated prior to initiating restraints. Thus, a thorough assessment is necessary in the following situations: in patients who are at high risk for application of physical restraints or siderails, prior to and during restraint reduction efforts, or in situations where the provider is assessing the continued need for restrictive devices. In restrained NH residents, an assessment should be conducted at least quarterly by the primary care provider to determine necessity for continued use.

Multidisciplinary collaboration with physical and occupational therapists, nurses, dieticians, and social workers is an important part of any evaluation regarding the use of restraints and siderails. The following section describes clinical approaches that reduce the likelihood of restrictive device use.

Promote Mobility

Maintaining physical activity in hospitalized elders and NH residents is crucial to preventing the harmful effects of immobility. Careful consideration is warranted when ordering bed rest. The ability to move around in bed and to transfer and ambulate safely is also important to prevent falls and injuries (Capezuti *et al.*, 1999b). The assessment should include the patient's ability to perform the skills necessary for safe mobility and transfer, including the need for assistance and assistive devices (e.g. walkers, canes). If there are problems, then a physical or occupational therapist should be consulted. Rehabilitation therapists may suggest transfer devices to enable or assist in safe transfer and promote stability when standing, which may include a trapeze, transfer pole or bar, or raised 1/4 or 1/2 length siderail directly attached to or adjacent to the top of the bed. These may also serve as assistive bed mobility devices.

Certain activities by nursing staff promote mobility, such as encouraging or assisting patients with changing position in bed, transferring out of bed to chair, and ambulating. Organized group walks around the nursing unit at specific times during the day promote mobility, provide diversion, and involve the patient in his/her recovery. Bed and toilet seat height should be adjusted to the patient's lower leg height in order to promote safe transfers.

Facilitate Observation

Patients at risk for falls or treatment interference should be located in rooms closer to the nurses' station to facilitate observation. Increased time spent out of rooms in hallways, at the nurses' station or in "day" rooms with other patients facilitates surveillance. Encourage family and friends to visit, especially during mealtimes and treatments, and at night to provide both meaningful distraction and assistance to staff. Providing communal dining when possible serves both this purpose and an opportunity for socialization.

Volunteers or paid "companions" can be an alternative when families are unable to stay with the patient (Jenson *et al.*, 1998). This, however, can incur significant cost and must be evaluated in relationship to the potential harm of leaving a patient alone. Patients at high risk for restraint, (i.e. confused persons unable to safely transfer/ambulate unassisted, who are agitated and have removed treatment devices, restraints, or have gotten out of bed with raised siderails) are also those most likely to suffer a restraint/siderail-related injury. When these patients are restrained, they require frequent observation, especially in a new environment. Thus, these patients may need to be targeted for "one-on-one" companions if other means of increased staff surveillance are not available.

An open intercom, "nursery", or "baby" monitor will promote audio contact between staff and patients. Video monitoring may be an option in some hospitals as well as motion-sensor lights or alarms in rooms that alert staff that the resident is ambulating in their room unassisted. Elopement control devices are used for "wanderers" who may walk into unsafe areas. They work similarly to department store tag devices. An identification tag placed on the resident's wrist or ankle will signal the detection monitoring device when the resident walks by it, thus, setting off the alarm (Connell, 1996).

Devices such as alarms are useful; however, staff must be available to respond quickly. There are various types of alarms: pressure-sensor activated, cord activated, and patient worn (Health Devices, 2004). Pressure-sensor activated alarms sound as shifts in weight occur on a pad placed over the mattress or chair cushion. Alarms worn by patients (usually on the thigh) are sensitive to resident position changes (e.g. from lying to standing). A call bell or similar device attached to clothing will sound when the resident rises and disconnects the cord from the socket. Alarms require individualization of delay time to minimize number of "false" alarms. Also, the occurrence of "nuisance" sounds may increase agitation in confused patients. Models that sound at the nurses' station, light a hallway call system, or activate a staff pager, reduce nuisance alarms (Health Devices, 2004). Some alarms include a voice "alarm", that is, a tape recorder that can play an individualized message addressing the resident by name and calmly instructing the resident to remain in his/her chair until the nurse arrives to provide assistance.

Offer Activities

It is not surprising that patients will attempt to ambulate without assistance or remove tubes when isolated in a room without meaningful activities. Television is not the solution; it may actually incite agitation. Recreation or activities therapists, if available, should be consulted. Family members can be encouraged to bring in favorite music or videotapes, hobby materials (e.g. knitting), or other items that the patient may enjoy. Staff or volunteers can also provide activities based on the patient's interest and cognitive level, for example, towels to fold, magazines to read, and stuffed animals to hold. Activities also serve to distract patients from "investigating" or disturbing tubes, monitor, leads, and dressings (Happ, 2000a). A well-tested hospital model employing volunteers focuses on reduction of delirium risk factors by, among others, promoting mobility and providing meaningful activities. The Hospital Elder Life Program has demonstrated significantly reduced cognitive and functional decline in at-risk older hospitalized patients (Inouye *et al.*, 1999; Inouye *et al.*, 2000; Rizzo *et al.*, 2001).

Maintain Continence

Often patients attempt to ambulate unassisted because of an urgent need to void. Assess the patient's ability to safely use a bedside commode or urinal, which may reduce the distance traveled to the bathroom and thus reduce falls. Query the patient or nursing staff regarding a change in toileting patterns including nocturia, bowel and bladder incontinence, which may require further evaluation by a continence specialist.

Promote Comfort

Comfort needs include equipment individualized to a patient's medical/functional condition and appropriate pain management. Providing comfortable and individualized seating is a major challenge, especially in the NH setting. In the NH, most patients spend the majority of their day in a wheelchair (Capezuti and Lawson, 1999). The prevalence of wheelchairs in NHs exceeds 50% and many patients spend their time in chairs that do not fit, and are uncomfortable (Brechtelsbauer and Louie, 1999). Wheelchairs were originally designed for transport only, not for long periods of sitting. Their sling-back seats do not provide the appropriate support. Seating problems such as poor back support; wheelchair being too tall, heavy, or wide; foot rests too high; and the hammock effect of the sling, are all associated with pain and agitation (Rader *et al.*, 2000). All these effects increase the risk for falling and use of physical restraints, since the patient may be uncomfortable and attempt to transfer unsafely.

Many products are available to adapt the chair to the individual resident's seating needs. Other adaptations for the wheelchair include a wedge cushion inserted under the resident's buttocks and thighs, which tilt the resident backward. A wedge seat prevents the resident from sliding forward. Similarly, leaning to the side is corrected with lateral supports or cushions. Stroke victims with hemiplegia (one-sided weakness) are at risk for shoulder subluxation if the weakened arm slips off the side of the chair. This can be prevented with devices attached to a wheelchair: an arm trough, elevated armrest, lateral arm support, or half tray. Patients who spend considerable time in a wheelchair are to be referred to a physical or occupational therapist for a seating evaluation (Rader *et al.*, 2000; Rader *et al.*, 1999).

The patient's comfort in bed can be improved with an overlay mattress cushion, air mattress, or sheepskin mattress pads (Capezuti *et al.*, 1999b). Pillows and leg separator cushions can be used to facilitate positioning. Heel pads and/or bed cradles are good choices for those with significant peripheral vascular disease or pressure ulcers. Refer to a Wound, Ostomy, and Continence (WOC) Nurse or physical therapist for device recommendations.

Chronic and acute pain is common in older adults; however, many are inadequately treated. Pain management includes both administration of analgesics and other treatments (e.g. physical rehabilitation exercise, relaxation training, biofeedback, hot packs). Older adults with dementia have the same types of medical conditions as nondemented elders; however, evidence suggests that they are unlikely to receive pain treatment (Scherder *et al.*, 1999). Thus, routinely scheduled (not "PRN," whenever necessary) analgesia is strongly recommended (American Geriatrics Society, 1998). Since they may not be able to report or describe pain, observation of nonverbal signs of pain is necessary. These indicators of pain include facial grimacing, physical aggression, pacing, uncooperativeness, or restless behavior (Decker and Perry, 2003).

Investigate Mental Status Changes

A change in mental status is important to assess since impaired cognitive status is highly associated with increased risk of falling and use of restrictive devices (van Doorn *et al.*, 2003). New behavioral symptoms (e.g. physical aggression) should first trigger a comprehensive evaluation of potential physical and/or environmental causes prior to initiating any physical or chemical restraint. Behavior can be used to communicate a need, threat to self-esteem, a state of arousal, or anxiety (Strumpf *et al.*, 1998). Confused older adults may not be able to express verbally that they are experiencing pain or have the need to use, for example, the toilet, and will often act out with some form of behavior (e.g. anxiety, wandering) (Talerico *et al.*, 1995; Miller and Talerico, 2002). Complicated cases will require a geriatric psychiatry consultation.

Address Fall Risk

If a patient has been deemed at risk of falls or has fallen, then a thorough evaluation of amenable risk factors contributing to future risk should be conducted. Falls, especially sudden onset of repeated falls, may indicate underlying acute pathology, such as infection, hypoglycemia, or dehydration (Gray-Miceli *et al.*, 1994). Evaluation of fall risk is addressed by several professional associations and academic institutions: the American Geriatrics Society, The British Geriatrics Society and The American Academy of Orthopaedic Surgeons (2001), American Medical Directors Association and The American Health Care Association (1998) and the University of Iowa (Ledford, 1996) and Assessing Care of Vulnerable Elders (ACOVE) Project on Falls Prevention (Rubenstein *et al.*, 2001).

Medications are associated with an increased risk for falling. All types of psychoactive medications (hypnotics, antidepressants, anxiolytics, benzodiazepines, and antipsychotics) have consistently been linked to an increased risk for falling (Yip and Cumming, 1994) due to the risk for adverse side effects such as syncope and orthostasis (Thapa *et al.*, 1995; Beers, 1997; Leipzig *et al.*, 1999). Ray *et al.* (2000) identified benzodiazepine users in NH residents having a rate of falls 44% greater than those not taking benzodiazepines. Additionally, fall risk increased with a higher dose of benzodiazepine use. Those on antidepressants, both tricyclic antidepressants and selective serotonin-reuptake inhibitors have a higher risk for falls when compared to nonusers (Thapa *et al.*, 1998; Thapa *et al.*, 1995). Thus, prescription of these medications must be carefully balanced against the risk of falls and related injuries. A general rule of geriatric pharmacology is to minimize the number of medications, assess the risk and benefit of each medication, and use those medications with the shortest half-life, least centrally acting or least associated with hypotension, and at the lowest effective dose. A pharmacist may be consulted to uncover potential drug–drug interactions and to make suggestions regarding inappropriate drug usage.

Environmental modifications may reduce falls. For example, a nonskid mat placed at the side of the bed and/or toilet and raised-tread socks can reduce the likelihood of slipping (Capezuti *et al.*, 1998b). For those patients unable to stand safely but who may accidentally roll out of or unsafely exit from bed, bed bumpers on mattress edges, concave mattresses, pillows, "swimming pool noodles" or rolled blankets under the mattress edge demarcate bed perimeters (Capezuti and Lawson, 1999).

Reduce Injury Risk

Since falling onto hard surfaces may increase the likelihood of fractures, a bedside cushion such as an exercise mat or an egg crate foam mattress may be used to reduce impact (Capezuti *et al.*, 1999b). Hip protector pads are the best studied single intervention strategy for fall-related injury prevention among high-risk older adults. Hip protectors are pads held in place next to the greater trochanter that reduce the force transmitted in a fall (Cameron, 2002). There exists several, large-scale, randomized, and controlled clinical trials that demonstrate a strong association between reduced hip fracture rates and hip pad usage (Cameron *et al.*, 2001; Kannus *et al.*, 2000). Compliance with wearing the hip protectors, however, is a significant problem due to discomfort and poor fit (Parker *et al.*, 2002). Incontinent NH residents experience discomfort when wearing the garment (Wallace *et al.*, 1993; Ross *et al.*, 1993).

For residents with a history of climbing around or over siderails, reducing the risk of an entrapment injury is paramount. Since restraint-related deaths can occur in less than a few minutes, these devices necessitate increased, not decreased staff observation. Inspect bed frames, siderails, and mattresses to identify possible entrapment areas (Parker and Miles, 1997; Hospital Bed Safety Workgroup, 2003).

Address Treatment Interference

Discomfort caused by unstable tube placement can increase the chances of self-removal or disruption of tube performance. Commercial tube holders to stabilize Foley catheters, intravenous lines, and feeding, drainage, and endotracheal tubes should be used (Capezuti and Wexler, 2003). Waterproof tape can decrease accidental extubations (Tominaga *et al.*, 1995). Devices can be camouflaged by hiding them under cloth (e.g. abdominal binder), undergarments or clothing, sheets, or blankets, to divert the patient's attention from a treatment. Infusion sites can be covered with commercial holders, bandages, or stockinettes (Capezuti and Wexler, 2003). For confused patients who "pick" or who are seeking tactile stimulation, provide fabric, stuffed animals, or an activity apron. Finally, periodically assess the need for any treatment like bladder catheterization or intravenous fluids; determine if it can be discontinued or if a less invasive treatment can replace it (Strumpf *et al.*, 1998).

CONCLUSION

In summary, physical restraints and restrictive siderails play a limited role in providing medical care to frail older patients. Rather, use of restraints and siderails leads to the harmful effects of immobility. Several studies have demonstrated that restraints and siderails can be removed without negative consequences.

Primary care providers can reduce the use of physical restraints and restrictive siderails by conducting a careful assessment and implementing appropriate individualized interventions. The use of nonrestrictive measures has been correlated with positive patient outcomes and helps to promote mobility and functional recovery. Most of these products, however, have not been prospectively evaluated in large randomized clinical trials for their individual contribution to reduction of falls or treatment interference (Agostini *et al.*, 2001; American Geriatrics Society, The British Geriatrics Society and The American Academy of Orthopaedic Surgeons, 2001). Further research on the efficacy of individual interventions that replace restrictive devices and improve mobility is still needed (Capezuti, 2004).

KEY POINTS

- Immobility is correlated with functional decline, which is considered a profound marker of morbidity and mortality.
- There is strong support in the literature linking physical restraint and restrictive siderail use with the consequences of immobility.
- The continued use of both restraint and siderail usage is based on embedded practices of health care providers who for decades have linked these devices to patient safety and protection.
- Restrictive devices are associated with numerous negative outcomes, including strangulation and asphyxiation.
- Research demonstrates that restrictive devices can be safely eliminated.

KEY REFERENCES

- American Geriatrics Society, The British Geriatrics Society and The American Academy of Orthopaedic Surgeons. Guideline for the prevention of falls in older persons. *Journal of the American Geriatrics Society* 2001; **49**:664–72.
- Capezuti E, Maislin G, Strumpf N & Evans LK. Side rail use and bed-related fall outcomes among nursing home residents. *Journal of the American Geriatrics Society* 2002; **50**:90–6.
- McCusker J, Kakuma R & Abrahamowicz M. Predictors of functional decline in hospitalized elderly patients: a systematic review. *Journals of Gerontology. Series A, Biological Sciences and Medical Sciences* 2002; **57**:M569–77.
- Minnick AF, Mion LC, Leipzig R *et al.* Prevalence and patterns of physical restraint use in the acute care setting. *Journal of Nursing Administration* 1998; **28**:19–24.
- Neufeld RR, Libow LS, Foley WJ *et al.* Restraint reduction reduces serious injuries among nursing home residents. *Journal of the American Geriatrics Society* 1999; **47**:1202–7.
- Rubenstein L, Powers C & MacLean CH. Quality indicators for the management and prevention of falls and mobility problems in vulnerable elders. *Annals of Internal Medicine* 2001; **135**:686–93.

REFERENCES

Agostini JV, Baker DI & Bogardus ST. Chapter 26: Prevention of falls in hospitalized and institutionalized older people. In KM McDonald (ed) *Making Health Care Safer: A Critical Analysis of Patient Safety Practices. Evidence Report/Technology Assessment No. 43* 2001; Agency for Healthcare Research and Quality, Rockville.

Allen C, Glasziou P & Del Mar C. Bed rest: a potentially harmful treatment needing more careful evaluation. *Lancet* 1999; **354**:1229–33.

American Geriatrics Society. *Position Statement: Restraint Use. Developed by the AGS Clinical Practice Committee and Approved May 1991 by the AGS Board of Directors* 1991, Reviewed 1997 and 2002, http://www.americangeriatrics.org/products/positionpapers/index.html.

American Geriatrics Society. The management of chronic pain in older persons. *Journal of the American Geriatrics Society*, 1998; **46**:128–50.

American Geriatrics Society, The British Geriatrics Society and The American Academy of Orthopaedic Surgeons. Guideline for the prevention of falls in older persons. *Journal of the American Geriatrics Society* 2001; **49**:664–72.

American Medical Directors Association and The American Health Care Association. *Falls and Fall Risk: Clinical Practice Guideline American Medical Directors Association* 1998; American Medical Directors Association, Columbia.

Anonymous. Cotsides: protecting whom against what? *Lancet* 1984; **35**:383–4.

Bair N, Bobek MB, Hoffman-Hogg L *et al.* Introduction of sedative, analgesic, and neuromuscular blocking agent guidelines in a medical intensive care unit: physician and nurse adherence. *Critical Care Medicine* 2000; **28**:707–13.

Beers MH. Explicit criteria for determining potentially inappropriate medication use by the elderly: an update. *Archives of Internal Medicine* 1997; **157**:1531–6.

Berland B, Wachtel TJ, Kiel DP *et al.* Patient characteristics associated with the use of mechanical restraints. *Journal of General Internal Medicine* 1990; **5**:480–5.

Bloomfield SA. Changes in musculoskeletal structure and function with prolonged bed rest. *Medicine and Science in Sports and Exercise* 1997; **29**:197–206.

Bonten MJ, Hayden MK, Nathan C *et al.* Epidemiology of colonisation of patients and environment with vancomycin-resistant enterococci. *Lancet* 1996; **348**:1615–9.

Bourbonniere M, Strumpf NE, Evans LK & Maislin G. Organizational characteristics and restraint use for hospitalized nursing home residents. *Journal of the American Geriatrics Society* 2003; **51**:1079–84.

Braun JA & Capezuti EA. The legal and medical aspects of physical restraints and bed siderails and their relationship to falls and fall-related injuries in nursing homes. *DePaul Journal of Health Care Law* 2000; **4**:1–72.

Brechtelsbauer DA & Louie A. Wheelchair use among long-term care residents. *Annals of Long Term Care* 1999; **7**:213–20.

Brush BL & Capezuti E. Historical analysis of siderail use in American hospitals. *Journal of Nursing Scholarship* 2001; **33**:381–5.

Bryant H & Fernald L. Nursing knowledge and use of restraint alternatives: acute and chronic care. *Geriatric Nursing* 1997; **18**:57–60.

Cameron ID. Hip protectors: prevent fractures but adherence is a problem. *British Medical Journal* 2002; **324**:375–6.

Cameron ID, Venman J, Jurrle SE *et al.* Hip protectors in aged-care facilities: a randomized trial of use by individual higher-risk residents. *Age & Ageing* 2001; **30**:477–81.

Capezuti E. Preventing falls and injuries while reducing siderail use. *Annals of Long-Term Care* 2000; **8**:57–63.

Capezuti E. Building the science of falls prevention research. *Journal of the American Geriatrics Society* 2004; **52**:461.

Capezuti E, Bourbonniere M, Strumpf N & Maislin G. Siderail use in a large urban medical center. *The Gerontologist* 2000; **40**:117.

Capezuti E & Braun JA. Medico-legal aspects of hospital siderail use. *Ethics, Law, and Aging Review* 2001; **7**:25–57.

Capezuti E, Evans L, Strumpf N & Maislin G. Physical restraint use and falls in nursing home residents. *Journal of the American Geriatrics Society* 1996; **44**:627–33.

Capezuti E & Lawson WT. Falls and restraint liability issues. *Nursing Home Litigation Investigation and Case Preparation* 1999; Lawyers and Judges Publishing Company, Tucson.

Capezuti E, Maislin G, Strumpf N & Evans LK. Side rail use and bed-related fall outcomes among nursing home residents. *Journal of the American Geriatrics Society* 2002; **50**:90–6.

Capezuti E, Strumpf NE, Evans LK *et al.* The relationship between physical restraint removal and falls and injuries among nursing home residents. *Journals of Gerontology. Series A, Biological Sciences and Medical Sciences* 1998a; **53**:M47–52.

Capezuti E, Talerico KA, Strumpf N & Evans LK. Individualized assessment and intervention in bilateral siderail use. *Geriatric Nursing* 1998b; **19**:322–30.

Capezuti E, Strumpf N, Evans LK & Maislin G. Outcomes of nighttime physical restraint removal for severely impaired nursing home residents.

American Journal of Alzheimer's Disease and Other Dementias 1999a; **14**:157–64.

Capezuti E, Talerico KA, Cochran I *et al.* Individualized interventions to prevent bed-related falls and reduce siderail use. *Journal of Gerontological Nursing* 1999b; **25**:26–34.

Capezuti E & Talerico KA. Review article: physical restraint removal, falls, and injuries. *Research and Practice in Alzheimer's Disease* 1999; **2**:3–24.

Capezuti E & Wexler S. Choosing alternatives to restraints. In EL Siegler, S Mirafzali & JB Foust (eds) *A Guide to Hospitals and Inpatient Care* 2003; Springer Publishing Company, New York.

Castle NG. Nursing homes with persistent deficiency citations for physical restraint use. *Medical Care* 2002; **40**:868–78.

Castle NG, Fogel B & Mor V. Risk factors for physical restraint use in nursing homes: pre- and post-implementation of the nursing home reform act. *The Gerontologist* 1997; **37**:737–47.

Castle NG & Mor V. Physical restraints in nursing homes: a review of the literature since the nursing home reform act of 1987. *Medical Care Research and Review* 1998; **55**:139–70.

Catalano M, Quelle LS, Jeric PE *et al.* Survival of acinetobacter baumannii on bed rails during an outbreak and during sporadic cases. *Journal of Hospital Infection* 1999; **42**:27–35.

Centers for Medicare and Medicaid Services. *Code of Federal Regulations: 42 C.F.R. § 483.13 (a)* 1999.

Centers for Medicare and Medicaid Services. 2004, http://www.cms.hhs.gov/media/press/release.asp?Counter=947.

Chevron V, Menard JF, Richard JC *et al.* Unplanned extubation: risk factors of development and predictive criteria for reintubation. *Critical Care Medicine* 1998; **26**:1049–53.

Cohen-Mansfield J & Werner P. Environmental influences on agitation: an integrative summary of an observational study. *American Journal of Alzheimer's Disease and Other Dementias* 1995; **10**:32–7.

Connell BR. Role of the environment in falls prevention. *Clinics in Geriatric Medicine* 1996; **12**:859–80.

Covertino VA, Bloomfield SA & Greenleaf JE. An overview of the issues: physiological effects of bed rest and restricted physical activity. *Medicine and Science in Sports and Exercise* 1997; **29**:187–90.

Covinsky KE, Justice AC, Rosenthal GE *et al.* Measuring prognosis and case mix in hospitalized elders. The importance of functional status. *Journal of General Internal Medicine* 1997; **12**:203–8.

Decker SA & Perry AG. The development and testing of the PATCOA to assess pain in confused older adults. *Pain Management Nursing* 2003; **4**:77–86.

Department of Health and Human Services. *Siderails Guidance. February 4, 1997 and December 1999* 1997, 1999; Health Care Financing Administration.

Evans LK & Strumpf NE. Tying down the elderly: a review of the literature on physical restraint. *Journal of the American Geriatrics Society* 1989; **37**:65–74.

Evans LK, Strumpf NE, Allen-Taylor SL *et al.* A clinical trial to reduce restraints in nursing homes. *Journal of the American Geriatrics Society* 1997; **45**:675–81.

Everitt V & Bridel-Nixon J. The use of bed rails: principles of patient assessment. *Nursing Standard* 1997; **12**:44–7.

Fortinsky RH, Covinsky KE, Palmer RM & Landefeld CS. Effects of functional status changes before and during hospitalization on nursing home admission of older adults. *Journals of Gerontology. Series A, Biological Sciences and Medical Sciences* 1999; **54**:M521–6.

Frengley J & Mion LC. Incidence of physical restraints on acute general medical wards. *Journal of the American Geriatrics Society* 1986; **34**:565–8.

Frengley J & Mion L. Physical restraints in the acute care setting: issues and future directions. *Clinics in Geriatric Medicine* 1998; **14**:727–43.

Gray-Miceli DL, Waxman H, Cavalieri T & Lage S. Prodromal falls among older nursing home residents. *Applied Nursing Research* 1994; **7**:18–27.

Greenland P & Southwick WH. Hyperthermia associate with chlorpromazine and full-sheet restraint. *American Journal of Psychiatry* 1978; **135**:1234–5.

Grisso JA, Kelsey JL, Strom BL *et al.*, NE Hip Fracture Study Group. Risk factors for falls as a cause of hip fracture in women. *New England Journal of Medicine* 1991; **324**:1326–30.

Grisso JA, Schwarz DG, Wolfson V *et al.* The impact of falls on an inner city elderly African-American population. *Journal of the American Geriatrics Society* 1992; **40**:673–8.

Hamers JPH, Gulpers MJM & Strik W. Use of physical restraints with cognitively impaired nursing home residents. *Journal of Advanced Nursing* 2004; **45**:246–51.

Hanger HC, Ball MC & Wood LA. An analysis of falls in the hospital: can we do without bedrails? *Journal of the American Geriatrics Society* 1999; **47**:529–31.

Happ MB. Preventing treatment interference: the nurse's role in maintaining technologic devices. *Heart & Lung: Journal of Acute and Critical Care* 2000a; **29**:60–9.

Happ MB. Using a best practice approach to prevent treatment interference in critical care. *Progress in Cardiovascular Nursing* 2000b; **15**:58–62.

Happ MB, Kagan SH, Strumpf NE *et al.* Elderly patients memories of physical restraint use in the intensive care unit. *American Journal of Critical Care* 2001; **10**:367–9.

Health Care Financing Administration. *HCFA Interpretative Guidelines, Rev. 250. Part II. Guidance to Surveyors for Long-term Care Facilities* 1992, Tag numbers F221-222, pp 76–8, F320, 131–2.

Health Care Financing Administration. *HCFA's National Restraint Reduction Newsletter: Restraint Rates-January 1998* 1998.

Health Devices. Bed-exit alarms. A component (but only a component) of fall prevention. *Health Devices* 2004; **33**:157–68.

Hirsch CH, Sommers L, Olsen A *et al.* The natural history of functional morbidity in hospitalized older patients. *Journal of the American Geriatrics Society* 1990; **38**:1296–303.

Hospital Bed Safety Workgroup. Clinical guidance for the assessment and implementation of bed rails in hospitals, long term care facilities, and home care settings. *Critical Care Nursing Quarterly* 2003; **26**:244–62.

Inouye SK, Bogardus ST, Baker DI *et al.* The hospital elder life program: a model of care to prevent cognitive and functional decline in older hospitalized patients. *Journal of the American Geriatrics Society* 2000; **48**:1697–706.

Inouye SK, Bogardus ST, Charpentier PA *et al.* A multicomponent intervention to prevent delirium in hospitalized older patients. *New England Journal of Medicine* 1999; **340**:669–76.

Inouye SK & Charpentier PA. Precipitating factors for delirium in hospitalized elderly persons. Predictive model and interrelationship with baseline vulnerability. *Journal of the American Medical Association* 1996; **275**:852–7.

Inouye SK, Wagner DR, Acampora D *et al.* A controlled trial of a nursing-centered intervention in hospitalized elderly patients: The Yale Geriatric Care Program. *Journal of the American Geriatrics Society* 1993; **41**:1353–60.

Janelli LM. Physical restraint use in acute care settings. *Journal of Nursing Care Quality* 1995; **9**:86–92.

Jenson B, Hess-Zak A, Johnston SK *et al.* Restraint reduction: a new philosophy for a new millennium. *Journal of Nursing Administration* 1998; **28**:32–8.

Joint Commission on Accreditation of Healthcare Organizations. *Comprehensive Accreditation Manual for Hospitals (Restraint and Seclusion Standards Plus Scoring: Standards TX 7.1- TX 7.1.3, 191-193j* 1996; Joint Commission on Accreditation of Healthcare Organizations, Oakbrook Terrace.

Joint Commission on Accreditation of Healthcare Organizations. *Issue 8 sentinel event alert: preventing restraint deaths (November 18, 1998)* 1998, http://www.jcaho.org/pub/sealert/sea8.html.

Joint Commission on Accreditation of Healthcare Organizations. *Sentinel Event Alert: Bed Rail-related Entrapment Deaths* 2002, Issue 27, September 6, 2002, http://www.jcaho.org/about+us/news+letters/sentinel+event+alert/sea_27.htm.

Kannus P, Parkkari J, Siemi S *et al.* Prevention of hip fracture in elderly people with use of a hip protector. *New England Journal of Medicine* 2000; **343**:1506–13.

Karlsson S, Bucht G, Eriksson S & Sandman PO. Physical restraints in geriatric care in Sweden: prevalence and patient characteristics. *Journal of the American Geriatrics Society* 1996; **44**:1348–54.

Katz L. Accidental strangulation from vest restraints. *Journal of the American Medical Association* 1987; **257**:2032–3.

Kolanowski A, Hurwitz S, Taylor LA *et al.* Contextual factors associated with disturbing behaviors in institutionalized elders. *Nursing Research* 1994; **43**:73–9.

Lahmeyer HH & Stock PG. Phencyclidine intoxication, physical restraint, and acute renal failure: case report. *Journal of Clinical Psychiatry* 1983; **44**:184–5.

Ledford L. Prevention of falls research-based protocol. In MG Titler (ed) *Series on Evidence Based Practice for Older Adults* 1996; The University of Iowa Gerontological Nursing Interventions Research Center Research Dissemination Core (RDC), Iowa City.

Leipzig RM, Cumming RG & Tinetti ME. Drugs and falls in older people: a systematic review and meta-analysis: i. Psychotropic drugs. *Journal of the American Geriatrics Society* 1999; **47**:30–9.

Levine JM, Hammond M, Marchello V & Breuer B. Changes in bedrail prevalence during a bedrails-reduction initiative. *Journal of the American Medical Directors Association* 2000; **1**:34–6.

Ljunggren G, Phillips CD & Sgadari A. Comparisons of restraint use in nursing homes in eight countries. *Age & Ageing* 1997; **26**:43–7.

Lofgren RP, MacPherson DS, Granieri R *et al.* Mechanical restraints on the medical wards: are protective devices safe? *American Journal of Public Health* 1989; **79**:735–8.

Maccioli GA, Dorman T, Brown BR *et al.* Clinical practice guidelines for the maintenance of patient physical safety in the intensive care unit: use of restraining therapies–American college of critical care medicine task force 2001–2002. *Critical Care Medicine* 2003; **31**:2665–76.

Mahoney JE. Immobility and falls. *Clinics in Geriatric Medicine* 1998; **14**:699–726.

Mahoney JE, Sager MA & Jalaluddin M. New walking dependence associated with hospitalization for acute medical illness: incidence and significance. *Journals of Gerontology. Series A, Biological Sciences and Medical Sciences* 1998; **53**:M307–12.

Matthiesen V, Lamb KV, McCann J *et al.* Hospital nurses' views about physical restraint use with older patients. *Journal of Gerontological Nursing* 1996; **22**:8–16.

Mayer RA, Geha RC, Helfand MS *et al.* Role of fecal incontinence in contamination of the environment with vancomycin-resistant enterococci. *American Journal of Infection Control* 2003; **31**:221–5.

McCusker J, Cole M, Abrahamowicz M *et al.* Environmental risk factors for delirium in hospitalized older people. *Journal of the American Geriatrics Society* 2001; **49**:1327–34.

McCusker J, Kakuma R & Abrahamowicz M. Predictors of functional decline in hospitalized elderly patients: a systematic review. *Journals of Gerontology. Series A, Biological Sciences and Medical Sciences* 2002; **57**:M569–77.

Miles SH. Deaths between bedrails and air pressure mattresses. *Journal of the American Geriatrics Society* 2002; **50**:1124–5.

Miles SH & Irvine PI. Common features of deaths caused by physical restraints. *The Gerontologist* 1991; **31**:42.

Miles SH & Irvine P. Deaths caused by physical restraints. *The Gerontologist* 1992; **32**:762–5.

Miller LL & Talerico KA. Pain in older adults. *Annual Review of Nursing Research* 2002; **20**:2063–88.

Minnick AF, Mion LC, Leipzig R *et al.* Prevalence and patterns of physical restraint use in the acute care setting. *Journal of Nursing Administration* 1998; **28**:19–24.

Mion LC. Establishing alternatives to physical restraints in the acute care setting. A conceptual framework to assist nurses' decision making. *AACN Clinical Issues* 1996; **7**:592–602.

Mion LC, Frengley JD, Jakovcic CA & Marino JA. A further exploration of the use of physical restraints in hospitalized patients. *Journal of the American Geriatrics Society* 1989; **37**:949–56.

Mion L, Minnick A & Palmer R. Physical restraint use in the hospital setting: unresolved issues and directions for research. *Milbank Quarterly* 1996; **74**:411–33.

Morrison A & Sadler D. Death of a psychiatric patient during physical restraint. *Medicine Science and the Law* 2001; **41**:46–50.

Neufeld RR, Libow LS, Foley WJ *et al.* Restraint reduction reduces serious injuries among nursing home residents. *Journal of the American Geriatrics Society* 1999; **47**:1202–7.

Noskin GA, Stosor V, Cooper I & Peterson LR. Recovery of vancomycin-resistant enterococci on fingertips and environmental surfaces. *Infection Control and Hospital Epidemiology* 1995; **16**:577–81.

O'Connor B, Moore A & Watts M. Hess'sign produced by bedrail injury. *The Irish Medical Journal* 2003; **96**(10):313.

O'Keefe S, Jack IA & Lye M. Use of restraints and bedrails in a British hospital. *Journal of the American Geriatrics Society* 1996; **44**:1086–8.

Parker MJ, Gillespie LD & Gillespie WJ. Hip protectors for preventing hip fractures in the elderly. *Cochrane Database of Systematic Reviews* 2002; **2**.

Parker K & Miles SH. Deaths caused by bedrails. *Journal of the American Geriatrics Society* 1997; **45**:797–802.

Phillips CD, Hawes C, Mor V *et al.* Facility and area variation affecting the use of physical restraints in nursing homes. *Medical Care* 1996; **34**:1149–62.

Podnos YD, Cinat ME, Wilson SE *et al.* Eradication of multi-drug resistant Acinetobacter from an intensive care unit. *Surgical Infections* 2001; **2**:297–301.

Rader J, Jones D & Miller LL. Individualized wheelchair seating: reducing restraints and improving comfort and function. *Topics in Geriatric Rehabilitation* 1999; **15**:34–47.

Rader J, Jones D & Miller L. The importance of individualized wheelchair seating for frail older adults. *Journal of Gerontological Nursing* 2000; **26**:24–32.

Ray WA, Thapa PB & Gideon P. Benzodiazepines and the risk of falls in nursing home residents. *Journal of the American Geriatrics Society* 2000; **48**:682–5.

Retsas A & Crabbe H. The use of physical restraints in western Australia nursing homes. *Australian Journal of Advanced Nursing* 1997; **14**:33–9.

Rizzo JA, Bogardus ST, Leo-Summers L *et al.* Multicomponent targeted intervention to prevent delirium in hospitalized older patients: what is the economic value? *Medical Care* 2001; **39**:740–52.

Robbins L, Boyko E, Lane J *et al.* Binding the elderly: a prospective study of the use of mechanical restraints in the acute care hospital. *Journal of the American Geriatrics Society* 1987; **35**:290–6.

Robinson BE, Sucholeiki R & Schocken DD. Sudden death and resisted mechanical restraint: a case report. *Journal of the American Geriatrics Society* 1993; **41**:424–5.

Ross JE, Wallace RB, Woodworth G *et al.* The acceptance of elderly of a hip joint protective garment to prevent hip fractures: Iowa FICSIT trial. In *The Second World Conference on Injury Control* 1993; The Centers for Disease Control, pp 90–1.

Rubenstein L, Powers C & MacLean CH. Quality indicators for the management and prevention of falls and mobility problems in vulnerable elders. *Annals of Internal Medicine* 2001; **135**:686–93.

Sager MA, Franke T, Inouye SK *et al.* Functional outcomes of acute medical illness and hospitalization in older persons. *Archives of Internal Medicine* 1996; **156**:645–52.

Scherder E, Bouma A, Borkent M & Rahman O. Alzheimer patients report less pain intensity and pain affect than non-demented elderly. *Psychiatry* 1999; **62**:265–72.

Scott TF & Gross JA. Brachial plexus injury due to vest restraints. *New England Journal of Medicine* 1989; **320**:598.

Selikson S, Damus K & Hamerman D. Risk factors associated with immobility. *Journal of the American Geriatrics Society* 1988; **36**:707–12.

Shorr RI, Guillen MK, Rosenblatt LC *et al.* Restraint use, restraint orders, and the risk of falls in hospitalized patients. *Journal of the American Geriatrics Society* 2002; **50**:526–9.

Si M & Neufeld RR. Removal of bedrails on a short-term nursing rehabilitation unit. *The Gerontologist* 1999; **39**:611–4.

Skeen MB, Rozear MP & Morgenlander JC. Posey palsy. *Annals of Internal Medicine* 1993; **117**:795.

Slaughter S, Hayden MK, Nathan C *et al.* A comparison of the effect of universal use of gloves and gowns with that of glove use alone on acquisition of vancomycin-resistant enterococci in a medical intensive care unit. *Annals of Internal Medicine* 1996; **125**:448–56.

Slomka J, Hoffman-Hogg L, Mion LC *et al.* Influence of clinicians' values and perceptions on use of clinical practice guidelines for sedation and neuromuscular blockade in patients receiving mechanical ventilation. *American Journal of Critical Care* 2000; **9**:412–8.

Strumpf NE & Evans LK. Physical restraint of the hospitalized elderly: perceptions of patients and nurses. *Nursing Research* 1988; **37**:132–7.

Strumpf NE, Robinson JP, Wagner JS & Evans LK. *Restraint-Free Care: Individualized Approaches for Frail Elders* 1998; Springer Publishing Company, New York.

Strumpf N & Tomes N. Restraining the troublesome patient: a historical perspective on a contemporary debate. *Nursing History Review* 1993; **1**:3–24.

Sullivan-Marx EM & Strumpf NE. Restraint-free care for acutely ill patients in the hospital. *AACN Clinical Issues* 1996; **7**:572–8.

Sullivan-Marx EM, Strumpf NE, Evans LK *et al.* Predictors of continued physical restraint use in nursing home residents following restraint reduction efforts. *Journal of the American Geriatrics Society* 1999; **47**:342–8.

Talerico KA, Capezuti E, Evans L & Strumpf N. Making sense of behavior: individualized care based on needs of the older adult. *The Gerontologist* 1995; **35**:128.

Talerico KA & Evans LK. Responding to safety issues in frontotemporal dementias. *Neurology* 2001; **56**:S52–5.

Talerico KA, Evans LK & Strumpf NE. Mental health correlates of aggression in nursing home residents with dementia. *The Gerontologist* 2002; **42**:169–77.

Thapa PB, Gideon P, Cost TW *et al.* Antidepressants and the risk of falls among nursing home residents. *The New England Journal of Medicine* 1998; **339**:875–82.

Thapa PB, Gideon P, Fought RL & Ray WA. Psychotropic drugs and risk of recurrent falls in ambulatory nursing home residents. *American Journal of Epidemiology* 1995; **142**:202–11.

Thomas DR. Focus on functional decline in hospitalized older adults. *Journals of Gerontology. Series A, Biological Sciences and Medical Sciences* 2002; **57**:M567–8.

Tinetti ME & Ginter SF. Identifying mobility dysfunction in elderly patients-standard neuromuscular examination or direct assessment. *Journal of the American Medical Association* 1988; **259**:1190–3.

Tinetti ME, Inouye SK, Gill TM & Doucette JT. Shared risk factors for falls, incontinence, and functional dependence. *Journal of the American Medical Association* 1995; **273**:1348–53.

Tinetti ME, Liu WL & Ginter SF. Mechanical restraint use and fall-related injuries among residents of skilled nursing facilities. *Annals of Internal Medicine* 1992; **116**:369–74.

Tinetti ME, Liu WL, Marottoli RA & Ginter SF. Mechanical restraint use among residents of skilled nursing facilities: prevalence, patterns, and predictors. *Journal of the American Medical Association* 1991; **265**:468–71.

Todd JF. Hospital bed side rails. Preventing entrapment. *Nursing* 1997; **27**:67.

Tominaga GT, Rudzwick H, Scannell G & Waxman K. Decreasing unplanned extubation in the surgical intensive care unit. *American Journal of Surgery* 1995; **170**:586–9.

Tung A, Tadimeti L, Caruana-Montaldo B *et al.* The relationship of sedation to deliberate self-extubation. *Journal of Clinical Anesthesia* 2001; **13**:24–9.

van Doorn C, Gruber-Baldini AL, Zimmerman S *et al.* Dementia as a risk factor for falls and fall injuries among nursing home residents. *Journal of the American Geriatrics Society* 2003; **51**:1213–8.

van Leeuwen M, Bennett L, West S *et al.* Patient falls from bed and the role of bedrails in the acute care setting. *Australian Journal of Advanced Nursing* 2001; **19**:8–13.

Vogel CM & Bromberg MB. Proximal upper extremity compressive neuropathy associated with prolonged use of a jacket restraint. *Muscle Nerve* 1990; **13**:860.

Wagner L, Capezuti E, Boltz M *et al.* Cost of environmental recommendations to reduce restrictive siderail use in nursing homes. *The Gerontologist* 2003; **43**:116.

Wallace RB, Ross JE, Huston JC *et al.* Iowa FICSIT trial: the feasibility of elderly wearing a hip joint protective garment to reduce hip fractures. *Journal of the American Geriatrics Society* 1993; **41**:338–40.

Walter LC, Brand RJ, Counsell SR *et al.* Development and validation of a prognostic index for 1-year mortality in older adults after hospitalization. *Journal of the American Medical Association* 2001; **285**:2987–94.

Werner P, Cohen-Mansfield J, Koroknay V & Braun J. The impact of a restraint reduction program on nursing home residents. *Geriatric Nursing* 1994; **15**:142–6.

Werner P & Mendelson G. Nursing staff members' intentions to use physical restraints with older people: testing the theory of reasoned action. *Journal of Advanced Nursing* 2001; **35**:784–91.

Yip YB & Cumming RG. The association between medications and falls in Australian nursing-home residents. *The Medical Journal of Australia* 1994; **160**:14–8.

Zinn JS. Market competition and the quality of nursing home care. *Journal of Health Politics, Policy, and Law* 1994; **19**:555–82.

143

Centenarians

Thomas T. Perls *and* Dellara F. Terry
Boston University School of Medicine, Boston, MA, USA

AN OPTIMISTIC VIEW

The prevalent notion that "the older you get, the sicker you get" often leads the lay public to assume that those who achieve exceptional longevity must have numerous age-related illnesses that translate into a very poor quality of life. Among researchers and clinicians, the observation that the prevalence and incidence of dementia increases with age, leads many to assume that dementia is inevitable for those who survive to age 100 and older (Ebly *et al.*, 1994; Thomassen *et al.*, 1998). For example, the East Boston Study indicated that almost 50% of people over the age of 85 have Alzheimer's disease (Evans *et al.*, 1989; Hebert *et al.*, 1995). Over the past decade or so, however, significant light has been shed on this assumption with a number of nonagenarian and centenarian studies addressing the prevalence and incidence of dementia amongst the oldest old; these are summarized in Table 1.

As most of the studies noted in Table 1 indicate, dementia is not inevitable with very old age. Conservatively, approximately 20% of centenarians are cognitively intact. Among centenarians who have some form of cognitive impairment, in one study, over 90% of these individuals compressed the time that they experienced functional impairment well into their 90s (Hitt *et al.*, 1999). The Heidelberg Centenarian Study recently proposed that those who develop dementia at extreme age have a shorter period of functional decline prior to the end of their lives (Kliegel *et al.*, 2004). Thus, centenarians are of interest in the study of dementia not only for the fact that some of them escape dementia, but also because most of them markedly delay in clinically expressing the disease until very late in their exceptionally long lives.

COMPRESSION OF MORBIDITY VERSUS DISABILITY

The compression of functional impairment toward the end of life that is observed among centenarians would at first glance appear to be consistent with James Fries's compression-of-morbidity hypothesis (Vita *et al.*, 1998). Fries proposes that as the limit of human lifespan is approached, the onset and duration of lethal diseases associated with aging must be compressed toward the end of life (Fries, 1980). While we found that functional impairment was compressed toward the end of life among centenarians, we noted, however, that some centenarians had long histories of an age-related disease. Perhaps an unusual adaptive capacity or functional reserve allowed some of these persons to live a long time with what normally would be considered a debilitating, if not fatal, disease while delaying its attendant morbidity and death by as much as decades (Lee, 2003; Richards and Sacker, 2003; Scarmeas and Stern, 2003; Stern, 2003; Wilson *et al.*, 2003).

To explore this hypothesis in our centenarian sample, we conducted a retrospective cohort study exploring the timing of age-related diseases amongst individuals achieving exceptional old age (Evert *et al.*, 2003). Three profiles emerged from the analysis of health history data. Forty-two percent of the participants were "survivors," in whom at least one of the 12 most common age-associated diseases was diagnosed before the age of 80. Forty-five percent were "delayers," in whom one of these age-associated diseases was diagnosed at or after the age of 80, which was beyond the average life expectancy for their birth cohort. Thirteen percent were "escapers," who attained their 100th birthdays without diagnosis of any of the 10 age-associated diseases studied. That most centenarians appear to be functionally independent through their early 90s suggests the possibility that "survivors" and "delayers" are better able to cope with illnesses and remain functionally independent compared to the average aging population. Thus, in the case of centenarians, it may be more accurate to note a compression of disability rather than a compression of morbidity. As would be expected, this is not generally the case with illnesses associated with high mortality risks. When examining only the most lethal diseases of the elderly such as heart disease, non-skin cancer, and stroke, 87% of males and 83% of females delayed or escaped these

Principles and Practice of Geriatric Medicine, 4th Edition. Edited by M.S. John Pathy, Alan J. Sinclair and John E. Morley.

Table 1 Studies addressing the prevalence or incidence of dementia amongst the oldest old

Study	Comments
Dutch population–based centenarian study	10 centenarians in a population of 100 000 people were all noted to have clinically evident dementia (Thomassen *et al.*, 1999). Expansion of the study to a population of 250 000 led to finding 15 of 17 centenarians as having dementia (Blansjaar *et al.*, 2000).
Swedish population–based study of people age ≥77	The prevalence of dementia amongst the 94 subjects age ≥95 was 48% (30% for men and 50% for women) (von Strauss *et al.*, 1999).
Canadian Study of Health and Aging	Dementia prevalence of subjects age ≥95 ($n = 104$) was 58%. The rate of increase in prevalence slowed at very advanced ages (Ebly *et al.*, 1994).
Study of Japanese Americans in King County, Washington	Dementia prevalence for subjects age ≥95 was 74% (Graves *et al.*, 1996).
MRC-ALPHA Study, of older people in Liverpool	Dementia prevalence amongst centenarians was 47% (Copeland *et al.*, 1999).
Northern Italian Centenarian Study	Dementia was diagnosed in 62% of 92 centenarians (Ravaglia *et al.*, 1999).
Finnish population-based centenarian study	56% of 179 centenarians had cognitive impairment (Sobel *et al.*, 1995).
Meta-analysis of nine epidemiologic studies of dementia among people age ≥80	Prevalence of dementia leveled off at around age 95 at a rate of 40% (Ritchie and Kildea, 1995).
New England Centenarian (population-based) Study	Cognitive impairment prevalence was 79% (Silver *et al.*, 2001).
Danish Centenarian Study	Dementia prevalence was 67% (Andersen-Ranberg *et al.*, 2001).
Coordinated study of dementia prevalence among centenarians in Sweden, Georgia (US), and Japan	Dementia prevalences ranged from 40% to 63% (Hagberg *et al.*, 2001).
Heidelberg Centenarian Study	Cognitive impairment prevalence was 75% (Kliegel *et al.*, 2004).
French Centenarian Study	Dementia prevalence was 65% among female and 42% among male centenarians (Robine *et al.*, 2003).

diseases (relatively few centenarians were "survivors" with such diseases). These results suggest there may be multiple routes to achieving exceptional longevity. The survivor, delayer, and escaper profiles represent different centenarian phenotypes, and probably different genotypes as well. The categorization of centenarians into these and other groupings (for example, cognitively intact persons or smokers without smoking-related illnesses) should prove useful in the study of factors that determine exceptional longevity.

NATURE VERSUS NURTURE

The relative contribution of environmental and genetic influences to life expectancy has been a source of debate. Assessing heritability in 10 505 Swedish twin pairs reared together and apart, Ljungquist *et al.* (1998) attributed 35% of the variance in longevity to genetic influences and 65% of the variance to nonshared environmental effects. Other twin studies indicate heritability estimates of life expectancy between 25% and 30% (Herskind *et al.*, 1996; McGue *et al.*, 1993). A study of 1655 old order Amish subjects born between 1749 and 1890 and surviving beyond age 30 resulted in a heritability calculation for life span of 0.25 (Mitchell *et al.*, 2001). These studies support the contention that the life spans of average humans with their average set of genetic polymorphisms are differentiated primarily by their habits and environments. Supporting this idea is a study of Seventh Day Adventists. In contrast to the American average life expectancy of 78 years, the average life expectancy of Seventh Day Adventists is 88 years. Because of their religious beliefs, members of this religious faith maintain optimal health habits such as not smoking, a vegetarian diet, regular exercise, and maintenance of a lean body mass that translate into the addition of 10 years to their average life expectancy as compared to other Americans (Fraser and Shavlik, 2001). Given that in the United States, 75% of persons are overweight and one-third are obese (Fontaine *et al.*, 2003), far too many persons still use tobacco (Wechsler *et al.*, 1998) and far too few persons regularly exercise (Wei *et al.*, 1999), it is no wonder that our average life expectancy is about 10 years less than what our average set of genes should be able to achieve for us.

Of course, there are exceptions to the rule. There are individuals who have genetic profiles with or without prerequisite environmental exposures that predispose them to diseases at younger ages. There is also a component of luck, which good or bad, plays a role in life expectancy. And finally, there is the possibility that there exist genetic and environmental factors that facilitate the ability to live to ages significantly older than what the average set of genetic and environmental exposures normally allow. Because the oldest individuals in the twin studies were in their early to mid-80s, those studies provide information about heritability of average life expectancy, but not of substantially older ages, for example, age 100 and older. As discussed below, to survive the 15 or more years beyond what our average set of genetic variations is capable of achieving for us, it appears that people need to have benefited from a relatively rare combination of what might be not-so-rare environmental, behavioral, and genetic characteristics, which are often shared within families.

Studying Mormon pedigrees from the Utah Population Database, Kerber *et al.* (2001) investigated the impact of family history upon the longevity of 78 994 individuals who achieved at least the age of 65. The relative risk of survival (λ_s) calculated for siblings of probands achieving the 97th percentile of "excess longevity" (for males this corresponded with an age of 95, and for women with an age of 97) was 2.30. Recurrence risks among more distant relatives in the Mormon pedigrees remained significantly greater than 1.0 for numerous classes of relatives, leading to the conclusion that single-gene effects were at play in this survival advantage. The Mormon study findings closely agree with a study of the Icelandic population in which first-degree relatives of those living to the 95th percentile of surviving age were almost twice as likely to also live to the 95th percentile of survival compared with controls (Gudmundsson *et al.*, 2000). Both research groups asserted that the range of recurrent relative risks that they observed indicated a substantial genetic component to exceptional longevity.

To further explore the genetic aspects of exceptional old age, Perls *et al.* analyzed the pedigrees of 444 centenarian families in the United States that included 2092 siblings of centenarians (Perls *et al.*, 2002a). Survival was compared to 1900 birth cohort survival data from the US Social Security Administration. As shown in Figure 1, female siblings had death rates at all ages that were about one-half the national level; male siblings had a similar advantage at most ages, though diminished somewhat during adolescence and young adulthood. The siblings had an average age of death of 76.7 for females and 70.4 for males compared to 58.3 and 51.5 for the general population. Even after accounting for race and education, the net survival advantage of siblings of centenarians was found to be 16 years greater than the general population.

Siblings might share environmental and behavioral factors early in life that have strong effects throughout life. It would make sense that some of these effects are primarily responsible for the shared survival advantage up to middle age. Recent evidence of effects of early life conditions on adult morbidity and mortality points to the importance of adopting a life course perspective in studies of chronic morbidity and mortality in later life as well as in investigations of exceptional longevity (Barker, 1998; Blackwell *et al.*, 2001; Costa, 2000; Elford *et al.*, 1991; Elo, 1998; Hall and Peekham, 1997; Kuh and Ben-Shlomo, 1997; Mosley and Gray, 1993). Characteristics of childhood environment are not only associated with morbidity and mortality at middle age, but they have also been found to predict survival to extreme old age (Preston *et al.*, 2003, 1998). Stone (2002) analyzed effects of childhood conditions on survival to extreme old age among cohorts born during the late nineteenth century. Key factors predicting survival from childhood to age 110 plus for these individuals, most of whom were born between 1870 and 1889, were farm residence, presence of both parents in the household, American-born parents, family ownership of its dwelling, residence in a rural area and residence in the non-South; characteristics similar to those that had been previously shown to predict survival to age 85 (Preston *et al.*, 2003, 1998).

In general, however, environmental characteristics such as socioeconomic status, lifestyle, and region of residence, are likely to diverge as siblings grow older. Thus, if the survival advantage of the siblings of centenarians is primarily due to environmental factors, that advantage should decline with age. In contrast, the stability of relative risk for death across a wide age range suggests that the advantage is due more to genetic than to environmental factors.

Whereas death rates reflect the current death rate at a moment in time, survival probability reflects the cumulative experience of death up to that moment in a cohort's life history. Thus, a relatively constant advantage from moment to moment (as seen in the relative death rates) translates into an increasing survival advantage over a lifetime (as seen in the relative survival probabilities (RSP)). This increase is seen in Table 2, which shows the RSP of the male and female siblings of centenarians at various ages.

By the age of 100, the relative survival probability for siblings of centenarians is 8.2 for women and 17 for men. From the analysis of death rates, we know that the siblings' survival advantage does not increase as the siblings age. Rather, the siblings' relative probability of survival is a cumulative measure and reflects their life-long survival advantage over the general population born around the same time. The marked increase in relative survival probability and sustained

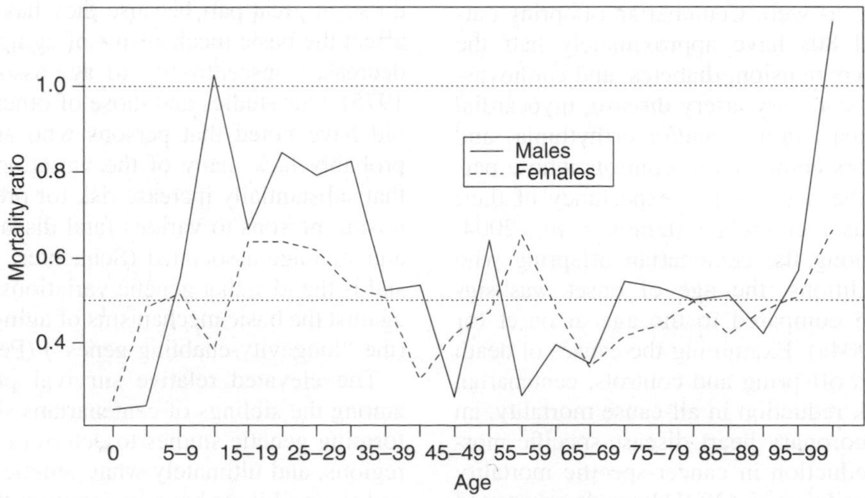

Figure 1 Relative mortality of male and female siblings of centenarians compared with birth cohort matched individuals (controls) from the general American population (survival experience of the controls comes from the Social Security Administration's 1900 birth cohort life table)

Table 2 Relative survival probabilities (RSP) with 95% confidence intervals (CI) of siblings of centenarians versus the US 1900 birth cohort

	Males			Females		
Age	RSP	Lower 95% CI	Upper 95% CI	RSP	Lower 95% CI	Upper 95% CI
20	1.00	1.00	1.00	1.00	1.00	1.00
25	1.00	0.99	1.01	1.01	1.00	1.02
60	1.18	1.15	1.21	1.12	1.09	1.14
65	1.29	1.25	1.33	1.16	1.13	1.19
70	1.48	1.42	1.53	1.24	1.21	1.28
75	1.68	1.60	1.77	1.36	1.31	1.41
80	2.03	1.90	2.16	1.54	1.47	1.60
85	2.69	2.47	2.91	1.83	1.73	1.93
90	4.08	3.62	4.54	2.56	2.39	2.74
95	8.35	6.98	9.71	4.15	3.73	4.57
100	17.0	10.8	23.1	8.22	6.55	9.90

survival advantage in extreme old age could be consistent with the forces of demographic selection, in which genes or environmental factors (or both) that predispose to longevity win out over those that are associated with premature or average mortality. The substantially higher relative survival probability values for men at older ages might reflect the fact that male mortality rates are substantially higher than female mortality rates at these ages and, thus, that men gain a greater advantage from beneficial genotypes than women do. Another possibility is that men require an even more rare combination of genetic and environmental factors to achieve extreme age than women do (Perls and Fretts, 1998). Either possibility could explain why men make up only 15% of centenarians.

CENTENARIAN OFFSPRING: FOLLOWING IN THE FOOTSTEPS OF THEIR PARENTS

The familiality of exceptional longevity demonstrated amongst centenarians and their siblings appears to extend to the offspring of centenarians as well. Centenarian offspring currently in their 70s and 80s have approximately half the relative prevalence of hypertension, diabetes, and cardiovascular disease (including coronary artery disease, myocardial infarction, congestive heart failure and/or arrhythmia) and cardiovascular risk factors compared to controls whose parents died at or before the average life expectancy of their birth cohort or to spousal controls (Atzmon *et al.*, 2004; Terry *et al.*, 2003). Among the centenarian offspring who did develop these conditions, the age of onset was significantly delayed when compared to the age at onset for controls (Terry *et al.*, 2004a). Examining the causes of death for deceased centenarian offspring and controls, centenarian offspring had a 62% risk reduction in all-cause mortality, an 85% risk reduction in coronary heart disease-specific mortality and a 71% risk reduction in cancer-specific mortality (Terry *et al.*, 2004b). Barzilai *et al.* (2001) have demonstrated that centenarian offspring, when compared to spousal controls, have favorable lipid profiles. These individuals have significantly larger HDL (high-density lipoprotein) and LDL (low-density lipoprotein) particle sizes compared to controls (Barzilai *et al.*, 2003). The larger particle sizes are associated with lower prevalences of cardiovascular disease, hypertension, and metabolic syndrome and are hypothesized to be predictive for longevity.

In addition to lipid profiles, another biomarker, heat shock protein 70 (HSP70), has been examined in the offspring of centenarians compared to spousal controls. Heat shock proteins, which help to chaperone, transport, and fold proteins when cells are exposed to a variety of stresses, may protect against or modify the progression of atherosclerosis. In a pilot study of 20 centenarian offspring and 9 spousal controls, Terry *et al.* (2004c) demonstrated a nearly 10-fold difference in levels of circulating HSP70.

GENETIC FINDINGS

Centenarians may be rare because a complex set of environmental and genetic variables must coexist for such survival to occur. The first genetic association with exceptional longevity, that has also withstood the test of time and numerous studies, has been the observation that the apolipoprotein E epsilon-4 (apo ε-4) allotype is rare amongst centenarians. Individuals who are homozygous for apo ε-4 have a 2.3–8 times greater risk of developing AD compared with the general Caucasian population (Corder *et al.*, 1993; Evans *et al.*, 1997). The allelic frequency of apo ε-4 drops off dramatically in the oldest age groups, presumably because of its association with Alzheimer's disease and vascular disease (Schachter *et al.*, 1994). Interestingly, the effect of apolipoprotein E allotype upon Alzheimer's disease incidence appears to decrease with age at these very old ages (Sobel *et al.*, 1995).

Richard Cutler, in what is now a classic paper in gerontology, proposed that persons who achieve extreme old age do so in great part because they have genetic variations that affect the basic mechanisms of aging and result in a uniform decreased susceptibility to age-associated diseases (Cutler, 1975). Our studies and those of others researching the oldest old have noted that persons who achieve extreme old age probably lack many of the variations (the "disease genes") that substantially increase risk for premature death by predisposing persons to various fatal diseases, both age-associated and non-age-associated (Schachter, 1998). More controversial is the idea that genetic variations might confer protection against the basic mechanisms of aging or age-related illnesses (the "longevity-enabling genes") (Perls *et al.*, 2002b).

The elevated relative survival probability values found among the siblings of centenarians support the utility of performing genetic studies to determine what genetic region or regions, and ultimately what genetic variations, centenarians and their siblings have in common that confer their survival advantage (McCarthy *et al.*, 1998). Centenarian sibships from the New England Centenarian Study were included in a genome-wide sibling-pair study of 308 persons belonging to 137 families with exceptional longevity. According to nonparametric analysis, significant evidence for linkage was noted for a locus on chromosome 4 at D4S1564 with an Maximum Lod Score (MLS) of 3.65 ($p = 0.044$) (Puca *et al.*, 2001). A detailed haplotype map was created of the chromosome 4 locus that extended over 12 million base pairs and involved the genotyping of over 2000 single-nucleotide polymorphism (SNP) markers in 700 centenarians and 700 controls. The study identified a haplotype, approximating the gene microsomal transfer protein (MTP) (Geesaman *et al.*, 2003). All known SNPs for MTP and its promoter were genotyped in 200 centenarians and 200 controls (young individuals). After haplotype reconstruction of the area was completed, a single haplotype, which was underrepresented in the long-lived individuals, accounted for the majority of the statistical distortion at the locus (~15% among the subjects versus 23% in the controls). MTP is a rate-limiting step in lipoprotein synthesis and may affect longevity by subtly modulating this pathway. Given that cardiovascular disease is significantly delayed among the offspring of centenarians and that 88% of centenarians either delay or escape cardiovascular disease and stroke beyond the age of 80, it makes sense that the frequency of genetic polymorphisms that play a role in the risk for such diseases would be differentiated between centenarians and the general population (Evert *et al.*, 2003; Terry *et al.*, 2003).

Dr. Nir Barzilai and his colleagues studying Ashkenazi Jewish centenarians and their families recently found another cardiovascular pathway and gene that is differentiated between centenarians and controls (Barzilai *et al.*, 2003). In Dr. Barzilai's study, controls are the spouses of the centenarians' children. They noted that HDL and LDL particle sizes were significantly larger among the centenarians and their offspring and the particle size also differentiated between subjects with and without cardiovascular disease, hypertension, and metabolic syndrome. In a candidate gene approach, the researchers then searched the literature for genes that impact upon HDL and LDL particle size and hepatic lipase and cholesteryl ester transfer protein (CETP) emerged as candidates. Comparing centenarians and their offspring against controls, one variation of CETP was noted to be significantly increased among those with or predisposed for exceptional longevity.

A PROPOSED MULTIFACTORIAL MODEL FOR EXCEPTIONAL LONGEVITY AND EXCEPTIONAL SURVIVAL PHENOTYPES

The fact that siblings of centenarians maintain half the mortality risk of their birth cohort from age 20 to extreme age suggests that multiple factors contribute to achieving exceptional longevity. For example, socio-demographic advantages may play key roles at younger ages, while genetic advantages may distinguish the ability to go from old age to extreme old age. Undoubtedly, exceptional longevity is much more complicated, with temporally overlapping roles for major genes, polygenic, environmental, and stochastic components. Such a scenario would be consistent with a threshold model, where predisposition for the exceptional longevity trait can be measured on a quantitative scale. Figure 2 illustrates the standard threshold model proposed by Falconer (1965) where it is predicted that the proportion of affected relatives will be highest among the most severely affected individuals. In the case of exceptional longevity, perhaps severity can be measured by additional years beyond a certain age (threshold) or by additional years of delay in age at onset for disease.

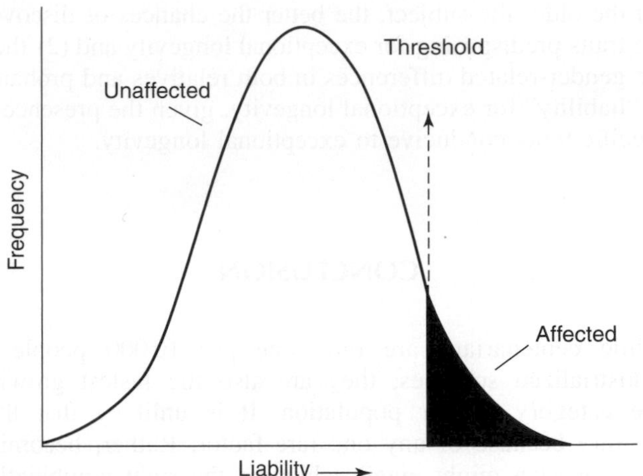

Figure 2 Threshold model of a multifactorial trait

Examples of phenotypes fitting the threshold model are early onset breast cancer or Alzheimer's disease, where relatives of patients who develop these diseases at unusually young ages, are themselves at increased risk or liability. Thus, a 108-year-old's "liability" or predisposition for exceptional longevity is further beyond the threshold than someone more mildly affected, as for example, a person who died at age 99. One interpretation of data indicating the higher relative survival probability of male siblings of centenarians compared to female siblings is that the males carry a higher liability for the trait, given the presence of the requisite traits. The model predicts that if a multifactorial trait is more frequent in one sex (as is the case with exceptional longevity which is predominantly represented by females), the liability will be higher for relatives of the less "susceptible" sex (males, in the case of exceptional longevity) (Farrer and Cupples, 1998). While we have not yet looked at relative survival probability of siblings of male versus female probands (something that certainly needs to be done), these elevated risks for male versus female siblings are interesting in this context. The model also predicts that the risk for exceptional longevity will be sharply lower for second-degree relatives compared to first-degree relatives, another observation we hope to test by having access to many expanded pedigrees. The ramifications of this model holding true for exceptional longevity (and/or exceptional survival phenotypes) include:

(1) the older the subject, the better the chances of discovering traits predisposing for exceptional longevity and (2) there are gender-related differences in both relatives and probands in "liability" for exceptional longevity, given the presence of specific traits conducive to exceptional longevity.

CONCLUSION

While centenarians are rare, one per 10 000 people in industrialized societies, they are also the fastest growing age category of our population. It is unlikely that they are rare because of any one rare factor. Rather, becoming a centenarian might entail achieving the right combination of genetic and environmental factors, much like winning the lottery requires the right combination of numbers. Each number by itself is not rare, but the right combination of five or six numbers certainly is. Complicating matters, the right combination of factors also likely varies from one person to the next, although there are similarities within families. One reason why the incidence of centenarians is growing may be understood by comparing with the analogy that the selection of lottery numbers is left less and less to chance. Better health-related behaviors and more effective public health and medical interventions make it significantly more likely for people to reach older age and for some to achieve extreme old age.

With the power of demographic selection, centenarians have already proven helpful in deciphering some polymorphisms and genetic loci associated, positively or negatively, with exceptional old age. The offspring of centenarians, who seem to be following closely in their parents' footsteps, might yield additional discoveries about phenotypic and genetic correlates of successful aging. Discovering genes that could impart the ability to live to old age while compressing the period of disability toward the end of life should yield important insight into how the aging process increases susceptibility to diseases associated with aging and how this susceptibility might be modulated (Hitt *et al.*, 1999; Perls *et al.*, 2002a). We anticipate that human longevity-enabling genes will be found to influence aging at its most basic levels, thus affecting a broad spectrum of genetic and cellular pathways in a synchronous manner. Another approach that researchers are in the early stages of understanding is differential gene expression in models known to slow the aging process, such as caloric restriction (Lee *et al.*, 1999). This may be another tool for discovering longevity-enabling genes. The centenarian genome should also be an efficient tool for ferreting out disease genes. Comparison of SNP frequencies implicated in diseases in centenarians and in persons with the diseases should show clinically relevant polymorphisms. The hope, of course, is that these approaches to gene discoveries will help identify drug targets and create drugs that would allow persons to become more "centenarian-like" by maximizing the period of their lives spent in good health.

KEY POINTS

- An optimistic view. Centenarians support the observation "the older you get, the healthier you've been".
- Compression of morbidity versus disability. Achieving exceptional old age likely requires a compression of disability, not necessarily morbidity, toward the relative end of life.
- Nature versus nurture. The majority of variation in average life expectancy is likely related to health-related behaviors. However, there appears to be a strong familial component to exceptional longevity and for truly extreme old ages, such as >103 years, specific genetic variations may play a prominent role.
- Centenarian offspring. Following in the footsteps of their parents. The offspring of centenarians are a valuable model for the study of environmental and genetic factors related to successful aging.
- Genetic findings. Reproducible genetic associations with exceptional longevity are still rare, reflecting the likely complex nature of gene–gene and gene–environment interactions that dictate the ability to survive to extreme old age.

KEY REFERENCES

- Barzilai N, Atzmon G, Schechter C *et al.* Unique lipoprotein phenotype and genotype in humans with exceptional longevity. *JAMA* 2003; **290**(15):2030–40.
- Evert J, Lawler E, Bogan H & Perls T. Morbidity profiles of centenarians: survivors, delayers, and escapers. *Journals of Gerontology. Series A, Biological Sciences and Medical Sciences* 2003; **58**(3):232–7.
- Hitt R, Young-Xu Y, Silver M & Perls T. Centenarians: the older you get, the healthier you have been. *Lancet* 1999; **354**(9179):652.
- Perls TT, Wilmoth J, Levenson R *et al.* Life-long sustained mortality advantage of siblings of centenarians. *Proceedings of the National Academy of Sciences of the United States of America* 2002a; **99**(12):8442–7.
- Schachter F, Faure-Delanef L, Guenot F *et al.* Genetic associations with human longevity at the APOE and ACE loci. *Nature Genetics* 1994; **6**:29–32.

REFERENCES

Andersen-Ranberg K, Vasegaard L & Jeune B. Dementia is not inevitable: a population-based study of Danish centenarians. *Journals of Gerontology. Series B, Psychological Sciences and Social Sciences* 2001; **56**:P152–9.

Atzmon G, Schechter C, Greiner W *et al.* Clinical phenotype of families with longevity. *Journal of the American Geriatrics Society* 2004; **52**:274–7.

Barker DJP. *Mothers, Babies, and Health in Later Life* 1998; Churchill Livingstone, London.

Barzilai N, Atzmon G, Schechter C *et al.* Unique lipoprotein phenotype and genotype in humans with exceptional longevity. *JAMA* 2003; **290**(15):2030–40.

Barzilai N, Gabriely I, Gabriely M *et al.* Offspring of centenarians have a favorable lipid profile. *Journal of the American Geriatrics Society* 2001; **49**(1):76–9.

Blackwell D, Hayward MD & Crimmins EM. Does childhood health affect chronic morbidity in later life? *Social Science & Medicine* 2001; **52**:1269–84.

Blansjaar BA, Thomassen R & van Schaick HW. Prevalence of dementia in centenarians. *International Journal of Geriatric Psychiatry* 2000; **15**:219–25.

Copeland JR, McCracken CF, Dewey ME *et al.*, The MRC-ALPHA Study. Undifferentiated dementia, Alzheimer's disease and vascular dementia: age- and gender-related incidence in Liverpool. *British Journal of Psychiatry* 1999; **175**:433–8.

Corder EH, Saunders AM, Strittmatter WJ *et al.* Gene dose of apolipoprotein E type 4 allele and the risk of Alzheimer's disease in late onset families. *Science* 1993; **261**(5123):921–3.

Costa D. Understanding the twentieth century decline in chronic conditions among older men. *Demography* 2000; **37**:53–72.

Cutler RG. Evolution of human longevity and the genetic complexity governing aging rate. *Proceedings of the National Academy of Sciences of the United States of America* 1975; **72**:4664–8.

Ebly EM, Parhad IM, Hogan DB & Fung TS. Prevalence and types of dementia in the very old: results from the Canadian study of health and aging. *Neurology* 1994; **44**(9):1593–600.

Elford J, Whincup P & Shaper AG. Early life experience and adult cardiovascular disease: longitudinal and case-control studies. *International Journal of Epidemiology* 1991; **20**:833–44.

Elo I. *Childhood Conditions and Adult Health: Evidence from the Health and Retirement Study* 1998; Population Aging Research Center Working Papers, University of Pennsylvania, Population Aging Research Center, Philadelphia.

Evans DA, Beckett LA, Field TS *et al.* Apolipoprotein E epsilon4 and incidence of Alzheimer disease in a community population of older persons. *JAMA* 1997; **277**(10):822–4.

Evans DA, Funkenstein HH, Albert MS *et al.* Prevalence of Alzheimer's disease in a community population of older persons. Higher than previously reported. *JAMA* 1989; **262**(18):2551–6.

Evert J, Lawler E, Bogan H & Perls T. Morbidity profiles of centenarians: survivors, delayers, and escapers. *Journals of Gerontology. Series A, Biological Sciences and Medical Sciences* 2003; **58**(3):232–7.

Falconer D. The inheritance and liability to certain disease estimated from the incidence among relatives. *Annals of Human Genetics* 1965; **29**:51–76.

Farrer L & Cupples A. Determining the genetic component of a disease. In J Haines & MA Pericak-Vance (eds) *Approaches to Gene Mapping in Complex Human Diseases* 1998; Wiley-Liss, New York.

Fontaine KR, Redden DT, Wang C *et al.* Years of life lost due to obesity. *JAMA* 2003; **289**:187–193.

Fraser GE & Shavlik DJ. Ten years of life: is it a matter of choice? *Archives of Internal Medicine* 2001; **161**(13):1645–52.

Fries JF. Aging, natural death, and the compression of morbidity. *New England Journal of Medicine* 1980; **303**(3):130–5.

Geesaman BJ, Benson E, Brewster SJ *et al.* Haplotype based identification of a microsomal transfer protein marker associated with human lifespan. *Proceedings of the National Academy of Sciences of the United States of America* 2003; **100**:14115–20.

Graves AB, Larson EB, Edland SD *et al.* Prevalence of dementia and its subtypes in the Japanese American population of King County, Washington state. The Kame Project. *American Journal of Epidemiology* 1996; **144**(8):760–71.

Gudmundsson H, Gudbjartsson DF, Frigge M *et al.* Inheritance of human longevity in Iceland. *European Journal of Human Genetics* 2000; **8**(10):743–9.

Hagberg B, Alfredson BB, Poon LW & Homma A. Cognitive functioning in centenarians: a coordinated analysis of results from three countries. *Journals of Gerontology. Series B, Psychological Sciences and Social Sciences* 2001; **56**:P141–51.

Hall A & Peekham CS. Infections in childhood and pregnancy as a cause of adult disease: methods and examples. *British Medical Bulletin* 1997; **53**:10–23.

Hebert LE, Scherr PA, Beckett LA *et al.* Age-specific incidence of Alzheimer's disease in a community population. *JAMA* 1995; **273**(17):1354–9.

Herskind AM, McGue M, Holm NV *et al.* The heritability of human longevity: a population-based study of 2872 Danish twin pairs born 1870–1900. *Human Genetics* 1996; **97**(3):319–23.

Hitt R, Young-Xu Y, Silver M & Perls T. Centenarians: the older you get, the healthier you have been. *Lancet* 1999; **354**(9179):652.

Kerber RA, O'Brien E, Smith KR & Cawthon RM. Familial excess longevity in Utah genealogies. *Journals of Gerontology. Series A, Biological Sciences and Medical Sciences* 2001; **56**(3):B130–9.

Kliegel M, Moor C & Rott C. Cognitive status and development in the oldest old: a longitudinal analysis from the Heidelberg Centenarian Study. *Archives of Gerontology and Geriatrics* 2004; **39**:143–56.

Kuh D & Ben-Shlomo B. *A Life Course Approach to Chronic Disease Epidemiology* 1997; Oxford University Press, Oxford.

Lee JH. Genetic evidence for cognitive reserve: variations in memory and related cognitive functions. *Journal of Clinical and Experimental Neuropsychology* 2003; **25**(5):594–613.

Lee CK, Klopp RG, Weindruch R & Prolla TA. Gene expression profile of aging and its retardation by caloric restriction. *Science* 1999; **285**:1390–3.

Ljungquist B, Berg S, Lanke J *et al.* The effect of genetic factors for longevity: a comparison of identical and fraternal twins in the Swedish Twin Registry. *Journals of Gerontology. Series A, Biological Sciences and Medical Sciences* 1998; **53**(6):M441–6.

McCarthy MI, Kruglyak L & Lander ES. Sib-pair collection strategies for complex diseases. *Genetic Epidemiology* 1998; **15**(4):317–40.

McGue M, Vaupel JW, Holm N & Harvald B. Longevity is moderately heritable in a sample of Danish twins born 1870–1880. *Journal of Gerontology* 1993; **48**(6):B237–44.

Mitchell BD, Hsueh WC, King TM *et al.* Heritability of life span in the Old Order Amish. *American Journal of Medical Genetics* 2001; **102**:346–52.

Mosley W & Gray R. Childhood precursors of adult morbidity and mortality in developing countries: implications for health programs. In J Gribble & S Preston (eds) *The Epidemiological Transition: Policy and Planning Implications for Developing Countries* 1993, pp 69–100; National Academy Press, Washington.

Perls T & Fretts R. *Why Women Live Longer Than Men* 1998, pp 100–7; Scientific American Press.

Perls TT, Wilmoth J, Levenson R *et al.* Life-long sustained mortality advantage of siblings of centenarians. *Proceedings of the National Academy of Sciences of the United States of America* 2002a; **99**(12):8442–7.

Perls T, Kunkel L & Puca A. The genetics of aging. *Current Opinion in Genetics & Development* 2002b; **12**:362–9.

Preston S, Elo IT, Hill ME & Rosenwaike I. *The Demography of African Americans, 1930 – 1990* 2003; Kluwer Academic Publisher.

Preston S, Hill ME & Drevenstedt GL. Childhood conditions that predict survival to advanced ages among African Americans. *Social Science & Medicine* 1998; **47**:1231–46.

Puca AA, Daly MJ, Brewster SJ *et al.* A genome-wide scan for linkage to human exceptional longevity identifies a locus on chromosome 4. *Proceedings of the National Academy of Sciences of the United States of America* 2001; **98**(18):10505–8.

Ravaglia G, Forti P, De Ronchi D *et al.* Prevalence and severity of dementia among northern Italian centenarians. *Neurology* 1999; **53**(2):416–8.

Richards M & Sacker A. Lifetime antecedents of cognitive reserve. *Journal of Clinical and Experimental Neuropsychology* 2003; **25**(5):614–24.

Ritchie K & Kildea D. Is senile dementia "age-related" or "ageing-related"? -evidence from meta-analysis of dementia prevalence in the oldest old. *The Lancet* 1995; **346**:931–4.

Robine JM, Romieu I & Allard M. French centenarians and their functional health status. *Presse Medicale* 2003; **32**:360–4.

Scarmeas N & Stern Y. Cognitive reserve and lifestyle. *Journal of Clinical and Experimental Neuropsychology* 2003; **25**(5):625–33.

Schachter F. Causes, effects, and constraints in the genetics of human longevity. *American Journal of Human Genetics* 1998; **62**(5):1008–14.

Schachter F, Faure-Delanef L, Guenot F *et al.* Genetic associations with human longevity at the APOE and ACE loci. *Nature Genetics* 1994; **6**:29–32.

Silver MH, Jilinskaia E & Perls TT. Cognitive functional status of age-confirmed centenarians in a population-based study. *Journal of Gerontology, Psychological Science* 2001; **56B**:P134–40.

Sobel E, Louhija J, Sulkava R *et al.* Lack of association of apolipoprotein E allele epsilon 4 with late-onset Alzheimer's disease among Finnish centenarians. *Neurology* 1995; **45**:903–7.

Stern Y. The concept of cognitive reserve: a catalyst for research. *Journal of Clinical and Experimental Neuropsychology* 2003; **25**(5):589–93.

Stone L. Early life conditions that predict survival to extreme old age, Paper presented at the *Annual Meeting of the Population Association of America*, Atlanta, 2002.

Terry DF, Wilcox MA, McCormick MA & Perls TT. Cardiovascular disease delay in centenarian offspring. *Journals of Gerontology. Series A, Biological Sciences and Medical Sciences* 2004a; **59**(4):M385–9.

Terry DF, Wilcox M, McCormick M *et al.* Reduced all-cause, cardiovascular and cancer mortality in centenarian offspring. *Journal of the American Geriatrics Society* 2004b; **52**:2074–76.

Terry D, McCormick M, Andersen S *et al.* Cardiovascular disease delay in centenarian offspring: role of heat shock proteins. *Annals New York Academy of Sciences* 2004c; **1019**:502–5.

Terry DF, Wilcox M, McCormick MA *et al.* Cardiovascular advantages among the offspring of centenarians. *Journals of Gerontology. Series A, Biological Sciences and Medical Sciences* 2003; **58**(5):M425–31.

Thomassen R, van Schaick HW & Blansjaar B. Prevalence of dementia over age 100. *Neurology* 1998; **50**:283–6.

Thomassen R, van Schaick HW & Blansjaar BA. Prevalence of dementia over age 100. *Neurology* 1999; **52**:1717.

Vita AJ, Terry RB, Hubert HB & Fries JF. Aging, health risks, and cumulative disability. *New England Journal of Medicine* 1998; **338**(15):1035–41.

von Strauss E, Viitanen M, De Ronchi D *et al.* Aging and the occurrence of dementia: findings from a population-based cohort with a large sample of nonagenarians. *Archives of Neurology* 1999; **56**(5):587–92.

Wechsler H, Rigotti NA, Gledhill-Hoyt J & Lee H. Increased levels of cigarette use among college students: a cause for national concern. *JAMA* 1998; **280**:1673–8.

Wei M, Kampert JB, Barlow CE *et al.* Relationship between low cardiorespiratory fitness and mortality in normal-weight, overweight, and obese men. *JAMA* 1999; **282**:1547–53.

Wilson R, Barnes L & Bennett D. Assessment of lifetime participation in cognitively stimulating activities. *Journal of Clinical and Experimental Neuropsychology* 2003; **25**(5):634–42.

PART III

Medicine in Old Age

Section 15

Diagnostic Interventions

144

Diagnostic Imaging and Interventional Radiology

J. Richard Harding

St Woolos and Royal Gwent Hospitals, Newport, UK

INTRODUCTION

Diagnostic imaging and interventional radiology in the elderly is little different from that of the adult population in general, but there are certain specific considerations. The problems and difficulties which can arise in diagnostic imaging and interventional radiology are not unique to the elderly; they are, however, more common in old age than in younger or middle-aged adults. Nevertheless, it is not unusual to occasionally encounter 80 or even 90 year olds who are fitter and more cooperative than some 50-year-old patients. Coupled with the increasing numbers of older people in the population at large plus the higher incidence and prevalence of many pathological conditions requiring investigation and treatment in this age-group, those difficulties which can arise assume an increasing importance; this justifies particular attention and care needed, in order to achieve a satisfactory investigation/intervention and to avoid undue distress or discomfort to the elderly patient. In particular, neoplastic disease and vascular disorders (cardiovascular, cerebrovascular, and peripheral vascular diseases) are more common in elderly patients than in younger or middle-aged patients.

Requests for radiological investigation of older patients, both for in- and outpatients, are received from many sources in addition to those from departments of geriatric medicine, but the potential problems are the same. Some nongeriatric clinical specialties have a high proportion of elderly patients (e.g. urology, gynecology, and general medicine), although referral of such patients can be from almost any clinical speciality (with the notable exceptions of obstetrics and pediatrics!). A large number of elderly referrals also emanate from general practice.

Appropriate choice of relevant investigation, with clear information/explanation to the patient and/or his/her relatives or carers can have a significant effect in alleviating or reducing unnecessary anguish in these patients, who are frequently already anxious, distressed, or in pain or discomfort as a result of their condition and age. Kindness and patience can pay dividends.

GUIDELINES TO GOOD PRACTICE IN RADIOLOGICAL IMAGING

The use of radiological investigations is an accepted part of medical practice, but there is no known safe radiation dose. In requesting any radiological investigation, it should be remembered that all X-rays are potentially carcinogenic and tetragenic. The patient's interest will be best served only if the likely disadvantages of the examination (inconvenience, discomfort, the risk of radiation to those X-rayed, and the benefits which might have to be foregone when resources are committed to the X-ray examination) are less than the anticipated benefits. Man-made radiation now accounts for 15% of the total radiation burden to the population, of which 97% is due to diagnostic medical exposures. No investigation should be requested unless it can be clinically justified and its result is likely to influence patient management. Many measures, including technical features of X-ray equipment design and radiographic technique, are utilized to reduce the radiation dosage to patients from necessary radiological examinations.

Some of the reasons for avoiding or reducing exposure to ionizing radiation from radiological examinations are not relevant in the elderly (e.g. avoiding radiation to the developing embryo or fetus in pregnant patients) or are of lesser significance than in younger patients (e.g. risks of mutation in germ cells), but it is, nevertheless, a sound and recommended practice to avoid unnecessary irradiation of patients and to keep that which is necessary to a minimum for the sake of the patient and the operator(s). Many elderly patients will still have a fairly long life expectancy,

Principles and Practice of Geriatric Medicine, 4th Edition. Edited by M.S. John Pathy, Alan J. Sinclair and John E. Morley.

so radiation-induced cancer cannot be dismissed. There is no threshold for the induction of such effects, any ionizing radiation is theoretically dangerous and its use must be justified, that is, the potential benefit must outweigh the small risks. Requests for radiological investigation should follow the guidelines published by the Royal College of Radiologists (RCR) in the booklet *Making the Best Use of a Department of Clinical Radiology: Guidelines for Doctors* (3rd edn) (RCR Working Party, 2003). These guidelines are not intended to replace clinical judgement but to support it in times of doubt or difficulty. The guidelines state that a useful investigation is one in which the result – positive or negative – will alter management or add confidence to the clinician's diagnosis. A significant number of radiological investigations do not fulfil these aims. Unnecessary investigations increase waiting time, waste limited resources (Audit Commission, 1995), lower standards, and may add unnecessarily to patient irradiation (The Ionising Radiation (Protection of Persons Undergoing Medical Evaluation or Treatment) Regulations 1988, (POPUMET); The Ionising Radiation (Medical Exposure) Regulations 2000, (IR(ME)R 2000); European Directive 97/43/Euratom (The Medical Exposures Directive). Such is the perceived risk of medical litigation that X rays are sometimes requested even when they are not considered clinically necessary by the referring doctor. If, as a result of careful clinical examination, it is decided that an X ray is not necessary for the future management of the patient and this is recorded in the patient's notes, it is unlikely that the decision will be challenged on medicolegal grounds. The position of clinicians following the guidelines will be further strengthened because it will have the support of the RCR. Apart from the medicolegal issue, the chief causes of the wasteful use of radiology are:

1. *Investigation when results are unlikely to affect patient management*: because the anticipated "positive" finding is usually irrelevant, for example, degenerative spinal disease (as " normal" as gray hairs from early middle age) or because a positive finding is so unlikely.
   DO I NEED IT?

2. *Investigating too often*: that is, before the disease could have progressed or resolved, or before the results influence treatment.
   DO I NEED IT NOW?

3. *Repeating investigations which have already been done*: for example, at another hospital, in an outpatient department, or in the accident and emergency department, or already requested by another member of the clinical team caring for the patient.
   HAS IT BEEN DONE ALREADY?

4. *Failing to provide appropriate clinical information and questions that the radiological investigation should answer*: Deficiencies may lead to the wrong radiographs being obtained (e.g. the omission of an essential view).
   HAVE I EXPLAINED THE PROBLEM?

5. *Performing the wrong investigation*: Imaging techniques are developing rapidly. It is often helpful to discuss the investigation with a radiologist before it is requested.
   IS THIS THE BEST INVESTIGATION?

Continued use of the RCR *Guidelines* leads to a reduction in the number of referrals for investigations and also to a reduction in medical radiation exposure (Roberts, 1988; National Radiological Protection Board and The Royal College of Radiologists, 1990; RCR Working Party, 1991; RCR Working Party, 1992; Roberts, 1992). Nevertheless, the primary objective of the RCR *Guidelines* is to improve clinical practice. Such guidelines work best if they are used in conjunction with clinicoradiological dialogue and as part of the audit process.

The *Ionizing Radiation* (POPUMET) *Regulations* (1988) require all concerned to reduce unnecessary exposure of patients to radiation. Health authorities, NHS trusts, and individuals using ionizing radiation must, by law, comply with these regulations. One important way of reducing radiation dose is to avoid repeating investigations unless there is a sound clinical reason to do so.

Table 1 shows the effective doses delivered by different examinations, the approximate equivalent number of chest

Table 1 Relative radiation doses and their equivalent natural radiation period

Examination	Effective dose (mSv)	Equivalent number of chest X rays (approx.)	Equivalent period of natural background radiation
Extremities[a] (e.g. knee)	0.01	0.5	1.5 days
Chest (single PA film)	0.02	1	3 days
Skull	0.1	5	2 weeks
Cervical spine	0.1	5	2 weeks
Dorsal spine	1.0	50	6 months
Lumbar spine	2.4	120	14 months
Hip	0.3	15	2 months
Pelvis	1.0	50	6 months
Abdomen	1.5	75	9 months
Biliary tract	1.3	65	7 months
Barium studies			
Esophagus	2.0	100	1 year
Stomach & duodenum	5.0	250	2.5 years
Small bowel	6.0	300	3 years
Large bowel	9.0	450	4.5 years
IVU	4.6	230	2.5 years
CT head[b]	2.0	100	1 year
CT chest or abdomen	8.0	400	4 years
Radionuclide studies[c]			
Lung ventilation (^{81m}Krypton)	0.1	5	2 weeks
Lung perfusion	1.0	50	6 months
Kidney	1.0	50	6 months
Thyroid	1.0	50	6 months
Bone	5.0	250	2.5 years
Myocardium (^{201}Thallium)	18.0	900	9 years

Source: Reprinted from *Clinical Radiology*, V39, Roberts CJ, Towards the more effective use of diagnostic radiology, pp 3–6, Copyright 1988, with permission from The Royal College of Radiologists.

[a]On the basis of a survey carried out in the mid-1980s. [b]On the basis of studies carried out in 1989. [c]Courtesy of Dr RA Shields, Manchester.

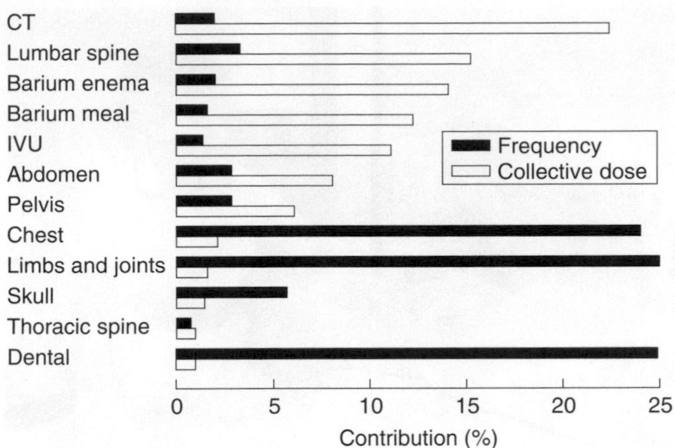

Figure 1 Frequency of, and collective dose from, different radiological investigations in the United Kingdom (Reprinted from *Clinical Radiology*, V39, Roberts CJ, Towards the more effective use of diagnostic radiology, pp 3–6, Copyright 1988, with permission from The Royal College of Radiologists)

radiographs, and the equivalent period of natural background radiation. The *effective dose* is a weighted sum of equivalent doses (in millisieverts, mSv) to a number of body tissues, where the weighting used for the different tissues depends upon the relative risks of fatal malignancy or severe hereditary defect for low radiation doses. The effective dose is the dose of uniform whole-body irradiation which would carry the same risk of malignant disorders as the examples listed, all of which involve nonuniform irradiation. Figure 1 shows the relative frequency of X-ray examinations and their contributions to the collective population dose. The dose imparted by computed tomography (CT) is high and should be minimized. In recent studies, the contribution of CT to the collective dose from all X-ray examinations has increased to one-third and is probably still rising (National Radiological Protection Board, 1992). In many situations, potentially less harmful imaging modalities such as ultrasound or magnetic resonance imaging (MRI) can be substituted for CT.

PROBLEMS IN RADIOLOGY – GENERAL CONSIDERATIONS

The problems which can arise in radiological examination of the elderly are mainly related to locomotor and communication difficulties resulting from the aging process and diseases occurring more commonly in old age. Complications which can occur in diagnostic imaging and interventional radiology relate not only to radiation but also to drugs used and procedures performed in the clinical radiology department (Ansell *et al.*, 1996).

For elderly outpatients, actually getting to the X-ray department can be difficult; such patients may be unable to use a car or public transport, or afford a taxi fare. Elderly patients may never have driven or have owned a car, or may have had to give up driving because of failing eyesight or musculoskeletal disabilities preventing driving or getting into or out of a car, or walking to it. Where car transport cannot be provided by a friend, relative or carer, or a taxi is unaffordable or inappropriate, the patient will be dependent upon a hospital car or the ambulance service. In cases of severe disability, ambulance transport is the only possibility. The patient may be unable to walk far and may require transfer into and out of the ambulance by wheelchair.

Suitable facilities at the hospital allow wheelchair access to departments, for example, wheelchair ramps alongside small flights of steps and adequate and appropriately sited provision of passenger lifts. This is easier to achieve in modern purpose-built hospitals and radiology departments than in those housed in older (e.g. Victorian) buildings, where such access was not originally planned.

Within the radiology department, the reception and waiting areas, changing cubicles, examination rooms, and toilets need adequate provision for wheelchair access. Modified changing cubicles are required, larger than normal, with extra-wide or double doors to accommodate not only the patient and wheelchair, but also a friend, relative, carer, nurse, or radiography helper for those patients who need assistance in dressing and undressing to change into an examination gown for radiographic procedures.

Problems can be encountered within the X-ray examination room in moving patients on and off the examination table. Most conventional radiographic imaging tables are quite high off the ground, the tabletop being anything between 24 and 28 inches above floor level; physically getting the less mobile patient on and off such tables, whether from a standing position or from a wheelchair, can present difficulties. This can be overcome by using specially designed elevating examination tables, which rise and lower hydraulically from a minimum height of 20 inches up to a maximum of 36 inches. Transfer of a patient to and from such variable-height tables is thus considerably easier than with conventional tables, and involves a minimum of lifting of the patient; some wheelchair patients are able to move themselves on and off such tables with only a little assistance (Figure 2). An additional advantage of this type of examination table is that it has a "floating" tabletop. Once the patient is lying on the table, it is not necessary to physically move him/her for radiographic positioning, as the entire tabletop is readily mobile longitudinally and laterally on release of electronic locks operated by foot switches. Thus, the patient and the part of the body to be radiographed can be easily positioned relative to the overhead X-ray tube without moving the patient relative to the tabletop, avoiding any potential discomfort. The precise position is delineated in the usual way for radiographic exposures by means of a light-beam collimator, which illuminates with visible light the shape, size, and position of the area on the patient to be radiographed. Some types of X-ray equipment (e.g. CT scanners) use low-power laser light beams for precise patient positioning.

For transferring patients on to examination tables, assistance from staff (radiographers, nurses, radiography helpers) is often required. Proper training of staff in patient-lifting techniques is essential to avoid injury to patients and staff.

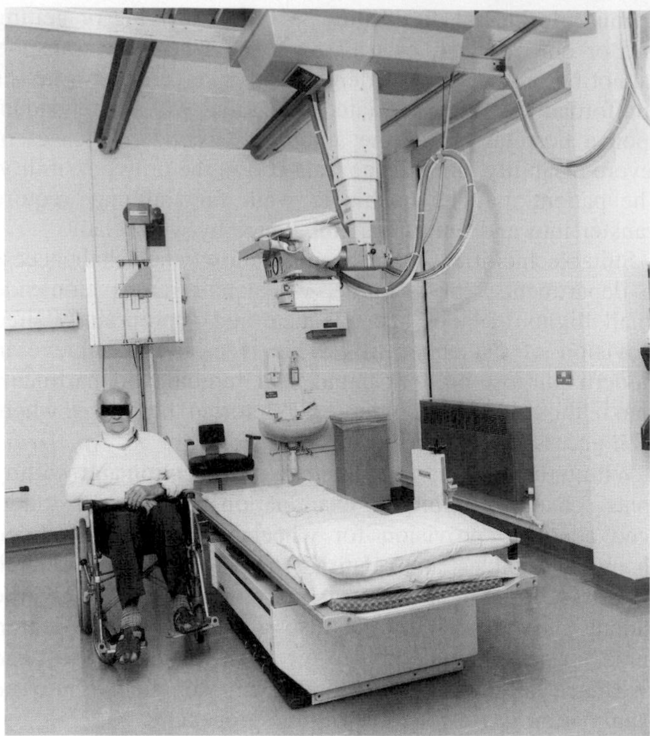

Figure 2 Elevating adjustable height, floating table top X-ray examination table

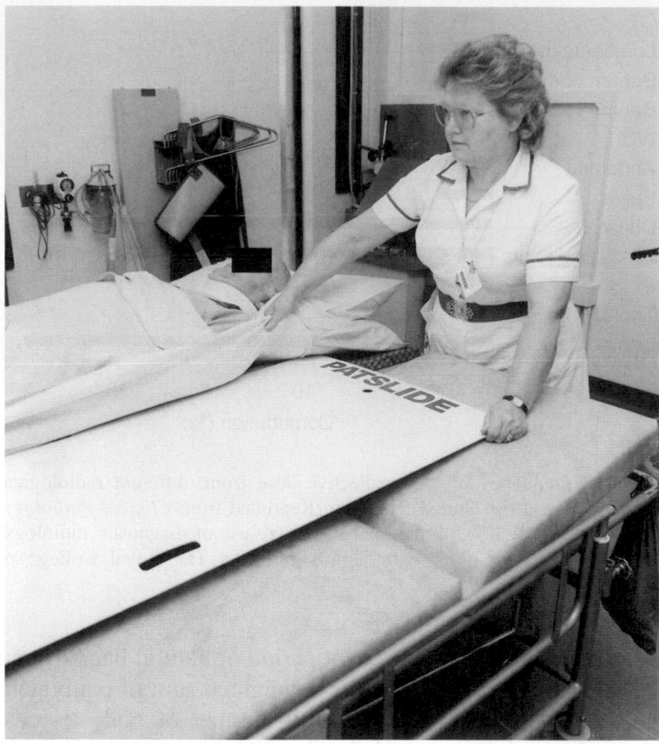

Figure 3 Placement of the Patslide® to transfer a patient from an X-ray examination table onto a hospital trolley

Lifting of patients without such training has the potential of back injury to the lifter and risks of the patients being dropped. Large numbers of back injuries currently occur to NHS staff as a result of lifting (Health and Safety Executive, 1992). Some hospitals and trusts have adopted "no-lifting" policies; all patient transfers and lifting being by mechanical aids – this has led to a significant reduction in the incidence of back injuries in staff (Royal College of Nursing, 1996). Mechanical lifting hoists are available for handling immobile patients. There are a variety of hoists available depending on patient's needs, but these hoists have tended to be used only in extreme cases as they have been felt to be cumbersome and time consuming to use. Newer battery-powered lifting hoists such as the Arjo Maxilift™ are much more versatile and user friendly, and are helpful for transfer of wheelchair patients onto examination tables.

Facilitation of transfer of patients from stretchers/trollies or inpatient beds on to examination tables can be helped using the Patslide®, a large, low-friction, semiflexible plastic sheet measuring about 5-feet long by 2-feet wide, that can be used to bridge the narrow gap between stretcher and examination table. The patient is rolled partly onto his/her side, the Patslide® positioned beneath the patient and a slide sheet, and the patient then rolled onto his/her back again and easily slid across it onto the examination table, because of the low coefficient of friction of the Patslide® surface plus the ease of maneuver of the slide sheet (Figure 3). Many hospital beds and stretcher trollies can be adjusted in height to ease such transfers, allowing a slight downhill slope for easier movement of patients both on and off. Slide sheets which aid the user to turn patients and to move them up and down the bed into a sitting position easily without causing discomfort to the immobile patient and without causing undue stress to either the patient or the carer can also help in the transfer of patients from hospital bed to trolley and then onto the X-ray table.

Some elderly patients are unable to stand without assistance, or to stand still enough or for long enough for erect radiographs to be obtained, for example, PA (posteroanterior) or lateral chest radiographs. These can be performed with the patient seated, using a special hydraulic examination chair with removable back and arm rests which can be left *in situ* except during the actual radiographic exposure (Figure 4). The seat can be raised, lowered, rotated, and locked in position with ease.

There are a variety of reasons why patients may need assistance getting on and off radiographic examination tables, including:

Immobility

- Joint stiffness and/or pain – arthritis, including osteoarthritis, rheumatoid arthritis, gout, ankylosing spondylitis, and other erosive arthropathies
- Muscle stiffness and pain – rheumatism, lumbago, and so on
- Neuralgia – sciatica, and so on
- Paralysis – stroke
- General weakness/debility
- Obesity

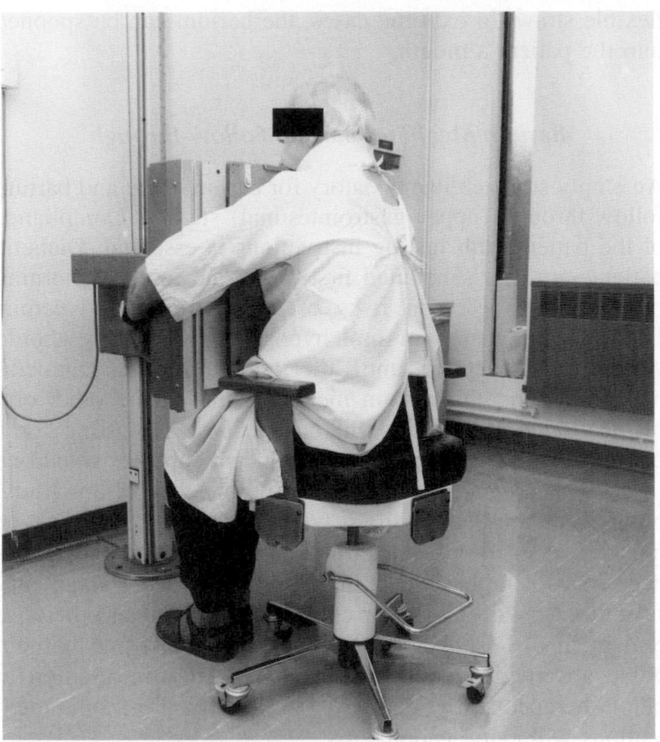

Figure 4 Use of hydraulic chair for erect chest radiographs for patients unable to stand

- Amputation
- Neurological disorders – Parkinson's disease, ataxias, multiple sclerosis
- Tendency to fall – vertigo, faintness

Inability to cooperate

- Deafness
- Blindness
- Failure to comprehend or remember instructions – dementia, lack of understanding of the language of communication

Unwillingness to cooperate

- Dementia – Alzheimer's disease, multi-infarct, and so on
- Psychological – depression, psychiatric illness, stubbornness, pride, dignity, shame, apprehension, claustrophobia.

Physiological handling of intravascular contrast media and of drugs used in radiology may be impaired in the elderly due to diminished renal and hepatic function; this must be allowed for in the choice and dosage of these agents.

IMAGING TECHNIQUES AND INTERVENTIONAL PROCEDURES – SPECIFIC PROBLEMS

Various problems can arise related to specific imaging investigations or interventional procedures. The following list is not intended to be exhaustive; it covers those examinations most frequently performed in elderly patients plus less common procedures where there are special considerations.

Plain Film Radiography

The general problems previously discussed, which can make getting on and off X-ray examination tables difficult, can also cause difficulties in patient positioning and radiographic exposure. Problems can be encountered in keeping patients still for sufficient time for the radiographic exposure; in these circumstances it is helpful to keep the exposure time as short as possible to minimize movement effects. This can be achieved by use of higher kilovoltage (kV) techniques when soft tissue contrast is not critical. Since radiographic exposure depends on the mAs (milliamp.seconds) setting, the use of as high a tube current as possible within the limits of the X-ray tube capacity and the generator output will shorten the time. For most X-ray sets, however, the mAs setting is combined in one control, so exposure time cannot be separately selected.

For abdominal exposures of the renal tract, kidney, ureter and bladder (KUB), the use of compression reduces the exposure, and hence the exposure time, by moving soft tissues not of interest out of the field of view. Bowel preparation can reduce the X-ray exposure for KUB radiographs by emptying the colon of feces (Hasan *et al.*, 1996). Immobilization devices such as sandbags, retaining straps and supports, and compression bands can be helpful in preventing involuntary movements.

The chest radiograph is useful in assessing heart size – clinical assessment can be misleading in the elderly patient (Mulkerrin *et al.*, 1991). Breath holding is important to avoid movement blur in radiographic examination of the chest or abdomen; achieving this can be difficult if the patient is unable to hear or understand instructions, has a very poor memory, or is unwilling or unable to cooperate for the reasons previously discussed. Shortage of breath may present similar problems in breath holding, even in cooperative patients. Breathlessness due to cardiac failure, airways obstruction (chronic obstructive airways disease – COAD – or asthma) can present problems, but fortunately the exposure for chest radiographs is short, typically 0.01 seconds. Anxious or agitated patients may have difficulty in keeping still; careful explanation and reassurance by the radiographer are essential.

Extremes of weight (i.e. gross obesity or emaciation) in some elderly patients can make correct radiographic exposure difficult. Emphysema necessitates relative underexposure of chest radiographs to avoid an overexposed "black" film. An abdomen distended by ascites or by a fecally overloaded colon from severe constipation, or the abdomen of a grossly obese patient requires relative overexposure. Exposure factors in plain film radiography are largely controlled automatically by means of automatic exposure control (AEC) ionization chambers, which are sensors that react to the amount of radiation passing through them *en route* to the film, terminating the exposure when sufficient; the skill of the radiographer is nonetheless paramount in obtaining good radiographic exposure as well as positioning.

For patients who are too unwell to be moved from the ward to the department of clinical radiology, portable radiographic examinations can be performed. These will seldom be of as good quality as departmental radiographs, owing to the limited power output of the portable X-ray machine, and particular difficulties arise in positioning the patient, achieving adequate film-focus distance, and controlling exposure. Portable exposures are best confined to chest radiographs, although a reasonable quality abdominal radiograph is possible, except in obese patients. Transfer of the patient to the radiology department in his/her hospital bed is a better alternative to portable radiography; even if the patient is still radiographed in bed, as higher-quality radiographs can be obtained.

Digital Radiography

In digital or "filmless" radiography, an X-ray image produced by an image intensifier is recorded digitally and stored in a computer memory, replacing the conventional X-ray film. (An image intensifier is a device for greatly enhancing the faint fluorescence of an input phosphor screen in response to radiation, by electron release and capture, causing much brighter fluorescence of an output phosphor screen viewed by a TV camera). The resulting image is viewed on a TV monitor. Hard copy can be made using a laser imager or other imaging devices (Harding and Roberts, 1996). The exposure time is usually shorter in digital radiography than in conventional radiography – this can be advantageous in patients who have difficulty in keeping still or in breath holding. Clinical Radiology Departments and hospitals generally are moving more and more towards computerised digital systems with paperless electronic requesting and reporting, and filmless PACS (picture archiving communication systems) without hard copy, and allowing simultaneous multi-site access to images by radiologists and clinicians.

Barium Studies of the Gastrointestinal Tract

Barium Swallow

The cooperation of the patient in drinking adequate volumes of barium quickly enough, and at the right time, is essential for diagnostic studies of the esophagus, and particularly for rapid sequence radiography (at 2, 3, or 4 frames per second) or videoradiography of the oropharynx and upper esophagus. Elderly patients are more likely to aspirate barium into the larynx, trachea, and bronchial tree during barium swallows and meals. This can lead to aspiration pneumonia requiring physiotherapy and can be fatal (Ansell, 1987).

Patients who are unable to stand can still have an erect barium swallow on an overcouch X-ray table by raising the footstep and sitting the patient on it. If there is difficulty in drinking from an ordinary cup, a feeding cup with a spout can be substituted, or the patient can drink through a large-bore flexible straw. In extreme cases, the barium can be spooned into the patient's mouth.

Barium Meal and Barium Follow-through

An empty stomach is mandatory for barium meal and barium follow-through (upper gastrointestinal) studies. Compliance of the patient with fasting instructions is essential. Diabetic patients are best scheduled first or second in early-morning barium lists to lessen risks of hypo- or hyperglycemia. Diabetics on insulin or oral hypoglycemic therapy should withhold these agents until after eating breakfast immediately following the barium meal. Patients taking other oral medication need to withhold this because of fasting for a barium meal or follow-through; pills and capsules should be taken with a small glass of water before the barium study, notwithstanding the requirements of fasting, and this must be made clear in the patient information/instruction sheet. It is necessary to emphasize the importance of taking a small cupful of water with tablets or capsules, as these can otherwise remain in the esophagus for long periods of time without being absorbed (Evans and Roberts, 1976). In addition to being therapeutically ineffective in this situation, some medications will cause esophagitis.

Orally ingested barium can subsequently cause severe constipation in susceptible elderly subjects (Ansell, 1987). This should be explained to the patient, relative, or carer, and the patient advised to eat plenty of high-fiber food, fruits, and so on after the barium meal, or to take a mild laxative.

Smooth-muscle relaxants are frequently administered to patients undergoing barium meals (and barium enemas) to allow adequate gaseous distension of the stomach (or colon) in double-contrast examinations, where fine mucosal detail can be evaluated. Buscopan (hyoscine *N*-butyl bromide, 20 mg intravenously) is often used, but should not be given to patients suffering from cardiac arrhythmias, coronary artery disease, or closed-angle glaucoma (Fink and Aylward, 1995), all of which are more common in the elderly. Glucagon 0.5 mg i.v. may be substituted in these patients (Goei *et al.*, 1995). An effervescent agent – sodium bicarbonate granules, powder, or tablets, sometimes with citric acid as an adjuvant – is swallowed before the barium to produce carbon dioxide gas for the double-contrast technique. The patient must refrain from burping or belching, or a double-contrast barium meal will not be possible.

A normally conducted barium meal means changing patient position from erect to prone and supine, and quite a lot of turning between prone and supine positions – patients have to be fit to undergo a barium meal! The examination can, however, be tailored with limited views and fewer changes of position in very ill patients.

Barium Enema

Bowel preparation for barium enema requires several days of dietary modification/restriction and strong oral laxatives on the day before the examination. This can make some patients unwell to the extent that outpatients will contact the radiology department requesting that the examination be cancelled or postponed; it is advisable to try to persuade these patients to attend regardless, as it is a pity to have undergone the fairly arduous preparation and then not to have the enema and, even worse, to have to undergo bowel preparation a second time. In particular, patients can feel unwell because of the bowel preparation during hot summer weather. Dehydration can occur; adequate fluid intake must be maintained. Migraine attacks may be precipitated in susceptible patients.

If a large or even moderate amount of fecal residue is present in the colon, a double-contrast examination is unlikely to be diagnostic; filling defects such as polyps or tumors can be missed, and ulceration can be difficult to evaluate. It is said that the radiologist who attempts a double-contrast barium enema on the inadequately prepared patient requires (and acquires) only a knowledge of feces! Such patients are better examined by a single-contrast technique using barium followed by water – this is far more likely to achieve a diagnostic result even without the superior mucosal detail afforded by double-contrast studies. A single-contrast examination is also more suitable for patients who have difficulty in retaining barium – it is quicker, less uncomfortable, and patients who cannot retain air insufflated for double-contrast examinations can often retain fluid in a barium/water examination. Multiple "spot" radiographs can be obtained on 100-mm cut film (as commonly used for barium meals) taken from the output phosphor screen of an image intensifier by a camera using a similar mirror arrangement to that in single-lens reflex cameras. This allows rapid alternation between a TV camera (during fluoroscopic screening) and a spot film camera (to record hard copy). There is the advantage of a shorter exposure time than with conventional radiographic film exposure, avoiding movement blur in restless or breathless patients, plus the added advantages of shortening the examination time, as 100 mm film changing is automatic and quick, and reducing radiation exposure compared with conventional film. In patients likely to have difficulty retaining barium, the use of a balloon retention barium enema catheter can help, but patient cooperation is still required – the inflated balloon catheter can be expelled rectally by uncooperative patients. The use of smooth-muscle relaxants makes the barium enema examination less uncomfortable for the patient, in addition to improving diagnostic quality. For patients with anal strictures or fistulae, in whom a normal-sized catheter cannot be inserted, a smaller Foley bladder catheter can be substituted.

Intravenous Urography (IVU)

Renal function declines in the elderly (Cox *et al.*, 1991). Higher doses of contrast medium may be required for opacification of the renal tract. Modern low-osmolality nonionic contrast media are much more patient-friendly than the older ionic contrast media, but there are still risks of allergy and precipitation of cardiac failure (Holtas and Tornquist, 1987; Harding, 1996a). Renal function of patients undergoing contrast examinations may become impaired, particularly if there is pre-existing renal disease (Trewhella and Dawson, 1990). Patients with diabetes are more likely to have some degree of impairment of renal function than the normal population and are said to be at greater risk of contrast nephropathy. Metformin (glucophage) therapy for non-insulin-dependent diabetes mellitus may occasionally cause severe life-threatening lactic acidosis in patients with impaired renal function, with mortality greater than 50% (Monson, 1993; Sirtori and Pasik, 1994). The combination of metformin and X-ray contrast media may have adverse affects because contrast media impair or further impair renal function and hence metformin excretion. Significant numbers of patients attending for diagnostic and interventional radiological procedures involving contrast medium administration, such as during IVU, will be taking metformin. All patients who are to receive intravascular X-ray contrast media (whether for IVU, vascular studies, or enhancement of CT scans) should be asked if they are diabetic and, if so, whether they are receiving metformin (glucophage) therapy. The advice of The Royal College of Radiologists is that if a patient is receiving metformin therapy, the drug should be stopped for 48 hours before and 48 hours after any X-ray contrast medium examination. This should be discussed fully with the patient's referring clinician or general practitioner (GP) – adjustment of the control of the patient's diabetes may be needed. Renal function should be checked 48 hours after the injection of X-ray contrast medium and prior to the resumption of metformin therapy. X-ray contrast medium–enhanced procedures in emergencies should continue to be carried out without delay. However, the patient's referring clinician or GP and the local renal physicians should be consulted. Obesity and constipation can obscure renal detail, although this can be overcome by tomography in patients able to cooperate with adequate breath-holding (tomography requires a longer exposure time than plain radiographs).

Vascular Radiology

Patient cooperation in keeping very still is essential for arteriography and venography, especially when digital subtraction is utilized. Digital subtraction angiography (DSA), previously known as *digital vascular imaging* (DVI), is similar to digital radiography, but may be included as an "add-on" to older fluoroscopic imaging equipment, as well as being built into digital radiographic equipment.

In DSA, summated TV frames early in a sequence of images during a dynamic vascular examination are subtracted pixel by pixel from later-summated TV frames, following intravascular injection of a radiographic contrast medium. This results in imaging only those structures in the field of view opacified by the contrast medium, with subtraction of overlying bony or gas-filled structures. This is analogous to a similar technique applied in the past using photographic subtraction of a plain radiograph taken before contrast medium injection from a later one in which the blood vessels were opacified by contrast medium. DSA is very sensitive and can satisfactorily image considerably diluted contrast medium. For example, faintly opacified arteries can be imaged following intravenous injection of contrast medium, which becomes diluted by mixing with blood during its passage through the right heart chambers, the pulmonary vascular system, and the left side of the heart before entering the systemic arterial circulation. This is a less invasive procedure than conventional arteriography and can be performed on an outpatient basis (Harding and Lenaghan, 1985). The image data may be recorded digitally, as in digital radiography, or on older systems may be recorded on magnetic recording tape in analog form. The subtraction images can be viewed dynamically on a TV monitor either as a continuous real-time image showing gradual appearance and disappearance of contrast medium in the blood vessels being studied, or as regularly upgraded static images at short time intervals. The optimal images can then be frozen for production of hard copy.

Very small amounts of patient movement during DSA can be compensated for on postexamination analysis by registering the position of the early mask relative to the contrast-filled images, or even utilizing a post-opacification mask, but larger amounts of movement make the technology unusable. For abdominal angiography breath holding is essential.

Vascular access for angiography by the Seldinger technique (Seldinger, 1953) requires local anesthesia to avoid excessive pain. Systemic intravenous sedation and analgesia may be needed in addition for apprehensive patients, but it must be remembered that older patients are frequently more sensitive to such agents because of diminished metabolic clearance, and a slowly administered, titrated lower dose is usually necessary, along with careful monitoring of pulse, respiration, blood pressure, and arterial oxygen saturation by pulse oximetry. If a patient is sedated to a semiconscious level, anesthetic assistance is the ideal; at the least, a trained and experienced nurse should be dedicated to the task of monitoring and caring for the patient (Skelly, 1996).

For some vascular procedures, and particularly for more difficult superselective arteriography and interventional vascular procedures, such as angioplasty, stenting, or embolization, a patient may be lying on the X-ray fluoroscopy table for several hours.

Many invasive vascular investigations are now being replaced by other noninvasive imaging modalities, for example, ultrasound, including Doppler and power Doppler, CT angiography, and MRI angiography.

ULTRASOUND

Ultrasound scanning uses a probe operated by the piezoelectric effect to emit ultrasound of frequency 3.5–10 MHz into the patient and receive returning echoes from internal structures, producing a real-time, gray-scale image displaying the echo intensity as a 2D image on a TV monitor. Doppler ultrasound allows flow within blood vessels to be displayed. In duplex Doppler, the 2D image and Doppler waveform are displayed simultaneously, allowing accurate placement of the sampling gate over the region of interest. Color flow Doppler assigns different colors (usually red and blue) to flow in different directions, so that adjacent arteries and veins are displayed in different colors superimposed on the monochrome ultrasound image.

Abdominal and pelvic ultrasound scanning needs the patient's cooperation in keeping still, turning into position, and breath holding including deep inspiration for examination of the liver, gallbladder, spleen, and kidneys. Adequate ultrasound examinations are more difficult to perform and interpret in obese patients, and also in very thin patients. Pelvic ultrasound for examination of the uterus, ovaries, and adnexa needs a full urinary bladder. Other ultrasound scans, for example, of the thyroid gland, breast, and testes, and arterial and venous Doppler ultrasound, do not usually present any special problems in the elderly.

NUCLEAR MEDICINE

Nuclear medicine imaging or gamma camera scanning produces images from γ-rays emitted by a radionuclide injected in to the patient. The most common radionuclide used is technetium (^{99m}Tc), which is tailored to image different structures or physiology by chelating it with compounds to target specific organs and/or physiological functions. The emitted γ-rays are detected by a gamma camera, which consists of a large lead-shielded crystal that scintillates when a γ-ray enters it. Groups of photomultiplier tubes behind the crystal detect and localize the scintillations and a computer analyzes the resulting electrical signals and reconstructs an image.

Nuclear medicine demonstrates physiology rather than anatomy. Because of the requirement to keep the radiation dose to the patient as low as possible, gamma camera scans typically need long imaging periods ranging from 5 to 30 minutes, during which the patient must remain absolutely still – this can be difficult for elderly patients. Patients with orthopnea due to cardiac failure can have difficulty lying flat for nuclear medicine examinations.

COMPUTED TOMOGRAPHY

Computed tomography (CT; computer-assisted tomography – CAT scanning) uses measurements of X-ray attenuation recorded by an array of detectors from a thin fan-beam of X rays. The X-ray source and detector array rotate circumferentially around the patient. This results in millions of measurements of X-ray attenuation, which can be used to reconstruct an image of an axial slice through the patient by computer analysis using a back-projection method. Images can be reformatted in other planes, for example, coronal and sagittal, by summating information from adjacent axial slices, and 3D reconstructions are possible. The latest generation of CT scanners use helical or spiral scanning instead of planar scanning of individual axial slices, resulting in decreased scanning time and allowing better dynamic imaging of blood vessels following contrast medium injection.

Patients must keep absolutely still during CT scans or image artefacts will occur. For examination of the thorax or abdomen, breath holding is necessary. It is possible to scan the entire thorax or abdomen during a single breath-hold in cooperative patients using helical scanning. CT angiography following intravenous contrast medium injection can produce diagnostic images, including 3D reconstructions, avoiding the need for conventional invasive arteriography.

MAGNETIC RESONANCE IMAGING

MRI uses the principles of nuclear magnetic resonance (NMR) to produce cross-sectional images without the use of ionizing radiation. The patient is placed in a very strong magnetic field, typically 0.5–1.5 tesla (5000–15 000 gauss; cf. the earth's magnetic field is 0.7 gauss). Radio frequency pulses are applied at the same frequency as the precession frequency of the protons (hydrogen atoms) present in the body, causing them to resonate, like tuning forks of the same frequency. Some of the protons which are aligned with the applied magnetic field will invert or "flip" as a result, and if the radio frequency pulse is long enough, the protons will all precess in phase rather than randomly. When the radio frequency pulse is removed the protons will revert to their former state; those which have inverted will return to their earlier alignment, and they will again precess randomly. This results in very small magnetic field changes which can be detected by receiving coils, amplified, and reconstructed into cross-sectional images in any plane (Harding, 1996b).

Examination sequences range from less than 1 minute to more typical times of 4 to 5 minutes, depending on the pulse sequence employed. During each examination sequence, complete freedom from movement is essential to avoid artefacts. Various immobilization devices and supports can aid this, often incorporated into surface coils, which give better visualization of localized body areas such as the head, neck, or knees.

MRI scanning can be a daunting experience for elderly patients, due to the confined space within the scanner and the noise generated during scanning when the magnetic field gradients are changing rapidly. For the patient, entering the aperture of the MRI scanner can be reminiscent of a coffin entering a crematorium – this certainly frightens some patients and about 5% of all patients refuse MRI scanning because of claustrophobia or fear. The noise during scanning with knocking and hammering sounds which can be similar to a pneumatic drill in operation, although not quite as loud, can be upsetting; ear plugs can minimize the problem, though this makes patient communication a little more difficult. Conventional headphones cannot be incorporated into ear muffs as they would be nonoperative in the high magnetic field within the scanner, tens of thousand times the strength of the earth's magnetic field.

There are various contraindications to MRI, most of which are more common than the average in elderly patients, for example, cardiac pacemakers, ferromagnetic implants such as some surgical clips, some prosthetic cardiac valve replacements, and cochlear implants.

THERMAL IMAGING

Thermography is not widely utilized in the United Kingdom, but is undertaken in some centers. It has the advantages of being noninvasive and free of risks. It can be performed by a contact technique using liquid crystal detectors or with a thermal imaging camera which detects infrared (IR) radiation emitted by the patient, displayed as an image on a TV monitor. Thermal imaging is mainly used in the investigation of back pain syndromes and vascular disorders. In the author's experience it has proved a very useful examination tool in the initial investigation of deep venous thrombosis (DVT) (Harding, 1995, and in the investigation of osteomyelitis complicating diabetic foot ulceration, where diagnostic thermographic changes occur before radiological abnomalities, enabling earlier aggressive therapy, with significant reduction in morbidity (Harding *et al.*, 1998, 1999)).

INTERVENTIONAL RADIOLOGY

Interventional procedures may be undertaken under X-ray fluoroscopic control, ultrasound, CT, or MRI guidance. The range of interventional radiological procedures is constantly increasing in scope and complexity (Watkinson and Adam, 1996; Wilkins *et al.*, 1989; Rickards and Jones, 1989; Harding, 1993). Careful selection of patients for interventional radiological procedures is essential, jointly decided between the radiologist and referring clinician.

Informed consent is essential before performing interventional radiological procedures, and is best obtained by the radiologist personally rather than by junior clinical medical staff who may not be familiar with the details of the procedure to be performed. Consent should be obtained before the patient comes to the radiology department. This gives the radiologist the opportunity to build a relationship with the patient and, although time-consuming, this is time well spent. The importance of good communication between the radiologist and the patient cannot be overstated. The radiologist can assess the apprehensions and likely reactions of the patient away from the pressures of the radiology department. The benefits and potential risks of the procedure can be explained under circumstances in which the patient is better able to concentrate and more likely to remember the points that have been made. It also gives the patient time to gain confidence in the radiologist, to ask questions, and to have a chance to reflect on what has been said before the procedure is performed. "Good communication is the greatest antagonist to litigation" (Oscar Craig, past President of the Royal College of Radiologists) (Allison and Allison, 1996).

Deep sedation and analgesia will be required for interventional radiological procedures, and for certain patients or procedures general anesthesia will be necessary. The patient sedated for interventional radiology will require careful clinical and electromechanical monitoring.

Clinical monitoring includes assessment of the level of consciousness, anxiety and/or pain, respiratory rate, depth and regularity, skin color, temperature and pulse rate, character, and regularity. Electromechanical monitoring includes pulse oximetry and blood pressure. ECG monitoring is a useful adjunct to pulse oximetry for patients at increased cardiovascular risk where myocardial ischemia and/or arrhythmia is present or may be precipitated. The elderly are particularly susceptible to both the wanted and unwanted effects of all benzodiazepine sedatives (Skelly, 1996).

- *Biopsy, and so on* – guided biopsy, aspiration cytology, and preoperative tumor localization.
- *Drainage* – percutaneous drainage of obstructed systems, collections, or abscesses.
- *Fistula creation, and so on* – deliberate creation of fistulae, ostomies, or shunts.
- *Stricture dilatation, and so on* – dilatation, stenting, or bypassing of strictures or recanalization of occlusions.
- *Embolization* – deliberate obliteration of occlusion of vessels or aneurysms.

Needle biopsy or aspiration cytology of masses under imaging guidance is used for diagnosis and staging in many parts of the body, for example, liver, pancreas, abdominal and pelvic lymph nodes, kidney, adrenal glands, spleen, retroperitoneum, lung, pleura, mediastinum, and musculoskeletal system. Preoperative breast tumor localization with a wire marker makes the surgical approach easier and more accurate.

Percutaneous drainage of abscesses or collections is frequently performed, including subphrenic and other intra-abdominal abscesses, intrahepatic abscesses, pyonephrosis, perinephric abscess, pelvic collections, and pancreatic cysts or pseudocysts. In the thorax, pleural, intrapulmonary, and mediastinal collections can be accurately drained under CT or ultrasound control.

Vascular procedures include percutaneous transluminal angioplasty and vascular stenting for arterial stenosis or occlusion, arterial thrombolysis for acute obstruction in peripheral limb arteries and coronary arteries, aspiration thromboembolectomy, and mechanical thrombectomy and venous thrombolysis. Percutaneous transcatheter embolization is used for deliberate occlusion of aneurysms or selective occlusion of blood vessels supplying arteriovenous malformations (AVMs) and fistulae, or varices. Emergency embolization for hemorrhage is most commonly required for gastrointestinal hemorrhage, massive hemoptysis usually from bronchial arteries, and trauma to kidney, liver, or pelvis. Pulmonary artery embolization is also occasionally performed, for hemoptysis is not responsive to bronchial (and nonbronchial systemic) embolization.

Dilatation and stenting can be undertaken in superior vena cava (SVC) obstruction. Complications relating to intravascular lines and, in particular, venous catheters are not uncommon, and can usually be easily remedied in the radiology department. Foreign bodies can be retrieved from the vascular system by percutaneous catheter techniques, for example, fragments of central venous catheters, inferior vena caval filters, metallic stents, and misplaced embolization coils.

Bronchial stenting for palliation of malignant tracheobronchial stenosis can be placed under a combination of direct (endoscopic) vision and radiological fluoroscopic screening.

The TIPS (transjugular intrahepatic portosystemic shunt) procedure is used to create a fistula between the portal and hepatic venous systems for the relief of portal hypertension with recurring variceal bleeding.

DVT can be prevented from causing pulmonary emboli by percutaneous insertion of devices into the inferior vena cava (IVC) under fluoroscopic control. IVC filters are not used in first-line prophylaxis against pulmonary embolic disease, but have a small but increasingly well-defined role in those patients who are unsuitable for conventional prophylaxis with anticoagulant therapy or who need temporary protection.

In the urinary tract, interventional procedures include percutaneous nephrostomy drainage and ureteric stenting for ureteric obstruction, percutaneous dilatation of ureteral strictures, percutaneous occlusion of ureteral fistulae, and percutaneous suprapubic cystostomy and urethral stenting for bladder outlet obstruction. Percutaneous nepholithotomy for renal calculi is used occasionally in selected cases, but has been largely superseded by extracorporeal shock wave lithotripsy (ESWL).

Biliary obstruction can be treated by percutaneous transhepatic biliary drainage or percutaneous cholecystostomy, which is also used for drainage of acute empyema of the gallbladder or for access for gallstone removal. Benign and malignant biliary structures can be dilated and stented percutaneously and calculi in the intrahepatic and extrahepatic tree removed. Interventional radiology may be combined with endoscopic procedures in the biliary tract.

In the gastrointestinal tract, interventional radiological procedures are performed in the treatment of esophageal structure by balloon dilatation and stenting. Percutaneous gastrostomy, transgastric jejunostomy, and percutaneous jejunostomy are used for enteral nutrition therapy or gastrointestinal decompression. Radiologically guided cacostomy can be used in colonic obstruction as a temporizing measure in high-risk surgical patients. Colonic strictures following surgical anstomosis can be dilated by balloon catheter techniques.

KEY POINTS

- An aging population is generally associated with multiple comorbid conditions.
- Good communication and an understanding approach is essential for successful investigation and intervention.
- Assessment of risk/benefit outcome is critical for successful resource utilization and clinical benefit for patients.
- Specific adaptations of radiology unit and equipment to facilitate management of older disabled patients are of cardinal importance.
- CT, MRI, Ultrasound, and barium studies are often essential investigations for older people, but require their cooperation.

KEY REFERENCES

- DH (Department of Health). *The Ionising Radiation (Medical Exposure) Regulations* 2000, (IR(ME)R 2000). Department of Health, Statutory Instrument 2000 No. 1059. The Stationery Office Limited, HMSO, London, ISBN 0-11-099131-1.
- European Union. *European Directive 97/43/Euratom (The Medical Exposures Directive)*; EU, Brussels.
- National Radiological Protection Board and The Royal College of Radiologists. *Patient Dose Reduction in Diagnostic Radiology* 1990; HMSO, London, ISBN 0-85951-327-0.
- RCR Working Party. *Making the Best Use of a Department of Clinical Radiology: Guidelines for Doctors* 2003, 5th edn; Royal College of Radiologists, London.
- Royal College of Nursing. *Introducing a Safer Patient Handling Policy* 1996, pp 1–7; Royal College of Nursing, London.

REFERENCES

Allison D & Allison H. Ethics and informed consent. In A Watkinson & A Adam (eds) *Interventional Radiology: A Practical Guide* 1996, pp 12–5; Radcliffe Medical Press, Oxford.

Ansell G. Alimentary tract. In G Ansell & RA Wilkins (eds) *Complications in Diagnostic Imaging* 1987, 2nd edn, pp 218–46; Blackwell Scientific Publications, Oxford.

Ansell G, Bettmann MA, Kaufman JA & Wilkins RA (eds) *Complications in Diagnostic Imaging and Interventional Radiology* 1996, 3rd edn; Blackwell Science, Oxford.

Audit Commission. *Improving Your Image: How to Manage Radiology Services More Effectively* 1995; HMSO, London, ISBN 0-11-8864-149.

Cox JR, Macias-Nunez JF & Dowd AB. Renal disease. In MSJ Pathy (ed) *Principles and Practice of Geriatric Medicine* 1991, 2nd edn, pp 1159–77; Wiley, Chichester.

DH (Department of Health). *The Ionizing Radiation (Protection of Persons Undergoing Medical Examinations or Treatment – POPUMET) Regulations* 1988; HMSO, London.

DH (Department of Health). *The Ionising Radiation (Medical Exposure) Regulations* 2000, (IR(ME)R 2000). Department of Health, Statutory Instrument 2000 No. 1059. The Stationery Office Limited, HMSO, London, ISBN 0-11-099131-1.

European Union. *European Directive 97/43/Euratom (The Medical Exposures Directive)*; EU, Brussels.

Evans KT & Roberts GM. Where do all the tablets go? *Lancet* 1976; **2**:1237–9.

Fink AM & Aylward GW. Buscopan and glaucoma: a survey of current practice. *Clinical Radiology* 1995; **50**:160–4.

Goei R, Nix M, Kessels AH & Ten Tusscher MPM. Use of antispasmodic drugs in double contrast barium enema examination: glucagon or buscopan? *Clinical Radiology* 1995; **50**:553–7.

Harding JR. Percutaneous antegrade ureteric stent insertion in malignant disease. *Journal of the Royal Society of Medicine* 1993; **86**:511–3.

Harding JR. Liquid crystal thermography in the investigation of deep venous thrombosis. In K Ammer & EFJ Ring (eds) *The Thermal Image in Medicine and Biology* 1995, pp 232–6; Uhlen Verlag, Vienna.

Harding JR. The characteristics of an ideal intravascular contrast medium. *RAD Magazine* 1996a; **22**(259):16.

Harding JR. Principles of magnetic resonance imaging. In L Paine (ed) *Hospital Management International* 1996b, pp 203–4; Sterling Publications, London.

Harding JR, Banerjee D, Wertheim DF *et al.* Infrared imaging in the long-term follow-up of osteomyelitis complicating diabetic foot ulceration. *Proceedings of the Engineering in Medicine & Biology Society, Institute of Electrical & Electronic Engineers* 1999; **21**:1104.

Harding JR & Lenaghan AE. The impact of digital subtraction angiography on a district general hospital. *The British Journal of Radiology* 1985; **58**:814.

Harding JR & Roberts SA. Laser imaging in clinical radiology. *Journal of Photographic Science* 1996; **44**:11–3.

Harding JR, Wertheim DF, Williams RJ *et al.* Infrared imaging in diabetic foot ulceration. *European Journal of Thermology* 1998; **8**:145–9.

Hasan AKH, Sutton D, Burne D & Menhinick S. Intravenous urography; the value of oral laxative. *International Uroradiology '96-Program and Abstracts* 1996, p 134; European Society of Uroradiology and the Society of Uroradiology.

Health and Safety Executive. *Manual Handling Operations Regulations 1992: Guidance on Regulations* 1992; HMSO, London.

Holtas S & Tornquist C. Renal complications of contrast media. In G Ansell & RA Wilkins (eds) *Complications in Diagnostic Imaging* 1987, 2nd edn, pp 37–52; Blackwell Scientific, Oxford.

Mulkerrin E, Saran R, Dewar R *et al.* The apex cardiac beat: not a reliable clinical sign in elderly patients. *Age Ageing* 1991; **20**:304–6.

National Radiological Protection Board. *Protection of the Patient in X-ray Computed Tomography* 1992; HMSO, London, ISBN 0-85951-345-8.

National Radiological Protection Board and The Royal College of Radiologists. *Patient Dose Reduction in Diagnostic Radiology* 1990; HMSO, London, ISBN 0-85951-327-0.

RCR Working Party. A multi-centre audit of hospital referral for radiological investigation in England and Wales. *British Medical Journal* 1991; **303**:809–12.

RCR Working Party. Influence of the Royal College of Radiologists' guidelines on hospital practice: a multicenter study. *British Medical Journal* 1992; **304**:740–3.

RCR Working Party. *Making the Best Use of a Department of Clinical Radiology: Guidelines for Doctors* 2003, 5th edn; Royal College of Radiologists, London.

Rickards D & Jones SN. Percutaneous interventional uroradiology. *The British Journal of Radiology* 1989; **62**:573–81.

Roberts CJ. Towards the more effective use of diagnostic radiology: a review of the work of the RCR Working Party on the more effective use of diagnostic radiology 1976–1986. *Clinical Radiology* 1988; **39**:3–6.

Roberts CJ. The RCR multi-centre guideline study: implications for clinical practice. *Clinical Radiology* 1992; **45**:365–8.

Royal College of Nursing. *Introducing a Safer Patient Handling Policy* 1996, pp 1–7; Royal College of Nursing, London.

Seldinger SI. Catheter replacement of the needle in percutaneous arteriography: a new technique. *Acta Radiologica* 1953; **39**:368–76.

Sirtori CR & Pasik C. Re-evaluation of biguanide, metformin: mechanism of action and tolerability. *Pharmacological Research* 1994; **30**:187–228.

Skelly A. Analgesia and sedation. In A Watkinson & A Adam (eds) *Interventional Radiology: A Practical Guide* 1996, pp 3–11; Radcliffe Medical Press: Oxford.

Trewhella M & Dawson P. Intravascular contrast agents and renal failure. *Clinical Radiology* 1990; **41**:373–5.

Watkinson A & Adam A (eds) *Interventional Radiology: A Practical Guide* 1996; Radcliffe Medical Press, Oxford.

Wilkins RA, Nunnerley HB, Allison DJ *et al.* The expansion of interventional radiology. Report of a survey conducted by the Royal College of Radiologists. *Clinical Radiology* 1989; **40**:457–62.

FURTHER READING

Gray JAM. Social and community aspects of ageing. In MSJ Pathy (ed) *Principles and Practice of Geriatric Medicine* 1991, 2nd edn, pp 181–94; Wiley, Chichester.

Monson JP. Selected side-effects. II. Metformin and lactic acidosis. *Prescribers' Journal* 1993; **33**:170–3.

PART III

Medicine in Old Age

Section 16

Infectious Disorders

145

Infectious Diseases

Ann R. Falsey
University of Rochester School of Medicine and Dentistry, Rochester, NY, USA

INTRODUCTION

It is at the extremes of age when susceptibility to infection and the complications thereafter are the greatest. With the rapid growth of the number of elderly persons in most developed countries, an understanding of the unique features of infectious diseases in the aged is essential. The many causes of increased morbidity and mortality from infections in the elderly are outlined in Table 1. Aging is associated with the presence of chronic diseases as well as declines in cellular and humoral immune function. In addition to the physiologic changes of aging, a segment of the older population lives in congregate settings such as group homes and long-term care facilities (LTCF), which present special issues related to the spread of infectious diseases.

The incidence of some infections, such as influenza, decreases with advancing age, yet the morbidity is substantially higher. However, many infections increase in both frequency and severity in older age-groups (Tables 2 and 3). It is also important to recognize that the specific types of organisms affecting older persons differ from those affecting younger age-groups and that older persons may not exhibit the typical clinical manifestations of infection that are observed in healthy young adults. Infections of specific organ systems will be discussed separately in their respective articles. This article will review the epidemiology, clinical manifestations, and general approach to infections in older persons. In addition, sexually transmitted diseases (STDs), severe acute respiratory syndrome (SARS), specific problems unique to LTCF, and current recommendations for vaccination in the elderly will be discussed.

EPIDEMIOLOGY OF INFECTIONS

Infections are among the most common causes of hospitalization and death in both community-dwelling and institutionalized older persons. The incidence of infection depends on the place of residence and functional status of the groups studied. Although 95% of older adults do not live in LTCFs, specific data on infection rates in community-dwelling elderly are limited. In a 2 year prospective study of 417 independent older persons, investigators found that 224 (54%) experienced a total of 494 infections (Ruben *et al.*, 1995). Respiratory tract, genitourinary and skin infections accounted for 53, 24, and 18% of the infections, respectively. Of note, 144 (35%) of these 417 persons were hospitalized 260 times. One hundred of the 260 admissions (38%) involved infection and, in half, infection was the primary diagnosis. In addition, hospitalized older persons have been shown to experience higher rates of nosocomial infections which are associated with a higher mortality rate (Emori *et al.*, 1991). The number of infections occurring in nursing homes approaches that of acute-care hospitals. The demographics of nursing-home populations are very different compared to those of community-dwelling older persons. Nursing-home residents are generally 85 years or older (40%), female (71%), and white (92%) (Verghese and Berk, 1990). Single day prevalence studies yield highly variable infection rates with upper limits of 32.7% and incidence rates up to 20 infections per 100 resident-months, resulting in approximately 1.5 million nosocomial infections per year in LTCF in the United States (Smith *et al.*, 1991). In addition to the chronic problems of respiratory, urinary tract, and skin infections, nursing homes are prone to epidemics of certain diseases, such as tuberculosis (TB), conjunctivitis, scabies, gastroenteritis, and influenza. Infection is the most common problem, necessitating transfer from nursing homes to acute-care hospitals, accounting for between 10 and 49% of all transfers.

Specific Infections

Bacterial Respiratory Infections

Pneumonia is one of the most important infectious causes of morbidity and mortality in persons of any age, but it is

Principles and Practice of Geriatric Medicine, 4th Edition. Edited by M.S. John Pathy, Alan J. Sinclair and John E. Morley.

Table 1 Causes of increased morbidity and mortality of infections in older persons

Immunosenescence
Diminished mobility
Physiologic change in organ systems
Poor circulation
Edema of soft tissues
Weakening of respiratory muscles
Depressed gag reflex
Obstructive uropathy
Changes in vaginal flora associated with diminished estrogen levels
Comorbid diseases
Cardiac
Pulmonary
Diabetes
Malignancies
Dementia
Peripheral vascular disease
Iatrogenic
Intravenous lines
Implantable cardiac devices: valves, pacemakers, defibrillators
Feeding tubes
Bladder catheters
Congregate living

Table 2 Infections that increase in frequency with age

Pneumonia
Tuberculosis
Urinary tract
Chronic bacterial prostatitis
Herpes zoster
Skin/soft tissue
Contiguous focus osteomielitis
Endocarditis
Bacteremia
Diverticulitis
Cholecystitis
Intrabdominal abscess
Clostridium difficile diarrhea

Adapted from Yoshikawa (1994).

Table 3 Increased mortality associated with infections in older persons

Infection	Relative risk of mortality of elderly compared to young adults
Pneumonia	3
Influenza	6–16
SARS	3–9
Pyelonephritis	5–10
Bacteremia	3
Appendicitis	15–20
Cholecystitis	2–8
Tuberculosis	10
Infective endocarditis	2–3
Bacterial meningitis	3
Herpes zoster	7
HIV	5

Adapted from Yoshikawa (1994).

in the young children and the elderly where its impact is greatest felt (*see* **Chapter 61, Respiratory Disease in the Elderly**). The incidence of pneumonia is 10 times greater in adults over 70 years compared to persons between 20 and 29 years old (Woodhead, 1994). In addition, the likelihood of requiring hospitalization for pneumonia rises dramatically with age; from 0.54 cases per 1000 among persons aged 35 to 44, to 11.6 cases per 1000 persons over age 75 (Marrie, 1994). The incidence of community-acquired pneumonia in all adult age-groups is highest during the winter months, and is likely due to winter respiratory viruses.

Pneumonia is the leading cause of nosocomial infection related deaths. In the National Nosocomial Infection Surveillance (NNIS) System study in the United States, pneumonia accounted for 18% of the infections and 48% of the deaths between 1986 and 1990 (Emori *et al.*, 1991). The risk of nosocomial infections increases from a relatively constant rate of 10/1000 discharges for persons under age 50 to 100/1000 over age 70 (Gross *et al.*, 1983). Other risk factors associated with nosocomial pneumonia in the elderly include neurologic disease, renal disease, dependency in activities of daily living, difficulty with oropharyngeal secretions, presence of nasogastric tubes, poor nutrition, intubation, and intensive care admission (Hanson *et al.*, 1992; Harkness *et al.*, 1990). Similar to the acute-care hospital, pneumonia is the second most common infection in chronic care facilities, but remains the most common cause of death (Niederman, 1993). The susceptibility to infection correlates strongly with the degree of functional impairment (Alvarez, 1990). Underdiagnosis of pneumonia is common because of nonspecific symptoms, the infrequent use of chest radiographs, and difficulty in obtaining sputum. Prevalence rates of lower respiratory tract infection in nursing homes range from 1.9 to 2.5% with incidence rates of approximately 47 per 100 resident-months (Garibaldi *et al.*, 1981).

The spectrum of pathogens that cause pneumonia in the elderly is broader than in young adults and includes nontypable *Hemophilus influenzae, Moraxella catarrhalis, Staphylococcus aureus,* and gram-negative bacilli. Nevertheless, *S. pneumoniae* remains the most common bacterial pathogen causing up to 60% of community-acquired pneumonias in the elderly (Woodhead, 1994). Lastly, the "atypical" pathogens *Mycoplasma pneumoniae* and *Chlamydia pneumoniae* are relatively uncommon in persons over age 65. Hospital-acquired pneumonia in the elderly is frequently caused by enteric gram-negative rods and accounts for as many as 60 to 80% of all cases (Niederman, 1993). The NNIS study showed that nosocomial pneumonia was due to Pseudomonas in 18%, Enterobacter sp. in 11%, *Klebsiella pneumoniae* in 8%, *E. coli* in 6%, and *S. aureus* in 15% of cases.

Viral Respiratory Tract Infections

Rates of upper respiratory tract infections, the majority of which are caused by viruses, decline with advancing age and average one infection per year. However, the rates of infection depend in large part on the place of residence with increased rates of infection observed in seniors living in congregate settings (*see* **Chapter 58, Epidemiology of Respiratory Infection**). A recent study by Hodder *et al.* (1995) showed that the overall rate of respiratory infections was 2.5/100 person-months in community-dwelling elderly in contrast to 10.8/100 person-months in an adult daycare setting. Rates of infection in nursing homes are highly variable due to the epidemic nature of most respiratory viruses.

Influenza virus is the most well recognized viral cause of serious illness in elderly persons. Although nonpandemic influenza attack rates are 20 to 30% in preschool and school-age children and drop to 10% for older adults, complications rates are highest in the elderly (Glezen and Couch, 1978). During epidemics of influenza H3N2, hospitalization rates are approximately 6 to 15/1000 for persons over age 65 (Glezen, 1982). Lower respiratory tract involvement with influenza also increases with age, rising from 4 to 8% in under age 50 up to 73% in persons over age 70 (Betts, 2000). The risk of death from influenza increases 39-fold by the presence of chronic medical conditions such as cardiovascular disease, diabetes, renal disease, anemia or immunosuppression, and the presence of both pulmonary and cardiovascular disease raises the mortality 870-fold.

Respiratory syncytial virus (RSV) is now recognized as the second most important respiratory viral pathogen in older persons with a disease burden similar to nonpandemic influenza (Thompson *et al.*, 2003). Outbreaks of RSV in nursing homes have been described with average attack rates of 20% and rates of pneumonia ranging from 5 to 67% and death ranging from 0 to 53% (Falsey and Walsh, 2000). Although the precise incidence is unknown, recent studies indicate that RSV is a cause of excess morbidity and mortality in community-dwelling elderly as well (Zambon *et al.*, 2001). In addition to influenza and RSV, a number of other viral pathogens such as coronaviruses, rhinoviruses, parainfluenza, and the newly described human metapneumovirus can also cause significant illness in older persons.

Urinary Tract Infection

Bacteriuria is the most common bacterial infection affecting older persons (Nicolle, 1997). The prevalence of bacteriuria in community-dwelling women under age 60 is <5%, which rises to 5 to 10% in women aged 60 to 70 years and 20 to 30% in those 80 years or above (Boscia *et al.*, 1986). For men, bacteriuria is rare before age 60 (<1%) but also becomes more common with increasing age. Bacteriuria is even more common in institutionalized older persons with prevalence rates of 30 to 50% in women and 20 to 30% in men, and correlates with functional disability, and is virtually 100% after 30 days with an indwelling urethral catheter (Warren *et al.*, 1982). Antimicrobial treatment of asymptomatic bacteriuria does not affect mortality and morbidity and is associated with adverse side effects, emergence of resistant flora and high relapse rates (*see* **Chapter 126, Urinary Incontinence** and **Chapter 127, Renal Diseases**).

Compared to the high incidence of asymptomatic bacteriuria, symptomatic urinary tract infection rates are relatively low. Despite this, they account for approximately 24% of all infections diagnosed in healthy older persons and are also the most common cause of bacteremia in both institutionalized and ambulatory elderly populations (Setia *et al.*, 1984). *Escherichia coli* is the most common pathogen in geriatric patients; however, the proportion of infections due to other gram-negative pathogens, such as Proteus, Klebsiella, Serratia, Enterobacter, and Pseudomonas, is higher than in younger groups (Baldassarre and Kaye, 1991). *Staphylococcus saprophyticus*, a common pathogen in young women, is unusual in older women. Of note, isolates from elderly men are frequently gram-positive organisms, such as Group B Streptococcus and *Enterococcus* sp (Boscia *et al.*, 1986).

Skin and Soft Tissue Infections

After the urinary and respiratory tract, the skin is the third most common site of infection in the elderly and the incidence of cellulitis, diabetic foot ulcers and other cutaneous infections all increase with age (Alvarez, 1990; Ruben *et al.*, 1995). In community-dwelling older persons, the incidence for all types of skin infections is 12.7/100 person years and the incidence of cellulitis is 3.2/100 person years (Ruben *et al.*, 1995). New skin infections occur at a rate of approximately 1.6 per 100 resident-months in nursing homes (Scheckler and Peterson, 1986).

Herpes Zoster

Varicella zoster virus remains latent in the dorsal root ganglion after primary infection and may reactivate at any time throughout life. The lifetime risk of zoster is approximately 10 to 20%; however, risk increases dramatically with advanced age (Straus *et al.*, 1988). The incidence of zoster in the general population is 215/100 000 but increases to 1424/100 000 in persons over age 75 (Donahue *et al.*, 1995). Approximately, 1% of persons over age 80 will develop herpes zoster each year with a significant risk of post herpetic neuralgia (Kost and Straus, 1996). Pain lasting over 1 year has been reported in 4, 22, and 48% of patients under age 20, over 55 and over 70 years, respectively (*see* **Chapter 148, Infections of the Central Nervous System**).

Infectious Diarrhea

Although the overall incidence of diarrhea in older persons in the general population is not increased, the impact of these illnesses is significant. A study of approximately 87 000 hospitalizations for gastroenteritis found that 85% of the 514 deaths were adults over the age of 60 with a case fatality of 3% in persons older than age 80 (Slotwiner-Nie and Brandt, 2001). Nursing-home residents are at highest risk for developing diarrheal illness because of outbreaks that tend to occur in closed populations. Outbreaks of Salmonella, *Escherichia coli* 0157:H7, rotavirus, Norwalk-like viruses, giardia, and cryptosporidiosis have all been reported in chronic care facilities. Lastly, age is associated with an increased risk of developing *C. difficile* colitis. Clusters of *C. difficile* have been reported from a number of nursing homes and control of outbreaks is very difficult because of the prolonged carrier state, hardy spores, and fecal oral contamination in demented and incontinent patients. Although more common, *C. difficile* colitis does not appear to have a worse clinical outcome with older age. Despite delayed diagnosis and higher white blood cell counts than younger persons, mortality was not significantly higher in older patients in several recent studies.

Meningitis

The incidence of meningitis in persons aged 60 or older is approximately 2 to 9/100 000 per year with a case-fatality rate of 35 to 81% (Miller and Choi, 1997). The spectrum of pathogens that cause meningitis in older persons is different from the ones that cause meningitis in healthy young adults (Schuchat *et al.*, 1997). Although *Streptococcus pneumoniae* is the most frequently isolated organism in all adult age-groups (32–68%), *Listeria monocytogenes* which is uncommon in young adults accounts for 10 to 25% of case of meningitis in the elderly. Viruses and *Neisseria meningitidis* that are common in children and young adults are uncommon in the elderly, whereas gram-negative bacillary meningitis occurs more frequently in older adults (Durand *et al.*, 1993). Although TB meningitis is not common at any age, the incidence of active TB rises with advancing age and therefore the diagnosis should be considered in any older person with "aseptic" meningitis (*see* **Chapter 148, Infections of the Central Nervous System**).

Bacteremia

Bacteremic illnesses increase in both frequency as well as mortality with advancing age (Richardson, 1993). The genitourinary tract accounts for 24 to 56% of cases of bacteremia with other sources including the abdomen, skin, and respiratory tract. The most commonly isolated species from community-dwelling elderly are *E. coli.* and *Klebsiella* sp., whereas other gram-negatives such as *Providencia stuartii, Proteus* sp., and *Pseudomonas* sp. are more frequently found in residents of long-term care. *S. aureus, Enterococcus* sp., and *S. pneumoniae* are the most common gram-positive bloodstream isolates. In LTCF, methicillin-resistant *S. aureus* can be a significant problem (Mylotte *et al.*, 2002). Mortality in bacteremic elderly patients varies from 9.1% in the community-dwelling elderly with gram-negative infections to 47.2% in elderly persons with nosocomial bacteremia (Richardson, 1993). Risk of death is increased in patients with nosocomial bacteremia, a nonurinary source, respiratory infection, *S. aureus* or inappropriate antibiotic treatment.

Infective Endocarditis

In the preantibiotic era, the most common endocarditis patient was a young person with rheumatic heart disease, whereas recent reviews show that the incidence of endocarditis now is substantially higher in patients over the age of 50 reaching a peak at 70 to 74 years (Selton-Suty *et al.*, 1997; Terpenning *et al.*, 1987; Wells *et al.*, 1990). With the decline of rheumatic heart disease, degenerative valvular lesions, such as calcified aortic valves and mitral annulus calcification, as well as mitral valve prolapse with redundancy are common predisposing conditions in the elderly persons (McKinsey *et al.*, 1987). In addition, nosocomial endocarditis due to invasive medical procedures is more common in older adults and accounts for 23% of cases (Terpenning *et al.*, 1987). α-Hemolytic streptococci and *S. aureus* remain the most frequently isolated pathogens; however, *Enterococcus* sp., *Streptococcus bovis,* and coagulase negative staphylococci are more common in elderly persons than in younger age-groups. As with almost all infectious diseases, mortality with endocarditis at older age is associated with increased mortality. Elderly patients with endocarditis have an approximately twofold higher risk of death compared to younger persons (Wells *et al.*, 1990). In addition, neurologic complications and permanent disability requiring subsequent long-term care are more common in older patients who survive an acute episode of endocarditis (*see* **Chapter 147, Infective Endocarditis in the Elderly**).

CLINICAL PRESENTATION

Most elderly patients exhibit typical clinical features of infectious processes. However, a significant proportion of older persons with serious infections may present with atypical or nonspecific signs and symptoms due to the effects of aging, dementia, and comorbid diseases (Table 4). This is particularly true for frail institutionalized persons whose cognitive impairment may prevent them from communicating specific focal symptoms. For instance, a number of studies have shown that elderly persons with pneumonia are less likely to complain of cough and pleuritic chest pain. Symptoms of dysuria, urgency, and frequency are often absent in elderly patients with cystitis, particularly in those who have indwelling catheters (Baldassarre and Kaye, 1991). In addition, flank pain and fever, which suggest pyelonephritis in young, healthy adults, are commonly absent in older patients. Underlying diseases, such as osteoarthritis, may mask the symptoms of a joint infection in the elderly adult. Similarly, meningismus may be difficult to detect in persons with cervical arthritis or parkinsonism, making it an unreliable diagnostic sign of meningitis in the elderly. Lastly, intra-abdominal processes are more likely to be overlooked in the

Table 4 Atypical symptoms of infection in older persons

Acute confusion
Change in functional status
Anorexia, weight loss
Weakness
Urinary incontinence
Falls
Tachypnea
Tachycardia
Hypotension
Hypothermia

Tuberculosis

In developed countries, LTCFs are a repository for TB. Today's octogenarians were infected 50 to 70 years ago when 90% of the adult population was exposed to TB. Endogenous reactivation of TB remains the leading cause of TB in older persons. However, exogenous reinfection or primary infection from a fellow resident with unsuspected TB within nursing homes has been well documented. A full discussion of TB in the elderly is beyond the scope of this article, but several general points regarding infection control in the LTCF should be made. First, all new admissions to an LTCF should have a two-step purified protein derivative (PPD) skin test and reactions should be documented in the chart (Zevallos and Justman, 2003). A positive PPD is classified as >10 mm of induration; however, >5 mm of induration is also considered positive in those who are in close contact with persons with infectious TB or who have chest radiographs suggestive of previous TB. Some authorities recommend PPD retesting annually or every 2 years for all residents with a negative PPD. At a minimum, nonreactors should be retested whenever a new active case of TB is diagnosed or suspected. Individuals with a positive PPD who were negative during the preceding 2 years and who have normal chest radiographs should receive isoniazid prophylaxis for 9 months under close supervision. Even for patients at advanced ages the benefits of such practice outweigh the risks. Previous recommendations included chemoprophylaxis for individuals with a positive PPD of unknown duration with certain high-risk conditions such as diabetes, renal failure, immunosuppression, chronic steroid use, and silicosis as well as those with abnormal chest radiographs. In 2000, the US Center for Disease Control and Prevention (CDC) with the American Thoracic Society revised the recommendations, such that any high-risk individual with a positive PPD should receive chemoprophylaxis regardless of age or duration of positive PPD. Residents of nursing homes are considered high risk. The decision to treat such individuals remains somewhat controversial. A high index of suspicion for active TB should be maintained by clinicians, because signs and symptoms may be atypical and the PPD negative in older persons. Employees of LTCFs are also at increased risk of infection with TB. They should have a PPD placed at the time of employment and also annually (Zevallos and Justman, 2003).

SPECIFIC INFECTIONS

Sexually Transmitted Diseases

Despite the perception among health-care providers that elderly adults are not at risk for STDs, many older adults remain sexually active and are at risk for STDs (Calvert, 2001). The Janus report on sexual behavior found that 69% of American men over the age of 65 and 74% of woman report some form of sexual activity at least weekly. Additionally, in a survey of persons between the ages of 80 to 100, 62% of men and 30% of women engaged in sexual intercourse. Because of cultural, social, and religious practices of older adults, they may be less likely to speak freely of STDs and thus, it is important for providers to be mindful of such issues. The finding of an STD in a nursing-home resident should always prompt an investigation because of concerns for elder abuse.

Human Immunodeficiency Virus

Human immunodeficiency virus (HIV) is a cause of enormous morbidity and mortality worldwide. While it is predominantly a disease of younger persons, data reported to the CDC in the United States indicates that approximately 10% of Acquired Immune Deficiency syndrome (AIDS) cases are in persons >50 years (Chiao *et al.*, 1999). Before 1989, 15% of AIDS cases in older persons were transfusion related. However, since 1996, the epidemiology of HIV in older adults has changed. Transfusion now only accounts for 2.4% of cases, whereas men who have sex with men accounts for the largest percentage at 36% and intravenous drug use (IVDU) accounts for 19%. Although IVDU is the second most common risk factor, it is significantly less than in individuals of ages between 13 and 49. Both heterosexual contact (14%) and unknown risk (26%) are significantly greater in adults over 50 years of age compared to younger age-groups.

Numerous studies indicate that older age is associated with a shortened interval between time of HIV diagnosis and the development of AIDS as well as time from onset of AIDS to death (Adler *et al.*, 1997). Hemophiliacs >55 years have a relative mortality of 4.7 after developing AIDS compared to younger counterparts. The reason for decreased survival in older AIDS patients is likely multifactorial and includes comorbidities, delay in diagnosis, and age-related immune dysfunction (Calvet, 2003). Studies by Adler *et al.* (1997) have demonstrated that destruction of T-cells of young and old patients progress at the same rate but older persons have an impaired ability to replace functional T-cells.

Clinical presentation of AIDS in older persons is similar to that in younger adults, but diagnosis remains challenging because common medical problems associated with aging may confuse or delay workup. Thus, patients may undergo extensive workups for cerebrovascular disease, Alzheimer's disease, malnutrition, cancer or depression before the diagnosis of HIV is even entertained. Although several studies have shown that the clinical presentation of AIDS in older patients is similar to the young and that pneumocystitis pneumonia (PCP) is the most common opportunistic infection in both groups, some differences are worth mentioning. 1996 CDC data indicates that older individuals are significantly more likely to develop wasting syndrome and HIV encephalopathy than are patients aged 13 to 49 years (Calvet, 2003). In addition, 14% of older adults develop malignancies; most commonly Kaposi's sarcoma or non-Hodgkin's lymphoma. HIV encephalopathy in older persons deserves special mention, given the prevalence of Alzheimer's and cerebrovascular disease in this population. HIV is associated with subacute encephalitis, which leads to a subcortical dementia in contrast to Alzheimer's disease which is a cortical disease often leading to aphasia and other manifestations of cortical dysfunction. The progression of HIV encephalopathy is expected to be relatively rapid with decline over months compared to the more slowly evolving Alzheimer's. In addition, HIV dementia is associated with pleocytosis in the cerebrospinal fluid (CSF) in 25% of cases, whereas CSF is normal in Alzheimer's disease. It is important to consider HIV in the workup of dementia since antiretrovirals may slow progression or improve symptoms.

The treatment of HIV infection in older age has not been well studied. Most trials of antiretroviral medications have excluded persons over age 60. A recent cross-sectional survey of HIV infected individuals taking highly active antiretroviral therapy (HAART) found that persons over age 55 tolerated therapy as well as younger subjects with no significant differences in adherence rates or the need for modification of treatment because of side effects (Manfredi *et al.*, 2003). However, older patients had lower mean drop in viremia (0.5 $\log_{10}$ vs 1.0 $\log_{10}$) and immune recovery was significantly slower and more blunted. Interestingly, other investigators found that compliance with HAART was better in persons >50 years compared to younger age-groups. At present, more studies of HAART in older age-groups are needed to evaluate efficacy; but age alone is not a sufficient reason to deny treatment.

Prevention of HIV is critical in all age-groups. A problem unique to older age-groups is that both health-care professionals as well as patients themselves do not perceive the risk appropriately. In AIDS behavioral studies in the United States, less than 7% of subjects who were sexually active, >50 years, and who resided in cities with a high prevalence of HIV had ever had HIV testing done (Calvet, 2003). Additionally, less than 11% of older people had ever discussed HIV testing with their doctor. As a result of decreased concerns about pregnancy, older adults are also much less likely to use condoms than younger people. Clearly, STD testing and safe sex practices need to be addressed in older age-groups.

Syphilis

Primary and secondary syphilis are not common in persons over age 55 accounting for only 4% of cases reported in the United States in 1997 (Calvert, 2001). Although uncommon, syphilis should be considered in any sexually active patient with an unexplained rash or a new genital ulceration. While early syphilis is not frequent, latent syphilis is primarily a problem of older age. A serum rapid plasma reagin (RPR) is typically included in a routine dementia workup. If the confirmatory specific *Treponema pallidum* antibody is positive, then all patients with infection for greater than 1-year duration should have a lumbar puncture performed. This includes most elderly adults with a positive RPR. It is particularly important to evaluate the CSF if any neurologic signs or symptoms are present (including deafness), the patient has co-infection with HIV or other signs of tertiary syphilis such as aortitis or gummas. Unfortunately, there is no gold standard for the diagnosis of neurosyphilis and CSF – venereal disease research laboratories (VDRL) are positive in only 50% of cases of neurosyphilis. Thus, even mild pleocytosis or elevation of protein may indicate CNS involvement and are indications for treatment. The optimal treatment of neurosyphilis is 18 to 24 million units of intravenous penicillin for 10 to 14 days. Follow-up is required to insure a response to therapy.

Herpes Simplex

Herpes Simplex virus type 2 (HSV-2) or genital herpes simplex is extremely common, affecting 22% of the adult population in the United States (Calvet, 2003). Seroprevalence for HSV-2 rises with increasing age, the highest prevalence being in previously married, black women aged 60 to 74 years. Approximately 70 to 80% of individuals with HSV-2 antibodies are not aware of their infection. Thus, HSV-2 should be kept in mind when evaluating perineal ulcers or rash even if the patient does not have a known history of genital herpes. The best method of diagnosis remains to be viral culture of early lesions. The virus is relatively hardy and grows rapidly; usually within 48 hours. However, a negative culture does not rule out the infection. Treatment includes acyclovir and the new formulations, famciclovir and valacyclovir, which offer improved oral absorption. Treatment may be initiated for primary infection to decrease symptoms or with recurrent disease to suppress outbreaks. Patients should be counseled that transmission can occur even if the patient has no symptoms, and therefore the use of condoms at all times is encouraged.

Gonorrhea

Infection with *Neisseria gonorrhea* is uncommon in the elderly and occurs at a rate of 4/100 000 in persons 65 years and older. There is no clear evidence that gonorrhea (GC) is more severe in elderly persons compared to the young although cases of disseminated GC in the elderly have been reported (Calvet, 2003). Diagnosis is usually made by urethral or cervical culture but can also be accomplished by polymerase chain reaction (PCR). Treatment of uncomplicated GC: a single dose of Ceftriaxone 125 mg IM, Cefixime 400 mg PO or an oral quinolone. Local resistance patterns and travel should be kept in mind when selecting therapy.

Severe Acute Respiratory Syndrome (SARS)

In March of 2003, the World Health Organization issued a global alert regarding a severe atypical pneumonia in China, Hong Kong, and Vietnam referred to as *Severe Acute Respiratory Syndrome* (SARS). A newly discovered coronavirus

(SARS-Cov) was subsequently identified as the cause of SARS (Peiris *et al.*, 2003). It is hypothesized that SARS-Cov is an animal virus, which crossed the species barrier into humans possibly from "game food" in southern China. Infected persons initially present with fever, myalgias, and rigors. Cough is common, but dyspnea and chest tightening may only present later in the illness. Unlike other common respiratory viruses, rhinorrhea and sore throat are uncommon. Diarrhea may occur in approximately 20% of cases. Laboratory findings include ground glass opacifications on chest radiographs, lymphopenia, and elevations of liver function tests. Although fever is present in over 90% of patients with SARS, afebrile cases of SARS can occur in the elderly. In one such case, an elderly adult presented with malaise and poor appetite with a hip fracture secondary to a fall but no fever.

The case-fatality rate during recent outbreaks was 9.6% (range 0–40%). Advanced age is the single most important risk factor for death; patients >60 years have a case-fatality rate of 45% and the relative risk of death is 1.5 to 1.8 per each decade of life increased (Christian *et al.*, 2004). Patients are most infectious later in the illness when symptoms progress, requiring hospitalization. Transmission is believed to be through direct or indirect contact of mucous membranes (eyes, nose, mouth) with infected secretions but spread via small particle aerosols has not been completely ruled out. Diagnosis can be made by viral culture, reverse transcriptase-polymerase chain reaction (RT-PCR) or serology; however, no test is very sensitive early in illness. Despite initial enthusiasm for high dose steroids and ribavirin, at present there is no specific therapy for SARS. Intensive work on antivirals and vaccines is ongoing.

VACCINATION

Vaccination is one of the most cost-effective strategies available to reduce the morbidity and mortality associated with a number of infectious diseases. Although vaccine response rates are diminished in older persons and cost effectiveness has been debated, three vaccines are recommended for all older persons: tetanus toxoid, pneumococcal vaccine, and influenza virus vaccine.

Tetanus–diphtheria Toxoid

The annual incidence of tetanus cases in developed countries is very low (Bentley, 1992). However, over 50% of the tetanus cases occur in persons over the age of 50, with 60% mortality. More than 90% of the deaths from tetanus are in persons over age 50 (Richardson and Knight, 1991). Because there is no natural immunity to tetanus, disease occurs almost exclusively in those who are inadequately or unimmunized. Since routine vaccination of school children and armed forces personnel did not begin until the 1940s, many elderly persons never received a primary series of tetanus toxoid immunization. In addition, the recommended booster doses every 10 years are frequently neglected in older persons. Studies from the United States, Britain, Germany, Denmark, and Sweden have shown that 45 to 80% of community-residing elderly and 30 to 50% of nursing-home residents lack immunity (Gergen *et al.*, 1995). Although commonly associated with accidental trauma, a significant number of tetanus cases occur in the setting of chronic skin ulcers, gangrenous extremities or recent surgery (Bentley, 1992). The current vaccine contains formaldehyde-denatured tetanus toxoid and diphtheria toxin (Td), and will provide protection to diphtheria as well as tetanus. Although studies have shown that the antibody levels achieved by older adults are lower than those of young adults, protective antibody titers are present in 100% of older persons after the third dose of primary immunization. Duration of antibody may also be somewhat diminished but booster doses are highly effective at raising antibody to protective levels. Vaccination is well tolerated by older persons and the only contraindication is a history of neurological or severe hypersensitivity reactions to previous Td. The current recommendations are that all older persons who are inadequately immunized or whose history of immunization is unknown receive primary immunization with Td. Although standard recommendations are for a single Td booster every 10 years after primary immunization, some authorities feel that a single booster given at age 65 is the most cost-effective practice (Balestra and Littenberg, 1993). All older patients evaluated for wounds should be questioned regarding immunization status, and Td immunization given as appropriate. In addition, immunity status should be determined prior to elective bowel surgery and for nursing-home patients with decubitus ulcers or vascular complications.

Pneumococcal Vaccine

Pneumococcal infections are an important cause of illness and death in older persons, thus making prevention of these infections by vaccination highly desirable. Approximately 30 to 50% of community-acquired pneumonias are due to *Streptococcus pneumoniae* (Fedson *et al.*, 1994). At least 16 000 cases of invasive pneumococcal disease occur yearly in the United States among people over age 65. Case-fatality rates are as high as 40% for bacteremia and 55% for meningitis, despite prompt diagnosis and treatment with appropriate antibiotics (Bentley, 1992). Vaccination has become even more important with the rapid increase and global spread of antibiotic-resistant pneumococci.

Pneumococcal vaccine contains purified capsular polysaccharide antigens from different serotypes of *S. pneumoniae.* The first vaccine, licensed in 1977, contained 14 of the 83 different serotypes. In 1983, an expanded 23-valent vaccine became available. Vaccine-associated reactions occur within 24 hours in 10 to 15% of elderly vaccinees and consist primarily of local discomfort. Fever of >100 °F occurs in approximately 2% of vaccinees and usually lasts less than 24 hours. Severe local and systemic reactions have been reported more often in younger persons and revaccinated individuals (Bentley, 1992). Pneumococcal vaccine and influenza vaccine may be administered simultaneously at different sites without affecting immunogenicity or side effects. Most healthy young adults maintain adequate antibody levels for 5 to 6 years. Several studies suggest that, while older persons respond to pneumococcal vaccine, they may have lower peak titers and antibody levels may diminish at a more rapid rate. Early studies involving small numbers of young individuals showed high rates of local Arthus-type reactions when subjects were revaccinated. More recent data indicate that older persons who received the 14-valent vaccine may be revaccinated with the 23-valent vaccine 6 years after primary vaccination with no significant side effects and a boost of antibody levels.

Much debate has been generated concerning the efficacy of pneumococcal vaccine in high-risk populations, particularly older persons. Pneumococcal vaccine was shown to be highly effective when tested in young healthy South African gold miners, a group in whom the incidence of disease is very high. However, the results of controlled trials in older persons in the United States have been inconclusive because of the small sample sizes used. Retrospective case-control studies have shown pneumococcal vaccine to be between 50 and 80% effective for the prevention of invasive pneumococcal disease in older persons (Fedson *et al.*, 1994). Vaccine efficacy has been shown to decrease progressively over time and is least efficacious in very elderly persons (>85 years). Yet, in the largest case-control study published, the 5-year efficacy in immunocompetent patients aged 65 to 74 was 71%, and in those 75 to 84 years of age the 3-year efficacy was 67% (Shapiro *et al.*, 1991). Analyses of the cost effectiveness of pneumococcal vaccine have estimated that routine vaccination of all persons over age 65 is a cost-saving procedure (Fedson *et al.*, 1994). The most recent analysis of the effectiveness of pneumococcal vaccine involved 47 000 adults over age 65 and confirmed a significant reduction in the risk of bacteremia associated with vaccination but did not show a beneficial effect for nonbacteremic pneumonia (Jackson *et al.*, 2004).

Pneumococcal vaccine is recommended for immunocompetent persons at increased risk of pneumococcal disease for a variety of chronic illnesses such as cardiovascular disease, pulmonary disease, diabetes mellitus, cirrhosis and, alcoholism (Table 7) (Center for Disease Control and Prevention, 1997). It is also recommended for patients with CFS leaks, and for persons aged 65 or older. Revaccination should be considered for those individuals at highest risk of fatal pneumococcal disease and who received the 23-valent vaccine over 6 years ago. It should also be considered for patients who have a rapid decline in antibody titers,for example, patients with nephrotic syndrome. Revaccination is also recommended for healthy elderly persons who received vaccine before age 65 and more than 10 years has passed. Routine revaccination of elderly persons is not currently recommended (Bentley, 1992). This is because of concerns about reduced immunogenicity of repeat vaccinations with polysaccharide vaccines. A recent study from Sweden examined the effect of revaccinating elderly adults after 5 years with pneumococcal vaccine (Torling *et al.*, 2004). Although there was a significant increase in the mean geometric antibody concentration, levels were lower than after primary vaccination. These issues have stimulated interest in the pneumococcal conjugate vaccines in adults (Abraham-Van Parijs, 2004). While these vaccines offer the advantage of stimulating T lymphocytes and memory, they include only seven antigenic types compared to 23 in the polysaccharide vaccines.

Table 7 Indications for pneumococcal vaccine

Primary vaccination
Over age 65 years
Ages 2–64 years
Chronic illnesses including CHF, COPD, diabetes, alcoholism, liver disease
Nephrotic syndrome, CSF leaks
Asplenia
Immunocompromised
Special ethnic groups including Native Americans and other groups with high rates of invasive pneumococcal disease
Revaccination (greater than 5 years since primary vaccination)
Patients with rapid decline in antibody levels
Asplenia
Nephrotic syndrome
Renal failure or transplantation
HIV
Other forms of immunosuppression
Over age 65
If primary vaccination took place under age 65
Vaccine status is unknown

Adapted from Center for Disease Control and Prevention (1997)

Influenza Vaccine

Influenza continues to be an important cause of excess morbidity and mortality throughout the world, especially in the elderly (Centers for Disease Control, 2004). The current vaccine contains two type A and one type B influenza virus strains representing the viruses predicted to circulate during the upcoming year. The vaccine is made from highly purified, egg-grown inactivated viruses in a trivalent preparation. Whole virus, subunits, and purified surface antigen preparations are available. Acute local reactions such as mild soreness at the vaccination site occur in approximately one-third of vaccinees. Systemic reactions, including fever, occur in less than 1% of vaccinees, and appear to be less severe in older persons. Influenza vaccine is contraindicated in persons with an anaphylactic or immediate hypersensitivity reaction to eggs.

The efficacy of influenza vaccine depends on the age and immunocompetence of the subjects as well as the match of the vaccine to the epidemic strain. In placebo-controlled trials of young healthy persons, efficacy rates for reducing influenza infection ranged from 67 to 92% (Bentley, 1992). Effectiveness in other populations, especially the elderly, has been more variable with occasional reports of vaccine failure. One of the few prospective, randomized, placebo-controlled trials of influenza vaccine efficacy, from the Netherlands, demonstrated that vaccination resulted in a

Table 8 Groups in which yearly influenza vaccination is recommended

Groups who are at increased risk for influenza-related complications
Persons > age 65
Residents of nursing homes and chronic care facilities
Persons with chronic cardiac or pulmonary disorders
Persons who have required regular medical follow-up during the preceding year because of chronic metabolic diseases (including diabetes), renal dysfunction, hemoglobinopathies or immunosuppression
Persons who can transmit influenza to high-risk groups
Physicians, nurses, and other health-care personnel
Employees of nursing homes with patient contact
Providers of home care
Household members of persons in high-risk groups

Adapted from Centers for Disease Control (2004).

58% reduction of influenza infection in vaccines (Govaert *et al.*, 1994). A recent three-year case-control study from the United States found influenza vaccine to be both efficacious and cost effective (Nichol *et al.*, 1994). Although vaccine recipients had more coexisting illnesses at baseline than those who did not receive the vaccine, vaccination was associated with a reduction in yearly hospitalization rates during the 3-year period for pneumonia and influenza by 48 to 57% and for all chronic respiratory conditions by 27 to 39%. Vaccination was also associated with a 37% reduction in the rate of hospitalization for congestive heart failure (CHF) when influenza A was epidemic. In the three influenza seasons studied, vaccination was associated with decreases of 39 to 54% in mortality from all causes. While effective in all older adults, benefit from influenza vaccine is greatest in those with high-risk conditions (Hak *et al.*, 2002). In addition, influenza vaccine is associated with a reduction in hospitalizations for cardiac disease and strokes in the elderly (Nichol *et al.*, 2003). In LTCFs, the efficacy of influenza vaccine in preventing uncomplicated influenza infection is low (28–37%) (Centers for Disease Control, 2004). However, the efficacy in reducing complications, including hospitalization (47%), pneumonia (58%), and death (76%), is substantial. Achieving a high rate of vaccination among nursing-home residents has been shown to reduce the spread of infection in such a facility, thus preventing disease through herd immunity.

A number of well-designed studies have shown influenza vaccine to be a highly cost-effective intervention and provide compelling evidence for increasing programs aimed at improving compliance with recommendations for annual influenza vaccination. Groups in whom vaccination is recommended are listed in Table 8.

KEY POINTS

- Infections are a leading cause of hospitalization and death in older persons.
- Susceptibility to infection in the elderly is multifactorial and includes diminished immune function, comorbid diseases, and congregate living residences.
- Signs and symptoms of infection in the elderly may be more subtle or atypical compared to young adults.
- LTCF have high prevalence rates of infection. Hand washing and antibiotic control are important measures for limiting the spread of resistant organisms in these facilities.
- Influenza and pneumococcal vaccine are beneficial and cost-effective methods to reduce morbidity and mortality associated with these infections in all groups of older adults.

KEY REFERENCES

- Jackson LA, Neuzil KM, Yu O *et al.* Effectiveness of pneumococcal polysaccharide vaccine in older adults. *The New England Journal of Medicine* 2004; **348**:1747–55.
- Kost R & Straus S. Postherpetic neuralgia – pathogenesis treatment and prevention. *The New England Journal of Medicine* 1996; **335**:32–42.
- Nichol KL, Nordin J, Mullooly J *et al.* Influenza vaccination and reduction in hospitalizations for cardiac disease and stroke among the elderly. *The New England Journal of Medicine* 2003; **348**:1322–32.
- Nicolle LE. Asymptomatic bacteriuria in the elderly. *Infectious Disease Clinics of North America* 1997; **11**(3):647–62.
- Slotwiner-Nie PK & Brandt LJ. Infectious diarrhea in the elderly. *Gastroenterology Clinics of North America* 2001; **30**:625–35.

REFERENCES

Abraham-Van Parijs B. Review of pneumococcal conjugate vaccine in adults: implications on clinical development. *Vaccine* 2004; **22**:1362–71.

Adler WH, Padmavathi V, Chrest FJ *et al.* HIV infection and aging: mechanisms to explain the accelerated rate of progression in the older patient. *Mechanisms of Ageing and Development* 1997; **96**:137–55.

Alvarez S. Incidence and prevalence of nosocomial infections in nursing homes. In A Verghese & SL Berk (eds) *Infections in Nursing Homes and Long-Term Care Facilities* 1990, pp 41–54; Karger, New York.

Arden NH. Control of influenza in the long-term-care facility: a review of established approaches and newer options. *Infection Control and Hospital Epidemiology* 2000; **21**:59–64.

Baldassarre JS & Kaye D. Special problems of urinary tract infection in the elderly. *The Medical Clinics of North America* 1991; **75**:375–90.

Balestra DJ & Littenberg B. Should adult tetanus immunization be given as a single vaccination at age 65? *Journal of General Internal Medicine* 1993; **8**:405–12.

Bentley DW. Vaccinations. *Clinics in Geriatric Medicine* 1992; **8**:745–60.

Bentley DW, Bradley SF, High F *et al.* Practice guideline for evaluation of fever and infection in long-term care facilities. *Journal of the American Geriatrics Society* 2001; **49**:210–22.

Betts R. Influenza virus. In GL Mandell, JF Bennett & R Dolin (eds) *Principles and Practices of Infectious Diseases* 2000, 4th edn, pp 1546–67; Churchill Livingston, New York.

Boscia JA, Kobasa WD, Knight RA *et al.* Epidemiology of bacteriuria in an elderly ambulatory population. *American Journal of Medicine* 1986; **80**:208–14.

Bradley SF. Issues in the management of resistant bacteria in long-term care facilities. *Infection Control and Hospital Epidemiology* 1999; **20**:362–6.

Bradley SF. Staphylococcus aureus infections and antibiotic resistance in older adults. *Clinical Infectious Diseases* 2002; **34**:211–6.

Calvert H. Sexually transmitted diseases. In T Yoshikawa & DC Norman (eds) *Infectious Disease in the Aging: A Clinical Handbook* 2001, 1st edn, pp 313–22; Humana Press, Totowa.

Calvet HM. Sexually transmitted diseases other than human immunodeficiency virus infection in older adults. *Clinical Infectious Diseases* 2003; **36**:609–14.

Center for Disease Control and Prevention. Prevention of pneumococcal disease: recommendations of the Advisory Committee of Immunization Practices (ACIP). *Morbidity and Mortality Weekly Report* 1997; **46**(RR-8):1–24.

Centers for Disease Control. Prevention and control of influenza: recommendations of the Advisory Committee on Immunization Practices (ACIP). *Morbidity and Mortality Weekly Report* 2004; **53**(RR-6):1–40.

Chiao KY, Ries KM & Sande MA. AIDS and the Elderly. *Clinical Infectious Diseases* 1999; **28**:740–5.

Christian MD, Poutanen SM, Loutfy MR *et al.* Severe acute respiratory syndrome. *Clinical Infectious Diseases* 2004; **38**:1420–7.

Donahue J, Choo P, Manson J & Platt R. The incidence of herpes zoster. *Archives of Internal Medicine* 1995; **155**:1605–9.

Durand M, Calderwood S, Weber D *et al.* Acute bacterial meningitis in adults. *The New England Journal of Medicine* 1993; **328**:21–8.

Emori TG, Banerjee SN, Culver DH *et al.* Nosocomial infections in elderly patients in the United States 1986–1990. *American Journal of Medicine* 1991; **91**(S3B):3B-289S–93S.

Falsey AR & Walsh EE. Respiratory syncytial virus infection in adults. *Clinical Microbiology Reviews* 2000; **13**(3):371–84.

Fedson D, Shapiro E, LaForce F *et al.* Pneumococcal vaccine after 15 years of use: another view. *Archives of Internal Medicine* 1994; **154**:2531–5.

Fendler EJ, Ali Y, Hammond BS *et al.* The impact of alcohol hand sanitizer use on infection rates in an extended care facility. *American Journal of Infection Control* 2002; **30**:226–33.

Garibaldi RA, Brodine S & Matsumiya S. Infections among patients in nursing homes: policies prevalence and problems. *The New England Journal of Medicine* 1981; **30**:731–5.

Gergen P, McQuillin G, Kiely M *et al.* A population-based serologic survey of immunity to tetanus in the United States. *The New England Journal of Medicine* 1995; **332**:761–813.

Glezen WP. Serious morbidity and mortality associated with influenza epidemics. *Epidemiologic Reviews* 1982; **4**:24–44.

Glezen WP & Couch RB. Interpandemic influenza in the Houston area 1974–76. *The New England Journal of Medicine* 1978; **298**:587–92.

Govaert TME, Thijs CTMCN, Masurel N *et al.* The efficacy of influenza vaccination in elderly individuals – a randomized double-blind placebo-controlled trial. *Journal of the American Medical Association* 1994; **272**:1661–5.

Gross PA, Rapuano C, Adrignolo A & Shaw B. Nosocomial infections: decade-specific risk. *Infection Control* 1983; **4**:145–7.

Hak E, Nordin J, Wei F *et al.* Influence of high-risk medical conditions on the effectiveness of influenza vaccination among elderly members of 3 large managed-care organizations. *Clinical Infectious Diseases* 2002; **35**:370–7.

Hanson LC, Weber DJ, Rutala WA & Samsa GP. Risk factors for nosocomial pneumonia in the elderly. *American Journal of Medicine* 1992; **92**:161–6.

Harkness GA, Bentley DW & Roghmann KJ. Risk factors for nosocomial pneumonia in the elderly. *American Journal of Medicine* 1990; **89**:457–63.

Hodder SL, Ford AB, FitzGibbon PA *et al.* Acute respiratory illness in older community residents. *Journal of the American Geriatrics Society* 1995; **43**:24–9.

Jackson LA, Neuzil KM, Yu O *et al.* Effectiveness of pneumococcal polysaccharide vaccine in older adults. *The New England Journal of Medicine* 2004; **348**:1747–55.

Knockaert DC, Vanneste LJ & Boobaers HJ. Fever of unknown origin in the elderly. *Journal of the American Geriatrics Society* 1993; **41**:1187–92.

Kost R & Straus S. Postherpetic neuralgia – pathogenesis treatment and prevention. *The New England Journal of Medicine* 1996; **335**:32–42.

Manfredi R, Calza L, Cocchio D & Chiodo F. Antiretroviral treatment and advanced age: epidemiologic laboratory and clinical features in the elderly. *Journal of Acquired Immune Deficiency Syndromes* 2003; **33**:112–4.

Marrie TJ. Community-acquired pneumonia. *Clinical Infectious Diseases* 1994; **18**:501–15.

McKinsey D, Ratts T & Bisno A. Underlying cardiac lesions in adults with infective endocarditis. *American Journal of Medicine* 1987; **82**:681–8.

Miller L & Choi C. Meningitis in older patients: how to diagnose and treat a deadly infection. *Geriatrics* 1997; **52**(8):43–55.

Mylotte JM, Tayara A & Goodnough S. Epidemiology of bloodstream infection in nursing home residents: evaluation in a large cohort from multiple homes. *Clinical Infectious Diseases* 2002; **35**:1484–90.

Nichol KL, Margolis KL, Wuorenma J & Von Sternberg T. The efficacy and cost effectiveness of vaccination against influenza among elderly persons living in the community. *The New England Journal of Medicine* 1994; **331**:778–84.

Nichol KL, Nordin J, Mullooly J *et al.* Influenza vaccination and reduction in hospitalizations for cardiac disease and stroke among the elderly. *The New England Journal of Medicine* 2003; **348**:1322–32.

Nicolle LE. Asymptomatic bacteriuria in the elderly. *Infectious Disease Clinics of North America* 1997; **11**(3):647–62.

Nicolle LE. Infection control in long-term care facilities. *Clinical Infectious Diseases* 2000; **31**:752–6.

Nicolle LE, Bentley DW, Garibaldi RA *et al.* Antimicrobial use in long-term-care facilities. *Infection Control and Hospital Epidemiology* 2000; **21**:537–45.

Niederman MS. Nosocomial pneumonia in the elderly patient chronic care facility and hospital considerations. *Clinics in Chest Medicine* 1993; **14**:479–90.

Norman DC. Fever in the elderly. *Clinical Infectious Diseases* 2000; **31**:141–51.

Peiris JSM, Yuen KY, Osterhaus AD & Stohr K. The severe acute respiratory syndrome. *The New England Journal of Medicine* 2003; **349**:2431–41.

Richardson J. Bacteremia in the elderly. *Journal of General Internal Medicine* 1993; **8**(2):89–92.

Richardson J & Knight A. The prevention of tetanus in the elderly. *Archives of Internal Medicine* 1991; **151**:1712–7.

Ruben FL, Dearwater SR, Norden CW *et al.* Clinical infections in the non-institutionalized geriatric age group: methods utilized and incidence of infections. The Pittsburgh good health study. *American Journal of Epidemiology* 1995; **141**:145–57.

Scheckler WE & Peterson PJ. Infections and control among residents of eight rural Wisconsin nursing homes. *Archives of Internal Medicine* 1986; **146**:1981–4.

Schuchat A, Robinson K, Wenger J *et al.* Bacterial meningitis in the United States in 1995. *The New England Journal of Medicine* 1997; **337**(13):970–6.

Selton-Suty C, Hoen B, Grentzinger A *et al.* Clinical and bacteriological characteristics of infective endocarditis in the elderly. *Heart* 1997; **77**:260–3.

Setia U, Serventi I & Lorenz P. Bacteremia in a long-term care facility. *Archives of Internal Medicine* 1984; **144**:1633–5.

Shapiro ED, Berg AT & Austrian R. Protective efficacy of polyvalent pneumococcal polysaccharide vaccine. *The New England Journal of Medicine* 1991; **325**:1453–60.

Slotwiner-Nie PK & Brandt LJ. Infectious diarrhea in the elderly. *Gastroenterology Clinics of North America* 2001; **30**:625–35.

Smith PW, Daly PB & Roccaforte JS. Current status of nosocomial infection control in extended care facilities. *American Journal of Medicine* 1991; **91**:3B-281S–5S.

Straus S, Ostrove J, Inchauspe G *et al.* Varicella-zoster virus infections. *Annals of Internal Medicine* 1988; **108**:221–37.

Terpenning M, Buggy B & Kauffman C. Infective endocarditis: clinical features in young and elderly patients. *American Journal of Medicine* 1987; **83**:626–34.

Thompson WW, Shay DK, Weintraub E *et al.* Mortality associated with influenza and respiratory syncytial virus in the United States. *Journal of the American Medical Association* 2003; **289**(2):179–86.

Torling J, Hedlund J, Konradsen HB & Ortqvist A. Revaccination with the 23-valent polysaccharide vaccine in middle aged and elderly persons previously treated for pneumonia. *Vaccine* 2004; **22**:96–103.

Verghese A & Berk S. Introduction and epidemiologic considerations. In A Verghese & A Berk (eds) *Infections in Nursing Homes and Long-Term Care Facilities* 1990, 1st edn, pp 1–11; S Karger, Basel.

Warren JW, Tenney JH, Hoopes JM *et al.* A prospective microbiologic study of bacteriuria in patients with chronic indwelling urethral catheters. *Journal of Infectious Diseases* 1982; **146**:719–23.

Wells AU, Fowler CC, Pegler-Ellis RB *et al.* Endocarditis in the 80's in a general hospital in Auckland [New Zealand]. *Quarterly Journal of Medicine* 1990; **76**:753–62.

Woodhead M. Pneumonia in the elderly. *The Journal of Antimicrobial Chemotherapy* 1994; **34**:85–92.

Yoshikawa T. Infectious diseases immunity and aging. In D Powers & J Morley (eds) *Aging Immunity and Infection* 1994, 1st edn, pp 1–11; Springer Publishing Company, New York.

Zambon MC, Stockton JD, Clewley JP & Fleming DM. Contribution of influenza and respiratory syncytial virus to community cases of influenza-like illness: an observational study. *Lancet* 2001; **358**:1410–6.

Zevallos M & Justman JE. Tuberculosis in the elderly. *Clinics in Geriatric Medicine* 2003; **19**:121–38.

146

Tuberculosis

Shobita Rajagopalan *and* Thomas T. Yoshikawa
Charles R. Drew University of Medicine and Science, Los Angeles, CA, USA

INTRODUCTION

In the year 2004, tuberculosis (TB) remained one of the leading infectious causes of illness and death worldwide. Estimates of morbidity and mortality from TB vary widely, but reliable sources report approximately two billion people currently infected with quiescent but viable tubercle bacilli, with two to three million deaths occurring from TB each year.

In the United States, during the past two decades, the excess in morbidity reflected a changing epidemiologic pattern. Human immune deficiency virus (HIV) infection, poverty, homelessness, substance abuse, and immigration from countries with a high prevalence of TB all contributed to TB morbidity. Overburdened public health TB services were not only unable to manage the resurgence in the 1980s but were also unprepared to cope with emerging multidrug resistance. Since the mid-1990s to the present, aggressive TB control, implementation, and enhanced resources have resulted in a substantial decline in the overall incidence of TB.

The geriatric population across all racial and ethnic groups and both genders are at substantial risk for *Mycobacterium tuberculosis* (*Mtb*) infection, perhaps because of both biological (compromised nutrition and immune status, underlying disease, medications, and possible racial predisposition) and socioeconomic factors (poverty, living conditions, and access to health-care). Most vulnerable are frail elderly residents of nursing homes and other long-term care facilities. Because of the highly communicable potential of *Mtb*, the inevitable endemic transmission between residents and from resident to staff has been demonstrated in such facilities. (For the purpose of clarity, TB infection, or latent TB, refers to contained and asymptomatic primary infection with a positive tuberculin skin test reaction, whereas TB disease indicates overt clinical manifestations of TB).

The Institute of Medicine report, *Ending Neglect: The Elimination of TB in the US,* which was undertaken through sponsorship from the Centers for Disease Control and Prevention (CDC), reviews the lessons learned from the neglect of TB between the late 1960s and the early 1990s and reaffirms commitment to a more realistic goal of elimination of TB in the United States (Institute of Medicine, 2000).

This chapter will review the epidemiology, pathogenesis and immunologic aspects, subtle clinical characteristics, diagnosis, management and prevention of *Mtb* infection in community-dwelling and institutionalized aging adults, as well as highlight the updated revised guidelines for targeted tuberculin skin testing and treatment of latent TB infection (LTBI).

EPIDEMIOLOGY

Developed nations including the United States and parts of Southeast Asia report an estimated 380 million persons infected with *Mtb*; about 80% of infected persons in Europe are 50 years of age or older (Rajagopalan, 2001). Population-based surveys of both TB infection and TB disease reveal that the overwhelming burden of disease and the highest annual risk for infection are borne by those living in developing countries.

In the United States, TB prevails among the foreign-born and minorities. From 1985 to 1992, TB incidence increased among all ethnic groups except non-Hispanic whites and Native Americans/Alaskan Natives. Among the different ethnic groups, Hispanics experienced the greatest increase in reported cases (74%) (Centers for Disease Control and Prevention, 1993). From 1992 to 2000, the overall incidence of TB in the United States declined by 45%, largely because of improved funding resources channeled into TB control programs, which allowed for the implementation of directly observed therapy (DOT). In 2000, the TB incidence ratio was 5.8 cases/100 000 population, the lowest ever recorded in this country (Centers for Disease Control and Prevention, 2002a). However, the percentage of cases among foreign-born persons increased from 27% in 1992 to 46% in 2000 (Centers for Disease Control and Prevention, 2002b).

Principles and Practice of Geriatric Medicine, 4th Edition. Edited by M.S. John Pathy, Alan J. Sinclair and John E. Morley.

TB also occurs with disproportionate frequency among the elderly (Reichman and O'Day, 1978; Narain *et al.*, 1985). Elders living in communal settings such as nursing homes or other long-term care facilities have a TB incidence rate approximately four times greater than the general population (Schultz *et al.*, 2001). The aggregate TB incidence rate for nursing home residents is 1.8 times higher than the rate seen in community-dwelling elderly (Hutton *et al.*, 1993). The enhanced efficiency of TB transmissibility within congregate settings such as prisons, nursing facilities (nursing homes), chronic disease facilities, and homeless shelters has raised concerns about TB infection and disease in the institutionalized elderly (Ijaz *et al.*, 2002; Rajagopalan and Yoshikawa, 2000). Positive tuberculin reactivity associated with prolonged stay among residents of long-term care facilities for the elderly has been demonstrated, implying an increasing risk of TB infection.

PATHOGENESIS AND IMMUNOLOGIC ASPECTS

The pathogenesis of TB infection and disease begins in most cases with the inhalation of the tubercle bacilli (Adler and Rose, 1996). The usual inoculum is no more than one to three organisms, which are taken up by alveolar macrophages and carried to regional lymph nodes. Spread may occur via the lymphohematogenous route with dissemination to multiple organs. From two to eight weeks after infection, cell-mediated immunity (CMI) and delayed-type hypersensitivity (DTH) responses develop, leading to the characteristic reactive tuberculin test and to the containment of infection. Chemoattractants cause monocytes to enter the area and become transformed into histiocytes forming granulomas. Although the bacilli may persist within macrophages, additional multiplication and spread is curtailed. Healing usually follows with calcification of the infected focus. Caseous necrosis may result secondary to the immune response. Erosion into a bronchiole causes cavity formation where bacilli can multiply and spread. Solid necrosis can result from production of hydrolases from inflammatory cells causing tissue liquefaction and creating a prime medium for microbial replication, generating up to 10 billion bacilli/ml.

Individuals who develop active disease either fail to contain the primary infection or develop reactivation as a result of relative or absolute immune suppression at a point remote from primary infection. This is most likely to occur in immunocompetent adults within the first 3 years after exposure. Factors related to progression of disease reflect a weakened immune status and include physiological states, for example, normal aging; associated intercurrent disease – particularly diabetes mellitus, malignancies causing primary immunosuppression or requiring toxic chemotherapy, or corticosteroid-dependant diseases such as asthma or collagen vascular disease; poor nutritional status particularly related to alcohol and drug abuse; smoking and HIV infection.

Although, it is likely that the increased frequency of TB in the elderly could partly be due to CMI that is impaired by senescence (shown in murine models), other concomitant age-related diseases (diabetes mellitus, malignancy), chronic kidney disease and renal insufficiency, poor nutrition, and immunosuppressive drugs may also contribute to this increase (Yoshikawa, 1992). In the elderly, approximately 90% of TB disease cases are due to reactivation of primary infection. Persistent infection without disease may occur in 30 to 50% of individuals. Some elderly persons previously infected with *Mtb* may eventually eliminate the viable tubercle bacilli and revert to a negative tuberculin reactor state. These individuals are thus at risk of new infection (reinfection) with *Mtb*. There are therefore three subgroups of older persons potentially at risk for TB: One subgroup never exposed to TB that may develop primary TB disease, a second subgroup with persistent and latent primary infection that may reactivate, and a third subgroup that is no longer infected and consequently at risk for reinfection.

SUBTLE CLINICAL CHARACTERISTICS

Clinicians must be aware that frail older persons with TB disease may not demonstrate the overt and characteristic clinical features of TB such as fever, night sweats, or hemoptysis. They may exhibit more subtle clinical manifestations of "failure to thrive" with anorexia, functional decline and low-grade fever, or weight loss (Perez-Guzman *et al.*, 1999). Although, several published works have attempted to delineate clear-cut differences between younger and older TB patients, such studies have provided quite variable findings. In a meta-analysis of published studies, comparing pulmonary TB in older and younger patients, evaluating the differences in the clinical, radiologic, and laboratory features of pulmonary TB, no differences were found in the prevalence of cough, sputum production, weight loss, fatigue/malaise, radiographic upper lobes lesions, positive acid-fast bacilli (AFB) in sputum, anemia or hemoglobin level, and serum aminotransferases (Perez-Guzman *et al.*, 1999). A lower prevalence of fever, sweating, hemoptysis, cavitary disease, and positive purified protein derivative (PPD), as well as lower levels of serum albumin and blood leukocytes were noticed among older patients. In addition, the older population had a greater prevalence of dyspnea and some underlying comorbid conditions, such as cardiovascular disorders, chronic obstructive pulmonary disease, diabetes mellitus, gastrectomy history, and malignancies. This meta-analytical review identified some subtle differences in clinical presentations of older TB patients, when compared with their younger TB counterparts. However, most of these differences can be explained by the already known physiologic changes that occur during aging.

The majority of older TB patients (75%) with *Mtb* disease manifest active disease in their lungs (Yoshikawa, 1992). Extrapulmonary TB in the elderly is similar to younger persons and may involve the meninges, bone and joint, and genitourinary systems, or disseminate in a miliary pattern (Mert *et al.*, 2001; Kalita and Misra, 2004; Shah *et al.*, 2001; Malaviya, 2003; Lenk and Schroeder, 2001). Infection of lymph nodes, pleura, pericardium, peritoneum, gall bladder, small and large bowel, the middle ear, and carpal tunnel have been described in the literature. Because TB can involve virtually any organ in the body, this infection must be kept in the differential diagnosis of unusual presentations of diseases, especially in the elderly. Thus, TB has been aptly described as "the great masquerader".

DIAGNOSIS

Clinicians caring for the elderly must maintain a high index of suspicion for TB when possible, in order to promptly recognize and treat infected individuals.

Tuberculin Skin Testing

The Mantoux method of tuberculin skin testing using the Tween-stabilized PPD antigen is one of the diagnostic modalities readily available to screen for TB infection, despite its potential for false-negative results (Markowitz *et al.*, 1993). In the elderly, because of the increase in anergy to cutaneous antigens, the two-step tuberculin test is suggested as part of the initial geriatric assessment to avoid overlooking potentially false-negative reactions (Tort *et al.*, 1995). The American Geriatrics Society routinely recommends two-step tuberculin testing as part of the baseline information for all institutionalized elderly (American Geriatrics Society, 1993). The two-step tuberculin skin test involves initial intradermal placement of five tuberculin units of PPD, and the results are read at 48 to 72 hours. Patients are retested within two weeks after a negative response (induration of less than 10 mm). A positive "booster effect", and therefore a positive tuberculin skin test reaction, is a skin test of 10 mm or more and an increase of 6 mm or more over the first skin test reaction. It is important to distinguish the booster phenomenon from a true tuberculin conversion. The booster effect occurs in a person previously infected with *Mtb* but who has a false-negative skin test; repeat skin test elicits a truly positive test. Conversion (not to be confused with the booster phenomenon) occurs in persons previously uninfected with *Mtb* and who have had a true negative tuberculin skin test, but who become infected within 2 years as demonstrated by a repeat skin test induration that is a positive 10 mm or more during this period. Several factors influence the results and interpretation of the PPD skin test. Decreased skin test reactivity is associated with waning DTH with time, disseminated TB, corticosteroids and other drugs, and other diseases as well as the elimination of TB infection. False-positive PPD results occur with cross-reactions with nontuberculous mycobacteria and in persons receiving the Bacillus Calmette-Guerin (BCG) vaccine, the latter having been administered to some foreign-born elderly persons, which has an unpredictable effect on the PPD skin test reactivity and is presumed to wane after 10 years. The use of anergy testing has been debated because of lack of a standardized protocol for selection of the number and type of antigens to be used, the criteria for defining positive and negative reactions, and administration and interpretation techniques (Slovis *et al.*, 2000).

QuantiFERON-TB (QFT) Testing

In 2001, the QuantiFERON-TB (QFT) test was approved by the US Food and Drug Administration (FDA) to aid in the detection of LTBI. This *in vitro* test measures by an enzyme-linked immunosorbent assay (ELISA), the concentration of interferon-gamma (IFN-γ) released from tuberculin PPD-sensitized lymphocytes in heparinized whole blood incubated for 16 to 24 hours. Interpretation of QFT results is stratified by estimated risk for *Mtb* infection in a manner similar to the tuberculin skin test using different induration cut-off values as shown in Tables 1(A) and (B) (Centers for Disease Control and Prevention, 2003a). The role for QFT in targeted testing has not yet been clearly defined and may be a useful alternative to tuberculin skin testing in the future for all infected individuals including the elderly.

Chest Radiography

Chest radiography is indicated in all individuals with suspected TB infection, regardless of the primary site of infection. In the elderly, 75% of all TB disease occurs in the respiratory tract and largely represents reactivation disease; 10 to 20% of cases may be as a result of primary infection (Woodring *et al.*, 1986). Although reactivation TB disease characteristically involves the apical and posterior segments of the upper lobes of the lungs, several studies have shown that many elderly patients manifest their pulmonary infection in either the middle or lower lobes or the pleura, as well as present with interstitial, patchy, or cavitary infiltrates that may be bilateral. Primary TB can involve any lung segment, but more often tends to involve the middle or lower lobes as well as mediastinal or hilar lymph nodes. Thus, caution must be exercised in dismissing the radiographic diagnosis of pulmonary TB in the elderly because of the atypical location of the infection in the lung fields.

Laboratory Diagnosis

Sputum samples must be collected from all patients, regardless of age, with pulmonary symptoms or chest radiographic changes compatible with TB disease and who have not been previously treated with antituberculous agents. In elderly patients unable to expectorate sputum, other diagnostic techniques such as sputum induction or bronchoscopy should be considered. Flexible bronchoscopy to obtain bronchial washings and to perform bronchial biopsies has been shown to be of diagnostic value for TB disease in the elderly; however, in the frail and very old patient, the risk of such a procedure must be carefully balanced against the

Table 1A Interim recommendations for applying and interpreting QuantiFERON-TB (Centers for Disease Control and Prevention. Guidelines for using the QuantiFERON-TB test for diagnosing latent *Mycobacterium tuberculosis* infection. *Morbidity and Mortality Weekly Report* 2003a; **52** (RR02): 15–8)

Reason for testing	Population	Initial screening	Positive results	Evaluation
Tuberculosis (TB suspect)	Persons with symptoms of active TB	Tuberculin skin testing (TST) might be useful; QFT not recommended	Induration ≥5 mm	Chest radiograph, smears, and cultures, regardless of test results
Increased risk for progression to active TB, if infected	Persons with recent contact with TB, changes on chest radiograph consistent with prior TB, organ transplants, or human-immunodeficiency virus infection, and those receiving immunosuppressing drugs equivalent of ≥15 mg day^{-1} of prednisone for ≥1 month[a]	TST; QFT not recommended	Induration ≥5 mm	Chest radiograph if TST is positive; treat for LTBI after active TB disease is ruled out
	Persons with diabetes, silicosis, chronic renal failure, leukemia, lymphoma, carcinoma of the head, neck, or lung, and persons with weight loss of ≥10% of ideal body weight, gastrectomy, or jejunoileal bypass[a]	TST; QFT not recommended	Induration ≥10 mm	
Increased risk for LTBI	Recent immigrants, injection-drug users, and residents, and employees of high-risk congregate settings (e.g. prisons, jails, homeless shelters, and certain health-care facilities)[b]	TST or QFT	Induration ≥10 mm; percentage tuberculin response ≥15 %	Chest radiograph if either test is positive; confirmatory TST is optional if QFT is positive; treat for LTBI after active TB disease is ruled out; LTBI treatment when only QFT is positive should be based on clinical judgment and estimated risk
Other reasons for testing among persons at low risk for LTBI	Military personnel, hospital staff, and health-care workers whose risk of prior exposure to TB patients is low, and US-born students at certain colleges and universities	TST or QFT	Induration >15 mm; percentage tuberculin response ≥30 %	Chest radiograph if either test is positive; confirmatory TST if QFT is positive; treatment for LTBI (if QFT and TST are positive and after active TB disease is ruled out) on the basis of assessment of risk for drug toxicity, TB transmission, and patient preference

[a]QFT has not been adequately evaluated among persons with these conditions; it is not recommended for such populations.

Table 1B QuantiFERON-TB testing: results and interpretation (Centers for Disease Control and Prevention. Guidelines for using the QuantiFERON-TB test for diagnosing latent *Mycobacterium tuberculosis* infection. *Morbidity and Mortality Weekly Report* 2003a; **52** (RR02): 15–8)

M–N[a] (IUmL)	T–N[b] (IUmL)	Avian difference (%)	Tuberculin response (%)[c]	Report and interpretation	Interpretation
≤1.5	All other response profiles	All other response profiles	All other response profiles	Interferon-gamma (INY-γ) response to mitogen is inadequate	Indeterminate
≥1.5	All other response profiles	All other response profiles	≤15	Percentage tuberculin response is <15 or not significant	Negative: *M. tuberculosis* infection unlikely
≥1.5	≥1.5	≤10	≥15 but <30	Percentage tuberculin response is 15–30	Conditionally positive: *M. tuberculosis* infection likely if risk is identified, but unlikely for persons who are at low risk
≥1.5	≥1.5	≤10	≥30	Percentage tuberculin response is ≥30	Positive: *M. tuberculosis* infection likely

[a]M–N is the IFN-γ responses to mitogen minus the IFN-γ responses to nil antigen. [b]T–N is the IFN-γ responses to purified protein derivative from *M. tuberculosis* infection. If T–N is <1.5 IUmL, the persons are deemed negative for *M. tuberculosis* infection, regardless of their percentage tuberculin response and percentage avian difference results. [c]A percentage tuberculin response cutoff of 15% is used for persons with identified risk for tuberculosis infection, whereas a cutoff of 30% is used for persons with no identified risk factors.

benefits of potentially making a definite diagnosis of TB (Patel *et al.*, 1993). In the case of pulmonary and genitourinary TB, three consecutive early morning sputum or urine specimens, respectively, are recommended for routine mycobacteriologic studies (Hanna, 1996; American Thoracic Society, 2000a). Sputum samples are examined initially by smear before and after concentration and then cultured for *Mtb*. Because routine mycobacterial culture methods may require up to 6 weeks for growth of *Mtb*, many laboratories now use radiometric procedures for the isolation and susceptibility testing of this organism; this method may identify the organisms as early as after 8 days. Sterile body fluids and tissues can be inoculated into liquid media, which also allow the growth and detection of *Mtb* 7 to 10 days earlier than in the solid media techniques. Histological examination of tissue from various sites such as the liver, lymph nodes, bone marrow, pleura, or synovium may show the characteristic tissue reaction (caseous necrosis with granuloma formation) with or without AFB, which would also strongly support the diagnosis of TB disease. Other diagnostic methods for TB that have been clinically evaluated include serology and nucleic acid amplification (NAA) tests such as polymerase chain reaction (PCR) and other methods for amplifying DNA and RNA (Centers for Disease Control and Prevention, 2000). The latter may facilitate rapid detection of *Mtb* from respiratory specimens; the interpretation and use of the NAA test results has been updated by the CDC. Similar techniques using DNA probes can be used to track the spread of the organism in epidemiologic studies and may be used to predict drug resistance prior to the availability of standard results; such methods are currently being used in some laboratories. The rapid diagnosis of TB is especially important in elderly patients, as well as HIV-infected persons, and patients with multidrug-resistant (MDR)-TB.

TREATMENT

Treatment of TB Disease

The recommended treatment regimens are for the most part based on evidence from clinical trials and are rated on the basis of a system developed by the United States Public Health Service (USPHS) and the Infectious Diseases Society of America (IDSA). There are four recommended regimens for treating patients with TB caused by drug-susceptible organisms. Although these regimens are broadly applicable, there are modifications that should be made under specified circumstances, which are described subsequently. Each regimen has an initial phase of 2 months followed by a choice of several options for the continuation phase of either 4 or 7 months. The recommended treatment algorithm and regimens are shown in Figure 1 and Table 2 (Centers for Disease Control and Prevention, 2003b).

Because of the relatively high proportion of adult patients with TB caused by organisms that are resistant to isoniazid (INH), four drugs are necessary in the initial phase for the 6-month regimen to be maximally effective. Thus, in most circumstances, the treatment regimen for all adults including the elderly with previously untreated TB should consist of a 2-month initial phase of INH, rifampin (RIF), pyrazinamide (PZA), and Ethambutol (EMB). If (when) drug susceptibility test results are known and the organisms are fully susceptible, EMB need not be included. If PZA cannot be included in the initial phase of treatment, or if the isolate is resistant to PZA alone (an unusual circumstance), the initial phase should consist of INH, RIF, and EMB given daily for 2 months. However, since most TB in the elderly is due to reactivation (from infection acquired prior to 1950), the organism will generally be sensitive to INH and other antituberculous drugs.

Treatment of MDR-TB is complex and often needs to be individualized, requiring the addition of a minimum of two additional antituberculous agents to which the organism is presumably susceptible, preferably in consultation with a TB expert who is familiar with *Mtb* drug resistance. Alternate drugs such as capreomycin, kanamycin, amikacin, ethionamide, and cycloserine, as well as the newer quinolones, may have to be used for treatment in such cases.

Monitoring of Response to Drug Therapy

Patients with active pulmonary TB should be monitored on a monthly basis with sputum examination until conversion to negative by culture is achieved; this usually occurs within 3 months in 90% of cases. Continued positive sputum cultures for *Mtb* beyond three months of initiation of therapy should raise the suspicion for drug resistance or noncompliance (if not on DOT); such patients should have sputum culture and susceptibility repeated and started on DOT pending results of these data. Follow-up chest radiography is indicated 2 to 3 months after initiation of drug therapy. Older patients are at greater risk for hepatic toxicity from INH. Although INH therapy poses a small but significant risk for hepatitis, the hepatitis is relatively low in frequency and mild in severity. It would appear, therefore, that with careful monitoring of the older patient, antituberculous chemotherapy is a relatively safe intervention in this population. It is recommended that clinical assessments as well as baseline liver function tests be performed before the administration of INH and RIF (and PZA) in older patients.

Monthly clinical evaluations and periodic measurements of the serum aminotransferase (SGOT) level should be performed in the elderly. If the SGOT rises to 5 times above normal or if the patient exhibits symptoms or signs of hepatitis, INH (as well as other hepatotoxic drugs) should be discontinued. After clinical symptoms improve or the SGOT level normalizes, or both, INH may be resumed at a lower dose (e.g. 50 mg kg^{-1} day^{-1}) and gradually increased to a full dose if symptoms and the SGOT level remain stable. In case of relapse of the hepatitis with the INH challenge, the drug should be replaced with an alternative regimen. There is some disagreement among clinicians regarding the monitoring of liver function tests in older patients on INH. Because frail, elderly patients may often be asymptomatic in the presence of worsening hepatitis and may not be able to communicate symptoms, laboratory monitoring seems prudent. The frequency of such monitoring (e.g. monthly or every 2 to 3 months) remains less clear. RIF, in addition to hepatitis, is also associated with orange discoloration of body fluids. EMB may cause loss of color discrimination, diminished visual acuity, and central scotomata; older patients receiving this drug should have frequent evaluation of visual acuity and color discrimination. Streptomycin is associated with irreversible auditory and vestibular damage and generally should

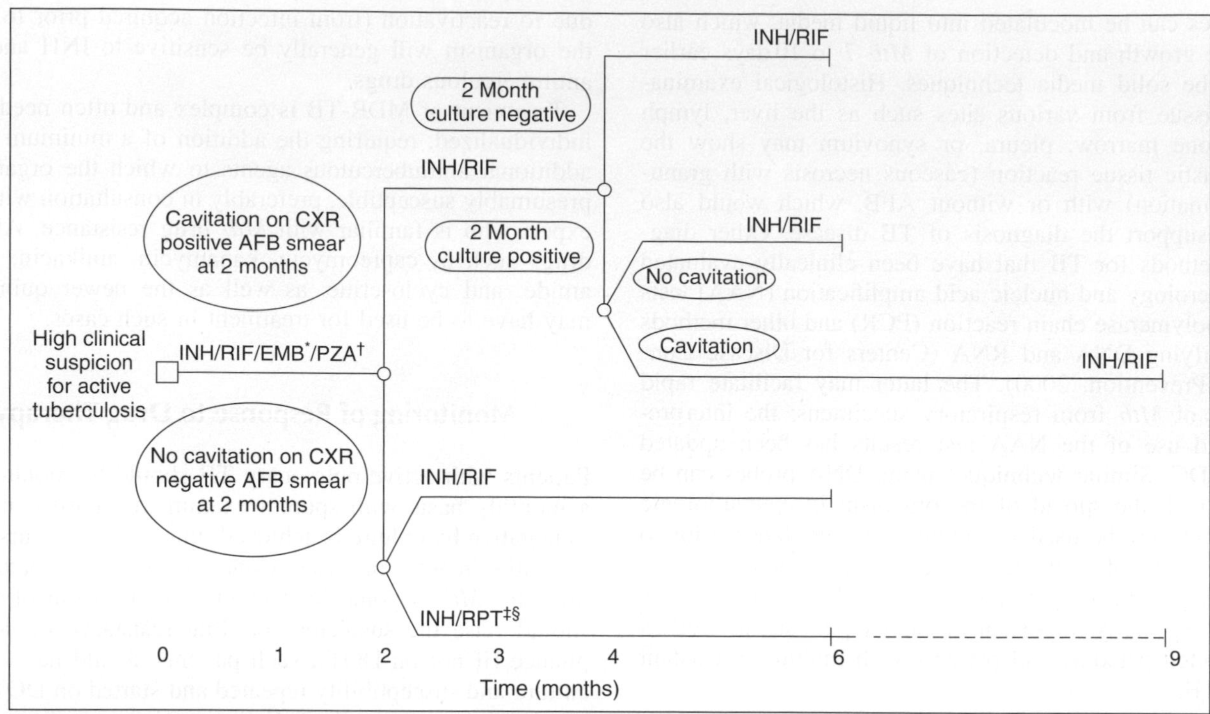

Patients in whom tuberculosis is proved or strongly suspected should have treatment initiated with isoniazid, rifampin, pyrazinamide, and ethambutol for the initial 2 months. A repeat smear and culture should be performed when 2 months of treatment has been completed. If cavities were seen on the initial chest radiograph or the acid-fast smear is positive at completion of 2 months of treatment, the continuation phase of treatment should consist of isoniazid and rifampin daily or twice weekly for 4 months to complete a total of 6 months of treatment. If cavitation was present on the initial chest radiograph and the culture at the time of completion of 2 months of therapy is positive, the continuation phase should be lengthened to 7 months (total of 9 months of treatment). If the patient has HIV infection and the $CD4^+$ cell count is <100/ml, the continuation phase should consist of daily or three times weekly isoniazid and rifampin. In HIV-uninfected patients having no cavitation on chest radiograph and negative acid-fast smears at completion of 2 months of treatment, the continuation phase may consist of either once weekly isoniazid and rifapentine, or daily or twice weekly isoniazid and rifampin,to complete a total of 6 months (bottom). Patients receiving isoniazid and rifapentine,and whose 2-month cultures are positive, should have treatment extended by an additional 3 months (total of 9 months).

[*] EMB may be discontinued when results of drug susceptibility testing indicate no drug resistance.
[†] PZA may be discontinued after it has been taken for 2 months (56 doses).
[‡] RPT should not be used in HIV-infected patients with tuberculosis or in patients with extrapulmonary tuberculosis.
[§] Therapy should be extended to 9 months if 2-month culture is positive.
CXR = chest radiograph; EMB = ethambutol; INH = isoniazid; PZA = pyrazinamide; RIF = rifampin; RPT = rifapentine.

Figure 1 Treatment algorithm for tuberculosis (Centers for Disease Control, American Thoracic Society & Infectious Disease Society of America, 2003b)

not be prescribed in the elderly. Adverse effects of PZA include hyperuricemia, hepatitis, and flushing. Dose adjustment of antituberculous drugs is necessary with streptomycin, when used in the presence of renal impairment; however, no adjustment is needed for INH, RIF, or PZA in most elderly patients.

Treatment of Latent TB Infection

Table 3 outlines the revised criteria for positive tuberculin skin test reactivity by size of induration requiring drug treatment (American Thoracic Society, 2000b). Drug therapy for latent TB (based on tuberculin skin test reactivity) considerably decreases the risk of progression of TB infection to TB disease. The recently revised recommended drug treatment of LTBI in adults including the elderly, is shown in Table 4 (Centers for Disease Control and Prevention, 2001). Since the LTBI treatment recommendations address adults in general, targeted skin testing and treatment of high-risk populations can be applied to the elderly. The INH daily regimen for 9 months has recently replaced the previously recommended 6-month schedule for treatment of LTBI. Randomized, prospective trials in HIV-negative persons have indicated that a 12-month regimen is more effective than 6 months of treatment; subgroup analyses of several trials indicate that the maximal beneficial effect of INH is likely to be achieved in 9 months, with minimal additional benefit gained by extending therapy to 12 months. Although the 9-month regimen of INH is preferred for the treatment of LTBI, the 6-month LTBI treatment course also provides substantial protection and has been shown to be superior to

Table 2 Drug treatment regimens of tuberculosis (Centers for Disease Control and Prevention. American Thoracic Society & Infectious Disease Society of America. CDC-ATS-IDSA Treatment of Tuberculosis. *Morbidity and Mortality Weekly Report* 2003b; **52** (RR11): 1–77)

Initial phase			Continuation phase				
Regimen	Drugs	Intervals and doses[c] (minimal duration)	Regimen	Drugs	Interval and doses[c,d] (minimal duration)	Range of total doses (minimal duration)	Rating[a] (evidence) [b] HIV – HIV[b]
1	INH RIF PZA EMB	Seven days per week for 56 doses (8 weeks) or days/week for 40 doses (8 weeks)	1a	INH/RIF	Seven days per week for 126 doses (18 weeks) or 5 days/week for 90 doses (18 weeks)[e]	182–130 (26 weeks)	A(I) A(II)
			1b	INH/RIF	Twice weekly for 36 doses (18 weeks)	92–76 (26 weeks)	A(I) A(II)[f]
			1c[g]	INH/RPT	Once weekly for 18 doses (18 weeks)	44–58 (26 weeks)	B(I) E(I)
2	INH RIF PZA EMB	Seven days per week for 14 doses (2 weeks), then twice weekly for 12 doses (6 weeks) or 5 days/week for 10 doses (2 weeks) then twice weekly for 12 doses (6 weeks)	2a	INH/RIF	Twice weekly for 36 doses (18 weeks)	62–58 (26 weeks)	A(II) B(II)[f]
			2b[g]	INH/RPT	Once weekly for 18 doses (18 weeks)	44–40 (26 weeks)	B(I) E(I)
3	INH RIF PZA EMB	Three times weekly for 24 doses (8 weeks)	3a	INH/RIF	Three times weekly for 54 doses (18 weeks)	78 (26 weeks)	B(I) B(I)
4	INH RIF EMB	Seven days per week for 56 doses (8 weeks) or 5 days/week for 40 doses (8 weeks)	4a	INH/RIF	Seven days per week for 217 doses (31 weeks) or 5 days/week for 155 doses (31 week)[e]	273–195 (39 weeks)	C(I) C(I)
			4b	INH/RIF	Twice weekly for 62 doses (31 weeks)	118–102 (39 weeks)	C(I) C(II)

Definition of abbreviations: EMB, Ethambutol; INH, isoniazid; PZA, pyrazinamide; RIF, rifampin; RPT, rifapentine.
[a]Definitions of evidence ratings: A, preferred; B, acceptable alternative; C, when A and B cannot be given; E, should never be given. [b]Definitions of evidence ratings: I, randomized clinical trial; II, data from clinical trials that were not randomized or were conducted in other populations; III, expert opinion. [c]When DOT is used, drugs may be given 5 days/week and the necessary number of doses adjusted accordingly. Although there are no studies comparing five with seven daily doses, extensive experience indicates this would be an effective practice. [d]Patients with cavitation on initial chest radiograph and positive cultures at completion of 2 months of therapy should receive a 7-month (31 weeks); either 217 doses [daily] or 62 doses [twice weekly] continuation phase. [e]Five-day-a-week administration is always given by DOT. Rating for 5 day/week regimens is AIII. [f]Not recommended for HIV-infected patients with CD4 cell counts <100 cells/μl. [g]Options 1c and 2b should be used only in HIV-negative patients who have negative sputum smears at the time of completion of 2 months of therapy and who do not have cavitation on initial chest radiograph (see text). For patients started on this regimen and found to have a positive culture from the 2-month specimen, treatment should be extended an extra 3 months.

Table 3 Skin test criteria for positive tuberculin reaction (mm induration) (American Thoracic Society. Diagnostic standards and classification of tuberculosis in adults and children. *American Journal of Respiratory and Critical Care Medicine* 2000a; **161:** 1376–95)

≥5 mm

1. HIV[a] positive persons
2. Recent contacts of person(s) with infectious tuberculosis
3. Persons with chest radiographs consistent with tuberculosis (e.g. fibrotic changes)
4. Patients with organ transplants and other immunosuppressed hosts receiving the equivalent of $>15\,\text{mg day}^{-1}$ prednisone for >1 month

≥10 mm

1. Recent arrivals (<5 years) from high-prevalence countries
2. Injection-drug users
3. Residents and employees of high-risk congregate settings: prisons, jails, nursing homes, other health-care facilities, residential facilities for AIDS[b] patients, and homeless shelters
4. Mycobacteriology laboratory personnel
5. High-risk clinical conditions: silicosis; gastrectomy; jejunoileal bypass; ≥10% below ideal body weight; chronic renal failure; diabetes mellitus; hematological malignancies (e.g. lymphomas, leukemias); other specific malignancies (carcinoma of the head or neck, and lung) (alcoholics are also considered high risk)

≥15 mm

1. Persons with no risk factors for TB

Chemoprophylaxis recommended for all high-risk persons, regardless of age. Persons otherwise low-risk tested at entry into employment, ≥15 mm induration is positive.
[a]HIV, Human-Immunodeficiency Virus; [b]AIDS, Acquired Immunodeficiency Syndrome.

Table 4 Revised drug regimens for treatment of latent tuberculosis infection in adults (including the elderly) (American Thoracic Society. Targeted skin testing and treatment of latent tuberculosis infection. *American Journal of Respiratory and Critical Care Medicine*; **161:** S221–47 (Adapted from CDC. Targeted tuberculin testing and treatment of latent tuberculosis infection. 2000; **49**(RR06). Interactions with human-immunodeficiency virus (HIV) – related drugs are updated frequently and are available at http/www.aidsinfr.nih.gov/guidelines). (Centers for Disease Control and Prevention. Update: fatal and severe liver injuries associated with rifampin and pyrazinamide for latent tuberculosis infection, and revisions in American Thoracic Society/Centers for Disease Control and Prevention – recommendations–United States. *Morbidity and Mortality Weekly Report* 2001; August 31, 2001; **50** (34): 733–5)

Drug	Interval and duration	Comments	Ratings HIV-negative	(Evidence) HIV-infected
Isoniazid	Daily for 9 months	In HIV-infected persons, isoniazid may be administered concurrently with nucleoside reverse transcriptase inhibitors (NRTIs), protease inhibitors, or, nonnucleoside reverse transcriptase inhibitors (NNRTIs)	A (II)	A (II)
Isoniazid	Twice weekly for 9 months**	Directly observed therapy (DOT) must be used with twice-weekly dosing	B (II)	B (II)
	Daily for 6 months	Not indicated for HIV-infected persons, those with fibrotic lesions on chest radiographs, or children.	B (I)	C (I)
Rifampin	Twice weekly for 6 months	DOT must be used with twice-weekly dosing.	B (II)	C (I)
	Daily for 4 months	Used for persons who are contacts of patients with isoniazid-resistant, rifampin-susceptible TB In HIV-infected persons, most protease inhibitors or delavirdine should not be administered concurrently with rifampin. Rifabutin with appropriate dose adjustments can be used with protease inhibitors (saquinavir should be augmented with ritonavir) and NNRTIs (except delavirdine). Clinicians should consult web-based updates for the latest specific recommendations	B (II)	B (III)
Rifampin plus pyrazinamide (RZ)	Daily for 2 months	RZ generally should not be offered for treatment of LTBI for HIV-infected or HIV-negative persons	D (II)	D (II)
	Twice weekly for 2–3 months		D (III)	D (III)

Strength of the recommendation: A. Both strong evidence of efficacy and substantial clinical benefit support recommendation for use. Should always be offered; B. Moderate evidence for efficacy or strong evidence for efficacy, but only limited clinical benefit supports recommendation for use. Should generally be offered; C. Evidence for efficacy is insufficient to support a recommendation for or against use, or evidence for efficacy might not outweigh adverse consequences (e.g. drug toxicity, drug interactions) or cost of the treatment or alternative approaches. Optional; D. Moderate evidence for lack of efficacy or for adverse outcome supports a recommendation against use. Should generally not be offered; E. Good evidence for lack of efficacy or for adverse outcome support a recommendation against use. Should never be offered.
Quality of evidence supporting the recommendation: I. Evidence from at least one properly randomized controlled trial; II. Evidence from at least one well-designed clinical trial without randomization for cohort or case-controlled analytic studies (preferably from more than one center), from multiple time-series studies, or from dramatic results from uncontrolled experiments; III. Evidence from opinions of respected authorities based on clinical experience, descriptive studies, or reports of expert committees.
The substitution of rifapentine for rifampin not recommended as rifapentine's safety and effectiveness not established for LTBI.

placebo in both HIV-positive and -negative persons. Hence, clinical judgment must be exercised based on local conditions, health departments or providers' experience, cost, and compliance issues. In a community-based study conducted in Bethel, Alaska, persons who took <25% of the prescribed annual dose had a threefold higher risk for TB than those who took more than 50% of the annual dose. A more recent analysis of study data indicated that the efficacy decreased significantly if less than 9 months of INH was taken (Comstock, 1999). In instances of known exposure to drug-resistant organisms, alternative preventive therapy regimens may be recommended. In addition, because of recent reports in 2001 of fatal and severe hepatitis associated with the 2-month RIF and PZA (R-Z) treatment regimen for LTBI, this regimen must be used with caution, especially in patients concurrently taking other medications associated with liver injury and in those with mild liver compromise (Centers for Disease Control and Prevention, 2001). R-Z is not recommended for persons with known underlying liver disease or for those who have had INH-associated liver injury. Persons being considered for treatment with R-Z should be informed about the potential hepatotoxicity and screened for liver disease or adverse effects from INH. To reduce the risk of liver injury associated with R-Z therapy, the American Thoracic Society (ATS) and CDC, with the endorsement of the IDSA, have prepared recommendations that supercede previous guidelines (Centers for Disease Control and Prevention, 2001).

Although these new recommendations do not specifically address aging adults, the concept of targeted skin testing and revised LTBI treatment guidelines for high-risk populations to include the elderly can be applied. Elderly persons receiving isoniazid should continue to be monitored for hepatitis and peripheral neuropathy induced by the drug.

INFECTION CONTROL ISSUES

The primary goal of an infection control program is to detect TB disease early and to isolate and promptly treat persons with infectious TB. Prevention of transmission of TB in any health-care environment is of utmost importance, both for patients and health-care workers. Enhanced awareness of drug-resistant TB has prompted public health agencies to institute strict TB identification, isolation, treatment, and prevention guidelines. The TB infection control program in most acute care as well as long-term care facilities should consist of three types of control measures: administrative actions (i.e. prompt detection of suspected cases, isolation of infectious patients, and rapid institution of appropriate treatment), engineering control (negative-pressure ventilation rooms, high efficiency particulate air [HEPA] filtration, and ultraviolet germicidal irradiation [UVGI]), and personal respiratory protection requirements (masks). The Advisory Committee for the Elimination of Tuberculosis of the CDC has established recommendations for surveillance, containment, assessment, and reporting of TB infection and disease in long-term care facilities; health-care professionals, administrators, and staff of such extended care programs should be made aware of these recommendations (Centers for Disease Control and Prevention, 1990).

KEY POINTS

- Tuberculosis (TB) is a significant infectious disease in the elderly that causes increased morbidity and mortality.
- Age-related decrease in adaptive immune responses in addition to underlying comorbid illnesses (diabetes, cancer, immunosuppression) may enhance susceptibility to TB.
- Frail older persons may not exhibit the classical symptoms and signs of TB, that is, fever, night sweats, weight loss, cough, and hemoptysis. TB must be treated as the "great masquerader" and considered in the differential diagnosis of unexplained malaise, anorexia and low-grade fevers, and nonspecific clinical manifestations of illness.
- Screening for TB utilizing the two-step tuberculin skin testing is routinely recommended in the initial assessment of elderly patients admitted to long-term care facilities (the utility of the QFT as an alternative for latent TB diagnosis in this setting needs to be further evaluated). Increased efficiency of transmission of TB between elderly residents of such facilities has been reported.
- Diagnosis and management of TB in the geriatric population is similar to younger patients; close monitoring for adverse reactions to drug therapy is important, particularly in patients taking multiple medications.

KEY REFERENCES

- American Thoracic Society. Diagnostic standards and classification of tuberculosis in adults and children. *American Journal of Respiratory and Critical Care Medicine* 2000a; **161**:1376–95.
- American Thoracic Society. Targeted skin testing and treatment of latent tuberculosis infection. *American Journal of Respiratory and Critical Care Medicine* 2000b; **161**:S221–47.
- Centers for Disease Control and Prevention. Control of tuberculosis in facilities providing long-term care to the elderly: recommendations of the Advisory Committee for the Elimination of Tuberculosis. *Morbidity and Mortality Weekly Report* 1990; **39**(RR-10):7.
- Centers for Disease Control and Prevention. Guidelines for using the QuantiFERON-TB test for diagnosing latent *Mycobacterium tuberculosis* infection. *Morbidity and Mortality Weekly Report* 2003a; **52**(RR02):15–8.
- Centers for Disease Control and Prevention, American Thoracic Society & Infectious Disease Society of America. Treatment of tuberculosis. *Morbidity and Mortality Weekly Report* 2003b; **52**(RR11):1–77.

REFERENCES

Adler JJ & Rose DM. Transmission and pathogenesis of tuberculosis. In WN Rom & SM Garay (eds) *Tuberculosis* 1996, 1st edn; Little, Brown and Company, New York.

American Thoracic Society. Diagnostic standards and classification of tuberculosis in adults and children. *American Journal of Respiratory and Critical Care Medicine* 2000a; **161**:1376–95.

American Thoracic Society. Targeted skin testing and treatment of latent tuberculosis infection. *American Journal of Respiratory and Critical Care Medicine* 2000b; **161**:S221–47.

American Geriatrics Society. *Two-Step PPD Testing For Nursing Home Patients On Admission* 1993; info.amger@americangeriatrics.org.

Centers for Disease Control and Prevention. Control of tuberculosis in facilities providing long-term care to the elderly: recommendations of the Advisory Committee for the Elimination of Tuberculosis. *Morbidity and Mortality Weekly Report* 1990; **39**(RR-10):7.

Centers for Disease Control and Prevention. Tuberculosis morbidity, 1992. *Morbidity and Mortality Weekly Report* 1993; **4**:696–7.

Centers for Disease Control and Prevention. Nucleic acid amplification tests for tuberculosis. *Morbidity and Mortality Weekly Report* 2000; **49**:593–4.

Centers for Disease Control and Prevention. Update: fatal and severe liver injuries associated with rifampin and pyrazinamide for latent tuberculosis infection, and revisions in American Thoracic Society/Centers for Disease Control and Prevention – recommendations–United States. *Morbidity and Mortality Weekly Report* 2001; **50**(34):733–5.

Centers for Disease Control and Prevention. *Reported Tuberculosis in the United States* 2002a; [database online: www.cdc.gov].

Centers for Disease Control and Prevention. Progress toward tuberculosis elimination in low-incidence areas of the United States: recommendations of the Advisory Council for the Elimination of Tuberculosis. *Morbidity and Mortality Weekly Report* 2002b; **51**:1–16.

Centers for Disease Control and Prevention. Guidelines for using the QuantiFERON-TB test for diagnosing latent *Mycobacterium tuberculosis* infection. *Morbidity and Mortality Weekly Report* 2003a; **52**(RR02):15–8.

Centers for Disease Control and Prevention, American Thoracic Society & Infectious Disease Society of America. Treatment of tuberculosis. *Morbidity and Mortality Weekly Report* 2003b; **52**(RR11):1–77.

Comstock GW. How much isoniazid is needed for prevention of tuberculosis among immunocompetent adults? *International Journal of Tuberculosis and Lung Disease* 1999; **3**:847–50.

Hanna BA. Diagnosis of tuberculosis by microbiologic techniques. In WN Rom & SM Garay (eds) *Tuberculosis* 1996, 1st edn, p 153; Little, Brown and Company, New York.

Hutton MD, Cauthen GM & Bloch AB. Results of a 29-state survey of tuberculosis in nursing homes and correctional facilities. *Public Health Reports* 1993; **108**:305–14.

Ijaz K, Dillara JA, Yang Z *et al.* Unrecognized tuberculosis in a nursing home causing death with spread of tuberculosis to the community. *Journal of the American Geriatric Society* 2002; **50**:1213–7.

Institute of Medicine. In L Geiter (ed) *Ending Neglect: The Elimination of Tuberculosis in the United States* 2000, pp 1–269; National Academy Press, Washington.

Kalita J & Misra UK. Tuberculous meningitis with pulmonary miliary tuberculosis: a clinicoradiological study. *Neurology India* 2004; **52**:194–6.

Lenk S & Schroeder J. Genitourinary tuberculosis. *Current Opinion in Urology* 2001; **11**:93–8.

Malaviya A. Arthritis associated with tuberculosis. *Best Practice and Research Clinical Rheumatology* 2003; **17**:319–43.

Markowitz N, Hansen NI, Wilcosky TC *et al.* Tuberculin and anergy testing in HIV-seropositive and HIV-seronegative persons. *Annals of Internal Medicine* 1993; **119**:185–93.

Mert A, Bilir M & Tabak F. Miliary tuberculosis: clinical manifestations, diagnosis and outcome in 38 adults. *Respirology* 2001; **6**:217–24.

Narain J, Lofgren J, Warren E & Stead WW. Epidemic tuberculosis in a nursing home: a retrospective cohort study. *Journal of the American Geriatric Society* 1985; **33**:258–63.

Patel YR, Mehta JB, Harvill L & Gatekey K. Flexible bronchoscopy as a diagnostic tool in the evaluation of pulmonary tuberculosis in an elderly population. *Journal of the American Geriatrics Society* 1993; **41**:629–32.

Perez-Guzman C, Vargas MH, Torres-Cruz A & Villarreal-Velarde H. Does aging modify pulmonary tuberculosis? A meta-analytical review. *Chest* 1999; **116**:961–7.

Rajagopalan S. Tuberculosis and aging: a global health problem. *Clinical Infectious Disease* 2001; **33**:1034–9.

Rajagopalan S & Yoshikawa TT. Tuberculosis in long-term care facilities. *Infection Control and Hospital Epidemiology* 2000; **21**:611–5.

Reichman LB & O'Day R. Tuberculosis infection in a large urban population. *American Review of Respiratory Diseases* 1978; **117**:705–12.

Schultz M, Hernandez JM, Hernandez NE & Sanchez RO. Onset to tuberculosis disease: new converters in long-term care settings. *American Journal of Alzheimer's Disease and Other Dementias* 2001; **16**:313–8.

Shah AH, Joshi SV & Dhar HL. Tuberculosis of bones and joints. *The Antiseptic* 2001; **98**:385–7.

Slovis BS, Plitman JD & Haas DW. The case against anergy testing as a routine adjunct to tuberculin skin testing. *Journal of the American Medical Association* 2000; **283**:2003–7.

Tort J, Pina JM, Martin-Ramos A *et al.* Booster effect in elderly patients living in geriatric institutions. *Medicina Clinica (Barcelona)* 1995; **105**:41–4.

Woodring JH, Vandiviere HM, Fried AM *et al.* Update: the radiographic features of pulmonary tuberculosis. *American Journal of Roentgenology* 1986; **146**(3):497–506.

Yoshikawa TT. Tuberculosis in aging adults. *Journal of the American Geriatrics Society* 1992; **40**:178.

147

Infective Endocarditis in the Elderly

Philippe Moreillon[1], **Alain Bizzini**[1] *and* **Yok Ai Que**[2]

[1] *University of Lausanne, Lausanne, Switzerland, and* [2] *Centre Hospitalier Universitaire Vaudois, Lausanne, Switzerland*

INTRODUCTION

The proportion of elderly people is increasing worldwide. In Switzerland, the percentage of people aged >65 years was below 2.5% in 1900, as compared to ca. 15% in 2000 (http://www.statistik.admin.ch). More global projections indicate that people of over 65 years will represent ca. 20% of the population in North America and Western Europe by 2030 (Lloyd-Sherlock, 2002). By this time, people over 65 years will represent 5–10% of the population in developing countries (Lloyd-Sherlock, 2002).

Elderly people are more prone to infections than younger adults. Thus, knowledge of infection in these people is important. This chapter addresses infective endocarditis (IE), focusing on relevant commonalities and differences between elderly and younger patients.

INCIDENCE

Despite continuous improvements in health care, the overall incidence of IE (2–6 per 100 000 population per year) has not changed over the past two decades (Bouza *et al.*, 2001; Hoen *et al.*, 2002; Moreillon and Que, 2004). This apparent paradox results from a progressive change in risk factors. Chronic rheumatic heart disease, which was a prime risk factor in the preantibiotic era, is now rare in industrialized countries (Normand *et al.*, 1995). This group of at-risk patients, which predominated in children and young adults, has been replaced by new at-risk groups, including intravenous drug users (IVDU), elderly people with valve sclerosis, patients with intravascular prostheses, patients exposed to nosocomial diseases and hemodialysis patients (Durack *et al.*, 1994; Bouza *et al.*, 2001; Abbott and Agodoa, 2002; Hoen *et al.*, 2002; Moreillon and Que, 2004). IVDU involve mostly young individuals (mean age 30–40 years) (Wilson *et al.*, 2002), whereas the other risk factors are more frequent in the elderly. As a result, the mean age of patients with IE has increased. It was 30 years in the 1950s, 50 years in the 1980s, and 55 to >60 years since the 1990s (von Reyn *et al.*, 1981; van der Meer *et al.*, 1992b; van der Meer *et al.*, 1992a; Hoen *et al.*, 2002; Moreillon and Que, 2004). In a literature review totalizing 3784 episodes of IE between 1993 and 2003, the incidence of IE was varied from <5 to >15 per 100 000 patients per year in individuals younger and older than 65 years, respectively (Hoen *et al.*, 2002; Moreillon and Que, 2004). Thus, the clustering of risk factors in elderly patients correlates with a >3-times increased incidence of IE.

DEMOGRAPHY

Several studies compared the characteristics of IE in elderly (age >65 years) and younger patients (Robbins *et al.*, 1980; Poupet *et al.*, 1984; Terpenning *et al.*, 1987; Werner *et al.*, 1996; Selton-Suty *et al.*, 1997; Gagliardi *et al.*, 1998; Netzer *et al.*, 1999). Besides the increased incidence in the elderly, demographic characteristics were not strikingly different. The reported predominance of IE in males over females persisted over age (ratio between 2/1–3/1) (Werner *et al.*, 1996; Selton-Suty *et al.*, 1997; Gagliardi *et al.*, 1998; Netzer *et al.*, 1999; Hoen *et al.*, 2002; Moreillon and Que, 2004), identifying the male gender as an independent risk factor.

Predisposing cardiac conditions and comorbidities varied somewhat. Preexisting cardiac conditions were less frequently known in older than in younger patients. In two studies, they were reported to be 20% versus 36% (Selton-Suty *et al.*, 1997), and 45% versus 62% (Poupet *et al.*, 1984) in older and younger patients, respectively. However, combining the results of several studies together indicates that this difference may not be generalized (Table 1).

Comorbidities were more frequent in older patients, but only to a minor extent. Diabetes was more frequent in one

Principles and Practice of Geriatric Medicine, 4th Edition. Edited by M.S. John Pathy, Alan J. Sinclair and John E. Morley.

Table 1 Clinical features of infective endocarditis in elderly (≥65 years) and younger (<65 years) patients. Data compiled from the literature

Clinical features	≥65 years[a,b]	<65 years[a,b]	Compiled from[a,c]
Symptoms			
– Fever	217/264 (82%)	360/404 (89%)	(1, 2, 3, 5, 6, 7)
– Asthenia	25/33 (75%)	34/68 (50%)	(1)
– Weight loss	40/86 (46%)	52/169 (31%)	(1, 5)
– Pleuritic pain	9/53 (17%)	22/101 (21%)	(5)
– Arthralgias	19/86 (22%)	43/169 (25%)	(1, 5)
Clinical signs			
– Cardiac murmur	120/167 (72%)	191/258 (74%)	(1, 2, 3, 5)
– Cutaneous signs and peripheral emboli	24/167 (14%)	51/258 (20%)	(1, 2, 3, 5)
– Palpable spleen	39/240 (16%)	131/418 (31%)	(1, 2, 3, 4, 5, 7)
– Neurologic signs	79/206 (38%)	73/247 (29%)	(2, 5, 6, 7)
Predisposing cardiac conditions	103/184 (56%)	250/426 (59%)	(1, 3, 4, 5, 6, 7)
Valve involved			
– Aortic	47/122 (38%)	99/254 (39%)	(4, 5, 6)
– Mitral	59/122 (48%)	98/254 (38.5%)	(4, 5, 6)
– Aortic and mitral	3/69 (4%)	24/153 (15%)	(4, 6)
– Other	18/122 (14%)	43/254 (17%)	(4, 5, 6)

[a]Only studies providing appropriate details were used. Vertical addition of patient numbers and percentages does not apply in the table. [b]Upper age limit varied between 65 and 70 years in some studies. [c]References used: 1, (Poupet *et al.*, 1984); 2, (Robbins *et al.*, 1980); 3, (Selton-Suty *et al.*, 1997); 4, (Werner *et al.*, 1996); 5, (Terpenning *et al.*, 1987); 6, (Gagliardi *et al.*, 1998); 7, (Netzer *et al.*, 1999).

study (Terpenning *et al.*, 1987; Selton-Suty *et al.*, 1997), but not in two others (Gagliardi *et al.*, 1998; Netzer *et al.*, 1999). Renal failure at admission was more frequent in two studies (Terpenning *et al.*, 1987; Netzer *et al.*, 1999), but not in a third one (Gagliardi *et al.*, 1998). On the other hand, the presence of an accompanying malignancy was uniformly more frequent in elderly than younger patients (Terpenning *et al.*, 1987; Gagliardi *et al.*, 1998; Netzer *et al.*, 1999).

How such patient characteristics may impact therapeutic decisions is unclear. A recent study attempted to establish a prognostic score for IE (Hasbun *et al.*, 2003). Parameters predicting mortality included alteration of the mental status, increased number of comorbidities, heart failure, bacterial pathogens (oral streptococci being associated to a better prognosis and *Staphylococcus aureus* to a worst prognosis), and absence of surgery. Neurological complications were one of the major predictors of mortality (Hasbun *et al.*, 2003; Poupet *et al.*, 1984). Age was not considered as a determinant.

Thus, age is only part of the prognostic evaluation. It should be considered in the patient's global context, including valve status and comorbidities.

RISK FACTORS

The key issues are preexisting valve lesions and transient bacteremia due to IE pathogens (see the section on Pathogenesis). On this basis, IE is commonly classified into four categories: (i) native valve IE, (ii) prosthetic valve IE, (iii) IE in IVDU, and (iv) nosocomial IE. In addition, the increasing incidence of IE in hemodialysis (Abbott and Agodoa, 2002) suggests that new categories may arise.

Classical risk factors include congenital heart disease and chronic rheumatic heart disease (Normand *et al.*, 1995). Most of these are primary features of children and young adults. Aortic bicuspid valves and congenital heart defects are more prevalent in younger than older patients with IE (Poupet *et al.*, 1984). On the other hand, the frequency of mitral valve prolapse is similar in both groups (Terpenning *et al.*, 1987; Selton-Suty *et al.*, 1997; Netzer *et al.*, 1999). Mitral valve prolapse is a relatively common (2–4% of the population) inheritable condition, which is linked to a dominant marker on chromosome 16. Only patients with valve regurgitation have an increased risk of IE.

Prosthetic valve endocarditis (PVE) occurs in 1–5% of cases, or 0.3–0.6% per patient-year (Sidhu *et al.*, 2001). A preexisting prosthesis is up to two times more frequent in elderly than in younger patients with IE (Poupet *et al.*, 1984; Terpenning *et al.*, 1987; Selton-Suty *et al.*, 1997). The issue of whether mechanical or bioprosthetic valves are more prone to infection remains unresolved (Sidhu *et al.*, 2001). PVE is classified as either early infection or late infection, depending on whether the symptoms of infection occur within 60 days after surgery or later. PVE peaks during the first 2 months after valve implantation and is often due to *Staphylococcus epidermidis*, and less frequently due to *S. aureus*. Progressive endothelialization of the prosthetic material over 2 to 6 months reduces the susceptibility of the implanted valve to infection. Late PVE is often due to other organisms including streptococci and sometimes gram-negative bacteria of the so-called HACEK group, including *Haemophilus* spp., *Actinobacillus actinomycetem comitans*, *Cardiobacterium hominis*, *Eikenella corrodens*, and *Kingella kingae*.

Intravenous drug users and HIV patients are at-risk groups constituted of relatively younger people. However, they may progressively increase in elderly patients in the coming years. In IVDUs, the tricuspid valve is infected in more that 50% of the cases, followed by the aortic valve in 25% and the mitral valve in 20%, with mixed right-sided and left-sided IE in a few cases (Wilson *et al.*, 2002). Most (60–80%) patients have no known preexisting valve lesions. The pathogens usually originate from the skin, which explains the predominance of *S. aureus* infections. *Pseudomonas aeruginosa* and fungi may also occur, and often produce severe forms of IE. In HIV patients, the mortality rate augments inversely to the CD4 counts. The risk is unaffected in patients with >500 CD4 cells mm^3, but increases by 4 times in those with <200 CD4 counts.

MICROBIAL ETIOLOGY

In the studies reviewed, *Staphylococcus* spp. and *Streptococcus* spp. were responsible for ≥80% of cases, and were rather similarly represented in both age-groups (Figure 1 and Table 2) (Robbins *et al.*, 1980; Poupet *et al.*, 1984; Werner *et al.*, 1996; Gagliardi *et al.*, 1998; Netzer *et al.*, 1999). Some studies reported an increase in the frequency of IE due to enteric streptococci, especially *S. bovis* biotype 1 (recently renamed *S. gallolyticus*), and *Enterococcus* spp. in elderly patients (Poupet *et al.*, 1984; Selton-Suty *et al.*, 1997; Hoen *et al.*, 2002). Figure 1 and Table 2 support this epidemiological profile.

One study reported that the increase in *S. gallolyticus* (formerly *bovis*) represented a shift from oral streptococci to enteric streptococci in the elderly, rather than an addition of the enteric species overall (Hoen *et al.*, 2002). Since *S. gallolyticus* IE is often connected to digestive neoplasia (Hoen *et al.*, 1994; Waisberg *et al.*, 2002), the association could mirror the greater frequency of tumors in elderly people (*see* **Chapter 128, Cancer and Aging**). Another intriguing fact is that several of the studies reporting an increase in IE due to *S. gallolyticus* in the elderly were from France (Selton-Suty *et al.*, 1997; Hoen *et al.*, 2002), suggesting the possibility of a local epidemiological feature. However, a recent review of the English literature confirmed the relation between IE due to *S. gallolyticus* and aging (Figure 1) (Moreillon and Que, 2004).

The frequency of negative culture IE varied between 5–15% and was equivalent in elderly and younger adults (Table 2) (Terpenning *et al.*, 1987; Selton-Suty *et al.*, 1997). Only one study reported a greater frequency of negative culture IE in elderly patients (ca. 20% vs 15% in younger patients) (Poupet *et al.*, 1984). Negative culture IE may occur

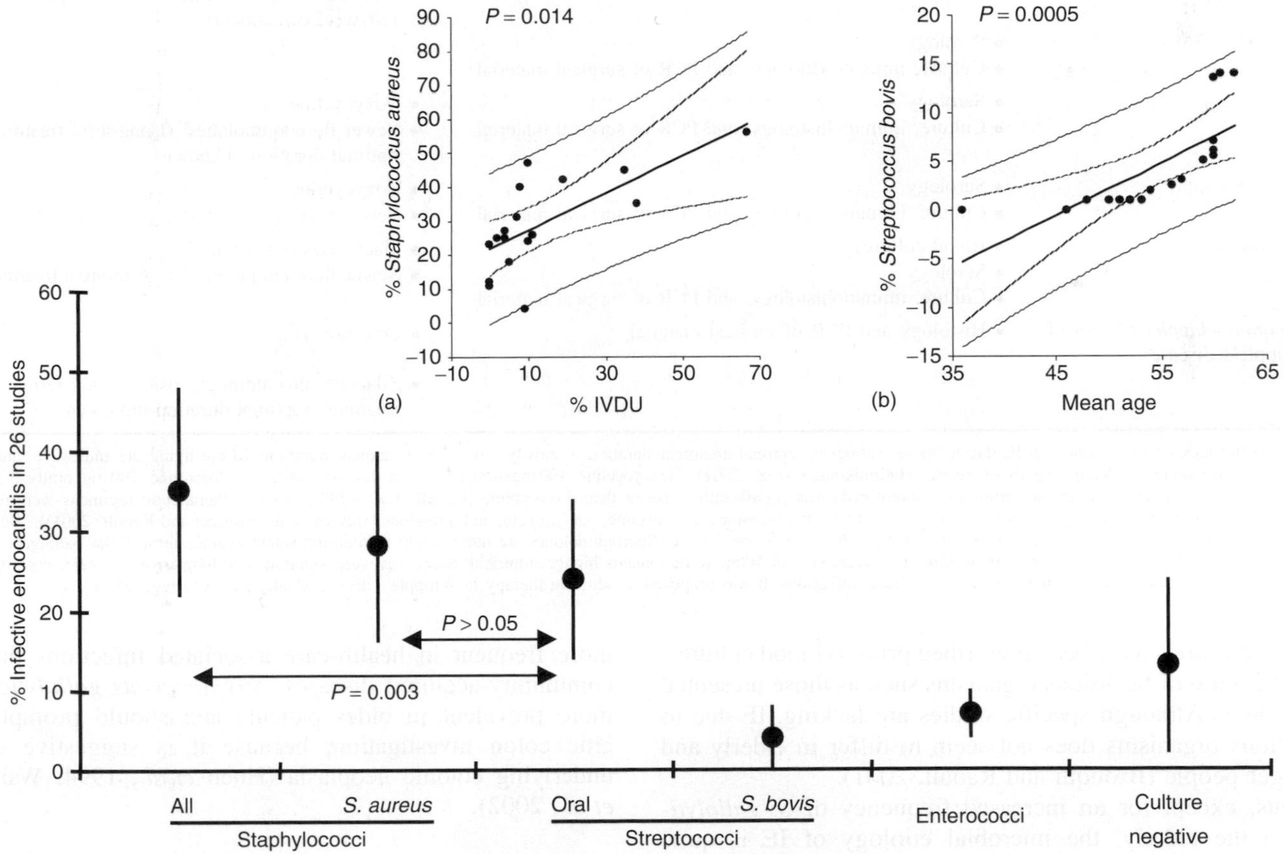

Figure 1 Percent of IE in 3784 episodes compiled from 26 studies published between 1993 and 2003 (Moreillon and Que, 2004). Insets present the linear regressions between the percent of *S. aureus* endocarditis and the percent of IVDU patients reported (a) and the percent of *S. bovis* (recently renamed *S. gallolyticus*) IE and the mean age of the study (b) plotted from 17/26 of the selected publications. Nine publications did not provide enough information to be included in this analysis. The *t*-test and linear regressions were used for statistical comparisons in the figure and the insets, respectively. $P < 0.05$ was considered significant (Reprinted with permission from Elsevier (*The Lancet*, 2004, **363**, 139–149))

Table 2 Microbiology of infective endocarditis in elderly (≥65 years) and younger (<65 years) patients. Data compiled from the literature

Microbial pathogens	≥65 years[a,b]	<65 years[a,b]	Compiled from[a,c]
Staphylococcus spp.	69/227 (30.5%)	139/396 (35%)	(1, 2, 3, 4, 5, 6)
–% *S. aureus*	48/64 (75%)	92/124 (74%)	(2, 3, 4, 5, 6)
–% Coagulase-negative	16/64 (25%)	32/124 (26%)	(2, 3, 4, 5, 6)
Streptococcus spp.	84/227 (37%)	119/396 (30.5%)	(1, 2, 3, 4, 5, 6)
Enterococcus spp.	26/151 (17%)	29/310 (9.5%)	(1, 3, 5, 6)
Gram-negative bacteria	12/186 (6.5%)	19/223 (8.5%)	(1, 2, 5, 6)
Others and Culture-negative	18/227 (8%)	30/396 (7.5%)	(1, 2, 3, 4, 5, 6)

[a]Only studies providing appropriate details were used to compare group of organisms. Vertical addition of patient numbers and percentages does not apply. [b]Upper age limit varied between 65 and 70 years in some studies. [c]References used: 1, (Poupet *et al.*, 1984); 2, (Robbins *et al.*, 1980); 3, (Selton-Suty *et al.*, 1997); 4, (Werner *et al.*, 1996); 5, (Terpenning *et al.*, 1987); 6, (Gagliardi *et al.*, 1998).

Table 3 Rare causes of infective endocarditis associated with negative blood cultures (Adapted from references (Brouqui and Raoult, 2001) and (Moreillon and Que, 2004))

Pathogens	Diagnostic procedure	Proposed therapy[a]
Brucella spp.	• Blood cultures	• Doxycycline plus rifampin or cotrimoxazole. (treatment for >3 months)[b]
	• Serology • Culture, immunohistology, and PCR of surgical material	
Coxiella burnetii (Agent of Q fever)	• Serology: IgG phase 1 >1/800 • Tissue culture, immunohistology, and PCR of surgical material	• Doxycycline plus hydroxychloroquine[c] • Doxycycline plus quinolone (>18 months treatment)
Bartonella spp.	• Blood cultures	• *β*-lactams or doxycycline plus aminoglycoside[d] (>6 weeks treatment)
	• Serology • Culture, immunohistology, and PCR of surgical material	
Chlamydia spp.	• Serology[e] • Culture, immunohistology, and PCR of surgical material	• Doxycycline • Newer fluoroquinolones[f] (Long-term treatment, optimal duration unknown)
Mycoplasma spp.	• Serology • Culture, immunohistology, and PCR of surgical material	• Doxycycline • Newer fluoroquinolones[f] (>12 weeks treatment)
Legionella spp.	• Blood cultures • Serology • Culture, immunohistology, and PCR of surgical material	• Macrolides plus rifampin • Newer fluoroquinolones[f] (>6 months treatment)
Tropheryma whipplei (Agent of Whipple's disease)	• Histology and PCR of surgical material	• Cotrimoxazole[g]
		• *β*-lactam plus aminoglycoside (Long-term treatment, optimal duration unknown)

[a]Owing to the lack of large series on IE due to these pathogens, optimal-treatment duration is mostly unknown. Treatment durations in the figure are indicative, and based on selected case reports. [b]According to reference (Hadjinikolaou *et al.*, 2001). [c]Doxycycline 100 mg orally twice a day and hydroxychloroquine 200 mg orally 3 times a day (hydroxychloroquine levels in the serum were monitored) was significantly superior than doxycycline (Raoult *et al.*, 1999). [d]Several therapeutic regimens were reported, including aminopenicillins and cephalosporins combined with aminoglycosides, doxycycline, vancomycin, and quinolones (reviewed in (Brouqui and Raoult, 2001)). [e]Beware of serologic cross-reaction with the more common IE pathogen *Bartonella* spp. [f]Newer fluoroquinolones are more potent than ciprofloxacin against intracellular pathogens such as *Mycoplasma* spp., *Legionella* spp., and *Chlamydia* spp. [g]Treatment of Whipple IE remains highly empirical. Successes were reported with long-term (>1 year) cotrimoxazole therapy. *γ*-interferon plays a protective role in intracellular infections. It was proposed as adjuvant therapy in Whipple's disease (Dutly and Altwegg, 2001).

when antibiotics have been prescribed prior to blood cultures, or in the case of fastidious organisms such as those presented in Table 3. Although specific studies are lacking, IE due to fastidious organisms does not seem to differ in elderly and younger people (Brouqui and Raoult, 2001).

Thus, except for an increased frequency of *S. gallolyticus* in the elderly, the microbial etiology of IE is quite comparable in older and younger patients. The prediction of a plausible pathogen depends on the patient's underlying conditions rather than on age. For example, coagulase-negative staphylococci are more frequent on prosthetic valve than on native valves. Antibiotic-resistant staphylococci are more frequent in health-care associated infections than in community-acquired diseases. *Streptococcus gallolyticus* is more prevalent in older patients and should prompt specific colon investigation, because it is suggestive of an underlying colonic neoplasia (Hoen *et al.*, 1994; Waisberg *et al.*, 2002).

MORTALITY

Mortality has been reported as being either much higher in elderly than younger patients (up to 45% vs 10–25%,

Table 4 Complications of infective endocarditis in elderly (≥65 years) and younger (<65 years) patients. Data compiled from the literature

Complications	≥65 years[a,b]	<65 years[a,b]	Compiled from[a,c]
Cardiac failure	65/130 (50%)	89/214 (42%)	(1, 6, 7)
Neurological symptoms	10/86 (11.5%)	13/150 (8.5%)	(1, 7)
Renal insufficiency	23/77 (30%)	19/132 (14%)	(1, 6)
Pulmonary complications	3/53 (6%)	17/101 (16%)	(5)
Arterial emboli	10/86 (12%)	14/277 (5%)	(1, 5)

[a]Only studies providing appropriate details were used to compare group of organisms. Vertical addition of patient numbers and percentages does not apply. [b]Upper age limit varied between 65 and 70 years in some studies. [c]References used: 1, (Poupet *et al.*, 1984); 2, (Robbins *et al.*, 1980); 3, (Selton-Suty *et al.*, 1997); 4, (Werner *et al.*, 1996); 5, (Terpenning *et al.*, 1987); 6, (Gagliardi *et al.*, 1998); 7, (Netzer *et al.*, 1999).

respectively) (Robbins *et al.*, 1980; Poupet *et al.*, 1984; Terpenning *et al.*, 1987), or rather similar (around 20%) in different age-groups (Werner *et al.*, 1996; Selton-Suty *et al.*, 1997; Gagliardi *et al.*, 1998; Netzer *et al.*, 1999). At least two variables might explain these differences. First, the heterogeneity of the cohorts studied, and second, the differences in diagnostic tools and diagnostic standards before and after the introduction of the validated "Duke" criteria for diagnosis of IE (Table 4) (Durack *et al.*, 1994; Li *et al.*, 2000).

Studies reporting a higher mortality included cases comprising notoriously severe prosthetic valve and nosocomial-acquired IE, which are more prevalent in elderly people (Robbins *et al.*, 1980; Terpenning *et al.*, 1987). In contrast, studies reporting equivalent mortalities included less severe cases of native valve and right-sided IE. Nevertheless, in one study, the increased mortality persisted after correction for the patient's heterogeneity (Terpenning *et al.*, 1987). Moreover, two recent studies including heterogeneous patients also reported quasi-comparable mortalities between different age-groups (Werner *et al.*, 1996; Selton-Suty *et al.*, 1997). Eventually, studies in which the patients were carefully matched, for example, for left-sided native valve IE, reported similar mortality rates in various age-groups as well (Gagliardi *et al.*, 1998; Netzer *et al.*, 1999). Thus, the reported variations in mortality may be due to additional factors.

Indeed, all the studies reporting a high mortality in older patients were completed before the application of the "Duke" diagnostic criteria, which were first introduced in 1994 (Durack *et al.*, 1994; Li *et al.*, 2000), and before echocardiography became routinely used for the purpose of IE diagnosis. In symmetry, all the studies reporting quasi-similar mortalities in all age-groups were performed after the introduction of these modern diagnostic tools. Diseased elderly patients may present confounding symptoms. Therefore, clinical diagnosis of infection may be difficult. In one earlier report, elderly patients with IE were mostly identified after secondary complications such as embolic stroke (Poupet *et al.*, 1984). Since stroke is associated with a poor prognosis (Gagliardi *et al.*, 1998; Netzer *et al.*, 1999; Hasbun *et al.*, 2003), earlier diagnosis and therapy might have improved the evolution of these patients. This may be particularly relevant in acute conditions such as *S. aureus* PVE in which a mortality rate of up to 47.5% was recently reported (Chirouze *et al.*, 2004). In consequence, prompt diagnosis, rather than age, emerges as a major determinant for IE prognosis.

PATHOGENESIS

The Valve Endothelium

The pathogenesis of IE has been reviewed (Moreillon *et al.*, 2002). The normal valve endothelium is very resistant to colonization and infection by circulating bacteria. On the other hand, mechanical lesions of this endothelium result in exposure of the underlying extracellular matrix proteins, the production of tissue factor, and the deposition of fibrin and platelets as a normal healing process. Such nonbacterial thrombotic endocarditis (NBTE) is an ideal *nidus* for bacterial adherence and colonization during transient bacteremia.

Endothelial damage may occur in several ways. Congenital cardiac abnormalities may cause turbulent blood flow, which in turn may provoke peeling of the endothelium. Valve scarring and calcification following rheumatic carditis or in the sclerotic valves of elderly patients result in endothelial lesions. Extrinsic intervention, such as prosthetic valve replacement or indwelling electrodes or catheters, also promote endothelial lesions. Recently, the presence of *Chlamydia pneumoniae* or cytomegalovirus in endovascular locations has been linked to atherosclerosis. Whether these organisms also trigger endothelial lesions that promote IE remains to be demonstrated.

Infective endocarditis can also occur without known or identifiable preexisting valve lesions. This is particularly true for *S. aureus*, which has emerged as the leading cause of IE in several recent surveys (Bouza *et al.*, 2001; Moreillon and Que, 2004). Local inflammation, which may occur in some circumstances (see the following text), triggers endothelial cells to express a variety of molecules, including integrins of the $\beta 1$ family (very late antigen or VLA) (Hemler *et al.*, 1990). Integrins are transmembrane proteins that can connect extracellular determinants to the cellular cytoskeleton. Integrins of the $\beta 1$ family bind circulating fibronectin to the endothelial surface. On their side, *S. aureus* and a few other IE pathogens carry fibronectin-binding proteins anchored to their walls. Hence, when activated endothelial cells bind fibronectin, they provide an adhesive surface to circulating staphylococci. Once adherent, *S. aureus* can trigger their active internalization by the host cells, in which they can either persist and escape host defenses and antibacterial agents, or multiply and spread to distant organs. This behavior is orchestrated by global regulators such as *agr* (for accessory gene regulator) and *sar* (for staphylococcal accessory regulator), which sense bacterial density and may trigger the secretion of hemolysins and toxins for the purpose of tissue invasion (Novick and Muir, 1999).

Thus, there might be at least two scenarios for primary valve colonization: one requiring a physically damaged endothelium, or NBTE, favoring infection by most types of organisms including viridans group streptococci, and one occurring on physically undamaged endothelia, caused by organisms capable of invading (e.g. *S. aureus*) and parasitizing (e.g. *Coxiella burnetii*, the agent of Q fever) the endothelium.

Infection of Presumably Undamaged Valve

It was believed that preexisting valve lesions were less frequently present in elderly than in younger patients with IE (Poupet *et al.*, 1984). This impression has not been confirmed in recent studies (Table 1). It relied on the detection of preexisting valve abnormalities by auscultation, as exemplified by an audible heart murmur. However, subtle valve abnormalities such as early degenerative valve lesions may pass undetected by auscultation.

Degenerative valve lesions are present in up to 50% of patients over 60 years with IE (Stehbens *et al.*, 2000) (*see* **Chapter 44, Cardiac Aging and Systemic Disorders**; **Chapter 46, Ischemic Heart Disease in Elderly Persons**). This condition involves local inflammation, microulcers, and microthrombi of the endothelium, which are quite similar to atherosclerosis (Stehbens *et al.*, 2000) (*see* **Chapter 53, Pathogenesis of Atherosclerosis**). An age-related increase in predisposing valve conditions was recently highlighted in a large (100 patients) echocardiography study (Croft *et al.*, 2004). The authors identified valve abnormalities that qualified for endocarditis prophylaxis (Dajani *et al.*, 1997; Moreillon, 2000) in up to 50% of patients aged more than 60 years. This may explain, at least in part, the increased risk of IE in the elderly.

The Role of Transient Bacteremia

Medical and surgical procedures in nonsterile anatomic sites may provoke transient bacteremia. Transient bacteremia also occurs spontaneously during normal activities such as chewing and toothbrushing. These bacteremia are usually of low grade and short duration (1–100 CFU/ml of blood for less than 10 minutes in the case of dental extraction). However, they may put patients with preexisting cardiac lesions at an increased risk of developing IE.

The fact that transient bacteremia occurs during normal activities probably explains why most cases of IE are not preceded by medico-surgical procedures (van der Meer *et al.*, 1992b; van der Meer *et al.*, 1992a; Strom *et al.*, 1998). Hence, even if antibiotic prophylaxis during procedures were effective, it would only prevent a limited number of IE cases. Good handling of potential portals of entry is primordial. These include at least the oral sphere (risk of *Streptococcus* spp.), the skin (risk of *Staphylococcus* spp.), the urinary tract (risk of *Enterococcus* spp.), and the related interventions (e.g. indwelling catheters).

Two increasingly frequent "health-care associated" bacteremia are of special concern: bacteremia in dialysis patients (especially hemodialysis) and nosocomial bacteremia. Elderly people are particularly exposed to such occurrences. IE is up to 3 times more frequent in hemodialysis patients than in the general population (Abbott and Agodoa, 2002). Moreover, >50% of the cases are due to *S. aureus*, which are often resistant to methicillin and multiple other drugs. Nosocomial IE accounted for 22% of 109 cases in one study (Bouza *et al.*, 2001). Many patients had debilitating conditions, but <50% had known cardiac predisposing factors. The predominant pathogens were staphylococci and enterococci, and were frequently associated with catheters and/or medico-surgical procedures (Bouza *et al.*, 2001). Another study estimated that up to 13% of nosocomial *S. aureus* bacteremia were responsible for subsequent IE (Fowler *et al.*, 1999). Mortality was greater than 50% (Bouza *et al.*, 2001). Therefore, recognition of such cases is important.

Microbial Pathogens and Host Defenses

Classical IE pathogens include *S. aureus, Streptococcus* spp. (primarily viridans group streptococci and *S. gallolyticus*), and *Enterococcus* spp. (primarily *E. faecalis*) (Figure 1, Table 2). These organisms share the ability to adhere to damaged valves, trigger local procoagulant activity, and nurture infected vegetations in which they can survive (reviewed in (Moreillon *et al.*, 2002)). They are equipped with numerous surface determinants that mediate adherence to host matrix molecules present on damaged valves (e.g. fibrinogen, fibronectin, platelet proteins). These determinants are mutually referred to as *MSCRAMM*, for microbial surface components recognizing adhesive matrix molecules. Damaged or inflamed endothelia carry multiple extracellular matrix molecules acting as specific ligands for MSCRAMMs.

After valve colonization, adherent bacteria escape host defenses. Complement is highly active against gram-negative bacteria, but not against gram-positive bacteria such as staphylococci and streptococci. In gram-negative bacteria, the final C5b-C9 membrane attack complex (MAC) of complement can perforate the lipopolysaccharide outer-membrane and kill the bacterium. Gram-positive bacteria do not have an outermost membrane. Instead, they have a thick peptidoglycan, which protects their inner plasma membrane from attack by MAC. This may explain the wide predominance of gram-positive over gram-negative bacteria in IE.

Although gram-positive bacteria are resistant to complement, they may be the target of platelet microbicidal proteins (PMPs). PMPs are peptides produced by activated thrombocytes that kill bacteria by a mechanism that is as yet incompletely understood. Microorganisms recovered from patients with IE are consistently resistant to PMP-induced killing, whereas similar bacteria recovered from patients with other types of infection were susceptible to PMP (Fowler *et al.*, 2000). Thus, escaping PMP-induced killing is a typical feature of successful IE pathogens.

Further infection involves promoting vegetation growth. Valve-adherent bacteria attract and activate circulating monocytes. Although activated, these monocytes fail to engulf their target organisms, a phenomenon referred to as *frustrated phagocytosis*. On the other hand, they produce cytokines that trigger local inflammation – and local deposition of fibronectin – as well as the production of tissue factor both by themselves and by neighboring endothelial cells.

Tissue factor is a 47 kDa integral membrane glycoprotein that activates coagulation by combining with factor VII and factor X, as well as platelets (Camerer *et al.*, 1996). Tissue factor is not produced by unperturbed endothelial cells or monocytes. However, it can be induced by various agonists including cytokines (IL-1) and bacterial components, and contributes to the vegetation's growth (Moreillon *et al.*, 2002) and thus, bacteria can encourage vegetation growth by subverting monocytes and endothelial cells to produce tissue factor.

A clear role for other host defenses remains uncertain. Experiment on immunization gave contradictory results and administration of granulocyte colony-stimulating factor did not influence the course of infection (reviewed in Moreillon *et al.*, 2002). Moreover, IE is not noticeably more frequent in immunocompromised patients than in those without immune defects. In established infection, bacteria are clustered in the amorphous platelet–fibrin vegetations. This explains why successful treatment of IE relies primarily on the ability of antibiotics to kill the bacteria *in situ*.

PROPHYLAXIS

Because of its severity, it is agreed upon that IE should be prevented whenever possible. Determining adequate prophylaxis implies establishing (i) the patients at risk, (ii) the procedures that might provoke bacteremia, (iii) the most effective prophylactic regimen, and (iv) a balance between the risks of the side effects of prophylaxis and of developing IE. Patients at risk and procedures inducing bacteremia have been identified by clinical studies (Strom *et al.*, 1998), and recommendations for prophylaxis have been proposed in several countries (Dajani *et al.*, 1997; Moreillon, 2000). On the other hand, the efficacy of prophylactic antibiotics is based on animal experimentation. Randomized, placebo-controlled studies do not exist in humans, because they would require too large a patient number and would raise ethical issues because of the severity of the disease. Case-control studies have suggested that IE prophylaxis was effective, but prevented only a limited number of cases (Strom *et al.*, 1998). Indeed, most cases of IE are not preceded by medical procedures (van der Meer *et al.*, 1992b; van der Meer *et al.*, 1992a; Strom *et al.*, 1998). Therefore, the primary prevention of IE should target infected foci responsible for spontaneous bacteremia (e.g. poor dental hygiene). Recommendations for IE prophylaxis are similar in elderly and younger people (Dajani *et al.*, 1997; Moreillon, 2000).

CLINICAL FEATURES

Infective endocarditis may follow an acute or subacute course. Clinical features reported in elderly and younger patients are reported in Tables 1 and 4. Although few differences exist, they are not large enough to portray a specific clinical profile of one or the other group.

Acute Infective Endocarditis

Acute IE is most frequently caused by *S. aureus*, followed by enterococci and certain streptococci, such as *Streptococcus milleri*. IE caused by *S. aureus* and other invasive pathogens can be devastating. Bacterial production of proteases and other exoproteins contributes to rapid destruction of valve leaflets and the development of abscesses located in the valve ring and the myocardium. Myocarditis and pericardial effusions are frequent. Patients are prostrated and have a high fever. Hypotension and shock may occur, caused both by the septic state and by cardiac failure. Cardiac vegetations may vary from a few millimeters in diameter to more than 1 cm. Large vegetations are frequent in acute staphylococcal and fungal IE and are more likely to detach and give rise to septic emboli. Complications in peripheral organs mainly result from embolic lesions; these may include skin abscesses (Janeway lesions), retinal emboli, cerebral abscesses, and splenic abscesses.

Major indications for urgent valve replacement include refractory cardiac failure due to valve destruction and persistent sepsis related to myocardial abscesses. A defect in atrioventricular conduction is often an early sign of septal invasion by a contiguous valve ring abscess, which usually requires urgent surgery.

Subacute Infective Endocarditis

Subacute IE is not usually due to *S. aureus*, but it may be due to any of the organisms listed in Figure 1 and Table 2. The course of subacute IE can mimic chronic wasting diseases. The duration between an identifiable event producing bacteremia (e.g. dental procedure) and the diagnosis of IE can vary from a few days to 5 weeks or more. Fever is almost always present (Table 1). Physical signs reflect the existence of cardiac or peripheral complications. These include a new or changing heart murmur and evidence of embolic events.

Immunologic stimulation during subacute IE causes hyperproduction of gammaglobulin. Rheumatoid factor is present in up to 50% of patients after 6 weeks of subacute infection; its level decreases after effective treatment. Immune phenomena may be the cause of petechiae, splinter hemorrhages, Osler nodes and Roth spots, arthritis, and glomerulonephritis. Osler nodes are small and painful nodular lesions on the pads of the fingers or toes or on the thenar or hypothenar eminences. They are caused by an allergic vasculitis. Although classic, they are not pathognomonic of subacute IE. Roth spots are rounded retinal hemorrhages with a white center. Focal or diffuse glomerulonephritis is present in most of the cases. Because these phenomena follow stimulation of the immune system, they are less common in acute IE.

Vascular Complications

Embolic lesions result from vegetation fragments breaking off the valve and lodging in arteries serving peripheral organs. Other types of vascular manifestations are the consequence of immune-related vasculitis. Mycotic aneurysms are found in up to 15% of cases, and are especially common in staphylococcal IE. They may arise either from direct invasion of the arterial wall by the infecting organisms, from septic embolization of the vasa vasorum, or from the deposition of immune complexes that may trigger local inflammation and weaken the arterial wall. Mycotic aneurysms tend to be located at the bifurcation points of vessels. They may either heal during antibiotic therapy or become clinically evident later, even months after the clinical cure of the disease. Therefore, the true incidence of mycotic aneurysms during IE is probably underestimated. In right-sided IE, embolization occurs in the pulmonary circulation and gives rise to pulmonary infiltrates and lung abscesses.

Neurologic Complications

Neurologic manifestations may occur in up to 40% of cases (Bouza *et al.*, 2001) (*see* **Chapter 72, Secondary Stroke**). However, because patients without neurologic symptoms do not undergo specific investigations, the true incidence of neurologic events during IE may be underestimated. Anatomic alterations include cerebral infarction, arteritis, abscesses, mycotic aneurysms, intracerebral or subarachnoid hemorrhage, encephalomalacia, cerebritis, and meningitis. Such complications occur most often in staphylococcal or streptococcal IE, but they are not restricted to IE caused by these pathogens. The frequency of stroke is similar between native valve and prosthetic valve IE (Cabell *et al.*, 2001). However, the frequency of both vegetations and stroke is significantly greater in patients with mitral valve IE than patients with aortic valve IE.

Controlling the infection is essential. Embolization sharply decreases within 1–2 weeks of effective therapy (Vuille *et al.*, 1994). Recurrent embolization may necessitate urgent valve replacement. This decision is difficult because anticoagulation during extracorporeal circulation and after valve replacement put the patients at an increased risk of secondary intracerebral hemorrhage. Therefore, the tendency is often to postpone emergency surgery and wait for the patient to stabilize. On the other hand, ongoing studies suggest that earlier intervention, within the first 72 hours of stroke, may be beneficial in selected patients (Piper *et al.*, 2001). The best approach to these challenging issues needs continuing investigation.

DIAGNOSIS

Infective endocarditis classically combines fever (Table 1), persistent bacteremia, and anatomic lesions of the valves. However, fever may be variable in elderly people (Norman, 2000), and blood cultures may remain negative in up to 10% of cases (Figure 1 and Table 2), often due to prior consumption of antibiotics. Clinical and microbiologic diagnosis of IE is difficult in such circumstances, or when changes in the valve status cannot be assessed owing to the lack of information on preexisting cardiac lesions (Durack *et al.*, 1994; Li *et al.*, 2000).

Fever

Fever may be present in ≥80% of both elderly and younger patients (Table 1), suggesting that the absence of fever in elderly patients is not an issue for IE. On the other hand, up to 20–30% of elderly patients have a blunted febrile response in the case of severe infection such as pneumonia and bacteremia (for review see (Norman, 2000)). The reason for the poorer febrile response in elderly patients is not entirely clear. Experimental models suggest that they both secrete less cytokines in response to infection, and respond less sharply to endogenous and exogenous pyogenes. The poor febrile response is a problem because it may both delay the diagnosis and give a false impression of security. Thus, other signs associated with infection, such as unexplained alteration of mental status, must be followed with scrutiny in elderly patients (Norman, 2000).

The Duke Criteria

In 1994, new diagnostic criteria based on both microbiologic data and echocardiographic imaging were proposed (Durack *et al.*, 1994). These so-called *Duke criteria* were validated worldwide, and were recently refined to more accurately detect IE in the case of negative blood cultures and *S. aureus* bacteremia (Table 5) (Li *et al.*, 2000). Today, all patients suspected of having IE should undergo at least one echocardiographic evaluation, including transesophageal echo in selected cases. However, a negative echo does not rule out IE when other criteria are positive.

Blood Cultures

The importance of blood culture cannot be overemphasized. It remains the best identification method and provides live bacteria for susceptibility testing. For the main etiologic agents, the first two blood cultures (drawn ≥30 minutes apart) will be positive in more than 90% of cases. Culture-negative IE is often associated with antibiotic consumption within the 2 previous weeks. It may also be due to fastidious or intracellular pathogens that are not easily detected by standard culture conditions. The diagnostic laboratory should be made aware of such possibilities, in order to take appropriate measures.

Culture-negative Infective Endocarditis

Identifying the pathogen in culture-negative IE requires special procedures. They comprise inactivating antibiotics in

Table 5 Modified "Duke" criteria for diagnosis of infective endocarditis (Adapted with modifications from references (Durack *et al.*, 1994; Li *et al.*, 2000) and (Moreillon and Que, 2004))[a]

Definition terminology used in the criteria
Major criteria
1. Blood culture
– Positive blood cultures (≥2/2) with typical IE microorganisms (viridans streptococci, *S. bovis*, HACEK[b] group, ***S. aureus*, or community-acquired enterococci in the absence of primary focus**)[c]
– Persistently positive blood cultures defined as 2 culture sets drawn >12 hours apart, or 3 or the majority of 4 culture sets with the first and last separated at least by 1 hour
– **Single positive culture for *Coxiella burnetii* or anti-phase I antibody titer >1 : 800**
2. Endocardial involvement
– Positive echocardiogram for IE (**transesophageal echo recommended in patients with prosthetic valves, patients rated as "possible" IE by clinical criteria, or complicated IE [paravalvular abscess]; transthoracic echo as first in other patients**):
(i) Oscillating intracardiac mass on valve or supporting structure, *or* in the path of regurgitant jets, *or* on implanted material, in the absence of an alternative anatomic explanation, *or*
(ii) Abscess, *or*
(iii) New partial dehiscence of prosthetic valve
– New valvular regurgitation (worsening or changing of preexisting murmur not sufficient)
Minor criteria
1. Predisposing cardiac condition or intravenous drug use
2. Fever: ≥38 °C (100.4 °F)
3. Vascular phenomena: major arterial emboli, septic pulmonary infarct, mycotic aneurysms, intracranial hemorrhage, conjonctival hemorrhage, Janeway's lesions
4. Immunologic phenomena: glomerulonephritis, Osler nodes, Roth spots, rheumatoid factor
5. Microbiology: positive blood cultures, but not meeting major criteria as mentioned above, serologic evidence of active infection with plausible microorganisms[d]
6. Echocardiogram consistent with IE but not meeting the major criterion noted above[e]
Diagnosis
Definite
• Pathology or bacteriology of vegetations, major emboli or intracardiac abscess specimen, *or*
• 2 major criteria, *or*
• 1 major and 3 minor criteria, *or*
• 5 minor criteria
Possible[f]
• **1 major and 1 minor criterion, *or* 3 minor criteria**
Rejected
• Firm alternative diagnosis, *or*
• Resolution of IE syndrome after ≤4 days of antibiotherapy, *or*
• No pathologic evidence at surgery or autopsy after ≤4 days of antibiotherapy
• Does not meet criteria mentioned above

[a]Modifications of the Duke criteria proposed by Li *et al.* (Li *et al.*, 2000) are highlighted in bold in the table. The revised criteria were validated against a retrospective cohort of pathologically demonstrated and/or prospectively followed endocarditis cases. The revision was intended to increase both the diagnostic specificity (diagnostic threshold) and the sensitivity for endocarditis due to *S. aureus* and difficult to cultivate organisms. [b]Includes *Haemophilus* spp., *Actinobacillus actinomycetemcomitans, Cardiobacterium hominis, Eikenella corrodens,* and *Kingella Kingae*. [c]Original Duke criteria state: "or community-acquired *S. aureus* or enterococci in the absence of primary focus" (Durack *et al.*, 1994). [d]Excludes single positive cultures of coagulase-negative staphylococci and organisms that do not cause endocarditis. [e]Appears in the original Duke criteria (Durack *et al.*, 1994), abandoned in the revised criteria (Li *et al.*, 2000). [f]Original Duke criteria state: "findings consistent with IE that fall short "Definite", but not "Rejected" (Durack *et al.*, 1994).

the culture media, prolonging incubation (≥2 weeks), serology, agglutination, indirect fluorescence, ELISA, complement fixation, and polymerase-chain-reaction (PCR) amplification of genes that are specific for bacteria, such as the genes of the 16S ribosomal RNA (Brouqui and Raoult, 2001; Houpikian and Raoult, 2002). PCR is useful to identify bacterial DNA in tissue samples, including valves, and peripheral emboli (Goldenberger *et al.*, 1997). It proved invaluable to detect poorly or noncultivable bacteria such as *Tropheryma whipplei* (Dutly and Altwegg, 2001). However, it may remain positive in spite of clinical cure even after prolonged antibiotic treatment. Thus, specific knowledge and careful interpretation is required to avoid erroneous conclusions.

Undiagnosed culture-negative IE is a problem because unusual pathogens may not respond to empirical β-lactam and aminoglycoside therapy. Table 3 lists the principal organisms of this group, and the proposed diagnostic procedures, and tentative therapy (Brouqui and Raoult, 2001).

MANAGEMENT

Treatment of IE involves several medical specialists including infectious disease experts, cardiologists, cardiovascular surgeons, and sometimes neurologists. In spite of this wide interest, no large-size and/or blinded studies exist on IE treatment. Most recommended therapies are based on

Table 6 Suggested treatment for native valve endocarditis due to streptococci, enterococci, and HACEK microorganisms (Adapted from references (Francioli *et al.*, 1995; Wilson *et al.*, 1995) and (Moreillon and Que, 2004))

Antibiotic	Dosage and route	Duration (week)	Comments
Penicillin-susceptible viridans streptococci and *Streptococcus bovis*:			
Penicillin G	6×2–3 million U day^{-1} IV	4	Preferred in patients older than 65 years or with impaired renal function
Ceftriaxone[a]	1×2 g day^{-1} day IV or IM	4	
Penicillin G with gentamicin	6×2–8 million U day^{-1} IV	2	Studies suggest that gentamicin 1 x/day might be adequate
	3×1 mg kg^{-1} day^{-1} IV or IM	2	
Ceftriaxone[a] with netilmicin	1×2 g day^{-1} IV or IM	2	
	1×4 mg kg^{-1} day^{-1} IV	2	
Vancomycin	2×15 mg kg^{-1} day^{-1} IV	4	Recommended for β-lactam allergic patients
Intermediate penicillin-resistant (MIC 0.1–1 mg l^{-1}) viridans streptococci and *Streptococcus bovis*:			
Penicillin G with gentamicin	6×3 million U day^{-1} IV	4	Studies suggest that gentamicin 1 x/day might be adequate
	3×1 mg kg^{-1} day^{-1} IV or IM	2	
Vancomycin	2×15 mg kg^{-1} day^{-1} IV	4	Recommended against highly resistant strains or for β-lactam allergic patients
Enterococcus spp.[b]:			
Penicillin G with gentamicin	6×3–5 million U day^{-1} IV	4–6	6-weeks therapy recommended for patients with >3 months symptoms
	3×1 mg kg^{-1} day^{-1} IV or IM	4–6	
Ampicillin with gentamicin	6×2 g day^{-1} IV	4–6	Studies suggest that gentamicin 1 x/day might be adequate
	3×1 mg kg^{-1} day^{-1} IV or IM	4–6	
Vancomycin with gentamicin	2×15 mg kg^{-1} day^{-1} IV	4–6	Monitor drug serum levels and renal function
	3×1 mg kg^{-1} day^{-1} IV or IM	4–6	
Microorganisms of the HACEK group[c]:			
Ceftriaxone[†]	1×2 g day^{-1} day IV or IM	4	
Ampicillin with gentamicin	6×2 g day^{-1} IV	4	Studies suggest that gentamicin 1 x/day might be adequate
	3×1 mg kg^{-1} day^{-1} IV or IM	4	

[a]Preferred for outpatient treatment. [b]Treatment of endocarditis due to vancomycin-resistant enterococci requires a careful assessment of susceptibility to alternative antibiotics, including the new streptogramin combination quinupristin/dalfopristin. [c]Includes *Haemophilus* spp., *Actinobacillus actinomycetemcomitans, Cardiobacterium hominis, Eikenella corrodens,* and *Kingella Kingae.*

experimental works, expert opinions, or small case-control studies (Francioli *et al.*, 1995; Wilson *et al.*, 1995; Moreillon and Que, 2004).

Bactericidal antibiotics are a cornerstone of therapy. Therapeutic schemes recommended for the most common pathogens are presented in Table 6 and Table 7 (Francioli *et al.*, 1995; Wilson *et al.*, 1995). High concentrations of antibiotic in the serum are desirable to ensure diffusion into the vegetations. Prolonged treatment is mandatory to kill dormant bacteria clustered in the infected foci. Outpatient and oral therapy is sometimes proposed (Rehm, 1998), but prolonged parenteral therapy is usually recommended.

The choice of an optimal regimen is based on antibiotic susceptibility testing. Minimal inhibitory concentrations of the principal drugs for the infecting pathogens should be determined. Resistant pathogens and culture-negative IE may fail to respond to standard treatment and this is discussed in the following text.

Penicillin-resistant Streptococci

Streptococci are becoming increasingly resistant to penicillin and other β-lactams, owing to a decreased β-lactam affinity of their membrane-bound penicillin-binding proteins (PBPs). Penicillin-resistant streptococci are classified as having either intermediate resistance (MIC of 0.1–1 mg l^{-1}) or high resistance (MIC over 1 mg l^{-1}).

Intermediately resistant streptococci may respond to standard therapy because β-lactam concentrations in the serum are much greater than the MIC for these bacteria. Peak serum levels of penicillin G, amoxicillin, or ceftriaxone are in the order of 100 mg l^{-1}, that is, 100–1000 times greater than the MIC of intermediately resistant streptococci (MIC = 0.1–1 mg l^{-1}). Nonetheless, potentiating the β-lactam activity by combining it with an aminoglycoside is recommended in such situations.

Alternative drugs must be considered against highly resistant streptococci. These include vancomycin, to which streptococci are still widely susceptible. In the future, newer quinolones with anti-gram-positive activity and quinupristin–dalfopristin may prove useful (Entenza *et al.*, 1995; Entenza *et al.*, 1999). Oxazolidinones are an alternative, but they are poor bactericides. Upcoming daptomycin and tigecycline require further experimental evaluation.

Methicillin-resistant and Vancomycin-resistant Staphylococci

All methicillin-resistant staphylococci carry a new, low-affinity PBP, called *PBP2A* that confers cross-resistance to most β-lactam drugs. In addition, methicillin-resistant staphylococci are usually resistant to most other drugs, leaving only vancomycin to treat severe infections.

Table 7 Suggested treatment for native valve and prosthetic valve endocarditis due to staphylococci (Adapted with modifications from references (Wilson *et al.*, 1995) and (Moreillon and Que, 2004))

Antibiotic	Dosage and route	Duration (week)	Comments
Native valves			
Methicillin-susceptible staphylococci			
Flucloxacillin, or oxacillin, or nafcillin	6×2 g day IV	4–6	The benefit of gentamicin addition is not
with gentamicin (optional)	3×1 mg kg^{-1} day^{-1} IV or IM	3–5 days	demonstrated
Cefazolin (or other first generation	3×2 g day^{-1} IV	4–6	Alternative for patients allergic to penicillins (not in
cephalosporins) with gentamicin (optional)	3×1 mg kg^{-1} day^{-1} IV or IM	3–5 days	case of immediate type penicillin hypersensitivity)
Vancomycin	2×15 mg kg^{-1} day^{-1} IV	4–6	Recommended for β-lactam allergic patients
Methicillin-resistant staphylococci			
Vancomycin	2×15 mg kg^{-1} day^{-1} IV	4–6	Recommended for β-lactam allergic patients
Prosthetic valves			
Methicillin-susceptible staphylococci[a]			
Flucloxacillin, or oxacillin, or nafcillin	6×2 g day^{-1} IV	≥ 6	Rifampin increases the hepatic metabolism of
with rifampin and gentamicin	3×300 mg day^{-1} orally	≥ 6	numerous drugs, including warfarin
	3×1 mg kg^{-1} day^{-1} IV or IM	2	
Vancomycin with rifampin and gentamicin	2×15 mg kg^{-1} day^{-1} IV	≥ 6	Recommended for β-lactam allergic patients
	3×300 mg day^{-1} orally	≥ 6	
	3×1 mg kg^{-1} day^{-1} IV or IM	2	
Methicillin-resistant staphylococci			
Vancomycin with rifampin and gentamicin	2×15 mg kg^{-1} day^{-1} IV	≥ 6	
	3×300 mg day^{-1} orally	≥ 6	
	3×1 mg kg^{-1} day^{-1} IV or IM	2	

[a]Rifampin plays a special role in prosthetic device infection, because it helps kill bacteria attached to foreign material. Rifampin should never be used alone, because it selects for resistance at a high frequency (ca. 10^{-6}).

Yet, vancomycin-resistance is developing. *S. aureus* and coagulase-negative staphylococci with intermediate resistance to vancomycin have emerged worldwide. The mechanism of intermediate resistance is mediated by chromosomal mutations affecting the synthesis of the cell wall (Hiramatsu, 2001). High vancomycin-resistance had emerged 15 years ago in enterococci, and could be transferred experimentally into *S. aureus* (Noble *et al.*, 1992). Recently, few highly vancomycin-resistant *S. aureus* were isolated in the clinics. Their vancomycin-resistant genes were also acquired from enterococci (Rep, 2002).

Treatment of IE caused by vancomycin-resistant staphylococci will require new approaches. At present, a few unconventional alternatives are available, including old and new β-lactams with relatively good affinity to PBP2A (Entenza *et al.*, 2002), quinupristin–dalfopristin combined with or without β-lactams (Entenza *et al.*, 1995; Vouillamoz *et al.*, 2000), antibiotic combination including cotrimoxazole (de Gorgolas *et al.*, 1995), and maybe oxazolidinones (Jacqueline *et al.*, 2002). Methicillin-resistant staphylococci are usually resistant to newer quinolones. Promising future drugs include daptomycin (Sakoulas *et al.*, 2003).

Multiple-drug-resistant Enterococci

These organisms are resistant to most available drugs, including vancomycin. Treatment of such bacteria relies on the combination of multiple drugs and the use of experimental antibiotics. It requires precise determination of antibiotic susceptibilities, testing for bactericidal activity, maybe determining the serum inhibitory and bactericidal titers, and monitoring drug levels in the serum. Although aminoglycoside-resistance is often present, these drugs may still synergize with cell-wall inhibitors, provided that the aminoglycosides MIC is ≤ 1000 mg l^{-1}. Streptomycin is worth testing because it may be active against enterococci that are resistant to other aminoglycosides. Salvage regimens suggested to combat highly aminoglycoside-resistant, but ampicillin-susceptible, enterococci include continuous infusion of high-dose ampicillin, alone or in combination with ceftriaxone, other β-lactam combinations, or oxazolidinones. Whenever envisioned, such an approach should be based on expert opinion. As for streptococci, upcoming daptomycin, and tigecycline require further studies (Kennedy and Chambers, 1989; Lefort *et al.*, 2003).

Culture-negative Endocarditis

Table 3 summarizes the treatment of IE due to rare pathogens. *Brucella* spp. IE responds to ≥ 3 months treatment with doxycycline (100–200 mg every 12 hours) plus cotrimoxazole (960 mg every 12 hours) or rifampin (300–600 mg day^{-1}) combined with or without streptomycin (16 mg kg^{-1} day^{-1}). Surgery may be required (Hadjinikolaou *et al.*, 2001). Cure is considered by an antibody titer returning to $<1:160$.

Coxiella burnetii IE is often treated with doxycycline combined with a fluoroquinolone for up to 3 years. Recurrences are common. Recently, a combination of doxycycline and hydroxychloroquine appeared more effective (Raoult *et al.*,

1999). Treatment success is considered when the anti–phase I antigen IgG titer is <1 : 800, and IgM and IgA titers are <1 : 50 (Raoult *et al.*, 1999).

Bartonella spp. IE responds to β-lactams (amoxicillin or ceftriaxone) combined with aminoglycosides (netilmicin or gentamicin) for at least 2 weeks, or β-lactams combined with other drugs (e.g. doxycycline) for a total of ≥6 weeks (Fournier *et al.*, 2001). Combination with surgery is reported in ≥90% of cases.

Treatment of IE due to *Chlamydia* spp., *Mycoplasma* spp., and *Legionella* spp., is unknown. These organisms are highly susceptible to newer fluoroquinolones *in vitro*. Therefore, fluoroquinolones should probably be part of the treatment.

IE due to *T. whipplei* is very rare. In non-IE Whipple's disease, cotrimoxazole (960 mg every 12 hours) given for ≥1 year is recommended (Dutly and Altwegg, 2001). Some authors recommend sequential treatment starting with penicillin plus streptomycin, or ceftriaxone plus gentamicin, for 2 to 6 weeks, followed by long-term cotrimoxazole. A recent review of 35 cases of Whipple IE supports this approach and suggests that surgical valve replacement might be a prerequisite for successful therapy (Fenollar *et al.*, 2001).

Surgery (*see* Chapter 51, Management of Acute Cardiac Emergencies and Cardiac Surgery; Chapter 52, Cardiac Surgery in the Elderly)

A detailed overview of surgical techniques is beyond the scope of this review. However, surgery is increasingly becoming important in the management of IE and was even associated with a better outcome in the prognosis scoring proposed overall (Hasbun *et al.*, 2003; Vikram *et al.*, 2003). Surgery encompasses both radical valve replacement and more conservative vegetectomy and valve repairs.

Surgery is necessary in 25 to 30% of cases during acute infection, and in 20 to 40% in later phases (Jault *et al.*, 1997; Alexiou *et al.*, 2000). The final outcome has little relation to the duration of prior antibiotic therapy. The principal indications comprise (i) refractory cardiac failure caused by valvular insufficiency, (ii) persistent sepsis caused by a surgically removable focus or a valvular ring or myocardial abscess, and (iii) persistent life-threatening embolization. The decision is multidisciplinary, and age is not a discriminatory feature (Hasbun *et al.*, 2003). Studies on the surgery of active IE report mortality rates of 8 to 16%, with actuarial survival at 5 years of 75 to 76% and at 10 years of 61% (Alexiou *et al.*, 2000).

CONCLUSION

The mean age of IE is increasing (Bouza *et al.*, 2001, Hoen *et al.*, 2002, Moreillon and Que, 2004). This correlates with an increase in risk factors that are more common in elderly (≥65 years) than in younger people. As a result, elderly people have a ≥3-times greater risk of acquiring IE than younger persons (Moreillon and Que, 2004). In spite of this evolution, demographic features, bacterial pathogens, and life prognosis appear not much different in both age-groups. Most patients have predisposing valve conditions as detected by echocardiography (Croft *et al.*, 2004). The major pathogens are *Staphylococcus* spp. and *Streptococcus* spp. (in ca. 80% of cases) and are similarly distributed in older and younger adults. One difference involves the partitioning of oral and enteric streptococci in older and younger patients (Hoen *et al.*, 2002). Elderly patients have an increased prevalence of IE due to *S. gallolyticus,* in relation with colon neoplasia, and a parallel decrease in IE due to oral streptococci (Hoen *et al.*, 2002; Moreillon and Que, 2004). This highlights that a genuine age-related modification of epidemiology. Aging has often been considered as an aggravating factor for life prognosis. However, recent reports suggest that this might not be true. Age-independent clinical and laboratory parameters are more predictive (Hasbun *et al.*, 2003). Moreover, prompt diagnosis and therapy is critical for clinical outcome. Thus, life prognosis should be considered in the patient's global context, rather than on age alone. On the other hand, studies on functional outcome are still missing.

KEY POINTS

- Age is not a primary determinant for life prognosis. Patients who are comparable for mental status, comorbidities, bacterial pathogen, cardiac conditions, and surgery have a similar chance of survival (Hasbun *et al.*, 2003, #613).
- The prognosis of IE depends on prompt diagnosis and therapy. Applying the modern Duke diagnostic criteria is critical (Durack *et al.*, 1994, #390; Li *et al.*, 2000, #1007).
- Degenerative valve sclerosis is a frequent predisposing condition in elderly people. It may be detected by echocardiography, while passing unnoticed in cardiac auscultation (Croft *et al.*, 2004, #867).
- *Staphylococcus* spp. and *Streptococcus* spp. are the principal pathogens of IE (in >80% of cases), and are similarly distributed in both elderly and younger patients.
- *S. gallolyticus* is more prevalent in elderly IE patients. It is frequently associated with a colon neoplasia and should prompt digestive investigations.

KEY REFERENCES

- Croft LB, Donnino R, Shapiro R *et al.* Age-related prevalence of cardiac valvular abnormalities warranting infectious endocarditis prophylaxis. *The American Journal of Cardiology* 2004; **94**:386–9.
- Gagliardi JP, Nettles RE, McCarty DE *et al.* Native valve infective endocarditis in elderly and younger adult patients: comparison of clinical

features and outcomes with use of the Duke criteria and the Duke Endocarditis Database. *Clinical Infectious Diseases* 1998; **26**:1165–8.

- Hoen B, Alla F, Selton-Suty C *et al.* Changing profile of infective endocarditis: results of a 1-year survey in France. *The Journal of the American Medical Association* 2002; **288**:75–81.
- Li JS, Sexton DJ, Mick N *et al.* Proposed modifications to the Duke criteria for the diagnosis of infective endocarditis. *Clinical Infectious Diseases* 2000; **30**:633–8.
- Selton-Suty C, Hoen B, Grentzinger A *et al.* Clinical and bacteriological characteristics of infective endocarditis in the elderly. *Heart* 1997; **77**:260–3.

REFERENCES

Abbott KC & Agodoa LY. Hospitalizations for valvular heart disease in chronic dialysis patients in the United States. *Nephron* 2002; **92**:43–50.

Alexiou C, Langley SM, Stafford H *et al.* Surgery for active culture-positive endocarditis: determinants of early and late outcome. *The Annals of Thoracic Surgery* 2000; **69**:1448–54.

Bouza E, Menasalvas A, Munoz P *et al.* Infective endocarditis – a prospective study at the end of the twentieth century: new predisposing conditions, new etiologic agents, and still a high mortality. *Medicine* 2001; **80**:298–307.

Brouqui P & Raoult D. Endocarditis due to rare and fastidious bacteria. *Clinical Microbiology Reviews* 2001; **14**:177–207.

Cabell CH, Pond KK, Peterson GE *et al.* The risk of stroke and death in patients with aortic and mitral valve endocarditis. *American Heart Journal* 2001; **142**:75–80.

Camerer E, Kolsto AB & Prydz H. Cell biology of tissue factor, the principal initiator of blood coagulation. *Thrombosis Research* 1996; **81**:1–41.

Chirouze C, Cabell CH, Fowler VG Jr *et al.* Prognostic factors in 61 cases of *Staphylococcus aureus* prosthetic valve infective endocarditis from the International Collaboration on Endocarditis merged database. *Clinical Infectious Diseases* 2004; **38**:1323–7.

Croft LB, Donnino R, Shapiro R *et al.* Age-related prevalence of cardiac valvular abnormalities warranting infectious endocarditis prophylaxis. *The American Journal of Cardiology* 2004; **94**:386–9.

Dajani AS, Taubert KA, Wilson W *et al.* Prevention of bacterial endocarditis. Recommendations by the American Heart Association. *The Journal of the American Medical Association* 1997; **277**:1794–801.

de Gorgolas M, Aviles P, Verdejo C & Fernandez Guerrero ML. Treatment of experimental endocarditis due to methicillin-susceptible or methicillin-resistant *Staphylococcus aureus* with trimethoprim-sulfamethoxazole and antibiotics that inhibit cell wall synthesis. *Antimicrobial Agents and Chemotherapy* 1995; **39**:953–7.

Durack DT, Lukes AS & Bright DK. New criteria for diagnosis of infective endocarditis: utilization of specific echocardiographic findings. Duke Endocarditis Service. *American Journal of Medicine* 1994; **96**:200–9.

Dutly F & Altwegg M. Whipple's disease and "*Tropheryma whippelii*". *Clinical Microbiology Reviews* 2001; **14**:561–83.

Entenza JM, Caldelari I, Glauser MP & Moreillon P. Efficacy of levofloxacin in the treatment of experimental endocarditis caused by viridans group streptococci. *The Journal of Antimicrobial Chemotherapy* 1999; **44**:775–86.

Entenza JM, Drugeon H, Glauser MP & Moreillon P. Treatment of experimental endocarditis due to erythromycin-susceptible or -resistant methicillin-resistant *Staphylococcus aureus* with RP 59500. *Antimicrobial Agents and Chemotherapy* 1995; **39**:1419–24.

Entenza JM, Hohl P, Heinze-Krauss I *et al.* BAL9141, a novel extended-spectrum cephalosporin active against methicillin-resistant *Staphylococcus aureus* in treatment of experimental endocarditis. *Antimicrobial Agents and Chemotherapy* 2002; **46**:171–7.

Fenollar F, Lepidi H & Raoult D. Whipple's endocarditis: review of the literature and comparisons with Q fever, Bartonella infection, and blood culture-positive endocarditis. *Clinical Infectious Diseases* 2001; **33**:1309–16.

Fournier PE, Lelievre H, Eykyn SJ *et al.* Epidemiologic and clinical characteristics of *Bartonella quintana* and *Bartonella henselae* endocarditis: a study of 48 patients. *Medicine* 2001; **80**:245–51.

Fowler VG Jr, McIntyre LM, Yeaman MR *et al.* *In vitro* resistance to thrombin-induced platelet microbicidal protein in isolates of *Staphylococcus aureus* from endocarditis patients correlates with an intravascular device source. *The Journal of Infectious Diseases* 2000; **182**:1251–4.

Fowler VG Jr, Sanders LL, Kong LK *et al.* Infective endocarditis due to *Staphylococcus aureus*: 59 prospectively identified cases with follow-up. *Clinical Infectious Diseases* 1999; **28**:106–14.

Francioli P, Ruch W & Stamboulian D. Treatment of streptococcal endocarditis with a single daily dose of ceftriaxone and netilmicin for 14 days: a prospective multicenter study. *Clinical Infectious Diseases* 1995; **21**:1406–10.

Gagliardi JP, Nettles RE, McCarty DE *et al.* Native valve infective endocarditis in elderly and younger adult patients: comparison of clinical features and outcomes with use of the Duke criteria and the Duke Endocarditis Database. *Clinical Infectious Diseases* 1998; **26**:1165–8.

Goldenberger D, Kunzli A, Vogt P *et al.* Molecular diagnosis of bacterial endocarditis by broad-range PCR amplification and direct sequencing. *Journal of Clinical Microbiology* 1997; **35**:2733–9.

Hadjinikolaou L, Triposkiadis F, Zairis M *et al.* Successful management of *Brucella mellitensis* endocarditis with combined medical and surgical approach. *European Journal of Cardio-thoracic Surgery* 2001; **19**:806–10.

Hasbun R, Vikram HR, Barakat LA *et al.* Complicated left-sided native valve endocarditis in adults: risk classification for mortality. *The Journal of the American Medical Association* 2003; **289**:1933–40.

Hemler ME, Elices MJ, Parker C & Takada Y. Structure of the integrin VLA-4 and its cell-cell and cell-matrix adhesion functions. *Immunological Reviews* 1990; **114**:45–65.

Hiramatsu K. Vancomycin-resistant *Staphylococcus aureus*: a new model of antibiotic resistance. *The Lancet Infectious Diseases* 2001; **1**:147–55.

Hoen B, Alla F, Selton-Suty C *et al.* Changing profile of infective endocarditis: results of a 1-year survey in France. *The Journal of the American Medical Association* 2002; **288**:75–81.

Hoen B, Briancon S, Delahaye F *et al.* Tumors of the colon increase the risk of developing *Streptococcus bovis* endocarditis: case-control study. *Clinical Infectious Diseases* 1994; **19**:361–2.

Houpikian P & Raoult D. Diagnostic methods current best practices and guidelines for identification of difficult-to-culture pathogens in infective endocarditis. *Infectious Disease Clinics of North America* 2002; **16**:377–92.

Jacqueline C, Batard E, Perez L *et al.* *In vivo* efficacy of continuous infusion versus intermittent dosing of linezolid compared to vancomycin in a methicillin-resistant *Staphylococcus aureus* rabbit endocarditis model. *Antimicrobial Agents and Chemotherapy* 2002; **46**:3706–11.

Jault F, Gandjbakhch I, Rama A *et al.* Active native valve endocarditis: determinants of operative death and late mortality. *The Annals of Thoracic Surgery* 1997; **63**:1737–41.

Kennedy S & Chambers HF. Daptomycin (LY146032) for prevention and treatment of experimental aortic valve endocarditis in rabbits. *Antimicrobial Agents and Chemotherapy* 1989; **33**:1522–5.

Lefort A, Lafaurie M, Massias L *et al.* Activity and diffusion of tigecycline (GAR-936) in experimental enterococcal endocarditis. *Antimicrobial Agents and Chemotherapy* 2003; **47**:216–22.

Li JS, Sexton DJ, Mick N *et al.* Proposed modifications to the Duke criteria for the diagnosis of infective endocarditis. *Clinical Infectious Diseases* 2000; **30**:633–8.

Lloyd-Sherlock P. Social policy and population ageing: challenges for north and south. *International Journal of Epidemiology* 2002; **31**:754–7.

Moreillon P. Endocarditis prophylaxis revisited: experimental evidence of efficacy and new Swiss recommendations. Swiss Working Group for Endocarditis Prophylaxis. *Schweizerische Medizinische Wochenschrift* 2000; **130**:1013–26.

Moreillon P & Que YA. Infective endocarditis. *Lancet* 2004; **363**:139–49.

Moreillon P, Que YA & Bayer AS. Pathogenesis of streptococcal and staphylococcal endocarditis. *Infectious Disease Clinics of North America* 2002; **16**:297–318.

Netzer RO, Zollinger E, Seiler C & Cerny A. Native valve infective endocarditis in elderly and younger adult patients: comparison of clinical features and outcomes with use of the Duke criteria. *Clinical Infectious Diseases* 1999; **28**:933–5.

Noble WC, Virani Z & Cree RG. Co-transfer of vancomycin and other resistance genes from *Enterococcus faecalis* NCTC 12201 to *Staphylococcus aureus*. *FEMS Microbiology Letters* 1992; **72**:195–8.

Norman DC. Fever in the elderly. *Clinical Infectious Diseases* 2000; **31**:148–51.

Normand J, Bozio A, Etienne J *et al.* Changing patterns and prognosis of infective endocarditis in childhood. *European Heart Journal* 1995; **16**(suppl B):28–31.

Novick RP & Muir TW. Virulence gene regulation by peptides in staphylococci and other Gram-positive bacteria. *Current Opinion in Microbiology* 1999; **2**:40–5.

Piper C, Wiemer M, Schulte HD & Horstkotte D. Stroke is not a contraindication for urgent valve replacement in acute infective endocarditis. *The Journal of Heart Valve Disease* 2001; **10**:703–11.

Poupet JY, Allal J, Thomas P *et al.* Infectious endocarditis in the elderly. *Revue de Medecine Interne* 1984; **5**:283–90.

Raoult D, Houpikian P, Tissot Dupont H *et al.* Treatment of Q fever endocarditis: comparison of 2 regimens containing doxycycline and ofloxacin or hydroxychloroquine. *Archives of Internal Medicine* 1999; **159**:167–73.

Rehm SJ. Outpatient intravenous antibiotic therapy for endocarditis. *Infectious Disease Clinics of North America* 1998; **12**:879–901, vi.

Rep MMWR. *Staphylococcus aureus* resistant to vancomycin – United States, 2002. *Morbidity and Mortality Weekly Report* 2002; **51**:565–7.

Robbins N, DeMaria A & Miller MH. Infective endocarditis in the elderly. *Southern Medical Journal* 1980; **73**:1335–8.

Sakoulas G, Eliopoulos GM, Alder J & Eliopoulos CT. Efficacy of daptomycin in experimental endocarditis due to methicillin-resistant *Staphylococcus aureus*. *Antimicrobial Agents and Chemotherapy* 2003; **47**:1714–8.

Selton-Suty C, Hoen B, Grentzinger A *et al.* Clinical and bacteriological characteristics of infective endocarditis in the elderly. *Heart* 1997; **77**:260–3.

Sidhu P, O'Kane H, Ali N *et al.* Mechanical or bioprosthetic valves in the elderly: a 20-year comparison. *The Annals of Thoracic Surgery* 2001; **71**:S257–60.

Stehbens WE, Delahunt B & Zuccollo JM. The histopathology of endocardial sclerosis. *Cardiovascular Pathology* 2000; **9**:161–73.

Strom BL, Abrutyn E, Berlin JA *et al.* Dental and cardiac risk factors for infective endocarditis. A population-based, case-control study. *Annals of Internal Medicine* 1998; **129**:761–9.

Terpenning MS, Buggy BP & Kauffman CA. Infective endocarditis: clinical features in young and elderly patients. *American Journal of Medicine* 1987; **83**:626–34.

van der Meer JT, Thompson J, Valkenburg HA & Michel MF. Epidemiology of bacterial endocarditis in The Netherlands. I. Patient characteristics. *Archives of Internal Medicine* 1992a; **152**:1863–8.

van der Meer JT, Thompson J, Valkenburg HA & Michel MF. Epidemiology of bacterial endocarditis in The Netherlands. II. Antecedent procedures and use of prophylaxis. *Archives of Internal Medicine* 1992b; **152**:1869–73.

Vikram HR, Buenconsejo J, Hasbun R & Quagliarello VJ. Impact of valve surgery on 6-month mortality in adults with complicated, left-sided native valve endocarditis: a propensity analysis. *The Journal of the American Medical Association* 2003; **290**:3207–14.

von Reyn CF, Levy BS, Arbeit RD *et al.* Infective endocarditis: an analysis based on strict case definitions. *Annals of Internal Medicine* 1981; **94**:505–18.

Vouillamoz J, Entenza JM, Feger C *et al.* Quinupristin-dalfopristin combined with beta-lactams for treatment of experimental endocarditis due to *Staphylococcus aureus* constitutively resistant to macrolide-lincosamide-streptogramin B antibiotics. *Antimicrobial Agents and Chemotherapy* 2000; **44**:1789–95.

Vuille C, Nidorf M, Weyman AE & Picard MH. Natural history of vegetations during successful medical treatment of endocarditis. *American Heart Journal* 1994; **128**:1200–9.

Waisberg J, Matheus Cde O & Pimenta J. Infectious endocarditis from *Streptococcus bovis* associated with colonic carcinoma: case report and literature review. *Arquivos de Gastroenterologia* 2002; **39**:177–80.

Werner GS, Schulz R, Fuchs JB *et al.* Infective endocarditis in the elderly in the era of transesophageal echocardiography: clinical features and prognosis compared with younger patients. *American Journal of Medicine* 1996; **100**:90–7.

Wilson LE, Thomas DL, Astemborski J *et al.* Prospective study of infective endocarditis among injection drug users. *Journal Infectious Diseases* 2002; **185**:1761–6.

Wilson WR, Karchmer AW, Dajani AS *et al.* Antibiotic treatment of adults with infective endocarditis due to streptococci, enterococci, staphylococci, and HACEK microorganisms. American Heart Association. *The Journal of the American Medical Association* 1995; **274**:1706–13.

148

Infections of the Central Nervous System

Michael Blank *and* Allan R. Tunkel
Drexel University College of Medicine, Philadelphia, PA, USA

MENINGITIS

Meningitis is defined as the inflammation of the meninges that is manifested by an increase in the number of white blood cells in cerebrospinal fluid (CSF), and may be a result of a wide variety of infectious and noninfectious etiologies. The following is an overview of the most common infectious causes of meningitis in the elderly, with emphasis on the epidemiology, etiology, clinical presentation, diagnosis, and management of these disorders.

Viral Meningitis

Epidemiology and Etiology

Viruses are the major causes of the aseptic meningitis syndrome, which has been defined as any meningitis (infectious or noninfectious) for which a cause is not apparent after initial evaluation and routine stains and cultures of CSF (Connolly and Hammer, 1990). The most common etiologic agents of the aseptic meningitis syndrome are the nonpolio enteroviruses (specifically Coxsackie and echoviruses), which accounts for 85–90% of cases in which a pathogen is identified (Connolly and Hammer, 1990). These viruses are worldwide in distribution and occur with a peak incidence in the summer and early fall. Other viral causes of the aseptic meningitis syndrome include arboviruses (e.g. St Louis encephalitis virus, the California encephalitis group of viruses, West Nile encephalitis virus, and the agent of Colorado tick fever), mumps virus, the herpesviruses (herpes simplex viruses types 1 and 2, varicella zoster virus (VZV), cytomegalovirus, Epstein–Barr virus, and the human herpesviruses 6 and 7), lymphocytic choriomeningitis virus, and the human immunodeficiency virus (HIV).

Clinical Presentation

Patients with viral meningitis often present with typical symptoms and signs of meningitis, including headache, meningismus, fever, and photophobia (Connolly and Hammer, 1990; Rotbart, 1995; Sawyer and Rotbart, 2004). Symptoms associated with the causative virus may also be present, such as vomiting and diarrhea with the enteroviruses, vesicular rash with herpes simplex virus (HSV), and a mononucleosis-like syndrome with primary HIV infection. The duration of illness in enteroviral meningitis is usually less than 1 week, with many patients reporting improvement after lumbar puncture, probably as a result of reduction of intracranial pressure.

Diagnosis

In enteroviral meningitis, lumbar puncture usually reveals a lymphocytic pleocytosis (100–1000 cells mm^{-3}), although there may be a predominance of neutrophils early in the course of infection; however, this quickly gives way to a lymphocytic predominance over the first 6–48 hours (Connolly and Hammer, 1990; Rotbart, 1995; Sawyer and Rotbart, 2004; Romero, 2002). However, in a recent retrospective chart review, 51% of 53 patients with aseptic meningitis and duration of symptoms for more than 24 hours had a neutrophil predominance in CSF, suggesting that a CSF neutrophil predominance is not useful as a sole criterion in distinguishing between aseptic and bacterial meningitis (Negrini *et al.*, 2000). CSF protein is elevated, while glucose may be normal or low, although these abnormalities, if present, are usually mild. Similar CSF abnormalities are usually observed in other causes of viral meningitis.

Viral cultures are rarely helpful in the etiologic diagnosis of the aseptic meningitis syndrome, except in cases of HSV meningitis. Acute and convalescent serum titers may be obtained to identify specific etiologic agents but are not helpful in acute diagnosis and management. The isolation of a nonpolio enterovirus from the throat or gastrointestinal tract is supportive evidence for the diagnosis of meningitis in the appropriate clinical setting, although viral shedding may occur for several weeks after initial infection, making it difficult to rule out past infection. Furthermore, the time

Principles and Practice of Geriatric Medicine, 4th Edition. Edited by M.S. John Pathy, Alan J. Sinclair and John E. Morley.

required for identifying an enterovirus from CSF using cell cultures is too long to be of clinical utility in establishing the diagnosis.

The polymerase chain reaction (PCR) has been shown to be useful in the diagnosis of meningitis due to HSV type 2 (Tedder *et al.*, 1994; Kojima *et al.*, 2002), and may be helpful in the identification of HIV in the CSF or plasma of patients with meningitis following primary infection. Reverse transcription-polymerase chain reaction (RT-PCR) has also been utilized for detecting enteroviral RNA, with sensitivity ranging from 86 to 100% and specificity from 92 to 100% in the diagnosis of enteroviral meningitis (Sawyer and Rotbart, 2004; Romero, 2002; Rotbart, 1990).

Therapy

Viral meningitis is usually a self-limited illness, and in the majority of cases only supportive therapy is indicated (Connolly and Hammer, 1990; Rotbart, 1995; Sawyer and Rotbart, 2004). However, this may change in the future. Pleconaril, a novel compound that integrates into the hydrophobic pocket of picornaviruses, has recently been shown to have beneficial effects on the clinical, virologic, laboratory, and radiologic parameters in patients with severe enterovirus infections (Romero, 2002; Rotbart and Webster, 2001). In cases associated with HSV infection (most often an initial infection with HSV type 2), treatment of the genital infection with acyclovir often results in resolution of the meningitis.

Bacterial Meningitis

Epidemiology and Etiology

Although numerous bacterial pathogens have been reported to cause meningitis in the elderly, certain agents are isolated more frequently.

Streptococcus pneumoniae is the most common cause of bacterial meningitis in the elderly. A contiguous (e.g. sinusitis, otitis media, or mastoiditis) or distant (e.g. endocarditis or pneumonia) site of infection is often identified. More serious pneumococcal infections occur in elderly patients and in those with underlying conditions such as asplenia, multiple myeloma, alcoholism, malnutrition, diabetes mellitus, and hepatic or renal disease (Musher, 1992). *S. pneumoniae* is also the most common etiologic agent of meningitis in patients with basilar skull fracture and CSF leak (Kaufman *et al.*, 1990). In the United States, the overall mortality rates for pneumococcal meningitis have ranged from 19 to 26% (Schlech *et al.*, 1985; Wenger *et al.*, 1990; Schuchat *et al.*, 1997). For this reason, the 23-valent pneumococcal vaccine is recommended for all patients over the age of 65 and for those in high-risk groups for serious pneumococcal infection.

Persons at risk for infection (including meningitis) with *Listeria monocytogenes* are the elderly ($\geq$50 years of age), those with underlying malignancy, alcoholics, those receiving corticosteroids, immunosuppressed adults (e.g. transplant recipients), and patients with diabetes mellitus and iron overload disorders (Lorber, 1997; Mylonakis *et al.*, 1998). Although *L. monocytogenes* is an unusual cause of bacterial meningitis in the United States, it is associated with high mortality rates (15–29%) (Schlech *et al.*, 1985; Wenger *et al.*, 1990; Schuchat *et al.*, 1997). Outbreaks of *Listeria* infection have been associated with the consumption of contaminated coleslaw, raw vegetables and milk, with sporadic cases traced to contaminated cheese turkey franks, alfalfa tablets, and processed meats; this points to the intestinal tract as the usual portal of entry.

Bacterial meningitis caused by aerobic gram-negative bacilli (e.g. *Klebsiella* species, *Escherichia coli*, *Serratia marcescens*, and *Pseudomonas aeruginosa*) is found in the elderly, occurring after head trauma or neurosurgical procedures, and in patients with gram-negative bacteremia (Tunkel and Scheld, 2005). Some cases have been associated with disseminated strongyloidiasis in the hyperinfection syndrome, in which meningitis caused by enteric bacteria occurs secondary to seeding of the meninges during persistent or recurrent bacteremias associated with migration of infective larvae; alternatively, the larvae may carry enteric organisms on their surfaces or within their own gastrointestinal tracts as they exit the intestine and subsequently invade the meninges.

Other bacterial species are less common causes of bacterial meningitis in the elderly (Tunkel and Scheld, 2005). *Neisseria meningitidis* may cause meningitis during epidemics (caused by serogroups A and C) or in sporadic outbreaks (serogroup B), although meningitis caused by this microorganism is more common in children and adults. Respiratory tract infections, with viruses such as influenza virus, may play a role in the pathogenesis of invasive meningococcal disease. There is an increased incidence of neisserial infections, including that caused by *N. meningitidis*, in persons with deficiencies of the terminal complement components (C5, C6, C7, C8, and perhaps C9), although the case fatality rates in these patients are lower than in those with an intact complement system (Ross and Densen, 1984). *Hemophilus influenzae* meningitis in elderly adults is associated with concurrent infections such as sinusitis, otitis media, and pneumonia, and underlying conditions such as chronic obstructive pulmonary disease, asplenia, diabetes mellitus, immunosuppression, and head trauma with CSF leak (Farley *et al.*, 1992). Meningitis caused by *Staphylococcus aureus* is usually found in the early postneurosurgical period or after head trauma, or in patients with CSF shunts; other underlying conditions include diabetes mellitus, alcoholism, chronic renal failure requiring hemodialysis, injection drug use, and malignancies (Schlessinger *et al.*, 1987). *Staphylococcus epidermidis* is the most common cause of meningitis in patients with CSF shunts (Kojima *et al.*, 2002). The group B streptococcus (*Streptococcus agalactiae*) may cause meningitis in adults (Domingo *et al.*, 1997; Dunne and Quagliarello, 1993); risk factors include age greater than 60, diabetes mellitus, cardiac disease, collagen vascular disorders, malignancy, alcoholism, hepatic failure, renal failure, and corticosteroid therapy, although no underlying disease was found in 43% of patients in one study (Dunne and Quagliarello, 1993).

Clinical Presentation

The classic symptoms and signs in patients with bacterial meningitis include headache, fever, and meningismus; these are seen in more than 85% of patients (Tunkel and Scheld, 2005; Tunkel, 2001). In a review of community-acquired meningitis in adults (Durand *et al.*, 1993), the classic triad of fever, nuchal rigidity, and change in mental status was found in only two-thirds of patients. Another review found the absence of fever, neck stiffness, and altered mental status effectively eliminated the likelihood of acute meningitis in adults (sensitivity of 99–100% for the presence of one finding in the diagnosis of acute meningitis) (Attia *et al.*, 1999). Other findings include cranial nerve palsies (~10–20%), seizures (~30%), and Kernig's and/or Brudzinski's signs. However, in a recent prospective study that examined the diagnostic accuracy of meningeal signs in adults with suspected meningitis, the sensitivity of Kernig's sign was 5%, Brudzinski's sign, 5%, and nuchal rigidity, 30% (Thomas *et al.*, 2002), indicating that the presence of these signs did not accurately distinguish patients with meningitis from those without meningitis. With disease progression, patients may develop signs of increased intracranial pressure such as hypertension, bradycardia, oculomotor nerve palsy, and coma.

However, elderly patients with bacterial meningitis, especially those with underlying conditions (e.g. diabetes mellitus or cardiopulmonary disease), may present insidiously with lethargy, confusion, anorexia, no fever, and variable signs of meningeal inflammation (Tunkel, 2001). In one review (Gorse *et al.*, 1989), confusion was very common in elderly patients on initial examination and occurred in 92 and 78% of those with pneumococcal and gram-negative bacillary meningitis, respectively. There may be a history of an antecedent or concurrent illness such as sinusitis, otitis media, or pneumonia. In the elderly patient, an altered or changed mental status should not be ascribed to other causes until bacterial meningitis has been excluded by CSF examination.

Clues to the causative agent in a patient with bacterial meningitis include the presence of a petechial or purpuric rash (*N. meningitidis*), rhinorrhea or otorrhea after a basilar skull fracture (*S. pneumoniae*), following neurosurgery or head trauma (staphylococcal spp. or aerobic gram-negative bacilli), or seizures, focal neurological deficits, ataxia, and cranial nerve palsies (*L. monocytogenes*) (Tunkel and Scheld, 2005; Tunkel, 2001).

Diagnosis

The diagnosis of bacterial meningitis rests with CSF examination following lumbar puncture (Tunkel and Scheld, 2005; Tunkel, 2001). CSF characteristics of bacterial meningitis include an elevated opening pressure in virtually all patients; values over 600 mmH_2O suggest the presence of cerebral edema, intracranial suppurative foci, or communicating hydrocephalus. The white blood cell count is elevated in untreated bacterial meningitis (usually 1000–5000 cells mm^{-3}) with a neutrophilic predominance, although lymphocytes may predominate in *L. monocytogenes* meningitis (~30% of cases). A CSF white blood cell count of <20 cells mm^{-3}, along with a high concentration of organisms, is indicative of a poor prognosis. An elevated protein (100–500 mg dl^{-1}) and decreased glucose (<40 mg dl^{-1}) are also typically observed; a CSF: serum glucose of $\leq$0.4 is found in the majority of patients with acute bacterial meningitis.

The CSF Gram stain provides rapid and accurate identification of the causative organism in 60–90% of patients with bacterial meningitis, with a specificity of almost 100%. Bacteria are observed in 90% of cases of meningitis caused by *S. pneumoniae*, but in only about one-third of patients with *L. monocytogenes* meningitis (Gray and Fedorko, 1992). CSF cultures are positive in 70–85% of patients overall. The probability of identifying the organism in CSF cultures may decrease in patients who have received prior antimicrobial therapy.

Several rapid diagnostic tests are available to aid in the etiologic diagnosis of bacterial meningitis (Tunkel and Scheld, 2005; Tunkel, 2001; Gray and Fedorko, 1992). Initial tests utilized counterimmunoelectrophoresis, although newer tests (staphylococcal coagglutination or latex agglutination) are rapid ($\leq$15 minutes) and more sensitive than counterimmunoelectrophoresis. Current latex agglutination tests detect the antigens of *H. influenzae* type b, *S. pneumoniae, N. meningitidis, E. coli* K1, and *S. agalactiae*. The overall sensitivity ranges from 50 to 100% (somewhat lower for *N. meningitidis* because of the limited immunogenicity of the group B meningococcal polysaccharide), although these tests are highly specific. However, the routine use of latex agglutination for the etiologic diagnosis of bacterial meningitis has recently been questioned, because results do not appear to modify the decision to administer appropriate antimicrobial therapy and false-positive tests have been reported (Tunkel *et al.*, 2004). Therefore, use of CSF latex agglutination is no longer routinely recommended in the determination of the microbial etiology in a patient with bacterial meningitis. Latex agglutination may be most useful for the patient who has been pretreated with antimicrobial therapy and whose CSF Gram stain and cultures are negative, although it must be emphasized that a negative test does not rule out infection by a specific meningeal pathogen.

PCR has also been studied on CSF specimens from patients with meningococcal meningitis, with a sensitivity and specificity of 91% in one study (Ni *et al.*, 1992). In another study, broad-based PCR demonstrated a sensitivity of 100%, a specificity of 98.2%, a positive predictive value of 98.2%, and a negative predictive value of 100% (Saravolatz *et al.*, 2003). Further refinements in PCR may demonstrate its usefulness in the diagnosis of bacterial meningitis in patients who already received antibiotics and when the CSF Gram stain, bacterial antigen tests and cultures are negative.

Antimicrobial Therapy

In patients suspected of having bacterial meningitis, blood cultures should be obtained and a lumbar puncture done immediately. If purulent meningitis is present, targeted antimicrobial therapy should be initiated on the basis of results of Gram staining (e.g. vancomycin and a third-generation cephalosporin if gram-positive diplococci are seen). However, if no etiologic agent can be identified or if there is a delay in the performance of the lumbar puncture, empiric antimicrobial therapy should be initiated on the basis of the patient's age and the underlying disease status (Tunkel and Scheld, 2005; Tunkel, 2001; Tunkel *et al.*, 2004). In patients who are immunosuppressed and have a history of central nervous system (CNS) disease, focal neurologic deficits, seizures or if papilledema is found on funduscopic examination, computed tomographic (CT) scan is recommended prior to lumbar puncture, with empiric antimicrobial therapy initiated before scanning. Empiric therapy for elderly patients with suspected community-acquired bacterial meningitis should include vancomycin, ampicillin, and a third-generation cephalosporin (see following text for specific recommendations). Once the meningeal pathogen is identified, antimicrobial therapy can be modified for optimal treatment (Table 1); recommended dosages for CNS infections are shown in Table 2.

For treatment of bacterial meningitis in elderly persons, choices of antimicrobial therapy should be based on prevalent trends in antimicrobial susceptibility. For meningitis caused by *S. pneumoniae*, therapy in recent years has been significantly altered by changes in pneumococcal susceptibility patterns (Tunkel and Scheld, 2005; Tunkel, 2001; Tunkel *et al.*, 2004). Numerous reports from around the world have documented strains of pneumococci that are of intermediate susceptibility (minimal inhibitory concentration (MIC) range of 0.1 to 1.0 $\mu g\,ml^{-1}$) and highly (MIC $\geq 2.0\,\mu g\,ml^{-1}$) resistant to penicillin G; susceptible strains have MICs $\leq 0.06\,\mu g\,ml^{-1}$. On the basis of these trends and because achievable CSF concentrations of penicillin are inadequate to treat these resistant isolates, penicillin can never be recommended as empiric therapy for patients with suspected or proven pneumococcal meningitis, pending results of susceptibility testing. As an empiric regimen, we recommend the combination of vancomycin plus a third-generation cephalosporin (either cefotaxime or ceftriaxone). If the isolate is susceptible to penicillin, high-dose intravenous penicillin G or ampicillin is adequate. If the isolate is relatively resistant to penicillin, only the third-generation cephalosporin needs to be continued. However, if the pneumococcal isolate is highly resistant to penicillin, the combination of vancomycin and the third-generation cephalosporin should be continued, because vancomycin therapy alone

Table 1 Specific antimicrobial therapy for meningitis

Microorganism	Standard therapy	Alternative therapies
Bacteria		
Streptococcus pneumoniae		
Penicillin MIC $<0.1\,\mu g\,ml^{-1}$	Penicillin G or ampicillin	Third-generation cephalosporin[a]; vancomycin
Penicillin MIC $0.1-1.0\,\mu g\,ml^{-1}$	Third-generation cephalosporin[a]	Meropenem; vancomycin
Penicillin MIC $\geq 2.0\,\mu g\,ml^{-1}$	Vancomycin plus a third-generation cephalosporin[a,b]	Third-generation cephalosporin plus a fluoroquinolone[c]
Enterobacteriaceae	Third-generation cephalosporin[a]	Aztreonam; fluoroquinolone; trimethoprim–sulfamethoxazole; meropenem
Pseudomonas aeruginosa	Ceftazidime[d] or cefepime[d]	Aztreonam[d]; fluoroquinolone[d]; meropenem[d]
Listeria monocytogenes	Ampicillin or penicillin G[d]	Trimethoprim–sulfamethoxazole
Hemophilus influenzae		
β-lactamase-negative	Ampicillin	Third-generation cephalosporin[a]; cefepime; chloramphenicol; aztreonam
β-lactamase-positive	Third-generation cephalosporin[a]	Cefepime, chloramphenicol; aztreonam; fluoroquinolone
Neisseria meningitidis	Penicillin G or ampicillin	Third-generation cephalosporin[a]; chloramphenicol; fluoroquinolone
Streptococcus agalactiae	Ampicillin or penicillin G[d]	Third-generation cephalosporin[a]; vancomycin
Staphylococcus aureus		
Methicillin-sensitive	Nafcillin or oxacillin	Vancomycin
Methicillin-resistant	Vancomycin	
Staphylococcus epidermidis	Vancomycin[b]	
Myobacteria		
Mycobacterium tuberculosis	Isoniazid plus rifampin plus pyrazinamide	Ethambutol[e]; streptomycin[e]; ciprofloxacin[e]
Spirochetes		
Treponema pallidum	Penicillin G	Doxycycline[f]; ceftriaxone[f]
Borrelia burgdorferi	Third-generation cephalosporin[a]	Penicillin; doxycycline
Fungi		
Cryptococcus neoformans	Amphotericin B[g]	Fluconazole
Candida species	Amphotericin B[g]	Fluconazole[f]
Coccidioides immitis	Fluconazole	Amphotericin B[h]

[a]Cefotaxime or ceftriaxone. [b]Addition of rifampin should be considered. [c]Fluoroquinolones with activity against *S. pneumoniae* should be used; see text for details. [d]Addition of an aminoglycoside should be considered. [e]Add to standard therapy in cases of suspected drug resistance; see text for details. [f]Value of these antimicrobial agents has not been established. [g]Addition of 5-flucytosine should be considered. [h]Intravenous and intraventricular administration.

Table 2 Maximal recommended dosages of antimicrobial agents for central nervous system infections in adults with normal renal and hepatic function[a]

Antimicrobial agent	Total daily dose	Dosing interval (hours)
Acyclovir	$30\,mg\,kg^{-1}$	8
Amikacin[b]	$15\,mg\,kg^{-1}$	8
Amphotericin B[c]	$0.6-1.0\,mg\,kg^{-1}$	24
Amphotericin B lipid formulation	$5\,mg\,kg^{-1}$	24
Ampicillin	12 g	4
Aztreonam	6–8 g	6–8
Cefepime	6 g	8
Cefotaxime	8–12 g	4–6
Ceftazidime	6 g	8
Ceftriaxone	4 g	12–24
Chloramphenicol[d]	4–6 g	6
Ciprofloxacin	800–1200 mg	8–12
Doxycycline	200–400 mg	12
Ethambutol[e,f]	$15\,mg\,kg^{-1}$	24
Fluconazole	400–800 mg	24
Flucytosine[e,g]	$100\,mg\,kg^{-1}$	6
Gentamicin[b]	$5\,mg\,kg^{-1}$	8
Imipenem	2 g	6
Isoniazid[e,h]	300 mg	24
Liposomal amphotericin B (AmBisome)	$5\,mg\,kg^{-1}$	24
Meropenem	6 g	8
Metronidazole	$30\,mg\,kg^{-1}$	6
Nafcillin	9–12 g	4
Oxacillin	9–12 g	4
Penicillin G	24 million units	4
Pyrazinamide[e,i]	$15-30\,mg\,kg^{-1}$	24
Rifampicin (rifampin)[e]	600 mg	24
Streptomycin[j,k]	$15\,mg\,kg^{-1}$	24
Tobramycin[b]	$5\,mg\,kg^{-1}$	8
Trimethoprim–sulfamethoxazole[l]	$10-20\,mg\,kg^{-1}$	6–12
Vancomycin[b,m]	$30-45\,mg\,kg^{-1}$	8–12
Voriconazole[n]	$8\,mg\,kg^{-1}$	12

[a]Unless indicated, therapy is administered intravenously. [b]Need to monitor peak and trough serum concentrations. [c]Can increase dosage to $1.5\,mg\,kg^{-1}$ per day in severely ill patients. [d]Higher dose recommended for pneumococcal meningitis. [e]Oral administration. [f]Maximum daily dosage of 2.5 g. [g]Maintain serum concentrations from 50 to $100\,\mu g\,ml^{-1}$. [h]Initiate therapy at a dosage of $10\,mg\,kg^{-1}$ per day. [i]Maximum daily dosage of 2 g. [j]Intramuscular administration. [k]Maximal daily dosage of 1 g. [l]Dosage based on trimethoprim component. [m]May need to monitor cerebrospinal fluid concentrations in severely ill patients. [n]Load with $6\,mg\,kg^{-1}$ IV every 12 hours for two doses.

may not be optimal therapy for patients with pneumococcal meningitis. Any patient who is not improving as expected, or has a pneumococcal isolate for which the cefotaxime/ceftriaxone MIC is $\geq 2.0\,\mu g\,ml^{-1}$ should undergo a repeat lumbar puncture to document sterility of CSF after 36–48 hours of therapy (Tunkel *et al.*, 2004); this may be especially important for patients who are also receiving adjunctive dexamethasone therapy (see following text). Some experts have also recommended the addition of rifampin for these highly resistant strains, although there are no clinical data to support this recommendation. In patients not responding, administration of vancomycin by the intraventricular of intrathecal route is a reasonable adjunct. Newer fluoroquinolones (e.g. moxifloxacin, gatifloxacin, gemafloxacin, garenoxacin) that have *in vitro* activity against *S. pneumoniae* may have utility in the treatment of pneumococcal meningitis (Tunkel *et al.*, 2004; Cottagnoud and Tauber, 2003). Trovafloxacin has been compared to ceftriaxone with or without vancomycin in children with bacterial meningitis (Saez-Llorens *et al.*, 2002), and both treatment groups had similar outcomes in terms of CSF sterilization and clinical success. Although trovafloxacin is no longer used because of concerns of liver toxicity, these data suggest the benefit of the newer fluoroquinolones in the treatment of bacterial meningitis. However, further clinical trials are needed before these agents can be recommended.

Adjunctive Therapy

Despite the availability of effective antimicrobial therapy, the mortality and morbidity from bacterial meningitis has not significantly changed over the past 20 years. Studies in experimental animal models of infection have demonstrated that a major factor contributing to increased morbidity and mortality is the generation of a subarachnoid space inflammatory response following antimicrobial-induced bacterial lysis (Tunkel, 2001). Administration of the anti-inflammatory agent dexamethasone was effective in attenuation of this inflammatory response, and led to several clinical trials examining the use of adjunctive dexamethasone in the therapy of bacterial meningitis. Most of these studies were conducted in infants and children with predominantly *H. influenzae* type b meningitis and supported the routine use of adjunctive dexamethasone in this patient population (Tunkel and Scheld, 2005; Tunkel, 2001).

Until recently, the use of adjunctive dexamethasone was not recommended in adults with bacterial meningitis. In a recently published prospective, randomized, double-blind trial in 301 adults with bacterial meningitis, adjunctive dexamethasone was associated with a reduction in the proportion of patients who had unfavorable outcomes and in the proportion of patients who died (de Gans and van de Beek, 2002); the benefits were most striking in the subgroup of patients with pneumococcal meningitis and in those with moderate-to-severe disease as assessed by the admission Glasgow Coma Scale score.

On the basis of these data and the apparent absence of serious adverse outcomes in the patients who received dexamethasone, the routine use of adjunctive dexamethasone ($0.15\,mg\,kg^{-1}$ every 6 hours for 2–4 days, given concomitant with or just prior to the first dose of an antimicrobial agent for maximal attenuation of the subarachnoid space inflammatory response) is warranted in adults with suspected or proven pneumococcal meningitis (Tunkel *et al.*, 2004; Tunkel and Scheld, 2002a). Adjunctive dexamethasone should not be used in patients who have already received antimicrobial therapy; if the meningitis is subsequently found not to be caused by *S. pneumoniae*, dexamethasone should be discontinued. However, the use of adjunctive dexamethasone is of particular concern in patients with pneumococcal meningitis caused by highly penicillin-resistant strains, since a diminished inflammatory response may significantly impair

CSF vancomycin penetration. In an experimental model of *S. pneumoniae* meningitis in rabbits, the concurrent use of dexamethasone with vancomycin decreased the penetration of vancomycin into the CSF and also decreased the rate of bactericidal activity of vancomycin. In patients with pneumococcal meningitis caused by strains that are highly resistant to penicillin or cephalosporins, careful observation and follow-up are critical to determine whether the use of adjunctive dexamethasone is associated with adverse clinical outcome in these patients.

Tuberculous Meningitis

Epidemiology and Etiology

Almost all cases of tuberculous meningitis are caused by *Mycobacterium tuberculosis*. Risk factors for the development of tuberculous meningitis include a history of prior tuberculous disease, advanced age, homelessness, alcoholism, gastrectomy, diabetes mellitus, and immunosuppression (Leonard and Des Prez, 1990). HIV infection has influenced the epidemiology of tuberculosis, in which extrapulmonary disease occurs in more than 70% of patients with AIDS, but in only 24–45% of patients with tuberculosis and less advanced HIV infection (Barnes *et al.*, 1991).

Clinical Presentation

Tuberculous meningitis often has a subacute, indolent presentation with a prodrome characterized by malaise, low-grade fever, headache, and personality changes (Leonard and Des Prez, 1990; Kent *et al.*, 1993); this is followed by a meningitic phase with worsening headache, meningismus, nausea, vomiting, and waxing-and-waning mental status. A history of prior clinical tuberculosis is obtained in fewer than 20% of cases. Up to 30% of patients have focal neurologic signs on presentation, usually consisting of unilateral or, less commonly, bilateral cranial nerve palsies (cranial nerve (CN) VI is the most frequently affected). Hemiparesis may result from ischemic infarction, most commonly in the distribution of the territory of the middle cerebral artery.

Diagnosis

CSF examination in patients with tuberculous meningitis often reveals a lymphocytic pleocytosis (5–500 cells mm^{-3}), although early in the course of disease there may be a mix of both lymphocytes and neutrophils (Leonard and Des Prez, 1990; Ogawa *et al.*, 1987). Following treatment with antituberculous drugs, a so-called "therapeutic paradox" may develop with a change in the white blood cell differential from a lymphocytic to a neutrophilic predominance. There is usually an elevated CSF protein (median of 150–200 mg dl^{-1}) and often a very low glucose (<20 mg dl^{-1}, although the median value is 40 mg dl^{-1}).

Because of the low number of organisms present in the CSF, acid-fast bacilli (AFB) smears are often negative (fewer than 25% of smears are positive). The sensitivity of smears of CSF was improved to 86% in one study by examination of up to four concentrated CSF specimens from repeated lumbar punctures (Kennedy and Fallon, 1979), although these results have not been duplicated.

On the basis of these poor results, several rapid diagnostic tests are under development to aid in the diagnosis of tuberculous meningitis. The most promising appears to be PCR, which can detect *M. tuberculosis* DNA in CSF specimens (Sinner and Tunkel, 2002; Zugar, 2004).

CT and magnetic resonance (MR) scanning may be useful to support the diagnosis of tuberculous meningitis (Leonard and Des Prez, 1990; Zugar, 2004). Hydrocephalus is frequently present at diagnosis or develops during the course of infection. The presence of basal cistern enhancement is also supportive evidence for the diagnosis. MR may be superior to CT in the identification of basilar meningeal inflammation and small tuberculoma formation.

Antimicrobial Therapy

Therapy for tuberculous meningitis is often initiated on the basis of the patient's clinical presentation, as cultures may take weeks to become positive and may remain negative in up to 20% of patients. In areas where drug resistance is not a problem, therapy with isoniazid, rifampin, and pyrazinamide for 2 months, followed by isoniazid and rifampin, should be adequate (Leonard and Des Prez, 1990; Sinner and Tunkel, 2002; Zugar, 2004). However, in areas with >4% isoniazid resistance, ethambutol or streptomycin should be added to the above regimen, and all four drugs continued until susceptibility results are available. Six months of therapy are used in most patients, although some authorities recommend a total treatment duration of 9 months for patients with tuberculous meningitis. In HIV-infected patients, therapy is continued for at least 12 months. For patients with suspected tuberculous meningitis caused by multidrug-resistant strains, at least five drugs should be used pending susceptibility testing. The fluoroquinolones (e.g. ciprofloxacin, ofloxacin) penetrate well into CSF and have good *in vitro* activity against *M. tuberculosis.* Most authorities recommend continuing therapy for a total of 18–24 months in patients with multidrug-resistant tuberculous meningitis.

Adjunctive Therapy

Corticosteroids have been shown to be of value as adjunctive therapy in tuberculous meningitis with resolution of fevers, improved mental status, and most importantly, the ability to treat or avert the development of spinal block (Leonard and Des Prez, 1990; Sinner and Tunkel, 2002; Zugar, 2004). Despite some controversy, most authorities recommend the use of corticosteroids in patients with tuberculous meningitis with extreme neurologic compromise, elevated intracranial pressure, impending herniation, or impending or established spinal block; some authors also recommend their use in patients with CT evidence of either hydrocephalus or basilar meningitis. Recommended therapy is prednisone 1 mg kg^{-1} per day slowly tapered over 1 month, although varying doses of dexamethasone or hydrocortisone have also been used. In a recent randomized, double-blind, placebo-controlled trial in Vietnam in patients with tuberculous meningitis, adjunctive dexamethasone improved survival in patients over 14 years of age (Thwaites *et al.*, 2004), although probably did not prevent severe disability.

Spirochetal Meningitis

Epidemiology and Etiology

Treponema pallidum (the etiologic agent of syphilis) disseminates to the CNS early during infection, with CSF abnormalities detected in 5–9% of patients with seronegative primary syphilis (Hook and Marra, 1992). The overall incidence of neurosyphilis has recently increased in association with HIV infection; in one report (Musher *et al.*, 1990), 44% of all patients with neurosyphilis had AIDS and 1.5% of AIDS patients were found to have neurosyphilis at some point during the course of their illness.

Approximately 10–15% of patients with Lyme disease will develop signs and symptoms of meningitis, usually early in the course of infection (Cadavid, 2004; Steere, 1989). Infection with *Borrelia burgdorferi* should be suspected in a patient with meningitis in association with other symptoms of Lyme disease, such as erythema migrans, malaise, myalgias, and arthralgias. Meningitis usually follows erythema migrans by 2–10 weeks, although only about 40% (range of 10–90%) of cases of Lyme meningitis are preceded by this characteristic rash. Illness occurs from May to November, with a peak incidence during the summer months.

Clinical Presentation

There are four categories of CNS involvement with *T. pallidum* (Hook and Marra, 1992; Marra, 2004). Syphilitic meningitis occurs within the first two years of infection, with symptoms of headache, nausea, vomiting, and less frequently fevers, meningismus, and mental status changes. Meningovascular syphilis (found in 10–12% of individuals with CNS involvement), occurring months to years after infection, results in focal neurologic findings as a result of focal syphilitic arteritis, which almost always occurs in association with meningeal inflammation; focal deficits may progress to a stroke syndrome with attendant irreversible neurologic deficits. Parenchymatous neurosyphilis (10–20 years after infection) manifests as general paresis and tabes dorsalis. Gummatous disease is very rare, and generally occurs more than 30 years following initial infection. Coinfection with HIV may alter the clinical course of syphilis, in which patients may be more likely to progress to neurosyphilis and show accelerated disease courses.

Symptoms of CNS infection with *B. burgdorferi* include headache, fever, meningismus, nausea, and vomiting (Cadavid, 2004; Steere, 1989). Up to 50% of patients will develop cranial nerve palsies, most commonly involving CN VII; facial nerve palsy is bilateral in 30–70% of patients, although the two sides are affected asynchronously in most cases. In untreated patients the duration of symptoms is 1–9 months and patients typically experience recurrent attacks of meningeal symptoms lasting several weeks, alternating with similar periods of milder symptoms. About half of the patients with Lyme meningitis have mild cerebral symptoms, consisting of somnolence, emotional lability, depression, impaired memory and concentration, and behavioral symptoms.

Diagnosis

CSF findings in patients with CNS syphilis are nonspecific, revealing a mononuclear pleocytosis (>10 cells mm^{-3} in most patients), elevated protein, and a normal or slightly decreased glucose (Hook and Marra, 1992; Marra, 2004). A reactive VDRL (venereal disease research laboratory) slide test in the CSF has a sensitivity of only 30–70% for the diagnosis of neurosyphilis (although the specificity is high), so treatment for neurosyphilis is indicated in the presence of any of the above abnormalities in association with the appropriate clinical setting. The fluorescent treponemal antibody absorption test (FTA-ABS), in the CSF has been examined as a possible diagnostic test for neurosyphilis; a nonreactive test effectively rules out the likelihood of neurosyphilis, although a positive test may result from the leakage of small amounts of antibody absorption from the serum into CSF, making it less specific than the CSF VDRL.

The best currently available laboratory test for the diagnosis of Lyme disease is the demonstration of specific serum antibody to *B. burgdorferi*, in which a positive test in a patient with a compatible neurologic abnormality is strong evidence for the diagnosis (Cadavid, 2004; Steere, 1989). It is currently recommended that when the pretest probability of Lyme disease is 0.20–0.80, sequential testing with enzyme-linked immunosorbent assay (ELISA) and Western blot is the most accurate method for ruling in or out the possibility of Lyme disease (American College of Physicians, 1997). A lymphocytic pleocytosis (usually <500 cells mm^{-3}) is observed in the CSF, along with an elevated protein and normal glucose in patients with Lyme meningitis. Antibodies and antigens to *B. burgdorferi* may be detected in the CSF by ELISA or Western blot, respectively, although antibody tests are not standardized with marked variability between laboratories. PCR may be a useful tool for the detection of *B. burgdorferi* DNA in CSF (Keller *et al.*, 1992), although PCR must still be considered experimental in the diagnosis of CNS Lyme disease (Connolly and Hammer, 1990).

Antimicrobial Therapy

Treatment for neurosyphilis is intravenous penicillin G 18–24 million units day in divided doses every 4 hours for 10–14 days (Marra, 2004). No large studies have been performed to evaluate alternative antimicrobial agents for the therapy of neurosyphilis; the tetracyclines, chloramphenicol, and ceftriaxone may have potential clinical utility based on case reports, clinical experience, and extrapolations from experimental animal studies.

Treatment of Lyme meningitis is intravenous ceftriaxone 2 g day for 2–4 weeks; the literature contains no agreement on the duration of therapy or on the minimal adequate dose of the antimicrobial (Cadavid, 2004; Steere, 1989). At present, there is no evidence to support treatment durations of longer than 4 weeks.

Fungal Meningitis

Epidemiology and Etiology

Cryptococcus neoformans is the most common fungal cause of clinically recognized meningitis with most cases seen in immunocompromised patients, including those with AIDS, transplant recipients, and in those receiving chronic corticosteroids (Tunkel and Scheld, 2002b). Other underlying conditions with an increased risk for cryptococcal disease include sarcoidosis, collagen vascular disorders (e.g. systemic lupus erythematosus), chronic renal and hepatic failure, and diabetes mellitus; *C. neoformans* meningitis has also been documented in apparently healthy individuals.

Meningitis due to *Candida* species is relatively rare and is often associated with disseminated disease. Risk factors include malignancy, neutropenia, chronic granulomatous disease, the presence of central venous catheters, diabetes mellitus, hyperalimentation, and corticosteroid therapy (Tunkel and Scheld, 2002b).

Coccidioides immitis is a fungus endemic to the semiarid regions and the desert areas of southwestern US. Lesser than 1% of infected patients develop disseminated disease, although, of those, one-third to one-half has meningeal involvement. Dissemination is associated with extremes of age, male gender, nonwhite race, and immunosuppression (e.g. corticosteroid therapy, organ transplantation, and HIV infection) (Tunkel and Scheld, 2002b; Ampel *et al.*, 1989).

Clinical Presentation

Clinical presentation of cryptococcal meningitis is different in non-AIDS and AIDS patients (Tunkel and Scheld, 2002b). In non-AIDS patients the presentation is typically subacute after days to weeks of infection with symptoms of headache and mental status changes, with or without fevers and meningismus. Ocular abnormalities (e.g. cranial nerve palsies and papilledema) occur in about 40% of patients. In contrast, AIDS patients may present with very minimal symptoms; the only clinical findings may be fever, headache and lethargy, and cranial nerve palsies are often absent.

Patients with *Candida* meningitis may present either abruptly or insidiously (Tunkel and Scheld, 2002b). Symptoms include fever, headache, and meningismus; patients may also have depressed mental status, confusion, cranial nerve palsies, and focal neurologic signs. The presentation is often similar to that observed with bacterial meningitis.

Meningeal infection with *C. immitis* most often follows a subacute or chronic course (Tunkel and Scheld, 2002b; Ampel *et al.*, 1989). Clinical findings include headache, low-grade fever, weight loss and mental status changes; disorientation, lethargy, confusion, or memory loss are seen in about 50% of patients. Signs of meningeal irritation have been reported in as many as one-third of patients.

Diagnosis

In most non-AIDS patients with cryptococcal meningitis, examination of the CSF reveals an elevated opening pressure, lymphocytic pleocytosis (range of 20–500 cells mm^{-3}), elevated protein, and normal or decreased glucose (Tunkel and Scheld, 2002b). AIDS patients with cryptococcal meningitis may have very low or even normal CSF white blood cell counts; 65% of patients have fewer than 5 cells mm^{-3} in CSF. India ink examination is positive in up to 50–75% of patients with cryptococcal meningitis, and the rate of positivity is even higher (~88%) in AIDS patients. As the India ink examination is difficult to perform and rates of positivity are dependent upon the experience of the laboratory, the latex agglutination test for cryptococcal polysaccharide antigen in the CSF should be performed and is both sensitive and specific for the diagnosis of cryptococcal meningitis, as long as samples are heated to eliminate rheumatoid factor. A presumptive diagnosis is indicated by a titer of $\geq 1:8$. The presence of cryptococcal antigen in the serum is also supportive evidence for the diagnosis, and may be detected in severely immunocompromised patients (i.e. those with AIDS); however, the value of the serum cryptococcal polysaccharide antigen for screening patients suspected of having meningeal disease has not been established. Routine and fungal cultures of the CSF are often positive.

Examination of the CSF in patients with *Candida* meningitis typically shows a mixture of neutrophils and lymphocytes, elevated protein, and decreased glucose. Yeast cells are seen on smear in approximately 50% of patients, with fungal cultures positive in most cases.

CSF examination in coccidioidal meningitis reveals a pleocytosis, occasionally showing a prominent eosinophilia (Tunkel and Scheld, 2002b; Ampel *et al.*, 1989). Unfortunately, only about 25–50% of patients have positive CSF cultures. Elevated serum concentrations of complement-fixing antibodies (titers in excess of 1 : 32–1 : 64) suggest dissemination. CSF complement-fixing antibodies are present in at least 70% of patients with early meningitis and from virtually all patients as disease progresses, although antibodies may fail to develop in the serum or CSF of patients with immunodeficiencies. When present, the antibody titers appear to parallel the course of meningeal disease.

Antimicrobial Therapy

The treatment of cryptococcal meningitis in non-AIDS patients is amphotericin B with 5-flucytosine for 4–6 weeks (Tunkel and Scheld, 2002b). The 4-week combination regimen can be used in the subset of patients who, at presentation, have no neurologic compromise, no underlying diseases, no immunosuppressive therapy, a pretreatment CSF white cell count $>20\,\mathrm{mm}^{-3}$, and a serum cryptococcal antigen titer of <1 : 32; and who, at 4 weeks, have a negative CSF India ink and CSF cryptococcal antigen titer <1 : 8. The optimal use of fluconazole in non-AIDS patients with cryptococcal meningitis is unclear. In a recently published report of 157 non-HIV infected with CNS cryptococcosis (Pappas *et al.*, 2001), patients were more likely to receive an induction regimen with amphotericin B and subsequent fluconazole, suggesting a role for fluconazole for consolidation therapy in this patient population. However, pending further data, non-AIDS patients should receive 4–6 weeks of amphotericin B plus 5-flucytosine.

Although the optimal therapeutic regimen for treating cryptococcal meningitis in AIDS patients has not been determined, the consensus is to use amphotericin B with or without 5-flucytosine for the initial 2 weeks of therapy or until a clinical response is obtained, followed by fluconazole at 400 mg day to complete a 10-week course. Doses of fluconazole up to 800 mg day have benefited some AIDS patients with cryptococcal meningitis who failed primary therapy or who relapsed (Berry *et al.*, 1992). Liposomal formulations of amphotericin B have also shown efficacy in AIDS patients with cryptococcal meningitis (Sharkey *et al.*, 1996; Leendera *et al.*, 1997). Chronic suppressive therapy with fluconazole (200 mg daily) is then continued indefinitely in patients with AIDS to prevent relapse.

Treatment of meningitis caused by *Candida* species is amphotericin B, with or without 5-flucytosine (Slavoski and Tunkel, 1995). Although there are no studies comparing the efficacy of single versus combination therapy, some investigators recommend combination therapy based on more rapid CSF sterilization and possible reduction of long-term neurologic sequelae in newborns. The efficacy of fluconazole in *Candida* meningitis has yet to be proven, but may be an acceptable alternative.

The previously recommended therapeutic regimen for coccidioidal meningitis was amphotericin B, administered both intravenously and intrathecally (Slavoski and Tunkel, 1995). Intrathecal administration may be via the lumbar, cisternal or ventricular route (i.e. through an Ommaya reservoir). The usual dosage is 0.5 mg 3 times weekly for 3 months, although 1.0–1.5 mg combined with hydrocortisone can be used. Antifungal therapy is discontinued once the CSF has been normal for at least 1 year on an intrathecal regimen of once every 6 weeks. Fluconazole has been examined in the therapy of coccidioidal meningitis, with one study revealing a response rate of 79%, although 24% of patients exhibited a persistent CSF pleocytosis despite the relative absence of symptoms (Galgiani *et al.*, 1993). On the basis of these results, fluconazole is recommended as first-line therapy for coccidioidal meningitis; therapy may need to be continued indefinitely.

Adjunctive Therapy

Increased intracranial pressure and hydrocephalus have been noted in AIDS patients with cryptococcal meningitis. Ventriculoperitoneal shunting, frequent high-volume lumbar punctures, acetazolamide, and corticosteroids have been used for these complications (Fessler *et al.*, 1998; Park *et al.*, 1999), although the precise roles of these measures remain to be established. Removal of CSF should be performed in patients with persistent elevated opening pressures after lumbar puncture; shunting procedures can ameliorate the sequelae of elevated intracranial pressure in AIDS patients with cryptococcal meningitis.

FOCAL CENTRAL NERVOUS SYSTEM INFECTIONS

Brain Abscess

Epidemiology and Etiology

Bacterial brain abscesses may be due to a single organism or may be polymicrobial in origin (Tunkel, 2005a; Mathisen and Johnson, 1997; Heilpern and Lorber, 1996). Clues to the likely etiologic agents may be found in the patient's history. Streptococci (aerobic, anaerobic, and microaerophilic) are identified in up to 70% of patients. They are normal inhabitants of the oral cavity, gastrointestinal tract, and female genital tract. Although streptococcal brain abscesses are seen most often in patients with otopharyngeal infections or infective endocarditis, they are isolated after neurosurgical or other medical procedures. Staphylococci are found in 10–15% of patients, usually those with a history of trauma or injection drug use. *Bacteroides fragilis* is identified in 20–40% of patients, often in mixed cultures. Enteric gram-negative bacilli are isolated in 23–33% of patients with brain abscess, often in patients with otitic foci of infection, septicemia, following neurosurgical procedures, or in those who are immunocompromised. Other bacteria (*S. pneumoniae, H. influenzae,* and *L. monocytogenes*) are seen much less frequently (<1% of cases). Patients with defects in cell-mediated immunity (e.g. patients with AIDS, transplant recipients and those receiving corticosteroids) have an increased incidence of brain abscess caused by *Nocardia* species.

Brain abscesses caused by *Aspergillus* species are seen in patients with hematologic malignancies and those with prolonged neutropenia; other risk groups include patients with Cushing's syndrome, diabetes mellitus, and hepatic disease (Tunkel, 2005a; Cortez and Walsh, 2004). Risk factors for development of cerebral mucormycosis include patients with diabetes mellitus (especially in association with diabetic ketoacidosis), hematologic malignancies, transplant recipients, and corticosteroid or deferoxamine use. Infection caused by either agent may result from direct extension of rhinocerebral disease or from hematogenous spread from a distant focus of infection.

Clinical Presentation

Symptoms in patients with bacterial brain abscess result from the presence of a space-occupying lesion, and include headache (~70% of cases), nausea, vomiting, and seizures (Tunkel, 2005a; Mathisen and Johnson, 1997; Heilpern and Lorber, 1996). Many patients also experience a change in mental status, ranging from lethargy to coma. Fever is found in only 45–50% of patients. The clinical presentation also depends upon the location of the abscess. Frontal lobe involvement may result in headache, drowsiness, inattention, hemiparesis, and/or motor disorders. Ataxia, nystagmus, and vomiting indicate a cerebellar lesion, while an abscess of the temporal lobe produces headache, aphasia, and visual field defects. Involvement of the brainstem may result in cranial nerve palsies, headache, fever, and vomiting.

Fungal brain abscesses often present with symptoms similar to those of bacterial brain abscess (see preceding text) (Tunkel, 2005a; Cortez and Walsh, 2004). However, some differences do exist. *Aspergillus* species have a tendency to invade blood vessels, and patients may present with signs and symptoms of cerebral infarction. In patients with rhinocerebral mucormycosis, symptoms may be referable to the eyes and sinuses in which patients present with headache, diplopia, and nasal discharge. Physical examination may show nasal ulcers or discharge, proptosis, and/or external ophthalmoplegia. Approximately 60% of patients will have orbital involvement, and there is an increased incidence of development of cavernous sinus thrombosis.

Diagnosis

Radiologic techniques, such as CT and MR, have revolutionized the diagnosis of brain abscess (Tunkel, 2005a; Mathisen and Johnson, 1997; Heilpern and Lorber, 1996). CT characteristically reveals a hypodense lesion with peripheral ring enhancement; there may also be a surrounding area of decreased attenuation due to cerebral edema. MR offers significant advantages over CT in the diagnosis of brain abscess, including early detection of cerebritis, detection of cerebral edema with greater contrast between edema and the brain, more conspicuous spread of inflammation into the ventricles and subarachnoid space, and the earlier detection of satellite lesions. Contrast enhancement with the paramagnetic agent gadolinium diethylenetriaminepentaacetic acid provides the added advantage of clearly differentiating the central abscess, surrounding enhancing rim, and cerebral edema surrounding the abscess.

In abscesses caused by *Aspergillus* species, radiographic studies (CT or MR) may show evidence of infarction with surrounding abscess formation. In mucormycosis, there may be bony erosion, sinus opacification, and evidence of cavernous sinus thrombosis.

CT has also been useful to permit stereotactic guided aspiration of brain abscesses to obtain tissue for microbiologic diagnosis (Tunkel, 2005a). Samples should be sent for Gram stain, aerobic and anaerobic culture, and smears and cultures for AFB and fungi. If there is a clinical suspicion of *Nocardia* infection, a modified AFB stain should also be done. Tissue should also be sent for histopathologic examination. Definitive diagnosis in fungal brain abscess is based on biopsy or resection of the lesion, with a characteristic appearance of the causative organism in microbiologic and histopathologic specimens.

Therapy

Empiric antimicrobial therapy for bacterial brain abscess should include agents active against streptococci, anaerobes, the Enterobacteriaceae, and staphylococci, although therapy can usually be chosen on the basis of the likely pathogenic mechanism of brain abscess formation (Table 3) (Tunkel, 2005a; Mathisen and Johnson, 1997; Heilpern and Lorber, 1996). Optimal therapy of brain abscesses includes surgical intervention with either stereotactic CT-guided aspiration, or craniotomy with resection or debridement; all lesions greater

Table 3 Empiric antimicrobial therapy of bacterial brain abscess

Predisposing condition	Usual bacterial isolates	Antimicrobial regimen
Otitis media or mastoiditis	Streptococci (anaerobic or aerobic), *Bacteroides* species, Enterobacteriaceae	Metronidazole + a third-generation cephalosporin[a]
Sinusitis (frontoethmoidal or sphenoidal)	Streptococci, *Bacteroides* species, Enterobacteriaceae, *Staphylococcus aureus*, *Hemophilus* species	Vancomycin + metronidazole + a third-generation cephalosporin[a]
Dental sepsis	Mixed *Fusobacterium* and *Bacteroides* species, streptococci	Penicillin + metronidazole
Penetrating trauma or postneurosurgical	*Staphylococcus aureus*, streptococci, Enterobacteriaceae, *Clostridium*	Vancomycin + a third-generation cephalosporin[a]
Lung abscess, empyema, bronchiectasis	*Fusobacterium, Actinomyces, Bacteroides* species, streptococci, *Nocardia asteroides*	Penicillin + metronidazole + a sulfonamide[b]
Bacterial endocarditis	*Staphylococcus aureus*, streptococci	Vancomycin + gentamicin

[a]Cefotaxime or ceftriaxone; ceftazidime or cefepime is used if *Pseudomonas aeruginosa* is suspected. [b]Sulfadiazine or trimethoprim–sulfamethoxazole; include if *Nocardia asteroides* is suspected.

Table 4 Antimicrobial therapy of brain abscess

Organism	Standard therapy	Alternative therapies
Actinomyces species	Penicillin G	Clindamycin
Aspergillus species	Voriconazole	Amphotericin B lipid complex, liposomal amphotericin B
Bacteroides fragilis	Metronidazole	Chloramphenicol, clindamycin
Candida species	Amphotericin B[a]	Fluconazole
Cryptococcus neoformans	Amphotericin B[a]	Fluconazole
Enterobacteriaceae	Third-generation cephalosporin[b]	Aztreonam, trimethoprim–sulfamethoxazole, fluoroquinolone, meropenem
Fusobacterium species	Penicillin G	Metronidazole
Mucormycosis	Amphotericin B	
Liposomal amphotericin B		
Amphotericin B lipid complex		
Nocardia asteroides	Trimethoprim–sulfamethoxazole or sulfadiazine	Minocycline, imipenem, meropenem, third-generation cephalosporin[b], amikacin
Pseudomonas aeruginosa	Ceftazidime[c] or cefepime[c]	Aztreonam[c], fluoroquinolone[c], meropenem[c]
Staphylococcus aureus		
Methicillin-sensitive	Nafcillin or oxacillin	Vancomycin
Methicillin-resistant	Vancomycin	
Streptococcus milleri, other streptococci	Penicillin G	Third-generation cephalosporin[b], vancomycin

[a]Addition of flucytosine should be considered. [b]Cefotaxime or ceftriaxone. [c]Addition of an aminoglycoside should be considered.

than 2.5 cm in diameter should be excised or stereotactically aspirated. Certain patients may be treated with medical therapy alone (Tunkel, 2005a; Carpenter, 1994), and these criteria include the presence of multiple abscesses, location in a surgically inaccessible area, clinical improvement with medical therapy alone, and abscess size ≤2.5 cm. Once culture results are available, antimicrobial therapy may be adjusted for optimal therapy (Table 4). Six to 8 weeks of intravenous therapy is recommended for treatment of bacterial brain abscess, often followed by several months of oral therapy (although the efficacy and necessity of this approach has not been established). Brain abscess caused by *Nocardia* species should be treated for up to 12 months, in conjunction with surgical resection.

The optimal therapy of fungal brain abscess requires a combined medical and surgical approach (Tunkel, 2005a; Cortez and Walsh, 2004). High-dose amphotericin B (0.8–1.25 mg kg^{-1} per day, with doses up to 1.5 mg kg^{-1} per day depending on the clinical response) with surgical resection or debridement is recommended for treatment of fungal brain abscess. The use of triazoles (fluconazole or itraconazole) is not recommended in fungal brain abscess based on the lack of clinical data on their efficacy. Voriconazole has recently been shown to be a useful agent in patients with *Aspergillus* brain abscess, and many authorities now consider this the agent of choice in patients with this infection.

Subdural Empyema

Epidemiology and Etiology

The most common predisposing conditions to cranial subdural empyema are otorhinologic infections; 50–80% of cases begin in the paranasal sinuses (Tunkel, 2005b; Silverberg and DiNubile, 1985). Other predisposing conditions include skull trauma, neurosurgical procedures, and infection of a preexisting subdural empyema; hematogenous dissemination occurs in only about 5% of cases. The bacterial species isolated from cranial subdural empyema include streptococci (~25–45%), staphylococci (~10–15%), and aerobic gram-negative bacilli (~3–10%); anaerobes (e.g. anaerobic and microaerophilic streptococci *Bacteroides fragilis*) have been recovered in up to 100% of cases; polymicrobial infections are common.

Clinical Presentation

Subdural empyema can present as a rapidly progressive, life-threatening infection with symptoms and signs related to the presence of increased intracranial pressure, meningeal irritation, and/or focal cortical inflammation (Tunkel, 2005b; Silverberg and DiNubile, 1985). A prominent complaint is headache, which is initially localized to the infected sinus or ear but becomes generalized as the infection progresses. Other clinical findings include vomiting, altered mental status (with progression to obtundation if treatment is not initiated), fever, and focal neurologic signs (usually within 24–48 hours with rapid progression). About 80% of patients have meningeal irritation, and seizures occur in more than half of cases. Without treatment, there is a rapid neurologic deterioration with signs of increased intracranial pressure and cerebral herniation. However, this fulminant presentation may not be seen in patients with cranial subdural empyema following cranial surgery or trauma, in patients who have received prior antimicrobial therapy, in patients with infected subdural hematomas, or in patients with infections metastatic to the subdural space.

Diagnosis

The diagnostic procedure of choice for cranial subdural empyema is either CT with contrast enhancement or MR imaging (Tunkel, 2005b). CT typically reveals a crescentic or elliptically shaped area of hypodensity below the cranial vault or adjacent to the falx cerebri; with extensive disease, there is often associated mass effect. Following the administration of contrast material, there is a fine, intense line of enhancement that can be seen between the subdural collection and cerebral cortex. Extensive mass effect, manifested as ventricular compression, sulcal effacement, and midline shift is invariably present. MR provides greater clarity of morphologic detail than CT and is particularly valuable in detecting subdural empyemas located as the base of the brain, along the falx cerebri, or in the posterior fossa. MR can also differentiate empyema from most sterile effusions and chronic hematomas, making it the diagnostic modality of choice for subdural empyema.

Therapy

The therapy of subdural empyema requires a combined medical and surgical approach because antimicrobial agents alone do not reliably sterilize these lesions and surgical decompression is needed to control increased intracranial pressure (Tunkel, 2005b; Silverberg and DiNubile, 1985). Drainage via burr hole placement is usually used in the early stages of subdural empyema when the pus is liquid, although it may not be adequate in 10–20% of patients. For patients requiring craniotomy, a wide exposure should be afforded to allow adequate exploration of all areas of suspected infection. In a recent report (Nathoo *et al.*, 2001), craniotomy appeared to be superior to burr hole and craniectomy drainage, as patients undergoing burr holes or craniectomy drainage not only required more frequent operations to drain recurrent or remaining pus, but also exhibited higher mortality rates and poorer outcomes.

Following the aspiration of purulent material, antimicrobial therapy is based on the results of Gram stain and predisposing condition. If the primary infection is paranasal sinusitis, otitis media or mastoiditis, therapy with vancomycin, metronidazole, and a third-generation cephalosporin (cefotaxime or ceftriaxone; or ceftazidime or cefepime if *P. aeruginosa* is suspected) is recommended pending organism identification. Parenteral therapy should be continued for 3–4 weeks and perhaps longer if an associated osteomyelitis is present (Tunkel, 2005b), although there are no firm data to support a specific duration of antimicrobial therapy in patients with subdural empyema.

Epidural Abscess

Epidemiology and Etiology

Epidural abscess refers to a collection between the dura mater and the overlying skull or vertebral column (Tunkel, 2005b). The etiologies of cranial subdural abscess are usually the same as for subdural empyema (see preceding text), whereas spinal epidural abscess usually follows hematogenous dissemination from foci elsewhere to the epidural space (25–50% of cases) or by extension from a vertebral osteomyelitis, local trauma, or infection (e.g. from penetrating trauma, decubitus ulcers, paraspinal abscess, back surgery, lumbar puncture, or epidural anesthesia). The likely infecting organisms in spinal epidural abscess are staphylococci (50–90%), streptococci (8–17%), and aerobic gram-negative bacilli (12–17%).

Clinical Presentation

Symptoms in patients with cranial epidural abscess are usually insidious with the presentation overshadowed by the primary focus of infection (e.g. sinusitis or otitis media) (Tunkel, 2005b; Danner and Hartman, 1987). Cranial epidural abscesses usually enlarge too slowly to produce sudden major neurologic deficits unless there is deeper intracranial extension. The typical complaint is headache; eventually focal neurologic signs, seizures, papilledema, and other signs of increased intracranial pressure may develop without appropriate therapy.

In contrast, spinal epidural abscess may develop rapidly within hours (following hematogenous dissemination) or pursue a chronic course over months (associated with vertebral osteomyelitis) (Connolly and Hammer, 1990). Initially, patients complain of focal vertebral pain (the most consistent symptom seen in 70–90% of patients), followed by root pain, defects of motor, sensory, or sphincter function, and finally paralysis. These symptoms and signs indicate the need for emergent evaluation, diagnosis, and treatment.

Diagnosis

MR imaging is the diagnostic procedure of choice for both cranial and spinal epidural abscess (Tunkel, 2005b). In cases of spinal epidural abscess, MR is recommended because it can visualize the spinal cord and epidural space in both the sagittal and transverse sections and can also identify accompanying osteomyelitis, intramedullary spinal cord lesions, and joint space infection (Hook and Marra, 1992).

Therapy

Recommendations for antimicrobial therapy for cranial epidural abscess are the same as for subdural empyema (see preceding text). Presumptive therapy for spinal epidural abscess must include an antistaphylococcal agent (i.e. vancomycin); coverage for gram-negative bacilli (e.g. ceftazidime or cefepime) must be included for patients with a history of a spinal procedure or injection drug use (Tunkel, 2005b). Antimicrobial therapy for an uncomplicated spinal epidural abscess should be continued for 3–4 weeks and for 6–8 weeks if osteomyelitis is present.

Surgical therapy for epidural abscess is aimed at drainage of the collection and for patients with neurologic changes to minimize the likelihood of permanent neurologic sequelae. Some patients with spinal epidural abscess have been treated with antimicrobial therapy alone (i.e. those with an unacceptably high surgical risk or those without neurologic deficits), although these patients must be carefully followed for clinical deterioration and for progression by radiologic studies (Tunkel, 2005b; Wheeler *et al.*, 1992; Baker *et al.*, 1992). Surgical decompression should be performed in patients with increasing neurologic deficit, persistent severe pain, increasing temperature, or peripheral white blood cell count. Surgery is not likely to be a viable therapeutic option in patients who have experienced complete paralysis for more than 24 hours, although some would perform surgical therapy in patients with duration of complete paralysis of less than 72 hours.

ENCEPHALITIS

Encephalitis is characterized by symptoms similar to those seen with acute meningitis, but patients with encephalitis are more likely to experience mental status changes and seizures. Numerous infectious and noninfectious etiologies may produce encephalitis. Most common are the herpesviruses that are also the most treatable. More recently, West Nile encephalitis has been reported in endemic areas and is discussed in the following section.

Herpes Simplex Virus

Epidemiology and Etiology

Herpes simplex virus accounts for approximately 10–20% of viral encephalitides, and occurs sporadically throughout the year, affecting all age-groups (Whitley, 2004); most cases are caused by HSV type 1. The disease is associated with significant morbidity and mortality (as high as 70% if untreated).

Clinical Presentation

Patients with HSV encephalitis often present with diminished levels of consciousness and focal neurologic signs, such as dysphasia, weakness, and paresthesias (Whitley, 2004; Whitley, 1990). Personality changes and fever are uniformly present, and approximately two-thirds of patients develop seizures, often involving the temporal lobes. The clinical course may be slow or progress with alarming rapidity, with progressive loss of consciousness leading to coma.

Diagnosis

CSF examination in HSV encephalitis reveals a lymphocytic pleocytosis in 97% of cases with biopsy-proven disease and an elevated protein (Whitley, 2004; Whitley, 1990). The presence of CSF red blood cells suggests the diagnosis but is not always present. About 5–10% of patients have normal CSF findings on initial evaluation. CSF viral cultures are positive in only ~4% of cases, making a definitive diagnosis difficult without performance of a brain biopsy. However, detection of HSV DNA in the CSF using PCR is both sensitive and specific, and is now the optimal method for the diagnosis of HSV encephalitis (Rowley *et al.*, 1990; Lakeman and Whitley, 1995).

Several noninvasive tests may also support the diagnosis of HSV encephalitis (Whitley, 2004; Cepelowicz and Tunkel, 2003). The electroencephalogram (EEG) may show a characteristic spike-and-slow wave activity with periodic lateralizing epileptiform discharges over the temporal and frontotemporal regions. CT with contrast administration may reveal a hypodense area with mass effect localized to the temporal lobes. MR is more sensitive than CT and is considered by many experts to be the most important and specific imaging technique. With the availability of these diagnostic modalities, brain biopsy is seldom indicated.

Antimicrobial Therapy

On the basis of its ease of administration and good safety profile, treatment with intravenous acyclovir 30 mg kg per day (in patients with normal renal function) in three divided doses for 14–21 days is recommended for patients with suspected HSV encephalitis (Whitley, 2004; Cepelowicz and Tunkel, 2003).

Varicella Zoster Virus

Epidemiology and Etiology

Herpes zoster is a consequence of reactivation of latent VZV, and a direct correlation exists between cutaneous dissemination and visceral involvement (including meningoencephalitis) (Tunkel and Scheld, 2002b; Cepelowicz and Tunkel, 2003). CNS complications associated with recurrent zoster infection result in significantly higher morbidity and mortality than primary varicella infection. This may be due to the advanced age and underlying illnesses of most patients with herpes zoster.

Clinical Presentation

Symptoms associated with CNS infection with VZV include headache, fever, vomiting, seizures, altered sensorium, and focal neurologic deficits (Tunkel and Scheld, 2002b; Cepelowicz and Tunkel, 2003). Encephalitis is the most common abnormality associated with herpes zoster, seen most commonly in patients of advanced age, following immunosuppression, and in those with disseminated cutaneous zoster. Some patients with ophthalmic zoster present with the distinctive CNS process of contralateral hemiplegia that usually occurs several weeks or more after zoster ophthalmicus; this finding is seen in up to one-third of CNS abnormalities in herpes zoster.

Diagnosis

CSF analysis in patients with herpes zoster encephalitis shows a lymphocytic pleocytosis and elevated protein, although these findings may be seen in up to 40% of zoster patients without CNS involvement (Tunkel and Scheld, 2002b; Cepelowicz and Tunkel, 2003). Viral cultures are rarely helpful diagnostically. In patients with zoster ophthalmicus with contralateral hemiplegia, a unilateral arteritis or thrombosis of involved vessels may be seen on cerebral angiography, and cerebral infarction may be seen on CT.

Antimicrobial Therapy

Although no clinical trials have established the efficacy of antiviral therapy in herpes zoster encephalitis, we believe intravenous acyclovir should be used in this setting.

West Nile Virus

Epidemiology and Etiology

West Nile encephalitis is an infection of the brain caused by West Nile virus (WNV), a flavivirus that is commonly found in Africa, West Asia, and the Middle East. The virus first appeared in the United States in 1999 with an outbreak of meningoencephalitis reported in New York City (Nash *et al.*, 2001). Mosquitos are the primary vectors of WNV, and anyone bitten by an infected mosquito can get the disease. It has been estimated that the risk to a person of getting infected with WNV from the bite of an *infected* mosquito is about 1% (Peterson and Marfin, 2002). Transmission can also occur via transplanted organs and infected blood products (Centers for Disease Control and Prevention, 2002). Most human infections with WNV are asymptomatic, but, in recent outbreaks, 1 in 5 infected persons developed West Nile fever and 1 in 150 developed CNS disease (Mostashari *et al.*, 2001); the elderly are much more likely to develop serious diseases. While the risk of infection with WNV may be small, the disease can be quite serious. Of those patients who develop symptoms serious enough to require hospitalization, 3–15% of cases are fatal.

Clinical Presentation

Patients with WNV encephalitis present with fever, headache, mental status changes, nausea, and vomiting (Campbell *et al.*, 2002; Marfin and Gubler, 2001). Severe generalized muscle weakness was a common feature in cases during the New York City outbreak, as well as in other outbreaks in the United States. Seizures are uncommon. Depressed deep tendon reflexes, diffuse muscle weakness, flaccid paralysis, and respiratory failure may also occur. The disease progresses to coma in about 15% of patients.

Diagnosis

CSF examination in patients with WNV encephalitis typically reveals a moderate lymphocytic pleocytosis (although no cells or neutrophils may be seen), elevated protein, and normal glucose. Testing for patients with encephalitis, meningitis, or other serious CNS infections can be obtained through local or state health departments. Public health laboratories usually perform an IgM antibody capture enzyme-linked immunosorbent assay (MAC-ELISA). Using this assay, virus-specific IgM can be detected in nearly all CSF and serum specimens received from WNV-infected patients at the time of their clinical presentation (Mostashari *et al.*, 2001). However, the serum IgM antibody may persist for more than a year and physicians must determine whether the detection of antibody is the result of a WNV infection in the previous year and unrelated to the current clinical presentation. The IgM in the CSF is specific for CNS infection, with almost all patients having detectable antibody by the first week of admission.

Treatment

There is no specific treatment for West Nile encephalitis (Peterson and Marfin, 2002; Campbell *et al.*, 2002). In more severe cases, intensive supportive therapy is indicated, often involving hospitalization, intravenous fluids, airway management, respiratory support, prevention of secondary infections (e.g. pneumonia, urinary tract infection), and good nursing care. Ribavirin in high doses and interferon α-2b were found to have some activity against WNV *in vitro*, but no controlled studies have been completed on the use of these agents for therapy of West Nile encephalitis. A multicenter controlled trial of intravenous immunoglobulin in the treatment of West Nile encephalitis is currently under way in the United States.

POSTPOLIO SYNDROME

Epidemiology

Any discussion of CNS infections in the elderly should include the postpolio syndrome. This syndrome does not appear to be because of persistent poliovirus infection, but rather is likely due to an age-related loss of surviving motor neurons, and their inability to innervate the enlarged motor neuron units seen in poliomyelitis patients (Modlin, 2004). In a study of the prevalence and risk factors for postpolio syndrome in a cohort of 551 former poliomyelitis patients in Allegheny County, Pennsylvania, 137 (~25%) developed symptoms of the postpolio syndrome between 32 and 39 years after the acute illness (Ramlow, 1992). Risk factors for the development of the postpolio syndrome were female sex, bulbar disease and the degree of postrecovery residual impairment. Despite the relatively high prevalence of this disorder, the majority of patients (80% in this study) did not require the use of new assisted devices to accomplish their activities of daily living, despite a subjective decline in their functional status.

Clinical Presentation

The postpolio syndrome is characterized by muscle weakness, muscle and/or joint pain, fatigue, and a decline in functional status occurring 30–40 years after acute poliomyelitis (Modlin, 2004). Some patients have progressive weakness and wasting in muscles that were not necessarily weak at the onset of poliomyelitis.

Diagnosis

Conventional electromyography (EMG) demonstrates chronic denervation; occasionally there may also be new or ongoing denervation manifested as fasciculations, fibrillations, and positive sharp waves (Modlin, 2004). Enlarged motor units consistent with highly increased fiber density can be demonstrated in 90% of patients on single-fiber EMG. However, the primary role of EMG is to exclude other causes of the patient's presentation.

Therapy

There is no definitive treatment for the postpolio syndrome, but symptomatic improvement may be obtained with analgesics such as paracetamol (acetaminophen) or nonsteroidal anti-inflammatory drugs, local heat application to affected muscles and joints, and a low-impact, nonfatiguing exercise program to prevent the development of muscle atrophy (Modlin, 2004). Patients may also benefit from rest periods, increased sleep time, and other energy conservation methods to overcome fatigue.

CREUTZFELDT–JAKOB DISEASE

Epidemiology

The most common human prion disease is sporadic, or classic, Creutzfeldt–Jakob Disease (CJD), with a worldwide incidence of approximately 1 case per million population (Janka and Maldarelli, 2004); however, among individuals aged 60–74 years, the incidence is 5 cases per million population (Holman *et al.*, 1996). Symptoms generally begin by age 60–70, with a mean age of onset of 60 years.

Clinical Presentation

Sporadic CJD is characterized by a rapidly progressive multifocal neurological dysfunction, myoclonus, and a terminal state of global severe cognitive impairment. About 40% of patients with sporadic CJD present with rapidly progressive cognitive impairment, 40% with cerebellar dysfunction, and the remaining 20% with a combination of both findings. The clinical picture rapidly expands to include behavioral abnormalities, higher cortical dysfunction, cortical visual abnormalities, cerebellar dysfunction, and both pyramidal and extrapyramidal signs (Collins *et al.*, 2004). Almost all patients with sporadic CJD develop myoclonus that involves either the entire body or a limb; myoclonus may be absent at disease onset, but appears with increasing severity as the disease progresses. After a rapidly progressive illness of 3–9 months, death usually occurs with the patient in an akinetic and mute state (Janka and Maldarelli, 2004).

Diagnosis

The clinical presentation, progressive nature, and failure to find any other diagnoses are the hallmarks of sporadic CJD. There are no available, completely reliable diagnostic tests for use before the onset of clinical symptoms in patients with sporadic CJD. During the course of disease, most patients develop a characteristic picture on EEG with periodic paroxysms of sharp waves or spikes on a slow background (Janka and Maldarelli, 2004; Chiofalo *et al.*, 1980). These periodic complexes have a diagnostic sensitivity and specificity of 67% and 87%, respectively, on a single EEG; if repeated recordings are obtained, more than 90% of patients show periodic EEG abnormalities. The triad of myoclonus, dementia, and EEG periodic sharp waves is a characteristic presentation of sporadic CJD.

Therapy

There is no treatment that can cure or control CJD. About 90% of patients die within 1 year (Janka and Maldarelli, 2004). Current treatment is aimed at alleviating symptoms and making the patient as comfortable as possible. Opiate drugs can help relieve pain; clonazepam and sodium valproate may help relieve involuntary myoclonus. Quinidine has been tested in an uncontrolled and unblinded study of patients with sporadic CJD; despite transient improvement in some patients, they reverted to their previous states and died of progressive disease (Follette, 2003).

KEY POINTS

- Empiric antimicrobial therapy, based on the patient's age and underlying disease status, should be initiated as soon as possible in patients with presumed bacterial meningitis; therapy should not be delayed while diagnostic neuroimaging tests are awaited.
- In elderly patients with bacterial meningitis, empiric antimicrobial therapy should consist of vancomycin,

ampicillin, and a third-generation cephalosporin (either cefotaxime or ceftriaxone), pending organism identification, and susceptibility testing.

- Adjunctive dexamethasone has been shown to reduce morbidity and mortality in adults with pneumococcal meningitis; this adjunctive modality should also be utilized in patients with tuberculous meningitis.
- The diagnosis of focal CNS infections (i.e. brain abscess, subdural empyema, epidural abscess) has been revolutionized by the development of neuroimaging studies; MR imaging has been especially useful in better detection of the extent of disease and early detection of cerebral edema.
- The therapeutic approach to focal CNS infections often requires a combined medical and surgical approach, because drainage of infected material can rapidly reverse neurologic symptoms and signs and antimicrobial therapy alone will not reliably sterilize these lesions.

KEY REFERENCES

- de Gans J & van de Beek D. Dexamethasone in adults with bacterial meningitis. *The New England Journal of Medicine* 2002; **347**:1549–56.
- Janka J & Maldarelli F. Prion diseases: update on mad cow disease, variant Creutzfeldt-Jakob disease and the transmissible spongiform encephalopathies. *Current Infectious Disease Reports* 2004; **6**:305–15.
- Romero JR. Diagnosis and management of enteroviral infections of the central nervous system. *Current Infectious Disease Reports* 2002; **4**:309–16.
- Thwaites GE, Bang ND, Duang NH *et al.* Dexamethasone for the treatment of tuberculous meningitis in adolescents and adults. *The New England Journal of Medicine* 2004; **351**:1741–51.
- Tunkel AR, Hartman BJ, Kaplan SL *et al.* Practice guidelines for the management of bacterial meningitis. *Clinical Infectious Diseases* 2004; **39**:1267–84.

REFERENCES

American College of Physicians. Guidelines for laboratory evaluation in the diagnosis of Lyme disease. *Annals of Internal Medicine* 1997; **127**:1106–8.

Ampel NM, Wieden MA & Galgiani JN. Coccidioidomycosis: clinical update. *Reviews of Infectious Diseases* 1989; **11**:897–911.

Attia J, Hatala R, Cook DJ *et al.* Does this adult patient have acute meningitis? *The Journal of the American Medical Association* 1999; **282**:175–81.

Baker AS, Ojemann RG & Baker RA. To decompress or not to decompress – spinal epidural abscess. *Clinical Infectious Diseases* 1992; **15**:28–9.

Barnes PF, Bloch AB, Davidson PT *et al.* Tuberculosis in patients with human immunodeficiency virus infection. *The New England Journal of Medicine* 1991; **324**:1624–50.

Berry AJ, Rinaldi MG & Graybill JR. Use of high-dose fluconazole as salvage therapy for cryptococcal meningitis in patients with AIDS. *Antimicrobial Agents and Chemotherapy* 1992; **36**:690–2.

Cadavid D. Lyme disease and relapsing fever. In WM Scheld, RJ Whitley & CM Marra (eds) *Infections of the Central Nervous System* 2004, 3rd edn, pp 659–90; Lippincott Williams & Wilkins, Philadelphia.

Campbell GL, Marfin AA, Lanciotti RS *et al.* West Nile virus. *The Lancet Infectious Diseases* 2002; **2**:519–29.

Carpenter JL. Brainstem abscesses: cure with medical therapy, case report and review. *Clinical Infectious Diseases* 1994; **18**:219–26.

Centers for Disease Control and Prevention. West Nile virus activity-United States, October 10–16, 2002, and update on West Nile virus infections in recipients of blood transfusions. *Morbidity and Mortality Weekly Report* 2002; **51**:929–31.

Cepelowicz J & Tunkel AR. Viral encephalitis. *Current Opinion in Infectious Diseases* 2003; **5**:11–9.

Chiofalo N, Fuentes A & Galvez S. Serial EEG findings in 27 cases of Creutzfeldt-Jakob disease. *Archives of Neurology* 1980; **37**:143–5.

Collins PS, Lawson VA & Masters PC. Transmissible spongiform encephalopathies. *Lancet* 2004; **363**:51–61.

Connolly KJ & Hammer SM. The acute aseptic meningitis syndrome. *Infectious Disease Clinics of North America* 1990; **4**:599–622.

Cortez KJ & Walsh TJ. Space-occupying fungal lesions. In WM Scheld, RJ Whitley & CM Marra (eds) *Infections of the Central Nervous System* 2004, 3rd edn, pp 713–34; Lippincott Williams & Wilkins, Philadelphia.

Cottagnoud P & Tauber MG. Fluoroquinolones in the treatment of meningitis. *Current Infectious Disease Reports* 2003; **5**:329–36.

Danner RL & Hartman BJ. Update of spinal epidural abscess; 35 cases and review of the literature. *Reviews of Infectious Diseases* 1987; **9**:265–74.

de Gans J & van de Beek D. Dexamethasone in adults with bacterial meningitis. *The New England Journal of Medicine* 2002; **347**:1549–56.

Domingo P, Barquet N, Alvarez M *et al.* Group B streptococcal meningitis in adults: report of twelve cases and review. *Clinical Infectious Diseases* 1997; **25**:1180–7.

Dunne DW & Quagliarello V. Group B streptococcal meningitis in adults. *Medicine* 1993; **72**:1–10.

Durand ML, Calderwood SB, Weber DL *et al.* Acute bacterial meningitis in adults. *The New England Journal of Medicine* 1993; **328**:21–8.

Farley MM, Stephens DS, Brachman PS *et al.* Invasive *Haemophilus influenzae* disease in adults: a prospective, population-based surveillance. *Annals of Internal Medicine* 1992; **116**:806–12.

Fessler RD, Sobel J, Guyot L *et al.* Management of elevated intracranial pressure in patients with cryptococcal meningitis. *Journal of Acquired Immune Deficiency Syndromes* 1998; **17**:137–42.

Follette P. Prion disease treatment's early promise unravels. *Science* 2003; **299**:191–2.

Galgiani JN, Catanzaro A, Cloud G *et al.* Fluconazole therapy for coccidioidal meningitis. *Annals of Internal Medicine* 1993; **119**:28–35.

Gorse GJ, Thrupp LD, Nudleman KL *et al.* Bacterial meningitis in the elderly. *Archives of Internal Medicine* 1989; **149**:1603–6.

Gray LD & Fedorko DP. Laboratory diagnosis of bacterial meningitis. *Clinical Microbiology Reviews* 1992; **5**:130–45.

Heilpern KL & Lorber B. Focal intracranial infections. *Infectious Disease Clinics of North America* 1996; **10**:879–98.

Holman RC, Khan AS & Belay ED. Creutzfeldt-Jakob disease in the United States, 1979–1994: using national mortality data to assess the possible occurrence of variant cases. *Emerging Infectious Diseases* 1996; **2**:333–7.

Hook EW III & Marra CM. Acquired syphilis in adults. *The New England Journal of Medicine* 1992; **326**:1060–9.

Janka J & Maldarelli F. Prion diseases: update on mad cow disease, variant Creutzfeldt-Jakob disease and the transmissible spongiform encephalopathies. *Current Infectious Disease Reports* 2004; **6**:305–15.

Kaufman BA, Tunkel AR, Pryor J & Dacey RG Jr. Meningitis in the neurosurgical patient. *Infectious Disease Clinics of North America* 1990; **4**:677–701.

Keller TL, Halperin JJ & Whitman M. PCR detection of *Borrelia burgdorferi* DNA in cerebrospinal fluid of Lyme neuroborreliosis patients. *Neurology* 1992; **42**:32–42.

Kennedy DH & Fallon RJ. Tuberculous meningitis. *The Journal of the American Medical Association* 1979; **241**:264–8.

Kent SJ, Crowe SM, Yung A *et al.* Tuberculous meningitis: a 30-year review. *Clinical Infectious Diseases* 1993; **17**:987–94.

Kojima Y, Hashiguchi H, Hashimoto T *et al.* Recurrent herpes simplex type 2 meningitis: a case report of Mollaret's meningitis. *Japanese Journal of Infectious Diseases* 2002; **55**:85–8.

Lakeman FD & Whitley RJ, The Infectious Diseases Collaborative Antiviral Study Group. Diagnosis of herpes simplex encephalitis: application of polymerase chain reaction to cerebrospinal fluid from brain-biopsied patients and correlation with disease. *The Journal of Infectious Diseases* 1995; **171**:857–63.

Leendera ACAP, Reiss P, Portegies P *et al.* Liposomal amphotericin B (AmBisome) compared to amphotericin B both followed by oral fluconazole in the treatment of AIDS-associated cryptococcal meningitis. *Acquired Immuno Deficiency Syndrome* 1997; **11**:1463–71.

Leonard JM & Des Prez RM. Tuberculous meningitis. *Infectious Disease Clinics of North America* 1990; **4**:769–87.

Lorber B. Listeriosis. *Clinical Infectious Diseases* 1997; **24**:1–11.

Marfin AA & Gubler DJ. West Nile encephalitis: an emerging disease in the United States. *Clinical Infectious Diseases* 2001; **33**:1713–9.

Marra CM. Neurosyphilis. In WM Scheld, RJ Whitley & CM Marra (eds) *Infections of the Central Nervous System* 2004, 3rd edn, pp 649–57; Lippincott Williams & Wilkins, Philadelphia.

Mathisen GE & Johnson JP. Brain abscess. *Clinical Infectious Diseases* 1997; **25**:763–81.

Modlin JF. Coffey. Poliomyelitis, polio vaccines, and the postpoliomyelitis syndrome. In WM Scheld, RJ Whitley & CM Marra (eds) *Infections of the Central Nervous System* 2004, 3rd edn, pp 95–110; Lippincott Williams & Wilkins, Philadelphia.

Mostashari F, Bunning ML, Kotsutani PT *et al.* Epidemic West Nile encephalitis, 1999, New York: results of a household-based seroepidemiological survey. *Lancet* 2001; **358**:261–4.

Musher DM. Infections caused by *Streptococcus pneumoniae*: clinical spectrum, pathogenesis, immunity, and treatment. *Clinical Infectious Diseases* 1992; **14**:801–9.

Musher DM, Hamill RJ & Baughn RE. Effect of human immunodeficiency virus (HIV) infection on the course of syphilis and on the response to treatment. *Annals of Internal Medicine* 1990; **113**:872–81.

Mylonakis E, Hohmann EL & Calderwood SB. Central nervous system infection with *Listeria monocytogenes*: 33 years' experience at a general hospital and review of 776 episodes from the literature. *Medicine* 1998; **77**:313–36.

Nash D, Mostashari F, Fine A *et al.* The outbreak of West Nile virus infection in the New York City area in 1999. *The New England Journal of Medicine* 2001; **344**:1807–14.

Nathoo N, Nadvi SS, Gouws E & van Dellen JR. Craniotomy improves outcomes for cranial subdural empyemas: computed tomography-era experience with 699 patients. *Neurosurgery* 2001; **49**:872–8.

Negrini B, Kelleher KJ & Wald ER. Cerebrospinal fluid findings in aseptic versus bacterial meningitis. *Pediatrics* 2000; **105**:316–9.

Ni H, Knight AI, Cartwright K *et al.* Polymerase chain reaction for diagnosis of meningococcal meningitis. *Lancet* 1992; **340**:1432–4.

Ogawa SK, Smith MA, Brennessel DJ *et al.* Tuberculous meningitis in an urban medical center. *Medicine* 1987; **63**:317–26.

Pappas PG, Perfect JR, Cloud GA *et al.* Cryptococcosis in HIV-negative patients in the era of effective azole therapy. *Clinical Infectious Diseases* 2001; **33**:690–9.

Park NK, Hospenthal DR & Bennett JE. Treatment of hydrocephalus secondary to cryptococcal meningitis by use of shunting. *Clinical Infectious Diseases* 1999; **28**:629–33.

Peterson LR & Marfin AA. West Nile virus: a primer for the clinician. *Annals of Internal Medicine* 2002; **137**:173–9.

Ramlow J *et al.* Epidemiology of the post-polio syndrome. *American Journal of Epidemiology* 1992; **136**:769–86.

Romero JR. Diagnosis and management of enteroviral infections of the central nervous system. *Current Infectious Disease Reports* 2002; **4**:309–16.

Ross SC & Densen P. Complement deficiency states and infection: epidemiology, pathogenesis and consequences of neisserial and other infections in an immune deficiency. *Medicine* 1984; **64**:243–73.

Rotbart HA. Diagnosis of enteroviral meningitis with the polymerase chain reaction. *The Journal of Pediatrics* 1990; **117**:85–9.

Rotbart HA. Enteroviral infections of the central nervous system. *Clinical Infectious Diseases* 1995; **20**:971–81.

Rotbart HA & Webster AD. Treatment of potentially life-threatening enterovirus infections with pleconaril. *Clinical Infectious Diseases* 2001; **32**:228–35.

Rowley A, Lakeman F, Whitley R *et al.* Diagnosis of herpes simplex encephalitis by DNA amplification of cerebrospinal fluid cells. *Lancet* 1990; **335**:440–1.

Saez-Llorens X, McCoig C, Feris JM *et al.* Quinolone treatment for pediatric bacterial meningitis: a comparative study of trovafloxaxin and ceftriaxone with or without vancomycin. *The Pediatric Infectious Disease Journal* 2002; **21**:14–22.

Saravolatz LD, Manzor O, VanderVelde N *et al.* Broad-range bacterial polymerase chain reaction for early detection of bacterial meningitis. *Clinical Infectious Diseases* 2003; **36**:40–5.

Sawyer MH & Rotbart HA. Viral meningitis and aseptic meningitis syndrome. In WM Scheld, RJ Whitley & CM Marra (eds) *Infections of the Central Nervous System* 2004, 3rd edn, pp 75–93; Lippincott Williams & Wilkins, Philadelphia.

Schlech WF III, Ward JI, Band JD *et al.* Bacterial meningitis in the United States, 1978–1981. The national bacterial meningitis surveillance study. *The Journal of the American Medical Association* 1985; **253**:1749–54.

Schlessinger LS, Ross SC & Schaberg DR. *Staphylococcus aureus* meningitis: a broad-based epidemiologic study. *Medicine* 1987; **66**:148–56.

Schuchat A, Robinson K, Wenger JD *et al.* Bacterial meningitis in the United States in 1995. *The New England Journal of Medicine* 1997; **337**:970–6.

Sharkey PK, Graybill JR, Johnson ES *et al.* Amphotericin B lipid complex compared with amphotericin B in the treatment of cryptococcal meningitis in patients with AIDS. *Clinical Infectious Diseases* 1996; **22**:315–21.

Silverberg AL & DiNubile MJ. Subdural empyema and cranial epidural abscess. *The Medical Clinics of North America* 1985; **69**:361–74.

Sinner SW & Tunkel AR. Approach to the diagnosis and management of tuberculous meningitis. *Current Infectious Disease Reports* 2002; **4**:324–31.

Slavoski LA & Tunkel AR. Therapy of fungal meningitis. *Clinical Neuropharmacology* 1995; **18**:95–112.

Steere AC. Lyme disease. *The New England Journal of Medicine* 1989; **321**:586–96.

Tedder DG, Ashley R, Tyler KL & Levin MJ. Herpes simplex virus infection as a cause of benign recurrent lymphocytic meningitis. *Annals of Internal Medicine* 1994; **121**:334–8.

Thomas KE, Hasbun R, Jekel J & Quagliarello VJ. The diagnostic accuracy of Kernig's sign, Brudzinski's sign, and nuchal rigidity in adults with suspected meningitis. *Clinical Infectious Diseases* 2002; **35**:46–52.

Thwaites GE, Bang ND, Duang NH *et al.* Dexamethasone for the treatment of tuberculous meningitis in adolescents and adults. *The New England Journal of Medicine* 2004; **351**:1741–51.

Tunkel AR. *Bacterial Meningitis* 2001; Lippincott Williams & Wilkins, Philadelphia.

Tunkel AR. Brain abscess. In GL Mandell, JE Bennett & R Dolin (eds) *Principles and Practice of Infectious Diseases* 2005a, 6th edn, pp 1150–63; Elsevier Churchill Livingstone, Philadelphia.

Tunkel AR. Subdural empyema, epidural abscess, and suppurative intracranial thrombophlebitis. In GL Mandell, JE Bennett & R Dolin (eds) *Principles and Practice of Infectious Diseases* 2005b, 6th edn, pp 1164–71; Elsevier Churchill Livingstone, Philadelphia.

Tunkel AR, Hartman BJ, Kaplan SL *et al.* Practice guidelines for the management of bacterial meningitis. *Clinical Infectious Diseases* 2004; **39**:1267–84.

Tunkel AR & Scheld WM. Corticosteroids for everyone with meningitis? *The New England Journal of Medicine* 2002a; **347**:1613–5.

Tunkel AR & Scheld WM. Central nervous system infection in the compromised host. In RH Rubin & LS Young (eds) *Clinical Approach to Infection in the Compromised Host* 2002b, 4th edn, pp 163–214; Kluwer Academic/Plenum Publishers, New York.

Tunkel AR & Scheld WM. Acute meningitis. In GL Mandell, JE Bennett & R Dolin (eds) *Principles and Practice of Infectious Diseases*, 2005, 6th edn, pp 1083–126; Elsevier Churchill Livingstone, Philadelphia.

Wenger JD, Hightower AW, Facklam RR *et al.* Bacterial meningitis in the United States, 1986: report of a multistate surveillance study. *The Journal of Infectious Diseases* 1990; **162**:1316–23.

Wheeler D, Keiser P, Rigamonti D *et al.* Medical management of spinal epidural abscess; Case report and review. *Clinical Infectious Diseases* 1992; **15**:22–7.

Whitley RJ. Viral encephalitis. *The New England Journal of Medicine* 1990; **323**:242–50.

Whitley RJ. Herpes simplex virus. In WM Scheld, RJ Whitley & CM Marra (eds) *Infections of the Central Nervous System* 2004, 3rd edn, pp 123–44; Lippincott Williams & Wilkins, Philadelphia.

Zugar A. Tuberculosis. In WM Scheld, RJ Whitley & CM Marra (eds) *Infections of the Central Nervous System* 2004, 3rd edn, pp 441–59; Lippincott Williams & Wilkins, Philadelphia.

PART IV

Health Care Systems

149

Geriatric Medicine Education in Europe

Antonio Cherubini[1], Philippe Huber[2] *and* Jean-Pierre Michel[2]

[1] Perugia University Medical School, Perugia, Italy, and [2] University Hospital of Geneva, Geneva, Switzerland

INTRODUCTION

The Council of Europe includes 45 state members, while the European community, limited until May 2004 to 15 countries, includes today 25 different countries, all with varying degrees of industrialization, economic benefits, and employment. These initial remarks highlight that it is really difficult to consider Europe as a homogeneous group of countries. The wide variation of demographic data is probably the best way of showing the disparity among the European countries (Economic Commission for Europe's Population Activities Unit, 2005):

- Birth rate: the highest is in Turkey (2.4/woman) and the lowest in Latvia (1.1/woman);
- Mortality rate during the first year of life: the highest is in Turkey (35.7/1000) and the lowest in Iceland (2.4/1000);
- Life expectancy at birth for men: the highest is in Iceland (79.9 years) and the lowest in Russia (61.3 years);
- Life expectancy at birth for women: the highest is in San Marino (83 years) and the lowest in Turkey (71 years).

However, in each developed European country, life expectancy at birth continues to increase: there is actually a 3-month "bonus" of life for each year of life (Oeppen and Vaupel, 2002). In 1999, Europe had a total population of 728 million inhabitants, of which 14% were over 65 years. Between 1999 and 2050, the expected increase of the 60+ and 80+ European population should reach 160% and 158%, respectively. In 2050, among 100 European inhabitants, 35 will be older than 65 years and 9 will be older than 80. The number of nonagenarians, centenarians, and supercentenarians (over 110 years) will continue to increase (Robine and Paccaud, in press). While the healthy life expectancy is longer than ever in developed countries, still many older subjects spend the last years of their life suffering from chronic diseases and increasing disability, which explains why a large percentage of patients requiring health care belong to this age-group.

One of the most efficient ways to cope with this programmed overflow of the older sick population with their specific medical and psychosocial needs would be to enhance the geriatric training of all categories of health-care professionals, and particularly medical doctors. It has been recently acknowledged that current medical education is failing to provide the knowledge and skills that are needed to manage chronic diseases that are common in the older population (Holman, 2004). It is unfortunate, therefore, that there is little evidence that European countries are responding adequately to this "Geriatric education imperative" (Besdine, 1989).

In 1994, a Group of European professors of medical gerontology provided an inventory of teaching activities in geriatrics in several European countries (Stähelin *et al.*, 1994). In this chapter, we aim to update this important review discussing the current status of geriatric medicine teaching at the undergraduate and postgraduate levels in various European countries, as well as the continuing medical and professional education activities.

UNDERGRADUATE GERIATRIC MEDICINE EDUCATION

Undergraduate geriatric medicine education remains a major area for development, and curricula have become available only recently in a number of European countries.

As part of a larger survey of geriatric medicine in Europe, the authors received information from 28 geriatricians, trained at the European Academy for Medicine of Aging (EAMA), and working in 14 different European countries. The results of this survey were, in general, difficult to analyze and interpret because of different curricula being taught within the medical schools surveyed. However, it is interesting to present these data because they can give some clues on the current status and also on the new trends in undergraduate geriatric education across Europe.

Principles and Practice of Geriatric Medicine, 4th Edition. Edited by M.S. John Pathy, Alan J. Sinclair and John E. Morley.

Western Europe

In Austria there are three medical schools, but no formal position on academic geriatric medicine exists, and consequently there is an inadequate level of teaching of the subject. In Belgium, among the existing 11 medical schools, only half have well-developed undergraduate geriatric teaching with academic positions in the biology of aging, geriatrics, and psychogeriatrics. Furthermore, Belgium is the first country that has established special interuniversity geriatric teaching activities to cover the training needs in geriatrics for all students in their last year of medical undergraduate study.

In the United Kingdom, every undergraduate medical school has a professorial department of geriatrics or a related subject. There is broad-based teaching in the science of aging, clinical geriatrics, and psychogeriatrics. These programs are well defined, based on both traditional and problem-based learning (PBL) approaches, and are usually integrated throughout the five years of medical course. France appears, today, as being one of the most advanced countries in undergraduate geriatric teaching, although geriatrics is not yet recognized as an independent speciality from internal medicine. However, there is at least one professorship in each French medical school ($N = 40$) with some of them still in the process of being appointed. Undergraduate teaching programs are based on a national core curriculum established by a group of French professors of geriatrics. The teaching activity is both traditional and problem-based, dealing with the geriatric giants as well as comprehensive geriatric assessment. The undergraduate teaching in geriatrics takes part of the last year of the medical course.

In Germany, undergraduate geriatric teaching is very often done under the leadership of internal medicine or other medical specialists who are not trained in geriatric medicine. In a few medical schools, the geriatric program is an independent one, or is sometimes linked with the public health and nursing programs.

In the Netherlands, the number of geriatric academic positions have decreased during the last five years, and unfortunately, the training is often embedded in the internal medicine and neurobiology curricula, although all students are still required to study this discipline. In Switzerland, only one of the five medical schools had a geriatric professorship in 2004. However, undergraduate teaching activities are developed in all the Swiss medical schools because of the involvement of promising nonacademic geriatricians. In Geneva, there is a well-developed and successful problem-based learning program, which takes place from the beginning to the end of medical studies (Table 1).

Table 1 New undergraduate geriatric core curriculum at the Geneva Medical School

The emergence of integrated problem-based undergraduate medical curricula is a real opportunity for the undergraduate teaching of geriatrics. The PBL approach allows integrating geriatrics vertically and longitudinally with the teaching of basic sciences and other clinical disciplines, since geriatrics is an intrinsically multidisciplinary and integrative field.

Most PBL curricula, for example, in Geneva, Switzerland, start with a preclinical curriculum in which the students acquire knowledge in basic sciences and participate in some kind of longitudinal Clinical Skills Program (Vu *et al.*, 1997). Geriatric objectives in basic sciences and clinical disciplines can be integrated in the problems of the PBL units. For instance, a problem in the "Cell growth and aging" unit of the Geneva curriculum describes the story of an old lady who is about to give up driving. This problem allows a discussion of the pathophysiology of cataract, theories of aging, cellular mechanisms of aging, as well as legal issues about evaluating the driving ability of older persons. Similarly, other geriatric objectives in basic sciences and clinical disciplines can be integrated in the problems of other PBL units (Huber *et al.*, 1998).

A longitudinal Clinical Skills Program that runs parallel to the PBL units allows an early and progressive acquisition of clinical skills relevant for geriatrics. For example, basic training in neuropsychological assessment can be coordinated with a problem concerning dementia.

Other types of PBL problems help further integrate basic sciences concepts, and to develop student's clinical knowledge and problem-solving abilities. This approach is especially relevant for addressing frequent clinical problems in older persons (stroke, dizzy spells, falls, malnutrition, dementia). Again, these problems can be coordinated with related seminars that emphasize the acquisition of important aspects of the geriatric assessment, such as functional assessment, evaluation of the social network, mental examination, or assessment of the nutritional status.

During the clinical phase, exposure to the inpatient and outpatient care of frail elderly subjects should be provided in an attempt to foster a positive and multidisciplinary approach to the care of the elderly. Exposure to normal and successful aging should be provided whenever it is possible. Finally, it is very important to stress that undergraduate geriatric curriculum must be mandatory and evaluated to ensure that the students receive geriatric clinical attachments for their daily clinical practice in the future.

Northern Europe

Finland, Norway, and Sweden have academic positions in geriatrics in each medical school, with an undergraduate geriatric program constituted by both traditional and problem-based teaching activities varying from a few hours to 44 hours in the 3rd and the 6th year of medical study. Geriatric patients staying in academic geriatric wards are accessible to every medical student, and this activity is always very well appreciated. The same is not true for the psychogeriatric and the long-term care/nursing home patients.

Southern Europe

In Italy, the majority of medical schools have at least one faculty member who is specialized in geriatric medicine, although in some of them the teaching of geriatrics is provided by nongeriatricians, mainly internal medicine physicians. All students receive a formal education in geriatrics during the last year of medical school, although the practical training is performed mainly within the acute care hospital, and only a few medical schools have implemented training in the community services, that is, in nursing homes.

In Greece, there is only one chair in geriatrics among six different medical schools, with the internal medicine departments providing optional geriatric teaching.

In Spain, geriatric medicine is mandatory for all medical students in the 3rd and 6th year of undergraduate training. However, there is only one medical school that has a professor of geriatric medicine, and in the vast majority of them, physicians, usually from the internal medicine department, with no formal education in geriatrics are in charge of teaching geriatric medicine. The students receive mainly formal lessons with little or no practical training, with the majority of training taking place in hospitals.

Eastern Europe

We have received updated information so far only from Hungary and Poland.

In Hungary, there is not yet any academic position in the biology of aging, geriatrics, or psycho geriatrics. However, an intermedical schools undergraduate geriatric program exists, due to the enthusiasm of a few well-trained (but not yet academic appointed) geriatricians. This 20-hour program takes place at the end of medical studies in each Hungarian medical school.

In Poland, the number of geriatric academic positions has increased considerably during the last few years. In each medical school where a geriatric academic position exists, a 30-hour undergraduate geriatric program has been introduced in the 5th year of study. Geriatric teaching is, however, not mandatory and no geriatric ward exists to train medical students in this speciality.

In summary, undergraduate geriatric training is better organized in Scandinavia, the United Kingdom, Belgium, France, and Italy, while the other countries have a less adequate educational system. In many countries, undergraduate training in gerontology and geriatrics is not well integrated in the medical curricula, particularly with basic and preclinical disciplines, being limited to the last year of training, with the risk of remaining isolated from the core educational contents.

It is interesting to note that a similar conclusion was arrived at by an independent report produced by a collaborative initiative of the World Health Organization and the International Federation of Medical Students' Association, which was released in 2002 (Keller *et al.*, 2002). The overall status of geriatric teaching in Europe is not considered "very promising" in this report, since in the majority of countries, particularly of central and southern Europe, there is a vast lack of structured geriatric teaching. Even in those universities that offer geriatric training, only a 20- to 40-hour course is usually provided, which includes the physiological, psychiatric, pharmacological, and pathological aspects of aging. Moreover, although the European Union of Medical Specialists – geriatric medicine section (GMS-UEMS) has produced an undergraduate curriculum in geriatric medicine in 1999, which has been approved by a number of national geriatric societies, there is no evidence that this curriculum has been implemented in EU countries (Geriatric Medicine Section of the European Union Medical Specialists, 2005).

The most important conclusion we can derive is that the lack of recognition of geriatric medicine as a distinct speciality in a majority of countries represents the most important cause of the unsatisfactory status of geriatric training at the undergraduate level in Europe. The main identified deficiencies were: lack of a sufficient number of academic geriatricians, lack of the adoption of a uniform curriculum, the short time devoted to geriatrics usually at the end of the medical training, and the inadequate organization of clinical training with older patients. The absence of gerontological education in the medical curriculum does not allow students to fully understand the complexity of older patients, while the limitation of practical training with geriatric patients to the acute hospital care undermines their capacity to appreciate the absolute need of interdisciplinary comprehensive assessment and continuity of care.

Another potential difficulty is the indifferent or negative attitude toward the care for older people expressed by medical students, which has been widely documented, particularly in studies from the USA (Coccaro and Miles, 1984; Reuben *et al.*, 1995). Improving knowledge about aging and older people by teaching gerontological and geriatric topics early in the curriculum as well as providing direct personal experience with healthy and active older people have been found to ameliorate the attitude and perception of medical students toward elderly subjects (Alford *et al.*, 2001).

GERIATRIC MEDICINE TEACHING AT THE POSTGRADUATE LEVEL

In many European countries, there are ongoing residency programs in geriatrics, with a well-defined curriculum. In some of them (e.g. Italy, Spain), geriatrics is an independent speciality, meaning that trainees enter a 4 to 5 year postgraduate training in geriatric medicine directly after medical school, while in others (e.g. Austria, Belgium, France, Germany, Netherlands, Switzerland, and United Kingdom), formal training in internal medicine or general practice may be required first, but often runs alongside training in geriatrics. Only in some of these countries, there is the requirement for an accreditation in geriatric medicine (Belgium, France, Ireland, the Netherlands, Switzerland, and United Kingdom). On the other hand there are some countries, such as Greece, Hungary, Luxemburg, and Portugal, which do not have any recognized geriatric training program (Hastie and Duursma, 2003). Although there is now an established geriatric curriculum produced by Geriatric Medicine Section of the European Union Medical Specialists (UEMS), 2005 the geriatric training programs remain extremely heterogeneous even within the same country; this is mainly because the training programs have been historically organized on the basis of the services which were locally available, and were not based primarily on the educational needs of the geriatric specialist. It is still of particular concern that in many countries geriatric training is hospital-based, and trainees do not have any access to community services, including nursing homes. It is now time that the organization of geriatric training is reconsidered, in order to restructure it with the aim of providing future specialists with the required knowledge and skills to practice twenty-first century geriatric medicine (Phelan *et al.*, 2003).

Concerning the geriatric education of postgraduate trainees in primary care or other specialities, there is evidence that it is nowadays extremely scanty or even completely ignored in the official curricula in many countries. This is certainly worrisome because primary care physicians as well as medical and surgical specialists are treating a large number of older patients, including the oldest, the very sick, and the most complicated and frail patients, but they are not adequately prepared to deal with their complex problems (Duursma *et al.*, 2004; Michel, 1997). Paradoxically, in several countries the geriatric training of nonmedical health-care professionals, especially nurses, is better organized than that of physicians. Finally, there is no well-organized continuous medical education program in geriatric medicine for the large number of physicians who did not get any formal exposure to geriatric medicine during their undergraduate and postgraduate training, and who still account for the majority of practicing medical doctors.

EAMA: A MODEL EXAMPLE OF GERIATRIC CONTINUOUS PROFESSIONAL TRAINING

The European Academy of Medicine of Aging (EAMA) (Stähelin *et al.*, 1994), organizes courses to train many of the future academic teachers of geriatrics in Europe. Part of the course deals with enhancing, updating, and improving the use of scientific knowledge by gathering data, gaining skills in critical interpretation of information, identifying deficiencies, learning how to establish priorities, and expressing important clinical messages. The first EAMA course (four residential 1-week sessions), started in January 1994 at the University Institute Kurt BOESCH (IUKB) in Sion (Switzerland), which significantly contributed to the launch of the course. In 2005, the course still has the same format. Each session includes state-of-the-art lectures by teachers and students, group discussions, and tutorial supervision of all student activities (Michel, 1997).

From 1995 to 2004, the weekly sessions have always addressed different topics and welcomed distinguished colleagues from all over the world, who played a key role in updating scientific knowledge and stimulating research ideas. EAMA recruits students from many European countries (Belgium, France, Germany, The Netherlands, Switzerland, United Kingdom, and several others including Eastern European countries such as Hungary, Poland, Russia), where geriatric societies select promising academic geriatricians, or students are nominated by senior academics in their own country. The Scientific committee also accepts outstanding non-European students (Argentina, Brazil, Israel, Lebanon, Mexico, Senegal, South Africa, and Tunisia) without exceeding a maximum number of 40 students per session to allow better supervision and interaction between students and teachers. This learning environment promotes a rich learning experience with cultural perspectives, multiple socioeconomical differences, and varied health-care organizations enhancing fruitful discussions on care and research issues. Geriatricians with many diverse perspectives interact on ethical issues and establish valuable networks.

The possibilities of exchanges were amplified by the launch of an EAMA virtual classroom located within the "www.healthandage.com/edu/eama" internet site. Since the first session, all the training activities of the teachers and students are evaluated. Students evaluate the performances of the teachers, the experts, and their colleagues, and vice versa. The comparison of evaluation results between students and teachers shows that students are stricter and more severe with their colleagues than the teachers themselves (Michel, 1997). The evaluation of the students' scores between the first and the last session of the third EAMA course showed that the scientific content of their lecture were enhanced, the formulation of taking home messages was more precise, and the techniques of oral presentation were better focused. In total, the score of the overall quality of the student's teaching performance between the first and the fourth session of the third course was increased by 31% (Swine *et al.*, 2004). The most impressive result of EAMA is the fact that 91% of the former students ($n = 167$) acquired professional promotion and 20% obtained an academic position.

The EAMA activities are now organized in close collaboration with the European Union Geriatric Medicine Society (EUGMS) and the International Association of Gerontology and Geriatrics – European Region (IAG-ER), allowing for an excellent and promising networking of the new generation of geriatricians.

The success of EAMA is officially recognized by their recent accreditation (2002) by both the Swiss Medical Federation and the European Union of the Medical Specialists – geriatric section. Another indicator of the success of the EAMA is the launch of similar initiatives in different parts of the world by former students: the "Academia Latino Americana de Medicina del Adulto mayor" (ALMA), the "Middle East Academy for Medicine of Aging" (MEAMA), the "Saint Louis University Geriatric Academy" (SLUGA) and, probably next year, the "European Nursing Academy for the Care of the Older" (ENACO).

CONCLUSION

Undergraduate and postgraduate training programs in geriatric medicine across Europe are varied in content and format and are often poorly developed. Restructuring of the educational process in order to equip future health-care professionals including physicians to provide specialist care to elderly patients is needed. Otherwise, we may see the progressive collapse of European health-care systems under the burden of the complexity and multiplicity of health-care needs of an increasing sick and disabled older population. It is therefore a priority for nongovernmental and professional organizations, such as EUGMS, UEMS, IAG-ER clinical section, and national geriatric societies, to try to influence the decision makers in both the health-care sector and the academic centers to address this urgent educational imperative.

Acknowledgment

The authors thank the EAMA students who provided them information concerning the geriatric teaching activities in their own countries.

KEY POINTS

- The European population is aging: while in 1999 14% of the subjects were older than 65 years, this percentage will increase by about 160% in the next 50 years. Whereas the majority of older people live healthy and independent lives, the risk of morbidity, ill health, and disability increases with age.
- The frail elderly population with its specific medical and psychosocial needs requires high-quality geriatric care: this can be provided only if appropriate geriatric training is guaranteed to all categories of health-care professionals and, particularly, doctors.
- There is little evidence that European countries are responding adequately to this "Geriatric education imperative". There is indeed an extreme heterogeneity in the provision of geriatric education, both at the undergraduate and the postgraduate level not only between different countries but also within the same country.
- In many European countries, undergraduate training in gerontology and geriatrics is not adequately developed and is not integrated into the medical curricula, particularly with basic and preclinical disciplines, being often limited to the last year of training and to the hospital setting.
- Postgraduate training in geriatric medicine is available in several European countries, but not at all in some others. In general, training is still limited to the hospital setting and does not include periods of training in the ambulatory, community and long-term care settings, where the majority of older patients are cured.

KEY REFERENCES

- Duursma S, Castleden M, Cherubini A *et al.* European Union Geriatric medicine Society Position paper on geriatric medicine and the provision of health care for older people. *The Journal of Nutrition, Health & Aging* 2004; **8**:190–5.
- Hastie IR & Duursma S. Geriatric Medicine Section of the European Union Medical Specialists Geriatric medicine in the European Union: unification of diversity. *Aging Clinical and Experimental Research* 2003; **15**:347–51.
- Huber P, Gold G & Michel JP. Innovation in an undergraduate geriatrics program. *Academic Medicine* 1998; **73**:579–80.
- Michel JP & the Group of European Professors of Medical Gerontology Raising the level of medical gerontology: Evaluation of the European Academy for Medicine of Ageing course. *Aging Clinical and Experimental Research* 1997; **9**:224–305.
- Stähelin HB, Beregi E, Duursma S *et al.* Teaching medical gerontology in Europe. *Age and Ageing* 1994; **23**:179–81.

REFERENCES

Alford CL, Miles T, Palmer R & Espino D. An introduction to geriatrics for first-year medical students. *Journal of the American Geriatrics Society* 2001; **49**:782–7.

Besdine RW. The maturing of geriatrics. *The New England Journal of Medicine* 1989; **320**:181–2.

Coccaro EF & Miles AM. The attitudinal impact of training in gerontology/geriatrics in medical school: a review of the literature and perspective. *Journal of the American Geriatrics Society* 1984; **32**:762–8.

Duursma S, Castleden M, Cherubini A *et al.* European Union Geriatric medicine Society Position paper on geriatric medicine and the provision of health care for older people. *The Journal of Nutrition, Health & Aging* 2004; **8**:190–5.

Economic Commission for Europe's Population Activities Unit. www.unece.org/ead/pau/a_home1.htm (accessed 20th February 2005).

Geriatric Medicine Section of the European Union Medical Specialists. www.uemsgeriatricmedicine.org (accessed 23rd February 2005).

Hastie IR & Duursma S. Geriatric Medicine Section of the European Union Medical Specialists Geriatric medicine in the European Union: unification of diversity. *Aging Clinical and Experimental Research* 2003; **15**:347–51.

Holman H. Chronic disease – the need for a clinical education. *The Journal of the American Medical Association* 2004; **292**:1057–9.

Huber P, Gold G & Michel JP. Innovation in an undergraduate geriatrics program. *Academic Medicine* 1998; **73**:579–80.

Keller I, Makipaa A, Kalensher T & Kalache A. *Global Survey on Geriatrics in Medical Curriculum Geneva* 2002; World Health Organization.

Michel JP & the Group of European Professors of Medical Gerontology Raising the level of medical gerontology: Evaluation of the European Academy for Medicine of Ageing course. *Aging Clinical and Experimental Research* 1997; **9**:224–305.

Oeppen J & Vaupel JW. Demography. Broken limits to life expectancy. *Science* 2002; **296**:1029–31.

Phelan EA, Paniagua MA & Hazzard WR. *Principles of Geriatric Medicine and Gerontology* 2003, 5th edn, pp 85–92; McGraw-Hill Companies, New-York.

Reuben DB, Fullerton JT, Tschann JM & Croughan-Minihane M, The University of California Academic Geriatric Resource Program Student Survey Research Group. Attitudes of beginning medical students toward older persons: a five-campus study. *Journal of the American Geriatrics Society* 1995; **43**:1430–6.

Robine J-M & Paccaud F. [La démographie des nonagénaires et des centenaires en Suisse] in press.

Stähelin HB, Beregi E, Duursma S *et al.* Teaching medical gerontology in Europe. *Age and Ageing* 1994; **23**:179–81.

Swine Ch, Michel JP, Duursma S *et al.* Evaluation of the European Academy for Medicine of Ageing "Teaching the teachers" program (EAMA course II 1997–8). *The Journal of Nutrition, Health & Aging* 2004; **8**:181–6.

Vu NV, Bader CR & Vassalli JD. The redesigned undergraduate medical curriculum at the university of Geneva. In AJJA Scherpbier, CPM van der Fleuten, JJ Rethans & AFW van der Steeg (eds) *Advances in Medical Education* 1997, pp 532–5; Klüwer Academic Publishers, Dordrecht.

Education in Geriatric Medicine in the United Kingdom

Robert W. Stout
Queen's University Belfast, Belfast, UK

INTRODUCTION

Geriatric medicine was first recognized as a speciality in the United Kingdom (UK) at the time of the introduction of the National Health Service (NHS) in 1948 (Evans, 1997; Barton and Mulley, 2003). Since that time, increasing numbers of specialists in geriatric medicine have been appointed, at first largely self-trained, but now having completed formal training programs, and usually having been first introduced to the subject as students. Education in geriatric medicine has developed alongside the clinical speciality.

MEDICAL EDUCATION

Medical education is conventionally divided into several phases. The first phase is the initial training leading to qualification as a doctor. In the United Kingdom, this is usually taken at undergraduate level but as some medical students are already graduates, the term used by the General Medical Council (GMC) – "basic medical education" – is preferable. Basic medical education is usually followed by a compulsory year as the most junior hospital doctor – "preregistration house officer". In the United Kingdom, in 2005, the house officer year will be replaced by a 2-year period of foundation training. This is followed by several more years of postgraduate or specialist training which combines supervised clinical experience and formal education and assessment. The remaining phase is "continuing professional development" and refers to the need for all doctors to continue educating themselves and updating their skills throughout their professional lifetimes; this will not be discussed further in this chapter.

HISTORY

Three phases in the development of basic medical education in geriatric medicine in the United Kingdom can be recognized. In the first 15 years of the speciality, education was largely informal and clinically based. The teachers were consultants in the speciality, they usually taught in their wards, and the teaching was based on the plethora of clinical signs found in their patients. Attendance at classes was often voluntary and specific time for geriatric medicine rarely appeared in curricula. Specialist training was also informal, largely based on experience gained in clinical practice, and sometimes took the form of a short attachment or "conversion course" for doctors already trained in general medicine or one of its specialities.

In 1965, the University of Glasgow appointed Professor (later Sir) W Ferguson Anderson to the first chair of geriatric medicine. Following this, chairs of geriatric medicine (sometimes with other titles) have been created in almost all universities with medical schools in the United Kingdom and in many other parts of the world. During the two decades following 1965, the academic discipline of geriatric medicine developed, and formal teaching courses were designed and published. Geriatric medicine became a required component of many medical school curricula, encouraged by the Recommendations on Basic Medical Education of the General Medical Council (General Medical Council, 1980) (Table 1). The state of education in geriatric medicine and gerontology at the end of these two decades was the subject of a comprehensive review published in 1985 (Stout, 1985).

The third phase was a revolution in medical education which started in the late 1980s culminating in the introduction of radically new medical curricula in the United Kingdom and many other countries. The exact role of geriatric medicine in these new curricula has not been described.

Principles and Practice of Geriatric Medicine, 4th Edition. Edited by M.S. John Pathy, Alan J. Sinclair and John E. Morley.

Table 1 The first published recommendations on teaching gerontology and geriatric medicine in the United Kingdom

United Kingdom (General Medical Council (1980))
The student should receive instruction in the special problems of diagnosis and treatment of illness in the elderly and in maintaining mental and physical health in old age. He should be introduced to the range of domiciliary and institutional services available for the care of the elderly

However, some of the "new" concepts in the revised curricula have already been in place in educational programs in geriatric medicine, and the change from the old to the new did not prove as difficult in this subject as it was in some other longer established disciplines.

Unfortunately, we now appear to be entering a fourth phase where some of the progress that has been made in introducing academic geriatric medicine in the United Kingdom is under threat. The threat arises from new imperatives on universities for quality assessments in both teaching and research. These have led medical schools to reorganize into smaller numbers of large academic units, and the smaller specialist departments, particularly those which have a broad clinical base and whose research is more applied and practice orientated, are not seen as a priority. As a result, a number of departments of geriatric medicine have ceased to exist. A survey of medical schools undertaken by the British Geriatrics Society in 2004 (Crome *et al.*, 2004) revealed that a considerable number of UK medical schools no longer had an academic department of geriatric medicine, and of those that had, only about one half had a professor as head of department. This contrasts with the state of academic geriatric medicine in 1996 when all UK medical schools had academic appointments in geriatric medicine, all but one at professorial level, several had more than one professor, and some also had professors of geriatric psychiatry. Of particular concern is, the poor recruitment into academic geriatric medicine and the lack of applicants for senior academic posts, including chairs. This is not unique to geriatric medicine, and is an extreme example of problems in UK academic medicine (Academy of Medical Sciences, 2002). Geriatric medicine, being one of the newer entrants into academic medicine, is particularly vulnerable. It is ironic that this should be happening at a time when the need for education and research in aging and the care of older people has never been greater.

THE APPROACH TO MEDICAL EDUCATION

Over the last two decades, medical education in the United Kingdom has become much more professionalized and most medical schools now have a department of medical education, usually staffed by a combination of people with medical qualifications who have taken a particular interest in education, and people with qualifications in education or related disciplines. Medical education departments play a major role in the design of curricula and provide training in techniques of delivering education and its assessment. They also coordinate the curriculum and it is no longer the case that individual disciplines, often identified by academic departments, are allocated a period of time in the medical curriculum and use it as they wish.

A number of issues have driven change in medical education. These include the following:

- much of what is learnt during the undergraduate period, frequently in the last few weeks before examinations, is rapidly forgotten;
- even if it was all remembered, much of it rapidly becomes out of date and is little used during the professional careers of medical graduates;
- much of the information that medical graduates use in practising their profession is acquired in the years following graduation;
- curricula did not always reflect the requirement for postgraduate education for whatever speciality the graduate enters; thus the aim of producing a doctor who could go into independent practice immediately after graduation is unrealistic;
- over the years, new knowledge and new subjects have developed and these tended to be fitted into the curriculum with very little thought on whether anything should be taken out;
- medicine is now practised in multidisciplinary teams, both in hospital and in the community, and preparation for working in teams needs to be included within the curriculum;
- new educational methods have been developed;
- the importance of assessment, both for students and for teachers.

The overall outcome of basic medical education is to produce graduates who have the knowledge and competencies to undertake the preregistration house officer year, have the basic framework of knowledge and skills to allow them to progress through postgraduate medical education in their chosen speciality, have an enquiring and reflective outlook on medical practice so as to be in a position to evaluate and, where appropriate, introduce new developments, and have the professional attributes expected of medical practitioners.

The first task in designing the new curriculum was to define the core knowledge and skills which were required of every medical graduate. This required hard reflective thinking on the part of medical educators and the acceptance by many that this might mean that their own particular subject would be taught in less detail than was previously the case. About two-thirds of the total curricular time is needed for a core education. (A European Directive rules that basic medical training, which includes the preregistration year, must be at least 6 years in duration, or 5500 hours of theoretical and practical instruction given in a university or under the supervision of a university.) Students also need to study some subjects in depth to allow them to see the boundaries of knowledge, to be introduced to methods of evaluation, literature searching, gathering and analyzing new data, and to study subjects of their own choosing, perhaps as a help to making career choices later. Thus, a series of student selected components (previously known as special study modules) have been introduced. The third feature of the new curriculum is integration. This includes vertical integration of the basic sciences with clinical subjects so that students learn at the same time, for example, the anatomy, physiology, and clinical examination of a system; and horizontal integration where overlapping subjects are taught together or in a coordinated fashion. Some components of the course should be taught on a multidisciplinary basis along with students of other health-care professions, including nursing and the allied health professions. New teaching methods have been introduced, including clinical skills centers in which students can learn clinical skills on lifelike models, and computer-aided and web-based teaching.

Integrated teaching is often system based using the anatomical and physiological systems of the body. Some medical schools in the United Kingdom use problem-based learning where the responsibility for their education is placed on the students who are presented with a clinical problem and then use their own initiative to acquire the appropriate knowledge of normal and abnormal structure and function. Problem-based learning is highly resource intensive, particularly in staff who act as facilitators rather than teachers, and not all medical schools have been able to introduce this method. Whichever method is used, the curriculum is student centered with the student carrying increasing responsibility for active learning rather than, as previously, being a passive recipient of what is delivered by teachers.

Assessment methods are now multiple and it is generally accepted that often several methods are necessary for assessing particular areas. While both the traditional essays and the multiple-choice question papers have a role in medical education, their role is specific and limited and it is inappropriate for them to be the only assessment methods. Continuous assessment by means of logbooks, portfolios, and records of achievement are used to test skills and attitudes. While knowledge and skills can be readily assessed, it is much more difficult to assess attitudes. Concern about doctors who have behaved inappropriately has focused attention on the attitudes of students, both on admission to the medical school and during the course, and increasing supervision of students through personal tutors and other similar schemes may identify the small number of students who have inappropriate attitudes.

University education, including medical education, is increasingly governed by bodies outside the universities. Since its foundation in 1858, the GMC has had responsibility for medical education in the United Kingdom. It has discharged this responsibility by publishing "Recommendations on Basic Medical Education" every decade and by inspecting the medical schools. The recommendations issued in 1993, under the title of "Tomorrow's Doctors" introduced radical change and set out the new educational principles mentioned above (General Medical Council, 1993). The GMC also introduced more rigorous inspections to ensure that medical schools complied with the recommendations. The latest edition of "Tomorrow's Doctors", issued in 2002 (General Medical Council, 2002), did not radically change the 1993 edition, but further emphasized the need to ensure that the standards of conduct for all medical practitioners set out in the GMCs document "Good Medical Practice" (General Medical Council, 2001) are infused throughout the curriculum. A number of GMC recommendations in "Tomorrow's Doctors" are relevant to the care of older people (Table 2). There are also recommendations on the principles of assessment and assessment procedures.

The Quality Assurance Agency (QAA) for higher education, which assesses teaching quality in higher education in the United Kingdom, has issued benchmark statements for each subject. These are a means for the academic community to describe the nature and characteristics of programs in specific subjects and represent general expectations about the standards for the award of qualifications at a given level. The benchmark statements are used by institutions in designing and evaluating programs, by external examiners, by the QAA when assessing the standards in universities, and by potential students and employers to help them understand programs of higher education. The benchmark statement for medicine (Quality Assurance Agency for Higher Education, 2002), although differing in style from "Tomorrow's Doctors", has essentially the same requirements. Some of educational outcomes are particularly relevant to the teaching of aging and the care of older people (Table 3). A further influential document, "The Scottish Doctor", produced by the Scottish Deans Medical Curriculum Group (2002), has a series of learning

Table 2 Recommendations on basic medical education relevant to the care of older people (General Medical Council, 2002)

1. Students must demonstrate respect for patients regardless of age (item 6c(ii))
2. Graduates must know about and understand the care of people with recurrent and chronic illnesses and people with mental and physical disabilities (item (16f))
3. Graduates must be aware of the importance of working as a team within a multiprofessional context (item (28f))
4. Graduates must understand the social and cultural environment in which medicine is practised in the United Kingdom and must understand human development and areas of psychology and sociology relevant to medicine including growing old (item (34))

Table 3 Benchmarks for medical education relevant to the care of older people (Quality Assurance Agency for Higher Education, 2002)

1. Graduates will demonstrate knowledge and understanding of
   (a) the different stages of the life cycle and how these affect normal structure and function (item 4.2(b))
   (b) impairment, disability, and handicap and the principles of rehabilitation (item 4.2(j))
   (c) epidemiological principles of demography and biological variability (item 4.2(o))
2. Core competencies: the graduate will be able to
   (a) undertake a relevant and systematic physical and mental examination in a sensitive manner appropriate for age. (item 6.2(1b))
3. Demonstration of competency:
   (a) Graduates should be capable of giving appropriate input into the multidisciplinary and multiprofessional teams involved in the management of patients in need of rehabilitation or palliative care, including the care of the dying (item 6.3(4))

outcomes, and the most extensive published description of assessment methods. These documents are all of great value in medical education and influential in curriculum development. In all cases, they look at the medical curriculum as a whole and do not mention specific disciplines or traditional university departments. Throughout all the documents, however, the principles of the care of older people appear and these allow the medical schools to ensure that education in aging and the care of older people is adequately represented in the curriculum.

It is essential that medical schools should have a lead for education in aging and the care of older people, whether as part of an academic department or in some other form, to ensure that the subject is adequately covered in the curriculum and that all doctors have basic knowledge of the subject. In addition to covering basic knowledge and skills, the course should enthuse students in the importance of the care of older people and encourage some to consider specializing in this branch of medicine.

BASIC MEDICAL EDUCATION

The Approach

The first task is to define a core curriculum – the essential knowledge, skills, and attitudes which all newly qualified medical practitioners must attain. This is expressed as outcomes. Because of its relatively recent introduction into medical education and the small amount of curricular time which is usually allocated to it, a core curriculum in geriatric medicine has already been defined (Stout, 1985).

The curriculum is "problem based", that is, learning is centered around clinical problems. Thus, when learning about the aging process, students might study the case history of an older person, or a life history, perhaps in written form or on video. In this way, the relevance of basic science to clinical practice can be demonstrated. The curriculum is "student centered" rather than "teacher driven". The emphasis is on learning rather than teaching and students are helped and guided to learn, with academic staff acting more as facilitators than teachers. Good clinical teachers are used to guiding students on how to learn from the patients they have seen.

Clinical teaching takes place in both the hospital and the community. Although teaching in the community is often considered to be the remit of general practice, other disciplines, such as psychiatry and geriatric medicine, extend beyond the hospital. The movement of teaching into the community is driven by two forces – the fact that much medical practice and the work of the majority of doctors takes place outside hospital, and changes in hospital practice, such as shortened lengths of stay, the increasing use of day procedures and the increasing specialization of hospital practice, which have changed the clinical profiles of hospitals in ways which make traditional clinical teaching difficult. Geriatric medicine with its hospital base and community outreach is well placed to lead new educational strategies combining hospital and community based clinical teaching. Multiprofessional education, with students of medicine, nursing, the allied health professions, and social work being taught together is also very appropriate for geriatric medicine.

CURRENT TEACHING OF GERIATRIC MEDICINE

Because of concern that the previous gains that had been achieved to ensure that aging and geriatric medicine were incorporated within the undergraduate curriculum were in danger of being lost, in 2004 the Education and Training Committee of the British Geriatrics Society undertook a survey of teaching geriatric medicine in UK medical schools. Questionnaires were sent to Deans or Heads of UK Medical Schools, members of the British Geriatrics Society Education and Training Committee, and Heads of Departments of Geriatric Medicine or their equivalent. Although the response was incomplete, the survey gave a useful snapshot of the place of geriatric medicine in UK medical curricula (Crome *et al.*, 2004). In all except one of the universities that responded, geriatric medicine is taught to all undergraduates. Human aging is also taught in many medical schools, most often as part of teaching in physiology, but also in social sciences and psychiatry. In most cases, the curriculum is organized and coordinated by a professor or senior lecturer in geriatrics although in some medical schools other academic staff or NHS consultants do this. Three-quarters of heads of departments felt that geriatric medicine should be taught as a separate subject although a few thought it could be linked to other subjects. Many also thought that nongeriatricians, including general physicians, general practitioners, psychiatrists, clinical pharmacologists, and therapists, could also teach geriatric medicine. Most felt that sufficient teaching time was allocated to the subject and that every student should be examined in geriatric medicine. In most cases, classical teaching methods of patient contact, lectures, and tutorials are used but about 50% of the medical schools that responded use problem-based tutorials. Geriatric medicine is taught in virtually all the clinical sites where it is practised. In about one-third of medical schools, undergraduates spend time in nursing home placements. One university was about to start a pilot program of multiprofessional education of medical and nursing students in geriatric medicine. There was a strong feeling that examinations should be clinically based, either during the course or at a final examination, and that geriatric medicine should be examined in association with other subjects. In most medical schools, geriatricians take part in the examination.

CURRICULUM DESIGN

Curriculum design must consider the educational outcomes, the educational program, assessment, and evaluation (Leinster, 2003a). Assessment differs from evaluation in that the former is concerned with the performance of the students, while the latter is a measure of how the program meets its objectives.

Educational Outcomes

Outcomes are statements of what students should be able to do at the end of a course of study which they could not do initially; they imply the testing of the effectiveness of the teaching course in terms of the achievement of these outcomes (Irwin *et al.*, 1976). Thus, an outcome describes what students should be able to do in order to demonstrate that they have acquired a required level of competence. Outcomes allow those involved in the different aspects of the curriculum, planning, teaching, learning, assessment, and evaluation, to have a framework within which they can design the teaching program and methods of assessment. Both teacher and student can be aware of the aims of the course and they are able to judge progress against these aims.

Outcomes in medical education cover knowledge, skills, and attitudes. In the past, attention was mainly paid to acquisition of knowledge – now more attention is paid to skills and attitudes. The whole can be incorporated into the concept of competence – the combination of knowledge, skills, and attitudes that enables the individual to practice medicine.

There are a number of reasons why a statement of educational outcomes is desirable. First, failure to state precise teaching outcomes permits and promotes unclear thinking and lowers the quality of learning. Second, identification of outcomes is a prerequisite for setting evaluative criteria. Third, only when outcomes are behaviorally stated, is it possible to determine whether they are trivial or not. When constructing outcomes, it must be emphasized that only outcomes which are intended and measurable are worth stating. Unanticipated outcomes from the course which distort the achievement of stated objectives require to be identified and incorporated into the stated outcomes. Thus, a process of "hard inventive thinking" is necessary in the construction of these outcomes (Irwin *et al.*, 1976).

Outcomes for basic medical education that have been subjected to "hard inventive thinking" are those from Queen's University Belfast (Stout and Bamber, 1979) (Table 4). Other lists of outcomes have been published, most notably those which were agreed at a World Health Organisation workshop in Edinburgh in 1982 (World Health Organisation, 1982) (Table 5). Although these outcomes were drawn up by a group of people who had experience in teaching gerontology and geriatric medicine, they were not subjected to the rigorous analysis suggested by specialists in education. Nevertheless, they correspond quite closely to the Belfast outcomes. Other published outcomes have been reviewed elsewhere (Stout, 1985). Common topics in all the published outcomes include:

demography of aging;
the aging process;
the presentation of disease in old age;
management of illness in older people;
attitudes to old age.

Any educational program in geriatric medicine must cover at least these topics.

The Educational Program

The educational program should be student centered and problem based. Geriatric medicine is ideal for problem-based learning as the essence of geriatric practice is the identification and resolution of problems presented by patients. The nonspecific nature of the problems allows wide-ranging discussion and hence a broad educational experience. The "giants of geriatrics" identified by Isaacs (1992) – immobility, instability, incontinence, and intellectual impairment – cover a wide range of diagnostic and management possibilities and would provide the basic list of problems on which the program would be based. A detailed medical undergraduate curriculum in geriatric medicine has been published by the British Geriatrics Society (British Geriatrics Society, 2004).

Teachers

Ideally, teachers of geriatric medicine should be engaged in clinical practice in the medical care of older people. In this way, they will have the knowledge, skills, and attitudes to the health care of older people that will be an example to the students. However, it is not sufficient for teachers to

Table 4 Educational outcomes in geriatric medicine of Queen's University Belfast (Stout and Bamber, 1979)

A Knowledge
The student should understand
1. the epidemiology of aging and its implications
2. the normal aging process and its relationship to disease and disability in old age
3. the pattern and presentation of disease in old age
4. the interaction of physical, mental, and social factors in the production of disease and disability in old age
5. the purpose, facilities, and organization of hospital care of elderly patients
6. the role, availability, and organization of community services in the care of elderly people
7. the prevention of dependency in old age
8. ethical issues in the care of elderly people

B Skills
The student should have the following skills:
1. the assessment of disease and disability in older people
2. the principles of management of elderly patients
   (a) the value and limitation of investigation procedures
   (b) the appropriate use of drugs
   (c) rehabilitation
   (d) continuing care
   (e) terminal care
   (f) the value of the multidisciplinary health-care team
3. Communication with older people, both those who are healthy and those who have communication difficulties

C Attitudes
The student should have an attitude of optimism in the care of elderly people

Table 5 WHO learning outcomes in gerontology and geriatric medicine (World Health Organisation, 1982)

1. A humane and positive attitude toward old people and to demonstrate the satisfaction and fulfillment which comes from professional involvement with the elderly and their families
2. An understanding of demographic factors and social changes in the aging of societies
3. An understanding of age-related changes in the context of human development and an appreciation of the causes of disability in old age; prevention and management of disability should be understood within both community and institutional settings
4. An understanding of the special features of presentation of disease in old age and the problems of therapy. The problems associated with drug therapy in old age require special consideration
5. An understanding of the principles of rehabilitation and their application to the elderly, a major objective being the attainment and maintenance of optimum physical, social, and mental function for each individual
6. An understanding of the importance of working as a member of a multidisciplinary team, with full understanding and appreciation of the roles and skills of physicians, nurses, rehabilitation therapists, social workers, and other team members
7. An understanding of the importance of acquiring skill in communicating effectively with the elderly and those involved in their care. This should be done in such a way as to lead to fuller understanding of the importance of the family and the social network of care
8. An understanding of the importance of protecting the liberty of the individual, so that the elderly may retain maximum choice and control over their own lifestyles and the manner in which they face death
9. An understanding of services available to old people and their families, with special emphasis on community aspects, and to stress the essential interdependence of these services and the need for effective cooperation between them and families and other carers
10. An understanding of principles and responsibilities of continuing care for elderly patients with irremediable disabilities, and of terminal care of dying patients

be skilled in their clinical discipline – they must also be trained in modern educational methods. Staff development is an essential component of every medical school, and the aim should be that all teachers, whether they hold positions in universities or in the health service, should have undertaken a course in educational methods.

For the effective teaching of geriatric medicine, an academic discipline is ideal. This allows academic teachers time to develop programs and teaching skills. It also allows teaching to take place in a setting of research, the essence of university education. "Academic geriatric program leaders must be excellent clinicians, consummate generalists, superb teachers and outstanding, fully competitive researchers. Anything less risks second-class status for geriatrics" (Hazzard, 1994). Close cooperation with related academic disciplines is essential, particularly with general (internal) medicine, general practice, psychiatry, and public health medicine.

The Teaching Setting

Geriatric medicine is a practical clinical subject and is best taught in a clinical setting. This will be the hospital and community facilities for the care of older people, and will include visits to care homes and the homes of older patients, for example, during assessment visits. Teaching should not be confined to statutory services – voluntary and private sector facilities can give a different view of old age. There is a danger that the use of medical and nursing settings, the most convenient for curriculum planners to organize, may give students a view of old age that emphasizes ill-health, disability, and dependency. It is essential that students gain a balanced view of old age, and learn that for many people old age is a time of good health and independence It is possible to use families of patients and attenders at community facilities to illustrate healthy old age. This concept can be introduced early in the medical course. As care in the community is one of the educational objectives for geriatric medicine, teaching cannot be confined to the hospital. Students must have the opportunity to learn about domiciliary care of dependent older people by observing it in action. As at least half of the medical students will become general practitioners, the care of older people outside the hospital is particularly relevant.

Analysis of clinical problems, with the student using all resources available, including the library and members of the health-care team acting as a resource of expertise, is the preferred learning technique. Thus the teaching setting must have space for discussion and for learning, and access to information and expertise.

Learning Systems

Surprisingly, the British Geriatrics Society survey (Crome *et al.*, 2004) showed lectures as a common teaching method. There should be little place for formal lectures in teaching a practical clinical subject. If used at all, lectures should be few in number, and should act as signposts or "roadmaps", giving an overview of the subject, putting it in context. Lectures should never be used to impart large amounts of factual information.

Student-centered, problem-based directed self-learning is ideally suited to education in geriatric medicine. Study guides direct the students' learning by providing sample case histories, key questions to be answered, and advice on how to obtain information, for example, from studying patients, consulting written information, for which references are given, or experts. Study guides also include self-assessments to allow students to measure their progress. Study guides can be conveniently combined with log-diaries. In these, students are provided with a list of experiences to be encountered and procedures to be undertaken and they keep a record of what has been achieved. They would normally be countersigned by a teacher.

Study guides and log-diaries allow students to take control of their own education, while giving them confidence that they are covering the right topics and neither omitting important material nor learning unnecessary detail. Although study guides and log-diaries are usually in written form, they can be computerized, and students may base their education on programs on personal computers.

Study guides and log-diaries do not remove the need for teachers, but require a different type of teaching. Instead of the teacher delivering information, teachers facilitate learning, with regular meetings of small groups of students reporting on their learning experiences, and being guided on future learning. Teachers function as catalysts and educational resources but do not necessarily control the teaching session. Changing from delivering information to facilitating learning is a major process and staff development is necessary before these teaching methods can be introduced.

The Content

Of the educational program in geriatric medicine is based on the outcomes described earlier in this chapter, modified according to time and facilities available and adapted to the needs of the entire medical curriculum. There is considerable scope for collaborative teaching in geriatric medicine. For example, the topic of rehabilitation may be covered in collaboration with specialists in rehabilitation medicine, rheumatology, orthopedic surgery, and psychiatry as well as in geriatric medicine. It is essential that there is coordination and central control of the curriculum so that important topics are neither inadvertently omitted nor duplicated in an unplanned way. Topics such as rehabilitation involve many disciplines and can be used for multidisciplinary learning as a preparation for working in a multidisciplinary team.

Evaluation

Evaluation of an educational program covers three aspects – the performance of the students in terms of the educational outcomes; the performance of the program in terms of the outcomes; the quality of the educational experience.

Assessment of Students

It may be regrettable but it is true that student learning is driven by assessments (Leinster, 2003b). Most students do not take seriously a program that does not have an assessment, and the students' expectations of the standard and content of the assessments has a major influence on their learning. Appropriate assessments are therefore an essential component of any educational program. The usual way of assessing educational outcomes is to test the students' knowledge and skills to appropriate standards (Leinster, 2004).

There is a wide variety of assessment methods available. The method chosen must be appropriate for the objective to be tested. Reproducibility and consistency in marking are other important attributes of any assessment method. When different attributes are to be tested, a combination of methods is often used. Traditional methods of assessment in medical education include written, both essay and multiple-choice papers, clinical and oral examinations. A written assessment of knowledge of geriatric medicine has been described (Lee *et al.*, 2004).

The objective structured clinical examination (OSCE) (Harden and Gleeson, 1979) combines clinical, oral, and written examinations in a test of clinical competence. All students sit the same examination. They move through a series of "stations", usually about 20, and spend about 5 minutes at each. At the stations, they may be asked to perform a procedure such as taking a clinical history, carrying out a clinical examination, or answering questions on treatment, photographs, medical images, or the results of laboratory investigations. Examiners are present at some stations and observe the students' performance, while students are left to write their answers at others. Simulated patients or plastic models can be used for testing clinical skills, as the OSCE is demanding on real patients. The OSCE requires careful preparation, the availability of suitable space and is intensive in its use of staff. However, large numbers of students can be examined in a relatively short time and the results are available almost immediately. It has the advantage of standardization and is relatively efficient in the use of examiners' time.

Separate assessments do not have to be held for each individual discipline in the medical curriculum, and there are both theoretical and practical reasons for combining assessments. By combining clinical subjects, the assessment can become more analogous to the clinical encounter where the doctor is faced with patients who are unclassified with respect to speciality and who may have multiple problems, physical, psychological, and social, involving many systems.

Assessment of the Educational Program

In the United Kingdom, the quality of university teaching is regularly assessed, both by the universities themselves and by external bodies. An important measure is the students' opinion of the course, assessed by questionnaire. It is important that students' opinions are sought on educational programs. Every part of the program will not be popular with every student. However, deficiencies which might otherwise remain undetected can be identified.

Attitudes

One of the educational outcomes is "to have an attitude of optimism in the care of older people". It is not possible to test this objective adequately in any form of assessment of student performance, and special surveys have to be undertaken. It has been shown in the past that many medical students, doctors, and other health professionals have negative attitudes toward old people. Well-designed educational programs in geriatric medicine may improve attitudes toward elderly people. Although a number of surveys of medical students' attitudes have been carried out, few have tested the influence of modern educational programs on attitudes.

The effect of teaching geriatric medicine on medical students' attitudes to older people was studied in Edinburgh (Deary *et al.*, 1993). Attitudes became more positive from first year to the clinical years, and improved further as a result of the geriatric medicine course. Although women had slightly lower scores for negative attitudes, the extent of the changes across the groups did not differ between the sexes. Contrary to the reports of some previous studies, the attitudes of the Edinburgh medical students were not unduly negative. Similar positive effects of a geriatric medicine course on attitudes to old people were reported in the United States (Bernard *et al.*, 2003).

The available evidence suggests that current educational programs in geriatric medicine have positive effects on the attitudes of medical students to old age. It is essential that any innovative programs should be tested for their effects on attitudes.

SPECIALIST EDUCATION

Specialist education in geriatric medicine covers training in the discipline for those whose careers will be in other specialities, including general practice, and training for those who will practice geriatric medicine either exclusively or in combination with general (internal) medicine. Until relatively recently, training has largely consisted of gaining clinical experience in hospital departments practising high standards of care (hence the term "training" rather than "education"), but training is becoming more formal and curricula are being developed.

Educational outcomes, programs, and evaluation for specialist training in geriatric medicine have been described but have not been as carefully analyzed as those for basic medical education. Before entering higher training, the trainee will have completed the 2 foundation years immediately after graduation and spent 2 or more years as a Senior House Officer gaining experience in a variety of medical specialities, including geriatric medicine (Ives, 2003). In the United Kingdom, the responsibility for devising programs for higher medical training rests with the Joint Committee on Higher Medical Training (JCHMT) which has a series of Specialist Advisory Committees (SACs), one of which is for geriatric medicine. The JCHMTs curriculum for higher medical training for geriatric medicine (Joint Committee on Higher Medical Training, 2003) sets out the requirements for the 5-year training period in the speciality (Tables 6 and 7) against a specification of generic skills which are relevant to all medical specialities (Table 8). At the end of the training period, the trainee, who has achieved an appropriate level of knowledge, skills, and competence, will be awarded a Certificate of Specialist Training (CST), which is a prerequisite for appointment as a consultant in the NHS.

Table 6 Primary learning objectives for specialist training in geriatric medicine (Joint Committee on Higher Medical Training, 2003)

1. Perform a comprehensive assessment of an older person, including mood and cognition, gait, nutrition, and fitness for surgery in an inpatient, outpatient, day hospital, or community setting
2. Diagnose and manage acute illness in old age in an inpatient setting and community setting where appropriate
3. Diagnose and manage those with chronic disease and disability in an inpatient, outpatient, day hospital, and community setting
4. Provide rehabilitation with the multidisciplinary team to an older patient in an inpatient, outpatient, day hospital, and community setting
5. Plan the discharge of frail-older patients from hospital
6. Assess a patient's suitability for and provide appropriate care to those in long term (continuing care) in the NHS or community
7. Assess and manage older patients presenting with the common geriatric problems (syndromes) in an in- or outpatient setting (or where appropriate, in a community setting):
   Falls with or without fracture
   Delirium
   Incontinence
   Poor mobility
8. To demonstrate an appropriate level of competence in the following subspecialities:
   Palliative care
   Orthogeriatrics
   Old age psychiatry
   Specialist stroke care
9. To be familiar with basic research methodology, ethical principles of research, comprehensive scrutiny of medical literature and preferably to have personal experience of involvement in basic science or clinical (health services) research

Table 7 Core knowledge areas for specialist training in geriatric medicine (Joint Committee on Higher Medical Training, 2003)

Basic science and gerontology
Common geriatric problems (syndromes)
Presentations of other illness in older persons
Drug therapy
Rehabilitation in older persons
Discharge planning and ongoing care
Education
Research and audit
Ethical and legal issues
Management
Health promotion

Table 8 Generic skills for specialist training in all medical specialities (Joint Committee on Higher Medical Training, 2003)

- Good clinical care
- Communication skills
- Maintaining good medical practice
- Maintaining trust
- Working with colleagues
- Team working and leadership skills
- Teaching
- Research
- Clinical governance
- Structure and principles of management
- Information use and management
- Cross speciality skills

CONCLUSION

Geriatric medicine is an essential component of basic medical education. Educational programs must adapt to new educational philosophies, while other disciplines can learn from some of the innovations introduced by geriatric medicine. While basic medical education is well established, outcomes, programs, and evaluation of specialist training in the discipline require further study.

KEY POINTS

- Medical education has undergone radical change in recent years and department based teaching is no longer the norm.
- Education in aging and the care of older people is essential for all health and social care professionals.
- Geriatric medicine is an ideal subject for problem-based learning.
- Assessment methods must be chosen to test the desired educational outcomes.
- Academic geriatric medicine, combining education, clinical practice, research, and innovation must be strengthened.

KEY REFERENCES

- British Geriatrics Society. *The Medical Undergraduate Curriculum in Geriatric Medicine* 2004, www.bgs.org.uk.
- Crome P, Youngman L, McGrath A *et al. The Teaching of Geriatric Medicine in the UK Undergraduate Medical School Curriculum* 2004; British Geriatrics Society, www.bgs.org.
- Stout RW. Teaching gerontology and geriatric medicine. *Age and Ageing* 1985; **14**(suppl):1–36.
- Stout RW & Bamber JH. A new undergraduate teaching course in geriatric medicine. *Medical Education* 1979; **13**:363–7.

REFERENCES

Academy of Medical Sciences. *Clinical Academic Medicine in Jeopardy* 2002; *Recommendations for change* www.acmedsci.ac.uk

Barton A & Mulley G. History of the development of geriatric medicine in the UK. *Postgraduate Medical Journal* 2003; **79**:229–34.

Bernard MA, McAuley WJ, Belzer JA & Neal KS. An evaluation of a low-intensity intervention to introduce medical students to healthy older people. *JAGS* 2003; **51**:419–423.

British Geriatrics Society. *The Medical Undergraduate Curriculum in Geriatric Medicine* 2004, www.bgs.org.uk.

Crome P, Youngman L, McGrath A *et al. The Teaching of Geriatric Medicine in the UK Undergraduate Medical School Curriculum* 2004; British Geriatrics Society, www.bgs.org.

Deary IJ, Smith R, Mitchell C & MacLennan WJ. Geriatric medicine: does teaching alter medical students' attitudes to elderly people? *Medical Education* 1993; **27**:399–405.

Evans JG. Geriatric medicine: a brief history. *British Medical Journal* 1997; **315**:1075–7.

General Medical Council. *Recommendations on Basic Medical Education* 1980; General Medical Council, London.

General Medical Council. *Tomorrow's doctors. Recommendations on Undergraduate Medical Education* 1993; General Medical Council, London.

General Medical Council. *Good Medical Practice* 2001, www.gmc-uk.org.

General Medical Council. *Tomorrow's doctors. Recommendations on Undergraduate Medical Education* 2002, www.gmc-uk.org.

Harden RMcG & Gleeson FA. Assessment of clinical competence using an objective structured clinical examination. *Medical Education* 1979; **13**:41–54.

Hazzard WR. To build an academic geriatric program of distinction. Lessons from experience at three US and two British academic health centers. *American Journal of Medicine* 1994; **97**(suppl 4A):6S–7S.

Irwin WG, Bamber JH & Henneman J. Constructing a new course for undergraduate teaching of general practice. *Medical Education* 1976; **10**:302–8.

Isaacs B. *The Challenge of Geriatric Medicine* 1992; Oxford University Press, Oxford.

Ives DR. Educational objectives for SHOs in medicine for the elderly on medical rotation. *Age and Ageing* 2003; **32**:493.

Joint Committee on Higher Medical Training. *Higher Medical Training Curriculum for Geriatric Medicine* 2003, www.jchmt.org.uk/geriat/index.asp.

Lee M, Wilkerson L, Reuben DB & Ferrell BA. Development and validation of a geriatric knowledge test for medical students. *JAGS* 2004; **52**:983–988.

Leinster S. Curriculum planning. *Lancet* 2003a; **362**:750.

Leinster S. Assessment in medical training. *Lancet* 2003b; **362**:1770.

Leinster S. Setting standards. *Lancet* 2004; **363**:496.

Quality Assurance Agency for Higher Education. *Medicine*. Subject Benchmark Statement 2002, www.qaa.ac.uk.

Scottish Deans' Medical Curriculum Group. *The Scottish Doctor* 2002, www.scottishdoctor.org.

Stout RW. Teaching gerontology and geriatric medicine. *Age and Ageing* 1985; **14**(suppl):1–36.

Stout RW & Bamber JH. A new undergraduate teaching course in geriatric medicine. *Medical Education* 1979; **13**:363–7.

World Health Organisation. *Teaching Gerontology and Geriatric Medicine: Report on a Workshop* 1982; World Health Organization Publication ICP/ADR 045(2), Edinburgh.

FURTHER READING

Alford CL, Miles T, Palmer R & Espino D. An introduction to geriatrics for first-year medical students. *Journal of the American Geriatrics Society* 2001; **49**:782–7.

Galinsky D, Cohen R, Schneirman C *et al.* A programme in undergraduate geriatric education – the Beer Sheva experiment. *Medical Education* 1983; **17**:100–4.

Institute of Medicine. *Aging and Medical Education. Report of a Study by a Committee of the Institute of Medicine* 1978; National Academy of Sciences, Washington.

Powers CS, Savidge MA, Allen RM & Cooper-Witt CM. Implementing a mandatory geriatrics clerkship. *Journal of the American Geriatrics Society* 2002; **50**:369–73.

151

The Contribution of Family Doctors to the Primary Care of Older People: Lessons from the British Experience

Steve Iliffe

Royal Free & UCL Medical School, London, UK

Based in part on the chapter 'The Contribution of Family Doctors' by Steven Iliffe, Joseph J. Gallo and William Reichel, which appeared in *Principles and Practice of Geriatric Medicine*, 3rd Edition.

INTRODUCTION

Population aging, escalating costs in pensions, health carc, and long-term care has prompted the emergence of a new policy agenda for active aging and improved quality of life in old age in all industrialized countries. Family doctors are often seen as being well placed to implement some of the health-related elements of this new agenda, particularly around health promotion, disability reduction, and chronic disease management. Frequent contacts between older people and their family doctor, knowledge of the individual patients accumulated by their physicians over long periods of time, and the presumed skill of generalists in integrating biomedical, psychological, and social perspectives on illness and disability should, when combined, allow family doctors to function as community geriatricians. The role for the family physician and general practitioner is, therefore, potentially great.

However, actual experience of primary care for older people suggests that there are significant obstacles to systematic application of the new policy agenda, both in systems where general practitioners function as gatekeepers to specialist services (the Anglo-Scandinavian model) and in those where generalists and specialists compete in the community (the US and predominant European model). These obstacles include a broad range of attention across all age groups that can exclude older people, a largely reactive medical culture that favors the younger, less tolerant, and more articulate cohorts, high caseloads that militate against in-depth or complex assessments, and significant gaps in the knowledge and skills of practitioners that reduce the potential for multifaceted interventions. The actual role for family doctors in promoting healthier aging and the optimal division of labor between them and specialists in medicine for older people are both open questions.

In policy terms, this uncertainty is one example of a broader theme that preoccupies policy makers and health-care managers; should unmet need be met by creating new, dedicated, specialist outreach services, or by changing the practice and performance of existing disciplines? This article explores these issues, using the historic evolution of primary care for older people in the United Kingdom as an example. In my view, the British experience of encouraging primary care for older people has important lessons for family doctors everywhere, because both primary care and specialist medicine for older people are well-developed disciplines and function within a complex policy framework on aging.

In the United Kingdom, the government has made a commitment to improve services for older people through combating age discrimination, engaging with older people, better decision making for services for older people, better meeting of older peoples' needs, and promoting a strategic and joined up approach. A draft of policy initiatives not only set the tone for service reconfiguration but also specified objectives and timescales. The most important of these is the National Service Framework for Older People (NSFOP) (Department of Health, 2001a), an ambitious 10-year plan to transform health and social care services for an aging population (*see* **Chapter 161, Health and Care for Older People in the United Kingdom**). At the same time, a controversial and fundamentally flawed policy, the promotion

Principles and Practice of Geriatric Medicine, 4th Edition. Edited by M.S. John Pathy, Alan J. Sinclair and John E. Morley.

of annual "checks" for those people aged 75 and over through general practice, has ended. This shift in policy also acknowledges the obstacles to developing primary care for older people and seeks ways to overcome them. As a contribution to this debate, I will suggest three related areas where efforts to change service delivery within communities may produce rapid gains – health maintenance and promotion in primary care, fostering a culture of case management amongst family doctors, and a new, multidisciplinary approach to medication review.

LEARNING FROM POLICY MISTAKES

A new contract for general practice in the United Kingdom, introduced in April 2004, has quietly deleted the contractual obligation to offer annual assessments of health to all people aged 75 and over, ending 13 years of ill-conceived policy based on thin science. The "75 and over checks" were introduced in 1990, without plausible evidence of health gain from such an approach and despite the objections of family doctors, and in practice were widely ignored. The UK government became the first to introduce a nationwide primary care–based screening program for older citizens, and has been followed by others in Europe, mesmerized by the rising demographic tide. There is much to be learned from this policy error, and as always the devil is in the details of conception and implementation.

Experimentation with population screening and assessment by different methods like postal questionnaires, specialist nurses, case-finding computer software, and dedicated clinics, and the search for "at-risk" groups were reflected in the debates that occurred both in the Royal College of General Practice and in the Health Visitors Association in the 1970s and 1980s. Although general practitioners dominated the reporting of the approaches to primary care for older people, health visitors pioneered much of the actual work on the ground, and the underlying ideas came as much from community nursing as from medicine (Taylor and Buckley, 1987).

These early studies explored the best ways to provide anticipatory care for older people, and acknowledged the iatrogenic risks of treating unimportant abnormalities and medicalizing old age. Brief, nonintrusive strategies for predicting functional problems during routine consultations were sought and tested in randomized controlled trials. The preoccupation of doctors with disease to the detriment of its social consequences, the failure to take into account the adaptive powers of older people, and the tendency to underestimate the burden borne by carers were all identified as major obstacles to progress in developing more effective primary care for older people. Medical and social problems overlapped in ways that were often puzzling to clinicians; screening led to an increase in referrals to other agencies but without clear evidence of benefit in many instances, and with variations in referral rates determined as much by the referrer as by the patient's problems. Finally, at-risk groups proved harder to identify than anticipated, for more pathological events occurred outside the expected at-risk groups than in them. The generation of general practitioners and nurses which did this work introduced important ideas about how aging in its organic, social, and psychological dimensions affected people's health, how essential multidisciplinary teamwork was to providing appropriate care for ill older people (Williams, 1995), and ultimately how networking with community-based agencies was a more useful model than referral to specialist care (Williams and Wallace, 1993).

Several such trials took place in the 1980s in the United Kingdom, Denmark, and the United States. Different trials used very different interventions and outcome measures, but there are some common features (Stuck *et al.*, 1993):

- a rise in morale amongst elderly people involved in screening programs;
- referrals to all agencies tended to increase, including to specialist medical care in some studies;
- the duration of in-patient stay fell in some studies, possibly through early intervention in disease processes;
- in-patient rates could increase through a greater use of respite care;
- reduction in mortality did occur in some trials, perhaps for the same reason that in-patient stays declined, but not in all;
- no trial up to 1990 demonstrated an improvement in older people's functional ability, and general practitioner workload only decreased in situations where alternative services were organized to bypass existing primary-care services.

In 1990, the UK government unilaterally changed the conditions of service for general practitioners, introducing a contractual obligation on members of primary health-care teams to offer annual assessments of health to patients aged 75 and over. These offers of assessment, which had to be made in writing, should be based on a home visit unless otherwise requested by the patient, and should include the following headings:

- *sensory function*
- *mobility*
- *mental condition*
- *physical condition including continence*
- *social environment*
- *medication use*

It was unclear what was intended when the contract for general practice was changed to include this obligation, but it was widely interpreted as a requirement to screen the 75 and over age group. As argued earlier, while there had been extensive research into the possible benefits of regular screening or assessment of older people, at the time of the introduction of the 75 and over checks there was still a lack of conclusive evidence that routine screening of whole populations was worthwhile. Nor was there a consensus on the best methods for such a screening approach, despite nearly 40 years of study (Harris, 1992). Many aspects of the elderly screening program built into the new GP contract therefore lacked a scientific basis, and its implementation was similarly ill-conceived. Undoubtedly the lack of a plausible evidence base and the lack of guidance on how to carry out the 75 and over assessments added to their unpopularity with general practitioners and led to piecemeal and often unenthusiastic implementation of the program (Brown *et al.*, 1992). Where assessment tasks were undertaken at all, they were delegated to practice nurses and were given low priority by the local health service administration (Chew *et al.*, 1994), which (with a few exceptions) provided neither leadership nor training for the program, nor policed its implementation.

In response to the criticisms of this policy, the UK's Medical Research Council (MRC) funded a trial (Fletcher *et al.*, 2002) comparing universal versus targeted assessments, and management by primary-care teams versus a multidisciplinary geriatric assessment team, in order to strengthen the evidence base. The MRC trial, therefore, was launched in a situation where evidence and policy were divorced and risked becoming the intellectual underpinning for shaky policy foundations in which there was little evidence of balanced equipoise in scientific thinking. Critics of the emphasis placed on the randomized control trial (RCT) as an evaluation technique might have used this study as an example of an experimental method applied to the wrong question. The trial team escaped from this awkwardness by developing a complex design that tested an idea not yet enshrined in UK policy, comprehensive geriatric assessment, as well as evaluating different forms of brief assessment.

COMPREHENSIVE GERIATRIC ASSESSMENT

The evidence base for the United States approach to comprehensive geriatric assessment is richer than that for the screening approaches used in the United Kingdom (Stuck *et al.*, 1993). In summary (Stuck *et al.*, 2004), reductions in nursing home admissions appear to depend on multiple follow-up home visits. A recent meta-analysis of home-based visiting programs that offered health promotion and preventative care to older people suggested that it was associated with a reduction in mortality and admission to institutional care (Elkan *et al.*, 2001). Programs with several visits per year reduced admissions by about a third. This is probably related to the timely detection of new problems: repeated annual assessments detected on average two new medical and one new psychosocial problem per person per year. Programs offered to the younger old (from 65 to 74 years) reduced mortality by 24%, whereas in older study populations no mortality reduction was seen. Finally, programs based on multidimensional assessments prevent deterioration in functional status, which indicate that the reduction of nursing home use is not related to a shift of long-term care from institutions to the community, but to a genuine preservation of functional ability. However, it was uncertain which components of the home visiting activity were beneficial or which populations were most likely to benefit (Egger, 2001).

THE MRC TRIAL

The MRC Trial of the Assessment and Management of Older People in the Community randomized 109 general practices and investigated whether universal assessment was more effective than targeted assessment, and whether it mattered who subsequently cared for the patients in whom problems were identified – a geriatric or primary-care team. In the targeted arm, only persons who reported a prespecified range of problems were invited to have a detailed multidimensional assessment, whereas in the universal arm everyone was invited to undergo the detailed assessment. The specificity of the screening questionnaire was high, but the sensitivity was below 50% for all dimensions: at least half of the problems were missed at the screen. The results on mortality and hospital admissions were disappointing, with few differences after 3 years of follow-up. Universal assessment was associated with a 17% reduction in institutional admissions, but this failed to reach prespecified levels of statistical significance. There were small gains in quality of life, and specialist assessment seemed to offer little benefit over family doctor assessment, a gratifying result for primary care offset by the limited gains made by any form of assessment. The findings are compatible, therefore, with previous trials of preventive home visits in older persons (Stuck *et al.*, 2002a). The following seem reasonable conclusions to draw from this study, the largest trial of primary care-based geriatric assessment ever conducted: (1) a simple screening questionnaire does not identify a target group effectively (2) preventive multidimensional geriatric assessment does reduce the risk of nursing home admissions, (3) programs based on single assessments are less effective than those with repeated assessments and long-term follow-up and (4) the primary-care team can manage problems as well as the geriatric team.

Where does this leave primary care for older people? We now know that management follow-up after assessment matters, even if we do not know how to target those most likely to benefit. There is still a need for a shorter, practical, primary-care friendly tool that builds on existing information, focuses on unmet needs (Crome and Phillipson, 2000), and can be used to trigger a comprehensive assessment process. Readers can judge for themselves whether this was not known two decades ago, while family doctors can now think about how they can incorporate comprehensive assessment and management packages into their workload. Here the latest policy development in the United Kingdom may help them, if only by offering a framework for thinking and experimentation.

THE NATIONAL SERVICE FRAMEWORK FOR OLDER PEOPLE (NSFOP)

The NSFOP is the key policy guidance for health and social care services and outlines a 10-year program of action. It advocates coordination of services to support independence and promote health, specialized services for key conditions, and a cultural change that fosters treatment of older people and their carers with respect, dignity, and fairness. Addressing ageism in public services is seen as an integral component of the modernization of health and social care services, and rooting out age discrimination is the first standard in the NSFOP. Through out the document "older people" are regarded as a heterogeneous group, with particular emphasis on the needs of ethnic elders, and it advocates that all services reflect the diversity of the population they serve, including the needs of carers.

The NSFOP addresses four themes with eight standards flowing through them. Amongst other functions, these standards address conditions particularly significant for older people, which are not covered in other National Service Frameworks: stroke, falls, and mental health problems associated with old age. The themes and standards are shown in BOX 1.

BOX 1

Theme 1: Respecting the Individual

Standard One: Rooting out Age Discrimination

National Health Services (NHSs) will be provided, regardless of age, on the basis of clinical need alone. Social care services will not use age in their eligibility criteria or policies, to restrict access to available services.

Standard Two: Person-centered Care

NHS and social care services should treat older people as individuals and enable them to make choices about their own care, achieved through: the single assessment process (SAP); integrated commissioning arrangements; integrated service provision; and including community equipment and continence services.

Theme 2: Intermediate Care

Standard Three: Intermediate Care

Older people will have access to a new range of intermediate care services at home or designated care settings, to promote their independence by providing NHS and LA services to prevent unnecessary hospital admission and rehabilitation services to enable early hospital discharge and prevent admission to long-term residential care.

Theme 3: Providing Evidenced-based Specialist Care

Standard Four: General Hospital Care

Older people's care in hospital is delivered through appropriate specialist care and by hospital staff who have the right set of skills to meet their needs.

Standard Five: Stroke

The NHS will take action to prevent strokes, working in partnership with other agencies where appropriate. People diagnosed with having had a stroke are managed by a specialist stroke service, and with their carers, participate in a multidisciplinary program of secondary prevention and rehabilitation.

Standard Six: Falls

The NHS, working in partnership with councils, acts to prevent falls and reduce resultant injuries in older people. Older people who have fallen receive treatment and rehabilitation and, with their carers, receive advice on prevention through a specialist falls service.

Standard Seven: Mental Health Services

Older people who have mental health problems can access integrated mental health services, provided by the NHS and councils to ensure effective diagnosis, treatment, and support for themselves and their carers.

Theme 4: Promoting an Active, Healthy Life

Standard Eight: the Promotion of Health and Active Life in Old Age

The health and well-being of older people is promoted through a coordinated program of action led by the NHS with support from councils. This standard is linked to the national public health agenda cited earlier.

The NSFOP creates opportunities for enhancing the quality of primary care for older people, and general practitioners and primary-care nurses with a specialist interest in aging and health may catalyze change at local level. In particular, the SAP, designed to ensure that older people receive *"appropriate, effective, and timely response to their health and social care needs in an integrated way"* (Brown *et al.*, 2003) calls for the introduction of a comprehensive assessment process. However, the lessons from previous policy and implementation in this arena raise two issues that still need to be addressed. The first is how to target clinical attention on the often complex problems of comorbidity to maximum effect in an aging population that is not homogeneous but is as diverse as younger cohorts, without lapsing into a culture that delegates the tasks to insufficiently trained nurses who follow a check-list approach to health needs assessment.

The second issue is the problem of collaboration across professional and agency boundaries. Although the MRC trial suggests that generalists perform as well as specialists, long-term management of complex problems in older people will inevitably rely on good working relationships between disciplines and organizations. There are many challenges in implementing a public-service policy that advocates collaboration between sectors to address both broad quality of life issues as well as prevention of ill health. The complexities of health and social care partnership working at an organizational level are well documented (Balloch and Taylor, 2001), as are those at the service delivery level (Manthorpe and Iliffe, 2003), constituting a *"pessimistic tradition"* (Hudson, 2002) in inter-professional working. There is a risk that the well-intentioned plans of the NSFOP could remain aspirations for lack of careful thought about how to change services in a policy environment that tries to innovate at ever greater speed.

How can this be prevented? Expanding on arguments summarized elsewhere (Iliffe and Drennan, 2005), I propose that three areas of activity now deserve particular attention in primary care; a systematic evidence-based approach to promoting well-being in older people, the development of a case-management culture, and the organization of medication reviews using the expertise of doctors, local pharmacists, and primary-care nurses. Our knowledge in these three areas varies from a reasonably high level of certainty in the clinical domains of health maintenance and promotion to considerable uncertainty in both case management and medication review. Although these activities can be put to test in Britain in a way that may not yet be possible, across whole populations at least, in other countries, this next round of experimentation in primary care for older people can draw upon international experience and also inform it. In particular, we may be able to answer questions about how much of these tasks can be undertaken by generalists working in primary care, and how much will depend on specialist activity in the community.

HEALTH PROMOTION

The NSFOP explicitly demands for the first time that the NHS and local authorities in partnership agree on programs to promote health in the aging and to prevent disease in older people. These programs were expected to improve access for older people to "mainstream" health promotion services and also develop *"wider initiatives involving a multisectoral approach to promoting health, independence, and well-being in old age"*.

Policy makers, researchers, and practitioners have neglected health promotion and illness prevention with older people (Victor and House, 2000) and the evidence base for preventive services and anticipatory care for older people is small and inconclusive. While the evidence base is being extended, family doctors have little choice but to take a "best buy" approach to health promotion with older people, focusing on the most tractable clinical problems. Given the effort required for population screening and the relatively limited benefit gained, targeted case-finding and health promotion activities combined with techniques of case management may be an effective way forward, emphasizing the diagnostic role of the family doctor in case-finding, and the case-management role of the primary-care nurse. Case-finding is different from population screening because it relies on the encounters between older people and their family doctors to identify unmet needs. In turn, this requires the physician to routinely incorporate enquiries about health needs into consultations, just as blood pressure checks (for younger adults) are now part of routine practice. Information obtained routinely then needs to be incorporated into medical records, in a way that both prompts later review and stimulates the collection of a full profile of health-related behaviors, risks, and needs over time and in the course of sequential encounters. Advocates of whole population screening conclude that their approach has been shown to be beneficial, and they are right that the trials do demonstrate some positive (if modest) outcomes and some potential health service savings. The weakness of their argument is that the external validity of trials of complex interventions is relatively poor, since mainstream services do not perform over the long term in the same way as practitioners engaged in short-term and often highly reinforced research trials. Reengineering services toward screening whole populations of older people may not prove to be cost effective at all, while modification of routine practice, although difficult to achieve quickly, may be more durable and effective.

The case-finding approach needs to be limited in its scope – nobody can do everything – and the clinical domains discussed here are common, important, and tractable problems (Iliffe *et al.*, 2005) identified in the preparation of an evidence base for a European study of health risk assessment in older people (Stuck *et al.*, 2002b). Eighteen clinical domains where the evidence for beneficial intervention seems strong enough to warrant changing clinical practice are shown in Table 1. These 18 domains can be used to guide service development, structure continuing professional education, and frame audits of clinical activity. They are offered as a provisional program of clinical development, knowing that the evidence base for interventions with older populations is evolving and that questions about identifying those most likely to benefit remain unanswered.

CASE MANAGEMENT

Identifying cases and initiating health promotion and maintenance activities are unlikely to have sustained beneficial effects on health in later life if they are not followed by

Table 1 Health risk assessment, prevention, and health maintenance for patients aged 65 and over

Domains	Primary prevention
Hypertension case-finding	Yearly measurement
Hyperlipidemia case-finding	5-yearly screen/use Coronary Risk Prediction chart to quantify risk
Diabetes mellitus: early detection	3-yearly screen with fasting blood glucose (FBG)
Colon cancer screening	Annual screening by fecal occult blood test
Prostate cancer screening	Screening in asymptomatic men not recommended
Dental care review	Recommend annual dental check
Visual loss case-finding	Recommend yearly eye test
Hearing loss case-finding	Annual whisper test as minimum, or use of brief hearing function questionnaire
Exercise promotion	Recommend regular exercise for cardiovascular fitness, balance, muscle strengthening or stamina
Nutrition assessment	Basic dietary advice about high fiber/low fat diets
Physical function assessment	Periodic functional assessment for patients with comorbidity using simple instruments like Timed Up And Go
Pain management	Routine enquiry at each patient encounter
Regular medication use	Regular review for $\geq$3 medications
Injury prevention/falls	Annual falls risk assessment and referral for deeper assessment and intervention
Urinary incontinence; case-finding	Routine enquiry about symptoms
Depression/dementia; case-finding	Assess patients $\geq$75 years with symptoms using standardized instruments
Smoking cessation	Cessation counselling for all smokers
Alcohol overuse; case-finding	Routine enquiry about quantity and frequency of consumption

systematic management of the cases so identified. Case-management techniques can improve access to health and social care services (Pacala *et al.*, 1995), enhance quality of life (Marshall *et al.*, 1999), and reduce admission to institutions (Stuck *et al.*, 1995). This latter finding has attracted much attention, with the success in reducing hospital admissions for exacerbations of chronic disease through case management run by Kaiser Permanente in the United States prompting another round of experimentation in Britain. As a result, small partnership projects to promote health in older people using case-finding and case-management strategies have merged across the United Kingdom, while a national demonstration project in nine areas has examined how the American chronic disease management program for nursing-home residents at high risk of hospitalization (Kane *et al.*, 2003) can be translated to English primary-care settings. The national demonstration project hinges on the development of a new advanced primary-care nurse role involving coordination of proactive care for older people. Better monitoring and education of high-risk older people and engagement of existing general practitioner and community nursing services appear to reduce recurrent hospital admissions enough to make the UK government want to roll out the case-management method to all areas by 2008. These projects could identify the necessary components of case management in the United Kingdom setting and help promote the emergence of a case-management culture in primary care, without necessarily setting up a new specialist services that bypasses the slow rate of change in established primary care.

This is a potentially exciting and productive development in primary care, but will it become part of normal care in a well-established system? Can a method developed in the United States, which has poorly developed primary-care provision and little if any system of health care in the NHS sense, be imported to the United Kingdom? How will the existing roles of general practitioners, practice nurses, and other community nurses fit alongside the new roles of advanced primary-care nurses? Will case management actually work in the sense of identifying and supporting vulnerable older people? And are there more benefits to health-care providers through reduced hospital admission than there are to older people with multiple problems?

The precedents for a change in work culture of this magnitude, and in the provision of services to an older population, are ambiguous. General practitioners have rarely been involved in developing case-management approaches (Leedham and Wistow, 1992), and apart from community psychiatric nurses, the role of nurses in care management was peripheral in the 1990s (Bergen, 1994) except for a few primary-care nurses functioning as care managers with access to a budget for social care either as part of the district nursing, social work, or general practice team. On the other hand most general practitioners and primary-care nurses would probably argue that most of their practice is based on a case-management model, and there is evidence that district nurses and health visitors use many elements of case management in their daily practice. A recent survey of practice nurses reported that they were more likely to use all the elements of case management where they were involved in chronic disease management than in single tasks delegated by the general practitioner (Evans *et al.*, 2005).

The recipients of case management and the elements of the case manager's role change according to the organizational and funding context. In a range of different contexts, case-management schemes for older people have addressed health promotion and independence (Storfell *et al.*, 1997), the management of single diseases (Goodwin *et al.*, 2003), the management of multiple chronic medical conditions, residents of nursing homes (Kane and Huck, 2000), or on the management of both health and social care. The eligibility criteria for an older person to receive case management are determined by the purpose of case management. For example, health maintenance organizations (HMOs) in America are keen to lower costs to the individual and the organization through preventable hospital admissions (Dixon *et al.*, 2004). Reports of American nurse care management schemes, which use comparisons of health care utilization before and after the introduction of the scheme for small cohorts of high-risk enrollees to the HMO, demonstrated decreased costs through reduced utilization of emergency room facilities and duration of patients' stay in the hospital and high levels of patient satisfaction (Quinn *et al.*, 1999). These findings are important for advocates of case management in primary care, but we need to be cautious because other evidence is less supportive. For example, a review of nine randomized control trials of case-management programs for any age group in primary care concluded that they improved some clinical outcomes, patient satisfaction, quality of life and functional status but did not reduce costs (Ferguson and Weinberger, 1998).

How case management is actually done also varies greatly. There appear to be two main models of the case manager's role: case managers holding budgets to finance care packages for the user (the brokerage model used by social services in the United Kingdom), and case managers providing services themselves and coordinating other agencies' service, as key workers. The different models variously employ nurses, nurse practitioners, social workers, or other health-care professionals as case managers, and also vary to the degree that the case managers work with doctors. Some models have regular structured reviews of the patients with primary-care doctors or specialist geriatric physicians (Quinn *et al.*, 1999); others have no specified relationship beyond the ability to refer to a primary-care doctor (Ritchie *et al.*, 2002). In some instances, case management has been incorporated as one element of a service redesign to integrate acute, primary, and long-term care (Johri *et al.*, 2003).

WHO BENEFITS MOST?

The evidence of impact is difficult to interpret and extrapolate to different health and social care systems, given the plethora of roles, aims, involvement of other professionals and differing types of services. Three randomized control studies in Italy, (Bernabei *et al.*, 1998) Canada, (Gagnon *et al.*, 1999) and the United States (Marshall *et al.*, 1999) provide more evidence about the impact of case-management approaches in different settings. The Canadian study reported no significant differences in quality of life, satisfaction with care, functional status, or hospital admissions between those receiving case management and those not, possibly because of the weak link between the nurse care manager and the patients' primary physician. The Italian and American studies reported that the intervention group receiving case management experienced less functional decline and were more independent for longer periods. The Italian study reported that hospital admission was lower in the intervention (case management) group than in the control and that use of family doctors was higher in the control group and overall costs were reduced in the intervention group. This study included an integrated model of care between primary and secondary care providers, with weekly multidisciplinary reviews of each patient's case. The American study reported that the use of the emergency department and hospital admission rates and health care costs were higher in the case-management group than the control group, possibly because the nurse and social work care manager were acting as advocates for older people.

While there is a growing body of knowledge internationally, it is still not clear which elements and services are most effective in which settings, and it is by no means certain that case management will reduce health service utilization and costs for the older population. Increased, coordinated use of case-management techniques between general practitioners and primary-care nurses could help address the interplay of comorbidity in a timely way, before older people become users of emergency services or start on a trajectory of repeated hospital admissions, but this does need to be demonstrated in well-designed studies. If case management is introduced widely in the absence of evidence from such studies, the error of the 75 and over checks may be repeated, potentially at higher economic cost to the health service. While this policy issue is being resolved, practitioners can use one component of case management virtually without extra resources, which is likely to be beneficial to patients and professionals alike; regular review of medication use in older people with multiple disorders.

MEDICATION REVIEW

The iatrogenic effects of prescribed medicines are a known factor in increased risk of hospital admission, and medication reviews are core components of case management. Medication management for older people is a major issue for the NHS, both in terms of the population health consequences and the resource utilization. Prescriptions in primary care for people aged over 60 account for about £4000 million of England's NHS budget annually (National Statistics Office, 2002), while the iatrogenic effects of prescribed medication are estimated to account for between 5 and 17% of all hospital admissions of people over 65 (Department of Health, 2001b). Multiple diseases, complicated medication regimes, transfer of prescribing between general practitioners and specialists, unreviewed repeat prescribing are all known risk factors for medication problems irrespective of the age of the patient. At the same time, it is recognized that there is under-prescribing for older people for common conditions such as COPD, depression, and hypertension (Royal College of Physicians, 2000). Population studies reveal that about 50% of people prescribed medication for long-term conditions do not take the medicine as prescribed (Carter *et al.*, 2003). Current estimates based on return-to-pharmacy schemes for unused medicines indicate that each Primary Care Trust in the United Kingdom may be spending about £1 million per annum on prescribed medicines that are wasted (Department of Health, 2001b).

Shared decision making on medicines between professional and patient, known as *concordance*, has been advocated to address some of these issues. The target of annual medication review for all people over 75 advocated by the NSFOP, with more frequent reviews for people at risk of medicine related problems, is another solution (Department of Health, 2001a). Medication review activities can take one of four forms (Task Force, 2003): (1) opportunistic, unstructured questions about medicines with patient, (2) technical review of a patient's prescriptions, (3) review of medicines with the patient's full medical records, and (4) face-to-face review of medicines and conditions with the patient.

However, the best approach to medication review for older people in general practice remains unclear. Older people are not a homogeneous group, and some studies indicate that not all older people would welcome the opportunity to formally review their medications with GPs or others (Knapp *et al.*, 2003; Zermansky *et al.*, 2001). Population and general practice studies report that between 20 and 42% of older people were not prescribed any medication while between 17 and 27% of patients over 75 were prescribed three or more medications. In contrast to hospital medicine, prescribing in general practice for older people is characterized by greater uncertainty about diagnoses, where people often present with multiple symptoms that are not easy to attribute and coexist with several known medical problems. Prescribing in these situations may be "realistic" in the sense it is aimed a symptom relief in the absence of diagnosis, or even at hypothesis-testing to reach a diagnosis, without being rational in the clinical-pharmacological sense (Cartwright and Smith, 1988).

The pattern of prescribing is likely to become more complicated as appropriately qualified nurses prescribe independently from a limited formulary of prescription-only medicines (Department of Health, 2002). This development is likely to contribute to the development and regulation of individual patient clinical management plans, and also permit a greater role for pharmacists in managing repeat prescription for people with chronic conditions. In the face of primary-care workforce and workload problems, the skills of pharmacists and nurses in primary care will be increasingly used in medication reviews with older people, potentially achieving therapeutic benefits with neutral cost implications (Krska *et al.*, 2001). However, this is an under-researched area, with little published literature on the effectiveness or cost consequences of nurse involvement in medication review for older people (Krska and Ross, 2002). Policy is clearly driving a greater role for pharmacists, practice nurses, district nurses, and nurse practitioners in medication reviews, alongside general practitioners. It is less clear what educational, organizational, and decisions support mechanisms are required for the different professional groups in situations where clinical risk judgments are complex or what the impact of review by different professional groups is on older people.

CONCLUSION

The proactive management of chronic diseases in adults is one the main challenges facing primary care, and health systems generally. In England and Wales, the NSFOP provides an impetus for primary care to address the health promotion and health care needs of older people with multiple pathologies and disabilities, and may be rekindling an enthusiasm for experimentation and innovation in primary care for older people. The great advantage of the national service framework is that it sets out not only objectives but also a research and development agenda, since there is much still unknown about how to enhance the quality of care for an aging population. Specialist and generalist disciplines can rebalance their division of labor, if transfer of skills into primary care can occur and hospital services become more effective in their management of late-life disorders. The lessons from the poor implementation of previous policies suggest that a cautious and selective approach building on existing skills while enhancing organizational capability is the best way to steer between policy imperatives and the evidence base. From my perspective there are three areas where focused activity in general practice could result in improved health care for older people: evidence-based health screening and health promotion, an increased culture of case management, and multidisciplinary strategies for medication review.

The 18 clinical domains that are described here as a core program for general practice-based care for older people constitute the easiest of the three areas of innovation. Clinical skills can be enhanced, educational skills can be built around the domains, and information systems modified to facilitate clinical thinking and the documentation of practice. Specialists in medicine and nursing for older people have obvious roles to play in promoting professional development in such domains, without necessarily having to provide services themselves, or at least not in the longer term. A transfer of skills from specialist to generalist domains is realistic, given the limited number of the clinical domains and their cultural familiarity to primary care, and may be facilitated by contractual changes for family doctors that resource and provide incentives for primary care for older people.

Case management is not so easy to introduce, partly because in general practice systematic review of patients with long-term problems is largely restricted to single domains like hypertension, diabetes, and asthma, and has yet to develop for complex patients with multiple pathologies and disabilities. Exploring this area needs time and energy, but can be given a positive impetus by specialist services where expertise already lies. The introduction of case management across the United Kingdom by 2008, possibly utilizing the expertise and personnel of US HMOs, will create a nationwide experiment in the application of case-management methods, worthy of carefully evaluation.

Medication review should be easy, and in the United Kingdom it is now part of the remuneration package for family doctors; it may prove more complex to implement than expected as pharmacists and nurses acquire new roles in evaluating medication use and become more engaged with clinical decision making. Again, specialists in medicine for older people can have an effect on primary-care development by promoting discussion about the problems of medication use with their colleagues in primary care, perhaps using critical incident methods to examine iatrogenesis as a factor in hospital admission. Case management as a tool could begin around medication review and expand out into domains like functional ability and quality of life as practitioners become familiar with the approach.

Although we should not expect progress to be as rapid in these three areas as it has been in the development of condition-specific services for stroke and falls prevention, or even in service reconfigurations like intermediate care, lasting changes in primary care for older people appear possible, given long-term commitment.

KEY POINTS

- Experience from the poor implementation of the 75 and over checks suggests that cautious and selective approach to promoting primary care for older people, and building on existing skills while enhancing organizational capability, is more realistic than a sudden and dramatic leap forward.
- The existing evidence base suggests that health promotion for older people is realistic in 18 clinical domains.
- A transfer of skills from specialists to generalists is feasible, given the limited number of the clinical domains and their cultural familiarity to primary care, and may be facilitated by contractual changes for family doctors.
- The culture of case management is less well established in general practice, but current policies support its growth, which can begin around regular medication review.
- Multidisciplinary strategies for medication review, particularly in managing complex cases, will assist general practitioners by bringing relevant expertise to bear on complex problems of comorbidity and disability.
- Pharmacists and nurses will acquire new roles in evaluating medication use and become more engaged with clinical decision making, as part of this evolution.

KEY REFERENCES

- Bernabei R, Landi F, Gambassi G *et al.* Randomised trial of impact of model of integrated care and case management for older people living in community. *British Medical Journal* 1998; **316**:1348–51.
- Elkan R, Kendrick D, Dewey M *et al.* Effectiveness of home based support for older people: systematic review and meta-analysis. *British Medical Journal* 2001; **323**:719.
- Stuck AE, Beck JC & Egger M. Preventing disability in older people. *Lancet* 2004; **364**(9446):1641–2.
- Stuck AE, Egger M, Hammer A *et al.* Home visits to prevent nursing home admission and functional decline in the elderly: systematic review and meta-regression analysis. *The Journal of the American Medical Association* 2002a; **287**:1022–8.
- Stuck AE, Elkuch P, Dapp U *et al.*, for the Pro-Age Pilot Study Group. Feasibility and yield of a self-administered questionnaire for health risk appraisal in older people in three European countries. *Age and Ageing* 2002b; **31**:463–7.
- Taylor RC & Buckley EG. *Preventive Care of the Elderly: a Review of Current Developments*, occasional paper 35 1987; Royal College of General Practitioners, London.

REFERENCES

Balloch S & Taylor M. *Partnership Working: Policy and Practice* 2001; The Policy Press, Bristol.

Bergen A. Case management in the community: identifying a role for nursing. *Journal of Clinical Nursing* 1994; **3**(4):251–7.

Bernabei R, Landi F, Gambassi G *et al.* Randomised trial of impact of model of integrated care and case management for older people living in community. *British Medical Journal* 1998; **316**:1348–51.

Brown L, Tucker C & Domokos T. Evaluating the impact of integrated health and social care teams on older people living in the community. *Health & Social Care in the Community* 2003; **11**:85–94.

Brown K, Williams E & Groom L. Health checks on patients 75 years and over in Nottinghamshire after the new GP contract. *British Medical Journal* 1992; **305**:619–21.

Carter S, Taylor D & Levenson R. *A Question of Choice – Compliance in Medicine Taking – A Preliminary Review* 2003; The Medicines Partnership, London.

Cartwright A & Smith C. *Elderly People: Their Medicines and their Doctors* 1988; Routledege, London.

Chew CA, Wilkin D & Glendinning C. Annual assessments of patients aged 75 years and over: general practitioners and nurses views and experience. *British Journal of General Practice* 1994; **44**:263–7.

Crome P & Phillipson C. Assessment of need. *Age and Ageing* 2000; **29**:479–80.

Department of Health. *National Service Framework for Older People* 2001a; The Stationary Office, London.

Department of Health. *Medicines for Older People: Implementing Medicines – Related Aspects of the NSF for Older People* 2001b; HMSO, London.

Department of Health. *Extended Independent Nurse Prescribing – a Guide to Implementation* 2002; Department of Health, London.

Dixon J, Lewis R, Rosen R *et al. Managing Chronic Disease: What Can We Learn from the US Experience?* 2004; Kings Fund Publications.

Egger M. Commentary: when, where, and why do preventive home visits work? *British Medical Journal* 2001; **323**:719.

Elkan R, Kendrick D, Dewey M *et al.* Effectiveness of home based support for older people: systematic review and meta-analysis. *British Medical Journal* 2001; **323**:719.

Evans C, Drennan V & Roberts J. Practice nurse involvement in care management. *Journal of Advanced Nursing* 2005; (in press).

Ferguson JA & Weinberger M. Case management programs in primary care. *Journal of General Internal Medicine* 1998; **13**:123–6.

Fletcher A, Jones DA, Bulpitt CJ & Tulloch AJ. The MRC trial of assessment and management of older people in the community: objectives, design and interventions. *BioMed Central Health Services Research* 2002; **2**:21.

Gagnon AJ, Schein C, McVey L & Bergman H. Randomized controlled trial of nurse case management of frail older people. *Journal of the American Geriatrics Society* 1999; **47**(9):1118–24.

Goodwin JS, Satish S, Anderson ET *et al.* Effect of nurse case management on the treatment of older women with breast cancer. *Journal of the American Geriatrics Society* 2003; **51**(9):1252–9.

Harris A. Health checks for the over-75s; the doubt persists. *British Medical Journal* 1992; **305**:599–600.

Hudson B. Interprofessionality in health and social care: the Achilles' heel of partnership. *Journal of Interprofessional Care* 2002; **16**(1):7–17.

Iliffe S & Drennan V. Assessment of older people in the community: from '75 & over checks' to National Service Frameworks. *Reviews in Clinical Gerontology* 2005; forthcoming.

Iliffe S, Harari D & Swift C Primary care for older people; back to the drawing board? In *New Developments in General Practice* 2005; RCGP Publications.

Johri J, Beland F & Bergman H. International experiments in integrated care for the elderly: a synthesis of evidence. *International Journal of Geriatric Psychiatry* 2003; **18**:222–35.

Kane RL & Huck S. The implementation of the EverCare demonstration project. *Journal of the American Geriatrics Society* 2000; **48**(2):218–23.

Kane RL, Keckhafer G, Flood S *et al.* The effect of Evercare on hospital use. *Journal of the American Geriatrics Society* 2003; **51**(10):1427–34.

Knapp P, Raynor DK, House AO & Petty DR. Patients' views of a pharmacist-run medication review clinic in general practice. *The British Journal of General Practice* 2003; **53**(493):607–13.

Krska J, Cromarty JA, Arris F *et al.* Pharmacist-led medication review in patients over 65: a randomized, controlled trial in primary care. *Age and Ageing* 2001; **30**(3):205–11.

Krska J & Ross S. Medication review: whose job is it? *International Journal of Pharmacy Practice* 2002; **10**:R86.

Leedham J & Wistow G *Community Care and General Practitioners*, Paper 6 1992; University of Leeds, Leeds; 2004; Nuffield Institute of Health Services Studies, London.

Manthorpe J & Iliffe S. Professional predictions: June Huntington's perspectives on joint working, 20 years on. *Journal of Interprofessional Care* 2003; **17**(1):85–94.

Marshall BS, Long MJ, Voss J *et al.* Case management of the elderly in a health maintenance organization: the implications for program administration under managed care. *Journal of Healthcare Information Management* 1999; **44**(6):477–91.

National Statistics Office. *Prescription Dispensed in the Community: Statistics for 1991 to 2001: England* 2002; Department of Health, London.

Pacala JT, Boult C, Boult LB *et al.* Case management of older adults in Health Maintenance Organizations. *Journal of the American Geriatrics Society* 1995; **43**:538–42.

Quinn JL, Pryblo M & Pannone P. Community care management across the continuum: study results from a medicare health maintenance plan. *Care Management Journals* 1999; **1**(4):223–31.

Ritchie C, Wieland D, Tully C *et al.* Coordination and Advocacy for Rural Elders (Care): a model of rural case management with Veterans. *The Gerontologist* 2002; **42**(3):399–405.

Royal College of Physicians. *National Sentinel Clinical Audit of Evidence Based Prescribing for Older People* 2000; RCP, London.

Storfell JL, Mitchell R & McCormack G. Nurse managed health care: New York's community nursing case management demonstrations project. *Journal of Advanced Nursing* 1997; **27**(10):21–7.

Stuck AE, Aronow HU, Steiner A *et al.* A trial of annual in-home comprehensive geriatric assessments for elderly people living in the community. *The New England Journal of Medicine* 1995; **333**(18):1184–9.

Stuck AE, Beck JC & Egger M. Preventing disability in older people. *Lancet* 2004; **364**(9446):1641–2.

Stuck AE, Egger M, Hammer A *et al.* Home visits to prevent nursing home admission and functional decline in the elderly: systematic review and meta-regression analysis. *The Journal of the American Medical Association* 2002a; **287**:1022–8.

Stuck AE, Elkuch P, Dapp U *et al.*, for the Pro-Age Pilot Study Group. Feasibility and yield of a self-administered questionnaire for health risk appraisal in older people in three European countries. *Age and Ageing* 2002b; **31**:463–7.

Stuck AE, Siu AL, Wieland GD *et al.* Effects of a comprehensive geriatric assessment on survival, residence and function; a meta-analysis of controlled trials. *Lancet* 1993; **342**:1032–6.

Task Force on Medicines Partnership and the National Collaborative Medicines Management Services Programme. *Room for Review: A Guide to Medication Review: The Agenda for Patients, Practitioners and Managers* 2003; Medicines Partnership: London.

Taylor RC & Buckley EG. *Preventive Care of the Elderly: a Review of Current Developments*, occasional paper 35 1987; Royal College of General Practitioners, London.

Victor C & House K. *Promoting the Health of Older People: Setting a Research Agenda* 2000; Health Education Authority, London.

Williams I. *Caring for Older People in the Community* 1995; Radcliffe, Oxford.

Williams EI & Wallace P. *Health Checks for People Aged 75 and Over*, occasional paper 59 1993; Royal College of General Practitioners, London.

Zermansky AG, Raynor DK, Vail A *et al.* "No thank you": why elderly patients declined to participate in a research study. *Pharmacy World & Science* 2001; **23**(1):22–7.

152

Carers and the Role of the Family

Jo Moriarty

King's College London, London, UK

Carers are among the unsung heroes of British life...Caring for carers is a vital element in caring for those who need care.

(Her Majesty's Government, 1999)

Carers must think of themselves first – because if they have to give up, there will be no carer.

(Aged and Community Care Division of the Australian Department of Health and Ageing, Undated)

Taking care of oneself is essential if the best care is to be provided to another person. Caregivers must learn how to balance their own needs with the needs of someone who needs care.

(US Department of Health and Human Services Administration on Aging, 2004)

INTRODUCTION

These opening statements encapsulate how better understanding of the role played by carers has become embedded into the political mainstream. In some ways, they represent the considerable progress that has been made since the UK Government's 1981 White Paper which lamented the declining numbers of single women describing them as the "*natural*" carers of older people (Department of Health and Social Security, 1981). In others, they indicate the way in which carers continue to be seen as a "resource" (Twigg and Atkin, 1994), and providing them with help is seen as the best way of ensuring that they will continue to care, a response typified in the observation that:

In a number of countries...carers are slowly becoming a central point in the strategic analysis of long-term care systems.

(Jacobzone, 1999, p20)

Nevertheless, despite the increasing recognition given to people providing unpaid care for a family member or friend, there are still reports that many carers continue to be unaware of their rights (Seddon and Robinson, 2001) or do not know whom to contact should they need help (Carers UK, 2005).

SCOPE

This chapter will give an overview of recent research looking at the role played by carers and other family members in the care of older people. It will draw on the evidence from the substantial literature on caring that has its theoretical basis in a number of disciplines, including medicine, nursing, psychology, sociology, and gerontology. These range from qualitative studies describing the experience of caregiving to large-scale surveys or complex intervention studies. It will reflect the fact that, while early literature was dominated by research undertaken in North America and the United Kingdom, there is now a growing number of studies from different parts of the world. However, as will emerge later in the chapter, while the literature on caring is extensive, its quality is uneven, and there continue to be areas where uncertainties remain about the best ways of providing support for carers.

The successful care of older people is dependent upon the ability of services to contribute in ways that either enhance pre-existing sources of support or establish changes in the way in which they operate (for example, when they have become inadequate to meet a person's needs). In order to provide clear and responsive solutions, professionals need a clear understanding of what help is provided in the family, by whom, and in what circumstances. This chapter will attempt to summarize these issues and to set the background of those older people who are seen by geriatric medical services in a wider context. It will also explore the interaction between family care and the utilization of health and social care services. This is where the links with the other chapters in

Principles and Practice of Geriatric Medicine, 4th Edition. Edited by M.S. John Pathy, Alan J. Sinclair and John E. Morley.

this book will emerge most strongly. Finally, it will end by taking stock and raising issues about how support for family carers can be improved in the future.

DEFINITIONS OF CARING

The term "carer" or "caregiver" was first developed to describe the unpaid work that people, generally women, undertook while looking after relatives or friends needing support because of age, disability, or illness. These early studies were associated with feminists (Finch and Groves, 1983; Lewis and Meredith, 1988), although contemporary research undertaken independently by psychiatrists also highlighted the effects of providing care for family members (Bergmann *et al.*, 1978; Grad and Sainsbury, 1968). Conceptually, as Twigg and Atkin (1994) have pointed out, definitions of caring go beyond merely providing assistance with tasks such as shopping or bathing that people are unable to carry out independently by themselves. Caring takes place within pre-existing relationships (Finch, 1989; Qureshi and Walker, 1989) and there are likely to be strong ties of affection or obligation. Intensity is also an issue and it has become customary to distinguish between "heavily involved" carers – those providing care for 20 hours a week or more, and those who are less involved (Parker and Lawton, 1994). The failure of some researchers to incorporate these variations into their sampling and analytical frameworks has resulted in one of the most frequent criticisms within the caring literature, namely, the lack of differentiation between participants with differing relationships and with differing levels of caring responsibility (Schulz *et al.*, 1997). Furthermore, many people caring for family members or friends, particularly those who are older, do not define themselves as carers (Milne *et al.*, 2001) making it harder for policies aimed at supporting them to reach all those for whom they are intended.

Legal Frameworks

While the existence of legislative structures to support carers do not, in themselves, guarantee that carers will receive all the help that they need (Montgomery and Holzhausen, 2003–2004), it is also important to acknowledge the effects of the differing legal frameworks where family support is given and received. In the United Kingdom (UK), the Carers (Recognition and Services) Act (1995) gave carers the right to have their needs assessed. This was strengthened by the Carers (Equal Opportunities) Act (2004) which placed a duty on local authorities to tell carers about their rights and to consider carers' employment, education, or leisure commitments when carrying out carer assessments. Local authorities themselves were given powers to enlist the help of health, housing, and education authorities in providing support for carers. In Germany, the *Pflegeversicherung* (long-term care insurance) has given carers an annual right to respite care (Schunk, 1998) while, in Finland, carers are entitled to cash benefits in return for a contractual agreement to provide a certain amount of care (Martimo, 1998). These systems of support must also be considered within the context of the overall balance between state provision and family support. The extent to which families are held legally responsible for an older member's care varies throughout the European Union (Millar and Warman, 1996; Zechner, 2004).

Changes to the Way "Caring" is Conceptualized

More recently, some commentators, especially those associated with the disability movement (Morris, 1997) have challenged the assumptions underpinning the word "caring", criticizing its construction of people needing assistance in their daily lives as a "dependant" or "receiver of care". Researchers on caring (Forbat, 2005; Nolan *et al.*, 2001; Nolan *et al.*, 2003) have also advocated the need for new paradigms that reflect the realities of the reciprocities between carers and those for whom they provide support. Thus, while "caring" remains a useful shorthand word to describe the range of support that is given in the context of relationships of kinship or affinity, it remains a term that is not value free and is interpreted in a variety of ways.

WHO CARES FOR OLDER PEOPLE?

Reliable international estimates of the numbers of carers in the population are rare, but in 2001, a question on caring was included in the decennial UK census for the first time and the Office for National Statistics, the government department responsible for official statistics in the UK, reported that in England and Wales, around one in ten people (5.2 million) was caring for someone who was either "sick, disabled, or elderly" (sic). More than half of these carers were aged 50 and over. Around one in five cared for over 50 hours per week, at least two hours a week more than the maximum 48-hour week for people in paid employment laid down by the European Working Time Directive. Furthermore, in the majority of cases, family carers are the only people providing care; 80% older people rely on help from family and friends only (Pickard *et al.*, 2000).

In 1985, a question on caring was included for the first time in the *General Household Survey* (GHS), an annual survey covering a representative sample of private households in the United Kingdom (Green, 1988). Since then, it has been repeated at intervals, enabling researchers to build up information on caring in the United Kingdom over time. In 2000, the last time that the question was included, the largest group of carers (38%) comprised adult children caring for a parent. A further 14% were caring for a parent-in-law. While proportionally more people cared for other relatives (21%), friends or neighbors (21%), than spouses (18%), these figures conceal the importance of spousal care in supporting older people living in the community. Here, wives caring for husbands or husbands caring for wives accounted for almost half of those caring for 20 hours a week (Maher and Green, 2002).

Carers' Age and Gender

The peak ages for caring occurs between the ages of 45 and 64, when almost a quarter of the people define themselves as having caring responsibilities, followed by those aged 65 and over, of whom 16% have caring responsibilities (Maher and Green, 2002). This highlights a consistent finding that the majority of older people are receiving care from another older person. There are now three times as many people in their 90s living in the United Kingdom than there were 30 years ago (Office for National Statistics, 2004). This means that carers, whether they are spouses or adult children, are increasingly likely to be in the older age-group themselves. Furthermore, older carers are much more likely to be caring for 20 or more hours a week and to be the sole carer of the person for whom they provide support (Arber and Ginn, 1991; Milne *et al.*, 2001; Parker and Lawton, 1994). As later sections will show, this has important consequences for identifying which carers are likely to experience difficulties in continuing with their caring role.

Contrary to many popular stereotypes, the overall proportions of men and women carers in the population are fairly similar (14 and 16% respectively) (Maher and Green, 2002). However, these overall figures mask important variations. The majority of men carers care for a spouse or partner living in the same household. Women are more equally divided between those caring for a husband or partner and those caring for a parent. Finally, women are more likely than men to be the sole or main carer (Maher and Green, 2002) and to be involved in giving personal care, such as helping with washing or dressing (Parker and Lawton, 1994).

The Impact of Social and Demographic Change (*see* Chapter 9, The Demography of Aging; Chapter 10, Social and Community Aspects of Aging)

While results from the GHS have been broadly consistent over the last decade (Maher and Green, 2002), less is known about the effects of demographic and social changes on the numbers of carers in the longer term. This is partly because many of the seminal studies from the late 1980s and early 1990s (Arber and Ginn, 1991; Parker and Lawton, 1994; Qureshi and Walker, 1989) have yet to be repeated. More importantly, there is still great uncertainty about how increases in the proportion of older people in the population (Office for National Statistics, 2004), changes in adult children's proximity to their parents (Shelton and Grundy, 2000), and women's increased participation in the labor market (Twomey, 2002) will influence family structures and kinship roles (Harper, 2003). However, one projection is that there will be an increase in the number of spouse carers but a decline in adult children providing care to parents living in the same household (coresident care) (Comas-Herrera *et al.*, 2003; Pickard *et al.*, 2000).

Another factor that has only recently been given attention in gerontological literature is the impact of the widespread international migration from the 1960s onwards (Harper and Levin, 2003). Older populations in North America, Australasia, and Europe have become increasingly ethnically diverse. Cultural competence, the ability of professionals to provide care that matches the needs and preferences of a diverse patient population, is seen as an important way of reducing health inequalities (Betancourt *et al.*, 2003). This is especially important for professionals working in settings such as cardiology, stroke, or diabetes, where they are likely to find comparatively high proportions of patients whose ethnicity is Black or South Asian (Riste *et al.*, 2001; Sica, 2004). While carers from a minority ethnic group may face issues similar to those experienced by their majority-culture counterparts, they are often additionally disadvantaged by professionals' stereotyped assumptions about the levels of support that they will have available from within their social networks (Adamson and Donovan, 2005; Katbamna *et al.*, 2004). This highlights the importance of approaches to older people and their families that are sensitive to differing cultural and ethnic backgrounds.

In order to understand how ethnicity influences caring, it is important to first appreciate the impact of caring itself.

THE IMPACT OF CARING UPON PEOPLE'S LIVES

Psychological Health

While it is difficult to demonstrate direct causal relationships between caring and psychological health, there is strong evidence that some carers are in poorer psychological health than their age- and gender-matched counterparts in the general population. A study using data from the first 10 waves of the British Household Panel Survey (BHPS), a nationally representative sample of more than 5000 private households in England, Scotland, and Wales, found that as measured by the 12-item General Health Questionnaire (GHQ) (Goldberg and Williams, 1988), a well validated screening measure for identifying psychological health problems such as anxiety and depression, between 15 and 17% of men and 20 and 25% of women without any caring responsibilities scored 3 or more on the GHQ-12. These scores are viewed as indicating that they were experiencing symptoms associated with psychological difficulties. By contrast, around 5% more men and women carers had scores that came within this range. More importantly, average scores were considerably higher among carers caring for a person in the same household and carers caring for more than 20 hours a week. This was especially true of coresident women carers or women caring for more than 20 hours per week of whom over a third appeared to be experiencing psychological distress (Hirst, 2003).

Buck *et al.* (1997) found that 39% of their sample of over 700 carers and former carers, identified using a random stratified sample of people aged 65 and over in four parts of the United Kingdom, scored above the cut point for probable psychological illness on the GHQ-30 (Goldberg and Williams, 1988), in comparison with 31% in the general population (Cox *et al.*, 1993). They also identified that some carers who had ceased to care, continued to experience psychological difficulties, even though the person for whom they cared had moved into long-term care.

A third study (Livingston *et al.*, 1996) using a representative community sample of people aged 65 but using a different measure of psychological health, the shortened version of the Comprehensive Assessment and Referral Evaluation (Gurland *et al.*, 1984), suggested that being a carer was not in itself a risk factor for poor psychological health but that where carers lacked social support, they were at greater risk of experiencing depression.

Physical Health

As mentioned earlier, given that many carers are old themselves, they are likely to experience health problems in their own right. A study of dementia caregivers suggested that carers with long-term health conditions themselves were at risk of greater carer stress (Bruce *et al.*, 2005). Furthermore, there is some evidence that with improved health technology, many carers are undertaking tasks that in the past would have been undertaken by nurses or health-care assistants (Schulz and Martire, 2004) and that carers are providing more intensive care over longer periods (Hirst, 2002). Specific problems often cited by carers include the difficulties of assisting someone to dress if they have arthritis or back pain from lifting (Henwood, 1998; Levin *et al.*, 1994). Even where carers are receiving assistance from other family members or friends and services, they are still likely to be providing most assistance with activities of daily living (ADLs), such as washing, and instrumental activities of daily living (IADLs), such as shopping (Moriarty and Webb, 2000).

Social Support

Social isolation and loneliness are frequently reported by carers who may no longer have the time to meet up with family members and friends, or to pursue hobbies or other interests. Carers not only report feelings of loss and social isolation in their relationships with others, their relationship with the person for whom they care may also have altered. Others have argued that levels of *received* (or enacted) social support may not be as important as how carers *perceive* they are supported. Thus, if a carer does not feel supported, then he or she may express feelings of distress even if others are providing help. By contrast, good overall levels of perceived social support are associated with increased carer well-being (Chappell and Reid, 2002; Lynch, 1998).

However, although deficits in social support have long been associated with increased rates of depression, the extent to which the experience of caring, social support, and depression interact are more uncertain, mainly because of the way in which different studies have conceptualized and operationalized social support in different ways (Miller *et al.*, 2001). The lack of a confiding relationship has been associated with increased carer depression (Waite *et al.*, 2004). Unlike carers who are adult children (who may have supportive relationships with a husband, wife, or partner), spouse carers often have lower levels of social support and this may be why they tend to report poorer social support and higher levels of depression (Murray *et al.*, 1997). The impact of these changes may be reduced when the relationship between the carer and the person for whom they care has been good (Braithwaite, 2000).

Financial Aspects

Carers are also likely to be financially disadvantaged. Extra expenditure may be required to pay for equipment, services, heating, and clothing. In addition, carers may give up paid employment, forgo promotion prospects, or retire early. While women are still more likely to be affected more severely than men, particularly in terms of being able to build up savings and a pension in retirement (Ginn and Arber, 1996), this is an issue for both men and women (Carmichael and Charles, 2003). In addition to the actual costs that carers may incur through direct expenditure and loss of paid employment, economic evaluations are increasingly seeking to include some element of the opportunity costs of caring, in terms of identifying what carers might have done, had they not been caring or to include a calculation of replacement care costs representing the sums needed, had a carer not been available (Netten, 1996). This latter sum is considerable. One recent estimate suggests the average costs of so-called *informal care* at over £14 000 per year per recipient, almost three times as much as the costs of formal care from health and social care services.

Factors Relating to the Person Cared for

Carers find some aspects of caring more difficult to cope with, than others. In particular, feeling unable to deal with behavioral changes, such as wandering, night time disturbance, or aggression, are rated as especially hard to deal with (Chappell and Reid, 2002; Clark *et al.*, 2004; Draper *et al.*, 1995). Being unable to leave the person for whom they care alone has also been associated with poorer psychological health (Resource Implications Study of the Medical Research Council Cognitive Function and Ageing Study, 1999).

IDENTIFYING CARERS IN NEED OF SUPPORT

The research cited above suggests that it should be possible for health professionals to identify carers who are at greater risk of experiencing greater difficulties in their caring role than others. In summary, these are likely to be

- coresident carers (Hirst, 2003);
- carers caring for more than 20 hours per week (Hirst, 2003);
- spouse carers, especially those lacking social support (Murray *et al.*, 1997) or those who have recently ceased to care (Buck *et al.*, 1997);
- carers coping with behavioral changes in the person for whom they care (Chappell and Reid, 2002);
- carers caring for an older person with depression or dementia (Murray *et al.*, 1997; Ory *et al.*, 1999).

This is not to imply that other carers will not require support, but it may help differentiate between the larger numbers of carers who may not need substantial help beyond acquiring information and practical support and those who would benefit from more sustained support.

Screening Measures for Carers

The interest in caregiver research has resulted in a considerable number of screening measures designed to capture carers' experiences. While measures such as Burden Interview (Zarit *et al.*, 1980) and the Relatives' Stress Scale (RSS) and Behavior and Mood Disturbance Scale (Greene *et al.*, 1982) were used extensively in early research, they have become less popular since we have acquired a broader conceptual understanding of caring. Measures that have been developed to screen carers (as opposed to those for whom they care) include the Carers' Assessment of Managing Index (CAMI), Carers' Assessment of Difficulties Index (CADI), and the Carers' Assessment of Satisfactions Index (CASI) (Nolan *et al.*, 1998), the Carers of Older People in Europe (COPE) (McKee *et al.*, 2003), and the Carers' Checklist (Hodgson *et al.*, 1998). These are among the few standardized measures to assess carers' needs that have been used in routine practice, as opposed to research settings (Moriarty, 2002).

WHAT HELP DO CARERS WANT FROM SERVICES?

The diversity to be found among carers themselves and in the sort of help that they provide means that there is no single service solution that will meet all their needs and preferences. Carers' cultural backgrounds may influence their ways of responding to caring. For example, US research suggests that carers from minority ethnic groups are more likely to use religion as a way of coping with caring variations and so professionals need to be aware of the different ways in which people deal with caring (Aranda and Knight, 1997; Connell and Gibson, 1997; Kuuppelomaki *et al.*, 2004). Furthermore, there are still uncertainties about the effectiveness of services to support carers. On the whole, intervention studies remain comparatively rarer in the United Kingdom than in the United States. In the United Kingdom, literature is better on studies looking at the process and at indicating what the carers' priorities in terms of services are – for example, a systematic review on supporting carers of people with cancer and those receiving palliative care concluded that we know more about the feasibility of interventions than their effectiveness (Harding and Higginson, 2003). Nevertheless, it is possible to identify a number of consistent messages. Not surprisingly, these broadly reflect the areas where carers may experience problems.

Information

The difficulty in accessing appropriate information and at the right time is a constant theme within carer research (Henwood, 1998). However, a Cochrane review of information provision for patients and carers following stroke concluded that few information giving strategies had been evaluated comprehensively (Forster *et al.*, 2005). Nevertheless, carers' accounts suggest that they value information that is delivered quickly and given in both verbal and written forms. This information may deal with information on prognosis, symptoms, and treatment (Low *et al.*, 1999; Mant *et al.*, 1998, Wachters-Kaufmann *et al.*, 2005), but carers also require information on other services, benefits, and legal issues, such as power of attorney (Moriarty and Webb, 2000). At the same time, it is important to realize the limitations of written information; not all carers use the information that they receive (Murphy *et al.*, 1995) and so it is important to review what they have received at a later date to see whether it has been useful.

Carer Education and Support

A number of studies have suggested that some carers benefit from programs aimed at helping them understand the problems faced by the person for whom they care and in developing strategies for coping with them. These include cognitive behavioral therapy (CBT) for carers of people with dementia (Marriott *et al.*, 2000), a psychoeducational program to help deal with behavioral problems (Ostwald *et al.*, 1999), and help with moving and handling techniques and simple nursing tasks for patients who have had a stroke (Kalra *et al.*, 2004). There is increasing interest in the use of information and communication technology (ICT) (Eisdorfer *et al.*, 2003), video (Hanson *et al.*, 1999), and telephone contact (Grant *et al.*, 2004) to supplement other support.

In addition to carers' groups designed as a way of delivering specific interventions, some carers appreciate attending general support groups (McFarland and Sanders, 2000). However, it has been suggested that people from managerial and professional backgrounds are overrepresented in their attendance (Wettstein *et al.*, 2004). It is not known whether this reflects their service preferences or whether they find it easier to make arrangements for substitute care and travel than other groups of carers.

Respite Services

Respite is the term used to describe a range of services giving carers a break, ranging from one or two hours in the home to overnight care in care homes or specialist units. A number of studies have looked at the impact of respite services, but the results present a mixed and sometimes contradictory picture (Arksey *et al.*, 2004). Partly, this is because the outcome measures used most often (changes in carers' psychological health and reductions in admissions to long-term care) may not be amenable to change from the provision of comparatively small amounts of help. Carers themselves rate respite services highly when they are felt to be of sufficient quality and meet the preferences of both themselves and the person for whom they care. Carers and service providers have different perspectives about what constitutes respite. This means that it is important that respite care is offered in a form that is meaningful to carers. In this sense, respite should be seen as an outcome, not a service (Chappell *et al.*, 2001).

Understanding the Needs of Carers at Different Times

It is becoming increasingly common to view caring as a trajectory, particularly when carers are caring for people with long or progressive conditions. (Wiles *et al.*, 1998). This means that the needs of carers will vary at different times. In addition to the support they need at the beginning of caring, carers also need continuing help; for example, many carers feel guilty when they experience negative feelings about caring but would be reluctant to admit this to the person for whom they care or to other family members and friends (Adamson and Donovan, 2005). Carers who have been bereaved or those caring for a person in long-term care may continue to experience feelings of distress (Buck *et al.*, 1997; Moriarty and Webb, 2000). Carers may also be reluctant to use services; in addition to the rationing of services by service providers, some carers are reluctant to use services in case they are denying them to others (Arksey, 2002).

DISCUSSION

Although there is now extensive literature on carers, much of it remains limited and there continues to be a need for more focused studies that are better able to demonstrate what sort of services help which sort of carers in which circumstances. It is noticeable that while there are many studies looking at carers' psychological health, few look at their quality of life (Low *et al.*, 1999). There are issues about the cross-national relevance from studies based upon service systems that may be very different. Furthermore, there is a need for new forms of evaluation (Qureshi, 2004) and forms of evaluation that take account of the outcomes that are important to carers, not just to service providers or researchers (Nicholas, 2003; Qureshi, 2003).

Nevertheless, as this chapter has shown, there are areas in which there is some degree of clarity. Many carers caring for older people are themselves old and are providing considerable amounts of assistance. Although the majority of carers will not experience difficulties with their caring role, a substantial number will and this is usually influenced by the amount of care that they provide and the emotional context in which it is given. Interventions increasingly use a combination of methods and may be based upon the use of new technologies. The amount and type of care that will be required to sustain older people in the future is uncertain. What is certain is that most family members continue to wish to play a part in its provision. The challenge for services is in responding to the diversity of caregiving arrangements and in providing help that is acceptable to both carers and to those for whom they care.

KEY POINTS

- Carers provide the majority of support to older people needing help with their daily lives. Many of these are spouses with health problems of their own.
- It is possible to identify carers at greater risk of needing support themselves.
- The sort of support that carers need will vary at different timepoints while they are giving care.
- Services need to be more focused upon the sort of help that carers themselves define as useful.

KEY REFERENCES

- Arksey H. Rationed care: assessing the support needs of informal carers in English social services authorities. *Journal of Social Policy* 2002; **31**:81–101.
- Braithwaite V. Contextual or general stress outcomes: making choices through caregiving appraisals. *The Gerontologist* 2000; **40**:706–17.
- Hirst M. Caring-related inequalities in psychological distress in Britain during the 1990s. *Journal of Public Health Medicine* 2003; **25**:336–43.
- Low JTS, Payne S & Roderick P. The impact of stroke on informal carers: a literature review. *Social Science & Medicine* 1999; **49**:711–25.
- Parker G & Lawton D. *Different Types of Care, Different Types of Carer: Evidence from the General Household Survey* 1994; HMSO, London.

REFERENCES

Adamson J & Donovan J. 'Normal disruption': South Asian and African/Caribbean relatives caring for an older family member in the UK. *Social Science and Medicine* 2005; **60**:37–48.

Aged and Community Care Division of the Australian Department of Health and Ageing. *Carer Information Pack: Taking Care of*

Yourself (Undated); Department of Health and Ageing, Canberra http://www.health.gov.au/internet/wcms/publishing.nsf/e11ffa331b366c54ca2569210006982f/ageing-carers-carerkit.htm/$file/takecare.pdf.

Aranda MP & Knight BG. The influence of ethnicity and culture on the caregiver stress and coping process: a sociological review and analysis. *The Gerontologist* 1997; **37**:342–54.

Arber S & Ginn J. *Gender and Later Life: a Sociological Analysis of Resources and Constraints* 1991; Sage Publications, London.

Arksey H. Rationed care: assessing the support needs of informal carers in English social services authorities. *Journal of Social Policy* 2002; **31**:81–101.

Arksey H, Jackson K, Croucher K *et al. Review of Respite Services and Short-Term Breaks for Carers for People with Dementia* 2004; NHS Service Delivery and Organisation (SDO) Programme, London.

Bergmann K, Foster EM, Justice AW & Matthews V. Management of the demented elderly patient in the community. *The British Journal of Psychiatry* 1978; **132**:441–9.

Betancourt JR, Green AR, Carrillo JE & Ananeh-Firempong O. Defining cultural competence: a practical framework for addressing racial/ethnic disparities in health care. *Public Health Reports* 2003; **118**:293–302.

Braithwaite V. Contextual or general stress outcomes: making choices through caregiving appraisals. *The Gerontologist* 2000; **40**:706–17.

Bruce DG, Paley GA, Nichols P *et al.* Physical disability contributes to caregiver stress in dementia caregivers. *The Journals of Gerontology Series. A, Biological Sciences and Medical Sciences* 2005; **60**:345–9.

Buck D, Gregson BA, Bamford CH *et al.* Psychological distress among informal supporters of frail older people at home and in institutions. *International Journal of Geriatric Psychiatry* 1997; **12**:737–44.

Carers (Equal Opportunities) Act 2004. 2004; The Stationery Office, London.

Carers (Recognition & Services) Act 1995. 1995, Chapter c 12; HMSO, London.

Carers UK. *Back Me Up: Supporting Carers When they Need it Most* 2005; Carers UK, London.

Carmichael F & Charles S. The opportunity costs of informal care: does gender matter? *Journal of Health Economics* 2003; **22**:781–803.

Chappell NL, Reid R & Dow E. Respite reconsidered: a typology of meanings based on the caregiver's point of view. *Journal of Aging Studies* 2001; **15**:201–16.

Chappell NL & Reid RC. Burden and well-being among caregivers: examining the distinction. *The Gerontologist* 2002; **42**:772–80.

Clark PC, Dunbar SB, Shields CG *et al.* Influence of stroke survivor characteristics and family conflict surrounding recovery on caregivers' mental and physical health. *Nursing Research* 2004; **53**:406–13.

Comas-Herrera A, Pickard L, Wittenberg R *et al. Future Demand for Long Term Care 2001–2031: Projections of Demand for Long Term Care for Older People in England* 2003; Personal Social Services Research Unit, Canterbury.

Connell CM & Gibson G. Racial, ethnic and cultural differences in dementia caregiving: review and analysis. *The Gerontologist* 1997; **37**:355–64.

Cox B, Blaxter M, Huppert F *et al. The Health and Lifestyle Survey* 1993; Dartmouth, Aldershot.

Department of Health and Social Security. *Growing Older, Cmnd 8173* 1981; HMSO, London.

Draper BM, Poulos RG, Poulos CJ & Ehrlich F. Risk factors for stress in elderly caregivers. *International Journal of Geriatric Psychiatry* 1995; **11**:227–31.

Eisdorfer C, Czaja SJ, Loewenstein DA *et al.* The effect of a family therapy and technology-based intervention on caregiver depression. *The Gerontologist* 2003; **43**:(4): 521–31.

Finch J. *Family Obligations and Social Change* 1989; Polity Press, Oxford.

Finch J & Groves D (eds) *A Labour of Love: Women, Work and Caring* 1983; Routledge and Kegan Paul, London.

Forbat L. *Talking about Care: Two Sides to the Story* 2005; The Policy Press, Bristol.

Forster A, Smith J, Young J *et al. Information Provision for Stroke Patients and their Caregivers* 2005; The Cochrane Library (Oxford).

Ginn J & Arber S. Patterns of employment, gender, and pensions: the effect of work history on older women's non-state pensions. *Work Employment and Society* 1996; **10**:469–90.

Goldberg D & Williams P. *A User's Guide to the General Health Questionnaire* 1988; The NFER-Nelson Publishing Company Limited, Windsor.

Grad J & Sainsbury P. The effects that patients have on their families in a community care and a control psychiatric service – a two year follow-up. *British Journal of Psychiatry* 1968; **114**:265–78.

Grant JS, Glandon GL, Elliott TR *et al.* Caregiving problems and feelings experienced by family caregivers of stroke survivors the first month after discharge. *International Journal of Rehabilitation Research* 2004; **27**:105–11.

Green H. *Informal Carers: a Study Carried out on Behalf of the Department of Health and Social Security as Part of the 1985 General Household Survey* 1988; HMSO, London.

Greene JG, Smith R, Gardiner M & Timbury GC Measuring behavioural disturbance of elderly demented patients in the community and its effects on relatives: a factor analytic study. *Age and Ageing* 1982; **11**:121–6.

Gurland B, Golden RR, Teresi JA & Challop J. The SHORT-CARE: an efficient instrument for the assessment of dementia, depression and disability. *Journals of Gerontology* 1984; **39**:166–9.

Hanson EJ, Tetley J & Clarke A. A multimedia intervention to support family caregivers. *The Gerontologist* 1999; **39**:736–41.

Harding R & Higginson IJ. What is the best way to help caregivers in cancer and palliative care? A systematic literature review of interventions and their effectiveness. *Palliative Medicine* 2003; **17**:63–74.

Harper S. Changing families as European societies age. *European Journal of Sociology* 2003; **44**:155–84.

Harper S & Levin S. *Working Paper Number WP503: Changing Families as Societies Age: Care, Independence and Ethnicity* 2003; Oxford Institute of Ageing, Oxford.

Henwood M. *Ignored and Invisible? Carers' Experiences of the NHS* 1998; Carers' National Association, London.

Her Majesty's Government. *Caring about Carers: a National Strategy for Carers* 1999; Department of Health, London.

Hirst M. Transitions to informal care in Great Britain during the 1990s. *Journal of Epidemiology and Community Health* 2002; **56**:579–87.

Hirst M. Caring-related inequalities in psychological distress in Britain during the 1990s. *Journal of Public Health Medicine* 2003; **25**:336–43.

Hodgson C, Higginson I & Jefferys P. *Carers' Checklist: An Outcome Measure for People with Dementia and their Carers* 1998; Mental Health Foundation, London.

Jacobzone S. *Labour Market and Social Policy – Occasional Papers No 38: Ageing and Care for Frail Elderly Persons: An Overview of International Perspectives* 1999; Organisation for Economic Co-operation and Development, Paris.

Kalra L, Evans A, Perez I *et al.* Training carers of stroke patients: randomised controlled trial. *British Medical Journal* 2004; **328**:1099–104.

Katbamna S, Ahmad W, Bhakta P *et al.* Do they look after their own? Informal support for South Asian carers. *Health and Social Care in the Community* 2004; **12**:398–406.

Kuuppelomaki M, Sasaki A, Yamada K *et al.* Coping strategies of family carers for older relatives in Finland. *Journal of Clinical Nursing* 2004; **13**:697–706.

Levin E, Moriarty J & Gorbach P. *Better for the Break* 1994; HMSO, London.

Lewis J & Meredith B. *Daughters Who Care: Daughters Caring for Mothers at Home* 1988; Routledge, London.

Livingston G, Manela M & Katona C. Depression and other psychiatric morbidity in carers of elderly people living at home. *British Medical Journal* 1996; **312**:153–6.

Low JTS, Payne S & Roderick P. The impact of stroke on informal carers: a literature review. *Social Science & Medicine* 1999; **49**:711–25.

Lynch SA. Who supports whom? How age and gender affect the perceived quality of support from family and friends. *The Gerontologist* 1998; **38**:231–8.

Maher J & Green H. *Carers 2000* 2002; The Stationery Office, London.

Mant J, Carter J, Wade DT & Winner S. The impact of an information pack on patients with stroke and their carers: a randomized controlled trial. *Clinical Rehabilitation* 1998; **12**:465–76.

Marriott A, Donaldson C, Tarrier N & Burns A. Effectiveness of cognitive–behavioural family intervention in reducing the burden of care in carers of patients with Alzheimer's disease. *British Journal of Psychiatry* 2000; **176**:557–62.

Martimo K. *Community Care for older People in Finland*. In C Glendinning (ed) *Rights and Realities: Comparing New Developments in Long-Term Care for Older People* 1998, pp 67–82; The Policy Press, Bristol.

McFarland PL & Sanders S. Educational support groups for male caregivers of individuals with Alzheimer's disease. *American Journal of Alzheimer's Disease* 2000; **15**(6):367–73.

McKee KJ, Philp I, Lamura G *et al.* The COPE index – a first stage assessment of negative impact, positive value and quality of support of caregiving in informal carers of older people. *Aging and Mental Health* 2003; **7**:39–52.

Millar J & Warman A. *Family Obligations in Europe* 1996; Family Policy Studies Centre, London.

Miller B, Townsend A, Carpenter E *et al.* Social support and caregiver distress: a replication analysis. *Journal of Gerontology: Series B, Psychological Sciences and Social Sciences* 2001; **56**:S249–56.

Milne A, Hatzidimitriadou E, Chryssanthopoulou C. *Caring in Later Life: Reviewing the Role of Older Carers* 2001; Help the Aged, London.

Montgomery A & Holzhausen E. Caregivers in the United States and the United Kingdom: different systems, similar challenges. *The Generations* 2003–2004; **27**:61–7.

Moriarty J. *Assessing the Mental Health Needs of Older People: Systematic Review on the Use of Standardised Measures to Improve Assessment Practice* 2002; Social Care Workforce Research Unit, London.

Moriarty J & Webb S. *Part of their Lives: Community Care for People with Dementia* 2000; The Policy Press, Bristol.

Morris J. Care or empowerment? A disability rights perspective. *Social Policy and Administration* 1997; **31**:54–60.

Murphy B, Schofield H & Herrman H. Information for family carers: does it help? *Australian Journal of Public Health* 1995; **19**:192–7.

Murray JM, Manela MV, Shuttleworth A & Livingston GA. Caring for an older spouse with a psychiatric illness. *Aging and Mental Health* 1997; **1**:256–60.

Netten A. The costs of informal care. In C Clark & I Lapsley (eds) *Planning and Costing Community Care* 1996; Jessica Kingsley Publishers, London.

Nicholas E. An outcomes focus in carer assessment and review: value and challenge. *British Journal of Social Work* 2003; **33**:31–47.

Nolan M, Davies S & Grant G (eds) *Working with Older People and their Families* 2001; Open University Press, Maidenhead.

Nolan M, Grant G & Keady J. *Assessing the Needs of Family Carers: a Guide for Practitioners* 1998; Pavilion Publishing, Brighton.

Nolan M, Lundh U, Keady J & Grant G (eds) *Partnerships in Family Care* 2003; Open University Press, Maidenhead.

Office for National Statistics. *Social Trends 34* 2004; The Stationery Office, London.

Ory MG, Hoffman R III, Yee JL *et al.* Prevalence and impact of caregiving: a detailed comparison between dementia and nondementia caregivers. *The Gerontologist* 1999; **39**:177–85.

Ostwald SK, Hepburn KW, Caron W *et al.* Reducing caregiver burden: a randomized psychoeducational intervention for caregivers of persons with dementia. *The Gerontologist* 1999; **39**:299–309.

Parker G & Lawton D. *Different Types of Care, Different Types of Carer: Evidence from the General Household Survey* 1994; HMSO, London.

Pickard L, Wittenberg R, Comas-Herrera A *et al.* Relying on informal care in the new century? Informal care for elderly people in England to 2031. *Ageing and Society* 2000; **20**:745–72.

Qureshi H. Evidence in policy and practice: what kinds of research designs? *Journal of Social Work* 2004; **4**:7–23.

Qureshi H. A response to dempster and donnelly 'outcome measurement and service evaluation–a note on research design': the importance of understanding social care outcomes. *British Journal of Social Work* 2003; **33**:117–20.

Qureshi H & Walker A. *The Caring Relationship: Elderly People and their Families* 1989; MacMillan, Basingstoke.

Resource Implications Study of the Medical Research Council Cognitive Function and Ageing Study. Informal caregiving for frail older people at home and in long term care institutions: who are the key supporters? *Health and Social Care in the Community* 1999; **7**:434–44.

Riste L, Khan F & Cruickshank K. High prevalence of type 2 diabetes in all ethnic groups, including Europeans, in a British inner city: relative poverty, history, inactivity, or 21st century Europe? *Diabetes Care* 2001; **24**:1377–83.

Schulz R & Martire LM. Family caregiving of persons with dementia: prevalence, health effects, and support strategies. *American Journal of Geriatric Psychiatry* 2004; **12**:240–9.

Schulz R, Newsom J, Mittelmark M *et al.* Health effects of caregiving: the caregiver health effects study: an ancillary study of the cardiovascular health study. *Annals of Behavioral Medicine* 1997; **19**:110–6.

Schunk M. The social insurance model of care for older people in Germany. In C Glendinning (ed) *Rights and Realities: Comparing New Developments in Long-Term Care for Older People* 1998, pp 29–46; The Policy Press, Bristol.

Seddon D & Robinson CA. Carers of older people with dementia: assessment and the Carers Act. *Health and Social Care in the Community* 2001; **9**:151–8.

Shelton N & Grundy E. Proximity of adult children to their parents in Great Britain. *International Journal of Population Geography* 2000; **6**:181–95.

Sica D. Optimizing hypertension and vascular health: focus on ethnicity. *Clinical Cornerstone* 2004; **6**:28–38.

Twigg J & Atkin K. *Carers Perceived: Policy and Practice in Informal Care* 1994; Open University Press, Buckingham.

Twomey B. Women in the labour market: results from the spring 2001 LFS. *Labour Market Trends* 2002; **110**:109–28.

US Department of Health and Human Services Administration on Aging. *National Family Caregiver Support Program Resources: Taking Care of Yourself* 2004; Administration on Aging, Washington.

Wachters-Kaufmann C, Schuling J, The H & Meyboom-de Jong B. Actual and desired information provision after a stroke. *Patient Education and Counseling* 2005; **56**:211–7.

Waite A, Bebbington P, Skelton-Robinson M & Orrell M. Social factors and depression in carers of people with dementia. *International Journal of Geriatric Psychiatry* 2004; **19**:582–7.

Wettstein A, Schmid R & Konig M. Who participates in psychosocial interventions for caregivers of patients with dementia? *Dementia and Geriatric Cognitive Disorders* 2004; **18**:80–6.

Wiles R, Pain H, Buckland S & McLellan L. Providing appropriate information to patients and carers following a stroke. *Journal of Advanced Nursing* 1998; **28**:794–801.

Zarit SH, Reever KE & Bach-Peterson J. Relatives of the impaired elderly: correlates of feelings of burden. *The Gerontologist* 1980; **20**:649–55.

Zechner M. Family commitments under negotiation: dual carers in Finland and Italy. *Social Policy and Administration* 2004; **38**:640–53.

FURTHER READING

Karlsson M, Mayhew L, Plumb R & Rickayzen B. Future costs for long-term care: cost projections for long-term care for older people in the United Kingdom. *Health Policy* (in press).

153

Nursing Home Care

David R. Thomas *and* John E. Morley

Saint Louis University Health Sciences Center and Saint Louis Veterans' Affairs Medical Center, St Louis, MO, USA

INTRODUCTION

Nursing home facilities are more unique than similar. The care of elderly persons in institutionalized setting varies by country, region, societal, and cultural factors. Approaches to long-term care in various countries include chronic geriatric hospitals, short-stay rehabilitation centers, residential living centers, and institutionalized skilled nursing homes. The nomenclature of a facility varies across settings, including "nursing home" in the United States and "care home" in the United Kingdom. A "nursing home" in the United States may refer to a specialized center for persons on ventilators, with acquired immunodeficiency syndrome, or with dementia who need skilled nursing care. A "care home" in the United Kingdom generally refers to a home registered under the Care Standards Act providing personal and residential care for older people, and also includes homes that provide nursing care (nursing homes). Not only is the classification confusing, but the public, and often the professional, view of nursing homes involves a number of misperceptions.

Misperception: Most older adults will live for many years in a nursing home and eventually die there. Truth: Fewer than 5% of older adults in United States and fewer than 10% in United Kingdom reside in resident and nursing home settings.

Misperception: Once a person enters a nursing home, he or she stays there for good. Truth: Many older adults who enter a nursing home will recover and leave (short-stay residents), while fewer older adults will remain in a nursing home once admitted (long-stay residents).

Misperception: Nursing homes are warehouses for older persons with little or no stimulation: Truth: A good home provides a social environment that often is very comforting for older persons who may have been isolated in previous living environments.

Misperceptions: No one likes living in a nursing home. Truth: Many residents prefer the reassurance of medical care, socialization, and a safe environment, and find the experience positive.

Facility Demographics

In the United States, there are approximately 18 000 nursing homes with a bed capacity of 1.9 million. The number of residents in the current statistical period was 1.6 million, with a bed occupancy rate of 87% (National Center for Health Statistics, 1999). Ownership of most nursing homes in the United States is by for-profit entities, while only 7% are owned by governmental entities (Figure 1). In the United States, most nursing homes have between 50 and 199 beds (79%) and only 8% had more than 200 beds. The average size of nursing homes was 107 beds.

Fifty-six percent of nursing homes are affiliated with other nursing homes in a chain ownership. These facilities accounted for 56.9% of all beds, 56.5% of all residents, and 61% of all discharges. Most nursing homes (62%) are located in a metropolitan statistical area (Gabrel, 2000). The distribution of nursing homes is uneven, with the Midwest and South census regions having 34 and 32% of facilities and 32 and 33% of all beds, respectively.

The nursing home industry employs a large number of persons in various occupations. The number of employees by occupation is given in Figure 2. The rate of staffing does not appear to vary much by type of nursing home ownership. A major problem for patient care in nursing homes is the high staff turnover rate. A vacancy rate of 19% for nurses has been reported (American Nursing Association, 1991). Turnover rate for nursing assistant has been reported to be as high as 93% (Caudill and Patrick, 1991). These high vacancy rates disturb continuity and force continuous training of new personnel.

Nursing home care is expensive. The per diem rates for private-pay individuals and for Medicare and Medicaid reimbursement is shown in Table 1. In the United States, the primary source of payment for nursing home care is Medicaid, a means-tested governmental source (see Figure 3). There are regional variations in nursing home charges and reimbursement (see Figure 4). The national costs of nursing home care was $53 billion in 1990, and was the fastest

Principles and Practice of Geriatric Medicine, 4th Edition. Edited by M.S. John Pathy, Alan J. Sinclair and John E. Morley.

Table 1 Average daily charge for private-pay residents by level of care of facility and for Medicare residents by selected nursing home characteristics: United States, 1997

	Level of care			Certification	
	Skilled	Intermediate	Residential	Medicare	Medicaid
Proprietary	$132.25	103.49	100.87	228.14	91.04
Voluntary nonprofit	147.47	118.01	80.91	201.45	116.49
Government and other	129.01	99.21	N/A	150.52	99.71

Source: Gabrel CS. An overview of nursing home facilities: Data from the 1997 National Nursing Home Survey. Advance data from vital and health statistics; no. 311. Hyattsville, Maryland: National Center for Health Statistics. 2000.

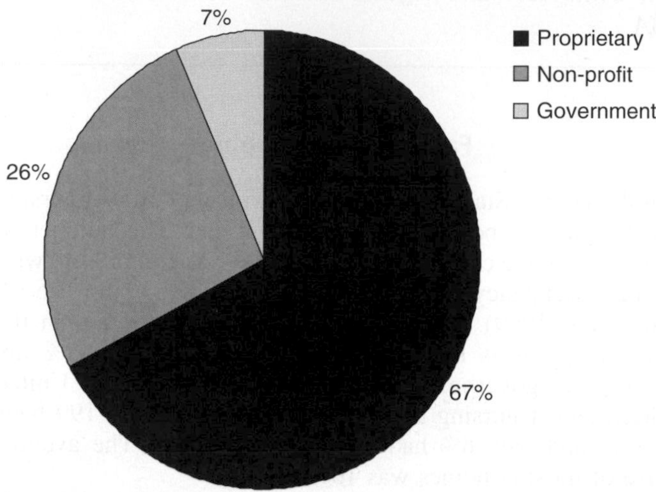

Figure 1 Percent distribution of nursing home facilities by ownership: United States, 1997. *Source*: Gabrel CS. An overview of nursing home facilities: Data from the 1997 National Nursing Home Survey. Advance data from vital and health statistics; no. 311. Hyattsville, Maryland: National Center for Health Statistics. 2000

growing component of major health-care expense in the national budget (Levit *et al.*, 1991). The projected cost for the year 2000 well exceeds $140 billion, and may exceed $700 billion by the year 2030 (Sonnenfeld *et al.*, 1991).

Nursing homes in other cultural settings differ considerably. For example, the Dutch experience demonstrates that among persons older than 65 years, approximately 20% had a short stay in an inpatient hospital department and 96% were discharged to their own home situation. Only 7% lived permanently in special institutions for chronic care, including residential care or nursing home care. Persons with physical disability or with progressive dementia, who have impaired activities of daily living (ADLs) and who need more complex continuing care beyond the range of home care services in a residential homes, are admitted to a nursing home. The number of nursing home beds is 3.6 per 1000 persons (in 2003), with a total of 330 nursing homes with approximately 26 000 beds designed primarily for persons with physical problems and 32 000 beds in psychogeriatric wards for persons with dementia. Nursing home care is covered by a mandatory national insurance system, the Exceptional Medical Expenses Act. In addition to the funds from this national insurance,

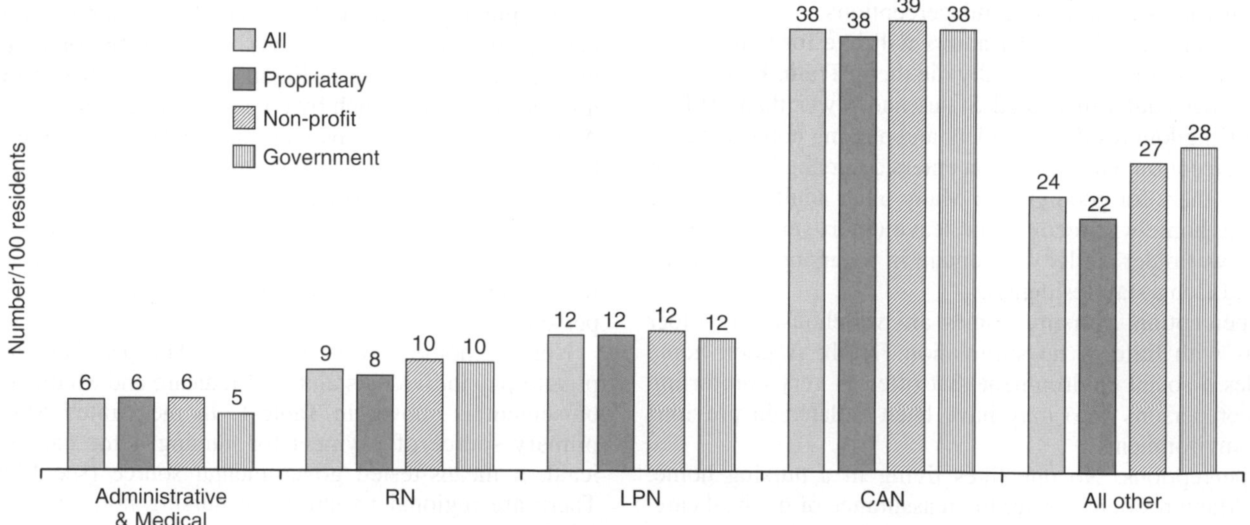

Figure 2 Number per 100 residents of full-time equivalent employees by occupational categories and selected nursing home characteristics: United States, 1997. Administrative & medical includes dentists, dental hygienists, physical therapists, speech pathologists and/or audiologists, dieticians or nutritionists, podiatrists, and social workers; N = registered nurse; LPN = licensed practical nurse; CNA = certified nursing assistant. *Source*: Gabrel CS. An overview of nursing home facilities: Data from the 1997 National Nursing Home Survey. Advance data from vital and health statistics; no. 311. Hyattsville, Maryland: National Center for Health Statistics. 2000

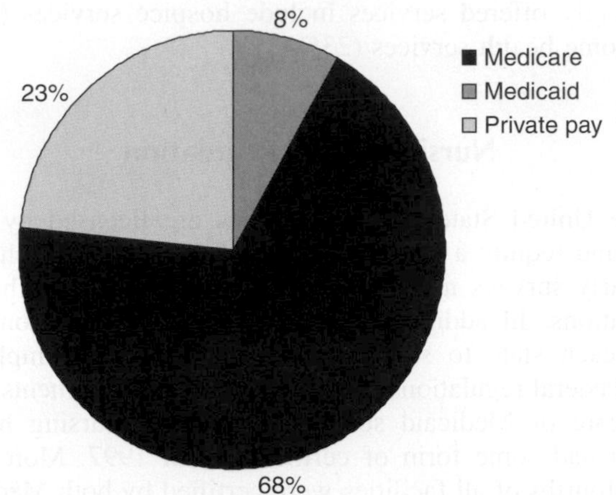

Figure 3 Nursing home payment *Source*: United States, 1997. *Source*: Gabrel CS. An overview of nursing home facilities: Data from the 1997 National Nursing Home Survey. Advance data from vital and health statistics; no. 311. Hyattsville, Maryland: National Center for Health Statistics. 2000

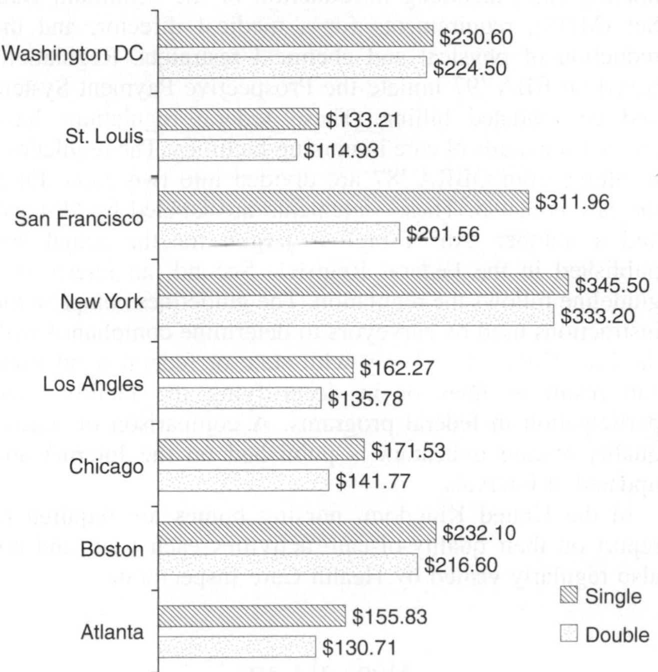

Figure 4 Average daily rate for a single-occupancy or double-occupancy nursing home accommodation: United States 2003. *Source*: The MetLife Market Survey of Nursing Home and Home Care Costs, August 2003

income- and household-dependent out-of-pocket payments are obligatory for persons admitted to nursing homes (Schols *et al.*, 2004).

In the United Kingdom, the number of patients in private or voluntary homes has risen from 18 200 in 1983 to 148 500 in 1994 (Black and Bowman, 1997). The number of institutional care beds for older persons has doubled to 563 000 between 1980 and 1995. National Health Service beds accounted for less than 10% of the total in 1995 compared with 23% in 1980, while private and voluntary (not for profit) residential and nursing homes increased to 76% (Kavanagh and Knapp, 1997).

Persons in the United Kingdom receiving long-term care provided in care homes are required to meet financial means testing. Those who have assets, including the value of their homes, above a limit (£18 500 in 2002) are required to pay the care home's fees in full. Those with assets below the limit make a copayment that is usually less than the full fee. For those with the lowest income and assets, this payment may be met from Income Support, the UK's means-tested welfare benefit. Almost all older people who own their home would be required to meet care home fees in full.

Means testing dates back to 1948 in the United Kingdom, and has changed little in the many years. However, the growing numbers of older persons and increasing home ownership has stressed the means test. Local public authorities are responsible for payment for long-term care for older persons who meet means test requirements, whether in a care home or in the person's own home. For care services delivered at home, the value of an older person's home is disregarded in determining how much he or she contributes. An older home owner is, therefore, likely to incur considerably more – and the public budget correspondingly less – of the cost of care in a residential setting than of equivalent cost care at home. The result is a financial incentive for public authorities to arrange for a home owner's care to be provided in an institution rather than in the person's own home. The financial incentive works in the opposite direction for older home owners themselves. Whether the likelihood of entry to a care home is increased or decreased by the level of an individual's economic resources would seem to depend on whether individual choice or the policy of the local public authority dominates (Hancock *et al.*, 2002).

Resident Demographics

In the United States, 43% of persons who were 65 years of age in 1990 will enter a nursing home in their lifetime. Of these, 55% will stay at least for 1 year, and 21% will stay for 5 years or longer (Kemper and Murtaugh, 1991). Nursing home use is strongly associated with age, even after adjusting for disability. This suggests that the future need for nursing home care will increase as the population increases in life expectancy. By the year 2030, the need for nursing home beds in the United States is projected to increase to 5 million (Zedlewski *et al.*, 1989; Doty, 1992).

Most nursing home admissions are for short-stay residents. About 2.5 million residents are discharged after an average length stay of 272 days. Long-stay residents remain in the nursing home for an average of 873 days.

Residents in nursing homes do not reflect the general population demographics. Ninety-one percent of nursing home residents are older than 65 years, but 46% are 85 years old or above. This raises the mean age for all current nursing home residents to 81 years (Figure 5). Most nursing home residents are women (72%), and these women are older

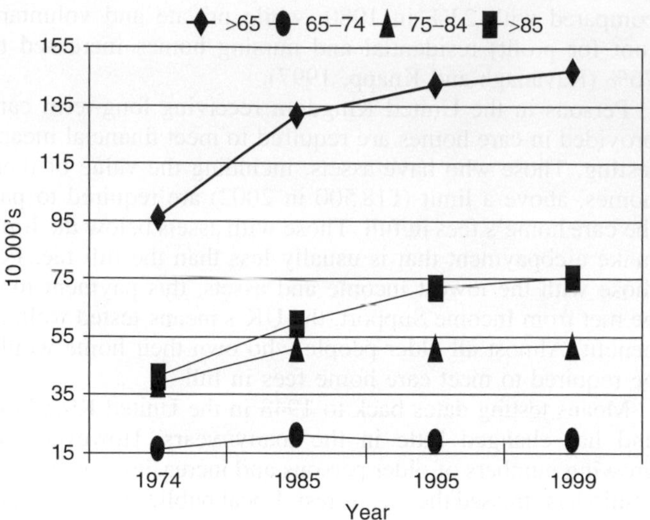

Figure 5 Nursing home residents 65 years of age and over: United States, 1973–1974, 1985, 1995, and 1999. *Source*: National Center for Health Statistics. Health, United States, 2004. With Chartbook on Trends in the Health of Americans. Hyattsville, Maryland: 2004

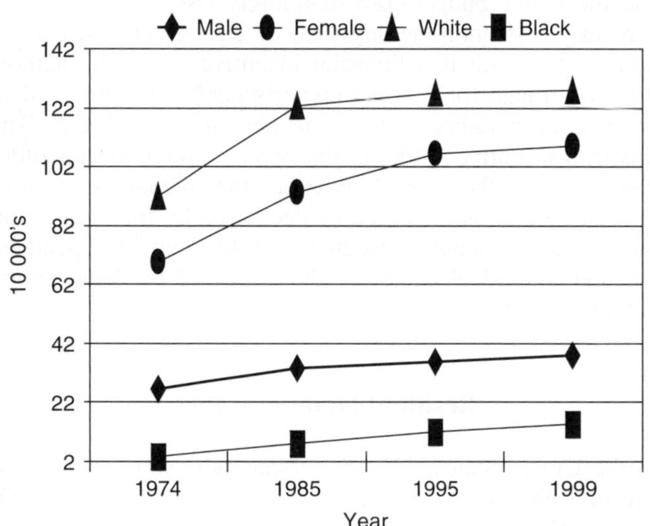

Figure 6 Nursing home residents 65 years of age and over: United States, by sex, and race 1973–1974, 1985, 1995, and 1999. *Source*: National Center for Health Statistics. Health, United States, 2004. With Chartbook on Trends in the Health of Americans. Hyattsville, Maryland: 2004

(mean age 83 years) compared to men (mean age 76 years). Racial demographics are only slightly different from the general population: 87% white and 12% black (Figure 6).

Nursing homes provide extensive services to residents. Almost all nursing homes reported providing nursing services (100%), medical services (97%), and personal care services that included ADLs (97%). Nonmedical services most frequently offered by nursing homes include nutrition (99%); social services including assistance to residents and their families in handling social, environmental, and emotional problems (98%); and physical therapy (97%). The least frequently offered services include hospice services (72%) and home health services (23%).

Nursing Home Regulation

In the United States, nursing homes are licensed by each state and require a certificate of need to operate. Each state regularly surveys nursing homes for compliance with state regulations. In addition, the Federal government contracts with each state to survey nursing homes for compliance with Federal regulations if the home receives payments from Medicare or Medicaid sources. Nearly all nursing homes (96%) had some form of certification in 1997. More than three-fourths of all facilities were certified by both Medicare and Medicaid. Only 4% of the 18 000 nursing homes were not certified.

Federal regulations are contained in two Congressional acts, the Omnibus Budget Reconciliation Act of 1987 (OBRA '87) and the Balanced Budget Act of 1997 (BBA '97). OBRA '87 had a major impact on general nursing care, including introduction of the Minimum Data Set (MDS), requirements for a medical director, and the reduction of physical and chemical restraints. Regulations based on BBA '97 initiate the Prospective Payment System and consolidated billing. These federal regulations have created standards of care in nursing facilities. The regulations resulting from OBRA '87 are divided into two parts. First, the law is stated. These statements are labeled by "F-tags" and a number. An "F-tag" is jargon for the actual law published in the Federal Register. Second, an interpretive guideline follows the regulation. The guidelines comprise the instructions used by surveyors to determine compliance with the law. Failure to comply with state or federal regulations can result in fines or in decertifying the facility from participation in federal programs. A comparison of federal quality-of-care indicators is published on the Internet and updated at intervals.

In the United Kingdom, nursing homes are required to report on their quality-of-care activities each year, and are also regularly visited by Health Care Inspectorate.

Medical Care

Care of residents in a nursing home is overseen by a physician. Each nursing home is required to have a physician Medical Director, who oversees the quality-of-care in the facility. Each resident is seen by their physician, who either visits them in the facility or arranges for clinic visits. The frequency of visits is dictated by medical necessity, but cannot be less frequent than once every 30 days for the initial 3 months following admissions, or less than once in every 60 days thereafter. Physician extenders or nurse practitioners may also see residents in a facility, but may not be used to meet this minimum standard.

The number of physicians who see residents in a facility is small. Only 1 in 10 primary care physicians provide care in a nursing home. Seventy-seven percent of all physicians report spending no time in a nursing home. Only 15% of specialists spend any time in a nursing home. Among physicians who report seeing patients in a nursing home, a majority spent less than 2 hours per week with residents (Katz *et al.*, 1997). Contributing to this minimal involvement, over one-third of surveyed physicians report inadequate training in geriatric syndromes such as falls, incontinence, dementia, nutrition, and chronic pain (Darer *et al.*, 2004).

Medical care in nursing homes focuses on chronic disease and geriatric syndromes, owing to resident comorbid conditions. Functional impairment is the final common pathway of most chronic disease, especially in older persons with multiple advanced disorders (Thomas, 2002a). Nursing home residents in the United States are becoming older, increasingly female, and more functionally impaired (Figures 5–7).

An estimated 59% of adults with five or more ADLs impairments will be admitted to nursing homes (Guralnik *et al.*, 1994). In general, functional status declines with time. Older adults in nursing homes with substantial functional impairment show poorer function at the end of the 6 months than those with higher function (Buttar *et al.*, 2001), and a shorter life expectancy in the nursing home than institutionalized adults of the same age who are less impaired (Donaldson *et al.*, 1980). Functional status is the most sensitive clinical indicator with which to follow disease progression or response to therapy in the elderly. The MDS as well as standardized brief clinical instruments are used to assess functional status. Improvement in function rather than cure of disease is the major therapeutic goal of nursing home care.

Other chronic conditions affect the care of residents in long-term care facilities. Between 45 and 70% of the estimated 1.6 million nursing home residents fall annually (Thappa *et al.*, 1996). Of these, 30–40% will fall two or more times and 11% will sustain a serious injury as a result of the fall (Rubenstein *et al.*, 1994). Urinary incontinence affects approximately half of nursing home residents (Ouslander and Schnelle, 1995). Dementia of various types is present in over 60% of typical nursing home residents (Jakob *et al.*, 2002; Rovner *et al.*, 1990), many of whom exhibit behavioral disturbances (Thomas, 2002b). The prevalence of pressure ulcers is higher in long term care settings (Thomas, 2001). In Medicare-certified nursing home beds, one-fourth of residents receive enteral feeding (Shaughnessy and Kramer, 1990; Haddad and Thomas, 2002). Weight loss and undernutrition frequently complicate the care of older adults (Thomas *et al.*, 2002). The prevalence of chronic conditions and interacting comorbid conditions increase the medical complexity of caring for nursing home residents. Several guidelines for the evaluation and management of common clinical problems in the nursing home have been published (Ouslander and Osterweil, 1994; Evans *et al.*, 1995). Table 2 provides some clinical characteristics of residents in nursing homes in the United States.

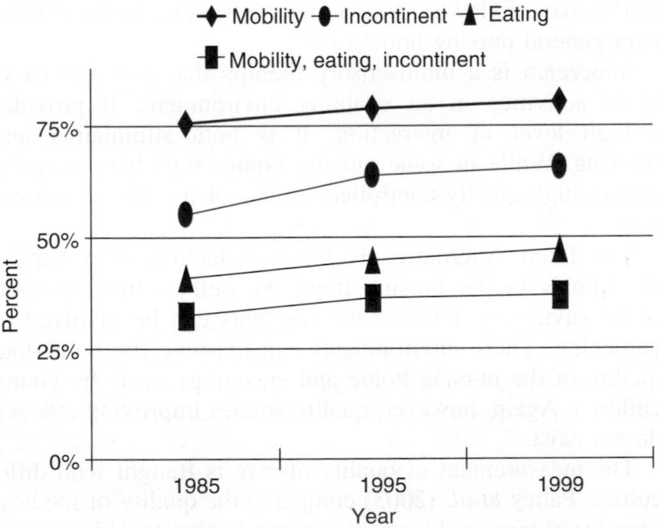

Figure 7 Nursing home residents 65 years of age and over: United States, by functional status 1985, 1995, and 1999. *Source*: National Center for Health Statistics. Health, United States, 2004. With Chartbook on Trends in the Health of Americans. Hyattsville, Maryland: 2004

Table 2 Some characteristics of residents in nursing homes in the United States in 2005

Condition	Residents (%)
Catheters	6.4
Contractures	30.5
Depression	45.5
Dementia	46.6
Urinary incontinence	55.8
Bowel incontinence	45.8
Behavioral symptoms	30.5
Pressure ulcers	7.3
Tube feedings	6.6
Significant weight loss	10.9
Influenza vaccinations	63.2
Pneumonococcal vaccinations	35.4
Fracture incidence	3.0
Dehydration	0.5
Moderate to severe pain	7.8
Nine or more medications	61.3
Urinary tract infection	9.5

COMPARISON OF NURSING HOMES IN DIFFERENT COUNTRIES

In 1997, *Age and Ageing* published a supplement comparing nursing homes in multiple different countries utilizing the data collected by the Resident Assessment Instrument (Fries *et al.*, 1997; Berg *et al.*, 1997; Ljunggren *et al.*, 1997; Sgadari *et al.*, 1997; Schroll *et al.*, 1997). Most of the data was collected in the early 1990s. These findings are summarized in Table 3. Some recent data collected using the Resident Assessment Instrument in the United States from 2005 is also included in the table. As can be seen, there is a large variability between countries.

Iceland and Denmark have over 50% of their nursing home population over 85 years of age, while in Italy and Japan, it is under 40%. Sweden and the United States have

Table 3 Comparisons between nursing homes across countries

Data collected	Denmark 1992–1993	Italy 1992–1994	Japan 1993	Sweden 1990–1993	Iceland 1994	France 1993	USA 1993	USA 2005
Age <65	4.2	4.5	4.6	3.8	1.8	10.2	6.5	
65–84	45.7	56.1	60.3	52.6	46.6	45.5	53.9	
85+	50.1	39.3	35.2	43.5	51.5	44.3	47.2	–
Length of stay								
≤30 days	2.6	–	0	22.8	0.7	3.8	20.9	–
>2 years	49.4	–	48.5	30.8	60.6	43.8	45.7	
Cognitively intact	21.8	15.3	32.7	19.7	28.5	11.0	18.5	53.4
Low ADLs	49.0	55.0	42.0		38.0		48.0	
Residents receiving rehabilitation	23.0	14.0	30.0	–	31.0	–	11.0	17.2
Restraints	2.2	16.6	4.5	15.2	8.5	17.1	16.5	7.6
Incontinence								
Urine	52.2	54.4	42.9	61.6	56.5	65.2	46.4	55.8
Bowel	22.4	45.3	30.6	39.5	23.0	55.5	29.5	45.8
Participate in activities	52.0	20.0	43.0	–	44.0	–	50.0	–
Nursing time per patient	–	–	84.4	133.7	–	–	118.3	–

over 20% of the nursing home population staying for less than 30 years, while none of the Japanese population stay for such a short time period. Except in Japan, under one-third of residents are cognitively intact. In the United States, this has changed remarkably in the 10 years since the survey, with now over half of the patients being cognitively intact. This almost certainly represents the shift from shorter length of stay in hospitals and more rapid discharge to nursing homes for rehabilitation. Of interest is that in the 1990s more residents in Japan and Iceland were receiving therapy than were residents in the United States, despite the fact that these two countries had the smallest number of residents staying for less than 30 days.

There was a low rate of physical restraint use in Denmark and Japan. The use of physical restraints has halved in the United States in the last decade. In Spain, 39.6% of residents were restrained. As all the evidence shows that restraints do more harm than good, it is extremely puzzling why nursing homes continue to use this abusive form of maltreatment. Of the five countries where social engagement was measured, only Italy had a very low level (20%). The other countries varied between 43 and 52%.

In the United States, it is now regulated that all residents have at least some form of social engagement every week.

Nursing time spent with each resident (patient) is highest in England and Wales at 155.5 minutes and lowest in Japan (84.4 minutes). In the United States, only 7.5% of the care was given by registered nurses compared to 53.2% in England and Wales. Registered nurses in Japan, Sweden, and Spain provided between 14 and 18.2% of the care.

Overall, these studies stress the differences between patient-mix and care in different countries. Asian nursing homes in Taiwan showed a moderate level of satisfaction with care, with a monotonous pace of life, inadequate privacy, and lost items being the major problems. The average Functional Index Measure (FIM) score was 49.2, which is similar to those seen in the United States in residential care facilities. 74.7% of patients had severe cognitive impairment. Physical restraint use was as high as 54%. Pressure ulcers varied from 5.3 to 12.1%. The prevalence of stool impaction was 29.4% (Yeh *et al.*, 2003). As the MDS is more widely used throughout the world, it will become possible to compare nursing homes throughout the world and to develop a gold standard for high-quality nursing homes.

Special Nursing Home Programs

Special Care (or Needs) Units have been developed in the United States to take care of persons with behavioral problems associated with dementia. These are usually locked units and have a higher staffing-to-resident ratio. Many also offer a higher level of recreational therapy. Some of these offer special programs such as pet or music therapy. Overall, studies have failed to show a major advantage of these units over general nursing home care.

Snoezelen is a multisensory therapy that provides easy-to-do activities in an enabling environment. It provides a high level of interaction. It is both stimulating and relaxing. While in some nursing homes staff have found it useful, high-quality-controlled studies of its efficacy do not exist.

The Eden Alternative is the introduction of a variety of animals to the nursing home as well as the provision of an environment where the residents can be involved in gardening. These environments can improve the home-like quality of the nursing home and encourage visits by young children. Again, however, quality studies improving efficacy do not exist.

The measurement of quality-of-care is fraught with difficulties. Fahey *et al.* (2003) compared the quality of medical care for elderly residents in nursing homes to elderly people living at home in the Bristol area. They found that in the nursing home only 74% of those persons with heart disease and 62% of those with diabetes mellitus had their blood pressure measured within the previous year.

Table 4 Example of facility quality measure/indicator report

Facility name ____________
City/State ____________
Provider number ____________
Login/Internal ID ____________

Run date ____________
Report period ____________
Comparison group ____________
Report version number ____________

		Facility				Comparison group		
Measure ID	Domain/Measure description	Num	Denom	Observed percent(%)	Adjusted percent(%)	State average(%)	National average(%)	State percentile
Chronic care measures								
	Accidents							
1.1	Incidence of new fractures	6	198	3.0	–	2.2	2.0	74
1.2	Prevalence of falls	33	215	15.3	–	15.2	13.0	55
	Behavior/emotional patterns							
2.1	Residents who have become more depressed or anxious	27	215	12.6	–	12.9	16.0	55
2.2	Prevalence of behavior symptoms affecting others: Overall	34	215	15.8	–	19.5	18.7	42
2.2-HI	Prevalence of behavior symptoms affecting others: High risk	26	115	22.6	–	23.5	21.8	51
2.2-LO	Prevalence of behavior symptoms affecting others: Low risk	8	93	8.6	–	8.2	8.0	63
2.3	Prevalence of symptoms of depression without antidepressant therapy	14	215	6.5	–	4.4	5.4	78
	Clinical management							
3.1	Use of 9 or more different medications	105	215	48.8	–	63.1	61.3	14
	Cognitive patterns							
4.1	Incidence of cognitive impairment	1	107	0.9	–	10.9	12.9	23
	Elimination/Incontinence							
5.1	Low-risk residents who lost control of their bowels or bladder	49	123	39.8	–	35.7	47.1	64
5.2	Residents who have/had a catheter inserted and left in their bladder	13	215	6.0	5.1	7.6	8.0	39
5.3	Prevalence of occasional or frequent bladder or bowel incontinence without a toileting plan	51	51	100.0	–	27.5	44.5	100[a]
5.4	Prevalence of fecal impaction	0	215	0.0	–	0.2	0.1	0
	Infection control							
6.1	Residents with a urinary tract infection	13	215	6.0	–	9.6	9.5	33
	Nutrition/Eating							
7.1	Residents who lose too much weight	36	208	17.3	–	10.0	10.9	89
7.2	Prevalence of tube feeding	26	215	12.1	–	4.7	7.2	92[a]
7.3	Prevalence of dehydration	1	215	0.5	–	0.6	0.5	74
	Pain management							
8.1	Residents who have moderate to severe pain	15	215	7.0	5.5	8.6	7.8	45
	Physical functioning							
9.1	Residents whose need for help with daily activities has increased	26	193	13.5	–	16.1	18.3	47
9.2	Residents who spend most of their time in bed or in a chair	16	215	7.4	–	3.2	5.5	92[a]
9.3	Residents whose ability to move in and around their room got worse	9	158	5.7	6.2	15.1	17.1	18
9.4	Incidence of decline in ROM	4	214	1.9	–	7.1	8.6	18
	Psychotropic drug use							
10.1	Prevalence of antipsychotic use, in the absence of psychotic or related conditions: Overall	28	188	14.9	–	22.8	21.9	21

ROM, range of motion.
Dashes represent a value that could not be computed.
[a]Above or below national average.

In contrast, in the United States, it is the expectation that blood pressure is measured monthly and in persons in Bristol living at home the rate of measurement was 96%. Only 38% of residents in nursing homes had been prescribed a β-blocker following a myocardial infarction. Nursing home residents were less likely than people living at home to have received a pneumonococcal vaccination, though the rate of nursing home vaccination was similar.

In the United States, studies using the MDS have demonstrated that residents who are incontinent are unlikely to be on a documented scheduled toileting regimen (Schnelle *et al.*, 2003). Troyer (2004) found that Medicaid residents had a slightly higher death rate than privately funded residents. Much of this difference was associated with the resident and also the market they were in. Stevenson (2005) found that consumer complaints concerning nursing homes, when made to State Survey agencies, were associated with low nurse aide staffing levels and the number of deficiencies found on the state survey. Persons who receive potentially inappropriate medications in the nursing home have a much higher chance of subsequent hospitalization or death (Lau *et al.*, 2005). Finally, it should be recognized that general practitioners who work in nursing homes will have a higher death rate in their patients than those who work only in the community, making it essential to establish a different standard for these practitioners (Mohammed *et al.*, 2004).

The big picture as given by the recounting above can be reduced to statistics for a single facility so that it can assess its quality and improve its care. Facilities in the United States can use their data as reported in the On-Line Survey Certification and Reporting (OSCAR) and the MDS Quality Indicator data to compare their facility to others in their region, state, and the nation (Table 4).

The best method to improve care is to put in place a Continuous Quality Improvement plan where data is collected and presented to the interdisciplinary team leaders and staff representatives monthly. When an unacceptable variation in the data is seen, a plan is put in place to determine the reason and to fix the problem. The same data is evaluated each month to allow the team to determine their success at fixing the problem. The differences between continuous quality improvement and old-fashioned quality assurance programs are delineated in Table 5. Areas in the nursing home that are highly amenable to continuous quality improvement programs are set out in Table 6. Examples of monitoring of data in the nursing home for prescribing and efficacy of therapies are given in Tables 7 and 8. The keys to Continuous Quality Improvement resulting in improved nursing home care are administrative buy in, team empowerment to fix the problem, and continuous collection and feedback of data.

Table 5 Comparison between quality assurance and continuous quality improvement

Quality assurance	Continuous quality improvement
Retrospective	Prospective/continuous
Lays blame	No blame
Administrator lead	Team lead
Opinion driven	Data driven
Problem focused	Customer focused
Snapshot	Continuous
Resistant to change	Seeks change

Table 6 Problems in the nursing home most amenable to quality improvement

Depression
Polypharmacy
Pressure ulcers
Undernutrition
Falls
Incontinence
Osteoporosis
Behavior problems
Lost items
Food quality
Customer satisfaction
Skin tears

Table 8 Measurement of quality in a skilled nursing facility utilizing the Functional Index Measure (FIM)

Level of function	Home	Discharge to hospital	Residential care facility
At home prior to event	106	82	106
On admission	77	55	53
At discharge	96	64	69

Table 9 The most frequent legal allegations of malpractice against nursing homes

1. Fall
2. Negligent care
3. Pressure ulcers
4. Lack of care
5. Abuse/assault
6. Dehydration/malnutrition
7. Elopement/wandering

Legal Issues in the Nursing Home

There has been a marked increase in lawsuits against nursing homes in the United States over the last 5 years. In many cases, these are frivolous and rely on the fact that the fear of large awards by a jury and the cost of litigation make the nursing home chains settle without going to court. The largest awards are made for elopement (average $860 000) and pressure ulcers (average $293 000). Table 9 lists the most frequent allegations against nursing homes.

Visualizing the Resident

Communication between all the members of the interdisciplinary team and the physician is often limited. The Geronte is a visual communication device originally developed in France. This single sheet provides a snap shot of the problems the resident has. Problem areas can be colored in by any staff member (Figure 8).

Table 7 Pharmacy quality assurance report for an academic skilled nursing facility

	Jan	Feb	Mar	Apr	May	Comparison group[a]
Routine meds(n)	9.2	9.4	9.4	9.3	9.7	9.8
PRN meds(n)	1.9	1.8	1.6	1.5	1.5	6.5
Antipsychotics(%)	11	7	5	6	4	12.2
Anxiolytics(%)	9	8	11	15	9	22.0
Sedative/hypnotics(%)	14	7	8	11	9	24.4

[a]Comparison group is to skilled nursing beds in the same city.

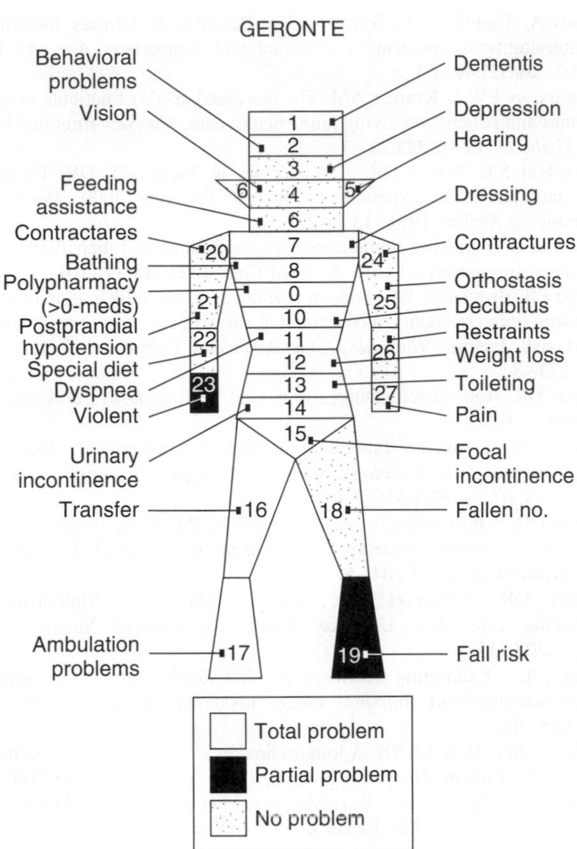

Figure 8 A visual communication device: the Geronte as used by LifeCare Centers of St. Louis and the Division of Geriatrics, Saint Louis University

KEY POINTS

- Nursing home facilities are more unique than similar.
- The Minimum Data Set provides a method to compare nursing homes worldwide.
- Nursing homes have short-stay residents who are predominantly there for rehabilitation and long-term residents who require custodial care.
- The introduction of special programs, for example, the Eden Alternative, increased involvement of physicians and Continuous Quality Improvement methods have improved quality of care in nursing homes.

KEY REFERENCES

- Doty PJ. The oldest old and the use of institutional long-term care from an international perspective. In R Suzman, DP Willis & KG Manton (eds) *The Oldest Old* 1992, pp 251–67; Oxford University Press, New York.
- Fries BE, Schroll M, Hawes C *et al.* Approaching cross-national comparisons of nursing home residents. *Age and Ageing* 1997; **26**(S2):13–8.
- Gabrel CS. An overview of nursing home facilities: data from the 1997 national nursing home survey. *Advance Data from Vital and Health Statistics* 2000; No. 311, National Center for Health Statistics, Hyattsville.
- Kavanagh S & Knapp M. The impact on general practitioners of the changing balance of care for older people living in institutions. *British Medical Journal* 1997; **315**:441–2.
- Ouslander JG & Osterweil D. Physician evaluation and management of nursing home residents. *Annals of Internal Medicine* 1994; **120**:584–92.

REFERENCES

American Nursing Association. Staff shortages hurting nursing homes the most. *The American Journal of Nursing* 1991; **91**:85–90.

Berg K, Sherwood S, Murphy K *et al.* Rehabilitation in nursing homes: a cross-national comparison of recipients. *Age and Ageing* 1997; **26**(S2):37–42.

Black D & Bowman C. Community institutional care for frail elderly people. Time to structure professional responsibility. *British Medical Journal* 1997; **315**:441–2.

Buttar A, Blaum C & Fries B. Clinical characteristics and six-month outcomes of nursing home residents with low activities of daily living dependency. *The Journals of Gerontology. Series A, Biological Sciences and Medical Sciences* 2001; **56**:M292–7.

Caudill ME & Patrick M. Costing nurse turnover in nursing homes. *Nursing Management* 1991; **22**:61–4.

Darer JD, Hwang W, Pham HH *et al.* More training needed in chronic care: a survey of US physicians. *Academic Medicine* 2004; **79**:541–8.

Donaldson LJ, Clayton DG & Clarke M. The elderly in residential care: mortality in relation to functional capacity. *Journal of Epidemiology and Community Health* 1980; **34**:96–101.

Doty PJ. The oldest old and the use of institutional long-term care from an international perspective. In R Suzman, DP Willis & KG Manton (eds) *The Oldest Old* 1992, pp 251–67; Oxford University Press, New York.

Evans JM, Chutka DS, Fleming KC *et al.* Medical care of nursing home residents. *Mayo Clinic Proceedings* 1995; **70**:694–702.

Fahey T, Montgomery AA, Barnes J & Protheroe J. Quality of care for elderly residents in nursing homes and elderly people living at home: controlled observational study. *British Medical Journal* 2003; **326**:580–3.

Fries BE, Schroll M, Hawes C *et al.* Approaching cross-national comparisons of nursing home residents. *Age and Ageing* 1997; **26**(S2):13–8.

Gabrel CS. An overview of nursing home facilities: data from the 1997 national nursing home survey. *Advance Data from Vital and Health Statistics* 2000; No. 311, National Center for Health Statistics, Hyattsville.

Guralnik JM, Simonsick EM, Ferrucci L *et al.* A short physical performance battery assessing lower extremity function: association with self-reported disability and prediction of mortality and nursing home admission. *The Journals of Gerontology. Series A, Biological Sciences and Medical Sciences* 1994; **49**:M85–94.

Haddad RY & Thomas DR. Enteral nutrition and tube feeding: a review of the evidence. *Gastroenterology Clinics of North America* 2002; **18**:867–82.

Hancock R, Antony A, Jagger C & Matthems R. The effect of older people's economic resources on care home entry under the United Kingdom's long-term care financing system. *The Journals of Gerontology. Series B, Psychological Sciences and Social Sciences* 2002; **57B**:S285–93.

Jakob A, Busse A, Riedel-Heller SG *et al.* Prevalence and incidence of dementia among nursing home residents and residents in homes for the aged in comparison to private homes. *Zeitschrift fur Gerontologie und Geriatrie* 2002; **35**:474–81.

Katz PR, Karuza J, Kolassa J & Hutson A. Medical practice with nursing home residents: results from the national physician professional activities census. *Journal of the American Geriatrics Society* 1997; **45**:911–7.

Kavanagh S & Knapp M. The impact on general practitioners of the changing balance of care for older people living in institutions. *British Medical Journal* 1997; **315**:441–2.

Kemper P & Murtaugh CM. Lifetime use of nursing home care. *The New England Journal of Medicine* 1991; **324**:595–600.

Lau DT, Kasper JD, Potter DE *et al.* Hospitalization and death associated with potentially inappropriate medication prescriptions among elderly nursing home residents. *Annals of Internal Medicine* 2005; **165**:68–74.

Levit KR, Lazenby HD, Cowan CA & Letsch SW. National health care expenditures. *Health Care Financing Review* 1991; **13**:29–54.

Ljunggren G, Phillips CD & Sgadari A. Comparisons of restraint use in nursing homes in eight countries. *Age and Ageing* 1997; **26**(S2):43–7.

Mohammed MA, Rathbone A, Myers P *et al.* An investigation into general practitioners associated with high patient mortality flagged up through the Shipman inquiry: retrospective analysis of routine data. *British Medical Journal* 2004; **328**:1474–7.

National Center for Health Statistics. *The National Nursing Home Survey* 1999.

Ouslander JG & Osterweil D. Physician evaluation and management of nursing home residents. *Annals of Internal Medicine* 1994; **120**:584–92.

Ouslander JG & Schnelle JF. Incontinence in the nursing facility. *Annals of Internal Medicine* 1995; **122**:438–49.

Rovner BW, German PS, Broadhead J *et al.* The prevalence and management of dementia and other psychiatric disorders in nursing homes. *International Psychogeriatrics / IPA* 1990; **2**:13–24.

Rubenstein LZ, Josephson KR & Robbins AS. Falls in the nursing home. *Annals of Internal Medicine* 1994; **121**:442–51.

Schnelle JF, Cadogan MP, Yoshii J *et al.* The minimum data set urinary incontinence quality indicators: do they reflect differences in care processes related to incontinence? *Medical Care* 2003; **41**:909–22.

Schols JMGA, Crebolder HFJM & van Weel C. Nursing home and nursing home physician: the Dutch experience. *Journal of the American Medical Directors Association* 2004; **5**:207–12.

Schroll M, Jonsson PV, Mor V *et al.* An international study of social engagement among nursing home residents. *Age and Ageing* 1997; **26**(S2):55–9.

Sgadari A, Topinkova E, Bjornson J & Bernabei R. Urinary incontinence in nursing home residents: a cross-national comparison. *Age and Ageing* 1997; **26**(S2):49–54.

Shaughnessy PW & Kramer AM. The increased needs of patients in nursing homes and patients receiving home health care. *The New England Journal of Medicine* 1990; **322**:21–7.

Sonnenfeld ST, Waldo DR, Lemieux JA & McKusick DR. Projections of national health expenditures through the year 2000. *Health Care Financing Review* 1991; **13**:1–27.

Stevenson DG. Nursing home consumer complaints and their potential role in assessing quality of care. *Medical Care* 2005; **43**:99–101.

Thappa PB, Brockman KG, Gideon P *et al.* Injurious falls in nonambulatory nursing home residents: a comparative study of circumstances, incidence, and risk factors. *Journal of the American Geriatrics Society* 1996; **44**:273–8.

Thomas DR. Age-related changes in wound healing. *Drugs & Aging* 2001; **18**:607–20.

Thomas DR. Focus on functional decline in hospitalized older adults. *The Journals of Gerontology. Series A, Biological Sciences and Medical Sciences* 2002a; **57A**:M567–8.

Thomas DR. Who's going to cause me trouble? Predicting behavioral disturbances in demented patients. *Journal of the American Medical Directors Association* 2002b; **3**:204–5.

Thomas DR, Zdrowski CD, Wilson MM *et al.* Malnutrition in subacute care. *The American Journal of Clinical Nutrition* 2002; **75**(2):308–13.

Troyer JL. Examining differences in death rates for medicaid and non-medicaid nursing home residents. *Medical Care* 2004; **42**:985–91.

Yeh S-H, Lin L-W & Lo SK. A longitudinal evaluation of nursing home care quality in Taiwan. *Journal of Nursing Care Quality* 2003; **18**:209–16.

Zedlewski SR, Barnes RO, Burt MK *et al.* *The Needs of the Elderly in the 21st Century* 1989; The Urban Institute, Washington.

Clinical Audit of Health Care

Jonathan M. Potter *and* **Michael G. Pearson**
Royal College of Physicians, London, UK

"The time has come for everyone in the NHS to take clinical audit very seriously"
Dame Deirdre Hine, Chair, Commission for Health Improvement
Sir Michael Rawlins, Chairman, National Institute for Clinical Excellence

Principles for best practice in clinical audit (NICE, 2002a)

DEFINITION

Clinical audit is a tool for improving the quality of care. A more detailed definition endorsed by the National Institute of Clinical Excellence (NICE) (NICE, 2002a) is as follows:

"a quality improvement process that seeks to improve patient care and outcomes through systematic review of care against explicit criteria and the implementation of change. Aspects of the structure, process and outcomes of care are selected and systematically evaluated against explicit criteria. Where indicated, changes are implemented at an individual, team or service level and further monitoring is used to confirm improvement in healthcare delivery."

The following chapter will expand on the components of this definition.

BACKGROUND

The concepts of measuring the outcome of clinical care are not new. Florence Nightingale recognized that some patients did better than others and worked out that ward hygiene mattered. But a combination of disinterest and sometimes outright resistance to criticism has prevented progress until quite recently. Ernest Codman, a surgeon in the eastern United States, suggested in 1917 that outcomes of surgery should be measured and went further to suggest that lay people could take part in the assessments. When his data pointed to colleagues functioning less well than others, he was excluded from the New England Medical Association. Professor Avedis Donabedian introduced the modern era of a more rigorous approach to improving quality in health care with his seminal works in the 1960s–1980s (Donabedian, 1966, 1988). He developed the concept of measuring structure (what is needed to provide a good service), process (what is done to provide a good service) and outcome (what is expected of a good service) as key elements to evaluating quality of care.

The 1980s saw the realization that health-care demands were in danger of exceeding the national capacity to supply. Resource management, including an important role for audit (Department of Health and Social Services. NHS Management Enquiry team, 1983), examined service function and costs. The Royal Colleges were promoting medical audit as part of good professional practice (Royal College of Physicians, 1989). As time passed, medical audit became clinical audit, recognizing that care is a multidisciplinary process, but audit remained a local activity with modest impact on the service. In the 1990s the National Health Service (NHS) commissioned a series of projects to devise clinical indicators of good practice. These were developed and published by the National Centre for Health Outcomes Development (NCHOD), for example, on urinary incontinence (Brocklehurst *et al.*, 1999) and fractured proximal femur (Fairbank *et al.*, 1999). Despite much endeavor, the outcomes of these activities were very limited and there was no coordination of them and no system for ensuring that action would follow if deficiencies were found.

In 1997, the new Government introduced a sea change in the role of quality management in the NHS with the White Papers *The new NHS; modern and dependable* (Department of Health, 1997) and *A first-class service: quality in the new NHS* (Department of Health, 1998). Quality of care was no longer to be the preserve of individual professionalism but became a matter of management responsibility. The Government sought to improve quality health care by:

- Continual improvement in the overall standards of clinical care

Principles and Practice of Geriatric Medicine, 4th Edition. Edited by M.S. John Pathy, Alan J. Sinclair and John E. Morley.

Table 1 National developments to implement the quality agenda in health care

Setting standards
• National Institute of Clinical Excellence (NICE)
• National Service Frameworks (NSFs)
• National Clinical Governance Support Team (NCGST)
Delivering improvements in care
• Modernization Agency
• National Information Strategy
Monitoring standards
• Commission for Health Improvement (CHI)
• Performance Frameworks
• Patient Councils

- Reducing unacceptable variations in clinical practice
- The best use of resources so that patients receive the greatest benefit

These aims were to be achieved by:

- Setting, delivering, and monitoring quality standards
- Making quality of care a management responsibility rather than just a professional commitment.

To execute these changes the Government established bodies and programs as indicated in Table 1.

In an unrelated move the Department of Health also commissioned a series of National Sentinel Audits, of which audits for stroke (Rudd *et al.*, 1999) and evidence-based prescribing in older people (Batty *et al.*, 2004) were the most successful.

In the United Kingdom, a series of high profile incidents and consequent inquiries (Department of Health, 2001; Shipman, 2003) have made the concept of clinical governance, that is, effective regulation, a nationally important issue. Without a measurement of care quality, it is hard if not impossible to assess whether the nationally produced and evidence-based guidelines commissioned by NICE are being implemented. And nor can those charged with assessing or inspecting services reach objective conclusions without reliable and robust quality measures. Clinical audit is thus a national necessity and not an option.

HOW EFFECTIVE IS CLINICAL AUDIT?

With the national commitment to evidence-based medicine, guidelines, and audit, what is the evidence that audit can alter practice? In primary care, several clinical effectiveness programs have indicated significant changes in practice amongst general practitioners (Cranney *et al.*, 1999; Feder *et al.*, 1995). A systematic review of audit and feedback in improving immunization rates demonstrated a −4 to +49% improvement in rates and the conclusion that in clinical practice audit and feedback were well worthwhile (Bordley *et al.*, 2000). Lim and Harrison (1992) showed that audit improved care markedly at 1 month but by 6 months the effect had worn off completely. In a systematic review of 85 studies, Jamtvedt *et al.* have found that audit with feedback resulted in changes ranging from 9% decrease in compliance with prescribed practice to a 71% increase in compliance (Jamtvedt *et al.*, 2004). The factor that was most associated with improvement was baseline degree of noncompliance. They conclude that audit and feedback can be effective in improving professional practice; however, the effects are generally small to moderate. Johnston *et al.* reviewed the barriers and facilitating factors for effective clinical audit (Johnston *et al.*, 2000). They found that audit was a valuable tool for improving care. Barriers and facilitating factors that have been identified are shown in Table 2.

Table 2 Barriers and facilitating factors to the success of clinical audit

Facilitating factors
Practical mechanisms for making data collection easy
Modern medical record systems
Information technology linking routine data collection to audit
Dedicated staff
Protected time
Supportive organizational environment
Sound leadership
Monitoring of the effectiveness of the audit program
Barriers
Lack of resources
Lack of expertise in project design or analysis
Small sample size
Incomplete data collection
Lack of coordinated plan for audit
Organizational impediments.
Lack of implementation mechanism
Inadequate management buy-in.

The reviews indicate that, after 40 years of medical and clinical audit, the secrets of success in improving the quality of care are still elusive. Results from recent well constructed national audits – including the National Sentinel Audit of Stroke and the Myocardial Infarction National Audit Programme (MINAP) – which have addressed the issues raised in Table 2 – do indicate that improvements in service can be achieved (Rudd *et al.*, 2001; Birkhead *et al.*, 2004). There are several additional factors to those in Table 2 that have contributed to their success including very careful piloting to ensure that data collection is reliable and repeatable, that analysis includes appropriate interpretation from a multidisciplinary group, and that feedback is rapid, that is, while staff are still in the same posts. Conclusions must have credibility with those who have to implement them. The following sections discuss some of the factors necessary to achieve credible outputs.

THE AUDIT CYCLE

Critical phases of the audit cycle (Pruce and Aggarwal, 2000) are shown in Figure 1.

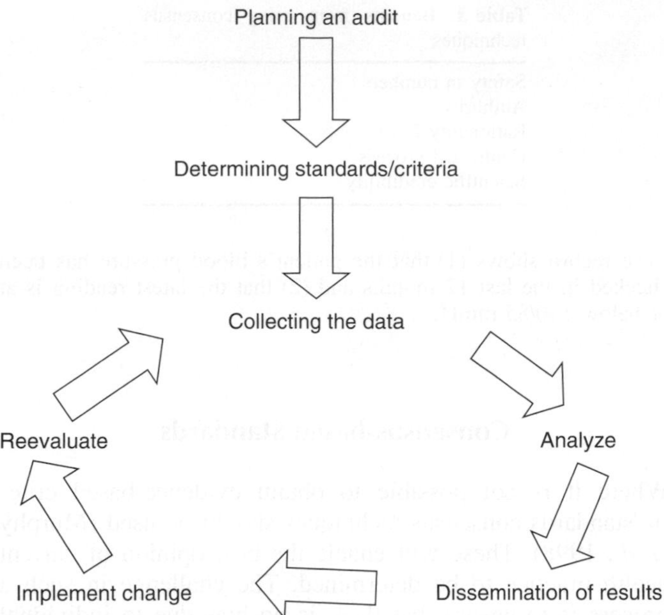

Figure 1 The audit cycle

PLANNING AN AUDIT

Identifying What is to be Reviewed

Any topic is suitable for audit. Pragmatically, it is sensible to focus on topics where there is a perceived inadequacy or variation in patient care or service provision. It is worth considering issues where there is a national priority to improve care, such as topics related to National Service Frameworks (NSFs) or the inspection criteria of the Healthcare Commission. Professionals with specialized areas of interest may wish to perform an audit of local practice. Results might be used as part of the clinical governance mechanism to explore aspects of care where there are concerns over the quality of care or where there have been significant numbers of complaints. A more powerful audit model is to perform the same audit in a number of sites and to use the combined data as a "benchmark" so that local performance can be assessed against the standards being achieved by one's peers elsewhere in the country.

Commitment to Audit

The recommendations of the Bristol Inquiry (Learning from Bristol: the Report of the Public Inquiry into Children's Heart Surgery at the Bristol Royal Infirmary 1984–1995) (Department of Health, 2001) emphasized the importance of clinical audit within the system of local monitoring of performance and the need for trusts to fully support such activity – including access to time, facilities, advice and expertise. These recommendations, welcomed by the government, echo the findings of systematic review, that clinical audit will only be successful if it is adequately resourced and it becomes part of routine practice. Commitment is not just a clinical matter. It is essential that health-care organizations as a whole seriously embrace these recommendations so that when results are available clinicians and managers are both willing to respond and jointly plan appropriate changes.

The planning phases need to look ahead to how the conclusions will be used. This ranges from the need to include variables that allow for useful interpretation of the results as well as quality consideration to ensure the results are valid and reliable. The huge potential of audit for improving care can only be realized if the outcomes of each study are accepted as valid by all parties and thus utilized as the basis for reviewing and adapting practice.

Skills for Carrying out Audit

The infrastructure required includes access to skilled personnel (with dedicated time for the project) to carry out the work and systems to facilitate audit. Expertise is required in establishing a sound methodology for the work (see the following text) including an understanding of such issues as the size of population required for study, identifying relevant data for collection, reliability and feasibility of data collection, data analysis, data presentation and implementation of change. A multidisciplinary team is required that can effectively plan, carry out and disseminate the results of audit work (Grant *et al.*, 2002). Even apparently simple tasks such as setting out a questionnaire are in practice quite difficult. Poorly phrased or ambiguous questions result in uninterpretable data. Therefore, most projects should be performed by nonclinical staff with experience and expertise both in the technical aspects and in project management. They need support from professional health-care workers to ensure the clinical acceptability and credibility and hence the validity of the study. If at all possible, there should be a wider steering group that is multidisciplinary and includes lay representation.

Modern audit has been made possible by the widespread availability of computing systems. They include software that can facilitate data collection, code and encrypt patient identifiable data and do sophisticated analysis – but they are not a substitute for the human skills and experience referred to in the preceding section.

Patient and User Input

Health services exist to serve the public and any assessment of care quality should include patient and users as full partners in the assessment process. Feedback from service users may shed a useful light on where services are inadequate, and also on the users' perspective of what is important as opposed to the views of management and professionals. Kelson (1999) has provided useful advice as to how user involvement can be achieved.

DETERMINING STANDARDS/CRITERIA

Explicit standards or criteria of best practice must be established against which to audit. While various definitions exist for a "criterion" and a "standard" in the context of audit, whichever term or definition is used, the important step is to establish a statement or statements of the level of practice against which health care is to be assessed.

There are two approaches (1) define a gold standard criterion and assess against that absolute target or (2) collect comparative data and assess relative performance against the benchmark created by what one's peers are doing. In theory, the gold standard is preferred but often the evidence needed to set that standard is lacking. Furthermore, gold standards can rarely command 100% compliance, for example, the top level aim for Chronic Obstructive Pulmonary Disease (COPD) might be 100% of patients have spirometry but the practical criterion might be set at 95% to allow for those who cannot do the procedure, who decline or who miss appointments. Similarly, the NSF target for thrombolysis is set at 75% meeting the "door to needle" target to allow for those who, for example, were not diagnosed until 12 hours after the infarct.

Evidence-based Standards

Where possible, such statements of best practice should be derived from evidence-based research. The methods used by such bodies as the Cochrane Collaboration (Cochrane, 2004), the Scottish Intercollegiate Guideline Network (SIGN) (SIGN, 2004) and the National Institute for Clinical Excellence (NICE, 2004a) all ensure a high degree of credibility in the recommendations derived. The process calls for careful attention to literature searching, critical appraisal and peer review. From such recommendations evidence-based audit standards/criteria can be determined.

Example: The NICE Clinical Guideline on "Chronic Obstructive Pulmonary Disease" (COPD) (NICE, 2004b) has as an evidence-based recommendation that "The presence of airflow obstruction should be confirmed by performing spirometry. All health professionals managing patients with COPD should have access to spirometry and be competent in the interpretation of the results".

The audit criterion proposed to complement the recommendation is:

"Percentage of patients with a diagnosis of COPD who have had spirometry performed."

Criteria may be derived from authoritative guidance such as the NSFs. For example, the NSF for Coronary Heart Disease has as a milestone:

"By April 2003 every practice should have clinical audit data no more than 12 months old available that describe: advice and treatment to maintain blood pressure below 140/85".

The NICE commissioned "Audit of the management of post-MI patients in primary care" (NICE, 2002b) included an audit review criterion:

"The record shows (1) that the patient's blood pressure has been checked in the last 12 months and (2) that the latest reading is at or below 140/85 mmHg".

Table 3 Benefits from using consensus techniques

Safety in numbers
Authority
Rationality
Controlled process
Scientific credibility

Consensus-based Standards

Where it is not possible to obtain evidence-based criteria/standards consensus techniques should be used (Murphy *et al.*, 1998). These will enable the best opinion of current health practice to be determined. The challenge in such a process is to ensure that there is no bias due to individual personalities or professions and to ensure that the views of all interested parties are included. Benefits of such approaches are shown in Table 3.

Approaches include the following:

Consensus panels: the use of panels who receive expert advice and representation and who then formulate a statement of best practice.

Nominal group techniques: relevant parties are brought together to discuss recommendations. Chairing has to be skilled to ensure that all view points are heard and to ensure that a full range of options are considered. Voting is in a blinded fashion so that personal views are expressed.

Delphi exercises: postal questionnaires are sent to a large range of individuals with a relevant interest. Statements of practice are proposed and voted on. Recommendations are refined and recirculated so that the recommendations move toward a consensus of the views of the group.

Selection of Gold Standard

In practical terms, health-care settings will need to determine what aspect of care they wish to audit. They will then need to seek the most appropriate standard(s) against which to audit that has the authority of being derived from one of the approaches above. Such standards may be derived from published guidelines, a NSF or a professional organization (Royal College of Physicians, 2004).

Types of Criteria/Standards Used

The Donabedian principle of measuring structure, process and outcome remains the basis for selecting the type of audit standards/criteria.

1. *Structure*: Measures of the facilities and resources available to a health-care setting will reflect the potential to provide high-quality care. It is difficult for staff to provide a high-quality service unless they have the resources to do it. Equally, it has to be recognized that high-class care is not guaranteed in premium facilities. Facilities have to be matched with staff who are provided with training and the expertise to carry out the appropriate care.

Example: For coronary heart disease, if a hospital does not have access to immediate coronary angiography it is not possible to provide the highest quality care for people with acute coronary syndromes.

Measures of "structure" can include facilities, staffing levels, skill mix, access to training, standard use of protocols, mechanisms for advice and information for patients and relatives.

Data relating to "structure" are the easiest of the audit measures to obtain. Such data form the basis of accreditation schemes and systems of this type are widely used internationally and in some parts of the United Kingdom as an indication of service quality.

2. *Process*: Audit criteria/standards of "process" explicitly define key aspects of care that should be provided if high-quality care is to be achieved. Aspects of process measured may include the history, examination, investigation, treatment, and follow-up care. The process may also include the involvement of carers. Processes of care need to be clearly defined to ensure reliable comparison between different sites and different data collection episodes.

Example: In stroke care, a swallow assessment is important as a process. The audit has to define what constitutes an appropriate swallow assessment and what detail within the records reliably reflect what was carried out.

Process data may be collected retrospectively by reviewing a selected number of cases. Such an approach has significant problems in ensuring that there is no selection bias in the notes that are retrieved. A planned retrospective audit such as the National Sentinel Audit of Stroke (assessing the care of 40 *consecutive* stroke patients in all hospitals in England, Wales and Northern Ireland) reduces the risk of bias. A more ideal, but organizationally more challenging approach, is to obtain prospective data with data collection part of routine practice as in the MINAP (Birkhead *et al.*, 2004).

In practice, measurement of process provides a useful reflection of whether care matches up with expected best practice. Data related to process can be more difficult to retrieve than measures of structure but tend to be easier to collect than outcome measures and have the added benefit that they are not dependent on case mix.

Structure, process and outcome are all interrelated. Data from the National Stroke audit has demonstrated that settings where good structures are in place presage better processes of care and lead to better outcomes. It is rarely apparent, however, at the outset, which will be the most sensitive measures. Increasing clinical audit experience will help provide an indication of the structures and processes that are important in determining high-quality care.

There are problems, however (Lilford *et al.*, 2004). If specific processes are identified as the markers for quality, departments and services wishing to be seen to provide high-quality care may concentrate purely on the selected process to the detriment of overall care.

3. *Outcome*: Ideally, the quality of health care should be evaluated by the outcomes it achieves.

Example: For urinary incontinence, does appropriate assessment and treatment of patients result in a reduction in the prevalence of incontinence? (Brocklehurst *et al.*, 1999)

Outcomes may be recorded as outcome "measures", for example, prevalence of a condition or death at 30 days or as an outcome "indicator", for example, percentage of asthma patients given a steroid inhaler on discharge. The latter is a process proxy that is linked to risk of readmission (Slack and Bucknall, 1997) but is not in itself an outcome.

Outcome "measures" can be difficult to utilize. Consideration needs to be given as to whether an outcome "measure" is a true measure or a surrogate measure. For the treatment of osteoporosis, reduced fracture rate is more important than increased bone density, although the latter is easier to measure. Terms must be clearly defined to permit comparative audit. For example, the number of people with incontinence (numerator) in a given population (the denominator) is difficult to determine. It is difficult to clearly define comparable denominator populations within which the prevalence of incontinence is to be measured. Case mix must be allowed for in comparing practice between settings. One setting may have a high proportion of older people in whom an increased level of morbidity, for example, incontinence, would be expected. Comparison with a setting containing a younger population would require case mix adjustment. A precise definition of incontinence will be required to allow comparative data collection. When the frequency of the outcome measure is very low, for example, death at 3 months after hip fracture – the large number of cases needed to be studied renders the outcome measure impractical.

Outcome "indicators" provide an alternative to outcome "measures" and have the potential advantage of being (1) measurable and (2) having face validity for those involved in treatment, that is, it is not surprising that giving out an effective therapy works. While it is important to determine whether outcome measures can be used, in practice it may be more pragmatic to use outcome indicators.

Whether "measures" or "indicators" are used, it is important to be clear from whose perspective the outcome is being considered; is it that of the professionals, the management, the patients, or the carers? For stroke, professionals may seek the best neurological recovery, the patient may seek the best functional recovery, and the management may seek the most cost-effective recovery, all of which will be measured in different ways.

For these various reasons, league tables relying on outcome measures have generated some bizarrely anomalous results and are mistrusted. One District General Hospital which was a beacon site for Stroke care had a very high stroke death rate (Hospital SMR was approximately 120) but the district SMR was only 94. As a beacon site, the hospital was keeping all patients with transient ischemic attacks and mild strokes out of hospital or in intermediate care facilities – thus the hospital SMR was based upon a different population compared with other hospitals. If public scrutiny of outcome measures is to occur, great care will be required to adjust for the potential confounding factors (Lilford *et al.*, 2004).

COLLECTING THE DATA

Important considerations in collecting data are shown in Table 4.

Defining Terms

Consistency in data collection requires accurate definition of terms. In stroke audit, patients should be managed in a stroke unit. How is a stroke unit defined? Answers to audit questions may not be straightforward. Patients with stroke should have a CT scan, however, if moribund it may not be appropriate. In collecting data a "No but..." option will allow for such specific exclusions. The appropriate data to collect from notes may not be clear. If a blood pressure measurement is required during a hospital stay, is it the first recorded measure, the mean, or a measure at some specific time point that is required? How does the data collector deal with a comment such as "Blood pressure normal" rather than a specific measure.

It is essential that these issues are clearly addressed or there will be considerable variability in the audit data collected from different sites and between different auditors. Advice sheets or books addressing these issues are extremely helpful to audit teams and should, where possible, be backed up with recourse to the audit developer to clarify specific issues if necessary. The development of standardized or national data sets are also helpful as they establish key data to be collected and identify the problems that may arise in data collection.

Table 4 Considerations with regard to clinical audit data collection

Define terms	
Define population to be studied	Numerator
Define reference population	Denominator
Case mix adjustment	
Define sample size	
Define sampling strategy	
Define data source	
Define data analysis	
Confidentiality	
Data Protection	
Pilot	
• reliability	
• validity	
• acceptability	

Defining Populations

Outcome measures are often expressed as prevalence rates. Good health care for urinary incontinence should reduce the prevalence of incontinence. How is the population with urinary incontinence to be measured (the numerator)? Is this the population within a ward, a hospital, a general practice list, a Primary Care Trust? Is the prevalence to be determined per 1000 population, per number entering a service or on a GP list (the denominator)? In making comparisons with other health-care settings it will be important that both the numerator and denominator are comparable. Again, clear advice to the auditing team from the audit developer is essential.

Case Mix Adjustment

Comparisons between settings will require case mix adjustment. When planning a project, the ways in which data will be presented, and to whom, should suggest what objections are likely to be raised to the results. Usually, these will be because a particular confounding factor has not been considered. Adding the appropriate extra variables increases the work of the project but ensures that the results/comparisons are accepted as valid. For urinary incontinence when comparing between care in different nursing homes, it will be important to be aware of the physical dependency and cognitive function of people whose care is being assessed. Differences in the numbers of people with dementia and with relevant physical disability such as stroke, will have an important impact on the prevalence and management of continence. There are many potential factors to take into consideration in case mix adjustment. In practical terms, it is sensible to collect only case mix data that are relevant to the planned presentation and use of the data.

Sampling

The sample size must be determined to ensure that meaningful results are obtained. Numbers will vary according to the measure being audited. These are statistical considerations that will not be described in detail but intended to ensure that the results of a project are robust enough to justify changing care practice and are not simply chance findings. In the National Sentinel Audit of Stroke, 40 case notes are retrospectively reviewed. If analyzed alone, it would be hard to reach many conclusions but when compared with 8000 cases from other hospitals, the statistical power is greatly increased. For outcome measures, a power calculation is required depending on the degree of change expected. If the desire is to see whether the management of osteoporosis is satisfactory using fractured femur as an outcome measure, many thousands of cases will need to be studied. If the outcome measure is the appropriate prescribing of bisphosphonates to prevent osteoporosis, meaningful results can be obtained with small numbers of subjects and can be achieved within hospital departments or general practices.

It may not be possible or practical to obtain all records and some method of randomization may be required. This may be achieved by collecting all cases over a limited period of time – or by the use of random numbers. Care must be taken to ensure that all randomly identified cases are obtained so that no systematic bias influences the findings. It may, for example, prove difficult to obtain notes when a person has died. Exclusion of such patients may have an important bearing on the evaluation of quality of care.

Data Source

Data are usually obtained from patient records. The difficulty in obtaining reliable data retrospectively from patient records is familiar to most health-care professionals. Unless there has been a predetermined data set incorporated into the records systems, there will be inherent difficulties in obtaining reliable data. The problem is more likely to arise with retrospective data collection. Processes and outcomes of care may occur without being recorded. The data required may not be readily accessible. Different departments and practices use different data record systems.

In order to increase the likelihood of reliable data collection, it is better to limit the numbers of items to be collected and to give careful consideration to what is most reliably available in the record systems to be reviewed.

For the future, standardized data collection systems in routine practice, for example, standardized admission clerking sheets, will simplify data collection. Furthermore, the goal should be to incorporate required audit data items into routine collection so that prospective real-time audit data collection becomes possible.

Consent and Confidentiality

Issues of consent and confidentiality are complex. The General Medical Council makes it very clear that patients have a right to have their medical data handled confidentially but also makes it clear that doctors must keep good records and should actively evaluate the services they deliver.

The Data Protection Act in the United Kingdom and parallel European legislation provide important safeguards to individuals to ensure that any data (paper or electronic) held on them is handled in a responsible manner that reflect their wishes. Local audit, that is, the evaluation of care quality within the clinician team is therefore part of direct medical care and does not require specific patient consent. Many patients have care from different parts of the health-care system, for example, diagnosis of a tumor in a district hospital followed by referral to a tertiary center for radiotherapy. Within cancer networks both secondary and tertiary units form part of the cancer team, such that when evaluating the effectiveness of care both parts are important. The concept of the "domain of care" is more useful than simply considering the institution. A guidance document (Information Commissioner, 2001) from the UK information commissioner has described the issues posed by the Data Protection Act and supports the above approach. It also identifies that the analysis of clinical care quality includes both clinical issues (process and outcome) and administrative issues (how the service was delivered). However, while it is permissible to collect data from the records of identified individuals, it is not permissible to identify those individuals in any of the resulting reports or analyses without the specific consent of that individual.

However, an important feature in the Data Protection Legislation is that patients receiving care should be made aware of how their data are to be used. It has not been routine practice in the United Kingdom to provide information leaflets for patients but it is likely to be so in future. If an individual wishes to "opt out" of allowing their data to be used, they have the right to be removed from the system.

Many audit studies would like to combine data from more than 1 unit and thus require local units to submit data to a central analysis system. This can only be done under three very specific conditions

- If the locally collected data are fully anonymized, that is, all identifiers such as name, date of birth, post code, are removed then the data may be transmitted to a center to be aggregated and analyzed.
- If some of the identifiers are retained within the data but encrypted or "pseudonymized" in such a way that no one in the central team can "read" the original, then the data are treated as "effectively anonymized". This may be useful if it is required at a later stage to link the data on an individual across more than one database – an activity that can be performed within the machines via the encrypted identifiers, and without needing central staff to break the code.
- If specific consent has been obtained from each patient to permit the transmission and use of their data.

Each local organization within the health service has an individual – the Caldicott guardian – responsible for monitoring how personal data are handled and shared and anyone setting up an audit that requires for data to be shared beyond the "clinical domain" should check with that local person to ensure that all necessary precautions have been taken.

Those collecting data must also consider other aspects of confidentiality such as the need to store data files in a secure filing cabinet or on a secure computer, and that data protection duties extend not only to the rights of the patient but also the rights of the clinicians delivering the services.

Pilot

It is essential to pilot an audit project. This will indicate whether the data required can be reliably obtained. It will provide an opportunity for testing interrater reliability of data by asking more than one person to collect similar data. The acceptability of the audit can be assessed. Are the number of items to be collected reasonable, can they be readily found from the records, is there sufficient time to collect the required data, do the collection staff have the expertise to interpret the records in the notes? The validity of the audit can be checked to see whether the pilot results obtained represent a reasonable reflection of practice.

DISSEMINATION AND CHANGE

Clinical audit can only be justified if, when deficiencies are found, there is a mechanism for stimulating change to improve future care. But change is notoriously difficult within NHS systems. The size and complexity of NHS systems are a problem and so too is the lack of clear lines of responsibility. Much research has centered on the mechanisms that can facilitate alterations in clinical practice (Johnston *et al.*, 2000) and some key factors are outlined in Table 5. Unless these factors are addressed at the outset, it is unlikely that improvements in practice, and hence the benefit of audit, will be realized.

Commitment

The clinical team may accept the findings of an audit but be unable to improve care because they do not have the authority to alter the budget or personnel configuration appropriately. Change requires the active cooperation of both clinical team and management. Each audit project should therefore plan how to ensure that the results will have sufficient credibility (data reliability, numbers, case mix control) and that clinicians will embark on the discussions needed to create change. And the planning must also consider whether the right data are being collected that will convince local management that change is needed. Good planning should ensure that the audit topic is considered important and that the aims are shared by all parts of the organization before the data collection even begins.

Identifying the Cause of Problems

Where results of the audit diverge from accepted best practice, the reasons need to be investigated. A simple rule is "investigate before you castigate". It is important not to presume that the divergence is the "fault" of individuals or their morale could be unnecessarily sapped. Good staff may be handicapped by inadequate organization or poor facilities and resources available for service delivery. Or the problem may relate to poor or outdated clinical practice. Once a cause has been identified, an action plan can be drawn up to address the problems.

Table 5 Factors associated with facilitating practice change

Strong commitment to the project
- From management
- From clinicians

Identifying what the problems are
Using effective educational techniques

Educational Methods

Current evidence suggests that there is considerable variation in the effectiveness of differing educational methods. Most recent systematic reviews indicate that multifaceted intervention is not necessarily needed so long as one of the more successful targeted approaches is used. Details of the effectiveness of differing interventions are shown in Table 6.

Simple feedback of results may not be enough. In the National Sentinel Audit of Evidence Based Prescribing, change depended on the activities of local working groups. Within the overall project's 150 centers there was no overall improvement – but in one center there was significant change. This center adopted an active and multifaceted approach and showed what might have been more widely possible (Batty *et al.*, 2001). In contrast, the National Sentinel Audit of Stroke incorporated active regional feedback of data to multidisciplinary teams of clinicians and managers and demonstrated significant changes between audit cycles (Rudd *et al.*, 2001).

Sharing of Data

Access to audit data has become an increasingly important issue. "Medical" and "clinical" audit were both, in origin,

Table 6 Effectiveness of differing educational interventions on clinical practice

Effective
- Educational outreach visits (Thomson O'Brien *et al.*, 2004a)
- Reminders (manual or computerized)
- Multifaceted interventions (including two or more of the following: audit and feedback, reminders, local consensus processes, marketing)
- Local opinion leaders (Thomson O'Brien *et al.*, 2004b)
- Local consensus processes (inclusion of participating practitioners in discussions to ensure they agree that the chosen clinical problem is important and the approach to managing the problem appropriate)
- Patient-mediated intervention (any intervention aimed at changing the performance of health-care professionals for which specific information was sought from or given to patients)

Ineffective
- Educational material (distribution of recommendations for clinical care, including clinical practice guidelines and electronic publications)
- Didactic educational meetings, for example, lectures (Davis *et al.*, 1999).

Source: Adapted from Pruce D, Aggarwal R. National Clinical Audit – a handbook for good practice (Pruce and Aggarwal, 2000).

a professional process for improving the quality of care. With the advent of clinical governance derived from the NHS White Paper *The new NHS: modern and dependable* (Department of Health, 1997), audit has become very much part of the management process. Clinical data is increasingly required and used in monitoring the quality of services provided and the individual performance of clinicians. Audit data from multicenter projects are now made available at local Hospital and Primary Trust level, to strategic health authorities and nationally to the Department of Health and to regulators such as the Healthcare Commission. It may be better to consider multicenter audit not just as an assessment of local quality against a benchmark, but as a form of clinical performance management.

Information should also, whenever possible, be shared with the public. Results need to be presented in a manner that is understandable and will not include all the details of interest to clinicians. Such data may well in future be included in legal arguments over services and fitness to practice.

While this more open use of data is inevitable and will help drive the benefits of audit, it challenges those performing the audit process (managers and clinicians alike) to ensure that audit data are a true and fair reflection of the service and practice under review.

REAUDIT AND SUSTAINING IMPROVEMENT

Reaudit must be carried out to "close the loop" and assess whether changes in service have resulted in improvement and to ensure that improvements are maintained.

Ideally, with audit data incorporated within routine data collection, prospective monitoring of performance can be maintained. Where recurrent "snap shot" audits are required, it can be challenging for services to keep coming back to the audit of one particular subject.

In general practice, several clinical effectiveness programs have been developed which have achieved recurrent audit with sustained improvements in practice for example, the Primary Care Clinical Effectiveness (PRICCE) project (Bandolier, 2005). The essence of these programs has now been incorporated into the new general practice contract requiring general practitioners to achieve quality standards.

While the primary care experience is linked in part to financial benefits which would be difficult to replicate in the secondary care setting, the apparent success of these programs would suggest that a lesson could be learnt which might be applied to the secondary care system.

CONCLUSION

There is good evidence that clinical audit performed well can identify substandard care, can stimulate changes that improve care, and can confirm sustained improvement. Although the principles have been known for many years, audit has not been taken seriously by the professions and the health service has invested very little in quality of care assessments.

The advent of computing makes data collection relatively easy in every clinical setting and as electronic patient records are introduced in the next decade, so the opportunities will mushroom. Clinicians need to take the opportunities that now exist to contribute to well-designed and targeted clinical audit programs. Subjects should be chosen which are of priority importance locally and nationally and where there is evidence that current practice is suboptimal. Clinicians should get involved with the intention of seeking sustained improvements in the service they provide. All clinicians should seek to ensure that their job specification includes time for audit, and this should be seen as a duty and not an optional extra. Health-care management needs to be committed wholeheartedly to the process. The commitment must firstly be to providing the infrastructure in terms of well-established audit departments whose strategy is an integral part of the Trust strategy. There should be investment in systems for simplifying data recording and retrieval and there should be a commitment to routine audit data collection. Management also needs to demonstrate willingness to review and improve facilities, resources and staffing if such is required to improve services. Success breeds success. The realization that audit can induce change and improvement would strongly encourage commitment to the process.

KEY POINTS

- The time has come for everyone in the NHS to take clinical audit very seriously.
- Personnel, resources and information technology for audit must be built into organizational structures.
- Audit data collection must become part of routine clinical data collection.
- Managerial and clinical commitment to changes in practice to enhance care is a prerequisite for audit to be beneficial.
- Increasing public scrutiny of audit results places a responsibility on managers and clinicians to ensure the validity of data.

KEY REFERENCES

- Batty GM, Grant RL, Aggarwal R *et al.* National clinical sentinel audit of evidence-based prescribing. *Journal of Evaluation in Clinical Practice* 2004; **10**:273–9.
- Department of Health. *A First Class Service: Quality in the New NHS* 1998; HMSO, London.
- Donabedian A. The quality of care. How can it be assessed? *The Journal of the American Medical Association* 1988; **260**:1743–8.
- NICE. *Principles for Best Practice in Clinical Audit* 2002a; Radcliffe Medical Press, Oxford.
- Rudd AG, Lowe D, Irwin P *et al.* National stroke audit: a tool for change? *Quality in Health Care* 2001; **10**:141–51.

REFERENCES

Bandolier. 2005, PRICCE project, http://www.jr2.ox.ac.uk/bandolier/ImpAct/imp01/EASTKENT.html.

Batty GM, Grant RL, Aggarwal R *et al.* National clinical sentinel audit of evidence-based prescribing. *Journal of Evaluation in Clinical Practice* 2004; **10**:273–9.

Batty GM, Husk J, Swan J & Grant R. What it takes to change prescribing. *Age and Ageing* 2001; **30**:79.

Birkhead JS, Pearson M, Weston C *et al.* Improving care for patients with acute coronary syndromes; initial results from the National Audit of Myocardial Infarction Project (MINAP) *Heart* 2004; **90**(9):1004–9.

Bordley WC, Chelminski A, Margolis PA *et al.* The effect of audit and feedback on immunisation delivery: a systematic review. *American Journal of Preventive Medicine* 2000; **18**:343–50.

Brocklehurst J, Amess M, Goldacre M *et al.* (eds). *Health Outcome Indicators: Urinary Incontinence. Report of a Working Group to the Department of Health* 1999; National Centre for Health Outcomes Development, Oxford.

Cochrane Library. *Structure of a Cochrane Review* 2004, http://www.cochrane.org/reviews/revstruc.htm.

Cranney M, Barton S & Walley T. Addressing barriers to change: an RCT of practice – based education to improve management of hypertension in the elderly. *The British Journal of General Practice* 1999; **49**:522–6.

Davis D, Thomson O'Brien MA, Freemantle N *et al.* Impact of formal continuing medical education: do conferences, workshops, rounds, and other traditional educational activities change physician behavior or health care outcomes? *The Journal of the American Medical Association* 1999; **282**(9):867–74.

Department of Health. *The New NHS: Modern and Dependable* Cm 3807, 1997; HMSO, London.

Department of Health. *A First Class Service: Quality in the New NHS* 1998; HMSO, London.

Department of Health. *Learning from Bristol: the Report of the Public Inquiry into Children's Heart Surgery at the Bristol Royal Infirmary 1984–1995.* Command paper CM 5207, 2001; HMSO, London.

Department of Health and Social Services. NHS Management Enquiry team. The Griffiths report. *National Health Service Management Enquiry* 1983; HMSO, London.

Donabedian A. Evaluating the quality of medical care. *Milbank Memorial Fund Quarterly: Health and Society* 1966; **44**(3 suppl 1):166–206.

Donabedian A. The quality of care. How can it be assessed? *The Journal of the American Medical Association* 1988; **260**:1743–8.

Fairbank J, Goldacre M, Mason A *et al.* (eds). *Health Outcome Indicators: Fractured Proximal Femur. Report of a Working Group to the Department of Health* 1999; National Centre for Health Outcomes Development, Oxford.

Feder G, Griffiths C, Highton C *et al.* Do clinical guidelines introduced with practice based education improve care of asthmatics and diabetic patients? A randomised controlled trial in general practice in east London. *British Medical Journal* 1995; **311**:1473–8.

Grant R, Batty G, Aggarwal R *et al.* National sentinel clinical audit of evidence based prescribing for older people: methodology and development. *Journal of Evaluation in Clinical Practice* 2002; **8**:189–98.

Information Commissioner. 2001, http://www.informationcommissioner.gov.uk/cms/DocumentsUploads/the_complete_audit_guide.pdf.

Jamtvedt G, Young JM, Kristoffersen DT *et al.* Audit and feedback: effects on professional practice and health care outcomes (Cochrane Review). *The Cochrane Library* 2004, issue 1; John Wiley & Sons, Chichester.

Johnston G, Crombie IK, Davies HT *et al.* Reviewing audit: barriers and facilitating factors for effective clinical audit. *Quality in Health Care* 2000; **9**:23–36.

Kelson M. *A Guide to Involving Older People in Local Clinical Audit Activity: National Sentinel Audits Involving Older People* 1999; College of Health, London.

Lilford R, Mohammed MA, Spiegelhalter D & Thomson R. Use and misuse of process and outcome data in managing performance of acute medical care: avoiding institutional stigma. *Lancet* 2004; **363**:1147–54.

Lim KL & Harrison BD. A criterion based audit of inpatient asthma care. Closing the feedback loop. *Journal of the Royal College of Physicians of London* 1992; **26**:71–5.

Murphy MK, Black NA, Lamping DL *et al.* Consensus development methods and their use in clinical guideline development. *Health Technology Assessment, NHS R& D HTA Programme* 1998, vol. 2, issue 3; Department of Health, London.

NICE. *Principles for Best Practice in Clinical Audit* 2002a; Radcliffe Medical Press, Oxford.

NICE. *Audit of the Management of Post-MI Patients in Primary Care* 2002b; National Institute of Clinical Excellence, London.

NICE. *Guideline Development Methodology* 2004a, http://www.nice.org.uk/Docref.asp?d=106883.

NICE. National clinical guideline on management of chronic obstructive pulmonary disease in adults in primary and secondary care. *Thorax* 2004b; **59**(suppl 1):1–232.

Pruce D & Aggarwal R. *National Clinical Audits. A Handbook for Good Practice* 2000; Royal College of Physicians, London.

Royal College of Physicians. *Medical Audit: A First Report. What, Why and How?* 1989; Royal College of Physicians, London.

Royal College of Physicians. *Clinical Effectiveness Forum* 2004, http://www.rcplondon.ac.uk/college/ceeu/ceeu_guidelinesdb.asp.

Rudd A, Irwin P, Rutledge Z *et al.* The national sentinel audit for stroke: a tool for raising standards of care. *Journal of the Royal College of Physicians of London* 1999; **33**:460–4.

Rudd AG, Lowe D, Irwin P *et al.* National stroke audit: a tool for change? *Quality in Health Care* 2001; **10**:141–51.

Shipman. *Shipman Inquiry Reports* 2003, http://www.shipman-inquiry.org.uk/reports.asp.

SIGN. *SIGN Methodology* 2004, http://www.sign.ac.uk/methodology/index.html.

Slack R & Bucknall CE. Readmission rates are associated with differences in process of care in acute asthma. *Quality in Health Care* 1997; **6**:194–8.

Thomson O'Brien MA, Oxman AD, Davis DA *et al.* Educational outreach visits: effects on professional practice and health care outcomes (Cochrane Review). *The Cochrane Library* 2004a, issue 1; John Wiley & Sons, Chichester.

Thomson O'Brien MA, Oxman AD, Haynes RB *et al.* Local opinion leaders: effects on professional practice and health care outcomes. (Cochrane Review). *The Cochrane Library* 2004b, issue 1; John Wiley & Sons, Chichester.

155

Improving Quality of Care

Julie K. Gammack[1,2] ***and*** **Carolyn D. Philpot**[1]

[1] Saint Louis University School of Medicine, St Louis, MO, USA, and [2] Geriatric Research Education and Clinical Center, St Louis, MO, USA

INTRODUCTION

Throughout most of history, medical care was delivered to an individual patient by an individual clinician. Public health services were rarely available and infection control practices were poorly understood. Institutional care was uncommon and reserved for those with means to afford the medical services. Over the last century, medical care has drastically changed through the development of antibiotics, immunizations, and new surgical techniques. The world's population is now growing rapidly, is aging, and requires more health services. Population-based medicine has become a priority as cost, volume, and efficiency have become critical issues in meeting the growing health-care demands of the medical consumer.

From providing services to meeting standards of practice, the health-care industry is under increasing pressure to provide the highest level of services to the greatest number of recipients. In an era of limited health-care dollars, practitioners often must do more with less, yet, medical advances and fear of litigation drive the cost of care upward. For these reasons, efficient, high-quality care is of increasing importance. Consumer groups, medical societies, and health-care organizations have been at the forefront in promoting quality in health care. With a collective voice, these groups have promoted change in the health-care system. Although slower than many other industries, the health-care establishment has recognized the importance of delivering quality goods and services.

With the advent of computers, the growth of the pharmaceutical industry, and advances in diagnostic technologies, the level of medical sophistication has risen dramatically. Clinicians and patients now have a multitude of therapeutic options that were unavailable only a few years ago. As with other industries, however, quantity of services does not automatically equate to quality of services. It is necessary to critically evaluate not only medical treatments and techniques but also the process by which medicine is delivered to the health-care consumer. Defining quality, measuring performance, and changing ineffective practices must now become routine activities as medicine moves toward more efficient and effective methods of health-care delivery.

THE HISTORY OF QUALITY

The History of Quality in Business

In 1906, the International Electrotechnical Commission (IEC) was established to provide uniformity to the electrotechnical field. (see Appendix 1 for organizational abbreviations) The IEC promoted quality, safety, performance, reproducibility, and environmental compatibility of materials and products. This was the first organization to develop international standards of business practice.

The International Federation of the National Standardizing Association (ISA) was another organization, focused on mechanical engineering, which set standards for industry and trade from 1926 to 1942. After ISA dissolved, a delegation of 25 countries convened to create a new organization to unify the standards of industry and production practices. In 1947, this organization, the International Organization for Standardization (ISO), was established in the United Kingdom to oversee the manufacturing and engineering trades.

The ISO is a federation of nongovernmental bodies now representing 148 countries across the world. The ISO has developed international standards by which trade, technology, and scientific activities can be measured. Companies may choose to be certified by the ISO-9000 quality management system. This certification ensures a minimum standard by which business processes, quality management, and safety are maintained International Organization for Standardization (2004). ISO certification is especially important for international and intercontinental business to ensure a uniform delivery of goods and services. The health-care industry is

Principles and Practice of Geriatric Medicine, 4th Edition. Edited by M.S. John Pathy, Alan J. Sinclair and John E. Morley.

one of many fields that may be evaluated in the ISO method. Although used in some countries to evaluate medical practices, it is not widely accepted as a suitable model for the health-care system.

Around the same time, that ISO was created, Dr W. Edwards Deming, a physicist and statistician from the United States, developed a new process for quality improvement in business. Through this process, all members of a work unit were responsible for continuous monitoring and improvement of products along all steps of production. High frequency errors were identified, corrected, and the resulting outcome monitored for improved quality. Any step in the production process could and would be a continuous target for revision. In this method, focus was shifted from the specific error of an individual to the systemic faults that allowed an error to go unnoticed or proceed uncorrected. The workforce was thus empowered to identify problems and institute a plan of correction. Deming introduced this process, now known as *Continuous Quality Improvement* (CQI) and also referred to as *Total Quality Management* (TQM), in Japan where it quickly led to a revolution in the efficient manufacturing of high-quality goods.

Deming knew that successful management of a complex process or problem required the focused attention of a team of individuals. Although each member was uniquely skilled in a task, the team worked together in developing solutions. The TQM process is well suited for quality improvement in the complex health-care environment, but has not historically been embraced by the medical establishment. The narrow view that blame for errors be placed on a single individual and that physicians be allowed autonomous control over medical processes has hindered the acceptance of TQM. This view is changing as organizations realize that medical errors and inefficiencies are usually the result of systemic problems that require multifactorial solutions.

The Evolution of Quality in Health Care

One of the first efforts to standardize medical delivery occurred in 1917 with the "Minimum Standard for Hospitals" program set forth by Drs. Franklin Martin and John Bowman of the American College of Surgeons (ACS). A one-page, five-point set of criteria was crafted to assess the quality of hospitals (Shaw *et al.*, 2003) (see Table 1). In 1918, only 89 of 692 hospitals surveyed met the minimum criteria.

Table 1 "The Minimum Standard" – American college of surgeons 1917

1. That physicians and surgeons privileged to practice in the hospital be organized as a definite group or staff.
2. That membership upon the staff be restricted to physicians and surgeons who are
   (a) full graduates of medicine in good standing and legally licensed to practice
   (b) competent in their respective fields
   (c) worthy in character and in matters of professional ethics.
3. That the staff initiate and, with the approval of the governing board of the hospital, adopt rules, regulations, and policies governing the professional work of the hospital.
4. That accurate and complete records be written for all patients and filed in an accessible manner in the hospital.
5. That diagnostic and therapeutic facilities under competent supervision be available for the study, diagnosis, and treatment of patients.

The ACS was responsible for hospital accreditation until 1952 when the Joint Commission on Accreditation of Hospitals (JCAH) was established to take on this responsibility. Led initially by Dr. Arthur W. Allen, the JCAH published standards for hospital accreditation in 1953. The JCAH initiatives were also incorporated outside the United States, with Canada offering its own accreditation through the Canadian Commission on Hospital Accreditation in that same year. Over the next two decades, the JCAH grew to include the review of long-term care facilities in 1966 and subsequently, mental health, dental, ambulatory care, and laboratory facilities. In 1987, JCAH was renamed the Joint Commission on Accreditation of Health care Organizations (JCAHO) to encompass the variety of services and activities offered Joint Commission on Accreditation of Health care Organizations (2004).

JCAHO has been a world leader in health-care accreditation and a prototype for further development of organizations that monitor and measure the quality of health-care delivery. Over the past two decades, the interest and efforts in health-care quality have grown exponentially. A variety of national and international organizations have evolved to assist the heath-care industry in meeting new consumer and regulatory demands for high-quality services and programs.

Organizations Leading Health Care Quality Improvement

In the United States, the Agency for Health care Research and Quality (AHRQ), previously the Agency for Health Care Policy and Research (AHCRP), is a leader in health-care quality initiatives. Founded in 1989, this agency of the United States Department of Health and Human Services (DHHS) has a mission to improve the health-care quality, safety, efficiency, and effectiveness for all Americans. AHRQ awards millions of dollars in grants to further evidence-based–outcomes research related to health-care quality improvement. Federal legislation authorizes AHRQ to coordinate health partnerships, support research, and advance information and technology systems. Of the many projects that are overseen by AHRQ, the United States Preventive Services Task Force (USPSTF) and Consumer Assessment of Health Plans (CAHPS) are most prominent.

The USPSTF is a 15-member, private-sector panel of experts, first convened by the United States Public Health Service in 1984 to develop and assess evidence-based preventive service measures. The hallmark publication of this taskforce titled "Guide to Clinical Preventive Services" was published in 1989, with a second edition released in 1996 U. S. Preventive Services Task Force (2003). Although clinicians and health-care societies do not always agree upon the details, these guidelines are frequently cited as "best evidence" and considered to represent the "standard of care" in preventive medicine services.

CAHPS is an organizational databank of health-care information used by consumers, employers, and health plans in evaluating heath-care systems and services. Surveys and reporting instruments are used to collect and present information on health-care providers such as Medicare and the Federal Employees Health Benefits Program. In the private sector, the National Committee for Quality Assurance (NCQA) reviews the quality of managed care health plans. Established in 1990, this nonprofit group also accredits the health-care organizations. The NCQA has recently partnered with AHRQ in support of the CAHPS program.

The Institute of Medicine (IOM) is another leader in the development of quality health care in America. This nonprofit organization was chartered in 1970 as a segment of the National Academy of Sciences. The mission of the IOM is to work outside the governmental framework in providing an independent, scientifically based analysis of the health-care system. "Quality of Care" was defined by the IOM in 1990 as, "the degree to which health services for individuals and populations increase the likelihood of desired health outcomes and are consistent with current professional knowledge" (Richardson and Corrigan, 2002).

IOM formally launched the first of three phases of a quality initiative plan, beginning in 1996 with an intensive review of the state of health care in America. In a statement declaring "The urgent need to Improve Health Care Quality", the IOM began focusing on ovcrusc, undcrusc, and misuse in medical care. During Phase Two, the Quality of Health Care in America Committee convened and has since published several reports, including "To Err is Human: Building a Safer Health System" and "Crossing the Quality Chasm: A New Health System for the twenty-first century".

More recently, the committee has lobbied for an error reporting system and legislation to protect those who report errors in an effort to promote quality improvement strategies. Twenty "Priority Areas for National Action" have also been established based on diseases or conditions that may be best managed using clinical practice guidelines.

The IOM has established six "Aims for Improvement" in health-system function. Health care should be (1) safe, (2) effective, (3) patient-centered, (4) timely, (5) efficient, and (6) equitable. The Committee has also identified "10 simple rules for (health-care system) redesign" which change the focus of health care from provider driven to consumer/system driven care.

In the United Kingdom, the National Health Service (NHS) has received annual reviews since the Commission for Health Improvement was established in 1999 by the national government. In April 2004, this organization was replaced by the Health-care Commission, which is charged with the task of reviewing and improving the quality of health care in the NHS and in the private sector. The Health-care Commission collects data on patient satisfaction and the health-care process on both a local and national level. This data is available for public inspection.

In Australia, evaluation and accreditation of medical practice takes place through the Australian Council for Health Care Standards (ACHS). Established in 1974, ACHS is an independent body comprising health-care leaders, governmental representatives, and consumers. ACHS accredits programs using a standardized model called the *Evaluation and Quality Improvement Program* (EQuIP). EQuIP sets standards in two broad categories: (1) patient-care services across the continuum of care and (2) the health-care infrastructure The Australian Council on Healthcare Standards (2002). ACHS also provides a Performance and Outcomes Service (POS) that measures the quality of patient care in health-care organizations. Using Clinical Indicators that quantitatively and objectively measure care, the POS compares individual performance to national aggregate data. Outlying data generates a "flag", which can alert the organization to quality control problems.

Australia is also home to The International Society for Quality in Health Care (ISQua). This nonprofit organization, representing 70 participating countries, provides services and information on health-care quality to medical providers and consumers. ISQua hosts an annual international summit to discuss performance indicators and promote a multidisciplinary approach to quality improvement programs. Participants include health policy leaders, researchers, health-care professionals, and consumer organizations. ISQua has established international standards for national health-care accreditation bodies, through their Agenda for Leadership in Programs for Health care Accreditation (ALPHA). The ISQua also supports the International Journal for Quality in Health Care, a peer-reviewed journal in its 15th year of publication.

Models for Evaluating Quality

The approach to quality in health care bears many similarities to quality improvement in the commercial sector by focusing on key issues of safety, effectiveness, consumer satisfaction, timely results, and efficiency. Within Europe, there is much diversity in the oversight and governmental mandates for quality of health-care practice. Most legislation surrounds the health system and hospital accreditation process, with less emphasis placed on individual clinical practices. On the basis of the established health care and payer system, each country may address quality control quite differently.

To better understand the most common methods of measuring health-care quality, a survey of European External Peer Review Techniques (ExPeRT) was initiated (Heaton, 2000). The results of this ExPeRT Project revealed four commonly used quality improvement models: health-care system accreditation, ISO certification (both discussed previously in this chapter), the European Foundation for Quality Management (EFQM) Excellence Model, and the Visitatie peer review method.

The EFQM was founded in 1988 by presidents of leading European companies and has used the "Excellence Model" for assessing the quality of an organization (Heaton, 2000).

The framework for this TQM approach includes nine criteria by which an organization is evaluated on "what it does" and "what it achieves". A Quality Award is presented after a process of self-assessment and internal review. Over 600 companies have been granted EFQM awards, and research indicates that the companies who employ these quality management principles demonstrate substantial financial and employee growth (Singhal and Hendricks, 2001).

The Visitatie model originated in The Netherlands and focuses on medical practice specifically, rather than on business practice broadly. Visitatie is a peer review process that uses practice and practitioner-derived guidelines to evaluate patient care. Emphasis is placed on individual and team performance, not organizational structure or outcomes. Unlike other methods, Visitatie does not result in a certification or accreditation award. Because the focus is on improving care through peer feedback, there is no "pass/fail" or punitive outcome. This model is becoming popular across Europe as a method for personal and peer review of medical care (Heaton, 2000).

Quality Improvement in Geriatrics

The elderly population is prone to adverse outcomes, especially when health-care delivery is fragmented. Research has demonstrated that adverse health events are more likely to occur in the elderly population and that the risk of adverse hospital events is twice as high for individuals over age 65 (Leap *et al.*, 1991; Miller *et al.*, 2001). Preventive medicine for seniors includes identifying patient safety issues that can lead to functional decline and poor-health outcomes. Identifying risk factors for decline and providing early intervention is effectively approached through a health care team-based TQM process.

Quality in health care has evolved from a reactive Quality Assurance (QA) model (Figure 1), to a proactive TQM model (Figure 2). Instead of focusing on compliance and adherence to external regulations or standards (QA model), TQM focuses on the continuous process of improving care relative to current internal practices. TQM involves not only change in practices on an individual level but also change in process on a larger scale that can benefit a broader population.

In the TQM team process, each discipline reports data collected on patient care since the previous team meeting, as well as areas of ongoing concern or newly identified issues. The team discusses markers (indicators) of quality and establishes targets to achieve by the next meeting. The team then develops a plan for achieving these targets. A method of measuring performance and collecting data is established. An individual or subcommittee is then assigned to carry out the quality improvement protocol and provide a progress report at the next meeting. If the goals are achieved, data continues to be tracked over time to identify trends in performance and to maintain the established goals. If previously established quality targets are not met, barriers or obstacles are explored.

Geriatricians are in a unique position to take a lead in the health-care quality improvement process. Interdisciplinary

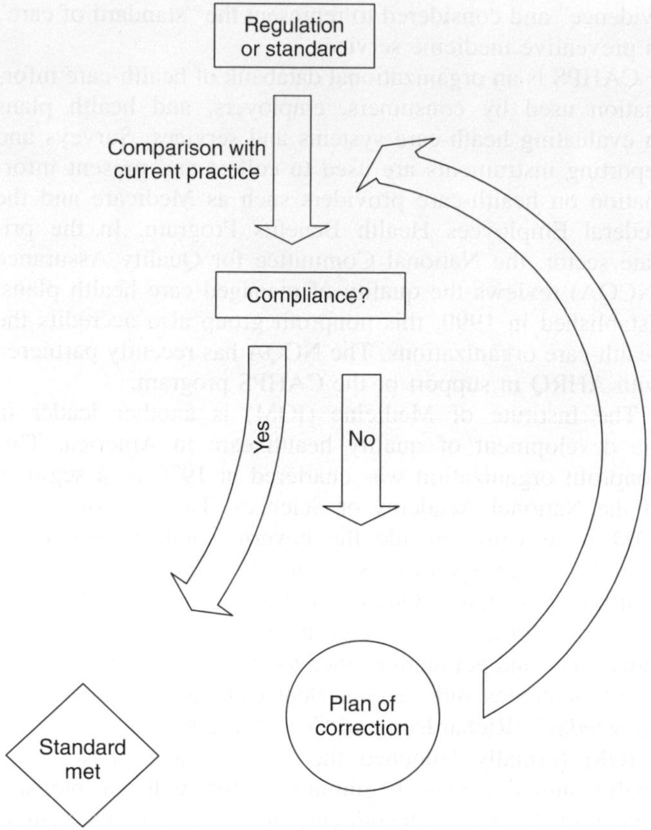

Figure 1 Quality assurance model

management and teamwork are at the core of geriatrics training and practice. Geriatricians are comfortable entrusting responsibility to team members and sharing in the problem-solving process. This is a requirement for the success of TQM programs. Geriatricians are also more likely than other physicians to have experienced the TQM process, as this is a routine activity in long-term care facilities. Through TQM, data on events such as falls and dehydration are tracked and shared with the staff at regular intervals. Trends are then discussed and solutions proposed when outlying results are identified.

Quality Indicators

In the United States, markers for quality in nursing home care, termed "*Quality Indicators*" (*QIs*), have been developed and tracked by the federal government through the completion of the required Minimum Data Set (MDS) resident evaluation questionnaire (Center for Health Systems Research and Analysis 1999; Zimmerman *et al.*, 1995) (*see* Table 2). Sentinel event and prevalence rates for 24 outcomes such as dehydration, decubitus ulcers, and falls are obtained from data on the MDS. Facilities are compared with local and national data for these markers. Outlying rates on the markers are "flagged" which may prompt investigation or oversight by the state nursing home regulatory board.

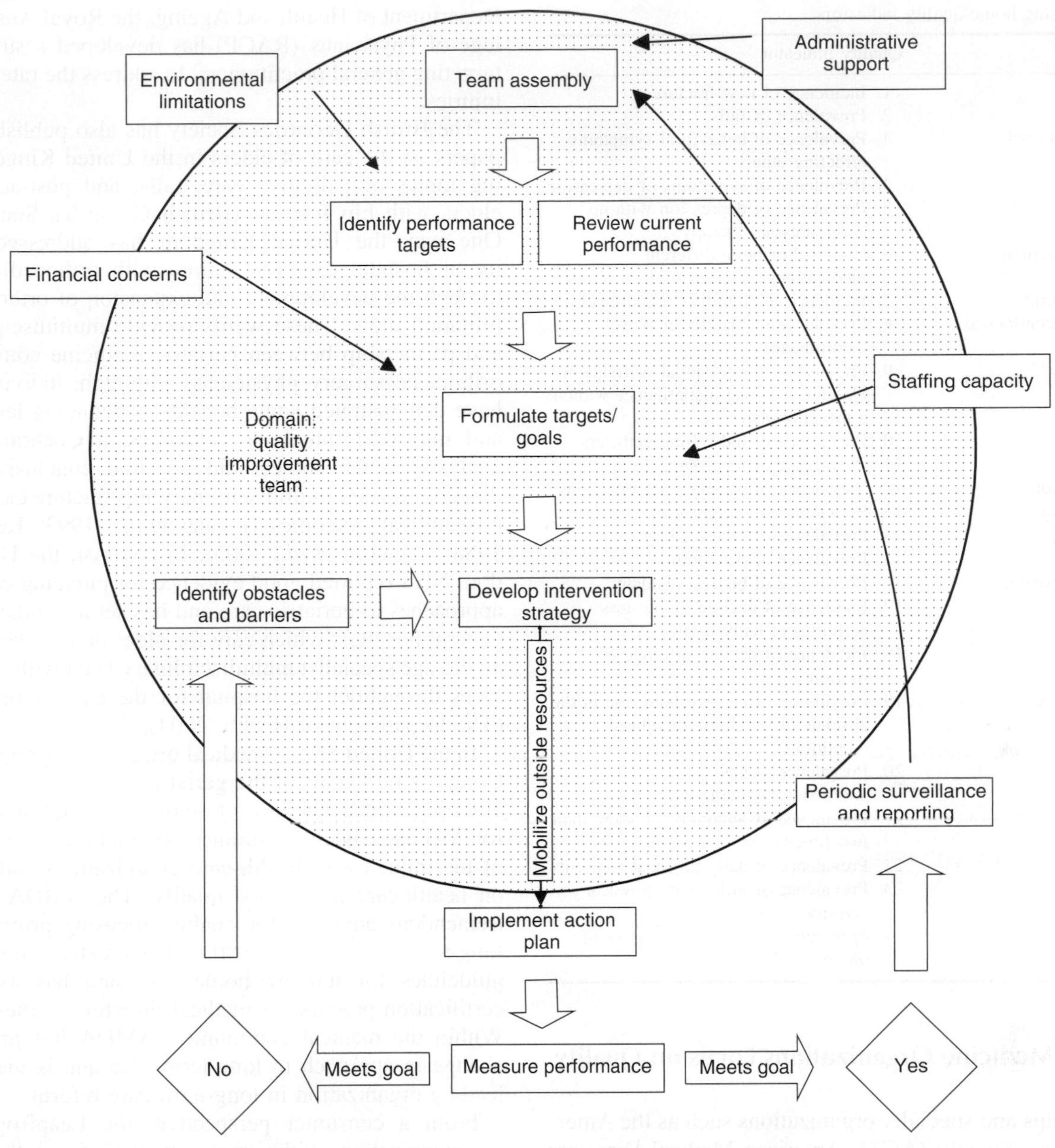

Figure 2 Total quality management (continuous quality improvement) model

The accuracy and utility of data extracted from the MDS has been debated, but quality indicators continue to serve as triggers for further assessment and care plan changes in the nursing home resident. Schnelle and colleagues have published a tremendous body of literature on the care process and health outcomes in nursing homes on the basis of information obtained from the MDS (Bates-Jensen *et al.*, 2004; Schnelle *et al.*, 2004; Cadogan *et al.*, 2004; Saliba and Schnelle, 2002). In some cases, the quality indicators are strongly associated with a positive or negative clinical outcome (Schnelle *et al.*, 2004; Cadogan *et al.*, 2004). In other cases, the indicators do not predict an event that might be expected on the basis of the provided data (Bates-Jensen *et al.*, 2004; Schnelle *et al.*, 2004).

The existing quality indicators do not adequately address quality of life and provision of daily care services. To address these issues, an expert panel of geriatricians convened and developed an additional set of quality indicators that complements the existing MDS-derived indicators. These measures may better track the quality of day-to-day care in nursing facilities (Saliba and Schnelle, 2002). The quality indicator domains include (1) preferences for daily life activities (2) frequency and form of activities of daily living (ADL) assistance (3) activity (4) assistive devices (5) goals of care and (6) communication. Although considered markers of quality care, many of these QIs are successfully achieved only in "the best nursing homes". Thus, although a target to strive for, these QIs may not be attainable for the average facility.

Table 2 Nursing home quality indicators

Domain	Quality indicator
Accidents	1. Incidence of new fractures
	2. Prevalence of falls
Behavior/Emotional patterns	3. Prevalence of behavioral symptoms affecting others
	4. Prevalence of symptoms of depression
	5. Prevalence of depression with no antidepressant therapy
Clinical management	6. Use of 9 or more different medications
Cognitive patterns	7. Incidence of cognitive impairment
Elimination/Incontinence	8. Prevalence of bladder or bowel incontinence
	9. Prevalence of occasional or frequent bladder or bowel incontinence without a toileting plan
	10. Prevalence of indwelling catheters
	11. Prevalence of fecal impaction
Infection control	12. Prevalence of urinary tract infections
Nutrition/Eating	13. Prevalence of weight loss
	14. Prevalence of tube feeding
	15. Prevalence of dehydration
Physical functioning	16. Prevalence of bedfast residents
	17. Incidence of decline in late-loss activities of daily living
	18. Incidence of decline in range of motion
Psychotropic drug use	19. Prevalence of antipsychotic use in the absence of psychotic or related conditions
	20. Prevalence of any antianxiety/hypnotic use
	21. Prevalence of hypnotic use more than two times in the last week
Quality of life	22. Prevalence of daily physical restraints
	23. Prevalence of little or no physical activity
Skin care	24. Prevalence of Stage 1 to 4 pressure ulcers

Geriatric Medicine Organizations Focus on Quality

Interest groups and specialty organizations such as the American Geriatrics Society (AGS), American Medical Directors Association (AMDA), British Geriatric Society (BGS), and Australian Society for Geriatric Medicine (ASGM) have taken a leadership role in bringing global quality improvement initiatives to the aging population. These organizations work within the health-care framework and governmental regulations unique to each country. Whereas national physician organizations focus efforts widely across the health-care system, these specialty groups address aging-specific health-care issues.

The ASGM has established a series of position papers that outline standards for geriatric care in Australia. One area of growing interest is in reduction of falls and fall-related injuries (Australian Society for Geriatric Medicine, 2004). Fall-related hospitalizations have increased to 0.8–1.4/year/100 adults aged 65–74, and accounted for 38.29 deaths/year/100 000 elders in 1996 (Australia Institute of Health and Welfare, 1997). With funding from the Australian Government Department of Health and Ageing, the Royal Australian College of Physicians (RACP) has developed a strategic plan, targeting general practitioners, to address the rate of falls and injuries.

The British Geriatrics Society has also published position papers on the care of elders in the United Kingdom including topics of palliative care, falls, and post-acute care of elders with hip fracture (British Geriatrics Society, 2004). One way the United Kingdom has addressed the quality of hospital care for seniors with orthopedic trauma is through the development and expansion of orthopedic rehabilitation units. These wards provide multidisciplinary care and partnership between geriatric medicine consultants and orthopedic surgery physicians. Although, individual studies have demonstrated some benefits in reducing length of stay and improved functional outcomes, a Cochrane Database analysis on the subject did not find conclusive evidence that coordinated multidisciplinary hip fracture care improved postsurgical outcomes (Incalzi *et al.*, 1993; Kennie *et al.*, 1988; Cameron *et al.*, 2003). In contrast, the United Kingdom NHS reported good evidence for pursuing collaborative approaches to geriatric care and has set a standard that, "All general hospitals which care for older people have identified an old age specialist multidisciplinary team with agreed interfaces throughout the hospital for the care of older people" (The Department of Health, 2004).

In the United States, medical organizations regularly lobby Congress on behalf of the geriatric medicine profession and elderly patients. The institution of a prescription drug benefit for Medicare health insurance beneficiaries is one example of the influence of health-care organizations and consumers on health-care policy and quality. The AMDA has been a tremendous advocate for quality, focusing primarily on the long-term care setting. AMDA has created clinical practice guidelines for nursing home care and has established a certification process for medical directors in these facilities. Within the medical community, AMDA has pressed for a change in approach to long-term care and is viewed as the leading organization in long-term care reform.

From a consumer perspective, the Leapfrog Group is an organization with great potential for influencing the quality of health-care plans and services. Founded by Fortune 500 executives, this group of over 150 companies aims to improve patient safety by lobbying for computerized physician ordering systems, appropriate patient referrals to subspecialty hospitals, and uniform critical care staffing in intensive care units. The Leapfrog Group represents 34 million health-care consumers and uses its health-care benefit purchasing power to influence the insurance industry in delivering health care that meets these quality standards (The Leapfrog Group for Patient Safety, 2004).

QUALITY IN THE NURSING HOME

When trying to improve quality of care, one must first characterize quality. Quality is the degree to which an outcome measures up to the expected gold standard. In health-care delivery, a quality process or intervention is measured against a standard practice that is administered to an individual patient, in a given situation, with a particular problem. Deviations from the standard of care affect the quality of care. Patients and their families expect health services to meet or exceed the standard of care, but may not understand what constitutes a reasonable standard.

To maintain the highest quality of care, continuous system-wide observation, evaluation, and monitoring are needed. Health-care managers are responsible for establishing performance standards for their staff and ensuring that these standards are met. The employees should feel comfortable providing feedback to the supervisors when aspects of health-care delivery require improvement. Managers must work with facility administrators to negotiate the resources necessary to allow the staffing team to carry out daily duties in an effective manner. Many quality improvement teams use the term "continuous quality improvement" to describe this process because maintaining quality is an ongoing activity.

Identifying the Problem

Areas of concern are brought to the attention of the health-care manager through a variety of avenues. In the long-term care setting, a nursing home administrator collects and catalogs this information through direct or indirect contact with residents, their families, and the facility staff. Administrators should also expect feedback and performance reports from the medical director and attending physicians working within the facility. At times, areas of concern may also come from the community or neighborhood hospitals.

All areas of concern are important. Substandard performance must be identified and immediately corrected. Good communication between all members of the facility is essential to ensure a positive resolution to a perceived problem. In one illustrative example, a husband is concerned about the care of his elderly wife in the nursing home because when he visits early each morning she is still in bed. After talking to the husband, it is learned that the wife was always an early riser. For years, they have had coffee first thing in the morning together. Because she is not assisted out of bed in the early morning to have coffee with her husband, he feels that she is receiving poor nursing care. Once these care expectations were identified and a solution communicated to the nursing staff, the patient was able to again enjoy the special morning time with her husband. The husband's perception of the nursing care improved and positive interactions at the facility could then ensue. Through good communication and problem solving, both husband and wife are now satisfied with the quality of care they receive.

Identifying a problem shortly after it occurs and promptly initiating a plan of correction is paramount. Timeliness often affects outcome. First impressions are very important when a patient first enters a long-term care facility. Every effort must be made to ensure that the transitional period is a positive experience. Positive experiences might include having a greeter meet residents when they first enter the facility. The greeter may be another nursing home resident or a nurse to assist them with the admissions process. A knowledgeable staff member should be available to answer questions for new residents and their families. Having a room ready upon arrival is also important in making the resident feel welcome. After acclimating to the facility, it is important for the residents to have periodic meetings to discuss the plan of care. These meetings help maintain a good line of communication and empower the resident to be a participant in the health-care process.

The Nursing Home Administrator

The nursing home administrator is responsible for the overall care within a facility and must handle all areas of concern that arise. Problems should be examined and categorized to better understand the origin of the difficulty. This information can alert the administrator to potential problems or areas of concern that need to be addressed. Nursing home administrators should be visible and accessible to families and residents, as well as staff, when responding to facility concerns. Most concerns fall into one of three categories: nursing care, laundry/housekeeping, and food. When complaints increase, the facility administrator must investigate and take steps to correct the problem.

Nursing Care

There are many interrelated components that impact the care provided by facility nursing staff. One of the most important areas, besides ensuring skill proficiency in the nursing staff, is the organization and function of nursing "systems". Systems of nursing practice must be in place in order to deliver high-quality care. Two examples of these "systems" include the structure of the nursing staff and the function of the nursing staff. Critical components of these systems include staffing patterns, delegation of work assignments, supervision, and evaluation of performance. Educational programs for the nursing staff should also be provided on an ongoing basis. The nursing assistants as well as the licensed nurses need to learn and review basic skills as well as specialty techniques necessary for the care for their residents. Ensuring a smoothly running system requires responsibility, good communication, respect, and clearly defined expectations. Nurses and administrators must view their interactions as two-way streets in order to build and maintain well-functioning nursing systems within a facility.

To maintain high-quality care, nurses must be able to identify residents "at risk" for unwanted outcomes. This can be performed during weekly multidisciplinary "high risk" needs assessment meetings for problems such as skin breakdown, falls, and confusion. Because mental status may change quickly and without notice in older adults, medical status must be assessed frequently. Nursing managers should periodically review high-risk individuals to help assure optimal care. Routine nurse manager oversight can address these and other potential problems before serious issues occur.

Laundry/Housekeeping

A second common area for concern in the provision of quality in long-term care facilities is its cleanliness. The administrator must convey to all of the staff that everyone be a participant in keeping the facility clean. All employees, from the director of nursing to the office assistant, should feel empowered to properly dispose of unattended waste or reduce clutter at the nursing stations. When trash and clutter are observed throughout the facility, the public perception is that care in other ways may also be substandard. Unpleasant odor is another factor that implies a lack of cleanliness. When the scent of urine or feces is present, even if transient, there may be a perception of poor patient care. Once a foul odor is identified, it must quickly be extinguished. Excessive rubbish and unpleasant odors imply to residents and families both a lack of concern and a lack of proper staffing in the facility.

Laundry, when done at the facility, is a service that frequently generates complaints. Laundry that is lost or not returned in a timely manner reduces patient dignity and increases care costs for residents and families. Lost clothing may be minimized by individually marking each item with a permanent marker or tape, or by placing a person's clothing in a special washing garment bag. Laundry problems may be best curtailed by encouraging residents to have clothing marked and by educating families on the laundering process. Some clothing does not withstand the rigor of industrial laundering and is best cleaned by the resident's family.

Food

It is difficult to please everyone when serving a large amount of food on a daily basis. A common complaint from nursing home residents is that their food is cold when it should be hot and that is not presented to them in a timely manner. Using a buffet-style dining system or a menu selection process can increase resident satisfaction. Allowing residents to participate in food choice improves interest in meals and adequate caloric consumption. Residents also need to participate in choosing the types of meals they receive. This can be done by interviewing the resident or by discussing meal plans at "Resident Council Meetings". Having an occasional "special" meal is also pleasurable and gratifying.

Quality Improvement Meetings

Members of the quality improvement team should include pharmacy, lab, attending physicians, the medical director, nursing, therapy, dietary, maintenance, activities, social service, medical records, and administration. Many long-term care facilities meet only on a quarterly basis to discuss various issues of quality care. This is not frequent enough. Monthly meetings help improve the communication of information and remind everyone of quality initiatives and areas for improvement.

Pharmacy should present the monthly number or percentage of residents on antipsychotics, anxiolytics, and antidepressants. By reassessing the continued need for psychotropic medication in nursing home residents, dosing and prescribing reduction frequently occurs. Pharmacy should also report the incident and type of medication errors and assist in developing methods to reduce errors. To minimize possible drug–drug interactions, a goal of nine medications or less per resident should be a target at the facility.

The laboratory service provider should report the number of microbial cultures performed during that month with those that were negative as well as positive. Organisms that are identified are reviewed along with antibiotic sensitivity patterns. Timeliness of the cultures reported to the facility and institution of appropriate antibiotics are reviewed. Trends in organisms, antimicrobial sensitivity, and clustering of infections should be assessed. Laboratory services should also investigate unnecessarily prolonged return of blood work reports and the effectiveness of data transmission to the nursing facility.

Each month, nursing should present the number of residents who developed decubitus ulcers, have indwelling foley catheters, and received physical restraints. To reduce the rate of injuries and falls, each facility should strive to be restraint-free (Capezuti *et al.*, 1998). The rate of facility-acquired decubitus and indwelling foley catheters, should be under five percent. If rates rise above five percent, action should be taken to justify or remedy this trend. Weight loss and excessive gain should be reported every month, including a probable cause and a plan of correction. Awareness is key and all disciplines can participate in weight loss prevention protocols.

Incident reports should be reviewed monthly. Investigation of resident incidents should include type, location where the incident took place, time of day (during which shift), weekend versus weekday, and degree of injury or impact. Trends or patterns in this data should be noted and a plan for incident reduction implemented. Employee incidents should also be evaluated. An increase in employee incidents and injuries is often directly related to employee dissatisfaction.

Patient census should be reviewed at each meeting along with admissions, transfers to and from the hospital, discharges to home/another facility, and deaths. When looking at nursing home admissions, one should also look at the source of their admission. Was the new admit from a hospital, and if so, which hospital? Are admissions trending up or down? What days and times are the hospital admissions arriving at the nursing home? Transfers to the hospital or emergency department should also be tracked. Was the transfer preventable? Are certain shifts or floors more likely to transfer residents out for urgent evaluation? This valuable information allows the nursing home administrator and director of nursing to identify staffing or skill deficiencies within the facility.

When providing therapy to the long-term care resident, the therapist needs to keep a record of the functional level prior to therapy, the number of days in therapy, the functional level when therapy was discontinued, and disposition upon discharge. It has been demonstrated that extending therapy for a few more days often improves overall outcome. Therapy services can use this information as a marketing tool. The department may display, in a graphic format, the functional level of residents prior to illness, upon initiation of therapy, and upon discharge of therapy.

The quality improvement process that is discussed and monitored during team meetings should be documented in an organized and systematic manner using a standardized reporting process (Table 3). Topics relevant to patient-care quality (e.g. falls) are selected by the team. Indicators of quality (e.g. fall rate, injurious falls, number of fractures) are identified and a target rate for the facility is established (e.g. <5 percent of falls resulting in injury). Data on patient outcomes is collected within the facility and compared with the established indicator target. If current standards fail to meet the target, areas for improvement (e.g. reducing nighttime falls) are identified and a plan of action established (e.g. scheduled toileting at bedtime). During the follow-up phase, data on the indicators is again collected to determine if the intervention has resulted in successful achievement of the established goals.

QUALITY IN ACUTE-CARE PRACTICES

Hospital Accreditation

The internationally recognized JCAHO mission is to provide accreditation and performance review for the safety and quality of health-care facilities. Established over 50-years ago, this independent nonprofit organization reviews not only hospitals, but also a variety of health-care facilities such as nursing homes, home-care organizations, health-care networks, outpatient centers, and clinical laboratories. Accreditation is a marker of quality valued by the community and used to promote the excellence of an institution.

Accreditation takes place after undergoing an on-site survey by a team of medical and business professionals. All aspects of care are reviewed, including compliance with safety procedures, patient-care processes, and the work environment. Hospital accreditation is valid for three years. JCAHO uses standardized performance criteria that were developed with the expertise and guidance of health-care leaders in academic medicine, business, and governmental agencies.

In an ongoing effort to improve the accreditation process, JCAHO implemented the ORYX initiative in 1997. This project integrates performance and health outcome measure in the evaluation of patient safety and delivery of health-care services. Accredited organizations are required to collect data on health outcomes and submit this information to JCAHO as a part of the evaluation process.

In other parts of the world, the hospital evaluation process may take place through national regulatory organizations. In Europe, hospital accreditation was first introduced in Spain through the Catalan Hospital Accreditation Programme (CHAP) in 1981 Clinical Accountability, Service Planning, and Evaluation (CASPE) (2004). Due to financial setbacks, this program was not continuously active until 1991. In the United Kingdom, a sustained accreditation program has been in place since 1990. Results of a 2001 survey indicate that 11 European countries have formally implemented hospital accreditation programs and nine have programs under development (Shaw, 2002).

In the United Kingdom, two independent and nongovernmental agencies provide health facility accreditation services. The Health care Accreditation Programme (HAP) was first developed to oversee the National Health Service hospitals but has grown to include public and community health-care centers. The Health Quality Service (HQS) oversees the accreditation of both public and private-sector institutions. Accreditation reports are available for public inspection in the United Kingdom and a handful of other countries, but in general are not available to health-care consumers in Europe. Although the majority of accredited programs are hospital-based, evaluations of community and outpatient care centers are evolving in several European countries.

Both JCAHO and HQS offer international accreditation services. In 1999, JCAHO initiated an international program for accreditation. To address the international differences in health-care delivery, a 16-member task force developed "international consensus standards" for the Joint Commissions International. This task force represents the health-care concerns, values, and governments of countries on six continents. HQS offers consultation services to European countries that are developing quality and accreditation programs. Two organizations, the European Societies for Quality in Health Care and the International Society for Quality in Health Care have just begun efforts to unify health-care accreditation throughout Europe and worldwide.

The Hospital Environment

It has long been known by geriatricians that the hospital is a dangerous place for frail, elderly individuals who are at high risk for iatrogenic complications. If immobility, delirium, and nutrition are not addressed upon hospitalization, unwanted morbidity, and functional decline can rapidly occur (Inouye *et al.*, 1998a; Inouye *et al.*, 1998b). Altering the hospital environment to improve outcomes in the elderly has become a focus of research and a measure of quality in health care. *US News and World Report* magazine ranks United States hospitals and medical programs each year. Among a host of factors used to evaluate quality, hospital-based geriatric services are included in this calculation (O'Muircheartaigh *et al.*, 2004).

Table 3 Continuous quality improvement report

Topic______________________ Dept.______________

Report Date______________________ Initial Report______________ Follow-up

I. Process Planning

Reason for selecting topic

Starting Date

Frequency of Monitoring

Sampling Population

Source of Information Records Survey Observation Other

Method for Data Collection

II. Indicators and Data Presentation

Indicator	Goal (Frequency or %)	Data (Numerical)	Data (Percent)

Interpretation of Data and Comparison to Established Goals:

III. Analysis and Plan of Improvement

A. Areas for Improvement	Obstacles or Barriers

B. Action Plan	Key Personnel	Initiation Date	Completion Date

IV. Follow-up and Re-evaluation

Indicator	Date to Re-evaluate	Key Personnel	Date for Follow-up Report

Report Prepared and Reviewed by:

Name	Title	Date

Over the past decade, several geriatric services have been developed with demonstrated benefit in reducing the risk of hospital-related morbidity and mortality. These programs have largely targeted the prevention of delirium and reduction in functional decline. Hospitals are increasingly aware that reducing adverse events in the elderly is important not only for maintaining a positive public reputation, but also in reducing health-care costs.

Acute Care for the Elderly (ACE) units have been shown to decrease discharge to nursing homes and to improve functional outcomes at hospital discharge (Landefeld *et al.*, 1995; Counsel *et al.*, 2000). The general principles of ACE units include an interdisciplinary care approach, tailoring the hospital environment to reduce iatrogenesis, maximizing functional status, daily geriatric assessments with an actively involved, specially trained nursing staff, and proactive discharge planning. The implementation of ACE units in hospitals is growing.

The Geriatric Evaluation and Management Unit (GEMU) is another multidisciplinary care model linked closely to the inpatient hospitalization setting. GEMUs provide subacute care and rehabilitation in a setting that bridges hospital to home. The goals of GEMU care include maximizing functional, social, and medical status through comprehensive geriatric assessment. Patients who would otherwise require nursing home placement receive dedicated medical and therapy services to regain lost independence. The GEMU model has demonstrated benefit in reducing rehospitalization, improving physical and cognitive functioning, reducing mortality, and increasing the likelihood of living at home after discharge (Stuck *et al.*, 1993). These outcomes are indicators of the quality and benefit of a multidisciplinary approach to care of the older adult.

QUALITY IN THE COMMUNITY SETTING

Home Care

Medical care in the home has shifted from the historical single-provider model of the early 1900s to a team-based service with the advent of home health-care organizations. This multidisciplinary approach has expanded the access and availability of health-care services to homebound individuals. Australia has taken home care to an even higher level of sophistication with the "Hospital in the Home" approach. This model provides hospital-like services to individuals at home who are acutely ill but unwilling to enter the hospital or for whom hospitalization is unlikely to provide any measurable health benefit. The quality of care for Hospital in the Home as measured by cost, patient satisfaction, and medical outcomes is at least equivalent to traditional hospital care (Board *et al.*, 2000; Caplan *et al.*, 1999).

Patient care in the home is of increasing complexity and acuity. For organizations to meet the quality care standards expected by consumers, home-care services must be broad in scope and efficient in delivery. The success of Hospital in the Home and growth of home care is in part due to the advancement of portable medical technologies. Mobile radiology and laboratory services have expanded the diagnostic capabilities of home-care providers. The availability of intravenous access services and infusion devices have allowed more frail and debilitated elders to receive necessary intravenous therapies without transfer to the hospital or nursing home setting. Portable electrocardiogram monitors and serum analysis systems, although not in widespread use, now allow providers a more efficient and expedited evaluation of the home-care patient.

To address the question of how home health services improve the quality of medical care, the AHRQ, through the Centers for Medicare and Medicaid Services (CMS) in the United States, has developed a Home Health Quality Initiative project. CMS currently provides financial reimbursement for more than half of the home-care expenditures for seniors Basic Statistics About Home Care (2000). A set of 11 quality measures was selected to evaluate home-care agency services. These measures were based on outcomes data from the Outcome and Assessment Information Set (OASIS) national standardized home-care database. Quality measures are functionally based, such as improvement in toileting or improvement in bathing, but also include the utilization of emergency or hospital services Centers for Medicare and Medicaid Services (2003). Using the reported outcomes on these quality measures, certified home-care agency evaluations can now be reviewed online by the medical consumer.

Home monitoring and telemedicine systems are of increasing interest in the care of chronically ill seniors. A variety of products that record patient information, transmit data to a monitoring center, or give patient reminders are now commercially available. Remote medical monitoring systems can intermittently or continuously monitor vital signs and disease symptoms using noninvasive and minimally intrusive sensors. These systems use Internet, radio, or phone-line transmission of medical information to a hardware- or software-based system that acquires, stores, and processes the data. Medical staff can examine the data in real time or at periodic intervals. Alert parameters can be programmed to immediately notify the provider, of abnormal findings. These systems are used almost exclusively in association with home health-care services. Initial studies suggest that for chronic disease management, electronic home-monitoring systems can reduce hospitalization rates, and length of stay, and improve disease control (Kornowski *et al.*, 1995; Mehra *et al.*, 2000; Maiolo *et al.*, 2003; Rogers *et al.*, 2001).

The most basic home-care technologies include personal alarm systems and emergency response telephones that make a voice connection between the patient and the response center. This "lifeline" monitoring system uses a self-activated call button that is often worn as a necklace or bracelet. More expansive and complex systems are being designed to monitor the home and activity of frail elders. The "smart home" technology utilizes sensors placed throughout the home to track "normal" daily activity and report potential emergencies by detecting deviations from typical activity patterns. These devices may improve the safety and security of older adults living at home, but conjure up unsettling images of an Orwellian world where "Big Brother" is watching.

Database Analysis in the United States

Large, centralized health-care organizations, such as health maintenance organizations (HMO) and the Department of Veterans' Affairs Medical Centers (VAMC) in the United States, frequently use health database analysis to track costs, utilization of services, and patient-care outcomes. Data from these organizations is used for epidemiology studies and for population-based research on disease and health-care services. Although cost containment may be a driving force in the monitoring of health statistics, these organizations have the infrastructure to use health-care data for quality improvement purposes.

Because laboratory, radiology, and pharmacy services are usually provided within the organization, utilization statistics may be readily available to the clinical and administrative providers. Often this information is tracked electronically within the organization. Practice patterns can be monitored and feedback sent to clinicians or departments to improve the delivery of patient care. Appointment backlogs, vaccination rates, and cancer screening rates may be targeted by the organization. Goals for improving the delivery of health care can be set and trends measured after instituting a plan of improvement.

There is growing interest in a disease-based team approach to improve health outcomes. Common disorders that require regular monitoring or result in high use of urgent care services, such as diabetes and asthma, are often the target of these efforts. Using nationally developed practice guidelines or internally developed clinical care protocols, centralized health-care organizations have the infrastructure to implement care processes to improve health outcomes.

Although clinical practice guidelines are not universally agreed upon in every detail, they are generally considered to represent a reasonable and achievable standard of care supported by current evidence-based research. Thus, adherence to practice guidelines may serve as a marker for quality care within an organization or clinical patient base. Pharmacy and clinical laboratory databases are used to provide individual feedback to clinicians on decision-making behavior, compliance with national guidelines, and improvement in patient outcomes over time. The use of database monitoring to generate electronic reminders that prompt screening and disease management have demonstrated improvement in practitioner adherence to health-care standards (Bentz *et al.*, 2002; Kitahata *et al.*, 2003; Filippi *et al.*, 2003).

Although database analysis offers much statistical information, ongoing problems include limitation of content, relative inaccessibility to information, lack of automated data, and data mismatches (Fink, 1998; Mullooly *et al.*, 1999). This could be improved through new financial and technical support to HMOs interested in outcomes-based research.

Health Care Audit in the United Kingdom

In the United Kingdom, population-based review is conducted through a process called *clinical audit*. The National Health Service has used this method of quality improvement for over 15 years. Clinical audit is a "systematic, critical analysis of the quality of medical care including the procedures used for diagnosis and treatment, the use of resources, and the resulting outcome and quality of life for the patient". Department of Health (1989) Clinical audit has evolved from a clinician-targeted to a system-targeted review that evaluates the outcomes of a quality improvement process.

Clinical audit is an internal method whereby a clinical practice, such as the frequency of ophthalmologic evaluation in diabetic patients or rate of influenza vaccination, is measured using medical record review. Performance markers are compared with accepted standards, practice guidelines, or previously established audit goals. If performance falls below expectations, a plan for practice revision is established and implemented. Follow-up audit is conducted to assess the success in achieving the targeted practice goals.

Clinical audit is a dynamic process that requires attention to changes in population demographics, health resources, and advances in medical knowledge. Comparison of audit results between clinical sites or regions must account for this heterogeneity. The geriatric population itself is a heterogeneous group. For the elderly, important clinical outcomes are linked less to chronological age than to functional ability. A clinical audit outcome measure of cancer screening rates in a healthy 75-year-old population, for example, may be quite different from a chronically ill and debilitated 75-year-old cohort.

The success of a clinical audit requires a well-structured approach, appropriate time, and appropriate resources. Too frequently, a problem is identified through the clinical audit, but a plan of correction is not implemented or the outcome of the correction is never evaluated. This may be due to a lack of experience and time on the part of the auditors, who are often junior clinicians within the organization. Resources must be available if an organization plans to undergo a systematic review of a clinical issue with the intent to implement a meaningful change in clinical practice.

Large-scale clinical audits can require significant administrative support. Charts must be collected, data extracted, and statistical evaluation performed. A protocol for change in practice must be developed with the input and agreement of clinical practitioners. Piloting the proposed change may be necessary to troubleshoot unforeseen barriers before implementing the plan on a larger scale. After an appropriate duration of practice, the clinical issue must be reevaluated to determine if the new protocol has had an impact on the targeted outcome of the program.

It is important that a clinical audit be viewed as a quality improvement activity and not as a means to emphasize personal shortcomings or to generate punitive action. The audit should focus on areas in need of general improvement and methods to achieve practice goals of the group or within the organization (Dickenson and Sinclair, 1998).

Clinical audit itself is not research, although it may generate research questions. Because an audit reveals epidemiological and demographic information about a clinical practice, the results may lead to publication of health-care trends or results of a quality improvement process. In an era of increasing attention to patient confidentiality and ethical research practices, approval to conduct an audit may be required by an organization. This is especially true in the United States, where academic centers and many health-care organizations have institutional review boards to ensure the safety and confidentiality of patient information.

FUTURE INITIATIVES IN HEALTH-CARE QUALITY

With the advent of high technology, the perception of quality has expanded to encompass the use and accessibility of electronic and computer-based devices in health care. Medical diagnosis, treatment, and documentation have advanced in sophistication to a point where electronics is standard and necessary for patient-care practices. Health-care services, communication, and reimbursement are expedited with the use of high technology. Individuals and organizations without Internet access, electronic medical records (EMRs), or access to innovative diagnostic/therapeutic devices may be viewed as "behind the times". Health-care consumers have an increasing expectation, well-founded or not, that technology-based initiatives provide superior quality and better medical outcomes.

High Technology in Medical Education

The use of technology has fundamentally altered the format of medical education. Computers have changed the classroom environment and augmented the quality of medical presentations. Lectures now efficiently utilize multimedia resources with the ability to present complex content using sophisticated instructional formats. Internet-ready classrooms allow an educator to conduct a search of the literature and access clinical information in real time.

Online, as opposed to live, in-class lectures are available at some medical schools. In one study, students expended 50 minutes less time to complete an on-line lecture activity than the live lecture group, but demonstrated equal post-lecture knowledge (Spickard *et al.*, 2002). Many studies have failed to demonstrate the superiority of Internet-based or computer-assisted tutorials over the traditional lecture and textbook format (Buzzell *et al.*, 2002; Vichitvejpaisal *et al.*, 2001; Williams *et al.*, 2001; Seabra *et al.*, 2004). Thus, an "electronic professor" does not replace the need for live interaction with medical educators. Like any instructional tool, electronic and computer-based programs must be used in the right context, for the right group, and with the appropriate level of "real life" interaction.

Subjects with a high degree of visual-spatial complexity such as gross anatomy and histology have seen remarkable benefit from the growth of digital teaching tools. Three-dimensional views and electronically created images have assisted students in understanding anatomical and physiological relationships. Trainees are being exposed to new technologies from the classroom through the clinical years. Teaching tools that did not exist just a few years ago are readily being incorporated into the educational environment.

New methods of medical education using simulation models are of increasing interest in reducing the incidence of procedural complications. In some studies, surgeons who received virtual reality simulator training for laparoscopic procedures demonstrated significant improvement in skill performance over those without this training (Grantcharov *et al.*, 2004; Jordan *et al.*, 2000). Other research has failed to demonstrate a difference in procedure time and patient discomfort between medical residents trained using a virtual reality-based procedural simulator and traditional bedside teaching techniques (Gerson and Van Dam, 2003). As the use of technology in diagnosis and treatment expands, so will the use of technology-based teaching tools in hopes of improving the quality of medical training.

In an effort to improve the efficiency and safety of patient care, handheld Personal Digital Assistant (PDA) devices have become increasingly popular in medical practice and medical education. Some medical schools and residency programs are providing trainees with these devices preprogrammed with educational tools and reference databases. PDAs have demonstrated benefit in reducing adverse medical events and improving the accuracy of medical documentation. Data is most supportive in the reduction of medication errors and identification of medication side effects (Collins, 2004; Carroll *et al.*, 2004).

Because PDAs now have wireless and Internet access capability, the potential for remote-site electronic access to a central patient-care database is being explored at some institutions. This access can be especially useful for the geriatric medicine practitioner performing house calls, nursing home care, and rural community-based care. These sites traditionally have limited access to electronic resources. Several institutions within the United States, including the VAMC system, have employed technologies that allow practitioners to use portable devices for remote-access to patient information. Patient confidentiality has been addressed through the use of encryption programs that prevent unauthorized access by wireless users.

PDA programs can be used to track and store patient information. This is especially useful in the immediate and accurate retrieval of patient records during after hours, off site, and telephone consultation with patients and other medical providers. The applications to patient safety are of growing importance in the quality improvement process at all sites of care. The use of PDAs and other portable electronic equipment will continue to grow as the demand for immediate and accurate medical information increases.

Electronic Medical Records

Electronic documentation of patient information is also of increasing importance in the delivery of quality medical care.

The hospital setting currently makes greatest use of electronic records, given the volume of information that must be collected and shared among medical practitioners. Whether data is entered electronically by practitioners or accessed in a read-only format, the EMR facilitates communication and access to information. Electronic charting has been shown to reduce documentation time and to improve the accuracy of assigning diagnostic codes (Stengel *et al.*, 2004). The use of computer technology in patient management has repeatedly been associated with a reduction in the frequency of many types of medical errors (Bates and Gawande, 2003).

Many electronic record systems operate via an Internet-based access system that allows users to enter and access data through any Internet-ready computer. Other institutions use on-site computer systems that require users to access data through terminals or workstations networked for this purpose. This system limits access but is potentially a more secure means of maintaining patient confidentiality.

The VAMC in the United States exclusively uses an EMR. This Computerized Patient Record System (CPRS) is the largest EMR in the world. All medical orders, laboratory tests, medical progress notes, medications, and other data are entered and viewed electronically by all medical providers. The system can be accessed remotely by those providers located off of the main medical campus. Alerts, prompts, and predesigned order sets have reduced the occurrence of medical errors and improved the efficiency of medical care within the VAMC system. Those countries with national health-care systems or large health provider groups (such as the VAMC) may be at best advantage to use an all-electronic record system, given the need for a well-structured system to oversee the design and support this form of health information system.

Telemedicine

With the advancement of digital data transfer, the Internet, and wireless-based technologies, rapid relay of visual and audio transmissions have led to the development of telemedicine programs between remote geographic locations. Videoconferencing has extensive educational and clinical applications for the health-care systems. Training can be provided in real time using interactive video technology that allows remote classrooms sites to see, hear, and speak with the instructor. Telemedicine allows primary and specialty-care providers to interact with patients and clinicians in geographically isolated or underserved segments of the population.

In a Singapore hospital pilot project, geriatric specialists conducted telerounds with two off-site homes for the elderly (Pallawala and Lun, 2001). This project was considered a success and was viewed favorably by both patients and clinicians. Improving access to health-care resources is an area of ongoing interest in the quality improvement process. As the technology improves and hardware costs decline, telemedicine will become an increasingly popular means of providing a broader array of health-care services to a larger segment of the patient population.

CONCLUSION

"Quality of Care" has been defined as, "the degree to which health services for individuals and populations increase the likelihood of desired health outcomes and are consistent with current professional knowledge". Quality in health care has become a priority as cost, volume, and efficiency have become critical issues in meeting the growing health-care demands of the medical consumer. Over the past two decades, the interest in health-care quality improvement has grown dramatically. Consumer groups, medical societies, and health-care organizations have actively promoted quality in health care. These national and international associations work within the health-care framework and governmental regulations unique to each country to help meet consumer and regulatory demands for high-quality medical services.

Based on the established health care and payer system, each organization may address quality control quite differently. Health-care facility accreditation is a common means of marking quality and promoting the excellence of an institution. Other groups may choose certification using established standards such as the ISO-9000 process. At the level of the individual provider, performance may be assessed through audit or comparison of practices with established clinical guidelines.

The TQM process is well suited for the complex health-care environment. This method is used to critically evaluate not only medical treatments and techniques but also the process by which medicine is delivered to the health-care consumer. Quality improvement may then involve change in practice on an individual level and change in operation on a larger scale that benefits a broader population. Using quality indicators and outcome measures that quantitatively and objectively measure care, outlying data can be used to alert the organization to quality control problems.

Geriatricians are in a unique position to influence the health-care quality improvement process. Interdisciplinary care and TQM are already familiar practices for most medical practitioners. As medical directors, geriatricians have taken a leadership role in improving institutional and rehabilitation practices. The quality of care for the elderly has been enhanced through new initiatives such as ACE and GEMU models and home-care technologies. Using new technologies, electronic databases and Internet resources, care for the older population stands to broaden in scope and sophistication in coming years. Geriatricians will continue to be strong advocates for care practices that improve the process and outcomes of medical care for a growing and aging population.

KEY POINTS

- The process of standardizing health-care quality has evolved over the last 100 years.

- The Joint Commission on Accreditation of Health care Organizations (JCAHO) has accredited hospitals and health-care facilities for over 50 years.
- Continuous Quality Improvement, also known as *Total Quality Management*, is a team-based approach used to evaluate and institute system-wide changes.
- Database analysis and health-care audit are two methods of evaluating quality on a population-based scale.
- The use of computers and electronic communication systems have improved medical efficiency and reduced medical errors.

KEY REFERENCES

- Dickenson E & Sinclair AJ. Clinical Audit of Health Care. In J Pathy (ed) *Principles and Practice of Geriatric Medicine* 1998, 3rd edn; John Wiley & Sons, Chichester, pp 1575–81.
- Heaton C. External peer review in Europe: an overview from the ExPeRT Project. *International Journal for Quality in Health Care* 2000; **12**(3):177–82.
- Richardson WC & Corrigan JM. The IOM quality initiative: a progress report at year six. Shaping the future. *Newsletter of the IOM* 2002; **1**(1):1–8.
- Stuck AE, Siu AL, Wieland GD *et al.* Comprehensive geriatric assessment: a meta-analysis of controlled trials. *Lancet* 1993; **342**:1032–6.
- Zimmerman DR, Karon SL, Arling G *et al.* Development and testing of nursing home quality indicators. *Health Care Financing Review* 1995; **16**(4):107–27.

REFERENCES

About USPSTF. U.S. Preventive Services Task Force. AHRQ Publication No. 00-P046, 2003, Agency for Healthcare Research and Quality, Rockville, http://www.ahrq.gov/clinic/uspstfab.htm.

Australia Institute of Health and Welfare. *National Health Priority Areas: Injury Prevention and Control Report* 1997, AIHW, Cat No. PHE 3 Canberra, http://www.aihw.gov.au/publications/health/nhpaipc97/nhpaipc97.pdf.

Australian Society for Geriatric Medicine. *Position Statements* 2004, Sydney, http://www.asgm.org.au/posstate.htm.

Basic Statistics About Home Care. *Sources of Payment for Home Care 1999 and 2000[a]: from Health Care Financing Administration, Office of the Actuary, National Health Expenditures: 1980–2010* 2000, Table 3, http://www.nahc.org/Consumer/hcstats.html, November 2001.

Bates DW & Gawande AA. Improving safety with information technology. *New England Journal of Medicine* 2003; **248**(25):2526–34.

Bates-Jensen BM, Alessi CA, Cadogan M *et al.* The minimum data set bedfast quality indicator: differences among nursing homes. *Nursing Research* 2004; **53**(4):260–72.

Bentz CJ, Davis N & Bayley B. The feasibility of paper-based tracking codes and electronic medical record systems to monitor tobacco-use assessment and intervention in an Individual Practice Association (IPA) Model Health Maintenance Organization (HMO). *Nicotine Tobacco Research* 2002; **4**(Suppl 1):S9–17.

Board N, Brennan N & Caplan GA. A randomised controlled trial of the costs of hospital as compared with hospital in the home for acute medical patients. *Australian and New Zealand Journal of Public Health* 2000; **24**(3):305–11.

British Geriatrics Society. *What's New at the BGS?* 2004, London, http://www.bgs.org.uk/homepages/new.htm.

Buzzell PR, Chamberlain VM & Pintauro SJ. The effectiveness of web-based, multimedia tutorials for teaching methods of human body composition analysis. *Advances in Physiology Education* 2002; **26**(1–4):21–9.

Cadogan MP, Schnelle JF, Yamamoto-Mitani N *et al.* A minimum data set prevalence of pain quality indicator: is it accurate and does it reflect differences in care processes? *Journals of Gerontology Series A-Biological Sciences and Medical Sciences* 2004; **59**(3):281–5.

Cameron ID, Handoll HHG, Finnegan TP *et al. Coordinated Multidisciplinary Approaches for Inpatient Rehabilitation of Older Patients with Proximal Femoral Fractures. Cochrane Methodology Review* 2003, Issue 4; John Wiley & Sons, Chichester, http//www.cochrane.org/reviews.

Capezuti E, Strumpf NE, Evans LK *et al.* The relationship between physical restraint removal and falls and injuries among nursing home residents. *Journals of Gerontology Series A-Biological Sciences and Medical Sciences* 1998; **53A**(1):M47–52.

Caplan GA, Ward JA, Brennan NJ *et al.* Hospital in the home: a randomised controlled trial. *Medical Journal of Australia* 1999; **170**(4):156–60.

Carroll AE, Tarczy-Hornoch P, O'Reilly E *et al.* The effect of point-of-care personal digital assistant use on resident documentation discrepancies. *Pediatrics* 2004; **113**(3 Part 1):450–4.

Center for Health Systems Research and Analysis. *Facility Guide for the Nursing Home Quality Indicators National Data System* 1999, http//www.cms.hhs.gov/medicaid/mds20/qifacman.pdf.

Centers for Medicare and Medicaid Services. *Home Health Quality Initiative Overview* 2003, http://www.cms.hhs.gov/quality/hhqi/HHQIOverview.pdf.

Clinical Accountability, Service Planning and Evaluation (CASPE). *Spain Summary Report* 2004, London, http://www.caspe.co.uk/expert/spain.htm.

Collins MF. Measuring performance indicators in clinical pharmacy services with a personal digital assistant. *American Journal of Health-System Pharmacy* 2004; **61**:498–501.

Counsel S, Holder C, Liebenauer L *et al.* Effects of a multi-component intervention on functional outcomes and process of care in hospitalized older patients. *Journal of the American Geriatrics Society* 2000; **48**:1571–81.

Department of Health. *Secretaries of State for Health, Wales, and Northern Ireland, and Scotland* Working for Patients. Medical audit. Working Paper 1989; HMSO, London.

Dickenson E & Sinclair AJ. Clinical Audit of Health Care. In J Pathy (ed) *Principles and Practice of Geriatric Medicine* 1998, 3rd edn; John Wiley & Sons, Chichester, pp 1575–81.

Filippi A, Sabatini A, Badioli L *et al.* Effects of an automated electronic reminder in changing the antiplatelet drug-prescribing behavior among Italian general practitioners in diabetic patients: an intervention trial. *Diabetes Care* 2003; **26**(5):1497–500.

Fink R. HMO data systems in population studies of access to care. *Health Services Research* 1998; **33**(3 Pt 2):741–59.

Gerson LB & Van Dam J. A prospective randomized trial comparing a virtual reality simulator to bedside teaching for training in sigmoidoscopy. *Endoscopy* 2003; **35**(7):569–75.

Grantcharov TP, Kristiansen VB, Bendix J *et al.* Randomized clinical trial of virtual reality simulation for laparoscopic skills training. *British Journal of Surgery* 2004; **91**(2):146–50.

Heaton C. External peer review in Europe: an overview from the ExPeRT Project. *International Journal for Quality in Health Care* 2000; **12**(3):177–82.

Incalzi RA, Gemma A, Capparella O *et al.* Continuous geriatric care in orthopedic wards: A valuable alternative to orthogeriatric units. *Aging-Clinical and Experimental Research* 1993; **5**:207–16.

Inouye SK, Peduzzi PN, Robison JT *et al.* Importance of functional measures in predicting mortality among older hospitalized patients. *JAMA* 1998a; **279**(15):1187–93.

Inouye SK, Rushing JT, Foreman MD *et al.* Does delirium contribute to poor hospital outcomes? A three-site epidemiologic study. *Journal of General Internal Medicine* 1998b; **13**(4):234–42.

International Organization for Standardization. 2004, About ISO, http://www.iso.org/iso/en/aboutiso/introduction/index.html#four.

Joint Commission on Accreditation of Healthcare Organizations. *A Journey Through the History~of the Joint Commission* 2004, Oakbrook Terrace, http://www.jcaho.org/about+us/history/index.htm.

Jordan JA, Gallagher AG, McGuigan J *et al.* A comparison between randomly alternating imaging, normal laparoscopic imaging, and virtual reality training in laparoscopic psychomotor skill acquisition. *American Journal of Surgery* 2000; **180**(3):208–11.

Kennie DC, Reid J, Richardson IR *et al.* Effectiveness of geriatric rehabilitative care after fractures of the proximal femur in elderly women: a randomized clinical trial. *British Medical Journal* 1988; **297**:1083–6.

Kitahata MM, Dillingham PW, Chaiyakunapruk N *et al.* Electronic human immunodeficiency virus (HIV) clinical reminder system improves adherence to practice guidelines among the University of Washington HIV Study Cohort. *Clinical Infectious Diseases* 2003; **36**(6):803–11.

Kornowski R, Zeeli D, Averbuch M *et al.* Intensive home-care surveillance prevents hospitalization and improves morbidity rates among elderly patients with severe congestive heart failure. *American Heart Journal* 1995; **129**:762–6.

Landefeld C, Palmer R, Kresevic D *et al.* A randomized trial of care in a hospital medical unit especially designed to improve the functional outcomes of acutely ill older patients. *New England Journal of Medicine* 1995; **332**:1338–44.

Leap LL, Brennan TA, Laird N *et al.* The nature of adverse events in hospitalized patients. Results of the harvard medical practice study II. *New England Journal of Medicine* 1991; **324**:277–84.

Maiolo C, Mohamed EI, Fiorani CM *et al.* Home telemonitoring for patients with severe respiratory illness: the Italian experience. *Journal of Telemedicine and Telecare* 2003; **9**(2):67–71.

Mehra MR, Uber PA, Chomsky DB *et al.* Emergence of electronic home monitoring in chronic heart failure. *Chemical Heritage* 2000; **6**:137–9.

Miller MR, Elixhauser A, Zhan C *et al.* Patient safety indicators: using administrative data to identify potential patient safety concerns. *Health Services Research* 2001; **36**:110–32.

Mullooly J, Drew L, DeStefano F *et al.* Quality of HMO vaccination databases used to monitor childhood vaccine safety. *American Journal of Epidemiology* 1999; **149**(2):186–94.

O'Muircheartaigh C, Burke A, Murphy W. *U.S. News and World Report's America's Best Hospital. The 2004 Index of Hospital Quality* 2004, http://www.usnews.com/usnews/health/hosptl/methodology/methodology_2004.pdf, Accessed August 13, 2004.

Pallawala PM & Lun KC. EMR-based TeleGeriatric system. *Medinfo* 2001; **10**(pt 1):849–53.

Richardson WC & Corrigan JM. The IOM quality initiative: a progress report at year six. Shaping the future. *Newsletter of the IOM* 2002; **1**(1):1–8.

Rogers MA, Small D, Buchan DA *et al.* Home monitoring service improves mean arterial pressure in patients with essential hypertension. A randomized, controlled trial. *Annals of Internal Medicine* 2001; **134**(11):1024–32.

Saliba D & Schnelle JF. Indicators of the quality of nursing home residential care. *Journal of the American Geriatrics Society* 2002; **50**:1421–30.

Schnelle JF, Bates-Jensen BM, Levy-Storms L *et al.* The minimum data set prevalence of restraint quality indicator: does it reflect differences in care? *Gerontologist* 2004; **44**(2):245–55.

Seabra D, Srougi M, Baptista R *et al.* Computer aided learning versus standard lecture for undergraduate education in urology. *Journal of Urology* 2004; **171**(3):1220–2.

Shaw CD. *Accreditation in Europe: Survey 2001* 2002; CASPE Research, London, http://www.forumq.at/Downloads/Shaw%20-%20APE%20summary%2007-2002.pdf.

Shaw P, Elliott C, Isaacson P *et al. Quality and Performance Improvement in Health Care. A Tool for Programmed Learning* 2003, 2nd edn; American Health Information Management Association, Chicago, Also available on the World Wide Web http://library.ahima.org/xpedio/groups/public/documents/ahima/bok1_020002.pdf.

Singhal V & Hendricks K. *Quality Award Winners also Improve Financial Performance* 2001, Atlanta, http://www.efqm.org/model_awards/downloads/3%20page%20summary.pdf.

Spickard A, Alrajeh N, Cordray D *et al.* Learning about screening using an online or live lecture: does it matter? *Journal of General Internal Medicine* 2002; **17**(7):540–5.

Stengel D, Bauwens K, Walter M *et al.* Comparison of handheld computer-assisted and conventional paper chart documentation of medical records. *Journal of Bone and Joint Surgery* 2004; **86A**(3):553–60.

Stuck AE, Siu AL, Wieland GD *et al.* Comprehensive geriatric assessment: a meta-analysis of controlled trials. *Lancet* 1993; **342**:1032–6.

The Australian Council on Healthcare Standards. *Who We Are* 2002; Ultimo New South Wales, Australia, http://www.achs.org.au/.

The Department of Health. *Standard Four-General Hospital Care* 2004, London, http://www.dh.gov.uk/PolicyAndGuidance/HealthAndSocialCareTopicc/OlderPeoplesSebvices/fc/en.

The Leapfrog Group for Patient Safety. *Fact Sheet*. April 2004, Washington, http://www.leapfroggroup.org/FactSheets/LF_FactSheet.pdf, Accessed June 29, 2004.

Vichitvejpaisal P, Sitthikongsak S, Preechakoon B *et al.* Does computer-assisted instruction really help to improve the learning process? *Medical Education* 2001; **35**(10):983–9.

Williams C, Aubin S, Harkin P *et al.* A randomized, controlled, single-blind trial of teaching provided by a computer-based multimedia package versus lecture. *Medical Education* 2001; **35**(9):847–54.

Zimmerman DR, Karon SL, Arling G *et al.* Development and testing of nursing home quality indicators. *Health Care Financing Review* 1995; **16**(4):107–27.

Appendix 1: Health-care quality organizations

Abbreviation	Organization	Origin	Created
ACHS	Australian Council for Health Care Standards	Australia	1974
AGS	American Geriatrics Society	United States	1942
AHRQ	Agency for Health care Research and Quality	United States	1989
AMDA	American Medical Directors Association	United States	1978
ASGM	Australian Society for Geriatric Medicine (Previously Australian Association of Gerontology and Australian Geriatrics Society)	Australia	1960s
BGS	British Geriatric Society	United Kingdom	1947
CAHPS	Consumer Assessment of Health Plans	United States	1999
CHAP	Catalan Hospital Accreditation Programme	Spain	1981
CMS	Centers for Medicare and Medicaid Services (Previously Health Care Financing Administration: HCFA)	United States	2001 (HCFA 1977)
EFQM	European Foundation for Quality Management	Europe	1988
HAP	Health care Accreditation Programme	United Kingdom	1990
HC	Health care Commission	United Kingdom	2004
HQS	Health Quality Service (Previously Kings Fund Organisational Audit: KFOA	United Kingdom	1998 (KFOA 1989)
IEC	International Electrotechnical Commission	United States	1906
IOM	Institute of Medicine	United States	1970
ISA	International Federation of the National Standardizing Association	Europe	1926
ISO	International Organization for Standardization	United Kingdom	1947
ISQua	The International Society for Quality in Health Care	Australia	1985
JCAH	Joint Commission on Accreditation of Hospitals	United States	1951
JCAHO	Joint Commission on Accreditation of Health care Organizations	United States	1987
NCQA	National Committee for Quality Assurance	United States	1990
NHS	National Health Service	United Kingdom	1948
RACP	Royal Australian College of Physicians	Australia	1938
USPSTF	U. S. Preventive Services Task Force	United States	1984
VAMC	Department of Veterans Affairs Medical Centers (Previously Veterans Administration: VA)	United States	1989 (VA 1930)

Resident Assessment Instrument/ Minimum Data Set

Brant E. Fries[1], Catherine Hawes[2], John N. Morris[3] *and* Roberto Bernabei[3,4]

[1] University of Michigan and Ann Arbor Veterans' Affairs Medical Center, Ann Arbor, MI, USA, [2] Texas A&M University System Health Science Center, College Station, TX, USA, [3] Hebrew Rehabilitation Center for Aged, Boston, MA, USA, and [4] Università Cattolica del Sacro Cuore, Rome, Italy

INTRODUCTION – COMPREHENSIVE GERIATRIC ASSESSMENT

Care of frail elderly individuals requires attention to a broad range of potentially interrelated problems. With advancing age, individuals are likely to have several chronic medical problems and conditions that need to be managed, and the need to take multiple prescriptions that have to be reviewed, and whose side effects need to be identified, monitored, and controlled. At the same time, appropriate care will also address issues of functionality – both physical and cognitive – to help maintain independence or assure that necessary assistance is available. In addition, an older person's well-being may be affected by the individual's social environment: whether she (the more likely gender) is isolated, able to get out (of her room in a nursing facility, of her home), and is able to interact reasonably successfully and often with others. Physical environment also plays a role in either helping frail elders maintain independence or placing them at risk, and must be evaluated. These are only some of the issues that may be part of a comprehensive geriatric assessment.

It would be impossible to address all of the potential issues that affect the health, functioning, and psychosocial well-being of a frail elder in a single assessment tool. One possible solution is to develop a tool that will permit the identification and codification, within a reasonable time frame, of sufficient information to allow a professional to identify problems or risk factors that serve as the basis for additional assessment and clinical interventions or care planning. This compromise is a "Minimum Data Set" (MDS). It is also important that the assessment items be standardized: rather than locally accumulated "baskets" of information, uniform information should be obtained using scientifically tested items. These items then begin to support a "language" for understanding and discussing long-term care.

While the driving force for developing an MDS is to support clinical decision-making around the care of an individual person at one point in time, it is easy to expand these notions to following individual's trajectories over time – how has the person come to this point in time? Are the problems we see now new or are they persistent manifestations of problems that have already been addressed? Knowing what a person was like, just prior to the onset of a hip fracture or stroke, can be critical in developing goals for recovery and clinical interventions. Thus, for a frail elder, an MDS can provide a structure for basic information that identifies the need for additional assessment that will ultimately generate the critical information needed to arrive at care decisions.

Beyond decision making for the individual, these same data have a spectrum of applications that greatly enrich the value of an MDS. These include monitoring quality, measuring outcomes, determining eligibility for services, setting payment levels based on acuity, evaluating programs, and developing policy.

In this chapter, we discuss one particular family of Minimum Data Sets, anchored on the United State's National Nursing-Home Resident Assessment Instrument (RAI), often referred to as the MDS. In particular, we address the design, development, and testing of the Nursing-Home MDS, other allied MDSs for other care sectors (such as home-care), applications of MDS data beyond care planning, implementation of these instruments in the United States and abroad, and finally, issues and future opportunities.

Principles and Practice of Geriatric Medicine, 4th Edition. Edited by M.S. John Pathy, Alan J. Sinclair and John E. Morley.

DEVELOPMENT OF THE NATIONAL NURSING-HOME RESIDENT ASSESSMENT INSTRUMENT/MINIMUM DATA SET

A long series of documented abuses in nursing homes increasingly prevalent in the 1960–1970s began to focus attention on the deplorable status of nursing-home care. A series of legal actions in the late 1970s and early 1980s confirmed the responsibility of the US Government, as a principal payer, to assure the quality of such care. Thus, in 1982, Congress requested from the Institute of Medicine (IOM) a study of the existing regulations, and recommended changes that would strengthen the regulations and enhance the ability of nursing facilities to ensure satisfactory care for their residents (IOM, 1986). The IOM report suggested a series of reforms of the "Conditions of Participation," the standards or requirements that nursing homes must meet in order to be eligible for federal and state funds for care of Medicare and Medicaid beneficiaries. The reforms recommended by the IOM were comprehensive and included provisions addressing standards, the inspection process, and enforcement, and recommended increased aide training, minimum staffing by registered nurses, and assurance of quality of care, quality of life, and the rights of residents.

A 2-year study, including a series of hearings, led to the IOM report (1986), in which one of the central conclusions was that the development of a uniform, comprehensive resident assessment system was essential for improving the quality of care in the nation's nursing homes. The Committee viewed comprehensive functional assessment as the cornerstone of individualized care planning that would focus on helping each resident attain and maintain their maximum practicable functioning and well-being.

Spurred by the legal requirements of court cases and pressure from advocates, many of the IOM recommendations were passed into law as part of the Omnibus Budget Reconciliation Act of 1987 (OBRA '87). One mandate was that the Health Care Financing Administration (now the Centers for Medicare & Medicaid Services – CMS) fund the development and then the implementation in 1991 of the "National Nursing-Home Resident Assessment Instrument/Minimum Data Set."

The new instrument system was designed to support care planning. To accomplish this, it consists of several parts. The first is the Minimum Data Set (MDS), the assessment itself, containing the core items necessary for a comprehensive assessment of the residents of nursing homes. On the other hand, it also includes items that only supported care planning, no matter how urgent or attractive other items were. The domains covered are shown in Table 1. Items are also described in greater detail in an accompanying *RAI Training Manual* (Morris *et al.*, 1996).

The MDS also provides "triggers". These are individual items or combinations of MDS elements which identify residents for whom specific Resident Assessment Protocols (RAPs) – the second part of the system – should be completed. The triggers were developed to identify current problems or the potential for improved function, as well as

Table 1 MDS 2.0 Domains

Identification and background information	Health conditions
Cognitive patterns	Oral/nutritional status
Communication/Hearing patterns	Oral/dental status
Vision patterns	Skin condition
Mood and behavior patterns	Activity pursuit patterns
Psychological well-being	Medications
Physical functioning and structural problems	Special treatments and procedures
Continence in last 14 days	Discharge potential and overall status
Disease diagnoses	Assessment information

Table 2 Resident assessment protocols (RAPs)

Delirium	Cognitive loss/dementia
Visual function	Communication
Activities of daily living function/rehabilitation	Urinary incontinence and indwelling catheter
Psychosocial well-being	Mood state
Behavioral symptoms	Activities
Falls	Nutritional status
Feeding tubes	Dehydration/fluid maintenance
Dental care	Pressure ulcers
Psychotropic drug use	Physical restraints

predictors of who is likely to have a problem in the future; thus, they indicate those people who have or are at risk of developing a problem. There are 18 RAPs, each addressing a major problem in the care of nursing-home residents. Table 2 lists the nursing-home RAPs. These assessment protocols are not intended to automate care planning or to create "cookie cutter" care plans that look the same for all clients. Instead, they are intended to help the clinician focus on key issues identified during the assessment process, so that the provider and the client can explore whether and how to intervene and develop an individualized plan of care. Each RAP has a structured framework – guidelines – for conducting additional assessment. This additional assessment is intended to clarify the nature of the problem or risk factor, to identify underlying causes, such as diseases or side effects of a medication, and to explore the potential for treatment or management of the condition and the medical causes. This information is used by the facility, ideally a multi disciplinary team including the resident's physician, to develop an individualized plan of care to address the targeted problem.

The intent of the protocol is educational rather than prescriptive. Each RAP organizes the information from MDS items that can be used to inform the care planning process and identifies additional assessment items and background information that might be needed. Thus, RAPs provide a formal context in which information about residents, their strengths, preferences, and needs, can be linked to care plan options. The guidelines, in essence, also ask the care planners to consider whether one problem may masquerade as another: have you considered that loss of communication attributed to dementia might actually be caused in this patient by a loss of hearing? Could this be a side effect of a particular medication and have you considered a "drug holiday" or a change in therapeutic dose? While not telling the clinical staff what to do, the guidelines challenge and help the care planner think through the process of care for the individual elder. Overall, the RAPs are critical in that they help clinical staff understand how they can use the assessment data. Together, the MDS assessment, RAPs, and their triggers form the RAI system.

Several approaches were employed in the development of the MDS to improve the validity and reliability of the assessment process and resulting data. These included design decisions such as the following:

- To assess residents' performance and function rather than potential function. For example, rather than ask whether a resident could dress, the MDS asks how they dress, with an included possible response that the activity did not occur in the past seven days.
- To describe manifested conditions or behavior rather than interpretations of the condition or behavior. Thus, the MDS asks whether the resident had "sad, pained, or worried facial expressions" or "crying/tearfulness" rather than asking whether the resident was sad.
- To include full definitions of items and responses on the form. For example, rather than just have an item refer to "eating", it's better to indicate what is meant, directly on the form. The MDS assessment form includes the definitions and response categories that address what to do if the resident is fed by others, gets nutrition through a tube, or feeds himself, but does so while dropping food on his clothing and the table Thus, the MDS uses the definition – "How resident eats and drinks (regardless of skill). Includes intake of nourishment by other means (e.g., tube feeding, total parenteral nutrition)". Another example is diagnoses, where those recorded should be "only those diseases that have a relationship to current Activity of Daily Living status, cognitive status, mood and behavior status, medical treatments, nursing monitoring, or risk of death (do not list inactive diagnoses)".
- To include examples and exclusions that deal with common confusion about how to respond for an item. To return to the eating example, should a person be considered dependent in eating if they require someone to open a milk carton or carry their tray to a table? The MDS identifies such assistance as "set-up help" and has a special response code for this. Such information needs, however, to be part of the assessment system and clearly indicated on the form (instrument) or in training material.
- To include time delimiters. For example, an assessor might be confused about how to score the resident who was unable to dress herself on the day of the assessment (due to a flare-up of his arthritis) but dressed independently the rest of the week. The lack of such specification would make the information unreliable, so the MDS contains time frames that are carefully specified for each item.
- To cover many domains and focus on function. Any assessment of elders must go beyond medical conditions and diagnosis to physical and mental function, as well as psychosocial well-being and measures of involvement. Further, the MDS attempts to address not only individuals' weaknesses, but also their strengths and preferences. The "down side" is that an assessment instrument can get excessively long, and a balance between length and comprehensiveness has to be found: not every item, scale, or even domain can be included, for this would be unwieldy. While not small (with close to 400 items), the MDS was the smallest instrument that would balance these competing goals
- To use all possible sources of information. There are distinct advantages to self-reported assessments, not only because they can usually be accomplished with less cost but also because, more importantly, they capture subjective feelings and opinions of the subject. However, some information is not provided well by the elder, such as diagnoses or the use of health services. The elder cannot be trained in accurate assessment or may bias a response because of embarrassment, avoidance, or lack of knowledge or perspective. The best scenario, used in the MDS, is to combine the two methods, collecting information both directly from the elder and from all others knowledgeable about the elder, including family, health care professionals (e.g., physicians, nurses, social workers, therapists, and nurse aides) and nonprofessionals, such as a spouse, adult, child, or neighbor who helps the elder. Further, it uses information in the medical record and the clinician's own observations of the resident, and asks the clinician conducting the assessment to use all appropriate sources in making decisions. When the information gathered from these multiple sources is contradictory, the assessor should use his or her best judgment of which is the most appropriate.
- To use "items" rather than "questions". To gather information on a particular topic, the MDS describes the information needed rather than posing a specific question. There are several advantages to this approach. This provides assessors with the greatest flexibility and encourages them to use multiple sources of information, including their own observations. While items are ordered on the instrument, without a fixed "script", there is no fixed order in which information is gathered, making the assessment process simultaneously more efficient and more accurate.

The approach taken to the development of the RAI included highly systematic development of the conceptual framework, basic reliability testing of the instrument and training materials, extensive field testing, design of data flow systems, and detailed planning of the implementation. A wide range of clinicians and researchers was included at every stage of the process. The professionals came from a wide spectrum of clinical disciplines including nursing, social work, medicine, physiotherapy, occupational therapy, speech therapy, recreational activity, and nutrition. Also represented were consumers, resident advocates, providers, representatives of the nursing-home industry, and regulators and measurement specialists.

The RAI system was implemented in 1990–1991 throughout the United States, in all nursing facilities that participate in the Medicare or Medicaid programs – 98% of all nursing homes in the country. Facilities must use the MDS/RAI to assess all residents (regardless of who pays for their care) upon admission and to develop their plan of care. It is also used to assess residents annually after admission and upon any significant change in their health status. A reduced "Quarterly Assessment" is performed to monitor the effects of care and the need for modifications to the care plan. The MDS assessment itself takes approximately two hours to complete for a new admission, about three-quarters of that time for an annual reassessment, and half that time for the reduced quarterly assessments, all excluding the time to develop the care plans. The average nursing-home resident triggers on approximately eight of the RAPs around which care planning must be considered. A care plan intervention may not be implemented for all triggered RAPs for a variety of reasons. For example, the multidisciplinary care planning team may set priorities among the existing problems and address a few in order of importance. Alternatively, the clinicians may conclude that addressing one area, such as depression, may also resolve another, such as nutritional risk, if they conclude that the resident's leaving food uneaten is a sign of the depression. The federally mandated nursing-home survey system, as part of ensuring compliance with acceptable standards of care, audits MDS assessments and their use by facilities in care planning. Some states also audit MDS data if it is used for payment or eligibility determinations.

A revised RAI was implemented in 1996, and beginning June 1998, facilities were required to submit computerized assessments to CMS that developed a national archive for research and monitoring purposes.

The MDS has been tested multiple times for inter-rater reliability. The tests conducted throughout the country have included inter-rater reliability among trained nurse assessors in nursing homes, facility versus research staff, nursing homes that are large and small, and those run for profit and those that are voluntary. These tests have demonstrated high levels of item reliability (as measured by the kappa statistic) in the initial MDS (Hawes *et al.*, 1995) and even higher with the revised instrument (Morris *et al.*, 1997). The most recent evidence comes from an extensive study performed for CMS as part of a six-state study of quality indicators. A reliability study collected dual assessments of a total of 5758 residents in 209 facilities. In each instance, a research nurse independently assessed a resident who had recently been assessed by facility staff. The two assessments were quite close. For example, for the MDS items describing cognitive and physical functional and clinical areas, the average Kappa reliability obtained was 0.79, which was very close to the average of 0.84 which was obtained when similar cases were scored by two research nurses. In fact, only about 4% of facilities were found to have deficient reliability scores. The general conclusion was that the MDS is being completed with reasonable consistency in American nursing homes (Morris *et al.*, 2002).

Field testing has addressed not only item reliability but also how users assess the reasons for any misclassification, misunderstandings of items and instructions, and the "value" of individual items for the care planning process. Additionally, research has addressed the validity of items and scales; we shall discuss this work later.

The structure of the RAI system and its direct use in clinical care planning has enabled it to achieve many of its goals. Its introduction in the United States led to observable changes in the quality and outcome of care. The evaluation examined the care of a sample of 2000 nursing-home residents in 255 facilities in 10 states, at two points in time in 1990 and 1991 before the RAI implementation, with a comparable cohort of residents in those facilities at two points in time during 1993. This evaluation demonstrated several significant changes in process and outcome quality, including:

- an increase in the comprehensiveness and accuracy of the information available in residents' medical records (Hawes *et al.*, 1997);
- an increase in the comprehensiveness of care planning, with care plans in the post-RAI period addressing a greater percentage of residents' health problems, risk factors, and their potential for improved function (Hawes *et al.*, 1997);
- an improvement in a wide array of other care processes that affect residents' quality of care and quality of life, including increased involvement of families and residents in care planning, increased use of advance directives, increased use of behavior management programs, increased involvement in activities, and decreased use of problematic interventions, such as indwelling urinary catheters and physical restraints (Hawes *et al.*, 1997; Teno *et al.*, 1997);
- a significant reduction in decline among residents in such areas as physical functioning in Activities of Daily Living (ADLs), cognitive status, and urinary continence (Phillips *et al.*, 1997); and
- a significant reduction in the number of nursing-home residents who were hospitalized, with no increase in mortality (Mor *et al.*, 1997b).

Currently, there are two ongoing efforts to revise the RAI. The first, funded by CMS, will revise the RAI for use in the United States, including adding items that can address issues of quality of life and satisfaction (Kane *et al.*, 2003). There is a separate effort by the initial RAI designers, in concert with an international research consortium, to develop an integrated suite of assessment instruments for the broader field of long-term care. We describe this latter effort next.

OTHER MINIMUM DATA SETS FOR LONG-TERM CARE

The success of the RAI/MDS for nursing homes encouraged the development of parallel assessment systems for other long-term care sectors. The inter*RAI* group, a nonprofit cross-national consortium of researchers including the developers of the original (nursing home) RAI, have developed a suite of instruments (interRAI, 2004), including:

- inter*RAI* LTCF – Long-term care facility (new version of the RAI)
- inter*RAI* HC – Home care
- inter*RAI* PC – Palliative care (institutional and community-based)
- inter*RAI* PAC – Post-acute care (institutional and community-based)
- inter*RAI* AL – Assisted living and residential care facilities
- inter*RAI* AC – Acute care – to address chronic care problems of individuals in hospitals with acute needs
- inter*RAI* MH – Mental health (psychiatric institutional care, short- and long-term)
- inter*RAI* CMH – Community mental health
- inter*RAI* CHA – Community health assessment (screener for lighter-care individuals in community settings)

Development is also proceeding on two additional instrument systems:

- inter*RAI* ID – Intellectual disability - persons with mental retardation and developmental disabilities
- inter*RAI* PWD – Persons with disability (younger individuals, usually under age 55, in both community and institutional settings)

Each instrument includes both an assessment – a Minimum Data Set – and applicable care planning guidelines (Clinical Assessment Protocols, like the RAPs for the RAI, discussed earlier). Each also has been tested for reliability and validity of items.

Although each instrument in the interRAI family of Minimum Data Sets has been developed for a particular population, they are designed to work together to form an integrated health information system (Hirdes *et al.*, 1999). In particular, all share a common language, that is, they refer to the same clinical concept in the same way across instruments. Using common measures enable clinicians and providers in different care settings to improve continuity of care, as well as to integrate care/support for each individual. Common language also allows families, advocates, and public payers to track the progress of program participants across settings and over time. Such information can yield important findings regarding what works to improve an individual's quality of life. On the other hand, specific items have been developed for each specific application. For example, the home-care instrument documents the individual's capability to perform more integrative activities (instrumental ADLs such as shopping, managing medications, housekeeping, etc.), environmental problems, and caregiver support; the palliative care instrument adds information on the individual's ability to address unfinished business and increased detail about pain control; the acute care instrument looks back to functional capability before the precipitating event of the stay, and so forth.

Table 3 Client assessment protocol (CAP) areas

Functional performance	Health problems/syndromes
ADL rehabilitation potential	Cardio-respiratory
Instrumental Activities of Daily Living (IADLs)	Dehydration
Health promotion	Falls
Institutional risk	Nutrition
Sensory performance	Oral health
Communication disorders	Pain
Visual function	Pressure ulcers
Mental health	Skin & foot conditions
Alcohol dependence & hazardous drinking	*Service oversight*
Cognition	Adherence
Behavior	Brittle support system
Depression and anxiety	Medication management
Elder abuse	Palliative care
Social function	Preventive health measures
Continence	Psychotropic drugs
Bladder management	Reduction in formal services
Urinary incontinence & indwelling catheter	Environmental assessment

As an example, the list of care planning areas addressed by home-care instrument (inter*RAI* HC) is shown in Table 3.

Thus, the suite of instruments provides a balance between common measures across the long-term care continuum and specialized measures for particular care environments. In 2005, the "harmonization" of all of the inter*RAI* instruments will be complete. This will assure that all items on multiple instruments have exactly the same wording and the same time frames, and will incorporate the experience of over a decade of their use to eliminate assessment items that have not worked and add new domains that need to be addressed. In the process, many of the instruments have been substantially shortened and divided into modules so that certain domains (e.g., mental health problems in home-care population) are only assessed in detail for individuals who meet specified triggering criteria.

APPLICATIONS OF MDS DATA

Although the sole primary function of the MDS is to support care planning, a variety of other applications of MDS data are valuable. Two – case-mix payment and quality measurement – have attracted the most interest, but other applications represent important capabilities that are available directly from secondary use of data already collected primarily for clinical purposes. The applications discussed here can apply to all of the instruments listed in the previous section, although not all have been developed for each instrument.

Scales and Profiles

The multitude of individual items in an MDS can make it difficult to describe major domains, such as depression or cognitive impairment. There is great advantage to have a single measure (index or categories), which can have direct clinical utility in a summary report about an individual. However, such a measure can also be used in a profile of program participants to provide epidemiological insight into the status of a target population, in an outcome measure (for example, for measuring quality or program evaluation), or as a covariate in a research study. An additional advantage is that scale development represents a criterion validation of MDS items, by comparing them with known and trusted external measures.

For the nursing home and home-care MDS, the following represent some of the scales that have been developed and validated:

- *Activities of Daily Living Hierarchy*: The ADL Hierarchy Scale groups the various activities of daily living according to the stages of the disablement process. Early-loss ADLs (e.g., dressing) are assigned lower scores than late-loss ADLs (e.g. eating). The ADL Hierarchy Scale provides six categories ranging from no impairment to total dependence (Morris *et al.*, 1999).
- *Cognitive Performance Scale*: The Cognitive Performance Scale (CPS) combines six items on memory impairment, level of consciousness, and executive function/daily decision-making, to produce a scale with seven levels from intact to very severe impairment. A variety of validation studies have demonstrated that the CPS is highly correlated with the Folstein Mini-Mental Status Examination (Morris *et al.*, 1994).
- *CHESS Scale*: The Changes in Health, End-stage Disease and Signs and Symptoms (CHESS) scale was designed to identify individuals at risk of serious decline. It can serve as an outcome indicator where the objective of care and services is to minimize problems related to declines in function. CHESS, originally developed for use in the nursing home, has been adapted for use with the MDS-HC. It uses six items to create a five-point scale. In both the nursing home and home-care populations, there is clear differentiation of all six levels of CHESS scores, and higher levels are predictive of adverse outcomes like mortality, hospitalization, pain, caregiver stress, and poor self-rated health (Hirdes *et al.*, 2003).
- *Depression Rating Scale*: The count of seven MDS depression items has been validated in a comparison of the DRS with the Hamilton Depression Rating Scale and the Cornell Scale for Depression. Compared to DSM-IV major or minor depression diagnoses, the DRS was 91% sensitive and 69% specific at a cutoff score of 3 out of 7 (Burrows *et al.*, 2000).
- *IADL Involvement Scale*: This scale is based upon a sum of seven items: meal preparation, ordinary housework, managing finances, medications, phone use, shopping, and transportation. Individual items are summed to produce a scale that ranges from 0 to 42, with higher scores indicating greater difficulty in performing instrumental activities.
- *Pain Scale*: The Pain Scale was originally developed for use in nursing homes and later translated for use with the MDS-HC. The scale uses two items to create a four-level score that has been shown to be highly predictive of pain in nursing-home residents as measured on the Visual Analogue Scale (Fries *et al.*, 2001).

Reports that combine these scales, potentially with individual items (such as diagnoses or services received) and other measures (e.g., case-mix categories; see the following text) can be useful both at the individual (clinical) level and when summarized for programs or populations. At the individual level, a summary profile can provide a "cover sheet" for a patient's chart or a "transfer document" that would follow a patient to another care setting: hospital, nursing home, and so on. For example, the Province of Ontario, Canada is experimenting with the "Personal Health Profile" that provides a one-page abstract of the home-care MDS, outlining key clinical points of interest to a nursing home admitting this individual. There is value also at an aggregate level, to describe those enrolled and cared for in a program. For example, the State of Michigan has used profiles of its home- and community-based programs to understand differences among the several agencies statewide providing services, and to compare those maintained with home care and those in nursing homes.

Case mix

Case mix is the identification of individuals' characteristics related to the cost of their care. In this application, the goal is to use MDS items in a system that can measure which individual uses more care and to measure the cost of this care. Initially, case-mix development was aimed at improving our understanding of the cost differences between nursing homes. Rapidly, it became clear that facilities varied in the range and distribution of types of residents for whom they cared, and that a method for relating resident characteristics to resource use was central to understanding underlying differences in the cost structures of nursing homes. Moreover, with the successful US implementation of the Diagnosis-Related Groups (Fetter *et al.*, 1991) case-mix system for acute care hospitals in the mid-1980s, the development of case-mix classification systems for all types of institutional providers became of immediate interest for the design of government payment systems. It was recognized that payment systems that recognize varying care needs of patients will, all other things being equal, promote more equitable provision of resources appropriate to patient needs.

The most used (MDS-based) nursing-home case-mix system is the Resource Utilization Groups (RUGs). The latest version, RUG-III, is part of the federal system for paying nursing homes under Medicare as well as almost a half of all state-funded systems in the United States; it is also used in Catalonia (Spain) and is to be implemented in three Canadian provinces and Iceland.

RUG-III (Fries *et al.*, 1994) is the algorithm that used 107 MDS items to group the nursing-home residents to explain resource use – per diem wage-weighted hours and minutes spent by facility staff caring for residents. The system incorporates up to three dimensions in describing a resident. The first dimension indicates one of the seven major types of nursing-home residents (Special Rehabilitation, Extensive Care, Special Care, Clinically Complex, Cognitively Impaired, Behavioral Problems, and Reduced Physical Functions, in decreasing order of resource use). The second dimension is an ADL index, a summary measure of functional capability, produced by combining four ADL measures (toileting, eating, transfer, and bed mobility). Although ADLs are the most effective measures in explaining resource use, they demonstrate even greater statistical power within defined major types of residents. Also, four ADLs are sufficient; additional ADLs provide little marginal information about resource use. The final dimension describes particular services (such as nursing rehabilitation) or problems (such as behavior). In combination, a total of 44 mutually exclusive RUG-III groups are formed.

Associated with each of the RUG-III groups is a case-mix index, a relative measure of the cost of caring for an individual in this group. Across the 44 groups, there is over a nine-to-one difference in this measure.

This range of resource use argues well for the appropriateness of incorporating case mix in payment systems. Nevertheless, the design of such payment systems is considerably more complex than simply the technical incorporation of case-mix. A few of the issues that need to be addressed include determination of the cost centers to be adjusted by case mix; whether the system will be historic cost-based or pricing; the design of incentives, for example, for discharge, admission of heavy care residents, or other desired facility behaviors.

While most focus historically has been on the use of case mix solely for payment system design, it can assist in facility management (e.g., helping identify trends in the types of residents admitted), staffing decisions (e.g., balancing wards compared to the staff assigned), comparing facilities, and serving as a single measure to best capture the differences in the mix of patients across facilities in statistical analyses (e.g., as a case-mix adjustor for quality indicators).

The use of RUG-III for cross-national comparisons has been greatly enhanced by a series of studies in different European and Pacific-rim nations, demonstrating that it appropriately distinguished the types of resident and that the relative relationship represented by the case-mix indexes holds across nations and care settings, the ratio of care times between residents from two RUG-III groups will be the same (Carpenter *et al.*, 1997). RUG-III thus is an important MDS scale for international comparisons.

There are case-mix systems developed as well for home care, assisted living, and mental health. The home-care system – RUG-III/HC – is a close parallel to the nursing-home RUG-III, thus permitting case-mix comparison of these two populations (Björkgren *et al.*, 2000).

Quality of Care

The MDS addresses quality of care issues in several manners. First, it has been mandated, designed, and implemented to help clinical staff better understand the needs of the residents under their care. With a comprehensive picture of the clinical, functional, social, and mental needs of their residents, staff can use the RAP system to focus on key problem areas and put in place an appropriate plan of care. Thus, the MDS can help *produce* quality of care. Second, items in the MDS can be combined to measure characteristics and outcomes of care that form the indicators of quality of care. In the United States, the CMS and others have moved to the use of MDS-derived Quality Indicators as both a teaching tool to advance quality and as a consumer tool to help families make better choices. We discuss this second use here in more detail.

At the facility level, what stands out is the challenge of simultaneously providing good to superior care in multiple outcome areas. Most of the problems assessed in the MDS do not necessarily relate to one another. Thus, if a facility gears up to provide superior pressure ulcer or restraint reduction care, these efforts will not by themselves carry over into good care in the areas of mood, pain, and delirium. To be a good to superior facility, staff will have to have reasonable clinical knowledge in a wide variety of areas. To achieve this objective will require lower staff turnover, a commitment to education, an active quality care initiative (e.g., a multiple problem CQI effort), staff buy-in at the highest levels, a true focus on the resident as the key to one's business effort, and accurate assessment of resident performance.

Key to this effort has been the emergence of validated quality indicators (QIs), constructed from resident-level clinical data from the MDS resident assessments and aggregated to the facility level. These QIs characterize the performance of nursing facilities on key measures of quality. According to this logic, facilities, state surveyors, purchasers of care, and family members can use performance measures to guide their understanding of the performance characteristics of different facilities. When problematic scores are found, families may be best advised to seek alternative homes for their loved ones, surveyors can focus on those clinical areas in which the home appears to be most deficient, and facilities can use these same data to target care problems for continuous quality improvement efforts.

Measures of nursing-home quality have been proposed and used by researchers in the past, but generally only for a small number of facilities or in select groups of facilities (Mor *et al.*, 1997a). Also, these measures were based upon aggregate data obtained about a nursing home, to compare the rate of events between facilities with various characteristics (Zinn, 1994). Two major efforts have developed quality indicators (QIs) based on the MDS and the appropriate case-mix adjustment mechanisms. The initial work by Zimmerman and colleagues (Zimmerman *et al.*, 1995) has more recently been expanded to a national study to design and validate nursing-home QIs: the CMS-funded MEGA Study (Morris *et al.*, 2002).

Multiple steps were involved in creating and validating QIs: relevant clinical events were identified (e.g., a fall, a stage 2 or higher pressure ulcer, or a decline in ADLs); the interval over which the events were to be measured was established (e.g., 90 days); the occurrence of these events among nursing-home residents over the specified time period was evaluated (e.g., too low a rate of occurrence would have negated the utility of an indicator); appropriate covariate adjustors were identified, to ensure that differential admission policies across facilities was not the cause for inter-facility variation in the rates; and, finally, the indicators were demonstrated valid, in that they were driven by facility processes of care rather than just measuring random occurrences.

The MEGA study QIs are multidimensional, encompassing clinical, functional, psychosocial, and other aspects of resident health and well-being. While single, simple composite measures would be attractive, this does not seem to be an adequate representation of quality. The MEGA team recommended that CMS utilize several QIs from each domain for purposes of public reporting, quality monitoring, and performance improvement.

In total, the MEGA study identified or created 45 quality indicators. Only two QIs had very low prevalence ("New insertion of indwelling catheter" and "Failure to improve and manage delirium" were below 5%); other QI rates ranged between 5 and 92% in nursing facilities. Of the remaining indicators, 13 of the chronic care indicators and four of the post-acute care indicators were judged to have quite a substantial process of care validation.

The chronic care quality indicators with the highest level of validity include (note: some represent multiple QIs, for high, low, or combined risk residents):

- Prevalence of indwelling catheter
- Bladder/bowel incontinence
- Urinary tract infections
- Infections
- Inadequate pain management
- Pressure ulcers
- Late-loss ADL worsening
- ADL worsening
- Locomotion worsening
- Improvement in walking
- Worsening bladder continence.

Four post-acute care quality indicators are highly valid, including:

- Failure to improve and manage delirium
- Inadequate pain management
- Failure to improve during early post-acute period
- Improvement in walking.

Quality indicators have several potential uses including: by facilities in management, for example in a continuous quality assurance system; by government agencies in targeting poor quality facilities for more intense quality of care surveys; by nursing-home organizations in identifying best care practices; and by consumers in identifying the best nursing homes for their loved ones. As an example of the last application, the CMS website now displays MDS-based QIs for all US nursing homes. There is ongoing research to determine whether the availability of such information actually affects consumer decisions.

Eligibility

MDS-HC data can also be used in screening systems intended to identify appropriate care pathways for clients. One issue that has most concerned policymakers has been the rising demand for long-term care services and the resulting costs. As a result, policymakers, advocates, and providers have been faced with the increasingly difficult task of prioritizing target population and allocating increasingly scarce public resources in a fair and equitable manner. Even in the absence of a financial objective, decisions need to be made as to the best setting for caring for an individual.

The data contained in an MDS – nursing home, home care, and so on – can support systematic, standardized methods for such screening and resource allocation activities. While some may be concerned about such use, there are two major advantages. First, the criteria can be developed objectively and scientifically, and are subject to scrutiny and refinement. Second, these systems should never be used without an appeal mechanism to address unusual cases. While appeals could be seen as a way to avoid the whole eligibility system, with both screening and assessment data these decisions can be tracked and used to distinguish between inappropriate "overrides" and potential improvements in the eligibility algorithms.

Several different screening tools currently available include:

MAPLe (Method for Assessing Priority Level): This screening system defines five priority levels that relate to the risk of adverse outcomes. Clients in the low priority level have no major functional, cognitive, behavioral, or environmental problems. Thus, they can be considered self-reliant. The high priority level is based on the presence of ADL impairment, cognitive impairment, wandering, behavior problems, and the client's status on the nursing-home risk CAP. Clients in the high priority level are nearly nine times more likely to be admitted to a long-term care facility than are the low priority clients. MAPLe also predicts caregiver stress (Hirdes *et al.*, 2002).

MI Choice: This 32-question screening tool is derived from the MDS-HC instrument and was developed for the Michigan Department of Community Health. The scoring algorithm groups individuals in one of five levels of care: nursing home, home care, intermittent personal care, homemaker, and information and referral services. The screen can be used over the phone to identify persons who are not likely to meet health, cognitive, and functional criteria for home care or institutional services. This enables expensive in-person assessment resources to be targeted to persons who have been identified by the screener as more likely to qualify as medically eligible for assistance. During the assessment process, MI Choice can also serve as a complement to the assessor's clinical insights and the individual's preferences about the most appropriate care setting (Fries *et al.*, 2002).

Resource utilization groups (RUG-III, RUG-III/HC): As described earlier, these are case-mix systems, identifying client groups that reflect the relative cost of services they are likely to consume. However, they can also enable decision-makers to identify groups of people who can be considered presumptively eligible for a particular service or benefit. In the US Medicare Prospective Payment System, certain RUG-III categories are determined to meet the Medicare eligible requirements (rehabilitation of skilled nursing services). RUG-III/HC will be used in Michigan to determine eligibility for nursing home or equivalent home- and community-based care.

Outcome Measures and Program Evaluation

Many MDS items or scales, taken from an individual assessment or from the contrast of two assessments of the same individual over a period of time, can serve as outcome measures. Three representative examples of the many possible ones include:

- The presence of any fall in the past 90 days is a negative outcome that is included in the nursing home and other MDSs. Similarly, hospitalization, the presence of pain, decubitus ulcers, loneliness, environmental problems, elder abuse, and so on, are all potentially useful inputs.
- Decline in continence when comparing the level on one assessment to a prior assessment 90 days earlier. One could similarly track declines (or improvements!) in isolation (how much of the time alone during the day), stamina, compliance with medication, and so on.
- Decline in cognition can also be detected as the change in a scale (e.g., the Cognitive Performance Scale) from one assessment to the next. Similarly, one could track overall ADL or IADL function, body mass index, depression, and so on.

An example is the report by Landi *et al.* (1999), which demonstrated a decline from 44% to 26% in the number of clients hospitalized from five home-care agencies in two Italian provinces, using comparisons before and after the implementation of the RAI-HC. Also, Gambassi found that ACE inhibitor therapy (vs. digoxin) for congestive heart failure improved survival and ADL function even for patients over age 85, individuals systematically underrepresented in randomized trials.

The research to derive quality indicators, which are designed around these same outcome measures, can often provide risk adjustment to be sure that populations are compared on similar grounds.

Research

Archives accumulated from the use of MDS assessments can provide data for a range of research topics from clinical and epidemiological to policy. Assessments can be considered by themselves to understand the constellation of clinical problems of individuals; linked with other assessments of the same individual to represent longitudinal trajectories; accumulated by facility, program, region, or nation; and, potentially linked with cost or other identifying characteristics (e.g., census level information to provide a regional "denominator" number of elderly persons, or nonprofit ownership of a facility). The breadth of domains in the MDS assessments provide appropriate measures for many areas of interest, as well as critical covariates to adjust for sample or population differences.

As of 2004, over 400 research articles were listed on the interRAI website. A few examples of these include:

- cross-national comparison of antidepressant use in nursing-home residents
- racial differences in the use of nursing homes
- accelerated decline in centenarians
- the effect of funding changes (e.g., the Balanced Budget Act of 1997) on access to post-acute care.
- risk factors (including race, age, and dementia) in the detection of pain.

There are several advantages to the use of MDS data for research. First, the data meets reasonable reliability standards. Second, there are a large number of observations available, making even rare population numerous, and permitting stratification or control group selection even on multiple characteristics. Third, there are a large number of facilities or agencies represented so that even if this is the appropriate level of analysis (e.g., for contrasting facilities or programs), there are sufficient numbers for strong statistical power. Fourth, the full population is represented and sampling error is eliminated. Fifth, when MDS systems are implemented as part of clinical care, then multiple assessments of the same individual are performed, and longitudinal trajectories and outcome measures can be developed. Finally, multiple years' worth of data are accumulated, so that temporal trends can be visualized.

Multiple Uses of MDS Data

The advantages listed earlier are the result of MDS systems being implemented as part of the standard care process in a setting. In the past, these types of "administrative" data sets, produced as a by-product of the delivery of care, have had low esteem in health policy research. Much of their reputation was well deserved. They have traditionally had most of the following characteristics:

- poor definitions in the instruments, leading to unreliability and lack of validity;

- no "owner" who gains value from the data and is able to promulgate accuracy;
- perceived as "paperwork" and "busy-work" by (overworked) staff who have no personal or professional stake in data accuracy and often never see them used for any discernable purpose;
- little monitoring of data quality or the completeness of assessments;
- no external audit of a facilities' assessments.

The MDS avoids many of these problems by its direct link to managing the care of nursing-home residents. With a central "core" based in clinical care, and performed by professionals responsible for the care of the resident, there are strong incentives to provide accurate information. This provides the foundation for the assessment and its accuracy: which responsible clinician wouldn't do the best job possible in the care they provide? However, once these data are available, motivated and collected for this primary purpose, all the other uses described earlier are valuable yet virtually free by-products.

The addition of alternative uses for the data makes those involved with an assessment system into interested "owners". For example, if the data are used for case-mix payment, quality assurance, staffing decisions, and so on, then facility management will be invested in assuring that the assessment is performed. Further, such multiple uses of the data can directly encourage their accuracy. For instance, consider an assessment item such as pressure ulcers. It is an indicator of a resident whose care is expensive, both for the care of the ulcer and for the other conditions that such a sick patient would have. Therefore, a facility paid under a case-mix payment system (e.g., one based on RUG-III) would get more money if a pressure ulcer was reported. But pressure ulcers are often also used as one of the indicators of poor quality of care, thereby encouraging under-reporting. Use of the MDS item on pressure sores simultaneously for both case-mix and for quality provides counterbalancing forces to encourage accurate assessment of this item. There are, of course, also substantial threats to the accuracy of MDS data. Multiple uses, while potentially providing offsetting incentives, also provide potential bias if individuals cannot see (or are not convinced of) them. The time to complete the MDS is substantial, especially for qualified staff who are often in short supply, potentially resulting in poor assessment or missing data. Staff turnover and inadequate training may mean that assessments are poorly done or incorrectly computerized. While many of these can be addressed through training, auditing programs, improved staffing and careful research methodology, they remain a concern for any research effort.

IMPLEMENTATIONS OF MDS INSTRUMENTS

The MDS instruments have been adopted for use in multiple settings around the world. A limited selection of these includes:

- the nursing-home MDS has been adopted as the national assessment system for Iceland;
- in addition to the mandate that all nursing homes use the MDS, 10 US states have adopted the MDS-HC (home care) and applications for determining eligibility;
- the Province of Ontario, Canada, has adopted the nursing-home, home-care, and mental health MDS instruments province-wide; six other Canadian provinces/territories have or are planning to adopt these instruments as well;
- the General Assembly of Spitex (the Swiss home-care association) has decided to implement the MDS-HC across the entire nation by the end of 2006;
- the MDS-HC has been adopted for use throughout Hong Kong and is one of three recommended assessment systems for home care in Japan;
- both the MDS and MDS-HC are being implemented nationwide in Estonia;
- the MDS-HC is used throughout two regions of Italy.

Several of these implementations are discussed in Fries and Fahey (2003). With these multiple implementations, cross-national data are becoming available to compare, on a common measurement basis, care provided to elderly persons around the world. Prior studies have been handicapped by the lack of detailed information about individuals, measured in a consistent manner. An example of such new studies includes the results of the Aged in Home-Care Project (*AdHOC*) which collected information on 3785 individuals residing in 11 European nations. These data showed that the provision of formal care to people with similar dependency varies extremely widely, with very little formal care in Italy, and more than twice as much as the average across all levels of dependency in the United Kingdom (Carpenter *et al.*, 2004).

KEY POINTS

- Resident Assessment Instrument/Minimum Data Set provides comprehensive assessment of elderly residents in nursing homes.
- MDS provides basis for individualized care planning.
- Other Minimum Data Sets available for home- and community-based and institutional settings, for post-acute, palliative, and mental health.
- Data can be used for multiple purposes, including case-mix measurement, quality indicators, eligibility, and policy research.
- RAI/MDS assessment systems have been implemented in multiple nations, enabling cross-nation comparisons.

KEY REFERENCES

- Fries BE & Fahey CJ (eds). *Implementing the Resident Assessment Instrument: Case Studies of Policymaking for Long-Term Care in Eight*

Countries 2003; Milbank Memorial Fund, New York, 5th November, http://www.milbank.org/reports/interRAI/ResidentAssessment_Mech2.pdf.

- Fries BE, Schneider D, Foley WJ *et al.* Refining a case-mix measure for nursing homes: resource utilization groups (RUG-III). *Medical Care* 1994; **32**:668–85.
- Hirdes JP, Fries BE, Morris JN *et al.* Integrated health information systems based on the RAI/MDS series of instruments. *Healthcare Management Forum* 1999; **12**:30–40.
- Morris JN, Nonemaker S, Murphy K *et al.* A Commitment to change: revision of HCFA's RAI. *Journal of the American Geriatrics Society* 1997; **45**:1011–6.

REFERENCES

Björkgren MA, Fries BE & Shugarman L. Testing a RUG-III based case-mix system for home health care. *Canadian Journal on Aging* 2000; **19**(suppl 2):106–25.

Burrows AB, Morris JN, Simon SE *et al.* Development of a minimum data set-based depression rating scale for use in nursing homes. *Age and Ageing* 2000; **29**:165–72.

Carpenter GI, Gambassi G, Topinková E *et al.*, Community Care in Europe: The Aged in HOme Care project (AdHOC). *Aging Clinical and Experimental Research* 2004; **16**:259–269.

Carpenter GI, Ikegami N, Ljunggren G *et al.* RUG-III and resource allocation: comparing the relationship of direct care time with patient characteristics in five countries. *Age and Ageing* 1997; **26**(suppl 2):61–6.

Fetter RB, Brand DA & Gamache D (eds). *DRGs: their Design and Development* 1991; Health Administration Press, Ann Arbor.

Fries BE & Fahey CJ (eds). *Implementing the Resident Assessment Instrument: Case Studies of Policymaking for Long-Term Care in Eight Countries* 2003; Milbank Memorial Fund, New York, 5th November, http://www.milbank.org/reports/interRAI/ResidentAssessment_Mech2.pdf.

Fries BE, Schneider D, Foley WJ *et al.* Refining a case-mix measure for nursing homes: resource utilization groups (RUG-III). *Medical Care* 1994; **32**:668–85.

Fries BE, Simon SE, Morris JN *et al.* Pain in U.S. nursing homes: validating a pain scale for the minimum data set. *The Gerontologist* 2001; **41**:173–9.

Fries BE, Shugarman LR, Morris JN *et al.* A screening system for Michigan's home- and community-based long-term care programs. *The Gerontologist* 2002; **42**:462–74.

Hawes MC, Morris JN, Phillips CD *et al.* Reliability estimates for the minimum data set for nursing facility resident assessment and care screening (MDS). *The Gerontologist* 1995; **35**:172–8.

Hawes C, Phillips CD, Morris JN *et al.* The impact of OBRA-87 and the RAI on indicators of process quality in nursing homes. *Journal of the American Geriatrics Society* 1997; **45**:977–85.

Hirdes JP, Fries BE, Morris JN *et al.* Integrated health information systems based on the RAI/MDS series of instruments. *Healthcare Management Forum* 1999; **12**:30–40.

Hirdes JP, Frijters DH & Teare GF. The MDS-CHESS scale: a new measure to predict mortality in institutionalized older people. *Journal of the American Geriatrics Society* 2003; **51**:96–100.

Hirdes JP, Poss J, Curtin Telegdi N & Chase M. Method for Assigning Priority Levels (MAPLe) for community and institutional services, *Montreal: Annual Scientific and Educational Meeting of the Canadian Association on Gerontology*, Montreal, 2002.

Institute of Medicine, Committee on Nursing Home Regulation. *Improving the Quality of Care in Nursing Homes* 1986; National Academy Press, Washington.

interRAI September 24, *An Overview of the interRAI Family of Instruments*, 2004; http://www.interrai.org.

Kane RA, Kling KC, Bershadsky B *et al.* Quality of life measures for nursing home residents. *Journals of Gerontology Series A-Biological Sciences & Medical Sciences* 2003; **58**:240–8.

Landi F, Gambassi G, Pola R *et al.* Impact of integrated home care services on hospital use. *Journal of the American Geriatrics Society* 1999; **47**:1430–4.

Mor V, Morris JN, Lipsitz L & Fogel B. Systems for long-term care outcome measurement. *Nutrition* 1997a; **13**:242–4.

Mor V, Intrator O, Hiris J *et al.* Impact of the MDS on changes in nursing home discharge rates and destinations. *Journal of the American Geriatrics Society* 1997b; **45**:1002–10.

Morris JN, Fries BE, Mehr DR *et al.* MDS cognitive performance scale. *Journal of Gerontology: Medical Sciences* 1994; **49A**:M174–82.

Morris JN, Murphy K, Nonemaker S *et al.* *Resident Assessment Instrument Version 2.0* 1996; Government Printing Office, Washington.

Morris JN, Nonemaker S, Murphy K *et al.* A Commitment to change: revision of HCFA's RAI. *Journal of the American Geriatrics Society* 1997; **45**:1011–6.

Morris JN, Fries BE & Morris SA. Scaling ADLs within the MDS. *Journal of Gerontology: Medical Sciences* 1999; **54A**:M546–53.

Morris JN, Murphy K, Mor V *et al.* *Validation of Long-Term and Post-Acute Quality Indicators*, Report to CMS under Contract Number 500-95-0062, 2002.

Phillips C, Morris JN, Hawes C *et al.* The impact of the RAI on ADLs, continence, communication, cognition, and psychosocial well-being. *Journal of the American Geriatrics Society* 1997; **45**:986–93.

Teno J, Branco K, Mor V *et al.* The early impact of the patient self-determination act in long-term care facilities: results from a 10 state sample. *Journal of the American Geriatrics Society* 1997; **45**:939–44.

Zimmerman DR, Karon SL, Arling G *et al.* Development and testing of nursing home quality indicators. *Health Care Financing Review* 1995; **16**:107–27.

Zinn JS. Market competition and the quality of nursing home care. *Journal of Health Politics, Policy and Law* 1994; **19**:555–82.

157

Nursing (UK)

Nicky Hayes

King's College Hospital NHS Trust, London, UK

INTRODUCTION – OVERVIEW OF CHAPTER

This chapter explains the characteristics and principles of older people's nursing and explores the scope of its application across the spectrum of care: from prevention of ill health, through acute illness and rehabilitation to continuing care. Nurses are involved with care provision for older people in a wide range of settings – primary care and community care home, hospital, mental health center, acute and rehabilitation wards, A&E, intermediate-care services, outpatients, day hospital, and nurse-led clinics. While many nurses work within the National Health Service (NHS), within older people's services, many also work in the independent sector. This is a significant care provider and employer, due to the majority provision of long-term care beds now being sited outside the NHS. In 2000, 70 895 qualified nursing staff were working in nursing homes, private hospitals, and clinics, the majority being in general nursing homes (UKCC, 2002). As well as being diverse in application to care settings, nursing older people is characterized by its flexibility, breadth, and overlap with other roles – coordinator, manager, essential caregiver, therapist, specialist carer, and educator are just some of the many aspects of specialist nursing across these areas of practice.

Over recent years, nursing older people has emerged from being a somewhat underrated and stigmatized area of nursing service into a recognized skilled speciality. This chapter examines how this process has been supported by professional articulation, development of nursing curricula and professional qualifications, extended roles and responsibilities, and publication of specialist standards and competencies. New roles such as the older people's specialist nurse, matron, and consultant nurse have provided a boost to clinical leadership and the retention of skilled practitioners within the nursing speciality. It will also be shown how the principles of caring for older people are applicable to nurses in many settings and specialities, not just to those nurses who work in older people's services, or have a title of older people's specialist nurse. It will be concluded that older people's nursing has many future opportunities, as well as challenges ahead, including extension of specialist practice, strengthening of nurses' roles in clinical leadership and research, and involving older people and carers further in care and service development. Underpinning all contemporary and future practice are the fundamental principles of caring for older people: use of a multidisciplinary, person-centered, evidence-based approach, which applies understanding of the impact of the aging process to the individual's wellness, illness, and recovery.

BACKGROUND – THE DEVELOPMENT OF OLDER PEOPLE'S NURSING

Since the work of Dr Marjorie Warren in the 1930s, and the emergence of geriatric medicine as a speciality, a parallel revolution has occurred in older people's nursing.

Nursing older people was once seen by some as an unattractive career option, associated with negative stereotypes of services that warehoused and institutionalized dependent older people. This stereotype was partly reinforced by the prolonged use by the NHS of former workhouse facilities for community hospitals and rehabilitation units, which were a physical reminder of the past for both patients and staff. The perceived unpopularity of work with older people has been found to be associated with these "impoverished environments" in which older people receive care, rather than negative attitudes towards older people themselves. The majority of students and qualified nurses now consider work with older people to be challenging and stimulating, and a highly skilled job (Nolan *et al.*, 2002).

Challenges to development of the speciality have particularly applied in the independent sector. While older people's nursing in the NHS is increasingly recognized and developed, the capacity for specialist nurses to further develop, and lead effective health-care practices in care homes has been limited by lack of investment in access to specialist

Principles and Practice of Geriatric Medicine, 4th Edition. Edited by M.S. John Pathy, Alan J. Sinclair and John E. Morley.

training and development. Nurses in the independent sector have limited opportunity for formal, funded professional development in comparison with that which is available to NHS nurses, yet it is in care homes that many of the most frail and medically complex older people in our society are cared for. The lack of investment is partly reflected in the issues underpinning complaints which arise against practitioners in this sector: the UKCC (2002) identified organizational issues such as low staffing levels, poor skill mix, and lack of leadership or direction that were common to the majority of complaints against nurses working in the independent sector. Professional issues, such as, lack of training and career progression are also a common feature. The introduction in 2001 of NHS-funded nursing for care home residents may be an opportunity for Primary Care Trusts to increase training and support to care homes, and help redress this imbalance and impact on the quality of service delivery. A further challenge to the independent sector is to increase published evidence of good practice and innovation from practitioners who work there, particularly in the nursing homes for older people.

Until fairly recently, there has been a relative lack of national standards, competencies, and research base within the nursing speciality. The skills and value of any speciality can only be recognized if there is an evidence base to support it and the practitioners are sufficiently articulate, empowered, and supported. Through nurse leadership, promotion of positive attitudes to aging, modernization of facilities and developments in nurse education, standards, policy and politics, and any stigma that might have existed of "geriatric nursing" has been gradually eroded.

The significant policy drivers which have recently emerged, the NHS Plan (Department of Health, 2000) and the National Service Framework for Older People (NSF) (Secretary of State for Health, 2001), set out principles and standards which rule out ageist policy and practice in all sectors. With this precedent firmly established, the major challenges and opportunities for older people's nurses lie in further development of specialist education, maintaining an appropriate focus on the essential areas of patient care, and developing and retaining a workforce with the required knowledge and skills. These issues will be more fully explored in the sections that follow.

DEVELOPMENT OF THE SPECIALIST NURSING ROLES

As already noted, nurses care for older people in a wide range of settings, yet many would not necessarily consider themselves to be older people's specialists. With the majority of hospital and primary care patients being aged over 65, it can be argued that most nurses require some knowledge of caring for older people. It is vital that skills are not just learnt in the classroom but that nurses who have contact with this patient group can also learn from experts in practice and then implement what they have learnt, with appropriate support and leadership. This is one reason for development of the specific role of the older people's specialist nurse (and other senior roles such as consultant nurse and matron within the NHS); by strengthening clinical leadership and clinical expertise in caring for older people, good practice will be role modeled and promoted. Clinical leadership helps ensure that knowledge and skills acquired through both pre- and postregistration education and professional development can be implemented and further developed.

The development of the role of older people's specialist nurse (OPSN) in all areas of care delivery has been strongly supported by both the Royal College of Nursing and the British Geriatrics Society, who published a joint statement in 2001 (RCN & BGS, 2001). Their statement points to the increasing complexity of health and social care for older people, and the difficulty in providing smoothly coordinated care focused on older people as individuals. It clearly articulates the potential value that this type of role can contribute to older people's care. This includes:

- expert clinical practitioner working alongside older people and their families;
- key resource to provide leadership for nursing and contribute to cross-boundary working;
- key contribution to implementation of the National Service Framework for Older People and the Single Assessment Process;
- working as part of a specialist multidisciplinary team, sharing a vision and accountability for comprehensive service delivery, and development of good practice.

Some NHS Hospital Trusts and Primary Care Trusts have now started to develop these roles, an example of which, older people's specialist nurse in Care Home support, is summarized in BOX 1.

BOX 1 Role of the OPSN in a Care Homes Support Team

The post of OPSN within a Care Homes Support Team was developed in three South London Primary Care Trusts in 2003.

The OPSNs work within a wider multidisciplinary support team, which includes dedicated sessions from Consultant Geriatricians, a Consultant Old Age Psychiatrist and a pharmacist. Eight posts, at senior nursing grades, were created and subsequently fulfill a variety of roles across primary care and in 40 nursing homes that include:

- undertaking initial determinations of NHS-funded nursing care in care homes (also known as the *RNCC*), and subsequent reviews including full continence assessments;

- holding a case load of selected older people who are resident in nursing homes within the three local boroughs;
- advising care providers on care planning and delivery;
- acting as a specialist skills' resource to care providers;
- identifying and triggering referrals to specialist care services;
- leading on behalf of the specialist interdisciplinary team on issues of clinical governance and monitoring of care.

When undertaking patient reviews, including determination of the RNCC, the OPSNs undertake an assessment of the residents' mental state and falls risk, and collect a range of health outcome measures. They provide advice to the Care Home staff on the resident's care plan, and specific clinical needs such as tissue viability and wound management. They contribute to a review of the resident's medication, in conjunction with the team's full-time pharmacist. The review is conducted when possible, and when wished by the resident, with the resident's family carer so that communication and support may be optimized. Working closely with the consultant members of the team, the OPSNs also contribute to the review of residents who receive fully funded NHS care both in Care Homes and their own homes. Finally, they are engaged in a range of practice development activity, benchmarking, audit and research in the Care Homes across the three boroughs.

The OPSN role described here provides a good example of how appropriately skilled and experienced nurses make skilled independent judgments and provide advice to care providers while contributing to multidisciplinary management of the older person. The roles of these particular nurses have a majority clinical focus, but are broad enough to include elements of activities such as research and audit, which help drive practice forward and develop the speciality.

The development of consultant nurse roles, was set out in the key document, *Making a Difference* (DoH, 1999). This strategy is applicable to nursing in all specialities, and has been highly influential in professional nursing development within the NHS. These leadership roles will help ensure that the standards of care for older people are maintained and developed both within and beyond specialist older people's services.

Consultant nurses' posts have four key role components (NHSE, 1999):

- professional leadership and consultancy
- expert practice
- practice development, research, and evaluation
- education and development.

There are, at the time of writing, 54 consultant nurse posts for older people in England, 23 of which are in acute trusts, 21 in primary care trusts, 8 in mental health trusts and 2 which span both mental health and acute trusts (Sturdy, 2004). The difference between the consultant role and that of specialist nurse is predominantly one of level of working – the consultant role has a greater leadership and strategic component, while retaining a 50% clinical component. Although there are no national criteria for the academic or professional level of a specialist nurse post, the nurse consultants are required to be qualified to at least master's level, and to have substantial experience within the speciality. Both types of roles contribute to the further development and leadership of the nursing speciality, and work well in partnership with each other. In the case of the OPSN team described above, overall clinical leadership and direction, and clinical supervision of the team, are provided by a consultant nurse.

UNDERPINNING PRINCIPLES OF NURSING PRACTICE WITH OLDER PEOPLE

Whether working as part of the multiprofessional team in delivering care for older people during an acute illness or in a period of maintenance of good health, or in any other stage in the continuum of health, the fundamental principle of nursing older people is the same: the use of a person-centered approach. The use of a person-centered approach in nursing means that individuality, choice, and rights are recognized and respected, when making assessments, planning, and delivering care. A prerequisite for person-centered care is also that nurses invest in care-giving out of choice, that they want to work with older people, value interdependence, and respect personhood (Mulrooney, 1997). This approach combines with recognition of the central importance of helping older people to meet their essential care needs, which includes assisting patients with intimate care and comfort. In order to deliver care using these holistic principles, all nurses are trained to use the nursing process. This is a problem-centered approach, which works through the four stages of:

- assessment
- planning
- implementation
- evaluation.

High-quality assessment of older people's needs depends upon good teamwork and the use of valid and reliable assessment tools. Older people's nurses work in an interdisciplinary way to contribute to the overall assessment of the patient, and are familiar with the use of a range of standardized and validated tools to support assessment of the person's physical, psychological, and social status. Some of the areas that nurses need to address when assessing the older person may be described within these three domains:

Physical
Tissue viability
Continence
Constipation and bowels
Pain
Rest and sleep
Foot health
Oral health
Prevention of ill health and promotion of good health
Falls risk and safety needs
Mobility
Eating, drinking, and nutrition
Self-care ability
Hygiene needs
Wound care
Administration of medicines

Social
Carers' needs
Recreation
Social networks and support
Transport
Communication
Appearance
Ethnicity and culture
Education and intellectual needs

Psychological
Mental health problems including dementia, depression, and delirium
Cognitive function
Behavior
Spiritual needs
Sexuality.

While these principles, domains, and processes underpin nursing care of older people in all areas, nurses also utilize specific knowledge and skills to enable them to care effectively for older people with different intensities or acuteness of care need. The older people's nurse is able to distinguish normal from abnormal aging, and recognizes the impact of the aging process upon health, illness, treatment, and recovery. They also understand the management of complex problems, physical, psychological and social, and are prepared to encounter these frequently and work closely with the multiprofessional team to achieve solutions to them. Nurses who are skilled in working with older people also work closely with colleagues from social care and at the interfaces between services, ensuring that transfers of care are managed properly. The next section explores the application of older people's nursing to four care areas: acute care, continuing care in care homes, working with older people and their carers in the community (with the specific example of admiral nurses), and rehabilitation and intermediate care.

Acute Care of Older People

During an acute phase of illness, older people need care by nurses who are not only skilled in the technical aspects of nursing but who can also apply knowledge of the impact of aging process in response to acute treatments and recovery. This particularly includes knowledge of how older people may respond differently to drug treatment, infection, injury, and pain than younger people. A particularly vital concern during acute illness is recognition of delirium, a condition which is often underrecognized by general nurses (Inouye *et al.*, 2001), but which the specialist nurse will understand as a reversible acute confusional state rather than an irreversible dementia, and will also recognize it as a condition that may persist beyond the acute phase of treatment. Patients who are acutely or chronically confused have specific health and safety needs including psychological management, falls and injury prevention, nutrition, and communication. In an acute setting, nurses need to be vigilant for these differences, and the implications for care planning in terms of patient and carer support.

The scope of nursing older people within acute care was described and critiqued in a report in 2001 from the Standing Nursing and Midwifery Advisory Committee (SNMAC). The report "Caring for Older People: a Nursing Priority" (SNMAC, 2001), formulated a number of standards of care for older people and their carers during an acute phase of illness, covering the following care domains:

- respect for older people's dignity;
- promotion of choice, involvement, and independence of older people and carers;
- facilitation of communication with older people and carers;
- individualized care and its management;
- continence;
- dementia;
- mental health;
- mobility;
- nutrition and hydration;
- pain management;
- palliative care;
- pressure damage prevention and management.

These domains offer a useful framework for identifying the fundamental care needs of older people in hospital, and describing the scope of nursing in this setting. The standards may be used to audit care, although in most hospitals, it has been the *Essence of Care* benchmarking (DoH, 2001b), which has been more widely implemented. The *Essence of Care* is relevant to all care areas, and will be described in more depth later.

In hospital care, the SNMAC report also strengthened the case for further development of speciality nursing roles. They identified that when there were obstacles to the delivery of high-quality care, this could be due to lack of clinical leadership, management and role modeling, inadequate training and preparation of nurses for working with older people, and deficiencies in the physical environment and resources (SNMAC, 2001). These are undeniable challenges in ensuring that acute care is appropriately tailored to older people's needs. The publication of the SNMAC report and the NSF helped to drive further improvement in acute care of older people in hospital, particularly for nursing in terms of leadership and in specific clinical areas of concern such as the feeding, hydration, and nutrition of older patients. Protected mealtimes for hospital patients are one example of this.

Quality improvement initiatives in acute care have particularly been related to the requirements of Standard 4 "General Hospital Care" of the NSF for Older People. This standard is as relevant to nurses as to all other health and social care professionals. The NSF supports the strengthening of clinical nurse leadership within interdisciplinary older people's services in general hospitals, including the role of the specialist nurse. The specialist nurse in an acute hospital may be ward or department based, or have a role in working at the interface with other areas, providing outreach expertise. The value to this type of role has been demonstrated in a recent evaluation of the introduction of OPSNs within an inpatient setting in Nottingham. This study provides evidence that the role can provide rapid assessment and review of patients with appropriate identification of transfer of care, discharge, referrals, and review (Harwood *et al.*, 2002).

The milestones set by the NSF also impact on training and preparation of staff who work with older people in acute settings: NHS Trusts are required to carry out a skills audit of all staff within the organization. Nurses being by far the largest proportion of the workforce has enabled trusts to review the training needs across the organization and put action plans in place to ensure that all staff have at least the minimum knowledge and skills to care for older people.

Continuing Care in Care Homes (*see* Chapter 153, Nursing Home Care)

Continuing care can be interpreted as the delivery of care services in any setting, including the client's own home, care homes, and other long-stay facilities. When older people require continuing care in their own home, NHS nurses provide registered nursing through the community nursing service, unless the older person prefers and has the means to privately employ a registered nurse. Care assistants, and often family caregivers or other informal carers otherwise deliver the majority of care. There is a similar skill mix in Care Homes with Nursing, where independent care providers employ registered nurses and care assistants, but care assistants under supervision from the registered nurses deliver the majority of care.

Masterson (1997) identified the function of nursing in continuing care is to provide

- specialist practice skills,
- assessment and review of needs,
- health promotion and health maintenance,
- partnership working with clients and carers.

Although this guidance (produced for the nursing regulatory body, the United Kingdom Central Council for Nursing, Midwifery & Health Visiting (UKCC)) predates the NSF for older people, the principles it sets out resonate with the NSFs person-centered and proactive approach to health and social care. Nurses have the key role to play in delivery of care and in ensuring that older people's continuing care needs are regularly and appropriately reviewed, reversible health problems are identified, and chronic health problems are appropriately managed so that the remaining function may be optimized. For them, this guidance is highly relevant. There may be only one registered nurse on duty for each shift within a Care Home with Nursing, and the responsibilities upon that practitioner are considerable, requiring them to lead the care team and ensure that care is properly delivered. Unlike acute or many subacute hospital settings, there is reduced access to medical cover and therapy input. Consequently, the skilled practitioner in continuing care manages the maintenance care of clients, while being alert to changes in health and well-being. They understand the implications of these changes, particularly when residents may be at the end of their life or in a condition in which hospital admission may be inappropriate. Particular skills relate to the mental health of nursing home residents, the proportion who have dementia being around 62% (Matthews and Dening, 2002). Safety issues related to wandering and challenging behaviors amongst this group of residents are managed frequently in nursing homes.

Some of the challenges to the development of specialist nursing in Care Home settings in the independent sector were raised at the beginning of this chapter, particularly in relation to investment in training and support for nursing. Some of the underlying reasons for these challenges can be further understood within Masterson's identification of the requirements for an effective nursing contribution to continuing care:

- appropriate education, induction, and clinical supervision;
- an organizational culture which is committed to continuing care;
- positive attitudes expressed by nurses and health visitors toward older people;
- supportive and committed management processes;
- respect for the contribution of other members of the care team;
- appropriate delegation and supervision.

The squeeze on resources within "for-profit" organizations that provide continuing care for older people means that it may be difficult to meet all of these conditions for registered nurses to make an effective contribution. For example, there is no obligation within the legal requirements of the National Minimum Standards for Care Homes for Older People (Secretary of State for Health, 2003) for independent care providers to make provision for clinical supervision for registered nurses. Standard 30 of the Standards does require staff to be trained and competent to do their jobs, and to have a minimum of three paid days training per year, but it does not specify the content of this. The requirement applies to registered nurses and health-care assistants, 50% of the latter group of carers being required to have received training to National Vocational Qualifications (NVQ) level 2 or equivalent – a basic standard which is below that of entry level to nurse training. In fact, only 42% of registered nurses working in nursing homes receive paid study time from their employers (UKCC, 2002). This suggests that while the employers clearly do have responsibilities for developing and training their staff they may interpret this creatively. Furthermore, there is no requirement for them to take account of specific published standards such as the SNMAC standards or the guidance of the NSF when determining the content or appropriateness of the training provided or supported. Registered nurses also have a professional obligation to ensure that they are fit to practice and to account for this to the Nursing and Midwifery Council when renewing their professional registration on a 3-yearly basis.

There is now a role for NHS nurses to support long-term care, which is delivered by the independent sector, through the requirement for determination of the level of NHS-funded nursing care (RNCC). The guidance on NHS-funded nursing care was issued in June 2001 (Department of Health, 2001). Originally referred to as *free nursing care* it sets out the NHS responsibility for provision of free nursing and health care whether the patient is in hospital, nursing home, or at home. Nursing Home residents must now have a determination of the level of NHS-funded nursing care undertaken by a designated NHS nurse prior to transfer to a Nursing Home, followed by reviews at 3 months and 1 year posttransfer. The NHS is also responsible for provision of continence products, which should only be supplied once a full assessment of the resident's continence has been completed. A registered nurse must carry out both these NHS responsibilities.

The determination of the level of NHS-funded nursing care is a high-level clinical judgment that requires a review of the risk, complexity, predictability and stability, and the resident's care needs (Department of Health, 2001a). To carry out the determination, a high level of knowledge, skill, and experience is required, with a recommendation by the Department of Health (DoH) that the designated nurses should include nurse specialists, nurse consultants, district nurses, discharge liaison nurses, and community psychiatric nurses. This has acted as a major catalyst for the provision of specialist nursing input to care home residents, based on the statutory requirement for the reviews to be carried out.

Working with Older People and their Carers in the Community (*see* Chapter 152, Carers and the Role of the Family)

A majority of older people never need long-term care in a Care Home, and probably would choose not to do so. Indeed only 4% of the population aged over 65 live in residential care settings, and the Royal Commission on Long Term Care recommended that more care should be given to people in their own homes, and more services should be offered to people who have an informal carer (Secretary of State for Health, 1999). While local authorities have responsibility for provision of personal and social care in people's own homes, the nursing needs of older people who live at home are met through community nursing services. This constitutes a high proportion of community practitioner's caseloads. Consequently, community nurses have a large role to play in the management of chronic diseases and have high levels of clinical skills in particular areas such as, continence management and tissue viability. The need for community nurses to have skills in caring for older people is becoming increasingly reflected in district nurse training courses (Ryder, 1994), although this is not a core curriculum requirement.

The introduction of the Single Assessment Process as part of the NSF for Older People (Secretary of State for Health, 2001) has brought a focus on the assessment of older people within health and social care. Primary care nurses' roles in assessment and care of older people in the community have a place at both overview and specialist levels of assessment, including working interprofessionally with both health and social care practitioners in comprehensive old age assessment of people who may need admission to a Care Home.

With the increasing prevalence of dementia with old age, specialist support for patients and their informal carers is a priority if community-based care is to be sustained, although primary care nurses have been found to have low understanding and confidence in identifying dementia and dealing with coexisting behavioral and mental health problems (Bryans *et al.*, 2003). This suggests that there is still progress to be made in the education and training of community nurses. Another approach is the development of specialist supporting nursing roles, such as admiral nurses. These are specialist mental health nurses, who work in the community, with families, carers, and supporters of people with dementia. In contrast to many community mental health teams, the service works primarily with the caregiver, focuses exclusively on dementia and offers continuing involvement including emotional support, information giving, and coordination of practical support. A Competency framework for admiral nurses has been developed (Traynor and Dewing, 2002) and the core competency areas are shown in BOX 2.

BOX 2 Core competency areas of Admiral Nurses

1. Therapeutic work (interventions)
2. Sharing information about dementia and carer issues
3. Advanced assessment skills
4. Prioritizing work
5. Preventative work and health promotion
6. Ethical and person-centered care
7. Balancing the needs of the carer and the person with dementia
8. Promoting best practice.

The identification of a specialist skill set and competencies is important for measuring and maintaining the quality of the service and ensuring the professional development of the practitioners. An evaluation of the service itself has identified a significant impact on the anxiety and insomnia of carers of people with dementia, although it did not find any difference in the outcomes for the person with dementia, in terms of institutionalization (Woods *et al.*, 2003). This is an example of a specialist competency framework; by contrast, a national competency framework covering older people's care will be discussed later.

Rehabilitation and Intermediate Care

"The nursing role in rehabilitation is key to the government's agenda of modernization of the NHS" and "rehabilitation should be part of every nurse's role" – two quotes from the Royal College of Nursing's Rehabilitation Workbook (RCN, 2000). Although the use of a rehabilitation approach is widely acknowledged, in publications such as this, as being important to the care of older people, definition and clarification of the nursing's role in rehabilitation has still been slow to emerge. It may be suggested that general nursing initially struggled to identify it's specific therapeutic component in rehabilitation, possibly because of an underlying tension between perceptions of the concepts of *caring* and *treating* – although it may be rather simplistic to make this distinction, nurses have conventionally tended to consider themselves as providing the former, while therapists and Doctors carry out the latter. It was not until the 1990s that nursing researchers began to analyze and clarify nursing's role within the multiprofessional rehabilitation team, and explore the overlap between the role of a nurse and a therapist.

Waters (1991), identified three domains of nursing's role in rehabilitation, which she identified as the three constructs of "general maintenance", "specialist" and "carry-on". This implies a caring role that meets essential needs, while adding specific specialist skills and an understudy component to ensure that therapy interventions are continued as part of planned care. Nolan *et al.* (1997) further identified a role for nurses in creating and sustaining a suitable environment for rehabilitation. More recently Long *et al.* (2001) identified six core nursing roles in rehabilitation, which are:

- assessment
- coordination and communication
- technical and physical care
- therapy integration and therapy carry-on
- emotional support
- involving the family.

These roles are closely associated with the 24-hour presence of nurses in inpatient units and the breadth and flexibility of nursing practice in all settings. Although the therapy carry-through, or "understudy" role of rehabilitation nurses, has been identified through the nursing literature, identification of specific therapeutic nursing skills in rehabilitation have been more elusive, but might also be suggested to include pain management, continence promotion and management of incontinence, falls prevention, health education, and the promotion of rest and sleep.

Patient reenablement, choice and empowerment are integral to the rehabilitation process, and nurses have embraced this approach to help older people regain optimum function and independence. A good example of this, allied to a specific aspect of nursing, is the practice in some units of offering older patients the opportunity to participate in patient's self-administration of medicines – a relinquishing of the traditional role of nurses in drug administration in favor of a partnership – an educative approach which is endorsed by the NSF for Older People (Medicines Management). A further example is the involvement of nurses in delivery of exercise programs for older people. Individualized, tailored exercise has an effective contribution to make in improving strength and balance in older people and reducing falls (Day *et al.*, 2002). Research by Robertson *et al.* (2001) has demonstrated a role for nurses in delivery of these programs, and this is another area in which UK nurses are beginning to develop practice and expand their roles in rehabilitation (Nursing Times, 2004).

Recent developments in intermediate-care services have brought more focus to health and social care roles in providing focused, time-limited rehabilitation services that are delivered both in the community and in bed-based services. Some of these services have been developed and led by nurses, particularly in nurse consultant roles. Although at the time of writing, these services are relatively new, some evaluation has been carried out. For example, evaluation of one nurse-led intermediate-care unit found it to be a safe alternative to conventional management (Steiner *et al.*, 2001). Inpatient stay in this type of unit has been found to be longer than on general medical wards (Griffiths *et al.*, 2001). Obviously, nurse-led units require multidisciplinary input and would not be effective in providing a rehabilitation service without the input of other professions including medicine, therapy, and pharmacy.

EDUCATION AND PREPARATION FOR NURSING OLDER PEOPLE

The Nursing and Midwifery Council (NMC) is the regulatory body for Nursing and Midwifery in the United Kingdom that specifies the requirements of preregistration nursing programs (NMC, 2002). The basic qualification of registered nurse in the United Kingdom is awarded on completion of 4600 hours of training within a 3-year course, 50% of which must be in clinical practice. The minimum academic standard of this training program is a diploma in higher education. The required core competencies of registered practitioners include a range of transferable skills within the following domains:

- professional and ethical practice
- care delivery and care management
- personal and professional development.

There are no competencies that explicitly address the care of older people, although multidisciplinary working is specified. Registered nurses are competent to practice with either adult child, or person with mental health or learning disabilities according to the particular branch program they undertook in the second part of the preregistration program. All preregistration nursing courses do include some practice contact with older people, although practice placements are designated as "adult" rather than specifically "older adult". It has been suggested that a positive learning environment is onc which ensures that students, staff and patients have a sense of security, belonging, continuity, purpose, achievement, and significance – this framework of "six senses" has been suggested by Professor Mike Nolan (Nolan *et al.*, 2002), who has made significant contribution to the development of postregistration curricula within the speciality of nursing and rehabilitation of older people.

Although there are Standards for Specialist Education and Practice (UKCC, 2001) likewise these do not specify educational requirements or qualifications for working with older people after initial registration. Employers, according to the duties and requirements of the post, determine this locally. Many specialist courses in the care of older people are available at degree and postgraduate level, offered at Universities throughout the United Kingdom. The English National Board (ENB) for Nursing framework for postregistration courses previously specified an outline curriculum for courses on nursing older people including the ENB 941 course, which was well known to practitioners until recently. These courses are no longer run since the Nursing and Midwifery Council absorbed the functions of the ENB in 2001. Postregistration course curricula are now determined and validated locally by education providers. There continue to be calls for greater emphasis on the care and rehabilitation of the older adults in nurse education. Long *et al.* (2001), for example, call for rehabilitation to be an ongoing thread through the preregistration curriculum, and at the postregistration level, a nationally recognized and accredited postregistration qualification in rehabilitation. This type of course should be multiprofessional.

While there is no nationally recognized qualification for the role of the older people's specialist nurse, an outline specification for preparation for the role has been published by the Royal College of Nursing and British Geriatrics Society (RCN & BGS, 2001). Specification for preparation for the role of older people's specialist nurse includes:

- sufficient and sound clinical experience working with older people;
- specialist postregistration development in the distinct and special aspects of older people's health and social needs;
- attributes and competencies which enable the nurse to respond expertly to the needs of the older person and professional colleagues;
- postregistration development in understanding the specific issues of later life, for example, the social and gerontological literature on older people's experiences of later life, the range of living circumstances and personal and social networks.

This provides a basis for development of specific posts within the many care areas in which specialist nurses may practice. A further route by which nurses may develop their skills and competency is through the Nursing and Midwifery Council (NMC) Higher Level Practice standards, which are described in BOX 3. Competency statements were developed around the NMC's seven higher-level practice standards, at each of the three levels of competency. These are generic and offer a framework for individual professional development.

BOX 3 The NMCs seven higher-level practice standards (UKCC, 2002a)

1. Providing effective health care
2. Leading and developing practice
3. Improving quality and health outcomes
4. Innovation and changing practice
5. Evaluation and research
6. Developing self and others
7. Working across professional and organizational boundaries.

The experience that nurses gain in practice with older people is recognized as a vital component of their expertise, although there has been a great increase in expectation of academic achievement of nurses who wish to specialize or work in more senior clinical roles. This is currently taken to its highest level in the requirements for nurse consultants to be qualified to at least masters' degree level.

BENCHMARKING AND MEASURING QUALITY OF NURSING CARE OF OLDER PEOPLE

The work of investigators such as Norton *et al.* (1962, 1975) were formative in raising issues around the care of older people in hospitals and continuing care. Since then, continued awareness of standards of care has been ensured through publications, some of which have already been mentioned, including statutory bodies such as SNMAC, UKCC, and professional organizations such as the RCN. Voluntary organizations such as Help the Aged have also contributed to public and professional awareness of care issues through campaigns such as the "Dignity on the Ward" campaign (Help the Aged, 2000). While the care of older people in hospital is the concern and responsibility of all staff, from porters to the Chief Executive, nurses have a strong contribution to make to ensuring that good practice is achieved and quality of care continuously improved, including in the core, or essential areas of care, such as nutrition, rest and elimination, and particularly in acute settings (SNMAC, 2001). This is why expertise in specialist older people's nursing has to include expertise in the fundamentals of nursing practice.

In the NHS, quality monitoring and initiatives within nursing practice fit within the broader framework of clinical governance, which has been defined as:

> "A framework through which NHS organisations are accountable for continually improving the quality of their services and safeguarding high standards of care by creating an environment in which excellence in clinical care will flourish."
>
> (Scally and Donaldson, 1998)

One of the key mechanisms that have recently emerged for monitoring and improving quality of nursing care in all care settings is the *Essence of Care* benchmarking (DoH, 2001b). The *Essence of Care* was designed to support the measures to improve quality that were set out in "A First Class Service" (DoH, 1998) and to contribute to clinical governance at a local level. The benchmarking tool has high relevance for nursing older people as it focuses on the fundamental or essential care needs of patients, which form the basis of nursing practice. These are:

- principles of self-care;
- personal and oral hygiene;
- food and nutrition;
- continence and bladder and bowel care;
- pressure ulcers;
- safety of clients/patients with mental health needs in acute mental health and general hospital settings;
- record keeping;
- privacy and dignity.

Standards of care in the independent sector are regulated through the National Minimum Standards for Care Homes for Older People (Secretary of State for Health, 2003). The specific clinical content of these standards covers basic requirements for:

- privacy and dignity;
- death and dying;
- service user plan;
- health care – including personal care, pressure sore prevention, continence management, psychological monitoring, falls prevention, and nutrition;
- medication.

The standards cover a similar range of domains to the *Essence of care*, that is, fundamental patient care. It can be suggested from this observation that in order for care providers to monitor and improve their service delivery effectively, a system such as the *Essence of Care* or equivalent quality improvement framework would complete the circle. The benchmarking process engages frontline staff in exploring and agreeing the level of quality they have achieved, evidencing it, and forming action plans for improvement. The process is, however, time consuming and consequently the same tensions apply to quality assurance in care homes as to the issues of professional development and training.

Competency frameworks are a further tool that can be used to ensure that nurses have the skills to deliver good care. As mentioned earlier, there are general professional competency frameworks through the professional bodies, which apply to all student and registered nurses. When services rely on a high proportion of unqualified care assistants, as is the case in independent sector Care Homes, it is particularly important that there are frameworks to ensure that care assistants demonstrate competence to provide care for older people too, and that the minimum care standards can be met. One approach to guiding this is the use of nationally developed competency frameworks which apply to all formal carers, both qualified and unqualified. For health and social care workers in older people's care, the national occupational standards database now offers this. Developed by the organization Skills for Health (2004), the framework addresses the skills and underpinning knowledge that is needed across a wide range of older people's care, and is being linked to NVQ and the Agenda for Change (a system of pay review within the NHS, implemented in 2004, applies to nurses and other staff although not to medical staff). It has relevance across all sectors of care delivery, and can be linked to staff training, induction, and performance appraisal.

A challenge arising from development of competency frameworks is that they work well at basic levels of practice but because of the reductionist process of defining competence, it can be argued that it is difficult to develop a competency framework that adequately describes the detail of practice at an expert level. Nursing practice is by its nature extremely complex and in the literature it has been theorized that nurses use many sources of knowledge, including intuitive, personal, and ethical knowledge (e.g. Carper, 1978) and deal with multiple tasks and demands when providing care. For example, the older people's specialist nurses in a Care Homes Support Team, which were described earlier, draw on extensive knowledge of both normal and abnormal aging, assessment and evidence-based practice, and interpret this within a setting that is both the person's home and a caregiving environment. They make high-level clinical judgments about resident's care needs and advise residents, carers, GPs, and other multidisciplinary team members. They combine these skills with a leadership role in practice development and clinical governance activity. It may not be possible to explain expert practice in terms of easily understood tasks but there remains a responsibility for practitioners to exercise professional accountability for their actions, and to demonstrate that their actions are effective. This is achieved by expert nurses through a combination of appraisal, peer review, clinical supervision, and collection of appropriate activity data.

THE FUTURE FOR OLDER PEOPLE'S NURSING – FUTURE CHALLENGES AND OPPORTUNITIES

This chapter has had scope to discuss in depth only a few of the issues relating to the present and ongoing development of older people's nursing. There are particular challenges in continuing care and the independent sector, but now that there is NHS recognition of its responsibility to fund registered nursing in care homes, it is to be hoped that there will be widespread recognition of the related obligation to support nursing development and help promote good practice. Generally, nursing is challenged to ensure sustained development of practice and the nursing contribution to older people's services in all sectors. In particular, evidence-based nursing practice requires a strong research base, and nursing needs to continue to develop its contribution, both into nursing aspects of care and also within multidisciplinary enquiry. With nurses increasingly acquiring graduate and postgraduate qualifications, there has never been a better time for this, although there needs to be access to adequate and substantial research funding, for which there is already intense competition within health care.

Nursing leadership in older people's services is at its strongest yet, but is challenged to champion and lead at all levels from local to international, and to continue to raise the profile of the speciality and ensure that it's value and professionalism are recognized. There is an associated opportunity for further development of nurse-led services and extension of older people's nurses' roles into areas such as prescribing and chronic disease management. Whatever the advances in roles, however, older people's nurses will always need to be experts at partnership working and multidisciplinary practice.

At the center of practice are older people and nurses who have much to learn from patients and clients and informal carers. The person-centered approach of nursing and strong emphasis on psychosocial as well as physical care identifies potential for nurses to further involve service users in developing services and evaluating the quality of care. A major challenge with this is the involvement of people with dementia and to find further ways to ensure that even when their ability to communicate is restricted, their needs, views, and feelings will be recognized and heeded. This particularly applies to care at end of life, and nurses are ideally placed to hear and help patients and carers express their views and choices. Older people's nurses face many ethical and moral issues in their work, and will always be able to offer a strong contribution within the interdisciplinary team, to supporting older people and their carers when these issues arise, and helping to maintain a focus on quality of life.

CONCLUSION

It is to be hoped that this chapter has provided a flavor of the skill and potential of older people's nursing, and the advances that have occurred in leadership and specialist skills development. The discussion has attempted to be realistic, by acknowledging some of the antecedents and challenges to contemporary nursing of older people, particularly those facing continuing care and the independent sector of care provision for older people. The scope of nursing older people, from essential care to expert practice, has nonetheless been illustrated. Issues have been explored around the development of practice in areas such as acute, continuing and primary care, and a number of policy, politics, and professional drivers have been identified. These continue to drive standards, competency development, education and professional development within the speciality, and older people's nurses and their professional leaders have embraced and responded to them. Older people's nurses have much to take professional pride in, and continue to have a tremendous contribution to make to health care in the future. The caveat remains that nursing will always need to stay patient-centered and focused on meeting essential care needs and quality of life, and share with medical and therapy colleagues a multidisciplinary approach to care.

KEY POINTS

- Nursing older people has developed into a skilled speciality.
- New roles such as the older people's specialist nurse and consultant nurse provide professional leadership and expert practice.
- The principles of nursing older people are based on person-centered care, a focus on essential care needs and interdisciplinary working.
- Professional standards, benchmarking, and competencies promote quality of care for older people in all sectors.
- Much nursing care for older people is provided through the independent sector, for whom particular challenges apply.

KEY REFERENCES

- Department of Health. *Making a Difference – Strengthening the Nursing, Midwifery and Health Visiting Contribution to Health Care* 1999; HMSO.
- Harwood RH, Kempson R, Burke NJ & Morrant JD. Specialist nurses to evaluate elderly in-patients referred to a department of geriatric medicine. *Age and Ageing* 2002; **31**:401–4.
- Royal College of Nursing and the British Geriatrics Society. *Older People's Specialist Nurse: A Joint Statement Form the Royal College of Nursing and the British Geriatrics Society* 2001; RCN/BGS, London.
- Standing Nursing and Midwifery Advisory Committee. *Caring for Older People: A Nursing Priority* 2001; Department of Health, London.
- UKCC. *Standards for Specialist Education and Practice* 2001; UKCC, London.

REFERENCES

Bryans M, Keady J, Turner S *et al.* An exploratory survey into primary care nurses and dementia care. *British Journal of Nursing* 2003; **12**(17):1029–37.

Carper B. Fundamental patterns of knowing in nursing. *Advances in Nursing Science* 1978; **1**:13–23.

Day L, Fildes B, Gordon I *et al.* Randomised factorial trial of falls prevention among older people living in their own homes. *British Medical Journal* 2002; **325**:238.

Department of Health. *A First Class Service: Quality in the New NHS* 1998; Department of Health, London.

Department of Health. *Making a Difference – Strengthening the Nursing, Midwifery and Health Visiting Contribution to Health Care* 1999; HMSO.

Department of Health. *The NHS Plan: A Plan for Investment, a Plan for Reform* 2000; HMSO, London.

Department of Health. *Guidance on Free Nursing Care in Nursing Homes* 2001; Health Service Circular HSC, 2001/17.

Department of Health. *NHS Funded Nursing Care: Practice Guide and Workbook* 2001a; Department of Health, London.

Department of Health. *Essence of Care – Patient-Focused Benchmarking for Health Care Practitioners* 2001b; DoH, The Stationery Office.

Griffiths P, Harris R, Richardson G *et al.* Substitution of a nursing-led inpatient unit for acute services: randomized controlled trial of outcomes and cost of nursing-led intermediate care. *Age and Ageing* 2001; **30**:483–8.

Harwood RH, Kempson R, Burke NJ & Morrant JD. Specialist nurses to evaluate elderly in-patients referred to a department of geriatric medicine. *Age and Ageing* 2002; **31**:401–4.

Help the Aged. *Dignity on the Ward: Promoting Excellence in Care, Promoting Practice in Acute Hospital Care for Older People* 2000; University of Sheffield, The School of Nursing and Midwifery.

Inouye SK, Foreman MD, Mion LC *et al.* Nurses' recognition of delirium and its symptoms: comparison of nurse and researcher ratings. *Archives of Internal Medicine* 2001; **161**(20):2467–73.

Long A, Kneafsey R, Ryan J & Berry J. *Exploring the Contribution of the Nurse in the Multiprofessional Rehabilitation Team*, Research Highlights 45, 2001; ENB, London.

Masterson A. *The Nursing and Health Visiting Contribution to the Continuing Care of Older People* 1997; Central Council for Nursing, Midwifery and Health Visiting, London.

Matthews FE & Dening T. Prevalence of dementia in institutional care. *Lancet* 2002; **360**:225–6.

Mulrooney CP. *Competencies Needed by Formal Care Givers to Enhance Elder's Quality of Life: The Unitility of the 'Person – and Relationship-Centred Caregiving Trait'* 1997; Sixteenth Congress of the International Association of Gerontology, Adelaide.

NHSE. *Nurse, Midwife and Health Visitor Consultants. Establishing Posts and Making Appointments*, HSC 1999/217 1999; NHSE, Leeds.

Nolan M, Booth A, Nolan J & Mason H. *Preparation for Multi-Professional/Multi-Agency Health Care Practice. The Nursing Contribution to Rehabilitation within the Multidisciplinary Team. Literature Review and Curriculum Analysis*, Research highlights 28, 1997; ENB, London.

Nolan M, Brown J, Davies S *et al. Longitudinal Study of the Effectiveness of Educational Preparation to Meet the Needs of Older People and their Carers: The Advancing Gerontological Education in Nursing (AGEiN) Project*, Research Highlights 48, 2002; ENB, London.

Norton D, McClaren R & Exton-Smith AN. *An Investigation into Geriatric Nursing Problems in Hospital* 1962; National Corporation for the Care or Older People.

Norton D, McClaren R & Exton-Smith AN. *An Investigation into Geriatric Nursing Problems in Hospital* 1975; Churchill Livingstone, Edinburgh.

Nursing and Midwifery Council. *Requirements for Pre-Registration Nursing Programmes* 2002; Nursing and Midwifery Council, London.

Nursing Times. Nurse-led workouts boost elderly care. *Nursing Times* 2004; News feature, July, 100, 30, 4.

RCN. *Rehabilitation: The Role of the Nurse. A Workbook.* 2000; RCN, London.

Robertson MC, Gardner MM, Devlin N *et al.* Effectiveness and economic evaluation of a nurse delivered home exercise programme to prevent falls 1. *British Medical Journal* 2001; **322**:697.

Royal College of Nursing and the British Geriatrics Society. *Older People's Specialist Nurse: A Joint Statement Form the Royal College of Nursing and the British Geriatrics Society* 2001; RCN/BGS, London.

Ryder E. Gerontology within district nurse education. *Journal of Advanced Nursing* 1994; **20**(3):430–6.

Scally G & Donaldson LJ. Clinical governance and the drive for quality improvement in the new NHS in England. *British Medical Journal* 1998; **317**:61–5.

Secretary of State for Health. *With Respect to Old Age: Long-Term Care – Rights and Responsibilities* 1999; The Stationery Office.

Secretary of State for Health. *National Service Framework for Older People* 2001; DoH.

Secretary of State for Health. *National Minimum Standards for Care Homes for Older People* 2003; The Stationery Office, London.

Skills for Health. *National Occupational Standards Database* 2004; Older People's Units. Accessible on line at http://195.10.235.25/standards database/index.htm.

Standing Nursing and Midwifery Advisory Committee. *Caring for Older People. A Nursing Priority* 2001, Department of Health, London.

Steiner A, Walsh B, Pickering R *et al.* Therapeutic nursing or unblocking beds? A randomised controlled trial of a post-acute intermediate care unit. *British Medical Journal* 2001; **322**(7284):453–60.

Sturdy D. Consultant nurses – changing the future? *Age and Ageing* 2004; **33**:327–8.

Traynor V & Dewing J. *Admiral Nurses Competency Project: Final Report* 2002; RCN Institute, London.

UKCC. *Standards for Specialist Education and Practice* 2001; UKCC, London.

UKCC. *The Professional, Educational and Occupational Needs of Nurses and Midwives Working Outside the NHS* 2002; UKCC, London.

UKCC. *Report of the Higher Level of Practice Pilot and Project* 2002a; Nursing and Midwifery Council, London.

Waters KR. *The Role of the Nurse in Rehabilitation of Elderly People in Hospital*. Unpublished PhD Thesis, University of Manchester, 1991.

Woods RT, Wills W, Higginson IJ *et al.* Support in the community for people with dementia and their carers: a comparative outcome study of specialist mental health service interventions. *International Journal of Geriatric Psychiatry* 2003; **18**(9):857.

158

Geriatric Occupational Therapy: Focus on Participation in Meaningful Daily Living

Karen F. Barney

Saint Louis University, St Louis, MO, USA

OVERVIEW

Humans as Occupational Beings

The science underlying the occupational therapy profession views humans as *occupational beings* (Clark *et al.*, 1997). In other words, *who we are* is often determined by *what we do*. What we do are the *activities (occupations)* that comprise our lives. Thus, the focus of occupational therapy interventions with and for older adults is to address their unique needs and preferences for *what they need and want to do*, typically in the face of age-related changes and acute and/or chronic conditions. These potential or actual changes in the ability to perform necessary and desired activities *(occupations)* in which they find meaning impact how elders conduct their everyday lives and present a threat to their overall health and identity (Clark *et al.*, 2001; Csikszentmihalyi, 1997). Typically, the identity and sense of well-being of the elders is expressed through their participation in the activities/occupations that comprise their roles, habits, and routines. These patterns of participation represent who they have been throughout their lives, who they are today, and who they may yet become. Participation in society to the extent needed and desired by elders is fundamental to their perception of the quality of personal life, and also a basic component of the World Health Organization's (WHO) latest disability model, the International Classification of Functioning, Disability and Health (ICF) (2001 (*see* **Chapter 10, Social and Community Aspects of Aging**).

Scope of Occupational Therapy Services

Occupational therapy (OT) services are provided at three different levels: (1) directly with individuals and/or family/caregiver(s), (2) consultation and administration with community organizations, and (3) consultation and/or administration with governmental and/or international agencies. Historically, the majority of services have been provided for individual patients and clients, however, a growing number of community level OT services have been established during the past 30 years.

Overall, OT services are designed to sustain or improve the everyday activity related well-being and quality of life of older adults. In addition, services aim to enable families, nongovernmental organizations, and government agencies to mobilize efforts that promote the health of elders, prevent deterioration, restore functions that are impaired by organic disease, impairment or disability, and/or provide compensatory techniques necessitated by age or disability-related changes. In providing services, OT personnel collaborate with older adults and organizations in order to sustain or improve the ability of elders to perform necessary and meaningful activities, taking into consideration their overall health status, personality, lifestyle, family, and other support systems. Thus, whether administered an individual, a group, or a population, OT interventions aim to ensure a quality of life commensurate with the elders' priorities, as well as those of their family members, carers, and their communities (*see* **Chapter 155, Improving Quality of Care**).

OT assessment and intervention services are provided collaboratively with or on behalf of older adults who are at risk for or experience limitations due to disease, acute or chronic illness, injury, developmental disability, and/or the aging process. For example, a person who has sustained a stroke may receive OT services in order to relearn how to dress or to feed herself or himself. These services are provided throughout the continuum of care, to address the full range of daily activity (occupation) and participation needs of older clients or patients, as shown in Figure 1 (*see* **Chapter 160, Geriatric Day Hospitals**).

The levels and forms of OT services span from the needs of older adults living in the community to the

Principles and Practice of Geriatric Medicine, 4th Edition. Edited by M.S. John Pathy, Alan J. Sinclair and John E. Morley.

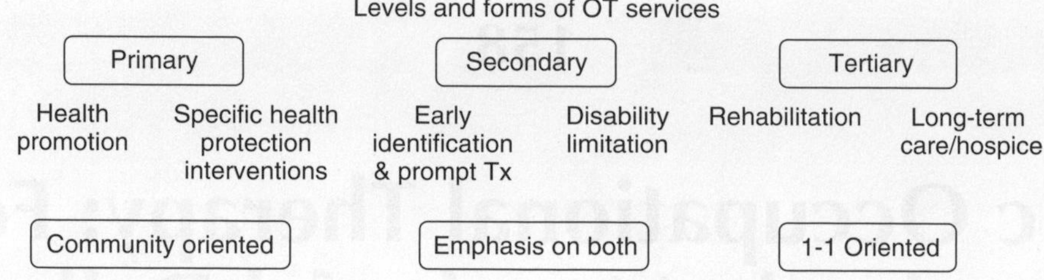

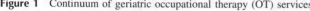

Figure 1 Continuum of geriatric occupational therapy (OT) services

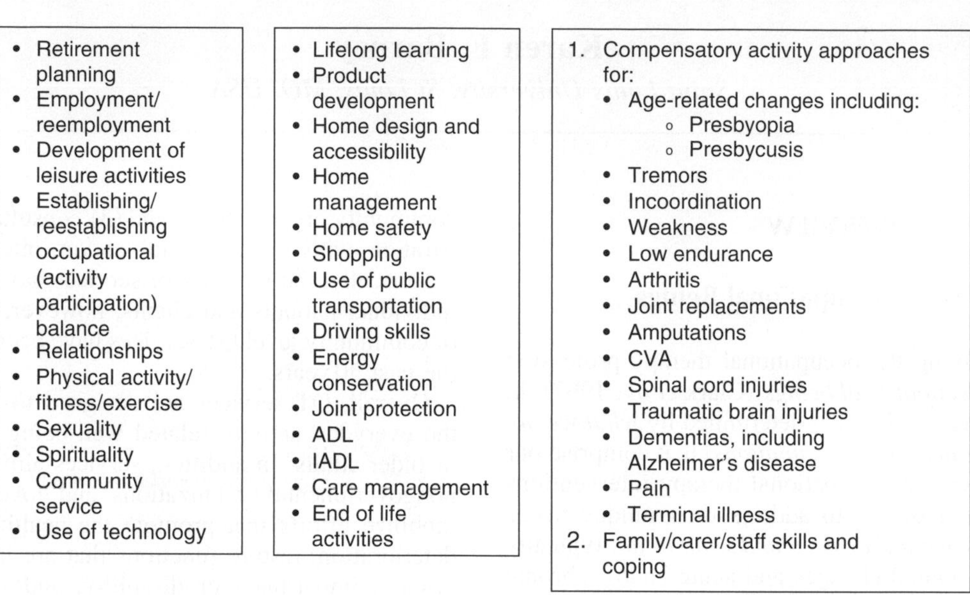

• Retirement planning • Employment/ reemployment • Development of leisure activities • Establishing/ reestablishing occupational (activity participation) balance • Relationships • Physical activity/ fitness/exercise • Sexuality • Spirituality • Community service • Use of technology	• Lifelong learning • Product development • Home design and accessibility • Home management • Home safety • Shopping • Use of public transportation • Driving skills • Energy conservation • Joint protection • ADL • IADL • Care management • End of life activities	1. Compensatory activity approaches for: • Age-related changes including: o Presbyopia o Presbycusis • Tremors • Incoordination • Weakness • Low endurance • Arthritis • Joint replacements • Amputations • CVA • Spinal cord injuries • Traumatic brain injuries • Dementias, including Alzheimer's disease • Pain • Terminal illness 2. Family/carer/staff skills and coping

Figure 2 Geriatric occupational therapy services

needs of those experiencing end-of-life circumstances. Thus, primary, secondary, and/or tertiary settings are included in this continuum of OT services. Primary care OT interventions include provision of health promotion and health protection services within communities. Examples of this type of services include programs on home safety to prevent falls and other injuries and driving retraining as elders experience age-related changes in function. Secondary care OT interventions include individual, group, and/or community approaches for management of health conditions such as arthritis and Alzheimer's disease. Figure 2 displays the categories of services that OTs provide to older adults, their family members, and/or carers:

This topical list depicts typical OT services and is not completely exhaustive. Professional OT services are provided in a range of settings throughout the continuum of care, as shown in Figure 3:

OT services are coordinated with the providers of health care and other services, including physicians, nurses, physical therapists, speech therapists, social workers, community and public health agencies, and others, whenever indicated and available. When services are provided on an individual basis, family members and/or other available support systems often become an integral component of the OT service team, to ensure successful intervention outcomes (*see* **Chapter 152, Carers and the Role of the Family**).

CONCEPTUAL FOUNDATIONS OF GERIATRIC OCCUPATIONAL THERAPY

With a simultaneous focus upon intrinsic and extrinsic factors that impact elders' participation in necessary and meaningful activities, OT personnel work in partnership with the individual or organizational client to promote the enablement of the elders to pursue a meaningful quality of life at all levels of care.

Person–Environment–Occupation–Performance/ Participation

Occupational therapists assess the patient's/client's abilities and occupational performance (enactment of movement, tasks, activities, and routines). These occupational performance abilities relate to the activities (known as *occupations*) that are important to the older individual in the context of their daily lives and environment. OT

- Individual homes/apartments
- Senior centers
- Senior housing
- Retirement centers
- Naturally occurring retirement communities
- Elder continuum of care centers
- Learning centers
- Shopping centers
- Parishes, temples, and congregations
- Private practices
  - Home modification services
  - Care management
  - Lifestyle redesign programs
  - Reemployment services
  - Driving skills
- Local, regional, and/or national private or public agencies

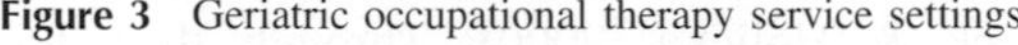

- Acute care
- Sub acute care
- General medicine services
- Rehabilitation
- Adult day services
- Group homes
- Assisted living
- Intermediate care
- Skilled care
- Palliative care
- Hospice care

Figure 3 Geriatric occupational therapy service settings

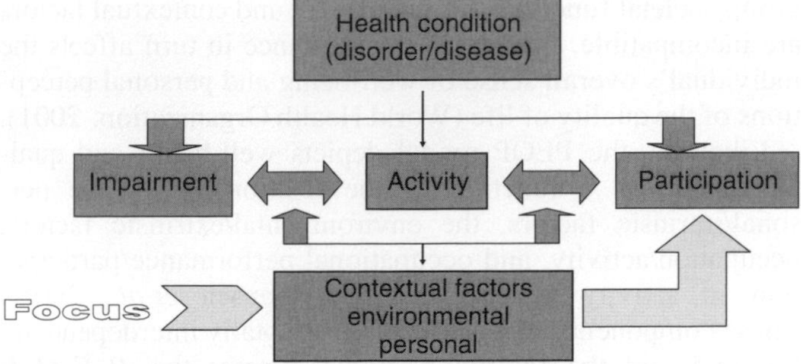

Figure 4 World Health Organization (WHO) International Classification of Function (ICF) model. (Adapted from Figure 1, International Classification of functioning, disability and health, World Health Organization, 2001)

interventions center on enabling elders to pursue the activities, tasks, habits, and routines that are personally important and meaningful to them. All of these activities and occupational components contribute to the elders' perception of their quality of life. Figures 4 and 5 compare the WHO ICF (World Health Organization International Classification of Function) model and the OT person–environment–occupation–performance/participation (PEOP) model (Christiansen *et al.*, 2005).

The WHO ICF is the currently accepted model for systematically grouping consequences associated with health conditions. Level of ability, function, and/or disablement is seen as a dynamic interaction between the individual's health condition and their personal environmental contextual factors. These intrinsic and extrinsic factors affect the individual's ability to pursue the needed and desired activities that comprise their lives and to participate in individual and

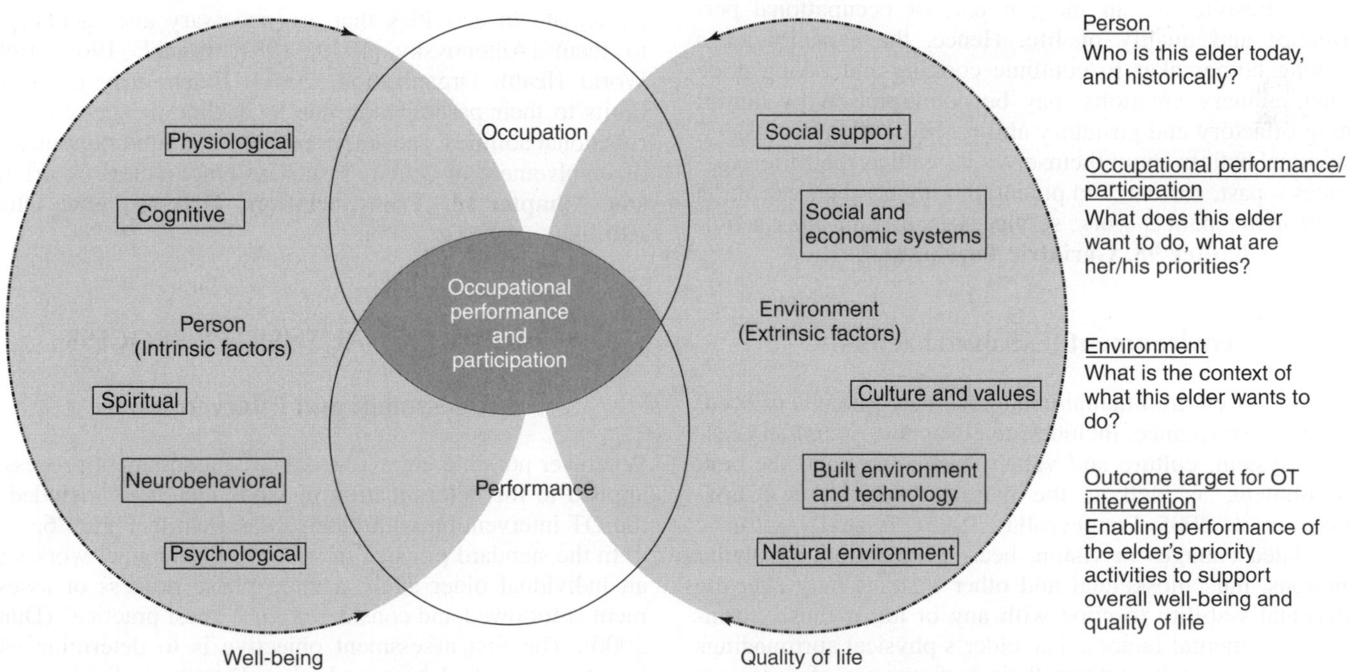

Figure 5 Person-environment-occupation-performance/participation (PEOP) model (Christiansen *et al.*, 2005) applied to geriatric OT practice (Copyright Slack, Inc.)

group societal functions. If impairment and contextual factors are incompatible, this set of circumstance in turn affects the individual's overall sense of well-being and personal perceptions of the quality of life (World Health Organization, 2001).

Likewise, the PEOP model depicts well-being and quality of life as a function of the relationship of the personal/intrinsic factors, the environmental/extrinsic factors, occupation/activity, and occupational performance/participation in activity and society (Christiansen *et al.*, 2005). These components are shown as being totally interdependent. Figure 5 and the following model express the *P-E-O-P* relationship:

$$Elder\ Quality\ of\ Life = f(Personal\ Attributes + Environmental\ Factors + Occupations + Participation)$$

Where "elder quality of life" is dependent upon and a function of the *person's* unique health status and functional abilities, plus the degree to which their *environment* supports the *occupations* that they need and want to pursue and allows them to *perform/participate* in society, to the extent they desire.

Person (Intrinsic Factors)

Occupational therapists assess and intervene to enable elders to cope with normal and inherent age-related changes known as *intrinsic factors*. These factors include physiological, cognitive, spiritual, neurobehavioral, and psychological components of human function. The older adult's level of motivation, as well as roles, habits, and routines that comprise her/his lifestyle are an integral part of occupational performance and quality of life. Hence, the capacity for a life-long homemaker to continue cooking and taking pride in her culinary creations may be compromised by diminishing olfactory and gustatory ability. In addition, the elders' individual beliefs about themselves, as well as their life experiences – past, current, and potential – impact their execution of self-maintenance, work, service, leisure, and other activities (*see* **Chapter 98, Geriatric Psychiatry**).

Environment (Extrinsic Factors)

Extrinsic, or environmental/contextual determinants of occupational performance, include social support, social and economic system, culture and values, technology and the built environment, as well as the natural environment (Christiansen *et al.*, 2005; Fougeyrollas, 1995). Typically, intrinsic age-related changes in vision, hearing, olfaction, vestibular functions, musculoskeletal and other systems may alter the individual's ability to cope with any or all of these extrinsic environmental factors. The elder's physical surroundings may not adequately support their performance of necessary and desired activities because of age-related changes that they experience. Thus, in order for elders to continue to live independently and participate as fully as possible, the inherent changes in sensory and other systems, as well as in cognition, may require changes in their physical environment and other external support systems.

Occupation

What we do consists of occupation(s). Occupations, better known as *activities*, including all abstract and observable types, comprise the everyday lives of people of all ages around the world (American Occupational Therapy Association, 2002). They also assist individuals in understanding who they are, as humans often define themselves by what they do. When young adults are asked, "What do you do?" they may respond by stating their role as student, the type of worker/vocation they pursue, or by their role as homemaker, or parent. When elders are asked the same question, they may respond differently, depending upon what is important to their sense of identity at this later point in life. Nevertheless, occupation/activity in all conceivable forms is the fabric of our existence.

Participation

Active involvement in daily life and various life situations comprise *participation*. This concept includes the ability to perform roles at home, work, and in the community. Various factors may hinder an individual's ability to function in one or more of these environments, due to lack of support, attitudes, physical, social, or societal barriers (Fougeyrollas, 1995; Whiteneck & Holicky, 2000). Through their life span individuals encounter different forms of access to participate in activities that are necessary and meaningful to them (Antonovsky, 1979, 1987; Frankl, 1963, 1997; World Health Organization, 2001). Elders may encounter limits to their participation due to decline in age-related or functional abilities, ageism, or policies that limit continuation of involvement in activities such as employment or driving (*see* **Chapter 13, Transportation, Driving, and Older Adults**).

OCCUPATIONAL THERAPY PROCESS

Assessment and Intervention

Wherever possible, an evidence-based assessment process is applied to the determination of what should be included in the OT intervention with elders, as shown in Figure 6.

In the standard practice in which OT personnel work with an individual older adult, a three phase process of assessment is followed and considered to be "best practice" (Dunn, 2000). The first assessment objective is to determine who has this individual been and what does the individual need and want to do, both in a short and long-term period. The second objective focuses on identifying where and how the

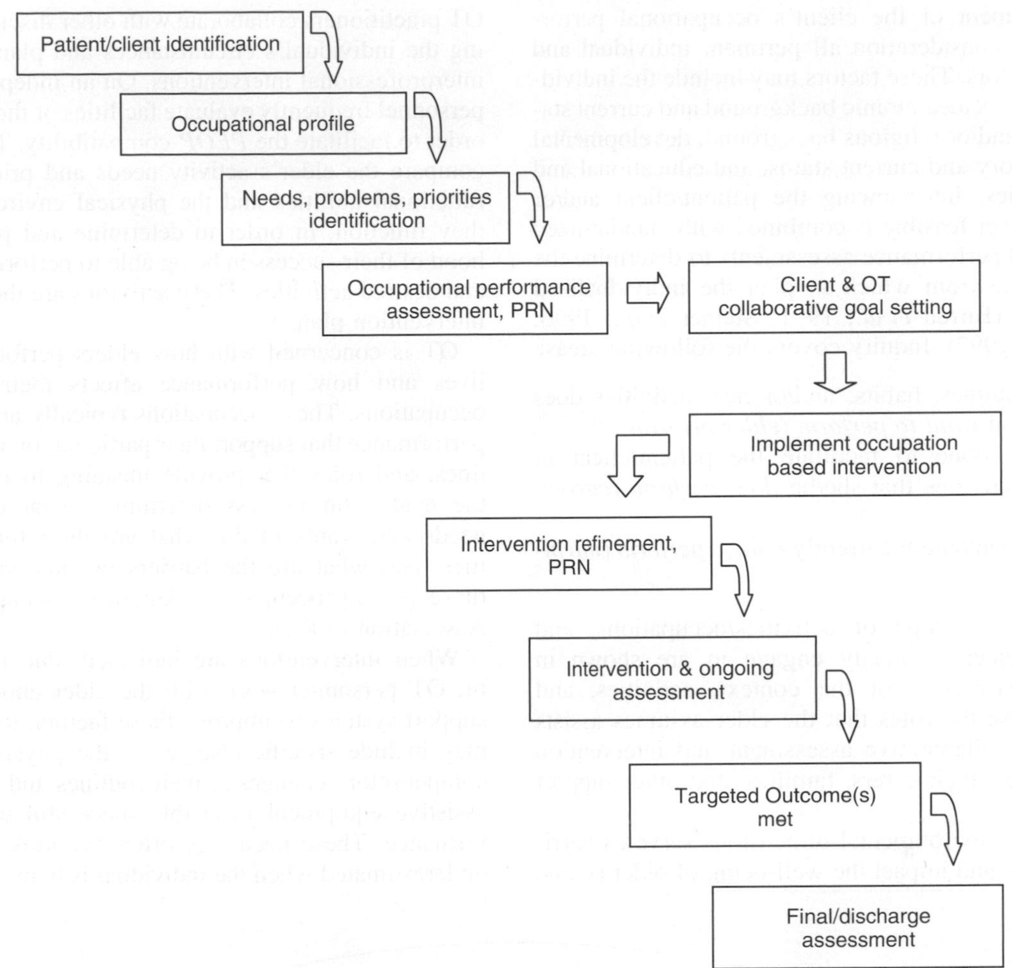

Figure 6 Geriatric occupational therapy assessment & intervention process

activities, tasks, routines, or other occupations can and/or should be done. The third area of concentration in assessment is to determine the biological, psychological, and/or social barriers to the elder's achievement of her/his desired activities. Other individuals or groups may also contribute to the compilation of information on occupational performance issues for the elderly (American Occupational Therapy Association, 2002; Christiansen *et al.*, 2005) (*see* **Chapter 19, Preventive Geriatrics**; **Chapter 57, Cardiac Rehabilitation in Older People**; **Chapter 170, Management of the Dying Patient**; **Chapter 131, Multidimensional Geriatric Assessment**; **Chapter 132, Function Assessment Scales**; **Chapter 153, Nursing Home Care**).

Occupational Profile

The initial step in the OT assessment process determines the client's occupational history and experiences, patterns of daily living, interests, values, and needs. The client's problems and concerns about performing daily and other relevant life activities are identified, the client's priorities are determined, and plans of care and/or management focus on these collaboratively determined priorities (Law *et al.*, 1997). The approach is top-down and client-centered, where enabling participation in personally and culturally relevant and meaningful activities is the focus of planning (Christiansen *et al.*, 2005; Kielhofner, 1995).

Occupational Performance Assessment

This step in the evaluation process specifically determines the client's biopsychosocial assets, needs, problems, or potential problems, based upon results of reliable and valid instruments. Preferably, performance of selected activities is observed in order to identify what supports and what hinders performance. Ideally the assessment process takes place in the elder's usual environment, typically at home, since performance in an unfamiliar environment may be different. Performance skills, performance patterns, context or contexts, activity demands, and client factors are all considered, but only aspects that are specifically relevant to the desired activities may be assessed. Targeted outcomes are identified, based upon the elder's expressed interests and needs.

An OT assessment of the client's occupational performance takes into consideration all pertinent individual and environmental factors. These factors may include the individual's age, gender, socioeconomic background and current status, racial/ethnic and/or religious background, developmental status, health history and current status, and educational and vocational histories. Interviewing the patient/client and/or the family whenever feasible is combined with standardized and agency-based performance assessments to determine the individual's profile from which to plan the individualized intervention plan (Birren *et al.*, 1991; Steiner *et al.*, 1996; Stewart & Ware, 1992). Inquiry covers the following areas:

1. What roles, routines, habits, and/or new activities does the patient/client *want to perform (elder priorities)*?
2. What may be done to facilitate the patient/client in the range of activities that she/he *does perform (current activities)*?
3. What is the patient/client currently *able to perform (intrinsic ability)*?

The environment, scope of activities/occupations, and roles in which elders typically engage in are shown in Figure 7. The knowledge of the context, activities, and those that comprise the roles that the elder assumes assists OT personnel in collaborative assessment and intervention with elderly clients, their carers, families, and other support systems.

Where multiple environmental dimensions serve as barriers to participation and impact the well-being of older adults, OT practitioners collaborate with other disciplines in evaluating the individual's circumstances and planning appropriate interprofessional interventions. On an independent basis, OT personnel frequently evaluate facilities or the elder's home, in order to facilitate the *PEOP* compatibility. These evaluations compare the elder's activity needs and priorities with their functional abilities and the physical environment in which they function, in order to determine and predict the likelihood of their success in being able to perform their necessary and desired activities. These activities are then targeted in the intervention plan.

OT is concerned with how elders perform in their daily lives and how performance affects their engagement in occupations. These occupations typically are components of performance that support their participation in the habits, routines, and roles that provide meaning to their lives. Thus, the evaluation process determines what the patient/client needs and wants to do, what are their functional capabilities, and what are the barriers or supports to performing those priority occupations American Occupational Therapy Association (2002).

When interventions are indicated, due to a poor *PEOP* fit, OT personnel work with the elder and family or other support systems to improve these factors. Recommendations may include specific changes to the physical environment, compensatory changes in their routines and activities, and/or assistive equipment to enable successful occupational performance. These needs are often overlooked completely or underestimated when the individual is being discharged from

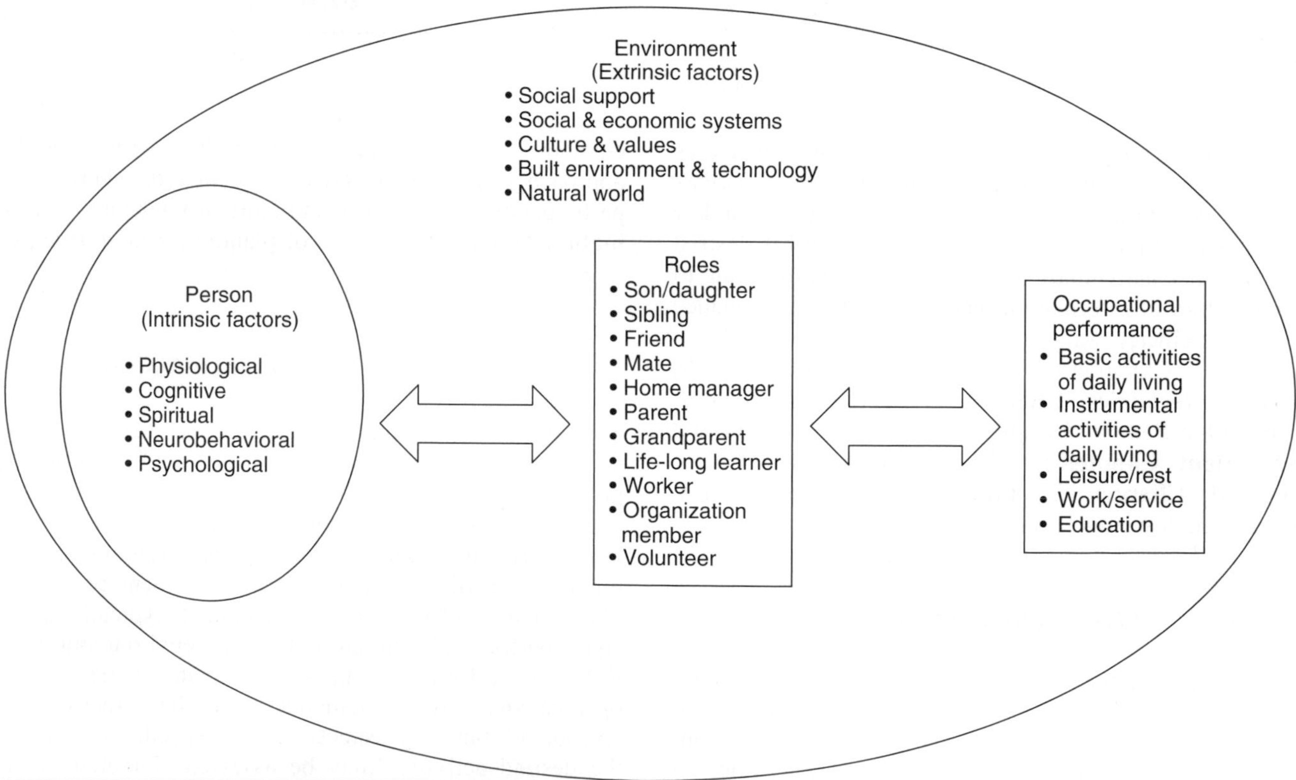

Figure 7 Geriatric occupational therapy assessment & intervention components

one level of medical care to another or to their home. When this insight is lacking, the gaps in environmental support may put the older adult at increased risk for dependency, as well as falls and other injuries (*see* **Chapter 18, Smart Homes**; **Chapter 100, Depression in Late Life: Etiology, Diagnosis and Treatment**; **Chapter 112, Gait, Balance, and Falls**).

Case 1: An 86-year-old Caucasian woman, Grace, was admitted to a local acute-care hospital following a right hip fracture sustained when she fell from a chair while trying to change a light bulb. She was scheduled for a hip replacement.

OT Intervention: During her hospitalization, OT personnel met Grace and completed an occupational profile that informed the therapist about this elderly woman – in particular, her lifestyle, and the activities that she needed and wanted to do. She was provided with a long-handled reaching device to enable her to more easily reach items in her hospital room and at home, once she was discharged. The OT learned that Grace enjoyed knitting and recommended that her daughter bring her mother's current knitting project to the hospital during her stay. Knowing that her right hip mobility would likely be limited for the weeks during her recovery from the hip replacement surgery, the OT worked with Grace on donning her socks, using a sock-aid, and continually reinforcing postsurgical hip precautions. During her hospital stay and immediately prior to discharge, the OT reviewed all activities of daily living (ADL) and instrumental activities of daily living (IADL) implications, as well as other high priority activities that Grace identified during her initial occupational profile. Grace agreed to have the OT arrange for her to have an elevated toilet seat, a tall shower stool, a handheld shower, and grab bars for her home toilet and shower areas for her use following discharge from the hospital. Additional recommendations were made regarding the height of the furniture that Grace would use at home for sitting, eating, and knitting. Grace's daughter agreed to obtain extensions for the legs of Grace's favorite easy chair, so that she would be able to sit and rise from the chair easily. At the time of discharge, Grace's daughter stated that she felt that her mother was well prepared to manage at home during the remainder of her recovery, and most important. . .. Grace agreed.

Case 2: A 65-year-old African man, Kwesi, who completed initial acute-care and rehabilitation treatment for a cerebral vascular accident (CVA) with left side hemiparesis and mild expressive aphasia was referred for continued OT upon discharge to his home. His wife and the OT collaborated with Kwesi in determining the priorities of his current activities and target goals. At this point, he was dependent upon his wife for assistance with toileting, bathing, and dressing, and was not performing IADL tasks that he had assumed prior to his CVA. These activities, plus rejoining his men's group were very important to him. Therefore, over the next several weeks his OT worked with him to upgrade his independence. Since organizing and sequencing the steps within those activities was still difficult, the OT provided him and his wife with strategies to enable him to relearn the steps that were problematic. The OT also worked with his wife to help her realize more success and improved coping with her husband's condition, as well as having more time for the activities that were important to her. Throughout this process the OT coordinated the intervention plan with Kwesi's physician and other health-care providers.

Intervention

Development of the Intervention Plan

OT personnel individually tailor the interventions to the patient/client's needs in order to promote optimal outcomes. The intervention plan is thus developed collaboratively with the patient, so that appropriate strategies, specific interventions, and targeted outcomes are included and mutually agreed upon. Therefore, the approach utilized to increase functional level in ADL, IADL, as well as self-esteem, socialization, and a sense of personal competence in whatever is pursued is unique to each patient/client.

Intervention Implementation Via Client-centered Care

Utilizing goal-directed activities that are meaningful to the patient/client, OT assists the individual to adapt to the physical and social environment. This approach promotes mastery of essential living skills, as well as those skills that represent the patient/client's other priority interests. As a group, elders exemplify highly diverse lifestyles and interests. Therefore, OT personnel identify modalities and activities that are motivating to the patient because they are relevant to her/his particular lifestyle. Collaboration with the patient/client, known as *client-centered care*, facilitates and enables the mobilization of the individual's internal psychological resources. This process then promotes greater participation in the intervention, which in turn, optimally assists in restoring or enhancing function where functional change or decline has occurred or is threatened. All interventions are continually documented, monitored, reevaluated, and adapted or discontinued, based upon the client's overall status.

OT interventions may include any or all of the following:

Use of Occupation to Enhance Quality of Life

1. *Health promotion*: Most individual's lives are comprised of a variety of self-maintenance, productive, leisure, and/or service activities. Thus OT personnel utilize occupations (activities), tasks, roles, routines, and/or habits, as therapeutic agents in achieving long- and short-term goals toward adaptation and habilitation, restoration of function, and/or enhancing the individual's quality of life. Many health promotion programs are provided in the community, however, OT personnel integrate health promotion perspectives in services throughout the continuum of care (Hay *et al.*, 2002; Rothman & Levine, 1992) (refer to Figures 1 and 3).

End of Life: The latter applies also to OT's promotion of quality of life and independence in daily occupations with terminally ill patients, to the extent possible for as long as possible. OT also facilitates maintenance of ADL, pain management, joy, life review, and other meaningful closure activities at the end of life by assisting the elder and their family members to participate in meaningful activities with terminally ill individuals (*see* **Chapter 170, Management of the Dying Patient**).

2. *Community level instruction and patient/client education*: In community settings, OT personnel provide health promotion and other training programs for the elders, family members, carers, and agency employees (Hay *et al.*, 2002; Rothman & Levine, 1992). The content is tailored to the needs of the target group, just as when interventions are implemented for individuals. Subjects covered include those identified or related to those given in Figures 2 and 7.

In acute or subacute care, rehabilitation, and home health care, collaborating with the older patient/client in basic skills training or retraining in functional occupations (e.g. ADL and/or IADL) are standard components of OT practice. Interventions may also focus on making positive transitions in overall lifestyle based on physical, emotional, and/or retirement and service needs of elders (Clark *et al.*, 1997, 2001). Furthermore, the OT personnel collaborate, wherever indicated, with other health-care providers in the rehabilitation team, as well as community agencies to promote optimal patient/client outcomes (Mullins *et al.*, 1997; Reilly, 2001).

Since older adults and their support systems may not be aware of age-related physiological and psychological changes, OT may also employ education or training in these areas to facilitate adaptation to deterioration of function and adjustments in relationships. Topics may include the use of compensatory strategies, recommendations for equipment, and other methods to compensate for loss in function and ensure the ability to participate in meaningful occupations. Health promotion teaching strategies may include the following (Hay *et al.*, 2002):

- prevention of physical deterioration through the use of age-appropriate approaches for participation in activities:
  - body mechanics
  - joint protection
  - energy conservation
  - activity and exercise guidelines
- prevention of psychosocial deterioration through the use of occupation:
  - adjustment of lifestyles to accommodate age-related, role, and other changes in life
  - the role of purposeful, balanced activities in maintaining health
  - overall time management
  - self-esteem, empowerment, mastery strategies
  - interpersonal skills and socialization activities
  - an emphasis on positive aspects of living in promoting a healthy lifestyle.

3. *Remediation strategies for functional decline*: OT interventions to compensate for sensorimotor occupational performance deficits focuses on enabling the elder to participate in the activities identified for maintenance of function and/or improvement. These activities include sitting and standing balance, strengthening, endurance, range of motion, and coordination. Therapeutic approaches employed in all of these occupational performance skills areas are related in the intervention process to ADL and IADL participation, including related tasks and roles performed by and meaningful to the individual.

Furthermore, comorbidities that the older adult experiences are simultaneously factored into the intervention approaches. Interventions are individualized to accommodate cognitive, behavioral, and affective changes that occur following a stroke and/or other neurological conditions, as in dementias or Parkinson's disease. When oral-motor dysfunction, muscular rigidity, joint pain, bradykinesia, or other symptoms impede direct intervention, OT practitioners utilize facilitatory techniques and positioning approaches. These interventions focus on enabling the elder to participate in functional, meaningful activities that accomplish the desired mobilization and overall rehabilitation goals. OT personnel also develop therapeutic programs in a wide variety of settings, which are shown in Figure 3.

4. *Physical environment adaptations*: Because of normal age-related changes, OT consultation and implementation of specific environmental adaptations and modifications may be indicated for most elders, in order to facilitate their continued participation in the activities that are important to them. Where individual or comorbid conditions limit participation, personally relevant physical environmental modifications may be recommended. Additional railings, ramps, grab bars, and assistive devices may be indicated, in order to promote accessibility and independence in mobility and the ability to pursue the elder's necessary and desired occupations. OT interventions also include methods to compensate for cognitive, memory, and psychological changes. These compensatory accommodations that can be implemented in existing or new facilities may make the difference between the elders' dependence and their meaningful participation. OT personnel also provide suggestions for environmental adaptations relative to therapeutic programming and activities for persons with dementia, including cognitive integration, orientation, memory, safety, and pursuit of meaningful activities.

5. *Technological aids and devices*: Low- as well as high-technological assistive devices may be recommended to enhance the elder's occupational performance and participation in solitary, group, or community activities. Low vision aids as well as assistive devices for hearing loss are examples of equipment that may be recommended for use if sensory deficits result in occupational performance deficits. OT personnel often recommend assistive devices for individuals who demonstrate limitations in sensorimotor function, range of motion, strength, coordination, and endurance. Different

types of assistive devices may be suggested for persons who demonstrate occupational performance deficits in their cognitive abilities. Overall, devices are recommended only if they support improved participation in the activities that are important to the elder and/or her/his family or other support system.

Intervention Review

As noted earlier and depicted in Figure 6, OT interventions are continually reviewed and refined, as indicated. Periodic reassessment of the client's status, including ongoing inputs from the elder and/or her/his carers, family members, and other support systems are integrated into any alterations in the intervention plan. When the targeted outcomes are met or it is determined that the elder may not be able to achieve the outcomes despite refinement of the intervention plan, the elder undergoes a final assessment process and is discharged or discontinued from OT services.

Outcomes (Engagement in Activity to Support Participation)

Outcomes – Outcome assessment information determines the extent to which the targeted goals and objectives of the intervention were met. This information is used to plan future actions with the client, discontinuation of services, and to evaluate the service program.

CONCLUSION

OT focuses on the elder's participation in the activities that comprise their lives and that are important to them. The aims of interventions are to (1) collaborate with the older adult to plan client-centered care, (2) tailor the approaches to meet the elderly patient's/ client's activity needs, and (3) address the elder's continued participation in society in a manner that is appropriate and meaningful to that individual, thus affecting her/his overall well-being and quality of life. Fundamental concerns of OT practitioners include supporting the elder's autonomy in setting priorities and making decisions regarding her/his participation and maintaining a level of mastery and control over her/his environment and lifestyle. OT personnel foster an enabling therapeutic relationship with older adults of all ability levels throughout the continuum of care. The emphasis of OT on the elder's ability to participate in meaningful occupations promotes cost-effective care, individual competence, and optimal quality of life (Clark *et al.*, 1997, 2001).

KEY POINTS

- Humans throughout their lives are *occupational beings*. Thus, *who we are* is typically framed by *what we do*. OT is patient/client centered, collaborative, and focuses on what the individual *needs* and *wants to do*.
- OT services aim to sustain or improve the elders' ability to perform necessary and meaningful activities (*occupations*), whether they are long term and historically a part of the elder's life or newly acquired interests and roles.
- OT identifies the strengths and priorities of the patient/client and partners with the individual and their family members or other support systems to ensure their participation in the occupations that sustain their overall health and quality of life.
- OT interventions focus on supporting age-related changes and/or comorbidities that affect the elder's ability to participate in desired activities/occupations. Interventions thus target the individual's biopsychosocial occupational performance abilities and often include adaptive approaches and assistive devices that compensate for any existing occupational performance deficits.
- OT services are provided throughout the continuum of care, from primary care health promotion and wellness approaches to interventions in tertiary, long-term care, and hospice settings.

KEY REFERENCES

- American Occupational Therapy Association. *The Occupational Therapy Practice Framework* 2002; The American Occupational Therapy Association, Bethesda.
- Christiansen CH, Baum CM & Bass-Haugen J (eds). *Occupational Therapy: Performance, Participation, and Well-Being* 2005; SLACK, Thorofare.
- Clark F, Azen SP, Zemke R *et al.* Occupational therapy for independent-living older adults: a randomized controlled trial. *Journal of the American Medical Association* 1997; **278**:1321–6.
- Csikszentmihalyi M. *Finding Flow: The Psychology of Engagement with Everyday Life* 1997; Harper Collins Publishers, New York.
- World Health Organization. *International Classification of Functioning, Disability and Health (ICF)* 2001; World Health Organization, Geneva.

REFERENCES

American Occupational Therapy Association. *The Occupational Therapy Practice Framework* 2002; The American Occupational Therapy Association, Bethesda.

Antonovsky A. *Health, Stress and Coping* 1979; Jossey-Bass, San Francisco.

Antonovsky A. *Unraveling the Mystery of Health: How People Manage Stress and Stay Well* 1987; Jossey-Bass, San Francisco.

Birren JE, Lubben JE, Rowe JC & Deutchman DE (eds). *The Concept and Measurement of Quality of Life in the Frail Elderly* 1991; Academic Press, San Diego.

Christiansen CH, Baum CM & Bass-Haugen J (eds). *Occupational Therapy: Performance, Participation, and Well-Being* 2005; Slack, Inc, Thorofare.

Clark F, Azen SP, Zemke R *et al.* Occupational therapy for independent-living older adults: a randomized controlled trial. *Journal of the American Medical Association* 1997; **278**:1321–6.

Clark F, Azen SP, Carlson M *et al.* Embedding health-promoting changes into the daily lives of independent-living older adults: long-term follow-up of occupational therapy intervention. *The Journals of Gerontology. Series B, Psychological Sciences and Social Sciences* 2001; **56B**:P60–3.

Csikszentmihalyi M. *Finding Flow: The Psychology of Engagement with Everyday Life* 1997; Harper Collins Publishers, New York.

Dunn W. *Best Practice Occupational Therapy in Community Service with Children and Families* 2000; SLACK, Thorofare.

Fougeyrollas P. Documenting environmental factors for preventing the handicap creation process: Quebec contributions relating to the ICIDH and social participation of people with functional differences. *Disability and Rehabilitation* 1995; **17**:145–53.

Frankl VE. *Man's Search for Meaning* 1963; Simon & Schuster Publishing, New York.

Frankl VE. *Man's Search for Ultimate Meaning* 1997; Plenum Publishing Corporation, New York.

Hay J, LaBree L, Luo R *et al.* Cost-effectiveness of preventive occupational therapy for independent-living older adults. *Journal of the American Geriatrics Society* 2002; **50**:1381–8.

Kielhofner G. *A Model of Human Occupation: Theory and Application* 1995, 2nd edn; Williams & Wilkins, Baltimore.

Law M, Polatajko H, Baptiste W & Townsend E. Core concepts of occupational therapy. In E Townsend (ed.) *Enabling Occupation: An Occupational Therapy Perspective* 1997, pp 29–56; Canadian Association of Occupational Therapists, Ottawa.

Mullins LL, Balderson BHK, Sanders N *et al.* Therapists' perceptions of team functioning in rehabilitation contexts. *International Journal of Rehabilitation & Health* 1997; **3**:281–8.

Reilly C. Transdisciplinary approach: an atypical strategy for improving outcomes in rehabilitative and long-term acute care settings. *Rehabilitation Nursing* 2001; **26**:216–20.

Rothman J & Levine R. *Prevention Practice: Strategies for Physical Therapy and Occupational Therapy* 1992; WB Saunders Company, Philadelphia.

Steiner A, Raube K, Stuck A & Aronow H. Measuring psychosocial aspects of well-being in older community residents: performance of four short scales. *The Gerontologist* 1996; **36**(1):54–62.

Stewart AL & Ware JE. *Measuring Functioning and Well-Being: The Medical Outcomes Study Approach* 1992; Duke University Press, Durham.

Whiteneck G & Holicky R. Expanding the disablement model. In M Brabois, S Garrison, K Hart & L Lehmkuhl (eds) *Physical Medicine and Rehabilitation: The Complete Approach* 2000; Blackwell Science, Malden.

World Health Organization. *International Classification of Functioning, Disability and Health (ICF)* 2001; World Health Organization, Geneva.

Systems of Health Care: the United Kingdom, the United States, and Australia

Julie K. Gammack[1], Gideon A. Caplan[2] *and* Krishnendu Ghosh[3]

[1] *Saint Louis University School of Medicine, St Louis, MO, USA and Geriatric Research Education and Clinical Center, St Louis, MO, USA,* [2] *Prince of Wales Hospital, Randwick, New South Wales, Australia, and* [3] *University Hospital, Coventry, UK*

INTRODUCTION

The extraordinary growth in life expectancy at birth in nearly all countries of the world reflects an ongoing revolution in longevity. This revolution encompasses both survival of individuals to older ages and changing age profiles of the entire population. The impact of the longevity revolution has been pervasive and profound. The demographic trend of an increased life expectancy has already changed the age profile of many countries and is continuing to be felt throughout the world. This trend has resulted in significant health-care changes, both on an individual and at societal level.

Developed nations across the world have approached the aging population and need for expanded health services in a variety of ways. Home health, hospital-based, and nursing home care have experienced a profound increase in complexity over the last quarter century. This complexity of care is reflected in the expansion of funding arrangements, number of service providers, and geographic service areas. Governments have expanded health care spending and broadened the scope of medical care. The development of health insurance programs has allowed a greater number of individuals to access medical services.

Institutes of higher learning have evolved to support the growing fields of gerontology and geriatric medicine. Educating the medical providers, workforce, and community on the needs of older adults has become an area of profound interest within and outside of the academic environment. It is important to draw older people into the processes of developing the services and new technologies that they themselves and others of their generation will use. By developing these new health-care opportunities, the greatest gains may be made in health, independence, and quality of life in old age.

OVERVIEW OF HEALTH-CARE DEMOGRAPHICS

United Kingdom

In the last 30 years, the population of the United Kingdom (UK) has grown 6.5% from 55.9 million in 1971 to 59.6 million in 2003. This population growth has occurred substantially more in the older age-groups. The percentage of people over age 65 has increased from 13% in 1971 to 16% in 2003, whereas the proportion younger than age 16 has dropped over the past 30 years. Projections for 2031 predict an increasingly rapid aging of the population with those over age 85 doubling from 1.9 to 3.8% of the UK population (Office for National Statistics, 2004).

Health-care spending in the United Kingdom has grown more quickly than other economic expenditures, reaching 7.7% of the gross domestic product (GDP) in 2002. Government, household, and charitable health-care costs reached £80.6 billion in 2002, compared with £74.8 billion the previous year (Office for National Statistics, 2003). Public health expenditures increased by £5.1 billion (8%) in 2002 compared with £700 million (5%) in private health expenditures. Despite a more rapid rate of growth, the proportion of publicly funded health expenditures has remained unchanged at 83%.

All individuals residing in United Kingdom are entitled to receive treatment from the National Health Service (NHS), which is free at the point of delivery. The NHS, established in 1948, is the third largest employer in the world after Chinese Army and Indian Railways respectively. Dr Tom Wilson was appointed the first consultant geriatrician in 1948 at Cornwall, which marked the introduction of this new medical speciality.

Principles and Practice of Geriatric Medicine, 4th Edition. Edited by M.S. John Pathy, Alan J. Sinclair and John E. Morley.

By late 2002, there were 1037 consultant geriatricians in United Kingdom, representing one consultant per 55 000 UK residents (Working Party Report, 2005). The British Geriatric Society (BGS) has recommended a ratio of one geriatrician per 50 000 of the population (one geriatrician for each 4000 people over age 75). This ratio does not include the increasing involvement of geriatricians in unselected acute medicine activities. In 2002, 88.6% of consultant geriatricians engaged in acute medicine compared with 30% in 1995. Geriatrics is currently the largest speciality under the Royal College of Physicians.

United States

The United States (US) spends 13% of the GDP, 1.8 trillion dollars, on health-care expenditures. This is more than any other industrialized nation (American Hospital Association and the National Chronic Care Consortium, 2002). Health-care expenditures have doubled in the past 10 years; however, 15% of population does not have health insurance. The provision of health care is equally split between private insurance, governmental programs (medicare/medicaid), and private or out-of-pocket payers.

The number of hospitals and length of hospital admission have dropped consistently since peaking in the early 1970s. Outpatient encounters have tripled since that time (American Hospital Association, 2004). Despite this trend, hospital expenditures have risen 60% in the last 10 years. About one-third of health-care resources are spent on hospitalization and one-quarter on physician services. Individuals, aged 65 or older, utilize one-quarter of outpatient encounters, half of hospitalization days, and one-third of the total health-care expenditures.

Currently 13% of the US population is age 65 or older. This population is projected to reach 20% by 2040 (U.S. Census Bureau, 2005). These trends have caused great concerns both economically and socially. The health-care budget cannot sustain the current growth rate of medical expenditures. Methods to provide cost-effective, quality health care for an aging population are being addressed on a system-wide level. Research funding, educational efforts, and clinical care models are being developed to better serve the health-care needs of the geriatric population.

Australia

Australia has an aging population comparable to most developed countries. In 2001, 13% of the 20 million residents were age 65 and over. With a life expectancy of 76.7 for males and 82.0 for females, it is estimated that one-quarter of the Australian population will be over age 65 by the year 2051. At that time, the projected life expectancy will be 83.3 for males and 86.5 for females. In this population, dementia is the leading cause of disease burden by a factor of two. Dementia accounts for 16.7% of years of life lost to disability. Currently, over 160 000 Australians have dementia and this rate is predicted to increase over 250% by 2041. While vascular disease and cancer remain the two leading causes of death, mortality rates from these diseases in older people have decreased markedly over the last decade.

While the health of the Australian population has generally been improving, the health of indigenous people, the Aborigines and Torres Strait Islanders (ATSI) has not improved at the same rate. These groups suffer death rates of two to three times that of the general population. The leading causes of death in these individuals remain vascular disease, respiratory illness, injury, and cancer. While aged care services for most Australians are targeted toward the population over age 70, for ATSI people these same services are provided for those over age 50.

Australia spent 9.5% of the GDP on health care in 2002 (AUD $72.2 billion). Although health spending has grown as the population has aged, this is mainly attributed to spending on new technology and pharmaceuticals, rather than on the increasing number of older individuals. The percentage of GDP spent on health care is lower than the US, comparable to Canada and European countries, but higher than the UK. The Australian health system is tortuous in its complexity, particularly for the consumer. The services and care for older adults have been particularly complicated.

DEVELOPMENT OF GERIATRIC MEDICINE

United Kingdom

For various historical reasons, specialist geriatric services developed as an integral part of the NHS in the United Kingdom earlier than in any other area of Europe. Margery Warren established geriatric medicine in Britain in the late 1930s. Her message was the need for assessment and rehabilitation of elderly disabled people, education of medical students, and research into the problems of aging and old age (Warren, 1943, 1946). This derived from her work in the workhouse infirmary associated with the West Middlesex Hospital in London. Her methods (careful medical and social assessment, medical treatment, and rehabilitation) were described in a series of publications (Warren, 1943, 1946, 1949). The general conclusion was that elderly patients should be treated in a special block in general hospitals because

- geriatrics is an important subject for the teaching of medical students;
- geriatrics should be an essential part of the training of student nurses;
- general hospital facilities are necessary for correct diagnosis and treatment;
- research on diseases of aging can only be undertaken with the full facilities of a general hospital.

These were visionary proposals in 1943.

The emerging recognition of the needs of older people in an aging society led to a number of major surveys and resulted in the collection of planning data for the introduction of new health-care services. Curran and colleagues (1946) published data on about 1000 males over age 65 and females over age 60 and who lived in poorer areas of Glasgow, all of whom received home visits. A social and medical survey of people in England over age 65 was also performed by the Nuffield Foundation in 1943. The results were published in two reports – "Old People" (1947) and the "Social Medicine of Old Age" (1948) (Nuffield Foundation, 1947; Sheldon, 1948). The British Medical Association (BMA) set up a working group in 1947 to review care of the elderly and infirm and to make general health-care recommendations (British Medical Association, 1947). Of the 21 BMA members, four were active in the new speciality of geriatrics (Amulree, Brooke, Cousin, Warren).

Dr Trevor Howell, originally a general practitioner (GP), became interested in elderly medicine after becoming responsible for Chelsea pensioners. He was appointed consultant physician at Battersea and subsequently opened one of the first geriatric units there (Adams, 1975; Irvine, 1986–1987; Howell, 1974). In 1947, he called a meeting to bring together physicians who had a special interest in older people and skills in rehabilitation, incontinence management, and domiciliary assessment.

This meeting launched the Medical Society for the Care of the Elderly. These pioneering physicians persuaded the Minister of Health to appoint more geriatricians as part of the hospital consultant expansion of the new NHS. The society was renamed the British Geriatrics Society in 1959 to emphasize the scientific basis of elderly medicine. The efforts of this society resulted in a revolution in the delivery of health care and services for the elderly.

During the 1960s and 1970s, remarkable improvements occurred in the medical care of patients who were managed on geriatric units. There was a rapid increase in the number of consultant geriatrician appointments in the 1960s from a total of four geriatricians in 1947, to over 300 by 1973. The NHS has recognized the value of geriatrics as an emerging speciality, and has invested significant time and resources to improve services and standards of care for older people.

During the 1980s and much of 1990s, the trend in United Kingdom was for geriatric practice to become more closely identified with acute general internal medicine and to be less involved with rehabilitation and long-term care. The improved access to acute diagnostic facilities for older people was welcomed. The rise in consumerism and desire for choice, have resulted in the public having a higher expectation of all services. Inadequacies and inequalities in the health care of older people have had a major influence on current heath policy.

A campaign started by a national newspaper and an older people's charity (Help the Aged) led the government to commission an independent inquiry into the care of older people. As a result of the finding, a National Service Framework (NSF) containing standards of care for older people was published on 27 March 2001 in order to apply to the NHS for implementation.

Through the NHS, the NSF for older people has been developed with guidance from an External Reference Group (ERG), cochaired by Dr Ian Philp (now the National Director of Older People's Services) and Ms. Denise Platt, Chief Inspector of the Social Services Inspectorate. The ERG brought together older people and their caregivers, health and social services professional staff, NHS and social services managers, and partner agencies.

The frameworks are designed to improve the quality of health care by setting standards for the structure, process, and intended outcomes of key medical conditions. These frameworks establish minimum practice standards and eliminate unacceptable care patterns. The NSF is a 10-year health-care improvement program implemented through local health and social care partners, and national underpinning programs. Progress is monitored through a series of milestones and performance measures, and is overseen by the NHS Modernization Board and the Older People's Services.

Using the NSF targets, the NHS and social care services treat older people as individuals and enable them to make choices about their own care. The NSF for older people is different from its predecessors (NSFs for cancer care, mental health, and coronary heart disease) in that it focuses on a population rather than on a set of conditions. The focus is larger and more complex, as older people consume about 50% of health and social care expenditures. This is the first framework to establish standards for social as well as health care (Philp, 2002). The NSF has established new national standards, service models, and social services for all older people, whether they live at home, in residential care or in hospital. This is achieved through the single assessment process, integrated commissioning arrangements, and integrated provision of services.

United States

In the United States, geriatrics came into the medical consciousness through the writings of Dr Ignatz Nascher. Although born in Austria, he was raised in the United States and received his medical degree from New York University. In 1909 at the age of 46, Dr Nascher published his first article on geriatrics titled *Longevity and Rejuvenescence*. In this work, he proposes that "geriatrics" be added to the medical vocabulary and that it be considered a distinct aspect in medicine. Over the next 5 years, he authored more than 30 articles on aging and the first American geriatrics textbook titled *Geriatrics: The Diseases of Old Age and Their Treatment*. This text focused dually on the physiology and pathophysiology of aging. Nascher touched on a multitude of topics including organ system physiology, pharmacology, diseases of aging, and psychosocial aspects of medicine. With an optimistic view, he wrote in 1926 that, "Geriatrics is now firmly established as a special branch of medicine..."

Unfortunately, geriatrics was not yet widely accepted and the growth of this speciality was quite slow through the 1930s and 1940s. The mid-1900s were notable for the establishment of two medical societies. Malford W. Thewlis founded the American Geriatrics Society in 1942, and the Gerontological Society (now called The Gerontological Society of America) was established in 1945.

Research in aging was championed by Dr E. Vincent Cowdry who received his Ph.D. in anatomy from the University of Chicago in 1913. During his 65-year career spent predominantly at Washington University School of Medicine, Dr Cowdry focused his research efforts on cancer and the cytologic changes of aging. During the later half of his career he authored several books including *The Problems of Ageing: Biological and Medical Aspects* (1939), *The Care of the Geriatric Patient* (1958), and *Aging Better* (1972).

Geriatrics in the United States developed as much through the establishment of governmental socioeconomic programs as it did from the work of prominent physicians. In 1861, a military pension plan was established to support the civil war era veterans. After the civil war, many states established veterans homes to provide disability and medical care services. These services were consolidated through the development of the veterans administration in 1930. By 1935, a rapidly increasing population of impoverished older adults led to the formation the Social Security Board which reorganized in 1946 to become the Social Security Administration. This program provides a retirement benefit to individuals upon leaving the workforce. Although state and federal subsidies for health-care services were sporadically available in the 1920s, the first private hospital insurance plan (Blue Cross) was not provided until 1933. Further discussion and development of government sponsored health insurance for the elderly spanned five presidential administrations and over three decades.

In 1950, through efforts by President Truman, the Federal Security Administration held a national conference on aging to assess the challenges posed by the changing population. No immediate programs were initiated, but this conference spurred the development of an advisory committee on aging and eventually led to the first White House Conference on Aging in 1961. The conference resulted in the expansion of social security benefits and support for the later development of medicare and medicaid. In 1965, insurance was finally guaranteed to older adults, the disabled, and the impoverished through the passage of medicare and medicaid programs.

During the mid-1900s, the US government was the primary financial sponsor of health-care research and scientific programs. The National Institute of Health (NIH) was formed in 1930 and later became a consortium of institutes and centers dedicated to health-care research. The National Institute on Aging (NIA) was formally established out of the NIH in 1974, but the roots of the NIA can be traced back to the 1940s and 1950s with the unit on aging, gerontology branch, and a section on aging as subsections of NIH programs.

The NIA receives substantial funding for the advancement of aging research. Through NIA support, the 32 Alzheimer's Disease Centers, 9 Claude D. Pepper Older American Independence Centers, and numerous Edward R. Roybal Centers for Research on Applied Gerontology sponsor investigations into the biological, behavioral, and clinical aspects of aging. During the last quarter century, there has been a growth in the private support of geriatric medicine research and education. Hundreds of millions of dollars have been provided by The John A. Hartford, Donald W. Reynolds, and other agencies dedicated to the care of the aging population.

Australia

The speciality of geriatric medicine in Australia is generally considered to have started in 1950 when the Hospital Commission of New South Wales (NSW) requested the Royal Newcastle Hospital to survey the known people with multiple sclerosis in the Hunter Valley, with a view to setting up a hospital clinic for those patients. Dr Richard Gibson and Miss Grace Parbery, a social worker, were appointed to conduct the survey and identified the need for medical, nursing, and domestic care at home for the chronic sick in general. It took another 5 years to institute these outreach services and subsequently hospital rehabilitation services as well. Rudimentary services started soon after in other states but the independent origins led to different patterns of development.

Australia was founded in 1901 as a federation of six states each of which had slightly different history and health system. Each state government retained control of existing health services, mainly hospitals. Over the years, the growth of national government taxation revenue has resulted in the introduction of new health-care programs, mainly nonhospital services. Many of these services were developed in response to genuine health-care deficiencies but as a result, Australia has a dually administered health system through a partnership of the national and state governments. The Australian national government generally retains primary control over the newly established health-care services or programs. The national government pays for community health, nursing home, and visits to doctors offices, but the level of control over these programs varies.

The Australian government pays for visits to doctors under the medicare scheme of universal health insurance. Medicare is partially funded by a 1.5% levy on income tax and a 1% surcharge from those earning at least AUD $50 000. Additional revenue for the physician may be generated from the patients, who are responsible for paying when the physician decides to charge an extra fee. Medicare reimburses physicians 85% of the established *Schedule Fee*, an amount derived from a survey of fees in the early 1970s. The schedule fee has been underadjusted for inflation over time, with a resulting 30% drop in reimbursement rates. This has prompted some physicians to pass on increasing copayment fees to their patients. At this time, the percentage of GP consultations entirely paid for by medicare has declined to about 70%.

Most medical care for older people is administered by GPs. Medicare disproportionately rewards GPs for shorter office-based consultations, which favors younger, single problem patients. General practice has also seen a shift toward corporatization, where companies employ GPs in multidoctor practices and generally discourage nonoffice work. These trends have resulted in a decrease in the number of GPs who perform home or nursing home visits. In 1999 a range of longer, better-remunerated consultations were introduced to encourage adequate consultations with frail, older people, including annual health assessments, multidisciplinary care planning, and case conferencing. These have recently been augmented to also cover residential aged care; however, these measures have not been adequately assessed to determine whether they provide any benefit.

The Australian government under the Pharmaceutical Benefits Scheme (PBS) pays for medications with some copayments charged to patients. Rapid increases in the cost of the PBS of around 15% per year have led to a variety of measures to decrease costs. One method is to limit the number of new drugs coming onto the PBS. Patients have also been required to pay the full cost of many new drugs. In other situations, drug companies will negotiate to cap payments for a new pharmaceutical agent on the basis of the projected medication expenditures for that agent.

Geriatric medicine is a relatively new, but growing speciality. A survey of all specialist consultant physicians found that there were 185 practicing geriatricians in 2003. One-third also practice general medicine. This provides Australia with approximately one geriatrician per 5900 people aged 75 and over (Dent, 2004; Australian Medical Workforce Advisory Committee, 1997). Because geriatric medicine attracts a higher proportion of female specialists in Australia, and over a lifetime, females work approximately 75% of the hours of male graduates, access to geriatricians is more limited than what is actually calculated. The demand for geriatricians is increasing, but not currently met by the supply of trainees. The profession, health-care industry and the government continue to grapple with this problem.

HOME HEALTH CARE

United Kingdom

The practice of seeing patients in their own homes has been an essential component of geriatric practice since its early stages when consultants inherited large panels of patients with long waiting lists. Home visits are usually ordered by a GP via a referral to the geriatric consultant who carries out the visit. Within the NHS, house calls are part of the consultant's contracts and are called *domiciliary assessment visits*. Nurses, therapists, and other health providers are also important members of the home care team.

The NSF has established numerous standards of care for older adults that relate to home health care (HHC): fall prevention, mental health evaluation, and health promotion. These standards can be incorporated into a multidisciplinary care plan or addressed by an individual medical provider in the home. Through the Health Act 1999, the National HealthCare Corp (NHC) has been establishing new partnerships to allow health authorities to improve HHC and social services. Local strategic partnerships have been formed between the public, private, and community sectors to provide a single and uniform framework through which the NSF mission can be achieved. Through these partnerships, community equipment services will be modernized, integrated home care services will be expanded, and higher standards of quality will be set for the residential care of older adults. Research on the impact of the continuity of care process on patient outcomes is being conducted through the NSF.

Health-care Standard: Falls

The aim of this standard is to reduce the number of falls that result in serious injury and to ensure effective treatment and rehabilitation for those who have fallen. The NHS, working in partnership with health-care councils, takes action to prevent falls and reduce resultant fractures or other injuries in the older population. Older individuals who have fallen receive effective treatment and rehabilitation and, with their caregivers, receive advice on prevention through a specialized falls service.

Some health care trusts and councils are already making significant progress toward the 2005 milestone of an integrated falls service. Although overall progress with integrated falls services has been heterogeneous, there has been considerable growth in certain individual components. For example, a recent Help the Aged survey of 94 primary care trusts found that, although only a few were on their way to an integrated service, most were in the process of developing falls prevention programs.

There are a number of important collaborations in place to promote the falls prevention program. The Healthy Living collaborative focuses on falls services, while other organizations are involved in falls program partnerships. In these areas, organizations and older people have come together to make small but effective changes in health-care delivery to prevent falls and improve services for those who have fallen.

The National Institute for Clinical Excellence has produced guidelines on falls prevention in 2004 and has been asked to produce osteoporosis prevention guidelines by 2005. The institute is also undertaking an appraisal on osteoporosis drug treatments. These guidelines and the appraisal will be very significant in the development of falls services.

Health-care Standard – Mental Health in Older People

The aim of this standard is to promote good mental health in older people and to treat and support those older people with dementia and depression. Older people who have mental health problems have access to integrated mental health services. The NHS and health-care councils ensure effective diagnosis, treatment, and support for patients and their caregivers. About 5% of the population over age 65 has dementia and about 10–15% of the population over age 65 has depression. This represents a large numbers of individuals who need high quality treatment and support to maximize their quality of life. Improving mental health services is a significant target area for the NSF. It is hoped that the widespread introduction of the single assessment process will result in earlier detection of dementia and depression.

Underdetection of mental illness in older adults is widespread, in part due to the nature of depressive symptoms and the fact that many older people live alone. Older people from minority and ethnic populations are at high risk of being underdiagnosed and undertreated for mental illnesses. Mental health services should be community-oriented, comprehensive, accessible, and individualized. Primary care groups and trusts should take responsibility for planning and delivery of mental health services in the local community.

Health-care Standard – The Promotion of Health and Active Life in Older Age

The aim of this standard is to extend the healthy life expectancy of older people. The health and well-being of older people is promoted through a coordinated program of action led by the NHS with support from local councils. There is significant progress toward the targets of increasing influenza immunization rates, reducing smoking, and improving management of blood pressure.

In an update from Department of Health (2004), older people expressed a willingness to stop smoking and take advantage of health screening and immunizations to stay healthy. Recently published "Better health in old age" report by Professor Ian Philp, National Director for Older People's Health, is an update on the 2001 NSF. According to the report, the services for older people are improving but must continue to expand to meet the needs of an increasingly aged population. The report also reveals that life expectancy has increased. Men reaching age 65 in 2002 can expect to live for another 16 years compared to 14.6 years in 1993. Women reaching age 65 in 2002 can expect to live for another 19 years compared to just over 18 years in 1993. Overall mortality rates for people over age 65 have fallen and death from suicide has dropped from 11.8 per 100 000 population in 1993 to 8.8 per 100 000 population in 2003.

United States

For most of history, medical care has been provided in the home by a physician. In the mid-1900s, 40% of all patient–physician encounters took place at home. With the growth of hospital and office-based care, by 1980, fewer than 1% of health-care visits took place at home (Leff and Burton, 2001). HHC began growing again in the 1980s as new models of home assessment developed and the delivery of home care evolved into an organized, multidisciplinary business. The current HHC model primarily utilizes nursing, therapy, and personal care providers to deliver health-care services. Physician house calls still remain underutilized as a means of caring for frail older adults.

Home visits are an effective method for delivering medical assistance for the aged and chronically ill and homebound individuals. House calls have most often demonstrated benefit in chronic and relapsing diseases such as congestive heart failure and emphysema. Regular visits by a medical professional can improve disease control and reduce hospitalizations (Rich *et al.*, 1995; Stewart *et al.*, 1999). This translates to a societal cost savings, which has prompted medicare, medicaid, and private insurance agencies to continue the funding of home care services.

Medicare and medicaid provided 50% of HHC coverage in the United States between 1990 and 1997. HHC expenditures grew almost sixfold to $18 billion. The growth of HHC utilization prompted a change in reimbursement from a fee for service to a prospective payment system reimbursement model. For each 60-day certification period, agencies are reimbursed around $2000 per enrollee, adjusted for geographic region and intensity of care provided. This has reduced the enrollment length and frequency of HHC visits, but has not significantly impacted the ability of physicians to access HHC services. Currently, 2.5 million visits are performed by 7000 agencies.

To qualify for HHC, an agency must receive a physician order, document that a recipient is homebound (a definition that has remained vague) and provide a skilled intervention by a nurse or a therapist. Common uses of HHC include medication management, disease assessment, wound care, home safety evaluation, physical and occupational therapy, and patient/family education. The average number of visits per enrollee is 36 (Centers for Medicare and Medicaid Services, 2005).

When personal care is needed at home, aides can be hired for in-home assistance with laundry, housekeeping, meal preparation, and personal care needs. Medicare does not pay for personal care aides, nor do most private insurance plans. Individual case management and social services are available to seniors based on resources and needs. Services such as meals-on-wheels, transportation, and legal aid are often provided on a sliding fee–scale basis. The availability of these services varies by community.

Hospice care is another service traditionally provided in the home, although there is a growing use of hospice in the nursing home setting. In 2003, 900 hospice agencies provided care to 290 000 individuals. 55% of these patients were served at home; 23% resided in nursing homes. The average length of service was 55 days but 30% of hospice recipients died within 7 days of enrollment. This suggests that hospice services are largely underutilized for those deemed to have "less than 6 months to live." (National Hospice and Palliative Care Organization, 2003). In addition to nursing, hospice provides therapy, social service, and family support in the home. Hospice agencies are not capable of providing continuous 24-hour personal care.

British physician Dame Cicely Saunders first coined the term *hospice* in 1967. The Dean of Yale School of Nursing, Florence Wald, subsequently adopted this care model in the United States. It was not until 1979 that the Health Care Financing Administration (HCFA) funded 26 hospices as a demonstration program. In 1982, hospice care was added as a benefit under the medicare and medicaid programs and has since become a standard benefit provided by all health insurance plans. To qualify for hospice a physician must certify an estimated life expectancy of 6 months or less. Eighty percent of hospice recipients are age 65 or older and just over half are female. Half of the hospice enrollees have a terminal diagnosis of cancer. Cancer diagnoses have dropped 10% in the last 3 years due to a rise in use of hospice care for nonmalignant terminal illnesses such as dementia and emphysema.

Australia

Home care services have become increasingly complex in the types of care provided, the funding arrangements, and number of service providers. The health-care needs of patients are also more complex due to greater functional and physical dependency. Medical care at home has traditionally been provided by GPs for patients who were too acutely or chronically unwell to attend office visits. However, the relatively poor reimbursement by medicare and the increasing demand for home visits has led many GPs to abandon them altogether. Because many aged care assessment teams (ACATs) now include a geriatrician or other medical officer, they may provide medical home visits as part of an initial assessment, but not as part of routine care.

Government sponsored community services existed as early as the 1940s, including emergency housekeeper service and meals-on-wheels, delivered by women volunteers on bicycles. The Australian government began funding home nursing services in 1956. Although the management and structure varies considerably between states, there is general availability of visiting registered nurses to provide nursing services in the home. Most commonly these services are time limited and based on the individual needs of the client and family. There are separate but generally parallel services for war veterans and individuals in the private sector.

Home and Community Care (HACC) services expanded in 1969 to support housekeeping or other domestic assistance, senior citizens centers, and welfare officers. Home care was further enhanced with the passage of the Home and Community Care Act in 1985 to include personal care such as bathing and dressing. Demand almost perpetually outstrips supply, because of underfunding, lack of gate keeping at entry, and inadequate exit strategies for maintenance services. A common assumption by service providers is that clients will not significantly improve and thus need prolonged enrollment in the program. Home care recipients assume that services are difficult to access and thus attempt to retain services long term rather than reaccess assistance at a later date.

HACC also funds meals-on-wheels, transportation, home maintenance and modification, counseling, social support, center-based day care, allied health services, provision of aids, respite care, and laundry. HACC services are not exclusively for older people, with 21% of their clients being under age 65, but usage rates do increase with age. For people aged 65–74, 47 per 1000 use HACC services, whereas 144 and 255 people per 1000 aged 75–84 and 85+ were using these services. The most commonly used service is domestic assistance (usually housekeeping). In 2002, 6.6 million hours of domestic assistance, 2.9 million hours of social support, 1.5 million hours of respite care, and 11 million meals were provided under the HACC program. The program was jointly funded by the state (40%) and national government at $1.2 billion in 2003.

ACATs are a network of 128 regionally based multidisciplinary teams that provide comprehensive geriatric assessment at home or in hospital, facilitate access to the best possible combination of services at home, and determine eligibility for residential and complex community care. ACATs often provide health advice and support for the common conditions, which afflict older people, such as dementia and incontinence. ACATs may assume the additional therapeutic role of rehabilitative therapy. ACATs assess approximately 1 in every 10 people over age 70 every year. ACATs have a key role in assessing older people at home in complex situations, such as when elder abuse is suspected or if guardianship is being considered. If residential placement is recommended, the ACAT works with the client and their caregiver to negotiate entry. Staffing varies but generally includes nursing and allied health, social workers, physiotherapists, occupational therapists, and psychologists. Increasingly ACATs have access to a geriatrician, particularly when they are colocated with a hospital aged care service, and sometimes even a psychogeriatrician. In nonmetropolitan areas, the medical officer is usually a GP (family medicine practitioner) with an interest in aged care (Lincoln Gerontology Centre, 2000–2001).

Referral to ACAT is from any source, including self-referral. ACATs perform a standardized initial assessment using a minimum data set, with subsequent assessments according to identified problems. Occasionally, ACATs must assess younger people with disabilities for eligibility to enter residential aged care if no suitable alternatives exist.

The shift away from institutional care has led to ever more complex packages of care being introduced into the community. The Community Options Program was established in the late 1980s to provide case management and brokerage funds in the community to a small group of clients that is up to 10 times the average level of funding for other HACC clients, and also as recognition of the wide range of services available in the community.

Community aged care packages (CACPs) were introduced in 1992 and support people at home with up to 14 hours of care per week as a substitute for admission to a hostel. Assistance with personal care such as bathing, domestic assistance with laundry, shopping, meal preparation, gardening, and transportation outside the home are provided. The median length of time on the program is just under a year. Two-thirds of people who leave the program are admitted to residential care or die. By December 2003, about 28 000 people were receiving this type of care and the government plans to increase availability to 18 CACP per 1000 persons over age 70. More than half (56%) of all recipients live alone and only 8% live with their children. Recipients pay up to $5.59 per day, with the Australian government providing $32.04 per day per recipient.

Extended Aged Care at Home (EACH) packages were introduced in 1998 to support people at home who are eligible for nursing home placement. Each client receives an average of 16.1 hours of care per week. These recipients tend to be younger (32% under age 75) and more cognitively intact (31% diagnosed with dementia, compared to 80% in nursing homes) than most nursing home residents. Most services are available upon request, although often for a small fee. The more complex packages of care require ACAT assessment of need (Aging and Aged Care Division, 2002).

Although the spectrum of home care appears broad and comprehensive, it is also cumbersome and complex. In practice, 17 separate programs are funded by the Australian government and delivered by a myriad of 4000 different service providers. The result is a complex health delivery system with patchy coordination and insufficient communication, particularly for consumers and their caregivers. In theory, one assessment by ACAT should be sufficient for any other service but, in practice, each service provider makes its own assessment.

That this plethora of providers does not meet the needs of older disabled people and their caregivers was demonstrated by a study of dementia sufferers in Victoria. Data revealed that over 40% of demented individuals do not make use of any community or respite services despite high levels of caregiver strain and little support from family and friends (Thomson *et al.*, 1997). When asked why they did not make use of various community services, 77–88% of individuals stated that the services were not needed. In reality, some caregivers were not managing well as evidenced by poor self-reported health and high levels of strain. Since 1972, caregivers have been subsidized by a domiciliary nursing care benefit to care for a disabled person at home who would otherwise require institutional care. The patient must be over the age of 16 and certified by a medical practitioner to require continuing care.

NURSING HOME CARE

United Kingdom

The NHS has allocated an additional £900 million annually, beginning in 2003, for the expansion of intermediate and nursing home care services. This provides for an additional 5000 beds and 1700 facilities. The NHS is working toward providing nursing care without cost to residents of nursing homes and to protect individuals from losing their home or other resources in order to pay for the costs of nursing home care. The average cost of residential and nursing care homes is between £300–400 per week.

Around 63% of older people permanently entering nursing homes come directly from the hospital. Integrated care services provided via a team of medical professionals are a most effective means of providing a comprehensive plan of care. The comprehensive team approach requires a collaborative effort between the hospital-based consultant geriatrician and the GP providing day-to-day care in the nursing home setting. Consultant geriatricians have been criticized for a relative lack of attention to the long-term care and community-based care needs of the frail elderly population.

In a survey of 810 (38% response rate) consultant geriatricians, one-third of clinical time was spent in emergency care services, one-third in general geriatric/rehabilitation services, and only one-eighth was spent on community-based/intermediate care services (British Geriatrics Society, 2004). Only 14% would change their job description, if allowed, to perform more community-based work, and 60% reported that this was the least important of their four core clinical activities. Given the nursing home needs of the UK population, the BGS recommends that senior consultant geriatricians be allowed to choose career progression pathways into community-based and nursing home care positions.

The NSF has established a specific standard for intermediate care of older adults. The goal is to provide integrated services, to promote faster recovery from illness, to prevent unnecessary acute hospital admissions, to support timely discharge and to maximize independent living. Older people will have access to a new range of intermediate care services at home or in designated care settings. The NHS Plan set out a major new program to promote independence for older people by developing a range of services that are delivered in partnership between primary and secondary health care, local authority services, and the independent sector. One of the critical elements in this program is the development of new intermediate care services.

Nursing homes would develop close association with the geriatric department. Admission to geriatric department was to be directly from the patients' own homes, or in some cases, transfer from other hospital wards for rehabilitation and resettlement. It was hoped that this department would be able to absorb older patients from acute medical wards and also relieve the surgical wards of their elderly patients after the postoperative phase and there must be sufficient beds in the nursing homes to absorb the patients who would be transferred to them from hospital or home.

United States

The number of nursing homes in the United States has dropped slowly since the early 1980s, although the total number of residents in nursing homes has increased almost 10% during that time. In 2002, 16 000 facilities were licensed, with an average capacity of 100 residents. 70% of nursing home residents are female and 90% are Caucasian. The average length of stay is 2–3 years. Despite common misconceptions of the elderly population, less than 5% of citizens over the age of 65 reside in nursing homes. Less than 20% of adults over age 85 live in nursing homes.

Most nursing homes certify a portion of their beds (25–35%) for postacute care, skilled nursing services. These residents receive intensive nursing, therapy, and medical services after an acute medical illness with the hope of regaining lost function. Medicare funds most of the skilled nursing care in the United States but private insurance also covers postacute rehabilitation services. Medicare beneficiaries receive up to 100 days of skilled nursing care before other insurance or private pay must shoulder costs. The average length of skilled nursing care is 27 days.

Medicare and most private insurers do not pay for nonskilled (custodial) care in nursing homes. The bulk of custodial care is paid for by medicaid once individuals have "spent down" their personal resources to the point of qualifying for this jointly state-federal sponsored health-care coverage. The medicaid qualification level varies by state. An individual generally must have a monthly income less than or equal to the federally designated poverty level ($776/month) and net personal resources of only a few thousand dollars. The average yearly cost of nursing home care is roughly $55 000. Nursing home insurance is becoming available but in general it is costly and not widely purchased by the general population (The National Nursing Home Survey, 2002).

Nursing home care has improved dramatically in the past 20 years. The Omnibus Budget Reconciliation Act (ORBA), passed in 1987, was instrumental in changing the management and oversight of nursing home care in the United States. Unfortunately, previous abuses have resulted in a highly regulated and punitive system of ensuring the quality of institutional patient care. Nursing homes are surveyed annually by the state regulatory agency. Deficiencies and fines are applied liberally and are a matter of public record. The state has the authority to immediately close down any facility that is found to have practices that place residents in "immediate jeopardy" of harm. Areas that are frequently cited include unnecessary use of physical restraints and psychotropic medication, weight loss, development of pressure ulcers, and fall related injuries.

As length of stay in hospitals shortens and the severity of illness of newly admitted residents increases, nursing homes have become more comprehensive in providing medical and therapy services. Most facilities offer intravenous antibiotics and fluids. Gastric tube feeding, suctioning, and oxygen treatment are routine. Facilities contract with mobile laboratory and radiology agencies. Physical, occupational, and speech therapists, nutritionists, and consulting pharmacists are on-staff or consult on a frequent basis.

Nurses are being challenged to perform more sophisticated care and more rigorous assessments while faced with limited staffing ratios and a high rate of nursing turnover.

Assisted living facilities are assuming some of the role that nursing homes played 20 years ago. "Well" elderly who require only some assistance with daily activities live semiindependently in studio-type apartments with or without a kitchenette. Facilities vary in size from several dozens to over one hundred residents in a single building. A licensed nurse is usually available during most of the day and may pass meds, perform assessments, inject insulin, check glucoses, and perform other skilled tasks based on resident needs. The provision of meals, light housekeeping, and social activities are usually included in the cost of room and board.

The cost of care is partly based on the level of services designated by the patient/family. Assisted living costs are highly variable but range from $24 000 to $36 000 or more per year. Almost universally, the cost of assisted living is incurred out-of-pocket by the resident and/or family. Despite being less costly, most long-term care insurance providers will not reimburse assisted living as an alternate to nursing home care. Assistance with activities of daily living (ADLs), instrumental activities of daily living (IADLs), safety checks, and other personal care are provided by 24-hour/day nursing assistants at the facility. At this time 800 000 residents reside in 30 000 assisted living facilities. Most assisted living residents receive medical care in the office of medical providers as opposed to on-site as in nursing homes. There are currently very few governmental regulations or requirements in assisted living facilities.

Australia

The development of residential aged care dates back to the poor houses of the nineteenth century. In NSW, the first state, government asylums for the aged and destitute were built to house the aged poor. By 1890, these homes had become "practically hospitals for chronic and incurable diseases as well as homes for the infirm and indigent". However the introduction of pension plan in 1909 allowed more aged poor to continue living in the community and institutional care was used only for marked disability or poverty (Dickey, 1983). Essentially all residential care was provided by the charitable and public sectors until the mid-1950s, but not-for-profit organizations still provide 63% of all residential care places.

In 1954, there was a swing back to residential aged care when the Australian government passed the Aged Persons Homes Act that provided subsidies to charities (and later to private operators) that built or purchased homes for needy older people. This prompted a surge in construction of nursing homes that continued for three decades. In the early 1970s, a quota of 50 nursing home beds per 1000 population of age 65 and over was introduced. An intermediate level of care, called *hostel*, was announced in an attempt to reduce the number of nursing homes being built, particularly by the private sector. Hostels were aimed at people who needed assistance with IADLs while nursing homes were designed for people who needed assistance with basic ADLs.

A 1978 survey found that 30% of nursing home residents could easily be treated at home with minimal services (Bennett and Wallace, 1983). In 1986, a government review pointed out that the cost of institutional care had risen tenfold in 10 years, from $100 million to $1 billion per annum, and the percentage of the Department of Health's budget paid to nursing homes had increased from 9 to 25% over 20 years. By the mid-1980s nearly 90% of all aged care funding was going to residential care. The rate has now been reduced to about 75% with a commensurate increase in community care.

In 2004, there were 175 000 allocated residential care sites and 30 000 community care sites.

On the basis of the truism that most people prefer to remain in their own homes, the government changed the quota for nursing home beds to 72.6 per 1000 people over age 70. In 1985, the multidisciplinary ACATs were charged with developing more stringent entry criteria, which resulted in a 35% decrease in admissions to nursing homes. HACC services were also strengthened in order to maintain people at home (Warne, 1987). Over the years, the government has changed the ratio of nursing homes and hostel places to increase the availability of home support, but this has been complicated by the growth of the population over age 70. Individuals over age 85 are most likely to require nursing home placement and are the fastest growing segment of the population. A decrease in funding for residential care has caused many facilities to close down. Ninety of licensed residential care centers are now allocated per 1000 population over age 70. These transformations have meant significant increases in disability in hostel care, as well as increased average disability in nursing homes.

A further series of reforms took place in 1997 with the introduction of the Aged Care Act. The two levels of care were unified under one legislative framework with an integrated Resident Classification Scale (RCS) and quality assurance framework. The levels were renamed high (nursing home) and low (hostel) care. The 1997 reforms also introduced a small amount of deregulation and emphasized greater contributions to the cost of health and welfare services by those with the capacity to pay.

In general, the provision of residential aged care remains a controversial issue in Australia. Approximately one in three people who reach 65 years of age will spend some time in residential aged care, but whether the cost should be met more by the community or by the individual and their family is a matter of equity, ethics, and finances.

HOSPITAL CARE

United Kingdom

The BMA set up a working group in 1947 to review care of the elderly and infirm. As per their recommendations, specialist geriatric departments were gradually established over the years in general hospitals, including teaching hospitals in the NHS. A geriatric department is comprised of wards reserved exclusively for elderly patients undergoing evaluation, active treatment, and rehabilitation. A common goal is to discharge patients from such wards either to their own homes or to other appropriate accommodations. Patients requiring ongoing nursing care for irremediable conditions are referred for nursing home admission.

For those aged 65 and over, various hospital admission policies are set up with some departments admitting according to need (i.e. those patients presenting with the "geriatric syndromes" or with mixed medical and social problems) for which the geriatric department was specially adapted. Others are admitted on an age-related basis, varying from 65 to 85 and over (Kafetz *et al.*, 1995; Brocklehurst and Davidson, 1989). These policies apply to emergency admissions while "cold" admissions referred by GPs through outpatient or domiciliary consultation usually include anyone aged 65 or over (British Geriatrics Society, 1995; Grimley, 1983).

Over time, acute-care admission policies have shifted toward an integration of geriatric medicine with general medicine for emergency admissions via a common Medical Admission Unit (MAU). This Newcastle Model (British Geriatrics Society, 1995) has been partially driven by the need to reduce junior doctors' hours of work and the problem of outliers – patients of one consultant being admitted to many different wards of the hospital when their wards are full. Accommodation of these difficulties has produced more rational and economic use of beds and staff.

Two-thirds of acute hospital beds are occupied by people over age 65. Hospitals therefore need to ensure that they are meeting the particular needs of older people, many of whom have a variety of health and social problems. The NSF places great emphasis on quality hospital care for older adults and has established a number of milestones, such as multidisciplinary team care, to measure progress. Nearly three-quarters of hospitals now have specialist multidisciplinary teams for the care of older people. Over 80% of these teams have a nurse leader, often a modern matron, with special responsibility for the care of older adults.

Health-care Standard – General Hospital Care

The aim of this standard is to ensure that older people receive the specialist help they need in the hospital and that they receive the maximum benefit from the hospital services. Hospital care for older adults is delivered through appropriate specialist consultation and by hospital staff who have the right set of skills to meet the needs of the patient. The hospital environment and support services should be targeted to anticipate the care requirements of the older adult.

Health-care Standard – Stroke Management

The aim of this standard is to reduce the incidence of stroke in the population and ensure that those who have had a stroke have prompt access to integrated stroke care services. The NHS will take action to prevent strokes by working in partnership with other agencies where appropriate. People who are thought to have had a stroke must be provided access to diagnostic services, be treated appropriately by a specialist stroke service, and be allowed to participate in a multidisciplinary program of secondary prevention and rehabilitation.

Outcomes for stroke patients are better when they are cared for by specialist stroke teams within designated stroke units. Lengths of stay on these teams are also shorter on average. Since the publication of the NSF for older people, many more speciality stroke services have been established and more are planned. There have been significant increases in the number of stroke physicians, the proportion of patients being treated in specialist stroke units, and the number of patients returning home after hospital treatment. There have also been important improvements in the care process. For example, 83% of patients are receiving brain scans to improve stroke diagnosis, far more than in the past. Ninety percent of hospitals which treat people with stroke now have stroke units, up from 82% in April 2004. More than one million bed days are being saved a year because of reductions in delayed discharge.

A variety of programs have been developed to improve stroke care. The NHS Modernization Agency has developed a "clinical governance development program", which seeks to engage frontline staff in radical reassessments of care delivery. The Sentinel Stroke Audit is also underway to measure the delivery of stroke care based on Royal College of Physicians' clinical practice guidelines. Despite these initiatives, stroke care across the country remains heterogeneous. Although 90% of hospitals have stroke units, only 36% of patients who have had a stroke are spending time in these units. Clearly, there is still much to do to ensure that the NSF standard for stroke management is met.

United States

Hospitals in the United States are evolving to provide speciality services for the aging patient with the hope of improving patient outcomes and reducing adverse health events. Programs such as adult day care, palliative care, and HHC, offered through the hospital system, address a wide variety of needs for elderly patients both during and after hospitalization. The American Hospital Association (AHA) publishes the prevalence of these services annually. In 2000, geriatric services, home health services, and skilled nursing care units were offered in over 35% of US hospitals (American Hospital Association and the National Chronic Care Consortium, 2002). In the subsequent 3 years, the frequency of all of these services has declined by up to 3% with current data illustrated in Table 1. The only geriatric programs, which have increased significantly, are palliative care and case management with 22.2 and 75.5% of hospitals having these services respectively in 2003 (Health Forum LLC/American Hospital Association, 2005). It is interesting that neither an acute care for the elderly (ACE) unit nor a stroke unit are used as markers in this consumer-evaluation model, but both are accepted by the field of geriatric medicine as beneficial interventions.

ACE Units

The ACE unit is a growing model for comprehensive and multidisciplinary care of the older hospitalized adult. Characteristics of most ACE units include an association with a university hospital, 20-bed unit, initiated in the late 1990s and open to admissions from a variety of medical services (Siegler *et al.*, 2002). The "ACE" concept and term were developed in the early 1990s with key elements of the model being (1) environment alterations, (2) patient-centered care, (3) interdisciplinary planning for discharge, and (4) medical care review, which are outlined in detail in Table 2 (Landefeld *et al.*, 1995). The goal of this model is to reduce the functional impairments which so often develop in acutely ill, hospitalized elders. This "dysfunctional syndrome" is outlined in Figure 1.

Two philosophical differences are employed in the ACE model of care. First, care management is shifted toward a

Table 1 Healthcare facilities and services trends

Special services offered	Number of hospitals	Percentage of hospitals
Skilled nursing care unit	1650	33.4
Intermediate care unit	506	10.2
Adult day care services	400	8.1
Assisted living	263	5.3
Case management	3733	75.5
Geriatric services	1998	40.4
Home health services	1848	37.4
Hospice	1153	23.3
Meals-on-wheels	633	12.8
Psychiatric-geriatric services	1505	30.4
Retirement housing	184	3.7
Palliative care program	1098	22.2

Source: Reproduced by permission of Health Forum.

Table 2 Key elements and illustrative features of the intervention program

Key element	Illustrative features
Prepared environment	Carpeting, handrails, uncluttered hallways Large clocks and calendars Elevated toilet seats and door levers
Patient-centered care	Daily assessment by nurses of physical, cognitive, and psychosocial function Protocols to improve self-care, continence, nutrition, mobility, sleep, skin care, mood, cognition (implemented by the primary nurse and based on the daily assessment) Daily rounds by the multidisciplinary team, led by the medical and nursing directors with the primary nurse, social worker, nutritionist, physical therapist, and visiting-nurse liaison
Planning for discharge	Early, ongoing emphasis on the goal of returning home Assessment of plans and needs for discharge by a nurse at the time of admission Early involvement of a social worker and home health-care nurse, if indicated
Medical care review	Daily review by the medical director of medicines and planned procedures Protocols to minimize the adverse effects of selected procedures (e.g. urinary catheterization) and medications (e.g. sedative-hypnotic agents)

Source: Reproduced by permission of the Massachusetts Medical Society from Landefeld CS, Palmer RM, Kresevic DM *et al.* (1995) A randomized trial of care in a hospital medical unit especially designed to improve the functional outcomes of acutely ill older patients. *NEJM*, **332**, 1338–44.

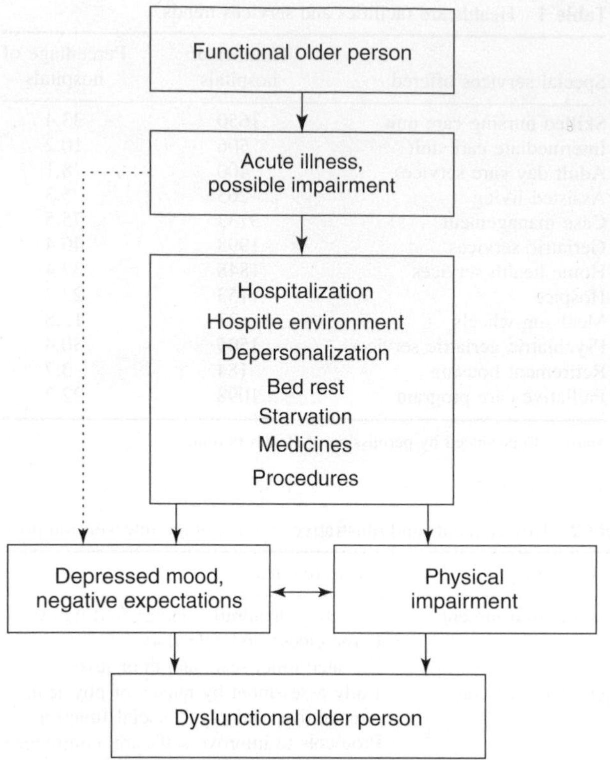

Figure 1 Conceptual model of the dysfunctional syndrome (Reprinted from *Clinics in Geriatric Medicine*, vol 14(4), Palmer RM, Counsell S, Landefeld SC, pp 831–49, Copyright 1998, with permission from Elsevier)

biopsychosocial rather than a biomedical model. Hospitalization and discharge planning focus on the relationship between the patient and the social structures that are needed for effective treatment. Barriers to successful recovery and risks for ongoing functional decline are identified early in the hospitalization. Appropriate interventions such as reduction in polypharmacy, nutritional assessment, social support evaluation, and physical and occupational therapy assessment are initiated for each patient. Discharge plans ensure that the patient transitions to an appropriate environment and with appropriate social services in place.

Second, a functional-based rather than disease-based approach is used in medical decision-making. Many elders suffer from multiple, chronic medical conditions that will not be cured. Goals of care focus on maximizing function in the context of disease management rather than solely marking improvement by measures of disease severity. With this method, functional status and quality of life measures become the markers for successful recovery from illness.

The implementation of an ACE unit has consistently resulted in improved functional status and increased discharge to home compared with usual care wards (Landefeld *et al.*, 1995; Asplund *et al.*, 2000; Counsell *et al.*, 2000). Despite the additional interventions applied by the multidisciplinary team, the total cost of hospital care is not higher on the ACE unit. The benefits of teamwork in caring for the complex and ill elderly adult translates to a more efficient and thorough treatment plan for both the hospital and the patient without incurring excess cost.

Stroke Units

Death from cerebrovascular disease is the third leading cause of death and more than two-thirds of strokes occur in patients over the age of 65. Despite long-standing use of stroke units outside of the United States, and strong evidence demonstrating the morbidity and mortality benefit of this strategy (Stroke Unit Trialists' Collaboration, 1997, 2002), comprehensive stroke management models are just beginning in the US health-care system. Previous literature on the benefit of an organized inpatient stroke care team comes almost universally out of the United Kingdom and northern Europe. For over 20 years, patients with acute stroke have been managed on a dedicated stroke unit: either on a discrete stroke ward or stroke team working exclusively in the care of stroke patients. Focus of the stroke unit can include acute stroke care, subacute rehabilitation, or a combination of strategies.

To improve the consistency and quality of stroke care across the United States, the "Brain Attack Coalition" (BAC) was convened in 2000 to establish recommendation for hospital care of stroke patients. The BAC recommended a two-tier organization for hospital-based stroke care: Primary Stroke Centers (PSCs) and comprehensive stroke centers (CSCs). This group outlined the major criteria of a PSC which are listed in Table 3 (Alberts *et al.*, 2000). PSCs provide the basic emergency evaluation and stabilization, while complex cases requiring speciality imaging and intervention should be referred to CSCs. A recent state-based survey of medical facilities indicates that less than 20% of hospitals have either a stroke unit or have the infrastructure to become a PSC (Camilo and Goldstein, 2003). Furthermore, the prevalence of key stroke services has not significantly changed over the past 5 years.

The stroke units of Europe are more similar in design to the US ACE unit, whereas stroke centers in the United States

Table 3 Major elements of a primary stroke center

Patient care areas
Acute stroke teams
Written care protocols
Emergency medical services
Emergency department
Stroke unit[a]
Neurosurgical services
Support services
Commitment and support of medical organization; a stroke center director
Neuroimaging services
Laboratory services
Outcome and quality improvement activities
Continuing medical education

Source: From 'Recommendation for the Establishment of Primary Stroke Centers' by Alberts, MJ *et al. JAMA*, **283**(23), 3102–3109. Copyright 2000, American Medical Association. All rights reserved.

[a]A stroke unit is only required for those primary stroke centers that will provide ongoing in-hospital care for patients with stroke.

Table 4 Comparison of geriatric complications. Geriatric complications – number (%) of patients and 95% confidence intervals

	Hospital in the home	Hospital	P
Confusion	0	10 (20.4%) 9.1%, 31.7%	0.0005
Falls	1 (2.0%) −1.8%, 5.8%	2 (4.1%) −1.4%, 9.6%	ns
All bowel complications	0	11 (22.5%) 10.7%, 34.1%	0.0003
Constipation	0	7(14.3%) 4.5%, 24.1%	0.013
Fecal incontinence	0	4 (8.2%) 0.5%, 15.9%	ns
All urinary complications	1 (2.0%) −1.8%, 5.8%	8 (16.3%) 6.0%, 26.6%	0.01
Urinary incontinence	1 (2.0%) −1.8%, 5.8%	6 (12.2%) 3.0%, 21.4%	ns
Urinary retention	0	2 (4.1%) −1.4%, 9.6%	ns
Phlebitis	2 (3.9%) −1.4%, 9.2%	3 (6.1%) −0.6%, 12.8%	ns
Pressure area/skin tear	1 (2.0%) −1.8%, 5.8%	3 (6.1%) −0.6%, 12.8%	ns

Source: From Caplan G. *et al.*, Hospital in the home: a randomised controlled trial. *MJA* 1999; 170: 150–160. Copyright 1999. The Medical Journal of Australia – reproduced with permission. ns, not significant.

are modeled after a "trauma center" concept. In contrast to the physical model of stroke and ACE units, the PSC represents a "process model" that focuses on delivery of care and availability of personnel and speciality services. Like trauma centers, stroke centers rely on a network of coordinated resources within a facility. The challenge for the future will be to meet the growing need for acute stroke care in the aging population.

Australia

In 1993, a government survey of 942 Australian hospitals found that 32% operated a geriatric service. These were almost exclusively based in the public sector, and usually consisted of visiting care services (Dorevitch and Gray, 1993). Only 13% of programs included a geriatrician. Replication of the survey in 2001 found that 31% of 778 hospitals had a geriatrician providing inpatient care (Gray *et al.*, 2002).

The distribution of geriatric services varies between states. Those states with more acute geriatric medical beds typically provide care to patients admitted through the emergency department. New South Wales, Western Australia, and South Australia have the highest ratio of acute geriatric beds (0.67–0.85 beds per 1000 people over age 70 in 2002). In Victoria and Western Australia there are more designated aged care rehabilitation beds (0.62–0.63 per 1000 people) than in the other states. The extent of geriatric services vary by hospital, with 11% reporting a day hospital, 7% having bed-based psychogeriatric services, and only 4% having orthogeriatric services. Orthogeriatric services provide coordinated orthopedic and geriatric management for older traumatic and elective orthopedic patients.

The type of geriatric services available to patients tends to mirror the hospital environment. Where the hospital focuses on acute-care and managing emergency admissions, more attention is devoted to improving assessment and management of older people in the emergency department and on acute hospital wards. Where the hospital has developed a stand-alone rehabilitation center, more emphasis is placed on managing chronic conditions, such as dementia, Parkinson's disease and incontinence. However, with time the scope of available services is increasing and differences between states are receding.

Stroke units are becoming increasingly popular, although geriatrician involvement is not universal. A recent study found that only 40% of all strokes were treated in stroke units (Lee *et al.*, 2003). Hospital in the home for older patients is increasing in popularity, but is essentially in its infancy as a model of health care. This service provides patient-centered care in the patient's home or a residential care facility, while decreasing the risk of hospital associated adverse events. Major geriatric complications were less likely to occur in the hospital in the home model compared with the traditional hospital model and are listed in Table 4 (Caplan *et al.*, 1999). Public hospitals, which are the majority, are under the control of state governments.

Only about 30% of hospitals are private and these concentrate on elective procedures. Almost all large and teaching hospitals are public, so that the vast majority of acute and more complicated medical or surgical work is done in public hospitals. Admission to a public hospital as a public patient is free to Australian residents. However, if a patient wants a choice of doctor, they must enter as a private patient. Owing to recent tax incentives, about 50% of the population has private insurance for hospital care. Public hospitals receive about half their budget from the national government and half through the state governments.

This dichotomy of control of the health system has led to lack of coordination, and incentive to cost-shift between the hospital and nonhospital sectors. There are also limited health services run by local government (the third tier), religious and charitable organizations, individuals, and private commercial interests.

ACADEMIC GERIATRICS

United Kingdom

The first academic chair of geriatric medicine was established in 1965 in Glasgow, Scotland. The first professor of elderly medicine was William Ferguson Anderson (1914–2001).

A pioneer of geriatric outreach clinics, he established a famous partnership with the GP of Rutherglen Health Centre.

Every medical school in United Kingdom now has a Department of Geriatric Medicine with at least one professor of medicine in geriatrics. Recently, the Royal College of Physicians has mandated that the membership examination contain questions from geriatrics medicine and rehabilitation. Knowledge of geriatrics has become a requirement for physicians-in-training.

Like other physicians, geriatricians must complete a period of general professional training (GPT) in acute medical specialities before starting higher training in their chosen speciality. The primary purpose of training is to promote the development of a physician who has the appropriate level of knowledge, skills, and competence to work independently and effectively as a consultant in geriatric medicine.

Applicants for higher medical training (HMT) should have completed a minimum of 2 years' GPT in approved posts at Senior House Officer (SHO) level and obtained the Diploma of Membership of the Royal Colleges of Physicians (United Kingdom or Ireland). A period of experience in geriatric medicine at SHO grade is considered desirable but not essential, before entry to HMT. The duration of HMT in geriatric medicine is 4 years. Those who wish to obtain dual certification with general (internal) medicine will require at least one extra year. HMT will require experience in both teaching hospital(s), or other major centers with academic activity, and district general hospitals.

Application for the certificate of completion of specialist training (CCST) can be made after successful training. CCST is granted by Joint Committee of Higher Medical Training (JCHMT) of Royal College of Physicians. CCST is mandatory requirement for specialist status, registration with the specialist register of General Medical Council (GMC), and to be eligible for substantive or honorary consultant post in United Kingdom. There are currently 466 specialist registrars geriatrics trainees in England, Wales, and Northern Ireland according to Consultant Census 2001–3/JCHMT database, October 2004.

A period of supervised (clinical or laboratory) research of good quality is considered a highly desirable part of specialist registrar training in geriatric medicine. A relevant research period may contribute up to 12 months toward the total duration of the training program. Each trainee is encouraged to have experience of participating in research whether it is laboratory-based (basic science) or clinical (health services) research.

United States

The development of academic geriatric programs and medical training has lagged behind the demand for a larger and more skilled geriatric medicine health-care workforce. This is in part due to the lack of universal acceptance of geriatrics as a unique discipline within the medical profession. With the increasing age, functional impairment, and psychosocial complexity of older adults, the mantra that "I'm a geriatrician because most of my patients are elderly," is fading, but slowly.

In 1982, Mount Sinai School of Medicine established the first Department of Geriatrics. At this time 80% of medical schools have some form of a geriatrics program. The vast majority of programs are organized as divisions or sections within a Department of Internal or Family Medicine. Few institutions have the financial capability of supporting independent departments of geriatric medicine. Two-thirds of programs have been in existence for less than 20 years. Fifty percent of these programs have less than six faculty members. Two-thirds of program directors have been in that position for less than 8 years. The first professorship in geriatric medicine was granted at Cornell University in 1977.

Dr Les Libow at Mount Sinai School of Medicine offered the first geriatric medicine fellowship program in 1966. Since that time the number of trainees and training sites remained fairly limited until the early 1980s. In the 1970s, the Veterans Administration (VA) was charged with the task of increasing the understanding of aging and passing this knowledge to health-care providers. Funding was provided in 1975 for the first VA Geriatric Research Education and Clinical Center (GRECC). Twenty-two GRECCs have since been established. GRECCs began offering geriatric medicine fellowship training opportunities in 1978.

In 1988 the Accreditation Council for Graduate Medical Education began accrediting geriatric medicine fellowship training programs. Sixty-two Internal Medicine and 16 Family Medicine programs offered fellowship training at that time. 1988 was also that year when an examination became mandatory to attain the Certification of Added Qualification (CAQ) in geriatrics after at least 2 years of fellowship training. To be eligible for CAQ, physicians must have completed US residency training and be board certified in either Internal or Family Medicine.

Until the mid-1990s, most fellows in geriatric medicine engaged in 2 or more years of training. Extended training was vital for the development of an academic and research career in geriatrics. In 1995, the training requirement for CAQ in geriatrics was reduced to 1 year. Although this may have partly achieved a desired goal of an increase in the total number of fellowship trained geriatricians, it has not resulted in a greater number of physicians adequately prepared to embark on a successful academic career. Over the last 10 years, the number of accredited programs has grown to 125 with roughly 400 first-year fellowship training positions. Unfortunately, almost one-third of fellowship slots go unfilled each year (Warshaw *et al.*, 2002a,b).

Australia

In NSW, geriatric medicine originated in the Royal Newcastle Hospital, an acute public hospital and later became an acute speciality hospital. Lidcombe Hospital in NSW was another early center of geriatric medicine that evolved away from the mainstream, having originally been an asylum which developed into an acute hospital, but retained a large group of long stay chronic patients. Many of the doctors involved there went on to be national leaders in geriatric medicine. In Victoria, South Australia, and Queensland the speciality started in chronic hospitals, which developed out of the poor houses, and continues as a rehabilitation hospital model, though it now also interacts with acute hospitals. In Victoria, the Mount Royal Hospital was a custodial institution for elderly people where the state hospital and charities commission decided to open a geriatric center, aimed at rehabilitation. Though the initial director was only part-time, the center flourished and also became a center for aging research.

The Australian Association of Gerontology formed in the early 1960s as a multidisciplinary organization interested in later life, and the doctors involved went on to form The Australian Society for Geriatric Medicine (ASGM) to meet the special needs of medical practitioners. Many geriatricians take a leading role as advocates for older people together with consumers and other service providers.

The first full professor of geriatric medicine was appointed at the University of Melbourne in 1975, though early professorships were often in "community medicine and geriatrics". Now each medical school boasts of at least one Professor and there are research institutes dedicated to age-related research in the larger states.

The Royal Australasian College of Physicians (RACP) recognizes geriatric medicine as a speciality. Trainees must complete 3 years of advanced training in geriatric medicine, though 1 year of this may include working in another speciality or in full-time research. Advanced training can only be undertaken after successfully completing the demanding written and oral basic physicians examination, which is generally attempted 4–5 years postgraduation from medical school. Only about two-thirds of candidates are successful in this exam. Almost all basic physician trainees, who later go on to various internal medicine subspecialities, have some exposure to working in geriatric medicine. This is most beneficial for attracting trainees for advanced training. However, workforce issues are as much a problem in terms of shortages in the supply of doctors for older people, as well as nurses and allied health professionals.

Many other research institutes also have some interest in age-related research. Clinical research is also conducted in many teaching hospitals. Most research funding derives from the National Health and Medical Research Council that does not yet have a section devoted to aging. However, in 2002 the Australian government released a national strategy for aging research and identified national research priorities which included "promoting and maintaining good health" whose goals include "aging well, aging productively". This led to the establishment of two research networks designed to encourage and seed fund collaborative interdisciplinary research into aging.

CONCLUSION

In the next 50 years, the population demographic in developed countries will change substantially. Up to a quarter of the citizens will be over age 65 with the highest growth rate in age seen in the oldest age-groups. Older adults are the highest consumers of health-care resources and are usually supported, at least in part, by local and national governmental medical programs. With health-care costs rising, countries like the United Kingdom, United States, and Australia are exploring alternate means of caring for the aging population.

Home care encompasses a wide variety of programs and services, most of which are not physician-directed. Traditional physician house calls dropped substantially in the early 1900s and despite a recurrence in interest, are still a minority of the home care encounters performed today. The provision of medical and nonmedical services allow individuals to remain independent and in their homes for a longer period of time. Many services are community based and thus help individuals maintain a connection with society.

Nursing home care increased substantially during the mid-1900s. As the aging population expanded, health expenditures increased tremendously. In an effort to control escalating long-term care costs, intermediate care settings have evolved to allow individuals more autonomy in a less costly setting. Resources and supervision are provided to individuals on an as-needed basis in most of these facilities. For individuals in need of comprehensive supervised care, nursing homes still provide the maximal degree of therapy, social work, and nursing support.

Hospital care has evolved to focus more on the delivery of quality health care to the elderly individual. Stroke units are well established as an effective model for managing hospitalized older adults. ACE units are now growing in the same manner. It is apparent that quality care for complex elderly patients requires a team of medical providers working together toward common goals.

Academic geriatrics has grown substantially over the past 50 years with most medical schools and academic centers establishing a department or section of geriatric medicine. The role of geriatricians, relative to GPs, is still evolving in the care of the older adult. As the older population expands there is an ongoing need to training physicians, both generalists and specialists, in the principles of geriatric medicine.

KEY POINTS

- The elderly will account for over 20% of the United Kingdom, United States, and Australian population in the next half century.
- Services for the elderly have grown most extensively in the realm of home health care.
- Geriatric wards, stroke units, and acute care for the elderly (ACE) units are well-developed and are effective models of hospital care for the elderly.
- The growth of nursing home care has slowed and is shifting to "intermediate care" service models.

- Geriatrics as a unique field of medicine has developed over the past half century.

KEY REFERENCES

- Caplan GA, Ward JA, Brennan N *et al.* Hospital in the home: a randomised controlled trial. *The Medical Journal of Australia* 1999; **170**:156–60.
- Kafetz K, O'Farrell J, Parry A *et al.* Age related geriatric medicine: relevance of special skills of geriatric medicine to elderly people admitted to hospital as medical emergencies. *Journal of the Royal Society of Medicine* 1995; **88**:629–33.
- Landefeld CS, Palmer RM, Kresevic DM *et al.* A randomized trial of care in a hospital medical unit especially designed to improve the functional outcomes of acutely ill older patients. *The New England Journal of Medicine* 1995; **332**:1338–44.
- Stroke Unit Trialists' Collaboration. Collaborative systematic review of the randomised trials of organised inpatient (stroke unit) care after stroke. *British Medical Journal* 1997; **314**:1151–9.
- Warne RW. Issues in the development of geriatric medicine in Britain and Australia. *The Medical Journal of Australia* 1987; **146**:139–41.

REFERENCES

Adams GF. Eld health–origins and destiny of British geriatrics. *Age and Ageing* 1975; **4**:65–8.

Alberts MJ, Hademenos G, Latchaw RE *et al.* Recommendation for the establishment of primary stroke centers. *The Journal of the American Medical Association* 2000; **283**(23):3102–9.

American Hospital Association. *Hospital Statistics* 2004, 154–61; Table 7, Health Forum LLC, Chicago.

American Hospital Association and the National Chronic Care Consortium. *Healthcare Trends and Chronic Care: A Snapshot* 2002, April, 1–6.

Asplund K, Gustafson Y, Jacobsson C *et al.* Geriatric-based versus general wards for older acute medical patients: a randomized comparison of outcomes and use of resources. *Journal of the American Geriatrics Society* 2000; **48**:1381–8.

Australian Medical Workforce Advisory Committee. *The Geriatric Medicine Workforce in Australia: Supply and Requirements 1996–2007* 1997; AMWAC Report 1997.5, AMWAC, Sydney.

Bennett C & Wallace R. At the margin or on average: some issues and evidence in planning the balance of care for the aged in Australia. *Community Health Studies* 1983; **7**:35–41.

British Geriatrics Society. *Acute Medical Care of Elderly People* 1995; British Geriatrics Society Compendium Document 12.2, Appendix 1, British Geriatrics Society, London.

British Geriatrics Society. Unpublished Data, *Current Views of Geriatricians in England and Wales* 2004.

British Medical Association. *The Care and Treatment of the Elderly and Infirm* 1947, Report of a Special Committee of the British Medical Association.

Brocklehurst JC & Davidson C. Interface between geriatric and general medicine. *Health Trends* 1989; **21**:48–50.

Camilo O & Goldstein LB. Statewide assessment of hospital-based stroke prevention and treatment services in North Carolina. *Stroke* 2003; **34**:2945–50.

Caplan GA, Ward JA, Brennan N *et al.* Hospital in the home: a randomised controlled trial. *The Medical Journal of Australia* 1999; **170**:156–60.

Counsell SR, Holder CM, Liebenauer LL *et al.* Effects of multicomponent intervention on functional outcomes and process of care in hospitalized older patients: a randomized controlled trial of Acute Care for Elders (ACE) in a Community hospital. *Journal of the American Geriatrics Society* 2000; **48**:1572–81.

Curran M, Hamilton J, Orr JS *et al.* The care of the aged: observations based on experience in Glasgow outdoor medical service. *Lancet* 1946; **1**:149–52.

Dent O. *Clinical Workforce in Internal Medicine and Paediatrics in Australasia* 2004; The Royal Australian College of Physicians.

Dickey B. Care for the aged poor in Australia, 1788–1914. *Community Health Studies* 1983; **8**:247–55.

Dorevitch M & Gray L. *National Survey of Hospital Geriatric Services: A Study of Hospital-based Geriatric Services in Australia* 1993; Australian Government Publishing Service, Canberra.

EACH Update Newsletter 2002, Aging and Aged Care Division. Issue 1; http://www.health.gov.au/internet/wcms/Publishing.nsf/Content/ageing-commcare-each-eachnews.htm/$file/each1.pdf, accessed 6 Apr 2005.

Gray L, Dorevitch M, Smith R *et al. Service Provision for Older Australians in the Acute-aged Care Sector: Final Report 2002* 2002, http://www.health.gov.au/minconf.htm, accessed July 2004.

Grimley EJ. Integration of geriatric with general medical services in Newcastle. *Lancet* 1983; **3**:1430–3.

Health Forum LLC/American Hospital Association. *Hospital Statistics* 2005, pp 151–64; Table 7, Healthcare InfoSource, Chicago.

Howell TH. Origins of the BGS. *Age and Ageing* 1974; **3**:69–72.

Irvine RE. *Forty Years On* 1986–1987, BGS Annual Report.

Kafetz K, O'Farrell J, Parry A *et al.* Age related geriatric medicine: relevance of special skills of geriatric medicine to elderly people admitted to hospital as medical emergencies. *Journal of the Royal Society of Medicine* 1995; **88**:629–33.

Landefeld CS, Palmer RM, Kresevic DM *et al.* A randomized trial of care in a hospital medical unit especially designed to improve the functional outcomes of acutely ill older patients. *The New England Journal of Medicine* 1995; **332**:1338–44.

Lee AH, Somerford PJ & Yau KKW. Factors influencing survival after stroke in Western Australia. *The Medical Journal of Australia* 2003; **179**:289–93.

Leff B & Burton JR. The future history of home care and physician house calls in the United States. *The Journals of Gerontology. Series A, Biological Sciences and Medical Sciences* 2001; **56A**(10):M606–8.

Lincoln Gerontology Centre. *Aged Care Assessment Program National Minimum Data Set Report* 2000–2001, http://www.health.gov.au/internet/wcms/publishing.nsf/Content/.

Medicare Home Health Agency Utilization by State 2005, Calendar Year 2000, Centers for Medicare and Medicaid Services. http://www.cms.hhs.gov/statistics/feeforservice/hhautil00.pdf, Accessed March 7, 2005.

National Hospice and Palliative Care Organization. *NHPCO National Data Set. National Trend Summary 2000-2003* 2003, http://www.nhpco.org/files/public/NDS00_03TrendsStats101904.pdf, Accessed March 7, 2005.

National Statistics Online – Ageing 2004, Office for National Statistics. General Register Office for Scotland and Northern Ireland Statistics and Research Agency http://www.statistics.gov.uk/cci/nugget.asp?id=949, Accessed March7, 2005.

National Statistics Online–Total UK Health Expenditure 2003, Office for National Statistics. General Register Office for Scotland and Northern Ireland Statistics and Research Agency http://www.statistics.gov.uk/cci/nugget.asp?id=669, Accessed March 7, 2005.

Nuffield Foundation. *Old People* 1947; Oxford University Press, Oxford.

Philp I. Developing a national service framework for older people. *Journal of Epidemiology and Community Health* 2002; **56**:841–2.

Rich MW, Beckham V, Wittenberg C *et al.* A multidisciplinary intervention to prevent the readmission of elderly patients with congestive heart failure. *The New England Journal of Medicine* 1995; **333**:1184–9.

Sheldon JH. *The Social Medicine of Old Age* 1948; Oxford University Press, Oxford.

Siegler EL, Glick D & Lee J. Geriatric nursing. *Optimal Staffing for Acute Care of the Elderly (ACE) Units* 2002; **23**(3):152–5.

Stewart S, Marley JE & Horowitz JD. Effects of a multidisciplinary, home–based intervention on unplanned readmissions and survival among patients with chronic congestive heart failure: a randomized controlled study. *Lancet* 1999; **28**:613–20.

Stroke Unit Trialists' Collaboration. Collaborative systematic review of the randomised trials of organised inpatient (stroke unit) care after stroke. *British Medical Journal* 1997; **314**:1151–9.

Stroke Unit Trialists' Collaboration. Organised inpatient (stroke unit) care for stroke. *The Cochrane Database Systematic Review* 2002; (1):CD000197, Copyright 2004.

The National Nursing Home Survey. 1999 Summary. *Vital and Health Statistics* 2002; **13**(152):http://www.cdc.gov/nchs/data/series/sr_13/sr13_152.pdf, Accessed February 21, 2005.

Thomson C, Fine M & Brodaty H. *Carers' Support Needs Project: Promoting the Appropriate Use of Services by Carers of People with Dementia* 1997; Research consultancy for the New South Wales Ageing and Disability Department as part of the New South Wales Action Plan on Dementia.

Total Population by Age 2005, Accessed March 8, http://www.census.gov/population/projections/nation/summary/np-t3-f.pdf. U.S. Census Bureau. National Population Projections. Summary Files, August 02, 2002.

Warne RW. Issues in the development of geriatric medicine in Britain and Australia. *The Medical Journal of Australia* 1987; **146**:139–41.

Warren MW. Care of chronic sick: a case for treating chronic sick in blocks in a general hospital. *British Medical Journal* 1943; **ii**:822–3.

Warren MW. Care of the chronic aged sick. *Lancet* 1946; **I**:841–3.

Warren MW. The role of a geriatric unit in a general hospital. *The Ulster Medical Journal* 1949; **18**:3–12.

Warshaw G, Bragg E, Shaull R *et al.* Survey of geriatric medicine fellowship programs, *Presented at the Association of Directors for Geriatric Academic Programs Annual Meeting*, Washington, 2002a.

Warshaw G, Bragg E, Shaull R *et al.* Survey of geriatric medicine in academic medical centers, *Presented at the Association of Directors for Geriatric Academic Programs Annual Meeting*, Washington, 2002b.

Working Party Report. *Consultant Physicians Working with Patients* 2005, 3rd edn; Royal College of Physicians, London.

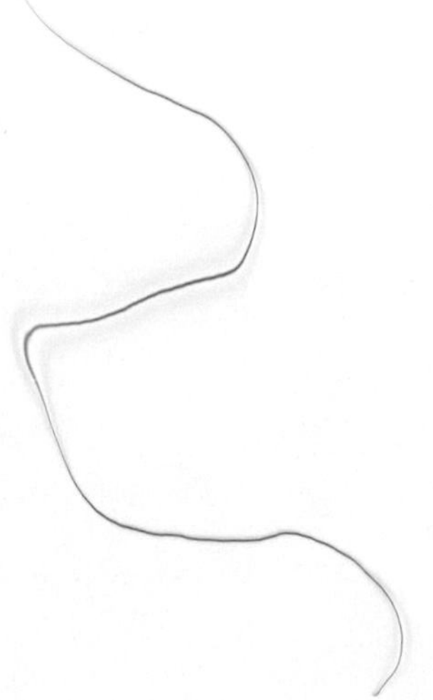

160

Geriatric Day Hospitals

Neil D. Gillespie[1] ***and*** **Irene D. Turpie**[2]

[1] *University of Dundee, Dundee, UK, and* [2] *McMaster University, Hamilton, ON, Canada*

INTRODUCTION

Geriatric Day Hospitals (DHs) are key components of specialized health services for the elderly throughout the world. They usually provide a community-based rehabilitation service for older persons and a bridge between hospital and community care, but have different contributions to make to the health care of older persons in various health-care settings. While the main emphasis of DHs relates to rehabilitation of the older person, the precise function varies depending on the health-care setting. The role of the DHs can vary from a predominantly diagnostic and assessment center to a more supportive and holistic facility used to optimize patient function with a wide variety of techniques and professional disciplines. In recent years, DHs have evolved to include preventative approaches to disease management.

Patients attending a DH present with a wide range of health and social problems. But the multidisciplinary nature of the care enables the best management of multiple pathology while minimizing disability and handicap.

Dr Lionel Cosin developed the concept of the first DH in 1957 in the Cowley Road Day Hospital in Oxford, United Kingdom as an extension of ward-based multidisciplinary assessment. Other Geriatric Medicine pioneers such as Professor John Brocklehurst and Dr John Dall further developed its role and persuaded local authorities to add vital transport services and diagnostic facilities.

The DH evolved at the same time as specialized services for the elderly and has continued to evolve, although its predominant role still revolves around the effective assessment, treatment, and rehabilitation of community living older adults with multiple health-care needs. The concept of Geriatric DHs was exported from Britain to other European countries, Canada, Asia, the United States, and Australia (where they are called *Community Rehabilitation Centres*). New Zealand DHs are usually sited in urban areas and serve geographically defined populations. There have been few attempts to provide such services to persons in rural settings (Rockwood *et al.*, 2000). The first DHs were set up in response to the clinical needs of frailer older people who could be effectively assessed and treated without the need for inpatient hospitalization. As a result, DHs were designed to function in response to many different parameters, but in general, the population of patients served is ambulant. Psychogeriatric DHs also exist, but are not as abundant as those with rehabilitative or medical purposes. They are not considered further in this chapter.

Day Hospital services have the potential to decrease hospital admission and prevent institutionalization, although, this has only been substantiated in communities where there is no comprehensive geriatric care system.

REFERRAL AND FUNCTION

While some patients are referred to DH following inpatient hospital treatment, family doctors form the usual referral source, often at the instigation of home-care health personnel. There are still few referrals from hospital specialists to DHs, although this is increasing.

Referral to DH rather than the outpatient clinic may be appropriate for a number of reasons, not least of which is transportation. This is usually provided without charge in the United Kingdom while other countries have nominal payments.

Most DH services concentrate on predominantly rehabilitative aspects of care, although others now focus on medical management in frail older people of specific diseases such as gastrointestinal disease, cardiovascular disease, and problems related to bone diseases including falls. Family doctor's involvement is also important. All DHs provide only periodic care and any medical management change must be quickly shared with the primary care physician.

One of the most useful aspects of DH assessment is the provision of adequate time and several viewpoints in the assessment of the older patient, not so readily

Principles and Practice of Geriatric Medicine, 4th Edition. Edited by M.S. John Pathy, Alan J. Sinclair and John E. Morley.

available in a short outpatient clinic consultation. A particular strength is the tailored nature of care to the older patient with consideration of transport issues, meal provision, and mobility problems. The contributions of each member of the multidisciplinary team, especially the physiotherapist and occupational therapist are important for many patients.

In those DHs, which provide investigation and medical management, the greater amount of time allocated to patient assessment relative to conventional outpatient clinics means that investigations such as X rays and ultrasound can be performed on the same day enabling rapid therapeutic decisions to be made with minimum inconvenience to the patient. While patients may often derive intangible benefits from the social aspects of attending a DH, this is generally not the primary objective of DH nor has its impact on health been measured in clinical trials.

In most communities, day centers, programs, and clubs provide social and maintenance care specifically tailored to the needs of the older individual. Although the differences between each of these facilities from DH may be clear to those who work within specialized services for the elderly, they are not so readily apparent to the general public and even other health-care professionals. In contradistinction to the day centers, DHs have a defined role in assessing and improving management and health and have a greater number of health professionals available. It is important to note that day centers and day programs are seen as increasingly important in *maintenance of function* in elderly patients.

Patients with "*geriatric giants*" (Table 1) are referred to DH, with the possible exception of patients with a dementia of such severity that they cannot benefit from the services provided or are apt to wander away in nonsecure premises and for whom a medical DH is not appropriate. In recent years with the advent of newer treatments for Alzheimer's disease (and the likelihood of other complicating coexistent conditions), more patients with dementia are being *referred* for medical assessment give the likelihood of other complicating coexistent conditions. Patients frequently have visual and mobility problems and the provision of arranged transport by ambulance or some other means can have a major impact on the older patient's access to treatment facilities. In general, most DHs provide assessment and treatment of the common general internal medicine conditions of old age (Table 2).

The optimum period of attendance for DH is not clear and has never been addressed in a formal clinical trial. But patients generally attend for 6 weeks, as this time framework should enable the assessment and treatment of most of the appropriate conditions. The relative merits of longer attendance are not clear and longer periods of attendance are unlikely to contribute to significant health-care benefits.

Patients may attend DH for 6 to 12 weeks for rehabilitation, usually 10 to 20 visits, but this may vary in individual day hospitals. At each visit they will have specified periods of treatment, although this has never been standardized in practice or by comparison in clinical trials, with therapy predominantly directed toward specific goals. Many DHs strive for shorter admission periods. The ideal length of stay has never been firmly established nor the ideal amount of therapy.

Day Hospitals are best situated in easily accessible situations, avoiding congestion at elevators and allowing easy drop off, of the attendees. There should be generous toilet facilities and adequate space for the physiotherapist and the occupational therapist and the other professionals (nutritionist, speech pathologist, social worker, nurse, nursing aides, and recreational therapist as example) who may form the team. Increasingly, medical students, other learners, and postgraduate trainees spend time in DHs and students appreciate the wide array of pathology and the willing cooperation of patients. Day Hospitals are often sited in contiguity to inpatient rehabilitative services, which has the advantage of sharing the staff and reinforcing the continuity of care. They can also be sited in Centers for Ambulatory Care where there is more of an emphasis on the community aspects of management or in other sites such as shopping malls, but with an association to a larger health facility.

Table 1 Conditions frequently managed and assessed in DH

Geriatric giants
Incontinence
Autonomic instability
Adverse drug reactions
Cognitive impairment
Falling

Poor mobility/falls
1. Stroke/TIA
2. Parkinson's disease
3. Osteoarthritis
4. Osteoporosis
5. Cardiac arrhythmias
6. Postural Hypotension

Breathlessness and fatigue
1. Heart failure
2. Chronic obstructive pulmonary disease
3. Chest infection

Anemia secondary to
1. Gastrointestinal blood loss
2. Chronic disease
3. B_{12} deficiency
4. Malignancy
5. Other causes

Symptoms caused by depression/dementia
1. Hypothyroidism
2. Vasculitis

Table 2 Some indications for referral to DH

- Postdischarge surveillance
- Rehabilitation following recent illness, for example, stroke, hip fracture
- Investigation and management of medical conditions, for example, anemia, heart failure, arthritis, Parkinson's disease, other neurological conditions.
- Falls assessment
- Assessment by speech and language therapist, dietician, physiotherapist, or occupational therapist.
- Nursing procedures, for example, catheter insertion/change
- Respite

FUNCTION

The key function of DH is access to comprehensive multidisciplinary assessment followed by instigation of appropriate treatment for older adults living in the community. Part of the comprehensive assessment process includes a team review with treatment programs tailored to individual patient's requirements. The integrated treatment plan and time for adjustment and socialization are important for older persons as they recover from illness and improve their overall function from the point of referral. In this regard, the simple aspects of rehabilitation such as encouragement, listening, socialization, and education are important, not only for conditions associated with immobility such as stroke or depression but also for other more "organic" conditions of old age such as diabetes or heart disease. It is likely that the socialization and company provided are helpful, although this has never been measured as an outcome. Educating the patient is an important role.

Most DHs with a rehabilitation focus set specific achievable goals for each patient, often in collaboration with the patient and/or family members. Discharge takes place when those goals have been attained or as near to them as the patient is likely to get. Often the person is discharged to a day center or to a community exercise or activity program.

In the current climate of rigorous economic health evaluation, many regions are trying to more clearly define and focus the functions of their DHs, one of the main driving forces being to decrease acute-care admission and prevent institutionalization. This has led to an important trend over recent years in the United Kingdom. The *medicalization* of DH services has resulted in more patients attending for specific medical therapy and interventions than 10 years ago (Table 2). In addition to conventional rehabilitation, patients may be referred for assessment and treatment of heart failure or for multidisciplinary assessment following a fall.

Journey of Care

A typical schedule for patients attending DH may include:

1. transport;
2. initial assessment, medical evaluation/assessment by other team members;
3. establishment of goals to be met by patients during admission;
4. investigations, ideally on the same site, but if not, may be able to facilitate or assist with preparation for diagnostic tests;
5. variable number of sessions per week (usually 2, lasting 4 or 5 hours);
6. therapies including transfers, mobilizing, exercise, improved balance and strengthening, kitchen practice, recreational therapy, health education, and midday meal provided;
7. team review;
8. discharge with connection to community programs, if appropriate.

Within this framework, DH patients receive the synergistic benefits of multidisciplinary assessment and treatment. Although there may be overlaps between the different modalities of treatment, if the patient can attend regularly and has rehabilitative potential, progress is made in a relatively short period of time.

For example, the older patient who has recently fallen and suffered a loss of confidence as a result of several falls may have his/her balance and walking assessed and evaluated by a physiotherapist while during the same attendance he/she be assessed for potential arrhythmias, medication, and other medical triggers for falls. In addition, stroke prevention issues can be addressed if the patient has coexistent hypertension and atrial fibrillation. Input from a pharmacist, physician, or from the nursing staff to check patients' adherence with their pharmaceutical regime and to improve their understanding may help minimize drug interactions and may prevent problems such as postural hypotension or difficulties associated with anticoagulation. Further assessment by the occupational therapist may reveal functional or cognitive aspects not immediately apparent in the conventional medical assessment process. The information is shared at a case conference enabling a consistent and realistic overall management scheme for the patient. Sometimes the specific requirements of each patient may not be immediately apparent, but over the time, will become clearer with the predominant issues influencing overall function becoming more readily apparent.

EVALUATION

Several studies over the years have assessed the effectiveness of the DH services throughout the world with differing degrees of emphasis. Most have been designed to answer specific questions relevant to specific cohorts of patients, including the effect of treatment on morbidity, readmission to hospital and mortality. In the early years of DH services, cost effectiveness was less of an issue, but in modern health-care economics, this is an important consideration in the evaluation of any health-care service.

Evidence for the effectiveness of DHs from clinical trials is weak, although intuitively, many health professionals who work with frail elderly patients and their families believe that DH services contribute significantly to all aspects of care. The details of selected illustrative clinical trials are discussed below.

A meta-analysis (Forster *et al.*, 1999) considered 12 randomized controlled trials selected by predetermined criteria (2867 participants) and prespecified outcome measures which were death, institutionalization, disability, global "poor outcome", and use of resources. The researchers also divided the comparative analysis of the included studies into three preselected groups: DH versus comprehensive care (inpatient and outpatient comprehensive geriatric assessment), DH versus domiciliary care (delivered in the patient's own home), and thirdly, DH versus no comprehensive care. The main conclusion was that DH patients showed trends in reduction in hospital bed use and placement in institutional care, but that there was no reported difference in mortality and subsequent deterioration. No cost saving was noted in any of the studies, although Long Term Care (LTC) placement and its substantial associated costs were reported for only two of the studies. Finally, it was noted that patients who underwent DH treatment regimes fared better than those patients who did not receive any form of comprehensive medicine for the elderly intervention.

Tucker *et al.* (1984) evaluated the impact of DH referral from both hospital and community care in a cohort of 120 patients in New Zealand at the inception of a DH service. Patients attended for on average 3 weeks for two sessions per week following an initial assessment of activities of daily living. Participants were randomized to DH care or standard care in their local health network. Overall function was improved in patients receiving DH care, although this function was not maintained in the medium term following discharge. Mood was improved over a 5-month period. Although this intervention was effective, there was difficulty in maintaining the benefit for a longer period of time without the need for rereferral.

In another study from Canada, Eagle *et al.* (1991) evaluated DH care compared with the usual care provided by the same group of geriatricians. The patient group was frail older patients referred to geriatricians, who included the patients into the study, if they felt that they would benefit from geriatric assessment. The study group attended DH for 2 days week^{-1} for approximately 3 months. The control group was followed by the same geriatricians in geriatric outpatient clinics or if indicated in a geriatric inpatient unit. A total of 113 patients were studied. Outcome measured using the Barthel Index (Mahoney and Barthel, 1965), a Quality of Life Index (Guyatt *et al.*, 1993), was similar between the two cohorts of patients. In this study, the DH intervention was no better than usual geriatric care and there was no cost saving. Both groups deteriorated during the follow-up period. It should be noted that many of the patients were too cognitively impaired to complete a complex quality of life questionnaire.

Hui *et al.* (1995) in Hong Kong in another randomized clinical trial noted improvements in the Barthel Scores in stroke patients who received DH input as part of their intervention package after being discharged from hospital. More recent work has evaluated the 3-month follow-up of patients discharged from Geriatric DH. Although the number of patients included in the evaluation is small, there was no evidence of sustained improvements in mobility or functional status at 3 months following discharge from Geriatric DH. This is perhaps not surprising, as previous studies have not shown large benefits to such a group of patients. In one DH evaluation, those patients with the greatest disability as measured on the SF12 scale (Rand Corporation and Ware, 1979) and who were able to attend a DH derived the greatest benefit (Lewis *et al.*, 2000), a finding which needs further study. Other work has attempted to evaluate the economics of geriatric DH care and found, following a cost-benefit analysis, that benefit relating to a geriatric DH exceeds the cost of the program.

DEVELOPMENTS

Despite the lack of definitive evidence relating to clinical effectiveness, DH services continue to flourish throughout the world. In terms of factors shaping the development of DH services, and other medical services for older people, the Community Care Act in the United Kingdom has had a significant influence as the redesign and modernization of many services has focused on the need to deliver health care in more of a community setting. As a result, the number of hospital-based long-term care beds are decreasing with more older people being managed in both residential and nursing homes. In principle, reduction of long-term beds makes initial sense, but has resulted in a trend for an increase in the numbers of frailer older people referred to secondary health-care facilities.

One of the increasing roles for DH is the management of conditions which require some of the services usually associated with hospitalization in the short term, but which do not require all the high-tech facilities in an acute-care center.

In principle, therefore, prevention of decompensation is an important function of community-specialized programs for the elderly. Maintenance therapy has in the past been provided in day centers and in some DHs. There is little to be gained by patients attending DH for prolonged periods of time following initial assessment and treatment. With advances in investigative and radiological technology, there are opportunities for DHs to provide additional integrated services for older patients. For example, neurovascular clinics for the management of those patients who have had a transient ischemic attack (TIA) are becoming more widespread and integrated services for patients with Parkinson's disease and incontinence are already established on a fairly widespread basis. Newer initiatives include falls clinics, which have ready access to bone densitometry and facilities for the management of heart failure including echocardiography. More established roles for DH in some countries include provision of blood transfusions, preparation for gastrointestinal investigations and medication reviews by a clinical pharmacist.

Additional newer services provided by DHs make use of the increasing role of extended nursing duties. These include visits to the patients' homes to monitor International Normalized Ratio (INR)s or attach a 24-hour ECG tape if required. Further roles could relate to optimizing medication adherence, although it is important to act in conjunction with services already provided by district nursing teams.

In reality, the roles for DH are considerable, but it is important to achieve the balance between medical and nursing care as well as the social aspects of care. When patients require predominantly nursing and medical care as well as the input of therapists, they should attend DH usually for a period of 4 to 6 weeks. Rehabilitative services may require a longer period. However, when patients are benefiting mainly in terms of social interaction that is the point at which they are best encouraged attending day centers and luncheon clubs.

Exercise plays an important role in the prevention of illness and the optimization of function. Many studies highlight the benefit of exercise in old age and patients attending DHs should be encouraged to attend exercise programs whether they are based in the DH itself or in another location. In addition to preventing cardiovascular disease and promoting well being, there is evidence that balance can be improved and falls decreased as a result of increased muscle strength and improvements in coordination (Gillespie *et al.*, 2001).

Most DHs have a considerable emphasis on holistic approaches to care. While this is important, it is still important that a diagnosis be established so that appropriate and effective treatments can be offered. While the use of specific therapies and drug treatments is likely to continue to increase, the multidisciplinary nature of care must be protected. Day Hospital provides a means by which effective, sometimes complex models of care can be delivered to an older population in a way acceptable to the patient.

Important changes are occurring in United Kingdom DHs and are being watched with interest elsewhere in the world. The concept of expanded comprehensive interdisciplinary assessment at the same time as management of significant medical problems is attractive and may avoid the hospitalization that is so often hazardous to the frail elderly.

Heart failure clinics improve management of chronic heart failure (Rich *et al.*, 1995). In older patients with heart failure, managed in a multidisciplinary setting, similar if not identical to many DH facilities, hospital admissions for heart failure are reduced with overall cost savings. This type of effective disease-specific intervention may be justifiable on a widespread basis in caring for the elderly in complex illness. Multiple pathology is the norm in the very old and multifaceted assessment and management are required. Epidemiological studies have confirmed the high prevalence of congestive heart failure (CHF) in specific cohorts of older people, but such patients with CHF often have cognitive impairment and mobility problems. Contributions from geriatricians, nursing team members, pharmacists, and other therapists combine synergistically to improve the overall quality of care. In addition to providing effective multidisciplinary management for older patients with established heart failure, DH patients can be prescreened for suspected cardiac disease.

A recent report highlighted the ability of brain natriuretic peptide (BNP) to incrementally detect cardiac disease in a cohort of older patients attending DH.[1] Screening older patients at DH with BNP may result in detection of cardiac disease and be useful in the assessment of older patients with vague symptoms who may have underlying cardiac disease (Hutcheon *et al.*, 2002).

DISCUSSION

When evaluating various forms of treatment, the randomized controlled trial is the benchmark for assessing efficacy. This is not the only valid means of evaluating DH care as qualitative evaluations and descriptive studies have some uses in these types of patients.

Traditionally, Barthel Index and Clifton Assessment Procedures for the Elderly (CAPE) (Pattie and Gilleard, 1979) scores have been used to evaluate geriatric medicine interventions. However, these instruments may be too insensitive to measure health-care benefits provided by DH care. Newer rating scales which concentrate on a population of less-frail, more ambulant older patients may be more useful in demonstrating some of the benefits on quality of life for DH patients. Disease-specific health-questionnaires may have a role as well as other general health-care questionnaires. A number of newer quality-of-life and health-care evaluation questionnaires for older people are currently being developed and may have a role in future studies. Goal attainment scaling allows the specific goals to be set by the patient and therapist and works well in showing response to change, although it does not function as well for comparison between patient groups (Rockwood *et al.*, 2003). The more recent health promotion aspects of DH care may reduce institutionalization and disability, but this has not been demonstrated as yet. Evaluation of these new uses should be a priority area for DH research.

Although the benefits of attending a DH may seem small, it is likely that small differences in management can result in significant benefits in function for the older patient. Maintenance of any benefits is important, but the reality is that many of the patients have multiple medical problems, which will wax and wane over a period of time with the chronic nature of their illness often the major limiting functional issue. Continued attendance at a day program may maintain function, but the ability to continue to attend may depend on health status.

In the nontrial world of routine clinical practice, the reality is that patients may benefit from different aspects of a comprehensive Geriatric Medicine Service at different times, as often they have multiple problems varying in severity over a given time course with differing and fluctuating health-care needs. Day Hospitals are heterogeneous and it is impossible to quantify the physiotherapy and other services patients receive either in the DH or in their own homes. There is no strong evidence for the amount and duration of therapy that is needed. In all of the published studies, outcomes important to patients are rarely considered. Minimization of handicap may be more important to a patient than disability or hospitalization. For example, if one can walk independently and without apprehension using a walking aid, this is a better outcome than the same disability without the ability to walk confidently. Focusing on the minimization of handicap rather than disability may also provide more positive outcomes. Such measures have not been used in the controlled DH trials.

Mortality as an outcome may not be as important to many older adults as it is to younger individuals and avoiding institutionalization is of great importance to most elders. Quality of life issues, mood improvements, and the social impact on health of lonely older adults attending DH and subsequently connected to other programs should be included as outcomes.

One key question is whether DH services provide any additional benefit to conventional geriatric medicine assessment. The outpatient nature of DH care is likely to be more appealing to those patients who are more mobile and who could derive benefit from therapy while remaining in their own homes. In the comparisons of heterogeneous groups of patients, it is difficult to demonstrate the particular benefits of various service types. It is easier to demonstrate the benefits of a particular type of therapy provided to specific patients with defined disease states.

Staff who work in DHs like working there. They enjoy the ongoing patient contact and the hours of work. However, they must also be able to adapt to change, as DH attendance is an intervention in itself and, thus, may change when different evidence becomes available.

Patient preference is another relevant patient issue. Many patients who have considerable mobility problems prefer treatment to be delivered in their own homes. But this should be weighed up with the issues associated with the social benefit of encouraging older patients to mix where possible and the negative health effects of loneliness. Outreach services from tertiary centers may be effective in the management of the older patients discharged from hospital. In some cases, patients are managed by teams who contributed to their care while the patients were still in hospital.

Other ways of potentially evaluating and justifying the continuation and development of DH services include assessment of specific intervention programs as well as additional activities in the DH facility including exercise programs and fitness regimes.

The latter have proven to be effective in promoting a more active lifestyle for older patients and thus facilitating the postponement of disability. Exercise in older patients is increasingly being recognized as useful for patients with heart failure, falls and balance problems, as well as a means of maintaining mood and DHs provide an ideal site to start this process.

CONCLUSIONS

Day Hospital services have been in existence for over 50 years and have developed to include many newer features. As with most aspects of specialized health services for the elderly, the multidisciplinary nature of the care is of crucial importance. While the benefits of this type of care are clear to those involved in the management of patients, the evidence base is less compelling for a number of reasons including the difficulties of obtaining suitable controls for evaluation in randomized trials, the broad diversity of the patients, the actual professional services provided and the patients' expectations.

Not surprisingly, DH care does best when compared with no care at all. It is difficult to compare DH care with other forms of care, as the unique nature of this multidisciplinary care is its strength. Day Hospitals are in a time of development as health care changes its focus to provide more community care and the numbers of frail elderly continue to increase. Some of the more disease-specific components of a DH service including management of chronic diseases such as Parkinson's disease, heart failure, diabetes, and gastrointestinal blood loss are easier to evaluate. However, the benefits in situations such as poor mobility, falls, and incontinence are less easy to measure, but nonetheless just as important to patients. If responses to treatment are slow, referral to other appropriate services may be necessary to ensure optimum function and a DH should be part of a continuum of specialized geriatric services and a key component of medicine for the elderly services. Day Hospital bridges the gap between comprehensive inpatient geriatric assessment and community-based care of the older patient.

Although most DHs have a considerable emphasis on holistic approaches to care, it is important to establish a clear diagnosis in individual patients so that appropriate and effective treatments are offered. While the use of specific therapies and drug treatments is likely to increase, the multidisciplinary nature of care must be protected. Day Hospital provides a means by which effective and sometimes complex models of care can be delivered to an older population in a way acceptable to the patient of the twenty-first century.

NOTE

[1] BNP a cardiac neurohormone is elevated in heart failure and other cardiovascular conditions and can be easily detected by a simple blood test.

Acknowledgment

The authors would like to acknowledge the advice of Dr J Dall in the preparation of this article.

KEY POINTS

- Geriatric DHs are key components of specialized health services for the elderly throughout the world.
- They usually provide a community-based rehabilitation service for older persons and a bridge between hospital and community care.
- The DH role can vary from a predominantly diagnostic and assessment center to a more supportive and

holistic facility using a wide variety of techniques and professional disciplines.

- Randomized trials have suggested that DH attendance reduces hospital bed use and placement in institutional care.
- Day hospital services are likely to expand and diversify in the future.

KEY REFERENCES

- Eagle DJ, Guyatt GH, Patterson C *et al.* Effectiveness of a Geriatric Day Hospital. *Canadian Medical Association Journal* 1991; **144**:699–704.
- Forster A, Young J & Langhorne P. Systematic review of day hospital care for older people. *British Medical Journal* 1999; **318**:837–41.
- Lewis DL, Turpie ID, MacLeod JC *et al.* A prospective evaluation of a Geriatric Day Hospital. *Annals (Royal College of Physicians and Surgeons of Canada)* 2000; **33**:348–52.
- Tucker MA, Davison JG & Ogle SJ. Day Hospital rehabilitation-effectiveness and cost in the elderly: a randomized controlled trial. *British Medical Journal* 1984; **289**:1209–12.

REFERENCES

Eagle DJ, Guyatt GH, Patterson C *et al.* Effectiveness of a Geriatric Day Hospital. *Canadian Medical Association Journal* 1991; **144**:699–704.

Forster A, Young J & Langhorne P. Systematic review of day hospital care for older people. *British Medical Journal* 1999; **318**:837–41.

Gillespie LD, Gillespie WJ & Cumming R. Interventions for preventing falls in the elderly. *Cochrane Database of Systematic Reviews* 2001; **3**:CD000340.

Guyatt G, Eagle J, Sackett B *et al.* Development and testing of a questionnaire to measure quality of life in the frail elderly. *Journal of Clinical Epidemiology* 1993; **1**(46):1433–44.

Hui E, Lum CM, Or KH & Kay RC. Outcomes of elderly stroke patients. *Stroke* 1995; **26**:1616–9.

Hutcheon SD, Gillespie ND, Struthers AD & McMurdo MET. B-Type natriuretic peptide in the diagnosis of cardiac disease in elderly day hospital patients. *Age and Ageing* 2002; **31**:295–301.

Lewis DL, Turpie ID, MacLeod JC *et al.* A prospective evaluation of a Geriatric Day Hospital. *Annals (Royal College of Physicians and Surgeons of Canada)* 2000; **33**:348–52.

Mahoney F & Barthel D. Functional evaluation: the Barthel index. *Maryland State Medical Journal* 1965; **14**:56–61.

Pattie AH & Gilleard CJ. *Manual of the Clifton Assessment Procedures for the Elderly (CAPE)* 1979; Hodder and Stoughton Educational, Sevenoaks.

Rand Corporation & Ware JE, The Rand Mental Health Inventory. In *Measuring Health: A Guide to Rating Scales and Questionnaires* 1979, 2nd edn, pp 213–19; Oxford University Press, New York.

Rich MW, Beckham V, Wittenberg C *et al.* A multi-disciplinary intervention to prevent the readmission of elderly patients with congestive heart failure. *The New England Journal of Medicine* 1995; **333**:1190–5.

Rockwood K, Stadnyk K, Carver D *et al.* A clinimetric evaluation of specialized geriatric care for rural dwelling, frail older people. *Journal of American Geriatric Society* 2000; **48**(9):1080–5.

Rockwood K, Howlett S, Stadnyk K *et al.* Responsiveness of goal attainment scaling in a randomized controlled trial of comprehensive geriatric assessment. *Journal of Clinical Epidemiology* 2003; **56**(8):736–43.

Tucker MA, Davison JG & Ogle SJ. Day Hospital rehabilitation-effectiveness and cost in the elderly: a randomized controlled trial. *British Medical Journal* 1984; **289**:1209–12.

Health and Care for Older People in the United Kingdom

Clive Bowman *and* **Catherine Dixon**
BUPA Care Services, Leeds, UK

INTRODUCTION

The provision of health and care for older people in the United Kingdom is difficult to understand without a sense of its history, in particular the funding and management arrangements. This chapter seeks to provide an overview of these to enable an understanding of contemporary services (2004). The need for a continuity of service provision means this is an account of evolutionary development not revolution. Two key factors shape health and care needs (however determined) and resources (money, facilities, and most importantly people).

A lack of substantive information regarding population needs and evidence to underpin policy development is a recurring weakness in the United Kingdom. Two drivers, namely, the will to improve services (often prompted by the scandal of inadequacy) and cost containment have been consistent features. Continued changes to operational structures and practices have been introduced in an attempt to improve performance and control the threshold of access to services. There has been a tendency to add layers of services to cover cracks and plug holes rather accepting a coherent strategy of development, which has complicated matters. Lengthy periods of underinvestment have been followed by crises of provision and hurriedly conceived initiatives and investment.

The evolving nature of the older population in the United Kingdom are addressed elsewhere (*see* **Chapter 9, The Demography of Aging**), and the evolution of the health and care needs and the socioeconomic context in which they occur are clearly fundamental. Before the arrival of effective medical treatments, the patterns of disease and disability were quite different. Epidemic infections such as tuberculosis have been controlled and the burden of morbidity and mortality from diseases variously associated with lifestyle and environmental factors are now being impacted upon by improvements in prevention, screening, and various interventions. Concurrent improvements in general health and living standards have meant that within the overall improvement in the health of older people, the "geriatric" population is now significantly older and impaired through diseases (such as the Alzheimer's disease) that currently are characterized by limited treatment opportunities and progressive dependency. These new patterns of dependency have other implications; partners, peers, and friends are of limited ability to care. Similarly, the family support from children is changing; offspring are typically fewer in number, older, and often living geographically distant. These changes need to be considered in the context of the relatively low esteem and attractiveness of a career in care for younger people. It follows that care will become increasingly costly and whilst an increasing proportion of older people have considerable wealth, typically related to the value of their homes, there are present real and further future problems regarding the adequacy of income in later life. Simply, people retiring in mid to late fifth decade with increasing longevity have put pension funds under stress. The difficulties of funding retirements that are sometimes exceeding the contributory working life beneficiaries has been compounded by the poor performance of many of the pension fund investments.

AN OVERVIEW OF HEALTH AND CARE IN THE UNITED KINGDOM

The origins of current approaches to the provision of health and care can be traced to the Poor Law policies from 1597 and 1601. A key objective of these was to exert a control on societal order and reduce the numbers of vagrants and "masterless men". Before effective medical treatment, care was "the" option for the incapacitated.

Principles and Practice of Geriatric Medicine, 4th Edition. Edited by M.S. John Pathy, Alan J. Sinclair and John E. Morley.

Much of the early provision was privately funded, often by wealthy philanthropists (e.g. industrialists). During the latter years of the nineteenth century, public involvement increased; for example, local parishes were enabled to form unions with workhouses becoming designated specifically for children, the aged, and infirm. Seeking admission to a Poor Law institution was not a soft option, and amongst many onerous commitments and selection procedures was a common requirement that applicants adopted the status of "pauperism", effectively being without personal means. Pauperism was commonly associated with a loss of the democratic right to vote. A Royal Commission (a British non-party political tool for gathering information and providing guidance for policy makers) was convened between 1832 and 1834 to consider the Poor Law system. It drew on extensive factual and subjective evidence (how many and what sort of people were in care) and in 1834 a new Poor Law was passed. As the nineteenth century progressed, the need for individuals to seek refuge under the Poor Law increasingly was as a result of illness and disability for which "infirmaries" were established by Poor Law authorities. The rules of Poor Law institutions were often well intentioned but in retrospect misguided; a typical example was observed in rules of a work house in north Somerset from the late 1800s that forbade inmates to be fed salmon more than thrice weekly (at that time, salmon was abundant and cheap, but considered to be of poor nutritional value).

The law requiring people to be classified as paupers before gaining entry to the infirmaries was abolished in 1885. The Poor Law was ultimately superseded by the local government act in 1929 and resulted in the transference of the functions of the old boards of guardians of the infirmaries to the county and borough councils. From 1930 to 1948, three forms of health-care provision could be recognized:

- Municipal hospitals: maternity hospitals, hospitals for infectious diseases like smallpox and tuberculosis, as well as hospitals for the elderly, mentally ill, and mentally handicapped, which were formed from the Poor Law infirmaries.
- Private health care: hospitals were fee-paying or voluntary; primary care was mainly fee-paying or insurance-based.
- Charity and the voluntary sector.

Older people were generally treated in municipal hospitals with the lingering vestiges of the Poor Law while most general hospitals evolved from the voluntary hospitals. Municipal hospitals had a lowly status that was unhelpful for older people, and commonly, clinical equipment consisted of discarded items from the general hospitals. There is a delightful irony in that some of the most distinguished teaching hospitals in the United Kingdom that evolved from large old infirmaries retain the name of Infirmary, with modern generations having little awareness of the historical stigma associated with the name.

In 1942, Sir William Beveridge pronounced "five evils" that overshadowed Britain – want, disease, ignorance, squalor, and idleness. Beveridge recommended a series of actions of which the welfare state was and is the most enduring and important for the United Kingdom, whether it is from a perspective of the vision, controversy, cost, or value. Beveridge was originally only asked to sort out the web of insurance services that were hindering development. In this, the rationalization of many small organizations unified to become the British United Provident Association (BUPA), which has continued to grow from insurer to extend into the provision of a wide range of health provisions including a large portfolio of facilities for the care for older people. The National Health Service (NHS) became reality on 5 July 1948. The key principles of the NHS were as follows:

- health care provided free at the point of use, although prescription changes and dental charges were subsequently introduced;
- universal eligibility, even for people temporarily resident or visiting the country. Anybody could be *referred* to any hospital, local or more distant;
- funding almost 100% from central taxation. The rich therefore contribute more than the poor for similar benefits.

The inception of the NHS coincided with a period of rapid medical development. Previously untreatable infections could be treated and often cured with newly developed antibiotics, while other drugs broadened the scope of medical effectiveness (for example, new diuretics for heart failure, anesthetic agents, and medication for the management of mental illness). While welcome, these early new developments ensured that balancing costs and expectations became embedded early and have remained an enduring feature of the NHS.

At the outset the NHS was, for administrative purposes, divided into three streams of activity, hospital services, family practitioner services (doctors, dentists, opticians, and pharmacists who remained self-employed contractors), and local authority health services (community nursing, midwifery, health visiting, maternal, and infant welfare clinics, immunization, and the control of infectious diseases). A "unified" structure was introduced in 1974 with three main levels of management, at district, area, and regional level. The 1974 organization proved wanting, being excessively managerially driven. In 1982, area health authorities were abolished to improve matters, but this also had a negative consequence on the integration and coordination of health and social services authorities.

Providing services for older people in the community (non-hospital settings) has remained contentious often because of an uncertainty in distinguishing health care from care (Timmins, 2001). Care services may be exemplified by home help support (cleaning, shopping, washing, and the like). Some health-care support is well defined, for example, visiting services for leg ulcer care, but there are substantial areas of overlap that remain disputed, illustrated by whether assistance with personal care such as bathing is a health intervention or an act of care. The significance of this becomes clear when it is recalled that health care remains free at the point of delivery, but that care is means-tested. Where services have not been well integrated and local arrangements remain unclear, these issues have often proved quite intractable!

In the early 1980s, the realization that long-term care provision was quite inadequate led to a freeing up of benefits for older people who needed or "chose" to enter care. Care homes mushroomed outside the usual restraint of planning and while many homes were laudable in their aims and the standards of care provided, a large proportion of facilities were provided from largely redundant boarding houses in seaside resorts and the like. Needs and means assessments were perfunctory, and care homes proliferated on the largesse of an inadequately managed benefits system. Concurrently, a lack of commitment was evident for NHS long-term care competing with new treatment technologies.

During the late 1980s and 1990s, an attempt to make the health service less monolithic and more responsive to needs resulted in a policy that created an internal market splitting purchasers and providers. General practitioners were encouraged to become "fund holders", a driving force was to reduce waiting lists for elective treatment. The internal market of the NHS and Community Care Act 1990 produced some of the biggest changes in the welfare state since the Second World War, with local authorities having overall responsibility for community care. From April 1993, local authorities became responsible for the assessment of people's needs and care management. This included the allocation of funds for places in nursing and residential homes as well as other services such as domiciliary care. Furthermore, local authorities were mandated to encourage and promote the development of private and voluntary agencies by purchasing care or services from them. The intention was that a "mixed economy of care" would bring better services as a result of increased competition from a variety of providers. An objective was to remove the financial incentive for people to be placed in care homes and promote the development of domiciliary support and other services that enable people to stay in their own homes. The budgets of local authorities were limited, and commonly older people were provided with levels of care that were "just" adequate with little capacity to address increasing dependence.

Community care enabled the frailest old to largely escape the outdated facilities that lingered from the Poor Law and promoted more home care and more domestic institutional care in new care homes. The infrastructure of geriatric medicine remained largely centered in hospitals, and the clinical responsibility for the most frail and vulnerable defaulted to over-stretched primary care (general practitioners). The internal market brought some change to traditional waiting lists, but it did not extend into acute and emergency systems or chronic disease management. Many older people whose needs could have been more proactively managed avoiding acute episodes were managed reactively by acute services with increasing numbers of older people being uncharitably termed *bedblockers*.

Following the election of "New Labour" in 1997, a new "third way" of running the NHS – driven by performance and benefiting from partnership – was sought. This was largely based on a more collaborative approach than the overt competition of the internal market. It is premature to determine whether the substantial investment to support this will produce lasting benefit to the health service. A series of National Service Frameworks (NSFs) have accompanied the modernization program including one for older people, that signaled objectives with varying levels of expectation regarding achievement. Published in 2001, the NSF for older people provided an extensive program that sought to (NSF, 2005)

- tackle age discrimination, to make it a thing of the past, and ensure older people are treated with respect and dignity;
- ensure older people are supported by newly integrated services with a well coordinated, coherent, and cohesive approach to assessing individual's needs and circumstances and for commissioning and providing services for them;
- specifically address those conditions which are particularly significant for older people – stroke, falls, and mental health problems associated with older age; and
- promote the health and well-being of older people through coordinated actions of the NHS and councils.

The NSF sought to make progress through a series of eight standards that were linked to targets (milestones); these were:

1. Age discrimination: People should be treated equitably on the basis of needs rather than by age.
2. Person-centered care: Interventions should have the best interests of the individual as the central objective.
3. Intermediate care: In recognition that older people may require longer to recover or rehabilitate following illness, a range of services are to be provided to enable them to achieve the best possible outcome and minimize the risk of inappropriately being admitted to long-term care. The expectation was of a host of new services, but much of what has been reported has been a renaming of existing services.
4. General hospital care: Older people's care in hospital is to be delivered through appropriate specialist care and by hospital staff who have the right set of skills to meet their needs.
5. Stroke: The NSF was perhaps most explicit in making clear expectations for community and hospital approaches to stroke by April 2004, but audit by the Royal College of Physicians indicates a significant failure to achieve the milestone.
6. Falls: The aim of this standard is to reduce the number of falls which result in serious injury and ensure effective treatment and rehabilitation for those who have fallen. The NSF sought that services should be operational by April 2005.
7. Mental Health in older people: Older people who have mental health problems should have access to integrated mental health services provided by the NHS and councils to ensure effective diagnosis, treatment, and support, for themselves and their carers. The lack of specification and significant means of audit has rendered this

little more than a well-reasoned recommendation in many areas.
8. Promotion of health and active life in older age: Health and well-being of older people is to be promoted through a co-coordinated program of action led by the NHS with support from councils. While there have been sporadic initiatives, Thai Chi and other commendable exercise initiatives remain rare.

The principles of the NSF were to apply to the care of older people wherever they were receiving care across the spectrum of health and social services, in their own home, a care setting, or in a hospital. Unlike other framework programs such as those for heart disease and cancer, new investment was notably absent and targets somewhat fuzzy. For many older people awaiting planned interventions such as cataract surgery or joint replacement modernisation initiatives have significantly improved, though it is unlikely that the NSF can claim any significant part in this. The vulnerable old, particularly those needing ongoing care, have simply not benefited. Indeed, while the hearts and minds of enthusiastic practitioners found a rallying point in the NSF, the lack of managerial targets have undermined its success. Much work has been focused on avoiding "inappropriate" admission to hospital and facilitating discharge from hospital to reduce "bedblockers" rather than questioning and addressing the causes and underlying trends in needs.

The concerns and uncertainty that surrounded long-term care led to the establishment of a Royal Commission by the new Labour government to provide guidance with regard to long-term care policy, as reported in 1999. The principal recommendation concerned funding and establishing processes to provide understanding of needs and assurance in care provision:

- The costs of long-term care should be split between living costs, housing costs, and personal care. Personal care should be available after assessment, according to need and paid for from general taxation: the rest should be subject to a co-payment according to means.
- The Government should establish a National Care Commission to monitor trends including demography and spending, ensure transparency and accountability in the system, represent the interests of consumers, and set national benchmarks, now and in the future.

(Royal Commission on Long Term Care, 1999)

Though there was a broad welcome for the Commission's report, the policy response was partial, in no small part due to the fact that not all the Commission supported the majority findings and a minority report was appended. The lack of unanimity regarding funding liability undermined political commitment. In spite of the Commission's concerns regarding the complexity of processes and administration, the route to care and responsibilities have increased. In England, the present policy is broadly outlined by an illustrative example of an older person sustaining a stroke with severe disability, for which hospital assessment and circumstances determine that long-term care in a care home would be the most appropriate care option. Firstly, it should be determined whether the individual warrants fully funded NHS care. It remains a matter of concern that the criteria for this are less than transparent, and fully funded care remains exceptional. More generally, living, housing, and personal care costs will be provided to a locally agreed level on the basis of means-testing.

The local authority has a statutory duty under the National Assistance Act 1948 to pay for the costs of care, provided that the individual is assessed as needing it and is unable to pay. The local authority also has an obligation to offer the individual a choice of a care home. If the care home of choice costs more than the local authority would usually pay, if no other home is available or the needs of the individual are such that the home is suitable to provide the care, then the local authority must meet the full cost of the care (subject to any contribution paid by the resident as a result of a means test). If the care home costs more than the local authority would usually pay for the care, under limited circumstances the resident may pay the difference between the cost of the care and the amount the local authority is prepared to pay. More usually a third party, a relative or a charity, may pay the difference. The payment is generally referred to as a *top-up* or *third party contribution*.

Under the Health and Social Care Act 2001, the responsibility for purchasing nursing care was transferred from local authorities to the NHS. Primary Care Trusts undertake an assessment of the individual's nursing care needs. If the individual is assessed as needing nursing care he/she will be allocated a band of low, medium, or high, subject to need. Payment is made directly to the nursing home subject to the band the individual falls into. The lack of consistency and clarity regarding eligibility for fully funded nursing care has led to a large number of complaints which the Health Service Ombudsman has investigated and have been the subject of several critical reports.

At the time of writing this chapter, further change in English health and care provision is likely. Health services are undergoing a radical change led by changing control of financial flows, with health commissioning increasingly vested with primary care and assessment and provision of means-tested personal care with social services. Increasingly, both sides can see the futility of parallel tracks and the confusion it creates for everyone and generally are keen for change. The Royal Commission report of 1999 recommended the establishment of a Care Commission; in practical terms this has been largely interpreted as a need for increasing regulation (see later in this chapter). What evidence exists indicates that the mental and physical disability of people in care is very high and is increasingly a consequence of neurodegenerative diseases and other forms of brain failure that require high levels of care.

An emerging trend is for new forms of housing that provide assisted living to become viable alternatives to care homes with externally sourced care being increased to meet even the highest levels of dependency. While choice is welcome, many professionals are becoming concerned that this trend reflects more about encouraging a greater personal responsibility for resourcing care through self-funding.

GERIATRIC MEDICINE IN THE UNITED KINGDOM

The specialty of geriatric medicine has its roots in the Poor Law infirmaries that had been run by municipal authorities, with the early physicians emerging from the posts of the medical superintendents. Some of the pioneers in the specialty were remarkable individuals, physicians with vision, conviction, commitment and ability. Marjory Warren is rightly acclaimed for her work and influence from the West Middlesex hospital proselytizing key lessons such as diagnosing and treating remedial conditions and promoting rehabilitation. Warren wrote a number of influential papers that are exemplified by an enduring pragmatism; for example, in 1946, she wrote of the inadequacy of existing geriatric services (Warren, 1946)

> "In the past, with no comprehensive geriatric service, most hospitals in a desire to have a quick turnover, have tried to reduce to a minimum the number of admissions of chronic sick cases, and of these chronic sick less interest and attention have been given to the aged than to others, with the result that they have been lamentably neglected from a medical point of view".

The early physicians were astonishingly effective in making improvements to the quality of life experienced by institutionalized older people and undertaking research regarding the big issues that afflicted their patients. The limitations imposed by the basic facilities that these clinicians worked within cannot be overstated. The relative lack of support along with the lack of recognition of their contribution is even more outstanding. A number of names are venerated and listing them invariably leads to important omissions, so readers are recommended to the paper by (Barton and Mulley, 2003).

The specialist medical society, now the British Geriatrics Society was founded in 1947 the stated purpose of this being "the relief of suffering and distress amongst the aged and infirm by the improvement of standards of medical care for such person, the holding of meetings and the publication and distribution of the results of such research" and it defined geriatric medicine (geriatrics) "is that branch of general medicine concerned with the clinical, preventive, remedial and social aspects of illness in older people. Their high morbidity rates, different patterns of disease presentation, slower response to treatment and requirements for social support call for special medical skills".

The Society appointed Lord Amulree as its first President in 1948 and it gradually developed, holding its first Autumn Scientific Meeting at the Royal College of Physicians (London) in 1966. In 1972, the journal *Age & Ageing* was launched. The society now boasts a membership of over 2000, hosts two major scientific meetings for members each year, it has a number of special interest groups, and its journal has an enviable international status.

Many of the early geriatricians found themselves responsible for literally hundreds of beds with long waiting lists for admission. A principal role was triage and an attempt to avoid institutionalization by recognizing and treating or rehabilitating remedial cases. A feature from the early days of geriatric medicine was the collegiate working and interdependence with a wide range of health professionals. Nursing was fundamental to the specialty, but other disciplines developed with the specialty particularly, physiotherapy and occupational therapy. As time progressed, the range of professionals and as their professionalism has increased, the maintenance of a led team has become increasingly difficult.

A recurring theme of the specialty has been the classification of patients, initially by ability (ambulant, bedridden, incontinent, simply confused and demented – requiring special care); then the specialty became increasingly defined by age. The retirement age of 65 initially marked the arbitrary transition from status as a medical patient to geriatric responsibility, itself having echoes to the old Poor Law. Subsequently, as the aging population evolved and the ability of general medicine extended, the defining age increased. Age-related services have in many places given way to integrated or needs-based approaches, and where they persist, the age qualification may be as high as 85. Integrated services typically include acute care for older people with general medicine and often provide "slower stream" resources for older people with complex or rehabilitation needs.

In 1984, Professor James Williamson from Edinburgh reviewed, in a lecture to the British Geriatrics Society, three phases of development of geriatric care, The Warren phase, The Community Care phase and a Preventative phase. Williamson voiced uncertainty regarding the specialties' future.

- *The Warren phase* is hallmarked by the understanding that there was potential for recovery and rehabilitation in many people who were typically consigned to institutional long-term care, that for those who did need long-term care had specialist needs in terms of facilities and equipment, and that surplus or discarded equipment from general hospitals were insufficient.
- *The Community care phase* is characterized by the recognition that intervention in the community was likely to avoid dependence, and that ongoing support often of a simple nature such as domestic support (cleaning, shopping) and ensuring heating could avert a need for more costly care. At this time, the institution widely known as the *day hospital* came into being. The driving force for this was primarily a crisis in staffing long-term care wards and realization that nurses and carers with family commitments may be available for day time employment, and that similarly some families would be able to provide care and support for their elders during the evening and night but not during the day when they were employed. The "day hospital" at its inception was fundamentally a provision of care and refuge. It was a product that typified the pragmatic, essentially practical, approach of the specialty, and soon day hospitals extended from providing refuge

to assessing, treating, and rehabilitating community-based older people.

- *Preventative phase* is built on the recognition that many older people underreported illness, and that screening could improve well-being and independence. This period during the mid-1960s coincided with a surge of development both in primary care and geriatric medicine, with academic recognition in universities and associated momentum in practice development.

Geriatric medicine in the United Kingdom enjoyed an international reputation and many countries developing services for older people visited to learn from the UK experience. British geriatricians have consistently taken the view that only by timely detection and intervention can admission to long-term care be minimized. Unsurprisingly, the notion that resources allocated for screening, diagnosis and early treatment would reduce the need for care found ready political support from successive governments responsible for financing.

The explosion of care homes and the shift of long-term care from the NHS to facilities deemed to be in "the community" led to geriatric services losing responsibilities for long-term care becoming fire fighters of acute disease in addition to general rehabilitation. Progressive geriatricians developed "disease"- and "presentation"-based practices targeting conditions that occur more commonly in later life (for example, Parkinson's disease, falls and continence). With some notable exceptions the admission to long-term care and continued oversight slipped from the grasp of geriatric medicine and the frailest old became increasingly disenfranchised from the specialty that had evolved primarily in response to their needs, and the clinical leadership and advocacy dissipated.

Many geriatric services had limited access to district hospital facilities until the mid- to late 1990s. This often meant that frail older people often acutely ill frequently had to travel to undergo simple X-ray examination. The widespread integration or establishment of geriatric services within acute hospitals has largely brought to an end these anomalies. Improvements in living standards cannot be overlooked, because as recently as the mid-to-late 1980s, many geriatricians could rely on admitting older people with hypothermia throughout winter as a consequence of inadequate heating. This has become a real rarity with hypothermia and its management almost disappearing from the skill set of geriatric departments.

The changing landscape of provision with entry to long-term care determined largely by social services departments and the level of nursing care to be commissioned determined by primary care arguably led to a loss of focus of geriatric medicine. Previous responsibilities to long-term care were replaced by a new commitment to acute care, and patterns of provision varied widely from hospital to hospital diminishing the clarity of purpose for the specialty.

In 1972 Bernard Isaacs, then a consultant at the Glasgow Royal Infirmary (later Professor of geriatric medicine at the University of Birmingham), published a book with colleagues entitled, "Survival of the unfittest: a study of geriatric patients in Glasgow" outlining serious deprivation for many older people and in particular describing a "Geriatric Hard Core" (Isaacs *et al.*, 1972):

> "The hard core is a black circle in the heart of the aging population. It is growing rapidly as the number of people who survive into advanced old age grows; as they outlive their spouses and friends; as their economic and social resources dwindle; and as the strength of their bodies and the clarity of their minds become eroded by undiagnosed and untreated disease".

Isaacs and colleagues described geriatric medicine as not being the medicine of the hard core, but that it might define the approaches of doctors that practice in this domain. The transfer of commissioning to primary care and the national service framework for older people (as described earlier) has effectively set a new framework within which geriatric medicine will need to reinvent itself. Some Primary Care Trusts have recognized the loss of specialist geriatric support and made appointments of "Community Geriatricians", often experienced consultants keen to be reengaged with their patients.

THE REGULATORY MAZE

Regulation of health and care has a tradition of developing in response to crises and scandal, which lead to new standards to be met by health and care providers.

The Health Advisory Service (HAS) was created in the early 1960s in response to a scandal regarding the care of people with learning difficulties in the Ely Hospital in Cardiff, a body that oversaw the "Cinderella" services, namely, psychiatric and geriatric health services. The HAS undertook programmes of service reviews that reported to health authorities, not only did the HAS point out deficiencies but it also commented positively on examples of good and innovative service provision. Perhaps the greatest strength of the HAS was that its director presented an annual report to government. Its directors and assessors were appointed on secondment from consultancies or academe either related to geriatric or psychiatric care. Many of the critical HAS reports were in respect of health service provided long-term care.

The HAS lost touch with a significant part of its constituency of older people with the shift of long-term care provision from the NHS to local authority social-services-commissioned care. Whether the HAS failed to respond to the changes in provision or was unable to do so, its role as a statutory entity for developing standards of care waned. It persists, though it now has the characteristics of a consultancy rather than a statutory centrally funded body that inspected and reported on services.

Central bodies and regulatory authorities have been established, for Health Services, the Commission for Health Audit and Inspection (CHAI) was founded in 2000 to be succeeded in 2004 by the Healthcare Commission which in addition incorporated aspects of the Audit Commission. Concurrently, social care was regulated initially by the National

Care Standards Commission (NCSC) that has been superseded by the Commission for Social Care Inspection (CSCI) that has incorporated the social services inspectorate. Both the Healthcare Commission and the CSCI are, at the time of writing, still relatively immature bodies. Serious gaps in regulation persist, for example, regulators of care hold providers to account, but there is a discontinuity with commissioners of care not being regulated by CSCI. This means that if inadequate care is purchased for an individual, it is the provider that presently remains accountable. It remains to be seen whether collaborative working between the two regulatory commissions will be forthcoming. The disjointed monitoring and regulation of health and care has proved problematic. An example that has attracted much public concern is the use, misuse, and abuses of medication, particularly neuroleptic agents. CSCI have increasingly inspected the storage, administration, and documentation of medication in care homes. However, the Healthcare Commission has (at the time of writing, late 2004) not actively been involved in the acts of prescribing or dispensing.

Concern regarding the abuse and mistreatment of older people receiving care has led to complex procedures for vetting potential employees and the establishment of a register of miscreants who have been determined unfit to work with vulnerable adults. Paradoxically, these arrangements were introduced into care provided by independent and charitable providers but not as yet to NHS workers, yet perhaps the most shameful case has been that of Dr Harold Shipman, the NHS GP who systematically murdered hundreds of his predominantly older patients.

The regulation of services for older people has become a major industry not only with CSCI and the Healthcare Commission but also the health and safety executive, not to mention advisory organizations such as NICE (National Institute of Clinical Effectiveness) SCIE (Social Care Institute for Excellence) and various Royal Colleges relating to professional groups. It is seemingly inevitable that the next step in developing regulation will be a degree of convergence of CSCI and the Healthcare Commission.

RESEARCH AND DEVELOPMENT

The early pioneers of geriatric medicine undertook much research in often extraordinarily testing circumstances. Dr Thomas Wilson, the first appointed NHS geriatrician (to Redruth in Cornwall) was typically innovative. Wilson reported various forms of bladder dysfunction in the Lancet, which have largely stood the test of time, having access to little more than red rubber tubing and manometers in surroundings that were extremely basic.

Development of the care for older people relies upon sustained programs of longitudinal research that can inform changing needs and provide authoritative reference regarding the effectiveness of various innovative approaches. In general medical specialties of interventional and therapeutic medicine there is a great pressure for evidence – for example, pharmaceutical innovations have a limited patent life, so companies need to ensure that products have an active evidence-base and they also have to have a "pipeline" of further new products to maintain their momentum; standing still is not an option. The scenario is very different when considering the provision of caring services. The most obvious pipeline is of older people!

Tension whether research should be clinically led or more socially orientated often leads to suboptimal parallel streams of work that is variously duplicated (clearly the correct approach is "integrated").

The care of older people has not been an area of major investment in relation to the size of the resources consumed by older people. Additionally, this chapter has described how geriatric medicine has become remote from the frailest and more concerned with acute care. The processes through which universities in the United Kingdom appraise the value of academic departments are largely centered on financial performance (grants won). Collectively, these factors have undermined academic geriatric departments in the United Kingdom generally and substantive research into frailty and care has become very limited.

CONCLUDING OBSERVATIONS

Geriatric care emerged from the Poor Laws and in many ways has contributed to the successful care of the aging in the British population. The needs and opportunities for health and care continue to change. The dual drivers of improving standards and managing resources remain key determinants of change and value. The population of older people in the United Kingdom generally is likely to continue to improve in health and life quality. An important and growing section will require high levels of care, and the difficulty of finding people willing to undertake caring roles is likely to be a continuing challenge. In 1962, Peter Townsend concluded his famous survey of residential institutions and homes for the aged in England and Wales with a statement that seems as pertinent today as then (Townsend, 1962):

> "It may be worth reflecting, if indeed a little sadly, that possibly the ultimate test of the quality of a free democratic and prosperous society is to be found in the standards of freedom, democracy and prosperity enjoyed by its weakest members".

KEY POINTS

- Care of older people in the United Kingdom has a tradition rooted in philanthropy that has evolved through the welfare state to an increasing personal responsibility.
- The needs of the aging population are changing with the social deprivation of poverty being replaced

by disability related to the chronic diseases of aging.

- A key focus of geriatric medicine in the United Kingdom has been a proactive approach to minimize the numbers of people entering care. Processes and practice in care have received relatively little attention.
- A tension between increasing standards of care and resource management has been a consistent feature in the United Kingdom.
- Regulatory zeal has been disproportionate to research, commissioning, and, in particular, investment in training.

KEY REFERENCES

- Barton A & Mulley G. History of the development of geriatric medicine in the UK. *Postgraduate Medical Journal* 2003; **79**:229–34.
- The National Service Framework for Older People. Can be accessed by 2005, http://www.dh.gov.uk/PublicationsAndStatistics/Publications/PublicationsPolicyAndGuidance/PublicationsPolicyAndGuidanceArticle/fs/en?CONTENT_ID=4003066&chk=wg3bg0.
- Timmins N. *The Five Giants: A Biography of the Welfare State* 2001; HarperCollins, London, A remarkably perceptive and informed understanding of the British Welfare State.
- With respect to Old Age: A report by the Royal Commission on Long-term Care The Stationary Office 1999, Cm4192-1 The Royal Commissions report contains a mine of factual information regarding care and its funding; it is also available at http://www.royal-commission-elderly.gov.uk.

REFERENCES

Barton A & Mulley G. History of the development of geriatric medicine in the UK. *Postgraduate Medical Journal* 2003; **79**:229–34.

Isaacs B, Livingstone M & Neville Y. *Survival of the Unfittest* 1972; Routledge & Kegan Paul Ltd, London.

The National Service Framework for Older People. Can be accessed by 2005, http://www.dh.gov.uk/PublicationsAndStatistics/Publications/PublicationsPolicyAndGuidance/PublicationsPolicyAndGuidanceArticle/fs/en?CONTENT_ID=4003066&chk=wg3bg0.

Timmins N. *The Five Giants: A Biography of the Welfare State* 2001; HarperCollins, London, A remarkably perceptive and informed understanding of the British Welfare State.

Townsend P. *The Last Refuge* 1962; Routledge & Kegan Paul Ltd, London.

Warren M. Geriatrics: a medical problem *The Practitioner* 1946; **157**:384–390.

With respect to Old Age: A report by the Royal Commission on Long-term Care The Stationary Office 1999, Cm4192-1 The Royal Commissions report contains a mine of factual information regarding care and its funding; it is also available at http://www.royal-commission-elderly.gov.uk.

FURTHER READING

Commission for Social Care Inspection. Website http://www.csci.org.uk, 2005, These organisations reports and websites generally provide a window on how things are!.

Healthcare Commission. 2005, Website http://www.chai.org.uk/homepage/fs/en.

Tallis R. *Hippocratic Oaths, Medicine and its Discontents* 2004; Atlantic Books, London Raymond Tallis, a professor of Geriatric Medicine at the University of Manchester and noted philosopher has produced an eminent if somewhat grumpy critique of contemporary medicine and healthcare.

The British Geriatrics Society. 2005, Website: http://www.bgs.org.uk.

Geriatrics in the United States

John E. Morley[1,2] ***and*** **Julie K. Gammack**[1,3]

[1] *Saint Louis University School of Medicine, St Louis, MO, USA,* [2] *Saint Louis Veterans' Affairs Medical Center, St Louis, MO, USA, and* [3] *Geriatric Research Education and Clinical Center, St Louis, MO, USA*

INTRODUCTION

Modern geriatrics was developed in England starting with the innovative work of Majorie Warren and her colleagues. However, it took workers in the United States into the 1980s and beyond to provide a scientific basis for the theories of geriatric care. The United States can also claim the honor of naming the discipline "geriatrics". Ignatz Leo Nascher, who was born in Vienna, obtained his medical degree from New York University in 1885. He coined the term geriatrics from *geronte*, a group of men over 60 years who ran the legislative council (*gerousia*) of Athens. The birth of geriatric psychiatry can be traced back to Benjamin Rush who, in 1805, wrote an article entitled, "On the Condition of the Body and Mind in Old Age" (Morley, 2004). Geriatrics in the United States at the start of the twenty-first century is extremely fragmented, but still provides some of the most innovative high-quality care. In many cases, however, geriatric medicine still functions on principles of care that were in vogue 50 years ago.

DEMOGRAPHY

At the start of the twentieth century there were 3.1 million persons over the age of 65, representing 4.1% of the total population of the United States. By 2000, there were 34.9 million older persons, representing 12.6% of the total population. It is estimated that by the middle of the twenty-first century 20% of the population will be 65 years and older (Figure 1). There has been a particularly dramatic growth in the old-old with over 4.5 million persons being over the age of 85.

Table 1 lists the major causes of death in persons 65 and over (National Vital Statistics Report, 2005). While heart disease remains the leading cause of death, the age-specific death rate for both heart disease and cerebrovascular accidents has declined by over 50% in the last 50 years. In contrast, the rate of malignancy-associated deaths has risen by 30% in older males and nearly 10% in older females. The leading causes of hospitalization include heart disease, pneumonia, cancer, strokes, and fractures in older persons. These lists of deaths and hospitalizations are in contrast to the common chronic conditions seen with great frequency in older persons (Table 2). The United States (US), like most developed nations, is seeing a "squaring off" of the life expectancy curve, meaning individuals are living longer and dying at a greater frequency in the older years. This then means that older individuals are living longer with a greater number of chronic medical conditions.

The United States spends 13% of the gross domestic product (GDP), 1.8 trillion dollars, on health-care expenditures. There are 271 000 hospital discharges per year for persons 65 to 74 years of age and 482 000 for those over the age of 65. The number of US hospitals and length of hospital admission have dropped consistently since peaking in the early 1970s, but the number of outpatient encounters has tripled since that time (American Hospital Association, 2004). The average number of visits made to a physician each year increases from 1.6 at 15 to 24 years of age to 5.2 at 65 to 74 years of age and 6.8 at 75 years and older. The majority of these visits in persons 65 and older are for the management of chronic problems as opposed to persons under 45 years where most visits are for acute problems. Individuals aged 65 or older utilize one-quarter of outpatient encounters, half of hospitalization days, and one-third of the total health-care expenditures.

Approximately half of all physician contacts for older persons occur in the physician's office (Xakellis, 2004). The most common providers are internists and family physicians. Hospitalized older persons are most likely to be cared for by internists, while geriatricians (internal or family medicine trained) most commonly provide nursing home and home care. In contrast, over half of the outpatient visits of older persons are to specialists (Bragg and Warshaw, 2005). Nearly half of the practice of ophthalmologists, cardiologists, and

Principles and Practice of Geriatric Medicine, 4th Edition. Edited by M.S. John Pathy, Alan J. Sinclair and John E. Morley.

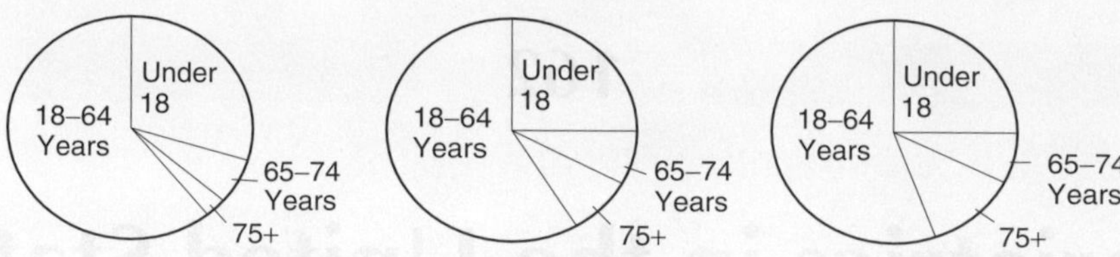

Figure 1 Percent of population in four age-groups: United States, 1950, 2000, and 2050. (*Sources*: US census bureau, 1950 and 2000 decennial censuses and 2050 middle series population projections)

Table 1 Causes of death in persons 65 years and older compared to the whole population in 2000

	Percent of all Deaths	
Cause of Death	Persons 65 and older	All ages
Heart disease	32.4	29.0
Malignant neoplasms	21.7	22.9
Cerebrovascular disease	8.0	6.8
Chronic lower respiratory tract disease	5.9	5.1
Influenza and pneumonia	3.1	2.6
Diabetes mellitus	3.0	3.0
Alzheimer's disease	3.0	2.2
Nephritis, nephritic syndrome, and nephrosis	1.8	1.6
Accidents	1.8	4.2
Septicemia	1.4	1.3

Table 2 Common chronic conditions per 1000 persons 65 years or older

Condition	Male	Female
Arthritis	411.2	534.5
Hypertension	298.0	410.8
Heart disease	311.3	238.0
Hearing impairment	386.8	243.2
Cataracts	140.1	194.3
Deformity or orthopedic impairment	156.5	158.4
Chronic sinusitis	109.6	122.5
Diabetes	121.8	84.3
Tinnitus	117.4	66.1
Visual impairment	103.8	70.0

urologists consists of patients 65 years of age and older. For this reason, 27 of the allopathic residency programs in the United States include special requirements for geriatrics in their training program.

Despite these health-care trends, older Americans in many ways are much better off than in the past. Seventy-two percent of the older population has graduated from high school compared to 17% in 1950. Overall, the net worth of older person households increased by 82% in the last 20 years. In 1959, 35% of older persons lived in poverty and by 2002 it was 10%. At age 65, the average life expectancy is 19.4 years for females and 16.4 years for males. Health screening and preventive medicine is accessible and funded by the vast majority of insurance plans. Figure 2 demonstrates the percentage of the different segments of the population who received influenza and pneumococcal vaccinations. The prevalence of chronic disabilities has decreased from 25% in 1984 to 20% in 1999.

HISTORICAL BACKGROUND

The development of social systems for geriatric care can be traced to 1861 with the military pension system for veterans of the Civil War. This was the precursor of the Veteran's Administration, formalized in 1930, which has had a major role in the development of scientific geriatrics as well as in providing outstanding care for older veterans. Other early care for old persons was provided in nursing homes run mainly by religious organizations, for example, Lafon Asylum of the Holy Family in New Orleans opened in 1842, or by poorhouses or rural poor farms.

By 1935, a rapidly increasing population of impoverished older adults led to the formation the Social Security Board which was reorganized in 1946 to become the Social Security Administration. This program provides a retirement benefit to individuals upon leaving the workforce. Although state and federal subsidies for health-care services were sporadically available in the 1920s, the first private hospital insurance plan (Blue Cross) was not provided until 1933. Further, discussion and development of government sponsored health insurance for the elderly spanned five Presidential administrations and over three decades.

Several important organizations developed in the 1940s and helped in establishing the discipline of geriatric medicine. The Club for Research in Aging was founded in 1939 with support of the Josiah Macy Jr Foundation. This group set the foundation for the Gerontological Society of America in 1945 with first President William MacNidder establishing the publication *The Journal of Gerontology* in the following year. The American Geriatrics Society (AGS) was organized in Atlantic City in 1942 by Malford W. Thewlis, with first President Lucien Stark presiding in 1943. The affiliated Journal of AGS was established in 1953. Both organizations have continued to sponsor these peer-reviewed publications.

Several decades later, in 1978, The American Association of Geriatric Psychiatry was established which spurred the development of fellowship training and certification in geriatric psychiatry in 1990. The American Medical Directors Association (AMDA) was also formed in 1978 and has become a leader in quality improvement initiatives in long-term care. AMDA has developed numerous clinical practice guidelines, training programs, and quality standards for nursing home care. This organization also administers and maintains the only recognized medical director certification program in the United States.

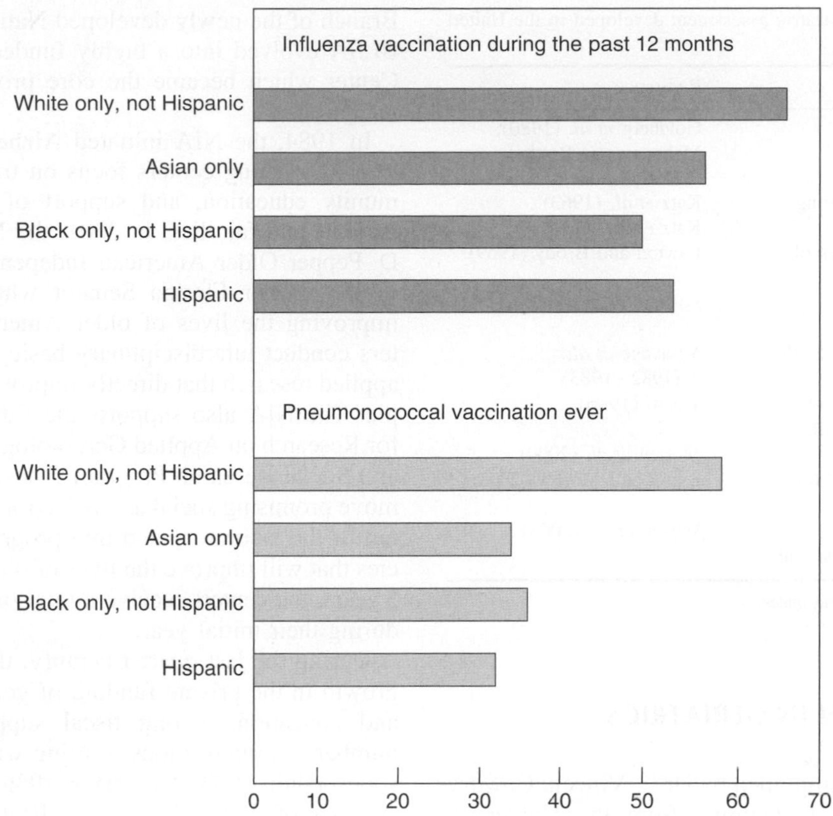

Figure 2 Influenza and Pneumonococcal vaccination among adults 65 years of age and over by race and hispanic origin: United States, 2000–2002

In 1950, through the efforts of President Harry S. Truman, the Federal Security Administration held a national conference on aging to assess the challenges posed by the changing population. No immediate programs were initiated, but this conference spurred the development of an advisory committee on aging. In 1958, Congressman John Fogarty, a Democrat from Rhode Island, called for the first White House Conference on Aging which took place in 1961. The major focus of the 1961 Conference was health care and significant outcomes included expansion of Social Security benefits and support for the later development of government funded health-care financing. In 1965, insurance was finally guaranteed to older adults, the disabled, and the impoverished through the passage of Medicare and Medicaid programs.

Subsequent White House Conferences have been held nearly every decade since 1960. Of importance, the 1971 White House Conference on Aging recommended the creation of a separate National Institute on Aging. Recent Conferences have emphasized health-care coordination and maximizing the effectiveness of existing programs for the elderly.

Geriatric Research, Education and Clinical Centers (GRECCs) were authorized by the federal government with the first sites established in 1975. The GRECC mission is to focus attention on the aging veteran population, to increase the basic knowledge of aging, and to transmit knowledge to health-care providers and improve quality of care to rapidly aging communities. GRECCs are based at Veterans Affairs Medical Centers (VAMC) and have played a major role in the development of scientific research and, in particular, in translational research and education in geriatrics. There are currently 21 GRECC sites across the United States.

The Veterans Administration (VA) also funded geriatric medicine fellowship programs beginning in 1978. 275 fellows were funded between 1980 and 1991. The purpose of the fellowship training program was to develop a cadre of physicians committed to excellence in geriatric research, education, and clinical care with the skills to become leaders of local and national geriatric medicine programs. In 2000, the VA established a Special Fellowship Program in Advanced Geriatrics at seven sites to develop academic and health systems leaders who are committed to leading this discipline in the twenty-first century.

As the discipline of geriatric medicine has evolved over the latter half of the twentieth century, US scientists and clinicians have been extraordinarily successful in developing assessment tools for older persons, which have gained worldwide acceptance (Table 3). Two new tools that have been recently developed are the Saint Louis University Mental Status Exam (SLUMS); (Banks and Morley, 2003) and the Simplified Nutritional Assessment Questionnaire (SNAQ; Wilson *et al.*, in press). These tools, provided in Table 4 and 5, are more refined than previously developed screening instruments.

Table 3 Screening tools for geriatric assessment developed in the United States

Date	Scale	Reference
1955	Barthel Index	Goldberg *et al.* (1980); Mahoney and Barthel (1965)
1963	Activities of daily living	Katz *et al.* (1963) Katz *et al.* (1970)
1969	Instrumental activities of daily living	Lawton and Brody (1969)
1975	Mini-mental status examination	Folstein *et al.* (1975)
1983	Geriatric Depression Scale	Yesavage *et al.* (1982–1983)
1986	Performance-orientated assessment of mobility	Tinetti (1986)
2000	ADAM	Morley *et al.* (2000)
2003	St Louis University Mental Status test	Banks and Morley (2003)
2005	Simplified Nutrition Assessment Questionnaire	Wilson *et al.* (2005)

ADAM, Androgen deficiency in aging males.

RESEARCH IN GERIATRICS

Research in aging was championed by Dr E. Vincent Cowdry who received his Ph.D. in anatomy from the University of Chicago in 1913. During his 65-year research career, spent predominantly at Washington University School of Medicine, Dr Cowdry focused on the cytologic changes of aging and cancer. He led both the Departments of Cytology and Anatomy at Washington University and was a strong proponent of interdisciplinary investigations in gerontology. During the later half of his career he authored several books including The Problems of Ageing: Biological and Medical Aspects (1939), The Care of the Geriatric Patient (1958), and Aging Better (1972).

During the mid-1900s, the US government was the primary financial sponsor of health-care research and scientific programs. The National Institute of Health (NIH) was formed in 1930 and later became a consortium of Institutes and Centers dedicated to health-care research. The National Institute on Aging (NIA) was formally established out of the NIH in 1974 and allocates significant funding to the advancement of aging research.

The roots of the NIA can be traced back to the 1940s and 1950s with the Unit on Aging, headed by Dr Edward J. Stiegliz, the Gerontology Branch, and the Section on Aging subsections of NIH programs. The first NIA director, Dr Robert N. Butler, was appointed in 1976 with Dr Nathan W. Shock directing scientific programs for the Institute.

Dr Shock was already well known to the geriatrics research community for his involvement in the Baltimore Longitudinal Study of Aging (BLSA) which he established in 1958. The BLSA originated through a 1-year grant to the NIH from the Josiah Macy Jr Foundation to develop a gerontology unit in the Baltimore City Hospital in 1940. Dr Shock was named chief of this unit, which later became the Gerontology Branch of the newly developed National Heart Institute. The BLSA evolved into a highly funded Gerontology Research Center which became the core program of the NIA at its inception.

In 1984, the NIA initiated Alzheimer's Disease Centers. The 32 existing centers focus on translation research, community education, and support of programs designed for patients and families. In 2001, the NIA funded nine Claude D. Pepper Older American Independence Centers, in honor of the former Florida Senator who devoted his career to improving the lives of older Americans. The Pepper Centers conduct interdisciplinary basic science and clinical and applied research that directly improves the lives of older people. The NIA also supports the Edward R. Roybal Centers for Research on Applied Gerontology through the Behavioral and Social Research Program. These centers are designed to move promising social and behavioral basic research findings out of the laboratory and into programs, practices, and policies that will improve the lives of older people. Supported for 5 years, the centers receive a total of $1.8 million in funding during their initial year.

During the last quarter century, there has been significant growth in the private funding of geriatric medicine research and education. Strong fiscal support has come from a number of organizations, starting with the Macy Foundation sponsorship of Dr Cowdry's 1939 textbook. Hundreds of millions of dollars have since been provided by charitable agencies dedicated to the care of the aging population.

Founded in 1929, The John A. Hartford Foundation is committed to health care, training, research, and service system innovations that will ensure the well-being and vitality of older adults. The mission of the Foundation is to increase the nation's capacity to provide effective, affordable care to its rapidly increasing older population. The Foundation is the leading philanthropic organization in the United States dedicated to the interests of aging and health. Since the early 1980s the Foundation has granted hundreds of millions of dollars to physicians, scientists, nurses, social workers, and other health-care providers for education, training, and research activities.

The Donald W. Reynolds Foundation, established in 1954 by media entrepreneur Donald Worthington Reynolds, is committed to improving the quality of life of America's growing elderly population through better training of physicians in geriatrics. The Foundation launched its Aging and Quality of Life Program in 1996. Its goal remains improving the quality of life for America's elderly by preparing physicians to provide better care for them when they become ill. The first Reynolds Center at the University of Arkansas was established with a grant of nearly $20 million. Since that time, 21 other centers have been funded with over $70 million in awards. In 1990, The Reynolds Foundation also began supporting the Association of Directors of Geriatric Academic Programs (ADGAP) to encourage the growth of training programs in geriatric medicine.

The Brookdale Foundation, originally endowed by the Schwartz Family, shares a common outlook and focus on the needs and challenges of America's elderly population.

Table 4 (SLUMS) Examination goes here

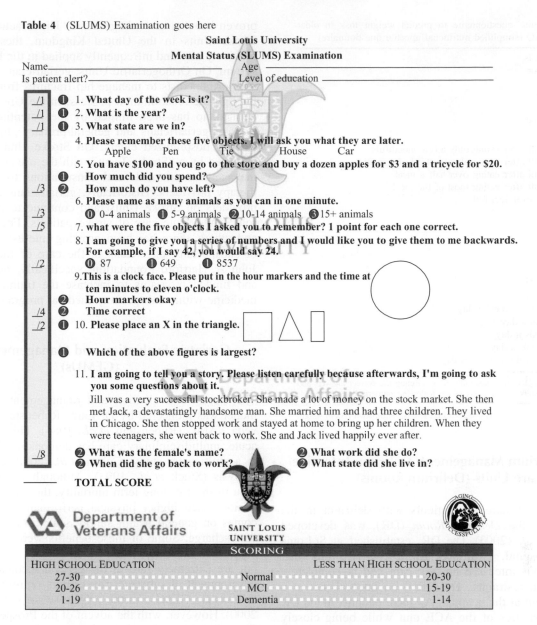

Saint Louis University
Mental Status (SLUMS) Examination

Name______ Age ______
Is patient alert?______ Level of education ______

Score	Points	Item
/1	1	1. **What day of the week is it?**
/1	1	2. **What is the year?**
/1	1	3. **What state are we in?**
		4. **Please remember these five objects. I will ask you what they are later.** Apple Pen Tie House Car
		5. **You have $100 and you go to the store and buy a dozen apples for $3 and a tricycle for $20.**
	1	**How much did you spend?**
/3	2	**How much do you have left?**
		6. **Please name as many animals as you can in one minute.**
/3		0 0-4 animals 1 5-9 animals 2 10-14 animals 3 15+ animals
/5		7. **what were the five objects I asked you to remember? 1 point for each one correct.**
		8. **I am going to give you a series of numbers and I would like you to give them to me backwards. For example, if I say 42, you would say 24.**
/2		0 87 1 649 1 8537
		9. **This is a clock face. Please put in the hour markers and the time at ten minutes to eleven o'clock.**
	2	**Hour markers okay**
/4	2	**Time correct**
/2	1	10. **Please place an X in the triangle.**
	1	**Which of the above figures is largest?**
		11. **I am going to tell you a story. Please listen carefully because afterwards, I'm going to ask you some questions about it.** Jill was a very successful stockbroker. She made a lot of money on the stock market. She then met Jack, a devastatingly handsome man. She married him and had three children. They lived in Chicago. She then stopped work and stayed at home to bring up her children. When they were teenagers, she went back to work. She and Jack lived happily ever after.
/8	2	**What was the female's name?**
	2	**When did she go back to work?**
	2	**What work did she do?**
	2	**What state did she live in?**
___		**TOTAL SCORE**

Department of Veterans Affairs

SAINT LOUIS UNIVERSITY

AGING SUCCESSFULLY

SCORING		
HIGH SCHOOL EDUCATION		LESS THAN HIGH SCHOOL EDUCATION
27-30	Normal	20-30
20-26	MCI	15-19
1-19	Dementia	1-14

The Foundation is committed to enhancing the training of a new generation of leaders in geriatrics and gerontology. The Brookdale National Fellowship Program, which began in 1985, sought those who had the professional expertise, capacity, and potential to become leaders in the fields of geriatrics and gerontology. Brookdale National Fellows conduct research which, it is hoped, leads to a society that is more knowledgeable and more responsive to issues related to aging.

SPECIAL PROGRAMS FOR OLDER PERSONS

Acute Care for the Elderly (ACE) Units

Since the original demonstration of the efficacy of these hospital-based units (Landefeld *et al.*, 1995; Palmer *et al.*, 1994; Miller, 2002), a number of university and community hospitals have established ACE units. The key features of the ACE Unit include (1) geriatric-sensitive environmental alterations, (2) patient-centered care, (3) interdisciplinary planning for discharge, and (4) medical care review. The goal of this model is to reduce the functional impairments that so often develop in acutely ill, hospitalized elders. Barriers to successful recovery and risks for ongoing functional decline are identified early in the hospitalization. Social and environmental factors that may impact independence and health are addressed by the hospital team. The quality of ACE units is variable across the country. For success, hospitals must commit to both the philosophy and care process of the ACE unit. Appropriate resources must be allocated, including recruitment and training of staff, time, and space for daily team meetings, and willingness to change the hospital environment for acutely ill elders.

Table 5 Appetite questionnaire to predict weight loss in older persons – SNAQ (simplified nutritional appetite questionnaire)

1. My appetite is
   (a) very poor
   (b) poor
   (c) average
   (d) good
   (e) very good
2. When I eat
   (a) I feel full after eating only a few mouthfuls
   (b) I feel full after eating about a third of a meal
   (c) I feel full after eating over half a meal
   (d) I feel full after eating most of the meal
   (e) I hardly ever feel full
3. Food tastes
   (a) very bad
   (b) bad
   (c) average
   (d) good
   (e) very good
4. Normally I eat
   (a) less than one meal a day
   (b) one meal a day
   (c) two meals a day
   (d) three meals a day
   (e) more than three meals a day

Instructions: Complete the questionnaire by circling the correct answers and then tally the results on the basis of the following numerical scale: A = 1, B = 2, C = 3, D = 4, E = 5.
Scoring: If the mini-CNAQ is less than 14, there is a significant risk of weight loss.

Acute Delirium Management: Delirium Intensive Care Units (Delirium Rooms)

A new model of care for patients with delirium in the hospital, called the *Delirium Room* (DR), was developed by Flaherty *et al.* (2003) The DR, established at St.Louis University Hospital, is a specialized four-bed unit that provides 24-hour intensive nursing care and is completely free of physical restraints. The DR is an integral part of a 22-bed ACE unit at the hospital. As such, patients in the DR benefit from features of the ACE unit while being closely managed by nurses and physicians who are acutely aware of the dangers to delirious older adults. This setting has shown to be effective in managing patients with delirium.

Another approach to delirium, through the use of a delirium consultation team, was pioneered by the geriatricians at Yale University (Inouye *et al.*, 1999). A standardized hospital protocol was implemented for the management of six risk factors for delirium: cognitive impairment, sleep deprivation, immobility, visual impairment, hearing impairment, and dehydration. Addressing these six factors led to a reduction in the incidence of delirium in hospitalized elders.

Geriatric Care for Speciality Conditions

A number of special care units have been developed to allow physician comanagement or multidisciplinary management of hospitalized older adults. Despite longstanding use, and proven benefits of Orthogeriatric "Hip Fracture" Units and Stroke Units in the United Kingdom, these models are relatively new and infrequently applied in the US health-care system. On Orthogeriatric Units, geriatricians work together with orthopedists to manage hip fractures from acute injury through the rehabilitation process. In the United States, this partnership has been limited by the potentially competing roles of geriatricians and general/primary physicians in the care of hospitalized elders. On Stroke Units, patients are managed by a "Stroke Team" with the use of reflexive care management protocols and consultations to physician and therapy providers. Historically, geriatricians have not been providers on Stroke Units, and continue to have a limited role in the acute care of stroke patients. For these reasons and others, there has been growing interest in the training of subspecialty physicians in the care of the elderly. The John A. Hartford Foundation, specifically, has emphasized and funded programs to increase the training of geriatric medicine within subspecialty medical programs.

Geriatric Evaluation and Management Units (GEMUs)

The Geriatric Evaluation and Management Unit (GEMU) model was pioneered by Dr Larry Rubenstein at the Sepulveda VAMC (Rubenstein *et al.*, 1984). This model of subacute, multidisciplinary care has demonstrated effectiveness in a multicenter study (Cohen *et al.*, 2002) and in a meta-analysis (Stuck *et al.*, 1993). Although no difference was seen in short or long-term mortality, the GEMU process has demonstrated higher physical performance and better outcomes on general health survey scales for patients at time of discharge. Some of these benefits were still apparent at 1-year follow-up. GEMUs are commonly found in the VA, but are extremely rare in the general medical setting. The development of subacute care centers represents an attempt to translate GEMUs to the private sector (Makowski *et al.*, 2000). However, with the advent of the Prospective Payment System, the majority of these units are too costly to provide this level of specialized nursing care.

Program of All-Inclusive Care for the Elderly (PACE)

This model was developed out of the On-Lok program in San Francisco, which supplied social and medical support for predominantly the older Chinese community living in the downtown area. The 26 existing programs now provide care for older persons who are frail enough to meet the requirements to enter a nursing home (Gross *et al.*, 2004). The mission of PACE (Program of All-Inclusive Care for the Elderly) is to allow the older person to continue living at home rather than being institutionalized. Each PACE site provides comprehensive medical and social services to around 200 participants. Care is provided through participation in an adult day health center, but inpatient and home care is provided as needed. Services are available 24 hours a day through the interdisciplinary care team. The PACE program provides near daily contact with enrollees by providing medications, meals, social services, recreational services, and transport, as well as routine health-care services. Each PACE site is federally funded via capitated payments from the Centers for Medicare and Medicaid Services and is expected to achieve a revenue-neutral status within several years of operation. In the United States, PACE represents one of the few comprehensive, all-inclusive systems of geriatric care.

Assisted Living Facilities (ALF)

Assisted care centers developed out of the "retirement community" model which traditionally accommodates only fully independent older adults. Assisted living facilities (ALFs) provide a bridge for older persons who are not yet impaired enough to require nursing home care, but cannot live alone. Also called Residential Care Facilities, these sites tend to provide minimal supervision in the medical area and instead focus on social and personal care needs. ALFs tend to be expensive, and because services are purchased in an *a la carte* fashion, potentially do not fully address the care needs of an older individual. To this point, ALFs are relatively unregulated by state or federal agencies. The quality of care and supervision is thus extremely variable, yet ALFs are a rapidly growing model of quasi-health care for seniors. Reimbursement for physician care provided on-site at ALFs is significantly lower than home care or office visits, despite the increasing level of chronic care delivered in these settings. Physicians are thus reluctant to focus care efforts at these sites and instead encourage patients to make the often difficult trip to a medical office. Given these issues, the American Geriatrics Society (AGS) in a 2005 position paper (AGS Health-care Systems Committee, 2005) has suggested the need to improve the quality of geriatric care at ALFs.

Nursing Homes

Four percent of persons over 65 years of age are in nursing homes. There are approximately 18 000 nursing homes with an average of just over 100 beds per nursing home. Fifty percent of nursing home residents are 85 years and over and 75% are female. At any time, approximately half of nursing home residents are receiving posthospital skilled care with a focus on rehabilitation. Federal sources (Medicaid and Medicare) account for 68% of the payment sources. Approximately 66% of nursing homes are owned by the propriety (for profit) sector, 30% by charitable nonprofits and the rest by the Federal and State governments (i.e. Veteran's Administration and Old Soldiers' Homes).

In 1986, the Institute of Medicine issued a report entitled, "Improving Quality of Care in Nursing Homes" and pointed out the shortcomings in nursing home care. In 1987, the Office of Budget Reconciliation Act (OBRA) created a number of regulations for nursing homes including the mandating of physician administrative services, nursing aide training, restraint and psychotropic drug reduction, and guidelines for reducing polypharmacy. Dr Mark Beers developed a list of drugs that should not be used in older persons – the so-called "Beers list" (Beers *et al.*, 1992). This list was revised in 2003 (Fick *et al.*, 2003) and despite its relative controversy, is applied to nursing home care by state survey agencies.

OBRA '87 also resulted in the development of the Minimum Data Set for Nursing Home Residents. This is now utilized to determine reimbursement for nursing homes and to provide a report card on nursing home quality that is available to the public on the Internet. Nursing homes are surveyed at least twice a year by teams of inspectors from the state. Poor performance can lead to fines or even closure of the nursing home. Many nursing homes in the United States have developed well-organized Continuous Quality Improvement (CQI) programs. CQI has led to extraordinary changes in quality of care in nursing homes in the United States. The focus on nursing home CQI was led by Schnelle and Ouslander (Schnelle *et al.*, 1993) and the Division of Geriatric Medicine at St Louis University (Morley and Miller, 1992; Miller *et al.*, 1995).

A specialized innovation in nursing homes has been the Eden Alternative. This model attempts to de-emphasize the medicalization and place emphasis on the home aspect of nursing homes. These nursing homes encourage pets in the facility and provide gardens for the residents. Empowerment of the residents to take initiative is an important component of this model.

Home Care

Physician-delivered home care was first implemented by the Homeopathic Medical Center in 1875. Originally, home care services were mainly obstetrical, then pediatric, but by 1975, 62% of visits were to the elderly. Under the guidance of Knight Steel, the center became a model for geriatric home care at what had become the Boston University Medical Center (Steel, 1987).

Over the past half-decade, the frequency of physician home visits has dropped significantly. In the mid-1900s, 40% of all patient–physician encounters took place at home. By 1980, less than 1% of health-care visits took place at home (Leff and Burton, 2001). Medicare and Medicaid provide 50% of home care coverage in the United States. The growth of home care services in the 1990s prompted a change in reimbursement from a fee for service to a prospective payment system reimbursement model. For each 60-day certification period, agencies are reimbursed around $2000 per enrollee. Over the last half century, home care in the United States has been predominantly delivered by nurses, social workers and physical therapists. Home visits in the United States have been shown to delay functional decline and improve health outcomes (Stuck *et al.*, 1995; Stuck *et al.*, 2002; Fabacher *et al.*, 1994). Recently, demonstration projects utilizing telemedicine in the home appear to be showing a new approach to home care.

Prescription Drug Financing: Medicare Part D

Medicare has not historically provided reimbursement for prescription medication. Medicaid does cover the costs of most medications for those elders who meet financial eligibility, generally those with an income at or below the federally established poverty level. Some seniors have supplemental insurance for prescription medication; however most pay substantial out-of-pocket medication costs. Medicare Part D, established under the presidency of George W. Bush, is a prescription medication benefit developed for Medicare eligible seniors. This program will begin on January 1, 2006, as the result of the Medicare Prescription Drug Improvement and Modernization Act of 2003. In an article titled "Understanding the Incomprehensible", Marshall (2004) attempts to explain Medicare Part D: "This act requires a basic premium of $420 a year and does not pay for the first $750. It then pays 75% of the next $2000 but nothing of the next $2850 (the truly incomprehensible part) and then pays 95% thereafter under most circumstances. This certainly is not a free drug benefit for seniors and as can be seen, is an incomprehensible bureaucratic policy!" Clearly, Medicare Part D will provide some prescription drug relief to seniors; however the long-term financing of health care and medication costs is in its infancy.

GERIATRIC EDUCATION

The development of academic geriatric programs and medical training has lagged behind the demand for a larger and more skilled geriatric medicine health-care workforce. This is in part due to the lack of universal acceptance of geriatrics as a unique discipline within the medical profession, and also reflects the declining trends in primary care residency training. Over the past 5 years, the percentage of internal medicine residency training positions filled by US medical graduates has dropped from 58 to 55%. The percentage of family medicine residency positions filled by US medical graduates has dropped from 57 to 41%. (National Residency Matching Program, 2005) The rising indebtedness of medical trainees and insecurity of Medicare/Medicaid reimbursement to physicians has compounded the problem. As a result, geriatric medicine fellowship training positions have become increasingly difficult to fill, with one-third remaining vacant in 2003. Over half of fellowship positions are filled by international medical trainees who have little guarantee of being employed in the United States as a geriatrician upon graduation. The number of fellows-in-training has remained essentially constant at 350 over the past 5 years despite the addition of 15 new fellowship training programs and 140 new positions available to trainees.

Dr Les Libow at Mount Sinai School of Medicine offered the first geriatric medicine fellowship program in 1966. The first professorship in geriatric medicine was granted at Cornell University in 1977. In the 1970s, the VA was charged with the task of increasing the education of health-care providers in geriatrics. Funding was provided in 1975 for the first VA Geriatric Research Education and Clinical Center (GRECC). Twenty-two GRECCs have since been established. GRECCs began offering geriatric medicine fellowship training opportunities in 1978.

In 1982, Mount Sinai established a Department of Geriatrics, the first of three to function as independent departments in the United States. Few of the 80% of medical schools with a geriatrics program have the current financial capability of supporting independent departments of geriatric medicine. Two-thirds of these geriatric programs have been in existence for less than 20 years. Two-thirds of geriatric medicine program directors have been in that position for less than 8 years and 50% have less than six faculty members.

In 1988, the Accreditation Council for Graduate Medical Education (ACGME) began accrediting geriatric medicine fellowship training programs. Sixty-two Internal Medicine and 16 Family Medicine programs offered fellowship training at that time. 1988 was also the year that an examination became mandatory to attain the Certification of Added Qualification (CAQ) in Geriatrics after at least 2 years of fellowship training. To be eligible for CAQ, physicians must have completed US residency training and be board certified in either Internal or Family Medicine.

Until the mid-1990s, most fellows in geriatric medicine engaged in two or more years of training. Extended training was vital for the development of an academic and research career in geriatrics. 1994 was the last year that a CAQ was offered for those who had not completed fellowship training in geriatrics. In 1995, the training requirement for CAQ in geriatrics was reduced to 1 year. Although this may have temporarily achieved a goal of more of fellowship trained geriatricians, it has not resulted in a greater number of physicians adequately prepared to embark on a successful academic career.

Despite the growth in the elderly population and the ACGME mandate for geriatric training in internal and family medicine residency programs, geriatrics continues to be underrepresented in the graduate medical education (GME) curriculum. Two-thirds of internal medicine programs reported 24 hours or less of geriatric medicine didactic training over the 3-year training cycle. Half of family medicine residency programs devote 24 hours or less to geriatric medicine didactic training (Warshaw website). It is thus of little surprise that, when surveyed, graduates of these programs report being unprepared to tackle the challenges of the aging population. Whereas 68% of graduating internal medicine residents feel "very prepared" to manage critically ill patients, only 52% feel very prepared to manage the elderly patient. Thirteen percent feel very prepared to manage nursing home patients (Blumenthal *et al.*, 2001). Forty-eight percent of graduating family medicine residents feel very prepared to care for the elderly and 27% to care for nursing home residents.

Other GME programs such as anesthesiology, obstetrics/gynecology, emergency medicine, urology, and physical medicine/rehabilitation now require geriatric medicine training. Internal medicine, family medicine, and geriatric medicine programs frequently provide the training for these disciplines. The John A. Hartford Foundation, a significant granter of geriatric medicine programs, has specifically targeted surgical and medical specialties, as well as subspecialties of internal medicine, to improve the education of trainees in these disciplines.

Even though most medical schools have some form of structured geriatric program, the vast majority of undergraduate medical education curriculum integrates geriatrics into other coursework rather than requiring a separate geriatrics experience. Less than 8% of geriatric academic time is spent on teaching medical students. Didactic lectures on geriatrics occupy a mean of 14.4 hours in the medical school curriculum (Eleazer *et al.*, 2005). Students may not recognize these integrated experiences in geriatrics, however. Thirty-five percent of all graduating medical students indicated that geriatrics was inadequately taught across the 4 years of medical school, as reported by the Medical School Graduation Questionnaire in 2004 (Association of American Medical Colleges, 2004).

As the older population expands there is an ongoing need to train physicians, both generalists and specialists, in the principles of geriatric medicine. The emphasis on geriatrics must begin in undergraduate medical education if interest in primary care geriatric fellowship training is to increase.

GERIATRICIANS IN PRACTICE

The role of geriatricians, relative to general practitioners, is still evolving in the care of the older adult. Geriatricians receive a certificate of added qualification in geriatric medicine by the American Boards of Family Practice or Internal Medicine for a period of 10 years (Warshaw and Bragg, 2003; Warshaw *et al.*, 2002). There have been just over 10 000 physicians certified as geriatricians. Recertification rates have been disappointingly low with 43% of internists and 61% of family practitioners recertifying. The Certificate of Added Qualifications (now subspecialty) in Psychiatry became available in 1991. Nearly 2600 psychiatrists have certified and the recertification rate is 65%. On the basis of these figures, there are currently 6615 certified geriatricians in the United States or one geriatrician for every 2510 American citizens. It is estimated that 36 000 geriatricians will be needed by 2030 in the United States, a number far above what is likely to be achieved with current training program enrollment.

As might be expected, geriatricians practice predominantly in the outpatient setting. Two-thirds reported weekly involvement in outpatient primary care and long-term care. One-quarter to one-third were regularly involved in the inpatient management of geriatric patients. (Medina-Walpole *et al.*, 2002).

A survey of past geriatric fellows identified a major deficit in administrative training especially in long-term care medical directorship and Medicare/managed care. Graduates also felt a need for further training in psychiatry, neurology, rehabilitation, and hospice/palliative care. This may explain why less than one-third of practicing geriatricians report regular clinical activity in the areas of rehabilitation services and hospice/palliative care. The perceived training deficits are due, at least in part, to the time constraints of a 1-year fellowship training program. (Medina-Walpole *et al.*, 2004). After just 1 year of training, less than half of graduated fellows report practicing "essentially all" geriatrics. One-third of graduated fellows practice "primarily geriatrics" in addition to another discipline (e.g. general internal medicine) and one-quarter practice "secondarily geriatrics" (Medina-Walpole *et al.*, 2002).

Another explanation for geriatrician practice patterns is salary and compensation. The average assistant professor in geriatrics earns $118 000 and a full professor $174 000. These are similar to the amounts earned by general internists and pediatricians. Chiefs of geriatric divisions earn an average of $212 000. Geriatricians in private practice, however, earned a mean of $155 276 which is less than pediatricians and general internists. In comparison, gastroenterologists, a procedure-orientated speciality, earned $351 614. Thus, with significant school loans to repay and the disparity in earning potential with other specialties, it is not surprising that geriatrics has problems recruiting physicians in the United States. Despite these factors, geriatricians have reported themselves to be among the most satisfied of all specialists (Leigh *et al.*, 2002).

Geriatricians frequently focus on end-of-life care and may elect to become certified in hospice and palliative medicine. This certification requires either fellowship training in palliative medicine or significant clinical experience in the field. A certification examination is required. Physicians who work extensively in the nursing home setting can become certified medical directors through the AMDA. This certification requires completion of coursework and evidence of good standing as a medical director, but at this time requires no examination. Neither of these certification programs requires fellowship training in geriatrics or CAQ in geriatric medicine.

Nonphysician practitioners are increasingly involved in the care of older adults. Gerontological nurse practitioners (GNP) have a Masters degree in nursing, focused on the care of the elderly. These practitioners have become leaders in improving care in nursing homes. GNPs frequently work in partnership with a physician in the outpatient and nursing home setting. In most states, GNPs are provided some degree of independence in prescribing medications. Some states allow GNPs to practice independently or with limited supervision by a physician. Physician assistants (PA) also provide care for older persons but generally have less independence in clinical practice. The scope and duration of medical training for PAs is more limited than GNPs and closer supervision by a physician is generally required.

LEGAL ASPECTS OF GERIATRICS

In the United States, patients expect to be fully informed of their diagnoses. They also have the right to choose their treatment even if it does not appear to be the best choice to the physician. Patient autonomy frequently overrides the principle of societal justice. All patients are encouraged to have a living will and/or a durable power of attorney for health care. The ability of a physician to withhold treatment or withdraw life-sustaining technology requires the patient to have made clear statements regarding medical decisions while in full control of their mental faculties. Unfortunately, patient wishes and legal directives are often vague or unknown. If a patient has no legally stated wishes or guardianship and cannot make decisions for him- or herself, care can be directed by the next of kin. Most states consider the spouse, followed by adult children, and then parents as the hierarchy for next of kin. Surrogate decision making by the next of kin can be a frustrating and inflammatory situation when the opinions on care differ between family members, physicians, and customary ethical standards.

When unexpected or negative medical outcomes develop, there is a tendency to blame a person or a group for purposes of financial reconciliation. It is increasingly recognized, however, that medical errors result from a series of system-wide problems and require system-wide solutions. Nonetheless, legal suits have become a way of life in the United States. Malpractice insurance premiums have driven physicians out of certain states and out of practice, in some cases. Obstetrical, surgical, and nursing home providers are especially vulnerable to malpractice claims and rising insurance costs. Many nursing homes cannot afford malpractice premiums and simply operate without insurance coverage for the facility or the medical director. Many physicians simply chose not to practice in the nursing home or in regions where malpractice premiums and claims are prohibitive. The legal system has become a game where the plaintiff's lawyer takes cases on contingency and a substantial share of the judgment. In many cases, these lawyers pay physicians substantial amounts to be expert, but not necessarily honest, witnesses. Fear of large jury awards has resulted in the majority of cases being settled out of court for between $100 000 and $200 000, regardless of the merits of the case. This ultimately contributes to "defensive medicine" practices and escalation in the cost of medical care.

CONCLUSION

In the next 50 years, the population demographic in the United States will change substantially. Geriatric care now and in the immediate future represents an incredibly expensive, inefficient, and inequitable practice of health care. Older adults are the highest consumers of health-care resources and are increasingly dependent on state and federal governmental medical programs. Unfortunately, the current medical system rarely provides the comprehensive health-care services required to maintain function and independence in the aging and frail population. Inpatient medicine must evolve to ensure a safe and multidisciplinary approach to care of the older adult. Home and intermediate care settings require greater attention from physicians and leadership from geriatricians. Outpatient medicine must utilize comprehensive approaches to support the wellness of aging adults. While the United States has been a leader in geriatric research, there is insufficient emphasis placed on the training of future leaders in geriatric medicine. As the "baby boomers" age, there is a growing need to make all physicians and health-care settings better equipped to care for the elderly population.

KEY POINTS

- Geriatricians in the United States have provided leadership in conducting controlled trials on systems of geriatric care.
- Geriatric care in the United States is extremely fragmented.
- The Veterans Administration has been the leader in geriatrics research and education.
- There is a shortage of trained geriatricians in the United States.

KEY REFERENCES

- Morley JE. A brief history of geriatrics. *The Journals of Gerontology. Series A, Biological Sciences and Medical Sciences* 2004; **59A**:1132–52.
- Warshaw GA & Bragg EJ. The training of geriatricians in the United States: three decades of progress. *The Journal of the American Geriatrics Society* 2003; **51**(7 suppl):S338–45.
- Warshaw GA, Bragg EJ, Shaull RW & Lindsell CJ. Academic geriatric programs in US allopathic and osteopathic medical schools. *The Journal of the American Medical Association* 2002; **288**:2313–19.

REFERENCES

AGS Health Care Systems Committee. Assisted living facilities: American geriatrics society position paper. *The Journal of the American Geriatrics Society* 2005; **53**:536–7.

American Hospital Association. *Hospital Statistics* 2004, pp 154–61; Health Forum LLC, Chicago.

Association of American Medical Colleges. *Medical School Graduation Questionnaire* 2004; Washington, DC, Accessed June 15, 2005, http://www.aamc.org/data/gq/allschoolsreports/2004.pdf.

Banks WA & Morley JE. Memories are made of this: recent advances in understanding cognitive impairments and dementia. *The Journals of Gerontology. Series A, Biological Sciences and Medical Sciences* 2003; **58**:314–21.

Beers MH, Ouslander JG & Fingold SF. Inappropriate medication prescribing in skilled-nursing facilities. *Annals of Internal Medicine* 1992; **117**:684–9.

Blumenthal D, Gokhale M, Campbell EG & Weissman JS. Preparedness for clinical practice. Reports of graduating residents at academic health centers. *The Journal of the American Medical Association* 2001; **286**:1027–34.

Bragg EJ & Warshaw GA. ACGME requirements of geriatrics medicine curricula in medical specialties: progress made and progress needed. *Academic Medicine* 2005; **80**:279–85.

Cohen HJ, Feussner JR, Weinberger M *et al.* A controlled trial of inpatient and outpatient geriatric evaluation and management. *The New England Journal of Medicine* 2002; **346**:905–12.

Eleazer GP, Doshi R & Wieland D. Geriatric content in medical school curricula: results of a national survey. *The Journal of the American Geriatrics Society* 2005; **53**:136–40.

Fabacher D, Josephson K & Pietruszka F. An in-home preventive assessment program for independent older adults: a randomized controlled trial. *The Journal of the American Geriatrics Society* 1994; **42**:630–8.

Fick Dm, Cooper JW & Wade WE Updating the Beers criteria for potentially inappropriate medication use in older adults: results of a US consensus panel of experts. *Archives of Internal Medicine* 2003; **163**:2716–2724.

Flaherty JH, Tariq SH, Raghaven S *et al.* A model for managing delirious older inpatients. *The Journal of the American Geriatrics Society* 2003; **51**:1031–5.

Folstein MF, Folstein SE, McHugh PR *et al.* Mini-mental state. A practical method for grading the cognitive state of patients for the clinician. *Journal of Psychiatric Research* 1975; **12**:189–98.

Goldberg RT, Bernad M, Granger CV *et al.* Vocational status: prediction by the Barthel index and PULSES profile. *Archives of Physical Medicine and Rehabilitation* 1980; **61**:580–3.

Gross DL, Temkin-Greener H, Kunitz S & Mukamel DB. The growing pains of integrated health care for the elderly: lessons from the expansion of PACE. *Milbank Quarterly* 2004; **82**:257–82.

Inouye SK, Bogardus ST Jr, Charpentier PA *et al.* A multicomponent intervention to prevent delirium in hospitalized older patients. *The New England Journal of Medicine* 1999; **340**:669–76.

Katz S, Downs TD, Cash HR & Grotz RC. Progress in development of the index of ADL. *Gerontologist* 1970; **10**:20–30.

Katz S, Ford AB, Moskowitz RW *et al.* Studies of illness in the aged: the index of ADL: a standardized measure of biological and psychosocial function. *The Journal of the American Medical Association* 1963; **185**:914–9.

Landefeld CS, Palmer RM & Kresevic DM. A randomized trial of care in a hospital medical unit especially designed to improve the functional outcomes of acutely ill older patients. *The New England Journal of Medicine* 1995; **332**:1338–44.

Lawton MP & Brody EM. Assessment of older people self maintaining and instrumental activities of daily living. *Gerontologist* 1969; **9**:179–86.

Leff B & Burton JR. The future history of home care and physician house calls in the United States. *The Journals of Gerontology. Series A, Biological Sciences and Medical Sciences* 2001; **56A**(10):M606–8.

Leigh JP, Kravitz RL, Schembri M *et al.* Physician career satisfaction across specialties. *Archives of Internal Medicine* 2002; **162**:1577–84.

Mahoney FI & Barthel DW. Functional evaluation: the Barthel index. *Maryland State Medical Journal* 1965; **14**:61–5.

Makowski TR, Maggard W & Morley JE. The life care center of St. Louis experience with subacute care. *Clinics in Geriatric Medicine* 2000; **16**:701–24.

Marshall CL. Understanding the incomprehensible: a guide to the new Medicare prescription drug benefit for case managers. *Lippincott's Case Management: Managing the Process of Patient Care* 2004; **9**:216–22.

Medina-Walpole A, Barker WH & Katz PR. The current state of geriatrics: a national survey of fellow-trained Geriatricians 1990–1998. *The Journal of the American Geriatrics Society* 2002; **50**:949–55.

Medina-Walpole A, Barker WH & Katz PR. Strengthening the fellowship training experience: findings from a national survey of fellowship trained geriatricians 1990–1998. *The Journal of the American Geriatrics Society* 2004; **52**:607–10.

Miller SK. Acute care of the elderly units: a positive outcomes case study. *Clinical Issues* 2002; **13**:34–42.

Miller DK, Coe RM, Romeis JC & Morley JE. Improving quality of geriatric health care in four delivery sites: suggestions from practitioners and experts. *The Journal of the American Geriatrics Society* 1995; **43**:60–5.

Morley JE. A brief history of geriatrics. *The Journals of Gerontology. Series A, Biological Sciences and Medical Sciences* 2004; **59A**:1132–52.

Morley JE, Charlton E, Patrick P *et al.* Validation of a screening questionnaire for androgen deficiency in aging males. *Metabolism: Clinical and Experimental* 2000; **49**:1239–42.

Morley JE & Miller DK. Total quality assurance: an important step in improving care for older individuals. *The Journal of the American Geriatrics Society* 1992; **40**:974–5.

National Residency Matching Program. *Positions Offered and Percent Filled by U.S. Seniors and All Applicants 2000–2004*; Updated 5/7/2004, http://www.nrmp.org/res_match/tables/table6_04.pdf. Accessed June 15, 2005.

National Vital Statistics Report 2005; **53**(17):9.

Palmer RM, Landefeld CS, Kresevic D & Kowal J. A medical unit for the acute care of the elderly. *The Journal of the American Geriatrics Society* 1994; **42**:545–52.

Rubenstein LZ, Josephson KR & Wieland GD. Effectiveness of a geriatric evaluation unit. A randomized clinical trial. *The New England Journal of Medicine* 1984; **311**:1664–70.

Schnelle JF, Ouslander JG, Osterweil D & Blumenthal S. Total quality management: administrative and clinical applications in nursing homes. *The Journal of the American Geriatrics Society* 1993; **41**:1259–66.

Steel K. Physician-directed long-term home health care for the elderly-a century-long experience. *The Journal of the American Geriatrics Society* 1987; **35**(3):264–8.

Stuck AE, Aronow HU, Steiner A *et al.* A trial of annual in-home comprehensive geriatric assessments for elderly people living in the community. *The New England Journal of Medicine* 1995; **333**:1184–9.

Stuck AE, Egger M & Hammer A. Home visits to prevent nursing home admission and functional decline in elderly people: systematic review and meta-regression analysis. *The Journal of the American Medical Association* 2002; **287**:1022–8.

Stuck AE, Siu AL & Wieland GD. Comprehensive geriatric assessment: a meta-analysis of controlled trials. *Lancet* 1993; **342**:1032–6.

Tinetti ME. Performance-oriented assessment of mobility problems in elderly patients. *The Journal of the American Geriatrics Society* 1986; **34**:119–26.

Warshaw GA & Bragg EJ. The training of geriatricians in the United States: three decades of progress. *The Journal of the American Geriatrics Society* 2003; **51**(7 Suppl):S338–45.

Warshaw GA, Bragg EJ, Shaull RW & Lindsell CJ. Academic geriatric programs in US allopathic and osteopathic medical schools. *The Journal of the American Medical Association* 2002; **288**:2313–19.

Wilson MMG, Thomas DR, Rubenstein LZ *et al.* Appetite assessment: simplified nutritional appetite questionnaire predicts weight loss in community dwelling adults and nursing home residents. *The American Journal of Clinical Nutrition* 2005; **78**:(In Press).

Xakellis GC. Who provides care to Medicare beneficiaries and what settings do they use? *The Journal of the American Board of Family Practice* 2004; **17**:384–7.

Yesavage JA, Brink TL, Rose TL *et al.* Development and validation of a geriatric depression screening scale: a preliminary report. *Journal of Psychiatric Research* 1982–1983; **17**:37–49.

FURTHER READING

The Institute for Health Policy and Health Services Research (IHPHSR) Association of Directors of Geriatric Programs (ADGAP) Database Project. American medical association and association of American medical colleges data from the national survey of graduate medical education programs. *Journal of the American Medical Association* 1992–2003.

Warshaw GA & Bragg EJ. *Longitudinal Study of Training and Practice of Geriatric Medicine IHPHSR ADGAP Database Project*. Figure 4.6: Survey of Program Directors of Family Medicine Residency Programs (Winter 2001) and Figure 4.2: Survey of Program Directors of General Internal Medicine Residency Programs (Winter 2002). Accessed June 15, 2005; http://www.adgapstudy.uc.edu/Reports/index.cfm.

163

Geriatrics and Gerontology in Japan

Yuko Suda[1] *and* **Ryutaro Takahashi**[2]

[1] *Toyo University, Tokyo, Japan, and* [2] *Tokyo Metropolitan Institute of Gerontology, Tokyo, Japan*

INTRODUCTION

The purpose of this chapter is to outline the trends of geriatrics and gerontology in Japan. The manuscripts on geriatric medicine and geriatric nursing were written by the coauthor, Takahashi, on the basis of reviewing the literature as well as conducting interviews with leading researchers in the areas. Following the same procedure, the manuscripts on geriatric psychiatry, epidemiological studies on aging, social gerontology, and psychological studies on aging were written by the author, Suda. These manuscripts were written first in Japanese and sent to the informants for proofreading, and eventually translated into English by the author.

GERIATRIC MEDICINE

Senior Citizens and Medicine

The longevity of Japanese men is 78.4 years. It is longer than that of those in other countries, with the exception of men in Ireland and Hong Kong who also have about the same longevities. The longevity of Japanese women is 85.3 years, which is the longest in the world. When viewed from a different perspective, more than half of Japanese men and three-quarters of Japanese women live for more than 80 years (The Ministry of Health, Labor and Welfare, 2004a).

Japan saw an increase of the older population within a very short time. The rate of increase of the population who were 65 years old and over was 7% in 1970. Within only 24 years, in 1994, the rate reached 14%. By comparison, France took 115 years, Sweden 85 years, England 47 years, and Germany 40 years to witness the same increase. Japan recently surpassed Italy and Sweden in terms of the rate of increase of the old population, and the rate is expected to reach 20% soon. The present high percentage of the old population is attributed to a progressively decreasing infant mortality rate and increasingly better health conditions among seniors (The Ministry of Health, Labor and Welfare, 2004a).

What is unique to Japan is that the longevity is significantly different between men and women. The difference is now about 7 years, and has been increasing over the past 20 years. This increasing difference of longevity between sex stems from the continuing decrease in longevities among men of younger age-groups since 1998. Especially, the increase in suicide deaths among men between the ages of 55 and 59 and above wields a serious impact on the overall longevity.

The primary causes of death among Japanese people are carcinoma, cardiovascular diseases, cerebral vascular diseases, pneumonia, accidents, and suicide. The differences by sex in the causes of death becomes distinct at the age of 80. The primary causes of death among men who are 80 years old and above are carcinoma (22.1%), pneumonia (17.3%), cardiovascular diseases (16.1%), and cerebral vascular diseases (14.2%). The primary causes of death among women who are 80 years old and above are cardiovascular diseases (20.7%), cerebral vascular diseases (17.0%), carcinoma (14.6%), and pneumonia (13.9%) (Cabinet Office, 2004).

Compared to other countries, the in-hospital days in Japan have been relatively long over the past few decades. However, the length of these days is becoming shorter in recent years (Table 1) as a result of the new reimbursement system introduced by the Ministry of Health, Labor and Welfare (MHLW).

The purpose of the new system is to control medical expenditures. Medical services in Japan are provided through the national public health insurance system. Formerly, the cost of care was reimbursed to hospitals or clinics on the basis of the treatment actually provided to patients. On the other hand, under the new system called the *Diagnosis Procedure Combination* (DPC) System, the payment from the national health insurance system is predetermined for each diagnosis and expected treatment for it. In addition, the reimbursement rate for acute care considerably drops when the in-hospital days of the patient exceed a certain period. In intermediate care, where patients do not need acute

Principles and Practice of Geriatric Medicine, 4th Edition. Edited by M.S. John Pathy, Alan J. Sinclair and John E. Morley.

Table 1 In-hospital days in recent years

Year	2003	2002	2001	2000	1999
In-hospital days	20.3	22.2	23.5	24.8	27.2

Source: Ministry of Health, Labor and Welfare (2004b).

care but are in need of certain medical interventions, the reimbursement rate for medical activities is set low, whereas better rates are given to rehabilitation and personal care.

The new system first had an impact on the 82 hospitals that were designated as hospitals to provide advanced acute care, such as university hospitals. In order for the hospitals to maintain the high-tech equipment and human resources necessary to provide advanced acute care, they had to control the in-hospital days in a cost-effective manner. Because providing intermediate care in these 82 hospitals reduced their cost-effectiveness, the task was delegated to other hospitals. The hospitals specialized for intermediate care then attempted to maintain the provision of medical services at a minimum, because medical activities did not bring in enough reimbursement. As a result, fewer and fewer hospitals are accepting senior patients who need both medical interventions and personal care, such as those suffering from chronic heart failure or chronic obstructive pulmonary diseases.

Despite these problems, MHLW seems to be determined to control the medical expenditures further. One of the new approaches under consideration is to establish a separate insurance system for seniors. But such a system is expected to increase the financial burden on seniors, and fierce controversies are aroused.

Origins and Primary Institutions of Geriatric Medicine

The origin of geriatric medicine in Japan dates back to the history of Yoikuin. In 1872, the heir prince of Russia was scheduled to visit Tokyo. It was an imminent task to sweep away the mentally or physically challenged and the homeless who were living on the streets. As a solution, Yoikuin, a private nonprofit organization, was established to institutionalize these people. As years went by, the function of Yoikuin gradually changed to a permanent shelter for the poor. Because poverty was primarily the problem of seniors in those days, the majority of the residents were seniors, and Yoikuin naturally built skills to care for them. Physicians were invited from the University of Tokyo, who provided medical care to the residents in exchange for using the facility of Yoikuin as a field for teaching students. The building of Yoikuin was burned down in the Tokyo Great Air Aid by the Allied Forces during the Second World War, and the new Yoikuin Nursing Homes were built in 1958.

In 1972, the Tokyo Metropolitan Geriatric Hospital, the first geriatric hospital in Asia, was built on the same campus as Yoikuin. The academic activities of the geriatric hospital were focused on clinicopathological studies. The number of autopsies conducted were over 8000. The efforts were especially focused on clarifying the mechanisms of the diseases which were common to the Japanese such as cerebral vascular diseases and cardiovascular diseases (Kameyama, 1979; Ohkawa *et al.*, 1986; Sugiura *et al.*, 1982).

Another important institution, Yokufukai, was established in 1925. The Kanto Great Earthquake had occurred 2 years before. The purpose of Yokufukai was to accommodate the victims from the disaster who were old and had no relatives or those who were mentally or physically challenged.

Fujiro Amako came to Yokufukai as the chief doctor in 1926. Amako established a system to organize and store detailed records on episodes and laboratory reports on the 500 residents in Yokufukai. The data were compared with autopsy data that were collected after the resident's demise. The outcomes from the comparisons were shared in the Clinicopathological Conference that was sponsored by Yokufukai. Years later, leading researchers in neuro-internal medicine, circulatory medicine, and other areas appeared in great numbers through these activities led by Yokufukai.

The project led by Toshio Ozawa deserves attention as well. In the mid-1980s, Ozawa evaluated the physical functional capacity of seniors living in a small town where the rate of increase of the old population was extremely high. The functional capacity examined included activities of daily living (ADL), cognitive functions, social interactions, and so forth. In those days, focusing on functional capacity rather than on diseases was innovative. The awareness of the importance of a comprehensive geriatric assessment was dramatically raised after this project. In 1993, Ozawa was appointed as the president of the Tokyo Metropolitan Geriatric Hospital (1983) where he established the Geriatric Evaluation and Management Unit, the first institution in Japan solely focusing on geriatric assessment (Ozawa, 1998).

In recent years, as a result of the combination of a staggering economy and policy changes of the Tokyo Metropolitan Government, Yoikuin Nursing Homes and the Tokyo Metropolitan Geriatric Hospital were dissolved. The function of the The Tokyo Metropolitan Institute of Gerontology (TMIG) was extremely constricted as well. In the meantime, the National Institute for Longevity Science was established in 1995. The institute was merged with a hospital in 2004 and its name was changed to the National Center for Geriatrics and Gerontology.

Academic Activities and Education

The first academic journal on geriatric medicine was the "Yokufukai Geriatric Journal" or "Acta Gerontologica Japonica" under another name, which was first issued in 1928. The "Nippon Ronen Igakkai Zasshi", the journal of the Japan Geriatric Society, was first issued in 1964, and 30–70 original papers have been published every year since then.

The first annual meeting of the Japan Gerontological Society was held in Tokyo in 1956. In 1959, the Society changed its function to an umbrella organization to unite two suborganizations: the Japan Geriatrics Society and the

Japan Socio-Gerontological Society. Recently, new academic associations joined the Japan Gerontological Society: the Japan Society for Biomedical Gerontology established in 1981, the Japanese Psychogeriatric Society organized in 1986, the Japan Society of Gerodontology joined in 1991, and the Japan Society of Care Management in 2003.

Examples of the distinguished outcomes obtained in this area are as follows:

- Tauchi and Sato (1968) clarified the changes by age in size and number of mitochondria of human hepatic cells.
- Uchida and Tomonaga (1989) found that the brain extract from Alzheimer's disease (AD) brains did not efficiently inhibit the abnormal sprouting responses. Uchida and colleagues also isolated a unique metallothionein-like protein that controlled the process. The metallothionein-like protein was named as *Growth Inhibitory Factor* (GIF). The study suggested that deficient GIF may induce abnormal sprouting responses in AD brains, which entailed the neuronal death accompanied by the accumulation of senile plaques, neurofibrillary tangles, and curly fibers.
- Yokode *et al.* (1995) clarified that cigarette smoke extract directly influenced cholesterol metabolism, which promoted the development of atherosclerosis.
- Seniors whose swallowing reflex and coughing reflex are weakened tend to suffer from deglutition pneumonia because they swallow viruses in the mouth with saliva while they are sleeping. Yoneyama and colleagues (2002) indicated that mouth hygiene was effective in preventing such infection.
- The Ethic Committee on Geriatric Medicine in Japan (2001) suggested possible roles geriatricians could undertake in terminal care.
- Yamauchi *et al.* (2003) discovered that calcitonin is effective in the treatment of osteoporosis.
- Hirai *et al.* (1980) and Kobayashi *et al.* (1981) identified that eicosapentenoic acid (EPA) influenced blood viscosity and platelets. EPA is contained in fish and the Japanese eat fish more frequently than people in many other countries. The study suggested the possible relation between food intake and the low prevalence rate of cardiovascular diseases in Japan.

The system to train geriatric practitioners was not established for many years. In 1912, Tatsukichi Irisawa, then professor of internal medicine of the University of Tokyo, wrote in his textbook that "geriatric medicine would be the indispensable part of medicine in near future" (The Japan Geriatrics Society, 2003). However, it was not until the beginning of the 1950s that geriatric medicine was finally included in the curriculum for the first time in Japan at the Medical School of the University of Tokyo. In 1962, the first division of geriatric medicine was initiated in the University of Tokyo, and the second was established in the University of Kyoto in 1968. As of 2004, 24 medical schools have a division of geriatric medicine, which is about 30% of the total number of medical schools in Japan.

One of the challenges faced by geriatric medicine is stemming from the conventional system of medical schools and their related institutions. Each medical school comprises divisions that are focused on their own specialities, and there are little interactions among them. Likewise, the Japan Geriatric Society is considered as a branch of the Japanese Society of Internal Medicine and is isolated from other associations such as the Medical Association on Respiratory System and the Medical Association on Digestive System. This condition is in contrast with the way geriatric medicine operates in other countries, where the importance of the holistic understanding of patients and collaborative relationships with experts in different areas seems to be more emphasized. As an attempt to claim for recognition as a unique and independent profession, the Japan Geriatric Society introduced the certified geriatric-physician system in 1988. However, there are no good job opportunities for the certified geriatric specialists even to this date.

In 2000, the Blue-Ribbon Committee on Aging, which was summoned by the Japan Science Council, expressed their concern on the poorly organized condition of geriatric medicine while the number of old patients was rapidly increasing. Even though they strongly recommended the improvement of the system for education, care-providing, and research on geriatric medicine, little progress was made.

Recent changes in the society brought about more difficulties. For example, the legal status of national universities changed from governmental to private-public organizations in 2004. Because the subsidies from the government are decreasing, attracting enough students and funds is an urgent task. As part of the effort, national medical schools are concentrating on distinguishing themselves in cutting-edge studies. Private medical schools are facing a different challenge. The private medical schools have accepted a far larger number of students compared to national medical schools so that they could provide medical training with reasonable tuition. However, the central government has been changing its policy recently to control the number of physicians. In response, the private medical schools are providing highly advanced training to their students so that their graduates of many numbers will still survive in the competitive job market. In the turmoil, both national and private medical schools are turning away from the areas where prominent achievement is hard to make in a short time, such as education for and practice of geriatric medicine.

GERIATRIC PSYCHIATRY

Geriatric psychiatry has been playing a leading role in the studies on dementia. The effort to clarify the prevalence rate of dementia started in the 1970s. Kazuo Hasegawa conducted a survey of a large sample in 1972 and 1973, and identified that the prevalence rate of memory problems among seniors living in a community was 4.5%. In the 1980s, many prefectures conducted similar surveys as Hasegawa did, and the conditions of seniors with memory problems were clarified nationwide in the beginning of the 1990s.

Table 2 Scales commonly used in Japan for screening of memory problems

Name of the scale	Sensitivity/specificity	Subjects used to develop the scale	Author
The Japanese version of MMSE	82.8%/93.3%	90 subjects without memory problems and 61 subjects with memory problems	Mori *et al.* (1985)
HDS-R	90%/82%	62 subjects without memory problems and 95 subjects with memory problems	Kato *et al.* (1991)

Source: Homma (2004).

Scales to screen those suffering from memory problems have been developed as well. In 1973, Hasegawa developed the Hasegawa Dementia Scale (HDS). It was truly innovative, considering that it was developed 1 year before the Mini-Mental Scale Examination (MMSE) was developed. These days, the Hasegawa Dementia Scale-Revised (HDS-R) (Kato *et al.*, 1991) is most commonly used. HDS-R is shorter than HDS and its usability has been improved. The largest advantage of HDS-R is that the questionnaire naturally fits in the context of Japanese culture, as it was developed in Japan. Its sensitivity and specificity in comparison with the Japanese version of MMSE is shown in Table 2.

A recent topic in relation to dementia is that the prevalence rate of Alzheimer's-type dementia is becoming higher than the prevalence rate of vascular dementia, whereas the latter was more commonly observed than the former until the early 1990s in Japan. As an attempt to delay the onset of Alzheimer's-type dementia, behavioral intervention programs are being developed. In order to detect memory problems at the early stage, educational programs for physicians to improve their skills are developed as well (Homma, 1998, 2004). For treatment, Akira Homma, with the TMIG, served as an organizer of clinical trials of donepezil (Aricept) and used it in a clinical setting for the first time in Japan.

Another important topic of geriatric psychiatry is depression. In Japan, seniors have the highest incident rate of suicide (Figure 1), and depression is considered to be one of the reasons. Efforts have been made to develop standardized scales to identify seniors suffering from depression, such as the Japanese version of the Geriatric Depression Scale (GDS) and the Japanese version of the Center for Epidemiological Studies Depression Scale (CED-D). However, depression among seniors still tends to be overlooked to this date.

Primary academic associations related to geriatric psychiatry are the Japanese Psychogeriatric Society and the Japan Dementia Care Society, both of which publish their own journals.

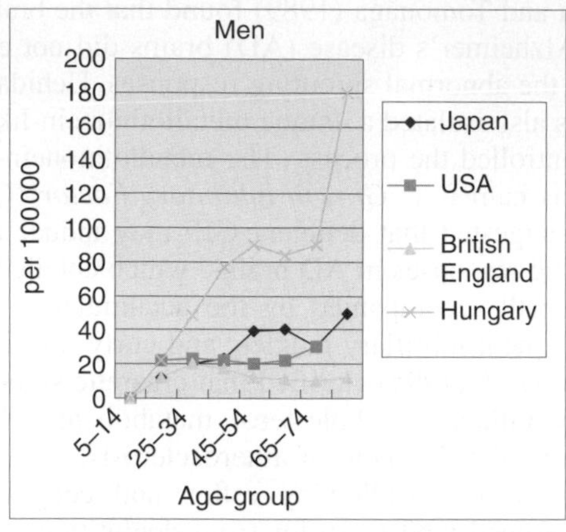

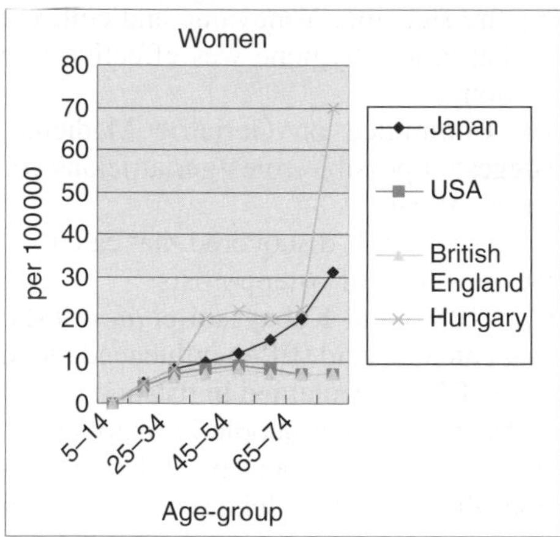

Figure 1 Comparison by country on suicide rate by age-group. *Source*: World Health Organization (1995)

EPIDEMIOLOGICAL STUDIES ON AGING

Background

The TMIG, which was established in 1972, undertook a crucial role in epidemiological studies on aging. TMIG was located on the same campus as Yoikuin Nursing Homes and the Tokyo Metropolitan Geriatric Hospital, and researchers from a wide range of areas, such as biology, medicine, epidemiology, psychology, psychiatry, sociology, nursing, and architecture, were engaged in studies on aging. In addition, the offices of primary academic associations related to aging were scated in TMIG, such as the Japan Geriatric Society, the Japanese Association of Geriatric Psychiatry, and the Japan Socio-Gerontological Society. Such an environment enabled TMIG to function literally as the center of aging studies in Japan.

Hiroshi Shibata, who led the Department of Epidemiology at TMIG from the 1970s to 1990s, recognized the importance of an interdisciplinary approach in aging studies from the beginning. He organized longitudinal projects of large samples, while involving different departments in TMIG such as the Department of Psychiatry, Sociology, and Psychology. Among the projects, the Koganei Study, which was conducted from 1976 to 1991, is especially well-known. The subjects were 500 seniors living in the Koganei City, located in the west part of Tokyo, and were followed every 5 years to examine their medical, behavioral, social, and psychological changes.

In 1997, the National Institute for Longevity Science initiated a comprehensive longitudinal study on aging. The subjects were 2300 people of ages 40–79 years, and their MRI-and CT-data were collected in addition to the data obtained through questionnaire surveys. The sample size and the comprehensiveness of the data collected were compatible to the Baltimore Longitudinal Study of Aging organized by the National Institute of Aging (NIA) in the United States (Shimokata *et al.*, 2000).

Related academic associations in the epidemiological studies on aging are the Japan Public Health Association and the Japan Socio-Gerontological Society.

Academic Studies

As the longevity is prolonged, functional capacity emerged as an important issue that influences the quality of life in the prolonged old age.

The first survey on functional capacity of the elderly with representative sample was conducted by the Tokyo Metropolitan Government in 1980. The survey reported that less than 5%, with the exception of dressing (5.5%), suffered from disability in each category of ADL such as locomotion, eating, dressing, bathing, and going to the toilet. On assessing hearing, vision, and communication ability, 79.6% of residents over 65 years and over were regarded as competent in daily living. The Tokyo Metropolitan Government is repeating the same study every five years since then. It has been reported that the age-adjusted ratio of disabilities is being improved (Shibata *et al.*, 2001) (Figure 2).

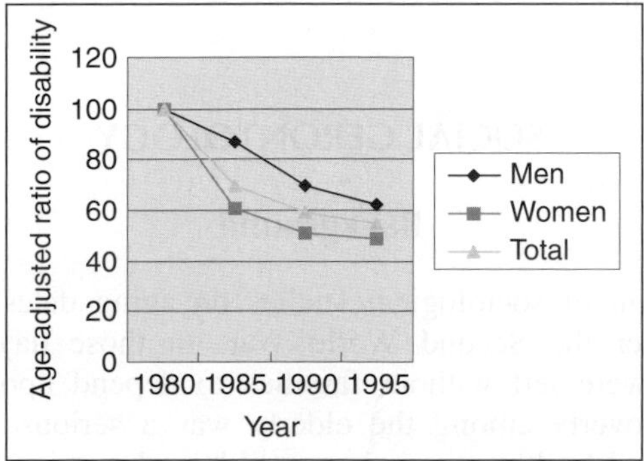

Figure 2 Age-adjusted ratios of disability in people >65 years old in Tokyo (Reproduced from Shibata H *et al.*, Functional capacity in elderly Japanese living in the community, *Geriatrics and Gerontology International*, 2001, **1**:8–13, with permission from Blackwell Publishing Ltd.)

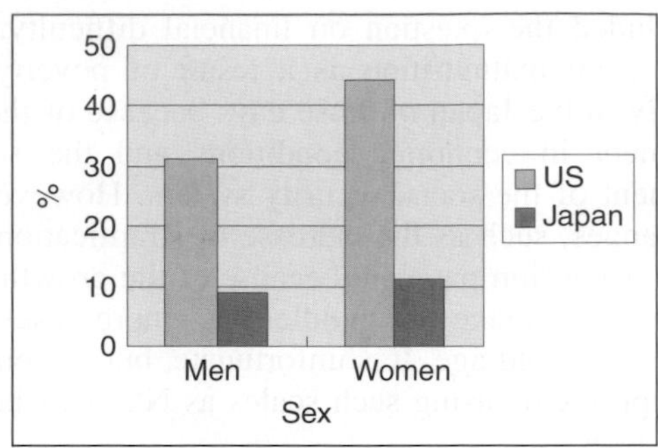

Figure 3 Prevalence rates of impaired functional capacity between the United States and Japan. Note: The data of the US sample were derived from America's Changing Lives Survey. The subjects in the Japanese counterpart were selected nationwide on the basis of a stratified two-stage random sample. In the case of incompetence in any one of three items of functional capacity (bathing, climbing stairs, and walking), they were regarded as disabled (Reproduced from Shibata H *et al.*, Functional capacity in elderly Japanese living in the community, *Geriatrics and Gerontology International*, 2001, **1**:8–13, with permission from Blackwell Publishing Ltd.)

In a cross-cultural study between the United States and Japan on functional capacity of those who were 60 years old and over, the Japanese were more likely to be competent than American seniors (Figure 3). Shibata *et al.* (2001) suggested that "this difference in the prevalence may result from a cross-cultural difference in responding to this type of interview. Otherwise, there may be some contributing factors to prevention of disability in Japan".

Factors related to functional capacity have also been examined. In the Koganei Study, the variables that predicted the functional capacity years later were: "history of hypertension" and "electrocardiogram (ECG) abnormalities" for men, "anxiety about present health status" and "being overweight" for women, and "low social activities at baseline" for both men and women.

In another study which was started by TMIG in 1991 as the Tokyo Metropolitan Institute of Gerontology-Longitudinal Interdisciplinary Study on Aging (TMIG-LISA), both ADL and instrumental activities of daily living (IADL) were related to the following variables examined 3 years before: "age (75 or older)", "less hand-grip strength", and "history of hospitalization in previous 1 year". The predictor for ADL alone was "lack of exercise". The predictors for IADL alone were "poor intellectual activities" and "poor social roles" (Shibata, 2000).

Psychological health is another issue that is closely related to the quality of life in old age. In the 1980s, the Japanese version of the Life Satisfaction Index (LSI) and the Philadelphia Geriatric Center (PGC) Morale Scale were developed. Recent studies report that the factor compositions of these scales are different between the United States and Japan (Ishihara *et al.*, 1999; Wada, 1979).

A number of studies on nutrition have also been conducted, focusing on the pattern of food intake. Developing the Japanese version of the Nutritional Screening Initiative (NSI) was once discussed in the 1980s. The problem was that the scale included the question on financial difficulty. Seniors suffering from malnutrition as a result of poverty existed only rarely in the Japan of those days because of the overall improvement in economic conditions and the successful management of the social security system. However, recent social changes, such as the increase of stratification and the decrease of pension payment because of the growth of older population, will make the middle class more susceptible to poverty in their old age. It is unfortunate, but screening malnutrition problems using such scales as NSI will be needed soon in Japan.

GERIATRIC NURSING

Background

In 1972, the Department of Geriatric Nursing was initiated in the TMIG. It was the first academic entity specialized for geriatric nursing in Japan. Because there were little professional publications on geriatric nursing in those days, the department started from organizing information in related areas through mass media such as newspapers. In practice, the department served as a pioneer in establishing the method of visiting nurse activities. The department also engaged in the development of assistive devices for frail seniors.

In 1989, the Branch of Geriatric Nursing was formed in the Japan Society of Nursing. Separate from this organization, the Japan Academy of Gerontological Nursing (JAGN) was established in 1996. The Branch of Geriatric Nursing is more attended by nurses engaged in practice in nursing homes and hospitals, and their discussions are focused on daily practice in the field. JAGN is more attended by those who work with universities or other academic institutions, and a wide range of academic interests are covered such as the development of nursing techniques for patients with geriatric diseases including dementia, developing methods for care in group home settings, improvement of community care systems, elder abuse, health promotion, and so forth.

In the 1990s, geriatric nursing was introduced in the educational system of nursing schools, as well as schools for midwives and public health nurses. Responding to these changes, universities for nurses followed the trend by introducing geriatric nursing in their curricula.

Recently, the Japan Society of Nursing introduced the system of the Certified Nurse Specialist (CNS). While the CNS in the United States stands for the Clinical Nurse Specialist, the CNS in Japan are those who have advanced skills in practice, consultation, and academic studies, and are specialized in certain areas such as geriatric nursing, oncological nursing, and psychiatric nursing. The idea of CNS was developed as a by-product of the discussion held in the 1970s, in which the possibility of introducing a similar system as the Nurse Practitioner (NP) in the United States was explored. The reason for abandoning the introduction of the NP system was based on the concern that the NP might be used as a cheap substitute for doctors. Thus, the CNS was created to emphasize the independence of nursing as a profession. The training to be a CNS is provided through 10 graduate schools of nursing. As of April 2004, there are 74 CNSs in Japan, among whom, five are specialized for geriatric nursing. The CNS in geriatric nursing are expected to serve as leaders in establishing care techniques in intermediary institutions for seniors as well as in visiting nurse programs.

Academic Studies

A wide range of topics are discussed in the area of geriatric nursing such as the role of visiting nurses in terminal care, team approach with other professionals in community care, the role of nurses in supporting victims of natural disasters, reminiscence, strategies in coping with senior patients who are not collaborative, and the effect of massage in the care for seniors.

In the past 10 years, the so-called geriatric syndrome, disability or decrease of functional capacity which are commonly observed among senior patients, has been an important issue. In dealing with the problems, care techniques have been developed for decubitus, other skin problems, eating or deglutition problems, and so on. Assessment tools to identify those who have high risk of falling, as well as the strategies to prevent falling, have also been developed.

Eminent progress is seen in the understanding of seniors with dementia. More understanding is being obtained on the meaning and rules for the way in which dementia patients wander and stop. Other behaviors such as touching, fingering, picking up, peering, and banging are also being paid attention to as possible avenues of communication with seniors having dementia. In addition, the effect of environment on memory control is identified through the studies on metamemory.

Effort has been made in developing scales and assessment tools such as the Japanese versions of the General Health Questionnaire (GHQ), the Oral Health Impact Profile (OHIP), and the Health-related Quality of life (SF-36). Other assessment tools include the ones to examine the quality of care in a short-stay setting, health-care needs of seniors with dementia living in community, and the seriousness of dried skin.

SOCIAL GERONTOLOGY

Background

The origin of sociological studies on aging dates back to soon after the Second World War. In those days, many seniors were left without families to depend upon. Especially, poverty among the elderly was a serious problem. Young and healthy men who could have become breadwinners in households had died during the war. Those who survived were occupied with supporting themselves and their children. Sociologists started to become interested in seniors through these problems, which provided leverage to the establishment of the Japan Gerontological Society in 1956. The public gradually started to pay attention to the predicament experienced by seniors as well, and social gerontology received attention from a wide range of people as an emerging area to respond to the issue.

Sociological studies on seniors in the late 1950s and in the beginning of 1960s were closely related to policies. Before 1963, when the Law of Social Welfare for the Elderly, a law similar to the Old Americans Act (OAA) in the United States, was installed, discussions were focused on what kinds of public services should be provided for the seniors in need. Once the services started to be provided through the law, the focus of studies turned to examining how the services were used, as well as identifying still-unmet needs and advocating for improvement (Maeda, 1975).

In the 1970s, as the Japanese economy expanded, needs among seniors changed from the "needs stemming from poverty" such as the needs for financial aid, food, and housing, to the "needs unrelated to poverty" such as the needs for in-home help services and opportunities for social activities (The Committee for Social Problems Related to Aging, 1974). Fumio Miura, with the National Institute on Social Policy at the time, served as a strong advocate for policy change in order to respond to the "new" needs among seniors. He especially undertook a crucial role in turning the focus of policy makers from institutional care to community care.

Social scientific approach to aging started in the late 1970s. Daisaku Maeda, the then Chief of the Department of Sociology at the TMIG, made an incomparable contribution to the process. Maeda launched an array of pioneering projects as well as introducing sophisticated research skills developed in other related areas. Maeda also established collaborative relationships with researchers and institutions in other countries on the basis of his many years of international experience.

After the TMIG's withdrawal from the leading role in the 1990s, social gerontological studies have been conducted by researchers belonging to the department of sociology or social work in universities. However, academic activities in this area are not as active as they used to be, nor can very few institutions organize longitudinal studies with large samples for many years as TMIG did. Several more years will be needed before ongoing separate activities can take a certain shape as a new trend.

Primary academic associations in this area are the Japan Socio-Gerontological Society and the Japan Society of Behavioral Science on Aging. Associations closely related to this area are the Society for the Study of Social Welfare, the Japan Society of Family Sociology, and the Japan Welfare Society Association.

Academic Studies

Seniors and Families

In Japan, caregiving (kaigo) has a connotation that "children as caregivers live together with old parents (doukyo)"

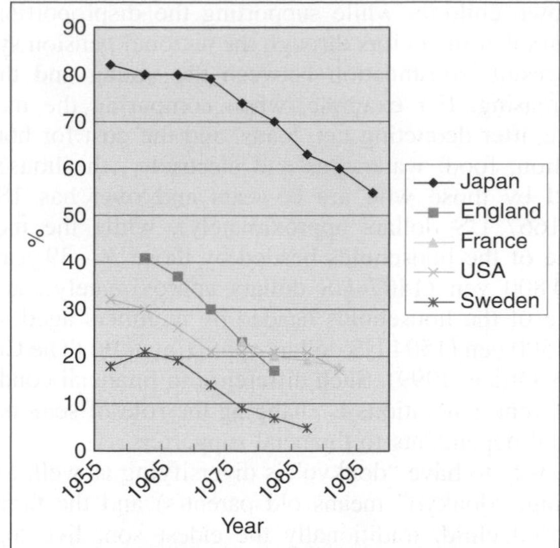

Figure 4 Percentage of those who are 65 years old and over living with their children *Source*: The Ministry of Health, Labor and Welfare (1996)

(Campbell, 2004). In the past few decades, however, the rate of seniors who have "doukyo" with their children is rapidly decreasing (Figure 4). This suggests not only the change of family structure but also the change in the notion of family and caregiving to old parents.

"Doukyo" has been considered as a sign that old parent(s) met their responsibility as parent(s) and children are fulfilling their responsibility of supporting their old parents in return by living together. It is also a sign of unchangeable love from children to old parents as well as the respect to relationships based on blood. When old parents are left alone without having "doukyo", the old parents feel ashamed while the children are considered immoral. However, the purpose of "doukyo" in these days is changing more for the convenience of the children; children save housing cost or daycare cost for their own children by having "doukyo" in the old parents' house (Naoi *et al.*, 1984; Okuyama, 1987).

One of the reasons for these changes of the "doukyo" culture lies in the improvement of financial conditions among seniors. Until the beginning of 1970s, it was said that "only one out of three old people, 60 years of age and over, could live on their own income" (Maeda, 1975). The situation stemmed from the fact that the compulsory retirement age was set between 55 and 57 in those days while the pension payment started between the age of 60 and 65. This yielded five to eight years during which retirees were left without an income. In addition, it was required to pay the premium for more than 25 years to receive the pension, and many retirees were not fulfilling the qualification. However, after the retirement age was increased to 60 years in the 1980s and the pension system became matured, the financial conditions of seniors dramatically improved. The seniors of these days obtained their houses before the so-called bubble economy when the prices were low, and they are now receiving full amount of pensions. In the meantime, younger generations suffer from expensive cost of housing and education of their own children while supporting the disproportionately large number of seniors through the national pension system. As a result, stratification between the young and the old is increasing. For example, when comparing the monthly income after deducting tax, loans, and the cost for housing, education, food, water, gas and electricity, the households headed by those who are 65 years and over has 183 400 yen (1667 US dollars approximately), while the monthly income of the households headed by those 30–39 years old is 154 800 yen (1407 US dollars approximately), and the income of the households headed by members aged 40–49 is 165 500 yen (1504 US dollars approximately) (The General Affairs Office, 1999). Such difference in financial conditions of different generations is changing the role of seniors from financial dependents to financial supporters.

The way to have "doukyo" is diversifying as well. Strictly speaking, "doukyo" means old parent(s) and the family of a married child, traditionally the eldest son, live together under the same roof and share the same income. However, in these days, some families live under the same roof while old parent(s) maintain their financial independence, or old parents and the young family use different entrances or kitchens to avoid intervening with each other's privacy. Other families live separately at a very short distance, such as living next door to each other while sharing most part of their lives.

Along with these changes of family, the notion of "successful aging" is changing as well. Kodama *et al.* (1995) identified two different groups among seniors in terms of their attitude toward aging: traditional seniors who expect to enrich their aging process through intimate relationships with family members, and "new" seniors who enjoy social activities outside home, appreciate independenc, and pursue their own preferences and beliefs.

Social Activities

When the compulsory retirement age was set several years before the beginning of the pension payment, the purpose of "work" after retirement was to earn money. As financial conditions among seniors improved, the meaning of "work" in old age changed to an opportunity to maintain an active life. Previous studies support the notion that "work" helps to maintain good health and morale (Wada, 1984). However, those studies are cross-sectional, and the cause-effect mechanism is still unclear.

One of the recent topics is the process of adaptation to retirement of male workers, and its influence on their relationships with their wives. As a custom of the Japanese society, men with full-time jobs seldom stay at home; they leave home early in the morning and come home late at night. They frequently work even during weekends or go out to entertain their clients by playing golf and pursuing other activities. These male workers are forced to change such a lifestyle by compulsory retirement, usually to a more family oriented one. Wives, who have been leading a separate life from their husbands for many years, are faced with a sudden "restart" of life as a married-couple. Therefore, retirement of male workers in Japan is a critical life event in which both husbands and wives are required to make a tremendous effort to readapt to each other. Previous studies indicate that husbands complain more about decrease in human relations because of retirement. However, as years go by, husbands express more satisfaction than their wives about their retired life (Sodei, 1988).

Lifelong learning is another important topic. Japanese municipalities are sponsoring the Senior University Program (Rojin Daigaku) in which invited speakers give lectures a few times a month, normally. Usually, participation is free of charge, and a qualification is not required. Popular topics discussed in the lectures are health problems common to seniors, tips for living a long life, and hobby-related topics such as gardening, and so forth. Recently, PC training has been introduced as well as lectures on the public long-term care system and the problems of the public pension system. Previous studies report that these learning activities bring about positive influence on seniors both physically and psychologically. However, the studies are not only cross-sectional but also no comparison is made between participants and nonparticipants. Thus, the effect of learning activities is still not clear in a strict sense.

Volunteer activities are also receiving attention as opportunities for seniors to contribute to society on the basis of their many years of experience in society. In the 1990s, many public organizations attempted to organize relatively healthy seniors as volunteers to support frail seniors in the community. However, according to Maeda and Adachi (1992), about 90% of seniors are reluctant to participate in such activities. The study indicated that seniors wished to interact with younger people. They also hope to enjoy their later life, rather than undertake such serious responsibilities.

Burden from Caregiving

The existing public-service system does not provide enough support for frail seniors to maintain their independence in the community. The Long-Term Care Insurance, a newly installed system that will be described in a later part of this chapter, is not exceptional. In the meantime, the shortage of nursing homes is serious, especially in metropolitan areas. For example, in Tokyo, it is said that it would take up to 20 years for a patient to enter a public nursing home because of an extremely long waiting list! In such a circumstance, the family has no choice but to undertake the primary role of caregiving, and there are many families at present that serve as primary caregivers for more than 10 years.

The majority of the primary caregivers are married daughters or daughters-in-law. Their spouses are usually occupied with their jobs, and their support cannot be expected. However, recently, more husbands have started serving as primary caregivers when their wives become frail. Young sons who cannot find jobs under the poor economy are also entering as caregivers. They continue to depend on their parents by living together, and caregiving turns out to be their primary "job" as the parents grow old.

Academic approach to family caregiving has been focused on the development of scales to measure the seriousness of the burden (Nakatani and Tojo, 1989; Mizoguchi *et al.*, 1995; Hattori, *et al.*, 2000). Standardized depression scales are also used to measure the burden of the family caregivers. The unique approach observed in Japan is to use the Chronic Fatigue Symptoms Index (CFSI) developed by Ogose (1991). CFSI was first developed to examine the chronic fatigue experienced by employees. However, it turned out to be widely used as a measurement to obtain comprehensive information on the burden experienced by family caregivers such as anxiety, depressive mood, exhaustion, irritation, general fatigue (low back pain, dim eyes, etc.), chronic fatigue (feeling tired when waking up in the morning, etc.), and physical symptoms (decrease of appetite, nausea, etc.).

As a new trend, some researchers are attempting to understand the positive aspects of caregiving experience (Nishimura, 2004). The viewpoint of social economists, in which caregiving is considered to be an exchange process, is gradually being introduced as well.

Social Services

Numerous "needs" surveys and studies on service use have been conducted in the past several decades. However, the system to provide long-term care for the elderly fundamentally changed in 2000, when the public Long-Term Care Insurance (LTCI), system, was installed. Many of the findings from the studies on public services conducted before 2000 are outdated.

Before LTCI, social services for the elderly were provided by tax through government or public agencies operating under a contract with the government. However, as the old population rapidly increased, the shortage of services turned out to be a serious problem since the availability of such public services was limited, and so was the amount of tax money to be spent for the services. In addition, the public-service system, operating on the basis of the Law of Social Welfare for the Elderly, which was established in 1963, was behind the times in many aspects. For example, the old system was not paying enough attention to the right of service users or accountability of government and public-service providers. LTCI was established as a resolution for the problems, through which a wide range of services are provided such as in-home help, a visiting nurse, day care, and institutional care. A semiprofessional position called *Care Manager* was also created in order to coordinate the services properly for each client. Half of the funds necessary to operate the system come from taxes and the rest are collected as premiums, which are compulsory payments for those who are 40 years and older. In addition, those who use services through the LTCI system are charged 10% of the entire actual cost of the services they use. LTCI promoted privatization as well. The government withdrew from service providing activities, while for-profit organizations, in addition to existing public agencies, were allowed to participate in the system as service providers. In this way, LTCI succeeded in increasing the amount of services provided as well as obtaining additional funds to support the expanded system.

Not many years have passed since LTCI has been installed, and solid outcomes based on sophisticated academic studies on LTCI are few, while anecdotal reports are uncountable. Basic statistics such as the number and health conditions of service users and the pattern of service use are collected in almost all municipalities, and are available to the public upon request.

Social Network/Social Support

Influenced by the trend of gerontology in the United States, numerous studies have been conducted on social networks and social support in Japan. The studies are focused on the development of scales, examination on the functions of social support, and the structure of support networks. Previous studies indicate that support networks of seniors in Japan primarily comprise of family members (Fukukawa *et al.*, 2002). This makes a contrast with the results in the United States, where seniors build intimate relationships both inside as well as outside of their families.

PSYCHOLOGY

Background

The founder of psychological studies on aging is Satokatsu Tachibana. His first paper on aging was published in 1926. Since then, he produced numerous papers in both domestic and international journals. In the 1960s, when geriatric psychiatry and social gerontology gradually obtained recognition from the society, psychology on aging was left behind. The turning point was 1972, when the Department of Psychology on Aging was established in the TMIG. The department undertook a leading role in defining psychological issues on aging and established methods to approach them.

The number of academic papers and presentations made in this area is increasing every year. Formerly, publications and presentations were made through the Japan Socio-Gerontological Society. Recently, academic communities that are not specialized in gerontology are more actively involved, such as the Association of Japanese Clinical Psychology, the Japanese Psychological Association, the Japanese Association of Educational Psychology and Japanese Society of Developmental Psychology. This trend indicates that old age is being considered as the final stage of personality development; thus psychological studies on aging is incorporated in developmental psychology rather than forming an independent area for it (Shimonaka, 2004, personal communication).

Academic Activities

Psychological studies on aging in the early days adopted the social psychological approach. Their interests were on the sources of happiness, loneliness, and subjective well-being of old people. The Department of Psychology on Aging at

TMIG conducted longitudinal studies on personality, self-image, anxiety, and cognition of the elderly. The primary findings from the longitudinal studies were that self-image became more positive while anxiety decreased as the subjects aged. It was also identified that widows recovered from the grief of losing their spouses within 2 years (Shimonaka and Nakazato, 1989; Sakaguchi, 2002).

How the society sees the seniors has been an important subject as well. "Nihon Shoki", the first history book published in Japan in 720, described seniors as heroes and heroines of wisdom who achieved longevity. However, in the sixteenth century, when Japan was divided into small provinces and there was constantly war among them, seniors became to be seen as useless drags. A saying which symbolized the negative image commonly shared about seniors in those days was, "Long life comes with a lot of shame". Buddhists advocated the idea of accepting "the shameful aging process" as a normal part of life instead of fighting against it. From the seventeenth to the end of the nineteenth century, there was no war inside the country. Under the peaceful environment, health promotion for a long life ("yojo-do") became popular. After the Second World War, democracy and individualism were introduced while industrialization and urbanization proceeded. As the extended family system was resolved in the process, the traditional culture of respecting seniors also eroded. As if to oppose the social changes, 15 September was designated in 1966 as a national day of "Respect for Seniors". In 1973, the Japan Railroad installed the system of "Silver Seat", in which certain seats in the trains were assigned for senior passengers to sit. In 1983, the Hyogo Prefecture passed the law to prohibit the use of word "old" to describe seniors in public, and "senior citizen" was adopted as an appropriate wording. In a short time, the same law was passed in the rest of the prefectures all over Japan. Shimonaka (1998) states that these movements could be interpreted as a way to "compensate for the loss of respect for seniors by installing formal systems".

Other topics in psychological studies on aging are as follows:

- clinical psychological approaches to deal with seniors with memory problems, such as, counseling, reminiscence (Matsuda *et al.*, 2002), and collage (Ishizaki, 2001);
- adaptation to a new task, such as institutionalization;
- caregiver's burden and coping problems;
- psychological characteristics such as cognitive functions and memory;
- grand parenting;
- influence of aging on personality and personal change at the terminal stage;
- stressful life events;
- personality traits commonly observed among centenarians.

Acknowledgments

We would like to express our deep appreciation to the following researchers who provided us with precious information. They are those who have literally been leading geriatrics and gerontology in Japan: (in alphabetical order) Homma, A. (Senior Researcher of the Tokyo Metropolitan Institute of Gerontology (TMIG)), Horiuchi, F. (Professor of Ibaragi Prefecture Medical University), Kanekawa, K. (Chancellor of Ishikawa Prefecture Nursing University), Meda, D. (Professor of Lutheren Theological University), Murai, J. (Former Associate Professor of Kyoto University), Ozawa, T. (Former President of the Tokyo Geriatric Hospital), Shibata, H. (Professor of Obirin University), Shichida (1999) K. (Professor of Nihon Sekijuji Musashino Nursing Junior College), and Shimonaka, Y. (Professor of Bukyo Gakuin University).

KEY POINTS

- Japan has experienced a rapid increase of old population in the past thirty years.
- Japanese geriatrics and gerontology studies have contributed to the understanding of the aging process, as well as the development of methods for effective interventions to the process.
- The constriction in the activities of the TMIG, in addition to the resolution of Yoikuin Nursing Homes and the Tokyo Metropolitan Geriatric Hospital, is wielding a serious impact on both practice and academic activities of geriatrics and gerontology in Japan.
- The future of geriatric medicine in Japan faces serious challenges. Especially, the poorly organized condition of the training system for geriatric practitioners raises a concern.
- The combination of the recent increase of stratification and the decrease of pension payment will make the middle class more susceptible to poverty in their old age. The issue of poverty among seniors was once overcome; however, it will surface again as a primary challenge of Japanese geriatrics and gerontology in the near future.

KEY REFERENCES

- Cabinet Office. *White Report on Aged Society* 2004; Cabinet Office.
- Homma A. *Guideline for Diagnosis, Treatment and Care for Alzheimer Patients: for Professionals Working in the Area of Geriatrics and Gerontology*, 2003 Block Grand Program Report of the Ministry of Health 2004; Labor and Welfare for Gerontological Science.
- Maeda D. Research in social gerontology in Japan. *Shakai Ronengaku* 1975; **5**:3–13.
- Shibata H, Sugisawa H & Watanabe S. Functional capacity in elderly Japanese living in the community. *Geriatrics and Gerontology International* 2001; **1**:8–13.
- Shimonaka Y. History and trend of psychological studies on aging in Japan. *Kyoiku Sinrigaku Nenpo* 1998; **37**:129–42.

REFERENCES

Cabinet Office. *White Report on Aged Society* 2004; Cabinet Office.

Campbell J. Doukyo & Kaigo. In Y Suda (ed) *The Ministry of Health, Labor and Welfare Research Fund Program: Preventing Premature Institutionalization of Frail Seniors, Supporting Families* 2004, pp 306–10; The Ministry of Health, Labor and Welfare Research Fund Program Report.

Fukukawa Y, Nakajima C, Tsuboi S & Niino N. Examining the structure of social network by age. *Rounen Shakaikagaku* 2002; **24**(2):153–60.

Hattori A, Ouchi A, Shibuya K *et al.* Measuring the burden of family caregivers using the Burn-out scale. *Nihon Ronen Igakkai Zasshi* 2000; **37**:799–804.

Hirai A, Hamazaki T, Terano T *et al.* Eicosapentaenoic acid and platelet function in Japanese. *Lancet* 1980; **2**(8204):1132–3.

Homma A. Epidemiological study on Alzheimer's type dementia. *Dementia Japan* 1998; **12**:5–9.

Homma A. *Guideline for Diagnosis, Treatment and Care for Alzheimer Patients: for Professionals Working in the Area of Geriatrics and Gerontology* 2003 Block Grand Program Report of the Ministry of Health 2004; Labor and Welfare for Gerontological Science.

Ishihara O, Shimonaka Y, Nakazato K *et al.* Stability of the morale measured by the revised PGC morale scale in give years. *Rounen Shakaikagaku* 1999; **21**(3):339–45.

Ishizaki J. The Innter World of Alzheimer's Patients Expressed in Collage. *Journal of Japanese Clinical Psychology* 2001; **19**(3):278–289.

Kameyama M. Pathogenesis of cerebral infarction-a clinical and pathological study. *Nippon Naika Gakkai Zasshi* 1979; **68**:468–75.

Kato C, Shimogaki H, Onodera A *et al.* Developing the short version of the Hasegawa dementia scale (HDS-R). *Ronen Igaku Zasshi* 1991; **2**(11):1339–47.

Kobayashi S, Hirai A, Terano T *et al.* Reduction in blood viscosity by eicosapentaenoic acid. *Lancet* 1981; **2**(8239):197.

Kodama Y, Koyano W, Okaura K & Ando T. Preferable lifestyle in old age among the middle-aged living in a city. *Rounen Shakaikagaku* 1995; **17**(1):66–73.

Maeda D. Research in social gerontology in Japan. *Shakai Ronengaku* 1975; **5**:3–13.

Maeda D & Adachi K. Analysis on attitude of healthy seniors toward volunteer activities for frail seniors. *Shakai Ronengaku* 1992; **38**:84–5.

Matsuda O, Kurokawa Y, Saito M & Maruyama K. Group-based Reminiscence Approach to the Elderly with Memory Problems. *Journal of Japanese Clinical Psychology* 2002; **19**(6):566–577.

Mizoguchi T, Iijima S, Niino N & Orimo H. Examining the caregiving burden using the cost of care index. *Nippon Ronen Igakkai Zasshi* 1995; **32**:403–9.

Mori E, Mitani Y & Yamatori S. The validity of the Japanese version of Mini-Mental State Examination when applied to neuro-patients. *Shinkei Shinri Gaku* 1985; **1**(2):82–9.

Nakatani Y & Tojo M. Burden experienced by family caregivers: developing the measurement and its validity. *Ronen shakaigaku* 1989; **29**:27–36.

Naoi M, Okamura K & Hayashi K. Living together with or separately from old parents: report from survey to middle-aged women. *Shakai Ronengaku* 1984; **21**:3–20.

Nishimura M. Caregiving relationship: reward and burden. In Y Suda (ed) *The Ministry of Health, Labor and Welfare Research Fund Program: Determining Factors to Delay Institutionalization of Frail Seniors and the Role of Families in the Process* 2004, pp 295–303; The Ministry of Health, Labor and Welfare Research Fund Program Report.

Ogose R. The validity and reliability of the Chronic Fatigue Symptoms Index (CFSI). *Rodo kagaku* 1991; **67**:147–57.

Ohkawa S, Inoue J & Sugiura M. A clinicopathologic study of dilated cardiomyopathy in the aged. *Journal of Cardiography* 1986; **9**(1 suppl):35–47.

Okuyama S. Plan on living together with or separately from old parents: survey to old parents and their children living in the mega-city. *Shakai Ronengaku* 1987; **26**:32–42.

Ozawa T. Comprehensive geriatric assessment. *Nippon Ronen Igakkai Zasshi* 1998; **35**:351–9.

Sakaguchi K. The link between positive-negative appraisals of bereavement and mental health after spousal loss. *The Japanese Journal of Psychology* 2002; **73**(5):425–30.

Shibata H, Sugisawa H & Watanabe S. Functional capacity in elderly Japanese living in the community. *Geriatrics and Gerontology International* 2001; **1**:8–13.

Shibata H. An overview of the Tokyo Metropolitan Institute of Gerontology-Longitudinal Interdisciplinary Study on Aging (TMIG-LISA, 1991–2001). *Journal of Aging and Physical Activity* 2000; **8**:98–108.

Shichida K. Challenges and future of the studies on geriatric nurse. *Nihon Ronen Kango Gakkaishi* 1999; **4**:6–10.

Shimonaka Y. History and trend of psychological studies on aging in Japan. *Kyoiku Sinrigaku Nenpo* 1998; **37**:129–42.

Shimonaka Y & Nakazato K. The process of psychological adaptation of seniors living in a nursing home. *Shakai ronengaku* 1989; **26**:65–75.

Shimokata H, Yamada Y, Nakagawa M *et al.* Distribution of geriatric disease-related genotypes in the National Institute for Longevity Sciences, Longitudinal Study of Aging (NILS-LSA). *Journal of Epidemiology* 2000; **10**((1):suppl) S46–55.

Sodei T. The influence of retirement to retired workers and their family. *Shakai Ronengaku* 1988; **10**(2):64–79.

Sugiura M, Matsuhita S & Ueda K. A clinicopathological study on vascular diseases in three thousand consecutive autopsies of the aged. *Japan Circulation Journal* 1982; **46**:337–45.

Tauchi H & Sato T. Age changes in size and number of mitochondria of human hepatic cells. *American Journal of Gerontology* 1968; **23**:454–61.

The Committee for Social Problems Related to Aging. Suggestion for social policies for the elderly. *Kikan Shakai Hosho Kenkyu* 1974; **10**(3):61–5.

The Ethic Committee on Geriatric Medicine in Japan. *Our Standpoint on Terminal Care for the Elderly* 2001, Also available on the World Wide Web: http://www.mhlw.go.jp/toukei/saikin.

The General Affairs Office. *Trend on Savings* 1999.

The Japan Geriatrics Society. *Progress Made and Future to Explore of Geriatric Medicine* 2003; Medical Review Press.

The Ministry of Health, Labor and Welfare. *White Report on Health and Welfare* 1996.

The Ministry of Health, Labor and Welfare. *Longevity of Japanese People: 2004 Summary of Life Tables* 2004a, Available on the World Wide Web: http://www.mhlw.go.jp/toukei/saikin.

The Ministry of Health, Labor and Welfare. *Hospital Report: 2004* 2004b, Available on the World Wide Web: http://www.mhlw.go.jp/toukei/saikin.

Tokyo Metropolitan Geriatric Hospital. *The Progress Made in the Past Ten Years* 1983.

Uchida Y & Tomonaga M. Neurotrophic action of Alzheimer's disease brain extract is due to the loss of inhibitory factors for survival and neurite formation of cerebral cortical neurons. *Brain Research* 1989; **48**(1):190–3.

Wada S. Social aging and adaptation to it: on the life satisfaction index. *Shakai Ronengaku* 1979; **11**:3–14.

Wada S. Employment of pension recipients and its effect. *Shakai Ronengaku* 1984; **19**:88–102.

World Health Organization. *Health Statistics Annual* 1995.

Yamauchi H, Suzuki H & Orimo H. Calcitonin for the treatment of osteoporosis: dosage and dosing interval in Japan. *Journal of Bone and Mineral Metabolism* 2003; **21**:198–204.

Yokode M, Nagano Y, Arai H *et al.* Cigarette smoke and lipoprotein modification. A possible interpretation for development of atherosclerosis. *Ann N Y Acad Sci.* 1995; **748**:294–300.

Yoneyama T, Yoshida M, Onrui T *et al.* Oral care reduces pneumonia in older patients in nursing homes. *Journal of American Geriatric Society* 2002; **50**:430–3.

FURTHER READING

Sugiyama Z, Takakawa T, Nakamura H *et al.* Developing the Japanese version of the PGC morale scale (1): its reliability and validity. *Shakai Ronengaku* 1981; **3**:57–69.

Care of the Elderly in Israel: Old Age in a Young Land

A. Mark Clarfield[1], Jenny Brodsky[2] *and* Arthur Leibovitz[3]

[1] *Ben Gurion University of the Negev, Beer Sheva, Israel, and McGill University, Montreal, QC, Canada,* [2] *JDC-Brookdale Institute, Jerusalem, Israel, and* [3] *Shmuel Harofeh Medical Centre, Beer Yaacov, Israel*

INTRODUCTION

Situated at the eastern end of the Mediterranean, Israel is a small country with a population of approximately 6.6 million covering only 20 700 square kilometers of territory. While still relatively young demographically (10% over age 65) in comparison to other developed states, from an absolute point of view, Israel has aged rapidly since the country obtained independence just over 50 years ago. Despite the pressures of waves of mass immigration, repeated war, and ongoing terrorism, an impressive set of institutions has been built to take care of the country's population in general and her elderly in particular (Clarfield *et al.*, 2000; Brodsky and Clarfield, 2001; Clarfield, 2000).

In this article, we will briefly describe Israel's demographic development, the organization and development of her health-care system, and the education of its formal caregivers. We will also touch on issues that make Israel unique from a gerontological point of view – such as the large proportion of Holocaust survivors among Israel's elderly and the situation of the Arab minority.

Demography

The population of Israel stands at just over 6.6 million, with nearly 80% being Jews and the rest Arabs (Muslim, Christian, and Druze). Israel has undergone a major increase in its relative proportion of elderly (65+) from less than 4% in 1948 to 10% in 2003 (Clarfield *et al.*, 2000; Brodsky *et al.*, 2004). Within the Jewish population, 11.3% are elderly, while in the non-Jewish population only 3.1% are over age 65 due to the much higher fertility rate among the latter group. Life expectancy at birth is among the highest in the developed world, especially for men, which stands at 77.5 years. Although, as would be expected, women have a higher life expectancy (81.5 years), Israel only ranks 16 in the world for women's life expectancy at birth while it ranks 6th for men (World Health Organization, 2004). This difference has yet to be adequately explained.

Despite the growth in the number of its older citizens, from a relative point of view, Israel is still one of the youngest of the world's developed countries primarily because of a relatively high fertility rate (2.9 children per woman in 2003). That said, the country has experienced an exponential increase in the absolute numbers of its older people due to a combination of both natural growth and immigration.

For example, while the general population increased 3.7 times during the past 50 years, the elderly population grew by a factor of 7.7, double that of the general population. The rate of increase of the older–old (aged 75 and over) is even more pronounced – 11.5. Thus, in Israel as elsewhere, not only has the general population been aging but the elderly population itself has been both increasing in numbers and growing older. The number of those aged 65 and older reached 670 000 at the end of 2003. It is projected that the proportion of elderly will remain stable up to 2010, but will rise to 12.7% of the total population by 2025 (numbering 1 176 000 persons) (Brodsky *et al.*, 2004).

Changes in levels of fertility and mortality alone cannot explain the rapid aging of Israeli society. Another unique characteristic that affects changes in the population's age structure is migration. Usually the elderly tend to be "reluctant movers" unless their motivation is strongly religious or emotional, or unless whole communities are on the move. The relatively high proportion of elderly persons in the waves of immigrants to Israel since the establishment of the country in 1948 is unique. On average, some 8% of all immigrants since 1948 were at least 65 years of age on arrival in Israel, and about 18% were between 45 and 64 (the middle-aged and

Principles and Practice of Geriatric Medicine, 4th Edition. Edited by M.S. John Pathy, Alan J. Sinclair and John E. Morley.

aging cohorts). This has been an important factor in the process and pace of the increase in the numbers and percentage of the elderly in the Israeli population.

Of special note is the recent reemergence of large-scale immigration, primarily from the former Soviet Union (FSU), which began at the end of 1989. From 1989 to 2002, almost one million immigrants arrived from the FSU, including 155 000 individuals aged 65 and over (approximately 12% of the current immigration cohort). Today these recent newcomers represent more than one-fifth of the country's elderly. The absorption of this particular aged population, which arrived without economic resources, presents new problems and challenges to Israeli society and to its current social and health-care systems (Brodsky *et al.*, 2004).

Clearly, while it is predicted that the percentage of old people will remain relatively stable over the next two decades, the significant absolute increase will continue to strain the capacities of the country's health and social services.

With respect to the Arab population, its high fertility has ensured that the proportion of those over age 65 has remained low and will not reach more than 6% even by the year 2020. However, from an absolute point of view, like Israel's Jewish citizens, the number of Arab Israelis will grow significantly with a projected increase of 66% between the end of the twentieth century and the year 2010 (Brodsky *et al.*, 2004).

Beyond the Arab-Jewish divide, Israel's population is even more heterogeneous, with each group having its own demographic history. Although Jewish citizens comprise four-fifths of the overall population, they constitute 94% of the elderly. Also, with respect to this group, almost all (90%) were born abroad, two-thirds of them in Europe. Given the aging of the survivors of the European Holocaust, this group makes up just under one half of Israel's elderly today. These people bring a special challenge to both caregivers and policymakers (Brodsky *et al.*, 2003; David and Pelly, 2003).

The Health-Care System

In 1995, Israel's National Health Insurance Law was promulgated (Chinitz, 1995). This progressive legislation, which ensures the provision of both acute and rehabilitative care (in-patient and out-patient), is available to all legal residents with almost no out-of-pocket costs. In addition, a generous drug-benefits plan is available to citizens of all ages. The health system is funded via a progressive payroll tax (with a ceiling of five times the average wage) paid by the employee. Unemployed, the elderly (≥60 years for women, ≥65 years for men), and those receiving disability and income support pay only a minimal tariff. These monies are transferred to the National Insurance Institute (*Bituach Leumi*), which then distributes them to each of the four sick funds according to a capitation mechanism. This system favors higher payments to the sick funds for those over age 65 and for those who suffer from a limited list of diseases (e.g. severe renal failure). The other half of the resources is supplied from general tax revenues.

Clinical care is organized and provided through one of four publicly financed and administered nonprofit sick funds (similar to American HMOs) mentioned earlier. These bodies are responsible for providing all of the acute and rehabilitative care to the whole population (Clarfield *et al.*, 2000; Clarfield, 2000).

DISABILITY AND LONG-TERM CARE SERVICES

Most relevant to the planning of long-term care services is the growth in the population of disabled elderly. Although the majority of older persons in Israel are independent, the changes that have taken place in the age, gender, and ethnic composition of Israel's elderly population have contributed to the increase in the absolute number and proportion of disabled elderly (who need assistance in personal care activities, such as dressing, washing, and eating). During the past two decades, the number of disabled elderly has grown 2.5 times, and in 2002, about 16% of older Israelis (including those living in institutions) were disabled in at least one activity of daily living (ADL). By the year 2010, the number of disabled elderly people is projected to increase by 31%, as compared to an expected 16% increase in the number of elderly. That is, the rate of increase of the disabled is double that of the total elderly population due to changes in its composition (Beer and Brodsky, 2002). On the other hand, there are initial indications that the new cohorts of elderly (especially the "young-old") are healthier than earlier ones (Clarfield *et al.*, 2004).

Institutional Long-term Care

Although the acute and rehabilitative side of care is highly socialized, with respect to institutional long-term care, the Israeli system is more analogous to the American Medicaid program (Clarfield *et al.*, 2000; Brodsky and Clarfield, 2001; Clarfield, 2000). Here, unlike that which pertains in acute and rehabilitative care, long-term institutional care is not covered by the above-described universal mechanism. Also, patients are placed at one of five levels of dependency with the institutions regulated by two Ministries: Health and Labour/Social Affairs. As is the case in the American system, those families that are able to purchase care from a licensed long-term institution (either for-profit or nonprofit) are expected to do so. However, given the high cost of such care, more than two-thirds of families turn to the Ministry of Health for a subsidy. (This can cover up to the entire cost of care, which is approximately 2500 USD per month.) However, co-payments are demanded according to a progressive system of accounting *by law* from the patient's spouse and children. Of interest is the fact that in the case of those categories of beds under the aegis of the Ministry of Labour and Social Affairs, even the resources and incomes of sons and daughters-in-law are included in the accounting of co-payments.

In comparison to most other industrialized countries, the majority of elderly people still lives or is cared for at home, with only 4.1% residing in a long-term care institution. Even among the disabled elderly, 78% still live in the community (Beer and Brodsky, 2002). It is clear that such a situation would be impossible without a great degree of family involvement, which is quite strong in Israel, an attitude fostered by both Judaism and Islam (Clarfield *et al.*, 2003). In addition, over the past decade, a number of formal services have been established, some quite innovative, meant to reinforce these social constructs and as such to help families cope with the burden of care.

Care at Home

Recent years have seen the rapid development of community and support services for the elderly who live at home. In the 1980s, forecasts of a significant growth in the number of disabled elderly raised fears that the cost of institutionalization would skyrocket if alternatives were not found. At the same time, an uneven distribution of funding for community and institutional services led to the desire for a more appropriate funding balance. All of these factors led to a range of efforts to develop community services (Naon and Strosberg, 1995).

Of the various models available, Israel chose to adopt the social insurance approach. In 1980, a 0.2% employee contribution to the National Insurance Institute was levied to create a reserve fund for implementing the law. By 1986, Israel's parliament, the Knesset, had completed the enactment of the Community Long-term Care Insurance (CLTCI) Law, and full implementation began in April, 1988.

The basic entitlement is for in-kind services, carefully delineated as a "basket of services" closely related to the direct care functions normally provided by families, such as personal care and homemaking. Benefits may also be used to purchase day care services, laundry services, absorbent undergarments for the incontinent, or an alarm system. Actual services are provided according to benefit levels set at 25% of the average market wage, with the severely disabled elderly receiving an additional 50% of this level (equivalent to about 10 or 15 hours of home care per week, respectively) (Brodsky and Clarfield, 2001; Naon and Strosberg, 1995).

Eligibility for benefits is not affected by any informal assistance an elderly person may receive from friends and/or family members. There is a means test for receiving benefits under the CLTCI law, but it is set at such a high level relative to the income status of the elderly that almost all of those who meet the clinical requirements are eligible for the entitlement. The less disabled elderly, who are not eligible for such services may still receive home care services from the social welfare system under a budget-restricted, income-tested program, which however provides fewer hours of care.

Home care (personal care and housekeeping services) is provided by semi-professional staff working for certified, licensed agencies. These agencies may be NGOs or for-profit agencies. The choice of a service provider is made by a local committee responsible for care planning, in consultation with the client and his family.

The first effect of the CLTCI law was to tremendously increase the resources earmarked for community care. This decision resulted in a more balanced allocation of public resources between institutional and community care. Prior to the law's implementation, expenditures for community services were limited, representing only 17% of public funds for long-term care (Naon and Strosberg, 1995). However, by 1994 (four years after the law's implementation) public funds for community care grew to constitute half of the public funding for long-term care.

This legislation has had a dramatic effect on the coverage of disabled elderly in the community. For example, the proportion of elderly receiving home care increased from 2% prior to implementation of the law to nearly 16–17% of the total elderly population (some 110 000 elderly in 2004).

Problems

Despite the range of services available, the situation in Israel results in many discontinuities between acute and long-term care as well as within the long-term care system. This problem among others was recognized more than 15 years ago and was studied comprehensively by the Netanyahu State Commission (Chinitz, 1995), which included a comprehensive examination of the whole health-care system. Among other things, this body recommended that within 3 years after the implementation of the National Health Insurance Law (in 1995), responsibility for long-term institutional care was meant to be transferred from the Ministry of Health to the patient's respective sick fund which, as mentioned earlier, already was responsible for acute and rehabilitative care for all ages. In this way, it was thought that one of the major discontinuities in the health-care system would be corrected. In addition, it was reasoned that following these changes, the sick funds would be more motivated to initiate programs that would encourage health promotion and prevention, geriatric assessment, and rehabilitation in order to keep the number requiring long-term institutional care (which would now be their fiscal responsibility) to an absolute minimum.

However, for many reasons (including primarily opposition from both the sick funds and the Treasury Ministry) this transfer of responsibility and jurisdiction has to date not come about (Clarfield *et al.*, 2000; Clarfield, 2000). Although the issue has been revisited several times since the Netanyahu State Commission (The National Institute for Health Policy and Health Services Research, 2002), this lack of implementation remains the single biggest barrier to taking the necessary steps required to improve integration of care for Israel's frail older population (Clarfield *et al.*, 2001).

Medical Education

There has been significant progress in geriatric education among all relevant health professionals over the last 20 years.

Geriatrics was recognized as a separate specialty by the Scientific Council of the Israeli Medical Association (IMA) in 1984. This act provided a professional basis for further progress and for the training of future generations of geriatricians of which there are now approximately 160 registered in Israel. (For comparison, this is almost the same number as, for example, in Canada, a country with five times Israel's population.)

There are three ways to specialize in geriatric medicine. In the first, somewhat analogous to the American model, after certification in either internal medicine or family medicine (5 years in both specialties), the physician is required to take an additional 2 years of geriatric training. Until several years ago, most geriatricians, especially those who now head the large geriatric centers or run academic departments, entered the field via the internal medicine route. However, of late there has been an increase in the number of candidates from family medicine.

In response to a perceived need for accelerating the number of physicians specializing in geriatrics, a "fast-track program" was initiated in 1993. This consists of a $4^1/_2$-year program, the first 2 years (post-internship) of which are in internal medicine followed by 2 years of geriatric fellowship and 6 months of research. There are 20 recognized geriatrics departments located in acute-care institutions or in one of the eight large geriatric teaching hospitals (which are analogous to American Veterans' Centers).

All training sites are inspected and accredited by the Israeli Medical Association. After successful completion of one of the aforementioned residency routes and after passing a two-stage board examination (including, as in Canada, an oral exam), the title "Specialist in Geriatric Medicine" is accorded (on recommendation of the IMA) by the Ministry of Health.

Unfortunately, most trainees in geriatric medicine, despite the demands of the formal syllabus, still have little exposure to normal aging, primary care, or community-based home care. Also, extensive out-patient work including formal geriatric assessment is still in its infancy in Israel.

Over the last 15 years, an interesting phenomenon has occurred. With the massive wave of immigration to Israel from countries of the FSU, approximately 9000 doctors came to the country, almost doubling the number of medical practitioners (Nire, 1999). Seizing an opportunity to kill two birds with one stone, the Ministry of Health and the Ministry of Absorption cooperated to fund training slots for many specialties, including geriatrics. Under the administration of an NGO, ESHEL (devoted to planning and development of services for the elderly in Israel), approximately 80 training slots for geriatricians have been funded throughout the country and these physicians are now beginning to practice.

In addition to the programs for the specialists in geriatric medicine there are two additional postgraduate programs that provide certificate training in geriatrics. One is held at Shmuel Harofe Hospital and has been offered annually since 1991. It began as a training course for immigrant physicians but for the last few years has been opened to all physicians interested in old-age medicine. More than 450 physicians, mostly from the long-term care sector, have taken this course.

The second setting for nonspecialist geriatric training is the postgraduate course provided by the Sackler School of Medicine of the Tel Aviv University. This program has been functioning since 1994 and is part of that faculty's continuing medical education curriculum. A postgraduate course in Geriatric Psychiatry is offered in the same educational framework.

With respect to undergraduate studies, geriatrics is offered by all four Israeli medical schools. Introductory lectures in geriatrics are given throughout the curriculum but the core teaching is based on a 2-week clerkship in one of the country's accredited geriatric units.

In some centers, there have been some innovative educational methods utilized. For example, at the Tel Aviv University, in accordance with a comprehensive approach to geriatrics, a special model has been developed as an assessment tool for medical students at the end of their clerkship. The tool combines summative with formative elements and provides an efficient way to assess the students according to what is referred to as the *five Cs*: clinical geriatrics, comprehensiveness, communication, coordination, and collaboration. A serious attempt is made to offer this evaluation in a nonthreatening and instructive manner. Another innovative approach has been the successful interdisciplinary model of teaching geriatrics to medical students created by combining geriatrics with epidemiology and preventive medicine.

With respect to the study of gerontology, two universities (Haifa and Ben Gurion University) have recently opened programs offering a Masters of Gerontology. These courses are not directed specifically toward physicians or nurses, although members of these professions do study in these programs.

SPECIAL ISSUES

Attitudes Toward Life and Death

In Israel, Judaism and to a lesser extent Islam have a strong formal and informal influence on the ethics and practice of health care. Of interest is the fact that the religion of Islam is also very close in many ways to Jewish philosophy on issues of end-of-life care (Clarfield *et al.*, 2003) as both religions place the highest value on the sanctity of life. For example in Judaism, one is enjoined to supersede all biblical commandments (except for three cardinal sins of idolatry, adultery, and murder) in order to save a life. Also, in addition to conventional medical care, rabbinical advice is often sought by those suffering from illness. In fact, the practice of consulting spiritual advisors in parallel with the conventional medical system has become quite widespread. Some might with justice consider this a form of alternative medicine. Both patient and family can receive advice (obviously of varying quality) according to which physician or medical center is considered to be expert in treating a particular disease (either in Israel or abroad). However, in many cases, this advice can interfere with appropriate medical decision-making. That said, one could consider this voluntary transfer of decision-making power to fall under the rubric of respect for patient autonomy.

Regarding end-of-life care, *Halacha* (Jewish law) explicitly forbids any act of euthanasia or assisted suicide and, as mentioned earlier, leans strongly toward the preservation of life. According to this system of belief, food and fluids should always be provided to the dying patient and their supply is not considered to be "extraordinary" (as it is for example under Catholic law). In addition, for example, it is forbidden to discontinue drugs or oxygen or to withhold blood transfusions or antibiotic therapy (Marcus *et al.*, 2001), even if the physician considers the patient to have an incurable illness.

That said, however, when a patient does indeed reach the stage of "active dying" (*goses*) it is in fact forbidden to do anything to extend life and thus prolong suffering. Of course the debate usually revolves around when a patient has reached the situation of being a *goses* and this is not easy to define. As a result of this complex set of beliefs, it is not unusual in Israeli long-term wards to see an extensive use of tube feeding (either gastrostomy or nasogastric) even in patients with end-stage dementia (Bentur *et al.*, 1996; Clarfield *et al.*, 2005).

The Arab Elderly

As mentioned earlier, all of Israel's citizens regardless of ethnicity or religion are eligible for the services described in this article. For the most part, while discrimination has been described in some spheres such as the allocation of budgets for education or municipal infrastructure, health services are available equally to all. With respect to aging, the Arab population is still relatively young. However, a significant increase, both relative and absolute is expected in the number of elderly Arabs in the coming years. For example, at the end of 2003 there were about 42 000 Arab elderly, but their number is expected to reach 119 200 by 2025. This will represent a nearly threefold increase in absolute numbers. As this population ages, the number and percentage of people with chronic diseases and related disabilities will rise significantly (Brodsky *et al.*, 2004).

While the Arab elderly are somewhat younger than their Jewish counterparts, they tend to be more disabled and therefore have greater medical and nursing needs. An extremely important measure of the need for formal services is functional ability, especially the ability to live independently. The percentage of Arab elderly who are disabled and need help with ADLs is two times higher than that of the Jewish elderly population. Concomitant with demographic changes are forces that affect the ability of informal support systems to provide care. For example, the rising number of Arab women in the labor force together with changes in elderly peoples' living arrangements has increased the need for formal services to share responsibility for the elderly with families. As services are developed, questions arise regarding the extent to which they have been adapted to the culture and norms of Arab society and meet that society's unique needs (Azaiza and Brodsky, 2003).

Holocaust Survivors

One of the noteworthy characteristics of the elderly population in Israel is that it includes a significant proportion of those who suffered through and survived the Holocaust. It is estimated that between 40 and 50% are such survivors, and the percentage of survivors among the elderly born in Europe reaches about 75% (Brodsky *et al.*, 2003).

During the first years after the World War II, a high prevalence of physical and mental impairments was noted, but many of theses unfortunates either died or were placed in a long-term institution. It is therefore possible to note that many of today's community-dwelling survivors are examples of successful coping. Most dealt (at least on the surface) with their Holocaust trauma, built families, and adjusted well in their social and occupational lives. However, with increased aging, this traumatized group have had to cope with new challenges brought on by the vicissitudes of aging. In addition, this process, often accompanied by loss of family members and friends, can also accelerate and intensify past crises.

There are a number of areas in which elderly survivors often suffer from special difficulties, (see the excellent manual published by The Baycrest Centre for Geriatric Care in Toronto for a complete clinical description (David and Pelly, 2003)). Compared to the European-born elderly who are not Holocaust survivors, some differences have been found in the physical and mental health of these two groups. For example, among Holocaust survivors, particularly among those who experienced incarceration in the European ghettos, were in hiding, or forced into slave and concentration camps, there is a higher prevalence of illnesses such as osteoporosis, disc disease, and fractures (Menczel and Marcus, 2003). This clinical picture may result, at least in part, from nutritional and general deprivation during their youth, which influenced their state in older age and their quality of life. Thus, in older age, Holocaust survivors need extra attention to their special social, mental, and health needs.

Gerontological Organizations

In addition to the formal medical and nursing services available, Israel has a large nonprofit and NGO infrastructure. Several national bodies such as the research-oriented Myers-Brookdale Institute of Gerontology and ESHEL, the organization for planning and development for services for the elderly (both daughter organizations of the American Joint Distribution Agency), have initiated many innovative new services and models of care for older people. For physicians there is an active Israel Geriatrics Society, as well as a large Israel Gerontological Society and a dynamic Alzheimers Association. Other groups have formed of late, including organizations for stroke victims and those who suffer from Parkinson's disease, among others.

CONCLUSION

While Israel is still somewhat younger than other developed countries from a relative point of view, the absolute number of elderly Israelis, both Arab and Jew, has grown enormously over the last several decades and will continue to do so for the foreseeable future. In many ways, the health-care system for the elderly is quite organized and functions well. However, the discontinuities involved in the transitions within acute care and from acute to long-term care and the very large number of actors and jurisdictions responsible for ongoing care and supervision of the frail elderly remain a serious problem. Much attention has been paid to this issue but a solution is not on the horizon.

The Jewish and Islamic nature of Israeli society and health-care makes the country an interesting social laboratory to examine how different communities under the same formal system look after their elderly people. Israel is in many ways a dynamic, albeit stressed society. Despite this, care of the elderly in many cases is fair to good and in some places, even excellent.

KEY POINTS

- Israel, while still relatively young by Western standards, is rapidly aging with the absolute number of elderly having increased logarithmically over the past 50 years.
- While acute and rehabilitative care are covered by universal health care, long-term institutional care remains poorly integrated with the main system of care resulting in fragmentation, especially for the frail.
- Israel's Jewish/Islamic social structure, the fact that so many of its elderly are Holocaust survivors, and that it is a country of immigration makes it an interesting natural gerontological laboratory.

KEY REFERENCES

- Brodsky J & Clarfield AM. An overview of home health care in Israel. *Journal of the American Medical Directors Association* 2001; **2**:264–8.
- Clarfield AM. Care of the elderly in Israel: present and future. *Clinical Geriatrics* 2000; **8**:29–37.
- Clarfield AM, Bergman H & Kane R. Fragmentation of care for the frail elderly – experience from three countries: Israel, Canada and the United States. *Journal of the American Geriatrics Society* 2001; **49**:1714–21.
- Clarfield AM, Paltiel A, Gindin Y *et al.* Country profile: Israel. *Journal of the American Geriatrics Society* 2000; **48**:980–4.
- Clarfield AM, Rosenberg E, Brodsky J & Bentur N. Healthy aging around the world: Israel too? *The Israel Medical Association Journal* 2004; **6**:516–20.

REFERENCES

Azaiza F & Brodsky J. The aging of Israel's Arab population: needs, existing responses and dilemmas in the development of services for a society in transition. *The Israel Medical Association Journal* 2003; **5**:383–6.

Beer S & Brodsky J. The elderly in Israel – population, disability rates and needs estimates for selected services: 1999–2010. *Reprint Series from 2001–2005 JDC-Eshel Seventh Five-Year Plan. Mashav – Planning for the Elderly – A National Data Base* 2002; JDC-Brookdale and ESHEL, Jerusalem [Hebrew].

Bentur N, Brodsky J & Habot B. *Complex Nursing Care Patients in the Geriatric Hospitalization System: A Prevalence Survey* 1996; JDC-Brookdale Institute of Gerontology, Jerusalem #RR:257–296.

Brodsky J, Be'er S & Schnoor Y. *Holocaust Survivors in Israel: Current and Projected Needs for Home Nursing Care* 2003; JDC-Brookdale Institute and National Insurance Institute, Jerusalem.

Brodsky J & Clarfield AM. An overview of home health care in Israel. *Journal of the American Medical Directors Association* 2001; **2**:264–8.

Brodsky J, Schnoor Y & Be'er S (eds) The Elderly in Israel The 2003 statistical abstract. *Mashav – Planning for the Elderly – A National Data Base* 2004; Myers-JCD Brookdale Institute and ESHEL, Jerusalem. (also available at: www.jdc.org.il/mashav).

Chinitz D. Israel's health policy breakthrough: the politics of reforms and the reform of politics. *Journal of Health Politics, Policy and Law* 1995; **20**:909–32.

Clarfield AM. Care of the elderly in Israel: present and future. *Clinical Geriatrics* 2000; **8**:29–37.

Clarfield AM, Bergman H & Kane R. Fragmentation of care for the frail elderly – experience from three countries: Israel, Canada and the United States. *Journal of the American Geriatrics Society* 2001; **49**:1714–21.

Clarfield AM, Gordon M, Markwell H & Alibhai S. Ethical Issues in end-of-life geriatric care; the approach of three monotheistic religions: Judaism, Catholicism and Islam. *Journal of the American Geriatrics Society* 2003; **51**:1149–54.

Clarfield AM, Paltiel A, Gindin Y *et al.* Country profile: Israel. *Journal of the American Geriatrics Society* 2000; **48**:980–4.

Clarfield AM, Rosenberg E, Brodsky J & Bentur N. Healthy aging around the world: Israel too? *The Israel Medical Association Journal* 2004; **6**:516–20.

Clarfield AM, Monette J, Bergman H *et al.* *Enteral Feeding in End-Stage Dementia: A Comparison of Religious, Ethnic and National Differences in Canada and Israel* 2005; British Geriatrics Society (Abstract), Birmingham, UK.

David P & Pelly S (eds). *Caring for Aging Holocaust Survivors: A Practical Manual* 2003; Baycrest Centre for Geriatric Care, Toronto.

Marcus EL, Clarfield AM & Moses AE. Ethical issues relating to the use of antimicrobial therapy in older adults. *Clinical Infectious Disease* 2001; **33**:1697–705.

Menczel J & Marcus EL. Osteoporosis among holocaust survivors. *Revista Espanola de Geriatria y Gerontologia* 2003; **38**(suppl 1):1–77. [abstract 95]

Naon D & Strosberg N. *The Impact of the Community Long-Term Care Insurance Law on Patterns of Institutionalization* 1995; JDC-Brookdale Institute of Gerontology, Jerusalem.

Nire N. *The Employment of Immigrant Physicians from the Former Soviet Union in 1998: Summary of Findings from a Follow-Up Study* 1999; Myers-JDC – Brookdale Institute, Jerusalem. [Hebrew]

The National Institute for Health Policy and Health Services Research, Health Services under the responsibility of the State: Health Promotion and Prevention, Institutional Nursing Care and Mental Health, *Conference Report: Health Services Under the Responsibility of the Ministry of Health*, Dead Sea, June 2002; [Hebrew]

World Health Organization *The World Health Report 2004 – Changing History* 2004; World Health Organisation, Geneva.

165

Geriatric Medicine in China

Leung-Wing Chu

University of Hong Kong and Hong Kong West Cluster Geriatrics Service, Queen Mary Hospital, Fung Yiu King Hospital, Tung Wah Hospital and Grantham Hospital, Hong Kong

INTRODUCTION

The Elderly Population in China

In the past 50 years, China has made great achievements in controlling infectious diseases and improving public health. A direct indicator is the demographic transition from a young population into an aging population. The proportion of elderly people aged 60 and above has already crossed 10% in the year 1999. In the 5th National Population Census of 31 provinces, autonomous regions, and municipalities of mainland China in November 2000, the population was 1 265 830 000. There were 88 110 000 elderly persons aged 65 and over. This represents 7% of the population. The average life expectancy at birth is 69.6 years for males and 73.3 years for females. (Tables 1, 2, and 3) (National Bureau Statistics of China, 2004).

There are several special features regarding population aging in China. The number of elderly people in China is huge and represents 20% of the world's elderly population and 50% of the Asian elderly population. The growth in the elderly population is rapid. From 1982 to 1999, the proportion of elderly persons aged 60 and above increased from 7.64 to 10.1%. Such a demographic transition occurred within 18 years in China, whereas the same change takes a few decades in the developed western countries. China has now moved into an accelerated phase of population aging and is becoming an aging society in an underdeveloped economy. While the western countries have become both "old" and "rich", China has become "old" before getting "rich". This constitutes a burden to the economic growth. Another characteristic is the regional differences in the demographic transition. Population aging occurs more rapidly in the developed coastal cities than the underdeveloped inner rural areas within China. The urban cities showed higher proportions of elderly people than the rural areas. For example, Shanghai has the highest percentage while Qinghai province has the lowest percentage of elderly persons. Among the subgroups of the elderly population, the growth of the oldest-old population (aged 80 and above) is fast and at a rate of 5.4% per year. The oldest-old population in China has increased from 8 millions in 1990 to 11 millions in 2000 and will become 27.8 millions in 2020 (Lee, 2004; National Bureau Statistics of China, 2004). With an aging population, the prevalence of chronic diseases which include diabetes mellitus, hypertension, stroke, coronary heart disease, and chronic obstructive pulmonary disease has increased. For example, 1.5 million patients are newly diagnosed with stroke every year in China. Heavy medical expenses are required, and these diseases constitute an important burden of disease for China. Although the life expectancy of women is higher than men, the number of healthy elderly women is lower than that of healthy elderly men. Women survive longer, but are less healthy than men (Du and Guo, 2000; Lee, 2004; Ministry of Health of China, 2004; National Bureau Statistics of China, 2004; Woo *et al.*, 2002). The birth control and one-child policy has a great impact on the family size in China (Festini and de Martino, 2004). The size of the Chinese family has decreased from four- to five-person households to three- to four-person households in recent years. Family size is big in rural areas and small in city areas. This trend has been affecting the foundation of traditional family support of the elderly people in China.

As formal aged care services are quite limited, many older persons would mainly require their family members to support them. This is particularly true in rural areas. The functions of family support include financial support (income security), care-giving tasks (physical care) and comforting tasks (psychological care). Most of the younger persons in China still largely maintain that taking care of the elderly family members is their responsibility. However, more and more young people are unable to provide all the family support functions, and would require some assistance from the government, the policy makers, and community service providers (Du and Guo, 2000; Woo *et al.*, 2002).

Principles and Practice of Geriatric Medicine, 4th Edition. Edited by M.S. John Pathy, Alan J. Sinclair and John E. Morley.

Table 1 China population in 2000

	Mainland China (1 November 2000; 5th National Population Census)	Hong Kong SAR (30 June 2000)	Macau SAR 30 (September 2000)	Taiwan (December 2000)
Total population	1 265 830 000	6 780 000	440 000 441 600 (2002)	22 280 000 22 605 000 (Dec. 2003)
Number of elderly (65 years and over)	8 811 000	745 800	34 003 (2002)	1 895 000
% of elderly (65 years and over)	6.96% (increase by 1.39% compared with 1990 Census)	11%	7.7% (2002)	8.52%
Average life expectancy at birth, years	All = 71.4 Male = 69.6 Female = 73.3	Male = 78.2 Female = 84.1 (2001)	Male = 76.2 Female = 80.2 (2001) 78.6 for all (2002)	Male = 72.6 Female = 78.3

Note: Population of China in 2000: (including mainland China, Hong Kong SAR, Macau SAR, and Taiwan) was 1 295 330 000.

Table 2 China major cities' population in 2000

	Beijing (2000)	Shanghai (2000)	Hong Kong SAR (30 June 2000)
Total population	13 819 000	16 737 700	6 780 000 6 724 900 (2001)
Number of elderly (65 years and over)	1 155 000	1 924 836 (3 06 049 aged 80+ years)	745 800
% of elderly (65 years and over)	8.4% (increase by 2.1% compared with 1990 Census)	11.5% (65+: increase by 2.1% compared with 1990 Census; 80+ increase by 2.2% compared with 1990 Census)	11.1%

Table 3 Declining birth and death rates in mainland China

	Mainland China (Overall)		Beijing		Shanghai	
Year	Natural birth rate (per 1000 pop.)	Natural death rate (per 1000 pop.)	Natural birth rate (per 1000 pop.)	Natural death rate (per 1000 pop.)	Natural birth rate (per 1000 pop.)	Natural death rate (per 1000 pop.)
1949	36	20	–	–	–	–
1970	33.43	7.6	–	–	–	–
1980	18.21	6.34	–	–	–	–
1990	21.06	6.67	13.35	5.43	11.32	6.36
2001	13.38	6.43	6.1	5.3	5.02	5.97
2002	12.86	6.41	6.6	5.7	5.41	5.95
2003	12.41	6.40	–	–	–	–

Note: Natural Death Rate = Crude Death Rate

The Elderly Population in Hong Kong SAR, Macau SAR, and Taiwan

In 2004, 0.82 million persons in Hong Kong were elderly people aged 65 and over, which represented 11.7% of the total Hong Kong population. The proportion of the Hong Kong elderly will increase to 24% by the year 2031 (Census and Statistics Department HKSAR, 2002a). This increase will place an enormous demand for long-term care and health-care services for the elderly. The aging demographic change is related to a decrease in the number of births in Hong Kong (Census and Statistics Department HKSAR, 2002a; Chow and Chi, 1997; Chow, 2000; Hospital Authority HKSAR, 2003a; Hospital Authority HKSAR, 2003b). The elderly dependency ratio which is defined as the number of persons aged 65 years and over per 1000 persons aged between 15 and 64 years will increase from 382 in 2001 to 562 in 2031. The average life expectancy at birth was 78.2 years for Hong Kong men and 84.1 years for women in 2001 (Tables 1,2, and 4). Closely related to the health-care needs of the elderly is their life expectancy at and above 60 years. At the age of 60, the average life expectancy was 21.4 years for men and 26.0 years for women in 2001, and at the age of 80, the average life expectancy was 8.1 years and 10.6 years for men and women respectively. The increased life expectancy is related to the improvement in public health and nutrition, and is also related to an improved medical care for very elderly patients (Census and Statistics Department HKSAR, 2002b; Chow and Chi, 1997; Chow, 2000; Hospital Authority HKSAR, 2003a; Hospital Authority HKSAR, 2003b). However, improved survival may not mean normal health without disability or functional improvement.

Table 4 Declining birth and death rates in Hong Kong SAR, Macau SAR, and Taiwan

	Hong Kong SAR		Macau SAR		Taiwan	
Year	Natural birth rate (per 1000 pop.)	Natural death rate (per 1000 pop.)	Natural birth rate (per 1000 pop.)	Natural death rate (per 1000 pop.)	Natural birth rate (per 1000 pop.)	Natural death rate (per 1000 pop.)
1946	20.1	20.1	–	–	–	–
1956	37.0	37.0	–	–	–	–
1966	25.5	25.5	–	–	–	–
1976	16.9	16.9	–	–	–	–
1986	13.1	13.1	–	–	–	–
1990	12.0	5.2	20.5	4.4	15.5	5.6
1995	11.2	5.1	14.1	3.2	13.8	5.7
2000	8.1	5.1	8.8	3.1	11.7	5.7
2002	7.1	5.0	7.2	3.2	11.0	5.7
2003	6.9	5.4	–	–	–	–

Note: Natural Death Rate = Crude Death Rate

Elderly persons have multiple chronic diseases, functional impairments, and need for regular medical services (Chu *et al.*, 1998; Woo *et al.*, 1997).

Macau SAR is a small city of China. It has a population of 0.44 million people. The crude birth and death rates are both falling over the past decade and the population is also aging. In 2002, the elderly aged 65 and above constituted 7.7% of its population. The average life expectancy at birth for males and females are 76.2 years and 80.2 years respectively. (Tables 1 and 4) (Macau SAR Government, 2004).

Taiwan has also experienced a rapid demographic transition. The fertility rate has decreased from 5.9 children per woman in 1949 to 1.77 in 1997. Thus, the ratio of adult children to older parents will fall greatly in the coming years. A decline in the death rate has resulted in an increase of the average life expectancy at birth. From the year 1951 to 1998, the average life expectancy at birth has increased from 53.4 years to 72.0 years for males, and from 56.3 years to 77.9 years for females. These changes have led to an increase of the elderly persons (aged 65 and over) from 2.5% in 1950 to 8.1% in 1997. By projection, this percentage will increase to 9.86% in 2010 and 13.83% in 2020. The increase of the oldest-old group (i.e. 80 years and over) within the elderly population is very fast. In 1960, 9.2% of the elderly population belonged to the oldest-old group. By 2036, almost one-quarter (23.8%) of the elderly population will be in the oldest-old group (Barlett and Wu, 2000) (Tables 1 and 4).

POLICIES TOWARD AGING IN MAINLAND CHINA

Officially, the basic principle in China's aging policy is to maintain sustainable development by setting up a partnership of elderly support system involving the state, the community, the family, and the individual. The priorities in meeting the challenge of population aging in China are to develop China's economy, to set up an old age security system, to speed up the establishment of community-based old age care system, to set up legislative system in order to protect the rights of the elderly (i.e. the Law of Protecting the Rights of the Elderly of the People's Republic of China was enacted in 1996), to establish safety networks for the elderly, to raise the living standards of the elderly and to create an environment for healthy aging. In the past decade, China has set up five principles as the guidance for the work on aging. The principles are "Elderly people should be supported, have medical care, be contributive to the society, be engaged in life-long learning, and live a happy life". In 1994, the China Development Outline on the Work of Aging was formulated with a view to gradually upgrade the living standard of the elderly and to enrich their cultural life (Liang, 1995).

HEALTH OF THE ELDERLY IN MAINLAND CHINA AND HONG KONG SAR

In mainland China, the top killer diseases in the year 2003 included cancer, cerebrovascular diseases, respiratory diseases, heart diseases and injuries, and poisoning. Chronic diseases included hypertension, cerebrovascular diseases, and coronary heart disease. Diabetes mellitus is more common in the urban city areas than in the rural areas (Ministry of Health of China, 2004) (Table 5). All these fatal and chronic diseases occur predominantly in the elderly persons.

In the Hong Kong SAR, the top killer diseases in the elderly include cancer, heart diseases, and pneumonia while the chronic diseases include arthritis, hypertension, and diabetes mellitus (Chiu *et al.*, 1998; Chu *et al.*, 1998; Chu *et al.*, 2005; Lau and Lok, 1997; Leung and Lo, 1997; Woo *et al.*, 1997) (Table 6).

Health-care Services in Mainland China

China's health-care delivery system is organized in a three-tiered fashion. In the urban areas, this consists of street health stations, community health centers, and district hospitals. In the economically less developed rural areas, village stations, township health centers, and county hospitals are responsible

Table 5 Causes of death and common chronic diseases in China (all ages) (2003)

City	County
Top killer diseases in 2003:	Top killer diseases in 2003:
Male	*Male*
1. Cancer	1. Cancer
2. Cerebrovascular diseases (stroke)	2. Cerebrovascular diseases (stroke)
3. Respiratory diseases	3. Respiratory diseases
4. Heart diseases (incl. HT heart disease)	4. Heart diseases (incl. HT heart disease)
5. Injury and poisoning	5. Injury and poisoning
6. Diseases of the digestive system	6. Diseases of the digestive system
7. Endocrine, nutrition, and metabolic diseases (e.g. Diabetes mellitus (DM))	7. Endocrine, nutrition, and metabolic diseases (e.g. Diabetes mellitus (DM))
8. Kidney diseases (Nephritis, nephrotic syndrome, etc.)	8. Kidney diseases (Nephritis, nephrotic syndrome, etc.)
Female	*Female*
1. Cancer	1. Cerebrovascular diseases (stroke)
2. Cerebrovascular diseases (stroke)	2. Respiratory diseases
3. Respiratory diseases	3. Cancer
4. Heart diseases (incl. HT heart disease)	4. Heart diseases (incl. HT heart disease)
5. Injury and poisoning	5. Injury and poisoning
6. Endocrine, nutrition, and metabolic diseases (e.g. Diabetes mellitus (DM))	6. Diseases of the digestive system
7. Diseases of the digestive system	7. Endocrine, nutrition, and metabolic diseases (e.g. Diabetes mellitus (DM))
8. Kidney diseases (Nephritis, nephrotic syndrome, etc.)	8. Kidney diseases (Nephritis, nephrotic syndrome, etc.)
Common chronic diseases:	*Common chronic diseases:*
1. Hypertension (54.7%)	1. Hypertension (16.4%)
2. Diabetes mellitus (16.3%)	2. Gastroenteritis (10.5%)
3. Cerebrovascular diseases (13.0%)	3. Rheumatoid arthritis (8.7%)
4. Coronary heart disease (12.4%)	4. Chronic obstructive airway disease (7.3%)
5. Rheumatoid arthritis (8.4%)	5. Choleltih and cholecystitis (4.7%)
6. Gastroenteritis (9.8%)	6. Cerebrovascular diseases (4.4%)
7. Choleltih and cholecystitis (8.5%)	7. Intervertebral disc disease (4.0%)
8. Chronic obstructive airway disease (8.2%)	8. Peptic ulcers (3.8%)
9. Intervertebral disc disease (8.1%)	9. Coronary heart disease (2.0%)
10. Peptic ulcers (3.4%)	10. Diabetes mellitus (1.9%)

Note: Ministry of Health of China, 2004.

Table 6 Mortality and morbidity of the elderly in Hong Kong

Leading causes of death in the elderly in 2001:

1. Cancer
2. Heart diseases (incl. HT heart disease)
3. Pneumonia
4. Cerebrovascular diseases (stroke)
5. Chronic lower respiratory disease
6. Kidney diseases (Nephritis, nephrotic syndrome, etc.)
7. Diabetes mellitus (DM)
8. Injury and poisoning

Common chronic diseases:

1. Arthritis (34.2–61.4%)
2. Hypertension (32–33%)
3. Fracture (17.1%)
4. Peptic ulcers (13.5–15.4%)
5. Diabetes mellitus (10.7–12.4%)
6. Coronary heart disease (8.6–14.3%)
7. Hyperlipidemia (7.4%)
8. Dementia (6.1%)
9. Hyperthyroidism (6.1%)
10. Chronic obstructive airway disease (6.0–8.2%)
11. Stroke (3.8–6.3%)
12. Asthma (3.0%)

Note: Chiu *et al.*, 1998; Chu *et al.*, 1998; Chu *et al.*, 2005; Lau and Lok, 1997; Leung and Lo, 1997; Woo *et al.*, 1997.

for the health-care delivery. The doctors in the village stations receive only three to six months of training (i.e. not formal medical school training) after junior high school and receive an average of two to three weeks continuing education every year. Township health centers usually have 10 to 20 beds and are looked after by a physician with three years of medical school education after high school. They are assisted by assistant physicians and village doctors. County hospitals usually have 250 to 300 beds and are staffed by physicians with four to five years of medical training after high school. They are assisted by nurses and technicians (China Medical Association, 2004; Editorial Committee of China Health Annual, 2003; Ministry of Health of China, 2004).

The health-care cost for the elderly is an important problem for the poor and those in rural areas. If they cannot afford the cost of health-care, they will be denied access to care. In the olden days, the rural Cooperative Medical System (CMS) schemes primarily provided funding and organized prevention, primary care, and secondary health care for the rural population. After 1950, a mutual assistance mechanism was established to provide access to basic drugs and primary health care. During the Cultural Revolution (1966–1976), the CMS was given political priority. The rural CMS then organized health stations, paid village doctors to deliver primary health care, provided drugs, and partially reimbursed patients for services received at township centers and county hospitals. China's relative success in extending health care to the rural population has played a key role in improving the health status of the population. However, CMS suffered from problems of poor management and a small risk-pooling base, contributing to the downfall of these early cooperative financing schemes after the initiation of agricultural reforms in 1980. The CMS has disintegrated in most rural areas and currently fewer than 10% of China's villages have CMS. In addition, many village doctors have left for farming or become private practitioners. Township health centers and county hospitals are largely financed by fee-for-service and out-of-pocket payment. Access to health care in many areas is now principally governed by the ability to pay for it and not the need for health care. Many of the elderly persons in villages will become bankrupt if they have a major illness and have to be hospitalized. For example, the cost of an average hospitalization would exceed the average annual income of 50% of the rural population. At present, the insurance coverage level of the primarily village-based community financing schemes in rural areas is severely limited. Poverty after an illness and the related treatment expenses continue to be a serious problem for the rural elderly as most of them are poor. Therefore, they are often deprived of the needed medical care because of the inability to pay. Regarding the rural CMS, reform is needed. In May 1997, the State Council issued a special document emphasizing that CMS reform is a major direction for China's rural health reform (China Medical Association, 2004).

For elderly persons who are retired government officials or workers from large corporations, the health-care cost will be paid from either the Government Insurance Scheme (GIS) or Labor Insurance Scheme (LIS), which have been effective in ensuring equity of access to health care. In urban areas, GIS and LIS will pay for the health-care cost for most elderly persons. Exceptions are those who do not belong to these two groups, they have to be financed by fee-for-service and out-of-pocket payment. Access to health care for these persons is determined by their ability to pay. In recent years, the government and other enterprises are facing increasing difficulty in supporting GIS and LIS medical expenditures. With the rapid introduction of high-technology medical services, increasing incomes drive up the demand for health care. Without an effective controlling mechanism on the medical service consumers or providers, China now faces a serious problem of inflation in medical costs. The primary weaknesses of GIS and LIS programs are the relative inefficiency in health resource allocation and health-care provisions as well as the lack of risk pooling across enterprises or across local governments. Each organization under GIS and LIS systems is self-insured. If an enterprise is running a deficit, it will not be able to reimburse the medical expenses of the employee or the retired elderly employee, rendering the individual uninsured (Woo *et al.*, 2002; China Medical Association, 2004).

Health care for the elderly needs governmental provision and support. However, the distribution of health-care resources including health-care professionals in China is very uneven. Geographical variations exist between cities and rural areas as well as coastal and inland areas in China. The gap is still growing with 80% of health-care resources allocated to the cities, out of which two-thirds are allocated to big hospitals. Primary health-care organizations and rural areas are severely insufficient. The rate of health-care utilization is very low, which is largely related to inadequate supply and access. The level of health-care resources in megacities like Beijing and Shanghai may match those in developed countries. However, primary health care is not adequately developed. The charging system for health-care is by insurance from government for government officials and employees of large companies. These are also applicable to retired older persons who have previously worked in government institutes or major companies. Ordinary elderly people without these insurance support have to pay the medical costs out of their own pockets. The financial subsidy policy of the government is usually not available and this is not reasonable (Lee, 2004).

Health-care financing reforms have started in some pilot cities recently. In 1994, Jiujiang in Jiangxi Province and Zhenjiang in Jiangsu Province were selected as pilot reform cities. A combination of individual saving account and social risk pooling forms the basis for the financing of medical expenditures. This model emphasizes individual responsibility with social protection through citywide risk pooling for GIS and LIS. These reforms have met with some success in controlling the escalation in medical costs and in expanding coverage to those who were previously uninsured or underinsured. This was a successful experience. In 1996, it was decided that the pilot scheme is to be extended to over fifty cities in 27 provinces and administrative regions (China Medical Association, 2004).

Community Health Services for the Elderly in China

According to the Chinese National Committee on Aging, China has limited resources to set up comprehensive facilities to meet the increasing needs of the elderly. However, community service is found to be an attractive way to complement the role of the family in caring for the elderly persons. Over the past decade, there has been a great development in community service. By 1997, there were 930 000 community service facilities, 5055 community centers and 1.01 million community service stations in the whole country – urban and rural areas. 85% of these facilities primarily serve the elderly persons in the local community. 5.4 million volunteers have provided service. The community service embraces several groups of service providers including care services for daily living (e.g. home help, lunch, household work, shopping, escort etc), cultural activities (e.g. activity centers, life-long learning, universities of third age), legal assistance (i.e. when the legal right of an elderly member is violated), and day care services. Day care services are provided by either home for the elderly or day care centers. The latter also provide simple medical services like clinical checkup, intravenous saline treatment (as "health maintenance"), and family hospital beds. The medical service components are derived from the earlier street health stations and community health centers in the urban areas. "Doctors" in these centers usually receive basic training only and do not have formal geriatric medicine training (Zhang, 2003).

GERIATRIC MEDICINE IN CHINA AND HONG KONG SAR

Geriatric medicine has been defined as a branch of general medicine that deals with the clinical, rehabilitative, psychosocial, and preventive aspects of illness in elderly people. Despite an emphasis on the impact of the aging population, geriatric medicine has not been developed in China yet. Traditionally, there is a group of doctors who practice "Geriatrics" in China. They are responsible for the delivery of medical care to "old" and senior government officials in China. Most of these doctors are well trained and specialized in one particular organ-based specialty (e.g. cardiology, respiratory medicine, neurology). Their training and clinical practice in "geriatrics" in mainland China are different from geriatricians in other parts of the world. Their research works are primarily targeted at an organ-based approach which includes cardiac diseases in the elderly, dementia, osteoporosis, biological mechanisms of aging, and antiaging drugs. However, there is a lack of research in geriatric syndromes like falls or clinical models of geriatrics care for older persons.

MEDICAL EDUCATION AND TRAINING PROGRAMS IN GERIATRIC MEDICINE AND GERONTOLOGY

As the absolute number and the proportion of the elderly population in China increase progressively, services for the elderly would become a combined effort of the elderly individual, family members, professionals, and lay persons in Chinese society. Professional care in geriatric medicine and gerontology has an important role to play in any aging society. There is a great need to provide education and training programs in geriatric medicine and gerontology for doctors, nurses, social workers, and allied health professionals. This is grossly inadequate in China. There is only one undergraduate educational program on social gerontology at the tertiary education level at the People's University of China, which was started in 1994 (Du and Guo, 2000).

The curriculum of basic undergraduate medical training in the medical schools of China includes both the general and the shorter special diploma curricula. The duration of the general comprehensive curriculum is of 5 years usually, but may be 6 to 7 years in some schools. In terms of scope, these are comparable to primary medical training in other countries. In 1999, there were 21 university-based medical schools and 69 independent medical schools (Higher Education Office of China Ministry of Education, 2004).

High-school graduates may also study the special diploma programs, with training that usually last for 4 years. These medical programs are not comprehensive in training and each of them would focus on a special area only (e.g. oral health, hygiene, child health, physiology, pharmacology, chemistry, clinical medicine, physics, basic medical sciences, Chinese medicine, preventive medicine, medical imaging, acupuncture etc.). In 1999, there were 20 medical diploma schools and 15 colleges with medical diploma courses (Higher Education Office of China Ministry of Education, 2004).

Geriatric Medicine Educational Program in Mainland China

As described previously, geriatric medicine has been defined as a branch of general medicine that deals with the clinical, rehabilitative, psychosocial, and preventive aspects of illness in elderly people. Education in Geriatric medicine is lacking in most medical schools. In the undergraduate medical training in China, teaching of geriatric medicine is included in the curriculum of only 2.9% of the medical schools. Most doctors in China are not equipped with knowledge in geriatric medicine when they graduate from medical schools. This policy is not in keeping with the need of the aging population in mainland China and is different from many parts of the world. In Hong Kong SAR, United Kingdom, Europe, and other developed countries, geriatric medicine is included in the core teaching of the undergraduate medical curriculum. In the United States, 60% of medical schools have included geriatric medicine in the core or compulsory modules, while 40% has included this as an optional module (Higher Education Office of China Ministry of Education, 2004).

In mainland China, there is as yet no formal clinical postgraduate educational program for doctors or allied health professionals in geriatric medicine. This indicates that although China has paid great attention to family planning and population control, the university education system has not changed and prepared for the need of an aging society. Compared to the widespread availability of postgraduate medical training in geriatric medicine in overseas countries like United Kingdom, United States, Canada, Europe, New Zealand, and Australia, the absence of educational training program in geriatric medicine should be rectified (Chow and Chi, 1997; Chow, 2000; Chu and Lam, 1997; Higher Education Office of China Ministry of Education, 2004; Hong Kong College of Physicians, 2002; Woo *et al.*, 2002). China should establish the field of geriatric medicine and gerontology in the university training system at the undergraduate and graduate school levels.

Specialty status for doctors in China primarily follows their research degrees (e.g. master and Ph.D. degrees) as well as their publications in those specialty areas (e.g. geriatric cardiology, osteoporosis, basic science in aging mechanism, dementia). There is no formal clinical specialist training for physicians in a subspecialty (e.g. cardiology, neurology, or geriatric medicine). Thus, most professors in current geriatric departments in China usually have a research interest in diseases which are prevalent in old age (Luk, 2000; Zhu, 1993).

The Chinese Geriatrics Society has been publishing the Chinese Journal of Geriatrics since 1982. The papers published in the journal can be categorized into disease-based research findings, biological mechanisms of aging, and anti-aging interventions. There is a lack of publication on clinical geriatrics services, geriatric assessment, models of geriatric care and interdisciplinary interventions. The summary report of the fourth committee meeting of the Chinese Geriatrics Society of the Chinese Medical Association emphasizes mainly research works on aging, antiaging, antiaging drugs, longevity, geriatric cardiology, geriatric respiratory diseases, dementia and molecular biology, and so on. The report also describes future problems, which included epidemiology research in diseases in the elderly, basic science research, clinical research on common geriatric diseases and health promotion (Wong, 1999). Unfortunately, problems due to the lack of clinical service in geriatric medicine and the need to train specialists in geriatric medicine in China are not yet realized. The current trend of continued development of pure organ-based specialists to look after frail geriatric patients who have multiple problems would be detrimental to the quality of care and the health-care cost in most geriatric patients. This will perpetuate fragmentation of care, neglect of atypical presentations of diseases in the elderly, unnecessary investigations, iatrogenesis related to the duplication of drugs and potential interactions related to multiple medical care providers.

Clinical Service in Geriatric Medicine

Geriatric departments have existed in China for a long time. The traditional role of doctors in these departments is to provide hospital care for senior government officials (working or retired). The doctors with specialty skills in this group may range from neurologist, cardiologist, intensive care physicians, urologist, and so on. The focus is still on organ-based hospital specialists. This is very different from the practice of geriatric medicine in other parts of the world (Chu and Lam, 1997; Fox and Puxty, 1993; Hall and Rowe, 1998; Isaacs, 1992; Lindsay and Barker, 1998; Swift, 1998). (*See also* **Chapter 161, Health and Care for Older People in the United Kingdom**; **Chapter 162, Geriatrics in the United States**; **Chapter 163, Geriatrics and Gerontology in Japan**; **Chapter 164, Care of the Elderly in Israel: Old Age in a Young Land**) The principles of geriatric assessment and interdisciplinary intervention are not practiced. Geriatric rehabilitation is also not available in clinical service programs of these departments.

THE HEALTH AND LONG-TERM CARE SYSTEM FOR THE ELDERLY IN HONG KONG SAR

All Hong Kong citizens are entitled to have inexpensive health- and social care services. Moreover, for those who are on Comprehensive Social Security Allowance (CSSA) Scheme, the service fees are waived. The latter scenario is very common among frail elderly patients in the hospitals. Together with an escalating health-care cost and an aging demography, the Hospital Authority (HA) is now having an annual budget deficit of HK$601 million (Hospital Authority HKSAR, 2004a).

The Social Welfare Department (SWD) has all along been responsible for the policy and funding of social services. At present, the social services for the elderly are categorized into community support (nonresidential) and residential care services for the elderly (Social Welfare Department HKSAR, 2004). In the past, long-term care services for the elderly referred primarily to residential care services, which are largely provided by the Nongovernmental Organizations (NGOs). Over the past decade, the private old age home industry has been developing rapidly and private old age homes now form the main service group for residential care of the elderly in Hong Kong. Meals delivery and personal care services are the key nonresidential home care services available to the elderly living in their own homes. The great demand for long-term residential care services has been a problem for many years and the magnitude of this problem is on the increase. At present, institutional care is quite commonly utilized and approximately 8% of the elderly in Hong Kong now resides in residential care homes for the elderly (RCHEs) and the hospital infirmary (Social Welfare Department HKSAR, 2004; Hospital Authority HKSAR, 2004b). The majority of the RCHEs in Hong Kong are the low-quality private old age homes, and a minority are government-funded care and attention homes and self-financing homes.

HISTORY OF DEVELOPMENT OF GERIATRIC MEDICINE IN HONG KONG SAR

On the basis of the British model, Hong Kong established its first geriatric unit in 1975. In the initial 10 years, the development of geriatric medicine was slow. However, in recent years, the importance of geriatric service to the elderly community has been gradually recognized. At present, there is at least one geriatric service per hospital cluster (Tables 7 and 8).

LACK OF A SYSTEMATIC APPROACH IN ACUTE GERIATRICS CARE IN HONG KONG SAR

The fundamental and serious problem in the present organization of hospital care for the elderly is a lack of systematic approach in the acute care for the elderly. While

Table 7 Geriatric service in Hong Kong Hospital authority by hospital clusters

Year	Cluster	Hospital	Unit/Ward/Team
1994	Hong Kong	Queen Mary Hospital (QMH)	Geriatric Team
1994	(HK) West	Fung Yiu King Hospital (FYKH)	Geriatric Department
2002		Tung Wah Hospital (TWH)	Geriatric Team
2004		Grantham Hospital (GH)	Geriatric Department
1990	Hong Kong	Rutonjee and Tang Siu Kin Hospitals (RTSKH)	Geriatric Department
1995	(HK) East	Pamela Youde Nethersole Hospital (PYNEH)	Geriatric Team
1996		Tung Wah East Hospital (TWEH)	Geriatric Team
1995		Wong Chuk Hang Hospital (WCHH)	Geriatric Department
1995		Saint John Hospital (SJH)	Geriatric Department
1996		Cheshire Home Chung Hom Kok (CCH)	Geriatric Team
1974	Kowloon East	United Christian Hospital (UCH)	Geriatric Ward
2000		Tseung Kwan O Hospital (TKOH)	Geriatric Team
1991		Haven of Hope Hospital (HOHH)	Geriatric and Rehabilitation Unit
1975	Kowloon West	Princess Margaret Hospital (PMH)	First formal Geriatric Department
1978		Caritas Medical Center (CMC)	Geriatric Department
1982		Kwong Wah Hospital (KWH)	Geriatric Unit
1994		Yan Chai Hospital (YCH)	Geriatric Team
1995		Our Lady of Maryknoll Hospital (OLMH)	Geriatric Team
1995		Wong Tai Sin Hospital (WTSH)	
1993	Kowloon Central	Queen Elizabeth Hospital (QEH)	Geriatric Team
1995		Kowloon Hospital (KH)	Geriatric and Rehabilitation Unit
2003		Buddhist Hospital (BH)	Geriatric Team
1985	New Territories	Prince of Wales Hospital (PWH)	Geriatric Team
2001	(NT) East	Shatin Hospital (SH)	Geriatric Unit
1997		Alice Ho Miu Ling Nethersole Hospital (AHMLNH)	Geriatric Team
1998		Tai Po Hospital (TPH)	Geriatric Team
1990	New Territories (NT) West	Tuen Mun Hospital (TMH)	Geriatric Department

Table 8 Geriatric services in the Hong Kong West Hospital Cluster

Acute hospital care	QMH (Integrated Model) GH (Direct transfer from Emergency Room)
Convalescent care	FYKH TWH GH
Geriatric rehabilitation beds	FYKH TWH GH
Long-stay infirmary beds for geriatric patients	FYKH TWH
Predischarge program and post-discharge support	QMH, TWH, FYKH, GH
Geriatric Day Hospital as day rehabilitation center	FYKH TWH
Geriatric Specialist Clinics	QMH Geriatric Specialist Outpatient Department QMH Memory Clinic QMH Falls Clinic QMH Nutrition Clinic FYKH Continence Clinic
Hong Kong West (HKW)	Outreach Geriatric Doctor Clinics in over 60 old age homes (Subvented Care and Attention homes, private old age homes, day care centers)
Community Geriatric Assessment Team (CGAT)	Visiting Medical Officer (VMO) under CGAT-VMO program Central Infirmary Waiting List (CIWL) clients preadmission assessment Domiciliary visits – medical, nursing, physiotherapy, and occupational therapy Educational and training program to carers and community elders Health education programs with community partners

a multidisciplinary, multidimensional geriatric assessment is frequently practiced in the extended care hospital, there is a general lack of acute geriatrics service in most acute care hospitals in Hong Kong. At present, only three out of 14 acute care hospitals have designated acute geriatric wards in the whole of Hong Kong (Table 7).

The number of elderly in the acute care hospitals is a huge case load. To be cost-effective, acute care for the elderly has to be focused. To attain a cost-effective health-care model, targeting of the frail elderly patients in the acute geriatrics care program is necessary. The targeted geriatric patients would be physically, cognitively, and/or psychosocially frail. The settings of screening geriatric assessment would be at the sites where the frail elderly are present (i.e. medical, surgical, and orthopedic, and emergency room settings). Concurrent with acute treatment of the presenting medical diseases, geriatric assessment and intervention should be started simultaneously to prevent and revert functional decline.

The unit for development of acute care for the elderly should include several core elements of acute care for the elderly in its program: targeting of frail elders (i.e. in the emergency department, general medical, orthopedic, neurosurgical, and surgical wards with particular attention to those elderly who are residents from old age homes), comprehensive geriatric assessment, case-based conference by interdisciplinary team, and intervention. The interdisciplinary management should include a "Prehab" program to prevent functional decline with an appropriately designed acute care ward environment and then a "Rehab" program to revert functional decline and improve activity of daily living. Discharge planning (i.e. predischarge planning and postdischarge support with appropriate placement) with a case management approach should be implemented. Clinical outcomes must be optimized while unnecessary hospital admissions prevented (Palmer *et al.*, 1994).

Inadequate rehabilitation after acute illness in the frail elderly is also a problem and the waiting time for Geriatric Day Hospital (GDH) rehabilitation is long. Inadequate GDH transportation is another obstacle to provide adequate day rehabilitation for the frail elderly. Because of moderate disability, they usually require transportation support (e.g. Nonemergency Ambulance Transport) from home to GDH.

ISSUES IN PRIMARY HEALTH CARE IN THE ELDERLY IN HONG KONG SAR

For the general population, primary health care is largely provided by the private health-care sector, and the government is responsible for approximately 10% of this service. The latter is provided by the general outpatient clinic. In the elderly, the proportion of private doctor consultation is less than in the young and approximately 70% of them consult general outpatient clinic for primary health-care problems (Census and Statistics Department HKSAR, 2001). Most of the patients attending these clinics are either old or financially poor. Primary care providers are mostly private doctors who can manage episodic health problems well, but are inexperienced in detecting and managing chronic geriatric problems. For example, dementia is sometimes reassured as "normal aging phenomenon" without appropriate investigations and treatments.

Health promotion to improve lifestyles (e.g. quit smoking, healthy diet, exercise, etc), disease prevention (e.g. falls prevention and influenza vaccination for the elderly), and early chronic diseases identification and control are important. These measures would improve the health of the whole population and decrease geriatric health problems and the need for long-term care in the years to come. The Elderly Health Service (EHS) of the Department of Health provides health promotion program for the elderly members of their Elderly Health centers (Department of Health HKSAR, 2004). However, data regarding improvement of health status of the elderly in these programs have not yet been reported. Moreover, elderly citizens who are not members in these centers do not have access to these programs.

GERIATRIC HEALTH CARE AT RESIDENTIAL CARE HOMES FOR THE ELDERLY (RCHES) IN HONG KONG SAR

Those elderly living at home and alone constitute 12.4% of the over 65 year olds (11.2 and 13.6% for elderly men and women respectively) (Census and Statistics Department HKSAR, 2002b). While community and primary health cares are largely provided by private family doctors and general outpatient clinic (GOPC) doctors, specialist geriatric services at old age homes are provided mainly by Community Geriatric Assessment Team (CGAT) and partly by Community Health Nurses (CNS) (Leung *et al.*, 2000; Luk *et al.*, 2002). A new program of Visiting Medical Officers (VMOs) has been started in October 2003 to improve areas of infection control and provide *ad hoc* primary or geriatric medical care for frail elders in old age homes. Approximately 100 VMOs have been appointed as part-time HA staff to upgrade the previously inadequate primary and geriatric care in over 100 old age homes in the whole of Hong Kong (Hospital Authority HKSAR, 2004a).

SERVICE GAP AND DUPLICATION ISSUES FOR HEALTH AND LONG-TERM CARE OF THE ELDERLY

Multiple and continuous gaps in our traditional care models may lead to their "falling through the cracks" phenomenon (Coleman, 2003). The fragmentation of care would lead to frustration of the elders and caregivers and cause potential harm to patients, for example, being subjected to either "multiple repeated or similar drugs" (multiple doctors) or "no drugs" (waiting for new case appointment). The latter is a common transitional care problem for the elderly in Hong Kong.

In the community, the single frail elder commonly receives multiple health-care services (e.g. the private family doctor, VMO, orthopedic doctor, ophthalmologist, cardiologist, endocrinologist, etc.) as well as multiple social services (e.g. members of several multiservice or social centers for the elderly, home help services etc.). The current problems include fragmentation of care, service gaps, overlapping of services, poor communication, and coordination. It is believed that an integrated geriatric health and long-term care team across both health and social sectors would be able to overcome these undesirable issues substantially.

Unfortunately, the current financing and public policy do not facilitate this development. Moreover, the present public health and social policy still lead to unhealthy competition for clients as well as creating some important gaps in services for the elderly. At present, separate service providers are under different budget holders in the Department of Health's Elderly Health Service (EHS of DH), Hospital Authority (HA), Social Welfare Department (SWD) and Non-Government Organizations (NGOs). Most elders would use the public health and social long-term care services. Only a small proportion of the elderly population seeks services from private hospitals, clinics, and social services. In general, the objectives and policies of different service organizations differ. The policy on service directions may also be different. In terms of collaboration between different elderly service providers, a service purchase model among different organizations is in operation, but this has great limitations in breaking the gaps or eliminating service overlaps. For example, the frontline staff has difficulty in working together as an integrated team despite overlapping of services (e.g. EHS of DH and Geriatric Service of HA). Loose collaboration is the practice at present, which is not ideal.

For the interface issue between public and private health sectors, there is a slow development. Communications have improved and private doctors can obtain discharge summary of their patients from HA if they have preregistered. The recent public–private collaboration with VMOs in the Caritas Evergreen Home is one of the successful pilot projects implemented by the author in the Hong Kong West (HKW) Hospital Cluster (Chu *et al.*, 2004).

The present organization of health care for the elderly indirectly gives rise to an overuse of hospital-care services as against community-care services. The trend for cost containment would shift hospital care from acute to subacute hospital care, and shorten the length of hospital stay in the acute care hospital per episode of admission. This is a consequence of merely concentrating only on the activity figures. There is no cost incentive to decrease unnecessary hospital readmissions. Moreover, there has been an overemphasis on specialty-led and organ-based disciplines, which are all very costly.

Thus, alternative health and long-term-care service models for the elderly with an appropriate health-care financing policy are needed urgently. Effective solutions should be explored and implemented in the near future to avoid catastrophic incidents in both health and social care services for the elderly.

The financial issue of the health-care system for the elderly in Hong Kong is inadequate financial resource for public health care of the elderly. Most of the elderly in Hong Kong are poor and obviously would choose to use the public health-care services (under Hospital Authority and Department of Health) rather than the private sectors. The financial condition of current and next generation older persons is definitely not good or optimistic.

RECOMMENDATION FOR AN INTEGRATED HEALTH AND SOCIAL CARE DELIVERY SYSTEM IN HKSAR

A comprehensive long-term and geriatric health-care program is needed for the elderly in Hong Kong SAR. This program can be subdivided into regional teams. The geriatric health and social long-term services must be fully integrated. We need to move the present interface and collaboration models further. Financial incentives are crucial for the success of this model. Merging different organizational structures to form an integrated long-term and geriatric care team is a cost-effective and sustainable way of providing targeted care to the frail elderly among the elderly population of Hong Kong.

CONCLUSIONS

The population of China is rapidly aging. Declining birth and mortality rates as well as 25 years of one-child policy are the main reasons for the phenomenon of fast population aging in China, particularly in urban cities like Shanghai, Beijing, and Hong Kong SAR. The practice of geriatric medicine with an interdisciplinary intervention is the most suitable clinical management approach for frail-older persons in China. Unfortunately, this has not yet started in most parts of China except the Hong Kong SAR. To cope with the needs of the aging population in China, there is a definite and pressing need to develop clinical geriatric service together with geriatric medicine educational programs throughout China. Research in local clinical geriatrics care models is also essential for proper evaluation of their effectiveness. In Hong Kong SAR, further improvement in the practice of geriatric care is needed. The fragmentation of health and long-term care services need to be rectified in the near future. Integration of geriatric services with social long-term care services is recommended.

KEY POINTS

- The population of China is aging and the proportion of elderly aged 60 years and above is over 10%.
- Geriatric medicine has not been developed in most parts of China except the Hong Kong SAR.
- Clinical geriatric service with an interdisciplinary team approach should be developed in China. Research in these clinical geriatric care models has to be performed simultaneously.

- Educational programs in geriatric medicine at the undergraduate and graduate levels and clinical training programs for doctors are greatly needed in most parts of China.
- The issues of inadequate health-care insurance for older persons in China need to be addressed. Contributions from the government, the older persons, and family are needed.

KEY REFERENCES

- China Medical Association 2004, http://www.chinamed.org.cn/healthcare2.htm, (assessed in September 2004).
- Chu LW & Lam SK. Geriatric medicine in Hong Kong. In SK Lam (ed) *The Health of the Elderly in Hong Kong* 1997, pp 1–20; Hong Kong University Press, Hong Kong.
- Lee L. The current state of public health in China. *Annual Review of Public Health* 2004; **25**:327–39.
- Woo J, Kwok T, Sze FKH & Yuan HJ. Ageing in China: health and social consequences and responses. *International Journal of Epidemiology* 2002; **31**:772–5.
- Zhang WF. *The Ageing of Population and the Policies of China (Monograph)* 2003; Chinese National Committee on Ageing, Beijing.

REFERENCES

Barlett HP & Wu SC. Ageing and aged care in Taiwan. In DR Phillips (ed) *Ageing in Asia-Pacific Region. Issues, Policies and Future Trends* 2000, pp 210–22; Taylor and Francis, London and New York.

Census and Statistics Department, HKSAR. Special Topics Report No. 27, *Social data collected via the General Household Survey*, 2001; Census and Statistics Department, HKSAR, Hong Kong.

Census and Statistics Department, HKSAR. *Hong Kong Population Projections 2002–2031* 2002a; Census and Statistics Department, HKSAR, Hong Kong.

Census and Statistics Department, HKSAR. *Thematic Report – Older Persons* 2002b; Census and Statistics Department, HKSAR, Hong Kong.

China Medical Association 2004, http://www.chinamed.org.cn/healthcare2.htm, (assessed in September 2004).

Chiu HF, Lam LC, Chi I *et al.* Prevalence of dementia in Chinese elderly in Hong Kong. *Neurology* 1998; **50**(4):1002–9.

Chow N. Ageing in Hong Kong. In DR Phillips (ed) *Ageing in Asia-pacific Region. Issues, Policies and Future Trends* 2000, pp 158–73; Taylor & Francis, London and New York.

Chow N & Chi I. Aging in Hong Kong. In SK Lam (ed) *The Health of the Elderly in Hong Kong* 1997, pp 173–92; Hong Kong University Press, Hong Kong.

Chu LW, Chi I & Chiu A. Incidence and predictors of falls in the Chinese elderly. *Annals Academy of Medicine, Singapore* 2005; **34**:60–72.

Chu LW, Ho C, Chan F *et al.* A new model of primary medical and specialist care for the elderly in residential care homes for the elderly, A public-private interface collaboration project, presented at *The Hong Kong SARS Forum and Hospital Authority Convention*, Hong Kong, 8–11 May 2004.

Chu LW, Kwok KK, Chan S *et al. A Survey on the Health and Health Care Needs of Elderly People Living in the Central and Western District of the Hong Kong Island* [Report] 1998; Central and Western District Board of Hong Kong, Hong Kong.

Chu LW & Lam SK. Geriatric medicine in Hong Kong. In SK Lam (ed) *The Health of the Elderly in Hong Kong* 1997, pp 1–20; Hong Kong University Press, Hong Kong.

Coleman EA. Falling through the cracks: challenges and opportunities for improving transitional care for persons with continuous complex care needs. *Journal of the American Geriatrics Society* 2003; **51**(4):549–55.

Department of Health, HKSAR. *Annual Report 2001/2002* 2004; Department of Health, HKSAR, Hong Kong.

Du P & Guo ZG. Population ageing in China. In DR Phillips (ed) *Ageing in Asia-Pacific Region. Issues, Policies and Future Trends* 2000, pp 194–209; Taylor and Francis, London and New York.

Editorial Committee of China Health Annual. *China Health Annual 2003 [Chinese] (Zhongguo Weisheng Nianjian)* 2003; People Health Publisher. Beijing.

Festini F & de Martino M. Twenty five years of one child family policy in China. *Journal of Epidemiology and Community Health* 2004; **58**:358–60.

Fox RA & Puxty J. Geriatrics and the problem solving approach. In RA Fox & J Puxty (eds) *Medicine in the Frail Elderly. A Problem-oriented Approach* 1993, pp 1–13; Edward Arnold, London, Boston, Melbourne and Auckland.

Hall MRP & Rowe MJ. The United Kingdom. In MSJ Pathy (ed) *Principles and Practice of Geriatric Medicine* 1998, 2nd edn, John Wiley & Sons, pp 1523–34; Chichester, New York, Weinheim, Brisbane, Singapore and Toronto.

Higher Education Office of China Ministry of Education *Reform and Development of Higher Medical Education in China [Chinese]* 2004; People Health Publisher, Beijing.

Hong Kong College of Physicians. Guidelines for higher training in geriatric medicine. In Hong Kong College of Physicians (ed) *Guidelines for Higher Training in Internal Medicine* 2002, pp 82–6; Hong Kong College of Physicians, Hong Kong.

Hospital Authority, HKSAR. *Hospital Authority Statistical Report 2001/2002* 2003a; Hospital Authority, HKSAR, Hong Kong.

Hospital Authority, HKSAR. *Hospital Authority Statistical Report 2000/2001* 2003b; Hospital Authority, HKSAR, Hong Kong.

Hospital Authority, HKSAR. *Hospital Authority Annual Plan 2004–2005* 2004a; Hospital Authority, HKSAR, Hong Kong.

Hospital Authority, HKSAR. *HA Monthly Statistical Report on Central Infirmary Waiting List on 30 June 2004* 2004b; Hospital Authority, HKSAR, Hong Kong.

Isaacs B. The giants of geriatrics. In B Isaacs (ed) *The Challenge of Geriatric Medicine* 1992, pp 1–5; Oxford University Press, Oxford, New York and Tokyo.

Lau CP & Lok N. Prevalence of coronary heart disease and associated risk factors in ambulant elderly. In SK Lam (ed) *The Health of the Elderly in Hong Kong* 1997, pp 99–110; Hong Kong University Press, Hong Kong.

Lee L. The current state of public health in China. *Annual Review of Public Health* 2004; **25**:327–39.

Leung EMF & Lo MB. Social and health status of elderly people in Hong Kong. In SK Lam (ed) *The Health of the Elderly in Hong Kong* 1997, pp 43–61; Hong Kong University Press, Hong Kong.

Leung JYY, Yu TKK, Cheung YL *et al.* Private nursing home residents in Hong Kong- how frail are they and their need for hospital services. *Journal of the Hong Kong Geriatrics Society* 2000; **10**(2):65–9.

Liang HC. The health management of the aged in China, presented at *The 5th Asia Oceania Regional Congress of Gerontology*, Hong Kong, 19–23 November 1995.

Lindsay RW & Barker WH. The United States of America. In MSJ Pathy (ed) *Principles and Practice of Geriatric Medicine* 1998, 3rd edn, pp 1535–48; John Wiley & Sons, Chichester, New York, Weinheim, Brisbane, Singapore and Toronto.

Luk WW Geriatric health care of Shanghai in the 21st century, presented at *The 2000 Hong Kong-Shanghai Geriatrics Scientific Forum. Hong Kong Geriatrics Society and Renji Hospital of Shanghai*, Renji Hospital, Shanghai, 11–14 May 2000.

Luk JKH, Chan FHW, Pau MML & Yu C. Outreach geriatrics service to private old age homes in Hong Kong West Cluster. *Journal of the Hong Kong Geriatrics Society* 2002; **11**:5–11.

Macau SAR Government 2004, http://www.gov.mo/english/indicator/ (assessed in September 2004).

Ministry of Health of China. *China Health Statistics Abstract in 2004* 2004, http://www.moh.gov.cn/statistics/digest04/tt.htm, (assessed in September 2004).

National Bureau Statistics of China. *Bulletin of 5th National Population Census (No. 1)* 2004, http://www.stats.gov.cn/tjgb/rkpcgb/qgrkpcgb/2002033_15434.htm, (assessed in September 2004).

Palmer RM, Landefeld CS, Kresevic D & Kowal J. A medical unit for the acute care of the elderly. *Journal of the American Geriatrics Society* 1994; **42**(5):545–52.

Social Welfare Department, HKSAR 2004, http://www.info.gov.hk/swd/text_eng/ser_sec/ser_elder/, (Assessed on 12th July 2004).

Swift CG. The problem-oriented approach to geriatric medicine. In MSJ Pathy (ed) *Principles and Practice of Geriatric Medicine* 1998, 3rd edn, pp 251–68; John Wiley & Sons, Chichester, New York, Weinheim, Brisbane, Singapore and Toronto.

Wong ST. A summary report of the 4th committee meeting of the Chinese geriatrics society of the Chinese medical association. *Chinese Journal of Geriatrics* 1999; **8**(18):197.

Woo J, Ho SC, Chan SG *et al.* An estimate of chronic disease burden and some economic consequences among the elderly Hong Kong population. *Journal of Epidemiology and Community Health* 1997; **51**(5):486–9.

Woo J, Kwok T, Sze FKH & Yuan HJ. Ageing in China: health and social consequences and responses. *International Journal of Epidemiology* 2002; **31**:772–5.

Zhang WF. *The Ageing of Population and the Policies of China (Monograph)* 2003; Chinese National Committee on Ageing, Beijing.

Zhu HM. Epidemiology of bone fracture and its influence on life quality in the elderly. *Chinese Journal of Geriatrics* 1993; **12**(3):168–72.

FURTHER READING

Hong Kong SAR Government. 2004; http://www.info.gov.hk/censtatd/eng/hkstat/ (assessed in September 2004).

Aging in Developing Countries

Luis M. Gutiérrez-Robledo

Instituto Nacional de Ciencias Médicas y Nutrición "Salvador Zubirán", México D.F., Mexico

THE IMPLICATIONS OF POPULATION AGING IN DEVELOPING SOCIETIES

Population aging has become a prominent topic as aging has emerged as a global phenomenon in the wake of the now virtually universal decline in fertility and, to a lesser extent, of increases in life expectancy. The theme is of immediate concern in developed countries, where aging is already well advanced and will continue, with serious consequences on every single aspect of life. It is also gaining importance in developing regions, where a number of countries have started worrying about the implications of population aging. With people in the developing world living longer and having fewer children, developing countries will have to be ready to meet the new health challenge of demographic aging. Medical advances and preventive health measures have meant significant progress against communicable diseases, which were once the main health threat in many such countries. But at the same time, the number of people with chronic and degenerative conditions has risen. Mortality rates from communicable disease in children under a year old were cut in half over the last 50 years. A decline in fertility rates from 3.1 to 2.4 children per woman followed. This coincided with the aging of the general population. The net result is that today, people over age 85 make up the fastest growing population group in these countries, increasing at a rate of 3 to 5% per year in some of them. The population over 65 years of age is growing at a rate of about 2% per year while overall population is growing at a rate of 1.3% annually. Not only are more people old now, but more people will get older. At the start of the twenty-first century, the average life expectancy in the region of the Americas is up to 72.4 years (WHO, 2001a).

With more elderly people living longer, chronic diseases and external causes have edged out communicable diseases as the main causes of death in many developing countries. They now account for about two-thirds of all deaths. Cardiovascular disease, cancer, injuries, and physical disability have become more prominent health problems. Endocrine problems such as diabetes and the metabolic syndrome are particularly frequent. Caring for an older population will mean a shift in the kind of health problems needing treatment. Another critical component is being sure that they get health care in the first place. Older adults living in isolated areas are more likely to lack permanent access to health care. Inequalities in people's risk of getting sick and dying, corresponds to inequalities in the distribution of resources. New health-care policies will need to address both sets of concerns. In this setting, preventive health continues to be important in old age to limit risks from factors such as environmental degradation, tobacco use, lack of physical exercise, violence, mental health problems, poor diet, motor vehicle accidents, and drug abuse (WHO, 2001b).

A long life should be everybody's right, but for older people in developing countries today, longevity can be a double-edged sword. Many older people never expected old age to be so stressful and difficult. For those who are poor, aging often means new burdens and worries about making ends meet. At the Second World Assembly on Ageing, governments signed the new International Plan of Action on Ageing (UN, 2002). But agreeing to the plan is only the beginning of a process. The key issue is how the plan is implemented and monitored. The challenge now is to mainstream aging issues into development processes and related international commitments. So far, aging is marginal in development debates. The International Development Targets and the UN's Millennium Development Goals (UN, 2004) largely ignore the question of how increasing numbers of older people can escape chronic poverty and be included in planning for a better future of communities and nations.

DEVELOPING SOCIETIES WILL EXPERIENCE SHORTER TIME TO REACH AGING STAGE AND WITH LESS RESOURCES

It is not our intention to discuss demographic or health data in great detail, but a summary of statistics on population and

Principles and Practice of Geriatric Medicine, 4th Edition. Edited by M.S. John Pathy, Alan J. Sinclair and John E. Morley.

Table 1 Health-related and population-aging variables in developing and middle-income countries, compared with some developed countries estimates for 2000[a]

Countries	Developing and middle income																									Developed		
	Afghanistan	Argentina	Bangladesh	Bolivia	Brazil	Chile	China	Costa Rica	Côte d'Ivoire	Cuba	People's Republic of Korea	Ethiopia	Haiti	India	Indonesia	Iran (Islamic Republic of)	Kenya	Mexico	Nigeria	Morocco	Pakistan	Republic of Korea	South Africa	Tunisia	Turkey	United States of America	United Kingdom	Japan
Indicators																												
Adult mortality (per 1000) females	376	92	252	219	136	67	110	78	494	94	192	535	373	213	191	139	529	101	393	113	198	71	502	99	120	84	67	44
Adult mortality (per 1000) males	437	184	262	264	259	151	161	131	553	143	238	594	524	287	250	170	578	180	443	174	221	186	567	169	218	147	109	98
Annual population growth rate (%)	4.8	1.3	2.2	2.4	1.4	1.5	1	2.8	2.4	0.5	1.1	2.8	1.7	1.8	1.5	1.9	2.7	1.7	2.9	2	2.6	0.9	1.8	1.5	1.7	1.1	0.3	0.3
Dependency ratio (per 100)	86	60	72	77	51	55	46	60	83	44	48	93	80	62	55	69	86	61	93	63	83	39	60	55	56	52	53	47
Percentage of population aged 60+ years	4.7	13.3	4.9	6.2	7.8	10.2	10	7.5	5	13.7	10	4.7	5.6	7.6	7.6	5.2	4.2	6.9	4.8	6.4	5.8	11	5.7	8.4	8.4	16.1	20.6	23.2
Total fertility rate	6.9	2.5	3.7	4.1	2.2	2.4	1.8	2.7	4.9	1.6	2.1	6.8	4.2	3.1	2.4	3	4.4	2.6	5.7	3.2	5.3	1.5	3	2.2	2.5	2	1.7	1.4
Healthy life expectancy at age 60 (years) females	5.8	16	8	10	12.6	15.7	14.3	15.6	8.5	15.5	12.1	7.5	8.5	10.9	12.5	11.4	9.1	15	8.2	10	8.7	16	10.4	12.6	13.4	16.8	17.4	21.4
Healthy life expectancy at age 60 (years) males	7.1	13.2	8.8	9.8	10.7	13.1	11.8	14	8.6	14.5	11.1	7.7	7.8	9.9	11.6	11.3	9.3	14.5	8.4	9.9	9.8	12.3	9.1	11.4	11.2	15	15.3	17.6
Healthy life expectancy at birth (years) females	32.5	65.9	47.9	51.4	59.2	67.4	63.3	66.4	38.9	66.7	56	35.1	44.9	51.7	58.4	58.6	40.1	65.3	41.1	54.5	46.1	68.8	43.5	61.7	60.5	68.8	71.4	76.3
Healthy life expectancy at birth (years) males	35.1	61.8	50.6	51.4	54.9	63.5	60.9	64.2	39.1	65.1	54.9	35.7	41.3	52.2	56.5	59	41.2	63.1	42.1	55.3	50.2	63.2	43	61	56.8	65.7	68.3	71.2
Healthy life expectancy at birth (years) total population	33.8	63.9	49.3	51.4	57.1	65.5	62.1	65.3	39	65.9	55.4	35.4	43.1	52	57.4	58.8	40.7	64.2	41.6	54.9	48.1	66	43.2	61.4	58.7	67.2	69.9	73.8
Life expectancy at birth (years) females	45.1	77.8	60.8	63.6	71.9	79.5	73	78.8	48.4	77.5	67.2	44.7	56.1	62.7	67.4	69.9	49.6	76.2	51.4	70.4	60.7	78.3	52.1	73.4	72.5	79.5	79.9	84.7
Life expectancy at birth (years) males	44.2	70.2	60.4	60.9	64.5	72.5	68.9	73.4	46.4	73.7	64.5	42.8	49.7	59.8	63.4	68.1	48.2	71	49.8	66.1	60.1	70.5	49.6	69.2	66.8	73.9	74.8	77.5
Life expectancy at birth (years) total population	42.8	73.7	61.6	62.2	68.4	76.1	70.8	76.4	46.2	76.8	66.1	47.5	53	60.6	65.4	68.3	49.7	74.2	51.6	69.3	61.2	74.6	51.2	70.9	68.9	76.8	77	81.3
Percentage of total life expectancy lost females	27.8	15.2	21.2	19.1	17.6	15.2	13.2	15.7	19.7	14	16.7	21.4	20	17.5	13.5	16.2	19.1	14.3	20.1	22.7	24.1	12.1	16.5	15.9	16.5	13.4	10.6	9.9
Percentage of total life expectancy lost males	20.5	12	16.2	15.6	14.8	12.4	11.6	12.6	15.6	11.6	14.8	16.6	16.9	12.7	10.9	13.3	14.5	11.2	15.5	16.3	16.6	10.3	13.3	11.8	14.9	11.1	8.7	8.1
Social security expenditure as % of general health expenditure	0	59.5	0	66.7	0	71.8	50.7	90.2	0	0	0	1	0	0	7.5	40.6	0	67.7	0	7.6	39.6	77.3	0	57.3	28.4	33.9	0	83.5
Total expenditure on health as % of GDP	5	8.9	3.6	5.2	7.6	6.8	5.3	6.9	6.2	7.1	2.4	3.2	4.8	5.1	2.7	6.4	8.7	5.7	3	4.7	4.1	5.9	8.7	6.2	5	13.1	7.3	7.7

[a]These figures were produced by WHO using the best available evidence. They are not necessarily the official statistics of Member States.
Source: Table produced by the author from data available at the World Health Organization website: http://www3.who.int/whosis/menu.cfm?path=whosis,bod,burden_statistics&language=english.

aging for developing countries is given in Table 1. These data are drawn principally from the WHO World Health Report 2001a, Statistical Annex. The data are therefore presented on a broadly comparable basis.

As it can be shown from this data, all these countries are facing the rapid growth of an aging population, although, in practice, their cutoff ages for defining "older people" are not the same. Indeed, for various purposes internally (retirement ages, pensionable age, granting of certain benefits), individual countries specify different chronological ages. For example, the age requirement for entitlement to elderly services and care in both Thailand and Malaysia is 60 years of age, while in Hong Kong, Korea, and Singapore it is 65, and in Mexico 70. Hong Kong and Singapore both have lower retirement ages in some sectors, at 55 (increasing to 60) in Singapore, and at 60 in Hong Kong, in many companies and the public sector. Definitions aside, the chronological aging of the population in most countries is obvious: in Hong Kong, 11% of the population is aged 65+; in Singapore, Thailand, Korea, and Mexico, it is 7%; and in Peru or Malaysia, it is 4% – all substantial increases on the previous decades' figures.

The factors underpinning the increase in the aging populations are similar across the countries. A major reason for this demographic aging is a very low fertility rate. Added to this are gradually increasing life spans. The life expectancy at birth of males and females in Hong Kong is 77 and 82 years respectively, while comparable figures in Singapore are 76 and 80, and in Malaysia, 70 and 75, and in Mexico 70 and 74.

There are also quite high elderly dependency ratios in these countries, and while dependency rates are not perfect, they are often taken as an indication of potentially increasing burdens both on the economically active population and on governments and their economies, especially in the health and welfare sectors. In many ways, increasing dependency ratios, like increasing life expectancy, as they reflect population aging, show the success in social and economic policies, good health and nutrition, modern welfare services, and a good standard of living for the population.

Demographic aging in these countries is very much influenced by the previous explosive demographic growth, and the ensuing rapid fertility lowering (Liao, 1996). This has resulted in a fast and explosive population aging. Furthermore, the growth of the elderly in these regions happens in a context of poverty, large heterogeneity, and profound inequity. Besides, in all less developed nations, at the same time, the extraordinary growth of the young population and of those of working age has to be managed. Between the year 2020 and 2040, these countries will show age structures approaching those of the developed world today. Only 20 years are left to gather resources that can be devoted to the care of the elderly and to develop an infrastructure for the same purpose.

Current demographic trends (UN, 2003) show that the differences between regions are considerable at the present time: a 15-point gap exists between the percentage of elderly people for the least developed countries and the more developed regions in 2000. For example, Latin America is moving toward patterns similar to those of developed regions. In this context, it is clear that population aging of the kind that raises serious economic and social issues in the more developed countries is not such a distant prospect in many developing and middle-income countries and is already a matter of concern for many others, particularly in Asia and Latin America.

The social and economic dimensions of this phenomenon depend as well on dynamics of the younger population. If this population grows as fast as, or faster than the older population, then the needs of the aged will probably be disregarded. From this perspective, what matters is relative growth of both segments of the population. This data from the UN allows projections that show how, with few exceptions, the rates of increase of the aged population during more recent periods are higher than the increase of the total population, and that these rates have been increasing steadily. This shows how rapid aging in these countries has been present, though unnoticed, for a long time.

While in developed countries, the current reality is that of an aging population that is healthier and better educated than ever before, and of whom 60% are neither disabled nor dependent (Robine and Romieu, 1998), in developing countries the analysis of the situation reveals many problems that make it more difficult to care for an emerging aging population in which illiteracy, poverty, poor social and family support prevail and lead to a poor self-care capacity. In such a context, finding the means with which to accomplish a "compression of morbidity", helping an aging population with 13–16 years of additional life expectancy at age 65 to remain active and robust until the last years of life is the biggest challenge to public health for the twenty-first century (Gutiérrez-Robledo, 2002).

Furthermore, a disturbing hypothesis has been stated, suggesting that massive improvements in survival such as those occurring in Latin America during the sixties, and concentrated within a few years after birth are likely to induce important changes in the mean and variance of the frailty distribution of the elderly population (Palloni *et al.*, 2002). It is well known that this fact alone could account for increases in the prevalence of disability as well as for slower improvements in mortality at older ages than would otherwise be expected. So, elderly health status and functional limitations are likely to have worse distributions than those observed among the elderly in more developed contexts. If this hypothesis proves to be true, then the aging process in the region will be characterized not only by its rapidity and dimension but also by an "expansion of morbidity", leading to a huge demand on health services.

In such conditions, countries in the region would be facing the "failure of success": as their populations attain longer life expectancies, they will be unable to support their health status and avoid dependency because of lack of resources and specific services. Nevertheless, at the same time, they will be facing an opportunity for creative social planning. If policy makers understand the immediacy and implications of all these phenomena, and the connections between population aging, early life health status and economic growth, the actual lack of infrastructure would open the way to the development of alternative, community-based care systems.

The case of Sub-Saharan Africa's elderly population deserves special consideration. Even though population aging is not as large as in other regions of the world, it must be considered as a potential cause for concern, since the largest increase in the number of elderly in the world between 1980 and 2000 will occur in Asia and Africa. The most rapid growth is expected in western and northern Africa whose elderly populations are projected to increase by a factor of nearly 5 between 1980 and 2025. A distinct feature of the aging situation in Africa is that a large proportion of the elderly people live and work in the rural areas. It is estimated that by the year 2020, approximately 64% of Africa's elderly will live in areas defined as rural. Also of significance is the fact that most of these elderly will be women. Africa has experienced an unprecedented proliferation of political unrest and civil strife. These and other economic hardships have caused millions of Africans to flee their countries, and at present, African refugees top the list in the world. Elderly persons have special difficulties coping with the hazardous and stressful journeys and are overwhelmed with the process of adjustment to new life. Many who choose to remain suffer from hardship, as there is hardly anyone left young enough to cultivate food and provide care and protection.

There is no doubt that the greatest constraint facing African countries with respect to planning for aging is the dearth of data on populations over age 60 years. Several areas of research deserve higher priority in order to get a more general view of aging (Apt, 1995).

DEVELOPING SOCIETIES WILL EXPERIENCE DIFFERENT INTERGENERATIONAL TRANSFERS

The economics of aging has been analyzed mainly in developed countries. In the very different context of developing regions with large informal sectors, flexibility of labor participation patterns, large nonmonetized economy, and lack of institutionalized pension systems, analyses so far have been much less detailed. Attention has been focused principally on the negative consequences of aging such as the problems regarding economic support for older people who no longer participate in the labor force, or do so with low productivity; and problems regarding elderly health care, like the financing of facilities and services and their adaptation to changing needs. But the economics of aging in developing countries must be examined in the context of broader demographic changes, of which aging is only one single aspect. A balanced, comprehensive view of the implications of those changes is needed. During the demographic transition that these countries are now undergoing, the decline of fertility causes not only an increase in the proportion of older people, but also, conversely, a reduction in the proportion of younger people. Of particular interest is the proportion of people under 15 years of age, as they are also dependent, even though to a lesser extent. So, we must place projected aging within the context of overall age dependency. In recent decades, the most significant change in age structures in developing countries has been the reduction in the proportion of young people due to fertility declines: the proportion aged 0–14 has been declining in all the developing regions since 1970–1975. It will continue to decline, and the resulting reduction in numbers will be roughly as large as the increase in the number of older people. This shift, and possible reduction in the total burden of dependents per person in the active age-groups, in turn, opens opportunities to redirect investment in health and human development. The period during which the age dependency ratio declines has been described as a "window of opportunity". This shift implies changing needs and, therefore, requires adaptations in health and social investment programs. For instance, as the overall costs of education for the society decline during this process, resources could be diverted to partially solve the additional health costs of aging (Schulz *et al.*, 1991).

For some old people, life will be better in the twenty-first century, for many it will be worse, for most there will be, seemingly, little change. Human societies, of which the old are an integral part, are subject to economic, social, and political pressures. Two-thirds of the world's elderly in this century live in developing countries, the majority being very poor. The main underlying cause of ill health in most of these countries, poverty, will be relieved only very slowly – if ever. Poverty and economic crisis adversely affect mortality rates among the elderly, in women more than men, and the strength of that association has been increasing over time (Wang *et al.*, 1997). In 1992, tightening of the embargo on Cuba increased the mortality in people older than 65 by 15%. The 1995 economic crisis in Mexico had a similar effect (Cutler *et al.*, 2000). The elderly constitute a particularly vulnerable group in times of economic crisis. The health of the elderly in Latin America is likely to be particularly sensitive to economic trends, and the present supply of health services may not be wholly effective in preventing this response. Present trends indicate that the gaps between rich and poor will widen both within and between countries, and will be a long lasting, if not permanent feature of rapidly changing economies (Davies, 1999). As developing countries struggle to cope with their economic problems, the aged individual is marginalized. The manifestations of poverty are much more severe for the aged. Rural poverty leaves older people alone in the village to look after themselves, while the family migrates to urban areas in search of jobs. In the middle of competing priorities at the national and family levels, the welfare of the elderly is usually given low or no priority.

The current health of younger generations can impact on older persons in a number of ways if they are expected to be earners as well as carers. A specific issue occurs in some countries where there is an impact from the morbidity and mortality of intermediate generations, for example, from HIV/AIDS, which is likely to significantly affect Thailand, Myanmar, the Philippines, and perhaps China (HelpAge International, 2002). As has been noted, the most unfortunate older people can be those who live utterly alone or with young, dependent grandchildren, yet with no middle generation. Such a scenario is, unfortunately, increasingly common in some African countries and may appear in the Asia–Pacific region as well (Gorman, 1999).

DEVELOPING SOCIETIES WILL EXPERIENCE MORE NEGATIVE ATTITUDES TOWARD AGING POPULATIONS

Old age poverty is too often presented as a matter of special pleading rather than a basic human right. In economics, poverty among older people is accepted as a norm; in health, routine discrimination against older people is tolerated; while in personal security, violence against older people is perceived as no one's business.

Policy on aging has to be based on equal rights for older citizens. In practice, older people are not treated equally before the law – national and international legislation to protect people from violence is often not applied in cases of violence against older people. Older people report that they view old age with anxiety and fear, not only because of worsening poverty, but because of increasing dependence on others and consequent vulnerability to physical, sexual, and psychological abuse. Welfare services frequently discriminate against older people. Where health and social services are offered, they often exclude older people, whether formally, by setting age limits, or informally, through negative staff attitudes. Most poor people work into very old age and, therefore, have the same requirements as other groups for employment, credit, development assistance, education, and training schemes. Yet credit is often denied on grounds of age, and there is an upper age limit on most loan schemes. Poverty, social exclusion, and discriminatory attitudes toward old age violate the human rights of older people. The UN Principles for Older Persons, for instance, do not have the status of legally enforceable rights.

DEVELOPING SOCIETIES WILL EXPERIENCE GREATER EXPECTATION OF GOVERNMENTAL PROGRAMS BUT MORE PROBLEMS DELIVERING SERVICES TO THE AGING POPULATION

The elderly, with their greater need for health care, put considerable strain on systems of health care in all societies and provide additional urgency to the search for solutions. The ideal of healthy aging requires that the elderly share the general facilities available to the population at large, and also receive additional care to meet their special needs. These include the social and physical environments, the promotion of healthy lifestyles, and the provision of medical and nursing care. Few professionals choose to care for the elderly, and as the majority of the world elderly are women, their low status in developing countries will continue to be a major barrier to their health as they age. Poverty is the greatest single cause of ill health at all ages and while its reduction is not strictly a role of the health sector, it is certainly a prerequisite, for its persistence will continue to adversely affect any health intervention (Lloyd-Sherlock, 1997).

Global aging impacts on policy in two ways. First, good policies can easily be undermined if they fail to take account of the radical demographic shifts that are now under way. The changing shape of populations creates new opportunities and challenges. Appropriate policy recognizes the valuable human resource represented by increased numbers of older people, supports their role in enhancing the quality of our societies, and protects their right to live in decency to the end of their lives. Secondly, there are powerful economic, social and ethical grounds for a fundamental shift in policy and opinion on older people in aging societies. Countries cannot afford to ignore the contribution to economic and social development made by millions of older people. More importantly, as a matter of equity and citizenship, the needs of older people have to be addressed in the context of human rights. The neglect of older people's most basic rights, to food, shelter, health care, and a voice, must end. The price of neglecting older individuals and the challenges of aging populations is increasing poverty; not only for those who are now old but also for younger generations. An opportunity for all of us to manage our own future will be lost unless determined action is taken now (Phua and Yap, 1998).

EPIDEMIOLOGIC TRANSITION: THE EXPANSION OF CHRONIC MORBIDITY

In 1971, Abdel Omran first proposed the concept of epidemiological transition (Omran, 1971). Today, this approach in population studies is widely used. Nevertheless, this concept is probably outdated, as it has become clear that the evolution of the epidemiological profile in different regions of the world follows no single pattern. In Latin America's experience, this transition shows some particular characteristics such as multiplicity; there is not one single way to follow but several possible roads – and vulnerability of the transitional course (Palloni, 1990). In these countries, the improvement of living standards has not been uniform for the population as a whole and the vulnerability of the poor sector is growing as a consequence of economic programs that have not favored them. Negative consequences are manifest in a greater morbidity and mortality in those vulnerable groups. So, morbidity patterns are not uniformly shifting toward degenerative disorders as infections still take a heavy toll on our elderly – tuberculosis is a particular case as its incidence is rising – and the evolution of chronic and degenerative disorders suffers a heavier influence of nutrition in its pathogenesis and outcome as is the case with diabetes whose high prevalence is associated with an even higher prevalence of other coronary risk factors, both associated with an increased risk of functional impairment (Lerman *et al.*, 1998).

The aging process exposes individuals to increasing risks of illness and disability. The key factors affecting the health profile of the elderly are incidence and timing of onset of chronic illnesses and disability, magnitude of rates of recovery, and mortality. But in poor countries, lifetime exposure to health problems means that many people enter old age already in chronic ill health. People can be frail and functionally impaired much earlier. This is particularly so for women who, after years of hard physical labor, poor nutrition, and many pregnancies, are on the threshold of old age by the end of their reproductive years. For older people in the developing world, personal health consistently ranks alongside material security as *a priority* concern. Physical health is for many poor people their single most important asset, bound up with the ability to work, to function independently, and to maintain a reasonable standard of living. Illness in old age is, therefore, an ever-present threat. Many older people live in fear of illness, for they cannot afford to be ill. Despite its importance to older people, health care is inaccessible to many. Hospitals tend to be concentrated in urban centers, far from the rural areas where many older people in developing countries still live. Even those who live in cities and towns can often only reach health facilities by using public transport, which is expensive, crowded, and not adapted for easy access. Treatment is often unaffordable for older people, even where it is nominally free of charge. Where fee exemption policies exist, older people could not benefit because of lack of information, shortage of supplies, and poor management. The negative attitude of health staff toward the treatment of older people is also a powerful factor dissuading many from seeking treatment (Palloni *et al.*, 2002).

The challenges to health systems are twofold. The first is to postpone the onset of disease as long as possible, and the second, to provide adequate services when people develop fatal or disabling illnesses. The World Health Organization (Yach *et al.*, 2004) estimates that, by 2020, chronic diseases, along with mental health disorders and injuries will make up 70% of the health-care needs in developing and newly industrialized countries. Older people form a significant part of this caseload. If unchecked, chronic diseases might pose a serious threat to the future solvency of health care and social protection systems. The challenges for developing countries are particularly formidable because of the speed of population aging, and the prevalence of absolute poverty and infectious diseases. There is a third and more fundamental constraint. Health spending in many developing countries is a tiny fraction of what is needed to meet these challenges. Per capita spending on health care in many countries of Sub-Saharan Africa, for example, is under 3% of the GDP (see Table 1), and that is skewed toward urban areas. So, as life expectancies and the possibility of exposure to risks for chronic health problems rise, chronic conditions become more prevalent and this happens during a longer period of time. Chronic conditions presently comprise the major health burden in developed countries, and trends for developing countries forecast a similarly concerning situation. Noncommunicable conditions and mental disorders accounted for 59% of total mortality in the world and 46% of the global burden of disease in 2000. The disease burden will increase to 60% by the year 2020; heart disease, stroke, depression, and cancer will be the largest contributors. Low- and middle-income countries are the biggest contributors to the increase in the burden of disease from noncommunicable conditions. In China or India alone, there are more deaths attributed to cardiovascular disease than in all other industrialized countries combined. These diseases share key risk factors: tobacco use, unhealthy diets, lack of physical activity, and alcohol use, all of these very often, during a lifetime. The current burden of chronic diseases reflects past exposure to these risk factors, and the future burden will be largely determined by current exposures. Moreover, in developing countries, chronic diseases have not simply displaced acute infectious ones; rather, such countries now experience a polarized and protracted double burden of disease. Moreover, if these countries thrive successfully, as economic development occurs, tobacco use and obesity (and presumably other risk behaviors) will increase. Eventually, uptake of risk factors will lead to onset of disease. Mortality and morbidity from chronic disease would subsequently decline along with continued economic development. Thus far, only some of the Organization for Economic Cooperation and Development countries have achieved these declines, which have been associated with consumption behavior, while declining mortality from chronic diseases is associated with very high levels of social and economic development. Thus, in the absence of policy actions, consumption of tobacco, alcohol, and foods high in fat and sugar increases along with gross national product, followed by associated increases in chronic diseases decades later. This contrasts with infectious diseases, which generally decline with economic growth. Chronic disease risk rates do not begin to fall yet and demand an integrated approach to their prevention, surveillance, and control (WHO, 2002).

HEALTH AND WELL-BEING OF THE ELDERLY IN DEVELOPING AND MIDDLE-INCOME COUNTRIES

Information is still scarce in this setting. Some more data on the subject is available in the Latin-American region. In 1998, Pan American Health Organization (PAHO) conducted a multicentric Study on Aging, Health, and Well-being (SABE) (Peláez *et al.*, 2003; MIAH, 2004) in seven major cities of Latin America and the Caribbean. According to the SABE survey, the prevalence of chronic conditions vary in the region: hypertension was reported by one out of every two persons 60 years and older; the lowest percentage was reported in Mexico City (43%) and the highest in Sao Paulo (53%). One out of five persons reported having heart disease. In most cities, at least one out of three older adults reported having arthritis. Diabetes was highest in Bridgetown and Mexico City, with 22% of older persons reporting it. The percentage of persons reporting having had a stroke is over 8%. Older men were less likely to report having arthritis and hypertension, but were just as likely as women to report having heart disease and diabetes. In the United States, a study of a much older population found that about 45% of persons aged 70 years or older had hypertension, 21%

had heart disease, 58% had arthritis, and 12% diabetes. The prevalence of stroke in this age-group was 9%. In Canada, 33% of persons 65 years or older reported having hypertension, 16% had heart disease, 47% had arthritis, and 10% had diabetes.

The SABE survey found that approximately one out of every five persons 60 years and older, in the combined sample, reported having some difficulty with the basic activities of daily living (bathing, dressing, using the toilet, eating, getting in and out of bed, and walking across a room). Included in this number were those who needed assistance in order to perform an activity as well as those who were unable to do the activity at all. Since the data obtained by the SABE survey concerns only elders living at home, it is difficult to estimate the true levels of disability without comparable data obtained from long-term care facilities or group homes. Anyway, these are very high levels of prevalence of activities of daily living (ADL) and instrumental activities of daily living (IADL) impairment and point to needs that, in the changing social and political contexts of these countries, may well require practical solutions quite different from the traditional ones. From this data, it seems clear that disease is more prevalent, begins earlier, and disability spans for a longer period of time. So, the correlation between a growing life expectancy and compressing morbidity is not yet present in Latin America, for as we have shown, risk of morbidity is higher and morbidity tends to be more devastating, with a higher risk of functional impairment.

Some other questions about the epidemiological transition in these countries remain open: To what extent do the successive cohorts of elderly people become either frailer or more robust? Will the "emerging" morbidity and mortality causes be the same when compared with fully developed countries? Can treating chronic diseases reverse disability? Are the elderly able to benefit from health and social interventions in this context? Answers are urgently needed in order to develop adequate long-term policies.

Provision of Services and Care

In broad terms, services and care for older persons can be considered under three categories: social security, health care, and social services.

Social Security

To ensure that the basic needs of older persons are met, the governments of some developing countries provide direct financial assistance, although this tends to be very limited. For example, Hong Kong has an Old Age Allowance of approximately US$80 per month, as an asset and income-tested benefit for its citizens aged 65 and over, known colloquially as "fruit money" due to its minimal value. It also has a means-tested Comprehensive Social Security Assistance Scheme, starting at US$325 per month for older persons (aged over 60) with some disability, rising to $558 for poorer older people needing nursing care. Mexico City, likewise, aims to guarantee a minimum living standard for its older adults through its newly codified 2000 Basic Livelihood Security Law, which built on the existing public assistance law, and its small "Elder Pension". On the other hand, some societies emphasize on provident fund schemes to provide income security for their retired workers. For example, in Malaysia, formal sector workers participate in a range of government and private sector pension schemes, but these are not compulsory for the self-employed, amongst whom the participation rate is low. These people will, therefore, have to rely largely on their own resources in old age. Such is the case as well for many countries in Latin America (Gill *et al.*, 2004).

Health Care

Health care comprises a wide range of services, at the primary care level, ranging from clinics to increasingly specialized hospitals and institutions. In many of the developing countries, in addition to western-style allopathic medicine, with mainly a disease-oriented nature, there is also an important parallel, and sometimes connected, system of traditional medicine, particularly in Asian countries. Older persons in Latin America often find traditional sources of health care a great comfort and culturally acceptable. Such traditional health care is mainly available through the private sector.

When in need of formal conventional health care and services, older adults, in all the societies under discussion, tend to rely mainly on publicly provided government facilities, particularly for hospital and rehabilitative services. This is because few older persons have the resources or insurance to pay for private sector medicine, although there are exceptions, such as people with special coverage, retired armed forces personnel, and some civil servants in some countries as Mexico. By and large, however, the older population will at present rely on out-of-pocket primary care, or if in need of hospital care, they turn to the public sector.

Most developing countries provide at least basic hospital services for their older populations, even if these are sometimes crowded and difficult to access. Many have already implemented, as is the case for Mexico, or at least have plans to introduce, insurance schemes to lessen the financial burden of medical services. Korea and Malaysia have also recently developed such a scheme (Gutiérrez-Robledo, 2002; Philips and Chan, 2002).

The health status of the current and future cohorts of older persons in these countries is also very important. At present, as noted above, expectation of life at birth is generally extending. As it has been said, there is no compelling evidence as yet as to whether there is a compression of morbidity in these regions, or a longer life and a worsening health status; seemingly, this is unfortunately the case (Palloni *et al.*, 2002; Vita *et al.*, 1998). This is clearly a very important question for policy makers, and it will underpin decisions about the sort of community and institutional services that are needed. Indeed, it will influence the nature of the medical and nursing skills and the training needed in the future, as well as many other issues. As a result, research needs to be conducted and epidemiological data needs to be systematically gathered as soon as possible.

The solution to the health problems of older persons requires more than access to a physician. It requires a change in the culture of health, and a public health approach to health education, health promotion, early detection of problems, and appropriate resources to provide community-based care and rehabilitation. There is a need for human resources to be trained to understand the different health needs of an aging population. Systems should be flexible and should provide coordinated services that are organized according to population needs and community resources.

The study of health determinants reveals that there is a wide range of factors that contributes to the health of older adults or puts them in situations of risk. These determinants rarely exist separately and thus rarely benefit from one-dimensional solutions. Therefore, multiple sectors and partners must collaborate to address interrelated risk factors and safeguard factors that promote active aging and prevent or delay the onset of chronic disease. Main risk factors are: social isolation and poverty; malnutrition and sedentarism; stress, anxiety, and depression.

Social isolation and poverty contribute to morbidity and negative health outcomes and reduce the ability of older persons to access information and assistance, as needed. Multisectoral approaches should alleviate poverty, educate older persons to understand their rights, and promote health literacy. There is mounting evidence of the importance of active living and proper nutrition to help prevent and alleviate disease and chronic conditions, boost the positive effects of rehabilitation, reduce the potential for falls and injuries, and help manage other risk factors. Diet and exercise play a positive role in maintaining function and preventing disability. Screening for malnutrition and targeting the identified nutritional needs with a variety of community interventions for the neediest are cost-effective means of strengthening the capacity of elders to adhere to wellness prescriptions and practices. In addition, a variety of programs are essential to promote elder participation in organized physical activities and exercise. The prevalence of mental health problems among elders contributes to misuse of medications, alcohol abuse, and self-destructive behavior, and reduces the capacity of the individual to care and manage health problems before they become disabling or life threatening. Considerable improvements have been made in the treatment of depression and anxiety, but the lack of coordination of primary health care and community mental health services results in a situation in which the mental health needs of most elders are often not met. Local strategies designed for the timely detection and treatment of depression, anxiety, and dementia in older persons are to be developed, including training mental health and primary health workers, as well as peer group counselors, to address the mental health needs of elders (PAHO/WHO, 2002).

In most of these countries, health-care systems are still designed to provide acute illness care. They lack a population-based, community health orientation that is focused on enhancing the capacity of the individual and the community for improving health, detecting early problems, and handling and managing chronic diseases with the least costly and most effective approaches. Public Health in most developing countries has not developed an integrated community approach to promote health and well-being in the older population. Much of the work to be done requires multisectorial collaboration: to alleviate poverty, promote healthy eating, physical and social activity, and to provide a coordinated system of care for older persons. Primary health-care systems in these countries need tools and resources to reorient or reorganize services to meet the complex health needs of older persons. The current method of organizing and financing primary health care with existing human resources cannot respond to the health needs of aging persons, even if additional resources are added to the services. Primary health-care needs population-based approaches, including prevention, early detection, and patient empowerment for self-management of chronic diseases. It also requires networking with community resources and other disciplines. This approach also needs human resources that are capable of moving beyond curing acute episodes, to understanding the need for a collaborative process involving the treating physician, other members of the health-care team, the patient, and other partners in the management of complex health problems. Effective care also requires effective monitoring of adherence and patient education. Training of primary health-care teams for care of the elder should be considered a priority and provided with resources. Training programs should be developed for teaching self-care or self-management for elders and families dealing with chronic diseases or complex health problems (Barry, 2002). There are evidence-based educational programs that teach the necessary skills for self-care and provide models for psychological support for elders. These resources should be adapted to the needs of elders who are very poor and who have low levels of education. There is a need to integrate social and health-care services to promote a continuum of support for older persons in danger of loosing autonomy. The performance of primary health care can be improved if linkages are made to community resources relevant to health promotion, prevention, treatment, management, rehabilitation, long-term care, and palliative care of the elderly population (PAHO, 2002a).

For this purpose, explicit guidelines and protocols for screening and assessing the physical, functional, emotional, and cognitive health of elders should be developed or adapted as it has been done by the Merck Institute for Aging and Health (MIAH, 2005).

Norms and standards for community-based programs such as adult day-care services, home care, foster adult homes, and assisted living facilities need to be developed and implemented. The public sector, NGOs, and the private sector need to form alliances for the development of age-friendly community services (WHO, 2004). However, the state must guarantee a minimum standard of quality care to protect the dignity and well-being of disabled and frail older persons.

Countries are beginning to experience the challenges posed by the care of frail older persons, and need to learn from the mistakes of those who have in the past, prioritized the institutional approach to long-term care and are now searching for better models of community-based long-term care. For example, during the past decade, the Governments of Canada and the United States have explored the development of more appropriate, as well as cost-effective, community-based alternatives to nursing homes. This has led to increased funding for home care and community day-care services and has limited the growth of nursing homes. The costs related to long-term care and palliative care will become a major issue in most of the developing countries during the next decade. Foresight in developing appropriate community models while the demand is still relatively low will avoid major problems during the next two decades when the demand could overwhelm the system (Brodsky, 2002).

Countries with more lead time at their disposal now have the possibility of planning well ahead for the necessary adaptations. In this perspective, they should define long-term strategies to partly reorient public investment efforts as well as training programs, set up public mechanisms for welfare where feasible, and foster or assist with the development of targeted initiatives and institutions in the civil society.

Social Services

This third category of services involves provision of services and assistance in kind, as well as housing or specialist accommodation for older persons. The range and depth of services developed in the countries under discussion are varied according to their different contextual needs. Some social services, such as recreational services, are generic and serve all ages, while others are more focused on older persons and include services such as institutional care, day care, personal care, and home help services. Issues related to the status and morale of older persons are sometimes also covered, and can include promoting the employment of older persons. Unlike other countries, Mexico, Korea, and Singapore increasingly emphasize employment of elders, Singapore in part because of predicted potential labor shortages.

The need for specialist or adapted forms of accommodation to enable some older persons to continue living in the community and to avoid institutionalization is widely recognized. Therefore, given the nature of demographic aging in the countries in this chapter, with large percentage increases expected in the number of older persons, coupled with social changes that are diminishing family care abilities, it is not surprising that housing forms a major plank in most social services and welfare policies. These range from policies to promote aging *in situ* and community care, to the provision of long-stay residential and hospital units with day-round nursing care. Home care and associated support is clearly crucial here. Most countries, specifically aim part of their housing policy for older persons on strategies to enable families to keep living with or near elderly relatives. These strategies include allocation of housing units nearby for children and elderly parents, and more rapid allocation of public housing when older relatives are included. It is strongly predicted that these types of initiatives will gain in importance, as the public sector tries to maintain family care and coresidence or residence nearby, for older people and their younger relatives, and to foster traditional values such as filial piety. In addition, policies to enable unrelated older persons to live together are also being attempted and may well expand as widowhood and longevity increase (Sokolovsky, 2000).

Unanimously, all countries recognize the importance of the family that cares for older people, particularly long-term care and financial support. These still depend greatly on family and the informal sector, the governments, while setting the scene, are the last resort provider of care at the moment, although this is clearly changing. The traditional Asian value of "filial piety", a two-way duty of care and responsibility between parents and children, is emphasized, especially among the Chinese society. These values prevail as well under different manifestations in most countries in Latin America. This assumes that older people will be cared for by families and communities, which is encouraged and promoted as the norm of the society. The family is seen as the key caring unit of society, and in some countries this has been embodied in law, for example, in Singapore, in the Maintenance of Parents Act in 1995, and in Mexico in the Older Adult Law in 2000.

This reliance on family care is a great strength and something of which these societies may justifiably be proud. However, its uncritical acceptance, and more importantly, the continuing expectation that families in the twenty-first century will be able to continue their functions as carers for older persons has been identified as *a potential weakness* (Ng *et al.*, 2002). This is particularly so when children are made to feel guilty if they are not able to take full care of their parents, however old or frail, and when their own domestic and economic circumstances make such care difficult. In some cases, the unbending expectation that families will be the primary caregivers has been seen to have actually deterred the development of coherent policies and effective public services for older persons. As a result, there is now growing pressure for these expectations to be amended. There must be services and other forms of assistance available, so that families can continue to shoulder what may become an increasingly heavy burden if left to them. While families undoubtedly do still have a very important caring function in all the countries under discussion, the ability of older persons to choose where they would like to live and with whom is also important. This will grow with future older cohorts, who will be better educated and better off than many of today's older persons. If asked where they would like to live, many older persons state that they would like to do so with their children, but this is an ideal. In reality, many older persons prefer their independence, and for personal reasons do not actually want to live with their children and risk intergenerational conflicts.

A number of practical factors militate against the family's easy continuation of care. First, many families are split because of migration for work and because of social issues such as bereavement or divorce. Second, family sizes are decreasing and will be even smaller in the future, reducing the number of children to share the social and economic responsibilities of care for elderly parents (Arriagada, 2004). The combined effects of these two factors mean that many future older persons may not have any children living nearby on whom they can rely. Third, housing space is at a premium and, in most middle-income country's cities, dwellings large enough to accommodate multigenerational families are becoming rarer and very expensive. Fourth, economic circumstances and social choice mean that many more women, the traditional carers for elderly parents or parents-in-law, are working and are not available as constant free carers. Last but not least, as noted above, many older persons themselves would prefer the freedom to live independently, perhaps near their children and grandchildren. This aspect, the welfare of older persons, is very important. Many do not wish to live in the same house as their children and do not wish to be perceived as burdens on them, especially in hard economic times (Sokolovsky, 2000).

All these factors operate in various combinations in the countries covered by the chapter. They heavily underscore the urgent need for policies and provisions to be developed, which will help families and will not place crushing burdens on them. The family as a caring institution is a resource and needs nurturing and support.

POLICY ISSUES

Following the former considerations, several issues have been raised: How to strengthen the informal support of the family, which is weakening because of the evolution that we have described? Is there any possibility of developing a social security for those in the informal sector? How do these countries protect the interests of the aged as they restructure their economies in the era of globalization? Are there any lessons to be learned from developed countries in these issues?

Overcoming marginalization is a main issue, poverty is its main instigator; economically it implies being at the periphery; politically, it means being out of decision making; and socially, it means being cut off from the appropriate life and culture of the society. Empowering the elderly throughout and ensuring elderly people's participation in society as a need means the avoidance of marginalization. The crucial issue is the avoidance of poverty. Mutual support structures could provide older persons with more control over their own lives but such organizations will not be able to satisfy elderly people's basic needs. Improving social services is also an urgent need, for the aging situation will generate a tremendous demand for social services. Some of this will be very basic such as food and shelter, others not so basic, as is dealing with disabilities. In order to improve these services, the first step is probably to recognize aging as an emerging and significant issue; secondly, to consider that a large majority of elderly people will have neither savings nor access to social security benefits; and third, to recognize that their need of social services are high and ranging from basic to rehabilitative services. The development must be based on the existing informal support system for the aging and the existing social service infrastructure. In this context, adult day-care centers can be developed with little additional input. Most countries cannot afford to develop specialist geriatric services. Special provisions will have to be made in the existing health system in order to prepare primary care professionals in the field of geriatrics (Gutiérrez-Robledo, 2002).

Planning for the health care of the elderly in less developed nations is already a must as aging and health care are already significant emerging policy issues in these countries. National policies on aging are developed in a complex set of contexts: sociocultural, political, economic, and international. The international context, in particular, is becoming increasingly important, as research and knowledge of the types of services and provisions for older persons that exist in different parts of the world become known. Also very important is the sociocultural context, as most of the countries under consideration regard older persons with traditional respect, even if this is not always translated into care and resources. The family is also widely regarded as the main and acceptable, indeed expected, provider of care and financial support. This is both a strength and a weakness in the development of these policies.

The desired objectives of public policy on aging would be to promote an optimal physical and mental functioning, lowering the incidence of chronic diseases and disabilities throughout, making available enough resources specifically devoted to this purpose, promoting intergenerational transfers in every possible level, promoting elderly empowerment through the combat of poverty, their engagement in decision making and in productive activities. At the same level, optimal health care of the elderly would require universal access to primary medical care and population-specific interventions, with an emphasis on health promotion and disease prevention, as well as development of home and community care. In every level, patient participation must be encouraged (Walker and Naegele, 1999).

Although the details of care and service provisions are different among countries, the nature and philosophy reflected in their implementation are, in many ways, more or less similar in all. This fact offers some insights that may be useful for planning and improving the policies and care for aging populations.

Although the growth of the aging population, and the need for policies with a longer-term perspective, is apparent, not all countries have a clear policy on aging. From this perspective, the International Plan of Action on Ageing 2002 contains a number of important points to be considered, including the concept of "secure aging" and several priorities that could seem daunting and ambitious (UN, 2002). But such ambition reflects the neglect that population aging has faced until relatively recently. The well-being of older people is clearly linked to that of their families and the wider community. Sound policy needs to recognize that aging populations have the same potential for investment as other age-groups.

In the same line of thought, and in a much more specific perspective, the Merck Institute for Aging and Health, together with the Pan American Health Organization have proposed a set of goals on the basis of the available information for the Latin-American region. Many of these goals can be proposed as well for other developing and middle-income countries in different regions of the world (MIAH, 2004).

Health policy makers need to be aware that today's older persons are in many ways an interim generation. Future programs must anticipate the emergence of older persons in the coming decades who will know and demand their rights, unlike the present generation, many of whom are humble and regard the state as the paternalistic authority. Many of tomorrow's older persons will be fitter, better educated, and wealthier. They will expect and demand responsive, high-quality services and provisions. Any national policy on aging that does not take this into account will be fatally flawed. However, a major challenge for the coming decade is likely to be how to develop quality services for future generations in a setting of scarce resources and while dealing with the needs of poorer and often less healthy people.

KEY POINTS

- Developing societies will experience a shorter time to reach the aging stage, and with less resources.
- They will experience more negative attitudes toward aging populations.
- Medical advances and preventive health measures have meant significant progress against communicable diseases, but at the same time, the number of people with chronic and degenerative conditions has risen.
- The aging process in such a context exposes individuals to increasing risks of illness and disability.
- Future programs must anticipate the emergence of older persons in the coming decades who will better know and demand their rights.

KEY REFERENCES

- Gutiérrez-Robledo LM. Looking at the future of geriatric care in developing countries. *Journals of Gerontology MS* 2002; **57A**(3):M1–6.
- Lloyd-Sherlock P. *Old Age and Urban Poverty in the Developing World* 1997; Cambridge University Press, Cambridge.
- Merck Institute for Aging and Health. *The State of Aging and Health in Latin America and the Caribbean. State of Aging and Health Reports Series* 2004, Available online at www.miahonline.org/resources/reports.
- Palloni A. The meaning of the health transition. In S Caldwell, P Findley, G Caldwell *et al.* (eds) *What we know about Health Transition: The Cultural, Social and Behavioural Determinants of Health*, 1990; The Australian National University Printing service.
- United Nations. *Second World Assembly on Aging Proceedings* 2002; available at: http://www.un.org/esa/socdev/ageing/waa/index.html.

REFERENCES

Apt NA. International models. Health care of the elderly in Africa: focus on Ghana. *Caring: National Association for Home Care Magazine* 1995; **14**(1):42–5, 47–9.

Arriagada I. Transformaciones sociales y demográficas de las familias latinoamericanas. *Papeles de Población* 2004; **10**(40):71–96.

Barry P. The critical role of practicing physician education, Paper presented at *United Nations Second World Assembly on Aging*, Madrid, 2002.

Brodsky J. Conclusions. In J Brodsky, J Habib & M Hirschfeld (eds) *Long-Term Care in Developing Countries: Ten Case-Studies* 2002; World Health Organization collection on long-term care, Geneva.

Cutler DM, Knaul F, Lozano R *et al. Financial Crisis, Health Outcomes and Aging: México in the 1980's and 1990's* 2000; Working paper 7746, National Bureau of Economic Research.

Davies HM. Ageing and health in the 21st century: an overview. In *Ageing and Health, Proceedings of a WHO Symposium* 1999; WHO, WHO/WCK/SYM/99.1

Gill I, Packard TG & Yermo J. *Keeping the Promise of Social Security in Latin America. 2004 World Bank* 2004; Stanford University Press.

Gorman M. Development and the rights of older persons. In J Randel, T German & D Ewing (eds) *The Ageing and Development Report: Poverty, Independence and the World's Older People* 1999, pp 3–22; Earthscan, London.

Gutiérrez-Robledo LM. Looking at the future of geriatric care in developing countries. *Journals of Gerontology MS* 2002; **57A**(3):M1–6.

HelpAge International. *State of the World's Older People 2002* 2002; HelpAge International, London.

Lerman I, Villa A & Gutiérrez-Robledo LM. Diabetes and coronary risk factors. Prevalence in rural and urban elderly Mexican populations. *Journal of the American Geriatrics Society* 1998; **30**:250–5.

Liao TF. Measuring population aging as a function of fertility, mortality, and migration. *Journal of Cross-Cultural Gerontology* 1996; **11**(1):61–79.

Lloyd-Sherlock P. *Old Age and Urban Poverty in the Developing World* 1997; Cambridge University Press, Cambridge.

Merck Institute for Aging and Health. *The State of Aging and Health in Latin America and the Caribbean. State of Aging and Health Reports Series* 2004, Available online at www.miahonline.org/ressources/reports.

Merck Institute for Aging and Health. *The State of Aging and Health in Latin America and the Caribbean* 2005, website: http://www.miahonline.org/tools/.

Ng ACY, Phillips DR & Lee WKM. Persistence and challenges to filial piety and informal support of older persons in a modern Chinese society: a case study in Tuen Mun, Hong Kong. *Journal of Aging Studies* 2002; **16**:135–53.

Omran A. The epidemiological transition; a theory of the epidemiology of population change. *Milbank Memorial Fund Quarterly* 1971; **49**:345–67.

PAHO/WHO. *A Guide for the Development of a Comprehensive System of Support to Promote Active Ageing* 2002; HPF/HPE Publication, Pan American Health Organization, Washington.

Palloni A. The meaning of the health transition. In S Caldwell, P Findley, G Caldwell *et al.* (eds) *What we know about Health Transition: The Cultural, Social and Behavioural Determinants of Health*, 1990; The Australian National University Printing service.

Palloni A, Pinto-Aguirre G & Pelaez M. Demographic and health conditions of ageing in Latin America and the Caribbean. *International Journal of Epidemiology* 2002; **31**:762–71.

Pan American Health Organization. Health and aging. Paper presented to *The 26th Pan American Sanitary Conference* PAHO, (CSP26/13), 2002a; Washington, www.paho.org.

Peláez M, Palloni A, Alba C *et al. Survey on Aging, Health and Wellbeing, 2000* 2003; Pan American Health Organization (PAHO/WHO).

Philips D & Chan A National policies on ageing and long-term care in the Asia Pacific: issues and challenge. In DR Phillips & ACM Chan (eds) *Ageing and Long-Term Care: National Policies in the Asia-Pacific (Social Issues in Southeast Asia)* 2002; the Institute of Southeast Asian Studies and the International Development Research Centre.

Phua KH & Yap MT. Financing health care in old age. In N Prescott (ed) *Choices in Financing Health and Old Age Security* 1998, pp 33–42; World Bank Discussion Paper No. 392, The World Bank, Washington.

Robine JM & Romieu I. *Healthy Active Ageing: Health Expectancies at Age 65 in the Different Parts of the World REVES Paper n°318 (Réseau Espérance de Vie en Santé – Network on Health Expectancy and the Disability Process)* 1998; Date of contribution: May 1998, Contributed by Jean-Marie Robine and Isabelle Romieu for the World Health Organization, Division of Health Promotion Education and Communication.

Schulz JH, Borowski A & Crown WH. *Economics of Population Aging* 1991; Auburn House, New York.

Sokolovsky J. *Living Arrangements of Older Persons and Family Support in Less Developed Countries* 2000; The United Nations, New York.

United Nations. *Second World Assembly on Aging Proceedings* 2002; available at: http://www.un.org/esa/socdev/ageing/waa/index.html.

United Nations. Long–range population projections, *Proceedings of the United Nations Technical Working Group on Long-range Population Projections United Nations Headquarters*, New York, 2003.

United Nations. *Millennium Development Goals* 2004; http://www.un.org/millenniumgoals/.

Vita AJ, Terry RB, Hubert HB & Fries JF. Aging, health risks and cumulative disability. *The New England Journal of Medicine* 1998; **338**:1035–41.

Walker A & Naegele G (eds). *The Politics of Old Age in Europe* 1999; Open University Press, Buckingham.

Wang J, Jamison DJ & Bos E. Poverty and mortality among the elderly: measurement of performance in 33 countries 1960–1992. *Tropical Medicine and International Health* 1997; **2**(10):1001–10.

World Health Organization. *The World Health Report 2001* 2001a; Statistical Annex, http://www3.who.int/whosis/menu.cfm?path=whosis, burden_statistics.

World Health Organization. *Innovative Care for Chronic Conditions* (Meeting Report) 2001b; WHO, Ginebra, (WHO/MNC/CCH/01.01).

World Health Organization. *World Health Report 2002. Reducing Risks, Promoting Healthy Life* 2002; WHO Geneva, available at http//www.who.int/whr.

World Health Organization. *Towards Age-Friendly Primary Health Care* (Active ageing series) 2004; World Health Organization.

Yach D, Hawkes C, Gould L & Hofman K The global burden of chronic diseases: overcoming impediments to prevention and control. *Journal of the American Medical Association* 2004; **291**:2616–22.

FURTHER READING

World Health Organization *Developing Integrated Response of Health Care Systems to Rapid Population Aging* 2003; WHO, Geneva.

Geriatrics from the European Union Perspective

Alfonso J. Cruz-Jentoft[1] ***and*** **Paul V. Knight**[2]

[1]Hospital Ramón y Cajal, Madrid, Spain, and [2]Royal Infirmary, Glasgow, UK

INTRODUCTION

Europe has a landmass of 9 938 000 sq. km (3 837 000 sq. miles), 6.7% of the total land area on earth, with varied climate, cultures, and populations. Unlike the United States, it is not a federation of states with a unifying governmental structure. However, the European Union (EU) does provide a certain amount of integration between the Member States in terms of laws, trade, and governmental policies. There remain areas where each Member State has the final say.

The European Union is a complex structure with the Council of the European Union being the main decision-making body. The Council is where ministers from each Member State can commit their government to various EU policies. The Council of the European Union and the Parliament, where members are elected directly by voters in each state, are the bodies responsible for European laws. The European Commission, based in Brussels, Belgium, is the civil service of Europe split into various directorates, each of which has an appointed political head combined with an overall Commission President. The Commission has responsibility for proposing legislation, implementing agreed policy, enforcing EU law and representing the European Union at international level (http://europa.eu.int/abc/index_en.htm, 2005).

From 1 May 2004, the European Union expanded to 25 Member States, having been 15 prior to the expansion. Although various enlargements have occurred from the original six states over the last 30 years, this is the single biggest expansion since its inception, increasing its population by 20% and its land area by 23%. This expansion brings in states from the Baltic, Eastern, and Mediterranean Europe. The population of the European Union will now number some 450 million with 150 million aged over 50 years.

DEMOGRAPHY

The European Union compiles statistics, thorough its agency Eurostat (http://europa.eu.int/comm/eurostat/), from Member States regarding a number of population and health-related parameters. However, these are collated rather than collected, so there can be problems with the uniformity of their collection not only in terms of completeness but also their comparability.

Bearing the above in mind, it appears that Europe's population has been aging steadily. In EU15 (the Member States before the recent expansion), because of falling birth rates and rising life expectancy, the number of people aged 65 years and over is projected to increase from 61 million in the year 2000 to 103 million in 2050. The proportionate increase in the very old, aged 80 years and over, is even more dramatic, going from 14 million to 38 million in the same time period. In 2003, EU15 was thought to have 16.8% of its population 65 years and over. The expanded European Union (EU25) has a slightly lower figure of 16.3%. These global figures disguise major variations across the European Union, for instance, Ireland had only 2.6% aged 80 years and over in 2003, while Sweden had 5.3%. Similarly, although, life expectancy at 60 years is 19.6 years for males and 23.8 years for females in EU25 in 2003, this varies in males from 15.2 years in Latvia to 20.9 years in Sweden and for females from 20.4 years in Latvia to 24.3 years in Sweden (European Commission, 2004).

In parallel with these changes, the working population, at least in EU15, over the same time frame is projected to decrease significantly (see Figure 1). This demographic time bomb has considerable implications for health and social care across the European Union.

Principles and Practice of Geriatric Medicine, 4th Edition. Edited by M.S. John Pathy, Alan J. Sinclair and John E. Morley.

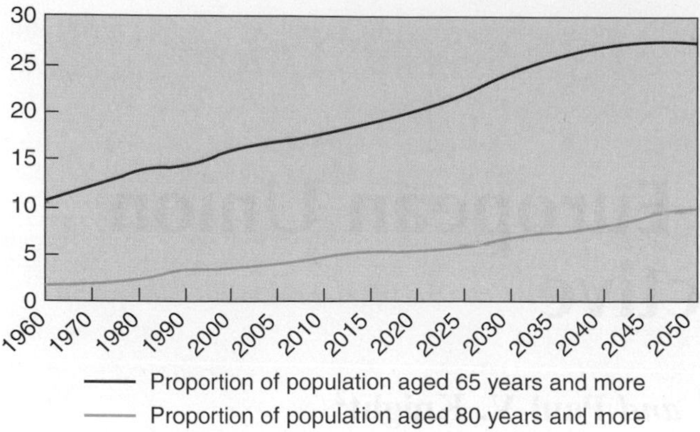

Figure 1 The aging EU population (Eurostat, population structure indicators (1960–1990), baseline scenario projection (2000–2050))

HEALTH AND HEALTH SYSTEMS

In EU15, all the of the Member States have systems in place that offer complete, or near complete, rights to health care for people residing within their borders. These are financed in two broad ways, either through general taxation, or utilizing systems based on occupational health insurance. Both systems limit their liability to pay the full cost of treatments such that expenditure borne by households amounts to between 20 and 30% in the majority of Member States. The difference is made up either through direct contributions or via supplementary private insurance, for example, France. It is however clear that public sector funding makes up a significant proportion of health expenditure in all the EU Member States: this proportion being lowest in Greece (56%) and rising to nearly 84% in the United Kingdom.

This reliance on a degree of financial participation may adversely affect some groups' access to health care as they are unable to afford the costs. This is particularly true of older people who may have both lowered incomes and considerable comorbidity. Thus, some Member States have enacted methods to target older people either by reducing their financial liability or ensuring that they are regularly screened by relevant health professionals.

In common with other developed countries, the Member States see the need to recruit staff appropriately trained in the needs of older people and also to create post-acute rehabilitation facilities to assist a multidisciplinary approach to treatment with the goal of reablement and settlement in the community. Unfortunately, often these rehabilitation sites are adrift from main acute centers in the mistaken belief that rehabilitation can wait till the conclusion of an acute episode of care.

In contrast, long-term care is seen mainly as a social risk. This seems to devalue it in many eyes and forgets that the primary reason for the need is multiple disabilities related to chronic ailments such as dementia and cerebrovascular disease. The responsibility for such care is often left to the family or untrained carers. Changes in epidemiology and demography make this an increasingly untenable situation. Almost all Member States are trying to share the costs of long-term care provision through insurance schemes and there is a move away from institutional to home-based care. In parallel, there is a drive to quantify quality standards for health care in general and long-term care in particular. As many states predict a need to increase health-care expenditure between 0.7 and 2.3 percentage points of gross domestic product (GDP) over the next 50 years, due to demographic changes, it can be seen that finance is a major issue for most governments. According to the Organisation for Economic Co-operation and Development (OECD) Health Data from the 4th Edition in 2002, it has been calculated that total health expenditure in EU15 in 2000 ranged from 6.6% in Finland to 10.6% in Germany. This contrasts with 13% in the same period in the United States.

The health needs of each country within the European Union still vary enormously (Whitehead, 1999) and will become more skewed with the generally poorer countries that have recently joined. For instance, the World Health Organization (WHO) standardized death rate per 100 000 population for ischemic heart disease varies from only 76.4 in France to 352.8 in Slovakia in 1999. Similarly, the incidence of tuberculosis ranges from only 4.8 per 100 000 population in Sweden to 88 in Latvia in 2001. This compares with 5.8 per 100 000 population in the United States in the same year.

HEALTH TRENDS

Life expectancy has been steadily growing in the European Union in the last century, and this trend has not stopped in recent years (Table 1). When a European citizen is 65 years old, he/she may expect to live more than 18 years into "old age". This means that diseases and disabilities of old age are steadily increasing. Changes in lifestyles, risk factor management and health care have pushed for a slow but steady reduction in the main cause of mortality in this age group: diseases of the circulatory system (a 24.9% reduction from 1990 to 2001). Stroke, a very frequent cause of disability in the elderly, has also decreased. However, mental health disorders (particularly dementing diseases and depression) seem to be increasing fast during the same time period, not only in mortality but also in morbidity.

One of the main problems researchers are faced with when studying illness in the elderly in the European Union is the lack of good morbidity data across Europe. Health statistics are available for communicable diseases, for health habits and lifestyles, and for disease-related mortality. However, there are no reliable data regarding geriatric diseases and syndromes (stroke, dementia, hip fracture, heart failure, diabetes, or other diseases) (Berr *et al.*, 2005). Data are fragmented, come from different years and sources, are gathered with different criteria, and are not systematically collected. Good age-specific data are especially sparse. Efforts have been recently undertaken by the statistical

Table 1 Health trends in 25 Member States of the European Union

	1990	2001
Basic demographic indicators		
Population, millions	44.04	45.22
% of population aged 65+ years	14.03	16.03
Mortality indicators		
Life expectancy at birth, years	75.54	78.19
Life expectancy at age 65, in years	16.63	18.17
SDR[a], diseases of circulatory system, 65+ per 100 000	2694.81	2022.07
SDR, ischemic heart disease, 65+ per 100 000	966.04	762.02
SDR, cerebrovascular diseases, 65+ per 100 000	720.23	529.12
SDR, malignant neoplasms, age 65+ per 100 000	1105.66	1049.17
SDR, mental disorders, and diseases of the nervous system and senses	134.92	179.01
Health-care resources		
Hospitals per 100 000	3.76	3.20
Hospital beds per 100 000	807.08	619.74
Acute-care hospital beds per 100 000	524.02	422.69
Physicians per 100 000	291.07	338.77
General practitioners per 100 000	96.44	97.82
Nurses per 100 000	730.44	773.87
Health-care utilization and costs		
Average length of stay, all hospitals	14.16	9.79
Average length of stay, acute-care hospitals only	9.55	6.99
Outpatient contacts per person per year	6.85	6.40
Total health expenditure, % of gross domestic product	7.27	8.81
Total health expenditure, $ per capita	1184.39	2030.81

World Health Organization, 2004.
[a]SDR, standardized death rate.

agencies of the United Kingdom and Belgium to define standards for the creation of a good database. However, research and progress in this area is urgently needed.

These changes have transformed the paradigm of health care. Health-care systems were once developed for the care of single, acute diseases, usually unexpected, with cure and self-sufficiency as usual outcomes. However, elderly patients usually have multiple, chronic morbidities (sometimes with acute exacerbations), where disease course can be expected, with dependency as a very frequent outcome. Unfortunately, health systems in Europe, very efficient for acute care, have only evolved slowly and in a very irregular and heterogeneous mode to be able to manage chronic diseases in dependent people. This lack of efficiency may explain why per capita health expenditure increases sharply after the age of 65 and even more sharply after the age of 80.

In the last two decades, the number of hospitals and hospital beds has been diminishing, especially those used for acute care, while the number of general practitioners, nurses, and primary care units has not grown at the same rate. Intermediate and long-term hospital beds have suffered a slower reduction, and rehabilitation and palliative care services for older people are scarce and irregularly distributed, not only between countries, but also within different areas of the same country.

Geriatric medical care is also extremely diverse within the European Union (Hastie and Duursma, 2003). Geriatric medicine is accepted in many European Countries, as a subspeciality of Internal Medicine. It is officially accepted by the European Union, but it is not yet available in every country: only 15 of the 25 countries have, in 2004, established the mechanism for mutual recognition of the speciality (Table 2). However, this list may not offer a fair picture of geriatric medicine in Europe. In some countries (Belgium, Germany), geriatric medicine has a wide distribution with hospital departments and specific geriatric training programs, even when mutual recognition has not been achieved. In other countries, geriatric medicine is not accepted as a separate speciality and is very poorly developed. European geriatricians are working hard to promote recognition of the speciality and development of geriatric medicine departments in every EU country.

One may expect that a medical speciality department would be somehow similar around Europe, so that similar up-to-date procedures will be applied to any patient admitted to a medical department of a hospital, that is, cardiology or gastroenterology. However, this is not true for geriatric medicine. Excellent geriatric departments exist in most EU countries, but citizens living in different places will have different access rights to these departments, and a significant proportion of older people in the European Union will not have access to geriatric medicine. This is not due to lack of evidence, as very solid evidence exists about the benefits of most levels of geriatric care, but to discrimination against old people by political decision makers. Primary care is universally available for the older population, but many general practitioners are not prepared to manage this special population due to a lack of academic

Table 2 Mutual recognition of geriatric medicine in the European Union

Belgique – België Belgien	
Česká republika	Geriatrie
Denmark	Geriatri eller alderdommens sygdomme
Deutschland	
Eesti	
Ελλάς	
España	Geriatria
France	
Ireland	Geriatrics
Italia	Geriatria
Κύπρος	Γηριατρική
Latvija	
Lietuva	Geriatrija
Luxembourg	
Magyarország	Geriátria
Malta	Ġerjatrija
Nederland	Klinische geriatrie
Österreich	
Polska	Geriatria
Portugal	
Slovenija	
Slovensko	Geriatria
Suomi – Finland	Geriatria – geriatric
Sverige	Geriatrik
United Kingdom	Geriatrics

leaders and continuing professional development in geriatric medicine.

The growing numbers of older people and the reduced ability of weaker family networks to care for them, when they depend on others, are also increasing the need for long-term care in different settings (home care, long-stay units or nursing homes). Such care has not been regularly covered by health systems, so it is not even a universal right within the European Union, in contradistinction to acute health care. In many cases, it depends on private systems or the recently termed "*medical-social sector*". Nursing home use and availability is also diverse across the European Union: rates are close to 10% for people 65 or older in some northern countries (Sweden, Holland) and lower than 3% in some Mediterranean countries (Spain, Portugal), with a gradient from north to south that is not only explained by economic reasons but also depends more on people preferences and family networks.

IMPACT OF THE EUROPEAN UNION

The public health policy and the promotion of a high level of human health is a relevant part of the EU Treaty. The prime responsibility for health systems, under the Treaty, falls to the Member States. Most recent developments in the care of older people, however, have been fostered by the European social policy agenda. In March 2000, the European Council in Lisbon set out a ten-year strategy (the Lisbon Strategy), a commitment to bring about economic, social, and environmental renewal in the European Union to make it the world's most dynamic and competitive economy. Under this strategy, social policies that ensure sustainable development and social inclusion are being fostered. These policies are based, in many cases, in an improved cooperation between Member States, respecting the principle of subsidiarity. The Lisbon Strategy is being reviewed yearly at the EU spring meetings. A major review in the area of health care of the elderly is scheduled for spring 2005.

Following the Lisbon meeting, the Gothëborg Council, (2001) asked for an initial report on orientations in the field of health care and care for the elderly, in conformity with the open method of coordination (a method used to improve coordination in some policy areas, allowing Member States to challenge common problems, defining their own national strategies, and benefiting from experiences of other Member States). This is a milestone, as never before have EU countries tried to establish a common strategy toward geriatric care.

This request resulted in a report from the Commission (COM 723 final, December 2001).[1] The report carefully analyzed the impact of demographic aging on health-care systems; expenditure, the growth of new technologies and treatments, an improved well-being and a better standard of living, the diversity of national systems, and the contribution of the European Union. Three long-term objectives were established: accessibility, quality, and viability. Access to health care is a fundamental right and an essential element of human dignity that must therefore be guaranteed for all EU citizens, regardless of income or wealth. The need for special protection is recognized for dependency and old age. Quality implies a search to reduce diversity and variation and look for "best practice" standards. Financial viability is needed to sustain health and social systems of care in the future.

Since then, Member States provide information on how they deliver the three suggested objectives. Their information was reflected in a joint report from the Commission and the Council on supporting national strategies for the future of health care for the elderly (March 2003). The European Parliament confirmed the validity of the three key objectives for the renovation of health care and long-term care.

Very recently, the Commission issued a new report (COM 304 final, April 2004) that sought to outline a common framework to support Member States in the reform and development of health care and long-term care using the open method of coordination. The report proposes common objectives for health-care provision that would add to similar ongoing coordinating processes in three social policy areas: pensions, social inclusion, and employment. The most relevant aspects of this document related to geriatric medicine are outlined in BOX 1.

BOX 1 Recent EU Action Lines Related to Geriatric Medicine[2]

- Health systems have a role in combating the risk of poverty and disease, contributing to social cohesion and fighting the consequences of demographic aging.
- The principles of accessibility of care for all (taking into account the needs and difficulties of the most disadvantaged groups and individuals), high-quality care for the population (which keeps up with the emerging needs associated with aging) long-term financial sustainability of this care have to be met.
- The provision and funding of health and long-term care are key elements of the economic and social modernization strategy of the European Union.
- To meet the challenges posed by demographic trends and technological progress, it is vital to have a sufficient number of trained professionals and to give them quality jobs.
- Demographic aging will mean more age-related illnesses and more people in long-term care; and a growing number of old people living alone. The response to the needs of this population group will include developing a wide range of services, including care at home, and specialized institutions, as well as closer coordination between care providers.
- The social protection systems need to be reformed in an integrated and coordinated way to meet these

challenges. Health and elderly care is one of the areas where coordination in the field of social protection should be streamlined.
- Access to high-quality care based on the principles of universal access, fairness, and solidarity must be ensured, providing a safety net against poverty or social exclusion associated with ill health, accident, disability or old age, for both the beneficiaries of care and their families. Particular attention will have to be paid to persons requiring long-term or expensive care, to those with particular difficulties accessing care and those on low incomes. Financial and physical accessibility of care systems for disabled persons has to be ensured, and specific care for elderly people offered, based in particular on closer coordination between the social services, primary carers, hospital services, and specialized institutions.
- The system should be properly funded in order to meet the new challenges posed by aging, changes in society and technological progress. Responsibility for the organization and funding of the health care and elderly-care sector rests primarily with the Member States.

Member States – including the new ones – will present "preliminary reports" covering the challenges facing their systems at national level, current reforms, and medium-term policy objectives by March 2005. They will be analyzed by the Commission, so that their views and contributions can be taken into account when the joint objectives of the streamlined social security process are established. This streamlining will lead in 2006 to an initial series of "development and reform strategies" in health care and long-term care for the period 2006–2009. The conclusions of the assessment of these strategies will be presented in the Joint report on social protection and social inclusion in 2007.

This acknowledgement of the European Commission is a promising step for geriatric care. Nevertheless, it must be remembered that the Commission can only suggest action lines, which have to be agreed and implemented by Member States. European and national organizations of geriatric medicine specialists have a long way to ensure that their older patients have the best multidisciplinary care in the most optimal setting.

CHALLENGES FOR THE EUROPEAN UNION

Although these recent advances are appealing, geriatric medical care in Europe is still challenged by governments, patients, colleagues, and other parties. Table 3 summarizes some of the challenges that have to be met in the future. Although, some of them depend on political compromise by decision makers, geriatricians will have to prove their ability to offer a broad research base, academic leadership, and efficient health care to their oldest patients Duursma *et al.*, (2004).

Table 3 Challenges for geriatric medical care in the European Union

- Demographic aging.
- High degree of variability in geriatric health-care systems between countries and within regions.
- Lack of resources allocated for acute health care, rehabilitation, and long-term care of elderly individuals.
- Competition with other specialities.
- Lack of social support systems and weak coordination with health-care systems.
- Urgent need for specific guidelines and evidence-based practice for older people and geriatric syndromes. Good research networks are also lacking.
- Lack of expertise and formal education in general geriatric medical care of primary-care physicians.
- Geriatric medicine is not officially accepted in some European states.
- Few academic leaders.
- Agism in patients, professionals, and politicians.

New EU countries face the special challenge of improving geriatric care in the face of competing interests by other national budget-demanding projects, with lower incomes than other EU countries. A change in the perception of aging as an opportunity, not as a problem, has to be fostered in many of these countries.

NOTES

[1] This and other related documents can be found in most European languages at http://europa.eu.int/.

[2] Extracted from "*Modernizing social protection for the development of high-quality, accessible and sustainable health care, and long-term care: support for the national strategies using the "open method of coordination"*". EU COM 304 final, April 2004.

KEY POINTS

- The European Union has 25 Member States.
- The demography of older people is varied and health trends differ.
- Systems of care are not fully developed in all Member States to cope with an increasing older population.
- There is a recognition of the need to give the population access to an appropriately trained health-care workforce.

KEY REFERENCES

- Duursma S, Castleden M, Cherubini A *et al.*, European Union Geriatric Medicine Society. Position statement on geriatric medicine and the provision of health care services to older people. *Journal of Nutrition Health Aging* 2004; **8**(3):190–195.

- European Commission. *The Social Situation in the European Union*. 2004, (Downloadable at http://epp.eurostat.cec.eu.int).
- http://europa.eu.int/abc/index_en.htm, accessed June 27, 2005.
- Hastie IR & Duursma SA. Geriatric medicine section of the European union of medical specialists. Geriatric medicine in the European union: unification of diversity. *Aging-Clinical and Experimental Research* 2003; **15**(4):347–351.
- Whitehead MM. Where do we stand? Research and policy issues concerning inequalities in health and in healthcare. *Acta Oncol* 1999; **38**(1):41–50.

REFERENCES

Berr C, Wancata J & Ritchie K. Prevalence of dementia in the elderly in Europe. *Eur Neuropsychopharmacol* 2005, [Epub ahead of print].

COM 723 final, December 2001 and COM 304 final, April 2004. Available in most European Languages at http://europa.eu.int/.

Duursma S, Castleden M, Cherubini A *et al*., European Union Geriatric Medicine Society. Position statement on geriatric medicine and the provision of health care services to older people. *Journal of Nutrition Health Aging* 2004; **8**(3):190–195.

European Commission. *The Social Situation in the European Union*. 2004, (Downloadable at http://epp.eurostat.cec.eu.int).

Gothëborg European Council. *Presidency Conclusions*. 2001, SN 200/1/01 Rev 1, conclusion #43. Available in most European Languages at http://europa.eu.int/.

Hastie IR & Duursma SA. Geriatric medicine section of the European union of medical specialists. Geriatric medicine in the European union: unification of diversity. *Aging-Clinical and Experimental Research* 2003; **15**(4):347–351.

http://europa.eu.int/abc/index_en.htm, accessed June 27, 2005.

Whitehead MM. Where do we stand? Research and policy issues concerning inequalities in health and in healthcare. *Acta Oncol* 1999; **38**(1):41–50.

FURTHER READING

Michel JP, Rubenstein LZ, Vellas BJ & Albarede JL. *Geriatric Programs and Departments Around the World* 1998; Serdi, Paris.

168

Delivery of Health Care in India

Om Prakash Sharma
Geriatric Society of India, New Delhi, India

HISTORICAL BACKGROUND

Ayurveda (Ray, 1994) was the system of medicine in the Indian subcontinent and its description is as old as *Sanatan Dharma (Hindu Religion). Dhanwantri,* the physician of Gods and Goddesses practiced only *Ayurveda*. The three other books (Upoddhat, 1994) in Ayurveda which became famous are *Charak-Samhita* (Upoddhat, 1994), *Sushurta-Samhita*, and *Kashyap-Samhita*. The Indian medicines were derived from *herbs*. Old age, old-age ailments, and antiaging measures (rejuvenation) have been described in the above medical literature.

After *Mahabharatha* (the great battle between members of two dynasties), the invasion of the Indian subcontinent by foreign powers began. This introduced other systems of medicine and led to cessation of researches and growth of *Ayurveda*. This continued under British rule, which lasted for 150 years. With the British Empire came the *System of Modern Medicine*, which is still the most popular system in India and is being followed by the majority of the society. This also has the blessings and support of the government.

With independence (1947), India inherited a population infested with diseases, poor sanitation, and an unplanned health support system. Diseases like *tetanus neonatorum, cholera, plague, puerperal sepsis, malaria, small pox, gastroenteritis,* and so on, used to take a heavy toll. Death in all age-groups was very common, but more so in neonates, infants, and children. The fury of epidemics was curtailed by the involvement of world bodies such as World Health Organisation (WHO). With education and also the improvement in per-capita income, the health scenario started improving. The death rate came down, life expectancy increased, and the population, especially that of older persons started rising. At present, approximately 86 million, that is, 8.6% of the total population is of geriatric age-group (above 60 years).

Indian scenario 1947 to 2003
(Life expectancy at birth)

1947: Life expectancy 34 years
2002: Life expectancy 64 years

Health awareness improved and so did the availability of medical facilities. Earlier, the attention was on bread earners only, but by the end of the last millennium, health of the elderly also became a topic of concern. Soon, medical men as well as lay public realized that what was earlier being discarded as old-age ailments and seen with a pessimistic attitude now needed changing. Medical and health needs of people aged more than 60 became an issue for which one looked toward the West for clues. This propagated development of geriatric medicine. A major turning point in the recognition of the potentials of the problem of aging in India was the "Vienna International Plan of Action on Ageing" adopted by the World Assemble on Ageing (United Nations, 1983). In 1982, the WHO had implemented several worldwide programs for the elderly by adopting the theme "Add life to years", which was followed by *Active Aging* and *Healthy Aging*. The Alma-Ata Declaration of WHO in 1978 introduced the notion of incorporating the needs of older persons within systems of primary care under the rubric of "Health for all" (United Nations, 1988) by the year 2000. A boom in the sociomedical activities came in 1999 by the declaration of Dr Koffi Annan in United Nations Assembly as the *International Year of Older Persons.*

DEMOGRAPHY OF AGING (PONNUSWAMI, 2003; KUMAR, 1997)

In India, persons 60 years and above are considered as elderly. At the beginning of this century, the number of

Principles and Practice of Geriatric Medicine, 4th Edition. Edited by M.S. John Pathy, Alan J. Sinclair and John E. Morley.

elderly was 12 million only, which doubled in the next 60 years, making their number 24 million by the year 1961. This number rose to 56 million by the year 1991. The figure for the year 2001 and projected figure for 2016 are 70 million and 112 million respectively. The decadal growth rates in 60+ age-group from 1951 to 1961 have remained above 26% and are about 5 to 8% higher than that for the total population. There has been a major increase in life expectancy at birth with a consequent impact at 60 years of age. Expectancy of life at birth has risen by more than 10 years from 49.7 years during 1970 to 1975 to 60.3 years during 1991–1995. Over this quarter century, life expectancy at 60 and 70 years has also shown significant rise from 13.8 and 8.9 years respectively to 16.2 and 10.6 years. In 1991 census data, it was observed that of the 78% of the elderly that lived in villages, there were 930 females to every 1000 males in 60+ age-group (see Figure 1), 34% of them were widowed (15% males and 54% females), 52% were illiterate, and 39% were working (60% males and 16% females).

Women normally outlive men and there are always more widows than widowers. From the point of view of geriatric management in India, we divide the above in three segments:

Young Elderly: 60–64 years
Middle Elderly: 65–70 years
Old Elderly: 71 years and above.

This division has been done because it influences all the three aspects relating to elderly care, that is, social, financial, and medical aspects. Considering that the young elderly are still fit to work and socially well adjusted in the younger generation, the age of retirement was raised (in the government jobs/PSUs) from 55 to 62 years in various capacities. The Supreme Court judges of India retire at the age of 65. This division is important from medical aspects also because people in the young elderly age-group were required to be absolutely fit and working, hence their medical and health needs had priority over the other two age sets.

Currently, there are 24 million elderly in the young elderly age-group and males outnumber females, contrary to the second and third groups.

HEALTH AND MORBIDITY

The leading cause of death in old age in India is cardiovascular diseases (CVD). Earlier in life, infections are still the leading causes of death, but among older people most deaths are due to noncommunicable diseases (Goha Roy, 1994). The Indian Council of Medical Research (ICMR) has attempted to compile data on morbidity from different sources.

- The total number of blind persons among the older population was around 11 million in 1996, 80% of them due to cataract (Angra *et al.*, 1997). The consequences of blindness are not limited only to physical disability that ensues, but also impinge on economic, social, and psychological domains of the affected individual's life. The calculated economic costs for maintenance of the blind is Rs 432 000 million, and loss of productivity is Rs 86 400 million over a decade. Nearly 60% of older people are said to have hearing impairment in both urban and rural areas. The hearing loss and resultant communication problems adversely affect the well-being of older people (Kacker, 1997).
- In 1996, the number of people with hypertension among the elderly population was nearly nine million. The prevalence rate of coronary heart disease among the urban population was nearly three times higher than the rural population and the estimated number of cases was around nine million in 1996 (Shah and Prabhakar, 1997).
- An estimated five million elderly people were diabetic and the prevalence rates were about 177 and 35 per 1000 for urban and rural dwellers respectively.
- A crude estimate of the prevalence rate of strokes is about 200 per 100 000 persons. Older persons surviving through peak years of stroke (55–65 years) with varying degrees of disability are already a major medical problem (Dalal, 1997).

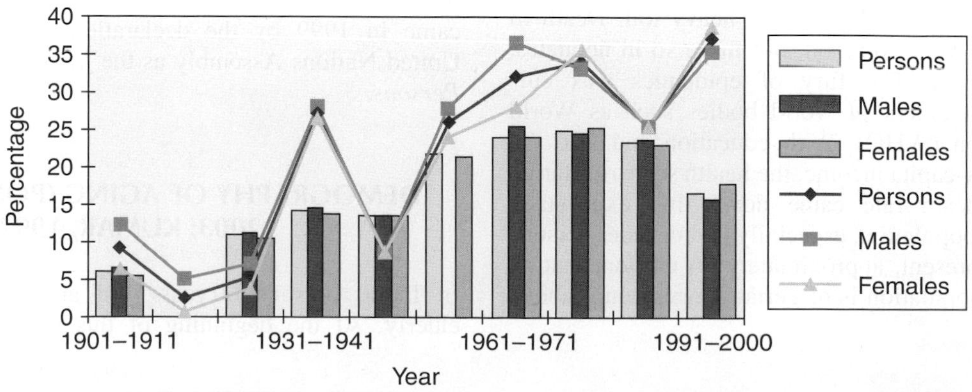

Figure 1 Decadal variation (percentage) in general population and elderly population (60+) by sex-wise – India (1901–2001)

- Population-based cancer registries were initiated by the ICMR in 1982. The number of older persons with cancer in 1996 was 0.35 million. The reports show that in coming years, as the number of aged increases, the problems associated with cancer in older age will require greater attention and resources.
- Age-related changes in the immune system render people susceptible to a variety of infections and tumors. Though tuberculosis-related mortality has declined, it is still not eradicated effectively and the prevalence rate is reported to be higher in the older age-group (Dey and Chaudhury, 1997). Adverse reactions and major side effects to anti-tuberculosis therapy have been reported in as much as 40% of the cases.
- Disabilities arising from aging assume greater significance as a large segment of this population is below the poverty line. Undernutrition is also common in this population (Srivastava *et al.*, 1996). Elderly people in low socioeconomic groups, in urban slums, or those living alone are at higher risk of poor dietary intake (Wadhwa *et al.*, 1997). The nutrients least adequately supplied in the diet of the aged Indian are calcium, iron, vitamin A, riboflavin, and niacin. Health is a key contributing factor to quality of life and is therefore closely associated to low socioeconomic conditions (Bali, 1997).

DISEASE PATTERN IN ELDERLY

Forty five percent of the elderly have a chronic disease. The 10 most common diseases are *hypertension, cataract, osteoarthritis, chronic obstructive airway disease, ischemic heart disease, diabetes, benign prostatic hypertrophy, dyspepsia, constipation, and depression.*

There is not much difference in the disease pattern between the rural and urban elderly. There are limited epidemiological studies about disease patterns in elderly. They are by Angra *et al.* on *cataract*, Dalal PM on *stroke*, Dey *et al.* on *infections*, Kacker SK on *hearing loss*, Srivastava *et al.* on *nutrition*, (Venkoba Rao, 1997) on *psychiatric problems*, and (Gupta, 1997) on *hypertension in elderly*.

Chronic diseases in elderly

Hypertension	*Cataract*	*Osteoarthritis*
Chronic obstructive airway disease	*Ischemic heart disease*	*Diabetes*
Benign prostate hypertrophy	*Dyspepsia*	*Constipation*
	Depression	

Rural elderly have apprehensions and apathy about contacting doctors of modern system of medicine. They mostly thrive on indigenous systems of medicine. Hence, they are usually brought to hospitals in the advanced stages of diseases. The five most common killer diseases in rural elderly are *bronchitis and pneumonia, ischemic heart disease, stroke, cancer, and tuberculosis.*

SOCIAL ISSUES AND HEALTH

Old age in India is associated with several social problems. They are social isolation, poverty, apparent reduction in family support, inadequate housing, impairment of cognitive functioning, mental illness, widowhood, bereavement, limited options for living arrangement toward end of life because of dependency due to physical or mental disease.

All these problems have an impact on the quality of life in old age and health care at the time of need. In traditional Indian societies, joint-family system used to take care of most of these social issues. In the INDO–UK Workshop in 1995, it was concluded that revival of the joint-family system would be the most befitting solution to the problems of elderly in India.

INDO – UK workshop 1995 (Sharma, 1999, 2004)

Joint-family system

However, with industrialization, urbanization, and disintegration of traditional joint family, older people in India are likely to face major social problems. In the absence of well-organized social support networks similar to that available in developed societies, the scenario appears gloomy. It is expected that in a not too distant future, the elderly in the organized sector will be opting more and more for living arrangements similar to that in developed societies namely old-age homes and senior citizen homes. For the elderly in the unorganized sector, the options remain limited due to poverty and destitution in the absence of family support. Nevertheless, family and the community provide the most important support for elderly persons in India. It is thus necessary to strengthen the traditional family system through community education and social interventions.

THE INFRASTRUCTURE

Social

In ancient times in India, the village was the unit and agriculture was the main profession. The system of joint family existed and it was not uncommon to see a family of four to five generations living together under the same roof. The head of the family was respected most and his opinion on account of his age, authority, and experience was considered valuable. The elderly were looked after well with devotion and dedication by the younger generation. The social support from the family was quite adequate and the need for support by the community or the government/ruler was rare. The financial, social, and emotional support was always provided by the younger family members and medical needs were also covered by them as and when required.

With industrialization and urbanization, the social problems started occurring in the form of migrations, leading to increasing numbers of nuclear families. The age-old joint-family system started cracking. Elderly people became unsupported in rural areas. In the urban area, the elderly suffered because of the changing economy. By the time people reached the age of retirement, they had exhausted their financial resources and savings in constructing a house, bringing up children, getting them educated, getting them married, and in fulfilling social obligations. The elderly who were not prepared for this transition became penniless and suffered the most especially when their children migrated for jobs and so on. The urban elderly were also divided economically into rich, middle class, and poor elderly.

The government came forward and made some *old-age homes* for the poor and destitute elderly. Old-age homes were also made by some Nongovernmental Organizations (NGOs) and individuals. The total number of old-age homes in India is about 2000. The government created some social schemes and brought out *constitutional and legal provisions*.

Constitutional Provisions (Ponnuswami, 2003; www.parliamentofindia.nic.in)

In the constitution of India, under various clauses, certain rights have been guaranteed to elderly citizens:

- Item 9 of the State List and Items 20, 23, and 24 of the Concurrent List relate to provision of old-age pension, social security, social insurance, economic and social planning, and relief to the disabled and the unemployed.
- Article 41, Directive Principles of State Policy (Fundamental Rights and directive Principles of State Policy, 1950), has particular relevance to old age social security. It directs that the State shall "make effective provision for securing the right to work, to education, and to public assistance in case of unemployment, old age sickness and disablement, and in other cases of undeserved want, within its limits of economic development and capacity".
- Article 41 is reinforced by Section 125 1(d) of the Code of Criminal Procedure, 1973 under which every person having sufficient means is required to provide for his parents who are unable to maintain themselves.
- Section 20 (3) of the Hindu Adoption and Maintenance Act, 1956, makes it obligatory on the part of the person to maintain his aged or infirm parents.
- Fundamental Right Article 16 (2) – Equal opportunity in matters of public employment.
- Article 21 – Protection of life and personal liberty. No person shall be deprived of his life or personal liberty except according to procedure established by law.
- Article 38 – State to secure a social order for the promotion of welfare of the people.
  - The State shall strive to promote the welfare of the people by securing and protecting as effectively as it may a social order in which justice, social, economic, and political, shall inform all the institutions of the national life.
  - The State shall, in particular, strive to minimize the inequalities in income, and endeavor to eliminate inequalities in status, facilities, and opportunities not only amongst individuals but also amongst groups of people residing in different areas or engaged in different vocations.
- Article 39(a) – Adequate means of livelihood.
- Article 39(b) – Right to ownership and control of material resources to subserve the common good.
- Article 39(c) – Ensures equal pay for equal work.
- Article 39(e) – Citizens not being forced by economic necessity to enter a vocation unsuited to their age or strength.
- Article 39A – Equal justice and free legal aid – The State shall secure that the operation of the legal system promotes justice, on a basis of equal opportunity, and shall, in particular, provide free legal aid, by suitable legislation or schemes or in any other way, to ensure that opportunities for securing justice are not denied to any citizen by reason of economic or other disabilities.
- Article 42 – Provision for just and humane conditions of work and maternity relief. The State shall make provision for securing just and humane conditions of work and for maternity relief.
- Article 43 – Living wage, etc., for workers – The State shall endeavor to secure, by suitable legislation or economic organization or in any other way, to all workers, agricultural, industrial, or otherwise, work, a living wage, conditions of work ensuring a decent standard of life and full enjoyment of leisure, and social and cultural opportunities and, in particular, the State shall endeavor to promote cottage industries on an individual or cooperative basis in rural areas.
- Article 44, Uniform civil code for the citizen – The State shall endeavor to secure for the citizens a uniform civil code throughout the territory of India.
- Article 47 – Raising the level of nutrition and the standard of living of its people and improvement of public health. The Concurrent List covers social security, social insurance, employment, invalidity, and old-age pension.
- Entry 24 in list III of schedule VII in constitution of India deals with welfare of laborers including condition of work, liability for workmen compensation, provident funds, invalidity, old-age pension and maternity benefits.
- Himachal Pradesh assembly passed Parents Maintenance Bill 1996, according to which, parents who are ignored by their children are to be given maintenance. In addition, to make it obligatory for errant wards not taking care of their aged parents, the bill aims at simplifying the procedure by authorizing the subdivisional officer (Civil) for fixing maintenance and additional commissioner as the appellate authority so that decisions can be taken and cases disposed of promptly, bringing justice and relief to older persons without loss of time.

Legal Provisions (Frontline from the Publishers of The Hindu, 2001)

As per the letter number F.No.20-76/99-SD, dated 3/11/99 of Ministry of Social Justice and Empowerment (SD Section), Government of India, the Honorable Chief Justice of India Shri R. K. Anand has advised chief justices of all the High Courts in the country to accord priority for the cause list for cases involving elderly persons and ensure their expeditious disposal.

- Section 88B of Finance Act 1992 (Income tax Act 1961) – Provides rebate of income tax to senior citizens who have attained the age of 65 at any time during the relevant previous year. From 1998 to 1999, tax rebate under Section 88B shall be as follows:
  - The amount of income tax before giving any rebate under Section 88, 88B and 88(1) or
  - Rs 10 000 or 40%, whichever is less (Rebate is available from assessment year 1998 to 1999 even if total income is above Rs 1 20 000).
- Section 80D (Finance Bill 1999) – An assessee is entitled to a deduction upto Rs 15 000 with effect from year 2000–2001, where assessee, his/her spouse, dependent parents, or any member of the family is a senior citizen (above 65 years), and medical insurance premium is paid to effect or keep in force an insurance in relation to him or her.
- Section 80DDB (Finance Bill 1999) – Provides a separate deduction to a resident assessee being an individual or Hindu undivided family member for expenditure incurred for medical treatment for the individual himself or his dependent relative, irrespective of disease. The deduction shall be limited to Rs 40 000 and in case of senior citizen, a fixed deduction of Rs 60 000 will be available.
- The Finance Act of 2000 provides a rebate of Rs 15 000 in income tax (as against Rs 10 000 in earlier years) for all senior citizens above the age of 65.
- Delhi Rent Control Act 1995 (Act No. 33 of 1995) – Section 24 explains the right to recover immediate possession of premises to accrue to members of the armed forces, and so on.
  - Where a person

    (1) is a released or retired person from any armed forces and the premises let out by him, his spouse, or his dependent son, or daughter are required for his own residence, (2) is a member of any of the armed forces and has a period of less than one year preceding that date of his retirement and the premises let out by him, his spouse, or his dependent son, or daughter, are required for his own residence after his retirement, he, his spouse, or his dependent son, or daughter, at any time, within a period of one year before the date of his retirement, apply to the Rent Authority for recovery of immediate possession of such premises. Section 25 explains the right to recover immediate possession of premises to accrue to Central Government and State Government employees. (3) is a retired employee of the Central Government or of a State Government and the premises let out by his spouse, or his dependent son, or daughter, are required for his own residence, such employee, his spouse, or his dependent son, or daughter, within one year from the date of his retirement or within a period of one year from the date of commencement of this Act, whichever is later, can apply to the Rent Authority for recovery of immediate possession of such premises. (4) is an employee of the Central Government or a State Government and has a period of less than one year preceding the date of his retirement and the premises let out by him, or his spouse, or dependent son, or daughter, are required by him for his own residence after his retirement, he, his spouse, or his dependant son, or daughter may at any time within a period of one year before the date of retirement apply to the Rent Authority for recovery of immediate possession of such premises.

Medical

Medical and health is a state subject. The Central Government as well as all the 28 State Governments have their own health ministries and Directorates of Health.

Flow Chart of Medical Infrastructure in India (see Figure 2)

Central Government

The Central Government has a Ministry of Health and Family Welfare and a Directorate of Health services; these bodies look after the medical and health needs of Central Government employees. They are also in charge of liaisons with world bodies like WHO, United Nations International Children's Emergency Fund (UNICEF), and so on, and control the funds of these bodies to the central as well as state health directorates.

Central Government Health Scheme (CGHS). This was started on 1 May 1954 on the pattern of National Health Service (NHS) of United Kingdom. The objective was to provide medical services to Central Government employees; however, certain other categories like journalists, judges, account services, post and telegraph, and autonomous bodies like the Delhi Police were also included in the scheme. CGHS covered the above category of people in 22 cities in India. There was a nominal contribution from the employees against which the services like consultation, investigations, medicines, in-hospital treatment, surgeries, and implants were provided. The employees were *referred* abroad in case suitable treatment was not available in this country. All the dependent family members and people retired from these services were included in this medical coverage. In the year 2000, the government took a bold decision to put many

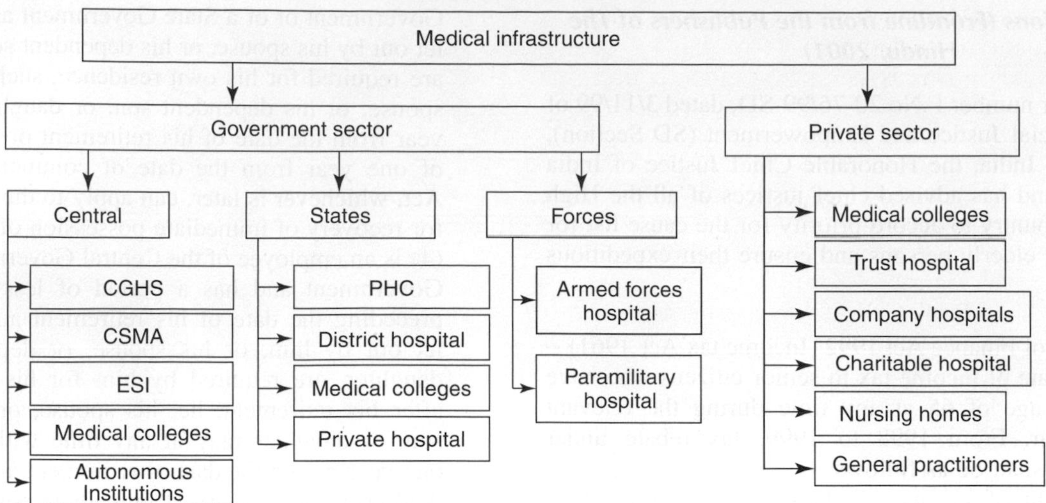

Figure 2 Medical infrastructure in India

private hospitals/institutions on the CGHS approved list for medical treatment.

Central Services Medical Assistance (CSMA). This was similar to CGHS but did not provide coverage for the retired and the elderly. It was limited to serving employees only, who, if posted at places outside the 22 cities, were allowed to opt for a nearby city where the CGHS infrastructure existed.

Employees State Insurance Corporation (ESI). Under the Ministry of Labour, this medical scheme was started to provide medical coverage for the labor class. Under this scheme, ESI hospitals and dispensaries were set up on a large scale. Elderly and retired persons continue to enjoy medical facilities under this scheme.

State Governments

All the 28 State Governments in India have the same three-tier system for providing health facilities. There are nearly 28 000 primary health centers (PHC) located in villages where primary care is provided free of cost. There are 575 district hospitals in these states where the patient is referred for secondary health care. In these states, there are hospitals attached to medical colleges as well as other hospitals that provide tertiary care. The State Government employees as well as the general public can avail treatment from all these places.

Public Sector Units. There are 258 public sectors under Central Government which have their offices, factories, refineries, plants, and so on, throughout the country. Their employees get medical aid from the hospitals and dispensaries owned by these public sector units (PSUs). There are provisions for referring them to government as well as private institutions in case of need.

Armed Forces and Paramilitary Forces

In each command, there is a command hospital and some smaller hospitals in the Indian Army. There are similar facilities for the Navy and Air Force. There is a large Research and Referral Center now being attached to a medical college under the Directorate of Armed Forces Health and Medical Services at New Delhi. There is already one medical college for armed forces at Pune. There are hospitals with paramedical forces like Border Security Force (BSF), Central Reserve Police Force (CRPF), Indo-Tibetan Border Police (ITBP), and so on.

Private Sector

In the last two decades, the private sector has developed considerably to provide health care and has exceeded the government infrastructure for health. There are tertiary care hospitals and research centers owned by various trusts, private companies, and also companies who have floated shares. Most of these large centers have been approved for treatment of government employees. There are also private nursing homes and clinics owned by private practitioners.

The private sector has become a significant partner with the government in health-care delivery.

Nursing

Nursing is an integral part of geriatric care. In India, the following courses in nursing have geriatrics as a part of teaching.

- Three-year diploma course for Nursing where the basic qualification is 10 + 2 (Schooling).
- Bachelors Degree in Nursing (B.Sc Nursing): This is a 4-year course.

- Masters Degree in Nursing (M.Sc. Nursing): This is a 2-year course after Bachelors Degree.
- M. Phil (Nursing): This is a 1-year course if done full time, but is a 2-year course if done part time.

The above facilities are available in RAK College of Nursing at New Delhi and also at Manipal Academy of Higher Education in Karnataka.

Ph.D. (Nursing): This is a 3 year course at Rajiv Gandhi University of Health Sciences, Bangalore; SNGT Women University, Mumbai; RAK College of Nursing, New Delhi; Jawahar Lal University, New Delhi; PGI, Chandigarh; and Punjab University.

PLANNING GERIATRIC SERVICES (WHO EXPERT COMMITTEE, 1974)

As per the health-care planning by Government of India in 1952, there was a three-tier system.

1. Primary care level (at village level)
2. Secondary care level (at district level)
3. Tertiary care level (in cities).

Primary care level is at the level of PHCs of which there are nearly 28 000 in this country. Health being a state subject, all these centers are funded and governed by states in India. However, the Central Government and world bodies do give them help from time to time under various programs. The doctors posted to PHCs are being encouraged to attend Continued Medical Education (CME) programs in geriatrics medicine.

Secondary care level is at the level of District Hospitals, which now number almost 600 and are also controlled by states in the above fashion. The specialists here are encouraged to upgrade themselves in geriatric medicine. Geriatric services are being introduced into these District Hospitals in the following manner:

Steps of geriatric care (WHO expert committee, 1974)	
1) Outpatient	*2) Inpatient*
3) Domiciliary	*4) Community*

At the tertiary care level, the centers are under control of the state, Central Government, NGOs, and other autonomous bodies. In the last two decades, private and corporate sectors have developed and improved substantially in health-care delivery and in the past one decade, the government has collaborated with the private sector, resulting in a better coordination between government and private sectors rather than rivalry/competition. Geriatric out patient departments (OPDs) and services are being conducted in these institutions.

With the rapid modes of transport, faster communication, changing economy, and so on, it is only arbitrary to keep these three distinctions. Beyond reasons related to administration and finances, secondary care level has largely merged into tertiary care level. I would therefore directly comment about such care levels which can be suitably modified depending upon resources and need.

DEVELOPMENT OF GERIATRIC MEDICINE

Government

Geriatric medicine has not been part of the undergraduate medical curriculum till recently. This gave no exposure to appropriate teaching in geriatric medicine to the medical and paramedical personnel produced in India till the late 1990s. "Vienna International Plan of Action on Ageing" adopted by the World Assemble on Ageing (UN, 1983) helped the initiation of geriatric services in India.

The Central Government in the year 1995 organized a workshop on geriatric care. This was a joint venture of the Government of India and the Government of Britain. The Ministry of Health and Family Welfare and ICMR participated on behalf of the Government of India. The problems were identified and the quantum was accessed and weighed against resources. It was concluded that revival of the joint-family system is the only solution to the geriatric situation in India at the moment.

In 1999, with WHO support, the Government of India carried out an exhaustive exercise to bring out learning material for medical and paramedical personnel. During the same exercise, an attempt was made to create resource personnel (medical) for geriatric care. Several government sponsored programs to create learning material for paramedics giving geriatric care were started. One such program was by NICE (National Initiative on Care of Elderly by the Ministry of Social Justice and Empowerment).

At this juncture, MCI introduced geriatric medicine into the medical undergraduate curriculum so as to give some exposure to MBBS students.

Institutions like the Medical College of Madras, which introduced an MD Degree in Geriatric Medicine, gave a lead to the teaching institutions, which was followed by Banaras Hindu University (BHU). The OPD services, geriatric units, and geriatric departments were started by many medical college hospitals as well as tertiary care hospitals. The doctors in government and armed forces were encouraged to undergo training in geriatrics.

NGOs

The main NGOs who played a significant role in sensitizing and updating doctors in India are the Geriatric Society of India (GSI), Indian Medical Association (IMA), and Indira Gandhi National Open University (IGNOU).

Geriatric Society of India (GSI)

The GSI was formed in the year 1980 with the main objective "to sensitize, train, and update Indian doctors in the field of Geriatrics". GSI organized CME programs at regional, national, and international levels. GSI organized its annual conferences jointly with the Association of Physicians of India (API) till 2002 when it finally separated from API for its independent scientific programs. GSI has organized International Conferences in the year 1999, 2001, and 2002. It has also awarded fellowships to the doctors who had made significant contributions in the field of geriatric medicine. The society supported Dr O.P. Sharma for bringing out the learning material "Geriatric Care in India". This became the first textbook on Geriatrics in India, which gives comprehensive coverage of Indian elderly in 77 Chapters spread over 750 pages. In the year 2004, Dr O.P. Sharma brought out another textbook "Geriatric Care" covering Geriatrics in 85 Chapters (Sharma, 2004). The society encouraged opening of OPDs for elderly care in government as well as nongovernmental institutions and gives technical help for this purpose. It also encourages medical and relief camps for elderly. GSI stimulates and supports research in the field of geriatric medicine.

Indian Medical Association (IMA)

IMA is the largest NGO of doctors in India. It works through its 1600 branches spread over the length and breadth of country. IMA, through its branches and through its academic wings (Indian College of General Practitioners, IMA Academy of Medical Specialities and IMA AKN Sinha Institute), is involved in CME activities. Geriatric medicine is a part of the activities of the CME. In 2002, the IMA AKN Sinha Institute started a PG Certificate Course in Geriatrics. Every year, about 250 doctors take up this course.

Indira Gandhi National Open University (IGNOU)

In 2001, IGNOU decided to start a Distant Education course in Geriatrics. It took one year to produce modules and the full course has now been commissioned. The first batch comprised 250 students.

Association of Physicians of India (API)

API is the voluntary body of physicians who carry out CME activities all over the country. API is considering geriatric medicine in all of its programs. The Indian College of Physicians is awarding scholarships under its Sponsored Training Program (STP) in geriatrics.

Medical Council of India (MCI) (Medical Council of India, 1995)

MCI is the watchdog of medical education in India. It had not included Geriatrics in the medical curriculum till late 1990s. Inspired by WHO declarations and repeated projections of rise in the number of elderly, MCI added Geriatrics in its revised undergraduate curriculum. The All Indian Institute of Medical Sciences (AIIMS) was one of the first few institutions to stress the teaching of geriatric medicine in the undergraduate curriculum. The example of the Madras Medical College is a lead in considering an MD in geriatric medicine. The department of Geriatric Medicine in BHU, Varanasi was one of the biggest to be set up in a medical institution.

NATIONAL POLICY OF THE AGED

A national policy for old persons was formulated in January 1999, which covers the dimensions of social, economic, and health security. The Union Ministry of Social Justice and Empowerment is the nodal agency for implementation. A national council for Older Persons has been constituted to implement the policies and programs for an aging population.

Key Elements of the Policy

1. To achieve integration between the young and old and develop a support system, formal and informal, to increase the potential of the families to take care of the aged persons.
2. Tapping human resources among elderly people.
3. Expansion of old-age pension scheme to include the private sector, subsidize health-care network with private sector involvement, increased standard tax deduction for senior citizens, legislations on parents' right to be supported by their children, regulatory authority to monitor pension funds, easy access to housing loans, and special provisions in the Indian Penal Code for protection of older persons.

The health services will be provided through primary, secondary, and tertiary-level government institutions, by nonprofit organizations including trusts and charitable institutions, and also private medical care.

Facilities for specialization in geriatric medicine will be provided in the medical colleges.

Hospices for chronically ill and deprived elderly will be set up.

Training and orientation will be provided to medical and paramedical personnel working at various levels of health-care facilities.

Primary health-care system to be strengthened and orientated to be able to meet the health needs of older persons.

There should be proper distribution of services in rural and urban areas and a much better health administration and delivery system.

High priority to health insurance to cater for the needs of different income groups in society with varying contributions and benefits.

Trusts, societies, and voluntary agencies promoted by way of grants, tax relief, lending at subsidized rates to provide free beds, medicines, and treatment to very poor elderly citizens with reasonable user charges for the rest of the population.

Private nursing homes and hospitals will be directed to offer discounts to older patients and public hospitals will have separate counters and convenient timings with facilities of geriatric wards.

Mobile medical unit of health services, special camps, and ambulance services will be encouraged to ensure accessibility and use of hospital services.

ELDERLY CARE COVERAGE

Elderly people obtain medical and health benefits from the following bodies:

1. Central Government – Central Government Health Scheme (CGHS)
2. State Government Health Services
3. Armed Forces Health Services
4. Public Sector undertakings
5. Employees State Insurance Corporation (ESI)
6. Mediclaim and Health Insurances

Retired personnel (age of retirement 60 years ± 2 years) have medical coverage ranging from partial to total coverage in Central Government, State Governments, armed forces, paramedical forces, industries, private entrepreneurs, and self-taken insurance coverage.

Health-Care Facility

- Sunday clinics at various hospitals in Delhi exist to enable senior citizens to get medical care easily.
- Geriatric ward and OPD (once a week) exist in municipal hospitals in Mumbai and Government hospitals of Chennai and Kerala.
- Free intraocular lens (IOL) is given for cataract surgery in Gujarat. However, in Maharashtra Rs 600 is to be paid.
- The mobile medicare unit (MMU) program is the program implemented by Help Age India to provide basic essential medicare at the doorstep of needy and underprivileged elderly in India.
- Free health-care checkup camps organized by government or social organizations.
- Medical Insurance Scheme (Mediclaim). This policy has been available since November 1999 to persons aged between five and 80 years. The sum insured varies from Rs 15 000 to 500 000 and premium varies from Rs 201 to Rs 16 185 per person per annum depending upon different quantums of insured services and age-groups. The cover provides for reimbursement of medical expenses incurred by an individual toward hospitalization/domiciliary treatment, hospitalization for any illness, injury, or disease contracted or sustained during the period of insurance.

Group Medical Insurance Scheme

The group Mediclaim policy is available to any group/association/institution/corporate body of more than 100 persons, provided it has a central administration point. The basic policy under this scheme is Mediclaim only.

Jan Arogya

The Jan Arogya scheme is primarily for the larger section of the population with an age limit of 70 years who cannot afford the high cost of medical treatment. The limit of cover per person is Rs 5000 per annum. The cover provides reimbursement of medical expenses incurred by an individual toward hospitalization/domiciliary hospitalization for any illness, injury, or disease contracted or sustained during the period of insurance.

Others

- The National Council for Older Persons has been constituted to provide guiding steps as well as feedback on the policies for welfare of elderly persons.
- Rupees 30 lakhs shall be provided to eligible institutions for construction of old-age homes/multiservice centers for older persons.
- Financial assistance up to 90% is provided to NGOs for establishing and maintaining old-age homes, day-care centers, MMUs, and for providing noninstitutional services to older persons.
- Special consideration has been given to elderly in telephone and banking services. Various helplines have been instituted.
- The National Consumer Redressal Commission (Legal aid Program), 5th Floor, A Wing, Janpath Bhawan, New Delhi, has been providing free legal aid in court or other matters.
- The National Institute of Social Defense, launched a project NICE in year 2000, which provides cost-free technical training on the care of elderly.

For success of various schemes and initiatives for the welfare of elderly people as described, effective implementation and continuous follow-up are required. Welfare of elderly citizens of rural areas requires reinforcement and strengthening of the ability and commitment of the family to provide care. Improvement in intergenerational relationships, care of destitute elderly, and promotion of productive aging (using wisdom and experience of elderly people) should be specially emphasized, besides efforts involving multiple sectors, thereby helping elderly individuals to live with dignity and self-esteem with the feeling of being wanted.

KEY POINTS

- The population of Elderly persons is rising significantly in India.
- There are both medical as well as social needs of Indian elderly which require attention.
- There is an urgent need to develop geriatric medicine.
- The infrastructure for Medical care of elderly persons needs expansion.
- The government and NGOs will join hands and become partners in geriatric care.

KEY REFERENCES

- Dalal PM. Strokes in the elderly: prevalence, risk factors and the strategies for prevention. *The Indian Journal of Medical Research* 1997; **106**:325–32.
- Kacker SK. Hearing impairment in the aged. *The Indian Journal of Medical Research* 1997; **106**:333–9.
- Kumar V. Ageing in India-an overview. *The Indian Journal of Medical Research* 1997; **106**:257–64.
- Sharma OP. *A textbook on Geriatric Care in India* 1999, ABN Publishers, New Delhi.
- Sharma OP. *A textbook on Geriatric Care* 2004, VIVA Books Private Ltd, New Delhi.
- Srivastava M, Kapil U, Kumar V *et al.* Knowledge, attitude and practices regarding nutrition in patients attending geriatric clinic at the AIIMS. In V Kumar (ed) *Ageing-Indian Perspective and Global Scenario* 1996, pp 407–9; All Indian Institute of Medical Sciences, New Delhi.

REFERENCES

Angra SK, Murthy GV, Gupta SK & Angra V. Cataract related blindness in India and its social implications. *The Indian Journal of Medical Research* 1997; **106**:312–24.

Bali A. Socio Economic status and its relationship to morbidity among elderly. *The Indian Journal of Medical Research* 1997; **106**:349–60.

Dalal PM. Strokes in the elderly: prevalence, risk factors and the strategies for prevention. *The Indian Journal of Medical Research* 1997; **106**:325–32.

Dey AB & Chaudhury D. Infections in the elderly. *The Indian Journal of Medical Research* 1997; **106**:273–85.

Frontline from the Publishers of The Hindu. Volume 18:Issue 22:Oct27-Nov 09, 2001.

Fundamental Rights and directive Principles of State Policy. Constitution of India (www.parliamentofindia.nic.in) 1950.

Goha Roy S. Morbidity related epidemiological determinants in Indian aged. An overview. In CR Ramachandran & B Shah (eds) *Public Health Implications of Ageing in India* 1994, pp 114–25; Indian Council of Medical Research, New Delhi.

Gupta R. Epidemiological evolution and rise of coronary heart disease in India. *South Asian Journal of Preventive Cardiology* 1997; **1**:14–20.

Kacker SK. Hearing impairment in the aged. *The Indian Journal of Medical Research* 1997; **106**:333–9.

Kumar V. Ageing in India-an overview. *The Indian Journal of Medical Research* 1997; **106**:257–64.

Ponnuswami I. Government policies and programmes of older persons in India. Paper presented at *The Fifth International Conference of IAHSA*, Sydney, 23–25 June 2003.

Ray PC. *History of Hindu Chemistry*, Kashyap Samhita Chowkhamba Sanskrit Sansthan 1994, Varanasi.

Schedule to the Indian Medical Council Act 1956, Medical Council of India, New Delhi 1995.

Shah B & Prabhakar AK. Chronic morbidity profile among elderly. *The Indian Journal of Medical Research* 1997; **106**:265–72.

Sharma OP. *A textbook on Geriatric Care in India* 1999, ABN Publishers, New Delhi.

Sharma OP. *A textbook on Geriatric Care* 2004, VIVA Books Private Ltd, New Delhi.

Srivastava M, Kapil U, Kumar V *et al.* Knowledge, attitude and practices regarding nutrition in patients attending geriatric clinic at the AIIMS. In V Kumar (ed) *Ageing-Indian Perspective and Global Scenario* 1996, pp 407–9; All Indian Institute of Medical Sciences, New Delhi.

United Nations. *Vienna International Plan of Action on Ageing* 1983; United Nations, New York.

United Nations. *World Demography Estimates and Projections* 1988, pp 1950–2025, United Nations, New York.

Upoddhat P3-6, Kashyap Samhita Chowkhamba Sanskrit Sansthan, 1994, Varanasi.

Venkoba Rao A. Psychiatric morbidity in the aged. *Indian Journal of Medical Research* 1997; **106**:361–9.

Wadhwa A, Sabharwal M & Sharma S. Nutritional status of the elderly. *The Indian Journal of Medical Research* 1997; **107**:340–8.

WHO Expert Committee. *Report on Planning and Organisation of Geriatric Services*, Technical Report Series Number 548, 1974; WHO.

169

Geriatrics in Latin America

Fernando Morales-Martínez[1] ***and*** **Martha Pelaez**[2]

[1] University of Costa Rica, San José, Costa Rica, and [2] Pan American Health Organization, World Health Organization, Washington, DC, USA

INTRODUCTION

The present status of geriatric medicine in Latin America reflects the demographic history of aging in the region and the diverse schemes for delivering health services to older adults. This chapter addresses these issues within the context of the various academic initiatives under development in the region and discusses the future outlook of geriatrics in Latin America.

Demography and Health Conditions in Latin America and the Caribbean

Latin America and the Caribbean are aging at an accelerated pace. Declining fertility rates combined with steady improvements in life expectancy over the latter half of the twentieth century have produced dramatic speed in the aging of the population. The number of persons 60 years and older in Latin America and the Caribbean is currently about 44 million. An expected annual rate of growth of 3.5% in this population during the first two decades of the century will bring the total of persons 60 years and older to close to 100 million. This number will grow to 168 million by the middle of the twenty-first century. Currently, older persons represent 8% of the total population in Latin America and the Caribbean. By 2025, 14% of the population in Latin America and the Caribbean will be 60 years of age and older (UN Population Aging). However, not all countries in the region are aging with the same momentum or have the same speed of growth. In Table 1, individual countries are presented with three indicators of aging: the proportion of the population above age 60, C(t), the mean age of the population, A(t), and an indicator of the availability of support among the younger generations, L(t). The first indicator is a conventional measure and needs little introduction. The second is also straightforward, *albeit* much less used, but of extreme utility to understand patterns of growth of the older population. The third, L(t), defined as a ratio of adult to older adults, is a crude indicator of kin availability and of constraints in the patterns of the living arrangements of older persons. Altogether, these indicators suffice to characterize the demographic nature of the growth of the older population (Palloni *et al.*, 2002).

A cross-sectional survey sponsored by the Pan American Health Organization (PAHO) during 2000, Aging, Health, and Well-being (SABE) in seven major cities of Latin America and the Caribbean documents that chronic disease is rapidly becoming the new epidemic of developing countries.[1] Hypertension was reported by one out of every two people 60 years and older; the lowest percentage was reported in Mexico City (43%) and the highest in Sao Paulo (53%). One out of five persons reported having heart disease, with the exception of elders in Bridgetown (12%) and in Mexico City (10%), where heart disease was reported less frequently. In most cities, at least one out of three older adults reported having arthritis. However, arthritis appeared to be most significant in Montevideo (48%), Buenos Aires (53%), and Havana (56%), where the proportion was closer to one out of every two elders. Diabetes was highest in Bridgetown and Mexico City, with 22% of older persons reporting it. The percentage of persons reporting having had a stroke is over 8%. Older men were less likely to report having arthritis and hypertension, but were just as likely as women to report having heart disease and diabetes.

In population studies, self-assessed health serves also as a summary measure of health that is well correlated with objective health indicators (Beaman *et al.*, 2003). In the SABE survey, the question: "Would you say that your health is excellent (=4), very good (=3), good (=2), fair (=1) or bad (=0)?" is consistent across cities, providing an aggregate value of the individual's objective health condition. Self-assessment of health is a relatively easy indicator that has been used in surveys throughout the world and is recognized as an important predictor of mortality (Idler and Benyamini, 1997). In SABE, the absolute levels of

Principles and Practice of Geriatric Medicine, 4th Edition. Edited by M.S. John Pathy, Alan J. Sinclair and John E. Morley.

Table 1 Values of the proportion of the population above age 60 [C(t)], the mean age of the population [A(t)], and the ratio of adults to older adults [L(t)] for 1950–2025: countries in Latin America and the Caribbean, and United States (calculations by Dr Alberto Palloni using the United Nations database, 1999)

Country	1950–1955			1990–1995			2020–2025		
	C(t)	A(t)	L(t)	C(t)	A(t)	L(t)	C(t)	A(t)	L(t)
Argentina	7.0	25.5	4.95	12.9	31.3	3.03	16.6	35.6	2.89
Bolivia	5.6	24.2	4.65	5.8	23.9	4.34	8.9	29.3	3.97
Brazil	4.9	23.5	5.16	6.7	27.4	4.31	15.3	35.0	3.24
Chile	6.9	25.4	4.52	9.0	29.6	3.72	18.2	36.2	2.69
Colombia	5.6	24.2	5.02	6.2	26.1	4.19	9.7	33.4	3.28
Costa Rica	5.7	24.3	4.22	6.4	26.4	4.27	14.3	33.8	3.09
Cuba	7.3	25.8	4.51	11.7	33.1	3.30	25.0	42.2	2.44
Dominican Republic	5.2	23.8	4.59	5.6	25.7	4.50	14.2	34.2	3.25
Ecuador	8.1	26.6	3.65	6.1	26.9	4.16	12.6	36.5	3.53
El Salvador	4.8	23.4	4.71	6.0	24.9	3.73	10.1	31.7	3.88
Guatemala	4.3	22.9	5.19	5.1	22.1	4.29	7.4	27.2	4.54
Honduras	3.9	22.5	5.40	4.5	22.3	4.57	8.6	29.4	4.17
Mexico	7.1	25.6	3.89	5.9	25.4	4.21	13.5	34.2	3.43
Nicaragua	4.1	22.7	5.15	4.3	21.7	4.61	8.4	28.4	4.35
Panama	6.5	25.0	4.34	7.3	27.1	3.89	10.5	35.2	3.13
Paraguay	8.9	27.4	3.54	5.4	24.7	4.32	9.4	29.9	3.79
Peru	5.7	24.3	4.66	6.1	27.0	4.29	12.6	36.8	3.56
Uruguay	11.8	30.2	3.37	16.5	34.2	2.69	18.4	37.3	2.57
Venezuela	3.4	22.0	7.00	5.7	25.6	4.61	13.2	33.2	3.32
Barbados	8.5	27.0	4.06	15.3	33.3	2.49	23.2	41.5	2.49
Jamaica	5.8	24.4	5.16	9.2	27.6	2.87	14.9	35.1	3.21
Trinidad	6.1	24.6	4.67	8.7	29.0	3.61	17.4	38.7	2.91
Puerto Rico	6.1	24.6	4.10	13.2	32.7	3.06	20.5	38.2	2.60
United States	12.5	30.8	–	6.6	35.6	–	24.7	40.6	–

Source: Aging in Latin America and the Caribbean, 2002. Unpublished article prepared for the Pan American Health Organization.

prevalence of poor/fair health is quite high, no city has a total summary score equal to 2.0 (Figure 1).

In addition to having poor health, one of every five persons 60 years of age and older in the research cities reported having some difficulty with the basic activities of daily living (bathing, dressing, using the toilet, eating, getting in and out of bed, and walking across a room). Included in this number were those who needed assistance in order to perform an activity as well as those who were unable to do the activity at all. The most common limitation among both men and women aged 60 years and older was walking across a room.

The majority of older persons living in urban centers in Latin America and the Caribbean have access to a primary health-care center. Over 50% of those interviewed by the SABE survey reported that they had visited an ambulatory care provider in the four months prior to the interview and at least 60% received a prescription. Of those who received prescription, over 80% had to pay for this prescription in Buenos Aires, Sao Paulo, and Havana; 69% in Montevideo, 38% in Mexico DF, and 20% in Bridgetown. Ten percent to 20% of elders who received prescriptions were unable to obtain the prescribed medication.

Trends in Health-care Delivery

The lack of health-care professionals trained to provide acute and chronic care for older persons in Latin America and the Caribbean is creating a major dilemma for the region. The two mega countries in the region, Brazil and Mexico, in combination have over 20 million persons 60 years old and over, approximately 42% of all elders in Latin America and the Caribbean. Brazil has only 20 hospitals with geriatric services and Mexico has a total of 12. The lack of organized services targeting the care of older people means that medical education continues to ignore the training of physicians in geriatric medicine. The lack of trained personnel to care for the complex and difficult conditions of older people results in a systematic exclusion of older adults from appropriate care. Therefore, when the health-care system cannot provide treatment, support or care for chronically ill and disabled older adults; families take refuge in homes for the elderly, or board and care homes that are staffed by untrained caregivers, and segregated from the mainstream of public health functions. In addition, because the majority of older adults do not have a pension and those who have a pension, it is not sufficient to cover the cost of living; the family typically finances the cost of private care. Therefore, the development of private nursing homes has lacked an economic incentive to develop professional solutions to the chronic care of older persons with disabilities.

The Evolution of Geriatric Medicine in Latin America

Costa Rica, Chile, Cuba, and Panama are the only countries that have a specialized geriatric hospital; these hospitals vary in the number of services provided and in the degree of complexity that they are able to handle. Costa Rica appears

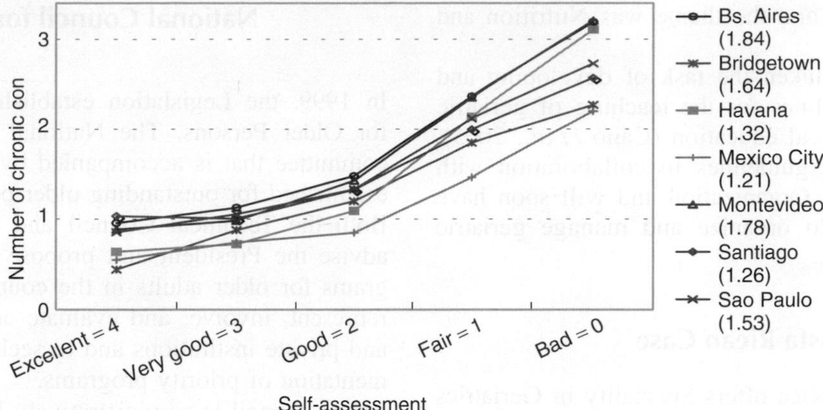

Figure 1 Self-assessed health according to number of chronic conditions (including depression) by city (*Source*: SABE Survey/PAHO – 2000 in Pelaez *et al.*, 2003. © PAHO)

Table 2 Availability of geriatric training and services in selected cities of Latin America

Country	Formal University training in Geriatrics[c]	Geriatric unit	Geriatric medicine department	Geriatric hospital	Day hospital	Home care
Argentina	Yes	Yes	Yes	No	Yes	Yes
Brazil	Yes	Yes	Yes	No	Yes	Yes
Costa Rica[b]	Yes	Yes	Yes	Yes	Yes	Yes
Colombia	Yes	Yes	Yes	No	Yes	Yes
Cuba	Yes	Yes	Yes	Yes[a]	Yes	Yes
Chile	Yes	Yes	Yes	Yes[a]	No	Yes
Ecuador	Yes	Yes	No	No	No	Yes
El Salvador	Yes	Yes	No	No	No	Yes
México	Yes	Yes	Yes	No	Yes	Yes
Panama	Yes	Yes	Yes	Yes[a]	No	Yes
Peru	Yes	Yes	Yes	No	Yes	Yes
Uruguay	Yes	Yes	Yes	No	No	No
Venezuela	Yes	Yes	No	No	Yes	Yes

Source: Survey done by Dr Fernando Morales-Martínez (2004).
[a]Inpatient service only (subacute care). [b]Costa Rica does have a geriatric hospital with a comprehensive service (Day hospital, outpatient home visiting, and inpatients). [c]Geriatricians with University training in recognized academic centers.

to offer the most comprehensive program. The teaching of Geriatrics has evolved during the past two decades in many countries of the region. Teaching University hospitals with Geriatric services are found in Argentina, Brazil, Chile, Costa Rica, Colombia, Cuba, México, Panama, Peru, Puerto Rico, Uruguay, and Venezuela. The teaching of Geriatrics in the medical education of general practitioners and family medicine has not become standardized, and if it occurs, it is not well documented. The development of geriatrics in nursing schools and allied health faculties is even less developed. Argentina, Brazil, Chile, Colombia, Costa Rica, Cuba, and México have developed training programs for some allied health professionals (see Table 2).

Latin American Academy of Medicine on Aging (ALMA)

Latin American Academy of Medicine on Aging (ALMA) (in Spanish *Academia Latinamerican de Medicina del Adulto Mayor*) was created in 2002 by a group of Geriatric Faculty Members from Latin American and Spain with the support of the Pan American Health Organization, the Merck Institute of Aging and Health, and the guidance of the European Academy of Medicine on Aging. The mission of ALMA has been adapted to meet the needs of Latin America. ALMA is the premier organization providing leadership in the development of health services for older adults; improving quality of care, and advocating for the training of health-care professionals in the basics of geriatric medicine. ALMA has a distinctive public health agenda in addition to the academic agenda for strengthening geriatric teaching in the region. ALMA has offered a yearly program since 2002, rotating through different Latin American countries. Each ALMA program includes an intensive course for teachers of geriatrics in a selected topic; a public health forum with public health authorities in the country where the course is delivered; and a primary care workshop on a topic of geriatric care. Thus, in each ALMA program, the message of Geriatric Medicine is provided to different audiences. The III program of ALMA was held in September 2004 in San José, Costa Rica, and the theme was Nutrition and Aging.

ALMA has also undertaken the task of developing and promoting uniform guidelines for the teaching of geriatric medicine in general medical education (Cano *et al.*, 2005). It is developing practice guidelines in collaboration with the Pan American Health Organization and will soon have an interactive web site to organize and manage geriatric knowledge for the region.

The Costa Rican Case

The University of Costa Rica offers Speciality in Geriatrics Medicine and Gerontology after graduating a medical doctor, with a 5 years duration program; the first 2 years are straight Internal Medicine and the following 3 years are Geriatrics and Gerontology within the National Geriatrics Hospital. At present, there are 43 geriatricians and 28 medical residents. The program graduates four geriatricians every year and admits six new medical residents every year.

Costa Rica is located in Central America and has a history of commitment to peace and health. The country has not had an army since the middle of last century and officially abolished the army by a new constitution in 1948. Instead, Costa Rica allocated a major portion of its budget to a program of universal education, universal access to medical services, and social security. All residents have a constitutional right to receive health care from a system of national hospitals providing curative care; provincial centers providing treatment and prevention programs, and community health centers providing primary health care to the whole population. Community health workers make home visits to local residents, maintain ties with families, conduct socioeconomic surveys, give talks in schools, and collaborate with community health committees, elected by local residents, to set priorities for communal health.

In 2004, infant mortality was 9.1 per thousand live births and life expectancy at birth was 78.5 years. General mortality was reduced by 38%. Life expectancy at 60 and 80 has continued to increase since the early 50s (Table 3).

Programs for the Elderly

In response to the challenges of an aging population, Costa Rica has made important progress in the development of public policies, plans, and programs to promote health, provide care, and strengthen the well-being of older adults.

Table 3 Life expectancy in Costa Rica

	1950		2000		2003	
	M	F	M	F	M	F
60 years	14.85	18.84	20.9	23.7	21.7	24.5
80 years	5.22	5.95	8.3	9.33	8.46	9.47

Source: Population Estimates, Instituto Nacional de Estadistica y Censos de Costa Rica. www.inec.go.cr and Centro Centroamericano de Poblacion, University of Costa Rica. www.ccp.ucr.ac.cr

National Council for the Elderly

In 1999, the Legislation established the National Council for Older Persons. The National Council is the technical committee that is accompanied by the Council of Notables established for outstanding older persons in the community. Both the Technical Council and the Council of Notables advise the President and propose policies, plans, and programs for older adults in the country. The council aims to represent, involve, and evaluate actions of public agencies and private institutions and to seek resources for the implementation of priority programs.

The council is administratively located in the Ministry of the Presidency. The President of the Republic designates the coordinator of the Council.[2] Representatives of the following Ministries form the Council: Health, Labor and Social Security, National Planning, Education, Joint Institute for Social Assistance, and representatives of the main nongovernmental agencies working with older adults in the country.

Medical care for older adults in Costa Rica includes preventive care, acute care, rehabilitation services, and long-term care facilities. Preventive care is directed primarily at the healthy elderly population (see Figure 2).

Acute care is provided in the first instance through a network of polyclinic and health centers. The first level refers patients either for outpatient assessment to the day hospital or to the outpatient department of the general hospital, or for inpatient care to the geriatric hospital. The majority of patients are discharged back to the community under the care of the staff in a polyclinic or health center, with additional service arranged prior to discharge as required. Follow-up care and respite care may be provided at the day-care center.

The National Council for Older Persons has a Secretariat to coordinate the activities of its representative institutions. The Secretariat is responsible for documenting initiatives relevant to the elderly: formulating a national plan with particular programs and specific strategies: analyzing and assessing existing programs; and developing new models of practice. The Secretariat also develops programs related to health and human services, education and employment, family support, and sanitary assistance.

The National Council and Technical Secretary employ a participatory planning process that involves public agencies, private institutions, and the local community. The planning process emphasizes the development of organizations and communities and includes a national campaign to increase public awareness, improve public attitudes, and recognize the rights of the elderly in society. The planning document itself emphasizes the involvement of public agencies and private institutions, collaboration in agency administration; participation in local community committees, development and dissemination of information on the social, political, economic, and psychological aspects of aging, education, and training at the community level, and research to promote health.

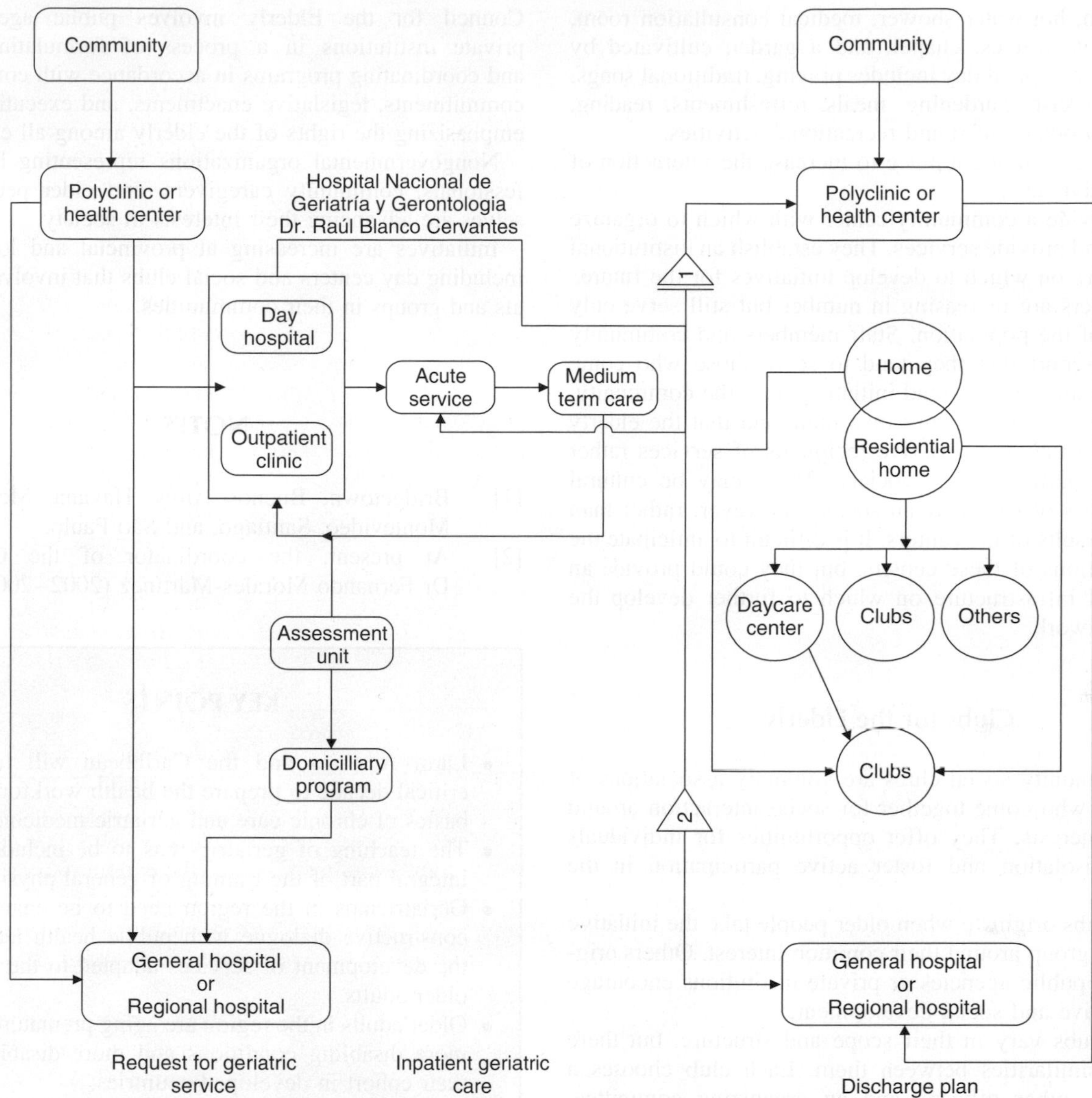

Figure 2 Scheme of graduated care of the elderly in Costa Rica

COMMUNITY INITIATIVES

Day-care Centers

Day-care centers are increasing in all areas of the country on the initiative of local communities with the support of public agencies and private institutions. The centers aim to provide care and resocialize disabled and disadvantaged older people into the community, especially those suffering from poverty, psychosocial problems, and family abandonment.

Day centers originate when residents take the initiative and form a local committee. The residents write a preliminary letter to public agencies and hold a meeting with interested individuals. They formulate a proposal for agency approval, develop a board of directors, and finalize plans for the center. They recruit volunteers to participate in programs and employ an administrator to coordinate the activities of the center. Some centers have as many volunteers as they have users of the facility.

Public agencies and private institutions support the development and maintenance of the center. They work with residents to construct the facility and employ the professional staff. They hold courses for volunteers on the problems of aging, recreational and cultural activities, social administration, and community organization. They hold courses for the elderly on the physical and psychological aspects of aging, group integration, and social interaction.

Day centers vary from one area to another, but there are some similarities among them. For example, one day-care center is located in a low-income area in a semiurban area outside San José. The facility includes a central room for social and recreational activities, a modern kitchen and dining room, hot-water shower, medical consultation room, administrative offices, chapel, and a garden cultivated by members. The typical day includes praying, traditional songs, physical exercise, gardening, meals, refreshments, reading, writing, and other social and recreational activities.

Day centers provide a place to increase the interaction of isolated individuals.

They provide a community center with which to organize programs and provide services. They establish an institutional infrastructure on which to develop initiatives for the future.

Day centers are increasing in number but still serve only a fraction of the population. Staff members and community volunteers report that they tend to serve those who come into them, rather than extend initiatives into the community, that they serve women more than men, and that the elderly perceive themselves as passive recipients of services rather than active participants in society. These may be cultural characteristics of Costa Rican society, however, rather than particular results of the centers. It is difficult to anticipate the future functions of these centers, but they could provide an institutional infrastructure on which to further develop the national network.

Clubs for the Elderly

These community social clubs are voluntary associations of individuals who come together for social interaction around common interests. They offer opportunities for individuals to reduce isolation and foster active participation in the community.

Some clubs originate when older people take the initiative and form a group around their common interest. Others originate when public agencies or private institutions encourage local initiative and social development.

Social clubs vary in their scope and structure, but there are some similarities between them. Each club chooses a coordinator, other officers, and an organizing committee. Each committee consults with members, assesses areas of common interest, and formulates an annual plan and weekly meeting agendas. Each coordinator meets with other coordinators in groups to report on activities and contribute to the network.

In some of the communities, women play strong social roles, while men experience isolation and would benefit from club participation. These older women participate actively in the community, but do not necessarily view themselves as a distinct organizational unit, or view the clubs as vehicles for organizing in the community. There is little such consciousness in Costa Rican society, but this could change in the future.

OPPORTUNITIES AND OBSTACLES

Costa Rica is developing a national network in response to the challenges of an aging population. The National Council for the Elderly involves public agencies and private institutions in a process of formulating policies and coordinating programs in accordance with constitutional commitments, legislative enactments, and executive decrees emphasizing the rights of the elderly among all citizens.

Nongovernmental organizations representing health professionals, community caregivers, and older people themselves are advancing their interests in society.

Initiatives are increasing at provincial and local levels, including day centers and social clubs that involve individuals and groups in their communities.

NOTES

[1] Bridgetown, Buenos Aires, Havana, Mexico City, Montevideo, Santiago, and São Paulo.

[2] At present, the coordinator of the Council is Dr Fernando Morales-Martínez (2002–2006).

KEY POINTS

- Latin America and the Caribbean will have one critical decade to prepare the health workforce in the basics of chronic care and geriatric medicine.
- The teaching of geriatrics has to be included as an integral part of the training of general physicians.
- Geriatricians in the region need to be engaged in a constructive dialogue with public health leaders for the development of services adapted to the needs of older adults.
- Older adults in the region are aging prematurely, have more disabling conditions and more disability than their cohort in developed countries.
- The Latin American Academy of Geriatric Medicine (Cano *et al.*, 2005) has become the premier organization for strengthening the teaching of geriatrics in Latin America.
- Costa Rica has shown that a coordinated and comprehensive approach to policy development needs to go hand in hand with the training of Geriatric physicians.

KEY REFERENCES

- Cano C, Gutierrez LM, Marin PP *et al.* Proposed minimum contents for medical school programs in geriatric medicine in Latin America. *Pan American Journal of Public Health*. Special Issue on Health, Well-being, and Aging in Latin America and the Caribbean 2005; **17**, Nos.5/6: 429–37.
- Idler EL & Benyamini Y. Self-rated health and mortality: a review of twenty seven community studies. *Journal of Health and Social Behavior* 1997; **38**:21–37.

- Palloni A, Pinto G & Pelaez M. Demographic and health conditions of ageing in Latin América and the Caribbean. *International Journal of Epidemiology* 2002; **31**:762–771.

REFERENCES

Beaman PE, Reyes-Frausto S & Garcia-Pena C. Validation of the health perceptions questionnaire for an older Mexican population. *Psychological Reports* 2003; **92**(3 Pt 1):723–734.

Cano C, Gutierrez LM, Marin PP *et al.* Proposed minimum contents for medical school programs in geriatric medicine in Latin America. *Pan American Journal of Public Health.* Special Issue on Health, Well-being, and Aging in Latin America and the Caribbean 2005; **17**, Nos.5/6: 429–37.

Idler EL & Benyamini Y. Self-rated health and mortality: a review of twenty seven community studies. *Journal of Health and Social Behavior* 1997; **38**:21–37.

Morales-Martínez F. *Survey on Geriatric Education Conducted with Key Informants from 11 Latin American Countries – Unpublished* 2004.

Palloni A, Pinto G & Pelaez M. Demographic and health conditions of ageing in Latin América and the Caribbean. *International Journal of Epidemiology* 2002; **31**:762–771.

Pelaez M, Wong R & Palloni A. *Health of Older Persons: Some findings from the PAHO Multicenter Survey SABE* 2003; Pan American Health Organization, Washington DC, ACHR 38/2003.7.

United Nations. *World Population Ageing: 1950–2050* 1999; United Nations Publications, New York.

FURTHER READING

Albala C, Ham-Chande R, Hennis A *et al.* The Health, Well-Being, and Aging ("SABE") survey: methodology applied and profile of the study population. *Pan American Journal of Public Health. Special Issue on Health, Well-being, and Aging in Latin America and the Caribbean* 2005; **17**, Nos.5/6:307–22.

Anzola E, Galinsky D, Morales-Martínez F *et al. La Atención de Las Personas Mayores. Un Desafío Para Los años Noventa* 1994; Organización Panamericana de la Salud, Washington.

Cambios demográficos en Costa Rica y Latinoamérica. *Hospital Nacional de Geriatría y Gerontología "Dr. Raúl Blanco Cervantes* 1991, San José, Costa Rica.

Chechoway B & Morales-Martínez F. En la Tercera Edad: new programmes to promote the health of older people in Costa Rica. *Ageing and Society* 1990; **10**:397–411.

Hospital Nacional de Geriatría y Gerontología "Dr. Raúl Blanco Cervantes". *La Historia Clínica Geriátrica* 1992; Caja Costarricense de Seguro Social, San José, Costa Rica.

Laake K & Morales-Martínez F. *Elementos Prácticos en la Atención de Las Personas Mayores* 1998; CENDEISSS, San José, Costa Rica.

Morales-Martínez F, Carpenter A & Williamson J. Dynamics of a geriatric day hospital, age and ageing. *Journal of the British Geriatric Society* 1984; **13**:34–41.

Morales-Martínez F. Long-term care services in Costa Rica. *Danish Medical Bulletin* 1987a; (Special Supplement Series 5), 38–40.

Morales-Martínez F. ?Qué es la geriatría? *Revista Gerontología en Acción (San José, Costa Rica)* 1987b; **1**(1):31–36.

Management of the Dying Patient

Ilora G. Finlay[1] *and* Saskie Dorman[2]
[1] *Cardiff University, Cardiff, UK, and* [2] *Velindre Cancer Centre, Cardiff, UK*

INTRODUCTION

Palliative care is the active total care of patients and their families by a multiprofessional team when the patient's disease is no longer responsive to curative treatment (World Health Organization, 1990). The focus is on quality of life, and care must address physical, emotional, social, and spiritual causes of distress.

Palliative care must begin early, to maintain quality of life for as long as possible. Any progressive disease process is continually evolving; new symptoms arise as the patient's physical condition worsens, so the patient needs constant reassessment and adjustment of all aspects of their management plan (Twycross, 1978). This continually changing situation means that palliative care is labor intensive both in terms of nursing and medical time (Twycross, 1978; Walsh and West, 1988).

The change in emphasis from cure to active palliation requires a change in attitude on the part of the carers (Finlay, 1976). In many instances, measures to control the disease may overlap with palliative care. The elderly patient often has coexisting pathologies which influence management (McQuay and Moore, 1984).

Growing awareness and acceptance of palliative care has allowed principles developed in the care of patients with advanced cancer to be applied to all patients with progressive life-threatening disease, irrespective of their diagnosis.

Patients who are terminally ill are often aware of their diagnosis and prognosis, but fear breaking the barrier of silence imposed by well-meaning family who believe the truth is devastating (Parkes, 1980). The patient can feel isolated and lonely, facing some "terrible, intangible, imminent death". All involved in the care of the patient need to understand the patient's and the family's perception of the disease process (Smith, 1993); for example, some patients think that everyone with cancer inevitably has pain, although only about 60% of patients with terminal cancer experience pain (Wilkes, 1984; Kane *et al.*, 1984). It is also important to know if the patient has had experience of similar disease in a close relative, since any horrifying experiences may compound the patient's own fears.

ASSESSMENT OF THE PATIENT

Is the Patient Terminally Ill?

The patient can be viewed as terminally ill when he or she is likely to die within the foreseeable future (usually under one year) from a specific progressing disease. The patient who is actively dying and is within the last days of life occupies a small subgroup. Many of the principles applicable to patients with a longer prognosis are important, even at this late stage; ethical dilemmas over stopping active treatments may need very careful consideration at this time.

It is tempting, but dangerous, to attribute to the prime pathology everything that occurs to patients once they are known to have a potentially terminal illness (Rees *et al.*, 1987). Intercurrent infections are particularly common to patients who are partially immunocompromised. Other diseases, such as myocardial ischemia, diabetes, Parkinson's disease, and hypothyroidism, may also occur. Each condition needs assessment and appropriate treatment; patients should not be denied the benefit of good general medical management simply because they happen to have a severe illness such as metastatic carcinoma.

The Problem List

At first, a problem list should evolve, which includes physical, emotional, social, and spiritual problems (see Table 1). The various components of each should be itemized: the patient may have several pains (Baines, 1989) and each pain should be separately recorded, for example, back pain, headache, myalgic pains, and abdominal colic. To maintain

Principles and Practice of Geriatric Medicine, 4th Edition. Edited by M.S. John Pathy, Alan J. Sinclair and John E. Morley.

Table 1 Example problem list from a patient with lung cancer

Physical
Pain in chest – rib metastasis
Pain L2/3 – lumbar vertebral metastases
Oral candida
Nausea – possible hypercalcemia
Dehydration
Constipation
Weakness
Anorexia
Emotional
Wife died 18 months ago, still grieving
Wife had breast cancer and similar back pain
Social
Lives alone, not coping with meals
No carers
Daughter over 100 miles away
Spiritual
"God's tested me too far"
Awareness
Knows "cancer"; expects to live "several years"
Believes stopping smoking has slowed disease

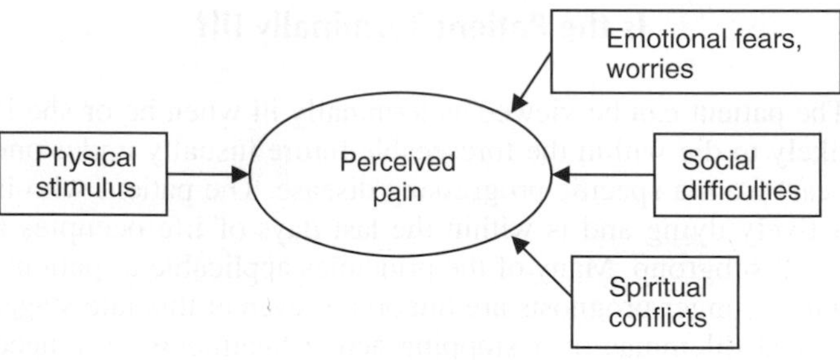

Figure 1 The components of pain

a holistic view, the patient's fears, disappointments, family tensions and conflicts, aims, and goals should be recorded. For example, if the patient feels that the diagnosis was delayed or missed initially, or feels that treatment was inappropriate, that information should also form part of the basic problem list.

Effective control of the physical aspect of a symptom cannot be achieved without attention to the social, emotional, and spiritual components of that symptom (Saunders, 1978) (see Figure 1).

ETHICAL CONSIDERATIONS

Many decisions in the management of the dying patient are less clear-cut than in those with a reasonable prognosis or chance of recovery. The four ethical principles of autonomy, beneficence, nonmaleficence, and justice create a framework within which each clinical decision can be formulated and tested.

Autonomy, usually taken simply to mean "self-governance", requires respect of the patient as a person in the context of the family which may have its own distinct identity and code of beliefs. Respect of autonomy means patients must be given information to make informed choices within the framework of their own language, vocabulary, and understanding. Patients' wishes for their future care, their values and their concerns, and the validity of any "advanced directive" (living will) must be confirmed and also clearly documented.

Nonmaleficence means that patients must not be burdened either by useless or futile distressing information, or by investigations or treatment which will not enhance their life.

Beneficence dictates that the predicted benefit must always outweigh the predicted risk. It is worth remembering that psychological benefit can validly outweigh physical risk in a holistic approach. This can mean that a drug or intervention is used for its positive effect, but in the knowledge that it may have some other adverse effects.

Within the principle of justice, the patient should have the best possible care within the resources available, but also these resources must be fairly allocated for the community they serve to derive maximum benefit.

Decisions such as feeding by artificial means, use of intravenous antibiotics and fluids, and the withdrawal of active treatments fall into the gray zone where an ethical framework becomes particularly helpful.

In patients with advanced neurological disease, feeding is often a problem. The evidence suggests that the dying, despite low fluid intake, often do not have biochemical markers of dehydration (Ellershaw *et al.*, 1995). For the few who experience thirst, this can be relieved by good mouth care and subcutaneous fluids, even at home (McQuillan and Finlay, 1995). It is essential that each case is assessed individually (Craig, 1996); rigid policies over hydration are unethical (Dunphy *et al.*, 1995).

SYMPTOM ANALYSIS

The diagnostic skills required in every patient encounter need to be applied to each symptom the patient presents, to ascertain the cause of that symptom (Baines, 1989). The patient who is terminally ill almost always has several symptoms. It is unusual for the patient to only have one site of pain; there are usually multiple pains, each in different sites and each with a different cause. The compilation of the problem list for the patient frequently elicits between 5 and 10 problems at first interview, although sometimes even more may be found.

The patient's perception of his or her own symptoms will be altered and exacerbated by fear, depression, insomnia, and worry (Twycross and Lack, 1983). For every symptom the four components (physical, emotional, social, and spiritual) should be defined (Saunders, 1978).

Some patients are "sick with worry" or experience "total pain", which requires care and counseling as a major adjunct to drug therapy. Patients all need time to talk about their fears (Maguire and Faulkner, 1988a,b) in a relaxed and peaceful environment; the professional's role is to sit and actively listen to the problems.

PAIN (*see* Chapter 78, Peripheral Neuropathy)

Pain is wherever the patient says it hurts. For each pain the site, duration, intensity, and probable cause should be noted (Thompson and Regnard, 1992). Table 2 lists causes of pain found in 500 admissions to a palliative care unit. Pain may be the first indicator of local recurrence of cancer, for example, pelvic pain from rectal or gynecological carcinomas. Radicular thoracic or cervical pain may precede leg weakness by hours or days in impending spinal cord compression. Pain is also a common feature of patients dying from illnesses other than cancer (Higginson, 1998). About 95% of pains are opioid sensitive; the remainder are usually neuropathic in origin, or there may be psychosocial issues exacerbating the pain (Woodruff, 2004).

The type of pain can be assessed and documented using the PQRST pnemonic (Twycross and Wilcock, 2001) (see Table 3). A diagram showing dermatomes can be very helpful to record the site of each pain (see Figure 2).

It is important to have a baseline assessment of each pain, so the response of the pain to analgesic interventions can be evaluated. Such reevaluation should occur every 24 hours until pain control is achieved. As a general rule, if no improvement in pain has been achieved within 48 hours, then specialist palliative medicine advice should be sought.

There are different rating scales for pain. All are subjective and nonlinear, but are a good working guide. Different patients find some easier than others, but useful ones are a 0–10 scale of 0 = "no pain" to 10 = "the worst pain imaginable", or a verbal rating scale "very severe/severe/moderate/mild/no pain" (Caraceni *et al.*, 2002).

Table 2 Causes of pains found in 500 admissions to a Marie Curie hospice unit

Tumor bulk
Visceral, caused by compression of adjacent cells
Bone: metastases with pathological fractures
Intrinsic and extrinsic esophageal tumor mass
Organ capsule stretching, particularly liver capsule pain
Pleuritic, from tumor nodules
Diaphragmatic, on inspiration, from diaphragmatic and liver metastases
Nerve compression
Radicular from spinal cord compression: thoracic, cervical
Headache from raised intracranial pressure
Rectal tenesmus
Skin metastases
Pains not caused directly by the cancer
Concomitant infection
Pleuritic chest pain
Mouth discomfort
Bladder spasms from cystitis
Infected pressure sores
Herpes zoster (shingles)
Oral herpes simplex
Aches associated with debility, but not directly attributable to neoplasm
Stiffness in a paralyzed limb
Arthritis
Neuropathic pain, postthoracotomy pain
Skin burning following radiotherapy
Causalgia
Angina
Reflux esophagitis
Peptic ulcer
Abdominal pain
Shoulder tip pain from perforation
Dyspepsia

Table 3 The PQRST characteristics of pain

P	Palliative factors	"What makes it better?"	Effect of medications, heat packs, and so on
	Provocative factors	"What makes it worse?"	Movement, eating, lying down, and so on
Q	Quality	"What exactly is it like?"	Burning, stabbing, dull ache, and so on
R	Radiation	"Where does it go to?"	
S	Severity	"How severe is it? How much does it affect your life?"	0–10 out of 10 mild/moderate/ severe/very severe effects on sleep, mobility, and so on
T	Temporal factors	"Is it there all the time or does it come and go? Is it worse at any particular time of day or night?"	Time since onset; constant or intermittent; duration of episodes of pain; time of day

Source: Copyright Twycross R. Wilcox A, 2001. *Symptom Management in Advanced Cancer*, 3rd edn; Radcliffe Medical Press, Oxford. Reproduced with the permission of the copyright holder.

Planning Analgesic Therapy

A few patients have good analgesia with regular paracetamol which is a Group I analgesic (Table 4), or with a nonsteroidal anti-inflammatory drug (NSAID). These may help as coanalgesics, particularly with opioids for bone pain. Elderly patients with an additional risk factor for peptic ulceration (previous history of ulceration or also taking steroids) require gastroprotection (Hawkins and Hanks, 2000), with a proton pump inhibitor or misoprostol. Cox-2 inhibitors were widely prescribed instead of conventional NSAIDs, but they do not eliminate the risk of peptic ulceration (Twycross *et al.*, 2003) and concerns about their safety have arisen recently.

A patient's perception of pain will be dramatically altered by fear and emotional or spiritual conflicts. The patient troubled by unresolved worries will not benefit fully from opioids without additional appropriate counseling. The patient must understand how treatment is aimed at the pain and be given realistic expectations by the prescriber.

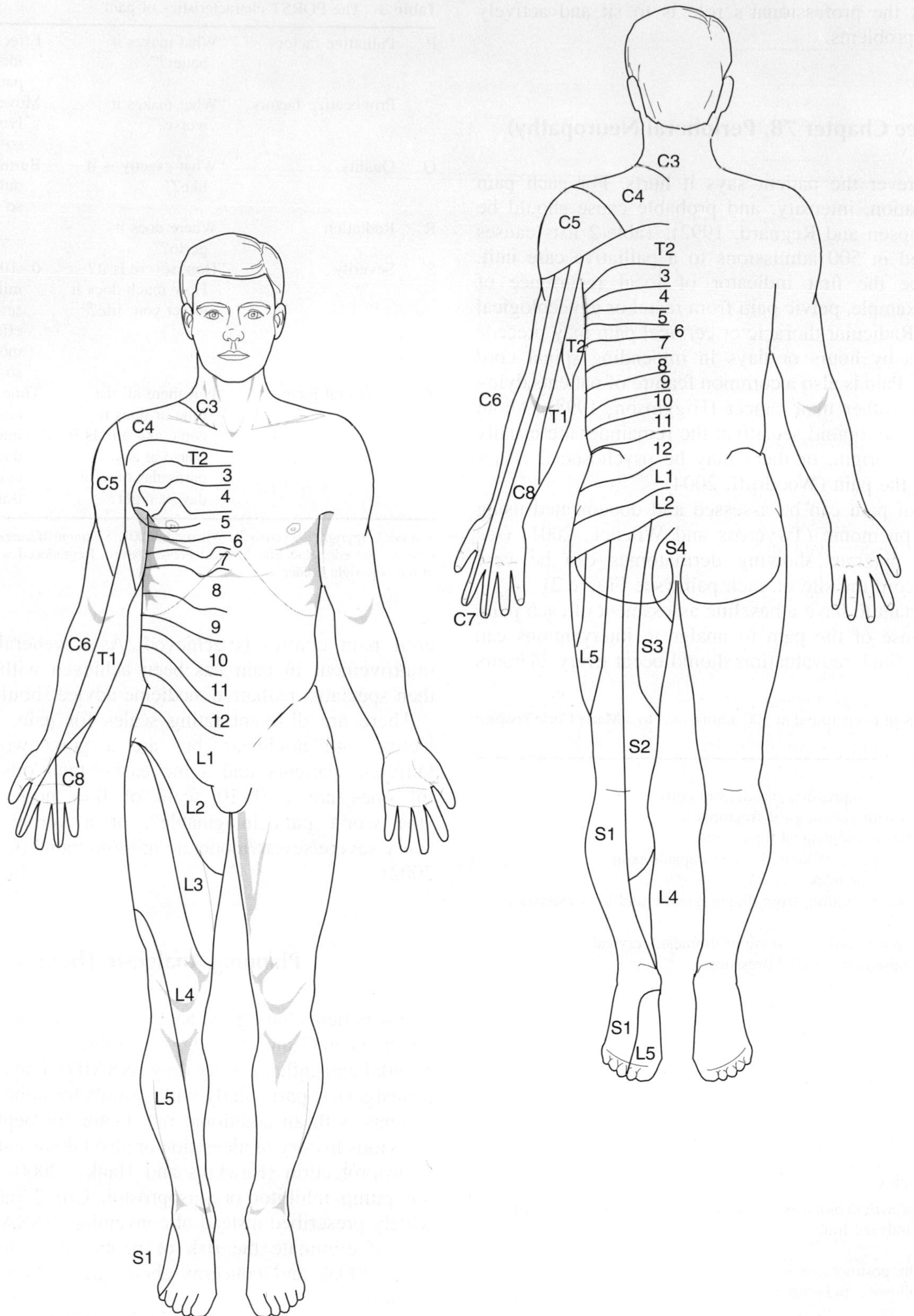

Figure 2 The use of a body chart allows quick and accurate documentation of the site and nature of a patient's pain. Dermatomes marked: C, cervical roots; T, thoracic roots; L, lumbar roots; S, sacral roots

Table 4 WHO classification of analgesics: the analgesic steps (World Health Organization, 1996)

Step 1	Step 2	Step 3
Nonopioid ± adjuvant	*Weak opioid* ± nonopioid ± adjuvant	*Strong opioid* ± nonopioid ± adjuvant
Paracetamol NSAIDs	Codeine Dihydrocodeine Dextropropoxyphene Tramadol	Morphine Diamorphine Oxycodone Hydromorphone Fentanyl Alfentanil Methadone Buprenorphine[a]

[a]Buprenorphine is a partial opioid agonist.

Starting Opioid Analgesia

Most patients with pain need a Group II (mild opioid) or Group III (strong opioid) drug. Co-codamol 30/500 is an effective analgesic given 6-hourly, containing paracetamol and codeine (a prodrug of morphine). However, some patients are poor cytochrome P450 2D6 metabolizers and for these patients, the analgesic effect of codeine is significantly impaired; this applies to 7% of Caucasians (Twycross *et al.*, 2003). Dihydrocodeine is very constipating and can cause dysphoria. Tramadol can be a useful mild opioid for some patients, but it is expensive in the United Kingdom (Joint Formulary Committee, 2005).

If pain is not completely controlled, a strong opioid should be started early rather than late. It is preferable to move to step 3 of the WHO analgesic ladder rather than use a variety of different weak opioids. Gaining control of the patient's pain promptly helps gain his or her confidence.

Morphine is the recommended first line Group III opioid, given orally if possible (Hanks, 2001). It is available as a solution (morphine hydrochloride or morphine sulphate) (Hillier, 1983) or in tablet form. The dose is titrated up in increments of 30–50% of the previous dose until pain control is achieved (Table 5) (Regnard and Davies, 1986). Opioids can be given to patients with cardiorespiratory disease (Abernethy *et al.*, 2003). An initial dose of 5- or 10-mg morphine solution 4-hourly is extremely safe. There is no maximal dose, but most pains are controlled by oral doses of 10–30 mg 4-hourly round the clock (Walsh and West, 1988).

Some patients can omit the 02.00 dose completely; some require a double dose at 22.00 to enable sleep through to 06.00. The patient can be maintained on slow release 12-hourly tablets or suspension (Twycross, 1978), by dose conversion from the normal release 4-hourly dose (Table 6).

Table 5 Incremental doses of oral morphine (Regnard and Davies, 1986)

5 mg → 10 mg → 15 mg → 20 mg → 30 mg → 45 mg → 60 mg → 90 mg → 120 mg, and so on at 30–50% increments

In very ill patients who are unable to swallow, or if vomiting prevents adequate absorption of oral medication, alternative routes of administration need to be used to maintain adequate pain relief. Several opioids are available for subcutaneous use in a syringe driver (Dover, 1987; Oliver, 1988); diamorphine is most commonly used in the United Kingdom as it is very soluble (high doses can be given in small volumes) (Twycross *et al.*, 2003). Compatibility data for various drugs given together by a syringe driver are available (Twycross *et al.*, 2003). Breakthrough additional opioid doses should be given subcutaneously as intramuscular injections are painful. Intravenous opioids should be avoided as tolerance appears to develop rapidly (Rogers *et al.*, 1985).

Side Effects of Opioids

About a third of patients develop transient nausea when commencing opioids; this responds to antiemetics acting at the chemoreceptor trigger zone, for example, haloperidol 1.5–5 mg at night, prochlorperazine 5 mg 8-hourly or levomepromazine 6 mg at night or 12-hourly (Twycross *et al.*, 2003, 1997).

Opioids are severely constipating. Unless the patient has true diarrhea before commencing opioids, a stimulant laxative with a softener must be given with the first dose and continued long term. Fecal softeners alone are insufficient. Senna liquid 10 ml (a stimulant) mixed with magnesium hydroxide 10 ml (a softener) given two or three times a day, or a combination laxative (e.g. co-danthramer) is usually effective at maintaining good bowel function. Polyethylene glycol 3500 (e.g. Movicol®) is also effective.

Some patients become drowsy or confused at very low doses of morphine; the elderly seem to be particularly at risk of this. For patients who do not tolerate morphine well, switching opioid may be helpful (Hanks, 2001). Oxycodone, available in solution or tablets in normal release and sustained release preparations, is a useful alternative to morphine. A parenteral preparation for subcutaneous use is also now available (Joint Formulary Committee, 2005).

Toxic morphine metabolites accumulate in renal failure. For patients with renal failure, fentanyl or alfentanil is preferable to morphine (Kirkham and Pugh, 1995), as these opioids are mainly metabolized to inactive compounds by the liver (Twycross *et al.*, 2003; Back, 2001). Fentanyl is not absorbed orally but can be given transdermally, subcutaneously, or transmucosally (Twycross *et al.*, 2003). It is available in transdermal patches which come in 25 μg hour^{-1} increments and need changing every 72 hours. Fentanyl is less constipating than morphine so laxatives may need to be adjusted. Occasionally, patients who have been on morphine for some time experience opioid withdrawal symptoms for about 24 hours when switching to fentanyl; these are controlled with doses of oral morphine. For patients who have variable, escalating, or unknown analgesic requirements, it is difficult to titrate transdermal fentanyl and it should not be used in these situations (Twycross *et al.*, 2003). For patients unable to take oral medications, a continuous subcutaneous

Table 6 Opioid dose regimes and approximate equivalent[a] morphine doses. (Adapted from Back, 2001 and Twycross *et al.*, 2003)

Drug		Examples	Example of dose regime[b]	24-hour total dose	Approximate equivalent[a] oral morphine 24-hour dose
Opioids given orally					
Codeine			60 mg 6-hourly	240 mg	24 mg
Tramadol			50 mg 6-hourly	200 mg	40 mg
Morphine sulphate	Normal release	Oramorph®	10 mg 4-hourly	60 mg	60 mg
Morphine sulphate	Slow release	MST Continus® Zomorph®	30 mg 12-hourly	60 mg	60 mg
Oxycodone	Normal release	Oxynorm®	5 mg 4-hourly	30 mg	45–60 mg
Oxycodone	Slow release	Oxycontin®	15 mg 12-hourly	30 mg	45–60 mg
Hydromorphone	Normal release	Palladone®	1.3 mg 4-hourly	7.8 mg	60 mg
Opioids given subcutaneously					
Morphine			5 mg 4-hourly	30 mg	60 mg
Diamorphine			5 mg 4-hourly	30 mg	60–90 mg
Oxycodone			5 mg 4-hourly	30 mg	60–90 mg
Opioids given by continuous subcutaneous infusion over 24 hours					
Morphine			20 mg over 24 hours	20 mg	40 mg
Diamorphine			20 mg over 24 hours	20 mg	40–60 mg
Oxycodone			20 mg over 24 hours	20 mg	40–60 mg
Fentanyl			400 μg over 24 hours	400 μg	60 mg
Alfentanil			2 mg over 24 hours	2 mg	60 mg
Opioid given transdermally (self-adhesive patch): change every 72 hours					
Fentanyl (patch)			25 μg hour^{-1}	600 μg	60–90 mg
Opioids given rectally (suppositories)					
Morphine hydrogel (nondissolving) suppositories m/r			50 mg once daily	50 mg	50 mg
Morphine (hydrochloride) suppositories			10 mg 4-hourly	60 mg	60 mg
Oxycodone (hydrochloride) suppositories			5 mg 4-hourly	30 mg	60 mg
Unsuitable opioids					
Pethidine		PO	50 mg 3-hourly	400 mg	50 mg
		IM	25 mg 3-hourly	200 mg	75 mg
Buprenorphine (partial opioid agonist)		SL	200 μg 8-hourly	600 μg	36 mg
		TD (patch)	35 μg hour^{-1}	800 μg	50 mg approx
Methadone		PO	Very variable pharmacokinetics; specialist supervision required		

m/r, modified release; PO, oral; IM, intramuscular; SL, sublingual; TD, transdermal.
[a]Equivalent doses are approximations only; doses must be carefully titrated for each individual patient. [b]Lower doses may be needed initially for frail patients or those who have not taken opioids before.

opioid infusion is easier to adjust. Fentanyl is available as oral transmucosal fentanyl citrate (OTFC) in "lozenges" which can be applied to the patient's oral mucosa to give additional doses of analgesia for breakthrough pain (Chandler, 1999). Many patients who are dying have a dry mouth and may be unable to use OTFC; sublingual fentanyl or alfentanil are other options for control of short-lived episodes of pain, but they should be prescribed only under specialist palliative medicine supervision.

Pain is a powerful respiratory stimulant. Significant respiratory depression does not occur at the dose the patient needs for analgesia. Patients should not be denied opioid analgesia for opioid-responsive pain. They can remain on opioids for many months. An increase in analgesic requirements indicates that the patient has more pain; it is not indicative of addiction (Portenoy, 1995).

Initial sedative effects wear off after two or three days. If the patient remains very drowsy, the opioid dose should be decreased and the patient reassessed, since the pain may be opioid resistant and the patient may be opioid toxic. Symptoms and signs of opioid toxicity include hallucinations, grimacing, hyperalgesia (the patient is extremely sensitive to painful stimuli, so may experience frequent breakthrough pain), allodynia (the patient appears to be in pain on being touched), pinpoint pupils, respiratory depression, and twitching or myoclonus. If untreated, seizures may follow (Woodruff, 2004).

Breakthrough Pain and Incident Pain

Breakthrough pains should be treated by a dose of morphine 50–100% of the 4-hourly morphine requirement and then the baseline dose increased accordingly; the pain must be regularly reassessed.

Patients who are taking opioids often also need Group I analgesics for other incidental pains, for example, headaches. They may benefit from coanalgesics such as NSAIDs, antidepressants, and steroids.

Others need a boost of analgesia for a specific activity causing incident pain, such as getting out of bed or dressing in the morning. A breakthrough dose given half an hour before moving can be helpful.

Difficult Pains

Bone Pain

Pain on movement is often poorly responsive to opioids alone. This includes bone pain, common in many malignancies, as well as joint pain (e.g. due to osteoarthritis).

Plain X-ray may not show metastases at an early stage; therefore, a combination of investigations may be required to localize a lesion. Where bone cortex is eroded, particularly mechanically important areas such as the neck of femur, the bone may be at risk of pathological fracture, and surgical pinning of the bone should be considered. Radiotherapy provides good analgesia in 80% of patients with pain from bone metastases, and should therefore always be considered (Woodruff, 2004). When multiple sclerotic bone metastases exist and the patient has a predicted prognosis of 6 weeks or more, strontium may be more effective and less debilitating than multiple doses of radiotherapy (Hoskin, 2004). Combinations of NSAIDs with opioids are a useful part of the management. Some bone pain, particularly due to metastatic breast cancer or myeloma, responds well to bisphosphonate infusion, even when the serum calcium is normal. Oral bisphosphonates do not seem to provide any analgesia. A trial of a bisphosphonates should be considered in difficult bone pain (Mannix *et al.*, 2000).

Some patients with advanced multiple metastases such as in myeloma can develop pathological bone fractures in sites where immobilization is impossible, such as the clavicle. A simple technique to provide analgesia can sometimes be effective: the fracture site is infiltrated with Depo-Medrone® (methylprednisolone acetate) 80 mg and bupivacaine hydrochloride 0.5%. This does not always require X-ray control and can provide adequate analgesia to allow the patient to be turned in the last days of life.

Neuropathic Pain

Neuropathic pains due to reversible damage from nerve compression or irreversible damage from neurodestruction (e.g. due to infiltration by tumor) or diabetic neuropathy are characterized by a burning or electric shock quality. They are often severe and are associated with altered sensation including allodynia or dysesthesia (Meyerson, 1990). Allodynia means the patient feels pain in response to a nonpainful stimulus; dysesthesia is an unpleasant abnormal sensation. Opioids can be helpful but are often needed in high doses and their use may be limited by side effects.

Neuropathic pain requires relief of any pressure on nerve fibers if possible. Tumor mass can be shrunk by radiotherapy and peritumor edema decreased by high-dose steroids (e.g. dexamethasone 8–16 mg day^{-1} in divided doses).

Low-dose amitriptyline (10–25 mg once or twice daily) appears to potentiate opioids through inhibition of serotonin reuptake and reduction in pain perception (Twycross *et al.*, 2003). Membrane-stabilizing anticonvulsants (e.g. carbamazepine) may help some patients, but tend to make the elderly very drowsy. Gabapentin is licensed for use in neuropathic pain, but again may be limited by drowsiness (Twycross *et al.*, 2003). It is safest to start tricyclic antidepressants or anticonvulsants at low doses and titrate up as tolerated by the patient.

Nerve blocks have a small place in the management of the terminally ill patient; the success rate of the block depends on the technique (Baines, 1981). Pain from pancreatic cancer can be dramatically relieved by celiac plexus block (Lipton, 1989), which may need to be repeated after a few months. Psoas compartment block may provide relief of hip pains. Epidural injection of steroids can improve pain from tumor infiltration at the spinal nerve root. Unfortunately, a few patients suffer deafferentation pain following neurolytic techniques. Therefore, in palliative care the drugs used tend to be temporary in action, such as bupivacaine with a depot steroid preparation.

Complex pain, such as sympathetically maintained pain, can be relieved by the appropriate nerve block (Cherny and Coley, 1994), although the place for nerve blocks in pain control is relatively small. Transcutaneous nerve stimulation provides a temporary partial blockade and often warrants a trial as it is so safe.

Ketamine was used as an anesthetic agent as it provides powerful analgesia (Fallon and Welsh, 1996), but it can cause severe dysphoria, hallucinations, a dramatic rise in blood pressure, and other side effects (Twycross *et al.*, 2003). It can be very effective in low-dose subcutaneous infusion in intractable neuropathic pain, when given with an antipsychotic or midazolam. It should only be used with palliative medicine supervision.

Similarly, methadone can provide good analgesia but its unpredictable half-life, which can be up to three days in some patients (Twycross *et al.*, 2003), makes it difficult to titrate in routine use.

CONSTIPATION

About half of all terminally ill patients are constipated, usually from a combination of anticholinergic drugs, opioids, poor fluid intake, and immobility associated with debility (Bruera *et al.*, 1994). High fiber preparations usually aggravate constipation as patients lack fluid, and they are unpalatable.

The use of magnesium hydroxide with senna, movicol, or co-danthramer for patients on opioids has been referred to. Lactulose is an effective stool softener in large doses (60–90 ml day^{-1}) with a mildly stimulant action (Regnard, 1988), but it can produce much flatus. In very severe

Table 7 Suitable laxatives

Osmotic laxatives	Stimulant laxatives	Fecal softeners	Rectally acting agents
Magnesium hydroxide	Senna	Docusate (capsules)	Bisacodyl suppositories (stimulant)
Polyethylene glycol 3500 (e.g. Movicol®)	Dantron (contained in co-danthramer)		Arachis oil (softener)
	Sodium picosulphate		Sodium citrate (e.g. Micralax Micro-enema®; osmotic)

constipation, higher doses of polyethylene glycol 3350 (e.g. Movicol® up to 8 sachets a day for up to 3 days) or sodium picosulphate ($5\,mg\,ml^{-1}$ up to three times a day) may be needed (Table 7) (Twycross *et al.*, 2003; Back, 2001). Occasionally, patients have fecal impaction which requires either high-dose Movicol® (Culbert *et al.*, 1998) or manual removal (a painful procedure which should only be done with adequate analgesia).

Bowel Obstruction

Ovarian and colon cancer often cause bowel obstruction at multiple sites, making surgery impossible (Baines *et al.*, 1985). Prevention is important: large doses of stool softener can maintain the stool as soft as toothpaste. Vomiting occurs in most patients with obstruction (Baines *et al.*, 1985), but does not become feculent until quite late; pain and distension are also often late signs. The diagnosis is clinical; abdominal X-rays seldom add anything to the picture in established obstruction and early films may show remarkably little.

When surgery is not possible, medical management of acute obstructive episodes requires antispasmodics such as hyoscine butylbromide for colic (Baines *et al.*, 1985), with an opioid for constant abdominal pain. An antiemetic acting at the vomiting center, for example, cyclizine, can control vomiting to some extent. Fecal softeners such as docusate should be given. A trial of corticosteroids may be tried although a systematic review on their effectiveness was not conclusive (Feuer and Broadley, 1999). Octreotide, generally only given under specialist supervision, may also be helpful to reduce the volume of intestinal secretions (Mercadente *et al.*, 1993).

The oral route cannot be used to give antiemetics, as gastric emptying is delayed and absorption is poor. Therefore, the subcutaneous route is preferable and a syringe driver is the drug delivery system of choice.

There is no evidence that a drip and suck regimen (with intravenous fluids and insertion of a nasogastric tube) is of help to these patients, and a nasogastric tube is irritating and nauseating. The obstructive episode should be managed to control symptoms even if sedation is an inevitable side effect. Unfortunately, acute obstruction with hard fecal matter in the bowel will resolve poorly so the mainstay of management is preventive palliation. A defunctioning colostomy can be distressing and difficult for the patient to come to terms with and should not be undertaken unless the patient's general condition indicates several months of active life and the patient fully understands the implications of surgery.

NAUSEA AND VOMITING

As for pain, the cause of the symptom must be determined. Vomiting may be the only sign of early bowel obstruction or hypercalcemia.

The stimulus to vomiting is triggered through different nuclei in the brainstem, and antiemetics differ with respect to efficacy at each site. The clinical circumstances can guide appropriate antiemetic therapy (Bentley and Boyd, 2001; Twycross and Back, 1998).

The chemoreceptor trigger zone, lying adjacent to the integrated vomiting center in the floor of the fourth ventricle, is stimulated by toxins, drugs, uremia, and hypercalcemia (Rousseau, 1995). Central dopamine antagonists at low dose (such as haloperidol 1.5–5 mg (Plotkin *et al.*, 1973) or levomepromazine 6 mg, once or twice daily (Twycross *et al.*, 1997)) are effective. They can be given orally or subcutaneously by syringe driver. Levomepromazine is slightly more sedative than haloperidol but can act as a mild coanalgesic with opioids; it is useful when other antiemetics fail. Buccal or rectal prochlorperazine are useful when the patient cannot swallow and a syringe driver is not available.

Cyclizine is an antihistamine that acts at the integrated vomiting center and is useful in combination with a central dopamine antagonist. It can be given as a continuous subcutaneous infusion by syringe driver (150 mg over 24 hours) but single injections tend to be painful and use in a syringe driver can cause painful inflammation at the syringe driver site.

Prokinetics such as metoclopramide or domperidone (available as tablets or suppositories) can be helpful in squashed stomach syndrome (Fallon and Hanks, 1994), for instance, when liver metastases cause extrinsic pressure on the stomach; they promote gastric emptying and duodenal peristalsis (Schulze-Delrieu *et al.*, 1981). Liver metastases can sometimes cause severe nausea which responds well to dexamethasone in low doses ($2–4\,mg\,day^{-1}$). $5HT_3$ antagonists are effective short term for chemotherapy- and radiotherapy-induced vomiting but are constipating and very much more expensive than the other antiemetics suggested above (Twycross *et al.*, 2003).

Hypercalcemia can be treated with intravenous fluids and a bisphosphonate, with dramatic relief from vomiting and other symptoms.

BREATHLESSNESS

Breathlessness is an extremely distressing symptom and is often inadequately relieved. It is a common symptom in end-stage cardiac and respiratory failure, as well as many cancers. It becomes more common as death approaches (Dudgeon *et al.*, 2001).

The common causes of breathlessness can usually be differentiated on history and medical examination.

Patients with acute cardiac failure may feel as though they are suffocating; they can respond promptly to intravenous furosemide, infusion of nitrates and parenteral diamorphine. Bronchospasm can be treated with nebulized bronchodilators; pneumonia causing breathlessness warrants antibiotics and physiotherapy. Pleural effusions can be drained relatively simply and painlessly. When bronchial occlusion by tumor is the main cause of breathlessness, it may be possible (dependent on the patient's condition) for an endobronchial stent to be inserted (Back, 2001).

Patients may benefit from treatment of symptomatic anemia. Oral iron is incorporated too slowly for it to be effective; its use requires the bone marrow to be functioning adequately and this may not be the case in anemia of chronic disease or in advanced malignancy. Transfusion of packed red cells is likely to yield most rapid symptomatic improvement. Erythropoietin may be an effective alternative in some patients, particularly in view of the limited supply of blood products (Mijovic, 2004). Transfusion is usually futile in the last few days of life.

Long-term oxygen therapy is beneficial to selected patients with chronic obstructive pulmonary disease (COPD), but oxygen alone is rarely adequate to control breathlessness in the dying patient (Shee, 1995).

Facial cooling (by a handheld or bedside fan, or a draught from an open window) can improve breathlessness. Having treated reversible causes, the sensation of breathlessness can be suppressed by opioids, sometimes at very low dose (Jennings *et al.*, 2001). In those already on opioids, the dose should be increased above that needed for analgesia to decrease the central drive to respiratory rate. The dose should be titrated as for pain control but in smaller increments, of 10–20%. For most patients, nebulized morphine is no better than nebulized saline for symptom relief (Jennings *et al.*, 2001).

Effective physiotherapy can teach patients to move efficiently and minimize breathlessness on exertion. Nurse-led breathlessness clinics have been shown to have a small but potentially significant effect in improving symptoms, using breathing control, relaxation, and activity-pacing techniques (Bredin *et al.*, 1999).

Breathlessness correlates better with psychological state than with objective measures of respiratory function (Ripamonti and Bruera, 1997); patients should be assessed for anxiety and depression and treated for these if appropriate.

Constipation should be avoided since the effort of defecating aggravates breathlessness.

The breathless patient who is unable to take oral medications in the last few days of life may respond well to parenteral opioids such as diamorphine 2.5–5 mg subcutaneously, with or without midazolam 2.5 mg subcutaneously. A syringe driver with diamorphine and low-dose midazolam may also be helpful.

FATIGUE

Fatigue is a very common and debilitating symptom of advanced disease, whether due to advanced malignancy or end-stage cardiac or respiratory failure. It is underreported and underrecorded (Kendall *et al.*, 2004), perhaps because patients and doctors feel that "nothing can be done".

Medical history, examination, and simple investigations should identify anemia, depression, and thyroid disease which can be treated. Several drugs (including sedatives, alcohol, β-blockers, many antidepressants, and antipsychotics) can cause excessive daytime somnolence or fatigue; antihypertensives may need to be rationalized dependent on the patient's cardiovascular and fluid status. Hypokalemia can cause muscle weakness and may respond to potassium supplements; if these are not effective, the patient may be deficient in magnesium (Twycross *et al.*, 2003).

Nonpharmacological management is important. Optimizing physical fitness, sleep hygiene, pacing activities, setting realistic and achievable goals can help the patient make the most of the time he or she has left.

CONFUSION

The elderly are particularly susceptible to acute confusion, possibly on a background of cognitive impairment due to dementia or cerebrovascular disease. Acute confusion is usually multifactorial; contributing factors include medications (anticholinergics, opioids, and benzodiazepines, amongst others), withdrawal from various drugs, urinary retention, constipation, hypoxia, uremia, urinary tract infections, and chest infections. Poor vision and hearing also predispose patients to acute confusional states (Caraceni and Grassi, 2003).

Hypercalcemia is an important cause of acute confusion which can respond dramatically to correction. It is often seen associated with tumors known to metastasize to bone, but may also be due to parathyroid-like hormone secretion by tumor (Ralston, 1994). Concomitant symptoms of anorexia, constipation, nausea, and dehydration may not be obvious since they are so common in patients who are terminally ill. Corrected serum calcium levels of over $3.5\,\mathrm{mmol\,l^{-1}}$ correspond to severe hypercalcemia (Heath, 1989; Iqbal *et al.*, 1988). Rehydration with intravenous 0.9% sodium chloride is the first line of treatment. If the hypercalcemia persists despite rehydration, intravenous bisphosphonates (e.g. pamidronate) can rapidly and effectively lower serum calcium levels (Kovacs *et al.*, 1995). Zoledronic acid can be tried if pamidronate is not effective (Twycross *et al.*, 2003). Steroids and oral bisphosphonates are of no benefit in patients with severe hypercalcemia. Treatment for hypercalcemia may need to be repeated after 3 or 4 weeks, but it should be recognized that hypercalcemia carries a poor prognosis and the patient with resistant hypercalcemia may require symptom control as they enter their terminal phase.

Confusion caused by cerebral metastases may temporarily respond well to high-dose dexamethasone (16 mg daily)

(Kirkham, 1988; Garde, 1965). If there is no response after 5 days, the steroid can be stopped abruptly.

The possibility of switching to an alternative opioid in patients who experience confusion on morphine has already been mentioned.

Low-dose antipsychotic medication such as haloperidol 0.5 mg (repeated after 30 minutes if not effective; higher doses in severe delirium with agitation) (Caraceni and Grassi, 2003) can help improve symptoms associated with confusion, such as hallucinations and paranoid thoughts.

Patients often have insight into their toxic confusional state, which is aggravated by fears. Patients should be nursed in a well-lit room with minimal background noise and be spoken to in clear simple terms to provide calming reassurance. Their experiences, whether real, hallucinatory, or paranoid, feel real and will be aggravated by a doctor or nurse seeming to be sceptical. It is more helpful to let the patient know that you understand that these disturbing experiences are happening and that you will try to do something about it.

DEPRESSION

The patient may undergo a process of grief, associated with awareness of the illness and loss of an independent lifestyle, compounded by fears and unresolved issues in life (Lichter, 1991). Grief has been described in terms of stages of anger, bitterness, bargaining, coming to terms, and reconciliation (Worden, 1983). In practice, these are not clear-cut, and people waiver in and out of conflicting emotional states (Stadeford, 1984). It is important to remember that the patient losing life's functions may be grieving deeply for his or her past and future.

The onset of deteriorating illness can reactivate grief from a previous bereavement. Awareness by all those looking after a patient will increase understanding of the patient's reaction to the current situation.

Depression is frequently missed but it is a treatable entity (Lloyd-Williams *et al.*, 2004). Antidepressants should be considered for those patients with early morning wakening, an anxiety state, feelings of excessive guilt or overwhelming pessimism about others (Regnard and Mannix, 1992). Other pointers such as weakness, tiredness, loss of appetite, or pessimism about self are often expected manifestations of the life-threatening disease process (Cody, 1990).

INFECTIONS

There is a tendency to feel that treatment should be avoided in patients who are deemed to be terminally ill. As a general rule, all treatments should be directed to making the patient more comfortable and not causing any distress.

Symptomatic cystitis should be treated empirically. Pneumonia causing pleuritic pain, cough, or other discomfort warrants antibiotics. Oral antibiotics can be taken relatively easily. Depending on patient choice and ease of venous access, intravenous antibiotics may also be used. Intramuscular injections are usually avoided because they are painful; they may be a last resort for a patient with septicemia (e.g. from a urinary tract infection) for whom oral antibiotics may be insufficient to relieve symptoms and venous access is impossible.

Patients with chronic illness causing immunocompromise are also susceptible to other types of infection. Herpetic infection may respond to antiviral agents. Fungal infections of the mouth and esophagus are common and very easily treated with imidazole antifungal agents such as fluconazole (Finlay, 1995); systemic fungal infections are extremely difficult to diagnose and carry a poor prognosis (Pizzo, 1993).

There seems little rationale in resuscitating a patient to allow him or her to die again only a short time later (Gillon, 1986). But it is unethical to withhold treatments which make a patient feel more comfortable during the last days of life, irrespective of whether they prolong life or not.

MOUTH CARE

Many patients have dryness of the mouth with debris over the teeth, gums, and tongue. Fresh pineapple sucked frequently is a useful debriding agent, although it can predispose to dental decay. Sodium bicarbonate is a useful mouthwash. Ill-fitting dentures should be relined to encourage comfortable eating. Dryness can be relieved by sucking crushed ice, particularly in the later stages of illness. Some patients derive benefit from artificial saliva and should be encouraged to take frequent sips (Trenter and Ceason, 1986).

Dryness is a frequent side effect of drugs, including opioids and anticholinergic medication.

Oral candidosis is found in over 80% of patients who are terminally ill, but does not appear to correlate directly with oral symptoms or signs (Finlay, 1986). Patients with candidosis involving the oropharynx or esophagus should receive systemic treatment with fluconazole for 3 to 4 days. Some strains of candida are now resistant to fluconazole; nystatin solution washed around the oral mucosa four times a day may be effective for these patients (Finlay, 1995).

DYSPHAGIA (*see* Chapter 73, Communication Disorders and Dysphagia)

Oral or esophageal candidosis should be treated if suspected. Imaging with contrast is only indicated for dysphagia not responding to antifungal treatment.

Neurological dysphagia can be helped by developing techniques whereby the head and neck are positioned to assist gravitational movement of food. These are usually idiosyncratic and take time to formulate with each individual patient. A speech therapist can advise on swallowing as well as communication.

Patients with esophageal obstruction may benefit from insertion of an endoesophageal stent (Woodruff, 2004).

ANOREXIA

As patients become frailer, they often lose the desire to eat. Food has great significance in social as well as nutritional terms: mealtimes may be a focus of household routine, and preparing food can be an expression of love. Close family members may feel rejected by the patient who no longer feels like eating their favorite meal. Food may also be the focus for anxieties about the patient's deteriorating condition; relatives may worry that "he should eat something or he will starve to death". Anorexia-cachexia syndrome, seen in many patients with cancer and some with severe COPD or cardiac failure, is not due to starvation *per se* but altered metabolism mediated by inflammatory cytokines (Strasser and Bruera, 2002).

It is helpful to explore the underlying worries about the patient who seems to be fading away before their eyes. Patients should be encouraged to eat what they fancy (often small portions are more appetizing) at times to suit them. Tastes often change in patients with advanced cancer. Calorie and protein supplement drinks may be of benefit but the patient should not be forced to drink supplements he or she finds unpalatable.

Good mouth care is vital to optimize oral intake. Treat oral candidosis and ensure any dentures fit well. Nausea has been discussed and can be treated with antiemetics dependent on the cause; prokinetics can improve gastric stasis.

Steroids are often used to augment appetite. However, in controlled trials, placebo treatment often has an effect, and the benefit seen in patients on corticosteroids is often short-lived (Woodruff, 2004; Jayasekera and Stone, 2004). Long-term steroid therapy is commonly complicated by side effects.

PRESSURE SORES AND OTHER WOUNDS (*see* Chapter 136, Pressure Ulceration)

Patients with terminal illness may be at risk of pressure sores for several reasons: poor mobility, malnutrition including vitamin deficiency, fragile skin, edematous tissues, and reduced sensation. Prevention is better than cure; optimizing mobility, pressure relieving cushions or mattresses, and frequent monitoring of pressure areas can all be helpful.

Painful open wounds may respond to topical morphine or diamorphine in gel (1 mg in 1 ml) (Back and Finlay, 1995), without systemic side effects.

Offensive odor can be reduced by topical metronidazole (0.75% gel) (Finlay *et al.*, 1996); charcoal dressings may absorb some of the odor (Woodruff, 2004), provided they are kept dry (they should not be in contact with an oozing wound). Wounds which ooze blood (e.g. fungating breast cancers) can be controlled by local radiotherapy (Woodruff, 2004) or electron therapy with minimal side effects. Oral tranexamic acid or topical application of weak adrenaline solution may also reduce bleeding.

LYMPHEDEMA

Input from a specialist lymphedema service can dramatically improve painful, heavy swollen limbs due to lymphedema. Meticulous skin care including hygiene and keeping the area well moisturized can help prevent inflammatory episodes. Massage by trained personnel can help drain lymphedema and compression bandaging can help to prevent fluid from reaccumulating; gentle exercise of affected limbs helps maintain lymphatic drainage (British Lymphology Society, 2001).

ASCITES

Ascites are commonly seen in patients with advanced ovarian or gastrointestinal cancers, as well as in end-stage cardiac or hepatic failure. For patients with symptomatic ascites and evidence of fluid overload, a trial of diuretics is indicated (Sharma and Walsh, 1995; Morris, 1984); protein-rich exudates may require paracentesis. Occasionally, patients benefit from insertion of a peritoneovenous shunt, if their general condition and prognosis allow it (Janu *et al.*, 1984). Guidelines for paracentesis in a palliative care setting have been developed (Stephenson and Gilbert, 2002).

HICCUP

The cause of hiccups may guide management; an H_2 blocker for dyspepsia or steroids for a subphrenic liver metastasis may help. Reduction of gastric distension (e.g. using metoclopramide as a prokinetic) may help. The acute attack may be stopped by direct pharyngeal stimulation; hiccups can also respond to nifedipine (Mukhopadhyay *et al.*, 1986; Lipps *et al.*, 1990) or baclofen (Bhalotra, 1990).

DISCUSSING THE DIAGNOSIS AND PROGNOSIS

It can be difficult to choose the correct time to inform the patient of an unfavorable prognosis (Buckman, 1984). The patient's family may exert enormous pressure that the patient should not be told, but lies to patients must be avoided (Gillon, 1985). Patients are aware that they are ill and not improving; imparting the truth should be done gently, answering the patient's questions honestly, without denying hope (Lancet, 1983). While the hope of cure is unattainable, there is hope of good symptom control, of going home, of achieving other goals, for example, grandchildren's weddings and birthdays; the physician must also give the patient reassurance of a commitment to care. Before directly answering questions, it is useful to explore with the patient at length his or her concept of what is wrong (Maguire and Faulkner, 1988a,b; Maguire *et al.*, 1993), using open questions such as "what did you really think was happening?" or "how do you think things are going?" Knowing the patient is looking forward to some event can be vital; the truth of progressive disease can be imparted with the hope that this goal will be reached. However, it is important that goals set are realistic hopes, so that the patient can trust in the physician's honesty.

However much the family pressurize, the patient should never be actively lied to. It is the patient's right to know what is happening and to know that confidentiality will be observed. The truth can be explored gently and the family included to avoid a conspiracy of silence. Once lied to, a patient will never believe the physician again.

A previous bad experience of a friend or a relative dying in distressing circumstances will be crucially important since fear of pain, incontinence, or confusion is common in patients desperate to maintain their dignity and personal integrity to the end.

There are no set rules on how a patient should be told a bad prognosis but the physician should feel emotionally comfortable with the conversation he or she is having with the patient. When patients are aware of being kept "in the dark" for a time, fears become accentuated; "the truth must be so awful that nobody has dared to talk to me about it". The more frightened a patient is, the less likely he or she is to talk about their fears (van Assendelft, 1986).

People have different concepts of words, for example, "tumor", "growth", "cancer", "malignancy", and so on. The patient's own "language" should be used as much as possible (McKillop *et al.*, 1988). After any information has been given, a follow-up conversation is important to discover what the patient has understood.

Much communication is done nonverbally; many cues are picked up by the patient unbeknown to the physician. The physician who avoids opportunities for the patient to ask questions indicates a refusal to answer questions. Creating the impression of having "all the time in the world" means the physician must shed the protective barrier of appearing busy, be prepared to sit down and tackle issues at the patient's own rate (Maguire, 1985). Other members of the team, for example, nursing staff, auxiliary nurses, social workers, domestics, and therapy staff, may seem to have more time and be more accessible key personnel to confide in; good communication within the team must be an essential part of planning for holistic patient care.

Predicting a prognosis is impossible (Christakis and Lamont, 2000). There is no accurate way of predicting life expectancy for a particular patient; time estimates are misleading (Maguire and Faulkner, 1988a,b). A specific time, for example, "three months" or "before Christmas", will be interpreted by patient and family as absolute fact and should be avoided. Some people view a fixed time prognosis as a death sentence. This can be avoided by explaining that the aim is to keep the patient "as well as possible for as long as possible" by adjusting treatment as necessary; problems cannot be specifically foreseen but realistic goals are achievable.

REQUESTS FOR EUTHANASIA

Occasionally, a patient will ask for something "to end it all". This is a sad request to hear, but must be dealt with calmly and sympathetically (Woodruff, 2004).

Some patients feel that they have become a burden on those close to them. Some think that physician-assisted suicide is the only way to end their physical, emotional, or spiritual distress. Others may be simply begging for help or attention. It is important to recognize that demoralized patients are more likely to ask for euthanasia (Kissane *et al.*, 2001), but respond well to excellent care (Chochinov, 1999; Chochinov *et al.*, 1995).

It is vital to look for the reasons underlying the request: look for poorly controlled physical symptoms, associated symptoms of depression, and for existential distress. Effective palliative care can reduce persistent requests for euthanasia to an absolute minimum – such requests are almost never seen to persist when specialist palliative care has been able to provide effective care for some time.

Research into why people ask for death (Chochinov *et al.*, 1995; Mak *et al.*, 2003; Filiberti *et al.*, 2001) has shown that key themes behind the request are as follows:

1. Fear – fear of a future worse than death; fear of becoming a burden.
2. Feeling of being a burden to family, loved ones, or society.
3. Anger and guilt and a sense of wanting control when the disease has taken control of their life.
4. Lack of an adequate environment of dignity-enhancing care (Chochinov, 2002).

Occasionally, patients are so distressed and exhausted that it is appropriate to offer sedation, usually for 24–48 hours. Such sedation using midazolam carefully titrated can then be lightened after one to two days, allowing the patient to reevaluate their position after rest and sleep.

AS DEATH APPROACHES

Not all physicians may feel confident or comfortable to recognize when death is approaching. When a patient's condition is deteriorating day by day, when they are unable to take more than sips of fluid, when they are too weak to get out of bed, their prognosis is likely to be measured in days.

As the patient becomes progressively weaker, the onset of a semicomatose state is often seen. At this stage, all measures must be directed at maintaining comfort and dignity rather than prolonging the dying phase. Rigorous review of medication is required; many drugs can be omitted with benefit (Ellershaw, 2004). Medications which are needed for control of symptoms can be given as subcutaneous injections or as a continuous subcutaneous infusion by syringe driver (Dover, 1987; Oliver, 1988). Fluid intake is often poor, but for those with thirst it can usually be relieved with oral care. "Routine observations" of blood pressure, temperature and oxygen saturation, blood tests, and other investigations become irrelevant and meddlesome and can be stopped (Ellershaw, 2004).

Doctors and nurses should discuss the aims of care with the family or next of kin (provided the patient does not object), so that they are aware that treatment is aimed at comfort and that futile measures will not be taken to attempt resuscitation. It may be helpful to reassure the relatives that "we will allow death to occur naturally" as a positive step, rather than that "treatment will be withdrawn" with negative connotations.

Secretions accumulate within the bronchial tree and cause "death rattle" which can be very distressing to relatives. Explanation of the cause of the sound, and reassurance that it is more distressing for the onlookers than for the patient, may help to alleviate some distress. Early administration of subcutaneous hyoscine or glycopyrronium can minimize the production of secretions, and should be repeated every 4 to 6 hours (Finlay, 1984), or given as a subcutaneous infusion over 24 hours. Repositioning can also drain secretions from the bronchial tree.

Relatives must have a clear explanation of what is happening and be warned that the cyclical pattern of Cheyne-Stokes breathing may occur.

The opioids are remarkably safe drugs. Many fear that a subcutaneous dose of diamorphine may "kill" the patient; the person who is dying should not have analgesia withheld, and well-planned doses will not hasten the end. It is sad to see a patient die of exhaustion when they have been denied adequate analgesia. The use of a syringe driver to administer a continuous infusion of opioid and other drugs (Dover, 1987) may often be easier for both relatives and nurses who find the process of repeated injections traumatic. If repeated subcutaneous injections are used, leaving a small "butterfly" needle *in situ* subcutaneously means that each dose can be given painlessly.

Restlessness in a patient who is dying has many potential causes, including urinary retention, pain, uremia, fear, and unresolved spiritual conflict. When reversible causes have been addressed, the patient may benefit from a benzodiazepine (e.g. midazolam) given subcutaneously, possibly by syringe driver.

The patient who appears comatose can still hear and relatives should be encouraged to continue talking to the dying person (Lamerton, 1979) and to each other. This may be an important time for apologies, reconciliations, or to express love and caring. Sensitive handling of the family at this stage can do much to avoid bitterness and anger developing later in their grief. The family benefit from knowing how to maintain comfort. For the patient at home, mouth care and turning regularly as part of pressure area care can be important physical care which the family can give.

It is important to ascertain any particular wishes they have for religious ceremony or customs around death.

A care pathway, giving guidance in the last few days of life, has been developed to improve care of the dying (Ellershaw, 2004). It is being implemented in many units throughout the United Kingdom and can guide care whether patients are dying in hospital, nursing home, palliative care unit, or at home.

EMERGENCIES

Most deaths are gentle and gradual. Occasionally, a sudden irreversible catastrophic event occurs such as massive hemorrhage, hemoptysis, massive pulmonary embolism, or stridor.

Death will occur within minutes whatever is done; the patient can be rendered unconscious using intravenous midazolam or other sedative drugs to relieve his or her terror. This is not any form of euthanasia; resuscitation attempts are futile and distress relatives and staff.

Whenever possible, such situations should be predicted and discussed with staff and relatives, but it is the one instance where the patient may benefit from ignorance.

BEREAVEMENT

The process of grief may begin before bereavement.

After a person has died, the family or close friends may find comfort from talking to the professional carers again about the person they have lost and often have questions about the way a person died which need to be answered to enable them to come to terms with their own loss.

The spouse of the elderly dying person is often at risk of complicated grief (Preston, 1989). After a lifetime together, often with increasing interdependence during retirement, the loss may result in a chronic or inhibited bereaved state (Stadeford, 1984). The primary care team may be key in providing long-term support and counseling (Charlton and Dolman, 1995). The effect of death on the other members of the family, particularly grandchildren, must also be considered; children may need permission to express their loss (Heegaard, 1988) and participate in the mourning process in the family (Preston, 1989).

WHAT CAN HOSPICE CARE OFFER?

The hospice movement was founded over 30 years ago in Britain and has developed into the speciality of palliative medicine. The philosophy of care is to provide a warm, emotionally safe environment in which the patient can receive treatment aimed at improving the quality of life.

Many patients who are terminally ill will never require the specialized services of an inpatient palliative care unit; their symptoms are easily controlled, they are psychologically at peace and have come to terms with their situation. However, it would be foolish, and even arrogant, for any one physician to feel that he or she is able to provide everything for a patient; hospice care should be used as an adjunct to the current medical team rather than a replacement. Facilities such as day care can provide occupational therapy, social company, and monitor symptom control while allowing the family time to attend to their own affairs (Anderson, 1987; Deans *et al.*, 1988). Home care support can complement, but not replace, the role of the primary care team for the patient cared for at home. A hospice does not have the noisy pressures of acute medical admissions (Soutar and Wilson, 1986), thereby providing a peaceful homely environment in which patient can be assessed in terms of their physical, emotional, social, and spiritual needs.

Just as other aspects require individual planning, so does spiritual input. Most people have individualistic beliefs and their own religious traditions must be respected by all concerned (Neuberger, 1994). The person nearing death has a greater need for spiritual counseling than for the ritualization of religion.

CONCLUSION

The patient approaching death has a right to expect some things from the attendant physician: a commitment to care, promoting quality rather than quantity of life, and helping to live actively and die with dignity.

KEY POINTS

- It may not be possible to cure a patient's progressive illness, but there is still much that can be done to enable as full and active a life as possible.
- Treatment should be tailored to suit the individual, within an ethical framework that allows fair allocation of resources.
- Look for the causes of symptoms; treat the reversible as well as giving symptomatic treatment.
- Consider all domains of distress: symptoms which are difficult to control may be compounded by fear or unresolved spiritual issues.
- If symptoms are not settling within 48 hours despite appropriate treatment, ask for help or advice from a palliative medicine specialist.

KEY REFERENCES

- Ellershaw JE. The management of the last 48 hours of life: The Liverpool Integrated Care Pathway for the Dying Patient. In A Hoy, I Finlay & A Miles (eds) *The Effective Prevention and Control of Symptoms in Cancer* 2004, pp 209–16; Aesculapius Medical Press, London, San Francisco, Sydney.
- Maguire P & Faulkner A. Communicate with cancer patients: 1. Handling bad news and difficult questions. *British Medical Journal* 1988a; **297**:907–9.
- Twycross R & Wilcock A. *Symptom Management in Advanced Cancer* 2001, 3rd edn; Radcliffe Medical Press, Oxford.
- Twycross RG, Wilcock A, Charlesworth S & Dickman A. *Palliative Care Formulary* 2003, 2nd edn; Radcliffe Medical Press, Oxford.
- Woodruff R. *Palliative Medicine* 2004, 4th edn; Oxford University Press, Melbourne.

REFERENCES

Abernethy AP, Currow DC, Frith P *et al.* Randomised, double blind, placebo controlled crossover trial of sustained release morphine for the management of refractory dyspnoea [see comment]. *British Medical Journal* 2003; **327**(7414):523–8.

Anderson R. The unremitting burden on carers. *British Medical Journal* 1987; **294**:63–74.

Back I & Finlay I. Analgesic effect of topical opioids on painful skin ulcers. *Journal of Pain and Symptom Management* 1995; **10**:493.

Back IN. *Palliative Medicine Handbook* 2001, 3rd edn; BPM Books, Cardiff.

Baines M. The principles of symptom control. In CM Saunders, DH Summer & M Teller (eds) *Hospice: The Living Idea* 1981, pp 99–118; Edward Arnold, London.

Baines M. Pain relief in active patients with cancer: analgesic drugs are the foundation of management. *British Medical Journal* 1989; **298**:36–7.

Baines M, Oliver DJ & Carter RL. Medical management of intestinal obstruction in patients with advanced malignant disease: a clinical and pathological study. *Lancet* 1985; **2**:990–3.

Bentley A & Boyd K. Use of clinical pictures in the management of nausea and vomiting: a prospective audit. *Palliative Medicine* 2001; **15**:247–53.

Bhalotra R. Baclofen therapy for intractable hiccoughs. *Journal of Clinical Gastroenterology* 1990; **12**:122.

Bredin M, Corner J, Krishnasamy M *et al.* Multicentre randomised controlled trial of nursing intervention for breathlessness in patients with lung cancer. *British Medical Journal* 1999; **318**:901–4.

British Lymphology Society, Strategy for Lymphoedema Care. [Online]. 2001 [cited 2005 July 6];[6 screens]. Available from: URL:http://www.lymphoedema.org/bls/membership/strategy.htm.

Bruera E, Suarez-Almazor M, Velasco A *et al.* The assessment of constipation in terminal cancer patients admitted to a palliative care unit: a retrospective review. *Journal of Pain and Symptom Management* 1994; **9**:515–9.

Buckman R. Breaking bad news: why is it still so difficult? *British Medical Journal* 1984; **228**:1597–9.

Caraceni A, Cherny N, Fainsinger R *et al.* Pain measurement tools and methods in clinical research in palliative care: recommendations of and Expert Working Group of the European Association of Palliative Care. *Journal of Pain and Symptom Management* 2002; **23**:239–55.

Caraceni A & Grassi L. *Delirium: Acute Confusional States in Palliative Medicine* 2003; Oxford University Press, Oxford.

Chandler S. Oral transmucosal fentanyl citrate: a new treatment for breakthrough pain. *The American Journal of Hospice & Palliative Care* 1999; **16**:489–91.

Charlton R & Dolman E. Bereavement: a protocol for primary care. *The British Journal of General Practice* 1995; **45**:427–30.

Cherny NI & Coley KM. Current approaches to the management of cancer pain a review. *Management of Cancer Pain* 1994; **2**:139–59.

Chochinov HM. Will to live in the terminally ill. *Lancet* 1999; **354**:816–9.

Chochinov HM. Dignity-conserving care – a new model for palliative care: helping the patient feel valued. *Journal of the American Medical Association* 2002; **287**:2253–60.

Chochinov HM, Wilson KG, Enns M *et al.* Desire for death in the terminally ill. *The American Journal of Psychiatry* 1995; **152**:1185–91.

Christakis NA & Lamont EB. Extent and determinants of error in doctors' prognoses in terminally ill patients: prospective cohort study. *British Medical Journal* 2000; **320**:469–72.

Cody M. Depression and the use of antidepressants in patients with cancer. *Palliative Medicine* 1990; **4**:271–8.

Craig G. Withholding artificial hydration and nutrition from terminally ill sedated patients; the debate continues. *Journal of Medical Ethics* 1996; **22**:147–53.

Culbert P, Gillett H & Ferguson A. Highly effective new oral therapy for faecal impaction. *The British Journal of General Practice* 1998; **48**:1599–600.

Deans G, Bennet-Emslie GB, Weir J *et al.* Cancer support groups – who joins and why? *British Journal of Cancer* 1988; **58**:670–4.

Dover SB. Syringe drivers in terminal care. *British Medical Journal* 1987; **295**:553–4.

Dudgeon DJ, Kristjanson L, Sloan JA *et al.* Dyspnea in cancer patients: prevalence and associated factors. *Journal of Pain and Symptom Management* 2001; **21**:95–102.

Dunphy K, Finlay I, Rathbone G *et al.* Rehydration in palliative and terminal care: if not – why not? *Palliative Medicine* 1995; **9**:221–8.

Ellershaw JE. The management of the last 48 hours of life: The Liverpool Integrated Care Pathway for the Dying Patient. In A Hoy, I Finlay & A Miles (eds) *The Effective Prevention and Control of Symptoms in Cancer* 2004, pp 209–16; Aesculapius Medical Press, London, San Francisco, Sydney.

Ellershaw JE, Sutcliffe JM & Saunders CM. Dehydration and the dying patient. *Journal of Pain and Symptom Management* 1995; **10**:192–7.

Fallon MT & Hanks GW. Control of common symptoms in advanced cancer. *Annals of the Academy of Medicine* 1994; **23**:171–7.

Fallon MT & Welsh J. The role of ketamine in pain control. *European Journal of Palliative Care* 1996; **3**:143–6.

Feuer DJ & Broadley K. Systematic review and meta-analysis of corticosteroids for the resolution of malignant bowel obstruction in advanced gynaecological and gastrointestinal cancers. *Annals of Oncology* 1999; **10**:1035–41.

Filiberti A, Ripamonti C, Totis A *et al.* Characteristics of terminal cancer patients who committed suicide during a home palliative care program. *Journal of Pain and Symptom Management* 2001; **22**:544–53.

Finlay IG. Care of the dying patient in general practice. *British Medical Journal* 1976; **291**:179–81.

Finlay IG. *Care of the Dying: A Clinical Handbook* 1984; Churchill Livingstone, London.

Finlay IG. Oral candida and symptoms in the terminally ill. *British Medical Journal* 1986; **292**:592–3.

Finlay I. Oral fungal infections. *European Journal of Palliative Care* 1995; **2**(suppl 1):4–7.

Finlay IG, Bowsyc J, Ramlau C & Gwiezdzinski Z. The effect of topical 0.75% metronidazole gel on malodorous cutaneous ulcers. *Journal of Pain and Symptom Management* 1996; **11**:158–62.

Garde A. Experiences with dexamethasone treatment of intracranial pressure caused by brain tumours. *Acta Neurologica Scandinavica. Supplementum* 1965; **13**:439–43.

Gillon R. Telling the truth and medical ethics. *British Medical Journal* 1985; **291**:1556–7.

Gillon R. Ordinary and extraordinary means. *British Medical Journal* 1986; **292**:259–61.

Hanks G. Morphine and alternative opioids in cancer pain: the EAPC recommendations. *British Journal of Cancer* 2001; **84**:587–93.

Hawkins C & Hanks GW. The gastroduodenal toxicity of nonsteroidal anti-inflammatory drugs. A review of the literature. *Journal of Pain and Symptom Management* 2000; **20**:140–51.

Heath DA. Hypercalcaemia of malignancy. *Palliative Medicine* 1989; **3**:1–11.

Heegaard M. *When Someone Special Dies* 1988; Woodland Press, Minneapolis.

Higginson I. Needs assessment and audit in palliative care. In C Faull, Y Carter & R Woof (eds) *Handbook of Palliative Care* 1998, pp 44–54; Blackwell Science, Oxford.

Hillier ER. Oral narcotic mixtures. *British Medical Journal* 1983; **287**:701–2.

Hoskin PJ. Bone pain: the evidentiary basis of current management strategies. In A Hoy, I Finlay & A Miles (eds) *The Effective Prevention and Control of Symptoms in Cancer* 2004, pp 71–9; Aesculapius Medical Press, London, San Francisco, Sydney.

Iqbal SJ, Giles M, Ledger S *et al.* Need for albumin adjustments of urgent total serum calcium. *Lancet* 1988; **2**:1477–8.

Jayasekera S & Stone P. The management of anorexia. In A Hoy, I Finlay & A Miles (eds) *The Effective Prevention and Control of Symptoms in Cancer* 2004, pp 195–200; Aesculapius Medical Press, London, San Francisco, Sydney.

Janu D, Price JE & Kettlewell MGW. Clinicopathological observations on metastases in man studied in patients with peritoneovenous shunts. *British Medical Journal* 1984; **288**:749–51.

Jennings AL, Davies AN, Higgins JPT & Broadley K. Opioids for the palliation of breathlessness in terminal illness (Cochrane Review). In *The Cochrane Library* 2001, Issue 3; Wiley, Chichester.

Joint Formulary Committee. *British National Formulary* 2005, 49th edn, British Medical Association and Royal Pharmaceutical Society of Great Britain, London.

Kane R, Wales J, Bernstein L *et al.* A randomised controlled trial of hospice care. *Lancet* 1984; **1**:890–4.

Kendall AH, Stone P & Andrews PLR. Pharmacological aspects of cancer-related fatigue. In A Hoy, I Finlay & A Miles (eds) *The Effective Prevention and Control of Symptoms in Cancer* 2004, pp 3–12; Aesculapius Medical Press, London, San Francisco, Sydney.

Kirkham SR. The palliation of cerebral tumours with high-dose dexamethasone: a review. *Palliative Medicine* 1988; **2**:27–33.

Kirkham SR & Pugh R. Opioid analgesia in uraemic patients. *Lancet* 1995; **345**:1185.

Kissane DW, Clarke DM & Street AF. Demoralization syndrome – a relevant psychiatric diagnosis for palliative care. *Journal of Palliative Care* 2001; **17**:12–21.

Kovacs CS, MacDonald SM, Chik CL & Bruera E. Hypercalcaemia of malignancy in the palliative care patient: a treatment strategy. *Journal of Pain and Symptom Management* 1995; **10**:224–32.

Lamerton RC. Cancer patients dying at home: the last 24 hours. *Practitioner* 1979; **223**(1338):813–7.

Lancet. Cancer care: the relative's view [Editorial], 1983; **2**:1188–9.

Lichter I. Some psychological causes of distress in the terminally ill. *Palliative Medicine* 1991; **5**:138–46.

Lipps D, Jabban B, Mitdrell MH & Daighan JD. Nifedipine for intractable hiccoughs. *Neurology* 1990; **40**:532.

Lipton S. Pain relief in active patients with cancer: the early use of nerve blocks improves quality of life. *British Medical Journal* 1989; **298**:37–8.

Lloyd-Williams M, Taylor F & Lawrie I. Assessment and management of depression in palliative care. In A Hoy, I Finlay & A Miles (eds) *The Effective Prevention and Control of Symptoms in Cancer* 2004, pp 183–94; Aesculapius Medical Press, London, San Francisco, Sydney.

Maguire P. Barriers to psychological care of the dying. *British Medical Journal* 1985; **291**:1711–3.

Maguire P & Faulkner A. Communicate with cancer patients: 1. Handling bad news and difficult questions. *British Medical Journal* 1988a; **297**:907–9.

Maguire P & Faulkner A. Communicate with cancer patients: 2. Handling uncertainty, collusion and denial. *British Medical Journal* 1988b; **297**:972–3.

Maguire P, Faulkner A & Regnard C. Eliciting the current problems of the patient with cancer – a flow diagram. *Palliative Medicine* 1993; **7**:151–6.

Mak YYW, Elwyn G & Finlay IG. Patients' voices are needed in debates on euthanasia. *British Medical Journal* 2003; **327**:213–5.

Mannix K, Ahmedzai SH, Anderson H *et al.* Using bisphosphonates to control the pain of bone metastases: evidence-based guidelines for palliative care. *Palliative Medicine* 2000; **14**(6):455–61.

McKillop WJ, Stewart WE, Ginsburg AD & Stewart SS. Cancer patients' conception of their disease and its treatment. *British Journal of Cancer* 1988; **58**:355–8.

McQuay H & Moore A. Be aware of renal function when prescribing morphine. *Lancet* 1984; **2**:284.

McQuillan R & Finlay I. Dehydration in dying patients. *Palliative Medicine* 1995; **9**:341.

Mercadente S, Spoldi E, Caraceni A *et al.* Octreotide in relieving gastrointestinal symptoms due to bowel obstruction. *Palliative Medicine* 1993; **7**:295–9.

Meyerson BA. Neuropathic pain: an overview. *Advances in Pain Research and Therapy* 1990; **13**:193–9.

Mijovic A. Blood transfusion in the treatment of weakness and fatigue in cancer. In A Hoy, I Finlay & A Miles (eds) *The Effective Prevention and Control of Symptoms in Cancer* 2004, pp 39–42; Aesculapius Medical Press, London, San Francisco, Sydney.

Morris JS. Ascites. *British Medical Journal* 1984; **289**:209.

Mukhopadhyay MD, Mark RO, Takeshi W & Wallace TI. Nifedipine for intractable hiccups. *The New England Journal of Medicine* 1986; **314**:1256.

Neuberger J. *Caring for Dying People of Different Faiths* 1994, 2nd edn, Mosby, London.

Oliver DJ. Syringe drivers in palliative care: a review. *Palliative Medicine* 1988; **2**:21–6.

Parkes CM. Terminal care: evaluation of an advisory domiciliary service at St. Christopher's hospice. *Postgraduate Medical Journal* 1980; **56**:685–9.

Pizzo PA. Management of fever in patients with cancer and treatment-induced neutropenia. *The New England Journal of Medicine* 1993; **328**:1323–4.

Plotkin DA, Plotkin D & Okum R. Haloperidol in the treatment of nausea and vomiting due to cytotoxic drug administration. *Current Therapeutic Research* 1973; **15**:599–602.

Portenoy RK. Pharmacologic management of cancer pain. *Seminars in Oncology* 1995; **22**:160–70.

Preston RJ. The consequences of bereavement. *The Practitioner* 1989; **233**:1137–9.

Ralston SH. Pathogenesis and management of cancer associated hypercalcaemia. *Cancer Surveys: Palliative Medicine: Problem Areas in Pain and Symptom Management* 1994; **21**:179–96.

Rees WD, Dover SB & Low-Beer TS. Patients with terminal cancer who have neither terminal illness nor cancer. *British Medical Journal* 1987; **295**:318–9.

Regnard C. Constipation: an algorithm. *Palliative Medicine* 1988; **2**:34–5.

Regnard C & Davies A. *A Guide to Symptom Relief in Advanced Cancer* 1986; Haigh and Hochland, Manchester.

Regnard CFH & Mannix K. Weakness and fatigue in advanced cancer – a flow diagram. *Palliative Medicine* 1992; **6**:253–6.

Ripamonti C & Bruera E. Dyspnea: pathophysiology and assessment. *Journal of Pain and Symptom Management* 1997; **13**:220–32.

Rogers HS, Li MKW & Hobbs KEF. Intravenous opioids in chronic cancer pain. *British Medical Journal* 1985; **291**:1124–5.

Rousseau P. Antiemetic therapy in adults with terminal disease: a brief review. *The American Journal of Hospice & Palliative Care* 1995; **12**:13–8.

Saunders CM. *Terminal Disease* 1978; Edward Arnold, London.

Schulze-Delrieu K, Summers RW & Finke D. Domperidone in reflux oesophagitis and gastric stasis. *Lancet* 1981; **1**:159.

Sharma S & Walsh D. Management of symptomatic malignant ascites with diuretics; two case reports and a review of the literature. *Journal of Pain and Symptom Management* 1995; **10**:237–42.

Shee CD. Palliation in chronic respiratory disease. *Palliative Medicine* 1995; **9**:3–12.

Smith N. Managing family problems in advanced disease – a flow diagram. *Palliative Medicine* 1993; **7**:47–58.

Soutar RL & Wilson JA. Does hospital noise disturb patients? *British Medical Journal* 1986; **292**:305–6.

Stadeford A. *Bereavement: Complicated Grief. Facing Death* 1984, pp 157–62; Heinnemann Medical Books, London.

Stephenson J & Gilbert J. The development of clinical guidelines on paracentesis for ascites related to malignancy. *Palliative Medicine* 2002; **16**:213–8.

Strasser F & Bruera E. Mechanism of cancer cachexia: progress on discntangling a complex problem. *Progress in Palliative Care* 2002; **10**:161–7.

Thompson J & Regnard C. Managing pain in advanced cancer – a flow diagram. *Palliative Medicine* 1992; **6**:329–35.

Trenter P & Ceason N. Nurse-administered oral hygiene. Is there a scientific basis? *Journal of Advanced Nursing* 1986; **11**:323–31.

Twycross R. Pain and analgesics. *Current Medical Research and Opinion* 1978; **5**:497–505.

Twycross R & Back I. Clinical management. Nausea and vomiting in advanced cancer. *European Journal of Palliative Care* 1998; **5**:39–45.

Twycross RG, Barkby GD & Hallwood PM. The use of low dose levomepromazine (methotrimeprazine) in the management of nausea and vomiting. *Progress in Palliative Care* 1997; **5**:49–53.

Twycross RG & Lack SA. *Symptom Control in Far Advanced Cancer: Pain Relief* 1983; Pitman, London.

Twycross R & Wilcock A. *Symptom Management in Advanced Cancer* 2001, 3rd edn; Radcliffe Medical Press, Oxford.

Twycross RG, Wilcock A, Charlesworth S & Dickman A. *Palliative Care Formulary* 2003, 2nd edn; Radcliffe Medical Press, Oxford.

van Assendelft AH. The doctor and the cancer patient. *Lancet* 1986; **1**:100.

Walsh TD & West RS. Controlling symptoms in advanced cancer. *British Medical Journal* 1988; **296**:477–81.

Wilkes E. Dying now. *Lancet* 1984; **1**:950–2.

Woodruff R. *Palliative Medicine* 2004, 4th edn; Oxford University Press, Melbourne.

Worden JW. *Grief Counselling and Grief Therapy* 1983; Tavistock, London.

World Health Organization. *Cancer Pain Relief and Palliative Care* Technical Report Series 804, 1990; WHO, Geneva.

World Health Organization. *Cancer Pain Relief* 1996, 2nd edn; WHO, Geneva.

Appendix

Conversion of SI Units to Standard Units

Appendix updated by D. Grammatopoulos

Clinical Biochemist, University of Warwick, Warwick, UK

BLOOD BIOCHEMISTRY

Investigation	SI units	Conversion factor	Standard units
Alpha-feto protein	0.0–20 μg/l	1.0	0.0–20 ng/ml
Ammon. Nitrogen	<40 μmol/l	1.4	15–45 μg/dl
Ascorbate	23–114 μmol/l	0.0176	0.4–2 mg/dl
Bicarbonate	24–30 mmol/l	1.0	24–30 m eq/l
Bilirubin (total)	2–17 μmol/l	0.059	0.12–1.0 mg/dl
Calcium	2.15–2.6 mmol/l	4.1	8.8–10.7 mg/dl
Cholesterol (WHO recommended range)	<5.2 mmol/l	38.6	<199 mg/dl
HDL Cholesterol	>1.0 mmol/l	38.6	>38.0 mg/dl
LDL Cholesterol	1.00–4.00 mmol/l	38.6	38–153 mg/dl
Chloride	98–107 mmol/l	1.0	98–107 m eq/l
Copper	12–21 μmol/l	6.4	76–134 μg/dl
Corticosteroid am	170–750 nmol/l	0.036	6.27 μg/dl
pm	50–200 nmol/l		2–8 μg/dl
Creatinine	50–120 nmol/l	0.013	0.65–1.2 mg/dl
Ferritin	18–300 μg/l	1.0	18–300 ng/ml
Fibrinogen	1.0–4.0 g/l	100	100–400 mg/dl
Folate	>1.4 μg/l	1.0	>1.4 ng/ml
Glucose (Random)	3.3–5.5 mmol/l	18	54–190 mg/dl
(Fasting)	<6.1 mmol/l		50–100 mg/dl
Iron	10.0–36 μmol/l	5.7	57–205 μg/dl
Iron binding capacity	45–70 μmol/l	5.6	250–390 μg/dl
Lactate	0.67–1.8 mmol/l	9.0	6–16 mg/dl
Lead	0.5–2.0 μmol/l	20	10–14 μg/dl
Magnesium	0.7–1.07 mmol/l	2.4	1.7–2.6 mg/dl
Osmolality	280–300 mmol/kg	1.0	280–300 m Osm/kg
Phosphorus	0.8–1.5 mmol/l	3.1	2.5–4.3 mg/dl

Investigation	SI units	Conversion factor	Standard units
Potassium	3.3–5.0 mmol/l	1.0	3.3–5.0 m eq/l
Protein (total)	58–80 g/l	0.1	5.8–8.0 g/dl
Albumen	38–50 g/l	0.1	3.8–5.0 g/dl
Globulin	18–36 g/l	0.1	1.8–3.6 g/dl
Immunoglobins			
Ig A	0.9–4.5 g/l	100	90–450 mg/dl
Ig M M	0.45–1.8 g/l		45–180 mg/dl
F	0.5–2.2 g/l		50–220 mg/dl
Ig G	7–19 g/l		700–1900 mg/dl
Sodium	136–145 mmol/l	1.0	136–145 m eq/l
Thyroxine	9.6–26.5 pmol/l	0.78	7.5–18.7 μg/dl
Transferrin	1.70–3.70 g/l	0.01	170–370 μg/dl
Triodothyronine (T3)	1.2–3.5 nmol/l	66	80–230 ng/dl
TSH	0.35–5.0 m U/l	1.0	0.35–5.0 μu/ml
Triglycerides	0.57–1.70 mmol/l	88.6	50–151 mg/dl
Urea	2.3–6.9 mmol/l	6	14–41 mg/dl
Vitamin B12	160–920 ng/l	1.0	160–920 pg/ml

URINE BIOCHEMISTRY

Investigation	SI units	Conversion factor	Standard units
Calcium	2.5–7.5 mmol/24 h	40	100–300 mg/dl
Creatinine	9–17 mmol/24 h	0.111	1.0–2.0 g/24 h
Hydroxyproline	0.08–0.25 mmol/24 h	125	10–35 mg/24 h
Phosphate	15–50 mmol/24 h	0.033	0.5–1.5 g/24 h
Potassium	25–100 mmol/24 h	1	25–100 m eq/24 h
Sodium	40–220 mmol/24 h	1	40–220 m eq/24 h

HEMATOLOGY

Investigation	SI units	Conversion factor	Standard units
Hemoglobin	11.5–16.5 g/l	1	1.15–1.65 g/dl
RBC	$3.80–5.80 \times 10^{12}$/l	0.001	$3.80–5.80 \times 10^{6}/mm^{3}$
WBC	$4.0–11.0 \times 10^{9}$/l	0.001	$4.0–11.0 \times 10^{3}/mm^{3}$
Platelets	$150–400 \times 10^{9}$/l	0.001	$150–400 \times 10^{3}mm^{3}$

Index

Notes

Abbreviations

CABG – coronary artery bypass grafting
COPD – chronic obstructive pulmonary disease
DIC – disseminated intravascular coagulation
MCI – mild cognitive impairment
MND – motor neuron disease
NIPPV – noninvasive positive pressure ventilation
NSAIDs – nonsteroidal anti-inflammatory drugs (NSAIDs)

American spelling have been used in this index, for example anemia
Cardiac Trials are indexed under their acronyms.
Page numbers in **bold** refer to boxes or tables
Page numbers in *italics* refer to figures

abarelix, prostate cancer 1514
abciximab 520
abdominal aortic aneurysm (AAA) 1003–5, 1360
abdominal pain
  acute pancreatitis 418
  colon cancer 1527
  gallstones 388
abdominal reflex, aging effect 747
abdominal X ray 418, 420, 1715
abducens nerve, aging 745
ablation procedures, atrial fibrillation 502, 504
Abmi hip screw *see* sliding hip screw (SHS)
Aborigines and Torres Strait Islanders 1890
Aβ-peptide *see* amyloid (Aβ-peptide)
abrasion, teeth *see* tooth, abrasion
abscess
  brain *see* brain, abscess
  dental 270
  epidural 1774–5
  intracranial 1225
  percutaneous drainage 1720
abuse, elder *see* elder abuse
acamprosate (Campral®) 165
acanthosis nigricans **1603**
acarbose 134
ACAS (Asymptomatic Carotid Atherosclerosis Study) 810
accessory muscles of respiration 672
  see also respiratory skeletal muscles
accident risk, Alzheimer's disease 1086–7
accommodation (housing) conversion 1089
Accreditation Council for Graduate Medical Education (ACGME) 1902, 1930
ACDOT-LLA study, diabetes **1437**
ACE inhibitors
  acute coronary syndromes 520
  aspiration pneumonia prevention 687
  atherosclerosis 620–1
  cardiac cachexia 642
  chronic renal failure 1500
  contraindications 574
  cough reflex 687
  diabetics 1439
  drug interactions 575
  in heart failure 574, 575, 576
    congestive heart failure 1565, 1863
    "escape", response 558
    rationale 557, 558
  hypertension therapy 518, 551
  peripheral vascular disease 627
  post-myocardial infarction 521, 522, **522**
  renal toxicity 1503
  stroke risk reduction 832
  ventricular arrhythmias 508
acenocoumarol 450
acephalic migraine 753–4
acetaminophen (paracetamol) 161, 986, 1350, **1652**
acetylcholine (ACh) 41, 971
  Alzheimer's disease 1076
  myasthenia gravis 900
acetylcholine receptors (AChR) 900
  antibodies, myasthenia gravis *see under* myasthenia gravis (MG)
acetylcholinesterase (AChE) 1076
  inhibitors 60
acetylsalicylic acid *see* aspirin
achalasia 360–1
acidosis, metabolic 1383
acitretin, psoriasis 1597
acoustic admittance 1221
acoustic neuroma (neurinoma) 1227–8, 1241, 1244
acoustic reflex test 1221
acoustic tympanometer 1221
acoustics 1219–20
acquired immune deficiency syndrome (AIDS) *see* AIDS
acquired lamellae, tooth enamel 261
acrodermatitis enteropathica (AE) 340
acromegaly 1399
  cause 1400
  clinical features 489, **1399**
  screening and treatment 1400–1
ACST (Asymptomatic Carotid Surgery Trial) 810, *810*
ACTH-producing tumors 1400
actigraphy 737
actinic cheilitis 263
actinic keratosis **1592**, 1600–1, *1600*
activated partial thromboplastin time (APTT) 446, 636
activated protein C resistance (APCR) 442–3, 634
ACTIVE (AF Clopidogrel Trial with Irbesartan for prevention of Vascular Events) 507
active neglect 182
activin, menopause 1416
activities, communication disorder assessment 1044–5, **1044**
activities of daily living (ADLs)
  Alzheimer's disease 1084, 1085, 1087
  anxiety association 1142
  assessment 1544, **1545**, 1554, 1861
    Health Maintenance Clinical Guidepath 205
    scales 1557, **1561**, 1574–5
  carers' assistance 852
  cervical spinal canal stenosis 994
  decline, reduced by exercise 136
  dementia 1141
  Down's syndrome 1186
  eye disorders 1205
  nursing home acquired pneumonia 666
  stroke rehabilitation 852–3, 854
Activities of Daily Living Hierarchy 1860
acupuncture, back pain 1361
acupuncture massage, back pain 1361
acute aortic syndrome 1006
acute care
  case-mix payment 1860–1
  nursing role (UK) 231–2, 1870–1
  quality improvement 1845–7, 1871
Acute Care for the Elderly (ACE) units, USA 1847, 1899–900, 1927
  delirium management 1928
ACUTE CHANGE IN MS (mental status) mnemonic **1112**, 1127
  delirium, drugs causing 1049–52, **1050**
acute coronary syndromes 516, 520
  see also angina pectoris; myocardial infarction, acute
acute exacerbation of COPD (AECOPD) 700–2
acute inflammatory demyelinating polyneuropathy (AIDP) 895
acute lymphoid leukemia (ALL) 469–70
acute myeloblastic/myelogenous leukemia (AML) 465–9
  clinical features/diagnosis 466
  hypoplastic 466, 468
  myelodysplasia transformation to 455, 457, 460, 466
  prognosis 467–8, 1510, **1510**
  treatment 466–8
  WHO classification 466, **466**

Acute Physiology and Chronic Health Evaluation (APACHE) II 419
acute promyelocytic leukemia (APL) 467, 1526
acute quadriplegic myopathy (AQM) 942
acute renal failure (ARF) 1498–9
acute subdural hematoma *see* subdural hematoma, acute
acute tubular necrosis (ATN) 1651
acute-care unit, Alzheimer's disease 1090
acyclovir 762, 895, 1594, 1732, 1776
A-δ primary afferents 982
adalimumab 1351
ADAM Questionnaire 118, **118**, 1424
adaptation, psychological, need for 54
Addison's disease 1391
adenosine echocardiograms 517
S–adenosyl methionine 388
adenoviruses 667
adequate intake (AI), nutrients 331
adhesive bridges 247, *248*, *249*
Adie's syndrome 972
adipocytokines, sarcopenia 918
adiponectin, sarcopenia 918
adipose tissue
  distribution
    central 281–2
    exercise role 129–30
  excess, prevention by exercise 129
  loss, cardiac cachexia 642
  mass, body composition optimization **126**
  physical activity inverse relationship 129
Admiral Nurses 1165, 1872–3
adrenal adenoma 544
adrenaline, aging effect 973
adrenergic blockade
  α-blockers *see* α-adrenoreceptor blockers (α-blockers)
  β-blockers *see* β-blockers (β-adrenoreceptor blockers)
  bladder 1462–3
adrenergic receptors
  α-adrenoceptors *see* α-adrenoceptors
  aging 61
  β-adrenoceptors *see* β-adrenoreceptors
  bladder 1462, **1462**
adrenergic stimulation, bladder 1462–3
α-1-adrenergic vascular tone 543
adrenocorticotropin (ACTH), tumors producing 1400
adrenomedullin (AM) 323
adult acne (rosacea) 1597–8, *1598*
adult protective services, US 181
advance directives 578, 1654, 1932
  ethical issues 1685–6
  Health Maintenance Clinical Guidepath 206
  NIPPV use 961
advanced sleep phase **734**
adverse drug reactions **218**
Advisory Committee for the Elimination of Tuberculosis 1747
advocacy 1683
aerobic exercise
  body fat changes 130
  bone health 127
  in cardiac disease 656–7
  cognitive function improvement 131, 132
  depression improvement 131
  diabetes management 135
  disease treatment by **134**
  heart failure management 578, 656–7
  recommendations for optimal aging **137**
  sarcopenia 922
  see also exercise training
aerobic gram-negative bacilli 1764, 1773
AFASAK (Danish Atrial Fibrillation, Aspirin, and Anticoagulant Therapy) 451
AFFIRM study 587
afterload, aging effect 567
afuzosin, benign prostatic hyperplasia 1472
age
  atrial fibrillation incidence *480*
  biological *vs* chronological 476
  chronological *vs* functional 202
  discrimination *see* agism
Age and Ageing 1919
age related disease 14, 37
  heart disease 476
  "normal" aging *vs* 14
  see also aging
age related hearing loss (ARHL) 1225–7, *1226*
age related macular degeneration (AMD) 39, 1206–7
  antioxidants 1206, 1671, 1672, 1673
  associated factors **1207**
  exudative (wet)/nonexudative 1206
  prevalence *1206*
  risk factors 1206, **1207**
  smoking 153
  surgery 1206
age-associated memory impairment (AAMI) 66, 1095
Aged Care Act, Australia (1997) 1898
aged care assessment teams (ACATs), Australia 1895, 1898
Aged in Home-Care Project (Ad*HOC*) 1864
Agency for Health Care Policy and Research (AHCPR) **1621**
Agency for Health Care Research and Quality (AHRQ) 1838, 1847
Age-Related Eye Disease study 1671, 1672
ageusia 1249
Aggrecan 991
aggressive behavior
  dementia and 1144
  Down's syndrome 1188
  in long term care patients 1155
aging
  adrenaline changes 973
  animals 13, 14
  anorexia of *see* anorexia of aging
  approaches to therapy 65–6
  biological perspective 13–8
  cancer 1509–17
  cellular damage mechanisms 15–6
    biochemical stresses and gene damage 15, 17
    DNA damage and repair 15
    interactions between mechanisms 16, 17, *17*, 37
    mitochondrial DNA mutations 15–6, 39
    protein damage 16
    telomere loss 15
  definition 14, 37
  demographics *see* demographics, of aging
  effects on tissues 14–5
  groupings (young-old to frail-old) 54
  "healthy"/"intrinsic" 487
  immune system 1590
  insulin signaling pathways affecting 16–7
  mechanisms 1589–90
  metabolic factors affecting 16–7
  models/theories
    antagonistic pleiotropy theory 14
    disengagement theory 1176
    disposable soma theory 14, 16
    evolutionary theory and 13–4
    free radical theory 37
    neuroendocrine theory 37
    neuroendocrine-immune theory 37
    "wear and tear" changes 37
  molecular deficit accumulation 14
  neurological signs 743–50, **744**
  neuropathology *see* neuropathology of aging
  neurotransmission changes 969–70, *970*
  noradrenaline effect 970, *970*, 973
  "normal" 14, 124, 125
    age related disease *vs* 14
  of organs 37–44, **44**
    see also specific organs
  parkinsonian features of 766
  physiology 37–46
    see also specific organs
  plasticity of nervous system 969
  psychology of *see* psychology of aging
  reasons for 13–4
  regulation of rate in *C. elegans* 17
  research 1926–7
  social/community aspects *102*, 104–14, *104*
    agism *see* agism
    effects 109–10, *109*
    elder abuse 111, 1921
    family structure 104
    housing problems 106–8, **107**, 229–30
    life course perspective 104, *105*
    lifestyle *see* lifestyle
    poverty *see* poverty
    relationships 109, *109*, 228–9
    religion/spirituality 110–1
    retirement 102–3, **102**, 108
  successful 1158–9
    health promotion *202*
    probabilities *482*
  see also specific systems/conditions
Aging and Quality of Life Program, USA 1926
Aging Male Survey 1424
aging male symptom (AMS) questionnaire 118, **119**
agism 108–9, **1802**, 1917
  ethical issues 1682–3
  psychiatric services provision 1164, 1169
agitation 1087, 1146, 1155
agnosias, stroke rehabilitation 855
agouti-related peptide (AgRP) 348
agranulocytosis 1409
AIDS 19–20
  autologous T cell transfusion 31
  clinical presentation 1731
  cryptococcal meningitis 1770–1
  developing countries 1968
  hyponatremia 1378
  prevalence 120
  weight gain induction 315–6
  see also HIV infection
air conducting hearing aids 1230–1
air conduction, sound 1220–1
AIRE study (Acute Infarction Ramipril Efficacy) 521, 522, 574
air-fluidized support systems 1614, **1614**, *1615*
airway
  management, ischemic stroke 818
  obstruction 693–4
  occlusion during sleep 737
  small, age related changes 695
akathisia 780
akinesia complex 766
alarms 1694
Alberta Road Test 145
albumin, serum, drug distribution 215–6
albuminuria 1502
alcohol 157–68
  abstinence 164, 386–7
  abuse *see* alcohol abuse
  addiction programme 164
  addiction specialist 164
  age differences in effect 159
  blood concentration 159, 162
  cardioprotective effects 157, 160
  congestive heart failure risk and 479
  consumption
    classification 158
    epidemiology 157–8
    hypertension management 550
    patterns 157
    sensible drinking guidelines 158–9, 166
    unit definition 159, 166
  dependence
    diagnosis 158, 162
    prevalence 158
  drug interactions 160–1, 166
  heart disease risk factor 477
  insomnia and 738
  medical consequences 159–60
  metabolism 159
  pharmacodynamic effects 159
  pharmacokinetic effects 159
  problem drinking diagnosis 162
  restriction, in heart failure 573
  stroke risk 802–3, 837
  tolerance 162
  withdrawal symptoms 164

alcohol abuse 157–68, 1153
  associated conditions 158, 164
  bone mass loss 1291
  diagnosis 162–3, **163**
    barriers 161–2
  differential diagnosis 163
  epidemiology 157–8
  medical consequences 159–60
  neurological assessment 162
  nutrient malabsorption **293**, 294
  oral cancer 243
  pancreatitis 417, 419
  physical examination 162
  prevalence 158
  screening 205, 1150
    questionnaires 162–3, **163**
  seizures and 871
  subarachnoid hemorrhage risk factor 1015
  suicide risk 164
  treatment 163–6
    barriers 161–2
    brief intervention 163
    detoxification 164
    initial approaches 163–4
    intervention 163–4
    long term 164–5
    motivational counseling 163, 164
    outcome 1199
    pharmacotherapies 165–6
    rehabilitation phase 164
    short term stabilization 164
  see also alcoholism
alcohol injection, trigeminal neuralgia 760
alcohol related peripheral neuropathy 894
alcohol related problems survey (ARPS) 163
alcohol use disorders identification test (AUDIT) 158
alcoholic brain damage 159
alcoholic dementia 158, **1085**, 1126
alcoholic hepatitis, acute 386
alcoholic liver disease 159, 386–8
Alcoholics Anonymous (AA) 164, 1198
alcoholism
  autonomic dysfunction 972
  early-onset 162, 165
  late-onset 162
  pharmacotherapies 165–6
  prevalence 158
  prognosis 157, 162, 165
  recent onset 162
  recurrence 166
  see also alcohol abuse
aldosterone 323, 557–8, **558**
aldosterone antagonists, heart failure 575
aldosteronism, primary 544
alefacept 1597
alemtuzumab 1515
alendronate
  hip fracture prevention 1341
  osteoporosis 1283, 1294
  Paget's disease of bone 1275, 1276
Alexander's law 1239
alfentanil, renal failure 2005
alginates 1622, **1622**
alien limb phenomenon 1120
alkalemia 1384
alkaline phosphatase
  bone-specific 1273
  serum, Paget's disease 1273, 1274
alkylating agents, myelodysplasia due to 455
allergic dermatitis, vulval 1455
ALLHAT (Antihypertensive and Lipid Lowering Treatment to Prevent Heart Attack Trial) 551
allodynia 2007
allopurinol 467, 1352
all-trans retinoic acid (ATRA) 459, 467
Alma-Ata Declaration 1983
alosetron 367
α-adrenergic agents 1463–4
α-adrenoreceptor, age related changes 1463
α-adrenoreceptor blockers (α-blockers)
  benign prostatic hyperplasia 1464–5, 1472
  diabetes mellitus 1439
  phosphodiesterase-5 inhibitor interaction 1472
  prostatitis 1480–1, **1481**
  side effects 1464–5
aluminum, osteoporosis 1291
alveolar hemorrhage 452
alveolitis
  cryptogenic fibrosing 717
  extrinsic allergic 716–7
  fibrosing 717–8
Alzheimer's Association Safe Return Program 1146
Alzheimer's disease (AD) 1073–81, 1083–91, 1168
  Aβ-peptide (amyloid) 1077, 1078, 1079
  accident risk 1086–7
  aging effect on cognitive function 48–9
  amyloid fibrils 64, 78
  amyloid hypothesis 1078
  amyloid peptide precursor (APP) 1076, 1077, 1078, 1079
  antioxidants 93
  anxiety 1142
  APOE4 gene association 111
  balance problems 1300
  behavioral symptoms 1087
  cardiovascular disease relationship 481
  cerebral metabolic rate 64
  characteristics 1114–5, **1115**
  cholinergic defect, treatment 65–6
  cholinergic neurons 60
  classification 1083, 1092–3
  clinical features 767, 788, 1083–4, 1092–3
  communication breakdown process
    clinical presentation 1040–1, **1040**, **1041**
    grammar application 1039, 1040
    language 1040
    sequencing 1039
    thinking 1038–9, 1040, 1041
    word finding 1039
    word sound assembly 1039
    word store 1040
  complications 1086–7
  dementia *see* Alzheimer-type dementia
  dental problems 255
  depression 1173, **1174**
  development risk 48
  diagnosis 1073, 1083–5, 1086, 1092–3
  diagnostic criteria 1135
  differential diagnosis 1084, **1084–5**
    frontotemporal dementia *vs* 1122, **1122**
  in Down's syndrome 1185, 1188, **1188**
  duration of disease 1086
  early-onset 1092
  evolution 1085–6
  excitatory amino acid-releasing neurons 62
  falls 1086–7
  follow-up 1087–8
  "frailty" gene 478
  GABAergic neurons 62
  genetics 48–9, 1076–7
  growth inhibitory factor etiological role 1937
  hallucinations 1140
  history 1073
  hormone replacement therapy 1451
  5-hydroxytryptamine 61
  incidence 59
  insomnia in 1145
  late-onset 478, 1092
  management (home/hospital) 1089–90
  mild cognitive impairment 1095
    progression predictors 1096–7, **1097**, **1098**, 1099
  mobility problems 1086–7
  natural history 1086
  nerve growth factor 64
  neurofibrillary tangles 1073–6, *1074*, 1077–8, 1078–9
  neuropathological changes 15, 71
    CA1 region 70
    cerebral amyloid angiopathy 77
    dendritic changes 71
    entorhinal cortex 70
    granulovacuolar degeneration 73
    Hirano bodies 72
    neuritic plaques 74
      see also senile plaques (below)
  neuropathological lesions 1073–6, *1074*, *1075*, *1076*
  olfactory dysfunction 1255
  oxidative stress 64
  paranoid delusions 1140
  physiopathological concepts 1078–9
  prevention 93
  protein synthesis capacity 63
  psychological symptoms 1087
  research 1168, 1937
  risk factors 1083
  senile plaques 64, 73, 1073–5, *1074*, *1075*, 1078–9
  serotonergic neuron dysfunction 62
  smoking 152–3
  synapse loss 63
  synaptophysin levels 63
  tau protein 1077–8, 1079
  treatment 1088–9
    palliative therapy 65–6
    primary care protocols 1164
  vascular dementia and 1106, 1114
  vitamin E supplements 334, 1671
  weight loss 1086
Alzheimer's Disease Centers, USA 1926
Alzheimer's International 1170
Alzheimer's Society 1165, 1168
Alzheimer-type dementia 1111
  development from MCI 1095, 1096, 1097
amantadine
  aspiration pneumonia prevention 688
  Huntington's disease 778
  influenza therapy/prevention 706, 1730, **1730**
  Parkinson's disease 772
  senile chorea 779
amaurosis fugax 806
ambient light sensors 191
ameloblastoma 270–1
American Academy of Anti-Aging Medicine 1667
American Academy of Neurology, driving guidelines 146
American Association of Anesthesiologists (ASA) 1647, **1648**
American Association of Cardiovascular and Pulmonary Rehabilitation (AACVPR) 728, 729
American College of Cardiology 1634–5
American College of Chest Physicians (ACCP) 728, 729
American College of Physicians, thyroid disease screening 1410
American College of Surgeons (ACS), hospital quality 1838, **1838**
American Diabetes Association 1439
American Geriatrics Society (AGS) 207, 1842, 1929
  falls prevention guidelines 1339
  history 2, 1924
American Heart Association (AHA) 1634–5
American Medical Association (AMA) 142, 144
American Medical Directors Association (AMDA) 1489, 1842, 1924
American Psychiatric Association 158
American Thoracic Society (ATS) 1746
American Thyroid Association 1410
American Urological Association (AUA) 1474
amino acid supplements, sarcopenia 923
aminoglycosides 1224, 1243, 1759
α-amino-3-hydroxy-5-methyl-4-isoxazolepropionic acid (AMPA)/kainate receptors 62
aminophylline 701–2, 705
aminotransferase, serum 1743
amiodarone
  after myocardial infarction 523
  atrial fibrillation 502, 503
  hepatitis due to 385
  peripheral neuropathy cause 894
  side effects **504**, 523
  ventricular arrhythmias 508, 510
amitriptyline 274, 987, 1594, 2007
ammonium sulfate precipitation technique 118

amnestic mild cognitive impairment 1095, 1152
amphetamine misuse *1192*, 1193, 1197
amphotericin B 1771, 1773
amphotericin lozenges 264, 267
ampicillin **1758**, 1759, 1766
ampulla (of semicircular canal) 1235
amputation
  diabetic foot 1313, 1315
  peripheral vascular disease 628
amputees
  phantom pain 1582–3
  prostheses 1576, 1581–2, *1582*
Amulree, *Lord* 3, 4–5, 6, 1919
amygdala-hippocampal complex 69
amyl nitrate, misuse *1192*
α-amylase 291–2
amylase, serum, pancreatitis 418, 420
amyloid (Aβ-peptide) 64
  aging neuropathology 64, 73, *73*
  Alzheimer's disease 1077, 1078, 1079
  dementia predictor in MCI 1097
amyloid angiopathy 76–8, *77*
amyloid associated with paraproteinemia 896
amyloid cardiomyopathy 487–8
amyloid hypothesis, of Alzheimer's disease 1078
amyloid precursor protein (APP) 49
  Alzheimer's disease 1076, 1077, 1078, 1079
  Down's syndrome 1185
amyloid/amyloid fibrils
  aging neuropathology 77
  Alzheimer's disease 78, *1075*, 1076, 1077
  cardiac deposition 487–8, 493
  choroid plexus 78
amyloidosis 441
  autonomic dysfunction 972
  cardiac 487–8
  primary, renal damage 1503
amyotrophic lateral sclerosis (ALS) 949
  see also motor neuron disease (MND)
anabolic steroids, cardiac cachexia 643
anal canal 395–6
anal gaping 398
anal sphincters 395–406
  aging 395–6
  artificial 403
  internal 395, 396
  muscle examination 409
  surgical repair 403
  tone 395
  see also external anal sphincter
anal surgery, fecal incontinence 397
"anal wink" 398
analgesia
  chronic pain 986–8
  hip fractures 1332
  Paget's disease of bone 1277
  terminally ill 2003–7
  WHO classification **2005**
analgesics
  adjuvant, chronic pain 987–8
  postpolio syndrome 1777
  tension-type headache 754–5
anarthria 844, 951, 960–1, 963
anastrozole, breast cancer 1514, 1536
Andorra, life expectancy 88, **88**
androgen(s)
  anorexia of aging 305
  brain cell osmolality 1371
  cardiac cachexia 642
  deficiency/deprivation
    complications 1514
    female sexual dysfunction 1662
    prostate cancer 1478, 1514
  myelodysplasia therapy 459
androgen deficiency of aging man (ADAM) *see* andropause
androgen replacement therapy (ART) 305
andropause 118–20, 206, 1421–2
  libido decline 119
  pathophysiology 1422
  symptom-screening tests 118, **118**, **119**, 1424
anemia 427–35
  aplastic 431–2, **432**
  causes **428**, 428–429
  of chronic disease 428, 429–30
    iron deficiency anemia *vs* 430, **430**
    treatment 432–3
  chronic renal insufficiency and 428, 429, 430
    treatment 432–3
  comorbid conditions 427
    heart failure 570–1, 572
  diagnosis by red cell morphology *429*
  differential diagnosis 428 32
  frailty 1565–6, *1568*
  hemolytic *see* hemolytic anemia
  iron deficiency *see* iron deficiency anemia
  macrocytic 429, 455
  microangiopathic hemolytic (MAHA) 446
  microcytic 429–30
  mortality risk 427
  myelodysplastic 429, 459, 468
  myelosuppression 1514
  normocytic 430
  nutritional 428
  prevalence 427–8
  sideroblastic 429
  treatment 427, 432–3, **432**
  vitamin B_{12} deficiency 429, 432
anesthesia 1647–57, **1654**
  cardiovascular morbidity 1648–9
  CNS morbidity 1649–50
  mortality 1647, *1648*
  myasthenia gravis 905
  postoperative dementia 1641–2
  renal morbidity 1636, 1650–1
  respiratory morbidity 1649
anesthetic drugs, renal injury 1650–1
aneurysm
  aortic *see* aortic aneurysm
  atrial septal, stroke risk 837
  saccular, subarachnoid hemorrhage 1018
  septic 1020
angiitis, primary 1126
angina bullosa hemorrhagica, oral 268
angina pectoris
  clinical features 515
  coronary artery narrowing 599
  hemodialysis 1500
  risk factors *see* ischemic heart disease, risk factors
  stable, therapy 519
  unstable, therapy 520
  valvular heart disease with 532
angiodysplasia 377
  gastrointestinal 372, 489
angiography
  aortoenteric fistula 377
  catheter 807–8, 1018–9
  coronary 586, 599, 1648
  gastrointestinal bleeding 376
  pulmonary embolic disease 714
angioplasty
  carotid 837
  coronary 519, 578–9, 599–600
  lower extremity 627–8
angiotensin I 1372
angiotensin II 557, 1372
  effects 543, **557**
  heart failure 557, 560
  hypertension 973
  receptors (AT_1 and AT_2) 322, 557
  thirst regulation 322, 323
angiotensin receptor blockers (ARBs) 574
angiotensin-converting enzyme (ACE) 557, 656, 1407
  inhibitors *see* ACE inhibitors
angle closure glaucoma 759
angular acceleration detection 1235
angular cheilitis (stomatitis) 264, *264*
anhedonia, Parkinson's disease 774
animals
  aging 13, 14
  defense systems 19
anismus *see* dyssynergic defecation
ankle jerk 746–7, 996
ankle-brachial index (ABI) 623
anorectal angle 396
anorectal manometry 399, 410
anorexia 313–4
  acute illness 313–4
  cachexia 314
  hospitalization 314
  terminally ill 2011
  TNF-α 917–8
  zinc deficiency 340
anorexia of aging 297–307
  causes 300–1, 919, 1566
  frailty 1566–7
  homeostasis loss 299
  medication induced 300
  pathological 299–300, **300**
  physical factors 300
  physiological 299, 300–1
  sarcopenia 919
anorexia-cachexia syndrome 2011
anosmia 1249
anosognosia 855
anosphrasia 1249
Antabuse-like reaction 161
antacids, anorexia-induction 300
antagonistic pleiotropy, theory 14
antegrade enemas 412
anterior circulation, infarction 816, 823
anterior pituitary *see* pituitary gland
anterior spinal artery 1001, 1002
  spinovascular insufficiency 1008
anterior spinal artery syndrome (ASAS) 1003, 1008, 1009
anterior spinal vein 1002
anthracycline 1514
anthraquinone laxatives 412
anthropometry 910, **911**
antiaging therapy 111, 1665–80, **1667**
  antioxidants 1667–8, 1670–4
  appeal of 1665–6
  current data 1669–70
  definition 1666
  hormones 1668, 1674–7
  impacts 1678
  means of testing 1670
  scientific basis 1667
  usage 1666–7
antiarrhythmic drugs 522–3, 1050
antibiotic sore mouth 264
antibiotics
  acute exacerbation of COPD 701
  acute pancreatitis 419
  aspiration pneumonia/pneumonitis 687
  atherosclerosis 621
  dysphagia in MND 961
  infected pressure ulcers 1623
  nutrient malabsorption **294**
  otitis media 1224
  pneumonia 687, 708
  prostatitis 1480, **1481**
  sepsis prophylaxis 1642
  terminally ill 2010
  see also antimicrobial therapy
antibodies
  age related changes 22–3, 26
  see also specific immunoglobulins
anticholinergic agents
  COPD 698
  dystonia 783
  Parkinson's disease 772
  salivary dribbling in MND 960
  side effects 783, 960, 1464
  stress incontinence 1464
  tardive dyskinesia 780
anticholinesterase inhibitors (AChEI)
  Alzheimer's disease 1088
  contraindications 1088–9
  memory clinic patients 1069
  myasthenia gravis 903
  side effects 1069, 1088, 1089
  vascular dementia 1115, *1116*
anticholinesterase test 902–3
anticoagulants/anticoagulation 449–54
  adverse effects 506, 637
  after myocardial infarction 521

age as contraindication? 506
atrial fibrillation 500, 505–7, 534, 605
bleeding risk 450–1
anticoagulation intensity and 451–2, *451*
intracranial bleeding 450–1
occult bleeding 452
polypharmacy 451, 506, 637
risk factors 451
sites 452, *452*
warfarin *see* warfarin, bleeding risk
cardiac surgery 603, 604–5
chronic subdural hematoma and 1031
compliance issues 452–3
duration 452
effectiveness in elderly 451
increased sensitivity with age 449–50
ischemic stroke 820
pulmonary embolic disease 714
response in elderly 449–50
risk–benefits and optimization 451–2, 453
spontaneous subdural hematoma and 1029
subarachnoid hemorrhage etiology 1020
underuse 451
vascular dementia 1107
venous thromboembolism 637
see also warfarin
anticonvulsants (antiepileptics) 873–5, **873**
diabetic neuropathy 893
dosages and half-life 873, **873**
level monitoring 875–6
neuropathic pain 987, 2007
osteoporosis risk 873
restless legs syndrome 781
withdrawal 876
anticytokine therapies 643
antidepressants
alcohol interaction 161
anxiety 1154
back pain 1363
delirium etiology 1051
depression 1150, 1178
dementia and 1124, 1138–9, **1138**
diabetic neuropathy 893
insomnia **739**
irritable bowel syndrome 367–8
motor neuron disease 962
Parkinson's disease 774
side effects 987
SSRIs *see* selective serotonin reuptake inhibitors (SSRIs)
tension-type headache 755
terminally ill 2010
tricyclic *see* tricyclic antidepressants
antidiarrheals 400
antidiuretic hormone (ADH) *see* vasopressin
antiemetics 1245, 2008
contraindications 1246
antiepileptic drugs *see* anticonvulsants (antiepileptics)
antiexcitotoxic agents 65
antifibrinolytic drugs 1022
antigen presenting cells (APC) 27
antigenic stimulation, chronic 19
antiglutaminergic agents 1089
antihistamines 161, 739, 1051
antihypertensive therapy
delirium etiology 1050
diabetics 1439
falls associated 477
in heart failure 578, **579**
ischemic stroke and 819
renal blood flow impairment 1496, 1502
subarachnoid hemorrhage 1023
vascular dementia 1107
anti-inflammatory agents **560**
see also nonsteroidal anti-inflammatory drugs (NSAIDs)
antimicrobial therapy
bacterial meningitis 1765–7, **1766**, **1767**
delirium etiology 1050
epidural abscess 1774
fungal meningitis 1771
spirochetal meningitis 1769–70
subdural empyema 1774
topical, wound cleansing 1621
tuberculous meningitis 1768
see also antibiotics
antimuscarinic drugs 1463, 1490
antineoplastic agents, peripheral neuropathy cause 894–5
Antioxidant Supplementation in Atherosclerosis Prevention (ASAP) 1671, 1673
antioxidants 331–6
age related macular degeneration 1206, 1671, 1672
alcoholic liver disease 388
antiaging therapy 1667–8, **1667**, 1670–4
cardiovascular disease 93
chemosensory dysfunction treatment 1257
clinical trial results 1673–4
with exercise, sarcopenia therapy 923
immune function restoration 32
neuroprotective therapy 65
vitamins 331–4, 1670–3
atherosclerosis 620
stroke risk reduction 836
antiparkinsonian drugs 1050
antiphospholipid syndrome, primary 443
antiplatelet therapy
NSAIDs contraindication 830
peripheral vascular disease 626
stable angina therapy 519
stroke risk reduction 822–3, 828, 830–1
antipsychotics (neuroleptics)
alcohol interaction 161
Alzheimer's disease 1087
atypical
bipolar affective disorder 1151
schizophrenia 1151
cough reflex suppression 689
in delirium 1056–7
delirium etiology 1051
dementia, delusions/hallucinations in **1140**
drug induced parkinsonism 768
dystonia 783
Huntington's disease 778
schizophrenia 1151
senile chorea 779
sensitivity reaction in Lewy body dementia 1119
swallowing reflex suppression 689
tardive dyskinesia induction 779
antiseptics, wound cleansing 1621
antispasmodics
delirium etiology 1050
irritable bowel syndrome 367
side effects 367
antispastic medications, cramp/spasticity in MND 960
antithrombin, deficiency 442, 445, 446, 633
antithrombotic therapy, ischemic stroke 820
antithyroid peroxidase antibodies (anti-TPO) 1411
anti-TNF therapy 643
antrum 363, 364–5
anxiety 1142
Alzheimer's disease 1084, 1087
assessment 984
chronic pain 982
COPD 700
dementia and 1142–3, **1143**
dental care 241
tremor 783
anxiety disorders 738, 1153–4
anxiolytics, Alzheimer's disease 1087
aorta 1001
acute occlusion 1006
ascending, atherosclerosis 596
coarctation 544–5
diameter 1003–4
dissection 606, 608, 1005–6
embolectomy 1006
spinovascular insufficiency 1003–6
surgery, spinal cord infarction after 1009
thoracic
aneurysms 606, *606*, 608, 1005
surgery 606–7, 608
thrombosis 1006
aortic aneurysm
abdominal 1003–5, 1360
investigations 1004
rupture 1004–5
spinovascular insufficiency 1003–5
surgical treatment 1004
symptoms/signs 1004
thoracic 606, *606*, 608, 1005
thoracolumbar 1005
aortic dissection 606, 608, 1005–6
aortic fenestration 1006
aortic intramural hematoma 1006
aortic regurgitation 530
angina with 532
management 588–9, **588**
valvuloplasty indications **534**
aortic sclerosis 487
aortic stenosis 481, 530
angina with 532
asymptomatic, valve replacement 601
calcific degenerative 600–1
clinical features 587
epidemiology 531
heart failure and 573
management 587–8
aortic valve replacement 587–8, **587**, 601
valvuloplasty indications **534**
aortic tube graft 1004
aortic valve
annular calcification 532
balloon valvotomy 602
bicuspid 481
incompetence 487
regurgitation *see* aortic regurgitation
replacement 587–8, 600–2, 607
in aortic regurgitation 588–9, **588**
in aortic stenosis 587–8, **587**
in asymptomatic aortic stenosis 601
bioprosthesis *vs* mechanical 587, 589, 603
indications **587**
mortality 588, 589, 601, *601*
"prophylactic" during CABG 601–2
size of prosthetic valve 601
stenosis *see* aortic stenosis
valvuloplasty 535, 573, 602
percutaneous balloon 602
aortoenteric fistula 377
aortoplasty, glue 1006
AP-1 1591
APACHE II (Acute Physiology and Chronic Health Evaluation) 419
apathetic frontotemporal dementia (FTD) 1121
apathetic thyrotoxicosis 1391, 1408
apathy, dementia and 1146
aphasia
classification 843
primary progressive 1039, 1040
progressive fluent 1123
progressive nonfluent 1121, 1122–3
apheresis, age related macular degeneration 1206
apnea *see* sleep apnea
apneustic breathing, stroke 678
apolipoprotein (Apo) 613
apolipoprotein E (ApoE) 49
Alzheimer's disease 1077, 1083
cerebral amyloid angiopathy 77
depression 1176
synaptic density 71–2
apolipoprotein E epsilon-4 (apo ε-4)
Alzheimer's disease 219, 1704
APOE4 gene and 111
centenarians 1704
heart disease risk factor 478
Lewy body dementia 1117
apomorphine, Parkinson's disease 772
apoptosis
Alzheimer's disease 1079
atherosclerotic plaque destabilization 620
bone marrow cells 22, *23*
heart failure mechanism 562
increased in myelodysplasia 457
motor neuron disease 957
necrosis *vs* 562

appetite questionnaire **1927**
appetite regulation 301–2, *301*
appetite stimulators **315**
apraxia
  corticobasal degeneration 1120
  in dementia 1040, 1137
  ignition 1301
  stroke rehabilitation 855
apraxic gait 1301
Aqueduct of Sylvius, CSF flow 789
arachnoid granulations 787
areca nut chewing 269
α-receptor blockers *see* α-adrenoreceptor blockers (α-blockers)
areflexic (paralytic) syncope
  clinical features 881–2
  diagnosis 882–3
  management 883
  mechanism 879, 880
arginine vasopressin (AVP) *see* vasopressin
argon laser iridotomy 1208
Argyll Robertson pupils 972
Aricept (donepezil) *see* donepezil
aripiprazole 1140
Arjo Maxilift™ 1714
arm weakness, in MND 962–3
aromatase inhibitors, breast cancer 1513–4
arrhythmias *see* cardiac arrhythmias
arsenic **341**
arsenic trioxide 469
arterial blood pressure *see* blood pressure
arterial disease, foot manifestations 1316
arterial dissection 1019
arterial stiffening, Osler's sign 545
arteriography, gastrointestinal bleeding 376
arteriosclerosis 542
  vascular dementia 1111
arteriovenous fistula
  dural/intradural 1008, 1020
  hemodialysis 1500
arteriovenous malformation (AVM) 1008, 1019–20
arthritides, frailty 1566
arthritis 1347–53, **1348**
  exercise effects **133**, 134, **134**
  heart failure comorbidity 571
  incidence, Latin America 1993
  investigations **1348**
  rehabilitation issues 1572, *1573*, 1580–1
  sexual dysfunction 120
  temporomandibular joint 273
  treatment 1350–2, **1350**
  see also individual types
arthroplasty
  cementing 1335
  displaced intracapsular hip fracture 1334–5, *1334*
    complications 1337, *1338*
  loosening 1337, *1338*
  refracture 1337
artificial vision 1209
ASAP study 1671, 1673
asbestos exposure 710, 712, 716
asbestosis 716
ascites, terminally ill 2011
ascorbic acid *see* vitamin C
aseptic meningitis, HIV-associated dementia 1126
aseptic meningitis syndrome 1763
aspartate aminotransferase (AST), serum, myopathies 936
Aspergillus, brain abscess 1771, 1772, 1773
asphyxiation, restraint complication 1692–3
aspiration 685, 844, 845
  dysphagia 844, 845
  silent 844
aspiration pneumonia 685–92
  development mechanisms 685–6, *686*
  diagnosis 686
  dysphagia 845
  motor neuron disease 961
  neuroleptic avoidance 689
  Parkinson's disease 775
  preventative strategies 687–9, *687*
  protective reflex absence 685
  stroke, following 821
  treatment 687
  vaccinations 689–90
aspiration pneumonitis 685, 686
  development mechanisms 686–7
  motor neuron disease 951
  treatment 687
aspirin
  acute coronary syndrome 520
  after CABG 600
  alcohol–drug interaction 161
  atrial fibrillation 505
  cancer prevention 1511
  chronic mitral regurgitation 589
  clopidogrel and 831
  functional platelet defects 439
  oral ulceration induction 266
  peripheral vascular disease 626
  post-myocardial infarction 521
  post-stroke 820
  secondary stroke risk reduction 828, 830, 831
  stroke risk reduction 822–3
  thromboembolic prophylaxis 636, 1332–3
assessment *see* geriatric assessment
Assessment and Management of Older People in the Community 1801, 1803
Assets and Health Dynamics of the Oldest Old Survey 348
Assisted Living Facilities (ALF), USA 107–8, 1897, 1929
assisted suicide 1951
assistive devices 1886–7
  chronic pain management 988
Association of Directors of Geriatric Academic Programs (ADGAP) 1926
Association of Physicians of India 1990
asteatotic dermatitis 1595–6, *1596*
asthma 702–5
  atmospheric pollution 703
  diagnosis and misdiagnosis 704
  epidemiology 702
  late-onset 702–3
  management 704–5
  mortality 703
  obstructive pattern 694–5
  pathogenesis 702–3
  presentation 703–4
  respiratory infection 705
  smoking 153
astrocytes, age related changes 76
asymmetrical neuropathy 891
Asymptomatic Carotid Atherosclerosis Study (ACAS) 810
Asymptomatic Carotid Surgery Trial (ACST) 810, *810*
AT877, subarachnoid hemorrhage 1023
ataxia telangiectasia 1590
ataxic breathing 678
ATBC Cancer Prevention Study 334, 1670–1, 1672
atenolol, hypertension therapy 547
atheroembolic disease, kidney 1502
atheroma/atheromatous plaques
  cardiac surgery morbidity and 595, 596
  carotid artery stenosis 805–6, *806*
  complex 611
  fibrous cap 611, 805
  ischemic stroke 815
  plaque formation mechanisms 611, 613–20
  plaque rupture 620, *620*, 805
  renal artery destruction 1496
  risk factors 805
atherosclerosis
  anatomy 611
  as autoimmune disease 32
  biochemical analysis 613
  blood vessel shear stress 617
  causes 91–2
  "cholesterol hypothesis" 613–6
  cholesterol insudation 615–6, *616*
  "endothelial activation hypothesis" 616–8
  fibrous tissue expansion 619
  fluid dynamics 616–7
  histological appearance 611–3, *612*
  hypertension 973
  immune deficiency 618–9
  immunohistochemistry 611
  inflammatory disease 618–9
  lesion classification 611
  leukocyte recruitment 618, *618*
  lipid deposition 613–6
  localization 616–8
  macrophages 616
  pathogenesis 611–22
  plaques *see* atheroma/atheromatous plaques
  tangential wall stress 616–7
  therapy 620–1
  type I-VIII lesions 611
  vitamin C supplements 1673
  vitamin E supplements 1671
  see also ischemic heart disease
Atherosclerosis Risk in Communities (ARIC) study 1434
athlete's foot *see* tinea pedis
atlantoaxial instability 992, 1187, **1187**
atlantoaxial posterior fixation system 995
atlas (C1), anatomy 991
ATM gene 1590
atrial ectopic beats 496
atrial fibrillation (AF) 494, 497–505
  chronic, exercise training 655
  clinical features 499
  consequences 498–9
  definition and classification 497, **498**
  dementia prevention in by warfarin 488
  epidemiology 449, 480, *480*, 497, 605–6
  etiology 497–8
  heart failure associated 573
  history and examination 499–500
  hyperthyroidism and 489
  investigations 500, **500**
  lone 498
  management 500–5, 605–6, 607
    aims 500
    anticoagulation 450, 451, 500, 505–7, 534, 605
    first detected episode 500
    new procedures 505, 535, 606
    pacing 502, 504–5
    thromboembolism prevention 500
    see also rate control, rhythm control (below)
  mortality 498
  nonvalvular 497–8
    intracranial bleeding with warfarin 450–1
    management 452
    prevalence and stroke risk 449
    stroke recurrence risk 831, *832*
  paroxysmal (PAF) 497, 500, 501
  permanent 497, 500
  persistent 497, 500
  rate control 500, 501–2
    nonpharmacological therapy 502
    pharmacological therapy 501–2
    vs rhythm control 500, **501**
  as respiratory disease complication 489
  rhythm control 500, 503–5
    DC cardioversion 503, 587
    nonpharmacological 504–5, 605–6
    pharmacological cardioversion 503–4
  secondary stroke risk 831–2, *832*
  stroke, ischemic 823
  stroke prevention 451, 452, 482
  as stroke risk factor 449, 451, 499, 801
  valvular 497, 533
atrial flutter 496, *497*
atrial natriuretic peptide (ANP) 499, 543
  brain water content regulation 1371
  heart failure 558, 657
  thirst regulation 323
atrial pacing 504–5, 576
atrial remodeling 498–9
atrial septal aneurysm (ASA) 837
atrial tachyarrhythmias 496–7
atrial tachycardia 496
atriopeptin 323

atrioventricular (AV) block 494–6
2:1 pattern 495, 496
first-degree 494–5
second-degree 495, 496
advanced 495, *495*
third-degree (complete) 495, 880–1
atrophic gastritis 285
atropine, salivary dribbling in MND 960
atypical antipsychotics *see* antipsychotics, atypical
atypical mycobacterial infection 710
audiometric testing 1228
AUDIT 163
audit *see* clinical audit
auditory brainstem response (ABR) 1227
auditory system 1219–33
auditory testing 205–6
aura, migraine 753, **753**
aural tumors 1241
Australia 1892–3
Community Rehabilitation Centres 1907
demographics 1890
home care 1895–6
hospital care 1901, **1901**
medical education/training 1902–3
memory clinics 1062
nursing home care 1897–8
quality of care 1839
siderail use 1691
Australian Association of Gerontology 1903
Australian Council for Health Care Standards (ACHS) 1839
Australian Society for Geriatric Medicine (ASGM) 1842, 1903
Australian Therapeutic Trial in Hypertension 547
Austria, medical education/training 1784, 1785
autoantibodies 32
increased with age 23, *23*, 31
peripheral neuropathy 891, **891**
autoimmune disease
endocrine 1391
fibrosing alveolitis 717–8
hearing loss 1228
autoimmune hemolysis 431, **432**
autoimmune hepatitis 384
diagnosis and treatment **384**, 386
autoimmune phenomena, age related 31–2, *31*
autoimmunity, in MND 959
autolytic debridement 1621
automated peritoneal dialysis (APD) 1501
"automatic processing" concept 1038, 1041
autonomic dysfunction
age related 41
diabetic neuropathy 892, 1315
Parkinson's disease 775
autonomic nervous system
abnormalities 969–80, **971**
cardiovascular *see* cardiovascular autonomic control
gastrointestinal function 978
pupillary abnormalities 972
temperature control *see* temperature control
urogenital function 978
neurobiology of aging 969–71
enteric system 971
neurotransmission 969–70, *970*
parasympathetic system 970
sympathetic modulation 970
sympathetic nerve activity 969–70, *970*
primary failure 971–2
secondary failure 972
autonomy 1653, 2002
autonomy (ethical) principle 1681–2, 1684, 1685, 1686
risk taking 232
autosomal dominant polycystic kidney disease (ADPKD) 1015
avascular necrosis, hip 1337, *1338*
AVID (Antiarrhythmics Versus Implantable Defibrillators) 510, 523
axial flaps, pressure ulcers 1624
axillary moisture assessment 324, 1637
axis (C1), anatomy 991
axodendritic expanse 62–3
azacitidine (5-axaciticine; 5-aza) 459, 469
azathioprine
bullous pemphigoid 1599
cryptogenic fibrosing alveolitis 717
dermatomyositis 938
Lambert Eaton myasthenic syndrome 906
mucous membrane pemphigoid 267
myasthenia gravis 904–5
rheumatoid arthritis 1351
azoles 1592, 1593

B cells
age related changes 20, 26, **40**
qualitative 26
quantitative **24**, 26
signal transduction 30
stem cell differentiation decline 23
transfusion 31
BAATAF (Boston Area Anticoagulation Trial for Atrial Fibrillation) 451
"Baby Boom" effect 59, *60*
baby monitors 1694
BAC (Brain Attack Coalition) 1900
Bacillus Calmette–Guérin (BCG) vaccine 690, 1741
back pain 1355–65
acute 1356
causes 1358–60
chronic 1356
chronic ambulatory peritoneal dialysis 1501
clinical evaluation 1356–64
red flags 1356
definitions 1355–6
differential diagnosis 1358, **1359**
episodes 1356
first onset 1356
flare-up 1356
health-care costs 1355
nonpharmacological intervention 1361–2
non-radiological investigations 1357–8
nonspecific lower back 1360
pharmacological interventions 1362–3
radiological investigations 1358
recurrent 1356
trigger points 1357
back schools 1362
baclofen 274, 960
bacteremia 1623, 1728, 1754
bacterial infections
acute exacerbation of COPD 700
brain abscess *see* brain, abscess
otitis media 1223
peripheral vestibular system 1240
see also specific bacterial infections
bacterial meningitis *see* meningitis, bacterial
bacterial overgrowth, small intestine 365
bacteriuria 1499, 1727
Bacteroides fragilis 1623, 1771
bad news, breaking 955, 1067
balance 1299–300
aging effect 745, 747–8
assessment 1305–6
disorders, screening 206
maintenance *1236*
peripheral sensation 1300
balance training 123, 129, **137**
Balanced Budget Act, USA (1997) 1820
balloon expulsion testing 410
balloon retention barium enema catheter 1717
balloon tamponade, variceal hemorrhage 377
balloon valvotomy, aortic valve 602
balloon valvuloplasty (percutaneous) 602
Baltimore Epidemiological Project (1996) 1435
Baltimore Longitudinal Study of Aging (BLSA) 281, 1926, 1939
Baltimore-Washington Cooperative Young Stroke Study 797
barbiturates 161, 1193
barium enema 1716–7
barium follow-through 1716
barium meal 1716
barium studies 1716–7
barium swallow 360, *360*, 1716
barium videofluoroscopy, dysphagia 359–60
baroreceptor(s)
peripheral 322
sensitivity 39, 543
in heart failure 555–6, 571
baroreceptor reflex (baroreflex)
aging effect 969–70, 975
analysis 974–5
dysfunction 39, 543
head-up tilt response 973
Barthel Index 227, **1575**, 1910, 1911
Bartonella, infective endocarditis **1752**, 1760
basal cell carcinoma (BCC) 1601, *1601*
basal ganglia
anatomy 770
infarcts 686, 688
Parkinson's disease 765, 770, *770*
bath water controls 192–3, *193*
bathing dependence 1141, 1144
Bazex syndrome **1603**
Beck Anxiety Inventory (BAI) 1150
Becker muscular dystrophy 943
bed rails *see* siderails
bed rest
back pain 1361
hip fractures 1333
bed sore *see* pressure ulcers/ulceration
bed-bound patients, pressure ulcers 1609
bed-occupancy sensors 191, *191*, 194, *194*
bed-occupancy systems, monitoring 193–4
bedside lamps, automatic 191, *191*
bedside swallow assessment 820
Beer Criteria 219
beer potomania 1373, 1377
behavior
aggressive *see* aggressive behavior
maladaptive (psychological) 54, *57*
Behavior and Mood Disturbance Scale 1813
Behavioral and Social Research Program, USA 1926
behavioral disorders/problems
Alzheimer's disease 1084, 1087
dementia *see* dementia, behavioral disorders
in Down's syndrome 1188
in long term care patients 1155
behavioral techniques
back pain 1362
heart disease prevention 649
smoking cessation 154
Behçet's disease 266
"behind the ear" (BTE) hearing aids 1231, *1231*
Belgium, medical education/training 1785
Bell's phenomenon, aging 745
beneficence (ethical) principle 1685, 1686, 2002
benign monoclonal gammopathies 896
benign paroxysmal positional vertigo (BPPV) 1238, 1241–2, *1241*, 1303
positional maneuvers 1246
benign prostatic hyperplasia (BPH) 1464–5, 1469–74, *1470*, 1499
comorbid conditions **1471**
dementia 1470
laboratory evaluation 1470–1
natural history 1469–70
overflow incontinence 1487
patient evaluation 1470, **1470**, **1471**
prevalence 1469
symptoms 1464, **1471**
treatment 1471–4, **1472**
combination therapy 1472
invasive surgery 1473–4
medical therapy 1464–5, 1472, **1472**
minimally invasive therapy 1465, 1473
testosterone replacement 1424
watchful waiting 1471–2
benoxaprofen, hepatotoxicity 385
benzhexol 960
benzodiazepines
alcohol interaction 161, 164
anxiety 1143, 1154
back pain 1363
biochemical testing 1195
delirium etiology 1051

benzodiazepines (*cont.*)
in dementia 1143, 1145
dependence 1193
fall-induction 1696
insomnia **739**, 1145
intoxication symptoms **1195**
migraine 754
misuse 1153, 1193
treatment guidelines 1197
motor neuron disease 960, 964
psychiatric comorbidity 1154, 1192
REM-sleep behavior disorder 738
restless legs syndrome 781
status epilepticus 876
withdrawal 1193, **1195**
bereavement 1150, 2013
complicated 1150
depression 1173, **1174**
Bernard–Soulier syndrome 439
β-adrenoreceptors 703
aging related reduction in heart 487, 530, 568
autoantibodies 556
β1-, β2- and β3- types 556
chronic activation, adverse effects 556, **556**
downregulation 543, 556
signaling pathways *556*, 556–557
β-agonists
β_2-agonists, in COPD 698
motor neuron disease 961
β-blockers (β-adrenoreceptor blockers)
acute coronary syndromes 520
atrial fibrillation 501–2
cardiac cachexia 642
contraindications 575
essential tremor 784
fasciculation in MND 960
glaucoma 1208
heart disease prevention 482
heart failure therapy 557, 574–5, 576
hypertension therapy 518, 548, 551
hyperthyroidism 1409
noncardiac surgical patients 1634
perioperative 1649
peripheral vascular disease 627
post-myocardial infarction 522, **522**, 523, 587
stable angina therapy 519
ST-elevated myocardial infarction 521
valvular heart disease 534
ventricular arrhythmias 508
betel quid, oral cancer etiology 269
Better Health in Old Age 1894
bevacizumab (Avastin) 1515
Beveridge, Sir William 1916
bidirectional nystagmus 1239
bile, age related changes 381
bile duct
obstruction, intervention 1720
stone removal 419
bile salts 292
bile-acid sequestrants, atherosclerosis 620
biliary electroshock, gallstones 389
biliary tract 381
diseases 388–90
biochemical testing
dementia predictor in MCI 1097–8
drug misuse 1195
bioelectrical impedance analysis (BIA)
muscle mass estimation 910, **911**
obesity assessment 347
biofeedback therapy 400–3, **401–2**, 1489
biofilm, dental *see* dental plaque
"biologic clock" 1589
biological age, chronological age *vs* 476
Biondi rings 78, *78*
biopsy
bone marrow 456
liver 386
lung, fibrotic disease 715
muscle *see* muscle biopsy
needle 1720
olfactory system 1254
renal, nephrotic syndrome 1502
salivary glands 272
skin, bullous pemphigoid 1599
transrectal ultrasound guided 1475
bipolar affective disorder 1150–1
misdiagnosis 1156
see also depression
bisoprolol, heart failure 574–5
bisphosphonates 136
absorption 1341
hip fracture prevention 1341
hypercalcemia of malignancy 1523
mechanism of action 1275, 1294–5
osteoporosis 1283, 1294–5, 1663
Paget's disease 1275–6
potency 1275
secondary resistance 1276
side effects 1275, 1283
bitemporal hemianopsia 1398
bite-raising appliances 246, *246*
Bitot's spots 332
black cohosh (*Cimicifuga racemosa*) 1419–20
black hairy tongue 265
blackout 879, 882
see also syncope
bladder
adrenergic receptors 1472, 1480
age related changes 1459–67
anatomy 1459–60, **1460**
capacity 1450
disease states 1461–2
female 1449–50, 1459
histology 1459, 1460–1
male 1459–60
pharmacology 1462
physiology 1460–1
receptors 1462, **1462**
surgical diseases 1460, 1463–5
base/neck/body 1460
compliance 1460
disinhibition in dementia 1462
external sphincter 1460
function 1460
overactive 1486–7, **1488**
management 1489, 1490
see also urge incontinence
wall blood flow 1460
bladder neck slings 1464, 1491
"bladder pacemaker" 1490
"blade of grass" lesion, Paget's disease 1270
blast cells, acute myeloid leukemia 465
bleeding
DIC 445, 446, *446*
disseminated intravascular coagulation 447
in myelodysplasia 458
postmenopausal 1451–2, **1451**, 1661
risk with anticoagulants *see* anticoagulants/anticoagulation
see also hemorrhage
blepharospasm 782
blindness
age related macular degeneration 1206
glaucoma 1207
monocular, subarachnoid hemorrhage 1017
smoking and 153
see also visual impairment
blood film 1525, 1526
blood gases 694
acute exacerbation of COPD 702
asthma 705
fibrotic lung disease 715
blood pressure
age related changes 542, *542*
ambulatory monitoring 545
diabetes mellitus 1437–9
elevated *see* hypertension
heart disease risk 476–7, 517–8
hypertension definition 541
hypertension therapy success marker 546
ischemic stroke, management 819
JNC recommendations 541
low *see* hypotension
management, subarachnoid hemorrhage 1023
measurement 203, 545
normal 541
postprandial 546
regulation 542, 1437–9
secondary stroke risk 832, *833*
sudden fall in, syncope 879–80, 882–3
variability, autonomic control 974–5, *975*
in very old, mortality inverse relation 549–50
blood products, DIC therapy 447
blood transfusions
acute myeloblastic leukemia 467
anemia 433
DIC 447
myelodysplasia 458, 469
blood urea nitrogen (BUN) 217–8, 324
blood vessels
aging effects 39–40, 76–8, *77*, 542
calcification 489
remodeling 612–3
shear stress, atherosclerosis 617
in skin, age related changes 1590–1
structure 611, *612*
Blue Cross, USA 1924
Blue-Ribbon Committee on Aging, Japan 1937
Bobath method, stroke rehabilitation 855
body, transcendence *vs* preoccupation 54
body charts, pain mapping *2004*
body composition
age related changes **125**, 280–1, 347, 912, **912**
disability risk factor 136
information need 282
optimization 125–30, **126**
testosterone replacement therapy 1423
body fat *see* fat (body)
body mass index (BMI)
aging 281
functional limitation/disability 920
heart disease risk *478*
limitations 1638–9
mortality 309
obesity assessment 347
stroke risk indicator 802
body sway 1300
body temperature 738
see also temperature control
body weight *see* weight
bone
alcohol abuse effect 160
biopsy, Paget's disease 1273
bowing, Paget's disease 1270
calcium metabolism 1261, 1262, 1264–5
conduction of sound 1220
deformity, Paget's disease 1270
formation markers 1273–4
fragility, osteoporotic fracture 1287–8
health, role of physical activity 126–7
see also exercise
loss *see* bone loss
macro-/microarchitecture, fractures 1287
mass, peak 1281
mechanical strength 1287
mineral density *see* bone mineral density (BMD)
osteoporotic fractures 1287
pain
Paget's disease 1270–1, 1277
palliative care 2007
remodeling 42
biochemical markers 1287–8, **1288**
osteoporotic fracture 1287–8
resorption 1270, 1274
scintigraphy
back pain 1358
osteomyelitis 1623, *1623*
Paget's disease 1271–3, *1272*
smokers 152
testosterone replacement therapy 1423
trabecular 1281, 1287
tumors, Paget's disease 1271
bone anchoring hearing aids 1232
bone conducting hearing aids 1230, 1232
bone densitometry 208, 1663
bone loss 1281
age related 42, 126, 283, 1265, **1265**
calcium metabolism 1262, 1264–5
hormonal causes 1289

mechanical causes 1291
"normal" aging *vs* age related disease 14–5
nutritional causes 283, 1289–91
postmenopausal women 152, 1264–5
toxic causes 1291–2
see also bone mineral density (BMD); osteoporosis
bone marrow
aspiration/biopsy, myelodysplasia 456
dysplasia 456
failure 1526
aplastic anemia 431–2
causes 428, **428**, 430
immune system aging 22
proliferative activity and apoptosis 22, 23, *23*
bone marrow transplantation 31, 468
see also stem cell transplantation
bone mineral density (BMD)
assessment 1282–3, 1286–7, 1341–2
exercise intervention trial 127, **128**
exercise modalities affecting 127
growth hormone therapy 1674
physical activity effect 126
postmenopausal women 1418
smokers 152
testosterone replacement 120, 1423, 1675
vitamin D supplements 337
bone-specific alkaline phosphatase 1273
Borg's scale 654
boron **341**, 1291
Borrelia burgdorferi 1769
bortezomib (velcade) 1515
"bottom half" parkinsonism 767
botulinum toxin 360–1, 783, 856, 960
bovine spongioform encephalopathy (BSE) 1125
bowel obstruction 1527, 2008
"boxcar" pattern 1525
BPH impact score **1471**
brachytherapy 1478, 1513
bradycardia 494–6, 501
after myocardial infarction 587
causes **494**
heart failure associated 573
bradykinesia 766, 1087
brain
abscess 758, 1771–3
therapy 1772–3, **1772**, **1773**
adaptation, hypernatremia 1380
aging of 41, 47–51, 59–67
approaches to therapy 65–6
cognitive function 48–9
external appearance 69
membrane structural markers 62–3
motor systems 47–8
palliative therapy 65–6
protein synthesis 63
alcoholic damage 159
atrophy 744–5, 1073
damage, in dysphasia 843
disease, cardiac features 488
free radical damage 63–4
hemorrhage 817, *817*
hyponatremia 1370–1
imaging *see* neuroimaging
infarction *see* cerebral infarction
injury, excitotoxic hypothesis 63
osmolality regulation 1370–2
posttraumatic subdural hematoma 1027
size:skull capacity ratio 1371
tissue loss, aging 60
tumor, headache 758
weight, aging 69
see also entries beginning cerebral
Brain Attack Coalition (BAC) 1900
Brain Bank Criteria, Parkinson's disease 765, 766, **766**
brain natriuretic peptide (BNP) 543, 558, *569*
cardiac disease/failure 569, 1911
"brain plasticity" 850
brain stem
ischemia, drop attacks 1303
neurons, Parkinson's disease 769
tumors, vestibular dysfunction 1244
brain-derived neurotrophic factor (BNDF) 131, 958
Brazil, demographics and service provision 1994, **1994**
breaking bad news 955, 1067
breakthrough pain 2006–7
breast cancer 1531–40, 1659–60
clinical features 1660
common types 1531
comorbidity 1531–2, 1537
emergencies 1520
estrogen deprivation 1513–4
HRT 1450–1
metastagenicity 1533
natural history 1533
presentation 1531
prognosis 1510–1, **1510**, 1660
prognostic factors 1536–7
quality of life 1532, 1537
risk factors 1485, 1533
screening 207, 1532–3, **1532**, 1659–60
sexual activity modification 115
staging 1531, **1532**
treatment/intervention 1532–3, **1533**
adjuvant endocrine 1535–6
advanced disease 1536
chemotherapy 1536
guidelines 1538–9
operable disease 1533–4
radiotherapy 1534–5
undertreatment justification 1531–2
variations in care 1537–8
vitamin A 333
breast-conserving therapy (BCT) 1534
breath holding 1715, 1719
breath tests, small intestine motility 365
breathing
pursed-lip 728
retraining 728
shallow, rapid during sleep 737
temporary cessation in sleep *see* sleep apnea
breathlessness *see* dyspnea (breathlessness)
breathlessness clinics 2009
Breslow depth 1602
Brief Pain Inventory 984
Bristol Activities of Daily Living Scale, dementia 1129
British Association of Psychopharmacology (BAP), drug misuse guidelines 1195, 1197
British Geriatrics Society (BGS) 1169, 1842, 1919
Education and Training Committee 1792
history 4, 5, 1891
recommendations 1890
British Health Checks model 201, 209–10, **209**
British Household Panel Survey 1811
British Medical Association (BMA) 3
British Ministry of Health 3
British Thoracic Society (BTS) 697, 709
British Tinnitus Association 1230
British United Provident Association (BUPA) 1916
Broca's aphasia 843
bronchial hemorrhage, pulmonary neoplasm 1521
bronchial irritability syndrome 703
bronchial stenting 1720
bronchiectasis 708
bronchitis
chronic *see* chronic obstructive pulmonary disease (COPD)
winter 697
bronchoalveolar lavage 715
bronchodilators
asthma 704
COPD 698, 701
bronchogenic carcinoma 710, 717, 1521
bronchoscopy 709, 711
bronchospasm, treatment 2009
bronzing, skin 1591, **1592**
The Brookdale Foundation 1926–7
Brooke, Eric 4
brown bowel syndrome 333
Brown–Sequard syndrome 993
Brucella, infective endocarditis **1752**, 1759
Bruegel's syndrome (Meige syndrome) 782
bruising, chronic DIC 447
bruxism 244–5
B-type natriuretic peptide *see* brain natriuretic peptide (BNP)
budgerigar fancier's lung 716–7
bulbar palsy 949
bulbar-onset motor neuron disease 951, 952, 954, 955
bulking agents, constipation 411
bullae, mucous membrane pemphigoid 267
bullous lesions, oral 266–8
bullous pemphigoid 1599, *1599*
bullous scabies 1595
bundle branch block 493, 507, **508**, 576
Bundle of His 494
Bunina bodies 956
BUPA (British United Provident Association) 1916
bupivacaine hydrochloride, pathological fractures 2007
buprenorphine 1195, 1197
bupropion 154, 697, 1139, 1178
contraindications 154
Burden Interview 1813
burning mouth sensation 271, 274–5, 1256
burns, immersion 184
bursae, foot 1323
bursitis, foot 1325
buscopan, barium meal 1716
buspirone, anxiety in dementia 1143

C terminal of atrial natriuretic peptide (CNP) 558
Ca 125, ovarian cancer 1456
CA1 region, aging 70, 72, *72*
cabergoline, restless legs syndrome 781
cachexia 314, 909
cancer 918
cardiac *see* cardiac cachexia
cacosmia 1249
Caenorhabditis elegans 16–7
caffeine, osteoporosis 1282
CAGE questions 162, **163**, 1150, **1150**, 1153
α-calcidol, hip fracture prevention 1341
calciferol *see* vitamin D
calcification, vascular 489
calci-mimetic drugs 1500
calcipotriene, psoriasis 1597
calcitonin gene related peptide (CGRP) 976, *976*
calcitonin therapy 997, 1276, 1283, 1523
calcitriol, hip fracture prevention 1341
calcium
dietary 1265–6
excitation–contraction coupling, heart 562–3, *562*
homeostasis/balance
aging 42, **42**, 970, 1261–7, **1262**, **1263**
normal 1261, **1262**
influx, pre-/post-synaptic 41
infusions, hyperkalemia 1383
intake, osteoporosis 1289
malabsorption 294
metabolism 1261
age related changes 1262–3, **1262**
bone loss 1264–5
primary *vs* secondary 1264
regulation 1261–2, *1262*, 1263–4, **1263**
motor neuron disease 958
osteoporosis 1662
renal tubular dysfunction 1497–8
resorption from bone 42
resting levels in heart failure 562–3
supplements 42, 1265–6, 1275
hip fracture prevention 1266, 1341
osteoporosis 283, 1283, 1293, 1294
calcium acetate, chronic renal failure 1500
calcium channel, L-type 562, 563
calcium channel antagonists (calcium blockers)
acute coronary syndromes 520, 521
chronic renal failure 1500
dihydropyridine, valvular heart disease 534
drug induced parkinsonism 768
heart failure 576
hypertension 551
nondihydropyridine, atrial fibrillation 502
post-myocardial infarction 522
ST elevated myocardial infarction 521

calcium channel antagonists (calcium blockers) (*cont.*)
  stable angina therapy 519
  subarachnoid hemorrhage 1023
calcium oxalate nephrolithiasis 335
calcium pyrophosphate deposit(s) 996
calcium pyrophosphate deposition disease (CPDD) 1349, 1352
calcium-regulating hormones 1263, **1263**
calculus 240
Caldicott guardian 1833
calisthenics, cardiac rehabilitation 654
call bells 1694
Callahan, Daniel 1683
caloric restriction **1667**, 1669
  antiaging therapy 1669
  immune function restoration 32
  obesity management 351
  programmed cell death 93
  prolonged 1669
  sarcopenia 925
Cambridge Heart Antioxidant Study 1671
Cambridge Mental Disorder of the Elderly Examination (CAMDEX) 1065
Campylobacter jejuni infection 895
Canada, life expectancy **88**
Canadian Amiodarone Myocardial Infarction Arrhythmia Trial 523
Canadian Consensus Conference on the Assessment of Dementia (CCCAD) 1129, **1129**
Canadian Implantable Defibrillator Study (CIDS) 510
Canadian Study of Health and Aging 476
Canadian Trial of Physiologic Pacing (CTOPP) 495, **496**
canalith repositioning maneuver 1246
canalithiasis 1241–2, *1241*
cancer 1509–17
  alcohol abuse and 160
  biological interaction 1509–11
  carers' support 1813
  cerebrovascular complications 1526–7
  in Down's syndrome 1188
  emergency medical services 1529
  epidemiology 1509, *1510*
  exercise effects **133**, **134**
  female 1659–60
  morbidity, India 1985
  mortality rates **170**, **173**, *179*
  oral side effects of drugs 255
  prevention *see* cancer prevention
  screening 1512
  thyroid nodules 1409–10
  treatment 1512–5
  see also malignant disease; *specific cancers (e.g. breast cancer)*
cancer anorexia-cachexia syndrome 314
cancer cachexia 918
cancer care, clinical audit 1833
cancer prevention 1511–2
  chemoprevention 1511–2, *1511*
  primary 1511–2
  secondary 1512
  selenium 335
  vitamin A supplements 333, 1672
  vitamin C supplements 1673
  vitamin E supplements 334, 1671
Cancer Prevention Study I and II 310, **311**
Cancer Research UK Breast Cancer Trial Group 1534
Candida infection
  meningitis 1770–1
  onychomycosis 1593
candidal leukoplakia 264, 268
candidosis
  acute atrophic (antibiotic sore mouth) 264
  acute pseudomembranous 263, *264*
  chronic atrophic (denture stomatitis) 263–4, *264*
  chronic hyperplastic 264, 268
  oral 263–4, **263**
    management 264
    terminally ill patients 256, 2010
cannabinoids, appetite stimulation 315
cannabis, misuse
  biochemical testing 1195
  epidemiology 1192, *1192*
  intoxication/withdrawal symptoms **1195**
  physical comorbidity 1193
capacity, ethical issues 1685
capecitabine, mucositis 1514
Capgras syndrome 1140
Caplan's syndrome 716
CAPRIE Study 626, 830–1, *831*
capsaicin 687, *762*, 763
captopril, hypertension 548
carbamazepine
  epilepsy 874, **874**
  manic episodes, dementia and 1139
  peripheral neuropathy in herpes zoster 895
  trigeminal neuralgia 274, 987
carbidopa-levodopa 737
carbocisteine 698
carbohydrates, absorption 42, 291–2
carbon dioxide, production (VCO_2), measurement 652
^{13}C isotope breath tests 364
carbon monoxide monitors 155, *155*
carboplatin, ovarian cancer 1456
carcinogenesis, aging 1510
carcinogens 1510
carcinoid tumors, lung 713
carcinomatous encephalomyelitis 1241
carcinomatous meningitis 1241
carcinomatous neuromyopathy 943
carcinomatous sensory neuronopathy 896
cardiac aging 39–40, **40**, 487–8, 487–91, *488*, 493, 542, 567–8
  diastolic/systolic function **40**
  myocardial cellular changes 529–30
cardiac amyloidosis 487–8
Cardiac Arrhythmia Suppression Trial (CAST) 504, 522–3
cardiac arrhythmias 493–513
  anticoagulation for 500, 505–7
  atrial fibrillation *see* atrial fibrillation (AF)
  atrial flutter 496, *497*
  atrial tachyarrhythmias 496–7
  atrial tachycardia 496
  AV block *see* atrioventricular (AV) block
  bradycardia 494–6
  cognitive decline associated 488
  confirmation and investigations 499–500
  electrocardiogram 872
  epidemiology 480, *480*
  escape rhythms 495
  hemodialysis 1500
  inappropriate medication use **220**
  post-myocardial infarction 508, 587
  preoperative detection 1648
  seizures 870
  ventricular *see* ventricular arrhythmia
  vitamin C toxicity 335
cardiac assessments, noncardiac surgery 1633–5
cardiac cachexia 490, 572, 639–45
  adipose tissue loss 642
  body composition changes 640
  "clinical" 639
  clinical implications 642–3
  definition 639
  epidemiology 639–40
  exercise 642
  immune abnormalities 640–1
  medication 642–3
  nutritional support 642
  prognosis 639–40
cardiac catheterization, in cardiogenic shock 586
cardiac disease *see* heart disease
cardiac emergencies, management 585–92
cardiac failure *see* heart failure
cardiac medications, adverse effects 385, 1050
cardiac muscle
  thyroid hormone responsiveness 1407
  see also myocardium
cardiac myocytes
  length increase in LV hypertrophy 561
  loss in heart failure 560, 561, 562
  regeneration 562
cardiac output 494, 576
  aging effect 487, 542
  reduced after myocardial infarction 585, 586, 587
cardiac pacing
  ablate and pace strategy 502
  atrial pacing 504–5, 576
  complications 495–6
  indications
    atrial fibrillation 502, 504–5
    AV block 495–6
    heart failure 576
    sick sinus syndrome 494
  permanent 502, 509
  physiological dual chamber (DDD/R) 495, **496**
  ventricular (VVI/R) 495, **496**
cardiac pain, impaired perception 488
cardiac rehabilitation 647–62
  benefits 649
  benefits of aerobic training 656–7
  comprehensive 657
  definition and aims 648–50, **648**
  delivery 648
  economic evaluation 658–9
  evidence-based results 652, 657–8
    cardiac surgery 657–8
    chronic heart failure 658
    coronary heart disease 657
  indications 648
  phases 650–1, **1578**
  program structure 650–5
    baseline assessment 651–2, **651**, 655
    exercise training *see* exercise training
  psychological aspects 1573
  secondary prevention strategies included 649–50
  utilization (international) 647–8
cardiac reserve
  aging effect 487, 488, 567
  assessment 652
cardiac resynchronization therapy (CRT) 576–7
cardiac sounds, physiological tinnitus 1228
cardiac surgery 585–92, 593–610
  age of patients 594
  anticoagulation management 603, 604–5
  assessment 596–8, **597**
  atrial fibrillation *see* atrial fibrillation (AF)
  benefits 597–8
  cardiac rehabilitation results 655, 657–8
  coronary bypass *see* coronary artery bypass grafting (CABG)
  costs and private *vs* socialized health-care 593
  exercise training after 655
  myocardial infarction complications 585–6
  open-heart surgery 593
  outcome 594–6, 1633
    cognitive dysfunction 489
    complications *595*
    morbidity 595–6, *595*
    mortality 593–4, 594–5, *594*
    neurological dysfunction 595–6
    renal dysfunction 596
  pre-/post-operative risk factors 595
  suboptimal timing, risks 598
  thoracic aorta 606–7
  transplantation 607
  valve surgery 600–3
    age trends 594, *594*
    aortic *see* aortic valve
    bioprosthesis *vs* mechanical 587, 589
    CABG with 594, 600, *601*, 604
    mitral *see* mitral valve
    prosthetic valve choice 600–7
    robotic surgery 536
    thromboembolism risk 603, *603*, 604
    warfarin use 603, **603**
    see also valvuloplasty
cardiac syncope 882
  clinical features and diagnosis 881, 882
  falls 1303
  management 883
  mechanism 880–1
cardiac tamponade, malignant 1524
cardiac transplantation 607, 608

Cardiff lifestyle improvement profile for people in extended residential care (CLIPPER) 1045
cardinal ligament, aging 1449
cardiogenic shock, management 586
cardiomyocytes, loss 530
cardiomyopathy
  dilated 509–10, 1674–5
  drug induced 1514–5
cardioprotective effects, of alcohol 157, 160
cardiopulmonary bypass, functional platelet defects 439
cardiopulmonary exercise test 652, 655
cardiopulmonary resuscitation (CPR) 1686
cardiorespiratory function, aging **124**
cardiovascular autonomic control 972–5
  blood pressure variability 974–5, *975*
  heart-rate variability 974–5, *975*
cardiovascular disease (CVD)
  β-carotene 1672
  delirium etiology 1052
  in Down's syndrome 1188
  heat strain effect 977
  hormone replacement therapy 1421
  HRT and 1451
  as leading cause of death 593
  mortality rates **170**, **172**, *177*, *178*
  pressure ulcer risk 1609
  selenium 335
  sexual activity 120
  stroke risk 801
  testosterone replacement therapy 1676
  vascular dementia 1104
  see also heart disease
Cardiovascular Health Study (CHS) 481, 517, 519
  body weight and mortality 310, **310**
  obesity and mortality 310, **311**
  peripheral vascular disease 624
  respiratory muscle strength 674
  weight loss and mortality 298, 311–2
cardiovascular risk assessment 1439, **1439**
cardiovascular system
  age related changes 39–40, 567–8, **568**, 1648
    see also cardiac aging
  alcohol manifestations 160
  in diabetic neuropathy 892
  immobility effects **1690**
  morbidity, postoperative 1648–9, **1648**
  restraints, effects **1690**
  signs of dehydration 324
  subclinical hyperthyroidism effects 1409
cardioversion, DC 503, 508, 587
care homes *see* nursing home care
Care Homes Support Teams, UK 1868–9, 1875
The Care of the Aged, the Dying, and the Dead 2
care planning, resident assessment *see* Minimum Data Set (MDS)
Care Programme Approach (CPA), NSF (UK) 1164
care resistiveness, dementia and 1143–4
caregiver(s) (carers) 1809–16
  burden on 1043, 1088
  delusions/hallucination care in dementia 1140
  demographics 1810–1
  dental health training programs 257–8
  depression risk 1156
  Down's syndrome 1185, 1186
  hearing impairment effects 1212
  involvement in activities 1044, **1044**
  Japan 1942–3
  legal frameworks 1810
  physical health 1812
  psychiatric care role 1156
  psychological health 1164–5, 1811–2
  respite services 1164–6, 1812–4, 1896
  role 852
  stamina, Alzheimer's disease 1089
caregiver support groups, Down's syndrome 1186
Carers (Equal Opportunities) Act, UK (2004) 1810
Carers (Recognition and Services) Act, UK (1995) 1164, 1810
Carers' Assessment of Difficulties Index (CADI) 1813
Carers' Assessment of Managing Index (CAMI) 1813
Carers' Assessment of Satisfactions Index (CASI) 1813
Carers of Older People in Europe (COPE) 1813
Caring for Older People: a Nursing Priority 1870
carisoprodol, back pain 1363
carnitine palmitoyl transferase-1 (CPT-1) 563
β-carotene 332–3, 1672
β-carotene and Retinol Efficacy Trial (CARET) 333, 1672
carotenoids 332, 1672
carotid angioplasty 837
carotid artery disease, cardiac surgery and 595, **595**
carotid artery hemorrhage, tumor erosion 1528
carotid artery stenosis 805–14
  atheroma 805–6, *806*
  causes 805–6
  endovascular intervention 811–2, *811*
  investigation 807–8, 836
  management 808–12
  presentation 806
  stroke prevention 808
  as stroke risk factor 801
  surgery
    asymptomatic patients 810–1
    endovascular treatment *vs* 811–2, *812*, **812**
    stroke risk 809, *809*, 810, *810*
    symptomatic patients 808–10
carotid bruits 807
carotid dissection 806
carotid Doppler ultrasound 807, **807**, 823, 836
carotid endarterectomy (CEA) 596
  stroke risk 823, 836, 1640
carotid sinus massage 882, 974
carotid sinus syncope 883
carotid sinus syndrome 882, 974
carpal tunnel syndrome 896–7
carvedilol 557, 574–5, 642
case management, primary care, UK 1803–5
case-mix 1860–1
CASH (Cardiac Arrest Study Hamburg) 510
CASS trial (Coronary Artery Surgery Study) 598
Catalan Hospital Accreditation Programme (CHAP) 1845
cataplexy, in multiple sclerosis 885–6
cataracts 1208–9
  antioxidants 333, 1671, 1672
  cortical 1208, **1209**
  diabetes mellitus 1207
  elective surgery trends *1632*
  formation 39
  risk factors **1209**
  vitamin C supplementation 336
catechol-*O*-methyltransferase (COMT) inhibitors 771–2
"Categorical Imperative" 1681
catheter angiography 807–8, 1018–9
cauda equina compression 996
cauda equina syndrome (CES) 1360
caudate, depression 1176
cavernous angiomas 1020
"caviar tongue" 263
Cawthorne Cooksey exercises 1246
CC5013 (Revimid) 469
CD-28 25, 29
CD-33 466, 467
CD-34 466
CD-56 466
CD-95 25
cecal dilatation 1527
cecal perforation 1527
cefixime, gonorrhea 1732
ceftriaxone
  gonorrhea 1732
  infective endocarditis **1758**, 1759
  meningitis 1767, 1770
  neurosyphilis 1770
celecoxib, arthritis 1351
celiac axis block 421
celiac disease 293, 717, 1187
celiac plexus block 2007
cell senescence **1667**, 1668–9
cell-mediated immunity (CMI), tuberculosis 1740
cellulitis 1623, 1727
centenarians 1701–8
  age related disease 1701–2
  dementia 1701, **1702**
  disability compression 1701–2
  "disease genes" 1704
  early life conditions 1703
  genetic findings 1704–5
  "longevity-enabling" genes 1704
  morbidity compression 1701–2
  multifactorial model for exceptional longevity 1705–6, *1705*
  nature *vs* nurture 1702–4
  offspring 1704
  sibling mortality 1703–4, *1703*, **1704**
  survival probability 1703–4
Center for Disease Control (CDC) 800, **801**
Center for Epidemiologic Studies Depression Scale (CES-D) 1173, 1176, 1177, 1938
Center for Medicare and Medicaid Services (CMS) 1560, **1560**, 1856, 1858
center of mass (COM)(center of gravity) 1300
Centers for Ambulatory Care 1908
Centers for Medicare and Medicaid Services (CMS) 1691
central adiposity, health 281–2
Central Government Health Scheme (CGHS), India 1987–8
central nervous system (CNS)
  aging effect 568, **569**
  alcohol–drug interaction effects 161
  dysfunction 686, 781
  infections 1763–80
    see also specific infections
central pontine myelinolysis 1379
Central Services Medical Assistance (CSMA), India 1988
central sleep apnea 737
central white matter, aging 75
cephalosporins, third generation 1766–7, 1774
cerebellar damage, dysarthria 843
cerebellar disease, vestibular dysfunction 1245
cerebellar hematoma 821
cerebellar hemorrhages 1244
cerebellar infarction 820
cerebellar lesions, kinetic tremor 783
cerebellopontine angle lesions 1244
cerebral amyloid angiopathy (CAA) 77–8, *77*
cerebral angiography 1776
cerebral blood flow 787
cerebral compensation 1237
cerebral cortex
  aging **61**, 70
  Alzheimer's disease 1074
  thyroid hormone response 1407
cerebral demyelinating lesions 1378–9, 1380
cerebral edema 820, 1382
cerebral hemisphere, bilateral damage 843
cerebral infarction 817, *817*
  ischemic stroke 815, 818
  silent 688, 1105
cerebral ischemia
  delayed, subarachnoid hemorrhage 1023–4
  global, subarachnoid hemorrhage 1021
  secondary 1022–3
cerebral metabolic rate, aging 64
cerebral tumor 758, 2009–10
cerebral vasculitis 1125–6
cerebrospinal fluid (CSF)
  diversion, shunting 790
  drainage, hydrocephalus 789
  elevated protein level 994
  examination, back pain 1357
  excess in ventricles *see* hydrocephalus
  infusion test 789, 791
  motor neuron disease 955
  outflow resistance 789
  pressure 788
  shunts, bacterial meningitis 1764
  volume changes in aging 69
cerebrovascular accident (CVA)
  bladder problems 1461
  fecal incontinence 398

cerebrovascular accident (CVA) (*cont.*)
  risk after cardiac surgery 595
  see also stroke
cerebrovascular disease (CVD)
  central vestibular system 1243–4
  classification 796–7, **796**, **797**
  dementia and *see* vascular dementia (VaD)
  diagnostic accuracy 797–8
  epilepsy and 869–70
  family history 803
  gait 1301
  genetics 803
  headache and 757
  incidence 799–800, *800*
  mortality data 798–9, *798*, *799*
  prevalence 799–800
  psychotropic medication risk 1157
  risk factors 800–3, **801**
  syncope in 880
  see also stroke; transient ischemic attack (TIA)
Certified Nurse Specialist (CNS) 1940
ceruloplasmin 340
cerumen (wax) 1222
cervical arteries 1001
cervical cancer 1455–6, 1660
  screening 207, 1512, 1660
  treatment 1455–6, 1660
cervical collar 962, 994, 995
cervical cord lesions 678
cervical dystonia (CD) 782
cervical intraepithelial neoplasia 1455
cervical myelopathy 993, 994–5
  gait 1301–2
  spondylotic 1363–4
cervical osteoarthritis 1187, 1347
cervical pain, osteoarthritis 1347
cervical spinal canal stenosis 991–5
cervical spine disorder, headache and 759, **759**
cervical spondylosis 992, 993, 1363–4
  age related 76
  dizziness 1303
  MND diagnosis pitfalls 952
  radiographic, headache 759
cervical spondylotic myelopathy 1363–4
cervical vertigo 1244
cervix, age related changes 1449
cetuximab 1515
CFTR (cystic fibrosis transmembrane conductance regular) gene 419
chair-bound patients, pressure ulcers 1609
chamomile, alcohol interaction 161
Changes in Health, End-stage Disease and Signs and Symptoms (CHESS) scale 1860
Charcot's triad 388–9
CHARISMA trial 831
Charlson Index 1532
CHARM-preserved trial 576
cheilitis
  actinic 263
  angular 264, *264*
chemonucleosis, prolapsed intervertebral disc 1360
chemoradiation, pancreatic cancer 422
chemosensory dysfunction/problems 1249
  evaluation and therapy 1256–7
chemotherapy 1514–5
  acute lymphoid leukemia 469
  acute myeloblastic leukemia 466–7
  appetite loss 300
  breast cancer 1536
  complications 1514
  leukostasis 1525
  in myelodysplasia 461
  myelodysplasia due to 455
  neurotoxicity 1514
  non-small cell lung cancer 711–2
  oral cancer 270
  oral effects 272
  ovarian cancer 1456, 1659
  pleural mesothelioma 712
  small cell lung carcinoma 712
  spinal cord compression 1521
chenodeoxycholic acid, gallstones 389
CHESS scale 1860
chest pain
  ischemic heart disease 515, 521
  noncardiac 362–3
chest physiotherapy, preoperative 1649
chest radiography
  cardiac tamponade 1524
  fibrotic lung disease 715
  heart failure 569
  preoperative 1635
  problems in 1715
  "reversed bat wing" appearance 715
  tuberculosis 1741
chewing, age related changes *242*, 243
Cheyne–Stokes respiration 678
chilblains, broken 1322
Chile, demographics and services 1994, **1994**
China 1953–64, **1960**
  Cooperative Medical System 1956–7
  demographics 1953–5, **1954**, **1955**, **1956**
  medical education/training 1958–9
  nursing home care 1961
  primary care 1961
  service provision, problems 1959–62
Chinese acute stroke study 820
Chinese Journal of Geriatrics 1959
Chlamydia, infective endocarditis **1752**, 1760
Chlamydia pneumoniae 1726
chloramphenicol, neurosyphilis 1770
chlordiazepoxide 161
chlorhexidine mouthwash 249, 262
chlorpromazine, delirium 1056–7
chlorpropamide, alcohol interaction 161
choking 844
cholecystitis 388, 389
  emphysematous 389–90
cholecystokinin (CCK)
  anorexia of aging 303–4, 1567
  chronic pancreatitis 421
  delayed gastric emptying 364–5
  function 303
cholelithiasis *see* gallstones
cholesteatoma 1223, 1240, 1241
cholesterol 613
  de novo synthesis *614*
  excretion 615
  ischemic heart disease risk 477, *477*, 518
  metabolism 613–5, *614*, *615*
  reverse transport 614–5, *614*
  screening 208
  serum, carotid artery stenosis 808
  stroke risk 802, 832–5, *833*, *834*, *835*
  total, target values in diabetes 1439
cholesterol crystals, atherosclerosis 611
cholesterol ester transfer protein (CETP) 478, 614
"cholesterol hypothesis", atherosclerosis 613–6
cholesterol uptake inhibitors 620
cholinergic crises 905
cholinergic neurons, aging 60, **61**
cholinesterase inhibitors 1119, 1137, 1138, 1152
chondrocalcinosis 1349
chondroitin sulfate 1350
chordae tendineae, ruptured 531, 589
chorea 777–80, **778**
  drug induced **784**
  senile 778–9
choroid plexus, aging 78, *78*
chromium 341–2, **341**
chromosomal translocations
  acute myeloblastic leukemia 467
  myelodysplasia 456
chromosomes, 5q deletion 456, 468
chronic ambulatory peritoneal dialysis (CAPD) 1500, 1501
chronic cycling peritoneal dialysis (CCPD) 1501
chronic disease
  demographics 88–95
  developing countries 1969–70
  medication adherence 862
  nutritional status 1985
  pressure ulcers 1609
  risk factors 132
chronic disease management program, USA 1804
Chronic Fatigue Symptoms Index (CFSI) 1943
chronic heart failure *see* heart failure, chronic
chronic inflammatory demyelinating polyneuropathy (CIDP) 895, 953
chronic myelogenous leukemia (CML) 1515
chronic obstructive pulmonary disease (COPD) 675–6, 696–702
  acute exacerbation 700–2
  cardiac manifestations 489
  care standards determination 1830
  epidemiology 696, 727
  frailty 1565
  histochemical analysis 676
  lung function abnormality 694–5, 697
  management 697–9, 727
    drug treatment 697–8
    mechanical ventilation 677
    nonpharmacological 699
  medication underprescribing 1805
  pathology 727
  presentation 696–7
  pressure ulcers 1609
  prevalence 696
  psychological factors 700
  psychosocial support 729
  pulmonary rehabilitation 699, 727–31
  rehabilitation 1579–80, **1579**
  respiratory muscles 675–6
chronic pain 981
  assessment 982–5
    "red flags" 984
  biopsychosocial concept 981
  control 981–90
  management 985–8
  mood disturbances 982
  treatment side effects, tolerance 986
chronic progressive external ophthalmoplegia (CPEO) 945–6, **946**
Chronic Prostatitis Symptoms Index **1481**
chronic renal failure (CRF) *see* renal failure, chronic
chronic subdural hematoma *see* subdural hematoma, chronic
chronic tension-type headache (CTTH) 755
chylomicrons 292, 613
Ciba Foundation 7
ciclopirox, onychomycosis 1325
ciclosporin 905, 1597
ciliary neurotrophic factor (CNTF) 958, 1569
cilostazol 627, 688
cingulate gyrus, spatial disorientation 1143
cinnarizine, vertigo 1245
ciprofloxacin 708, 1224
circadian rhythm disorders 735, 737, 738
circle of Willis 1243
circuit training, cardiac rehabilitation 654
circumvallate papillae 1250
cirrhosis
  alcohol association 159–60
  hepatitis C virus 383
  primary biliary (PBC) 390
citalopram 774, 1178, 1179
clamminess, syncope 881
Classification of Mental and Behavioural Disorders 1114
claw toes, diabetic foot 1314
Client Assessment Protocol (CAP) **1859**
client-centered care *see* person/client-centered care
Clifton Assessment Procedure for the Elderly (CAPE) 227, 1911
Clinical Accountability, Service Planning, and Evaluation (CASPE), Spain 1845
Clinical Antipsychotic Trials of Intervention Effectiveness (CATIE) 1152
clinical audit, perioperative 1655
clinical audit, UK 1827–36, 1848–9
  criteria 232
  definition 1827, 1848
  effectiveness 1828, **1828**
  phases 1828–35, *1829*
    data collection 1832–4, **1832**
    dissemination 1834–5, **1834**
    planning 1829
    standards/criteria determination 1830–2, **1830**

Clinical Dementia Rating (CDR) 146, 1085
clinical governance 1828, 1835, 1899
Clinical Lectures of the Diseases of Old Age 1
clinical psychology services 859–68, 1169, 1577
  CBT *see* cognitive behavioral therapy (CBT)
  ethical issues 866
  theoretical framework 860–2
  see also specific countries
clinical trials, study design 1292
clinicians, epidemiological data use 795
clobazam, epilepsy 875, 876
clobetasol, scabies 1595
clock face drawing 1065
clodronate, osteoporosis 1294
clonazepam 738, 781, 875, 1777
clonidine
  fecal incontinence 399
  hot flashes 1416
  medication overuse headache 756
  side effects 366
  withdrawal management 1195, 1197
clopidogrel
  acute coronary syndrome 520
  after myocardial infarction 521
  aspirin and 831
  atrial fibrillation 507
  peripheral vascular disease 626
  side effects 831
  stroke risk reduction 823, 830–1, *831*
Clopidogrel *versus* Aspirin in Patients at Risk for Ischemic Events (CAPRIE) trial 626, 830–1, *831*
Clostridium difficile 1727–8, 1730
clozapine, delirium 1056
Club for Research in Aging, USA 1924
cluster analysis, diet scores 286, **286**
cluster headache (periodic migrainous neuralgia) 274, 756–7, **756**
  chronic 756–7, **756**
coagulation
  activation 445, 634
  deep vein thrombosis risk 634
  defects
    acquired 440–1, **440**
    hereditary 439–40
  disseminated intravascular *see* disseminated intravascular coagulation (DIC)
  vitamin K 337
coagulation cascade *439, 443*
coagulation factors, increased 449
  see also individual factors
coagulation tests 437, **438**
coal workers' pneumoconiosis 715–6
coarctation of aorta 544–5
cobalamin 338
cobalt **341**
"cobblestone" tongue 271
cocaine, misuse 1193, 1197
cocaine-amphetamine-regulated transcript (CART) 303
coccidioidal meningitis 1770–1
Coccidioides immitis 1770
cochlea 1235
cochlear conductive presbycusis 1227
cochlear implants 1230, 1232
cochlear membrane breaks 1228
cochlear nerve abnormalities 1222, 1229
Cochrane Collaboration 843, 1830
Cockayne syndrome 1589–90
Cockcroft–Gault equation 430
co-codamol, palliative care 2005
codeine (methylmorphine) 400, 986
Codman, Ernest 1827
Codman-Hakim valve 790, *790*
"coffee ground" aspirates 376
cognition
  aging 59
  menopause 1418
  positive changes 57
  testosterone replacement therapy 1423
cognitive assessment
  driving capability assessment 144
  memory clinics 1065–6, **1066**
cognitive behavioral therapy (CBT) 861
  anxiety 1154
  carers' support 1813
  chronic pain management 988
  depression 1179
  drug misuse 1198
  insomnia 738–9
  with naltrexone 165
  stroke rehabilitation 863, 864–5
cognitive decline/dysfunction 59, 131, 1152–3
  cardiac conditions associated 488
  communication impact 842
  diabetes mellitus 1434–5
  etiology 1065
  fecal incontinence 397
  heart failure comorbidity 571, 572
  normal pressure hydrocephalus 792
  screening 164, 206
  see also cognitive impairment
Cognitive Dementia and Memory Services (CDAMS) Clinics, Australia 1062
cognitive disorders 1152–3
cognitive distortions, depression 1176
cognitive function
  aging effect 48–9, 744–5, **744**
  in Alzheimer's disease 1083–4, 1085, 1092
  dementia predictor in MCI 1097
  diseases affecting 48–9
  exercise effect 131–2
  heritability 49
  in multisystem atrophy 972
cognitive impairment
  communication effect 842
  depression and 1174
  food intake 285
  inappropriate medication use **220**
  restraint use 1691
  sarcopenia 921–2
  stroke related 863–4
  testosterone replacement therapy 1675
  see also cognitive decline/dysfunction; dementia
cognitive impairment, no dementia (CIND) 1152
cognitive neuropsychological model 843
Cognitive Performance Scale (CPS) 1860, 1863
cognitive processing, Parkinson's disease 773
"cognitive slowing", Alzheimer's disease 1039
cognitive therapy 1362
  see also cognitive behavioral therapy (CBT)
cognitive training, memory clinic patients 1068
cogwheel rigidity, Parkinson's disease 766
colchicine 388, 390, 412, 1351–2
cold exposure, hypothermia 977
colitis
  fecal incontinence 398
  infectious 374–5
collagen vascular disorders 1502, 1729
collapse, nonepileptic attacks 879
Colles fracture 1282
colon cancer *see* colorectal cancer
colonic transit
  aging effect 978
  measurements, constipation 409–10
colonoscopy 376, 399, 409
color flow Doppler ultrasound 1718
colorectal cancer
  acute cecal dilatation 1520
  folate supplements 338
  screening 207–8, 1512
colostomy 403, 1454, 2008
coma
  hyperglycemic hyperosmolar nonketotic 1433
  ischemic stroke 818–9, **819**
coma score
  Glasgow (GCS) 1029
  posttraumatic subdural hematoma 1028
comedones 1591, **1592**
Commission for Health Audit and Inspection (CHAI), UK 187, 1920
Commission for Health Improvement, UK 1168, 1857
Commission for Social Care Inspection (CSCI), UK 187, 1921
common bile duct, aging 381
common cold 667–8, 706
Common-Sense Model of Illness Representation 861
communication 841
  aging effects 841–2
  assessment of components/processes 1041–2, **1042**
  breakdown in dementia *see* communication disorders in dementia
  cognition impairment effect 842
  depression impact 842
  hearing impairment effect 841–2
  motor speech impairment effect 842
  nonverbal 2012
  process model 1037–8, *1038*
  with terminally ill patient 2012
  vision impairment effect 842
communication bus 189, *190*
  radio-based 189, 197
  smart home 189, 197
communication disorders 841–4, 846
  assessment/diagnosis 842–4
  see also specific diseases/disorders
communication disorders in dementia 1037–46, 1137
  assessment 1041–5
    activities 1044–5, **1044**
    carer's burden 1043
    carer's perception 1043
    components/processes 1041–2
    daily lifestyle 1043–4
    engagement opportunities 1044–5
    functional 1042–5, **1043**
    hearing 1043
    physical environment 1045, **1045**
    vision 1043
  interventions 1042–3, **1043**, **1044**
  normal process breakdown 1038–41
    grammar application 1039–40
    sequencing 1039–40
    thinking 1038–9
    word sound assembly 1039–40
    word store 1039–40
  speech muscles 1040
community acquired pneumonia
  causes 707
  epidemiology and risk factors 665
  hospitalization rate 665
  mortality 708
Community Aged Care Packages (CACPs), Australia 1895–6
community based care, mental health 1158
community care *see* home care
Community Care Act, UK (1990) 1910, 1917
Community Dental Service (CDS) 256, 257
Community Long-term Care Insurance Law (1988) 1949
Community Mental Health Teams for Older People (CMHT-OP), UK 1165
community nursing care 1872, 1873
Community Options Program, Australia 1895
community rehabilitation, orthogeriatrics 1343
community residences, Alzheimer's disease 1090
compensatory stepping 1300
competence
  elder abuse 186
  ethical issues 1685
complement 1754
complementary therapy
  glaucoma 1208
  sexual dysfunction 117, 118
complete heart block 495, 880–1
completed stroke 1244
compliance with medications 862
  anticoagulants 452–3, 637
  epilepsy 875
  failure *see* noncompliance with medication
  importance in heart failure 573
compound A 1650–1
compound muscle action potential (CMAP) 906
comprehension, dysphagia 843
Comprehensive Aphasia Test 843
Comprehensive Assessment and Referral Evaluation 1812

Comprehensive Geriatric Assessment 1435, **1435**
Comprehensive Podogeriatric Assessment Protocol (Helfand Index) 1316, **1318–20**
compression neuropathy 896–7
compression stockings 637, 1598
compression tip screw *see* sliding hip screw (SHS)
compression ultrasound 636
compression-of-morbidity hypothesis 1701
computed tomography (CT) 1718–9
  acoustic neuroma 1227
  Alzheimer's disease 1084
  aortic aneurysm 1004, 1005
  back pain 1358
  bacterial meningitis 1766
  brain abscess 1772
  brain tumor 1527
  dementia with parkinsonism 1117
  diaphragmatic structure 673
  epilepsy 873
  fibrotic lung disease 715
  HSV encephalitis 1775
  image artefacts 1719
  ischemic stroke 817
  memory clinic patients 1066–7
  muscle mass estimation 910, **911**
  myasthenia gravis 903
  normal pressure hydrocephalus 788, *788*, 791, 793
  Paget's disease of bone 1273
  pancreatic cancer 422, *422*
  pancreatitis 418, *418*, 420
  parkinsonism 767
  perimesencephalic hemorrhage 1019, *1019*
  radiation doses 1713, *1713*
  spinal canal stenosis 993–4, 997
  subarachnoid hemorrhage 1017–8, *1017*
  subdural empyema 1773–4
  subdural hematoma 1028, *1028*, 1031, *1031*
  tuberculous meningitis 1768
  vascular dementia 1105–6
  VZV encephalitis 1776
computed tomography angiography (CTA) 1018, 1719
Computerized Patient Record System (CPRS), USA 1850
computers
  aphasia/dysphasia therapy 843
  smart home 189
conductive deafness 1222–5, **1222**
  tinnitus 1229
Conference of the European Ministers for Transport (CEMT) 141
confidentiality, breaking, driving risk 147
confusion
  acute, causes 2009–10
  chronic subdural hematoma 1030
  opioid side effects 2005
  terminal illness 2009–10
Confusion Assessment Method (CAM) 1047–8, 1127, 1150
confusional arousals in sleep 734
congenital heart disease 481
  Down's syndrome 1188
  infective endocarditis 1750
congestive heart failure (CHF) 479–80
  apoptosis of cardiac myocytes 562
  cognitive decline 488
  cytokines 559, **559**
  epidemiology 479–80, *480*
  exercise effects **133**, 134, **134**
  frailty 1565, *1567*
  hyponatremia *1375*, 1378
  management 482, 1911
    ACE inhibitors 1863
  mortality rates 479, **479**
  renin-angiotensin-aldosterone system 557
  risk factors 479
  see also heart failure
conjugated equine estrogen (CEE) 1419
connective tissue disorders 806, 1349
"conscious effortful processing" concept 1038, 1041
consciousness loss
  hyperventilation attacks 884
  posttraumatic subdural hematoma 1028
  see also coma; syncope
constipation 407–15
  barium induced 1716
  chronic 407, 411
  clinical approach 409–10
  comorbidity 408
  definitions 407
  diagnostic tests 409–10, *410*
  drug induced 408, **408**, 412–3, 2005
  epidemiology 407–8
  etiology 408, **408**, **409**
  history 409
  impact 407–8
  Parkinson's disease 775
  pathophysiology 407–8
  physical examination 409
  primary/secondary 407
  quality of life 408
  self-reported 407–8
  terminally ill 2007–8
  treatment 410–2, **411**
constraint therapy, stroke rehabilitation 853
Consumer Assessment of Health Plans (CAHPS) 1838, 1839
contact sports, Parkinson's disease 769
contact tracing, tuberculosis 710
continence mechanism 396
continuing care *see* nursing home care
continuing professional development 1789
  see also medical education/training
continuous hyperfractionated accelerated radiotherapy (CHART) 711
continuous positive airway pressure (CPAP) 737
Continuous Quality Improvement (CQI) 1838
  features 1824, **1824**
  model **1841**
  programs 1929
  report **1846**
contractures, Alzheimer's disease 1087
contrast media 1715, 1717
contrast sensitivity, eye 1205, 1209
Coombs test 431
Cooperative Medical System schemes, China 1956–7
coordination, aging effect 746
COPD *see* chronic obstructive pulmonary disease (COPD)
copper 340–1, **341**
  osteoporosis 1291
cor pulmonale 699
core body temperature, circadian rhythm 738
Cornell Depression Inventory, Down's syndrome 1186
Cornell Depression Scale in Dementia 1129
Cornell Scale for Depression 1860
corns 1321–3
coronary angiography 586, 599, 1648
coronary angioplasty 519, 578–9, 599–600
  see also percutaneous transluminal angioplasty (PTA)
coronary arteries, stenosis 599
coronary artery bypass grafting (CABG) 585, **586**, 598–600, 607
  age of patients 594, *594*, 599
  antithrombotic therapy after 600
  benefits and effects 598–9
  cardiac rehabilitation results 657–8
  cost-effectiveness 599
  elective 599, 600
  indications 585, **586**, 599
  internal mammary artery as conduit 600, *600*
  mortality 594–5, 599, **599**, 607
  percutaneous coronary angioplasty *vs* 599–600
  stable angina therapy 519
  valve surgery with 594, 600, *601*, 604
    aortic valve replacement 601–2
coronary cataract 1208
coronary heart disease (CHD)
  cholesterol concentration 613
  diabetes mellitus 1439
  HRT 1418, 1419
  menopausal women 1418
  morbidity, India 1984
  peripheral vascular disease with 625, **625**
  testosterone replacement therapy 1422–3
  vitamin A supplements 333
  vitamin B_6 deficiency 339
  vitamin E supplements 334, 1670
  see also ischemic heart disease
coronary revascularization 519, 523–4
  complete *vs* incomplete 599
  indications 585, **586**
  see also coronary artery bypass grafting (CABG)
coronary thrombosis 520
coronaviruses 1732–3
corpectomy, cervical spinal canal stenosis 995
corpora amylacea, aging 76, *76*
cortical bone 1281
cortical implants, eye 1209
cortical-striatal-pallidal-thalamus-cortical pathway 1176
corticobasal degeneration (CBD) 1120
corticosteroids
  alcoholic liver disease 387–8
  as appetite stimulators 314–5
  aspiration pneumonitis 687
  asthma 704
  COPD 698, 701
  cryptogenic fibrosing alveolitis 717
  delirium etiology 1050
  giant cell arteritis 757
  large vessel vasculitis 1007
  myelodysplasia 459
  myopathy due to 940–1
  oral lichen planus 266
  osteopenia due to 135–6
  psoriasis 1597
  rheumatoid arthritis 1351
  transforaminal injection 994
  tuberculous meningitis 1768–9
  Wegener's granulomatosis 718
  see also steroids
corticotrophin releasing factor (CRF) 1176
cortisol
  age related changes 1390
  cardiac cachexia 642
  depression 1176
  endogenous overproduction 544
Cosin, Lionel 4, 1907
Costa Rica
  demographics **1994**, **1996**
  medical education/training 1994–5, **1995**
  service provision **1995**, 1996–8, 1997–8, *1997*
costal diaphragm 672
costs/expenditure
  for carers 1812
  resource allocation, ethics 1682–3
cotrimoxazole 1759
cotsides *see* siderails
couch potato syndrome 1392, *1392*
cough, smokers' 696
cough reflex 685, 1488
  ACE inhibitors and 687
  suppression 689
cough syncope 883
coughing, aspiration during swallowing 844
Council of the European Union 1685, 1977
counseling
  depression 1178
  drug misuse 1197–8
  terminally ill 2002–3
  tinnitus 1230
Cowdry, Edmund 1, 1892, 1926
COX-2 inhibitors
  arthritis 1350–1
  chronic pain 986
  gout 1352
  motor neuron disease 960
  postoperative pain **1652**
Coxiella burnetii **1752**, 1759–60
cramp, in MND 950, 960, 963
cranial arteritis (giant cell arteritis) 274, 757, 1007
cranial epidural abscess 1774–5
cranial mononeuropathy 892
cranial nerves, aging effect **744**, 745

cranial radiotherapy, prophylactic 712
cranioatlantoaxial instability 992
craniotomy 1029, 1032, 1774
crash fragility 141
crash risk 141–2
C-reactive protein (CRP) 709, 918, 1348
creatine 217–8, 1569
  supplements, sarcopenia 923
creatine kinase (CK), serum 936, 937
creatinine, serum 489, 1471
creatinine clearance (Ccr)
  age related changes 1496
  anemia in chronic renal insufficiency 430
  calculation 430
  chronic renal failure 1500
  reduction 570
creative thinking 56
creativity 56
CREDO trial (Clopidogrel for the Reduction of Events During Observation) 520
Creutzfeldt-Jacob's disease (CJD) 1124–5, **1125**, 1777
  clinical features **1085**, 1777
cricopharyngeal sphincter 845
Criteria for Therapeutic Shoes for Diabetics **1320**
critical-period programming 291
Crohn's disease 266, 398
crude rates definition 796
crural diaphragm 672
crusted (Norwegian) scabies 1595
cryotherapy 994, 997, 1478
cryptococcal meningitis 1770–1
Cryptococcus neoformans 1770
cryptogenic fibrosing alveolitis 717
cryptogenic organizing pneumonia 715, 718
crystallins 39
Cuba, demographics/service provision 1994, **1994**
Cullen's sign 418
cultural competency 112
cupulolithiasis *1241*, 1242
CURB65 score 708
CURE trial (Clopidogrel in Unstable Angina to Prevent Recurrent Events) 520
Cushing's disease 544, 1400
Cushing's syndrome 544, 942
cushions, pressure-relieving 1616, **1616**, *1617*
cutaneous reflexes, aging effect 747
cyanosis, cryptogenic fibrosing alveolitis 717
cyclic leg compression devices 1332
cyclizine, nausea/vomiting 2008
cyclo-oxygenase-2 enzyme inhibitors *see* COX-2 inhibitors
cyclophosphamide, large vessel vasculitis 1007
cyclophosphamide, methotrexate and 5-fluorouracil (CMF) 1536
cyclosporine 905, 1597
cyproheptadine 315
cyst(s)
  dental 270
  dentigerous 270
  epidermoid (epidermal inclusion) 1600, *1600*
  horn 1599, *1600*
  pineal 78
  thyroid 1410
cystadenomas, serous 421
cysticercosis 952
cystitis 324, 1409
cystoceles 1459
cystometric studies, bedside 1489
cytarabine, acute leukemia 467
cytocerebral syndrome 1050
cytochrome c oxidase, deficiency 16
cytochrome P450 217, **217**
cytogenetics
  acute leukemia 466, 469
  myelodysplasia 456, 468
cytokines
  age related changes 28–9, 31, 40, 305
  alcoholic liver disease 386, 388
  anorexia of aging 305, 1567
  antagonism 388
  atherosclerosis 618
  cardiac cachexia 640–1
  effect on skeletal muscle 38
  food intake levels 305, 314
  heart failure mechanism 559–60
  muscle strength loss 1569
  sarcopenia 916–8
  Th1/Th2 types 28, 29
cytopenia 455–6, 457, 1525
cytotoxic chemotherapy *see* chemotherapy

daf-2 gene 17, 1668
daf-16 gene 17
Danish Nurses Cohort study 1533
dantrolene, spasticity in MND 960
dapsone 267
darbepoietin 468–9, 1514, 1566
Darco shoe 1327
darifenacin, overactive bladder 1490
dark adaptation, eye 1205, 1209
DASH trial (Dietary Approaches to Stop Hypertension) 550
Data Protection Act, UK (1998) 1833
DATATOP trial 772
dauer larva 17
day care facilities, hospices 2014
day hospitals 5–6, 1907–13
  evaluation 1909–10
  psychiatric services 1166
  referral and function 1907–9, **1908**
daycare admission, surgical patients 1655
daytime sleepiness 734, 735, 736
  circadian rhythm disorder 738
DC cardioversion 503, 508, 587
D-dimers 446, 447, 636, 1526
deafness *see* hearing loss/impairment
death
  from Alzheimer's disease 1086
  causes 19, **20**, 515
  see also mortality
death rates *see* mortality rates
"death rattle" 2013
decibel (dB) scale 1219
decision-making
  age related changes 55
  health-care, preventive geriatrics and 202
decitabine 460, 469
decompensation, vestibular 1237, *1237*, *1241*
decompression surgery *see* surgical decompression
decompressive hemicraniectomy 820
deconditioning (functional decline) 1689
decongestants, delirium etiology 1051
decubitus ulcer *see* pressure ulcers/ulceration
deep brain stimulation (DBS) 783, 784
deep tendon reflexes, aging effect 746–7
deep vein thrombosis (DVT)
  age range 633
  clinical features 636
  diagnosis/investigations 636, 1719
  hip fractures 1332
  incidence 449
  management 452, 636–7
  "multiple hit model" 633, *635*
  pulmonary embolic disease 714
  recurrent, management 637
  risk factors 634, **634**
    acquired 634–5
    genetic 633–4
  stroke, following 820
defecation 396, 407
defecography 410
deferoxamine 458
DEFINITE (Defibrillators in Nonischemic Cardiomyopathy Treatment Evaluation) 510
degenerative conditions 14
degenerative dementia, non-Alzheimer type **1085**
degenerative joint disease *see* osteoarthritis (OA)
degenerative subluxation (spondylolisthesis) 996
deglutition 322, 845
  see also swallowing
dehydration 282–3, 321–7
  causes 283
  clinical 323–6
  clinical assessment 324–5
  daily fluid requirements 325
  delirium etiology 1053
  diagnosis 324–5
  drinking assistance 325
  dry mouth 271
  dysphagia 845
  hypertonic 324–5
  iatrogenic 323–4
  ischemic stroke and 819
  isotonic 324
  laboratory indices 324
  management 325–6
  mortality rates 283
  pressure ulcers 1609–10
  risk factors 323–4, **324**
dehydroepiandrostenedione sulphate (DHEAS) 1416, 1677
dehydroepiandrosterone (DHEA) 1393–4, 1677
  age related decline 33
  bone mineral density 1677
  cardiac cachexia 642
  female sexual dysfunction 116
  function 1677
  muscle mass 1568, 1677
  postmenopausal women 1416, 1421
  supplementation 924–5, 1421, 1677
delayed-type hypersensitivity (DTH) 1740
Delhi Rent Control Act (1995) 1987
delirium 1047–60, 1152
  adverse outcomes 1048
  awareness of 1048
  clinical features 1049
  comprehensive approach 1048–56
  dementia differentiation 1135
  dementia *vs* 1049, **1049**
  diagnosis 1048–9, **1049**, 1870
  etiology 1049–53, **1049**, **1050**
    medication 1049–52, **1050**
  evaluation 1048, 1049–53, **1049**, **1050**
  incidence 1047–8
  management 1048, 1054–6, **1054**, 1928
    home care *vs* hospitalization 1054
  misdiagnosis 1049
  Parkinson's disease 774
  pharmacological restraints 1056–7
  physical restraints 1056, 1692
  prevention 1048, 1054–6, **1054**
  risk factors 1054, **1054**
Delirium Index 1057
Delirium Room (DR) 1055–6, *1055*, 1928
delirium tremens 164
DELIRIUMS mnemonic 1049–53, **1049**
Delphi exercises 1830
Delta-like-1 (Notch ligand) 28
delusions 1139
  complex 1139–40
  dementia and 1139–41
  treatment 1140
demeclocycline 1379, 1523
dementia 1111–33
  activities of daily living dependence 1141
  agitation 1146
  alcohol related 158, 1126
  Alzheimer's *see* Alzheimer's disease
  anticoagulation for atrial fibrillation and 506
  anxiety and 1142–3, **1143**
  apathy 1146
  behavioral disorders **1128**, 1129, 1135–48
    conceptual framework 1136–7, *1136*
    physical causes 1136
    see also specific disorders
  bladder problems 1462
  cardiac conditions and 488
  cardiovascular disease relationship 481
  carers *see* caregiver(s) (carers)
  cerebral vasculitis 1125–6
  chronic pain assessment 985
  communication disorders *see* communication disorders in dementia
  cortical 1113, **1114**
  corticobasal degeneration (CBD) 1120
  delirium differentiation 1049, **1049**, 1135
  delusions and 1139–41
  depression and 1123–4, **1123**, 1173, 1174, 1177, **1177**

dementia (*cont.*)
diagnosis approach 1127, **1128–9**, 1129
driving and 145, 146
elopement 1146
epidemiology 1149
epilepsy and 869
etiology 1129
falls 1304
food intake reduction 300
food refusal 1144–5
frontotemporal lobular degeneration *see* frontotemporal lobular degeneration (FTLD)
functional impairment 1137–8
hallucinations and 1139–41
HIV-associated (HAD) 1126
Huntington's disease 777, 1125
insomnia 1145–6, **1145**
interference with others 1146
Lewy bodies in *see* Lewy body dementia
in long term care patients 1155
MCI development predictors 1096–7, **1097**, **1098**, 1099
MCI progression 1096
meaningful activities, initiation inability 1141–2, **1142**
medication induced 1127
memory clinics 1061
mood disorders and 1138–9, **1138**, **1139**
motor neuron disease 950, 951, 956
multiinfarct 506
multisystem atrophy 1120
neurofibrillary tangles 1076
neurological features 767
non-Alzheimer degenerative **1085**
nondegenerative **1085**
normal pressure hydrocephalus *see* normal pressure hydrocephalus (NPH)
paraneoplastic limb encephalitis 1126–7
with Parkinsonism 1115–7, **1116**
Parkinson's disease *see* Parkinson's disease dementia (PDD)
personality and 1137, **1137**
prevalence 1701, **1702**
Australia 1890
Japan 1937
USA nursing homes 1821
prevention in atrial fibrillation 488
prion diseases 1124–5, **1124**
progressive supranuclear palsy 1120
resistiveness to care 1143–4
reversible 1067
risk reduced by exercise 131, **133**
senile, Alzheimer's disease and 1073
sleep disorders 735–6
smart home technology 191, 195
smoking 152–3
spatial disorientation 1143
subcortical *see* subcortical dementia
vascular *see* vascular dementia
dementia care mapping 1045
dementia clinics *see* memory clinics
Dementia Services Development Centers 1170
dementing disorders 1152
demethylating agents, myelodysplasia 460
demographics
of aging 87–99, 101–4, **104**
chronic disease *see* chronic disease
dependency ratios *102*
developing countries 1965–8, **1966**
European Union 1977, 1978
life expectancy *see* life expectancy
mortality rates *see* mortality rates
sex ratios 103, *103*
see also specific countries
future changes 96
life expectancy *see* life expectancy
mortality rates *see* mortality rates
mortality selection 95–6
trajectories 95–6
world population trends 59, **60**, 157
see also specific countries
dendrites, aging neuropathology 71
dendritic arborization 60
dendritic cells (DC) 27
denial, alcohol problems 161
Denmark, nursing home care 1821, 1822, **1822**
dental abscess 270
dental care 275
access to 241
assessment guide **251**
barriers to 241–3
clinical 243–4, 244–53
dependent patients **250**
domiciliary treatment 241, 257, 275
history taking 244
medically compromised 275
periodontal treatment 247–9
professional training 258
prosthetic treatment 249–53
registration difficulties 241
restorative 244–7
soft tissue **250**, **251**, 253
special care patients 253–6, **255**
standard improvement recommendations **254**
terminally ill 2010, 2011
see also tooth
dental caries 245, *245*, 262
dental cysts 270
dental health, promotion 257–8
dental hygiene, inadequate 243, 244
dental hygienist 258
dental plaque 263
accumulation, dentures 245, *245*, 248
removal 262
dental problems, in Down's syndrome 1188
dental services 256–7
dental status 240–1
dentate gyrus, neuronal loss 70
dentigerous cyst 270
dentition *see* tooth (teeth)
denture(s)
aesthetics 250
cleaning procedures 252–3, **253**
construction 252
expectations of 242
full 250–2
hygiene *244*, 252–3
labeled 253, *253*
learning to wear 250–2
lifespan beliefs 242
naming 253
partial 244, 245, 250
reduced food intake 300
reduced saliva 252
retention 252
training appliances 250, *252*
denture stomatitis 263–4, *264*
denture-associated hyperplasia 265, 268
Department of Motor Vehicles (DMV) 147
depletion theory, depression 1176
Depo-Medrone® (methylprednisolone acetate) 2007
Deprenyl and Tocopherol Antioxidant Therapy of Parkinsonism (DATATOP) trial 1119–20
depressant drugs, withdrawal 1193
depression 1150, 1173–83
Alzheimer's disease 1084, 1087, 1173, **1174**
bereavement and 1173, **1174**
cardiac rehabilitation strategy 649
carers 1812
chronic pain 982
communication effect 842
comorbidity with medical illness 1173, 1174, 1175
COPD 700, 729
course 1174–5
delirium etiology 1052
dementia and 1119, 1123–4, **1123**, 1138, 1173, 1174, 1177, **1177**
diabetes mellitus 1435
diagnosis 1177, **1177**
Down's syndrome 1188
dysthymic disorder 1173, **1174**
epidemiology 1149, 1174
etiology 1175–7
general medical condition 1173–4, **1174**
exercise effects **133**, **134**
functional gastrointestinal disorders 367
genetic susceptibility 1176
heart failure comorbidity 571
HRT 1417
inappropriate medication use **220**
insomnia and 738
Lewy body dementia 1118
in long term care patients 1155
major 1173, **1174**
melancholia with 1173, **1174**
memory clinics 1067
menopause 1417
minor 1173, **1174**
MND 962
mortality, nonsuicide 1175
in Parkinson's disease 774, 1119
rating scales 1860
screening 206, 1545
service provision 1893–4
sexual dysfunction 120
sleep problems and 733, 738
stroke related 856, 862–3, 1573
subsyndromal 1173
subthreshold 1173, **1174**
subtypes 1173–4, **1174**
suicide 1175, **1175**
terminally ill 2010
treatment 1178–9
biological 1178–9, **1178**
exercise/training 129, 131
psychological 1179
underprescribing 1805
urinary incontinence 1487
vascular dementia 1115
weight loss 300
without sadness 1173
see also bipolar affective disorder
depsipeptide 460
dermal ulcer *see* pressure ulcers/ulceration
dermatitis
allergic, vulval 1455
asteatotic 1595–6, *1596*
seborrheic 1596, *1596*
stasis 1598, *1598*
dermatological conditions *see* skin disorders
dermatomyositis (DM) 937–8
pathological features 937–8, *938*
skin involvement 937, *938*, **1603**
dermatophyte test medium (DTM) 1593
dermis 37
aging 1590–1, **1590**
dermo-epidermal junction, aging 38
desipramine, depression 1178
desmoglein-I 267
desmopressin 439, 1371
desquamative gingivitis 265
detoxification, alcohol abuse 164
detrusor hyperreflexia 1461
detrusor instability (DI) 978, 1453
detrusor muscle contraction 1450, 1487
developing countries 1970–1
aging demographics 1965–8, **1966**
population aging 1965–76
chronic morbidity 1969–70
intergenerational transfers 1968–9
policy issues 1969, 1974–5
service provision 1971–3
social services 1973–4
developmental reflexes, aging effect 747
developmental stages (Erikson) 53–4
developmental tasks 53–4
DEXA *see* dual-energy X-ray absorptiometry (DXA)
dexamethasone
bacterial meningitis 1767
cerebral metastases induced confusion 2009–10
mucous membrane pemphigoid 267
spinal cord compression 1521, 1527
tuberculous meningitis 1769
dextropropoxyphene, chronic pain 986–7
diabetes insipidus 1372, 1373, 1374–5
causes 1374–5, **1402**
hypernatremia 1381
diabetes mellitus
alcohol association 160

autonomic dysfunction 972
barium meal/follow-through 1716
blood pressure regulation 1437–9
cardiovascular features 490
cardiovascular risk assessment 1439 **1439**
care homes *see* nursing home care
carotid artery stenosis 808
cataracts 1207
chronic pancreatitis 420
cognitive dysfunction 1434–5, **1435**
disability 1434
epidemiology 1432
fecal incontinence 397
frailty 1565, *1567*
functional assessment 1435, **1435**
gastrointestinal dysfunction 366
glucose control 1436–7
impact of 1432–40
incidence
developing countries 1970
Latin America 1993
ischemic heart disease 152, 477, 518–9
lipid regulation 1439–40
metabolic comas 1433
MND association 959
modes of presentation 1432, **1432**
morbidity, India 1984
nutrient absorption 293
onychomycosis 1593
pathogenesis 1432
peripheral neuropathy 891–3, **891**
peripheral vascular disease risk 624
pressure ulcers 1609
risk factors **1432**
sexual dysfunction 120
stroke risk 801, 835
taste dysfunction 1256
type 1, Down's syndrome 1187
type 2 1431–44
comorbid conditions 135
depression 1435
exercise therapy role 134–5
initial care plan **1436**
insulin regimes **1438**
management aims **1436**
muscle mass preservation 130
obesity 350
prevention, by exercise 132, **133**
resistance training 135, **135**
treatment literature review 1435–6, **1437**
weight loss 313
vitamin C supplements 1673
vitamin E supplements 1671
X-ray contrast media 1717
Diabetes Prevention Program (DPP) 132
diabetic amyotrophy 893
diabetic foot 1313–5, *1314*, **1315**, *1322*, 1433
falls 1301
risk factors **1433**
ulcers 1324
diabetic gastroparesis 366
diabetic ketoacidosis (DKA) 1383, 1433
diabetic nephropathy 1502
diabetic neuropathy 891–3, **891**
diabetic retinopathy (DR) *1206*, 1207, **1207**
Diagnosis Procedure Combination System, Japan 1935–6
Diagnostic and Statistical Manual of Mental Disorders (DSM)
alcohol abuse/dependence 158
Alzheimer's disease 1073, 1083, 1085, 1092–3
delirium 1047, 1048–9
dementia 1127, **1128**
depression 1173
drug misuse 1194, **1194**
vascular dementia 1103–4, 1114
diagnostic disclosure, memory clinics 1067–8, **1068**
diagnostic imaging 1711–22
good practice guidelines 1711–3
wasteful usage 1712
see also specific types
diagnostic related groups (DRGs) 1683
dialysis 1382, 1500–1
see also hemodialysis
3,4 diaminopyridine 906
diaphragm 672
hemispheric ischemic stroke 678
strength measurement 674
wasting 679
weakness, MND 961
diaphragmatic breathing 728
diarrhea 340
infectious 1727–8
diastolic blood pressure (DBP)
hypertension definition 541
low, adverse effects 542
orthostatic hypotension 973
diastolic J-curve 477
diastolic ventricular interaction (DVI) 564
diathermy, lumbar spinal canal stenosis 997
diazepam 161, 875, 876
diclofenac 1350, 1352
diet
age related macular degeneration 1206
cardiac rehabilitation 649–50
cataracts 1208
composition (normal diet) 291
diabetics in care homes 1441
heart disease risk factor 478
hypertension management 550
hypertension pathogenesis 543
osteoporosis 1282
stroke risk 802
see also healthy eating; nutrition
dietary fats *see* fat (dietary)
dietary fiber, constipation treatment 410
dietary guidelines 288–9, *288*
dietary intake
population differences 283–5
vulnerable groups 284–5, **284**
dietary patterns 286–7
dietary reference intakes (DRIs) 330–1, **331**
diethylstilbestrol, prostate cancer 1478
differential communication assessment 842
differentiating agents, myelodysplasia 459–60
diffuse plaques, aging neuropathology 73, *73*
digital hearing aids 1216, *1216*, 1231
digital (filmless) radiography 1716
digital rectal examination (DRE) 208, 376, 398–9
digital subtraction angiography (DSA) 1717–8
dignity, conceptualization 1682, 1685
"Dignity on the Ward" campaign 1874
digoxin
alcohol interaction 161
appetite loss 300
atrial fibrillation 501, 502
delirium etiology 1050
distribution/renal clearance 575
drug interactions 575
heart failure 501, 575, 576
mechanism of action 501
monitoring 575
renal impairment 1503–4
side effects/toxicity 501, 575
dihydrocodeine, palliative care 2005
24,25-dihydroxy-vitamin D 1497
1,25-dihydroxyvitamin D_3 (1,25$(OH)_2$D) 336, 1262
age related changes 1263, **1263**, 1265, 1497
dilated cardiomyopathy 509–10, 1674–5
diltiazem 502, 519
dilute Russell viper venom test (DRVVT) 443
dioctyl calcium sulphosuccinate 411
dioctyl sodium sulphosuccinate 411
diphenoxylate 400
dipsogenesis 322–3
dipyridamole 823, 830
dipyridamole-thallium imaging 516–7
direct antiglobulin test 431
direct diastolic ventricular interaction (DVI) 564
direct thrombin inhibitors (DTI) 507, 831–2
disability 1911
antiaging therapy 1666
cardiovascular disease and 481
diabetes mellitus 1434
diseases associated 136
functional assessment scales *1555*, 1559–60, **1559**
ICIDH definition 852, 1571
impairment 239–40
prevention/treatment by exercise 136–7
risk factors 136, *280*
service provision, Israel 1948–50
theoretical framework 1553, 1554, *1555*
disability allowances 964
disasters, impact on geriatric care 112–3, **112**
disease clustering, diabetes mellitus 135
disease count index 1532
disease-modifying antirheumatic drugs (DMARDs) 1351
disengagement theory of aging 1176
disequilibrium 1244, 1245
disinhibited frontotemporal dementia (FTD) 1121
diskectomy 995, 1360
diskitis 1359–60
Disposable Soma theory 14, 16
disseminated intravascular coagulation (DIC) 445–8
diagnosis 446, **446**, 1526
oncological emergency 1526
pathophysiology 445–6, *446*, **446**
symptoms 1526
triggers 445, **446**
distal splenorenal shunt 377
disulfiram (Antabuse®) 165
diuretics
heart failure 570, 575, 576
hyponatremia induction 1378
thiazide *see* thiazide diuretics
valvular heart disease 534
divalproex sodium 754, 1151
Diverter device 505
diverticulitis 1501
diverticulosis 293, 377
dizziness 1237
assessment 1306
causes **1237**
central vestibular origin 1238
character 1238
drug induced 1243, **1243**
falls 1303
peripheral labyrinthine origin 1238
vestibular disorders 1235
DNA
analysis, white oral lesions 269
damage 15, 1589–90
methylation changes in myelodysplasia 459
methylation inhibitors 459–60, 469
oxidative damage 64
repair 15
DNA probes, tuberculosis 1743
dobutamine, as positive inotropic drug 587
docetaxel, breast cancer 1536
dofetilide, atrial fibrillation 504
domiciliary treatment, dental care 241, 257, 275
domperidone 2008
Donabedian principle 232, 1830–2
Donald W. Reynolds Foundation 1892, 1926
donepezil 745, 1088, 1137, 1938
adverse effects 1069
dong quai (*Angelica sinensis*) 1420
do-not-resuscitate (DNR) orders 1654
do-not-resuscitate policies 1686
L-dopa *see* levodopa (L-dopa)
dopamine
acute renal failure 1499
age related changes 60–1
aspiration pneumonia prevention 688
drug induced parkinsonism 768
intravenous, as inotropic drug 587
Parkinson's disease 769
striatal synapse, aging **41**
dopamine agonists 686, 772, 781, 1400
dopamine D1 receptors *770*
dopamine D1-like receptors 30
dopamine D2 receptors 61, *770*
antagonists 768
dopamine depleting agents, Huntington's disease 778

dopamine receptor blockers
 drug induced parkinsonism 768
 dystonia 783
 Huntington's disease 778
 substance P 686
 tardive dyskinesia induction 779
dopaminergic neurons 60–1, **61**, 769
Doppler echocardiography 590
Doppler ultrasound 1718
 carotid artery disease 807, **807**, 823, 836
 peripheral vascular disease 623
dorsal kyphosis 533, 1450
"doughnut" cushions 1612
"doukyo" 1941–2
"Dowager's hump" (dorsal kyphosis) 533, 1450
Down Syndrome Medical Interest Group 1186
Down's syndrome 1168, 1185–9
 Alzheimer's disease and 1076, 1185, 1188, **1188**
 associated disorders 1186–8, **1186**
 behavior disorders 1188
 cancer and 1188
 cardiovascular disorders 1188
 celiac disease 1187
 dental problems 1188
 dermatological conditions 1187–8
 endocrinological disorders and 1186–7
 epilepsy 1188
 examination in 1186
 eye disorders 1188
 foot problems 1188
 genetics 1185
 gynecological problems 1188
 joint problems and 1187, **1187**
 otolaryngolic conditions and 1187
 pain 1186
doxazosin, benign prostatic hyperplasia 1472
doxorubicin, cardiomyopathy induction 1515
doxycycline 1480, 1598, 1759
dressing, interventions in dementia 1141
dressings
 foot 1326
 pressure ulcers 1621–2, **1622**
DRGs (diagnostic related groups) 1683
drinking assistance, dehydrated person 325
drip and suck regimen 2008
Driver and Vehicle Licensing Agency (DVLA), UK 147, 870, 1032–3
driver licensing authorities 146–7
driving 141–9
 capability assessment 142–5, *143*
  disease associated risks 145
  driver licensing authorities 146–7
  history taking 142
  important factors 142–5, **144**
  insurance authorities 146–7
  interventions 142, 146, **146**
  physician responsibility 146–7
 crash fragility 141
 crash risk 141–2
 epilepsy 876
 habits 145
 illness and 141–2
 license removal 147
 on-road capability test 144–5
 simulation 144, 159
 skills evaluation 142
 subdural hematoma, after 1032–3
 transient global amnesia 870
dronabinol 315, 1145
drop attacks 871, 1302–3
drug(s) 1191
 absorption 215, **216**
 adverse reactions **218**
 clearance/elimination 217–8
 compliance *see* compliance with medications
 distribution 215–7, **216**
 iatrogenic effects 1805
 metabolism 217
 noncompliance 546, 571
 prescribing *see* drug prescribing
 secondary hypertension due to 545
 sensitivity 218
drug history, back pain 1357
drug hypersensitivity syndrome 1599
drug induced conditions
 anorexia 300
 constipation 408, **408**
 dehydration 323–4, **324**
 dementia 1127
 dizziness 1243, **1243**
 driving and 142
 esophagitis 362
 falls 1304
 fecal incontinence 398
 fibrotic lung disease 718
 generalized gingival enlargement 262
 headache 759
 heat intolerance 977
 hepatitis 384–5, 386, 1743
 hypersalivation **273**
 hypokalemia, muscle weakness 941
 hyponatremia 1378
 insomnia 738, 1145
 lichenoid reaction 266
 lupus 1349
 migraine 753
 oral problems 255
 oral ulceration 266
 parkinsonism 768
 peripheral neuropathy 894, **894**
 psychiatric disorders 1154
 syncope 880
 taste dysfunction 1256
 tinnitus 1228–9, **1229**
 urinary incontinence 1488, **1488**
drug interactions
 ACE inhibitors 575
 alcohol and drugs 160–1, 166
 α-blockers 1472
 digoxin 575
 drugs and nutrients 293–4, **294**
 in heart failure 572, 575
 warfarin 604, **604**
drug misuse/abuse 1191–202
 assessment 1193–5, **1196–7**
  investigations 1195, **1195**, **1196–7**
 causes 1191
 clinician, importance to 1191
 dependence *vs* harmful use **1194**, 1194–5
 diagnosis criteria 1194, **1194**
 epidemiology 1192, *1192*
 intoxication symptoms **1195**
 mental health 1192–3
 physical comorbidity 1193
 policy 1199, **1200**
 prescription drugs 1150, 1153
 psychiatric comorbidity 1192–3
 seizures and 871
 treatment interventions 1195, 1197–9
 types 1191
 withdrawal
  management 1195, 1197
  symptoms 1195, **1195**
 see also intravenous drug users; *specific drugs*
drug prescribing 219–21
 inappropriate medication use 219, **220**
 recommendations **220**
 underuse of beneficial drugs 220–1
drusen 1206
dry mouth 271, **271**
 management 272
 terminally ill 2010
 see also xerostomia
dry skin *see* xerosis
'dual effect', physician-assisted suicide 965
dual photon absorptiometry (DPA) 1283
"dual tasking", aging 1300
dual-energy X-ray absorptiometry (DXA) 208
 bone mineral density 1283
 muscle mass estimate 910, *910*, **911**
 obesity assessment 347
 osteoporosis 1286–7
 sarcopenia 1568
Duchenne muscular dystrophy 943
Duke criteria, infective endocarditis 1756, **1757**
duloxetine 994
duodenum 363–5
duplex ultrasound 624, 636, 1718
dural arteriovenous fistulae 1008, 1020
dural artery 1001
dying patient management *see* palliative/end-of-life care
dynamic graciloplasty, fecal incontinence 403
dynamic hip screw *see* sliding hip screw (SHS)
dynamic tremor 783
dysarthria 843, 844, **844**
 brain region association 843
 in dementia 1040
 in MND 951, 960–1
dysesthesia 2007
dysexecutive syndrome 865
dysfunctional syndrome 1899, *1900*
dysgeusia 1249
dyskinesia
 Parkinson's disease 770
 spontaneous oral 778–9
 tardive 779–80
 while awake 780
dyslipidemia
 ischemic heart disease risk 518
 peripheral vascular disease risk 624
 treatment 626, 1441
dysosmia 1249
dyspareunia 1454, 1661
dyspepsia
 aspirin induced 830
 functional 367
dysphagia 359–60, 845–6
 assessment 845, **846**
 esophageal 359–60, **360**
 ischemic stroke 820–1
 management 845
 motor neuron disease 961
 oropharyngeal 359
 Parkinson's disease 366, 775
 stroke rehabilitation 851, 854–5
 symptoms 845
 terminally ill 2010–1
dysphasia 842–3
 brain region association 842–3
 stroke rehabilitation 855, 856
dysphoria, testosterone replacement therapy 1423
dyspnea (breathlessness)
 cardiac tamponade 1524
 chronic mitral regurgitation 589
 clinics 2009
 COPD 675
 cryptogenic fibrosing alveolitis 717
 extrinsic allergic alveolitis 716
 fibrotic lung disease 715
 heart failure 569, 677
 ischemic heart disease 515
 terminally ill 2008–9
dyspraxia 843–4
dyspraxia of speech 843–4
dyssynergic defecation 407
 biofeedback 413
 tests and examination 409, 410
dysthymia, treatment 1178
dysthymic disorder 1173, **1174**
dystonia **778**, 781–3
 classification 781–2, **781**, **782**
 drug induced **784**
 generalized 782, **782**
dystrophic axons, aging 72
dystrophinopathies 943
DYT1 gene, dystonia 782

EAA *see* excitatory amino acids (EAA)
ear disease
 middle-ear, chronic 1240
 otitis externa 1223, 1240
 symptoms 1222–32
 see also otitis media
early-life experiences, heart disease and 478–9
earwax (cerumen) 1222
East Anglia Hip Fracture Audit 1343
eccentric muscle contractions, sarcopenia 922
echinacea, alcohol interaction 161

echocardiography
  adenosine 517
  heart failure 570
  infective endocarditis 590
  transesophageal 500, 590
  transthoracic 500
  valvular heart disease 533
ecstasy, misuse *1192*
ectocervix, age related changes 1449
ectopic beats
  atrial 496
  ventricular 507, *507*
edema
  cerebral 1382
  diabetic foot 1315
  pulmonary 502, 515, 585–6, 589
  varicose veins 1315
Eden Alternative 1822, 1929
edentulousness, prevalence 240, **240**
edrophonium chloride 679, 902–3
education
  aging implications for 56
  Health Maintenance Clinical Guidepath 205
  heart disease prevention 649
  medical *see* medical education/training
  secondary prevention and 1576–7
Edward R. Roybal Centers, USA 1926
efalizumab, psoriasis 1597
effective dose **1712**, 1713
ego
  differentiation 54
  transcendence *vs* preoccupation 54
Ehlers–Danlos syndrome 441
elastosis 1591, **1592**
elder abuse 111, 181–8, 1154, 1921
  awareness 205
  competence 186
  definitions 182
  Down's syndrome 1186
  expert witnesses 185
  initial assessment 183–4
  institutional 186–7
  intervention 184–6
  laboratory investigations 184
  mental state assessment 184
  ongoing investigations 184–6
  perpetrator 182, 183
  police involvement 184–5
  prevalence 182, **182**
  recognition 183
  responsible agencies (UK) 187
  risk factors 182–3, 186
  spousal 182
  types of 182
  victim 182
  victim institutionalization 185–6
  victim testimony 185
  web sites 187
elderly, definition 487
elderly-onset rheumatoid arthritis (EORA) 1348
electric toothbrushes 249
electrical stimulation
  pressure ulcers 1625
  stroke related spasticity 856
electroacupuncture, back pain 1361
electrocardiogram (ECG)
  12-lead surveys 493, 494
  24-hour ambulatory 493
  Alzheimer's disease 1088
  atrial fibrillation 500
  cardiac arrhythmia 870
  cardiac tamponade 1524
  epilepsy 872
  exercise, preoperative 1648
  hyperkalemia 1383
  ischemic stroke 817
  memory clinic patients 1066
  monitoring, cardiac rehabilitation 655
  post fall 1305
  PR interval and prolongation 494–5
  preoperative 1648
  pulmonary embolic disease 714
  QRS interval prolongation 576
  resting, ischemic heart disease 516
  signal-averaged (SAECG) 517
  ST-segment depression 516
  syncope 882
  valvular heart disease 533
electroconvulsive therapy (ECT) 1157
  bipolar affective disorder 1151
  depression 1150, 1157, 1178
  psychotic depression 1179
electrodesiccation and curettage (ED&C) 1601, 1602
electroencephalogram (EEG)
  ambulatory, epilepsy 872
  cardiac arrhythmia 870
  Creutzfeldt-Jacob's disease 1124, 1125, 1777
  epilepsy 869, 870, 872, **872**
  HSV encephalitis 1775
  memory clinic patients 1066
  psychogenic nonepileptic attacks 885
  sleep disorder assessment 737, 872
  sleep structure measurement 734
  syncope 883
electrogastrogram (EGG) 364, 978
electrolyte balance 1023, 1369–87
  preoperative assessment 1637–8
electromyography (EMG)
  dermatomyositis 938
  dyssynergic defecation 410
  dystonia 782
  fecal incontinence 399
  inclusion body myositis 939
  motor neuron disease 954
  myasthenia gravis 902
  myopathies 936–7
  periodic limb movements in sleep 737
  postpolio syndrome 1777
  restless leg syndrome 737
  sleep disorder assessment 737
  spinal canal stenosis 994, 996
electron transport system (ETS) complexes 915
electronic barostat, gastric relaxation 364
electronic medical records *see* patient records
electrooculogram (EOG) 737
electrophysiology, dementia prediction 1097
electroshock therapy 1139
elopement, dementia and 1146
elopement control devices 1694
emergency department
  alcohol problem prevalence 158
  oncological emergencies 1519–20
emergency medical services, cancer 1529
emergency psychiatry 1154
emergency response telephones 1847–8
emollients, foot fissures 1326
emotional lability, motor neuron disease 951, 962
emotional support, end of life care 578
emotions, delirium etiology 1052
emphysema 1715
  senile 695
  see also chronic obstructive pulmonary disease (COPD)
emphysematous cholecystitis 389–90
Employees State Insurance Corporation, India 1988
empty sella syndrome 1399–400
empty sella turcica 1401
"empty" speech, Alzheimer's disease 1039
emptying drugs (motility agents) 1050
empyema, subdural 1773–4
ENABLE project 193, 194, 196
'enabling', alcohol abuse/interaction 161
enalapril, hypertension therapy 547
encephalitis 1775–6
  herpes simplex virus 1775
  varicella zoster virus 1775–6
  West Nile Virus 1776
encephalomyelitis, carcinomatous 1241
encephalopathy, hepatic 1126
encephalopathy, hyponatremic 1375, 1379–80
"enclosed fibers", muscle 672
end stage renal disease (ERSD) 1499–500
  dialysis 1500–1
  renal transplantation 1501
Ending Neglect: The Elimination of TB in the US 1739
endoaneurysmorrhaphy 1004
endocarditis, infective *see* infective endocarditis
endocrine diseases
  aging 1391–2
  cardiovascular features 489–90
  in Down's syndrome 1186–7
  frailty 1566
endocrine hormones 32–3
endocrine system, aging 43–4, **43**
endocrinology, aging 1389–95
  HYPER/HYPO-disease 1389
endocrinopathies, foot problems 1313–5
end-of-life care *see* palliative/end-of-life care
end-of-life issues, in MND 964–5
endograft, aortic aneurysm 1004
endometrial cancer 1456, 1659
  HRT and 1451, 1676
  presenting symptoms 1456
  risk factors 1451, 1456, 1659
  treatment 1456, 1659
endorgan hormones 1389
endoscopic retrograde cholangiopancreatography (ERCP)
  gallstones 389
  pancreatic cancer 422
  pancreatitis 418, *418*, 420
endoscopic third ventriculostomy 791
endoscopic ultrasound, gallstones 389
endoscopy
  aortoenteric fistula 377
  esophageal dysphagia 359
  esophagus 358
  noncardiac chest pain 362
"endothelial activation hypothesis" 616–8
endothelial cells 611, 973
endothelial dysfunction, age-associated 542–3
endothelial-derived relaxing factor (EDRF) *see* nitric oxide
endothelin
  aging effect 973
  essential hypertension role 973
  heart failure mechanism 558–9
endothelin antagonists 559
endothelin-1 558–9, **559**
endovascular treatment
  carotid artery stenosis 811–2, *811*
  limitations 811
  subarachnoid hemorrhage 1022, 1024
endpoint, clinical trials 1292
endurance training
  chronic heart failure 655
  obesity management 351
  for optimal aging **137**
  pulmonary rehabilitation 728
enemas **411**, 412
  barium 1716–7
energy
  availability, aging 64
  content of meals 973
  expenditure 348, 653
  intake *see* food intake
enflurane, renal injury 1650
engagement opportunities, communication 1044–5
ENT (ear, nose and throat) drugs 1051–2
entacapone, Parkinson's disease 771–2
enteral feeding
  acute pancreatitis 419
  contraindication in dementia 1145
  dysphagia after stroke 821
  surgical patients 1639
  undernutrition 314
  see also tube feeding
enteral tube, fluid replacement therapy by 326
enteric nervous system 357, 971
enteroceles 1459
enteroscopy, gastrointestinal bleeding 376
enterovirus, meningitis 1763
entorhinal cortex 70, 1074
entrapment neuropathies 893, 896–7, 963
environmental issues/problems 4, 229–30
  adaptations 1886
  housing 106–8, **107**, 229–30
environmental stress, hippocampal cell death 63

enzymatic debriding agents 1620
enzyme-linked immunosorbent assay (ELISA) 1769
eosinophilia, chronic pulmonary 715
eosinophilic pneumonia, chronic 718
Epidemiological Catchment Area (ECA) study 1193
epidemiology rates, definition 796
epidermal inclusion (epidermoid) cyst 1600, *1600*
epidermis 37
  aging **1590**
  photoaging 1591
epidermoid cyst 1600, *1600*
EPIDOS study (Epidemiology of Osteoporosis study) 126
epidural abscess 1774–5
epidural hematoma 1006–7
epidural injection 988, 1360, 2007
epilepsy 869–77
  Alzheimer's disease and 1087
  antiepileptic drugs 873–5, **873**
  complex partial seizure 872, 876
  diagnosis 869, 870
  differential diagnosis 870–1
  in Down's syndrome 1188
  driving and 145, 876
  drug resistant type, management 876
  epidemiology 869, **870**
  etiology 869–70, **870**
  falls 1303
  generalized 871–2, 873
  investigations 872–3, **872**
  localization related 871, 872, 873
  psychogenic nonepileptic attacks and 885
  seizure classification 871–2, **871**
  simple partial seizure 872
  status epilepticus 876
  subdural hematoma and 1032
  syncope misdiagnosis 883
  treatments 873–6, **873**
epinephrine (adrenaline), aging effect 973
episodic cluster headache 756–7, **756**
episodic dyscontrol 884
episodic memory 1037, 1038–9
episodic tension-type headache (ETTH) 755
epithelial cells, glandular, aging 695
epithelial nevus, oral 269
eplerenone 575
epoietin *see* erythropoietin, human recombinant
eptifibatide 520
epulis, fibrous 262
equilibrium apraxia 1301
erectile dysfunction 117–8, 1433
  autonomic function, aging effect 978
  brachytherapy side effect 1478
  cardiovascular disease 120
  causes 117, **117**
    drug induced 117, 1433
    external beam radiation therapy 1477–8
  diabetes mellitus 1433
  nitric oxide levels 119
  partner education 1421
  prevalence 117
  radical prostatectomy complication 1477
  screening 206
  testosterone replacement therapy 1423
  treatment **118**
"ergoreceptors" 656, 657
ergot derivatives, respiratory dysfunction 676–7
erosive osteoarthritis *see* osteoarthritis
erythema gyratum repens **1603**
erythrocyte glutathione reductase assay 336
erythrocyte sedimentation rate (ESR) 709, 1348
erythroderma **1603**
erythroid hyperplasia, myelodysplasia 456
erythroid series 465
erythroplakia 269
erythropoiesis, ineffective 431, 456, 457
erythropoietin 465, 1498
  deficiency 428, 430
  human recombinant 432–3
    anemia 1514, 1566, 2009
    inadequate response 433, **433**
    monitoring 433
    myelodysplasia therapy 459, 468–9
eschar 1618, 1620, *1620*
Escherichia coli 1727
escitalopram, depression 1178
esophageal dysphagia 359–60, **360**
esophageal motility
  age related changes 358–9
  evaluation 358
  ineffective 361
esophageal motility disorders 359–63, 366
esophageal spasm, diffuse 361, *361*, *362*
  management 362–3
esophageal sphincter 845
  lower *see* lower esophageal sphincter (LES)
  upper 358, 359
esophageal varices, bleeding 372
esophagitis 160, 372
esophagogastroduodenoscopy (EGD) 376
esophagus
  age related changes 978
  "cockscrew" appearance *362*
  "nutcracker" 362–3
  strictures, pill esophagitis 362
Essence of Care 1870, 1875
essential tremor (ET) 783
  aging 746
  clinical features 767
  pathophysiology 784
  treatment 784
Established Populations for Epidemiologic Studies of the Elderly (EPESE) 136
  body weight and mortality 310, **310**, 311, 312, **312**
  obesity and mortality 310, **311**
Established Populations for the Epidemiologic Study of the Elderly (EPESE) 1557
estimated average requirement (EAR), nutrient intake 330–1
estradiol 1416, 1450
Estratest 1421
estrogen
  brain cell osmolality 1371
  deep vein thrombosis risk 634
  deficiency 1289, 1662
  deprivation, breast cancer 1513–4
  esterified 1419
  hormonal fountain of youth 1394
  muscle mass 917
  osteoporosis 1283
  prostate cancer 1478
estrogen replacement therapy 523
  heart disease prevention doubt 478
  osteoporosis 1663
  stress incontinence 1464
  see also hormone replacement therapy (HRT)
estrone, menopause 1416
etanercept 643, 1351, 1597
ethambutol 709, 1743, **1745**, 1768
  side effects 1743
ethanol related myopathies 940
ethical issues 1681–7
  advance directives 1685–6
  agism 1682–3
  euthanasia 1684–5
  medical futility 1686–7
  perioperative care 1653–4
  predictive genetic testing 1687
  quality of life 1683–4, 1685
  rehabilitation, clinical psychology 866
ethnic groups, minorities *see* minority ethnic groups
ethosuximide, epilepsy 875
etidronate 1275, 1294
etoposide 712
etoricoxib 1351, 1352
Euro Score, cardiac surgery risk assessment 596, **597**, 607
Europe, hearing aid provision 1216
European Academy of Medicine of Aging (EAMA) 1783, 1786
European Association of Geriatric Psychiatry (EAGP) 1170
European Carotid Surgery Trial (ECST) 808–9, 1640
European Commission 1977
European Diabetes Working Party for Older People
  blood pressure regulation guidelines 1438
  diabetic care home resident treatment 1442
  diabetic care home residents 1441
  glucose regulation guidelines 1436–7, *1445*
European External Peer Review Techniques (ExPeRT) 1839
European Foundation for Quality Management (EFQM) 1839–40
European Myocardial Infarction Amiodarone Trial 523
European Organization for Research and Treatment of Cancer (EORTC) 1534
European Pressure Ulcer Advisory Panel (EPUAP) 1617, **1617**, **1621**
European Stroke Prevention Study-2 (ESPS-2) 830
European Union 1977–82, **1981**
  aging demographics 1977, *1978*
  health trends 1978–80, **1979**
  see also specific countries
European Union Geriatric Medicine Society (EUGMS) 1786
European Union of Medical Specialists – geriatric medicine section (GMS-UEMS) 1785
EuroQol questionnaire, cardiac surgery benefits 598, **598**, 607
euthanasia
  ethical issues 1684–5
  Israeli attitudes 1951
  MND and 949, 964
Evaluation and Quality Improvement Program (EQuIP), Australia 1839
evening primrose oil 1420
evidence-based medicine (EBM) 1292
  limitations 201
evidence-based practice 1830, 1876
  see also clinical audit
evolution, of longevity 14
evolution biology 13–4
evolutionary theory, aging and 13–4
EWPHE (European Working Party on High Blood pressure in the Elderly) trial **547**, 548, **548**
ex vacuo phenomenon, subdural hematoma 1030
examestane, breast cancer 1514
examination chairs, hydraulic 1714, *1715*
examination charges, dental care 241
examination tables
  elevating 1713
  radiology 1713, *1714*
excitatory amino acids (EAA) 63, 957–8
  EAAergic neurons, aging **61**, 62
excitotoxic damage, MND 958
excitotoxicity 63, 1079
executive function measurement 1065
exemestane, breast cancer 1536
exercise 123–40
  adipose tissue accretion and distribution 129–30
  aerobic *see* aerobic exercise
  aging effect on heart modifiable by 530
  capacity 124–5, **124**
    assessment 651–2
    maximal 696
  cardiac cachexia 642
  cognitive function 131–2
  depression and 1179
  disability prevention/treatment 136–7
  disease prevention by 132, **133**
  disease recurrence prevention 133
  disease treatment by 132–6
  falls prevention 1307
  heart disease protection 478, 519
  heart failure management 577–8, 658
    contraindications 578
    see also exercise training
  high-intensity, pulmonary rehabilitation 728
  hypertension management 550
  intensity
    body fat changes 129–30
    effect on bone health 127
  life expectancy increase 124
  "lifestyle" integration of 123
  limb skeletal muscle 673

muscle mass preservation 130, 913
neurotoxicity (of aging) prevention 131
osteoporosis 1293
psychological well-being and 131
recommendations for optimal aging **137**
role in bone health and fracture risk 126–9
exercise modality/intensity 127
fracture treatment 127, 129
postmenopausal women 127, **128**
secondary stroke risk reduction 837
tolerance
cardiac rehabilitation 649, 654, 656
reduced by beta-blockers 502
walking as *see* walking as exercise
see also exercise programs for elderly; exercise training
exercise ECG, preoperative 1648
exercise programs for elderly 519
cardiac rehabilitation *see* exercise training
delivery in day hospitals 1911
heart failure management 577
nursing role in delivery 1873
pulmonary rehabilitation 1580
see also exercise training; physical activity
exercise stress testing 516
6-minute walk test 652, 1305
for cardiac rehabilitation 651–2
ergometric 652
valvular heart disease 533
exercise therapy/rehabilitation
back pain 1361
chronic pain 988
intermittent claudication 627
maximal oxygen uptake 696
osteoporosis 1663
peripheral vascular disease 627
peripheral vestibular disorders 1246
pulmonary rehabilitation 728
see also exercise training
exercise training
aerobic *see* aerobic exercise
cardiac muscle benefit mechanism 564
cardiac rehabilitation 652–5, 1578–9
after cardiac surgery 655, 657–8
in chronic heart failure 655, 658
circuit training 654
continuous training 653
contraindications **655**
in coronary disease 656, 657
duration 653, 654
efficacy 652–3
frequency/intensity 653
interval training 653–4
modality and phases 653–4
progression 654
safety 652–3, 654–5
contraindications **655**
resistance *see* resistance/resistive training
strength exercises, cardiac rehabilitation 653
weight training, cardiac rehabilitation 653
exertional fatigue, heart failure 677
expiration, muscles 672
expressed prostatic secretion, prostatitis 1480
Extended Aged Care at Home (EACH) packages, Australia 1896
external anal sphincter 395–6
defecation 396
tone 395
external beam radiation therapy 1477–8
external fixation device, Paget's disease 1275
external ophthalmoplegia 944
Exton-Smith, *Professor* Norman 5
extracapsular hip fractures 1331, *1331*, 1333
extracellular fluid 1369
extracellular matrix (ECM), fibrous 619
extracellular space 1369
extrapyramidal motor symptoms (EPS) 1118
extrapyramidal system damage 843
extrinsic allergic alveolitis 716–7
eye
age related changes 39, **39**
movements, aging 745
eye disorders 1205–10
in Down's syndrome 1188
prevalence 1205, *1206*
vitamin A deficiency 332
vitamin E supplements 1671
see also entries beginning visual
eye drops, glaucoma 1208

facetectomy 995, 997
facial cooling, breathlessness 2009
facial nerve, taste 1250
facial pain
causes 267, 273, **273**, 274
psychogenic (atypical) 274
facial palsy 845, 1224–5, **1224**
facioscapulohumeral (FSH) muscular dystrophy 944, *944*
factor V Leiden 633
factor VIII
deficiency 439–40
increased levels 633
inhibitors, acquired 441
factor IX deficiency 439–40
"failure to thrive", tuberculosis 1740
fallopian tube, age related changes 1449
falls 1299–309
Alzheimer's disease 1086–7
assessment 1339–41, *1340*
clinical presentation 1302–4
consequences 1304–5
death 1304
delirium and physical restraints 1056
dementia and 1138
drop attacks 1302–3
drug induced 1304, 1696
antihypertensives 477
inappropriate medication use **220**
epidemiology 1299
extrinsic 1302
fear of 1300, 1304–5
foot problems 1301
fractures 1304–5
hip 1339–41, *1340*
future research 1308
hazard modification 1307
hazards causing 1302
at home 1299
intrinsic 1302, **1302**
"long lie" 1305
loss of consciousness 1303
management/prevention 1306–8
assistive devices 1308
day hospitals' role **1908**, 1909, 1910
exercise 1307
initiatives 1893
interdisciplinary assessment 233, *233*
medication 1307–8
NSF (UK) standard **1802**, 1917
restraints 1308, 1691–2, 1693
risk assessment 1544–5, **1545**
siderails 1692, 1693
orientation 1288
Parkinson's disease and 774–5
patient assessment 1305
posttraumatic subdural hematoma 1028
prevalence, nursing home care 1821
reflex actions 1288
rehabilitation 1306
risk factors 1288, **1288**, **1302**
sarcopenic obesity **921**
stroke patients 854
syncope and 883–4
falls clinics 1306
false ptyalism **273**
famciclovir 386, 895, 1594, 1732
familial hypercholesterolemia (FH) 615
familial motor neuron disease 951–2, 956
family history, back pain 1357
family structure, aging and 104
family therapy, drug misuse 1198
famotidine, arthritis 1350
farmer's lung 717
farnesyl diphosphate synthase 1294
farnesyl transferase inhibitors 460–1, 467, 469
fasciculation 746, 952, 954, 960
fasciocutaneous flaps 1624
faslodex, breast cancer 1514
fast twitch fibers 671
fasting 313
fast-tracking policy/guidelines 1332
fat (body)
abdominal, physical activity and 129
age related changes 347
caloric restriction 1669
exercise effect *see* exercise
redistribution 281
testosterone replacement therapy 120, 1423, 1675
fat (dietary)
absorption 42, 292
intake, heart disease risk factor 478
see also lipid(s)
"fat frail" 1568
fatigue 677, 2009
fat-specific insulin receptor knockout (FIRKO) 32
fatty acids, n-3 polyunsaturated 642
fatty liver, obesity 350
fatty streaks, atherosclerosis 611
Favre–Racouchot disease 1591, **1592**
fear, dental care 241
febrile response, diminished 1729, **1729**
fecal impaction 397, 413
fecal incontinence 395–406
causes 397, **397**
continence mechanism 396
diagnostic tests 399, **399**
drug induced 398
evaluation 398, **398**
history taking 398
physical examination 398–9
prevalence 396–7, **397**
risk factors 397, **397**
surgery induced 397
treatment 399–403, **399**, *400*
types 397–8
fecal mass examination 409
fecal occult bleeding, gastrointestinal bleeding 371
fecal occult blood testing 207
fecal retention 1053
fecal softeners 2008
feet *see* foot problems
female genital tract, age related changes 1449–50
female health issues 1659–64
female hypoactive sexual desire disorder 116–7
female sexual dysfunction (FSD) 115–7
doctor patient discussion failure 1662
hormonal changes 1662
management **117**, 1454
menopause/postmenopause 1416–7, 1661–2
pharmacological therapy 1454
physical changes 1662
prevalence 1661
psychological therapy 1454
psychosocial changes 1662
screening questions **1661**
femoral fractures 1270
femoral head cutout 1337, *1339*
femoral nerve block 1332
fenoprofen, arthritis 1350
fentanyl, renal failure 2005–6
ferritin 429, 430
FEV_1/FVC ratio, age related changes 696
fever 1729
infective endocarditis **1750**, 1756
ischemic stroke 819
pressure ulceration 1608
fever of unknown origin (FUO) 1729
fiber, constipation treatment 410
fibrates 615, 1440
fibrillary (immunotactoid) nephropathy 1503
fibrin, elevated 446
fibrin D-dimer 446, 447, 636, 1526
fibrinogen, depletion 446
fibrinogen degradation products (FDP), increased 446, 447
fibrinolysis, activation in DIC 445
fibroatheromas 611

fibroscope, spinal canal stenosis 994
fibrosing alveolitis 717–8
fibrotic lung disease 714–8
fila olfactoria 1250
financial abuse 184
finasteride 1472, 1475, 1512
fine-needle aspiration biopsy (FNAB), thyroid 1410
finitude 1682
  see also ethical issues
Finland
  community acquired pneumonia 665
  medical education/training 1784
Finnish Diabetes Study 132
A First-class service: quality in the new NHS 1827, 1875
fish oil (n-3 polyunsaturated fatty acid) 642
fissures, foot 1326
fistula
  arteriovenous *see* arteriovenous fistula
  labyrinthine 1238, 1240
  oro-antral 244
  vaginal discharge **1452**
fitness *see* physical fitness
5-day colon transit measurement 410, *410*
5q-syndrome 456, 468
five-chair rise 1305
flaccid paralysis, hyperkalemia 1383
flail arms motor neuron disease 950
flashes, hot *see* hot flashes
flecainide 504, 508
flexibility training, recommendations **137**
flexible bronchoscopy 1741–2
flexible sigmoidoscopy 399
"floating tabletop", radiology 1713, *1714*
flossing, teeth 249
flow volume loops, Parkinson's disease 676
flucinonide 266, 267
fluconazole
  meningitis 1771
  onychomycosis 1593
  oral candidosis 264, 2010
5-flucytosine, cryptococcal meningitis 1771
fludrocortisone 883, 892
fluid balance
  hip fractures 1332
  monitoring after stroke 819
  preoperative assessment 1637–8
fluid balance charts, dehydration assessment 325
fluid replacement therapy 325–6, **325**
  complications 325, 326
  hypernatremia 1382
  postoperative 1638
  subarachnoid hemorrhage 1023
fluorescein, chronic pancreatitis 420
fluorescent *in situ* hybridization (FISH) 456
fluorescent treponemal antibody absorption test (FTA-ABS) 1769
fluoride **341**
  mouthwash/topical 249
  osteoporosis 1291
fluoride gel 249
fluoroquinolones 1480, **1481**, 1767, 1768
5-fluorouracil, actinic keratosis 1601
5-fluorouracil, adriamycin and cytotax (FAC) 1536
5-fluorouracil, epirubicin and cyclophosphamide (FEC) 1536
fluoxetine 851, 1139, 1178
fluoxymesterone 315
flushing 1598
fluvoxamine 1178
foam cells (FC) 611, 616
foam dressings **1622**
focal atrophy (non-Alzheimer dementia) **1085**
focal dystonia 781–2, **782**, 783
α fodrin 32
folate/folic acid 337–8, **341**
  absorption 338
  aspiration pneumonia prevention 688
  deficiency 300, 338
  replacement 432
  stroke risk reduction 835–6
foley catheter use, nursing homes 1844
foliate papillae 1250
follicle-stimulating hormone (FSH) 1401, 1450
  perimenopausal period 1415, 1419
Folstein Mini-mental State 1545
Food and Drug Administration (FDA) (US) 1056, 1157
food intake
  changes over time 283–4, *283*
  frailty 1566–7
  obesity 348–9
  undernutrition 298–9
food refusal, dementia and 1144–5
food texture, dysphagia 845–6
foot drop, in MND 962
foot problems 1311–28
  associated risks **1312**
  bursitis 1325
  clinical assessment 1316–7
  dermatologic features **1321**
  diabetic neuropathy 893
  in Down's syndrome 1188
  endocrinopathies 1313–5
  falls and 1301
  fissures 1326
  joint diseases 1312–3, **1313**, **1314**, *1314*
  keratotic lesions 1317–24
  management 1326
  musculoskeletal findings *1314*, *1322*, **1323**, *1323*
  neurologic findings **1322**
  onychial findings **1321**, *1322*
  primary risk diseases **1312**
  secondary risk diseases **1313**
  toenails 1324–5
  ulceration risk **1323**, *1324*
  vascular findings **1317**
foot pumps, hip fractures 1332
footcare 1326–7
  peripheral vascular disease 627
footwear 1327
  bursitis 1325
  examination 1317
  fall prevention 1307
foraminectomy 994
forced expiratory volume in one second (FEV_1) 694
  FEV_1/FVC ratio 696
forced vital capacity (FVC) 676, 694
Fordyce's spots 263
forefoot problems 1317
forgetfulness 1039
  see also memory
fortified foods 288, 289
4 glass test, prostatitis 1480
Fox's sign, acute pancreatitis 418
fractional excretion of urea (FEU) 1498
fracture liaison nurse 1341
fractures
  age related risk **1282**
  falls 1304–5, 1306
  "fragility" **1287**, 1339
  osteoporosis *see* osteoporosis
  Paget's disease of bone 1270
  pathological 1525, 2007
  prevention, role of exercise 126–9
  risk 126, 1329
  see also specific bones (e.g. hip fractures)
"fragility" fracture **1287**, 1339
frail-old people 54
frailty 1565–70
  cardiovascular disease relationship 481
  causes *1566*
  definition 481, 1565, **1566**
  diseases resulting in 1565–6
  heart failure association 572
  oldest old 1156
  pathophysiology 279, *280*, 1565–9
  pathway *1566*
  preventive strategies **1570**
  renal tubules 1498–9
  testosterone replacement therapy 1423
  threshold 1565, *1566*
  tumor growth 1511
"frailty" gene 478
FRAMES, motivational interviewing in drug misuse 1198
Framingham Heart Study (FHS) 517, 541
  body weight and mortality 310, **310**
  cardiovascular disease as stroke risk factor 801
  diabetes and hypertension 1434
  hypertension as stroke risk factor 800
  obesity and mortality 310, **311**
  weight loss and mortality 312
France
  life expectancy **88**
  medical education/training 1785
  memory clinics 1062
  nursing home care **1822**
free flaps, pressure ulcers 1624
free hormone levels, age related changes 1390–1
free radicals *see* reactive oxygen species (ROS, free radicals)
free thyroxine (FT4) 1406
Frenchay Aphasia Screening Test 843
fresh frozen plasma infusion 373–4
friction, pressure ulcers 1607–8, *1608*, 1612
frictional keratosis 268
frontal bossing, Paget's disease 1271
frontal cortex, left, aphasia 1122
frontal lobe
  apraxic gait 1301
  weight changes in aging 69
"frontal release" signs, aging effect 747
frontotemporal dementia (FTD) 1121–2, **1122**
  apathetic 1121
  clinical features **1085**
  communication breakdown 1039, 1040
  diagnostic criteria 1136
frontotemporal lobular degeneration (FTLD) 1121–3
  frontotemporal dementia 1121–2, **1122**
  progressive nonfluent aphasia 1121, 1122–3
  semantic dementia 1121, 1123
frusemide (furosemide) 1378, 1499, 1522
frustrated phagocytosis, endocarditis 1754–5
"F-tags" 1820
fulminant liver failure, hepatitis A virus 383
function assessment scales 1553–63, 1575, **1575**
  disability *1555*, 1559–60, **1559**
  functional limitations 1558, **1559**
  health related quality of life 1560–2, **1560**, **1561**
  impairment 1557–8
  principles 1554–7
  theoretical framework 1553–4, *1554*, *1555*
functional capacity, noncardiac surgical patient 1634
functional decline/impairment 1689
  dementia and **1128**, 1129, 1137–8
Functional Index Measure (FIM) 1822
functional reach test 1306
fungal infections
  brain abscess *see* brain, abscess
  meningitis 1770–1
  otitis externa 1223
  terminally ill 2010
  toenails 1325
fungiform papillae 1250
funny turn, nonepileptic attacks 879
furosemide (frusemide) 1378, 1499, 1522

G proteins 556
GABA (gamma-aminobutyric acid) 62
GABAergic neurons **61**, 62
gabapentin
  cervical spinal canal stenosis 994
  epilepsy 874
  manic episodes, dementia and 1139
  neuropathic pain 987, 2007
  peripheral neuropathy in herpes zoster 895
  postherpetic neuralgia 987, 1594
  restless legs syndrome 781
  side effects 987
gag reflex 820, 845–6
gait 1300–2
  aging effect 747–8
  apraxic 1301
  muscle strength 1301
  reeducation 1306
  sarcopenic obesity **921**

testing, vestibular system disorders 1240
gait disorders/impairment
  lumbar spinal canal stenosis 996
  motor neuron disease 962
  normal pressure hydrocephalus 787–8, 792
  screening 206
  senile, gait pattern 1301
  vitamin E deficiency 333
galanin 303
galantamine 1088
gallbladder
  age related changes 292, 381
  diseases 388–90
  gangrene 389
  perforation 389
gallium nitrate 1276, 1523
gallstone ileus 389
gallstones 388–9
  acute pancreatitis 417, 419
  surgery 389, 419
gamma camera scanning 1718
Gamma nail 1335
gamma-aminobutyric acid (GABA), aging 62
gamma-knife radiotherapy 1401, 1513
gangrene
  gallbladder 389
  peripheral vascular disease 623
gas cooker monitors 194
gastric acid
  age related changes 42, 292
  reflux, tooth erosion 262
gastric angiodysplasia 372, 489
gastric distension 301–2, 364
gastric emptying 363
  age related changes 42, 302, 364
  appetite regulation 301
  delayed 364–5, **364**, 366
  measurement 363–4
  medications 364
gastric fundus 302, 363
gastric inhibitory peptide (GIP) 304
gastric motor function 363–5
  medication effects 364, **364**
gastric myoelectrical activity 978
gastric relaxation measurement 364
gastrinoma 421
gastritis
  alcohol association 160
  atrophic, vitamin B_{12} deficiency 285
  chronic, nutrient absorption 293, **293**
  gastrointestinal bleeding 372
gastroenteritis 1381, 1727
gastroesophageal reflux, aspiration pneumonia 689
gastroesophageal reflux disease (GERD) 363
  defenses against 358
  myotomy complication 360
  noncardiac chest pain 362
  predisposing factors 359
  symptoms and diagnosis 363
gastrointestinal angiodysplasia 372, 489
gastrointestinal bleeding 371–9
  acute 489
  aspirin, increased risk with 830
  causes 372–3, **372**
  clinical course/features 371–2
  drug history 375
  histological diagnosis 372–3, **373**
  history 374–5
  initial evaluation 373–4
  intravascular volume restoration 373–4
  lower tract **374**
    causes **373, 375**
    clinical presentation 371, **372**
    incidence 371
  management 373–7
  mortality 371, 450
  neoplastic lesions 373
  NSAIDs associated 450
  physical examination 375–6
  surgery 376
  ulcer bleeding 372, **372**
  underlying medical problems 371
  upper tract **374**
    causes **372, 375**
    clinical presentation 371, **372**
    incidence 371
    prevalence **375**
  variceal hemorrhage 377
gastrointestinal disease/disorders
  cardiac manifestations 489
  external beam radiation therapy and 1477–8
  functional 367–8
  neck pain 1363
gastrointestinal function 978
  motor *see* gastrointestinal motility
  sensory 357–69
gastrointestinal hemorrhage *see* gastrointestinal bleeding
gastrointestinal malignancies, in emergency room 1527
gastrointestinal motility 357–69
  control 357
  systemic disorders 365–7
  see also small intestine, motility
gastrointestinal tract
  age related changes 42, **42**, 292, 302, 408
    pathophysiology 357–8
  autonomic innervation 971, 978
  diabetic neuropathy features 892
  immobility effects **1690**
  interventional procedures 1720
  oncological emergencies 1527
  restraints effects **1690**
Gatterer, Edeltraut 1685
gaze stability 1239–40
GB virus type C (GBV-C) 384
gemcitabine, pancreatic cancer 422
gene therapy, lumbar spinal canal stenosis 997
gene(s)/genetics
  anomalies in glaucoma 1208
  contribution to aging process 13–4
  expression, aging 63
  heart disease risk factor 478
general anesthesia *see* anesthesia
General Assembly of Spitex 1864
general conversation, communication assessment 1041
General Health Questionnaire (GHQ) 863, 1811–2
General Household Survey, UK *170*
General Medical Council (GMC), UK 1789, **1790**, 1791
general practitioners (GPs)
  memory clinics *vs* 1063–4
  see also primary care
General *versus* local Anaesthetic for Carotid Surgery (GALA) study 836
generalized anxiety disorder (GAD) 1149, 1153
generalized epilepsy 871–2, 873
genetic testing
  Huntington's disease 1125
  predictive, ethical issues 1687
Geneva Medical School 1784, **1784**
genfitinib 1515
geniculate herpes 761
genital herpes 1732
genital prolapse 1449
genital tract, female, age related changes 1449–50
genitourinary system
  dysfunction in diabetic neuropathy 892
  effects of restraints **1690**
genuine stress incontinence (GSI) 1453
geotranscendence, depression 1176
geriatric assessment 1801
  ADLs *see* activities of daily living (ADLs)
  Alzheimer's disease 1088
  functional *see* function assessment scales
  health promotion 1801
  history 1544
  IADLs *see* instrumental activities of daily living (IADL) Scale
  interdisciplinary
    falls prevention 233, *233*
    problem-orientated 227–8, *228*, 230
    stroke rehabilitation 233, *233*
  multidimensional 1543–52
    components 1544–5, **1545**
    effectiveness 1547–50
    rationale 1543–4
    settings 1545–7
  multidisciplinary 1790, 1791
    problem-orientated 225, *225*, 227–8, 230–1
  primary care 1800–1
    see also specific countries
  problem-orientated 223–36
    categories 226–30
    evaluation 232–4, *233*
    implementation 230–2
    nurse role 231
    rationale 223–4
  psychiatric *see* psychiatric services
  psychological *see* clinical psychology services
  rehabilitation process 1574–6, **1575**
  screening tools *see* screening tools/programs
geriatric day hospitals *see* day hospitals
Geriatric Depression Scale (GDS) 206, 863, 984, 1150, **1575**
  dementia 1129
  depression 1177
  Down's syndrome 1186
  Japanese version 1938
Geriatric Evaluation and Management Unit (GEMU) 1847, 1928, 1936
Geriatric Hip Fracture Service 1343
geriatric medical education/training *see* medical education/training
geriatric orthopedic rehabilitation unit 1342–3
Geriatric Rehabilitation Following Fractures in Older People 1343
geriatric research 1926–7
Geriatric Research, Education and Clinical Centers (GRECCs) 1902, 1925, 1930
geriatric services 6
  see also specific countries; *specific services (e.g. memory clinics)*
Geriatric Society of India 1990
geriatric syndrome 1940
geriatrician, memory clinics 1064
Geriatrics 1
germ cell tumors, female 1456
Germany
  life expectancy **88**
  medical education/training 1784, 1785
germinal centers 21, *22*
Geronte visual communication device 1824, *1825*
gerontological evaluation *see* geriatric assessment
gerontological nurse practitioners 1931
Gerontological Society of America 2, 1924
"geropsychiatric" medications, delirium etiology 1050
Get up and go Test 1306
getting lost, dementia and 1143
ghrelin 304–5
  aging 1393, **1393**
  muscle mass 1568
  obesity 304, 348–9
  resistance 304
ghrelin analog replacement 1402
giant cell arteritis 274, 757, 1007
gingivae
  age related changes 262
  disorders 262–3
  enlargement 262
  hemorrhages 262
  recession 240, 248, 262
gingivitis
  chronic 262–3
  desquamative 265
  Down's syndrome 1188
Ginkgo biloba 1069
ginseng, menopausal symptoms and 1420
Girdlestone hip 1337
GISSI trial 521
Glandosane (Fresenius) sprays 272
Glanzmann's thrombasthenia 439
glare, eye 1205, 1209
Glasgow Coma Score (GCS) 1029
Glasgow Criteria, acute pancreatitis 419

Glasgow Hearing Aid Benefit Profile 1216
glasses, importance of maintenance 1043
glaucoma 1207–8
  angle closure 759
  associated factors **1208**
  facial pain 274
  headache and 759
  open-angle 759, 1207
  prevalence *1206*
  risk factors **1208**
  treatment 1208
Gleason grading system, prostate cancer 1475
glial fibrillary acidic protein (GFAP) 76
glial-derived neurotrophic factor (GDNF) 958
glibenclamide, contraindications 1436
gliosis 76, 956
global deterioration scale (GDS) 1040–1, **1040**, **1041**
Global Initiative for Chronic Obstructive Lung Disease (GOLD) guidelines 727, 729
globus pallidum (GPi), deep brain stimulation 783
glomerular filtration rate (GFR)
  age related changes 430, 978, 1495–6
  cardiovascular disease and 489
glomerular sclerosis 1495, 1499
glomerulonephritis 1502–3
  crescentic 1503
glomerulopathies, primary 1502–3
glomerulosclerosis, intercapillary 1502
glomus jugulare 1228
glomus tympanicum 1228
glossopharyngeal nerve, taste 1250
glossopharyngeal neuralgia, headache and 761, **761**
GLT-1, oxidative damage 64
glucagon, barium meal 1716
glucagon-like peptide-1 (GLP-1) 304
glucagonoma 421
glucocorticoids
  age related hippocampal damage 41
  effect on skeletal muscle 38
  excess 1283, 1289
  hypercalcemia of malignancy 1522
glucosamine, osteoarthritis 1350
glucose
  control, diabetic neuropathy 893
  hyperkalemia therapy 1383
  regulation 1436–7, *1445*
  utilization changes in heart failure 564
glucose, blood
  control, diabetes management 134
  fasting 208
glucose tolerance
  idiopathic peripheral neuropathy 897
  impaired 350, 1434
glucose-6-phosphate dehydrogenase deficiency 431, 959
glue aortoplasty, aortic dissection 1006
GLUT1 and GLUT4 563
glutamate, in MND 957–8
glutamate antagonist, riluzole 963
γ-glutamylcarboxylase 337
glutaraldehyde cross-linked collagen injections 403
glutathione 39
glutathione peroxidase 334
glutathione reductase assay 336
gluteus maximus transposition 403
glycerin suppositories, constipation 412
glycerol injection, trigeminal neuralgia 760
glycoprotein IIb/IIIa antagonist 520
glycopyrrolate 960
glycoxidation 16
Goal Planning Process 861
  patient-centered 865, 1576
gold salts, oral ulceration due to 266
Golytely 376
gonad function 1422–9
gonadotrophin releasing hormone (GnRH) 1401, 1450
  agonists/antagonists 1478
gonadotrophins, secretion 1401
gonorrhea (GC) 1732
Good Medical Practice 1791
Gore-Tex chordae 602–3
Goulstonian lectures 744
gout **1313**, 1348–9
  chronic tophaceous **1313**, 1348
  treatment 1351–2
Gracely Box Scale (GBS) 984
graciloplasty, fecal incontinence 403
Gradenigo's syndrome 1225
grammar application 1038
  Alzheimer's disease 1039, 1040
  assessment 1041
  dementia 1039–40
gram-negative bacilli, aerobic 1764, 1773
"granny battering" *see* elder abuse
granular myringitis 1223
granulocyte colony-stimulating factor (G-CSF) 465
  acute leukemia therapy 467
  myelodysplasia therapy 458–9, 469
granulocyte-macrophage colony-stimulating factor (GM-CSF)
  acute leukemia therapy 467
  myelodysplasia therapy 459
granulocytes 19, 26–7
granulosa cell tumor 1456
granulovacuolar degeneration 72–3, *73*
Graves' disease 1411
Graves' ophthalmopathy, myopathy 942
gray matter, aging neuropathology 70–5
"the great imitator" 1031
Greater Cincinnati and Northern Kentucky Stroke Study 803
Greece
  health expenditure 1978
  medical education/training 1785
Green bottle (*Lucilia sericata*) 1620
GRETA trial 1535
Grey Turner's sign 418
group therapy, drug misuse 1198
group training, memory clinic patients 1068
growth factors
  motor neuron disease 958
  myelodysplasia therapy 458–9
  pressure ulcers 1625–6
growth hormone (GH) 1393, **1393**, 1674–5
  cardiovascular features 489
  muscle mass 1568
  recombinant human (rhGH) 642–3
  secretion, age related changes 1402, 1674
growth hormone releasing hormone (GHRH) 28
growth hormone supplementation 1402, 1670, 1674–5
  aging acceleration 1675
  cancer risk 1675
  muscle mass 1674
  sarcopenia 923, 924
  side effects 1393, 1675
growth inhibitory factor 1937
guardrails *see* siderails
Guillain–Barré syndrome (GBS) 679, 895, 953, 972
gums *see* gingivae
gustatory system 1250–1, *1251*
  age related changes 1252, *1253*, 1256
  dysfunction *see* taste dysfunction
  functional tests 1251–2
gut function, age related changes 978
gut-brain-gut axis 971
guttate psoriasis 1597
gynecological cancer 1455–6
gynecology 1449–58
  common symptoms 1451, **1451**
  hormonal changes 1450
  problems, in Down's syndrome 1188
gyri, aging neuropathology 69

H2 blockers, delirium etiology 1050
habit training
  fecal incontinence 399
  urinary incontinence 1489
Hachinski Ischemic Score 1103
Haemophilus influenzae see Hemophilus influenzae
hair cells 1235, *1236*
Hallpike maneuver 1239, *1239*, 1242
hallucinations 1139
  Alzheimer's disease 1140
  dementia and 1139–41
  Parkinson's disease 774
  treatment 1140
hallux valgus *1314*, *1322*
halobetasol, scabies 1595
haloperidol
  cerebrovascular event risk 1157
  confusion 2010
  delirium 1056–7
  dementia, delusions/hallucinations in 1140
  nausea/vomiting 2008
  postoperative confusion 1650
Hamilton Depression Rating Scale 1860
hammertoes *1314*, *1322*
hand dexterity impairment 993
hand weakness 962–3
handicap 1911
  ICIDH definition 852, 1571
handwashing 689, 1729
Harvard Alumni Health Study 650
Hasegawa Dementia Scale (HDS) 1938
Hasegawa Dementia Scale-Revised (HDS-R) 1938, **1938**
Hashimoto's thyroiditis *31*
HDL-Atherosclerosis study 1671, 1672, 1673
head and neck neoplasms 1528
head and neck radiation 1411
head trauma
  bacterial meningitis 1764
  carotid dissection 806
  diabetes insipidus 1374–5
  Parkinson's disease 769
  smell loss 1254
  subdural hematoma after 1027, 1028
headache 751–63
  brain tumor 1527
  cerebrovascular disease and 757
  cervical spine disorder and 759, **759**
  chronic cluster 756–7, **756**
  chronic daily 755–6, **756**
  chronic subdural hematoma 1030
  classification 751, **752**
  clinical description 751–2
  cluster *see* cluster headache
  diagnosis 751–2, **752**
  giant cell arteritis and 757
  glaucoma associated 759
  glossopharyngeal neuralgia 761, **761**
  hypnic 757, **757**
  mass lesion associated 758
  medication induced 759
  migraine *see* migraine
  Parkinson's disease and 758–9
  pituitary adenomas 1400
  postherpetic neuralgia 761–3, **761**, *762*
  posttraumatic (PTH) 759
  prevalence 751, **752**
  primary 751, 752–7
  secondary 751, 757–9
  sinusitis associated 759
  subarachnoid hemorrhage 1016–7
  subdural empyema 1773
  tension-type *see* tension-type headache
  trigeminal neuralgia 759–61, **759**, *760*, **760**
Heaf skin test 709
Health Advisory Service (HAS), UK 8, 1920
Health and Retirement Survey 1434
Health and Social Care Act, UK (2001) 1918
Health care Accreditation Programme (HAP), UK 1845
Health Care Financing Administration, USA 1856
Health Care Financing Service 1691
health counseling, Down's syndrome 1186
health information systems, medical records *see* patient records
Health Maintenance Clinical Guidepath 201–9, 207–8
  categories of older persons 202, **203–4**
  details **203–4**, 204–9
  office visits 203
The Health of the Elderly at Home 3

Health Outcomes Survey (HOS), USA 1560, **1560**
health policy, primary care, UK 1799–801
Health Professionals Follow-up Study 802
health promotion
  geriatric assessment 1801
  NSF (UK) standard **1802**, 1803, 1894, 1917–8
  primary care, UK 1803, **1804**
  for successful aging *202*
Health Quality Service (HQS), UK 1845
health related quality of life (HRQoL) 1560–2, **1560**, **1561**
  see also quality of life
health status, life expectancy prediction 202
health-care audit *see* clinical audit
Healthcare Commission, UK 187, 1839, 1920, 1921
"Health-Care Guidelines for Individuals with Down Syndrome" 1186
health-care setting, alcohol problem prevalence 158
health-care systems *see specific countries*
Healthy Active Life Expectancy (HALE) 233
Healthy Diet Index (HDI) **285**, 286
healthy diet scores 286–7
  cluster analysis 286, **286**
healthy eating
  cardiac rehabilitation strategy 649–50
  mortality 286–7, *287*
Healthy Eating Index (HEI) **285**, 286
hearing
  acoustics 1219–20
  aging effect 745
  assessment in dementia 1043
  mean thresholds *1226*
hearing aids 1230–2
  air conducting 1230–1
  "behind the ear" 1231, *1231*
  bone anchoring 1232
  bone conducting 1230, 1232
  candidature 1231–2
  digital 1231
  earmolds 1230
  importance of maintenance 1043
  "in the canal" 1231
  "in the ear" 1231
  modular 1231
  patient expectations 1231
  provision 1215–6
  provision thresholds 1213
  settings 1231
  volume control 1231
hearing disorders
  epidemiology 1211–8
  predictions 1214, *1214*
  prevalence 1212–5, *1213*, *1215*
  rehabilitation 1216–7
  research requirements 1217
  service provision 1215–6
  see also hearing loss/impairment
Hearing Level Scale (dB HL) 1219–20
hearing loss/impairment 1222–32
  adaptations 1230
  age related 1225–7, *1226*
  amplification methods 1230–2
  assistive devices 1886
  asymmetrical 1227–8
  autoimmune 1228
  communication effect 841–2
  conductive *see* conductive deafness
  Down's syndrome 1187
  heart failure association 572
  management 1230–2
  measurement 1220–2
  morbidity, India 1984
  patterns 1227–8
  prevalence 841
  progressive bilateral 1227
  screening 1545
  sensorineural 1225–8, 1229
  statistics 1231, *1232*
  sudden 1228
  traumatic 1228
  ventriculoperitoneal shunt, following 792
  see also hearing disorders
heart
  aging *see* cardiac aging
  conducting system 494
    fibrosis 487, 493
  manifestations of systemic disease 488–90
  sounds, physiological tinnitus 1228
  see also entries beginning cardiac
Heart and Estrogen/Progestin Replacement Study (HERS) 115–6, 1418, 1419, 1676
Heart and Estrogen/Progestin Replacement Study Follow-up (HERS II) 1419, 1661
heart block *see* atrioventricular (AV) block
heart disease
  congenital *see* congenital heart disease
  dementia relationship 481
  in diabetes mellitus 152
  epidemiology 475–85, *476*, 647–8
  frailty relationship 481
  hypertension 151
  ischemic *see* ischemic heart disease
  Paget's disease of bone 1271
  prevention 481–2, *483*
  rheumatic *see* rheumatic heart disease
  risk factors 475–6
    see also under ischemic heart disease
  screening 1911
  secondary prevention 482, 648, 649–50
    see also cardiac rehabilitation
  smoking and 151–2
  valvular *see* valvular heart disease
  see also cardiovascular disease (CVD)
heart failure 567–83
  acute 1633–4, 2009
  chronic 555–66, 647
    aerobic training 656–7
    body composition 640
    cardiac cachexia 639–40
    cardiac rehabilitation 658
    exercise training 655
    neuroendocrine abnormalities 641–2, *641*
    prognosis 640, *640*
  clinical features 555, 569–73
  comorbidities 570–2, **571**
    hospital admissions due to 572, *573*
    prevalence 572, *572*
  congestive *see* congestive heart failure
  diagnosis 569–70
  diastolic 480, 487, 567–8
    management 576
    risk factors **480**
  diastolic ventricular interaction 564–5
  end-stage 578
  epidemiology 479, 480, 567
  etiology and precipitants 570, **570**, 573
  humoral alterations 557–60
  inappropriate medication use **220**
  LV remodeling *see* left ventricle, remodeling
  management 501, 555, 573–8
    beta-blockers 557, 574–5
    day hospitals' role 1910, 1911
    device therapy 576–7
    end of life 578
    exercise 577–8
    future prospects 579, **579**
    goals 573
    multidisciplinary care 577
    pharmacotherapy 573–6
    of precipitating factors 573
  mechanisms 555–66
  molecular/cellular adaptations 562–5
    altered gene expression 563–4
    altered myocardial energetics 564
    excitation–contraction coupling 562–3, *562*
    skeletal muscle changes 564, *564*
  mortality and causes 577, 578
  in myocardial infarction, management 586–7
  neural adaptations 555–7
  nonvalvular atrial fibrillation risk 497–8
  nutrition association 490
  pathophysiology 567–8
  prevention 578–9
  prognosis 578
  as progressive disorder 555
  renal conditions associated 489
  in respiratory diseases 489
  respiratory muscle weakness 677
  right-sided 589
  signs and symptoms 569
  systolic 480
    management 574–6, *576*
    risk factors **480**
  valvular heart disease with 573
Heart Outcomes Prevention Evaluation (HOPE) study 334, 832, 1420
Heart Protection Study 518, 834, *834*, *835*
heart rate
  aging effect 487, 530, 568, 975
  analysis 975
  in atrial fibrillation *see* atrial fibrillation (AF)
  exercise training in cardiac rehabilitation 653
  response to stress 530
  variability, autonomic control 974–5, *975*
heart valves
  age related changes 530–1
  bioprosthetic 587, 589, 603, 604
    anticoagulation for 605
    "first-generation" and "third-generation" 603, 605
  disease *see* valvular heart disease
  endothelium, endocarditis 1753–4
  mechanical 603
    anticoagulation for 605
  replacement 532, 600–3
    see also under cardiac surgery; valvular heart disease
  see also specific heart valves
heartburn 363
heart-lung machine 607
heat intolerance, medication induced 977
heat related deaths 112, *977*
  prevention **112**
heat shock proteins 619
  HSP70, centenarians 1704
"heat stress days" 977
heat stroke 977
heat therapy 994, 997
heavy metal screening, peripheral neuropathy 891
hedonistic homeostatic dysregulation (HDD) 1119
heel cups, bursitis 1325
heel protectors 1612, *1612*
Heidelberg Centenarian Study 1701
height, measurement 205
Helicobacter pylori infection 159, 363, 367, 489
  gastric cancer 93
heloma durum (corn) 1321–3
heloma miliare (seed corns) 1323
heloma molle (soft corns) 1323
heloma neurovascular 1317, 1322
Help the Aged 1874
Helsinki Aging Brain Study 1106
Helsinki Aging Study 549
hematemesis 371, 374
hematochezia, hemorrhoids 377
hematological emergencies 1525–6
hematoma *see individual hematomas*
hematopoietic growth factors, myelodysplasia 458–9
hematopoietic stem cells (HSCs) 23
  transplantation *see* stem cell transplantation
hematuria 1470–1
hemiarthroplasty, hip fractures *1334*, 1335, 1337
hemifield slide phenomenon 1398
hemiparesis, carotid artery stenosis 806
hemiplegic motor neuron disease 950
hemiplegic shoulder 856
hemispheric ischemic stroke 678
hemochromatosis, secondary 458
hemodialysis 1500–1
  hyperkalemia 1384
hemoglobin
  anemia definition 427
  DIC diagnosis 446
  increased by recombinant erythropoietin 433
  structural defects, anemia 430–1
  subtypes 430, 431

hemoglobin (*cont.*)
  synthesis defects, anemia 431
hemoglobin H (Hb H) disease 431
hemoglobinopathies 430–1
hemoglobinuria, paroxysmal nocturnal 432
hemolysis, autoimmune 431, **432**
hemolytic anemia 430
  autoimmune 431–2, **432**
  microangiopathic 446
hemophilia A/B 439–40
hemophiliacs, HIV/AIDS 1731
Hemophilus influenzae 707
  meningitis 1764, 1765, **1766**, 1767
  otitis media 1223
hemopoiesis 465, *466*
hemoptysis 708, 716, 1521–2
hemorrhage
  anticoagulant-associated *see* anticoagulants/anticoagulation
  bronchial, pulmonary neoplasm 1521
  carotid artery, tumor erosion 1528
  in chronic pancreatitis 420
  emergency embolization 1720
  gastrointestinal *see* gastrointestinal bleeding
  radical prostatectomy complication 1477
  see also bleeding
hemorrhagic spots, foot 1321
hemorrhagic stroke 802–3, 821
hemorrhoids, internal 375
hemosiderin 818, 1315, 1598
hemosiderinuria 432
hemostasis abnormalities/disorders 437–44
  stroke risk 802
  vitamin C deficiency 335
hemostatic system 445
Henoch–Schönlein purpura 441
heparin
  acquired coagulation defects 440
  arrhythmias after myocardial infarction 587
  deep vein thrombosis 636
  DIC and 447
  low-molecular weight *see* low-molecular-weight heparin
  prophylaxis, hip fractures 1332
  pulmonary embolic disease 636, 714
  ST elevated myocardial infarction 521
  stroke, following 820
  thromboembolic prophylaxis 1642
  venous thrombosis 442, 636
heparin induced thrombocytopenia (HIT) 438
hepatic disease 381–8
hepatic encephalopathy 1126
hepatitis 381–6
  acute alcoholic 386
  autoimmune *see* autoimmune hepatitis
  chronic 386
  drug induced 384–5, 386, 1743
  vaccinations 383, 386, *387*
  viral 381–4
    geographical distribution *382*
    screening 385
hepatitis A virus (HAV) 381–2
  geographical distribution *382*
  symptoms 383
  vaccination 383, *387*
hepatitis B virus (HBV) 383
  geographical distribution *382*
  hepatocellular carcinoma 388
  transmission 383
  treatment 386
  vaccination *387*
hepatitis C virus (HCV) 383
  alcohol association 159–60
  geographical distribution *382*
  hepatocellular carcinoma 388
  prevalence 383, 1156
  treatment 386
hepatitis D virus (HDV) 383
  coinfection 383
  superinfection 383
hepatitis E virus (HEV) 383–4
hepatitis F virus (HFV) 383
hepatitis G virus (HGV) 384
hepatocellular carcinoma (HCC) 388
hepatocytes, age related changes 381
herbal medications
  alcohol interaction 161
  medication review 205
  menopausal symptoms 1419–20
  psychiatric disorder induction 1154
herceptin 1515
hereditary hemorrhagic telangiectasia 441
hereditary motor neuropathies 954
Hereditary Motor Sensory Neuropathy (HMSN) type II 889, 897
Hereditary Neuropathy with Liability to Pressure Palsies (HNPP) 889
hereditary spastic paraparesis 953
hereditary spherocytosis 431
hernia, hiatus 359
heroin 1192, 1193
herpes simplex virus (HSV) infections
  encephalitis 1775
  lips 267
  meningitis 1763
  type 2 (HSV-2), genital 1732
herpes zoster (shingles) 895, 1593–4, *1593*, *1594*
  diagnosis 1594, *1594*
  disseminated 1594
  encephalitis 1775–6
  epidemiology 1727
  ophthalmic involvement 1594
  oral lesions 267
  peripheral neuropathy 895
  postherpetic neuralgia 761
  trigeminal 267
herpes zoster oticus 267, 1240
Hertz (Hz) 1219
hexamethylene bisacetamide 459
hiatus hernia 359
hiccups 678, 2011
hierarchical balance test 1557
high-density lipoprotein (HDL) cholesterol 518, 614, 802
highly active antiretroviral therapy (HAART) 1456, 1732
hip arthroplasty/replacement 1335, *1632*
  Paget's disease of bone 1277
hip fractures 1282, 1329–45
  basal 1331
  classification 1330–1, *1331*
  delayed diagnosis 1329–30
  diagnosis 1329–30
  displaced 1331, 1334–5, **1335**
  fall assessment 1339–41, *1340*
  fast-tracking policy/guidelines 1332
  imaging 1330, *1330*
  incidence, physical activity effect 126
  initial management 1331–3
  intracapsular 1331, *1331*
  male:female fracture ratio 1285
  medical care 1338–42
  mortality 1286, **1286**
  muscle loss 919
  nonunion 1333, 1335, 1337
  operative care 1333–5, *1334*, *1336*
  osteoporosis 1285
  postoperative care 1335–8
  preoperative nutrition 1639
  pressure ulcers 1609
  redisplacement 1337, *1337*
  repair 1333–5
  risk 1329
  secondary fracture prevention 1338–42
  smokers 152
  stable/unstable 1331
  surgical complications 1337–8, *1337*, *1338*, *1339*
  treatment costs 1329
  undisplaced 1330, 1331, 1333–4
  vitamin K deficiency 337
  wound healing complications 1337
hip protectors 1293, 1308, 1341, 1696
hippocampus
  aging, neurochemistry **61**
  aging neuropathology 71, 72, *72*
  Alzheimer's disease 1074
  neuronal loss/shrinkage 70
  spatial disorientation 1143
Hirano bodies 72, *72*, 956
Hirayama disease 949, 952–3
  see also motor neuron disease (MND)
histone deacetylase inhibitors 460
history-taking, difficulties 1357
HIV encephalopathy 1731–2
HIV infection 1456–7, 1731–2
  developing countries 1968
  doctor–patient discussion failures 1457
  incidence in elderly people 1457
  infective endocarditis 1750–1
  malignancy in 1731
  meningitis 1763, 1768, 1769
  motor neuron disease and 958
  opportunistic infections 1457
  prevention 1732
  risk factors 1456–7
  transfusion related 1731
  treatment 1732
  see also AIDS
HIV-associated dementia (HAD) 1126
HMG-CoA reductase inhibitors *see* statins
Hobson, *Professor* William 3
Hodgkin's disease, lung 713
Hoffman's reflex 993
Holland nail 1335
holocaust survivors 1951
Home and Community Care Act, Australia (1985) 1895
home care 5
  Alzheimer's disease 1089–90
  delirium and 1048, 1054
  quality issues 1847–8
  technological aids 1847–8
  see also specific countries
Home Health Quality Initiative, USA 1847
home help, Alzheimer's disease 1089
home nurse, Alzheimer's disease 1089
homeless population, mental health care 1158
homeothermy *see* temperature control
homocysteine 338
  muscle mass 1569
  peripheral vascular disease risk 624
  stroke risk 802, 835–6, *836*
  in vitamin B_{12}/folate deficiencies 339, 429
homocysteine theory 93–4
homocystinuria, homozygous 633
homonymous hemianopia 851
homophobia 121
homosexuals 120–1
Hong Kong 1971
Honolulu Heart Program 519, 801
Honolulu-Asia Aging Study 131
HOPE (Heart Outcomes Prevention Evaluation) study 522, 576
hormonal therapy, cancer 1513–4
hormone(s)
  anorexia of aging 301–5, **301**
  antiaging therapy **1667**, 1668, 1674–7
  appetite regulation 301–5, *301*
  energy homeostasis regulation 348–9, *349*
  fountain of youth 1392–4
  heart disease risk factor 478
  regulation
    aging 1389–91, **1391**
    feedback systems 1389, *1390*
  sarcopenia 916–8
  secretion, age related changes 43–4
hormone postreceptor responsiveness 1391
hormone receptor responsiveness 1391
hormone replacement therapy (HRT) 1419, 1450–1, 1661, 1676
  breast cancer risk 1450–1, 1533
  cancer development risk 1676
  cardiovascular disease 1451
  chemosensory dysfunction 1257
  endometrial cancer 1451
  ischemic heart disease and 523, 1419
  osteoporosis 1294, 1450, 1676
  sarcopenia 923–5

spinal cord ischemia 1003
vasomotor symptom relief 1450
venous thromboembolism 1451
horn cysts 1599, *1600*
Horner's syndrome 972
hosiery, footcare 1326
hospice care 2013–4
motor neuron disease 964
see also palliative/end-of-life care
hospital acquired pneumonia *see* nosocomial pneumonia
Hospital Advisory Service (HAS) (UK) 8
Hospital Anxiety and Depression Scale (HADS) 863
hospital care/hospitalization
acute *see* acute care
alcohol related 158
delirium management 1054–6
delirium prevalence 1152
dental care provisions 257
elder abuse 187
mental health services 1158
MND, final stages 964
NSF (UK) standard 1898
see also specific countries
Hospital In Patient Enquiry (HIPE), UK 7
Hospital Stroke Aphasic Depression Questionnaire (SADQ) 863
"hospital-at-home" schemes (UK) 232
hospital-at-home teams 701
hospitalization at home 1090
hospitalization in medium- or long-stay units 1090
host defense systems 19
see also immune system
hot and cold therapy 994
hot flashes 115, 1416, 1450, 1660–1
management 1419
rapid eye movement sleep 1418
HOT Study, diabetic treatment targets **1437**
House of Lords, physician-assisted suicide 965
housebound, oral health 241
housing problems 106–8, **107**, 229–30
Howell, Trevor 4, 1891
hugging, Down's syndrome 1185
human immunodeficiency virus (HIV) *see* HIV infection
human metapneumovirus 668
human papilloma virus 16 (HPV-16) 269, 1455
human papilloma virus 18 (HPV-18) 269, 1455
human T lymphotropic virus 1 (HTLV 1) 958
humoral immunity 21, 1590
Hungary, medical education/training 1785
huntingtin 778
huntingtin gene 47
Huntington's disease (chorea: HD) 777–80, 1125
aging effect on motor systems 47
dementia 777
dopamine levels 61
early-/late-onset 777
nigrostriatal neuron loss 61
predictive genetic testing 1687
psychiatric features 777, 778
treatment 778
Hutchinson's sign 1594
hydralazine, heart failure therapy 574
hydrocephalus
acute, subarachnoid hemorrhage 1021, *1021*
normal pressure *see* normal pressure hydrocephalus (NPH)
pineal cysts 78
stroke, following 820
hydrochlorothiazide 547
hydrocolloids 1622, **1622**
hydrocortisone 275, 1769
hydrofibre dressings 1622, **1622**
hydrogels 1622, **1622**
hydrogen breath tests 365
hydrogen peroxide 26
hydrotherapy, chronic pain 988
3-hydroxy-3-methylglutaryl coenzyme A (HMG CoA) 613
3-hydroxy-3-methylglutaryl coenzyme A (HMG CoA) reductase 613
inhibitors *see* statins
hydroxychloroquine 1351
5-hydroxytryptamine *see* serotonin (5-hydroxytryptamine (5-HT))
25-hydroxyvitamin D (25-OHD) 336, 917, 1262, *1262*
hyoscine 960
hyper fractionated radiation therapy 1513
hyperaldosteronism 544
hyperbaric oxygen therapy 1005
hypercalcemia
acute confusion 2009
of malignancy 1276, 1522–3
management 1276, 2009
oncological emergency 1522–3
Paget's disease of bone 1271
polyuria induced by 324
hypercementosis, teeth 244
hypercholesterolemia 617
familial 615
hyperfibrinolysis 446
hyperfiltration theory 43
hyperglycemia 420, 819, 893, 1432
hyperglycemic hyperosmolar nonketotic (HONK) coma 1433
hyperhomocysteinemia 338, 633
hyperkalemia 1383–4, 1497
hyperkeratosis 1320
nail groove 1325
hyperlipidemia 219
hypernatremia 1380–2, 1496
causes 1373, 1381
essential 1372, 1374, 1381–2
hypertonic dehydration 325
water depletion 1637
hyperopia, aging 745
hyperosmolar states 1370
hyperparathyroidism 943, 1289
hyperphosphaturia 1497
hyperpigmentation 1591, **1592**
hyperprolactinemia 1400
hyperreflexia 787
hypersalivation (ptyalism) 272–3, **273**
hypersecreting pituitary adenomas 1398, 1399
hypertension 541–54
alcohol association 160
assessment/risk stratification 546–7
carotid artery stenosis 808
chronic, orthostatic hypotension and 546
diabetics 1438
diagnosis 545–6, 1438
diastolic 490, 517
essential 541–2, 973
heart disease risk factor 476–7
heart failure associated 570, 573
prevention 573, 578
hemorrhagic stroke 821
high-risk group, management 546
inappropriate medication use **220**
incidence, developing countries 1970, 1993
intermittent office (IOH) 545
ischemic heart disease risk 476–7, 517–8, 519
isolated systolic (ISH) 477, 517, 541
management 551
low-risk group, management 546
morbidity, India 1984
nonvalvular atrial fibrillation 497–8
obesity 350
pathophysiology 542–3
peripheral vascular disease risk 624, 626
prevalence 541–2
pulmonary 729
renal damage 1501–2
risk factors 546–7
secondary 544–5, 973
sexual activity 120
stroke risk 795, 800–1, 819, 832, *833*
subarachnoid hemorrhage risk 1016
systolic 517
systolic–diastolic (SDH) 541–2
treatment 518, 550–1
benefits 551
stroke risk reduction 798, 822
treatment, clinical trials 547–50
trial characteristics **547**
trial results **548**
very old subjects 549–50
underprescribing 1805
very old subjects 549–50
vitamin C supplements 1673
vitamin E supplements 1671
weight loss 313
white-coat 545
see also blood pressure
Hypertension Detection and Follow-up Program (HDFP) 542
hyperthermia 977
hyperthermic ablation, atrial fibrillation 606
hyperthyroidism (thyrotoxicosis) 1408–9
apathetic 1391, 1408
clinical features 489–90, **1408**
diagnosis 1411
myopathy 942
patient referrals 1409
secondary hypertension due to 545
subclinical 489, 1409
thyrotropin-secreting tumors 1401
treatment strategy 1409
hypertonic dehydration 324–5
hypertonic sodium chloride 1379–80
hypertriglyceridemia 518, 1392
hyperuricemia, prevention 467
hyperventilation, stroke 678
hyperventilation attacks 884
hyperviscosity syndrome 1525
hypervitaminosis A 333
hypnic headache 757, **757**
hypnogram 734, *735*
hypnotic drugs
Alzheimer's disease 1087
dementia 1145, **1145**
insomnia 739, **739**
use in institutions 736
hypoalbuminemia 385
hypodermis 37
hypodermoclysis 326
hypodipsia 322–3, 1372, 1374
hypogastric arteries 1001
hypogeusia 1249
hypoglycemia 871, 885
hypogonadism
anemia association 428
Down's syndrome 1187
erectile dysfunction 117
male *see* andropause
obesity 350–1
pituitary adenoma 1399
prevalence 924
screening 206
secondary 118, 1401
hypokalemia 1384–5, 1497
myasthenia gravis 904
hyponatremia 1375–80, 1496
brain damage 1375
chronic 1375–7
clinical features 1375–7, **1375**, *1376*
congestive heart failure *1375*, 1378
drug induced conditions 1378
in heart failure 558
incidence/prevalence 1375
malignancy-associated 1379
management 1379–80
oncological emergency 1523
postoperative *1376*, 1377, *1377*
transient 1636
prophylactic measures 1379–80
risk factors 1375, *1376*
SSRI risk 1179
total body water estimation 1380
vasopressin 1370
hyponatremic encephalopathy 1375, 1379–80
hypoosmolar states, brain response 1370
hypopituitarism 1399, **1399**, 1400
hypopnea 737
hyposmia 1249

hypotension
  gastrointestinal bleeding 373
  ischemic stroke and 819
  orthostatic (postural, positional) 545–6
    autonomic control 973
    diabetic neuropathy 892
    heart disease risk 477
    motor manifestations 881
    Parkinson's disease 775, 972
    screening 203
    syncope 883
    volume depletion 1637
  postprandial 365, 545, 546
    autonomic control 973–4
hypothalamic-pituitary-gonadal-axis 1389
hypothalamo-pituitary axis 78–9
  control of thymic function 28, *28*
hypothalamus 1389
  aging neuropathology 71
  anterior portion lesions 28, 30
  damage in hypothermia 977
  neuroendocrine control 30
hypothermia
  autonomic nervous system 976–7, **977**
  management 1920
  perioperative 1651, **1651**
  primary/secondary 977, **977**
hypothyroidism 1391, 1407–8
  causes 1411
  clinical features 490, 1407, **1407**
  congenital, Down's syndrome 1186–7
  myopathy 942
  peripheral vascular disease risk 624
  secondary 1408
  subclinical 1408, 1411
  treatment 1408
hypotonic dehydration 325
hypovolemia, syncope 974
hypoxemia, postoperative delirium 1640–1
hypoxia
  acute exacerbation of COPD 702
  delirium etiology 1052
  hyponatremia 1375
  stroke 678
hysterectomy
  cervical cancer 1660
  constipation 408
  endometrial cancer 1456, 1659
  ovarian cancer 1456
hysteroscopy 1452, 1456
HYVET (Hypertension in the Very Elderly Trial) **547**, **548**, 550

ibandronate 1294
ibitumomab 1515
ibutilide 504
Iceland, nursing home care 1821, 1822, **1822**
ichthyosis, acquired **1603**
ictal state, delirium etiology 1053
"ideal medical model" 224
idiogenic osmoles 1370
idiopathic small fiber painful sensory neuropathy 897
ignition apraxia 1301
ileorectostomy 413
ileostomy, sexuality 1454
iliococcygeus muscle 396
illicit drug abuse 1153
image intensifiers 1716
imaging, diagnostic *see* diagnostic imaging
imatinib 1515
imiquimod 1601
immersion burns 184
immobility/immobilization 1689
  bone mass loss 1291
  deep vein thrombosis risk 634
  effects of **1690**
  frailty 1566
  pressure ulcer risk 1608–9
  reduced food intake 300
  restraints 1692
immune globulin, intravenous *see* intravenous immunoglobulin
immune risk phenotypes (IRP) 31
immune system 19–36
  acquired (specific) 19
    development 20
  aging 19–36, 40–1, **40**, 1590
    functional 20, *20*
    see also specific cell types
  cell-mediated, tuberculosis 1740
  cells 23–7
    see also specific cell types
  cytokine changes 28–9, 31, 40
  deficiency, atherosclerosis 618–9
  humoral responses 21, 22–3, 26, 1590
  impaired response, zinc deficiency 340
  lymphoid and hemopoietic tissues 20–2, *21*, *22*
  natural (innate) 19
  restoration of function 32–3
  senescence 20–3
    tumor growth 1511
  signal transduction 29–30, 33
  T-cell-dependent (cell-mediated) 20
immune thrombocytopenic purpura (ITP) 437–8
immunochemilumenescence (IMCA) assays 1411
immunoglobulin(s) 22–3
  intravenous *see* intravenous immunoglobulin
immunoglobulin A (IgA) 21, **22**
immunoglobulin A (IgA) nephropathy 1502
immunoglobulin E (IgE), asthma 703
immunoglobulin G (IgG) 22–3
immunological memory 19
immunomodulatory therapy 907
immunoradiometric (IRMA) assays 1411
immunosuppressed patients, dental care 275
immunosuppressive therapy 438, 459
impairment 1557–8
  disability 239–40
  theoretical framework 1553–4
implantable cardioverter defibrillator (ICD) 509, *509*, 510
  costs 577
  heart failure 577
implantable loop recorder, syncope 882
impotence *see* erectile dysfunction
"in the canal" (ITC) hearing aids 1231
"in the ear" (ITE) hearing aids 1231
incidence rate, definition 796
incident pain 2006–7
inclusion bodies, in anterior horn cells 956
inclusion body myositis (IBM) 939–40
incontinence
  costs 397
  day hospitals, management role 1910
  double 397
  fecal *see* fecal incontinence
  functional 1487, **1488**
  nursing home care 1821, 1823
  treatment, clinical audit 1827, 1831, 1832
  urinary *see* urinary incontinence
indapamide 832
independence, driving and 141
India 1983–92
  demographics 1983–4, *1984*
  hospital care 1989
  infrastructure 1985–9
    constitutional/legal 1986–7
    medical 1987–9, *1988*
    social 1985–7
  medical education/training 1989–90
  nurse education/training 1988–9
  nursing home care 1986
  policy issues 1990–1
  primary care 1989
Indian Medical Association (IMA) 1990
Indira Gandhi National Open University (IGNOU) 1990
INDO-UK Workshop 1985
infections/infectious diseases 1725–37
  age related frequency **1726**
  atherosclerosis etiology 91–2
  atypical symptoms 1728, **1728**
  back pain 1359–60
  cardiovascular features 490
  central vestibular system 1244–5
  chronic ambulatory peritoneal dialysis 1501
  clinical presentation 1728–9
  delirium etiology 1052–3
  epidemiology 1725–8
  increased risk, in myelodysplasia 455
  morbidity/mortality **1726**
  neck pain 1363
  oral mucosa 263–5
  pressure ulcers 1622–3, **1622**
  rates 1725
  skin 1591–5, 1727
  terminally ill 2010
  see also specific infections
infectious arthritis 1349
Infectious Diseases Society of America (IDSA) 1743
infective endocarditis (IE) 1749–62
  acute 1755
  blood cultures 1756
  clinical features **1750**, **1753**, 1755–6
    fever **1750**, 1756
  complications 1753, **1753**, 1756
  culture-negative 1751–2, **1752**, 1756–7
    management **1752**, 1759–60
  diagnosis 1756–7
  embolization 1756
  epidemiology 481, 1728, 1749–50
  management 590, 1757–60
    antibiotics 1758, **1758**, **1759**
    multiple-drug-resistant enterococci 1759
    penicillin-resistant streptococci 1757
  microbial etiology 590, 1751–2, **1752**
  mortality 1752–3
  nosocomial 1754
  pathogenesis 1753–5
  preexisting cardiac conditions 1749, **1750**
  prognostic scoring 1750
  prophylaxis 1755
  prosthetic valve 590, 1750
  risk factors 1750–1
  septic aneurysms 1020
  stroke risk 1756
  subacute 1755
  surgery 1760
  types 1750
  valve replacement indications 1755
  valvular heart disease with 590
  vegetation growth 1754–5
inferior cerebellar artery, occlusion 816
inferior hypophyseal arteries 1397
inferior vena cava (IVC) filter 636, 1720
infestations 1591–5
inflammation, in MND 959–60
inflammatory bowel disease 266, 374–5
inflammatory demyelinating polyneuropathy 895
inflammatory disorders, Paget's disease of bone 1271
inflammatory lower MND, diagnosis pitfalls 953
infliximab 1351
influenza vaccine 706, 1730, 1734–5
  efficacy 1734–5
  indications 206–7, **1735**
  pneumonia prevention 689–90
  schedule *387*
  USA 1924, *1925*
influenza virus 706, 1734
  chemoprophylaxis 1730, **1730**
  control 1729–30
  epidemiology 667, 1727
  treatment 706
informant questionnaire on cognitive decline in the elderly (IQCODE) 1065
information provision, patients and carers 1813
informed consent 1686
  Down's syndrome 1186
  dysphasia 843
  interventional radiology 1719
  surgical patients 1653
infrared (IR) thermal imaging 1719
inhibin 1415
injury prevention, Health Maintenance Clinical Guidepath 205
inotropic drugs, positive 587

insomnia **734**, 738–9, 1154–5
associated conditions 738
dementia and 1145–6, **1145**
drug induced 738
evaluation 738
inappropriate medication use **220**
perimenopause 1418
prevalence 733
psychophysiological 738
sleep hygiene 738, 739
sleep-state misperception 738
treatment 738–9, **739**
delirium etiology 1052
inspiration, muscles 672
inspiratory muscle training 728
Institute of Medicine (IOM), USA 1839, 1856
institutionalization
Alzheimer's disease 1089
caregiver impact 1156
institutions
meaningful activity planning in dementia 1141–2, **1142**
sleep in 736
Instrumental Activities of Daily Living (IADL) Scale 227, 1860
Alzheimer's disease 1085, 1087
assessment 205, 1544, **1545**, 1554, 1574–5
measurement scale 227, 1860
carers' assistance 852
dementia 1141, **1141**
Down's syndrome 1186
sarcopenic obesity 921
insulin
anorexia of aging 305
hyperkalemia 1383
postprandial hypotension 973–4
resistance 130, 135
signaling pathways 16–7
insulin pens 1436
insulin resistance syndrome 1392, *1392*
see also metabolic syndrome
insulin-like growth factor (IGF)
motor neuron disease 958, 963
muscle mass 1568–9
insulin-like growth factor-1 (IGF-1) 32, 1393
acromegaly screening 1401
bone mass 1290
sarcopenia 924
insulinoma 421
insurance authorities, driving capability 146–7
insurance companies, driving, informing of illness 146
Integrative Social Cognition Model 861
integrin 1753
intelligence
aging effects 49, 55, 744
crystallized/fluid 55
intensive care unit (ICU)
acute respiratory disease 718–9
delirium in 1047, 1152
oncological emergencies 1528–9
status epilepticus 876
interaction loss, communication difficulties 1042
intercostal arteries 1001
intercostal muscles, structure 672
interdental toothbrushes 249
interdisciplinary assessment *see* geriatric assessment
interface (direct) pressure, pressure ulcers 1606
interference with others, dementia and 1146
interferon-alpha 386
interferon-beta, hepatitis B virus 386
interferon-γ (IFNγ) 28, 29, 618–9
INTERHEART study 476, 477, 478, 493–4
interleukin(s), atherosclerosis 618–9
interleukin-1 (IL-1) 305, 314, **559**
interleukin-2 (IL-2) 28
interleukin-2R (IL-2R) 29
interleukin-4 (IL-4) 28
interleukin-5 (IL-5) 28
interleukin-6 (IL-6) 28
decreased production by macrophages 26
food intake levels 305
heart failure mechanism **559**
Paget's disease of bone etiology 1270
sarcopenia 917
sarcopenic obesity 918
interleukin-7 (IL-7) 23, 28
interleukin-10 (IL-10) 27, 28
interleukin-11 (IL-11), recombinant human 459
interleukin-18 (IL-18), heart failure **559**
intermediate care 1169, 1578
NSF (UK) standard **1802**, 1896, 1917
see also specific countries
intermediate density lipoprotein (IDL) 613
intermediolateral column cells 971
intermittent claudication 623, 627, 1316
intermittent decompensation 1237
intermittent neurogenic claudication 996
internal anal sphincter 395, 396
internal auditory artery ischemia 1241
internal carotid artery
dissection 806
occlusion 816
stenosis, ultrasound 807, **807**
internal fixation, intracapsular hip fractures 1333–4, *1334*
internal mammary artery, as conduit in CABG 600, *600*
International Association of Gerontology (IAG) 7, 1786
International Breast Cancer Group Trial IV 1535
International Classification of Diseases
alcohol abuse/dependence 158
Alzheimer's disease **1084–5**
drug misuse 1194, **1194**
stroke classification 796–7, **797**
vascular dementia 1103–4, 1114
International Classification of Diseases, Adapted for use in the United States (ICDA) 796
International Classification of Function (ICF) model 860, 1571–2, 1881–2, *1881*
International Classification of Impairments, Disabilities, and Handicaps (ICIDH) 852, 1571
stroke rehabilitation model 852, 854
International Classification of Sleep Disorders 733, 738
International Electrotechnical Commission (IEC) 1837
International Federation of the National Standardizing Association (ISA) 1837
International Headache Society (IHS) 751, **752**, 754, **756**, 759
International Normalized Ratio (INR) **442**, 1910
see also warfarin
International Organization for Standardization (IOS) 1837–8
International Plan of Action on Ageing, UN (2002) 1965, 1974
International Psychogeriatric Association (IPA) 1170
International Society for Quality in Health Care (ISQua), Australia 1839
International Stroke Trial (IST) 819, 820
International Study of Post Operative Cognitive Dysfunction (ISPOCD) 1641–2
Internet 111–2
antiaging therapy 1665
telemedicine 112, 1847, 1850
tinnitus information 1230
interneurons, cortical, aging 62
interpersonal therapy (IPT) 1179
interspinous implant 997
interstitial lung disease 714–8
interventional radiology 1719–21
informed consent 1719
intervertebral disk
age related disease 76
cervical spinal canal 991
degeneration 991–2, 1356
lumbar spinal canal stenosis 995, 996
prolapsed 1360
intestinal adaptation phenomenon 291
intestine
calcium metabolism 1261, 1262, 1264
obstruction 1527, 2008
see also small intestine
intra-aortic balloon pump 586, 589
intracapsular hip fractures, repair 1333–5
intracavernosal injections 118
intracellular adhesion molecule-1 (ICAM-1) 27, 618
intracellular space 1369
intracerebral grafting 772
intracerebral hematoma 451, 1021
intracerebral hemorrhage, recurrent 827–8
intracranial abscess 1225
intracranial bleeding
spontaneous 821
warfarin related 450–1
intracranial pressure (ICP)
chronic subdural hematoma 1030
headache and 758
normal 1027
normal pressure hydrocephalus 789, 790, 792
intraductal papillary mucinous tumor, pancreas 421
intradural arteriovenous (AV) fistulae 1008
intramedullary hip screw nail (IMHS) 1335
intramedullary nails, hip fractures 1335, *1336*, 1337–8
intraocular lens implants (IOL) 1209
intraocular pressure (IOP), increased 1206, 1208
intravascular SVC stents 1524
intravascular ultrasound (IVUS), atherosclerosis 611–2
intravenous drug users
HIV risk factor 1731
infective endocarditis 1750–1
see also drug misuse/abuse
intravenous fluid infusion 326
intravenous immunoglobulin
dermatomyositis 938
Guillain–Barré syndrome 679
immune thrombocytopenic purpura 438
myasthenia gravis 905
intravenous urography (IVU) 1717
intrinsic minus foot 1322
intrinsic positive end-expiratory pressure 675
intubation, acute exacerbation of COPD 702
intussusception, internal 410
iodine **341**
iodine-based dressings 1621
ionizing radiation, cardiovascular disease etiology 92
Ionizing Radiation (POPUMET) *Regulations* (1998) 1712
ipratropium 701
IQ, age related changes 55
see also intelligence
iridotomy surgery 1208
iron
absorption 292
chelation 458
deficiency, restless legs syndrome 781
overload 458, 469
supplementation 781
iron deficiency anemia 428, 429–30
alcohol association 160
anemia of chronic disease *vs* 430, **430**
angular cheilitis 264
iron sulfate 432
irritable bowel syndrome (IBS) 365, 367
constipation 367, 407
Isaacs, Bernard 1920
Isaacs' syndrome 906–7
ischemic heart disease 515–28
aerobic training benefits/effects 656
aortic stenosis with 532
cardiac rehabilitation results 657
clinical features 515
diagnostic techniques 516–7
epidemiology 475–9, 488, 515
exercise effects **133, 134**
frailty relationship 481
heart failure associated 570, 579
mortality rates 475, 517
WHO standardized 1978
risk factors 475–6, **476**, 517–9
age 476

ischemic heart disease (*cont.*)
  alcohol 477–8
  cholesterol 477, *477*, 518, 519
  diabetes mellitus 477, 518–9
  dyslipidemia 477, *477*, 518, 519
  genetics 478
  hormones 478
  hypertension 476–7, 517–8, 519
  left ventricular hypertrophy 518
  obesity and diet 478, 519
  physical inactivity 478, 519
  psychosocial factors 478–9
  smoking 153, 477, 517
 therapy
  ACC/AHA guidelines 520, 521
  acute coronary syndromes 520, 521
  coronary artery bypass surgery 585
  hormone replacement therapy 523
  stable angina 519
 see also angina pectoris; coronary heart disease (CHD)
ischemic nephropathy 1496, 1502
ischemic penumbra 815
ischemic stroke 815–21
 alcohol consumption association 803
 classification 796, **796**, 815–6
 clinical presentation 815–6, 823
 coexisting conditions 818, **818**
 differential diagnosis 816–7, **816**
 etiology 815, **816**
 investigations *817*, 817–8, **817**
 management 818–21
  airway 818
  anticoagulants 820
  antithrombotics 820
  arterial blood pressure 819
  coma 818–9, **819**
  dysphagia 820–1
  fever 819
  metabolic considerations 819
  neurosurgical 820
  nutrition 820–1
  oxygenation 818
  physical therapy 819–20
  progress monitoring 818
  thrombolytic therapy 820
  venous thromboembolic disease 820
 pathogenesis 815, **816**
 peripheral vascular disease 625
 prevention, secondary 822–3
 recurrent 827
 vascular dementia 1112
 see also stroke, acute
ISIS-2 trial 521
isoflavones, menopausal symptom management 1420
isoflurane, renal injury 1650
isoniazid (INH)
 hepatitis due to 385, 1743
 peripheral neuropathy cause 894
 side effects 1743
 tuberculosis 709, 1743, **1745**
  latent 1744, **1746**
 tuberculous meningitis 1768
isosorbide dinitrate 574
isotonic dehydration 324
Israel 1947–52
 demographics 1947–8
 geriatric services
  disability and long term care 1948–50
  home care 1949
  palliative/end-of-life care 1950–1
 gerontological organizations 1951
 medical education/training 1949–50
Israel Geriatrics Society 1951
Israel Gerontological Society 1951
Italy
 medical education/training 1784
 memory clinics 1062
 nursing home care 1821, **1822**
 obesity prevalence 348
itraconazole 264, 1325, 1593
ivermectin, scabies 1595

Jan Arogya scheme, India 1991
Janetta procedure 761
Japan 1935–45
 carers' role 1942–3
 epidemiology of aging 1938–40
 intermediate care 1935–6
 life expectancy 88, **88**, 1935
 medical education/training 1936–7
 nursing home care 1821, 1822, **1822**
 psychiatric services 1937–8
 psychological studies of aging 1939, 1943–4
 social gerontology 1940–3, *1941*
 suicide incidence 1938, *1938*
Japan Academy of Gerontological Nursing (JAGN) 1940
Japan Geriatrics Society 1936–7
Japan Gerontological Society 1936–7, 1941
jaws 270–1
 swelling 270–1
 tremor, aging 746
Jerusalem, obesity prevalence 348
jitter 902, 906
John A. Hartford Foundation 1892, 1926, 1931
Joint Commission on Accreditation of Health Care Organizations (JCAHCO) 1838, 1845
Joint Commission on Accreditation of Hospitals (JCAH) 1838
Joint Committee on Higher Medical Training (JCHMT) 1796, **1796**, 1902
joint contractures, Alzheimer's disease 1087
joint diseases 1347–53
 foot problems 1312–3, **1313**, **1314**, *1314*
 pressure ulcer risk factor 1608–9
 surgery 1352
joint problems, in Down's syndrome 1187, **1187**
joint subluxation, in MND 962, 963
Joseph Rowntree Foundation (JRF) 190
Josiah Macy Jr Foundation, USA 1924, 1926
justice, terminally ill 2002
juvenile rheumatoid arthritis, Down's syndrome 1187

Kant 1681–2
Kaplan index 1532
Kaposi's sarcoma 1731
Kegel exercises 399
Kennedy's disease 949, 951
 see also motor neuron disease (MND)
Kennedy's syndrome 953
keratinocytes, age related changes 1590, 1591
keratosis
 actinic **1592**, 1600–1, *1600*
 seborrheic 1599–600, *1600*
 sublingual 268–9
keratotic lesions 1317–24
 management 1323–4
Keshan disease 334
ketamine, neuropathic pain 2007
ketoconazole 1514, 1592, 1596
kidney
 aging 42–3, **43**, 1495, 1501–3
 calcium metabolism 1261
 drugs 1503–4
 mass, age related decrease 43
 see also entries beginning renal
kinesiophobia 984
kinetic tremor 783, **783**
knee joint
 arthroplasty 1277
 osteoarthritis 1347
knowledge, aging effect 49
Koganei Study 1939
Korenchevsky, Vladimir 7
Kuopio Study 1434

La (SS-B) autoantibodies 272
laboratory tests
 Alzheimer's disease 1084, 1088
 memory clinics 1066
labyrinthine fistula 1238, 1240
labyrinthitis 1224
lace-up shoes 1327
lactobacillus, vaginal 1417
lactulose, constipation 411, 2007
lacunar infarction 816, 823, 827
 recurrence rate 827
Lambert Eaton myasthenic syndrome (LEMS) 905–6
 clinical features 953–4
 respiratory muscle weakness 679
Lambeth Disability Screening Questionnaire **1575**
laminectomy 995, 997, 1521
laminoplasty 995, 997
lamivudine 386
lamotrigine, epilepsy 875
Lancet Sanitary Commission report (1869) 2
Langerhans cells 27, 1590, 1591
language
 Alzheimer's disease 1040
 mechanisms/neural basis 841
 thought relationship 1037–8
laparoscopic cholecystectomy, gallstones 389
LaPlace, law *561*
Laron's syndrome 992
larval therapy 1620, 1625, *1626*
laryngeal carcinoma, emergencies 1520
Lasegue (straight leg raising) test 1357
Lasèque's sign 996
laser endoscopic surgery 1513
laser photocoagulation, lung cancer 713
laser therapy
 cataracts 1209
 glaucoma 1208
 prostate resection 1473
laser trabeculoplasty, glaucoma 1208
laser-assisted *in situ* keratimileusis (LASIK) 1205
The Last Refuge 3
Late-Life Function and Disability Instrument (Late-Life FDI) 1558, 1559–60, **1559**
late-life migraine accompaniments 753–4
late-life psychoses 1151–3
 see also specific diseases/disorders
latent tuberculosis infection (LTBI)
 testing 1741, **1745**
 treatment 1744–6, **1746**
lateral pelvic tilt 1615–6, *1616*
lateral (sigmoid) sinus thrombosis 1225
latex agglutination 1765
Latin America 1993–9, **1995**
 demographics 1993–4, **1994**
 see also specific countries
Latin American Academy of Medicine on Aging (ALMA) 1995–6
Lausanne Technical Consensus statements 1170
Law of Social Welfare for the Elderly (1963), Japan 1943
lawsuits, nursing home care 1824, **1824**, 1932
laxatives 408
 combination use 413
 palliative care 2007–8, **2008**
 stimulant **411**, 412
L-dopa *see* levodopa (L-dopa)
lead pipe rigidity 746, 766
lead poisoning 954, 956
Leapfrog Group, USA 1842
learned helplessness, depression 1176
learning
 disabilities, psychiatric services 1168
 new things, Alzheimer's disease 1038–9
 optimal 55
learning theory models, drug misuse 1197
lecithin cholesterol acyl-transferase (LCAT) 614
leflunomide 1351
left atrial appendage (LAA) 499, 505
left ventricle 487
 afterload reduction 534
 dysfunction in heart failure 569
 hypertrophy 493, 516, 518, 530
  concentric, hypertension and 547
  stroke risk factor 801
  triggers and pathogenesis 560–1, **560**
 impaired filling, aging related 487
 increased loading 530
 pressure-volume relationship, age effect 567, *568*

remodeling in heart failure 560–2
apoptosis 562, 564
systolic dysfunction 479, 488–9, 588
wall thickness increase, heart failure 560–1
left ventricular ejection fraction (LVEF) 480, 521, 530, 567
assessment, cardiac rehabilitation **651**
left ventricular end-diastolic pressure (LVEDP) 564, 565, 588
left ventricular end-diastolic volume (LVEDV) 561
left-hemisphere stroke 120, 842–3
leg weakness, motor neuron disease 962
legal issues 1810, 1932
Legionella, infective endocarditis **1752**, 1760
Leiden study 549, 634, **634**
lenalidomide 460
lens, age related changes 39
lentigines 1591, **1592**
lentigo maligna melanoma 1602
leptin 304, 348
age related changes 304, 1423
congenital deficiency 304
obesity 304, 349, 351
resistance 304, 349
sarcopenia 918, 919
letrozol, breast cancer 1514
leukemia 465–71
acute lymphoid 469–70
acute myeloblastic *see* acute myeloblastic/myelogenous leukemia (AML)
acute promyelocytic 467, 1526
chronic myelogenous, treatment 1515
gingival 262
leukocyte(s)
counts, infectious arthritis 1349
diapedesis, atherosclerosis 618
recruitment, atherosclerosis 618, *618*
leukoplakia 268
leukostasis 465, 1525
leukotriene antagonist therapy 704
levator ani muscle 396
level of consciousness (LOC), delirium 1049
levetiracetam, epilepsy 875
levodopa (L-dopa)
augmentation 781
complications 771, **771**
delirium etiology 1050
dyskinesia 770
dystonia 783
gastrointestinal dysfunction 366
Parkinson's disease 768, 771, 1119
rebound 781
respiratory dysfunction 676
restless legs syndrome 781
swallowing reflex 688
levomepromazine 2008
Lewy bodies 74–5, *75*
parkinsonism 765, 766
Parkinson's disease 769, 1117
Lewy body dementia 1117–9
clinical features **1085**, 1118
diagnosis 1117–8, **1117**
diagnostic criteria 1136
management 1119
parkinsonism associated 765–6, 1116–7
pathogenesis 769
smart home communication system problems 195
spectrum of 1117, *1118*
lexical memory 1037–8
liaison psychiatric services 859
libido 1417, 1423
see also female sexual dysfunction (FSD)
lichen planus 265–6
oral lesions 265–6, *265*
lichen sclerosus (LS), vulval 1455
lichenoid reaction, drug induced 266
lidocaine, tinnitus 1230
life expectancy **103**, 1783
increased 124, 593
nature *vs* nurture 1702–4
prediction from health status 202
trends 59, **60**
European Union 1978, **1979**
industrialized countries 88–90, **88**, *90*
see also specific countries
life spans 13
animals 13, 14
lifestyle
active, exercise capacity preservation 124–5
daily, communication disorders 1043–4
disability risk factor 136
education 205
historical perspectives 1
hypertension pathogenesis 543, 546
physical activity 110, *110*
see also exercise programs
SENECA study 110
lifestyle modifications
cardiac rehabilitation 649–50, **650**
diabetes management 134–5
hypertension management 550
stroke risk reduction 822, 837
lifestyle scores, mortality 286–7, *287*
light chain nephropathy 1503
light faders *190*, 191, *191*
light treatment 738, 1179
lignocaine, for pain in MND 962
lignocaine patches, chronic pain 988
Lilliputian hallucinations 774
limb(s)
movement, psychogenic nonepileptic attacks 884
myoclonic jerks 881
limb-girdle dystrophies 943–4
limbic areas, Alzheimer's disease 1074
limb-onset motor neuron disease 950, 952, 962
lindane, scabies 1595
linear acceleration detection 1235
lip(s)
age related changes 263
cancer 269
varicose veins 263
lipase (serum), pancreatitis 418, 420
lipid(s)
oxidative damage 64
profiles
centenarian offspring 1704
testosterone replacement therapy 1423
regulation, diabetes mellitus 1439–40
see also fat (dietary)
lipid-lowering therapy
acute coronary syndromes 521
cardiac rehabilitation 650
see also statins
lipofuscin 39, 64, 72
motor neuron disease 956
sympathetic ganglia in aging 79
α-lipoic acid 1257, 1673
lipopolysaccharide (LPS) 26
lipoproteins (LPs) 613
lip-shave operation, actinic cheilitis 263
liquid nitrogen, actinic keratosis 1600–1
Lisbon Strategy 1980
Listeria monocytogenes 1728, 1764, 1765
lithium **341**, 757, 1139, 1151
lithostatine 419
liver 381–93
age related changes 217, 292, 381
biopsy 386
cholesterol 613
drug metabolism 217
failure, fulminant 383
fatty, obesity 350
function tests, alcohol abuse 162, 163
metastases, nausea 2008
thyroid hormone response 1407
transplantation 390, 1378–9, 1382
liver disease
alcoholic 159, 386–8
chronic, alcohol abuse 162
coagulation defects 440
hypernatremia 1382
hyponatremia 1378–9
"liver spots" 1591, **1592**
Liverpool Longitudinal Study, of mental health of community-dwelling elderly 1126
living will, paramedic treatment 1529
Llermitte's sign 993
Local Government Act, UK (1929) 2
localization related epilepsy 871, 872, 873
locked-in syndrome 678
locus ceruleus, aging 71, 74
lofexidine 1195, 1197
long term care (LTC)
mental health care 1149, 1158
psychiatric care role 1155–6
psychotropic medications 1157
long term care facilities (LTCF)
dental care provisions 256
infection rates/control 1725, 1729–31
methicillin-resistant *S. aureus* 1728
long term memory stores 1037
long term oxygen therapy (LTOT) 699
longevity 16
evolution of 14
see also life expectancy
Longevity and Rejuvenescence 1891
Longitudinal Study of Aging, obesity prevalence 348
long-stay units, Alzheimer's disease 1090
Long-Term Care Insurance, Japan 1942, 1943
loop diuretics, hyponatremia induction 1378
loperamide 366, 367, 400
lorazepam 876, 1056–7
Lord test 1306
loss of awareness, syncope 882
Loss of Protective Sensation (LOPS) criteria **1321**
loudness 1219–20
low back pain *see* back pain
low protein diet, renal failure 1500
low-air loss mattresses 1614, **1614**
low-density lipoprotein (LDL)
absorption 292
oxidation 613, 618
receptor (LDLr) 613–4
low-density lipoprotein (LDL) cholesterol
heart disease risk 477, 518, 519
target values, diabetes mellitus 1439
lower category benign breast disease (LCBBD) 1533
lower esophageal sphincter (LES) 359
bird's beak/rat's tail tapering 360, *360*
botulinum toxin injections 360–1
manometry 358, *358*
pressure reducing drugs 361
lower extremity angioplasty 627–8
lower extremity bypass surgery 627–8
lower respiratory tract infections 705–10
low-molecular-weight heparin 440
chronic DIC 447
surgery, with mechanical heart valves 605
venous thromboembolism 636, 637
Lucilia sericata (Green bottle) 1620
lumbar drain, normal pressure hydrocephalus 789, 791
lumbar infusion test 789
lumbar plexopathy 896
lumbar puncture
memory clinic patients 1066
meningitis 1763, 1765, 1767
normal pressure hydrocephalus 788–9
spinal hematoma etiology 1007
subarachnoid hemorrhage 1018
lumbar scoliosis 996
lumbar spinal canal stenosis 995–8, 1360
lumbar spondylolisthesis 996
lumbar spondylosis 952
lumbar supports, back pain 1361
lumbar-sacral osteoarthritis 1187
lumbosacral pain, osteoarthritis 1347
lung
aging 41, **41**, 1635
functional changes 568, **569**
biopsy, fibrotic disease 715
collapse/consolidation 694
disease *see* respiratory disease
fibrosis, diffuse, signs 694
hyperinflation, in COPD 675
obesity 350
transplantation 718

lung (*cont.*)
  volume, age related decline 41
  see also entries beginning pulmonary or respiratory
lung cancer 710–3
  mortality 1509
  non-small cell (NSCLC) 711–2
  prognostic changes with aging **1510**, 1511
  small cell 712, 905–6
  syndrome of inappropriate ADH 1379
lupus anticoagulant 443
luteinizing hormone (LH) 118, 1401, 1415, 1450
luteinizing hormone-releasing hormone (LH-RH) analogs 1514
Luxembourg, medical education/training 1785
lycopene 1672
Lyme disease 1769
lymph nodes, age related changes 21
lymphatics, skin, age related changes 1591
lymphedema, terminally ill 2011
lymphocytes
  age related changes **24**
  infiltrate into thyroid gland 1405
  receptors expressed 30
  see also B cells; T cell(s)
lymphocytic pleocytosis
  HSV encephalitis 1775
  meningitis 1763, 1768, 1769, 1770
lymphocytic thyroiditis 1411
lymphoid tissues, age related changes 21–2
lymphoma
  Hodgkin's 713
  non-Hodgkin's 713, 1510, **1510**

Maastricht Memory Clinic 1096
Maclachlan, Daniel 1
macrocytosis 429
macronutrients
  absorption 291–2
  intake levels over time 283–4
macrophages 19, 26, 616
maculae 1235
macular degeneration *see* age related macular degeneration (AMD)
MADIT (Multicenter Automatic Defibrillator Implantation Trial) 509, 523
Maeda, Daisaku 1941
maggots (larval therapy) 1620, 1625, *1626*
magic mushrooms, misuse 1192, *1192*
magnesium 1291
  renal tubular dysfunction 1497–8
  supplements 1497
magnesium hydroxide, constipation 411–2, 2007, **2008**
magnesium-containing laxatives 411–2
"magnetic gait" 767
magnetic resonance angiography (MRA) 807, 1018
magnetic resonance imaging (MRI) 1719
  Aqueduct of Sylvius CSF flow 789
  back pain 1358
  brain abscess 1772
  brain tumor 1527
  carotid dissection 806
  cervical spinal canal stenosis 992, 993, 994
  contraindications 1719
  dementia with parkinsonism 1117
  depression 1177
  disadvantages 818
  epidural abscess 1774
  epilepsy 873
  examination sequences 1719
  fecal incontinence 399
  hip fracture 1330
  HSV encephalitis 1775
  ischemic stroke 817–8
  lumbar spinal canal stenosis 997
  memory clinic patients 1066–7
  muscle mass estimation 910, *910*, **911**
  myasthenia gravis 903, *903*
  normal pressure hydrocephalus 788, 789, *789*, 791
  Paget's disease of bone 1273
  parkinsonism 767, 1117
  post-stroke 849–51, *850*, *851*
  restless legs syndrome 781
  sarcopenia 1568
  spinal cord compression 1521
  subarachnoid hemorrhage 1018
  subdural empyema 1773, 1774
  tuberculous meningitis 1768
  vascular dementia 1105–6
Maintenance of Parents Act, Singapore (1995) 1973
Making a Difference 1869
Making the Best Use of a Department of Clinical Radiology: Guidelines for Doctors (3rd edn) 1712
maladaptive beliefs, chronic pain 984
Malassezia, seborrheic dermatitis 1596
male climacteric (menopause) *see* andropause
malic enzyme 1406
malignant disease
  back pain 1359
  central vestibular system 1244
  deep vein thrombosis risk 446, 635
  DIC in 445
  fever of unknown origin 1729
  HIV related 1731
  neck pain 1363
  peripheral neuropathy 896
  peripheral vestibular system 1241
  sensory neuropathy 895–6
  see also cancer
malingering 884
malnutrition
  delirium etiology 1053
  dementia and 1144
  dysphagia 845
  pressure ulcers 1609–10
  sarcopenia 919
malondialdehyde 616
malpractice claims, nursing home care 1824, **1824**, 1932
mammography 1660
mandible, anginal pain radiating to 274
mandibular alveolus, aging 270
manganese **341**, 1291
manic episodes, dementia and 1139
mannitol, fecal incontinence 398
manometry
  achalasia 360, *361*
  diabetes mellitus 366
  diffuse esophageal spasm 361, *361*
  esophagus 358, *358*
  gastric emptying 364
  small intestine 365
Mantoux skin test 709, 1741
MAPLe (Method for Assessing Priority Level) 1862
"marche a petit pas" 748, 767, 1114
Marfan's syndrome 606
marijuana, glaucoma 1208
Massachusetts Male Survey 1424
massage therapy 994, 1361
mastectomy 1534, 1535–6
mastoid air cell infection 1224
mastoidectomy, cortical 1223–4
mastoiditis, acute/chronic 1224
MATCH study (Management of Atherothrombosis with Clopidogrel in High-risk patients) 831
material abuse 182
matrix metalloproteinases (MMPs) *561*, 1618–20
  atherosclerosis 619, 620
mattresses 1613–5, *1613*
  back pain, advice in 1361
  dynamic 1614, *1614*
  static 1613, *1613*, *1614*
maxillae, Paget's disease 271
maximal exercise capacity 696
maximal expiratory pressure (MEP) 673–4
maximal inspiratory pressure (MIP) 673–4
maximum free water clearance 1498
maximum oxygen consumption (VO_2 max) 124, 567, *568*
  age related decrease 41
  cardiac rehabilitation 652, 653, 656
  measurement 652
maximum voluntary ventilation, decline 571
Maze procedure 505, 535, 606
McGill Pain Questionnaire 984
meal delivery service 1089
meal patterns 284
Meals on Wheels, dementia 1141
MEALS-ON-WHEELS mnemonic **1568**
mean corpuscular volume (MCV) 163
meaningful activities, in dementia 1141–2, **1142**, 1146
measles, mumps, rubella (MMR) vaccination *387*
mechanical lifting hoists 1714
mechanical ventilation
  asthma 705
  effect on respiratory muscles 677
  motor neuron disease 961
  weaning 677
mechanogrowth factor (MGF) 1393, 1568–9
meclizine, delirium etiology 1051–2
median nerve, entrapment 896–7
median rhomboid glossitis 264
Medic Alert Program 1146
Medicaid 1894, 1929–30
Medical Council of India 1990
medical education/training
  continuing professional development 1789
  Europe 1783–7
    history 6–7
    postgraduate 1785–6
    undergraduate 1783–5, **1784**
  GMC (UK) recommendations 1789, **1790**, 1791
  Latin America 1994–5
  technology use 1849
  see also specific countries
medical futility, ethical issues 1686–7
Medical Research Council (MRC), UK
  antiepileptic drug withdrawal 876
  hypertension working party **547**, 548, **548**
  Trial of the Assessment and Management of Older People in the Community 1801, 1803
Medical Research Council Cognitive Function and Aging Study (MRC-FAS), 2001 1106
Medical Society for the Care of the Elderly 4, 8, 1891
Medical Therapy of Prostate Symptoms (MTOPS) trial 1465, 1470, 1472
Medicare (US) **1320**, 1894, 1929–30
Medicare Prescription Drug Improvement and Modernization Act, USA (2003) 1930
Medicare Prospective Payment System 1863
medication *see* drug(s)
medication overuse headaches (MOHs) 755–6
medication review 205
  hypertension management 547
  primary care, UK 1805–6
Mediclaim, India 1991
Mediterranean Diet Score (MDS) **285**, 286
medroxyprogesterone acetate, weight gain 315
medullary artery 1001
medullary artery of Adamkiewicz (MAA) 1001
medullary carcinomas, thyroid 1409–10
MEF2A (myocyte enhancer factor-2) 478
MEGA Study, USA 1861–2
megakaryocyte(s), myelodysplasia 456
megakaryocyte growth and development factor (MGDF) 459
megakaryocyte series 465
megestrol acetate 315–6, 1145, 1420
Meige syndrome 782
melancholia, with depression 1173, **1174**
melanocytes 38, 1590, 1591
melanoma 1602, *1602*
melanosis coli 412
melatonin 738, 1394
  effect on immune system 31, 33
melena, gastrointestinal bleeding 371, 374
memantine
  dementia 1089, 1138, 1152
  memory clinic patients 1069
  Parkinson's disease 1120
  vascular dementia 1115
membranous nephropathy (MN) 1502
memory 59
  aging effect 49, 55–6, 59
  cholinergic hypothesis 60

communication role 1037–8
long term/short term 55
mild cognitive impairment 1095
procedural 1038, 1044
semantic 1037, 1039
sensory 55
training 1067, 1068
working 1037, 1039
memory aids 1067, 1068, 1138
memory clinics 1061–71, 1167
Alzheimer's disease 1085
assessment 1063, 1064–7
benefits of 1062–3, **1062**
cognitive assessment 1065–6, **1066**
developments (global) 1062
diagnosis at 1063
diagnostic disclosure 1067–8, **1068**
effectiveness 1063–4
GP management *vs* 1063–4
history of 1061–2
information needs of patient 1067–8
interventions 1067–9
laboratory tests 1066
in local dementia services 1069
management 1063
medical examination 1065
multidisciplinary teams 1064
neuroimaging 1066–7
patient history 1065
rationale 1062–3, **1062**
referral to 1062, 1063
memory impairment/problems
Alzheimer's disease 1074, 1083–4
dementia 1137
prevalence, Japan 1937
screening tools 1938, **1938**
Mendelson syndrome *see* aspiration pneumonitis
Ménière's disease (syndrome) 1227, 1238, 1242–3
meningitis 1763–71
aseptic 1126, 1763
bacterial 1764–8
adjunctive therapy 1767–8
antimicrobial therapy 1765–7, **1766**, **1767**
carcinomatous, vestibular symptoms 1241
coccidioidal 1770–1
cryptococcal 1770–1
epidemiology 1728
fungal 1770–1
meningococcal 447
otitis media complication 1224, 1225
pathogens 1728
spirochetal 1769–70
tuberculous 1768–9
viral 1763–4
Menkes syndrome 340–1
menopausal transition (MT) 1415
menopause 115–6, 1415–21, 1450–1, 1660–2
age of onset 1415, 1660
cessation of menses 1415
clinical features 1416–8, **1416**
cognition 1418
definition 1415, 1450
diagnosis 1661
early, risk factors 1415
early symptoms 1660–1, **1661**
hormonal changes 1415–6
HRT *see* hormone replacement therapy (HRT)
induced 1415
male *see* andropause
osteoporosis 1418
perimenopausal evaluation 1419
perimenopausal syndrome management 1419–21
perimenopause 1415, 1660
postmenopausal health maintenance 1421
postmenopause 1415
premature 160, 1187
stages 1415
urogenital symptoms 1450
vasomotor symptoms 1450
menstrual periods, irregular 1660
mental capacity, ethical issues 1685
mental competence 843, 965
mental deterioration, hydrocephalus 787, 788
mental health
drug misuse association 1192–3
NSF (UK) standards 1163–4, **1545**, 1802, 1893–4, 1917–8
mental health services *see* clinical psychology services; psychiatric services
mental status tests 1087, 1127
see also Mini-Mental State Examination (MMSE)
mental vitality 53, 56, 57, 131
meperidine, delirium etiology 1052
Merck Institute for Aging and Health 1975
mercury, toxicity 266, 954
Merry Walker, dementia 1138, 1141
mesothelioma, pleural 712–3
metabolic abnormalities
delirium etiology 1053
ischemic stroke 819
metabolic acidosis 1383
metabolic comas, diabetes 1433
metabolic equivalent (MET) levels 1634
"metabolic fitness" 123
metabolic syndrome 129, 1392, *1392*
Down's syndrome 1187
metabolism, age related changes **125**
metacarpophalangeal (MCP) joints, arthritis 1348
metastases
breast cancer 1533
cerebral tumors 2009–10
oral cancer 270
peripheral vestibular system 1241
skin **1603**
spinal cord compression 1521
metatarsophalangeal (MTP) joints, gout 1348
metered dose inhalers (MDIs) 698
metformin 134, 351
methadone 1195, 1197
adverse effects 1193
biochemical testing 1195
chronic pain 987
maintenance treatment 1197, 1198
neuropathic pain 2007
reduction treatment 1198
methicillin-resistant staphylococci, infective endocarditis 1758–9
methicillin-resistant *Staphylococcus aureus* (MRSA) 1728, 1730
methionine 338
deficiency 94
Method for Assessing Priority Level (MAPLe) 1862
methotrexate 905, 938, 1007, 1351, 1597
methyl *tert*-butyl ether (MTBE), gallstones 389
methyl testosterone 1417, 1421
methyldopa 385, 1050
methylene-tetrahydrofolate reductase (MTHRF) deficiency 634
methylmalonic acid 429
methylnaltrexone 412–3
methylprednisolone, dermatomyositis 938
5-methyltetrahydrofolate 338
methyl-transferase inhibitors 459–60, 469
metoclopramide 366, 2008
metolazone 575
metoprolol 520, 574–5
metronidazole 894, 1598, 1730, 1774
metyrapone, Cushing's disease 1400
Mexico
demographics **1994**
Older Adult Law (2000) 1973
service provision 1994
MI Choice 1862–3
mice, aging 13, 14
micelles 292
Michigan Alcoholism Screening Test (MAST) 163
in geriatric patients (MAST-G) 163
miconazole, oral candidosis 264
miconazole nitrate, onychomycosis 1325
microadenomas, pituitary 1397–8, 1400
microangiopathic hemolytic anemia (MAHA) 446
microcytosis 429
MICRO-HOPE study, diabetic treatment **1437**
micronutrients
absorption 292
drug interactions **330**
effects of aging **294**
function **294**
microsomal transfer protein (MTP) 1705
microvascular flaps, pressure ulcers 1624
microwave thermotherapy 1473, 1482
micturition, autonomic function 978
micturition syncope 871, 880, 883
middle cerebral artery (MCA), occlusion 816
middle ear disease
chronic 1240
inflammation/infection *see* otitis media
midodrine, diabetic neuropathy 892
migraine 752–4
acephalic 753–4
aura, with/without 753, **753**
clinical features 753, **753**
differential diagnosis 754
equivalents 753–4, **754**
medication induced 753
nonepileptic attacks 885
phases 753
post-/prodrome 753
prevalence 751, 752, *752*
prevention 754, **755**
prognosis 752
treatment 754, **754**, **755**
vestibular dysfunction 1245
migrating motor complex (MMC) 365
mild cognitive impairment (MCI) 59, *60*, 1095–101, 1152
aging 744–5
amnestic 1095, 1152
classification 1099, *1099*
dementia predictors 1096–7, **1097**, **1098**, 1099
etiology 1095–6, **1096**
memory clinics 1061
outcome 1096, *1096*
prevalence 1095
progression prevention 1099
terminology 1095, **1096**
milk thistle (silymarin) 388
Millennium Homes project 190, 194–5, 197
Million Women Study, HRT and breast cancer 1451, 1533
milrinone, as positive inotropic drug 587
MINAP (Myocardial Infarction National Audit Programme) 1828
minerals 329–46
absorption 292
deficiency, prevalence 329–30
Mini Nutritional Assessment (MNA) 205, 1087
minimally modified LDL (MM-LDL) 618
Mini-Mental State Examination (MMSE) 864, 1065, 1087, 1546
Alzheimer's disease 1085
dementia 1150
depression 1177
Down's syndrome 1186
vascular dementia 1106
Minimum Data Set (MDS) 1855–65
applications 1859–64, 1929
case-mix payment 1860–1
quality of care 1840–1, 1861–2
research 1863
scales and profiles 1859–60
care pathways identification 1862–3
development 1856–8
domains **1856**, 1859–60
Resident Assessment Protocols 1856–7, **1856**, 1858
Minnesota tube 377
Minnesota Twin Study of Adult Development and Aging 49
minocycline, in MND 963
"minor cognitive motor disorder" 1126
minority ethnic groups
carers 1811, 1813
psychiatric services 1156, 1169
mirtazapine 778, 1139, 1178
misoprostol, constipation 412

Misuse of Drugs Act (1971) 1199, **1200**
Misuse of Drugs Regulations (2001) 1199, **1200**
mithramycin 1276, 1523
mitochondria 15–6
  dysfunction in MND 959
  function, aging effect 64
  reactive oxygen species formation 16
mitochondrial DNA (mtDNA)
  mutations 15–6, 39
  sarcopenia 915
mitral annular calcium 625, **625**
mitral regurgitation 530
  acute, management 589
  chronic 589, 607
    management 589–90
  epidemiology 531
  heart failure in 573
  ischemic 589, 602
  surgery 589
    indication 602
    Maze procedure 535
  survival/prognosis 589, 602, *602*
  valvuloplasty 536, 589–90, 602–3
    indications **534**
mitral stenosis 590
  valvuloplasty indications **534**
mitral valve
  myxomatous degeneration 531
  premature closure 588
  prolapse 531, 1188, 1750
  surgery 602–3
    indications 602
    in mitral regurgitation *see* mitral regurgitation
    in mitral stenosis 590
    repair 602–3
    replacement 573, 602–3
mixed dementia 1106, 1114
MMSE *see* Mini-Mental State Examination (MMSE)
mobile dental units 257
mobile feet 1317
mobility
  assessment 1545–6, **1545**
  motor neuron disease 962
  transportation impact 141
  see also rehabilitation
mobility impairment/problems
  Alzheimer's disease 1086–7
  dental care 241
  pressure ulcer risk 1608–9
  social effects 105
mobility related disability, obesity 350
mobilization, stroke, following 819–20
Mobitz types I/II second-degree heart block 495
Modernisation of NHS Hearing Aid Services (MHAS) program 1216
modified radical mastectomy (MRM) 1534
modified Romberg test 1305–6
modular hearing aids 1231
Mohs surgery 1601, 1602
moisture, pressure ulcer development 1608
molybdenum **341**
MONICA project (WHO) 799
monoamine(s), appetite regulation 302
monoamine oxidase-A (MOA-A) 61
monoamine oxidase-B (MOA-B) 61
monoaminoxidase inhibitors (MAOI) 771, 772
monoclonal antibodies 925, 1515, **1515**
monoclonal gammopathies, benign 896
monocular blindness, subarachnoid hemorrhage 1017
monocyte chemotactic peptide-1 (MCP-1) 618
monocytes, age related changes **24**, 40
monosaccharides, absorption 292
mood disorders
  Alzheimer's disease 1084
  dementia and 1138–9, **1138**, **1139**
  due to general medical condition 1173–4, **1174**
  Parkinson's disease 774
  stroke related 862–3
  see also depression
mood stabilizers 1139, **1139**
Moraxella catarrhalis, otitis media 1223
morbilliform drug eruptions 1598–9, *1599*
Mormons, life expectancy 1702–3
morphine
  acute coronary syndrome 520
  breakthrough pain 2006–7
  chronic pain 987
  dosages **2006**
  incremental doses **2005**
  palliative care 2005
  side effects 2005
mortality
  extrinsic, evolution of longevity and 14
  see also death
mortality rates 88–95, 796
  inverse relation to exercise level 124
  world-wide *169–80*, **174**
    all-cause **170**, **171**, **175**, *175*, *176*
    cancer **170**, **173**, *179*
    cardiovascular disease **170**, **172**, *177*, *178*
    see also specific countries
Morvan's syndrome 906
MOST (Mode Selection Trial) 495, **496**
motility agents, delirium etiology 1050
motivational counseling, alcohol abuse 163, 164
motivational interviewing, drug misuse 1197, 1198
motor cortex, aging 71
motor manifestations, syncope 881
motor neuron(s), age related changes 76
motor neuron disease (MND) 949–67
  breaking bad news 955
  bulbar-onset 951, 952, 954, 955
  clinical features/course 950–2
  definition 949–50
  diagnosis 950, 954–5
  diagnostic pitfalls 952–4
  differential diagnosis 952–4
  drug treatment 963
  end-of-life issues 964–5
  epidemiology 955–6
  etiology 956, 957–60
  excitotoxicity 63
  familial 951–2, 956
  flail arms 950
  frontotemporal lobular degeneration 1121
  hemiplegic 950
  hospice care 964
  insulin-like growth factor 963
  investigations 954–5
  limb-onset 950, 952, 962
  mortality 961–2, 964
  multidisciplinary team approach 964–5
  paraplegic 950
  pathology 956–7
  pathophysiology 949, 957–60
  prognosis 952
  respiratory failure 676
  terminology 949–50
  treatment, symptomatic 960–3
    arm weakness 962–3
    cramp 960
    depression 962
    dysarthria 960–1
    dysphagia 961
    fasciculation 960
    leg weakness 962
    pain 962
    respiratory failure 961–2
    salivary dribbling 960
    spasticity 960
motor neuropathy, diabetic foot 1314
motor speech disorder 842
  dysarthria *see* dysarthria
motor systems
  aging effect 47–8, **744**, 745–8
  diseases affecting 47–8
motor therapy, stroke rehabilitation 853
motor units 39, 671
motor weakness, cervical myelopathy 993
mouth, smokers 152
movement disorders
  aging effect 47–8
  non-parkinsonian 777–86, **778**
Movicol®, constipation 2008
MPTP induced Parkinson's disease 769
MRC (UK) *see* Medical Research Council (MRC), UK
mucolytic therapy, in COPD 698
mucosa, oral *see* oral mucosa
mucosal lymphoid tissue 21–2
mucositis 272, 1513, 1514
mucous membrane pemphigoid (MMP) 266–7, *267*
mucous membranes, elder abuse 184
mucus, nasal 1250
multichannel intraluminal impedance 358
multidisciplinary assessment *see* geriatric assessment
multidisciplinary team
  heart failure management 577
  stroke management 822
multidrug resistance p-glycoprotein (MDR-1) 455
multidrug-resistant tuberculosis (MDT-TB) 1743
multifocal atrial tachycardia (MAT) 496
multifocal glasses, falls 1303, 1308
multifocal motor neuropathy (MMN) 895, 953
multi-infarct dementia (MID) 1111, 1113
  see also vascular dementia (VaD)
multiorgan failure, in DIC 445
multiple endocrine neoplasia (MEN) 1409–10
multiple sclerosis (MS) 274, 678, 885–6
multisystem atrophy (MSA)
  autonomic dysfunction 971–2
  clinical features 767, 971
  dementia 1120
  parkinsonism 1116
  pathogenesis 769
  prevalence 971
Murphy's sign 388
muscarinic receptors 1462, 1490, **1490**
muscle
  aging 38–9, **39**, 672–3, 916
  atrophy 39, 130, 656, 745–6
    sarcopenia 914–5
  basal metabolic rate decrease 38
  biopsy *see* muscle biopsy
  body composition optimization **126**
  bulk, aging effects 745
  changes in heart failure 564, **564**
  composition measurement 912
  contractures, Alzheimer's disease 1087
  disorders *see* myopathies
  fibers *see* muscle fibers
  hypertrophy after exercise 130
  hypoperfusion in chronic heart failure 656
  mass
    aging effect 47, 347
    decrease *see* sarcopenia
    dehydroepiandrosterone 1677
    estrogen 917
    growth hormone effect 1568
    growth hormone supplementation 1674
    in vivo measurement 910, **911**
    insulin resistance and 130
    physical exercise 913
    preservation by exercise 130
    testosterone replacement 119–20, 916–7, 1423, 1568, 1675
  myasthenia gravis 899–900, 902
  overactivity 906
  oxidative capacity, aerobic training 657
  oxidative stress 914–6
  power 746, 902
  regenerative capacity decline 38
  strength 39, 746
    measurement 921
  structural organization 671–2
  tone, aging effect 746
  wasting 130, 909
  weakness 899–900, 906, 1777
muscle biopsy
  chronic progressive external ophthalmoplegia 946, *946*
  corticosteroid myopathy 941, *941*
  Cushing's syndrome *941*, 942
  dermatomyositis 938, *938*
  ethanol related myopathies 940
  inclusion body myositis 939–40, *939*, *940*
  myopathies 937
  polymyositis 939, *939*

muscle fibers 671–2
  apoptosis in sarcopenia 916
  type I (slow twitch) 38
  type II (fast twitch) 38, 39
muscle "quality" 912
muscle relaxants 161, 1052, 1363
muscle specific tyrosine kinase (MuSK) 901
muscle sympathetic nerve activity (MSNA) 969–70
muscles of mastication 270–1
muscular dystrophies 943–4
  Becker 943
  classification 943, **943**
  Duchenne 943
  facioscapulohumeral 944, *944*
  limb-girdle 943–4
  oculopharyngeal 944, *945*
musculocutaneous flaps, pressure ulcers 1624
musculoskeletal disorders 1580–3
  see also specific conditions
musculoskeletal function, aging 125
musculoskeletal system, immobility/restraints effect **1690**
MUSTT (Multicenter Unsustained Tachycardia Trial) 509
mutations, accumulation 14
  mitochondrial DNA (mtDNA) 15–6, 39
myasthenia gravis (MG) 899–907
  acetylcholine receptor (AChR) antibodies 900–1, **901**, 902
  anesthesia 905
  anticholinesterase test 902–3
  associated immune diseases 900, **900**
  classification 900, **900**
  clinical features 899–900, **900**, 954
  diagnosis 902–3
  differential diagnosis 903
  drugs, adverse effect 900, **900**
  electromyography 902
  incidence 899
  management 903–5, *904*
  ocular 905
  pathogenesis 900–2
  penicillamine induced 901
  prognosis 900
  respiratory muscle weakness 679
  seronegative 901
  striated muscle antibodies 901
  thymus 902
myasthenic crises 679, 905
myasthenic syndrome 679
mycobacterial infection, atypical 710
Mycobacterium tuberculosis 1739, 1768
  see also tuberculosis (TB)
mycophenolate mofetil 1599
Mycoplasma, infective endocarditis **1752**, 1760
Mycoplasma pneumoniae 707, 1726
mycotic aneurysms 1756
mycotic infection *see* fungal infections
myelin, aging neuropathology 75, 79
myeloblasts, myelodysplasia 456
myelodysplasia 455–64
  acute myeloid leukemia development 455, 457, 460, 466
  anemia in 429, 459, 468
  classification 457, **457**, **468**, 468
  clinical features 455–6, 468
  cytogenetics 456, 468
  diagnosis 456, 468
  epidemiology 455, 470
  International Prognosis Scoring System **458**, 468, **469**
  pathogenesis 456–7, 459, 465
  prognosis/prognostic factors 457–8
  stem cell defects 455, 461, 465
  supportive care 458–61, 466, 468–9
    differentiating agents 459–60, 469
    farnesyl transferase inhibitors 460–1, 469
    growth factors 458–9, 469
    immunosuppressives 459
    pyridoxine, androgens and vitamins 459
    thalidomide and lenalidomide 460, 469
    transfusions and iron overload 458, 469
  therapy related (drugs causing) 455, 456
  treatment 458, 468–9
    intensive 458, 461
    stem cell transplantation 461, 468
myelodysplastic anemia 429, 459, 468
myelodysplastic syndromes (MDS) 429, 433, 455, 465
myeloid series 465
  abnormalities in myelodysplasia 456
myeloma, renal disease 1503
myelopathy
  arteriovenous malformations 1008
  cervical *see* cervical myelopathy
  chronic, spinovascular insufficiency 1009–10
myeloproliferative disorders 439
myelosuppression, anemia 1514
myenteric plexus 357
mylotarg 467, 1515
myoblasts 38
myocardial infarction, acute (MI)
  anemia association 427
  asymptomatic 516
  cardiac rehabilitation cost-effectiveness 658–9
  clinical features 515–6, **516**
  heart failure and, management 586–7
  insulin resistance syndrome 1392
  mechanical complications, management 585–6, **586**
  mortality 586
    rates (Canada) **494**
  non-ST-elevation (NSTEMI), therapy 520
  postoperative 1633–4, 1649
  recognized *vs* unrecognized 515–6
  risk factors *see under* ischemic heart disease
  sexual activity resumption **121**
  "silent" 479, 515
  ST-segment elevation (STEMI) 520, 521
  therapy after 521–3, **522**
    antiarrhythmic drugs 522–3
    medical approach **524**
  ventricular arrhythmias after 508, 587
Myocardial Infarction National Audit Programme (MINAP) 1828
myocardial ischemia
  assessment for cardiac rehabilitation **651**
  coronary artery bypass surgery 598
  misdiagnoses 515
  referred pain 274
  silent 515, 625
myocardium
  age related cellular changes 529–30
  altered energetics in heart failure 564
  beta-adrenoreceptor subtypes 556
  extracellular matrix 530, 561, **562**
  hypertrophy 560–1
  interstitial fibrosis 561
  stiffness 487, 493, 1648
  see also cardiac myocytes
myocilin gene (MYOC), glaucoma 1208
myoclonic jerks, limb 881
myocytolysis 488
myopathies 935–47, **936**
  acquired **936**, 937–43
  acute quadriplegic (AQM) 942
  classification 935, **936**
  clinical assessment 935–6
  clinical features 935
  differential diagnosis 935
  drug induced 940–2
    acute rhabdomyolysis 941, **941**
    painful 941, **941**
    painless 940–1, **941**
    patterns **940**
    periodic weakness 941
  endocrine 942–3
  ethanol related 940
  extraocular muscle involvement 935
  idiopathic inflammatory 937–40
  inherited **936**, 943–6
  laboratory investigations 936–7
  metabolic 942–3
  muscle wasting 935
  overlap syndromes 937
  pain 936, 941, **941**
  paraneoplastic 943
  respiratory muscle weakness 936
  toxic 940–2
myosin, isoforms, switching in heart failure 563
myosin ATPase 672
myositis
  inclusion body 939–40
  statins 834
myostatin, sarcopenia 919
myostatin D, muscle growth inhibition 1569
myosteatosis 1568
myotomy 360, 363
myotonic dystrophy (DM) 944–5, *945*
myringitis 1223
myringitis hemorrhagica bullosa 1223

nails
  psoriasis 1597, *1597*
  see also toenails
naloxone 323, 1401
naloxone-3-glucuronide 413
naltrexone (ReVia®) 165
nandrolone 1393
napping during the day 735, 738
naproxen 923, 1350, 1352
narcolepsy, investigation 736
narcotics, delirium etiology 1052
Narcotics Anonymous 1198
narrow band UVA, psoriasis 1597
nasal sinus disease 1254
nasal-associated lymphoid tissue 21–2
Nascher, Ignatz 1, 1891, 1923
nasogastric feeding, post hip fracture 1333
nasogastric lavage, gastrointestinal bleeding 376
nasogastric suction, hypokalemia 1384
nasogastric tubes, aspiration pneumonia 689
nasopharyngeal carcinoma 275
National Alzheimer's Association, Switzerland 1062
National Assistance Act, UK (1948) 1918
National Cancer Institute Surveillance Epidemiology End Result Cancer registries 1538
National Care Standards Commission (NCSC), UK 1920–1
National Center for Geriatrics and Gerontology, Japan 1936
National Centre for Health Outcomes Development (NCHOD), UK 1827
National Committee for Quality Assurance (NCQA), USA 1839
National Confidential Enquiry into Perioperative Deaths (NCEPOD, 1999) 635, 1633, 1647
National Corporation for the Care of Old People, UK 2
National Eye Institute Age related Eye Disease Study (AREDS) 1206
National Health and Nutrition Examination Survey (NHANES) 93, 428, 542, 647
  stroke mortality 798
  vitamin deficiency 330
National Health and Nutrition Examination Survey (NHANES I)
  body weight and mortality 309–10, **310**
  obesity and mortality 311, **311**
  weight loss and mortality 311, 312, **312**
National Health and Nutrition Examination Survey (NHANES III) 912, 1434
National Health Service (NHS) (UK)
  alcohol pharmacotherapy 165
  Breast Cancer Screening programme 1532, **1532**
  GP contract, British Health Check model and 209
  hearing aid provision 1216
  history 2, 3
  principles 1916
  Single Assessment Process for elderly **209**, 210
National HealthCare Corp (NHC), UK 1893
National Highway Traffic Safety Administration, US 142, 144
National Institute for Clinical Excellence (NICE) (UK)
  Alzheimer's disease therapy 1061

National Institute for Clinical Excellence (NICE) (UK) (*cont.*)
  cholesterol target values, diabetics 1439
  clinical audit definition 1827
  COPD guidelines 696, 698
  evidence-based standards 1830
  guidelines, implementation 1828
  pressure-relieving devices guidelines 1612–3
  smoking cessation therapy 154–5
National Institute for Longevity Science, Japan 1936, 1939
National Institute for Mental Health, UK 1170
National Institute for Neurological Disorders and Stroke (NINDS) 796
National Institute for Social Work, UK 1164–5
National Institute of Health (NIH), USA 1892, 1926
National Institute of Mental Health (NIMH) 1152
National Institute of Neurological and Communicative Disorders and Stroke and the Alzheimer's Disease and Related Disorders Association (NINCDS–ADRDA) criteria 1073, 1083, 1106
National Institute of Neurological Diseases and Stroke-Society for Progressive Supranuclear Palsy (NINDS-SPSP) criteria 1120
National Institute of Neurological Disorders and Stroke and the Association Internationale pour la Recherche et l'Enseignement en Neurosciences (NINDS-AIREN) 1104, 1106, 1114, **1114**
National Institute on Aging (NIA), USA 1892, 1926
National Long Term Care Survey, USA (2004) 89
National Minimum Standards for Care Homes for Older People, UK 1871, 1875
National Nursing-Home Resident Assessment Instrument *see* Minimum Data Set (MDS)
National Osteoporosis Foundation 1282, 1421
National Sentinel Audit of Evidence Based Prescribing, UK 1834
National Sentinel Audit of Stroke, UK 1828, 1831, 1832, 1834
National Service Framework (NSF) for Coronary Heart Disease (UK) 1830
National Service Framework (NSF) for Older People (UK) 210
  drug misuse 1199
  memory clinics 1061
  orthogeriatrics guidelines 1343
  rationale 1891
  Single Assessment Process 230, 1165, 1894
  standards/targets 1801–3, **1802**, 1917–8, 1920
    falls management/prevention **1802**, 1917
    health promotion **1802**, 1803, 1894, 1917–8
    hospital care 1898
    intermediate care **1802**, 1896, 1917
    mental health 1163–4, **1545**, 1802, 1893–4, 1917–8
    person/client-centered care **1802**, 1917
    stroke rehabilitation **1802**, 1898–9, 1917
National Service Framework (NSF) for Stroke (UK) **1802**, 1898–9, 1917
National Study of Hearing 1212
National Treatment Outcome Research Study (NTORS) 1198
natriuretic peptides 558
  analogues 558
  see also atrial natriuretic peptide (ANP)
natural killer (NK) cells 19, 20, **24**, 26
nausea 2005, 2008
nebulizers, in COPD 698
neck
  immobilization, cervical spondylotic myelopathy 1363–4
  pain 1363–4
  stiffness, subarachnoid hemorrhage 1017
  trauma, carotid dissection 806
necrotic tissue, dry/moist 1618, *1620*
needle biopsy 1720
negative craving, alcohol abstinence 165
neglect 1154
  active 182
  oldest old 1156
Neisseria gonorrhea 1732
Neisseria meningitidis 1764, 1765, **1766**
neodymium:YAG (Nd:YAG) laser iridotomy 1208
neoplasia *see* cancer; malignant disease
neosphincter operations 403
neostigmine, constipation 412
neostriatum, Parkinson's disease 60–1
nephritis, acute interstitial 1503
nephropathy
  fibrillary (immunotactoid) 1503
  immunoglobulin A (IgA) 1502
  ischemic 1496, 1502
  light chain 1503
  membranous 1502
nephrotic syndrome 1502–3
nerve blocks, neuropathic pain 2007
nerve conduction studies, in MND 954
nerve growth factor (NGF) 64, 958, 970, 1079
  antibodies 972
nerve injury, taste dysfunction 1256
nerve roots, aging neuropathology 76
nervous system
  aging 41–2, **41**, **125**
  chronic renal failure 1500
Netherlands
  medical education/training 1784, 1785
  nursing home care 1818–9, 1980
neural presbycusis 1226–7
neuritic plaques, aging effect 73–4, *74*, 745
neurochemistry
  aging 59–67, **61**, 66
  essential tremor 784
neurocognitive dysfunction, cardiac surgery and 596
neurodegeneration, age-associated 63–4
neuroendocrine theory of aging 37
neuroendocrine-immune network 30–1, *30*
neuroendocrine-immuno theory of aging 37
neurofibrillary tangles 72, 74, 745
  Alzheimer's disease 1073–6, *1074*, 1077–8, 1078–9
neurofilament accumulation, in MND 957
neuroimaging
  brain imaging **817**
  dementia 1115, 1117, 1129
  dementia predictor in MCI 1097
  ischemic stroke 817–8, *817*
  memory clinics 1066–7
neuroleptic malignant syndrome 1051
neuroleptics *see* antipsychotics (neuroleptics)
neurological assessment, alcohol abuse 162
neurological disease/disorders
  dehydration 323, **324**
  neck pain 1363
  vestibular dysfunction 1245
neurological dysphagia, terminally ill 2010–1
neurological function, surgical patients 1640–2
neurological rehabilitation 1583
neurological signs of aging 743–50, **744**
  see also individual signs
neurological system, effects of restraints **1690**
neurologist, memory clinics 1064
neuroma, acoustic 1227–8, 1241, 1244
neuromelanin 64, 769
neuromuscular function, aging effect 47
neuromuscular junction disorders 899–907
  Lambert Eaton syndrome *see* Lambert Eaton myasthenic syndrome (LEMS)
  myasthenia gravis *see* myasthenia gravis (MG)
  peripheral nerve hyperexcitability 906–7
neuromyopathy, definition 954
neuromyotonia 906–7
neuronal connectivity, aging 62–3
neuronal loss 60, 70
  Alzheimer's disease 1076
  gastrointestinal tract 357
  Huntington's disease 778
neuronal membrane markers, aging 62–3
neuronal shrinkage in aging 70
neuro-ophthalmology, aging 745
neuropathic pain **983**, 2007
neuropathology of aging 69–84
  amyloid angiopathy 76–8, *77*
  blood vessels 76–8, *77*
  brain weight 69
  central white matter 75
  cerebral cortex 70
  choroid plexus 78, *78*
  corpora amylacea 76, *76*
  dendritic changes 71
  dystrophic axons 72
  external brain appearance 69
  gliosis 76
  granulovacuolar degeneration 72–3, *73*
  gray matter, microscopic changes 70–5
  gross changes 69
  Hirano bodies 72, *72*
  Lewy bodies 74–5, *75*
  lipofuscin 72
  nerve roots 76
  neurofibrillary tangles 74
  neuronal loss/shrinkage 70
  Nucleus Basalis of Meynert 70
  peripheral nerve 79
  pineal gland 78
  pituitary gland 78–9
  plaques 73–4, *73*, *74*
  spinal cord 76
  subcortical nuclei 70–1
  sympathetic ganglia 79
  synaptic density 71–2
  ubiquitinated deposits 72
  ventricular size 69
  see also individual pathologies
neuropathy
  asymmetrical 891
  compression 896–7
  idiopathic 897
  MND diagnosis pitfalls 953–4
  motor, diabetic foot 1314
  multifocal motor 895, 953
  see also polyneuropathy
neutropenia, leukemia 1526
neutropenic ulceration 266
neuropeptide Y (NPY) 303, 348
neuropeptides, enteric nervous system 971
neuroprotective therapy 65
Neuropsychiatric Inventory (NPI) 1087, 1129
neuropsychiatric manifestations
  Parkinson's disease 773–4, **773**
  vitamin B_{12} deficiency 339
neuropsychological function, aging effects 744
neuropsychological testing
  Alzheimer's disease 1084
  dementia 1127
  dementia prediction in MCI 1097
  driving capability assessment 144
  normal pressure hydrocephalus 789–90
neuroreflexology, back pain 1362
neurosurgery
  bacterial meningitis 1764
  cerebellar hematoma 821
  intracranial hemorrhage 821
  ischemic stroke 820
  Parkinson's disease 772, **772**
neurosyphilis 1129, 1245, 1732, 1769–70
neurotoxic agent exposure, MND 956
neurotransmission, aging effect 969–70, *970*
neurotransmitters
  anorexia of aging 301–5, **301**
  appetite regulation **301**, 301–5, *301*
  penile erection *117*
neurotrophic factors, aging 64
neurovascular tyloma 1317
neutron activation 910, **911**
neutropenia, in myelodysplasia 455, 457
New England Centenarian Study 1704–5
New Mexico Aging Process Study, body composition changes 912, **912**
The new NHS; modern and dependable 1827, 1835
"newly old" population, antiaging therapy 1665
NHS *see* National Health Service (NHS) (UK)
NHS and Community Care Act, UK (1990) 1910, 1917
niacin, cholesterol reduction 615
nicardipine 1023

nickel **341**
nicotinamide 1599, 1669
nicotinamide adenosine dinucleotide (NAD) 1669
nicotine replacement therapy 154, 697
nifedipine 534
"night owls" 735
nimodipine 1023
nitrates
  angina therapy 519, 520
  heart failure therapy 565, 576
nitric oxide (NO)
  actions *617*
  age-associated decline 542
  atherosclerosis *617*
  enteric system 971
  in heart failure 559, 657
  motor neuron disease 957, 958
  production 26, 617, *617*
nitric oxide synthase (NOS) 617
  inducible (iNOS) 559
nitrofurantoin 894
nitroglycerin 161, 519, 520
NKT cells 26
NMDA antagonists 1069, 1089, 1115
NMDA receptors, aging 62
Nocardia, brain abscess 1771, 1772, 1773
nociceptive pain **983**
nociceptive system, age related changes 982
nocturia 1461–2
nocturnal bruxism 261
nocturnal movements, pressure ulcers 1609
nocturnal myoclonus 780
nodular melanoma 1602
nodular scabies 1595
noise
  exposure, tinnitus 1228–9
  sleep effects 736
Nolan, *Professor* Mike 1874
"no-lifting" policies 1714
nonbacterial thrombotic endocarditis (NBTE) 1753
noncardiac chest pain (NCCP) 362–3
noncompliance with medication
  in heart failure 571
  hypertension therapy 546
  reasons 571, 572
nondegenerative dementia **1085**
nondirective counseling, drug misuse 1198
nonepileptic attacks 879–87
  differential diagnosis 879, **880**
  hyperventilation attacks 884
  hypoglycemia 885
  migraine 885
  misdiagnosis 879
  in multiple sclerosis 885–6
  panic attacks 884
  presentation 879
  psychogenic 884–5
  sleep phenomena 885
  syncope *see* syncope
  transient global amnesia 885
  witness accounts 879
non-Hodgkin's lymphoma 713, 1510, **1510**
noninvasive mechanical ventilation (NIV), COPD 677, 702
noninvasive positive pressure ventilation (NIPPV) 961
non-maleficence (ethical) principle 1684, 1685, 2002
nonorganic epileptic attack 871
non-rapid eye movement (NREM) sleep 734
nonshivering thermogenesis 976
non-small cell lung cancer (NSCLC) 711–2
"nonspecific neuropathy of late life" 889
nonsteroidal anti-inflammatory drugs (NSAIDs)
  alcohol–drug interaction 161
  antiplatelet therapy and 830
  arthritis 1350–1
  back pain 1363
  bone pain 2007
  chronic pain 986
  chronic pancreatitis 421
  delirium etiology 1050
  with exercise, in sarcopenia 923
  gastrointestinal side effects 1350
  heart failure association 571, 572
  hepatotoxicity 385
  migraine 754
  naltrexone interaction 165
  nephrotoxic effects 1351
  oral ulceration induction 266
  postoperative pain **1652**
  postpolio syndrome 1777
  pseudogout 1352
  renal toxicity 1503
  side effects 1350–1
  spinal canal stenosis 994, 997
  toxicity monitoring 1350
nontraumatic intracranial hemorrhage (NIH) stroke scale 797
nonvalvular atrial fibrillation (NVAF) *see* atrial fibrillation (AF)
noradrenaline (NA) *see* norepinephrine
noradrenergic nerves, aging 30, 61, **61**
norepinephrine (noradrenaline)
  aging effect 61, 970, *970*, 973
  drugs enhancing, stroke rehabilitation 851
  enteric nervous system 971
  increased in elderly 543
  increased in heart failure 555
  Parkinson's disease 769
  as positive inotropic drug 587
  reduced, by aerobic training 657
  thermoregulation 976
  thirst regulation 323
normal pressure hydrocephalus (NPH) 787–94
  clinical presentation 787–8
  dementia 1127
  diagnostic modalities 788–90
    aqueductal CSF stroke volume 789
    CSF infusion test 789, 791
    CT 788, *788*, 791, 793
    lumbar drain 789, 791
    lumbar infusion test 789
    lumbar puncture 788–9
    MRI 788, 789, *789*, 791
    neuropsychological testing 789–90
  differential diagnosis 788
  etiology/pathophysiology 787
  follow-up 793
  gait 1302
  idiopathic 787
  incidence 787
  long term care 793
  outcome/prognosis 792
  parkinsonism 1116
  secondary 787
  shunt responsiveness prediction 788, 789, 791
  treatment 790–2
    complications 791–2, *792*
    endoscopic third ventriculostomy 791
    patient selection 791
    ventriculoperitoneal shunting 790, *790*, *791*
Normative Aging Study 348
normotherapy (radiant heat), pressure ulcers 1625
North American Symptomatic Carotid Endarterectomy Trial (NASCET) 808–10, 1640
Northern Manhattan stroke study 801, 802
Norton's scale, Alzheimer's disease 1087
nortriptyline 987, 1178
Norway, medical education/training 1784
Norwegian (crusted) scabies 1595
nosocomial infections, siderail use 1692
nosocomial pneumonia 1726
  epidemiology 666–7
  incidence 707
  mortality 707–8
  prophylaxis 707
  risk factors 666–7, 707
novel translational repressor (NAT-1) 1407
nuclear cataract 1208, **1209**
nuclear medicine 1718
nucleic acid amplification (NAA) tests 1743
Nucleus Basalis of Meynert 70
Nuffield Foundation, UK 2, 7
number needed to treat (NNT) 1292, *1293*
Nun Study, mixed dementia 1114
nurse education/training
  India 1988–9
  UK 1873–4
nurse role
  acute care 231–2, 1870–1
  exercise programmes 1873
  home care 1872–3
  problem-orientated assessment 231
  rehabilitation 1873
  see also specific countries
nursery monitors 1694
Nurses Health Study 310, **311**, 333
Nursing and Midwifery Council (NMC), UK 1873, 1874
nursing care, Alzheimer's disease 1089
nursing home(s)
  acquired pneumonia 665–6, 707
  alcohol problem prevalence 158
  constipation prevalence 407
  fecal incontinence 396
  food intake 284–5, **284**
  infection rates 1725
  infectious diarrhea outbreaks 1727
  pressure ulcer prevalence 1605
  restraint usage 1690
  sexuality 121
  siderail use 1691
  tuberculosis 667, 1740
nursing home care 6, 1817–26
  diabetic patients 1440–2
    blood pressure regulation 1438
    deficiencies in care 1440, **1440**
    early detection importance 1441, **1441**
    glucose regulation guidelines 1436
    intervention studies 1441
    prevalence 1440–1
  European Union 1980
  foley catheter use 1844
  inter-country comparisons 1821–2, **1822**
  legal issues 1820, 1824
  malpractice claims 1824, **1824**, 1932
  physical restraints 1822, 1844
  quality improvement **1824**, 1842–5
    measurement 1822–4, **1823**, **1842**
  Resident Assessment Protocols *see* Resident Assessment Protocols
  resident visualization 1824–5, *1825*
  see also specific countries
"nutcracker" esophagus 361, 362–3
nutrient(s)
  deficiencies 281, **282**
    burning mouth sensation 274
  factors affecting intake 331, **332**
  high-risk (deficiency) 285–6
  see also specific nutrients
nutrient absorption 291–5
  age related changes 292–3, **293**
  disease modulation 293, **293**
  drug-nutrient interactions 293–4, **294**
  macronutrients 291–2
  micronutrients 292
  regulation 291
nutrition 279–90
  acute pancreatitis 419
  alcohol effects 160
  bone loss 283
  heart disease risk 92
  heart failure and 490
  hip fractures 1333
  ischemic stroke 820–1
  surgical outcome 1638–40
  see also diet
nutritional interventions 314
nutritional peripheral neuropathy 894
nutritional status
  aging effects 110, *110*
  assessment 1545, **1545**, 1610
  chronic disease 1985
nutritional supplements 314
  health indices 287–8
  preoperative 1654
  surgical patients 1639–40

nutritional support, cardiac cachexia 642
nystagmus, types 1239

oat cell carcinoma, lung 712, 905–6
  carcinomatous sensory neuronopathy 896
obesity 347–53
  assessment 347
  consequences in elderly 349–50, **349**
  deep vein thrombosis risk 634
  disease-specific risks 350–1
  energy intake/expenditure 348–9
  functional performance 920
  heart disease risk 478, 519
  management 351, **351**
    exercise and diet 129
    medication 351
    surgical 351
  mechanisms 348–9, **348**
  mortality 129, 310–1, **311**, 349–50
  nutrient utilization 349
  preoperative 1640
  prevalence 348
  sarcopenia *see* sarcopenic obesity
  sleep apnea 737
  stroke risk 802
OBRA '87 1820, 1856, 1897, 1929
obstructive sleep apnea 676, 737, 1418
  see also sleep apnea
obstructive uropathy 1499
occupational therapy 1879–88
  Alzheimer's disease 1089
  assessment and intervention 1882–7, *1883*
    components *1884*
    smart home technology 196–7
  cervical spinal canal stenosis 994
  driving assessment 144
  models 1880–2, *1881*
  motor neuron disease 963
  outcomes 1887
  Parkinson's disease 773
  person/client-centered care 1885
  scope of services 1879–80, *1880*
  settings *1881*
  see also rehabilitation
octreotide 377, 421, 974, 1401, 2008
ocular hypertension 1206, 1208
Ocular Hypertension Treatment Study (OHTS) 1208
ocular myasthenia 905
oculomotor nerve, aging 745
oculopharyngeal muscular dystrophy 944, *945*
odorant receptor genes 1249–50
odynophagia 359
Office for National Statistics (UK), drug misuse 1192
Ohm's law 542
oil of evening primrose 1420
olanzapine 778, 1056, 1057, 1140, 1157
Older Adult Law, Mexico (2000) 1973
Older Drivers Project 142
older people's specialist nurse (OPSN) role, UK 1871
older people's specialist nurse (OPSN) role (UK) 1868–9
oldest old, psychiatric care 1156
old-old people 54
olfaction, aging effect 745
olfactory anesthesia 1249
olfactory bulb (glomeruli) 1250
olfactory nerve 745, 1250
olfactory neuroepithelium 1249
olfactory receptor cells 1250
olfactory system
  age related changes 1252, *1253*
  anatomy 1249–50, *1250*
  biopsy 1254
  dysfunction *see* smell dysfunction
  functional tests 1251–2
olfactory vector hypothesis 1255
Omnibus Budget Reconciliation Act, USA (1987) 1820, 1856, 1897, 1929
On the feat of death poem 1159
oncological emergencies/urgencies 1519–30
  acute symptoms 1520–1
  CNS events 1526–7
  first time presentation 1520–1
Ondine curse 678
On-Line Survey Certification and Reporting (OSCAR) 1824
on-road capability test 144–5
onychauxis *1314*, *1323*, 1325
onychia *1322*, 1325
onychocryptosis (ingrown toenail) *1322*
onychodysplasia *1314*, *1322*
onychodystrophy *1314*
onychogryphosis (Ram's horn toenail) *1322*, 1325
onycholysis 1593, *1593*
onychomycosis *1322*, 1325, 1592–3, *1593*
  assessment **1319**
  treatment 1593
onychophosis 1325
open-angle glaucoma 759
  primary (POAG) 759, 1207
open-door expansive hinge laminoplasty 995
ophthalmic herpes 761
ophthalmoplegia, external 944
opiates/opioids
  anorexia of aging 302–3
  appetite regulation 302–3
  bone pain 2007
  chronic pain 987
  constipation-induction 412–3
  Creutzfeldt-Jacob's disease 1777
  dependence 1192
  dose regimens **2006**
  intoxication symptoms **1195**
  misuse, physical comorbidity 1193
  motor neuron disease 964
  palliative care 2005
  periodic limb movements of sleep 781
  postoperative pain **1652**
  potency 987
  restless legs syndrome 781
  side effects 2005–6
  withdrawal symptoms **1195**
optic nerve, aging 745
optimal discrimination score (ODS), audiometry 1222
oral cancer 243–4, 269–70
  clinical appearance 243, 269–70, *270*
  dietary deficiency 269
  etiology 269
  metastases 270
  prognosis 270
  risk factors 243, 266
  screening 243–4
  smoking 152
  treatment 270
oral disease 261–77
  examination 261
  gingival 262–3
  mucosal infections 263–5
  mucosal lesions 265–8, **265**
  periodontal ligament 262–3
  salivary gland disorders 271–2
  systemic effects 275
oral dyskinesia, spontaneous (SOD) 778–9
oral dyspraxia 844
oral hairy leukoplakia 268
oral health 239–60
  chair-side information 257
  demographics 239
  dental care *see* dental care
  dietary advice 249
  promotion 257–8
oral hemorrhage, tumor induced 1528
oral hygiene, aspiration pneumonia 688–9
oral mucosa
  age related changes 263
  bullous lesions 265–8, **265**
  dehydration 324
  infections 263–5
  red lesions **268**, 269
  ulcerative lesions 265–8, **265**
  white lesions 268–9, **268**
oral status 240–1
oral transmucosal fentanyl citrate (OTFC) 2006
oral ulceration 265–8
  drug induced 266
  recurrent 265–6, **265**
orchiectomy, prostate cancer 1478
orexins (hypocretins) 303
  deficiency 303
Organization for Economic Cooperation and Development (OECD) 141
oro-antral fistula 244
oromandibular dystonia (Meige syndrome) 782
oropharyngeal metering 322
oropharyngeal suction 960
Orpington prognostic scale, ischemic stroke 823
orthogeriatrics
  collaboration models 1342–3
  combined orthopedic care 1343
  hip fractures 1329–42
  supported discharge 1343
  traditional orthopedic care 1342
orthoses 1576, 1581
  arthritis 1350
  bursitis 1325
  foot 1327
orthostasis, diabetic neuropathy 892
orthostatic hypotension *see* hypotension, orthostatic
orthostatic tremor 783
ORYX initiative 1845
os odentoideum, cervical canal stenosis 994, 995
Osawa, Toshio 1936
oscillopsia 1238
oseltamivir, influenza 706, 1730, **1730**
Osler nodes 1755
Osler's maneuver 545
Osler's sign 545
osmolar threshold, thirst 1372
osmoreceptor cells 321
osmotic equilibrium 1369
osmotic laxatives 411–2, **411**
osmotic set point 1403
ossification of posterior longitudinal ligament (OPLL) 992
osteitis deformans *see* Paget's disease of bone
osteoarthritis (OA) 1347–8
  disability reduced by exercise 136
  Down's syndrome 1187
  foot manifestations **1314**
  investigations 1347–8
  joints involved 1347
  medication 1350–1
  surgery 1352
osteoblasts 1262, 1265
  Paget's disease of bone 1270
osteocalcin 1273–4, 1291
osteoclasts 1262, 1294
  Paget's disease of bone 1270
osteomalacia, muscle weakness 943
osteomyelitis
  diagnosis 1359, 1623, *1623*
  pain 1359
  pressure ulcers 1623
  thermal imaging 1719
osteopenia 571, 1187
osteophytes 1358
  cervical spinal canal stenosis 992, 994
  growth, spinal 1356
  osteoarthritis 1347
osteoporosis 42, 1285–97, 1662–3
  age related (type II) 1265, **1265**, 1418
  antiepileptic drugs, risk with 873
  bone loss pathophysiology 1288–92
  cardiovascular disease and 489
  clinical pathway 1295, *1295*
  cost 1662
  definition 283, 1450
  diagnosis 1286–8
  Down's syndrome 1187
  epidemiology 1281–4, 1285–6
  exercise effects **133**, **134**
  fractures 1282
    exercise effects 127, 129, **133**, **134**
    extraskeletal determinants 1288, *1288*
    management *1288*
    pathogenesis *1288*

protein 1290
reduction by statins 489
risk 1285, *1286*, 1418, 1662
sites 1450
skeletal determinants 1287–8
heart failure association 571
HRT and 1450, 1676
incidence 283, 1281–2
laboratory evaluation 1663
male:female fracture ratio 1285
management 1292–3, **1293**
strategies 1283–4
men 1282
menopause 1418
"normal" aging *vs* age related disease 14–5
postmenopausal (type I) 1264–5, **1265**, 1418, 1421
prevention 1292–5, 1893
primary 1662
prostate cancer treatment 1478–9
protein replenishment 1290–1, **1291**
racial variations 1281–2, **1282**
risk assessment guidelines 1282
risk factors 1282, **1283**, 1450, 1662–3, **1663**
screening 208
secondary 1662, **1663**
treatment 1341–2
treatment 1292–5, 1580, 1663
clinical audit 1831, 1832–3
exercise role 127–8
nonpharmacological 1284, *1284*
pharmacological 1293–4, **1293**
vitamin A 1672
vitamin D supplementation 93
vitamin K 1291
WHO diagnostic criteria 1287
osteoporosis circumscripta 1270, 1271
osteoradionecrosis, jaws 272
osteosarcoma, Paget's disease of bone 1271
osteosclerotic myeloma 896
otitic hydrocephalus 1225
otitis externa 1223, 1240
otitis media 1223–5
acute infective 1223
chronic 1223–4
conductive deafness **1223**
surgery **1223**
complications 1224–5
inflammatory 1223
otoconia 1235
otolaryngolic conditions, in Down's syndrome 1187
otolith organ 1235
otological surgery, indications 1246
otorhinologic infection 1773
otoscopy, otitis media 1224
ototoxicity, aminoglycosides 1243
ouabain 543
Outpatient Bleeding Risk Index 451
outpatient mental health services 1199
ovarian cancer 1456, 1659
symptoms 1659
treatment 1456, 1659
ovarian function 1415–21
ovary
age related changes 1449
androgen production 1415–6
palpable 1659
over the counter (OTC) drugs 205
delirium etiology 1051
over-dentures *246*, 247, *247*, *248*, 250, *250*
vertical dimension loss 246
overflow incontinence
fecal 397, **398**
urinary 1487, **1488**
surgery 1490–1
oxcarbazepine, epilepsy 875
Oxford Gerontological Institute 7
Oxfordshire Community Stroke Project (OCSP)
prognosis prediction 823, **823**
stroke classification 796, 797, 815–6
stroke incidence 800
stroke recurrence risk 802
oxidative radicals *see* reactive oxygen species (ROS, free radicals)
oxidative stress/damage 37, 1667–8, **1667**
age-associated neurodegeneration 63–4
to DNA 15
to mitochondrial DNA 16
Parkinson's disease 769–70
sarcopenia 914–6
skeletal muscle 914–6
telomere loss 15
oxybutynin 1490
oxycodone 987, 2005
oxygen
PaO_2 decrease with age 41
saturation measurements 702, 705
VO_2 max *see* maximum oxygen consumption (VO_2 max)
oxygen therapy
acute coronary syndrome 520
asthma 705
COPD 699, 702
hyperbaric 1005
long term 699
postoperative hypoxemia 1636
pulmonary embolic disease 714
ST-segment-elevated myocardial infarction 521
oxygenation, ischemic stroke 818
oxymetholone 315, 925
oxytocin 1402

p53 93, 1669
pacing (rapid walking), dementia 1146
pacing and pacemakers *see* cardiac pacing
paclitaxel, breast cancer 1536
Paget's disease of bone 1269–79
biochemical markers 1273–4
bone deformity 1270
bone pain 1270–1, 1277
cardiac disorders 1271
clinical presentation 1270–1
"cutting cone" lesions 1271
diagnostic evaluation 1271–3
diagnostic recommendations 1274
differential diagnosis 1274, **1274**
epidemiology 1269
etiology 1269–70
follow-up 1276–7
fractures 1270
genetics 1270
jaws 271
neurological symptoms 1245, 1271
pathophysiology 1270
prevalence 1269
radiology 1271–3
radionuclide bone scanning 1271–3, *1272*
retreatment 1277
skin manifestations **1603**
skull vault 271
surgery 1277
treatment 1274–6
tumors 1271
Paget's disease of cervical bodies 992
"paid companions" 1694
pain 981
abdominal *see* abdominal pain
aging 981–2
assessment 2003
postoperative 1652–3
preventive geriatrics 205
back *see* back pain
breakthrough 2006–7
chest *see* chest pain
chronic *see* chronic pain
components *2002*
delirium etiology 1053
dementia, expression in 1136
Down's syndrome 1186
facial *see* facial pain
frailty 1566
mapping *2004*
motor neuron disease 962
neck 1363–4
palliative care 2003–7, **2003**
phantom 1582–3
postoperative
management 1652–3, **1652**
reporting 1652
rating scales 1860, 2003
referred 1363
relief *see* analgesia; analgesics
restraint use reduction 1695
threshold 982
tolerance 982
see also specific anatomical regions
Pain Assessment in Advanced Dementia (PAIN-AD) 985
Pain Scale 1860
pain scores 1652
pain-associated behaviors 984
paired helical filaments (PHF) 1074, *1075*, 1078
palliative/end-of-life care 1682, 2001–16
bereavement 2013
care pathways 2013
carers' support 1813
Council of the European Union report 1685
emergencies 2013
ethical issues 1684–5, 2002
final days 2012–3
future challenges 1876
hospices 2013
life expectancy predictions 2012
lung cancer 713
pain, causes **2003**
pain management 2003–7
pancreatic cancer 422
patient assessment 2001–2
pleural mesothelioma 712
problem list 2001–2, **2002**
semicomatosed patient 2013
symptom analysis 2002–3
see also ethical issues; euthanasia; terminal illness; *specific countries*
pallor, syncope 881
palmomental reflex 787
pamidronate 1275, 1294, 1523
Pan American Health Organization (PAHO) 1970–1, 1975, 1993–4, *1995*
Panama, demographics/service provision 1994, **1994**
pancrealauryl test 420
pancreas
aging 417
calcification 420, *420*
pancreas divisum 419
pancreatic ascites 420
pancreatic cancer 421–2, *421*
imaging 422, *422*
pancreatic diseases 417–23
inflammatory 417–21
nutrient absorption 293, **293**
pancreatic duct ectasia 417
pancreatic enzyme secretion 292
pancreatic pseudocysts 420
pancreatitis
acute 417–9
alcohol association 160
chronic 419–21, *420*
sclerosing 421
pancytopenia 456, 466, 468
panic attacks 871, 884
panic disorder 1153
Pap tests 1659, 1660, 1661
papillae, tongue 1250
para-aminobenzoic acid (PABA) excretion test 420
paracetamol (acetaminophen) 161, 986, 1350, **1652**
paradoxical puborectis contraction *see* dyssynergic defecation
parahippocampal cortex, dendritic changes 71
paraldehyde 876
paralysis
flaccid, hyperkalemia 1383
pressure ulcer risk factor 1608
paralytic syncope *see* areflexic (paralytic) syncope
paramyxoviruses, Paget's disease etiology 1269–70
paranasal sinus disease 1254
paranasal sinuses, subdural empyema 1773
paraneoplastic limb encephalitis 1126–7

paraneoplastic neuropathy 953–4
paranoid delusions, Alzheimer's disease 1140
paraparesis, hereditary spastic 953
paraphilias 121
paraplegia 1003, 1004
paraplegic motor neuron disease 950
paraproteinemias 441, 896
paraproteins, motor neuron disease 959
parasomnias 733
parasympathetic nervous system
  aging 970
  ocular deficits 972
parasympathetic neurons, aging effect 970
parasympathetic tone, sick sinus syndrome 974
parathyroid glands, serum calcium sensitivity 1264
parathyroid hormone (PTH)
  age related changes 42, 1263, 1265
  calcium homeostasis 1261–2, *1262*
  end-stage renal failure 1499
  osteoporosis 1294, 1295
  sarcopenia 917
paratonia, aging 746, 747
parenteral feeding 419, 1639
Parents Maintenance Bill, India (1996) 1986
Parinaud's syndrome 78
PARK genes 770
parkin 770
parkin gene 48
parkinsonian gait 748, 788, 1087, 1301
parkinsonian syndrome, tremor 746
parkinsonism 765–76
  dementia and 1115–7, **1116**
  diagnosis 765–6
  driving and 146
  drug induced 768
  motor neuron disease 950
  see also Parkinson's disease
Parkinson's clinics 765
Parkinson's disease (PD) 765–76
  aging effect on motor systems 47–8
  autonomic dysfunction 775, 972
  classification 765
  clinical features 765, 766
  constipation 413
  definition 765
  diagnosis 765–6, **766**, 1117
    error rate 765
  differential diagnosis 766–7, **766**
  dopaminergic neuron loss 60–1
  dual tasking 1300
  epidemiology 768–9
  falls in 774–5, 1304
  familial 48
  gait 748, 788, 1087, 1301
  gastrointestinal dysfunction 366
  genetics 48, 770
  headache and 758–9
  incidence 47–8, 59, 768
  Lewy bodies 75, 1117
  lifetime risk 768
  management 765, 770–5, **771**
    day hospitals' role 1910
    drug treatment 770–2, 883
    goals 771
    neurosurgery 772, **772**
    nondrug interventions 772–3
    problems of 774–5
    psychiatry 773–4
    syncope and 883
    see also specific drugs
  MPTP induced 769
  neuropathological changes 71, 75, 1117
  nonfamilial 48
  olfactory dysfunction 1255
  oxidative stress 64
  pathogenesis 769–70
  pathology 769
  prognosis 768
  psychology 773–4, **773**
  pulmonary function 676–7
  rehabilitation 772–3, 1572
  risk factors 768–9
  sexual dysfunction 120
  smoking 153
  tremor, nicotine 153
  urodynamic findings 1461
  voiding symptoms 1461
Parkinson's disease dementia (PDD) 773–4, 1116–7, 1119–20
  management 1119
Parkinson's Disease Society 773
Parkinson's plus syndrome 767, 1117
paronychia 1325
parosmia 1249
paroxetine, depression 1139, 1178–9
paroxysmal movement disorders 885–6
paroxysmal nocturnal hemoglobinuria (PNH) 432
paroxysmal symptoms, in multiple sclerosis 885–6
pars flaccida retraction 1224
partial androgen deficiency of aging man *see* andropause
partial anterior circulation infarction (PACI) 816, 823
  recurrence rate 827
partial dentures 244, 245, 250
partial hip replacement 1335
PASE (Pacemaker Selection in the Elderly) **496**
passive infrared sensors, smart homes 191
passive neglect 182
passive smoking, stroke risk 802
patent foramen ovale (PFO) 837
paternalism, ethical issues 1686
pathological fractures 1525, 2007
patient controlled analgesia (PCA) 1653
patient records, electronic 230, 1849–50
  personal patient profiles 225
  problem-orientated 223–4
Patient Self Determination Act, USA (1991) 1685
patient–carer support groups 1044
patient-centered goal planning 865, 1576
patient-lifting techniques 1713–4
Patslide® 1714, *1714*
Patterson-Kelly syndrome (Plummer-Vinson syndrome) 264, 269
Pavlov ratio 991
PBN (α-phenyl-*N*-*tert*-butyl nitrone) 65
PCR *see* polymerase chain reaction (PCR)
PDA (Personal Digital Assistant) devices 1849
PDK2 563
peak expiratory flow rate (PEFR) 694
pedestrians, transport planning to assist 141
pedophilia 121
pedunculopontine nucleus, aging 71
peg-filgrastim 1514
pelvic floor dysfunction *see* dyssynergic defecation
pelvic floor exercises 1463
  stress incontinence 1453, 1463, 1489–90
  uterovaginal prolapse 1453
pelvic floor massage, prostatitis 1482
pelvic floor muscles, aging 1449, 1459
pelvic outlet dysfunction *see* dyssynergic defecation
pelvic ultrasonography 1718
pelvis, pressure ulcer development 1615–6
Pemberton, John 3
pemphigoid
  bullous 1599, *1599*
  mucous membrane 266–7, *267*
pemphigus vegetans 267
pemphigus vulgaris 267
penicillamine, anorexia induction 300
penicillamine induced myasthenia gravis 901
penicillin G **1758**, 1766, 1769
penicillin-resistant streptococci, endocarditis 1757
pentoxifylline 388, 557, 627
peptic ulcer disease 376
  gastrointestinal bleeding 372, **372**
peptide YY (PYY) 304
percutaneous balloon compression, trigeminal neuralgia 760–1
percutaneous balloon valvotomy (PBV) 590
percutaneous endoscopic gastrostomy (PEG) 855, 961
percutaneous transcatheter embolization 1720
percutaneous transluminal angioplasty (PTA) 1720
  stenosis 1007–8
  see also coronary angioplasty
performance-oriented mobility assessment (POMA) 1306
pergolide 737
pericardial effusions, malignant 1524
pericardiectomy 1524
pericardiocentesis 1524
perimenopause 1415, 1660
perindopril, secondary stroke reduction 832
Perindopril Protection Against Recurrent Stroke Study (PROGRESS) 832, *833*
perineal descent, excessive 409
perineum examination, fecal incontinence 398
periodic acid-Schiff stain (PAS) 780, 1593
periodic hypothermia 977
periodic leg movements during wake (PLMW) 780
periodic limb movement disorder (PLMB) 780–1
periodic limb movements in sleep (PLMs) **734**, 736, 737
  differential diagnosis 780
  treatment 781
periodic migrainous neuralgia *see* cluster headache
periodontal disease 240, 1188
periodontal ligament 262–3
periodontitis 152, 262–3
perioperative care, ethical considerations 1653–4
perioperative hypothermia 1651, **1651**
peripheral arterial disease (PAD)
  clinical features *1316*, **1317**
  muscle wasting 918
  prevalence 624, **624**
  risk factors 1316
  vascular studies 1316
  see also peripheral vascular disease (PVD)
peripheral arterial insufficiency, foot ulcers 1324
peripheral dual energy absorptiometry (pDXA) 1283
peripheral nerves
  aging neuropathology 79
  hyperexcitability 906–7
peripheral nervous system, aging **42**, **125**, 889
peripheral neuropathy 889–98
  alcohol related 159, 894
  autoantibody-associated 891, **891**
  autonomic dysfunction 972
  classification 889, 891, **891**
  clinical features 889
  dermatological changes 889, **891**
  in diabetes mellitus 891–3, **891**
  diagnosis 889, *890*
  entrapment neuropathies 893, 896–7
  falls 1301
  hereditary 889
  herpes zoster 895
  idiopathic neuropathies 897
  inflammatory demyelinating polyneuropathy 895
  malignancy 896
  nutritional 894
  sensorimotor 1433
  sensory neuropathies 895–6
  toxins 894–5, **894**
  uremia 893
  vitamin B_{12} deficiency 339
  Wernicke's encephalopathy 972
peripheral quantitative tomography (pQCT), bone density 1283
peripheral resistance, hypertension 973
peripheral vascular disease (PVD) 623–31
  amputation 628
  atherosclerotic disorders with 625, **625**
  critical lower limb ischemia 623
  exercise rehabilitation 627
  foot care 627
  gangrene 623
  medical management **628**
    ACE inhibitors 627
    antiplatelet drugs 626
    β-blockers 627
  morbidity/mortality 625–6
  muscle atrophy 1569
  noninvasive diagnosis 623–4
  pressure ulcers 1609, *1610*
  prevalence 624, **624**
  risk factors 624, 626

surgery 627–8
ulceration 623
walking distance increasing drugs 627
see also peripheral arterial disease (PAD)
periradicular injection 997
peristalsis, primary/secondary 358
peritoneal dialysis, hyperkalemia 1384
peritonitis 1501
periurethral sphincter collagen injections 1490
permethrin, scabies 1595
peroneal nerve, entrapment neuropathy 896, 897
persistent hypothermia 977
persistent pain, aging 981–2
persistent vegetative state (PVS), ethical issues 1685
personal alarm systems 1847–8
Personal Digital Assistant (PDA) devices 1849
personality
dementia and 1137, **1137**
developmental-stage models 53
personality disorders 1155
person/client-centered care
goal planning 865, 1576
NSF (UK) standard **1802**, 1917
occupational therapy 1885
principles 1869
Person-Environment-Occupation-Performance/Participation (PEOP) model 1880–2, *1881*, 1884
pethidine 987
petrositis 1225
Pflegeversicherung 1810
p-glycoprotein 455
phacoemulsification, cataracts 1209
phagocytosis 26
frustrated, infective endocarditis 1754–5
Phalen's sign 896
phantom pain 1582–3
phantosmia 1249
Pharmaceutical Benefits Scheme, Australia 1893
pharmacodynamics 218, **1514**
pharmacogenetics 218–9
pharmacogenomics 111
pharmacokinetics 215–7, **216**
age related changes **1514**
pharmacologic changes, aging 1514, **1514**
pharmacological restraints, delirium 1056–7
pharmacological stress testing 516–7
pharyngoesophageal function 42
pharynx, swallowing 844–5
phase-advanced sleep 735, 738
phase-delayed sleep 735
phasic muscle stretch reflexes 746–7
phenobarbitone, epilepsy 873, 876
phenol nerve blocks 856
phenylbutyrate, myelodysplasia therapy 459
phenytoin
cramp in MND 960
epilepsy 873, 874, **874**, 875–6
peripheral neuropathy in herpes zoster 895
status epilepticus 876
trigeminal neuralgia 274
pheochromocytoma 544
Philadelphia Geriatric Center Morale Scale **1575**, 1939
phobia 1149
phobic disorder 1153
phonemic cueing 1040
phonemic paraphasias 1041
phorbol myristate acetate (PMA) 29
phosphate, renal tubular dysfunction 1497–8
phosphate enemas 412
phosphatidyl-4,5-bisphosphate (PIP2) 29
phosphatidylcholine, alcoholic liver disease 388
phosphocreatine, heart failure 564
phosphodiesterase-5 inhibitors
α-blockers interaction 1472
contraindications 118
erectile dysfunction 118
pharmacokinetics **118**
side effects **118**
phospholambam 562, 563
phospholipase C (PLC) 29
phospholipids 613, 616
phosphosoda, constipation 412
photoaging 1591–2, **1592**
photodamage, vitamin C 1673
photodynamic therapy, actinic keratosis 1601
photoreceptors, density decrease with age 39
physical abuse 182
physical activities of daily living (PADLs) 1141
physical activity 110, *110*, 123
adipose tissue accretion/distribution 129–30
chronic adaptation 125
cognitive function improvement 131–2
definition 123
increased, cardiac rehabilitation 650
obesity management 351
role in bone health 126–7
threshold and optimal levels 124
see also exercise; exercise programs
physical fitness 123
dose–response relationship with health 123–4
physical inactivity
ischemic heart disease risk 478, 519
see also sedentary lifestyle
physical restraints 1690
dehydration 324
delirium 1056
effects of **1690**
elder abuse 186
nursing home care 1822, 1844
postoperative confusion 1650
see also restraints
physical therapy
arthritis 1350
ischemic stroke 819–20
normal pressure hydrocephalus 793
pressure ulcers 1625
prostatitis 1481–2, **1481**
physician assistants, USA 1931
physician role, alcohol abuse 161
physician-assisted suicide 2012
motor neuron disease 949, 964–5
Physicians Health Study 333
Physicians Plan for Older Drivers' Safety (PPODS) *143*
physiology of aging 37–46
see also specific organs
physiotherapy
back pain 1362
breathlessness 2009
motor neuron disease 963
Parkinson's disease 773
spinal canal stenosis 994, 997
stroke rehabilitation, Bobath method 855
uterovaginal prolapse 1453
phytotherapy, benign prostatic hyperplasia 1472
Pick's disease 1121
see also frontotemporal lobular degeneration (FTLD)
picture archiving communication systems (PACS) 1716
pill esophagitis 362
pilocarpine, dry mouth 271, 272
pineal cysts 78
pineal gland, age related changes 31, 78
pipe smokers, leukoplakia 268
piroxicam induced hepatitis 385
pitch 1219
pituitary adenoma 428, 544
pituitary apoplexy 1020, 1399
pituitary gland 1397–404
age related changes 44, 78–9, 1397
anatomy 1397
anterior
blood supply 1397
hormone secretions 1401–2, **1401**
anterior, disorders
clinical features 1397–400
treatment 1400–2
blood supply 1397
cell types **1398**
hormones **1398**, *1398*
posterior 1402–3
anatomy 1402
blood supply 1397
diseases 1402
pituitary stalk 1397
pituitary tumors 1397–9
nonfunctioning 1398–9
treatment 1400
pituitary-adrenal axis disorders, myopathies 942
plain radiography *see* X-ray
plantar calcaneal bursitis 1325
plantar responses, aging effect 747
plaque, dental *see* dental plaque
plaque psoriasis 1597, *1597*
plaques
aging neuropathology 73–4, *73*, *74*
atheromatous *see* atheroma/atheromatous plaques
senile, Alzheimer's disease 1073–5, *1074*, *1075*, 1078–9
plasma cell dyscrasias 896, 1503
plasma exchange 679, 905, 907
plasma volume 1369–70
plasmapheresis, hyperviscosity syndrome 1525
Plastazote insoles, bursitis 1325
plasticity, nervous system 969
platelet(s)
functional defects 439, **439**
growth factors released 43
number disorders 437–8
platelet counts
disseminated intravascular coagulation 1526
normal 437
thrombocytopenia 1526
platelet endothelial cell adhesion molecule-1 (PECAM-1) 618
platelet glycoprotein IIb/IIIa antagonist 520
platelet microbicidal proteins (PMPs) 1754
platelet transfusions 374, 458, 467
platelet-derived growth factor (PDGF) 91, 619, 1625
pleconaril, viral meningitis 1764
pleiotropy 14
antagonistic, theory 14
pleural effusion 420, 694, 2009
pleural mesothelioma 712–3
plicamycin (mithramycin) 1276, 1523
plication procedures, fecal incontinence 403
Plummer-Vinson syndrome 264, 269
pluripotent hemopoietic stem cell (PHSC) 465
pneumatic dilatation, achalasia 360
pneumococcal meningitis 1767
pneumococcal vaccine 1733–4
cost effectiveness 1734
indications 1734, **1734**
recommendations 207
revaccination 1734
USA, usage 1924, *1925*
vaccine-associated reactions 1733–4
23-valent, pneumonia prevention 690
pneumoconioses 715–6
pneumonectomy 711
pneumonia 706–8
aspiration *see* aspiration pneumonia
atypical 707
causes 706
chronic eosinophilic 718
cryptogenic organizing 715, 718
epidemiology 1725–6
nosocomial *see* nosocomial pneumonia
pathogens 1726
treatment 708
see also community acquired pneumonia
pneumonitis, aspiration *see* aspiration pneumonitis
pneumothorax, signs 694
poikilothermia 976
Poland, medical education/training 1785
polio virus, MND association 958
poliomyelitis 953
postpolio syndrome 1776–7
polyarteritis nodosa 953, 954
polycythemia 1424
polydipsia 1377–8
polydipsia-hyponatremia syndrome 1377
polydrug misuse 1191
polyethylene glycol (PEG), constipation 411, 2008, **2008**

polyethylene glycol (PEG)-based bowel preparation 376
polymerase chain reaction (PCR)
  infective endocarditis 1757
  meningitis 1764, 1765, 1768
  tuberculosis 1743, 1768
polymyalgia rheumatica 1566, 1580
polymyositis (PM) 939
polyneuropathy
  acute inflammatory demyelinating 895
  chronic inflammatory demyelinating 895, 953
  sensory, diabetes mellitus 892
  symmetrical 891
polypharmacy 215–21
  acute renal failure 1499
  anticoagulation risks 451, 506, 637
  dehydration 323–4
  driving and 145
  drug misuse 1191
  endocrine diseases 1391
  in heart failure 572
  medical errors 215
poly(ADP-ribose) polymerase (PARP) 15
polysomnography (PSG) 736–7
  see also electroencephalogram (EEG)
polyvinyl ring pessary 1453
pontine/medullary hemorrhages 1244
Poor Law Amendment Act, UK (1834) 1916
Poor Law Relief Act, UK (1601) 2, 3, 1915
population trends, USA 95–6
porcelain veneers *246*, 247
porphyria 954
portable radiographic examinations 1716
portocaval shunt 377
Portugal
  medical education/training 1785
  nursing home care 1980
positional nystagmus 1239, **1239**
positive pressure ventilation, in MND 676
positron emission tomography (PET)
  brain tumor 1527
  dementia predictor in MCI 1097
  dystonia 782
  normal pressure hydrocephalus 790
  Parkinson's disease 771
  restless legs syndrome 781
  stroke, neural imaging after 849–50
postacute-care facilities, delirium and 1047–8
Post-AV nodal ablation Evaluation (PAVE) trial 502
postencephalitic parkinsonism 769
posterior circulation infarction (POCI) 816, 823
  recurrence rate 827
posterior cortical cataract 1208
posterior longitudinal ligament 995
posterior pelvic tilt 1615, *1615*
posterior polar cataract 1208
posterior semicircular canal 1235
posterior spinal artery 1001–2
  occlusion/insufficiency 1009
posterior spinal vein 1002
posterior subcapsular cataract 1208, **1209**
postherpetic neuralgia 274, 1594
  headache and 761–3, **761**, *762*
postmenopausal bleeding (PMB) 1451–2, **1451**, 1661
postmenopausal women
  exercise intervention trials 127
  osteoporosis *see* osteoporosis
postoperative confusion (POC) 1649–50, **1650**
postoperative delirium 1152, 1640–1
postoperative dementia 1641–2
postoperative hypoxemia 1636
postoperative radiotherapy (PORT), lung cancer 711
postoperative stroke 1640, 1650, **1650**
postpolio syndrome 1776–7
postprandial hypotension *see* hypotension
postthrombotic leg syndrome 637
posttraumatic headache (PTH) 759
posttraumatic stress disorder (PTSD) 1154
posttraumatic subdural hematoma *see* subdural hematoma, posttraumatic
postural hypotension *see* hypotension, orthostatic
postural instability, Parkinson's disease 774
posture
  aging effect 747–8
  Alzheimer's disease 1086
postvoid residual (PVR) volumes 1488–9
potassium 94
  disorders 1382–4
  renal tubular dysfunction 1497
  replacement therapy, hypokalemia 1385
  supplements, myasthenia gravis 904
potassium channel blockers 503
  sotalol 503, 508, 510, 523
  see also amiodarone
potassium chloride, hypokalemia 1385
potassium hydroxide (KOH) test 1592, 1593, *1593*
^{40}K counting 910, **911**
Pott's disease 1360
poverty 105–6, *106*
  anorexia 299
  developing countries 1972
  food intake 285
power of attorney, homosexuals 121
PPARγ agonists, atherosclerosis 621
PQRST pneumonic, pain **2003**
Practical Management of the Elderly 5
practice guidelines, limitations 201
pragmatic dysfunction 842, 1039
preatheroma 611
pre-βHDL 614
Predementia Alzheimer's disease scale (PAS) 1098, **1098**, 1099
prednisolone/prednisone
  acute exacerbation of COPD 701
  bullous pemphigoid 1599
  cryptogenic fibrosing alveolitis 717
  dermatomyositis 938
  hypercalcemia of malignancy 1522–3
  immune thrombocytopenic purpura 438
  Lambert Eaton myasthenic syndrome 906
  mucous membrane pemphigoid 267
  myasthenia gravis 903–4, 905
  oral lichen planus 266
  rheumatoid arthritis 1351
  tuberculous meningitis 1769
pregabalin, epilepsy 874–5
pregnenolone 1394
prehypertension 541
preload, aging effect 567
premature aging syndromes 1589–90
premature menopause 160, 1187
premature ventricular contractions (PVC) 507
premature ventricular depolarization (PVD) 507
presbycusis 842, 1225
  aging 745
  cochlear conductive 1227
  neural 1226–7
  sensory 1226
  strial 1227
presbyesophagus 359
presbyopia, aging 745
prescription charges, Latin America 1994
presenilin 1 49, 1076, 1077
presenilin 2 49, 1076
Present Pain Intensity 984
pressure areas, hip fractures 1332
pressure sore status tool (PSST) 1617
pressure sores *see* pressure ulcers/ulceration
pressure ulcer scale for healing (PUSH) tool 1617
pressure ulcers/ulceration 1605–30
  age 1609
  assessment 1864
  bony prominences 1606–7, *1607*
  classification 1617–8, **1617**, *1618–9*
  complications 1623
  costs 1605
  definition 1605, 1655
  grades 1 and 2 **1617**, *1618*
  grades 3 and 4 **1617**, *1619*
  healing times 1617
  hip fractures 1332
  infections 1622–3
  litigation 1605
  management 1616–26
  mortality 1605
  nursing home care 1844
  pathogenesis 1605–8, *1607*
  patient repositioning 1612, 1616
  perioperative 1654–5, **1655**
  photography 1617–8
  postoperative care 1624
  pressure relief 1616–7
  pressure-relieving devices 1612–3
  prevalence 1605
    nursing home residents 1821, 1822
  prevention 1611–6
  risk assessment 1610–6
    scales 1610–1, **1610**, *1611*
  risk factors 1608–10, **1608**
  sites 1605, *1606*
  surgery 1623–4
  terminally ill 1609, 2011
pressure-relieving cushions 1616, **1616**, *1617*
pressure-relieving devices 1612–3
  selection **1611**, 1612
  staff education 1613
pressure-sensitive mats 191
pressure-sensor activated alarms 1694
presyncope 879
pretrigeminal neuralgia 760
prevalence rate definition 796
preventative care *see* health promotion
prevention of disease, primary/secondary 201
Prevention of Falls Network Europe (ProFaNE) 1308
preventive geriatrics 201–13
  decision-making issues 202
  models
    British Health Checks 201, 209–10
    Health Maintenance Clinical Guidepath 201–9
    see also both individual models
primary biliary cirrhosis (PBC) 390
primary care 6
  mental health services 1158
  substance abuse intervention 1153
  see also specific countries
Primary Care Clinical Effectiveness (PRICCE) project 1835
primary care physicians, dementia 1152
primary open-angle glaucoma (POAG) 759, 1207
primary progressive aphasia (PPA) 1039, 1040
primidone 784, 873
primitive reflexes, aging effect 747
Principles for Older Persons, United Nations 1969
printed materials, guidelines for preparation 56
prion diseases, dementia 1124–5, **1124**
prion protein (PrP) 1124
prison inmates, psychiatric care 1156
problem-orientated assessment *see* geriatric assessment
problem-orientated medical records (POMR) 223–4
Problems of Aging 1
procedural memory 1038, 1044
processing speed, aging effect 49
prochlorperazine 1245, 1246, 2008
professional training/education
  medical *see* medical education/training
  nursing *see* nurse education/training
Profile of Mood States 984
progesterone, brain cell osmolality 1371
progestins, breast cancer 1514
"Progetto Memoria" 1062
Program of All-Inclusive Care for the Elderly (PACE), USA 1928–9
Program to Encourage Active, Rewarding Lives for Seniors (PEARLS) 1179
PROGRESS (Protection Against Recurrent Stroke Study) 549, 1438
progress monitoring, ischemic stroke 818
progressive bilateral deafness 1227
progressive fluent aphasia 1123
progressive massive fibrosis (PMF) 715–6
progressive muscular atrophy (PMA) 949, 950
  see also motor neuron disease (MND)
progressive neurodegenerative disorders, MND *see* motor neuron disease (MND)

progressive nonfluent aphasia 1121, 1122–3
progressive supranuclear palsy (PSP) 1255
  clinical features 767
  dementia 1120
  parkinsonism 1116–7
prokinetic agents 412, 2008
prolactin (PRL)
  pituitary tumor hypersecretion 1399
  psychogenic nonepileptic attacks 885
  secretion, age related changes 1401–2
prolactinomas 1399, 1400
prolene suburethral sling insertion 1491
prolonged spontaneous tinnitus (PST) 1212
prompted voiding
  fecal incontinence 399
  urinary incontinence 1489
propionyl levocarnitine 627
propoxyphene, osteoarthritis 1350
propranolol 784, 960
proprioceptive neuromuscular facilitation (PNF) **137**
propylthiouracil, alcoholic liver disease 388
proscar longterm efficacy and safety study (PLESS) 1463
PROSPER study **1437**
prostaglandins, glaucoma 1208
prostate cancer 1474–9
  androgen deprivation 1514
  detection 1474
  disease progression treatment 1478–9
  disseminated intravascular coagulation 1526
  epidemiology 1474
  grade 1475
  natural history 1476
  screening 208, 1474, 1512
  staging 1476, **1476**
  symptoms 1474
  testosterone replacement therapy 1424
  treatment 1476–9, **1476**
    radiation therapy **1476**, 1477–8
    surgery **1476**, 1477
  vitamin E supplements 1474
  watchful waiting 1476–7, **1476**
Prostate Cancer Prevention Trial 1474–5
prostate diseases 1469–83
prostate gland
  adrenergic receptors 1472, 1480
  anatomy 1469, *1470*
  growth 1459
  hyperplasia *see* benign prostatic hyperplasia (BPH)
prostatectomy
  bladder dynamics 1460
  open, benign prostatic hyperplasia 1474
  overflow incontinence 1491
  radical 1477
    complications 1477
    observation *vs* 1512
  radical retropubic, prostate cancer 1477
prostate-specific antigen (PSA) 1474–5
  age-adjusted 1475, **1475**
  benign prostatic hyperplasia 1471
  finasteride induced reduction 1475
  normal range 1474
  prostate cancer screening 1474–5
  prostate size indicator 1472
  testosterone replacement 1675
  velocity 1475
prostatic massage, prostatitis 1480, 1481
prostatitis 1479–82
  acute bacterial 1479–80, **1479**
  chronic bacterial 1479, **1479**, 1480
  classification 1479, **1479**
  diagnosis 1480
  epidemiology 1479
  etiology 1479–80
  evaluation 1480, **1480**
  laboratory testing 1480
  minimally invasive therapy 1482
  nonbacterial 1479
  symptoms index 1480, **1481**
  treatment 1480–2, **1481**
prostheses 1576, 1581–2, *1582*
prosthetic valve endocarditis (PVE) 590, 1750
protamine infusion 374, 605
protein(s)
  absorption 292
  damage associated with aging 16
  osteoporosis 1293
  oxidative damage 64
  supplementation 923, 1290–1, **1291**, 1333
  turnover, age related changes 916
protein C deficiency 442, 445, 446, 633
protein kinase A (PKA) 556
protein kinase C (PKC) 29, 33
protein malnutrition/undernutrition, bone mass 1289–90, *1290*
protein S deficiency 442, 445, 446, 633
protein tyrosine kinase
  inhibitors, myelodysplasia therapy 469
  phosphorylation 29
protein-energy malnutrition
  adverse effects 298, **299**
  chronic 313
  pathological factors 299–300
  pressure ulcers 1610
  prevalence 298
  surgery 1654
  see also undernutrition
proteosome inhibition 1515
prothrombin time 337, 385
proton pump inhibitors (PPI) 362, 363, 376
proverb interpretation, assessment 1065
proximal diabetic neuropathy 893
proximal femoral nail (PFN) 1335
proximal tibial osteotomies 1277
proxy, incompetent surgical patients 1653–4
pruritus 1595–6
PSA *see* prostate-specific antigen (PSA)
psammona bodies 78, *78*
pseudo-achalasia 360
pseudoarteriosclerotic parkinsonism 767
pseudodementia, in depression 1123, 1177
pseudoephedrine, stress incontinence 1463
pseudogout 1349
  treatment 1352
pseudohypertension 545
pseudohypoparathyroidism 992
pseudomembranous colitis (PMC) 1730
Pseudomonas, otitis externa 1223
Pseudomonas aeruginosa, otitis externa 1240
pseudo-Pelger–Huët phenomenon 429, 456
pseudoseizures 884–5
pseudostatus epilepticus 884
psoas compartment block, hip pain 2007
psoralen and UVA (PUVA), psoriasis 1597
psoriasis 1597, *1597*
psychiatric disorders **983**, 1149–61
  see also specific diseases/disorders
psychiatric services 1168
  assessment 1545, **1545**
  see also specific countries
psychiatric setting, alcohol problem prevalence 158
psychiatrist, memory clinics 1064
psychiatry 1149–61
  best practice models 1157–8
  diagnostic interview 1150, **1150**
  emergencies 1154
  end-of-life care 1156–7
  epidemiology 1149–50
  prevention of disorders 1157, **1157**
  psychopharmacology 1157
  special populations 1155–6
    caregivers 1156
    ethnic minorities 1156
    long term care residents 1155–6
    oldest old 1156
    prison inmates 1156
  see also specific diseases/disorders
psychogenic nonepileptic attacks 884–5
psychogenic polydipsia 1377
psychological abuse 182
psychological aspects 1573–4
  carers 1164–5, 1811–2
  religion/spirituality 110–1
psychological disorders, pain **983**
psychological losses, of aging 54
psychological symptoms, Alzheimer's disease 1087
psychological therapies *see* psychotherapy
psychological well-being, exercise association 131
psychology, definition 53
psychology of aging 53–7
  creativity changes 56
  developmental tasks 53–4
  implications of changes for practice 56–7
  intelligence 55
  life stage perspective 53–4
  maladaptive behaviors 54, 57
  memory changes 55–6
  mental vitality 53, 56
  sensory losses 56
  successful 53
psychometric assessment 1554–7
  communication disorders 1042
  memory clinic patients 1065, **1066**
  see also function assessment scales
psychopharmacology 1157
psychophysiological insomnia 738
psychoses 1151–3
  acute, Parkinson's disease 773, 774
  see also specific diseases/disorders
psychosocial factors
  disability risk factor 136
  heart disease risk factor 478–9
psychosocial treatment
  dementia 1152
  heart disease secondary prevention 649
  schizophrenia 1151
  substance abuse 1153
Psychosocial Typology of Illness 861
psychotherapy
  bipolar affective disorder 1151
  dysthymic disorder 1178
  provision *see* clinical psychology services
  see also cognitive behavioral therapy (CBT)
psychotic depression, treatment 1179
psychotic manifestations, Alzheimer's disease 1087
psychotropic drugs
  alcohol interaction 161
  long term care residents 1157
  misuse 1192
  psychiatric disorder induction 1154
psyllium, constipation 411
ptosis, oculopharyngeal muscular dystrophy 944, *945*
ptyalism (hypersalivation) 272–3, **273**
public health workers, epidemiological data use 795
pubococcygeus muscle 396
puborectalis muscle 396
pudendal neuropathy 408
pulmonary artery embolization 1720
pulmonary artery pressure 533
pulmonary disease *see* respiratory disease
pulmonary edema 502, 515, 585–6, 589
pulmonary embolectomy 714
pulmonary embolic disease 713–4
pulmonary embolism 480
  after stroke 820
  age range 633
  clinical features 636
  diagnosis/investigations 636
  incidence 449
  management 452, 636–7
  models, left ventricular end-diastolic pressure 565
  mortality 635
pulmonary hypertension, rehabilitation 729
pulmonary pressures 533
pulmonary rehabilitation 727–31, 1579–80, **1579**
  breathing retraining 728
  contraindications 729
  COPD 699, 727–31
  end-of-life issues 728–9
  exercise therapy 728
  health-care utilization 730
  maintenance programs 730
  outcomes 729–30
  patient education 728–9
  patient selection 729
  program location 728

pulmonary rehabilitation (*cont.*)
program organization 699, 727–9
psychosocial support 729
pulmonary reserve, aging effect 568, **569**
pulse, syncope 882
pulse pressure, increased 517, 541
pulse rate, during postural changes 546
punched out lesions, gout 1348
pupillary abnormalities, aging and 972
pure autonomic failure 971–2
pure-tone audiometry (PTA) 1219, 1220–1
deafness classification 1220, **1221**
flat loss 1227
ski-slope loss 1227
strial presbycusis 1227
purified protein derivative (PPD) skin test 1731, 1740
purpura
Henoch–Schönlein 441
immune thrombocytopenic 437–8
senile 441
thrombotic thrombocytopenic 440–1
pursed-lip breathing 728
putamen, depression 1176
pylorus 363
pyramidal cells, aging 62
pyramidal neurons, Alzheimer's disease 1074
pyramidal tract degeneration, motor neuron disease 956
pyrazinamide
side effects 1744
tuberculosis 709, 1743, **1745**
latent 1746, **1746**
tuberculous meningitis 1768
pyrexia *see* fever
pyridinoline, bone resorption marker 1274
pyridostigmine, myasthenia gravis 903
pyridoxine 459, 709, 894
pyridoxine-5′-β-D-glucoside 339

Quality Assurance Agency (QAA), UK **1791**, 1791
quality of care 1837–53
definition 1842–3
improvement initiatives 1840
acute care 1845–7, 1871
community setting 1847–9
nursing home care *see* nursing home care
organizations 1838–9, 1842
measurement/evaluation
indicators 1840–1, **1842**, 1861–2
Minimum Data Set *see* Minimum Data Set (MDS)
models 1839–40, *1840*, **1841**
see also clinical audit
see also specific countries
quality of life
anemia effect 427
bath water controls 193
communication difficulties 1042
COPD 700
decline associated with immune system decline 31
enhancement strategies 1885–7
ethical issues 1683–4, 1685
health related (HRQoL) 1560–2, **1560**, **1561**
improvement by cardiac surgery 597–8
measurement 1910, 1911
smart homes 195–6
Quality of Life Index 1910
QuantiFERON-TB (QFT) test 1741, **1742**
quantitative sudomotor axon reflex test (QSART) 897
quantitative ultrasound (QUS), bone mineral density 1283
quetiapine 774, 1140, 1141
quinidine, Creutzfeldt-Jacob's disease 1777
quinine sulphate, cramp in MND 960
quinolone, gonorrhea 1732

race, stroke risk 803
radiant heat (normotherapy), pressure ulcers 1625
radiation **1712**
ionizing, cardiovascular disease 92
radiation colitis 377
radiation pneumonitis 711
radiation proctitis 377
radiation therapy *see* radiotherapy
radicular artery 1001
radiculopathy, cervical spinal canal stenosis 992–3, 994
radio, smart home communication system 194–5
radioactive iodine 1409, 1513
radioactive strontium 1513
radioactive sumerium 1513
radioactive yttrium 1513
radiofrequency ablation (RFA) 1513
radiofrequency denervation, back pain 1362
radiofrequency gangliolysis, trigeminal neuralgia 761
radiographically inserted gastrostomies (RIG) 961
radiography *see* X-ray
radioimmuno-precipitation assay (RIA), myasthenia gravis 902
radioisotope bone scan *see* bone, scintigraphy
radioisotopes 1513
radiologically guided cacostomy 1720
radiology
acute pancreatitis 418
Alzheimer's disease 1088
best practice guidelines 1711–3
doses **1712**, *1713*
Paget's disease of bone 1271–3
problems in 1713–5
see also X-ray
radionuclide cisternography 790
radionuclide studies *see* scintigraphy
radiotherapy 1513
bone pain 2007
breast cancer 1534–5
cervical cancer 1455–6
lung cancer 711, 712
myelodysplasia due to 455
oral effects 272
spinal cord compression 1521
superior vena cava syndrome 1524
raloxifene 1294–5, 1511
ramantadine, influenza 706
ramipril, stroke risk reduction 832
Ramsay-Hunt syndrome 267, 1240
RANK/RANKL/OPG regulatory system 1265
rape, elder abuse 121, 184
rapid eye movement (REM) sleep 734, 1418
rapid eye movement sleep behavior disorder (RBD) **734**, 736, 737–8
rapid plasma reagin (RPR), syphilis 1732
Ras MAP-kinase pathway, inhibitors 460–1
rate of perceived exertion (RPE) 125, 654
rationing (of resources), ethical issues 1682–3
Rawls's theory of justice 1683
reaction time, age related changes 55
reactivating therapy, memory clinic patients 1068
reactive oxygen species (ROS, free radicals) 14, 617, *617*, 915
heart failure 564
immune cell damage 32
mitochondrial source 16
motor neuron disease 954, 957
skin aging and 38
sunlight effect on formation 38
see also oxidative stress/damage
reading aloud, communication assessment 1041
reality orientation, communication disorders 1042
recall, of information 55
recognition, matching information 55
recombinant basic fibroblast growth factor (rh b-FGF) 1625
recombinant human growth hormone (rhGH) 642–3
recombinant platelet derived growth factor-BB (rh PDGF-BB) 1625
recombinant tissue plasminogen activator (rTPA) 820
Recommended Dietary Allowances (RDA) 330, 331
rectal columns (anal cushions) 395
rectal prolapse 409
rectocele 410, 1459
rectosphincteric incontinence 398
rectum 395
defecation 396
red blood cell
accelerated destruction, anemia 431
enzyme defects 431
membrane defects, anemia 431
precursors, myelodysplasia diagnosis 456, 457
red clover, menopausal symptom management 1420
"red eye of renal failure" 1500
5-α reductase inhibitors 1463, 1464–5, 1472
referred pain, neck 1363
reflex syncope
clinical features and diagnosis 882
mechanism 879, 880
warning symptoms 881
reflexes, aging effect 746–7
see also individual reflexes
refractive error 1205, *1206*
medical/social risk factors **1206**
refractory anemia with excess blasts (RAEB) 456, **457**, 461, 468
refractory anemia with excess blasts in transformation (RAEB-T) 456, **457**, 461
refractory cytopenia with trilineage dysplasia (RCTD) 457
regional analgesia, postoperative 1653
rehabilitation 1571–86, **1574**
activity and participation restrictions 1572–3, **1572**
aids and adaptations 1576
amputees 1581–3, *1582*
assessment 1574–6, **1575**
cardiac *see* cardiac rehabilitation
musculoskeletal disorders 1580–3
neurological 1583
nurse role 1873
Parkinson's disease 1572
patient-centered goal planning 865, 1576
principles 1574
psychiatric *see* psychiatric services
psychological aspects 1573–4
see also clinical psychology services
pulmonary 1579–80, **1579**
settings 1577–8
stroke 822
terminology/classifications 1571–2
see also occupational therapy
rehydration, hypercalcemia 2009
relationship issues 109, *109*, 228–9
Relatives' Stress Scale (RSS) 1813
religion, aging and 110–1
REM sleep 734, 1418
reminiscence, communication disorders 1042
renal artery blood flow 43, 544, 978
renal biopsy, nephrotic syndrome 1502
renal diseases 1495–506
cardiac features 489
end stage *see* end stage renal disease (ERSD)
medullary hypotonicity 1498
tubular frailty 1498–9
vascular alterations 1496
renal excretion, drugs 217–8, **217**
renal failure
acute 1498–9
analgesia 2005
chronic 1499–501
exercise effects **133**, **134**
hyperkalemia 1383
postoperative 1636–7
renal function
age related changes 217–8, 570, 572, 1650
aging effect 42–3, **43**, 543, 568, **569**
medication dosage adjustment 1514
postoperative 1636–8
renal impairment/dysfunction
after cardiac surgery 596
cardiovascular disease and 489
chronic insufficiency-associated anemia *see* anemia
drug toxicity 1503–4

peripheral neuropathy risk 894
pre-/postoperative 1636–7
see also renal function
renal replacement therapy (RRT) 1500–1
renal sympathetic activity, aging effect 978
renal transplantation 893, 1501, 1502
renal tubular dysfunction 1496–8
Rendu Osler-Weber syndrome 376
renin 322, 323
renin-angiotensin-aldosterone system (RAAS) 543, 557, 973
renovascular disease, secondary hypertension 544
renovascular renal failure 1496
repetitive chair stand test 1558
repetitive nerve stimulation (RNS) 902
repetitive transcranial magnetic stimulation (rTMS) 1179
Repose Bootee *1612*
Repose mattress 1613, *1613*
reserpine, delirium etiology 1050
reservoir incontinence 397–8
Resident Assessment Protocols 1821
Minimum Data Set 1856–7, **1856**, 1858
residential homes *see* nursing home care
resistance to CSF outflow (R_{CSF}) 789
resistance/resistive training
body fat changes 130
bone health 127
corticosteroid induced osteopenia reduced 135
depression improvement 129, 131
diabetes management 135, **135**
disease treatment by **134**
heart failure management 577–8
muscle mass maintenance/increase 130
obesity management 351
osteoporotic fracture treatment 129
recommendations for optimal aging **137**
respiratory muscle strength 674
sarcopenia 922
resource allocation, ethical issues 1682–3
Resource Utilization Groups (RUGs) 1860–1, 1863
'respiration-to-speech apraxia' 1040
respiratory depression, opioid analgesics 2006, 2009
respiratory disease 693–726
cardiac manifestations 489
delirium etiology 1052
obstructive pattern 694–5
restrictive pattern 695
sarcoid 718
signs 693–4
respiratory drive, reduction during sleep 737
respiratory dysfunction
peri-/postoperative 1635
postoperative care 1649
preoperative assessment 1635–6
respiratory failure, motor neuron disease 676, 961–2
respiratory function tests 694, 697
respiratory infections *see* respiratory tract infections
respiratory skeletal muscles
aging effects 671–83
muscle strength 673–4, 696
muscle structure 673, 695
endurance 674–5, 695–6
fatigue 674
oxygen consumption 675
structure 672
weakness and disease 675–80, **675**
respiratory syncope, mechanism 880, 881
respiratory syncytial virus (RSV) 667, 668, 706, 1727
respiratory system
age related changes 41, **41**, 695–6, 1649
anesthesia effects 1649
immobility effects **1690**
preoperative preparations 1649
respiratory tract infections
asthma 705
bacterial 1725–6
cardiac features 489
epidemiology 665–70, 1725–7
lower tract 705–10
undernutrition 680
upper tract 1254
viral 1726–7
vitamin E supplements 1671
respite families, Alzheimer's disease 1090
respite services, carers 1164–6, 1812–4, 1896
rest tremor 783, **783**
resting energy expenditure (TEE) 313
resting metabolic rate (RMR) 348
restless legs syndrome (RLS) **734**, 737, 780–1
restraints 1689–700
behavioral symptom control 1692
"best practice" 1693–4
complications 1692–3
fall prevention 1308, 1691–2, 1693
justification 1691–2
in nursing home care 1822, 1844
pharmacological 1056–7
physical *see* physical restraints
psychological effects **1690**, 1692
reduction in use approaches 1693–6
comfort promotion 1695
continence maintenance 1695
fall risk assessment 1695–6
injury risk reduction 1696
mental status change investigations 1695
mobility promotion 1694
observation 1694
patient activities 1694–5
reduction in use outcomes 1693
risk factors 1691–2
resuscitation
cardiopulmonary, ethics 1686
hip fractures 1332
posttraumatic subdural hematoma 1028
resveratrol 1669
reticulocyte count, increased 428
retina, age related changes 39
retinal pigment epithelium (RPE) 1206
retinoic acid 1511, 1512
retinoids 1672
retinol binding proteins (RBP) 332
retirement 102–3, **102**, 108
retirement homes, Alzheimer's disease 1088, 1090
retroperitoneal hemorrhage 452
reversible dementia 1067
rhabdomyolysis, acute 941, **941**
rhabdosphincter 1460
rheumatic heart disease 529, 590
chronic, infective endocarditis 1749, 1750
epidemiology 480–1
rheumatoid arthritis (RA) 1348
age related incidence *31*
extraarticular manifestations 1348
fibrosing alveolitis 717
foot manifestations **1313**
medication 1350–1
muscle wasting 918
radiological evaluation 1348
renal damage 1502
spinal canal stenosis 992, 996
rheumatoid factor (RF) 1348
rheumatological disorders, neck pain 1363
rhinophyma 1597
rhinoviruses 667–8, 706
ribavirin 386, 1776
riboflavin (vitamin B_2) 336, **341**
rifampin (rifampicin)
bacterial meningitis 1767
infective endocarditis 1759
side effects 1743
tuberculosis 709, 1743, **1745**
latent TB 1746, **1746**
tuberculous meningitis 1768
right ventricular end-diastolic pressure (RVEDP) 564, 565
rigid feet 1317
rigidity 746
Parkinson's disease 766
rimantadine, influenza prophylaxis 1730, **1730**
ring sideroblasts 456, 468
Rinne test 1220
risedronate 1276, 1283, 1294
risk management 232
risperidone
cerebrovascular event risk 1157
delirium 1056, 1057
dementia, delusions/hallucinations in 1140, 1141
rituximab 1515
rivastigmine, Alzheimer's disease 1088
Ro (SS-A) autoantibodies 272
robotic surgery, valvular heart disease 536
Roche European American Cataract Trial 1671, 1673
Rochester Study 1434
rocker soles 1327
rod-catch test 1305
rofecoxib 986, 1351, 1511
Romberg test 1240
root canals, age related changes 261
rosacea 1597–8, *1598*
Roth spots, infective endocarditis 1755
Rotterdam Study, diabetes and cognitive dysfunction 1434
Rowan Report, UK (2003) 1168, 1170
Royal Australasian College of Physicians (RACP) 1903
Royal College of General Practitioners 166
Royal College of Physicians, UK 7, 166
Royal College of Psychiatrists, UK 166, 1168
Royal College of Radiologists (RCR) best practice guidelines 1712
Royal Commission on Long Term Care 1872, 1918
royal jelly 94
"rule of threes", memory clinic information 1067–8
ryanodine receptor/calcium release channel (RyR2) 563

S14 gene, triiodothyronine 1407
S100 calcium binding protein 1185
SABE (Study on Aging, Health and Well-being) 1970–1, 1993–4, *1995*
saccular aneurysms 1018
saccule 1235
sacral nerve stimulation, fecal incontinence 403
sacral neuromodulation, urinary incontinence 1490
S-adenosyl methionine, alcoholic liver disease 388
safety rails *see* siderails
SAGE (Systemic Assessment of Geriatric Drug Use via Epidemiology) database 1440
Saint Louis University Mental Status Exam (SLUMS) 1186, 1925, **1927**
salbutamol 701, 705, 961
saline, intravenous
hypercalcemia of malignancy 1522
hyponatremia 1523
saliva
denture retention 271
dribbling in MND 960
flow rate assessment 271
oral health function 243
Saliva Orthana (Nycomed) aerosol sprays 272
salivary glands
age related changes 271
biopsy 272
disorders 271–2
salmon calcitonin, hypercalcemia of malignancy 1523
salt
depletion 1637–8
restriction, hypertension management 550
retention, in heart failure 557, *557*
see also saline, intravenous; sodium
sandals 1327
Sandhoff disease 953
Sans Everything: a Case to Answer 7–8
sarco-endoplasmic reticulum ATPase (SERCA2a) 562, 563
sarcoid lung disease 718
sarcopenia (muscle mass changes) 130, 672, 909–33, 1567–9
acute morbidity 918–9
anorexia 919
biochemistry *1569*
chronic disease associations 914, 918–9

sarcopenia (muscle mass changes) (*cont.*)
  class I and class II 913
  classification 912–3, *912*
  correlates/consequences 919–22
  cytokines 916–8
  definition 38, 909–10
  etiology 914–9, *915*
    "vicious loop" 920, **920**
  functional limitation/disability 920
  genetic susceptibility 919
  health-care costs 914
  heart failure association 568, **569**, 571, 577
  hormones 916–8
  incidence/prevalence 913
  malnutrition 919
  measurement 910–2
  mortality 922
  muscle denervation 916
  muscle fiber apoptosis 916
  muscle mass 921
  muscle mitochondrial damage 914–6
  muscle strength 921
  obesity *see* sarcopenic obesity
  oxidative stress 914–6
  prevention 922–5
  protein turnover 916
  risk factors 913–4
  sedentary lifestyle and 125
  testosterone 1568
  treatment 922–5
    exercise 922–3
    exercise plus other therapy 922–3
    hormone replacement 923–5
    outcomes 926, *927*
    pharmacological 925
  weight loss 298
"sarcopenic obese" 1568
sarcopenic obesity 350, 920–1
  balance **921**
  etiology 918, 926, *926*
  falls and gait **921**
  instrumental activities of daily living 921
  prevalence 920, *920*
Sarcoptes scabiei mite 1594
SARS *see* severe acute respiratory syndrome (SARS)
satellite cells 119, 1568
satiety, sensory-specific 301
scabicides 1595
scabies 1594–5, *1594*
  diagnosis 1595, *1595*
scalp hematomas, elder abuse 184
scarring, foot 1325–6
scavenger receptors, macrophages 616
SCD-HeFT (Sudden Cardiac Death in Heart Failure Trial) 508, 509
Schedule for the Evaluation of Individual Quality of Life (SEIQoL) 1684
schizophrenia 1151
Scientific Council of the Israeli Medical Association 1950
scintigraphy
  bone *see* bone, scintigraphy
  constipation 410
  esophagus 358
  gastric emptying 363, *364*
  thallium perfusion 516
scleroderma (systemic sclerosis) 366–7, 717, 1502
sclerosing pancreatitis 421
sclerosis, root canals 244
sclerotherapy, variceal hemorrhage 377
scoliosis, lumbar 996
SCOPE study (Study on Cognition and Prognosis in the Elderly) 549
Scottish Audit of Surgical Mortality 1633
The Scottish Doctor 1791–2
Scottish Intercollegiate Guideline Network (SIGN) 657, 1578, 1830
screening tools/programs 1869–70, 1925, **1926**
  cardiac disease 1911
  carers' support 1813
  depression 1545
  memory problems 1938, **1938**
  Minimum Data Set *see* Minimum Data Set (MDS)
  visual impairment 1545
  see also geriatric assessment; *specific instruments and diseases*
scurvy 94, 262, 335, 441
seating, pressure ulcer prevention 1615–6
sebaceous cyst (epidermoid cyst) 1600, *1600*
seborrheic dermatitis 1596, *1596*
seborrheic keratosis 1599–600, *1600*
secondary angle closure glaucoma 759
secondary autonomic failure 972
secondary hypothermia 977, **977**
sedation, in Down's syndrome 1186
sedatives, elder abuse 186
sedentary lifestyle
  cardiac disease 478, 519
  disability association, exercise effect 136
  diseases associated 132
  increased perception of effort and 125
  muscle mass loss 125
seed corns (heloma miliare) 1323
seed migration, brachytherapy 1478
SEER program, breast cancer 1509, 1537
segmental dystonia 782, **782**
seizures
  alcohol-withdrawal syndrome 164
  brain tumor 1527
  bupropion 154
  complex partial epileptic 872, 876
  epilepsy *see* epilepsy
  functional 884–5
  medications, delirium etiology 1052
  simple partial epileptic 872
  subarachnoid hemorrhage 1017
  tonic-clonic 870, 871
selective androgen receptor modulators (SARMs) 120, 1393, 1568, **1568**
selective estrogen receptor modulators (SERMs) 1513–4
  breast cancer prevention 1511–2
  hip fracture prevention 1341
  osteoporosis 1283, 1294–5
selective optimization with compensation, depression 1176–7
selective serotonin reuptake inhibitors (SSRIs)
  cardiac rehabilitation strategy 649
  delirium etiology 1051
  dementia and 1138–9
  depression 1138–9, 1178, 1417
  frontotemporal dementia 1122
  Huntington's disease 778
  hyponatremia risk 1179
  irritable bowel syndrome 368
  migraine 754
  motor neuron disease 962
  noncardiac chest pain 363
  Parkinson's disease 774
  side effects 1179
selegiline 334, 772, 1069
selenium 334–5, **341**
selenium sulfide, seborrheic dermatitis 1596
selenoproteins 334
self image, sexuality 115
self-help, smoking cessation 154
self-help groups, drug misuse 1198
sella turcica, enlarged 1399–400
semantic dementia 1121, 1123
semantic memory 1037, 1039
semicircular canals 1235
semipermeable film 1622, **1622**
semustine (methyl-CCNU), myelodysplasia due to 455
SENECA (Survey in Europe on Nutrition and The Elderly: A Concerned Action) 110, 284, **284**, 347
senescence 37
  motor neuron and muscle changes 39
  somatic *vs* germ line 14
Sengstaken–Blakemore tube 377
senile chorea 778–9
senile dementia, Alzheimer's disease and 1073
senile emphysema 695
senile hypofiltration 1495–6
senile osteoporosis (type II) 1265, **1265**, 1418
senile plaques, Alzheimer's disease 1073–5, *1074*, *1075*, 1078–9
senile purpura 441
senile vaginitis *see* vaginitis, atrophic
senna 412, 2007
sensorimotor function, aging effect 745–8
sensorineural deafness 1225–8, 1229
sensors, smart home 189, *190*, 197
sensory losses, age related 56
sensory neuronopathy, carcinomatous 896
sensory neuropathy 895–6
  diabetic foot 1314
sensory polyneuropathy, diabetes mellitus 892
sensory presbycusis 1226
sensory problems, pressure ulcers 1610
sensory system, aging effect **744**, 748
sentinel loop, acute pancreatitis 418
sentinel lymph node mapping 1513
Sentinel Stroke Audit 1899
sepsis 445, 447
  prophylaxis 1642
septic aneurysms 1020
Sepulveda Road Test 145
Seranoa Repens (Saw Palmetto) 1473
"series ventricular interaction" 564
SERMs *see* selective estrogen receptor modulators (SERMs)
serotonergic neurons, aging 61–2, **61**
serotonergic syndrome 986, 1051
serotonin (5-hydroxytryptamine (5-HT))
  age related loss 61
  HT_{1A} receptor antagonist 65
  Parkinson's disease 769
  postmenopausal women 1417
serotonin syndrome 986, 1051
serotonin-norepinephrine reuptake inhibitors (SNRI) 1464
serous labyrinthitis 1224
sertraline 774, 1157, 1178
serum testing, hepatitis 385
Seventh Day Adventists, life expectancy 1702–4
severe acute respiratory syndrome (SARS) 1732–3
  fatality rate 19, **20**
sevoflurane 1650–1
sex cord tumors, female 1456
sex differences
  anemia prevalence 427–8
  atrial fibrillation incidence *480*
  heart disease incidence *476*, *477*
  see also other specific disorders
sex hormone binding globulin (SHBG) 118, 1391, 1422
sex hormones
  deficiency, bone mass loss 1289
  effect on immune cells 32–3
  weight gain induction 315
sexual abuse 121, 184
sexual activity
  inhibiting factors 1454
  prevalence 115, 1416–7
  response to aging 1454
sexual disorders 1155
sexual dysfunction 1155
  female *see* female sexual dysfunction (FSD)
  male *see* erectile dysfunction
  management 1420–1
  urinary incontinence 1487
  zinc deficiency 340
sexual intercourse, death during 120
sexuality 115–22, 1453–4
  aging 115–22, **116**
  chronic illness 1454
  disease effect 120
  effects of surgery 1454
  nursing home 121
  older man 117–20
  older women 115–7, *116*
sexually transmitted diseases (STDs) 1731–2
SF-36 health survey questionnaire 1560–2, **1560**, **1561**
  cardiac surgery benefits 598
sharpened Romberg test 1305

shear forces
pressure ulcer development 1607, *1608*
reduction 1607, 1612
Sheldon, Joseph 3
sheltered housing, UK 107–8
SHEP study 542, 547, 549, 578
characteristics 547, **547**
diabetic treatment targets **1437**
ideal body weight 297
outcome **548**
weight loss 298
shingles *see* herpes zoster (shingles)
Shipman, Harold 111, 1921
shivering mechanism 1651
shivering thermogenesis 976
shock, cardiogenic, management 586
Shock, Nathaniel 2, 1926
Short Michigan Alcoholism Screening Test-Geriatric Version (SMAST-G) 1153
shorter alcohol related problems survey (shARPS) 163
short-stay centres, Alzheimer's disease 1090
shoulder-hand syndrome 856
shunt surgery, variceal hemorrhage 377
shunt tap, ventriculoperitoneal shunt infection 791, 792
Shy-Drager syndrome (SDS) 767
sick sinus syndrome 493, 494, 532, 568, 576, 974
sickle-cell disease 430–1
sideboards *see* siderails
siderails 1691
effects of **1690**, 1691
elder abuse 186
entrapment 1692–3, 1696
fall prevention 1692, 1693
see also restraints
sigmoidoscopy, flexible, colon cancer 207
signal transduction 29–30, 33
signal-averaged electrocardiography (SAECG) 517
sildenafil (Viagra) 118, **118**
contraindications 1472
postmenopausal women 1421
silent aspiration 821, 844
silent cerebral infarction 688, 1105
silent myocardial ischemia *see* myocardial ischemia
silica exposure 716
silicon **341**, 1291
silicone molding, foot orthoses 1327
silicosis 716
silver-based dressings 1621
silymarin (milk thistle) 388
Simplified Nutritional Assessment Questionnaire (SNAQ) 1925, **1928**
Simulated Presence Therapy, dementia 1142
simvastatin, secondary stroke risk reduction 834, *834*, 835, *835*
Single Assessment Process (SAP), UK 230, 1165, 1894
single photon densitometry, bone density 1283
single photon emission computed tomography (SPECT)
dementia predictor in MCI 1097
memory clinic patients 1066–7
normal pressure hydrocephalus 790
Parkinson's disease 765, 771
restless legs syndrome 781
single-energy X-ray (SXA) absorptiometry 208, 1283
single-fibre electromyography (SF-EMG) 902
sinoatrial node 494
age reduction in β-adrenoceptors 487, 530
loss of pacemaker cells 487, 493
sinus formation, foot 1325
sinus node bradycardia 974
sinus node dysfunction 493, 494, 532, 568, 576
sinus rhythm 822–3, 832
sinus tracts, pressure ulcers 1623
sinusitis, headache and 759
sir2 gene 1669
sit to stand functional strength test 1305
sitting position
aspiration pneumonia 689
ideal 1615, *1615*
six simple variables (SSV) model, ischemic stroke 823
6-minute walk test 652, 1305
sixth nerve palsy 1017
Sixty-Plus Reinfarction study 450
Sjögren's syndrome 1349
age related incidence *31*
auto-reactive T cells 32
diagnostic criteria **272**
dry mouth 272
fibrosing alveolitis 717
salivary glands 272
sensory neuropathy 895–6
symptoms 1349
skeletal muscle *see* muscle
skeleton, aging 42
skin
aging 37–8, **38**, 1590–1, **1590**
clinical changes 1590–1
components/cells **38**
histological changes 1590–1, **1590**
intrinsic/chronologic 1590–1
physiologic functions 1591, **1591**
sun exposure 1591–2, **1592**
vitamin D production 1662
assessment, pressure ulcer prevention 1611–2
chronic renal failure 1500
elder abuse 184
functions and structure 37
grafts, pressure ulcers 1624
peripheral neuropathy features 889, **891**
thinning 38
wrinkling 37
skin appendages, aging **1590**, 1591
skin disorders 1589–604
benign neoplasms 1599–600
in Down's syndrome 1187–8
infections 1591–5, 1727
infestations 1591–5
inflammatory 1595–9
internal malignancy features 1602, **1603**
malignant neoplasms 1600–2
premalignant neoplasms 1600–2
vitamin A deficiency 332–3
zinc deficiency 340
skin equivalents, pressure ulcers 1626
skull deformities, Paget's disease 1271
sleep 733
age effects 734–5, *735*
alcohol effects 159, 166
deprivation, EEG 872
enhancement, melatonin 1394
episodic events/phenomena 885
history taking 736
in institutions 736
loss, effects of 734
napping during the day 735, 738
non-rapid eye movement 734
phase-advanced 735, 738
phase-delayed *735*
rapid eye movement 734
rapid eye movement (REM) 1418
slow-wave 734
stages 734
structure 734–5, *735*
sleep apnea 696, **734**, 737, 1155
central 737
Down's syndrome 1187
investigation 736
obstructive 676, 737, 1418
screening 208–9
secondary hypertension due to 545
sleep diaries 736, *736*, 739
sleep disorders/disturbances 733–40, **734**
in Alzheimer's disease 1087
assessment 736–7, *736*
circadian rhythm disorders 735, 737, 738
classification 733
comorbid conditions 733
consequences 733–4
daytime sleepiness *see* daytime sleepiness
in dementia 735–6
etiology 733
insomnia *see* insomnia
menopause 1417–8
nocturia 1461
in Parkinson's disease dementia 1119
periodic limb movements in sleep **734**, 736, 737
prevalence 733
in progressive supranuclear palsy 1120
REM-sleep behavior disorder **734**, 736, 737–8
restless leg syndrome **734**, 737
sleep apnea *see* sleep apnea
sleep related breathing disorders 733–4, 737
sleep hygiene, insomnia 738, 739
sleep related breathing disorders (SRBD) 733–4, 737
stroke 678
sleep-aides 1155
sleep-state misperception insomnia 738
sleep-walking 734
sliding hip screw (SHS) 1334, 1335, *1336*
postoperative complications 1337–8, *1339*
slow twitch fibers 671
slow vital capacity (SVC) 694
slow-wave sleep 734
small cell lung carcinoma (SCLC) 712, 905–6
small intestine
aging 365
bacterial overgrowth 365
motility 365
aging 42, 365
diabetes mellitus 366
nutrient absorption 291
smart homes 189–98
activity prompts 192
applicability to the elderly 190
automated text messages 195
bath water control 192–3
behavior monitoring
difficulties 193–4
errors 194
future trends 197
carer emulation approach 192–3
communication systems 194–5
design 192–3
ethics 196
facilities required 189, *190*
future trends 197–8
infrastructure needed for introduction 196–7
links with outside world 196
occupational therapist' assessment 196–7
operational backup 196–7
quality of life 195–6
social isolation reduction 196
technical maintenance p0017:
usage 191–2
user friendliness 190–1
smell 1249–58
sense of 745
smell dysfunction
anorexia of aging 300–1
causes 1252–6
evaluation 1256–7
malingering 1252
management 1256–7
viral induced 1254
Smell Identification Test™ 1251–2, *1252*
smokers' cough 696
smoking 151–6
Alzheimer's disease 152–3
associated diseases 151–3
asthma 153
blindness 153
bone mass loss 152, 1291–2
bronchogenic carcinoma 710
cessation *see* smoking cessation
cognitive performance 152–3
COPD 696
dementia 152–3
heart disease risk 151–2, 477, 517
mouth, effects on 152
oral cancer 243, 269
oral candidosis 263
osteoporosis 1291–2
Parkinson's disease 768–9

smoking (*cont.*)
  peripheral vascular disease risk 624
  positive effects 153
  postmyocardial infarction 153
  prevalence 151, *151*
  stroke risk 152, 801–2, 837
smoking cessation 153–5
  "5A-strategy" 649
  asbestosis 716
  cardiac rehabilitation 649
  COPD 697
  cryptogenic fibrosing alveolitis 717
  elderly 154–5
  Health Maintenance Clinical Guidepath 205
  hypertension management 550
  methods 154
  peripheral vascular disease 626
  self-help 154
  silicosis 716
  time for effects to occur 153–4
  without external help 154
smooth muscle relaxants 362–3, 1716
SMS links, smart homes 196
Snoezelen 1822
social aspects *see* aging
social capital 478
  heart disease relationship 478–9
social class, tooth loss 240
social isolation
  alcohol abuse 161–2
  anorexia 299
social losses, of aging 54
The Social Medicine of Old Age 3
social network behavior therapy 1198
social problems, dementia **1128**, 1129
Social Security Administration, USA 1924
social services
  developing countries 1973–4
  role in elderly care 6, 1943
social support 1577
  assessment **1545**
  carers 1812
  depression 1177
  developing countries 1972
  networks 1943, 1985–6
social work, problem-orientated assessment 231
socioeconomic planners 795
socioemotional selectivity theory, depression 1177
sodium
  homeostasis, age related changes 1373
  reabsorption reduced by natriuretic peptides 558
  renal tubular dysfunction 1496–7
  retention, age related 543
sodium bicarbonate 1383, 1716
sodium chloride
  hypertonic 1379–80
  see also salt
sodium fluoride gel, dry mouth 272
sodium phosphate bowel preparation 376
sodium polystyrene sulfonate (Kayexalate) 1383–4
sodium sulfacetamide 1598
sodium valproate
  Creutzfeldt-Jacob's disease 1777
  epilepsy 874, **874**
  see also valproic acid
sodium-calcium exchange 543
sodium-calcium exchanger (NCX), heart failure 563
sodium-containing laxatives 411–2
soft corns (heloma molle) 1323
soft tissue infections 1727
solifenacin, overactive bladder 1490
SOLVD trial 574, 579
somatic senescence 14
somatosensory function, aging effect 748
somatostatinoma 421
sorbitol 398, 411
sotalol 503, 508, 510, 523
sound, frequency 1219
sound waves 1219
soy products, menopausal symptoms 1420
"Space Available for the Cord" (SAC) 991
SPACE study (on antioxidants in cardiovascular disease) 1671
spacers, COPD 698
SPAF study (Stroke Prevention in Atrial Fibrillation) 505
Spain
  community acquired pneumonia 665
  medical education/training 1785
  nursing home care 1822, 1980
spasmodic dysphonia (Meige syndrome) 782
spasmodic torticollis 782
spasticity
  motor neuron disease 960
  stroke related, management 855–6
spatial disorientation, dementia and 1137, 1143
Special Fellowship Program in Advanced Geriatrics, USA 1925
specialist nurses, memory clinics 1064
specialist nursing roles 1940
  Admiral Nurses 1165, 1872–3
  UK 1868–9, 1871, 1874
spectazole, tinea pedis 1592
speech apraxia, in dementia 1040
speech audiometer 1221
speech audiometry 1221–2
  performance-intensity curves 1222, *1222*
  rollover 1222, *1222*
speech discrimination loss 1226–7
speech disorders *see* communication disorders
speech impairment, dementia 1137
speech muscle activation/programming 1038, 1040, 1041
speech repetition, dementia 1043
speech signal distortion 842
speech therapy 773, 843, 1042
spherocytosis, hereditary 431
sphincter(s) *see specific sphincters*
sphincter training exercises, fecal incontinence 399
sphincteroplasty, anterior, fecal incontinence 403
sphincterotomy, complications, fecal incontinence 397
spinal angiography, aortic aneurysm 1005
spinal arteriovenous malformations 1020
spinal bulbar muscular atrophy (SBMA) 951
spinal canal
  diameter 991
  stenosis 1009
    cervical 991–5
    lumbar 995–8, 1360
    Paget's disease 1271
spinal cord
  aging neuropathology 76
  compression 1521
    cervical myelopathy 993
    osteoarthritis 1347
  infarction 1008–9
  injury, breathing disruptions 678
  ischemia 1003, 1008–9
    see also spinovascular insufficiency
  vascular disorders 1002–8
  vasculature 1001–2, *1002*
spinal epidural abscess 1774–5
spinal hematomas 1006–7
spinal manipulation therapy (SMT) 1361–2
spinal muscular atrophy 953
  distal 954
spinal root atrophy 956
spinal stenosis, Paget's disease 1271
spinal veins
  spinovascular insufficiency 1002, 1009
  thrombosis 1009
spine
  aging 991, 1356
  pathology, MND diagnosis pitfalls 952–3
spinovascular insufficiency 1001–13
  acute aortic occlusion 1006
  anterior spinal artery 1008
  aorta involvement 1003–6
  aortic aneurysm 1003–5
  aortic dissection 1005–6
  aortic intramural hematoma 1006
  arteriovenous malformations 1008
  chronic myelopathy 1009–10
  ischemic cord infarction 1008–9
  large vessel vasculitis 1007–8
  posterior spinal artery 1009
  spinal hematomas 1006–7
  spinal veins 1002, 1009
  spinal venous system 1002
  Takayasu's disease 1007–8
  vascular disorders of cord 1002–8
spiraling immobility 1689
spirituality, aging and 110–1
spirochetal meningitis 1769–70
spirometry
  acute exacerbation of COPD 700–1
  asthma 704
  fibrotic lung disease 715
  preoperative 1635
spironolactone, heart failure 575
splanchnic blood flow 973
spleen
  age related changes 21, *22*
  germinal centers 21, *22*
splenectomy 438
spondylolisthesis, lumbar spine 996
spondylosis
  cervical spine *see* cervical spondylosis
  lumbar spine 952
spontaneous oral dyskinesia (SOD) 778–9
spontaneous vestibular nystagmus 1239
sporadic Creutzfeldt-Jacob's disease (sCJD) 1124, 1777
sporadic olivopontocerebellar atrophy (SOPCA) 767
SPORTIF trial 831–2
SPORTIF III trial 507
sputum examination
  lung cancer 710
  tuberculosis 709, 1741–2, 1743
squamous cell carcinoma (SCC) 1601–2, *1602*
  oral ulceration 266
  premalignant conditions 361, 1455, 1600–1
  treatment 1602
squamous cell hyperplasia 1455
squamous papilloma, lung 713
squashed stomach syndrome 2008
SS-A (Ro) antibodies 1349
SS-B (La) antibodies 1349
stability limits 1300
standing, balance 1299–300
Standing Nursing and Midwifery Advisory Committee (SNMAC), UK 1870
Stanford type A/B aortic dissection 1005–6
stapedius muscle contraction, assessment 1221
staphylococci
  brain abscess 1771
  coagglutination, meningitis 1765
  infective endocarditis 1751, *1751*, **1752**
  otitis externa 1223
  subdural empyema 1773
Staphylococcus aureus
  infectious arthritis 1349
  infective endocarditis 1753
  meningitis 1764, **1766**
  methicillin-resistant (MRSA) 1728, 1730
  pressure ulcer infection 1623
  vancomycin-resistant 1759
Staphylococcus epidermidis
  infectious arthritis 1349
  meningitis 1764, **1766**
  prosthetic valve endocarditis 1750
Staphylococcus saprophyticus 1727
starvation 313
stasis dermatitis 1598, *1598*
statins (HMG-CoA reductase inhibitors) 615
  acute coronary syndrome 521
  atherosclerosis 620
  cardiac rehabilitation 650
  diabetes mellitus 1440
  dyslipidemia 626
  heart failure prevention 578
  ischemic heart disease prevention 518
    secondary 482
  myopathy induction 941–2
  osteoporotic fracture reduction 489
  side effects 834
  stroke risk reduction 833–5, *833*, *834*, *835*
  ST-segment elevated myocardial infarction 521

stationary ability, aging effect 747–8
status epilepticus 876
steatorrhea, chronic pancreatitis 420, 421
Steele Richardson Olszewski syndrome *see* progressive supranuclear palsy (PSP)
stem cell defects, myelodysplasia 455, 461, 465
stem cell therapy, in MND 963
stem cell transplantation
  in aplastic anemia 432
  myelodysplasia therapy 461
  nonmyeloablative 461
stent/stenting
  aortic 1005, 1006
  pancreatic cancer 422
  secondary stroke risk reduction 837
  thoracic aortic surgery 606–7
steroids
  acute quadriplegic myopathy 942
  appetite augmentation 2011
  chronic subdural hematoma 1032
  potency **1595**
  see also corticosteroids
sticky patches, atherosclerosis 615
stiff wing collar, carotid sinus syndrome 974
stimulant laxatives, constipation **411**, 412
stimulants
  adverse effects 1193
  intoxication symptoms **1195**
  misuse, epidemiology 1192
  withdrawal symptoms **1195**
Stokes–Adams attacks 880–1
stomach 363–5
  see also entries beginning gastric
stomatitis 264, *264*
  denture 263–4, *264*
STONE (Shanghai Trial of nifedipine in the Elderly) trial **547**, 548, **548**
stool examination 376, 409
stool softeners, constipation 411
stool water, hypokalemia 1384
STOP-Hypertension trial **547**, 548, **548**, 549
straight leg-raising test 1360
strangulation, restraint complication 1692
streptococci
  brain abscess 1771
  infective endocarditis 1751, *1751*, **1752**
  subdural empyema 1773
Streptococcus agalactidae, meningitis **1766**
Streptococcus bovis 1751, *1751*
Streptococcus gallolyticus 1751, *1751*
Streptococcus pneumoniae 707, 1726, 1728
  meningitis 1764, 1765, 1766, **1766**, 1767, 1768
  otitis media 1223
  vaccine 1733–4
streptomycin 1743–4, 1759, 1768
stress
  heart rate response 530
  neuroendocrine-immune network activation 30, *30*
  tremor 783
stress incontinence 1463–4, 1487
  causes 1487
  inappropriate medication use **220**
  injection therapy 1464
  pharmacologic management 1463–4
  surgery 1464, 1490–1
  symptoms **1488**
  taping procedures 1464, 1491
stress ulcers 377
strial presbycusis 1227
striated muscle antibodies 901
striato nigral degeneration (SND) 767
striatum
  aging neurochemistry **61**
  aging neuropathology 70–1
  dopamine, age related changes **41**
  Parkinson's disease 770
stroke 815
  acute 815–25
    care pathways 822
    clinical guidelines 822
    epidemiology 815, **816**
    hemorrhagic 821
    ischemic *see* ischemic stroke
    neurological complications **819**
    prognosis 823, **823**
    risk factors 815, **816**
    services organization 821–2
  aspiration pneumonia 686
  breathing patterns 678
  cardiac manifestations 488
  cognitive impairment 863–4
  completed, vertebrobasilar artery 1244
  dementia risk 1105
  dysphagia treatment 855
  epidemiology 795–804
  excitotoxicity 63
  exercise effects **133**
  hemorrhagic 802–3, 821
  HRT 1418
  incidence 59
  ischemic *see* ischemic stroke
  left hemisphere 120, 842–3
  magnetic resonance imaging (MRI) *851*
  mood disorders associated 862–3
  morbidity, India 1984
  MRI 849–51, *850*
  perioperative, cardiac surgery and 595
  postoperative 1640, 1650, **1650**
  prevention
    in atrial fibrillation 451, 452, 482
    day hospitals' role 1909
  prognosis 795
  psychiatric morbidity screening 863
  recurrence risk 802, 827, *828*
  rehabilitation *see* stroke rehabilitation
  risk after transient ischemic attack 827, *828*
  risk factors, atrial fibrillation 449, 451, 499, 801
  secondary 827–39
    atrial fibrillation as risk factor 831–2, *832*
    interventions to reduce risk 828–37, *829*
  smoking 152
  spasticity associated 855–6
  subarachnoid hemorrhage *see* subarachnoid hemorrhage
  vascular dementia related to 1103, 1104, 1105
  vitamin E supplements 1671
  wheelchair adaptations 1695
  see also cerebrovascular disease (CVD)
Stroke Aphasic Depression Questionnaire (SADQ) 863
Stroke Data Bank classification system 796
Stroke Drivers Screening Assessment 864
stroke rehabilitation 849–58
  ADLs 852–3, 854
  Bobath method 855
  clinical psychology services 862–6
  cognitive behavioral therapy 863, 864–5
  components 852–4
  constraint therapy 853
  environmental issues 865–6
  information provision, patients and carers 1813
  interdisciplinary assessment 233, *233*
  muscle tone management 855–6
  neurological basis of recovery 849–51, *850*
  NSF (UK) standard **1802**, 1898–9, 1917
  objectives 851–2
  problems 853, 854–7
  psychological aspects 1573
  quality of life measurement 1910
  recovery patterns 851
  resource allocation 1683
  sexual function 865
  standards 1831–2
stroke units 821–2, 1900–1, **1900**
strongyloidiasis, disseminated 1764
strontium ranelate, osteoporosis 1295
Study of Osteoporotic Fractures (2002) 1434
Study on Aging, Health and Well-being (SABE) 1970–1, 1993–4, *1995*
Sturdee, Edwin 3
subamrilic acetic acid (SAHA) 460
subarachnoid hematoma 1006–7
subarachnoid hemorrhage (SAH) 1015–25
  aneurysm clipping 1022
  assessment 1020–1
  blood pressure management 1023
  brain scanning 1017–8, *1017*
  causes 1018–20
  clinical condition at admission 1020–1
  clinical features 1016–7
  complications 1021–4
  delayed cerebral ischemia treatment 1023–4
  diagnosis 1016–8
  epidemiology 1015
  grading scales 1020, *1020*
  investigations 1017–8
  management **1022**
    complications 1021–4
    poor condition at admission 1020–1
  outcome 1016, **1016**
  quality of life studies 1016, **1016**
  rebleeding 1022
    early 1020–1
  risk factors 1015–6
  saccular aneurysms 1018
  secondary cerebral ischemia prevention 1022–3
  vasospasm treatment 1023, 1024
subarachnoid space, inflammatory response 1767
subcortical dementia 1113, **1114**
  HIV-associated dementia 1126
  Huntington's disease 1125
subcortical ischemic vascular dementia (SIVD) 1113–4
subcortical nuclei, aging neuropathology 70–1
subdural effusion, ventriculoperitoneal shunting 790, 791, 792, *792*
subdural empyema 1773–4
subdural hematoma 1027–33
  acute 1021, 1027–30
    spontaneous 1029–30
  chronic 1030–3
    investigation 1031, *1031*
    outcome 1031–2
  delirium etiology 1053
  driving 1032–3
  headache 758
  posttraumatic 1027–9
    investigation 1028, *1029*
  spinovascular insufficiency 1006–7
subdural space 1027
subiculum, neuronal loss in aging 70
subkeratotic hematoma *1316*
sublingual keratoses 268–9
submucous plexus 357
subperiosteal osseointegrated titanium implants 270
substance misuse 1153
  see also drug misuse/abuse
substance P 686, 687
substantia nigra
  aging neuropathology 71, 74
  dopaminergic neuron loss 60–1
  Parkinson's disease 765, 769, 770
subsyndromal depression 1173
subthreshold depression 1173, **1174**
subtrochanteric fractures 1331, *1331*
  surgery 1335, *1336*
subungual hematoma *1314*, *1323*
subungual hyperkeratosis 1593, *1593*
successful aging *see* aging, successful
sucralfate, pill esophagitis 362
sudden death, epidemiology 480
suggested immobilization test (SIT) 780
suicide 1154
  assisted 1951
  depression and 1175, **1175**
  epidemiology 1149
  incidence, Japan 1938, *1938*
  risk, alcohol abuse 164
  risk factors 1175
  see also physician-assisted suicide
sulci, aging neuropathology 69
sulfamethoxazole (Bactrim), prostatitis 1480
sulfasalazine, rheumatoid arthritis 1351
sulindac, arthritis 1350
sulphonylurea 1436–7
sulphur toxin, MND association 959
sun avoidance, actinic keratosis 1600

sundowning 1145, 1146
sunscreens, rosacea 1598
superficial reflexes, aging effect 747
superficial spreading melanoma 1602, *1602*
superior hypophyseal arteries 1397
superior semicircular canal 1235
superior vena cava obstruction 1720
superior vena cava syndrome 1523–4
superior vena cava thrombosis 1524
superoxide dismutase 334
superoxide dismutase type 1 (SOD 1) gene 951, 952, 957
supplementary feeding, pressure ulcer prevention 1610
support devices, smart home 189, 192, *192*, 197
support groups
  COPD 729
  pulmonary rehabilitation 729
SUPPORT study 578, 677, 1686
support surfaces, pressure ulcer prevention 1613–6
  characteristics **1614**
  mattresses 1613–5, *1613*
  Medicare/Medicaid categories 1614–5
  seating 1615–6
  selection **1611**
supported discharge, orthogeriatrics 1343
suppurative labyrinthitis 1224
suprachiasmatic nuclei
  aging neuropathology 71
  sleep problems in dementia 735
supranuclear palsy, progressive *see* progressive supranuclear palsy (PSP)
supraventricular tachycardia 507, **508**
sural nerve, aging effects 79
surgery
  aortic aneurysm 1004
  cancer 1513
  cardiovascular morbidity 1648–9
  choice of approach 1655
  chronic subdural hematoma 1032
  CNS morbidity 1649–50
  complications, nutrient malabsorption 293
  delirium, postoperative 1047
  elective, clopidogrel discontinuation 830
  epidural abscess 1774
  fecal incontinence 403
  fungal brain abscess 1773
  gastrointestinal bleeding 376
  non-small cell lung cancer 711
  obesity 351
  oral cancer 270
  outcome *see* surgical outcomes
  Paget's disease of bone 1277
  perioperative medical assessment 1631–45
  peripheral vascular disease 627–8
  pleural mesothelioma 712
  postoperative medical assessment 1631–45
  postoperative morbidity/mortality reduction 1654–5
  posttraumatic subdural hematoma 1028–9
  preoperative assessment 1651–2
  pressure ulcers 1623–4
  prolactinomas 1400
  pulmonary embolic disease 714
  renal morbidity 1650–1
  respiratory morbidity 1649
  spinal canal stenosis 994, 997
  spinal cord infarction 1009
  subarachnoid hemorrhage rebleed prevention 1022
  urinary incontinence 1490–1
surgical brain lesions (SBLs), dementia 1129
surgical decompression
  after stroke 820
  epidural abscess 1775
  lumbar spinal canal stenosis 997
  subdural empyema 1774
surgical outcomes 1631–3
  cardiac surgery *see* cardiac surgery
  emergency surgery 1633
  noncardiac surgery 1633–5
  nutrition 1638–40
surgical patients, effects of pain 1652–3
Surveillance, Epidemiology and End Result (SEER) program, breast cancer 1509, 1537
survival, evolutionary programming for 13–4
survival motor neuron 2 (SMN2) gene 951
swallowing 844–5
  disorders 359–61
  normal 844–5, *845*
  phases 844–5
  problems *see* dysphagia
swallowing reflex 685, 687, 689
sweating, thermoregulatory autonomic impairment 977
Sweden
  life expectancy 88, **88**
  medical education/training 1784
  nursing home care 1821–2, **1822**, 1980
  restraint usage 1690
Swedish Adoption/Twin Study of Aging 49
Swedish longitudinal Octogenarians (OCTO)-immune study 25, 31
Swedish Trial in Older Patients with Hypertension **547**, 548, **548**, 549
Switzerland
  medical education/training 1784, **1784**, 1785
  memory clinics 1062
symmetrical polyneuropathy 891
sympathetic ganglia, aging neuropathology 79
sympathetic nervous system
  activation, adverse cardiac effects 555, **556**
  activity 969–70
  age related changes 41
  hypertension 543, 973
  modulation 970
  ocular abnormalities 972
  overactivity in heart failure 555–6, **556**, 564
  syncope 974
  thermoregulation 976
sympathetic tone, sick sinus syndrome 974
symptomatic generalized epilepsy 872
symptomatic orthostasis, diabetic neuropathy 892
synapses, aging 60, 63
synaptic density, aging neuropathology 71–2
synaptophysin, aging 63
syncope 879–84
  areflexic (paralytic) *see* areflexic (paralytic) syncope
  assessment 1306
  atrial fibrillation 499
  cardiac *see* cardiac syncope
  cardiovascular autonomic control 974
  classification 879, **880**
  clinical manifestations 881–2
  diagnosis/investigations 882–3
  management 883–4
  mechanisms 879–81
  misdiagnosis 883
  postprandial hypotension 974
  seizures 870–1
  sinus node bradycardia 974
  trigger factors 881
  see also specific types
syndrome of inappropriate ADH (SIADH) 1179, 1374, 1389, 1402, 1403, 1523
  diagnostic features 1523
  lung cancer 1379
syndrome of reset osmostat 1382
syndromes of disuse 133
α-synuclein
  gene 48
  Lewy bodies in aging 75
  Lewy body dementia *1118*
  multisystem atrophy 767, 1120
  Parkinson's disease 769
syphilis 268, 1732
  tertiary 268
syphilitic glossitis 268
syphilitic meningitis 1769
syringe drivers, palliative care 2005, 2013
syringing, earwax 1222
syringomyelia 952
Syst-China (Systolic Hypertension in China) trial **547**, 548, **548**
systemic inflammatory response syndrome (SIRS) 417
systemic lupus erythematosus (SLE) 1349
  epidemiology 31, *31*
  joint manifestations 1349
  lupus anticoagulant 443
  renal damage 1502
systemic sclerosis, progressive 366–7, 1502
Syst-Eur (Systolic Hypertension in Europe) trial 547, **547**, **548**, 549
systolic blood pressure (SBP)
  DASH eating plan effect 550
  hypertension definition 541
  orthostatic hypotension 973
Systolic Hypertension in the Elderly Program *see* SHEP study

T cell(s) 23–6
  age related changes 23–6, 31, 40, **40**, 1590
    naïve and memory helper cells 25
    qualitative 26
    quantitative 23–4, **24**, *24*
    signal transduction 29–30
    subset changes 25–6, *25*, 28
  atherosclerosis 611
  auto-reactive 32
  $CD4^+$, regeneration *24*, 27
  CD4/8 ratio **24**, 25, 28
  $CD8^+$, decline with age 25
  $CD25^+CD4^+$ 26
  $CD28^-$, expansion 25
  cytokines released 28–9
  dysfunction, oxidative mechanism 32
  emigration from thymus 27–8
  extrathymic 27
  lectin induced proliferation 26
  memory 25
  NKT subset 26
  progenitors, decline with age 23
  Th1, atherosclerosis 618–9
  transfusion 31
T cell antigen receptor (TCR) 26, 29
Tachibana, Satokatsu 1943
tachycardia
  atrial 496
  broad complex, causes **508**
  supraventricular 507, **508**
  ventricular *see* ventricular tachycardia
  volume depletion 1638
tacrolimus, oral lichen planus 266
tadalafil (Cialis) 118, **118**, 1472
tagged red blood cell (TRBC) scanning 376
Tai-Chi, falls prevention 1307
tailor's bunion 1325
Taiwan, nursing home care 1822
Takayasu's disease 1007–8
talking about the past, Alzheimer's disease 1039
tamoxifen 1513, 1534, 1535–6
  breast cancer prevention 1511
  complications 1511–2
  primary biliary cirrhosis 390
  side effects 1513
tamsulosin, benign prostatic hyperplasia 1472
tandem position 1305
tangential wall stress, atherosclerosis 616–7
tap controls 190
tap water, wound cleansing 1621
tardive dyskinesia (TD) 779–80
targeted therapy, cancer 1515
Targon nail 1335
taste 1249–58
  thresholds 292
taste buds 1250–1, *1251*
taste dysfunction 1255
  anorexia of aging 300–1
  causes 1255
  evaluation 1256–7
  management 1256–7
tau protein 1077–8, 1079, 1097–8, 1121
Taxanes, breast cancer 1536
Taxol, ovarian cancer 1456
tazarotene, psoriasis 1597
technetium (^{99m}Tc) 1718

technology use 1847–8
  assistive devices 1886–7
  medical education/training 1849
  medical records *see* patient records
  telemedicine 112, 1847, 1850
teeth *see* tooth
Teflon injection, stress incontinence 1464
tegaserod 367, 412
telangiectasia, hereditary hemorrhagic 441
tele-alarm, Alzheimer's disease 1089
telecare 189
telehealth systems 198
telemedicine 112, 1847, 1850
telerehabilitation 198
telomerase 37, 1668
  absence 15
  inhibitors 1669
telomeres 1668–9
  DNA damage 1589–90
  functions 15
  loss 15, 37
temperature, core (body) 738
temperature control 975–7
  effector mechanisms 976
  hyperthermia 977
  hypothermia 976–7, **977**
  poikilothermia 976
  see also hypothermia
temporal (giant cell) arteritis 274, 757, 1007
temporal bone fractures 1241
temporal lobe
  tumors, "disequilibrium" 1244
  weight changes in aging 69
temporomandibular joint pain 273
teniposide, small cell lung carcinoma 712
tension-free vaginal tape (TVT) surgery 1464, 1491
tension-type headache 754–5
  chronic (CTTH) 755
  classification **756**
  episodic (ETTH) 755
  migraine associated 752
  prevalence 754
  treatment 754–5
terbinafine 1325, 1592, 1593
terminal care *see* palliative/end-of-life care
terminal illness 2001
  anorexia 2011
  constipation 2007–8
  Council of the European Union report 1685
  dental care 256, 2010, 2011
  depression 2010
  diagnosis/prognosis discussion 2011–2
  ethical considerations 2002
  euthanasia requests 2012
  patient perception (symptoms) 2002, 2003
  pressure ulcers 1609
  see also palliative/end-of-life care
terminology (in geriatric medicine), history 8
terrorism 112–3, **112**
tertiary contractions, esophagus 358
testicular function 1422–4
testicular-atrophy, alcohol association 160
testosterone
  age related changes 118, 315, 924, 1391, 1393, 1422, 1675
    females 116
    regulation **119**
  anorexia of aging 305
  appetite stimulation 315
  decline, muscle changes 38
  in depression 1176
  measurement 118–9, 1422
  obese men 350–1
  sarcopenia 1568
  tissue available 118–9
testosterone replacement therapy 1675–6
  behavioral effects 1423
  benefits 1422
  effects 119–20, **120**, **1393**, 1422–4
  female sexual dysfunction 116, **116**, 1417, 1420–1, 1454
  muscle mass 916–7, 1568, 1675
  osteoporosis 1283–4
  routes of administration 120, **120**, 1421, 1424
  sarcopenia 924
  sexual function 1675
  side effects 120, 1393, 1417, 1421, 1424, 1676
tetanus toxoid (TT) immunization 26, 207
tetanus–diphtheria vaccination 1733
  schedule *387*
tetracyclic antidepressants, back pain 1363
tetracycline 266, 1598, 1599, 1770
tetracycline mouthwash 268
thalamotomy 784
thalassemia 429, 431
  β-thalassemia 430, 431
thalidomide
  appetite stimulation 315
  Behçet's disease 266
  cancer treatment 1515
  myelodysplasia therapy 460, 469
thallium perfusion scintigraphy 516
theophylline, COPD 698, 701
theophylline "madness" 1050
theories (of old age) 1
therapeutic range, drugs 216
thermal imaging 1719
thermogenesis 976
Thermold shoe 1327
thermoplastics, foot orthoses 1327
thermoregulation *see* temperature control
thermoregulatory effector mechanisms 976
Thewlis, Malford 1, 1892
thiamine deficiency 972
thiazide diuretics 117, 1439
  hypertension therapy 518, 548, 551
thiazolidinediones (TZD) 351, 1436
thinking 1037
  Alzheimer's disease 1038–9, 1040, 1041
  assessment 1041, 1042
  dementia 1038–9
  frontotemporal dementia 1039
  language relationship 1037–8
  vascular dementia 1039
thioproline 32
third nerve palsy 1017
third ventricle, endoscopic ventriculostomy 791
thirst 1372
  age related changes 282–3, 321–3, 322, 1373, 1402
  evaluation 1372
  impairment 568, **569**
  mechanisms
    defective 1372
    homeostatic 321–2, **322**
  nonhomeostatic regulation **322**, 323
  regulation 1372
  stimuli 1372
  threshold 1498
thoracic aortic aneurysm 606, *606*, 608, 1005
thoracic cage, age related changes 695
thoracic/thoracoabdominal radiculopathy 893
thoracolumbar aortic aneurysm 1005
thoracolumbar spine fractures 995
thrombin inhibitor, direct (DTI) 507, 831–2
thrombocytopenia 458, 1525–6
  drug induced 438
thromboembolism
  atrial fibrillation association 499, 500
  cardiac valve replacement and 603, *603*, 604
  epidemiology 449, 633–5
  prophylaxis 1332, 1642
  venous *see* venous thromboembolism
thrombolytic therapy
  after myocardial infarction 578–9
  care standards determination 1830
  ischemic stroke 820
  in stroke, brain imaging 818
  ST-segment elevated myocardial infarction 521
  unstable angina pectoris 520
thrombophilia 442–3, **442**
  genetic 633–4
thrombopoietin, myelodysplasia therapy 459
thrombosis
  aorta 1006
  microvascular, in DIC 445, 446, *446*
  sites, ischemic stroke 815
  spinal vein 1009
  venous *see* venous thrombosis
  Virchow's factors 449
thrombotic disorders 441–2
thrombotic thrombocytopenic purpura 440–1
thrombus formation 613, 620
thrush 263, *264*
thymectomy, myasthenia gravis 905
thymic involution 20, 21, 23, 28, 30, 40
thymic peptides (hormones), immune function restoration 31
thymoma
  myasthenia gravis 902, 903, *903*
  thymectomy 905
thymulin 30
thymus
  age related changes 21, *21*, **27**, 27–8
  as 'aging clock' 24
  functional decline 27–8, **27**
  grafting to restore immune function 31
  hypoplasia 28
  myasthenia gravis 902
  role in immune function (normal) 23–4
  role in immune system aging 21, 27–8
thyroid disorders 1405–14
  myopathies 942
  risk factors 1411
  screening 1410–1, *1411*
thyroid gland
  adenomas 1409
  age related changes 1405
    clinical implications 1407–9
  cancer 1409–10
  cysts 1410
  dysfunction, cardiovascular features 489–90
  hormone action changes 1406–7, **1406**
  hormone clearance 1406
  hormone economy changes 1405–6, **1406**
  nodules *see* thyroid nodules
  weight increases 1405
thyroid hormone(s)
  age related decline 38
  mitochondrial function 94
  replacement 1408
  tissue metabolism 1407
thyroid hormone responsive protein (THRP) 1407
thyroid nodules 1405
  cancer 1409–10
  causes **1409**
  differential diagnosis **1409**
  patient workup 1410, *1410*
  prevalence 1409
thyroid stimulating hormone (TSH) 208, 1405–6
"thyroid storm" 1409
thyroiditis *31*
  Hashimoto's *31*
  lymphocytic 1411
thyrotoxicosis *see* hyperthyroidism (thyrotoxicosis)
thyrotropin releasing hormone (TRH) 1405
thyrotropin (TSH)-secreting tumors 1401
thyroxine (T4) 1390, 1406
  replacement therapy 490, 1408
tiagabine, epilepsy 875
tibial osteotomies, Paget's disease 1277
tibolone 116, 925, 1295, 1421
tics, drug induced **784**
tilt testing, syncope 882
tilt training, syncope 883
tiludronate, Paget's disease 1275
"Timed up and go" test 1305, 1306
tin **341**
tinea pedis 1591–2, *1592*
  moccasin distribution 1592
  potassium hydroxide test 1592, *1593*
Tinel's sign 896
Tinetti gait and balance scale test 1300
tinetti's test, Alzheimer's disease 1088
tinnitus 1228–30
  drug induced 1228–9, **1229**
  prevalence 1214–5, 1229
tinnitus maskers 1230
tirofiban, acute coronary syndromes 520

tissue engineering, pressure ulcers 1626
tissue factor, infective endocarditis 1755
tissue inhibitors of metalloproteinases (TIMPs) *561*
tiuxetan 1515
tizanidine, in MND 960
TNM staging, prostate cancer 1476, **1476**
tobacco
  erectile dysfunction 117
  oral cancer etiology 269
  see also smoking
tobacco-associated leukoplakia 268
tocopherol 333
α-tocopherol 1670–1
α-tocopherol and β-carotene Cancer Prevention Study (ATBC) 334, 1670–1, 1672
α-tocopherol transfer protein (α-TTP) 333
tocotrienols 333
toenails
  care 1326
  involution 1325
  plate thickening 1324–5
  problems 1324–5
toileting difficulties, interventions in dementia 1141
toileting schedules, urinary incontinence 1489
Tokyo Metropolitan Geriatric Hospital 1936
Tokyo Metropolitan Institute of Gerontology (TMIG) 1936, 1938, 1941
  Longitudinal Interdisciplinary Study on Aging (TMIG-LISA) 1939
tolbutamide, alcohol interaction 161
tolerable upper intake level (TUL), nutrients 331
tolterodine, urge incontinence 1490
"Tomorrow's Doctors" 1791
TONE (trial of nonpharmacologic interventions in the elderly) 550
tongue
  black hairy 265
  varicose veins 263
  wasting in MND 952, 954
tonic-clonic seizure 870, 871
tonic-clonic status epilepticus 876
tooth (teeth)
  abrasion 261–2
    cavity formation 246–7
    restorative care 245, *245*, 246–7
  age related changes 261
  attrition 261
    restorative care 245, *245*
  enamel, age related changes 261
  erosion 246, 262
    restorative care 246
  extraction 244–5
  food intake and 284
  loss 240
  pulp, age related changes 261
  root, retained 270
  sensitivity 273
    toothpaste 249
  socket infection 273
  unerupted 270
  wear 261–2
toothbrush, modification 249
toothpaste 249
topical negative pressure therapy (TNP) 1624–5
topiramate 754, 875
topoisomerase II inhibitors 455
toremifene 1513
Torg ratio 991
Torg–Pavlov ratio 991, 993
torsin A, dystonia 782
tositumomab 1515
total anterior circulation infarction (TACI) 816, 823
  recurrence rate 827
total body potassium, age related changes 1497
total body water (TBW) 1369–70
  age related changes 1498
  drug distribution 216
  measurement 1369–70
total energy expenditure (TEE) 313
Total Quality Management (TQM) 1838, 1840, **1841**
Townsend, Peter 3
toxic nodular goiters, radioactive iodine ablation 1409
toxins, peripheral neuropathy 894–5, **894**
trabeculations, bladder 1459
trabeculoplasty, laser, glaucoma 1208
tracheostomy 962, 1528
traction
  hip fractures 1333
  prolapsed intervertebral disc 1360
training *see* medical education/training
tramadol (hydrochloride) 986, 997, 2005
tranquilizer misuse 1192
transaminases, hepatitis 385
transcutaneous electrical nerve stimulation (TENS) 988, 1362
transdermal fentanyl patches 987
transdiaphragmatic pressure 674, 675
transentorhinal cortex, Alzheimer's disease 1074
transesophageal echocardiography (TOE) 500, 590
transfer coefficient (K_{CO}) 694
transfer factor (TL_{CO}) 694
transferrin, soluble receptor 430
transforming growth factor-β (TGF-β) 29
transfusion transmitted virus (TTV) 384
transient back pain 1355
transient global amnesia 870, 885
transient ischemic attack (TIA)
  headache 757
  management, neurovascular clinics 1910
  seizures 870
  stroke risk factor 802, 827, *828*
  syncope and 880
  vertebrobasilar artery 1243
  see also stroke rehabilitation
transient monocular blindness (amaurosis fugax) 806
transjugular intrahepatic portosystemic shunts (TIPS) 377, 1720
transmissible spongiform encephalopathies 1124–5, **1124**
transplantation
  organs *see specific organ transplants*
  stem cell *see* stem cell transplantation
transport/transportation 5–6
  driving *see* driving
  problems 1713
  system adaptation 141
transrectal ultrasound guided biopsy (TRUS) 1475
trans-scleral laser cyclophotocoagulation 1208
transtentorial herniation, respiratory patterns 678
transthoracic echocardiography (TTE) 500
transurethral incision of the prostate 1473
transurethral needle ablation (TUNA) 1473
transurethral resection of the prostate gland (TURP) 1465, 1473
transvaginal ultrasound measurement 1451–2, 1456, 1661
trastuzumab 1515
trauma
  hearing loss 1228
  neck pain 1363
  peripheral vestibular system 1241–2
  toenail plate 1324–5
traumatic alopecia, elder abuse 184
traumatic thoracolumbar burst fractures 996
traumatic ulcers, oral 265
trazodone 1139, 1143, 1145
treadmill exercise tests 516, 652
treadmill training, stroke rehabilitation 853
treatment interference 1692
  prevention methods 1696
  restraint use 1692
tremor 783–4
  aging effects 746
  anxiety 783
  classification 783, **783**
  definition **778**
  drug induced **784**
  essential *see* essential tremor (ET)
  Parkinson's disease 766
  position-specific 783
  postural 783, **783**
  stress 783
  task-specific 783
Treponema pallidum 1732, 1769
TRH stimulation test 1409
Trial of the Assessment and Management of Older People in the Community (MRC) 1801, 1803
triamcinolone acetonide 266
Trichophyton rubrum 1325
tricyclic antidepressants
  back pain 1363
  cervical spinal canal stenosis 994
  delirium etiology 1051
  depression 1139, 1178
  irritable bowel syndrome 367–8
  migraine prevention 754
  neuropathic pain 987
  noncardiac chest pain 363
  peripheral neuropathy in herpes zoster 895
trigeminal nerve
  demyelination 760
  olfactory role 1250
trigeminal neuralgia 273–4
  headache and 759–61, **759**, *760*, **760**
trigger points, back pain 1357
triglycerides 518, 519, 613
triiodothyronine (T3) 1406, 1407
  age related decline 38
  S14 gene 1407
trimethoprim, prostatitis 1480
triple H therapy, subarachnoid hemorrhage 1023–4
triple therapy regimen, renal transplantation 1501
trisomy 21 1185
  see also Down's syndrome
trochanteric fractures 1331, *1331*
  surgery 1335, *1336*
trochlear nerve, aging 745
Tropheryma whipplei **1752**, 1760
troponin, increased 488
troponin T, isoforms 563
trospium, overactive bladder 1490
Trotter's syndrome 275
trovafloxacin, bacterial meningitis 1767
trunk restraints, usage 1690
tube feeding
  Israeli attitudes 1951
  nursing home acquired pneumonia 666
  see also enteral feeding
tuberculin skin test 690, 709, 1741
  booster effect 709, 1741
  conversion 1741
  criteria **1745**
  false-negative 709
  false-positive 1741
  nursing home residents 667
  positive result 1741
tuberculoma 1244–5
tuberculosis (TB) 708–10, 1739–48
  chemoprophylaxis 709–10, 1731
  clinical characteristics 708–9, 1740–1
  comorbid conditions 1740
  contact tracing 710
  cryptic 709
  diagnosis 1741–3
  disseminated 709
  endogenous reactivation 1731
  epidemiology 667, 1739–40
  extrapulmonary 1740–1
  failure to diagnosis 708–9
  immunology 1740
  infection control 1731, 1746–7
  laboratory diagnosis 709, 1741–3
  latent *see* latent tuberculosis infection (LTBI)
  long term care facilities 1731
  miliary 708
  morbidity, India 1985
  necrosis 1740
  pathogenesis 1740
  radiological features 709
  reactivation 1740
  spinal 1360
  treatment 709–10, 1743–6, *1744*, **1745**
    response monitoring 1743–4
tuberculous meningitis 1768–9
tubotympanic otitis media 1223
tumor(s) *see* cancer; malignant disease
tumor biology, aging 1510–1, **1510**

tumor necrosis factor (TNF) 26
antagonists 557
heart failure mechanism 559, **559**, 564
tumor necrosis factor-α (TNF-α) 29
anorexia 917–8
antagonists, alcoholic liver disease 388
bone mass loss 1289
cardiac cachexia 640–1
chronic heart failure 640–1
decreased production 26
food intake 305, 314
muscle wasting 641, 917–8
sarcopenia 917–8
tunic adventitia 611
tunic intima 611
tunic media 611
tuning fork tests 1220, 1238
12-step programs, drug misuse 1198
two-step tuberculin test 1741
tympanic membrane inflammation/infection 1223
tympanogram 1221, *1221*
tympanometry 1221
tympanosclerosis 1224
type 2 diabetes *see* diabetes mellitus, type 2
Tzanck smear 1594, *1594*

ubiquitin 72, 769, 956, 1078
UK National Study of Disability, hearing disability 1214
UK Prospective Diabetes study (UKPDS) 134, **1437**
UKPACE (UK Pacing and Cardiovascular Events) **496**
ulcers/ulceration
diabetic foot 1315
foot **1319**, 1324
oral *see* oral ulceration
peptic *see* peptic ulcer disease
peripheral arterial disease 1316
pressure *see* pressure ulcers/ulceration
ulnar nerve, entrapment neuropathy 896, 897
ultrasonography
abdominal 1718
anal, fecal incontinence 399
aortic aneurysm 1004
back pain 1358
cholecystitis 388–9
deep vein thrombosis 636
gallstones 389
gastric emptying 364
pancreatic cancer 422
pancreatitis 418, 420
pelvic 1718
problems 1718
spinal disorders 1358
unconsciousness *see* consciousness loss
undernutrition 298
adverse effects 298, **299**
alcoholic liver disease 386–7
causes 298–300, 313
clinical assessment 1638–9
heart failure association 572
nutritional interventions 314
paradox 297
pathological 299–300, **300**
preoperative assessment 1638–9
prevalence 298, 329
reduced food intake 298–9
respiratory muscle weakness 679–80
see also protein-energy malnutrition
unerupted teeth 270
Uniform Data System for Medical Rehabilitation (UDSMR) 1575
unilateral auditory and vestibular failure 1241
United Kingdom (UK) 1915–22
clinical audit *see* clinical audit, UK
demographics 1889–90, **1994**
health expenditure 1978
home care 1893–4
"hospital-at-home" schemes 232
nurse role 1872–3
quality improvement 1848–9
hospital care 1898–9
history 5–6
nursing role 231–2, 1870–1
intermediate care
NSF standard **1802**, 1896, 1917
nursing role 1873
psychiatric services 1169
medical education/training 1784, 1785, 1789–97
approach 1790–2, 1901–2
basic **1791**, 1792–6, **1793**, **1794**
evaluation 1795
history 6–7, 1789–90, **1790**
Quality Assurance Agency benchmarks 1791, **1791**
specialist 1796, **1796**, 1902
memory clinics 1061
National Service Framework *see entries beginning* National Service Framework
nurse education/training 1873–4
nursing home care 1871, 1896
facility demographics 1819
psychiatric services 1168, 1871–2
regulation 1820
nursing practice 1867–77
education/training 1873–4
future of 1875–6
principles 1869–73
quality of care measurement 1874–5
specialist nursing roles 1868–9, 1871
primary care 1799–808, 1919–20
case management 1803–5
geriatric assessment 1800–1
health promotion 1803, **1804**
history 6, 1917
medication review 1805–6
MRC Trial 1801, 1803
nursing role 1872–3
policy 1799–801
quality improvement 1847–9
psychiatric services 1163–71, 1168
carers' support 1164–5
community mental health teams 1165–6
development 8, 1163–4
hospital-based 1166–7
international perspectives 1169–70
learning disabilities 1168
NSF standard 1163–4, **1545**, **1802**, 1893–4, 1917–8
nursing home care 1168, 1871
referral pathway 1167, *1167*
special groups 1168–9
voluntary organizations 1166
quality of care 1839
regulation 1920–1
services, development 2–8, 1890–1, 1915–20
problems 7–8
siderail use 1691
United Kingdom Central Council for Nursing, Midwifery and Health Visiting (UKCC) 1871
United Kingdom Parkinson's Disease Society 766, **766**
United Nations
International Plan of Action on Ageing (2002) 1965, 1974
Principles for Older Persons 1969
United States Department of Health and Human Services, drug misuse treatment 1199
United States of America (USA) 1923–33
ACE units *see* Acute Care for the Elderly (ACE) units
Assisted Living Facilities 107–8, 1897, 1929
chronic disease management program 1804
chronically disabled population 96, *97*
community acquired pneumonia incidence 665
demographics 1890, 1923–4, **1924**, *1924*, *1925*
geriatrics research 1926–7
home care 1848, 1894–5, 1929
hospital care 1899–901, **1899**, **1900**
life expectancy 88, **88**
medical education/training 1902, 1930–1
memory clinics 1061
National Vital Statistics System, stroke mortality 798, *798*
nursing home care 1819–25, **1822**, 1896–7
facility demographics 1817–8, *1818*, **1818**, *1819*
quality measurement **1929**
resident demographics 1819–20, *1820*, *1821*
special programs 1822–4
palliative/end-of-life care 1894–5
medical education/training 1931
quality of care 1838–9
restraint usage 1690
services, development 1891–2, 1924–5, **1926**
siderail use 1691
special programs 1927–30
tuberculosis prevalence 667, 1739
United States Preventive Services Task Force (USPSTF) 203, 207, 208, 1838
thyroid disease screening guidelines 1410
United States Public Health Service (USPHS), tuberculosis treatment 1743
University of Pennsylvania Smell Identification Test (UPSIT) 1251–2, *1252*, 1255
upper esophageal sphincter (UES) 358, 359
upper extremity training, pulmonary rehabilitation 728
urea 1370, 1498
uremia, peripheral neuropathy 893
urethra, female 1449–50, 1459
urge incontinence
dementia 1462
falls 1302
treatment 1490
see also bladder, overactive
urinalysis
benign prostatic hyperplasia 1470
prostatitis 1480
urinary incontinence (UI) 1453, 1485–93
assessment 206, 1453
brachytherapy side effect 1478
causes **1453**
classification 1486
clinical detection 1488–9, **1488**
complications/consequences 1487–8, **1488**
costs 1485, 1487
diagnostic evaluation 1489
drug induced 1488, **1488**
embarrassment 1487
functional 1487, **1488**
heart failure association 571
invasive procedures 1490–1
investigation 1489
management 1453, 1489–90
mixed 1486
nonpharmacological interventions 1489–90
normal pressure hydrocephalus 787, 788, 792
overactive bladder 1486–7
overflow *see* overflow incontinence
pathophysiology 1486
pharmacological therapy 1490
delirium etiology 1050
physical examination 1488
predisposing factors 1486
prevalence 1453, 1485
radical prostatectomy complication 1477
reversible, causes **1486**
risk factors 1485–6, *1486*
sex differences 1485
sexual activity modification 115
stress *see* stress incontinence
surgery 1453, 1490–1
urge *see* urge incontinence
urinary retention 1053, 1473, 1478
urinary tract
age related changes 1486
interventional procedures 1720
urinary tract infections 1499
dehydration 324
delirium etiology 1052–3
epidemiology 1727
estrogen withdrawal 1450
urine
acidification 1497
dilution 1498
osmolarity, dehydration 325

urine (*cont.*)
  testing, drug misuse 1195
urocortin, sarcopenia 925
urodynamic studies, urinary incontinence 1489
urogenital atrophy
  menopause 1417
  sexual dysfunction 115
urogenital function, aging and 978
ursodeoxycholic acid 389, 390
uterosacral ligaments, age related changes 1449
uterovaginal prolapse 1452–3
uterus, age related changes 1449
utricle 1235

vaccination 1733–5
  aspiration pneumonia prevention 689–90
vaccines *see individual vaccines*
vacuum assisted closure (VAC) therapy 1624–5
vacuum tumescence devices 118
vagina
  age related changes 1417, 1449
  atrophy, menopause 1417
  cancer 1660
  dryness 115
  pH changes 1417
vaginal discharge 1452, **1452**
vaginal pessaries, urinary incontinence 1490
vaginitis
  atrophic 1449, 1452, **1452**
    management 1420
  infective 1452, **1452**
vagus nerve, taste 1250
valacyclovir 1594, 1732
valdecoxib, arthritis 1351
valerian, alcohol interaction 161
validation, communication disorders in dementia 1042
valproic acid
  manic episodes, dementia and 1139
  myelodysplasia therapy 460
  see also sodium valproate
valvotomy, percutaneous balloon 590
valvular aortic stenosis 625, **625**
valvular heart disease 529–39
  clinical features 532–3
  consequences 529
  epidemiology 531–2
  heart failure in 573
  incidence/prevalence 529
  infective endocarditis with 590
  mild to moderate, outcome 531
  objective testing/investigations 533
  pathophysiology 529–31
  progressive nature 529, 532
  prophylactic surgery 536
  superimposed on heart disease 530–1
  treatment 534–6, 600–3
    goals 534
    open valve replacement/repair 535
    percutaneous replacement/repair 535–6
    percutaneous stent prosthesis 536
    pharmacological 534–5
    replacement 532
    robotic surgery 536
    see also under cardiac surgery
  see also specific heart valves
valvuloplasty 573
  aortic valve *see* aortic valve
  catheter-based balloon 535–6
  indications **534**
  open surgical 535
  percutaneous 535–6
vanadium **341**
vancomycin
  bacterial meningitis 1766–7, 1768
  Clostridium difficile 1730
  infective endocarditis 1758, **1758**
  subdural empyema 1774
vardenafil (Levitra) 118, **118**, 1472
variant Creutzfeldt-Jacob's disease (vCJD) 1125
variceal banding 377
variceal hemorrhage 377
variceal ligation 377
varicella zoster virus (VZV) 895, 1593, 1727
  encephalitis 1775–6
varicose veins
  deep vein thrombosis risk 634
  foot 1315
  lips 263
  tongue 263
vasa vasorum 611
vascular cell adhesion molecule-1 (VCAM-1) 618
vascular cognitive disorder (VCD) 1115
vascular cognitive impairment (VCI) 1115, 1152–3
vascular cognitive impairment no dementia (VCI-ND) 1115
vascular dementia (VaD) 1103–9, 1111–5
  Alzheimer's disease and 1106, 1114
  characteristics 1114–5, **1115**
  clinical presentation *1113*
  coexisting neurodegenerative pathology 1106, 1114
  communication breakdown process 1039, 1040
  diagnosis 1106–7, 1114–5
  diagnostic criteria 1103–4, 1135–6
  epidemiology 1104, **1104**
  management 1107, 1115
  nomenclature 1115
  prevalence 1111, 1112
  short telomeres 15
  speech apraxia 1040
  stroke related 1103, 1105
  subcortical white-matter lesions 1103, 1105–6
  subtypes 1112–4
vascular disease/disorders
  hemorrhagic 441, **441**
  peripheral vestibular system 1241
  pressure ulcers 1609, *1610*
vascular endothelial growth factor (VEGF) 460, 959
vascular impedance, increased with age 542
vascular insufficiency, in MND 959
vascular radiography 1717–8
vascular resistance, increased with age 542
vascular smooth muscle cells (VSMCs) 611, 619–20
vascular stenting 1720
vascular vestibular neuritis 1238, 1241
vasculitis
  foot ulcers 1324
  infective endocarditis 1756
  large vessel 1007–8
  renal damage 1502
  spinal cord/roots 953
vasoactive intestinal polypeptide (VIP) 976, *976*
vasoconstricting agents, hypertension 542
vasoconstriction, thermoregulation 976
vasodilatation
  nitric oxide mediated 617–8
  thermoregulation 976, 977
vasodilating agents, hypertension 542
vasopressin 322, 1370–1
  age related changes 322, 1389, 1402–3, 1498
  cerebral effects 1370–1
  elevated in heart failure 558
  regulation 1373–4
  release stimuli 1373
  renal collecting duct responsiveness 1402
  thirst regulation 1372
  V1/V2 receptors 558, 1374
  variceal hemorrhage 377
  vascular reactivity 1371
vasovagal syncope 974
  aging and 975
  clinical features 881
  diagnosis 882
  management 883
  mechanism 880
  myoclonic jerks 870–1
Velcro crepitations 694, 717
Venereal Disease Research Laboratory (VDRL) 1129
venlafaxine 1157
  depression 1139, 1178, 1179
  hyponatremia risk 1179
  menopausal symptom management 1420
venography, contrast, deep vein thrombosis 636
venous disease, foot manifestations 1315
venous embolism, oncological emergency 1527–8
venous stasis, deep vein thrombosis risk 634
venous thromboembolism (VTE) 633–8
  clinical nonrecognition problem 635–6
  epidemiology and pathogenesis 449, 633–5
  HRT and 1418, 1419, 1451
  ischemic stroke 820
  management 451, 636–7
  primary prophylaxis 635–6
  risk factors 633, **634**
    acquired 634–5
    genetic 633–4
  see also deep vein thrombosis (DVT); pulmonary embolism
venous thrombosis 441–2
  hip fractures 1332
  oncological emergency 1527–8
ventilation-perfusion isotope lung scanning 636
ventilation/perfusion mismatch, heart failure 571
ventilation/perfusion (V/Q) scan 714
ventilatory support
  acute respiratory disease 718–9
  see also mechanical ventilation
ventralis intermedius (VIM) nucleus, stimulation 784
ventricle (brain), size, aging effect 69
ventricle (heart)
  changes in atrial fibrillation 499
  compliance, loss 530
ventricular arrhythmia 507–10
  after myocardial infarction 508, 587
  assessment for cardiac rehabilitation **651**
  in ischemic heart disease 516
  primary prevention 508–10
    in dilated cardiomyopathy 509–10
    implantable cardioverter defibrillator 509, *509*, 510
  prognosis 507–8
  secondary prevention 510
  ventricular fibrillation 577, 587
  see also ventricular tachycardia
ventricular assist devices 607
ventricular contraction, premature (PVC) 507
ventricular depolarisation, premature (PVD) 507
ventricular ectopic beats 507, *507*
ventricular fibrillation 577, 587
ventricular tachycardia 507, *507*, **508**
  after myocardial infarction 587
  heart failure 577
ventriculomegaly 787, 788, *788*
ventriculoperitoneal shunting
  flow regulation 790
  infection from 791, 792
  normal pressure hydrocephalus 790, *790*, *791*
    responsiveness prediction 788, 789, 791
  programmable valves 790, *790*, *791*
verapamil 502, 519
verbal dyspraxia 844
verbal fluency, assessment 1065
verbal skills, age related changes 55
vertebrae 991, 995
  fractures 1282, 1285, 1359
vertebral arteries 1001
vertebrobasilar insufficiency 1238
vertebrobasilar ischemia 1243–4
  syncope 881
vertical dimension loss, mouth 242, *242*
  restorative care 246, *246*
vertical nystagmus 1239
vertigo 1303
  acute, management 1245
  cervical 1244
  definition 1237
  management 1245
  migraine 1245
  time course 1238
  see also benign paroxysmal positional vertigo (BPPV)
vertigo-provocative movements 1242
very low density lipoprotein (VLDL) 613
Vesnarinone Trial (VEST) 559

vestibular apparatus
  aging 1235–7
  anatomy 1235
  compensation 1237
  head position awareness 1236, *1236*
  physiology 1235–7
vestibular dysfunction, iatrogenic 1243
vestibular nuclear complex, aging 71
vestibular nuclei 1243
vestibular rehabilitation 1246
vestibular schwannoma 1227–8, 1241, 1244
vestibular system disorders 1235–47
  associated symptoms 1238
  central 1243–5
  diagnosis 1237–40
  examination 1238–40
  history 1237–8
  management 1245–6
  peripheral 1240–3
vestibulo-cochlear nerve, aging 745
vestibulo-ocular reflex (VOR) suppression 1240
Veteran's Administration, USA 1924, 1925
Veterans Administration Cooperative Study, hypertension 547
Veterans Affairs Medical Centers (VAMC) 1849, 1850, 1925
Viagra *see* sildenafil (Viagra)
videoconferencing 1850
videofluoroscopy, dysphagia/swallowing 821, 845–6
videotelemetry, epilepsy 872
"vigorous" achalasia 360
violence, in long term care patients 1155
viral infections
  acute exacerbation of COPD 700
  hepatitis *see* hepatitis, viral
  meningitis 1763–4
  motor neuron disease 958
  noninfluenza respiratory 667–8
  otitis media 1223
  Paget's disease of bone 1269–70
  parkinsonism 769
  taste dysfunction 1256
viral vestibular neuritis 1238, 1240
vision
  assessment, communication disorders 1043
  changes, pituitary adenomas 1400
  diseases impacting on 842
  falls 1303–4
  loss *see* visual impairment/loss
vision aids, age related macular degeneration 1206
Visitatie model 1840
visual acuity
  assessment 205–6
  diabetes mellitus 1433
  pituitary apoplexy 1020
  refractive error 1205
visual agnosia, semantic dementia 1123
Visual Analogue Mood Scale (VAMS) 863
visual communication device (Geronte) 1824, *1825*
visual impairment/loss
  activities of daily living 1205
  age related 39
  assistive devices 1886
  communication effect 842
  diabetic retinopathy 1207
  falls 1303–4
  heart failure association 572
  morbidity, India 1984
  screening 1545
  zinc deficiency 340
visual suppression, of vestibular responses 1240
visual system, aging effect 745
visual vertigo 1238
visuospatial dysfunction, stroke rehabilitation 855
vital capacity measurements 679
vitamin(s) 329–46
  absorption 292
  alcohol abuse treatment 164
  deficiency, prevalence 329–30, **330**
  drug interactions **330**
  myelodysplasia therapy 459
vitamin A 332–3, **341**
  absorption 332
  cancer prevention 333, 1672
  deficiency 285
    eye disorders 332–3
    prevalence 330, **330**
  function 332, 1672
  preformed 332
  recommended daily allowance 332, 1672
  supplements 1672
  toxicity 333, 1672
vitamin B
  deficiency, prevalence 330, **330**
  stroke risk reduction 835–6
vitamin B_1 **341**
vitamin B_2 336, **341**
vitamin B_3 **341**
vitamin B_6 339, **341**
  bone metabolism 1291
  deficiency 339
  supplementation 94
  toxicity 339
vitamin B_{12} 338–9, **341**
  absorption 292
  bone metabolism 1291
  deficiency 285, 338–9
    anemia 429
    myelodysplastic anemia *vs* 468
    peripheral neuropathy 894
    screening for 429
  function 338
  malabsorption 294
  replacement 432
vitamin C 335–6, **341**, 1672–3
  absorption 335
  bone metabolism 1291
  cancer prevention 1673
  deficiency 262, 285, 335
  function 335
  recommended daily allowance 1673
  side effects/toxicity 335–6, 1673
  supplements 336, 1673
vitamin D 336–7, **341**, 1392–3
  absorption 336
  age related changes 1263, **1263**
  calcium homeostasis 1261–2, *1262*
  daily intake 337
  deficiency 285–6, 336–7, 1392–3
    osteoporosis 1662
    prevalence 330, **330**
    risk factors 336–7
  metabolism disorders, myopathies 943
  osteoporosis 1289
  production 285, 292
  sarcopenia 917
  supplements 93, 337, 1265–6
    bisphosphonates use 1275
    fracture prevention 1266, 1341
    muscle strength/function 917
    osteoporosis 283, 1283, 1293
  synthesis 336
  toxicity 93, 337
vitamin D receptors (VDR), intestinal 1264
vitamin E 333–4, **341**, 1670–1
  absorption 333
  deficiency 333, 894
  with exercise, sarcopenia 923
  function 333
  immune function restoration 32
  MCI/dementia 1069
  supplements
    Alzheimer's disease 334, 1671
    cancer prevention 334, 1671
    coronary heart disease 334, 1670, 1671
    immune response 334
    long term effects 334
    side effects 1670
    stroke 1671
vitamin K 337, **341**
  absorption 337
  acquired coagulation defects 440
  deficiency 337
  osteoporosis 1291
  parenteral 374, 605
  toxicity 337
vitamin K antagonists 605
  see also warfarin
Vitamins in Stroke Prevention (VISP) study 836
VITAmins TO Prevent Stroke (VITATOPS) trial 836
Vitrathane insoles, bursitis 1325
VO_2 max *see* maximum oxygen consumption (VO_2 max)
vocabulary, aging effects 744
voice alarms 1694
voiding diary 1488
voiding reflex 1460
voltage-gated calcium channels (VGCC) 905, 906
voltage-gated potassium channels (VGKC) 906
volume depletion 1637–8
volume of distribution, drugs 216, **216**
volume overload 570
voluntary euthanasia, in MND 964
voluntary hospitals, UK history 2
voluntary organizations, UK 1166, 1874
vomiting
  bowel obstruction 2008
  hypokalemia 1384
  terminally ill 2008
Von Economo's encephalitis 769
von Willebrand factor 440
von Willebrand's disease 440
voriconazole, fungal brain abscess 1773
vulva
  age related changes 1449
  cancer 1456, 1660
  lesions, sexual intercourse 1454
vulval disorders 1455
vulvectomy 1456, 1660
vulvodynia (vulval pain) 1455

waist circumference measurement 281–2, 347, 350
waist to hip ratio 281–2, 802
Waldenström's macroglobulinemia 441
walking, aging effect 747
  see also gait
walking aids
  lumbar spinal canal stenosis 997
  Paget's disease of bone 1275
walking as exercise
  dementia risk reduced 131
  Health Maintenance Clinical Guidepath 205
  heart failure management 578
walking frames, wheeled 699
Wallenberg (lateral medullary) syndrome 1244
wander reminder 195, *195*
wandering off, dementia 1146
warfarin
  adjusted dose (INR 2–3) 505, **505**
  adverse effects 506
  after myocardial infarction 521, 587
  age related requirements 449
  arrhythmias after myocardial infarction 587
  atrial fibrillation 505, **505**
  bleeding risk 450, 506
    intracranial bleeding 450–1
  cardiac valve surgery 603, **603**, 604
    INR range 604, 605
  chronic mitral regurgitation 589
  complication risk 831
  contraindications **603**
  dementia prevention in atrial fibrillation 488
  dosing, management 604, 637
  drug interactions 506, **506**, 604, **604**
  duration 452
  hip fracture prophylaxis 1332
  International Normalized Ratio (INR) 440, 449, 450, 637, 1910
    target level 452
  low dose, atrial fibrillation 505
  pharmacokinetics/pharmacodynamics 216–7, 506
  prescribing considerations 637
  regular monitoring 506
  self-management 605
  simvastatin, enhancement by 835

warfarin (*cont.*)
  sinus rhythm and 832
  stroke prevention in atrial fibrillation 451, 452, 482
  stroke recurrence risk reduction 823, 831, *832*
  tailored induction doses 452
  under use 506
  venous thromboembolism 442, 637
  see also anticoagulants/anticoagulation
Warren, Marjory 2, 3–4, 1544, 1919
  geriatric care recommendations 1890–1
Washington University Road Test 145
wasting syndrome 1731
water
  balance 1369–87, 1373
  depletion 1637
  excretion 1402–3, 1462
  fluoridation 249
  metabolism, age related changes 1373
  retention 543
    pathophysiology in heart failure 557, *557*, 558
  total body *see* total body water (TBW)
water deprivation tests 1373
Waterlow risk assessment scale 1611, *1611*
web servers, smart homes 196
Weber test 1220
Wechsler subscales of cognitive function 49
Weed, Lawrence 223–4
"weekly planner", dementia 1044
Wegener's granulomatosis 715, 718
weight
  age related changes 280–1, 347
  ideal 297
  mortality associated 349–50, **349**
  plain radiography problems 1715
  population-based observations 309–10, **310**
  stability 282
weight cycling, in diabetes 135
weight loss 298, 309–19
  aging 281
  Alzheimer's disease 1086
  causes 313
  chronic pain management 988
  comorbid conditions 312–3
  dehydration indicator 324
  dementia and 1144
  diabetes management 134
  functional impairment assessment 1640
  hypertension management 550
  involuntary 313–6
  lifestyle modifications 312
  mortality 298, 309, 311–2, **312**
  pharmacological interventions 314–6, **315**
  screening and management 204–5
  voluntary 312, 313
weight-bearing
  bone mass maintenance 1291
  postoperative hip fractures 1335–6
weight-lifting 125, 127
Welsh Community Diabetes Study 1433, 1434
wen (epidermoid cyst) 1600, *1600*
Werner's syndrome 1590
Wernicke–Korsakoff syndrome 1126
Wernicke's aphasia 843
Wernicke's encephalopathy 972
Wertheim's hysterectomy 1455
West Nile virus encephalitis 1775, 1776
Western blot, Lyme disease 1769
wheelchair access, hospital 1713
wheelchairs
  adaptations 1695
  patient repositioning schedules 1616
whiplash injuries 1363
white blood cell counts, leukostasis 1525
white folded gingivostomatosis (oral epithelial nevus) 269
white matter
  aging 63
  depression 1177
  lesions, vascular dementia 1103, 1105–6
  normal pressure hydrocephalus 788, *789*
"white-coat syndrome" 545
Williamson, James 1919
Wilson, Thomas 1921
winter bronchitis 697
withdrawal delirium 1640–1
withdrawal of drugs *see* drug misuse/abuse, withdrawal
Women Health Initiative Memory Study (WHIMS) 1418
Women's Angiographic Vitamin and Estrogen study 1671
Women's Health and Aging Study (WHAS) 1434, 1557
Women's Health Initiative Memory Study (WHIMS) 1676
Women's Health Initiative (WHI) study
  HRT and breast cancer 1450–1
  HRT and cancer 1676
  HRT and coronary heart disease 115–6, 1418, 1419, 1421, 1661, 1676
  HRT and dementia 1418
  HRT and stroke 1418
  premarin side effects 1394
Worcester, Alfred 2
word finding, Alzheimer's disease 1039
word sequencing 1038
  Alzheimer's disease 1039
  assessment 1041, **1042**
  dementia 1039–40
word sound assembly 1038
  Alzheimer's disease 1039
  assessment 1041, **1042**
  dementia 1039–40
word store 1038
  Alzheimer's disease 1040
  assessment 1041, **1042**
  dementia 1039–40
workhouse infirmaries, UK history 2
World Federation of Neurological Surgeons (WFNS) 1020, *1020*
World Federation of Neurology 949–50
World Health Organization (WHO)
  acute myeloblastic leukemia classification 466, **466**
  alcohol abuse/dependence 158, 163
  Alma-Ata Declaration 1983
  analgesia steps **2005**
  ICF model 860, 1571–2, 1881–2, *1881*
  ICIDH *see* International Classification of Impairments, Disabilities, and Handicaps (ICIDH)
  memory clinics 1069
  MONICA project, stroke incidence 799
  myelodysplasia classification 457, **457**, 468, **468**
  osteoporosis diagnostic criteria 1287
  stroke definition 795, 815
  tuberculosis infection rate estimates 667
world population trends *see* demographics
World Psychiatric Association 1170
wound(s)
  characteristics **1620**
  cleansing 1621, **1621**
  debridement 1618–21
    autolytic 1621
    maggots 1620
    mechanical 1621
    sharp 1620, *1620*
  exudate 1618–20
  healing
    age related changes 38, **38**
    impaired 335, 340
  hematoma, postoperative hip fracture 1337
  infection, postoperative hip fracture 1337
  irrigation 1621
  management 1618
writer's cramp 782
writer's tremor 783
written aids, memory clinic patients 1068

xenobiotic metabolism 959
xerosis 1595–6
  foot *1314*, *1316*, *1322*, *1323*
xerostomia 243, 271, *271*
  dental caries 262
  drug induced **271**, 272
  oral candidosis 263
  radiotherapy induced 255, *255*, 272
ximelagatran, atrial fibrillation 507, 832
X-linked bulbospinal neuronopathy 953
X-ray
  Alzheimer's disease 1088
  asbestosis 716
  back pain 1358
  cervical spinal canal stenosis 992, 993, 994
  chronic subdural hematoma 1031
  "eggshell" calcification 716
  emphysema 1715
  exposure factors 1715–6
  higher kilovoltage (kV) techniques 1715
  hip fractures 1330, *1330*
  ischemic stroke 817
  lumbar spinal canal stenosis 997
  osteophytes 1358
  Paget's disease of bone 1271, *1272*, *1273*
  problems 1715–6
  silicosis 716
  spinal cord compression 1521
  tuberculosis 709

Yesavage Geriatric Depression Scale 1545
yoga, depression improvement 131
Yoikuin 1936
Yokufukai 1936

zanamivir, influenza 706, 1730, **1730**
Zarit scale 1088
Ziggbee radio bus 197
zinc 339–40
  absorption 339
  deficiency 32, 292, 340
  osteoporosis 1291
  therapy 1256
  toxicity 340
zinc pyrithione 1596
zoledronic acid 1276, 2009
zolendronate 1294, 1523
zoster *see* herpes zoster (shingles)
zoster sine herpete 267, 1593
Zung Self-rating Depression Scale 1545
Zutphen Study 1434